New Oxford Textbook of
Psychiatry

Project Administrator	Carole Sunderland
Project Editor	Roberta Nichols
Indexer	Linda English
Production Controller	Gill Watts
Development Editor	Kate Martin
Design Manager	Claire Walker
Typographer	Jonathan Coleclough
Illustrations	Technical Graphics Department, Oxford University Press
Publisher	Alison Langton

volume **1**

New Oxford Textbook of
Psychiatry

Edited by

Michael G. Gelder
Emeritus Professor of Psychiatry,
Warneford Hospital, University of Oxford,
Oxford, UK

Juan J. López-Ibor
Professor of Psychiatry,
Complutense University, Madrid, Spain;
President, World Psychiatric Association

and

Nancy Andreasen
Director, Mental Health Clinical Research Centre,
University of Iowa Hospital and Clinic,
Iowa City, USA

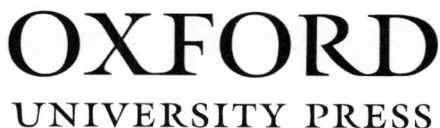

OXFORD

UNIVERSITY PRESS

Great Clarendon Street, Oxford OX2 6DP

Oxford University Press is a department of the University of Oxford.
It furthers the University's objective of excellence in research, scholarship,
and education by publishing worldwide in

Oxford New York

Auckland Bangkok Buenos Aires Cape Town Chennai
Dar es Salaam Delhi Hong Kong Istanbul Karachi Kolkata
Kuala Lumpur Madrid Melbourne Mexico City Mumbai Nairobi
São Paulo Shanghai Taipei Tokyo Toronto

Oxford is a registered trade mark of Oxford University Press
in the UK and in certain other countries

Published in the United States
by Oxford University Press Inc., New York

First published 2000
Reprinted 2003
First published in paperback 2003

A catalogue record for this title is available from the British Library

Library of Congress Cataloging in Publication Data
(Data available)
ISBN 0–19–852810–8 (set)
ISBN 0–19–852818–3 (volume 1)
ISBN 0–19–852819–1 (volume 2)

10 9 8 7 6 5 4 3 2 1

Only available as a set.

Printed in Italy

Preface

Three themes can be discerned in contemporary psychiatry: the growing unity of the subject, the pace of scientific advance, and the growth of practice in the community. We have sought to reflect these themes in the *New Oxford Textbook of Psychiatry* and to present the state of psychiatry at the start of the new millennium. The book is written for psychiatrists engaged in continuous education and recertification; the previous, shorter, *Oxford Textbook of Psychiatry* remains available for psychiatrists in training. The book is intended to be suitable also as a work of reference for psychiatrists of all levels of experience, and for other professionals whose work involves them in the problems of psychiatry.

The growing unity of psychiatry

The growing unity in psychiatry is evident in several ways. Biological and psychosocial approaches have been largely reconciled with a general recognition that genetic and environmental factors interact, and that psychological processes are based in and can influence neurobiological mechanisms. At the same time, the common ground between the different psychodynamic theories has been recognized, and is widely accepted as more valuable than the differences between them.

The practice of psychiatry is increasingly similar in different countries, with the remaining variations related more to differences between national systems of health care and the resources available to clinicians, than to differences in the aims of the psychiatrists working in these countries. This unity of approach is reflected in this book whose authors practise in many different countries and yet present a common approach. In this respect this textbook differs importantly from others which present the views of authors drawn predominantly from a single country or region.

Greater agreement about diagnosis and nosology has led to a better understanding of how different treatment approaches are effective in different disorders. The relative specificity of psychopharmacological treatments is being matched increasingly by the specificity of some of the recently developed psychological treatments, so that psychological treatment should no longer be applied without reference to diagnosis, as was sometimes done in the past.

The pace of scientific advance

Advances in genetics and in the neurosciences have already increased knowledge of the basic mechanisms of the brain and are beginning to uncover the neurobiological mechanisms involved in psychiatric disorder. Striking progress has been achieved in the understanding of Alzheimer's disease, for example, and there are indications that similar progress will follow in uncovering the causes of mood disorder, schizophrenia, and autism. Knowledge of genetics and the neurosciences is so extensive and the pace of change is so rapid that it is difficult to present a complete account within the limited space available in a textbook of clinical psychiatry. We have selected aspects of these sciences that seem, to us and the authors, to have contributed significantly to psychiatry or to be likely to do so before long.

Psychological and social sciences and epidemiology are essential methods of investigation in psychiatry. Although the pace of advance in these sciences may not be as great as in the neurosciences, the findings generally have a more direct relation to clinical phenomena. Moreover, the mechanisms by which psychological and social factors interact with genetic, biochemical, and structural ones will continue to be important however great the progress in these other sciences. Among the advances in the psychological and social sciences that are relevant to clinical phenomena, we have included accounts of memory, psychological development, research on life events, and the effects of culture. Epidemiological studies continue to be crucial for defining psychiatric disorders, following their course, and identifying their causes.

Psychiatry in the community

In most countries, psychiatry is now practised in the community rather than in institutions, and where this change has yet be completed, it is generally recognized that it should take place. The change has done much more than transfer the locus of care; it has converted patients from passive recipients of care to active participants with individual needs and preferences. Psychiatrists are now involved in the planning, provision, and evaluation of services for whole communities, which may include members of ethnic minorities, homeless people, and refugees. Responsibility for a community has underlined the importance of the prevention as well as the treatment of mental disorder and of the role of agencies other than health services in both. Care in the community has also drawn attention to the many people with psychiatric disorder who are treated in primary care, and has led to new ways of working between psychiatrists and physicians. At the same time, psychiatrists have worked more in general hospitals, helping patients with both medical and psychiatric problems. Others have provided care for offenders.

The organization of the book

In most ways, the organization of this book is along conventional lines. However, some matters require explanation.

Part 1 contains a variety of diverse topics brought together under the general heading of the subject matter and approach to psychiatry. Phenomenology, assessment, classification, and ethical problems are included, together with the role of the psychiatrist as educator and as manager. Public health aspects of psychiatry are considered together with public attitudes to psychiatry and to psychiatric patients. Part 1 ends with a chapter on the links between science and practice. It begins with a topic that is central to good practice—the understanding of the experience of becoming a psychiatric patient.

Part 2 is concerned with the scientific foundations of psychiatry grouped under the headings neurosciences, genetics, psychological sciences, social sciences, and epidemiology. The chapters contain general information about these sciences; findings specific to a particular disorder are described in the chapter on that disorder. Brain imaging techniques are discussed here because they link basic sciences with clinical research. As explained above, the chapters are selective and, in some, readers who wish to study the subjects in greater detail will find suggestions for further reading.

Part 3 is concerned with dynamic approaches to psychiatry. The principal schools of thought are presented as alternative ways of understanding the influence of life experience on personality and on responses to stressful events and to illness. Some reference is made to dynamic psychotherapy in these accounts, but the main account of these treatments is in Part 6. This arrangement separates the chapters on the practice of dynamic psychotherapy from those on psychodynamic theory, but we consider that this disadvantage is outweighed by the benefit of considering together the commonly used forms of psychotherapy.

Part 4 is long, with chapters on the clinical syndromes of adult psychiatry, with the exception of somatoform disorders which appear in Part 5, Psychiatry and Medicine. This latter contains more than a traditional account of psychosomatic medicine. It also includes a review of psychiatric disorders that may cause medical symptoms unexplained by physical pathology, the medical, surgical, gynaecological, and obstetric conditions most often associated with psychiatric disorder, health psychology, and the treatment of psychiatric disorder in medically ill patients.

Information about treatment appears in more than one part of the book. Part 6 contains descriptions of the physical and psychological treatments in common use in psychiatry. Dynamic psychotherapy and psychoanalysis are described alongside counselling and cognitive-behavioural techniques. This part of the book contains general descriptions of the treatments; their use for a particular disorder is considered in the chapter on that disorder. In the latter, the account is generally in two parts: a review of evidence about the efficacy of the treatment, followed by advice on management in which available evidence is supplemented, where necessary, with clinical experience. Treatment methods designed specially for children and adolescents, for people with mental retardation (learning disability), and for patients within the forensic services are considered in Parts 9, 10, and 11 respectively.

Social psychiatry and service provision are described in Part 7. Public policy issues, as well as the planning, delivery, and evaluation of services, are discussed here. Psychiatry in primary care is an important topic in this part of the book. There are chapters on the special problems of members of ethnic minorities, homeless people, and refugees, and the effects of culture on the provision and uptake of services.

Child and adolescent psychiatry, old age psychiatry, and mental retardation are described in Parts 8, 9, and 10. These accounts are less detailed than might be found in textbooks intended for specialists working exclusively in the relevant subspecialty. Rather, they are written for readers experienced in another branch of psychiatry who wish to improve their knowledge of the special subject. We are aware of the controversy surrounding our choice of the title of Part 10. We have selected the term 'mental retardation' because it is used in both ICD-10 and DSM-IV. In some countries this term has been replaced by another that is thought to be less stigmatizing and more acceptable to patients and families. For example, in the United Kingdom the preferred term is 'learning disability'. While we sympathize with the aims of those who adopt this and other alternative terms, the book is intended for an international readership and it seems best to use the term chosen by the World Health Organization as most generally understood. Thus the term mental retardation is used unless there is a special reason to use another.

In Part 11, Forensic Psychiatry, it has been especially difficult to present a general account of the subject that is not tied to practice in a single country. This is because systems of law differ between countries and the practice of forensic psychiatry has to conform with the local legal system. Although many of the examples in this part of the book may at first seem restricted in their relevance because they are described in the context of English law, we hope that readers will be able to transfer the principles described in these chapters to the legal tradition in which they work.

Finally, readers should note that the history of psychiatry is presented in more than one part of the book. The history of psychiatry as a medical specialty is described in Part 1. The history of ideas about the various psychiatric disorders appears, where relevant, in the chapters on these disorders, where they can be considered in relation to present-day concepts. The history of ideas about aetiology is considered in Part 2, which covers the scientific basis of psychiatric aetiology, while the historical development of dynamic psychiatry is described in Part 3.

Michael Gelder
Juan López-Ibor
Nancy Andreasen

Acknowledgements

We are grateful to the many colleagues who have advised us about certain parts of the book.

The following helped us to plan specialized parts of the book: Dr Jeremy Holmes (Part 3, Psychodynamic Contributions to Psychiatry); Professor Richard Mayou (Part 5, Psychiatry and Medicine); Professor Robin Jacoby (Part 8, Psychiatry of Old Age); Sir Michael Rutter (Part 9, Child and Adolescent Psychiatry); Professor William Fraser (Part 10, Mental Retardation); Professor Robert Bluglass (Part 11, Forensic Psychiatry).

The following helped us to plan certain sections within Part 4, General Psychiatry: Professor Alwyn Lishman (delirium, dementia, amnestic syndrome, and other cognitive disorders); Professor Griffith Edwards (alcohol use disorders); Dr Philip Robson (other substance use disorders); Professor Guy Goodwin (mood disorders); Professor John Bancroft (sexuality, gender identity, and their disorders); Professor Gregory Stores (sleep–wake disorders); Professor Keith Hawton (suicide and attempted suicide). In Part 6, Professor Philip Cowen advised about somatic treatments, Dr Jeremy Holmes about psychodynamic treatments, and Professor David Clark about cognitive-behavioural therapy. Dr Max Marshall provided helpful advice about forensic issues for Part 7. We also thank the many other colleagues whose helpful suggestions about specific problems aided the planning of the book.

Finally, we record our special gratitude to the authors and to the staff of Oxford University Press.

Contents
Volume 1

Contents
Volume 2

Part 7 Social psychiatry and service provision

Part 10 Mental retardation (learning disability)

Part 11 Forensic psychiatry

Contributors list

Susan Abbey Associate Professor of Psychiatry, University of Toronto, Ontario, Canada
Chapter 5.3.6

Gene G. Abel Professor of Clinical Psychiatry, Emory University School of Medicine, Atlanta, Georgia, USA
Chapter 4.11.3

Henry David Abraham Chief, Alcohol and Drug Treatment Services, Butler Hospital, Lexington, Massachusetts, USA
Chapter 4.2.3.4

Clive Adams Cochrane Schizophrenia Group, University of Oxford Department of Psychiatry, Warneford Hospital, Oxford, UK
Chapter 6.1.1.2

Zahir Ahmed Honorary Lecturer in Psychiatry, Division of Psychological Medicine, University of Wales College of Medicine, Cardiff, UK
Chapter 10.4

Hagop S. Akiskal Professor of Psychiatry and Director of the International Mood Center, University of California at San Diego, California, USA
Chapter 4.5.8

Stanley E. Althof Case Western Reserve University School of Medicine, Cleveland, Ohio, USA
Chapter 4.11.2

Lawrence Amsel Research Psychiatrist, Columbia University, New York, USA
Chapter 4.15.3

Adrian Angold Associate Professor of Child and Adolescent Psychiatry, Duke University Medical Center, Durham, North Carolina, USA
Chapter 9.1.4

Jules Angst Honorary Professor of Psychiatry and Honorary Doctor of Medicine, Zurich University Psychiatric Hospital, Zurich, Switzerland
Chapter 4.5.6

E. Arensman Senior Researcher, Department of Clinical Psychology, Vrije Universiteit, Amsterdam, The Netherlands
Chapter 4.15.2

Lesley M. Arnold Division of Women's Health Research, Department of Psychiatry, University of Cincinnati College of Medicine, Cincinnati, Ohio, USA
Chapter 4.13.1

Arnoud Arntz Doctor of Clinical Psychology and Experimental Psychopathology, Maastricht University, The Netherlands
Chapter 2.5.3

J.K. Aronson Clinical Reader in Clinical Pharmacology, University of Oxford, UK
Chapter 6.2.1

Roland Atkinson Professor and Head, Division of Geriatric Psychiatry, School of Medicine, Oregon Health Sciences University, Portland, Oregon, USA
Chapter 8.5.2

J.L. Ayuso-Mateos Professor of Psychiatry, Department of Medicine and Psychiatry, University of Cantabria, Spain
Chapter 5.3.5

Susan Bailey Consultant Child and Adolescent Forensic Psychiatrist, Salford NHS Trust and Maudsley NHS Trust; Senior Research Fellow, University of Manchester, UK
Chapter 9.4.1

Robert Baldwin Consultant, Old Age Psychiatrist, and Honorary Senior Lecturer, Manchester Royal Infirmary, UK
Chapter 8.5.4

James C. Ballenger Chairman and Professor, Medical University of South Carolina Institute of Psychiatry, Charleston, South Carolina, USA
Chapter 4.7.3

Demetrio Barcia Chairman of Psychiatry, Hospital General Universitario, Murcia, Spain
Chapter 4.1.1

David H. Barlow Center for Anxiety and Related Disorders at Boston University, Massachusetts, USA
Chapter 4.7.1

Jacqueline Barnes Royal Free and University College Medical School, University College London, and Tavistock Clinic, London, UK
Chapter 9.3.4

Arnd Barocka Professor of Psychiatry, University of Erlangen, Germany
Chapter 1.9

Christopher Bass Consultant in Liaison Psychiatry, John Radcliffe Hospital, Oxford, UK
Chapter 5.2.9

Per Bech Professor of Psychiatry and Head of Psychiatric Research Unit, WHO Collaborating Centre, Frederiksborg General Hospital, Hillerød, Denmark
Chapter 4.5.2

DeAnna A. Beckman Division of Women's Health Research, Department of Psychiatry, University of Cincinnati College of Medicine, Cincinnati, Ohio, USA
Chapter 4.13.1

Ruth M. Benca Associate Professor, Department of Psychiatry, University of Wisconsin-Madison, Madison, Wisconsin, USA
Chapter 4.14.5

Sidney Benjamin Senior Lecturer, University of Manchester, UK
Chapter 5.2.6

Peter Berner Universitätsklinik für Psychiatrie, Vienna, Austria
Chapter 1.9

T.P. Berney Consultant Psychiatrist, Prudhoe Hospital, Northumberland, UK
Chapter 10.6

German E. Berrios Consultant in Neuropsychiatry, Department of Psychiatry, University of Cambridge, UK
Chapters 2.1.1 and 4.3.1

J.M. Bertolote Chief, Mental Disorders Control Unit, World Health Organization, Geneva; Associate Professor, Department of Psychogeriatrics, University of Lausanne, Switzerland
Chapter 7.4

Dinesh Bhugra Senior Lecturer in Psychiatry, Institute of Psychiatry, King's College London, UK
Chapter 1.8

Michel Billiard Department of Neurology B, Gui de Chauliac Hospital, Montpellier, France
Chapter 4.14.3

Max Birchwood Director, Early Intervention Service, Northern Birmingham Mental Health Trust, and University of Birmingham, UK
Chapter 6.3.2.4

Alan H. Bittles Foundation Professor of Human Biology, Edith Cowan University, Perth, Australia
Chapter 8.1

Dora Black Honorary Consultant, Child and Adolescent Psychiatry, Traumatic Stress Clinic, London; Honorary Lecturer, University of London, UK
Chapter 9.3.5

S. Blairy Department of Psychiatry, University Clinics of Brussels, Erasme Hospital, Brussels, Belgium
Chapter 4.5.5.1

Sidney Bloch Professor of Psychiatry, University of Melbourne; Senior Psychiatrist, St Vincent's Hospital, Melbourne, Australia
Chapters 1.5 and 6.3.8

Robert Bluglass Emeritus Professor of Forensic Psychiatry, University of Birmingham; Honorary Consultant in Forensic Psychiatry, Reabank Clinic, Birmingham, UK
Introduction to Section 11 and Chapter 11.9

Bernhard Bogerts Department of Psychiatry, University of Magdeburg, Germany
Chapter 2.3.5

F. Borrell Associate Professor, Department of Medicine, Barcelona University; Director, Centro de Atencion Primaria, Area Basica de Salud 'La Gabarra', Cornellà de Llobregat, Spain
Chapter 1.10.2

Nick Bouras Consultant Psychiatrist and Senior Lecturer, Guy's Hospital, London, UK
Chapter 10.9

William R. Breakey Professor, Department of Psychiatry and Behavioral Sciences, Johns Hopkins University School of Medicine, Baltimore, Maryland, USA
Chapter 7.2

Chris R. Brewin Department of Psychology, Royal Holloway College, University of London, UK
Chapter 4.6.3

Ian Brockington Professor of Psychiatry, University of Birmingham, UK
Chapter 5.4

George W. Brown Professor of Sociology, Academic Department of Psychiatry, St Thomas's Hospital, London, UK
Chapter 2.6.1

E.T. Bullmore Institute of Psychiatry, King's College London, UK
Chapters 2.3.7 and 2.3.8

Jose Luis Carrasco Professor of Psychiatry, Hospital Fundacion Jimenez Diaz, Universidad Autonoma, Madrid, Spain
Chapter 4.12.3

Angela Cartagena-Rochas Mount Sinai School of Medicine, New York, USA
Chapter 4.6.4

D.J. Castle University of Western Australia, Fremantle, Australia
Chapter 4.3.5.1

M. Caterina Director, Department of Psychiatry, Ciudad Badia, Barcelona, Spain
Chapter 1.10.2

Nadia Chabane Chef de Clinique Assistant, University of Paris VII, France
Chapter 9.2.6

Jonathan Chick Senior Lecturer, Department of Psychiatry, University of Edinburgh, UK
Chapter 4.2.2.4

Daniel Chisholm Institute of Psychiatry, King's College London, UK
Chapter 7.7

Derek Chiswick Honorary Senior Lecturer in Psychiatry, University of Edinburgh, UK
Chapter 11.3

Sudhansu Chokroverty Professor of Neurology, New York Medical College; Clinical Professor of Neurology, Robert Wood Johnson Medical School, New Brunswick, New Jersey, USA
Chapter 4.14.6

Gary Christenson Associate Clinical Professor of Psychiatry, Department of Psychiatry, University of Minnesota; Director, Mental Health Clinic, Boynton Health Service, University of Minnesota, Minneapolis, Minnesota, USA
Chapter 4.13.2

Anthony Clare Clinical Professor of Psychiatry, Trinity College, Dublin, Ireland
Chapter 1.2

David M. Clark Professor of Psychiatry and Wellcome Principal Research Fellow, University of Oxford Department of Psychiatry, Warneford Hospital, Oxford, UK
Chapter 6.3.2.1

John Collinge Director, MRC Prion Unit, Imperial College of Science, Technology and Medicine, London, UK
Chapter 4.1.5

John E. Cooper Emeritus Professor of Psychiatry, University of Nottingham, UK
Chapter 1.10.1

F.-R. Cousin Psychiatrist, Centre Hospitalier Saint-Anne, Paris, France
Chapter 4.3.9

P.J. Cowen University of Oxford Department of Psychiatry, Warneford Hospital, Oxford, UK
Chapter 6.2.9.2

Tom K.J. Craig Professor of Community Psychiatry, Guy's, King's and St Thomas's Schools of Medicine, London, UK
Chapters 7.10.2 and 7.10.3

Paul Crits-Christoph Professor of Psychology in Psychiatry, University of Pennsylvania School of Medicine, Philadelphia, Pennsylvania, USA
Chapter 6.1.2

Michael Crowe Consultant Psychiatrist, South London and Maudsley NHS Trust; Honorary Senior Lecturer, Institute of Psychiatry, King's College London, UK
Chapter 6.3.7

D.G. Cunningham Owens Reader in Psychiatry, Department of Psychiatry, University of Edinburgh, UK
Chapter 4.3.7

Pinhas N. Dannon Psychiatric Medical Center, Sheba Medical Center, Tel Hashomer and Sackler School of Medicine, Tel Aviv University, Israel
Chapter 4.8

Anthony S. David Professor of Cognitive Neuropsychiatry, Institute of Psychiatry, King's College London, UK
Chapters 4.3.3.1 and 4.3.3.2

Kate Davidson Senior Research Psychologist, Department of Psychological Medicine, University of Glasgow, UK
Chapter 4.12.7

Giovanni de Girolamo National Institute of Health, National Mental Health Project, Rome, Italy
Chapters 4.12.4 and 4.12.5

K.W. de Pauw Consultant and Senior Clinical Lecturer, Department of Psychiatry, St James's University Hospital, Leeds, UK
Chapter 4.9

Shoumitro Deb Clinical Senior Lecturer in Neuropsychiatry, Division of Psychological Medicine, University of Wales College of Medicine, Cardiff, UK
Chapter 10.4

H. Dilling Professor of Psychiatry, Department of Psychiatry, Lübeck Medical University, Germany
Chapter 1.11

Otto Doerr-Zegers Professor of Psychiatry, University of Chile; Chief of Ward, Public Psychiatric Hospital, Santiago de Chile
Chapter 3.4

A. Došen Catholic University Nijmegen and Nieuw Spraeland, Oostrum, The Netherlands
Chapter 10.5.2

Patrizia Dotto Unit of Clinical Psychology, ASL 2, Lucca, Italy
Chapter 4.12.5

Jo Douglas Consultant Clinical Psychologist, Great Ormond Street Hospital for Sick Children, London, UK
Chapter 9.2.8

D. Colin Drummond Reader in Addiction Psychiatry, Department of Psychiatry of Addictive Behaviour, St George's Hospital Medical School, University of London, UK
Chapter 4.2.2.5

Graham Dunn School of Epidemiology and Health Sciences, University of Manchester, UK
Chapter 2.2

Nigel Eastman Senior Lecturer in Forensic Psychiatry, St George's Hospital Medical School, University of London, UK
Chapter 11.7

Anke Ehlers Department of Psychiatry, University of Oxford, UK
Chapters 4.6.1 and 4.6.2

Leon Eisenberg Maude and Lillian Presley Professor of Social Medicine and Emeritus Professor of Psychiatry, Harvard Medical School, Boston, Massachusetts, USA
Chapter 1.3.1

R.M. Epstein Associate Professor, Departments of Family Medicine and Psychiatry, Primary Care Institute, University of Rochester School of Medicine and Dentistry, Rochester, New York, USA
Chapter 1.10.2

Timo Erkinjuntti Chief, Memory Research Unit, Department of Clinical Neurosciences, Helsinki University Central Hospital, Helsinki, Finland
Chapter 4.1.9

Brigette A. Erwin Adult Anxiety Clinic of Temple University, Philadelphia, Pennsylvania, USA
Chapter 4.7.2

Colin A. Espie Professor of Clinical Psychology and Head of Department of Psychological Medicine, University of Glasgow, UK
Chapter 4.14.2

Rodolfo Fahrer Chairman and Professor, Department of Mental Health, School of Medicine, University of Buenos Aires, Argentina
Chapter 5.1

Christopher G. Fairburn Wellcome Principal Research Fellow and Professor of Psychiatry, University of Oxford, UK
Chapters 4.10.2 and 6.3.2.2

Peter Falkai Professor of Medical Psychology, Rheinische Friedrich-Wilhelms-Universität, Bonn, Germany
Chapter 2.3.5

Stephen V. Faraone Associate Professor of Psychology, Department of Psychiatry, Harvard Medical School at Massachusetts Mental Health Center, Boston, Massachusetts, USA
Chapter 4.3.8

Michael Farrell Senior Lecturer and Consultant Psychiatrist, National Addiction Centre, South London and Maudsley NHS Trust, London, UK
Chapter 4.2.3.5

David P. Farrington Professor of Psychological Criminology, University of Cambridge, UK
Chapter 11.2

Melanie J.V. Fennell Consultant Clinical Psychologist; Director, Oxford Diploma in Cognitive Therapy, University of Oxford Department of Psychiatry, Warneford Hospital, Oxford, UK
Chapter 6.3.2.3

Max Fink Emeritus Professor of Psychiatry and Neurology, State University of New York at Stony Brook; Professor of Psychiatry, Albert Einstein College of Medicine; Attending Psychiatrist, Long Island Jewish Medical Center, New York, USA
Chapter 6.2.9.1

Per Fink Director, Research Unit for Functional Disorders, Aarhus University Hospital, Risskov, Denmark
Chapter 5.2.3

Philip A. Fisher Research Scientist, Oregon Social Learning Center, Eugene, Oregon, USA
Chapter 9.5.4

Martine F. Flament Chargée de Récherche INSERM, CNRS UMR 7593, Paris, France
Chapter 9.2.6

Simon Fleminger Consultant Neuropsychiatrist, Maudsley Hospital, London, UK
Chapters 4.1.11 and 4.1.14

Jonathan Flint Department of Psychiatry, University of Oxford, UK
Chapter 2.4.2

Laurie M. Flynn Executive Director, National Alliance for the Mentally Ill (NAMI), Arlington, Virginia, USA
Chapter 7.9

Susan Folstein Professor of Psychiatry, Tufts University School of Medicine, Medford, Massachusetts, USA
Chapter 4.1.8

Peter Fonagy Freud Memorial Professor of Psychoanalysis, University College London; Director of Research, Anna Freud Centre, London, UK; Director, Child and Family Center and Clinical Protocols and Outcomes Center, Menninger Clinic, Topeka, Kansas, USA
Chapters 6.3.5 and 9.5.2

W. Fraser Division of Psychological Medicine, University of Wales College of Medicine, Cardiff, UK
Introduction to Section 10

David M. Fresco Adult Anxiety Clinic of Temple University, Philadelphia, Pennsylvania, USA
Chapter 4.7.2

Alexandra M. Freund Max Planck Institute for Human Development, Berlin, Germany
Chapter 2.5.1.2

Lutz Frölich Department of Psychiatry, University of Frankfurt, Germany
Chapter 5.6

Tom Fryers International Consultant in Public Health and Mental Health; Adjunct Professor in Community Medicine, New York Medical College, New York, USA; Visiting Professor of Rehabilitation, Queen's University, Kingston, Ontario, Canada
Chapter 10.2

K.W.M. Fulford Professor of Philosophy and Mental Health, University of Warwick; Honorary Consultant Psychiatrist, University of Oxford, UK
Chapter 1.5

Glen O. Gabbard Bessie Walker Callaway Distinguished Professor of Psychoanalysis and Education in the Kansas School of Psychiatry, Menninger Clinic, Topeka; Clinical Professor of Psychiatry of Kansas School of Medicine, Wichita, Kansas, USA
Chapter 3.5

J. Garrabé Psychiatrist, Centre La Verrière, MGEN, Le Mesnil Saint-Denis, France
Chapter 4.3.9

M. Elena Garralda Professor of Child and Adolescent Psychiatry, Imperial College School of Medicine, London, UK
Chapter 9.3.2

Ann Gath Formerly of University College London, UK
Chapter 10.8

John Geddes Senior Clinical Research Fellow; Honorary Consultant Psychiatrist, University of Oxford Department of Psychiatry, Warneford Hospital, Oxford, UK
Chapter 1.12

S. Nassir Ghaemi Harvard Bipolar Research Program, Massachusetts General Hospital, Consolidated Department of Psychiatry, Harvard Medical School, Boston, Massachusetts, USA
Chapter 4.5.1

Ian Gibbs Social Work Research and Development Unit, University of York, UK
Chapter 9.5.6

David Gill Research Fellow, Department of Psychiatry, University of Oxford, UK
Chapters 4.1.2 and 5.2.9

Christopher Gillberg Professor of Child and Adolescent Psychiatry, University of Göteborg, Sweden
Chapter 9.5.5

Madeline Gladis Assistant Professor of Psychology in Psychiatry, University of Pennsylvania School of Medicine, Philadelphia, Pennsylvania, USA
Chapter 6.1.2

Julia Gledhill Clinical Research Fellow, Imperial College School of Medicine, London, UK
Chapter 9.3.2

David Goldberg Director of Research and Development, Institute of Psychiatry, King's College London, UK
Chapter 7.8

Frederick K. Goodwin Professor of Psychiatry, George Washington University, Washington, DC, USA
Chapter 4.5.1

Guy Goodwin W.A. Handley Professor of Psychiatry, University of Oxford, UK
Chapter 4.5.5.2

Ian Goodyer Professor of Child and Adolescent Psychiatry, University of Cambridge, UK
Chapter 9.2.5

Kevin Gournay Professor of Psychiatry Nursing, Institute of Psychiatry, King's College London, UK
Chapter 6.4.2

P.M. Grasby Senior Lecturer, MRC Cyclotron Unit, Hammersmith Hospital, London, UK
Chapter 2.3.6

Richard Green Head, Gender Identity Clinic, and Visiting Professor of Psychiatry, Imperial College of Medicine at Charing Cross Hospital, London, UK; Emeritus Professor of Psychiatry, University of California, Los Angeles, California, USA
Chapters 4.11.4 and 9.2.12

Adrian Grounds University Lecturer in Forensic Psychiatry, Institute of Criminology and Department of Psychiatry, University of Cambridge, UK
Chapter 11.6

Michael Gunn Professor of Law and Head of Department, Department of Academic Legal Studies, Nottingham Law School, Nottingham Trent University, UK
Chapter 11.1

Lars Gustafson Professor of Geriatric Psychiatry, University Hospital, Lund, Sweden
Chapter 4.1.4

Jennifer Gutstein Department of Child Psychiatry, College of Physicians and Surgeons, Columbia University, New York, USA
Chapter 9.2.10

Robert Hale Consultant Psychotherapist, Portman Clinic, Tavistock and Portman NHS Trust, London, UK
Chapter 11.4.2

John N. Hall Department of Clinical Psychology and University Department of Psychiatry, Warneford Hospital, Oxford, UK
Chapter 1.10.3.2

Wayne Hall Professor of Drug and Alcohol Studies, University of New South Wales, Sydney, Australia
Chapter 4.2.3.8

Edwin Harari Consultant Psychiatrist, St Vincent's Hospital, Melbourne, Australia
Chapter 6.3.8

Richard Harrington University Department of Child and Adolescent Psychiatry, Royal Manchester Children's Hospital, Manchester, UK
Chapter 9.5.3

James C. Harris Professor of Psychiatry and Behavioral Sciences and Pediatrics, Johns Hopkins University School of Medicine, Baltimore, Maryland, USA
Chapter 9.2.7

Paul J. Harrison Clinical Reader in Psychiatry, University of Oxford Department of Psychiatry, Warneford Hospital, Oxford, UK
Chapter 4.3.5.2

Allison G. Harvey Department of Experimental Psychology, University of Oxford, UK
Chapter 4.6.1

Keith Hawton University of Oxford Department of Psychiatry, Warneford Hospital, Oxford, UK
Chapter 4.15.4

Richard G. Heimberg Adult Anxiety Clinic of Temple University, Philadelphia, Pennsylvania, USA
Chapter 4.7.2

Scott Henderson Director, Centre for Mental Health Research, Australian National University, Canberra, Australia
Chapter 2.7

George R. Heninger Professor, Department of Psychiatry, Yale University School of Medicine, New Haven, Connecticut, USA
Chapter 6.2.3

Thomas Herzog Department of Psychosomatic Medicine, University Hospital, Freiburg, Germany
Chapter 5.6

Peter Hill Professor of Child Mental Health, St George's Hospital Medical School, London, UK
Chapter 9.1.5

Mike Hobbs University of Oxford Department of Psychiatry, Warneford Hospital, Oxford, UK
Chapter 6.3.1

A.J. Holland Lecturer, Department of Psychiatry, University of Cambridge, UK
Chapter 10.1

Jimmie C. Holland Chair, Department of Psychiatry and Behavioral Sciences, Memorial Sloan-Kettering Cancer Center, New York, USA
Chapter 5.3.7

Sheila Hollins Professor of Psychiatry of Learning Disability, Department of Psychiatry and Disability, St George's Hospital Medical School, University of London, UK
Chapter 10.7

Jeremy Holmes Consultant Psychiatrist/Psychotherapist, North Devon District Hospital, Barnstaple; Senior Lecturer, University of Bristol, UK
Chapter 3.3.2

Suzanne Holroyd Associate Professor, Department of Psychiatric Medicine, University of Virginia School of Medicine, Charlottesville, Virginia, USA
Chapter 8.5.6

Geraldine Holt Consultant Psychiatrist and Senior Lecturer, Guy's Hospital, London, UK
Chapter 10.9

Allan House Professor of Liaison Psychiatry, University of Leeds, UK
Chapter 5.3.1

Robert Howard Senior Lecturer in Old Age Psychiatry, Institute of Psychiatry, King's College London, UK
Chapter 8.5.3

Jane Hubert Senior Lecturer in Social Anthropology, Department of Psychiatry and Disability, St George's Hospital Medical School, University of London, UK
Chapter 10.7

Frits J. Huyse Associate Professor in Consultation–Liaison Psychiatry, Free University, Amsterdam, The Netherlands
Chapter 5.8

Iulian Iancu Psychiatric Medical Center, Sheba Medical Center, Tel Hashomer and Sackler School of Medicine, Tel Aviv University, Israel
Chapter 4.8

Abel Ickowicz Assistant Professor of Psychiatry, University of Toronto; Staff Psychiatrist, Hospital for Sick Children, Toronto, Canada
Chapter 9.2.3

Matti Iivanaien Professor, Department of Child Neurology, University of Helsinki, Finland
Chapter 10.5.3

Leslie Iversen Department of Pharmacology, University of Oxford, UK
Chapter 6.2.7

Richard Ives National Children's Bureau, London, UK
Chapter 4.2.3.7

Assen Jablensky Professor of Psychiatry, University of Western Australia, Perth, Australia
Chapters 4.3.4 and 4.3.6

Robin Jacoby Clinical Reader in the Psychiatry of Old Age, University of Oxford, UK
Chapters 8.4 and 8.5.7

Kay Redfield Jamison Professor of Psychiatry, Johns Hopkins School of Medicine, Baltimore, Maryland, USA
Chapter 1.1

Martin Jarvis ICRF Health Behaviour Unit, Department of Epidemiology and Public Health, University College London, UK
Chapter 4.2.3.9

John G.R. Jefferys Department of Neurophysiology, Division of Neuroscience, University of Birmingham, UK
Chapter 2.3.9

Rachel Jenkins Director, WHO Collaborating Centre, Institute of Psychiatry, King's College London, UK
Chapter 7.1

Wolfgang G. Jilek Clinical Professor Emeritus of Psychiatry, University of British Columbia, Vancouver, British Columbia, Canada
Chapters 4.16 and 6.5

Andrew Johns Consultant Forensic Psychiatry and Honorary Senior Lecturer, Maudsley Hospital, London, UK
Chapter 11.4.4

Deirdre Johnston Clinical Assistant Professor, Department of Psychiatry and Behavioral Medicine, Wake Forest University School of Medicine, Winston-Salem, North Carolina, USA
Chapter 8.7

E.C. Johnstone Professor of Psychiatry and Head, Department of Psychiatry, University of Edinburgh, UK
Chapter 4.3.7

David P.H. Jones Senior Clinical Lecturer in Child Psychiatry, Park Hospital for Children, University of Oxford, UK
Chapter 9.3.1

A.F. Jorm Professor and Deputy Director, Centre for Mental Health Research, Australian National University, Canberra, Australia
Chapter 8.3

Peter R. Joyce Professor, Department of Psychological Medicine, Christchurch School of Medicine, Christchurch, New Zealand
Chapter 4.5.4

Markus Kaski Director, Rinnekoti Research Foundation, Espoo, Finland
Chapter 10.3

John Kellett St George's Hospital Medical School, London, UK
Chapter 8.5.8

David Kennard Head of Psychology and Psychotherapy, The Retreat, York, UK
Chapter 6.3.9

A.J.F.M. Kerkhof Professor of Clinical Psychology, Vrije Universiteit, Amsterdam, The Netherlands
Chapter 4.15.2

Otto F. Kernberg Professor of Psychiatry, Cornell University Medical College, New York; Training and Supervising Analyst, Columbia University Center for Psychoanalytic Training and Research, New York, USA
Chapter 3.2

Arthur Kleinman Presley Professor of Anthropology and Psychiatry, Harvard University; Chair, Department of Social Medicine, Harvard Medical School, Cambridge, Massachusetts, USA
Chapter 2.6.2

Ami Klin Yale University, New Haven, Connecticut, USA
Chapter 9.2.2

Martin Knapp Institute of Psychiatry, King's College London; London School of Economics, University of London, UK
Chapter 7.7

Israel Kolvin Emeritus Professor of Child and Family Mental Health, Tavistock Clinic and the Royal Free and University College Medical School, London, UK
Chapter 9.2.11

Michael D. Kopelman Division of Psychiatry and Psychology, United Medical and Dental Schools of Guy's and St Thomas's Hospitals, London, UK
Chapter 4.1.13

Malcolm Lader Professor of Clinical Pharmacology, Institute of Psychiatry, King's College London, UK
Chapter 6.2.2

Fergus D. Law Honorary Senior Registrar and Clinical Lecturer, Psychopharmacology Unit, University of Bristol, UK
Chapters 4.2.1 and 6.2.8

Paul Leber Director, Neuro-Pharm Group, LLC, Potomac, Maryland, USA
Chapter 6.1.1.1

Dusica Lecic-Tosevski Associate Professor of Psychiatry, School of Medicine, University of Belgrade, Yugoslavia
Chapter 4.12.3

Julian Leff Professor of Social and Cultural Psychiatry, Institute of Psychiatry, King's College London, UK
Chapter 1.3.2

Bernard Lerer Biological Psychiatry Unit, Hadassah-Hebrew University Medical Center, Jerusalem, Israel
Chapter 2.3.4

R.J. Levin Department of Biomedical Science, University of Sheffield, UK
Chapter 4.11.1

Peter F. Liddle Professor of Psychiatry, University of British Columbia, Vancouver, British Columbia, Canada
Chapter 4.3.2

Felice Lieh Mak Professor, Department of Psychiatry, University of Hong Kong, Hong Kong
Chapter 5.2.10

James Lindesay Professor of Psychiatry for the Elderly, University of Leicester, UK
Chapters 8.5.1 and 8.5.5

Per Lindqvist Director, Örebro Forensic Psychiatry Services, Sweden
Chapter 11.8

Jouko K. Lonnqvist Professor, National Public Health Institute, Helsinki, Finland
Chapter 4.15.1

Juan López-Ibor Chairman, Department of Psychiatry, San Carlos University Hospital, Complutense University, Madrid, Spain
Chapter 4.12.1

Armand W. Loranger Emeritus Professor of Psychiatry (Psychology), Cornell University Medical College, White Plains, New York, USA
Chapter 4.12.2

Simon Lovestone Institute of Psychiatry, King's College London, UK
Chapter 4.1.3

Ernest S.L. Luk Department of Psychological Medicine, Monash University, Melbourne, Australia
Chapter 9.5.8

Alexander McCall Smith Professor of Medical Law, University of Edinburgh, UK
Chapter 1.6

Susan L. McElroy Biological Psychiatry Program, Department of Psychiatry, University of Cincinnati College of Medicine, Cincinnati, Ohio, USA
Chapter 4.13.1

Peter McGuffin Director and Professor of Psychiatric Genetics, Institute of Psychiatry, King's College London, UK
Chapter 2.4.1

Paul R. McHugh Henry Phipps Professor of Psychiatry; Director, Department of Psychiatry and Behavioral Science; Psychiatrist-in-Chief, Johns Hopkins University School of Medicine, Baltimore, Maryland, USA
Chapter 1.7

I.G. McKeith Professor of Old Age Psychiatry, Institute for the Health of the Elderly, University of Newcastle upon Tyne, UK
Chapter 4.1.6

Kwame McKenzie Clinical Lecturer, Department of Psychological Medicine, Institute of Psychiatry, King's College London, UK; Visiting Scholar, Department of Social Medicine, Harvard University Medical School, Boston, Massachusetts, USA
Chapter 7.3

Mark W. Mahowald Director, Minnesota Regional Sleep Disorders Center, Hennepin County Medical Center; Professor of Neurology, University of Minnesota Medical School, Minneapolis, Minnesota, USA
Chapter 4.14.4

Mario Maj Institute of Psychiatry, University of Naples, Italy
Chapter 4.1.10

Andrea L. Malizia Honorary Consultant in Clinical Psychopharmacology, Psychopharmacology Unit, University of Bristol, UK
Chapter 6.2.9.3

Rosemarie Mallett Social Psychiatry Section, Institute of Psychiatry, King's College London, UK
Chapter 7.10.3

Ulrik Fredrik Malt Professor of Psychiatry (Psychosomatic Medicine), National Hospital, University of Oslo, Norway
Chapter 5.3.8

Anthony Mann Professor of Psychiatric Epidemiology, Institute of Psychiatry, King's College London, UK
Chapter 7.8

J. John Mann Professor of Psychiatry, Columbia University, New York, USA
Chapter 4.15.3

Karl F. Mann Professor of Psychiatry and Addiction Research; Chairman, Department of Addictive Behaviour and Addiction Medicine, Central Institute of Mental Health, Mannheim University of Heidelberg, Mannheim, Germany
Chapter 4.2.2.3

John C. Markowitz Associate Professor of Psychiatry, Weill Medical College of Cornell University; Director, Psychotherapy Clinic, Payne Whitney Clinic, New York Presbyterian Hospital, New York, USA
Chapter 6.3.3

John Marsden Lecturer, Institute of Psychiatry, King's College London, UK
Chapter 4.2.4

Jane Marshall Senior Lecturer in the Addictions, National Addiction Centre, Institute of Psychiatry, King's College London, UK
Chapters 4.1.12 and 4.2.2.2

Barbara Maughan MRC Child Psychiatry Unit, Institute of Psychiatry, King's College London, UK
Chapter 9.1.2

Richard Mayou Professor of Psychiatry, University of Oxford, UK
Chapters 4.1.2 and 5.2.1

Herbert Y. Meltzer Department of Psychiatry, Vanderbilt University School of Medicine, Nashville, Tennessee, USA
Chapter 6.2.5

J. Mendlewicz Department of Psychiatry, University Clinics of Brussels, Erasme Hospital, Brussels, Belgium
Chapter 4.5.5.1

Harald Merckelbach Professor of Experimental Psychology, Maastricht University, The Netherlands
Chapter 2.5.3

Harold Merskey Emeritus Professor of Psychiatry, University of Western Ontario, Canada
Chapter 5.2.4

Gillian C. Mezey Consultant and Senior Lecturer in Forensic Psychiatry, Traumatic Stress Service, St George's Hospital Medical School, London, UK
Chapter 11.5

R.H.S. Mindham Nuffield Professor of Psychiatry, University of Leeds, UK
Chapter 4.1.7

Carine Minne Consultant Psychotherapist, Portman Clinic, Tavistock and Portman NHS Trust, London, and Broadmoor Hospital, UK
Chapter 11.4.2

Alex Mitchell Lecturer in Psychiatry, University of Leeds, UK
Chapter 5.3.1

Richard F. Mollica Director, Harvard Program in Refugee Trauma; Associate Professor of Psychiatry, Harvard Medical School and Harvard School of Public Health, Cambridge, Massachusetts, USA
Chapter 7.10.1

Francisco Mora Professor and Chairman of Physiology and Medicine, Complutense University, Madrid, Spain; Professor of Physiology, Biophysics and Medicine, Iowa University, Iowa City, Iowa, USA
Chapter 2.1.2

Emanuel Moran Consultant Psychiatrist, Grovelands Priory Hospital, London, UK
Chapter 4.13.3

Paul E. Mullen Professor of Forensic Psychiatry, Monash University; Clinical Director, Victorian Institute of Forensic Mental Health, Monash University, Melbourne, Australia
Chapters 11.4.3 and 11.8

Christoph Mundt Psychiatric Hospital of the University of Heidelberg, Germany
Chapter 1.9

Alistair Munro Emeritus Professor of Psychiatry, Dalhousie University, Halifax, Nova Scotia, Canada
Chapter 4.4

R.M. Murray Institute of Psychiatry, King's College London, UK
Chapter 4.3.5.1

Juan C. Negrete Professor and Head, Addictions Psychiatry Program, University of Toronto, Canada
Chapter 4.2.2.1

Charles B. Nemeroff Reunette W. Harris Professor and Chairman, Department of Psychiatry and Behavioral Sciences, Emory University School of Medicine, Atlanta, Georgia, USA
Chapter 2.3.3

Jeffrey Newcorn Mount Sinai School of Medicine, New York, USA
Chapter 4.6.4

Michael E. Newman Biological Psychiatry Unit, Hadassah-Hebrew University Medical Center, Jerusalem, Israel
Chapter 2.3.4

Anula Nikapota Consultant in Child and Adolescent Psychiatry, Brixton Child and Adolescent Mental Health Team, Bethlem Maudsley NHS Trust, London, UK
Chapter 9.5.7

Russell Noyes Jr Department of Psychiatry, University of Iowa College of Medicine, Iowa City, Iowa, USA
Chapter 5.2.5

David J. Nutt Professor of Psychopharmacology and Head of Clinical Medicine, University of Bristol, UK
Chapters 4.2.1 and 6.2.8

Margaret Oates Senior Lecturer in Psychiatry, University of Nottingham, UK
Chapter 1.10.1

David R. Offord Professor of Psychiatry, McMaster University; Director, Centre for Studies of Children at Risk, Hamilton Health Sciences Corporation and McMaster University, Hamilton, Ontario, Canada
Chapter 9.1.3

Catherine Oppenheimer Consultant Psychiatrist, Warneford Hospital, Oxford, UK
Chapter 8.6

Candice A. Osborn Professor of Clinical Psychiatry, Morehouse School of Medicine, Atlanta, Georgia, USA
Chapter 4.11.3

Christopher M. Palmer Instructor of Psychiatry, Harvard Medical School, Boston; Assistant Psychiatrist, McClean Hospital, Belmont, Massachusetts, USA
Chapter 6.2.6

Gordon Parker Professor and Head, School of Psychiatry, University of New South Wales, Australia
Chapter 4.5.3

E.S. Paykel Department of Psychiatry, University of Cambridge, UK
Chapter 4.5.7

John B. Pearce Emeritus Professor of Child and Adolescent Psychiatry, University of Nottingham, UK
Chapters 9.4.2 and 9.5.1

R.C.A. Pearson Department of Biomedical Science, University of Sheffield, UK
Chapter 2.3.1

Keith J. Petrie Associate Professor, School of Medicine, University of Auckland, New Zealand
Chapter 5.7

Cynthia R. Pfeffer Weill Medical College of Cornell University, New York Presbyterian Hospital–Westchester Division, White Plains, New York, USA
Chapter 9.2.10

Katharine A. Phillips Associate Professor, Department of Psychiatry and Human Behavior, Brown University School of Medicine, Butler Hospital, Providence, Rhode Island, USA
Chapter 5.2.8

Pierre Pichot Académie Nationale de Médecine, Paris, France
Chapter 1.4

Malcolm Pines Institute of Group Analysis, London, UK
Chapter 6.3.6

Harrison G. Pope Jr Professor of Psychiatry, Harvard Medical School, Boston; Chief, Biological Psychiatry Laboratory, McClean Hospital, Belmont, Massachusetts, USA
Chapter 6.2.6

Robert M. Post Chief, Biological Psychiatry Branch, National Institute of Mental Health, Bethesda, Maryland, USA
Chapter 6.2.4

Graham E. Powell Psychology Services, London, UK
Chapter 1.10.3.1

Herschel Prins Professor, Midlands Centre for Criminology and Criminal Justice, University of Loughborough, UK
Chapter 11.4.1

Frederic M. Quitkin Professor of Clinical Psychiatry, Columbia University, New York, USA
Chapter 6.1.3

Shulamit Ramon Professor of Interprofessional Health and Social Studies, Anglia Polytechnic University, Cambridge, UK
Chapter 6.4.3

James Reich Associate Clinical Professor, Department of Psychiatry, Stanford Medical School, Palo Alto; Associate Clinical Professor, Department of Psychiatry, University of California Medical School at San Francisco, California, USA
Chapter 4.12.4

Burton V. Reifler Professor and Chair, Department of Psychiatry and Behavioral Medicine, Wake Forest University School of Medicine, Winston-Salem, North Carolina, USA
Chapter 8.7

Helmut Remschmidt Director, Department of Child and Adolescent Psychiatry, Philipps Universität, Marburg, Germany
Chapter 9.2.1

Katharine Rimes University of Oxford Department of Psychiatry, Warneford Hospital, Oxford, UK
Chapter 5.5

Ian Robbins Consultant Clinical Psychologist, St George's Hospital, London, UK
Chapter 11.5

Philip Robson Consultant Psychiatrist and Senior Clinical Lecturer, University of Oxford Department of Psychiatry, Warneford Hospital, Oxford, UK
Chapter 4.2.3.1

Gary Rodin Professor of Psychiatry, University of Toronto, Ontario, Canada
Chapter 5.3.6

Maria A. Ron Professor of Neuropsychiatry, Institute of Neurology, University College London, UK
Chapter 5.3.2

Robin Room Professor and Director, Centre for Social Research on Alcohol and Drugs, Stockholm University, Sweden
Chapter 4.2.2.6

W. Rössler Professor of Clinical Psychiatry and Psychology, University of Zürich, Switzerland
Chapter 6.4.1

Marjaneh Rouhani Department of Psychiatry and Behavioral Sciences, Memorial Sloan-Kettering Cancer Center, New York, USA
Chapter 5.3.7

James R. Rundell Professor of Psychiatry, F. Edward Herbert School of Medicine, Uniform Services University of the Health Sciences, Bethesda, Maryland, USA
Chapter 5.3.4

Gerald Russell Emeritus Professor of Psychiatry, Director of the Eating Disorders Unit, Hayes Grove Priory Hospital, Hayes, Kent, UK
Chapter 4.10.1

Paul Salkovskis University of Oxford Department of Psychiatry, Warneford Hospital, Oxford, UK
Chapter 5.5

Diana Sanders University of Oxford Department of Psychiatry, Warneford Hospital, Oxford, UK
Chapter 6.3.1

Russell Schachar Professor of Psychiatry, University of Toronto; Staff Psychiatrist, Hospital for Sick Children, Toronto, Canada
Chapter 9.2.3

Carlos H. Schenck Staff Psychiatrist, Minnesota Regional Sleep Disorders Center, Hennepin County Medical Center; Associate Professor of Psychiatry, University of Minnesota Medical School, Minneapolis, Minnesota, USA
Chapter 4.14

John Schlapobersky Group Analyst, Group Analytic Practice, London; Consultant Psychiatrist, Medical Foundation for Victims of Torture, London, UK
Chapter 6.3.6

Patricia Schreiner-Engel Associate Clinical Professor, Department of Obstetrics, Gynecology and Reproductive Science, and Department of Psychiatry, Mount Sinai School of Medicine, New York, USA
Chapter 4.11.2

J. Scott Professor of Psychiatry, University of Glasgow Gartnavel Royal Hospital, Glasgow, UK
Chapter 4.5.7

Stephen Scott Institute of Psychiatry, King's College London, UK
Chapters 9.1.1 and 9.2.4

Nicholas Seivewright Consultant Psychiatrist in Substance Misuse, Community Health Sheffield NHS Trust, Sheffield, UK
Chapter 4.2.3.3

David Shaffer Department of Child Psychiatry, College of Physicians and Surgeons, Columbia University, New York, USA
Chapter 9.2.10

Michael Sharpe Senior Lecturer in Psychological Medicine, University of Edinburgh, UK
Chapter 5.2.7

Gregory Simon Investigator, Center for Health Studies, Group Health Cooperative, Seattle, Washington, USA
Chapter 5.2.2

Andrew Sims Professor of Psychiatry, University of Leeds, UK
Chapter 1.9

Ian Sinclair Professor of Social Work, University of York, UK
Chapter 9.5.6

Phillip R. Slavney Eugene Meyer III Professor of Psychiatry; Director, General Hospital Psychiatry, Johns Hopkins University School of Medicine, Baltimore, Maryland, USA
Chapter 1.7

George Freeman Solomon Emeritus Professor of Psychiatry and Biobehavioral Sciences, University of California, Los Angeles, California, USA
Chapter 2.3.10

D. Souery Department of Psychiatry, University Clinics of Brussels, Erasme Hospital, Brussels, Belgium
Chapter 4.5.5.1

Elizabeth Spencer Senior Clinical Medical Officer, Early Intervention Service, Northern Birmingham Mental Health Trust, Birmingham, UK
Chapter 6.3.2.4

David A. Spiegel Center for Anxiety and Related Disorders at Boston University, Boston, Massachusetts, USA
Chapter 4.7.1

Ursula M. Staudinger Professor of Psychology, Dresden University of Technology, Dresden, Germany
Chapter 2.5.1.2

Alan Stein Royal Free and University College Medical School, University College London, and Tavistock Clinic, London, UK
Chapter 9.3.4

Barbara Stein Department of Psychosomatic Medicine, University Hospital, Freiburg, Germany
Chapter 5.6

Derek Steinberg Consultant Psychiatrist and Visiting Senior Tutor, Ticehurst House Hospital Children's and Adolescent Service, Wadhurst, UK
Chapter 9.5.9

William S. Stone Instructor in Psychology, Department of Psychiatry, Harvard Medical School at Massachusetts Mental Health Center, Boston, Massachusetts, USA
Chapter 4.3.8

Gregory Stores Department of Psychiatry, University of Oxford, UK
Chapters 4.14.1 and 9.2.9

Elizabeth A. Stormshak Assistant Professor, University of Oregon, Eugene, Oregon, USA
Chapter 9.5.4

Anthony Storr Emeritus Fellow, Green College, Oxford, UK
Chapters 3.1 and 3.3.1

James J. Strain Professor/Director, Behavioral Medicine and Consultation Psychiatry, Mount Sinai School of Medicine, New York, USA
Chapter 4.6.4

John Strang Professor; Director of the National Addiction Centre, Institute of Psychiatry, King's College London, UK
Chapters 4.2.3.2 and 4.2.4

Albert Stunkard Professor of Psychiatry, University of Pennsylvania, Philadelphia, Pennsylvania, USA
Chapter 4.10.3

J. Suckling Clinical Age Research Unit, Department of Health Care for the Elderly, King's College School of Medicine and Dentistry, University of London, UK
Chapters 2.3.7 and 2.3.8

Michele Tansella Professor of Psychiatry and Chairman, Department of Medicine and Public Health, Section of Psychiatry, University of Verona, Italy
Chapters 7.5 and 7.6

Mary Target Senior Lecturer in Psychoanalysis, Psychoanalysis Unit, University College London; Deputy Director of Research, Anna Freud Centre, London, UK
Chapter 9.5.2

Anita Thapar Professor of Child and Adolescent Psychiatry, University of Manchester, UK
Chapter 2.4.1

June Thoburn Professor of Social Work, University of East Anglia, Norwich, UK
Chapter 9.3.3

Anne E. Thompson Consultant Child and Adolescent Psychiatrist, Lincoln District Healthcare NHS Trust, Lincoln, UK
Chapter 9.4.2

Graham Thornicroft Professor of Community Psychiatry, Institute of Psychiatry, King's College London, UK
Chapters 7.5 and 7.6

Adolf Tobeña Professor of Psychiatry and Medical Psychiatry, School of Medicine, Autonomous University of Barcelona, Spain
Chapter 4.12.6

Bruce J. Tonge Professor and Head, Monash University Department of Psychological Medicine and Centre for Developmental Psychiatry, Monash Medical Centre, Clayton, Victoria, Australia
Chapter 10.5.1

Brian Toone Consultant, Maudsley Hospital; Honorary Senior Lecturer, Institute of Psychiatry, King's College London, UK
Chapter 5.3.3

Ming T. Tsuang Stanley Cobb Professor of Psychiatry and Head, Department of Psychiatry, Harvard Medical School at Massachusetts Mental Health Center, Boston, Massachusetts, USA
Chapter 4.3.8

Cynthia L. Turk Adult Anxiety Clinic of Temple University, Philadelphia, Pennsylvania, USA
Chapter 4.7.2

André Tylee Director, Royal College of General Practitioners Unit for Mental Health Education in Primary Care, Institute of Psychiatry, King's College London, UK
Chapter 7.8

Peter Tyrer Division of Primary Care and Health Sciences, Imperial College School of Medicine, London, UK
Chapter 4.12.7

Amy M. Ursano Department of Psychiatry, University of North Carolina at Chapel Hill School of Medicine, Chapel Hill, North Carolina, USA
Chapter 6.3.4

Robert J. Ursano Professor and Chairman, Department of Psychiatry, Uniformed Services University of the Health Sciences, F. Edward Herbert School of Medicine, Bethesda, Maryland, USA
Chapter 6.3.4

Marcel van den Hout Professor of Medical Psychology and Mental Health, Maastricht University, The Netherlands
Chapter 2.5.3

Jim van Os Senior Lecturer, Department of Psychiatry, University of Maastricht, The Netherlands; Honorary Senior Lecturer, Department of Psychological Medicine, Institute of Psychiatry, King's College London, UK
Chapter 7.3

Fred R. Volkmar Yale University, New Haven, Connecticut, USA
Chapter 9.2.2

Thomas A. Wadden Professor of Psychology in Psychiatry, University of Pennsylvania, Philadelphia, Pennsylvania, USA
Chapter 4.10.3

John Weinmann Professor of Psychology as Applied to Medicine, United Medical and Dental Schools, London, UK
Chapter 5.7

Myrna M. Weissman Professor of Epidemiology in Psychiatry, College of Physicians and Surgeons of Columbia University; Chief, Division of Clinical and Genetic Epidemiology, New York State Psychiatric Institute, New York, USA
Chapter 6.3.3

Sarah Welch Consultant Psychiatrist, South London and Maudsley NHS Trust, London, UK
Chapter 4.2.3.5

G. Clare Wenger Centre for Social Policy Research and Development, University of Wales, Bangor, UK
Chapter 8.2

Simon Wessely Professor of Epidemiological and Liaison Psychiatry, Institute of Psychiatry, King's College London, UK
Chapter 5.2.7

Kay Wheat Senior Lecturer in Law, Department of Academic Legal Studies, Nottingham Law School, Nottingham Trent University, UK
Chapter 11.1

Barbara A. Wilson OBE Medical Research Council Cognition and Brain Sciences Unit, Addenbrooke's Hospital, Cambridge, UK
Chapter 2.5.2

Adam R. Winstock National Addiction Centre, Institute of Psychiatry, King's College London, UK
Chapters 4.2.3.2 and 4.2.3.6

Michael G. Wise Professor and Vice-Chair, Department of Psychiatry, University of California Davis Medical Center, Sacramento, California, USA
Chapter 5.3.4

Richard Jed Wyatt National Institutes of Mental Health, Bethesda, Maryland, USA
Chapter 1.1

William Yule Professor of Applied Child Psychology, Institute of Psychiatry, King's College London, UK
Chapter 2.5.1.1

Anne Zachary Consultant Psychotherapist, Portman Clinic, Tavistock and Portman NHS Trust, London, UK
Chapter 11.4.2

Karl Zilles Brain Research Institute, University of Dusseldorf, Germany
Chapter 2.3.2

Joseph Zohar Psychiatric Medical Center, Sheba Medical Center, Tel Hashomer and Sackler School of Medicine, Tel Aviv University, Israel
Chapter 4.8

1

The subject matter of and approach to psychiatry

1.1 On being a patient

Kay Redfield Jamison and Richard Jed Wyatt

It is difficult to be a psychiatric patient, but a good doctor can make it less so. Confusion and fear can be overcome by knowledge and compassion, and resistance to treatment is often, although by no means always, amenable to change by intelligent persuasion. The devil, as the fiery melancholic Byron knew, is in the detail.

Patients, when first given a psychiatric diagnosis, are commonly both relieved and frightened—relieved because often they have been in pain and anxiety for a considerable period of time, and frightened because they do not know what the diagnosis means or what the treatment will entail. They do not know if they will return to the way they once were, whether the treatment they have been prescribed will or will not work, and, even if it does work, at what cost it will be to them in terms of their notions of themselves, potentially unpleasant side-effects, and the reactions of their family members, friends, colleagues, and employers. Perhaps most disturbing, they do not know if their depression, psychosis, anxieties, or compulsions will return to become a permanent part of their lives.

The specifics of what the doctor says, and the manner in which he or she says it, are critically important. Most patients who complain about receiving poor psychiatric care do so on several grounds: their doctors, they feel, spend too little time explaining the nature of their illnesses and treatment; they are reluctant to consult with or actively involve family members; they are patronizing, and do not adequately listen to what the patient has to say; they do not encourage questions or sufficiently address the concerns of the patient, they do not discuss alternative treatments, the risks of treatment, and the risks of no treatment, and they do not thoroughly forewarn about side-effects of medications.

Most of these complaints are avoidable. Time, although difficult to come by, is well spent early on in the course of treatment when confusion and hopelessness are greatest, non-compliance is highest, and the possibility of suicide substantially increased. Hope can be realistically extended to patients and family members, and its explicit extension is vital to those whose illnesses have robbed them not only of hope, but of belief in themselves and their futures. The hope provided needs to be tempered, however, by an explication of possible difficulties yet to be encountered: unpleasant side-effects from medications, a rocky time course to meaningful recovery which will often consist of many discouraging cycles of feeling well, only to become ill again, and the probable personal, professional, and financial repercussions that come in the wake of having a psychiatric illness.

It is terrifying to lose one's sanity or to be seized by a paralysing depression. No medication alone can substitute for a good doctor's clinical expertise and the kindness of a doctor who understands both the medical and psychological sides of mental illness. Nor can any medication alone substitute for a good doctor's capacity to listen to the fears and despair of patients trying to come to terms with what has happened to them.

Doctors need to be direct in answering questions, to acknowledge the limits of their understanding, and to encourage specialist consultations when the clinical situation warrants it. They also need to create a therapeutic climate in which patients and their families feel free, when necessary, to express their concerns about treatment or to request a second opinion. Treatment non-compliance, one of the major causes of unnecessary suffering, relapse, hospitalization, and suicide, must be addressed head-on. Young males, early in the course of their illness, are particularly likely to stop medication against medical advice, and the results can be lethal.[1,2] Unfortunately, doctors are notoriously variable in their ability to assess and predict compliance in their patients.[3]

Asking directly and often about medication concerns, scheduling frequent follow-up visits after the initial diagnostic evaluation and treatment recommendation, and encouraging adjunctive psychotherapy, or involvement in patient support groups, can make a crucial difference in whether or not a patient takes medication in a way that is most effective. Aggressive treatment of unpleasant or intolerable side-effects, minimizing the dosage and number of doses, and providing ongoing education about the illness and its treatment are likewise essential, if common-sense, ways to avert or minimize non-compliance.

Education is, of course, integral to the good treatment of any illness, but this is especially true when the illnesses are chronic or tend to recur. Patients and their family members should be encouraged to write down any questions they may have, as many individuals are intimidated once they find themselves in a doctor's office. Any information that is given orally to patients should be repeated as often as necessary (due to the cognitive difficulties experienced by many psychiatric patients, especially when acutely ill or recovering from an acute fitness) and, whenever feasible, provided in written form as well. Additional information is available to patients and family members in books and pamphlets obtainable from libraries, bookstores, and patient support groups, as well as from audiotapes, videotapes, and the Internet.[2,4] Visual aids, such as charts portraying the natural course of the treated and untreated illness, or the causes and results of sleep deprivation and medication cessation, are also helpful to many.[5–7]

Patients, when they are well, often benefit from a meeting with their family members and their doctor which focuses upon drawing up contingency plans in case their illness should recur. Such meetings may include what is to be done in the event that hospitalization is required and the patient refuses voluntary admission, a discussion of early warning signs of impending psychotic or depressive episodes, methods for regularizing sleep and activity patterns, techniques to protect patients financially; and ways to manage suicidal behaviour should it occur. Suicide is the major cause of premature death in the severe psychiatric illnesses,[8,9] and its prevention is of first concern. Those illnesses most likely to result in suicide (the mood disorders, comorbid alcohol and drug abuse, and schizophrenia) need to be treated early, aggressively, and often for an indefinite period of time.[2,4,10] The increasing evidence that treatment early in psychiatric illness may improve the long-term course needs to be considered in light of the reluctance of many patients to stay in treatment.

No-one who has treated or suffered from mental illness would minimize the difficulties involved in successful treatment. Modern medicine gives options that did not exist even 10 years ago, and there is every reason to be expect that improvements in psychopharmacology and diagnostic techniques will continue to develop at a galloping pace. Still, the relationship between the patient and doctor will remain central to the treatment as Morag Coate wrote 35 years ago in *Beyond All Reason*:[10]

> Because the doctors cared, and because one of them still believed in me when I believed in nothing, I have survived to tell the tale. It is not only the doctors who perform hazardous operations or give life-saving drugs in obvious emergencies who hold the scales at times between life and death. To sit quietly in a consulting room and talk to someone would not appear to the general public

as a heroic or dramatic thing to do. In medicine there are many different ways of saving lives. This is one of them.

References

1. Jamison, K.R., Gerner, R.H., and Goodwin, F.K. (1979). Patient and physician attitudes toward lithium: relationship to compliance. *Archives of General Psychiatry*, **36**, 866–9.
2. Goodwin, F.K. and Jamison, K.R. (1990). *Manic–depressive illness.* Oxford University Press, New York.
3. Sackett, D.L., Haynes, R.B., and Tugwell, P. (1985). *Clinical epidemiology: a basic science for clinical medicine.* Little, Brown, Boston, MA.
4. Wyatt, R.J. (1998). *Practical psychiatric practice. Forms and protocols for clinical use* (2nd edn). American Psychiatric Association, Washington, DC.
5. Post, R.M., Rubinow, D.R., and Ballenger, J.C. (1986). Conditioning and sensitization in the longitudinal course of affective illness. *British Journal of Psychiatry*, **149**, 191–201.
6. Wehr, T.A., Sack, D.A., and Rosenthal, N.E. (1987). Sleep reduction as a final common pathway in the genesis of mania. *American Journal of Psychiatry*, **144**, 201–4.
7. Suppes, T., Baldessarini, R.J., Faedda, G.L., Tondo, L., and Tohen, M. (1993). Discontinuing maintenance treatment in bipolar manic–depression: risks and implications. *Harvard Review of Psychiatry*, **1**, 131–44.
8. Harris, E.C. and Barraclough, B. (1997). Suicide as an outcome for mental disorders: a meta-analysis. *British Journal of Psychiatry*, **170**, 205–28.
9. Roy, A. (ed.) (1986). *Suicide.* Williams and Wilkins, Baltimore, MD.
10. Coate, M. (1964). *Beyond all reason.* Constable, London.

1.2 Public attitudes and the problem of stigma: psychiatry and the media

Anthony Clare

Introduction

The term stigma derives from the Greek and refers to bodily signs designed to expose something unusual and bad about the moral status of the signifier. Such signs were 'cut or burnt into the body and advertised that the bearer was a slave, a criminal, or a traitor',[1] someone to be avoided, especially in public. In Christian times, two metaphorical modifications were added. The first referred to physical, bodily signs of spirituality or grace, so-called stigmata, including eruptions and wounds on the body similar to those suffered by Jesus Christ.[2] The second referred to bodily signs of a physical disorder, as in the classical stigmata of leprosy or advanced alcoholic cirrhosis. However, the conventional contemporary use of the concept of stigma involves the notion of an attribute that is discrediting. History is replete with examples of stigmatization on grounds of race, ethnicity, gender, social status, nationality, and sexual orientation, as well as physical and mental functioning. The sociologist Erving Goffman, in a classic book devoted to the analysis of stigma,[1] points out that the person with a stigma is more often than not defined as somehow less than human, and that to explain and justify stigmatization human beings tend to construct a particular theory or ideology. The stigmatization of the mentally ill, for example, rests on theories of moral weakness, dangerousness, contamination, and culpability.

It has, however, been argued, most cogently by Sayce,[3] that the concept of stigma has not been useful as a rallying point for collective stategies to challenge prejudice and that the concept of stigma is itself stigmatizing. A New Zealand national strategy to combat discrimination against the mentally ill argues:[4]

> Years of research into public attitudes and stigma have not led to the development of effective models for change ... Whereas stigma attaches to the consumer, discrimination results from the actions of others. If placed in a human rights framework, there is clear evidence that widespread discrimination is exercised against people with mental illness. More importantly, that framework also offers a well-tested methodology for identifying and resolving discriminatory practices.

Most of us learn our expectations and stereotypes of mental illness behaviour during early childhood and, whilst much of the imagery involved is spurious, such expectations and stereotypes are continually reaffirmed and reinforced in ordinary social interactions. Much of the language of mental health has been absorbed into the public discourse in a manner which is quite explicitly stigmatizing—the use of such terms as 'psycho', 'nutter', 'maniac', and 'schizo' to demean and deni-

Table 1 Stigmatizing conceptions of the psychiatrically ill

Belief	Action required
Psychiatric illness not true illness	
Feigned illness	Sufferers to be held responsible for
Excessive complaining	actions and denied sick role
Avoidance of responsibilities	
Psychiatrically ill	
Are dangerous	Control, custody, discipline
Are contaminating	Isolation
Are weak	Reject/require 'pulling themselves together'
Are culpable	Hold them responsible, punish them

grate contaminates and degrades the entire field of mental health and has been the subject of much adverse criticism.[5]

The political abuse of psychiatry has given psychiatrists cause to be alert to the professional danger of being misused as agents of social control and contributors to the process of stigmatization of the mentally ill. Western psychiatry, as Littlewood and Lipsedge[6] have suggested, tends towards conservatism in its attitude to the social order, and others[7, 8] have argued for greater recognition to be paid to the social and cultural assumptions on which much psychiatric theory and practice are based and which can contribute to subtle stigmatization of psychiatric ill individuals within the mental health services.

Stigmatization of the mentally ill

At the heart of the stigmatization of the mentally ill and of those who care for them are a number of beliefs (Table 1).

The lack of objective, stable, and consistent markers of mental illness is a major contributory factor in the persistence of the belief that in some way mental illnesses are not true or real illnesses compared with so-called organic disorders. Nor is this a prejudice confined to a Western medicine disfigured by a simplistic Cartesian dualism. Raguram *et al.*[9] have shown that depressive symptoms are construed as much more socially disadvantageous than somatoform symptoms in a South India patient population, while Fabrega,[10] in a extensive review of the literature pertaining to psychiatric illness and its stigma in non-Western society, has concluded that, with the possible exception of Islam, the potential for condemnation and stigmatization of psychiatric illness seems to be present in most of these societies.

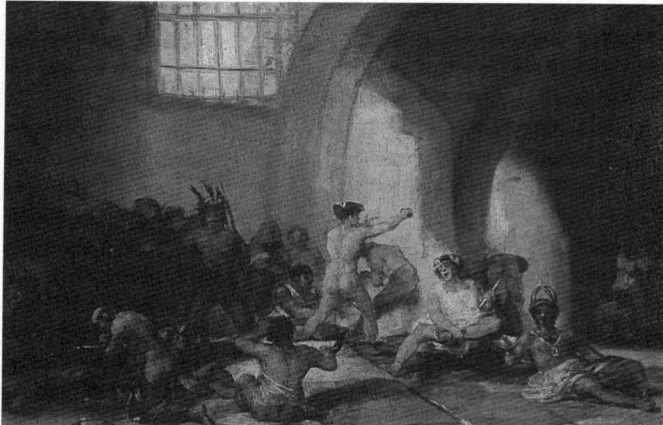

Fig. 1 Goya's *The Madhouse*

Of these various stereotypes, that of the psychiatrically ill as violent is perhaps the most tenacious and in part contributes to the virulence and persistence of other aspects of stigmatization. It is a long-standing perception. A substantial part of the history of psychiatry has been the history of confinement. Our images of madness, derived from that history, powerfully reinforce the notion of mental illness as a state of incipient, latent of actual violence. The very word 'bedlam', defined in the *Concise Oxford Dictionary* amongst other things as 'a place of uproar', derives from one of the earliest psychiatric institutions, Bethlem Hospital. The growth of the mental hospital, a spectacular phenomenon of the nineteenth century, did little to reduce the fear and the ignorance surrounding the mentally ill. Whatever the precise contribution of enlightenment values to their rise, the mental hospitals retained much of the aura of abuse, neglect, and cruelty which surrounded the madhouses of earlier epochs, so memorably captured in Goya's *The Madhouse* painted in the early years of the nineteenth century (Fig. 1). Goya depicts the mentally ill as isolated, locked in an inner world of hallucinations and delusions, 'tragic figures at war with one another and themselves'.[11]

Despite the clinical and therapeutic benefits provided by the asylums, the major drawback concerned their size, isolation, and institutional atmosphere. The asylum, referred to disparagingly and revealingly down through the years as 'the bin', helped ensure that the public image of mental illness would continue to include notions of custody, control, chronicity, containment, and fears of contamination and violence. Many such hospitals became overcrowded, poorly staffed, and cut off from the main body of medicine.

With the decline of the mental hospital and the simultaneous development of the acute psychiatric unit in the setting of the general hospital and the rise of what has come to be known as community psychiatry, hopes have risen that the stigmatization of the mentally ill might be reduced and eventually eliminated. Psychiatric illness has become more visible. The mentally ill are no longer locked away out of sight and out of mind. But in countries such as the United States and the United Kingdom, where the rundown of the mental hospital has not always been accompanied by development of sufficient alternative treatment facilities, there has been a rise in concern regarding the association of mental illness and violence[12–14] and a fear that much of the gain made in terms of the education of the general public and the greater involvement of the mass media in positive portrayal of mental

health issues may be offset by a demand for greater custody and control of the mentally ill within the community.[15]

Public attitudes

Public attitudes are clearly influenced by the media and are susceptible to change as media attitudes change. The media of course constitute a disparate collection which include not merely television and radio but the cinema, advertising, newspapers, magazines, and pamphlets. In a review of mass media coverage of mental health issues, Philo *et al.*[5] commented on the upsurge in the amount of research into public attitudes to mental illness which has been a feature of the past decade. This increase in interest relates at least in part to the implementation of community care legislation and the recognition of the need to create a more positive social climate in which it is acceptable to seek help without fear of discrimination and stigmatization. Several studies[16–18] provide information which cautiously suggests that public attitudes are changing for the better. More people admit to knowing someone in their family who has had a mental illness, believe in the importance and the usefulness of treatment, and would be happy to employ or live next to someone mentally ill. The role of voluntary organizations, including the National Association for Mental Health (MIND) and the National Schizophrenia Fellowship, in highlighting the plight of the mentally ill and the need for better and more accessible services, and in rewarding good practice in press reporting and broadcasting, is likewise an important positive one. While mental health professionals often avoid the media for fear of misquotation and oversimplification, there are examples of the successful use of the media to communicate information about mental health issues.[14,19,20]

However, concern remains regarding media coverage of mental illness. The first major study,[21] conducted by Nunally in 1961, indicated an essentially negative portrayal of the mentally ill in the media, and subsequent studies suggest that not a great deal has changed.[22–24] In a more recent summary,[25] Philo concluded: 'the results show clearly that ill-informed beliefs on, for example, the association of schizophrenia with violence, can be traced directly back to media accounts'.

One medium that has manifested a fascination with psychiatry and psychiatric illness since its beginnings is the cinema, and it too has been accused by critics of reinforcing powerful negative stereotypes of both psychiatrists and psychiatric patients.[26–29] In one study, involving 487 people who had a family member with severe mental illness, 85.6 per cent identified 'popular movies about mentally ill killers' as the largest single contributor to the stigma of that illness.[30]

To be set against such negative perceptions is the growing trend in published autobiographical accounts of serious mental illness which, in addition to being frank, factual, and detailed, are generally positive concerning the effectiveness of psychiatric intervention. A bibliography of such personal accounts, published in 1996, lists seven anthologies and 48 autobiographies of former patients published since 1980.[31] Some authors are noted writers, poets, and artists, capable of providing a vivid and sharp account of the inner world of mental illness. Several noted psychologists have also written of their own psychiatric ill-health, treatment, and recovery. Such accounts reveal that mental health care professionals themselves can behave in a discriminatory and stigmatizing fashion *vis-à-vis* colleagues with a history of psychiatric ill-health.[32,33]

Destigmatization

If the cardinal contributory factors to stigmatization are ignorance, fear, and hostility, then the antidotes are information, reassurance, and a vigorous antidiscriminatory campaign on the part of policy-makers and opinion-formers. It is generally accepted that if progress is to be made in the destigmatization of mental illness and the provision of more positive accurate images of psychiatric illness and psychiatry, the professionals involved in mental health issues together with patients, families, and support organizations will need to work closely with the media.[16] Experience in the United States suggests that a combination of approaches is needed. Journalists and broadcasters need to be persuaded that inaccurate reporting, stereotyped portrayals, and sensationalist use of discriminatory language and labels are no longer acceptable. In some parts of the United States, concerned individuals and groups have joined together to establish 'media watch' campaigns through which offensive reports and programmes are identified and responses to editors and producers organized. In the United Kingdom, complaints can be made to the Press Complaints Commission and to the Broadcasting Standards Council which has examined the whole issue of the stigmatization of the mentally ill in its revised Code of Practice.[34]

A number of systematic public education campaigns have been launched in recent years specifically to improve public perceptions and combat stigmatization in the mental health field. In the United Kingdom, the Royal Colleges of Psychiatrists and of General Practitioners launched a Defeat Depression Campaign in 1992 which aimed to increase public and professional awareness of depression and its treatment.[35] At the outset of the campaign, research had shown that most members of the public did not know what depression was. Many felt that physical illness was easier to sympathize with as it was easier to see. Most considered counselling the best way to treat depression and certain life events, such as bereavement, marital breakdown, and loss of a job, as most likely to cause it. Antidepressants were not clearly understood, and were clearly confused with tranquillizers and regarded as seriously addictive. Yet the survey did show that some 90 per cent of the public polled agreed that people who suffer from depression deserve more understanding and sympathy from their families, relatives, and friends than they receive at the moment. A similar number agreed that anyone can suffer from psychiatric ill-health, while over half claimed to have a close relative or friend who had suffered from depression. Research has also shown that lowered negative perceptions towards individuals with severe mental illness are associated with previous contact with this population and with the presentation of empirically based information, including information on the association between violence and mental illness.[36]

In 1996, the World Psychiatric Association convened the first meeting of experts from around the world, representing consumer groups, public health experts, sociologists, anthropologists and psychiatrists, and embarked on a major international antistigma programme, with the main focus being on the stigma associated with schizophrenia.[37] The goal of this programme is to increase awareness and knowledge of the nature of schizophrenia and treatment options, to improve public attitudes about those who have or have had schizophrenia and their families, and to generate action to eliminate discrimination and prejudice. Pilot initiatives in Spain, Canada, and Austria have commenced, and the programme is designed to involve local and national authorities, the media, voluntary and self-help groups, mental health care and educational professionals, and the psychiatrically ill.

References

1. Goffman, E. (1963). *Stigma: notes on the management of spoiled identity*, p. 11. Penguin, Harmondsworth.
2. Whitlock, F.A. and Hynes, J.V. (1978) Religions, stigmatization: an historical and psychophysiological enquiry. *Psychological Medicine*, **8**, 185–202.
3. Sayce, L. (1998). Stigma, descrimation and social exclusion: what's in a word? *Journal of Mental Health*, **7**, 331–43.
4. New Zealand Mental Health Commission (1997). *Discrimination against people with experiences of mental illness*. Discussion Paper for the Mental Health Commission. New Zealand Mental Health Commission, Wellington.
5. Philo, G., Secker, J., Platt, S., *et al.* (1994) The impact of the mass media on public images of mental illness: media content and audience belief. *Health Education Journal*, **53**, 271–81.
6. Littlewood, R. and Lipsedge, M. (1989). *Aliens and alienists: ethnic minorities and psychiatry* (2nd edn.). Unwin Hyman, London.
7. Boyle, M. (1993). *Schizophrenia: a scientific delusion?* Routledge, London.
8. Littlewood, R. (1992). Towards an intercultural therapy. In *Intercultural therapy* (ed. J. Kareem and R. Littlewood), pp. 3–13. Blackwell Science, Oxford.
9. Raguram, R., Weiss, M.G., Channabasavanna, S.M., and Devins, G.M. (1996). Stigma, depression and somatization in South India. *American Journal of Psychiatry*, **153**, 1043–9.
10. Fabrega, H. (1992). Psychiatric stigma in non-Western societies. *Comprehensive Psychiatry*, **32**, 6, 534–55.
11. MacGregor, J.M. (1989). *The discovery of the art of the insane*, p. 72. Princeton University Press.
12. Torrey, E.F. (1994). Violent behaviour by individuals with serious mental illness. *Hospital and Community Psychiatry*, **45**, 653–62.
13. Berlin, F.S. and Malin, H.M. (1991) Media distortion of the public's perception of recidivism and psychiatric rehabilitation. *American Journal of Psychiatry*, **148**, 1572–6.
14. Wolff, G., Pathare, S., Craig, T., *et al.* (1996) Public education for community care. *British Journal of Psychiatry*, **168**, 441–7.
15. Clare, A.W. (1994). *Violence, mental illness and society*. The Stevens Lecture. Royal Society of Medicine, London.
16. MORI (1979). *Public attitudes to mental illness*. Market and Opinion Research International, London.
17. Brockington, I.F., Hall, P., Levings, J., and Murphy, C. (1993). The community's tolerance of the mentally ill. *British Journal of Psychiatry*, **162**, 93–99.
18. Huxley, P. (1993). Location and stigma: a survey of community attitudes to mental illness. *Journal of Mental Health* **2**, 73–80.
19. Barker, C., Pistrang, N., Shapiro, D.A., *et al.* (1993). You in mind: a preventative mental health television series. *British Journal of Clinical Psychology*, **32**, 281–93.
20. Kay, R., Martin, B., Kelly, D., and Stark, C. (1997). Using the media during Mental Health Week. *Psychiatric Bulletin*, **21**, 451–3.
21. Nunally, J.C. (1961). *Popular conceptions of mental health: their development and change*. Rinehart and Winston, New York.
22. Matas, M., El-Guebaly, N., Harper, D., *et al.* (1986). Mental illness and the media: part II. Content analysis of press coverage of mental health topics. *Canadian Journal of Psychiatry*, **31**, 813–17.
23. Meagher, D., Newman, A., Fee, M., and Casey, P. (1995). The coverage of psychiatry in the Irish print media. *Psychiatric Bulletin*, **19**, 642–4.
24. Scott, J. (1994). What the papers say. *Psychiatric Bulletin*, **18**, 489–91.

25. Philo, G. (1997). Changing media representations of mental health. *Psychiatric Bulletin*, **21**, 171–2.

26. Gabbard, K. and Gabbard, G. (1980). From *Psycho* to *Dressed to Kill*: the decline of the psychiatrist in the movies. *Film/Psychology Review*, **4**, 157–68.

27. Domino, G. (1983). Impact of the film *One Flew Over the Cuckoo's Nest* on attitudes towards mental illness. *Psychological Reports*, **53**, 179–83.

28. Hyler, S.E., Gabbard, G.O., and Schneider, I. (1991). Homicidal maniacs and narcissistic parasites: stigmatization of mentally ill persons in the movies. *Hospital and Community Psychiatry*, **42**, 1044–8.

29. Schneider, I. (1987). The theory and practice of movie psychiatry. *American Journal of Psychiatry*, **144**, 996–1002.

30. Wahl, O.F. and Harman, C.R. (1989). Family views of stigma. *Schizophrenia Bulletin*, **15**, 131–9.

31. Sommer, R., Clifford, J.S., and Norcross, J.C. (1998). A bibliography of mental patients' autobiographies : an update and classificatory system. *American Journal of Psychiatry*, **155**, 1261–4.

32. Miles, S.H. (1998). A challenge to licensing boards: the stigma of mental illness. *Journal of the American Medicial Association*, **280**, 865.

33. Jamieson, K.R. (1996). *An unquiet mind*. Picador, Basingstoke.

34. Broadcasting Standards Council (1994). *Code of practice* (2nd edn). Broadcasting Standards Council, London.

35. Vize, C. and Priest, R. (1993). Defeat Depression Campaign—attitudes towards depression. *Psychiatric Bulletin*, **17**, 573–4.

36. Penn, D.L. and Martin, J. (1998). The stigma of mental illness: some potential solutions for a recalcitrant problem. *Psychiatric Quarterly*, **69**, 235–47.

37. Sartorius, N. (1997). Fighting schizophrenia and its stigma. A new World Psychiatric Association educational programme. *British Journal of Psychiatry*, **170**, 297.

1.3 Psychiatry as a worldwide public health problem

1.3.1 Psychiatry and health in low-income populations*

Leon Eisenberg

In 1995 my colleagues and I completed a report on world mental health.[1] It outlines the extent of the problems and the priorities for intervention among low-income populations. Our most prominent finding was the interconnectedness of health problems, such as depression, heart and lung diseases, sexually transmitted diseases, and other behaviour-related diseases, on the one hand, and of psychosocial pathologies, such as violence, alcoholism, abuse of women and children, and underlying social conditions such as war, poverty, and discrimination, on the other. They form self-perpetuating spirals.

At a press conference to launch the book on 15 May 1995, at the United Nations, Secretary General Boutros Boutros Ghali stated:

> This Report . . . reminds us of the great human suffering caused by mental illness . . . the international community has risen to many challenges in the past. Now it must do the same (for) mental health . . . The challenge is to combine concern for mental health . . . humanitarian assistance and protection efforts. Development policies must . . . protect and promote mental health

Disease burden

What metric is suitable for measuring the global burden of disease (**GBD**)? The statistic must incorporate morbidity and mortality and be sufficiently broad to include suffering and handicap. One answer is the disability-adjusted life-year (**DALY**).[2] The DALY is a statistic developed to summarize in a single number the impact of premature death, as well as the suffering and disability, resulting from specific disease conditions. Age at death, as well as death itself, is taken into account by subtracting the age at death from life expectancy remaining at that age to compute 'years of life lost'. In order not to undervalue years lost in developing countries, the figure for life expectancy is that of the developed world. To take suffering and disability into account, each surviving year is adjusted by the duration and severity of disablement (i.e. blindness or paralysis) resulting from disease. The focus is on health status; life is valued precisely the same whenever it is in jeopardy, and no financial data are included.

*This chapter first appeared in *Comprehensive Psychiatry*, **38**, 69–73, and is reproduced by permission of the publishers.

The burden of mental illness

Using the DALY as the basic statistic, the *World Development Report*[2] concludes that mental health problems make up 8.1 per cent of the total GBD. Of that 8.1 per cent, the largest contributors are depressive disorders, self-inflicted injuries. Alzheimer's disease and other dementia, and alcohol dependence, followed by epilepsy, psychoses, drug dependence, and post-traumatic stress disorder. Depressive and anxiety disorders account for between one-quarter and one-third of all primary-health-care visits worldwide.[3,4] When appropriately diagnosed and treated, suffering is alleviated, disability prevented, and function restored; when ignored, major losses persist.[5] By the year 2025, three-quarters of all elderly persons with dementia (about 80 million) will live in low-income societies. Mental retardation and epilepsy rates are three to five times higher in low-income societies compared with industrialized countries. In some Asian and African countries, up to 90 per cent of patients with epilepsy—a treatable condition for which cost-effective drug therapy is available—do not receive anticonvulsants.[6]

In addition to that 8 per cent, as much as an additional 34 per cent of the GBD is due to disorders that are behaviour related, such as violence, smoking and drinking, AIDS and other sexually transmitted diseases, motor vehicle and other unintentional injuries, and gastrointestinal diseases that stem from failure to follow sanitary practices. An estimated 5 to 10 per cent of all persons on Earth are affected by alcohol-related diseases. Narcotics and other illicit drugs constitute a large and rapidly increasing source of morbidity in poor and rich societies alike. Thus, more than one-third of the GBD is potentially preventable by changing behaviour, a challenge that will require large-scale interventions to influence social messages, as well as counselling for individuals.

The *World Health Report*[7] lists, in separate tables, the 10 leading causes of mortality, the 10 leading causes of morbidity, and the 10 leading causes of disability. No psychiatric disorder appears on the mortality list; neurotic, stress-related, and somatoform disorders together make up the third most important cause of morbidity. However, in terms of chronically disabled persons, mood disorders are the most important single cause; mental retardation is fourth, epilepsy sixth, dementia seventh, and schizophrenia ninth.

Even more striking is a recent analysis undertaken by Murray and Lopez[8] of the Harvard Center for Population and Development Studies. Depression was the fourth leading cause of DALYs in 1990, exceeded only by lower respiratory infections, diarrhoeal diseases, and perinatal conditions (Table 1).

Table 1 Top 10 causes of DALYs worldwide for both sexes in 1990

Disease or injury	DALYs (x 10³)	Cumulative %
All causes	1379 238	
1. LRI	112 898	8.2
2. Diarrhoeal diseases	99 633	15.4
3. Perinatal conditions	92 313	22.1
4. Depresssion	50 810	25.8
5. IHD	46 699	29.2
6. Stroke	38 523	32.0
7. Tuberculosis	38 426	34.8
8. Measles	36 250	37.4
9. Road traffic accidents	34 317	39.9
10. Congenital anomalies	32 921	42.3

LRI, lower respiratory infection; IHD, ischaemic heart disease.

Twenty-five years from now, depression will be second only to ischaemic heart disease as a cause of GBD (Table 2). Whereas ischaemic heart disease will account for 5.9 per cent of the total GBD, depression will account for 5.7 per cent. Despite the fact that neuropsychiatric conditions make up five of the 10 most important causes of long-term disability, despite the fact that depression alone is currently the fourth most important cause of DALYs, and despite the fact that depression will be the second leading cause 25 years from now, mental health is largely missing from the international health agenda.

Promising solutions

Despite widespread pessimism about mental disorders in public health circles, much can be accomplished by applying present means. We have unequivocal evidence for the effectiveness of pharmacological, psychosocial, and combined treatments in depression[9,10] and anxiety disorders,[11,12] as well as for specific interventions to prevent certain developmental disorders (iodinization of salt, environmental lead abatement, immunizations, perinatal care, and so on).[13]

The single most important issue is to give priority to mental health

Table 2 Top 10 causes of DALYs worldwide for both sexes in 2020

Disease or injury	DALYs (x 10³)	Cumulative %
All causes	1 388 836	
1. IHD	82 325	5.9
2. Depression	78 662	11.6
3. Road traffic accidents	71 240	16.7
4. Stroke	61 392	21.1
5. COPD	57 587	25.3
6. LRI	42 692	28.4
7. Tuberculosis	42 515	31.4
8. War	41 315	34.4
9. Diarrhoeal diseases	37 097	37.1
10. HIV	36 317	39.7

IHD, ischaemic heart disease: COPD, chronic obstructive pulmonary disease; LRI, lower respiratory infection.

around the world. In the words of Secretary General Boutros Boutros Ghali:

> ... Medical and social issues which are often viewed separately must be dealt with as a whole . . . the priority of mental health must be heightened . . . resources must expand . . . responsibilities must be recognized more completely.

Key clinical initiatives

A major commitment to upgrade the quality of mental health services

The care of the mentally ill should be specified in national and regional health plans and should receive adequate budgetary allocations. Primary health care must be 're-engineered' to improve the treatment of neuropsychiatric disorders. Improvements in mental health systems require rational drug policies for psychotropic medications and reliable provision of adequate drug supplies. The human rights of patients require protection in mental health legislation.

A small cadre of well-trained mental health professionals (including, in particular, psychiatric nurses) is essential to mental health programmes in order to design and implement training programmes, provide consultation to general health workers, and supervise the care of the chronically mentally ill. At the same time, major efforts are necessary to educate generalist physicians about psychiatric conditions, to improve behavioural science teaching in medical education, and to provide in-service training for practitioners.

Better mental health services for children and adolescents, including early detection and prevention

Priority should be given to providing effective services integrated within all forms of health care. Early detection of epilepsy and appropriate medication to control seizures will enable children with the disorder to participate fully in school, to prepare for work, and to avoid the burns, injuries, educational failure, and stigma associated with the disorder. Prevention of mental retardation can be achieved through birth planning, prenatal and perinatal care, hospital deliveries for difficult births, immunization, optimal nutrition (calories, protein, and micronutrients), home visits and day care, child safety measures, and school-based programmes on family life and sexuality.[13]

Public schools (state schools) are the principal social institution for furthering the cognitive and emotional development of children. Teachers can learn to recognize signs and symptoms of mental illness and child abuse, to manage early problems in the classroom, and to refer to those children requiring more assistance to mental health facilities.

Systematic efforts to assess the global burden of alcohol and drug abuse, to reduce demand, and to develop treatment and prevention programmes

In no other area of mental health is there such a lack of reliable systematic data on the severity, magnitude, and distribution of the problem needed to develop effective policy strategies as in the area of illicit drugs. International bodies must increase their capacity for meaningful data gathering. Governments must develop stronger policies to reduce demand. Public education is crucial to prevent the onset of use among the young. Traditional and non-traditional treatment approaches at the community and individual levels need implementation and rigorous evaluation.[14]

Support for research

Ignorance is always more costly than knowledge; research is all the more essential in difficult economic times.[15] Because mental health problems are common to developing and industrialized countries, knowledge can be transferred in both directions. Priority should be placed on strengthening the indigenous capacity for research among colleagues in developing countries. It is imperative that we encourage national-level interdisciplinary mental health policy research units and connect them with international networks of researchers. Such international networks can serve as a clearinghouse for relevant concepts, methods, and data.[16]

Psychosocial pathology

What of psychosocial pathologies and the social circumstances that underlie them? The 1995 report of the World Health Organization,[17] entitled *Bridging the Gaps*, provides a sobering introduction to the leading cause of mortality and morbidity:

> The world's most ruthless killer and the greatest cause of suffering on earth is . . . extreme poverty. It is the main cause of reduced life expectancy, of handicap and disability, and of starvation. Poverty is a major contributor to mental illness, stress, suicide, family disintegration and substance abuse . . . For many of the people in the world today, every step in life, from infancy to old age, is taken under the twin shadows of poverty and inequity and under the double burden of suffering and disease. For many, the prospect of a longer life may seem more like a punishment than a prize.

The external debt of developing countries grew 15-fold over the past two decades; in 1970 it was $100 billion, by 1980 it had increased to $630 billion, and by 1992 to more than $1500 billion.[18] Growing economic disparities between and within countries fuel conflict. The gulf between the poor and rich of the world is widening. The gap in per capita income between the industrial and developing world has tripled in the past 30 years. Developing countries, with 80 per cent of the world's people, control only 21 per cent of the global gross national product (**GNP**). Differences in economic and health status within countries are as great or greater than those between countries. Brazil, classified by the World Bank[2] as an 'upper-middle income country' has a per capita GNP of $2940, yet one in six Brazilians subsists on less than $1 per day, and one in three on less than $2 per day. The United States ranks in the upper 5 per cent of nations in average life expectancy, but the life expectancy of black men aged 15 to 44 years living in Harlem is lower than that of a male Bangladeshi of the same age.[19]

Of the 40 instances of armed conflict under way at the time of writing, not one is a significant war between states.[20] The goal is no longer the destruction of opposing armies, but the terrorization of civilian populations who constitute 'the enemy.' Such low-intensity warfare results from the political and economic legacies of the Cold War, from the disintegration of state authority and the breakdown of civil and political order, from illegitimate state institutions, from social cleavages based on religious, cultural, or ethnic origins, inflamed by power-seeking demagogues, and from widespread illiteracy, poor health, political repression, and economic deprivation in countries the world over.[21] There are 20 million officially recognized refugees worldwide, twice the number that there were 10 years ago; there are at least as many internally displaced persons. Refugees and internally displaced persons exhibit high rates of depression, anxiety disorders, post-traumatic stress disorder, and other forms of mental distress.

Hunger, deprivation, depression, and violence affect women disproportionately. Women bear more heavily the negative effects of economic restructuring on families. Selective abortion, female infanticide, differential triage of sick children in poor families, and maternal mortality have all taken a substantial toll on women's lives and mental health. Sen[22] has calculated that in Southeast Asia 100 million women are missing; that is, the only viable explanation for the high male-to-female ratio in the Southeast Asian population, in contrast with the female preponderance in the West, is the premature death of 100 million women. Child abuse in exploitative settings, in the commercial sex industry, among the hundreds of thousands of street children, in settings of ethnic and political conflict, and in families under stress is a major source of degradation and wretchedness for millions.

Recommendations

In addition to comprehensive health policy, it is essential to develop what Dr Julio Frenk[23] of Mexico calls 'healthy policies'. Explicit attention must be paid to the mental health consequences of social and economic decisions; for example, the imposition of 'structural adjustment' on the economy of the developing countries must be accompanied by corrective measures to blunt the impact on the poor. Policies that reduce poverty, encourage gainful employment, and provide universal basic education, primary health care, decent housing, and adequate nutrition are all prima facie goods. They are not merely a concession to an abstract vision of social justice—they have tangible effects on the health of individuals and communities.

Specific initiatives

Co-ordinated efforts to improve state gender policies, to interdict violence toward women, and to empower women

The years of education women receive is the single most important determinant of their own health, the health of their children, and the health of their families.[24,25] Policies that deny women full citizenship must be fought not only because they violate human rights, but also because they destroy health. Women must take leadership roles in governments, international agencies, and non-governmental organizations. Laws to ensure the protection of women against domestic violence—laws accompanied by effective enforcement—are foundation efforts for mental health.

Broad initiatives to control the causes and consequences of violence

Only far-reaching changes in international and national politics will reduce the frequency of armed conflicts. Peace and security initiatives must target violence as the major threat to social well being. Mental health concerns need to be more widely understood in peace and security programmes. The analysis of mental health issues, from the effect of racism on identity to the vicious cycles of revenge, is essential in preventing ethnic conflict.

References

1. Desjarlais, R., Eisenberg, L., Good, B., and Klein, A. (1995). *World mental health: problems and priorities in low-income countries*. Oxford University Press, New York.
2. World Bank (1993). *World development report—investing in health (world development indicators)*. Oxford University Press.
3. Eisenberg, L. (1992).Treating depression and anxiety in primary care. *New England Journal of Medicine*, **326**, 1080–4.
4. Ustun, T.B. and Sartorius, N. (1995). *Mental illness in general health care: an international study*. Wiley, New York.
5. Wells, K.B., Stewart, A., Hays, R.D., *et al.* (1996). The functioning and well being of depressed patients: results from The Medical Outcomes Study. *Journal of the American Medical Association*, **262**, 914–19.
6. Eisenberg, L. (1997). Sociocultural perspectives. In *Epilepsy* (ed. J. Engel and T.A. Pedley), pp. 41–6. Lippincott–Raven, New York.
7. World Health Organization (1996). *The world health report 1996: fighting disease, fostering development*. World Health Organization, Geneva.
8. Murray, C.J.L. and Lopez, A.D. (1996). *The global burden of disease and injury*, Vol. 1. Harvard University Press, Cambridge, MA.
9. Clarkin, J.F., Pilkonis, P.A., and Magruder, K.M. (1996). Psychotherapy of depression. *Archives of General Psychiatry*, **53**, 717–23.
10. Kupfer, D.J. and Thase, M.E. (1996). Recent developments in the pharmacology of mood disorders. *Journal of Consulting and Clinical Psychology*, **64**, 646–59.
11. Barlow, D.H. and Lehman, C. (1996). Advances in the psychosocial treatment of anxiety disorders. *Archives of General Psychiatry*, **53**, 727–35.
12. Lydiard, R.B., Brawman-Mintzer, O., and Ballenger, J.C. (1996). Recent developments in the psychopharmacology of anxiety disorders. *Journal of Consulting and Clinical Psychology*, **64**, 660–8.
13. Eisenberg, L. (1992). Child mental health in the Americas: a public health approach. *Bulletin of the Pan American Health Organization*, **26**, 230–41.
14. Crits-Chistoph, P. and Siqueland, L. (1996). Psychology treatment for drug abuse. Selected review and recommendations for national health care. *Archives of General Psychiatry*, **53**, 749–56.
15. Eisenberg, L. (1997). The social imperatives of medical research. *Science*, **198**, 1105–10.
16. Weissman, M.M., Eisenberg, L., Goldberg, D., *et al.* (1999). World mental health: epidemiologic strategies to address problems in underserved populations: task force report. *International Journal of Mental Health*, in press.
17. World Health Organization (1995). *Bridging the gaps*. World Health Organization, Geneva.
18. UNICEF (1996). *The state of the world's children in 1996*. Oxford University Press, New York.
19. McCord, C. and Freeman, H.P. (1990). Excess mortality in Harlem. *New England Journal of Medicine*, **322**, 173–7.
20. Carnegie Commission on Preventing Deadly Conflict (1996). *Report to the Board of Trustees*. Carnegie Corporation of New York, New York.
21. United Nations Development Program (1996). *Human development report 1996*. Oxford University Press, New York.
22. Sen, A. (1990). More than 100 million women are missing. *New York Review of Books*, **37**, 61–7.
23. Frenk, J. (1993). The new public health. *Annual Review of Public Health*, **14**, 469–90.
24. Caldwell, J.C. (1986). Routes to low mortality in poor countries. *Population Development Review*, **12**, 171–220.
25. Hobcraft J. Women's education, child welfare and child survival. *Health Transition Review*, **3**, 159–75.

1.3.2 **Transcultural psychiatry**

Julian Leff

Clinical relevance of transcultural psychiatry

With the mass movements of populations that have characterized the second half of this century, there can be few psychiatrists who do not encounter members of an ethnic minority group in their practice. The principles of transcultural psychiatry are obviously of relevance to this type of psychiatrist–patient interaction, but they are also of central importance even when the psychiatrist and patient share the same ethnic background. This is because within a particular ethnic group there are invariably many subcultures, for example based on religious affiliation, which encompass a diversity of beliefs. It is essential that the psychiatrist be aware of the common belief systems likely to be encountered, not simply to enhance rapport with patients and relatives, but in order to avoid serious mistakes in ascribing pathology to experiences that are accepted as normal by the subculture. For example, it is important to be aware that about half of recently bereaved people experience the image, the voice, or even the touch of the dead person[1] and that 2 per cent of the general population admit to hearing voices.[2] The political repercussions of ignorance of such subcultural phenomena are illustrated by the accusations of misdiagnosis of black patients which have come from both outside and within the profession.

There are two main streams of thought and enquiry that have shaped the development of transcultural psychiatry: social anthropology and psychiatric epidemiology. In a number of ways these disciplines are opposed; the former is concerned with qualitative data and emphasizes cultural relativity, while the latter relies on quantitative data and prioritizes a search for universal disease categories. The tools of the epidemiologist are standardized interview schedules which are linked with definitions of symptoms and signs, and rules for reaching a diagnosis. These have been introduced in an attempt to reduce the subjectivity of the psychiatrist's judgement to a minimum. By contrast, it is the person's subjective experience of illness that is the prime focus of the anthropologist. Consequently the use of standardized psychiatric interviews has been criticized by anthropologists as imposing a Western biomedical model of disease on the rich variety of experience of illness and distress. The conflict between these opposing approaches is probably unresolvable, and they are best viewed as contributing complementary material to our understanding of psychiatric morbidity.[3]

The contribution of psychiatric epidemiology

Cultural influences on the psychoses

Epidemiologists have been keen to discover whether psychiatric conditions are universal and appear with the same incidence across human populations. Universality would minimize the role of culture in shaping the form of a condition, while a uniform incidence would indicate that biological factors played a major role in aetiology. Schizophrenia has been the focus of many epidemiological surveys, especially the cross-national studies conducted by the World Health Organization (**WHO**). The International Pilot Study of Schizophrenia[4] showed that it was possible to conduct a psychiatric epidemiological study across a wide variety of cultures and languages.[5] The use of standardized assessment and diagnostic techniques revealed that the core symptoms of schizophrenia were subject to few cultural variations. The most striking difference in the form of the illness was that catatonic symptoms were relatively frequent in patients from developing countries, but rare in the other centres.

The success of this study led to an even more ambitious project—the Determinants of the Outcome of Severe Mental Disorders. The main aim was to collect epidemiologically based samples of psychotic patients making a first contact with health services in centres around the world. This was designed to allow the comparison of incidence rates, and subsequently of the outcome of patients in different cultures using relatively unbiased samples. It was found that the incidence of narrowly defined schizophrenia was remarkably uniform across a diversity of countries.[6] However, when patients with a broad diagnosis of schizophrenia but lacking the core Schneiderian symptoms were considered, the incidence rates across centres showed a threefold difference which was highly significant. This suggests that sociocultural factors are likely to play a much greater role in the aetiology of non-Schneiderian schizophrenia than in the narrowly defined form, although the nature of these factors remains to be determined.

Dramatic differences in outcome at a 2-year follow-up were found, with schizophrenic patients in developing centres faring considerably better than those in developed centres despite a paucity of psychiatric personnel and facilities. This was not explained by a higher proportion of cases with an acute onset in the developing centres, raising intriguing questions about the beneficial aspects of traditional cultures. Explanations that have been proposed include beliefs that the causes of illness are external to the patient, the low demands for productivity and punctuality in an agrarian economy, and the quality of traditional family life. Only the latter has been investigated, using the Expressed Emotion measure, and appears to make an important contribution since family carers in India are far less critical and more tolerant of patients with schizophrenia than their counterparts in Britain.[7]

Mania has been the focus of much less transcultural research than schizophrenia, but what little there is suggests that psychotic experiences are more common in Nigerian and African-Caribbean patients than in patients from European countries.[8,9]

Cultural influences on the neuroses

Variations in frequency across cultures

Whereas neither the form nor the incidence of psychoses vary much across cultures, neuroses show dramatic variations in both respects. So-called culture-bound syndromes are an extreme example of variation in frequency since it is claimed that they are confined to specific cultural groups (see Chapter 4.16). However, even with common conditions such as depression, the range of prevalence rates from studies across cultures is extremely wide. A review of 19 studies mostly conducted in developing countries found a difference in prevalence of neuroses of more than 300-fold from the highest to the lowest.[10] There are at least three plausible explanations. Unlike psychoses, there

is no clear boundary between depressive symptoms severe enough to constitute an illness and subclinical depression. Shifting the threshold for a depressive illness towards the milder end of the spectrum will automatically increase the prevalence rate. Few comparative studies of neuroses across cultures have been conducted with the rigour of the WHO projects on schizophrenia using standardized clinical interviews and diagnostic techniques. Higher prevalence rates usually result from surveys in which every subject is interviewed with a standard clinical schedule, rather than relying on key informants and non-standardized clinical judgements.

A second possibility is that the neuroses take markedly varied forms in different cultural groups, giving rise to problems of recognition and hence of counting. Early European clinicians in Africa claimed that depression did not occur among the indigenous people. This was probably due more to ethnocentric blinkers than to the existence of a different form of the condition. However, there is evidence that there is a greater focus on bodily symptoms in patients in developing countries. Somatization is by no means uncommon in patients in developed countries, particularly those of lower socio-economic status, but somatic symptoms are more likely to dominate the picture in patients in a developing country. This is determined partly by beliefs about illness and partly by mutual expectations of patients and doctors, issues which will be discussed later. The significance of somatic symptoms may well be missed by standardized interviews designed to detect the cognitive experiences of depression.

A third explanation assumes that the differences in prevalence are genuine and are ascribable to cultural influences on the origin and course of the neuroses. The emphasis on the measurement of prevalence of neuroses as opposed to incidence for the psychoses is due to the small proportion of new cases of the former that present to psychiatric services. Hence it is necessary to conduct population surveys, which are costly in terms of time and trained personnel—a prohibitive expense for most developing countries. The few population surveys that have been conducted in both developed and developing countries using the same methods of interviewing and case ascertainment have shown either no difference in the prevalence of neuroses[11,12] or a higher rate in the developing country.[13,14]

Variations in form across cultures

One of the most striking transcultural aspects of the neuroses is the great variation in the frequency of classical conversion hysteria. Whereas this condition is rarely seen in psychiatric and neurological services in developed countries today, it is still a common form of presentation in developing countries. Of the first 1000 patients attending the University Psychiatric Clinic in Cairo in 1966, 11.2 per cent were suffering from a hysterical condition.[15] Hysteria constituted 8.3 per cent of all first attenders at an outpatient clinic in Eastern Libya[16] and 8.9 per cent of outpatient contacts with the psychiatric service in Chandigarh, North India, in 1977.[17] Conversion hysteria used to be relatively common in Europe during the last century, as we can infer from Charcot's demonstrations in Paris and Freud's early clinical practice. It was also a frequent diagnosis in soldiers during both World Wars, but has subsequently become a rarity. Its disappearance from developed countries over the last 50 years contrasted with its persistence in developing countries poses an intriguing question about the influences at work. The most likely explanation is that there has been a shift in the presentation of neurotic distress from the bodily form of hysteria to the more cognitive forms of depression and anxiety, and that this process has occurred more rapidly in developed countries. There are important consequences of this interpretation for both help-seeking behaviour and the concept of depression.

Contributions of anthropology

Help-seeking behaviour

In general people seek help from healers who hold the same beliefs as they do. Traditional healers in developing countries have the advantage of sharing the same belief system about illness with their clients. Thus they can take for granted a great deal of common ground and do not need to embark on long explanations. Clients of traditional healers often present their distress in terms of somatic symptoms. Skilled healers are adept at understanding the relationship problems that underlie the client's bodily complaints, and their prescription of rituals is aimed at involving the client's social network and regularizing relationships. Problems in communication arise when the patient brings somatic symptoms to the Western trained doctor, who is incapable of recognizing the relationship difficulties that have prompted the complaints.

It would be a mistake to believe that traditional healers are confined to developing countries or to ethnic minority groups in developed countries. Alternative medicine flourishes where Western biomedicine is perceived by the public to be ineffective, and psychiatry is one of those areas. Patients with psychiatric conditions are very likely to seek help from acupuncture, spiritual healing, homeopathy, or herbal remedies, in addition to consulting the general practitioner or psychiatrist. A sympathetic enquiry will elicit a number of sources of alternative medicine in the neighbourhood of the psychiatric facility. The efficacy of these treatments for any psychiatric condition has not been established, but it is a sobering thought that rauwolfia, an effective herbal antipsychotic, was used by Indian traditional healers for hundreds of years before chlorpromazine was introduced.

The concept of depression

At the same time as the evidence for a biological basis for depression appears to be strengthening, the Western concept of depression has been criticized by transcultural researchers. Obeyesekere[18] considers that each culture has developed its own methods for dealing with painful emotions. The Bhuddists of Sri Lanka cope with the loss of a loved person by meditating on the illusory nature of the world of sense, pleasure, and domesticity. Among the Kaluli of New Guinea, the response to loss is anger and the expectation of being adequately compensated by society. Blame is externalized and society is expected to provide social support for the aggrieved individual.[19] In Iran most children learn to grieve in the context of religious ceremonies for Iranian martyrs. The response to personal loss is assimilated into the wider communal experience of historical tragedy.[20] Obeyesekere[18] refers to these coping measures as 'the work of culture' and views the construction of a disease known as depression as a Western cultural resource. Its incorporation into international classifications of diseases could be viewed as 'the imposition of Western cultural standards that are presented as universal and inseparable parts of an emerging new world order'.[21] If a biological basis for the neuroses was firmly established such a formulation could be readily dismissed, but the efficacy of non-biological treatments for depression and anxiety, such as cognitive therapy, marital therapy, and behaviour therapy, indicates that Obeyesekere's view deserves serious consideration. It represents a specific example of the general premise that Western biomedicine is itself a cultural construction and needs to be seen as one of many different ways of dealing with the experience of illness and distress.[22] The achievement of biomedicine in ridding the world of smallpox and other fatal diseases is undeniable, but in the field of psychiatry in particular we need to remain open to the ways other cultures have developed for helping people with what we would term psychiatric illness.

References

1. Rees, W.D. (1971). The hallucinations of widowhood. *British Medical Journal*, **4**, 37–41.
2. Schwab, M.B. (1977). A study of reported hallucinations in a southeastern county. *Mental Health and Society*, **4**, 344–54.
3. Ensink, K. and Robertson, B. (1996). Indigenous categories of distress and dysfunction in South African Xhosa children and adolescents as described by indigenous healers. *Transcultural Psychiatric Research Review*, **33**, 137–72.
4. World Health Organization (1973). *The international pilot study of schizophrenia*, Vol. 1. Geneva, WHO.
5. Westermeyer, J. and Janca, A. (1997). Language, culture and psychopathology: conceptual and methodological issues. *Transcultural Psychiatry*, **34**, 291–311.
6. Jablensky, A., Sartorius, N., Ernberg, G., *et al.* (1992). Schizophrenia: manifestations, incidence and course in different cultures: a World Health Organization ten-country study. *Psychological Medicine*, **20**, 1–97.
7. Wig, N., Menon, D.K., Bedi, H., *et al.* (1987). Expressed emotion and schizophrenia in North India. II. Distribution of expressed emotion components among relatives of schizophrenic patients in Aarhus and Chandigarh. *British Journal of Psychiatry*, **151**, 160–5.
8. Leff, J.P., Fischer, M., and Bertelsen, A. (1976). A cross-national epidemiological study of mania. *British Journal of Psychiatry*, **129**, 428–37.
9. Makanjuola, R.O. (1982). Manic disorder in Nigerians. *British Journal of Psychiatry*, **141**, 459–63.
10. Leff, J. (1988). *Psychiatry around the globe* (2nd edn). Gaskell, London.
11. Leighton, A.H., Lambo, T.A., Hughes, C.C., Leighton, D.C., Murphy, J.M., and Macklin, D.B. (1963). *Psychiatric disorder among the Yoruba*. Cornell University Press, Ithaca, NY.
12. Stanley, D. and Wand, R.R. (1995). Obsessive–compulsive disorder: a review of the cross-cultural epidemiological literature. *Transcultural Psychiatric Research Review*, **32**, 103–36.
13. Orley, J. and Wing, J.K. (1979). Psychiatric disorders in two African villages. *Archives of General Psychiatry*, **36**, 513–20.
14. Hollifield, M., Katon, W., Spain, D., and Pule, L. (1990). Anxiety and depression in a village in Lesotho, Africa: a comparison with the United States. *British Journal of Psychiatry*, **156**, 343–50.
15. Okasha, A., Kamel, M., and Hassan, A.H. (1968). Preliminary psychiatric observations in Egypt. *British Journal of Psychiatry*, **114**, 949–55.
16. Pu, T., Mohamed, E., Imam, K., and El-Roey, A.M. (1986). One hundred cases of hysteria in Eastern Libya: a socio-demographic study. *British Journal of Psychiatry*, **148**, 606–9.
17. Wig, N.N. and Pershad, D. (1975–1977). *Triennial statistical report*. Department of Psychiatry, Postgraduate Institute of Medical Education and Research, Chandigarh, India.
18. Obeyesekere, G. (1985). Depression, Buddhism and the work of culture in Sri Lanka. In *Studies in the anthropology and cross-cultural psychiatry of affect and disorder* (ed. A. Kleinman and B. Good), pp. 134–52. University of California Press, Berkeley, CA.

19. Schieffelin, E.L. (1985). The cultural analysis of depressive affect: an example from New Guinea. In *Culture and depression: studies in the anthropology and cross-cultural psychology of affect and disorder* (ed. A. Kleinman and B. Good), pp. 101–33. University of California Press, Berkeley, CA.

20. Good, B.J., Good, M., and Moradi, R. (1985). The interpretation of human depressive illness and dysphoric affect. In *Studies in the anthropology and cross-cultural psychiatry of affect and disorder* (ed. A. Kleinman and B. Good), pp. 369–428. University of California Press, Berkeley, CA.

21. Bibeau, G. (1997). Cultural psychiatry in a creolizing world: questions for a new research agenda. *Transcultural Psychiatry*, **34**, 9–41.

22. Kakar, S. (1995). Clinical work and cultural imagination. *Psychoanalytic Quarterly*, **64**, 265–81.

1.4 The history of psychiatry as a medical specialty

Pierre Pichot

Introduction

In 1918 Emil Kraepelin wrote:[1]

> A hundred years ago, they were practically no alienists. The care of the mental patients was nearly everywhere in the hands of head supervisors, attendants and administrators of the houses for the mentally ill and the role of the physicians was limited to the treatment of the physical illnesses of the patients.

He pointed out that, in the first decades of the nineteenth century, many of the books dealing with psychiatric themes were still written by medical doctors, such as Reil (who coined the word psychiatry), who had few contacts with mental patients or even by philosophers and theologians, and that only in the great scientific centres had specialists appeared 'who had decided to spend their life in the study and treatment of mental diseases'.

The history of psychiatry as a medical specialty has to be distinguished from the history of psychiatric medical knowledge which began in ancient Greece with the birth of medicine as a science. For more than 2000 years some physicians observed and treated mental illnesses, institutions were created in which the 'lunatics' and the 'insane' were received. But, as rightly pointed out by Kraepelin, the truth is that psychiatry was not really a medical specialty. One can argue about the precise date of the appearance of psychiatry as a specific field of medicine and of the psychiatrist as a specialist devoting his professional competence exclusively to the care of the mentally ill. Denis Leigh recognizes that 'some degree of specialization occurred [in England] among respectable physicians' in the middle of the eighteenth century when the monopoly of Bethlem was broken and new 'lunatic hospitals', such as St Luke's were opened.[2] On the other hand, the American historian Jan Goldstein stresses that in France the language, as an exact reflection of the underlying reality, began to use expressions such as *homme spécial* to describe a physician specializing in a branch of medicine such as psychiatry only around 1830.[3]

Pinel and the birth of psychiatry as a branch of medicine

Despite those divergences, it is generally accepted that the work of Philippe Pinel constitutes a turning point. His role has several aspects. He is known worldwide as the physician who 'liberated the insane from their chains' in a dramatic initiative he started in 1793 at the height of the French revolution, at the Bicêtre asylum, and completed 3 years later at the Salpêtrière asylum. However, the reality is more complex.

Pinel, who was born in 1745, had studied medicine, translated Cullen's books into French, and published scientific papers on various subjects. He acted as a physician in a small Parisian 'madhouse', the Pension Belhomme, in which wealthy lunatics were confined at the request of their families. At that time most of the Parisian insane were confined for a few weeks in the general hospital—the Hôtel Dieu. If their state did not rapidly improve, they were considered as incurable and send to Bicêtre or the Salpêtrière, built a century before, which also received other social deviants such as beggars and prostitutes. Pinel, who was known by his politically influential friends for his progressive scientific ideas, was appointed physician to Bicêtre. The division for the insane was under the direction of an overseer (*surveillant*), Pussin, who had already introduced humanitarian reforms in the care of the patients. Pinel's merit was to approve and systematically to develop Pussin's empirical measures and to propose an explicit scientific theory for their mode of action. Inspired by Crichton's views about the nature of the 'passions', by Condillac's psychology, and by the ideas of Jean-Jacques Rousseau, he created the *traitement moral* which he claimed to be effective with patients previously considered as incurably ill.

The improvement of the conditions in which the insane were cared for, supported and expanded by Pinel, was not an isolated French phenomenon. In Tuscany, Chiarugi had already in 1789 asserted that the basis of the extensive reforms he had introduced in the local asylum for the insane was that 'it is a supreme moral duty and a medical obligation to respect the mental patient as a person'. In England, where public opinion had been shocked by the inhuman treatment to which King George III had been submitted during his mental illness, a pious Quaker, William Tuke, deeply affected by the conditions in which the wife of a member of the Society of Friends had died in York lunatic asylum, decided to set up a special institution under the government of the Friends 'for the care and accommodation of their own members'. At the Retreat, opened in 1796 near York, physical restraints were largely abolished, and religious and moral values were emphasized in the relations with the patients.

Chiarurgi's reforms did not survive the upheavals caused by subsequent wars and the political divisions of Italy, and Tuke's creation of the Retreat had not been prompted by medical considerations but was the expression of religious humanitarian purposes. The role played by Pinel was decisive, not so much because of the changes he promoted in the conditions of the patients, although they had a profound influence, but because he made the study and treatment of mental disorders a branch of medicine.

In 1801 Pinel published the *Medico-philosophical Treatise on Mental Alienation*. In it he presented the various clinical manifestations he had observed, proposed a simple nosological system, largely borrowed from older authors, examined possible aetiological factors, and described his 'moral treatment' in detail. The book has remained a landmark in the history of psychiatry, even being considered by the philosopher Hegel as a 'moment of capital importance in the history of humanity'. For Pinel, insanity was a disease and the patient affected by it remained, despite the loss of his reason, a human being. Its study, like the rest of medicine, had to be 'a science which consists of carefully observed facts'. Goldstein[3] has shown that Pinel's main preoccupation was to prove this scientific nature of the new medical specialty by repudiating the previous practices of the 'empirics' and 'charlatans'— the two terms being practically synonymous. He had accepted the method Pussin had developed empirically, he transformed it in his moral treatment by providing a scientific theory of its mode of action. A curiously premonitory aspect of his emphasis on the necessity of a scientific methodology is to be found in his *Tables to Determine How Probable is the Curability of Alienation*, published in 1808. He provided statistical data on the efficacy of his therapeutic method according to the types of mental disorders and in comparison with spontaneous evolution, and concluded that medicine can only be a true science through the use of the calculus of probability!

Psychiatry as a profession: Esquirol and the clinical approach

If, because of the international influence of the ideas expressed in his book, Pinel is the founder of psychiatry as a medical discipline, he was not a psychiatric specialist in the strict meaning of the term. Although he retained his position at the Salpêtrière until his death in 1826 and is known today for his contributions to mental medicine, he had many other medical interests which gave him, in his time, a leading position among the Paris physicians; his *Philosophical Nosology*, published in 1796 and a classical reference for several decades, deals with general pathology. The case of his pupil and successor, Esquirol, who became the prototype of the psychiatric specialist was very different. At the Salpêtrière he was only in charge of the 'section of the insane'. He was later appointed medical director of the Charenton psychiatric asylum near Paris and owned in addition a small clinic, in which he treated his private patients. All his activities were exclusively dedicated to the study and treatment of mental disorders and the teaching of psychiatry. His book *On Mental Diseases* published in 1838, in which he collected his previous publications, acquired a fame as great as Pinel's *Treatise*. In 1913 Karl Jaspers recognized that the later great representatives of German psychiatry, such as Griesinger and Kraepelin, were strongly indebted to Esquirol. He, and the school he founded, effectively developed one of the basic tenets of the new medical specialty. For Esquirol, careful objective observation and analysis of the symptoms and the behaviour of the patients was fundamental. He originated the descriptive clinical approach, expanded by his pupils. Even more than Pinel, he was suspicious of unproved theories and, when he eventually suggested relations between pathogenic factors and syndromes, remained extremely cautious in his interpretations. Zilboorg, the psychoanalytically oriented historian of psychiatry, has accused

this predominantly descriptive approach of creating a 'psychiatry without psychology' because, lacking psychodynamic concepts, its attempted objectivity remained at an allegedly superficial level.[4] The truth is that it laid the foundations of the present description of the mental disorders. The 'atheoretical' descriptive approach adopted in the present nosological systems—both the American *Diagnostic and Statistical Manual* and the *International Classification of Diseases*— whose proclaimed purpose is to emphasize the medical character of psychiatry is, in this respect, a return to Esquirol's principles.

The social aspects of psychiatry and the asylum system

By the end of the eighteenth century it was recognized that the study of mental alienation was part of medicine. However, mental diseases were of such a nature that it was not possible to treat the insane in the same conditions as patients affected by other diseases. Their most obvious manifestations had social consequences. According to the prevailing philosophical view, the mentally ill were deprived of free will by their illness. In practice, they were unable to participate in the normal life of the society and were often considered as potentially dangerous. Because of this they had generally been confined in madhouses of various kinds. One of the aspects of the reforms initiated by Pinel had been to make more explicit the difference in nature between the socially deviant behaviour of the insane, which, being the consequence of an illness, belonged exclusively to medicine, and the other deviations which society had to control and eventually to repress. The implementation of this fundamental distinction during the first half of the nineteenth century helped to give psychiatry its specific shape as a profession by being at the origin of forensic psychiatry and by leading to the formulation of precise rules concerning the commitment of the insane to institutions of a strictly medical character.

The legal code promulgated by Napoleon in 1810 stipulated that 'no crime or delict exists if commited in a state of dementia', with the old term dementia being used as a synonym of Pinel's mental alienation. This legal provision, introduced in similar forms in other countries, opened an important domain of activity to the medical profession of psychiatrist. Because of their now recognized specialized knowledge, the alienists were to help the judges in determining whether the mental state of an individual convicted of a 'crime or delict' was normal or pathological, with decisive consequences on the subsequent decision. The title of Esquirol's *Treatise* mentions explicitly that it describes the mental diseases 'in their medical, hygienic and medico-legal aspects'. The conflict (which still exists) between the judges, usually supported by public opinion, who took a restrictive view of the concept of mental disease, and the psychiatrists, who tended to expand it to include new types of deviant behaviour, is illustrated by the violent controversies provoked by Esquirol's description of 'homicidal monomania'. They had an even more famous counterpart in England. J.C. Pritchard, an admirer of Esquirol, had isolated 'moral insanity' as a specific mental disorder in two books published in 1837 and 1842; in the second he examined its 'relations to jurisprudence'. Half a century later, in 1897, Henry Maudsley, who was in favour of the use of this diagnosis, recognized that this category, although internationally accepted by the psychiatrists, corresponded to:

... a form of mental alienation which has so much the look of vice and crime that may persons regard it as an unfounded medical invention'. Judges have repeatedly denounced it from the bench as a 'most dangerous medical doctrine', 'a dangerous innovation' which, in the interest of society, should be reprobated.

The general acceptance of the new medical concept of mental alienation implied the existence of adequate facilities for the treatment of the patients. The creation of new asylums—the term was retained— and the reorganization of the old ones was the answer. The French law of 1838 which fixed the detailed rules for the expansion of the new system to the whole country and for its functioning and financial support had a model character. Similar results were obtained in, for example, England with the Asylum Act 1828 and the Lunacy Act 1845. Outwardly the new system was the extension, under more humane conditions, of the previous institutional practices. However, it had radically original features. While recognizing the necessity of protecting society, it stressed the fact that the insane had a fundamental right to be protected and medically treated in a competent way. The deprivation of liberty for the patients which it still implied was strictly controlled to prevent possible misuse and anyway was justified, according to Esquirol and most contemporary psychiatrists, not only by the loss of free will, which was a consequence of the illness, but also by the therapeutic value of separation from a pathogenic milieu.

The asylum system became the central element of psychiatric care and was both the consequence and the determining factor of the emergence of psychiatry as a medical specialty to which it gave, until the end of the nineteenth century and even beyond, an original character. The asylums acquired a quasi-monopoly in the care of the mentally ill. The few private institutions reserved for the wealthier members of the population, which often belonged to alienists in charge of an asylum, were generally submitted to the same legal rules. Private practice with ambulatory patients, as existing today, was exceptional or dealt with cases which were not then considered to belong to mental alienation. As a result, the study of mental illness was predominantly restricted to the more severe forms of disorder. Another consequence was that the alienists in charge of patients committed to the asylums had a dual function, a fact that differentiated them from other hospital physicians. In addition to their medical duties, they were involved in the legal procedures which determined the conditions of admission, stay, and eventually release of the mentally ill. As superintendents, they also often had economic and financial responsibilities, being in charge of the material as well the medical aspects of the functioning of their institutions.

Despite the fact that the laws now strictly differentiated the nature of the limitations of liberty in asylums and in prisons, the participation of the alienist in a form of social control was eventually perceived negatively by the public, and often by other physicians, and contributed to accentuating the specificity of psychiatry inside medicine. During the third and the fourth decades of the nineteenth century, which saw the birth of the asylum system, the psychiatrists became really conscious of their identity as a professional group. In England, France, Germany, and the United States they founded societies and began to publish journals with specialized scientific goals. Such a description oversimplifies an evolution which was progressive and in some cases took different directions. The creation and the extension of the asylum system took many years; it did not reach its classical form until the last part of the century, as testified by the famous campaign conducted in

the United States during the 1840s by Dorothea Dix who complained that many of the mentally ill were still incarcerated in almshouses and prisons. The moral treatment practised in the institutions was eventually used to justify brutal measures, alleged to be therapeutic, and the behaviour of the attendants, who were not usually medically trained (significantly, they were known as *surveillants* in France), was too often of a purely repressive character. It was a long time before the proposals made in 1856 by the British psychiatrist John Conolly in his book *The Treatment of the Insane without Mechanical Restraints* were put into practice everywhere.

The biological and the psychological model

The clinical orientation of Pinel, Esquirol, and their followers was basically empirical. By concentrating on describing observable symptoms and abnormal behaviours, it avoided theoretical controversies. However, many believed that if psychiatry was to become a branch of the medical sciences and to progress, it had to adopt models similar to those accepted by the rest of medicine. According to the anatomoclinical perspective, which was now dominant, diseases were distinct entities. Each disease was defined by a characteristic pattern of symptoms provoked by a lesion or eventually a dysfunction of an organ to be discovered at autopsy. In 1821 Bayle, following this scheme, described the typical clinical symptoms and lesions of the brain in the general paralysis of the insane. Despite the disappointing results of the further anatomopathological studies (brain lesions were observed in only a small proportion of cases), there was increasing conviction that, with better investigation methods, mental disorders, like other diseases, could be explained by somatic causes. The degeneration theory, proposed in 1857 by Morel, which attributed many forms of insanity to the hereditary transmission of dysfunction of the nervous system produced by the noxious effects of environmental factors and whose influence lasted until Kraepelin, is another expression of this biological orientation whose aim was to give psychiatry an undisputed medical status.

The biological and the purely clinical approaches were concerned with different conceptual levels—the discovery of the causes of insanity and the description of its manifestations respectively. Therefore they could easily coexist. Even when the followers of Pinel and Esquirol expressed reservations about the applicability of the biological model to every type of mental disorder, they still believed in the medical nature of psychiatry. The situation created in the German-speaking countries by the school of the 'mentalists' (the term *Psychiker* by which they were known means 'psychologically oriented'), who were predominant during the first half the nineteenth century, was very different. Influenced by philosophical, religious, and romantic trends, those psychiatrists took a radical dualistic position, postulating the absolute difference between the physical body and the spiritual soul. The soul was the source of the whole psychic life and hence eventually of its abnormal aspect—insanity. A term such as disease, appropriate for the somatic illnesses, could only be used metaphorically in psychiatry. The sins of the patients were the origin of the mental disorders, and psychiatry belonged more to moral philosophy than to medicine. These ideas were developed in various related forms by the majority of the German psychiatrists of the period (Heinroth, Ideler, Langerman, and many others). Their ideological position had two consequences: scientific relations with other schools, such as the French and the English who saw in the publications of the mentalists obscure philosophical theories devoid of medical character, were largely cut off, and they provoked a violent reaction in Germany itself. The most extreme representatives of the contending group of 'somatists' (*Somatiker*), such as Jakobi and Friedreich, saw the mental disorders as symptoms of somatic diseases, not necessarily of the brain. In fact for them mental diseases as such did not exist. They defended aggressively their biological and sometimes bizarre hypotheses, such as the aetiological role of intestinal worms, against the mentalists. Finally, around 1850, they gained the upper hand. The publication in 1845 of *Pathology and Therapy of the Nervous Diseases* by Wilhelm Griesinger, an heir to their school who was also influenced by the French alienists, is a landmark in the history of the German psychiatry. With his appointment in 1865 as professor of psychiatry in Berlin, where he succeeded the mentalist Ideler, medical psychiatry was definitely established in Germany as a branch of the natural sciences.

The rise of neuropsychiatry

Romberg's *Lehrbuch der Nervenkrankheiten* symbolizes the birth of neurology as an autonomous medical specialty studying and treating the diseases of the nervous system. It was published 5 years after Griesinger's *Textbook* in which, adopting and expanding Bayle's anatomo-clinical model he had affirmed: 'Mental diseases are diseases of the brain'. If both psychiatric and neurological symptoms originated in the nervous system, some form of association between the two specialties was a logical step, at least at the conceptual level. One aspect of their complex relationship was the creation of neuropsychiatry which developed its most characteristic aspects in the German-speaking countries.

The universities acquired considerable power and influence in the second half of the nineteenth century. From the 1850s on, chairs were created for the teaching of the new common discipline and special institutions, the university clinics, were built with hospital beds for psychiatric patients (if their disorders became chronic they were sent to the nearest asylum), laboratories for research on neurophysiology and neuroanatomy, and special wards for the neurological cases—Griesinger's first move when he took over the chair of psychiatry at Berlin was the creation of neurological wards at the Charité. The leading neuropsychiatrists in charge of these institutions often performed research in both fields with equal competence, as shown by the work of Wernicke and Westphal, and later of Kleist and Bonhöffer, in Germany and of Meynert in Austria.

The concept of neuropsychiatry, appearing at a period during which the German school was progressively gaining influence, had a deep impact on psychiatric thought and on the psychiatric profession, even if its institutional driving force, the university clinic system, was not developed everywhere to the same extent as in Germany. For example, it was conspicuously absent in England, despite the fact that the theoretical position taken by the most important psychiatrist of the time, Henry Maudsley, was very close to that of Griesinger. The National Hospital in Queen's Square, London, founded in 1860, retained a virtual monopoly on the teaching of neurology for many decades, and psychiatry, taught essentially in hospitals, was not represented at university level until the 1930s. However, in most countries, neuropsychiatric institutions coexisted with the asylums where the alienists had the unenviable task of caring for chronic mental patients, often with inadequate means. The concept of neuropsychiatry reflected a basically biological perspective on the aetiology of the mental illnesses expressed in the creation of a new specialty associating competence in the two previously separated domains of medicine. However, it provoked ideological and professional tension between the 'pure' psychiatrists, mainly those in charge of asylums, and the neuropsychiatrists, predominantly involved in teaching and research. In the long term, this conflict was one of the factors which finally led, in the 1960s, to the almost complete administrative and institutional separation of the two specialties in countries such as France where they had been, at least formally, associated. But many traces of the old situation remain. The most influential scientific journal published in German, *Nervenarzt*, still deals equally with neurology and psychiatry, and the term 'neuropsychiatric' survives in the titles of many teaching and research institutions.

The neuroses and the birth of the psychotherapies

The study of the neuroses, in which the relations between psychiatry and neurology were also involved, resulted in completely different, but equally important, changes to psychiatry as a medical specialty. The term neurosis had been coined in 1769 by Cullen to describe a class of diseases he attributed to a dysfunction of the nervous system. In this very heterogenous group, two entities of very ancient origin, hysteria and hypochondriasis, had predominantly psychological manifestations. Since the affected patients were not usually commited to asylums, they were not normally studied by alienists, but by specialists in internal medicine such as Briquet who, in 1859, wrote the classical *Treatise on Hysteria*. Because of the assumed nature of the neuroses, the new discipline of neurology rapidly took an interest in them.

Charcot, the founder of the French neurological school, was responsible for the internal medicine wards at the Salpêtrière—they were not associated with the 'divisions of the insane' at the same hospital, the domain of the alienists. In about 1880 he became interested in hysterical patients which, because of their seizures, were admitted to the same ward as the epileptics. He developed a purely neurological theory of the disease which he described and studied using hypnosis. This was the former 'animal magnetism', long fallen into disrepute, but to which he gave a new scientific status. Charcot's descriptions of the *grande hystérie*, which he demonstrated on selected patients in his famous public lectures, were justly criticized later, but his international fame attracted students from all over the world. One of them was a young lecturer in neuropathology at the University of Vienna, Sigmund Freud, who, impressed by Charcot's lectures, decided to devote all his energies to the study and the treatment of the neuroses. Another was a French professor of philosophy (psychology was then a branch of philosophy), Pierre Janet, who had become interested in the psychological aspects of the neuroses. He was later to develop in parallel with Freud a psychopathological theory which, despite the traces it has left (the concepts of psychasthenia and the dissociative processes in hysteria) were not to be as internationally successful as Freud's psychoanalysis. Charcot's ideas were opposed by Bernheim, the professor of internal medicine at the Nancy Medical School and also an adept of hypnosis. He attacked the neurological interpretations of the

Salpêtrière and claimed that suggestion played a central role in the phenomena described by Charcot.

The general interest in the neuroses, which extended beyond medicine to *fin de siècle* literature, was an international phenomenon. In 1880 Beard, an American neurologist, described a new neurosis, neurasthenia, which soon aroused even more interest than Charcot's hysteria. Psychiatry had played almost no part in this evolution, but this was to change under the influence of three related developments: the changes which took place within the concept of neurosis, the birth of the psychotherapies, and the incorporation in the field of psychiatry of psychopathological manifestations, even if they were of minor intensity.

The transformation of the concept of neurosis is apparent in the position taken by Kraepelin in the 1904 edition of his *Textbook*. He introduced a chapter, 'The psychogenic neuroses', on the grounds that 'among the neuroses, to which belong epilepsy and chorea, one must isolate a sub-group characterized by the purely psychological cause of the apparition of the symptoms'. The disintegration of the old concept left to neurology, which from now on abandoned the generic term, diseases (such as epilepsy and chorea) whose somatic manifestations could be shown to express a dysfunction of a precise part of the nervous system. Psychiatry took charge of hysteria, hypochondriasis, neurasthenia, and the related phobic, obsessional, and anxious disorders, which constituted the new neuroses. This concept was justified by the psychological nature of the symptoms and the causes recognized even by a biologically oriented psychiatrist such as Kraepelin. This redrawing of the frontier between the neurological and psychiatric specialties also testified to the extension of the limits of psychiatry. Pinel's insanity, until then defined by the necessity of commitment to special institutions, was replaced by a broader concept. A new class corresponding to our present personality disorders had already appeared in the 1894 edition of Kraepelin's *Textbook*. It had been isolated for the first time in 1872–1874 by the psychiatrist Koch. Like the neuroses, the cases were rarely observed in asylums but nevertheless they were now considered as belonging to the psychiatric field of study.

This field was further modified by the birth of the psychotherapies. In fact, they had a long history. In 1803 one of the first German mentalists, Reil, had described under the name of 'psychic therapy' (*psychische Curmethode*) a number of procedures, including very violent somatic ones, which could influence the 'perturbed passions of the soul', and Pinel's moral therapy contained psychotherapeutic elements. However, psychotherapies as techniques whose formal rules were based on an explicit theory about their psychological mechanisms of action derived mainly from Mesmer's animal magnetism as rehabilitated by Charcot. The emergence of the psychotherapies, characteristic of the last decades of the nineteenth century, was intimately related to the renewed study of the neuroses. After he had abandoned hypnosis, Freud developed psychoanalysis, but many other techniques evolved during the same period, which were as well or even better known at the time although they were to have a less lasting success. One of these was the method of Janet, who still occasionally used hypnosis. In 1904 Dubois, a Swiss neuropathologist from Bern, introduced a technique influenced by Bernheim's theory of suggestion in *The Psychoneuroses and their Moral Treatment*, and claimed to produce a 'psychological re-education' by a combination of rational and persuasive elements. His international reputation brought him patients from all over the world. The 'rest cure', proposed in 1877 by the American neurologist

S. Weir Mitchell for the treatment of hysteria and later of neurasthenia, was combined with Dubois' method by Dejerine, Charcot's successor as professor of neurology in Paris.

This very incomplete summary illustrates the striking fact that, because of their intimate connections with the neuroses, the psychotherapies originated inside neurology. When the study and treatment of the neuroses were incorporated into psychiatry, the psychiatrists considered that they were an integral part of their activity and tried to retain the monopoly of their practice. They never completely succeeded. Already Freud had, according to his biographer Jones, 'warmly welcomed the incursion in the therapeutic field of suitable people from another walk of life than medicine'. The problem of the 'lay analysts', a source of conflict within the psychoanalytic movement, is only an aspect of a broader question which was later to involve the relations of the medical specialty of psychiatry with the new professional group of clinical psychologists.

From the beginning of the twentieth century to the Second World War

During the first half of the twentieth century psychiatry developed in many directions. Kraepelin's monumental synthesis established around 1900 a nosological system which, in its broad outlines, has remained valid until today. Without being radically altered it was completed, to mention only a few contributions, in 1911 by Bleuler's description of schizophrenia and in 1913 by Jaspers' psychopathological perspective, developed by the Heidelberg school and Kurt Schneider, and by other psychiatrists working in academic institutions. However, the old conflict between the 'mentalists' and the 'somatists' reappeared in a modified form. The mainstream of psychiatry had abandoned the extreme positions of the 'brain pathologists' of the Meynert–Wernicke type but, while recognizing a limited influence of psychological factors, admitted in a general way the biological origin of the more severe mental disorders—the psychoses. The empirical discoveries of biological treatments—of general paralysis by malaria therapy (Wagner von Jauregg in 1917), of schizophrenia by insulin coma (Sakel in 1933) or by chemically induced seizures (von Meduna in 1935), and of depression by electroconvulsive therapy (Cerletti in 1938)—not only helped to dispel the prevailing therapeutic pessimism, but provided supporting arguments. However, an opposing ideological current represented by psychoanalysis had arisen from the study of the neuroses. Its attention was concentrated on the study of complex psychopathological mechanisms postulated to be at the origin of the neurotic, and later also of the psychotic, symptoms, favoured psychogenetic aetiological theories, and advocated psychotherapy as the fundamental form of treatment. Psychoanalysis expanded steadily during this period and gained enthusiastic adherents in many countries. However, partly because of the suspicion and even hostility of many members of the psychiatric establishment, they remained isolated in close-knit groups with their own teaching system independent of the official medical curriculum, and the use of their therapeutic technique was restricted to a small number of mostly neurotic patients seen in outpatient clinics or, more often, in private practice.

The great majority of patients suffering from mental disorders were still confined in asylums, and the enormous increase in their number, mainly related to the social changes accompanying industrialization and urbanization although other factors have been invoked, was striking. In Great Britain it grew from 16 000 in 1860 to 98 000 in 1910, three times more rapidly than the population. A similar phenomenon was observed in all countries and persisted until the end of the 1940s despite the introduction of the first biological therapies. In the United States they were already 188 000 patients in mental hospitals in 1910, and by the end of the Second World War 850 000 were lodged in huge institutions which were overpopulated, understaffed, and could only provide custodial care. This obvious degeneracy of the asylum system, contrasting with the progresses in the scientific field, stimulated efforts to improve the practice of psychiatry and its institutional framework. Most of these improvements took place after 1920 and, although their results remained relatively limited, they were the forerunners of later more drastic changes.

The education of psychiatric specialists, which had varied widely from country to country, was improved and systematized. A convergence of evolution is apparent during this period which can be said, to some extent, to have seen the formal administrative recognition of psychiatry as a medical specialty. Educational programmes and controls of the level of competence were introduced which extended beyond psychiatrists in academic positions. A limited teaching of psychiatry became compulsory even in the general medical curriculum. In France, psychiatrists for public asylums and, in some cases, residents in psychiatry were selected by a competitive examination system. In England, the Board of Control recommended in 1918 that a leading position in a psychiatric institution could only be occupied by a physician who had obtained a Diploma in Psychological Medicine awarded by the Royal College of Physicians and by five universities. In the United States the moving force behind the reforms was Adolf Meyer, the Director of the Henry Phipps Clinic at Johns Hopkins University from 1913 to 1939, who organized a systematic residency system and promoted the creation of the Board of Neurology and Psychiatry. This Board was established in 1936 and awarded a diploma which it became necessary to hold to be recognized as a specialist.

The changes were reflected in the vocabulary. The term psychiatry, originating in the German-speaking countries and mostly used there, was adopted everywhere at the beginning of the century. In France, the health authorities officially substituted 'hôpital psychiatrique' for 'asile d'aliénés' and 'psychiatre' for 'aliéniste' in the 1930s. In England, a Royal Commission used the words 'hospital', 'nurse', and 'patient' instead of 'asylum', 'attendant', and 'lunatic' for the first time between 1924 and 1926. However, efforts were also made to dissociate, when possible, the social protection function of the institutions from their medical role by allowing them to admit patients under the same conditions as the general hospitals. In 1923 a special section was created in the Paris Sainte-Anne asylum which provided treatment to voluntary patients and had both hospital beds and a large outpatient department. In England the Mental Health Act 1930 made voluntary admissions to psychiatric hospitals possible; by 1938 they already constituted 35 per cent of all admissions.

Social considerations had always been evident in psychiatry, but their traditional expressions had mainly been of a negative nature, i.e. the confinement of patients in asylums. The new possibility of free admissions reflected an increase in tolerance towards the disturbing character of mental illness. At the same time a differently oriented and broader social perspective appeared. The concept of mental hygiene originated in the United States with the creation in 1919 by a former patient, Clifford Beers, of an organization whose internationally grow-

ing influence was manifested by well-attended congresses held in Washington in 1930 and in Paris in 1937. From its beginnings the movement was not purely medical and was influenced by various humanitarian philosophical trends. It emphasized the role of social factors, such as living conditions or educational practices, in the origin of mental disturbances and promoted their prevention and treatment by the close co-operation of psychiatrists and nurses with non-medical groups in the community. One of the institutional consequences of these ideas was the creation of the profession of social worker. They began their activity in Adolf Meyer's clinic (Adolf Meyer had been an early supporter of the mental hygiene movement whose principles converged with his own ideas), at the Sainte-Anne Hospital in Paris, in England where the London School of Economics opened a special training course in 1929, and elsewhere.

Contemporary with the emergence of psychiatric social work was the expansion of clinical psychology. The Binet–Simon scale for the measurement of intelligence, developed in 1905, was the first application to psychiatry of the new discipline of experimental psychology which had originated at the end of the previous century. This initial contribution led to the creation of a professional class of clinical psychologists who were initially concerned with the development and use of psychological assessment instruments and with theoretical research in a few psychiatric centres. Their number initially remained low; in 1945 the United States, where they were most numerous, had about 4000 psychiatrists but only 200 clinical psychologists.

The expansion of psychiatry after 1945

The Second World War coincided with a major transformation of the psychiatric specialty. The war had vividly demonstrated the frequency of mental disorders in the United States; they had proved to be the leading cause of medical discharges from the military service and the primary cause of almost 40 per cent of selective service rejections. The previously prevailing view that psychiatry was a minor and often somewhat despised medical discipline, concerned primarily with the custodial care of psychologically deviant and potentially troublesome individuals, was progressively dispelled. The preservation and the restoration of mental health—an expression from now on often used by national and international institutions—began to be considered by governments as an important task. The fundamental changes which took place after 1945 and shaped psychiatry as we know it today were the result of this new atmosphere and of the emergence of new perspectives in the three traditional domains— the psychological, the social, and the biological. Some appeared in slightly different forms at different times, their relative influence was submitted to variations, and eventually they came into conflict. The result has been an impressive expansion and increase of the efficacy of psychiatry, profound institutional transformations, and successive ideological waves which have had a major impact on the professional position of the psychiatrist.

The demographic data reflect the new importance of psychiatry in medicine. In the United States the proportion of psychiatrists in the medical profession was 0.7 per cent in 1920, 1.4 per cent in 1940, and 5.5 per cent in 1970, the rate of growth having doubled after the Second World War. In France at present there are 18 psychiatrists for 100 000 habitants; they constitute 6 per cent of all physicians. Similar levels were reached during the postwar decades in the developed countries and remain relatively stable today. Even before this spectacular increase in numbers, psychiatrists had been becoming conscious of the necessity to affirm the identity of their discipline. The First World Congress of Psychiatry, held in Paris in 1950, has been followed by periodic meetings and by the creation of the World Psychiatric Association to which almost every national society of psychiatry belongs. The health authorities of various countries have become conscious of the necessity to provide adequate financial means to support research and training in the discipline. In 1946 the United States government created the National Institutes of Mental Health for such a purpose, and similar efforts were made in many countries although the structures of the organizations formed were different. To promote the same goals at the international level, the World Health Organization, created immediately after the Second World War, had a Section (later Division) of Mental Health which, among other co-ordinating activities, tried to overcome the difficulties of communication between the national schools by establishing a common nosological language.

While the changes affected almost all countries, they were most spectacular in the United States. From the end of the nineteenth century until the 1930s, the concepts developed in the German-speaking countries had been the most influential. This disappeared with the advent of the National Socialist regime which, under cover of racist theories, expelled many of the leading psychiatrists from Germany and Austria, introduced compulsory sterilization for several varieties of mental illnesses, and promoted the voluntary killing in psychiatric hospitals of mentally retarded children and chronic patients. The United States, which had emerged from the Second World War as the most powerful country in the world, began to exert a widespread influence in psychiatry as in the rest of medicine. Because of the prestige of its research and teaching institutions and the worldwide influence of its scientific publications, reinforced by the progressive adoption of English as the language of international scientific communication, American psychiatry became a model in many countries, even though many of the theoretical trends and technical advances it adopted and developed had originated in Europe. However, in the United States, with a local colouring, they took on a special intensity.

The psychodynamic wave

An important factor in the spread of the doctrine of psychoanalysis was the emigration of a relatively large number of German and Austrian psychoanalysts to the United States from 1933 onwards. They had been compelled to leave their home countries for racial reasons—psychoanalysis had been condemned by the National Socialist regime as Jewish and Freud's books had been publicly burned. Many of the young psychiatrists trained in large numbers to answer the demands of the armed forces adopted psychoanalysis under the influence of some of those in charge of the programmes. For a generation, until the end of the 1960s, psychoanalysis became the dominant ideology in American psychiatry.

The American form of psychodynamism often deviated from Freudian orthodoxy, but it emphasized the role of psychogenetic factors, the value of the study of intrapsychic mechanisms, and the basic importance of psychotherapy, while giving little consideration to the traditional clinical approach and to nosology. The domination of this essentially psychological orientation, sometimes compared with the success of the German mentalist school during the first half of the nineteenth century, had important consequences. Although the dis-

orders of hospitalized psychotics were eventually interpreted according to psychoanalytic theory, psychotherapy was mostly used, as it has been since its beginnings,on ambulatory neurotic patients. As early as 1951–1952, 3000 of the 7500 American psychiatrists identified private practice as their main activity, and in 1954 the number of private psychiatrists exceeded that of their salaried colleagues for the first time, with a quarter of the former devoted exclusively to psychotherapy. However, with the initial encouragement of official institutions such as the Veterans Administration, the clinical psychologists began to engage in psychotherapeutic activities. The number of members of the Clinical Psychology Section of the American Psychological Association reached 20 000 in 1980 at a time when they were 26 000 psychiatrists in the United States. In public opinion, and to a certain extent in general medical opinion also, psychiatry was assumed to consist only of psychotherapy and psychology.

In most other countries the developments that occurred in the United States were not as intense, generally appeared later, and were modified by local traditions and influences. In the German-speaking countries they were delayed by the still powerful neuropsychiatric perspective and the temporary vogue for existential phenomenology. In the United Kingdom, the eclectic current fostered by the influential London Institute of Psychiatry during the decades following the war restricted the advance of psychodynamism; in 1956 *Time Magazine* could affirm, as a conclusion of a survey, that 'all of Great Britain [had] half as many analysts as New York City'. In France, the psychoanalyst Jacques Lacan gave the doctrine a special colouring. On the whole, however, the rise of psychodynamism was a general phenomenon, except in the communist countries where Freud's doctrine had been condemned on ideological grounds.

A reaction began in the 1960s with the successes of the new pharmacotherapies. Clinical psychologists had developed alternative radically different psychotherapeutic methods based on learning theories, especially the behaviour therapy introduced in 1958 by Wolpe, supported in the United Kingdom by Eysenck, and the cognitive therapy often associated with it. These methods competed successfully with the psychodynamic techniques and conquered a large part of the field. Psychodynamism did not disappear; many of its concepts retained their place in psychiatry and psychotherapeutic methods continued to be practised, but it lost its predominant ideological position. In addition to its theoretical contributions, when its influence on the professional aspect of psychiatry is considered from a historical perspective, it has been an important factor in the further expansion of the activity of psychiatrists in the treatment of relatively minor disorders and has also encouraged clinical psychologists to play an active and independent role in this field.

The social wave

At the end of the Second World War there was a great desire for social change; one of its aspects was the belief that everyone had a 'right to health' or at least the right to receive adequate medical care regardless of ability to pay. This resulted in the creation of the National Health Service in the United Kingdom in 1948 and the Social Security system in France, together with similar developments in other countries. The social perspective, which was one of the basic principles underlying these developments, initiated major institutional changes in psychiatry. They were the result of a number of factors—the necessity to give to the whole population an easy access to psychiatric care, and also the belief that social elements played an important role in the aetiology of the mental disorders and that they could greatly contribute to the healing process, with the aim of progressively reintegrating the patient in the community.

The most spectacular aspect of the new policy was the decline of the asylum system, still in a dominant position in psychiatry; in fact, the number of patients in psychiatric hospitals in the developed countries reached its peak in 1955. The criticisms of the 'degeneration' of the functioning of psychiatric hospitals and the segregation of patients in institutions often located far from their homes and families were not new. However, the previous partial improvements, such as the decrease in the number of compulsory commitments or the creation of outpatient departments, were replaced by the creation of completely new structures. Ideally, the country would be divided into geographical zones or sectors with a population of about 100 000, and each zone would have a multidisciplinary team of psychiatrists, nurses, clinical psychologists, social workers, and occupational therapists responsible for mental health. Visits and therapeutic interventions in the patient's home and easily accessible outpatient departments were to play an increasingly important role. If hospitalization was necessary, it should be as far as possible in small units located in a general hospital where the time of stay was to be reduced to the absolute minimum. Special institutions such as day hospitals, night hospitals, and specially adapted workshops would contribute to the progressive readaptation of the patient to the life in the community. The introduction of this 'community care', which was expected to work in close co-operation with general practitioners and various public and private institutions, would result in the disappearance of the traditional psychiatric hospital and to 'deinstitutionalize' psychiatry. The new system was introduced in various forms in most countries after 1969. In the United States the Community Mental Health Center Act was promulgated in 1967. In the United Kingdom, which had strong traditions of social psychiatry, plans for the implementation of community care were discussed in the 1960s, and in 1975 the Government White Paper *Better Services for the Mentally Ill* encouraged the formation of multidisciplinary 'primary care teams' which also included general pratitioners. In France, an official directive in 1960 created the *psychiatrie de secteur* which was expected to result in the progressive elimination of *hospitalocentrisme*. The World Health Organization (**WHO**) encouraged all its member countries to adopt similar practices.

Although in the last 40 years community care has become the official doctrine everywhere, except in Japan where the rate of hospitalization in mostly private hospitals has grown continuously, its implementation has not been easy despite the major therapeutic improvements brought about by pharmacotherapy. In some parts of the United States the sudden closure of public psychiatric hospitals combined with the inadequacies of the Community Mental Health Centers were for a time at the origin of an appalling lack of care for a number of mentally ill people. The expected 'fading out' of hospitalization has been slow. According to the WHO, in 1976 the number of mental health beds (including beds for the mentally retarded) per 1000 population was 6.5 in Sweden, 5.5 in the United Kingdom, 3 in France, and 2 in Germany. These figures have since decreased and the types of hospitalization have changed. In 1955, 77 per cent of the 'psychiatric care episodes' in the United States occurred in public psychiatric hospitals, compared with 20 per cent in 1990. In 1994, 1.4 million mental patients were hospitalized, but only 35 per cent in public psychiatric hospitals compared with 43 per cent in general hospitals and 11 per

cent in private psychiatric hospitals, which increased in number from 150 in 1970 to 444 in 1988. In France, where the total number of psychiatric patients treated in public institutions (including children) is now about a million, 60 per cent are seen exclusively on an ambulatory basis, but the number of hospital beds has only been reduced by half.

Reflecting the increasing influence of social perspectives, the organizational changes modified psychiatry as a profession. The increase in the number of psychiatrists in private practice was paralleled, in general to a lesser extent, by an increase in the public sector where their role was modified. In the traditional asylum the authority of the psychiatrist was unchallenged and limited only by the legal provisions related to the procedures of commitment. The nurses, and later the clinical psychologists, social workers, and occupational therapists, were 'paramedical auxiliaries' in a subordinate position. The creation of multidisciplinary teams, working in various settings, gave the psychiatrist a function of co-ordination made increasingly complex by the claims of professional autonomy made by the former auxiliaries. In some cases, such as in the American Mental Health Centers, the psychiatrists who were a small minority in the team and had less and less control over its functioning, resented what they considered to be the loss of their medical status.

The importance given to social factors was not limited to the system by which care was delivered. Sometimes, combined with radical ideological and political attitudes, it took more extreme forms. The criticisms, which first centred on the inadequacies of the existing institutions, extended to the concept of mental disease itself. The antipsychiatric movement claimed that mental diseases were artificial constructs which were not related to diseases in the medical meaning of the term. The allegedly pathological behaviours, such as those conceptualized as schizophrenia, were in fact normal reactions to an inadequate social system. The so-called treatments were techniques used by the ruling classes to preserve the social order of which they were the beneficiaries. The only solution was a drastic reform of society. Such theses varied in their content and in the arguments used. They were developed by authors such as Szasz, Laing, and Cooper in the English-speaking world, the philosopher Foucault in France, and the psychiatrist Basaglia in Italy. They reached their greatest influence in the 1960s and a few attempts were made to put their ideological principles into practice. Although they attracted much attention at the time, they were very limited and short lived. One of the few countries where this movement had a practical impact was Italy. Basaglia's strongly politically oriented theories were influential in the later legal reform of the antiquated asylum system, but, despite the apparently revolutionary character of some of the new administrative provisions, the changes made were very similar to those taking place in other countries.

The biological wave

Psychotropic drugs, such as opium, had been used since the origins of the medical treatment of psychiatric patients. During the nineteenth and the first half of the twentieth century, synthetic drugs such as the bromides, the barbiturates, and the amphetamines were developed. Some of them, especially the sedatives and hypnotics, had a real but in practice marginal value in alleviating some symptoms. They had never constituted an effective treatment of mental disorders. Modern psychopharmacology not only initiated what has been rightly called a therapeutic revolution in psychiatry but also gave a powerful new impulse to the biological perspective. Its date of birth is usually considered to be 1952 when the remarkable activity of chlorpromazine on the symptoms of schizophrenia and mania was discovered. This had been preceded in 1949 by the demonstration of the value of lithium salts in manic states. A few years later it was shown that the continuous administration of lithium salts prevented the recurrence of manic and depressive phases in the mood disorders. This was followed by the introduction of drugs acting on the depressive manifestations (imipramine and the monoamine oxidase inhibitors in 1957) and on anxiety (including chlorediazepoxide, the prototype of the benzodiazepines, in 1960). In one decade clinicians had empirically discovered the fields of application of the main classes of psychoactive drugs—the neuroleptics, the antidepressants, the anxiolytics, and the mood stabilizers—which had been synthesized by biochemists and previously tested by pharmacologists on animal models. The scale and rapidity of the spread of their use had major repercussions.

The first was a modification of the image of psychiatry. The layman generally expected a physician to prescribe drugs to treat the disease from which he suffered. In part because it did not conform to the expected therapeutic behaviour, psychiatry had been seen as an atypical and almost non-medical specialty. In addition to the specificity of the institutions in which it was generally practised, psychological techniques were unknown in the rest of medicine, and even the recently introduced biological techniques (the shock therapies and the lobotomy) had a somewhat strange and frightening character. The establishment of pharmacotherapy contributed strongly to modifying this perception, even if it did not completely remove the traditional prejudices.

The second consequence was even more important. There were, at least initially, controversies about the roles of pharmacotherapy and of the new social perspectives in the restructuring of the mental health care system. In fact, the number of inpatients in psychiatric hospitals began to decrease from 1955 on, and it seems obvious that the main cause was the therapeutic efficacy of the drugs. They reduced the mean length of hospitalization and eventually even made it unnecessary. Although some types of patients did not benefit from them and the mental state of others was only improved, many who had previously been condemned to long stays in the hospital were able to return to the community, with their treatment eventually being continued in rehabilitation settings and often on an ambulatory basis. Pharmacotherapy had made possible the practical implementation of social trends. In addition to this basic contribution to the 'deinstitutionalization' movement, pharmacotherapy was an essential factor in the growth of private practice. The success of psychotherapy had been one contribution to this, but the complexity of its techniques, the length of the treatment, its applicability to only a few types of disorder, and the uncertainty of the results limited its use to a relatively small number of selected patients, even in the United States during the period of the greatest popularity of psychodynamism. Pharmacotherapy could be used much more easily, on a much larger number of patients, and did not require a long and complex training. Some of the drugs, such as the anxiolytics, had an immediate symptomatic effect, and others (the antidepressants and the neuroleptics) could attenuate or suppress the pathological manifestations in a few weeks and, outside the acute phase requiring hospitalization, could be used on an ambulatory basis. It was not only private psychiatrists who were able to treat many of their patients successfully; general practitioners also began to prescribe psychotropic drugs on a large scale.

The third consequence was the explosive development of biological research in psychiatry. The first therapeutic discoveries were largely empirical, but new biochemical techniques allowed some of the modes of action of the drugs to be elucidated. From 1960 on, studies of the influence of these drugs on various aspects of neurotransmission in the brain stimulated hypotheses about the abnormal biochemical mechanisms considered to be the physical substrate of the mental disorders. Meanwhile new methods had been introduced for examination of morphological modifications of the living brain and even of the nature and localization of the biochemical processes taking place in its different parts. The discovery by Watson and Crick in 1953 of the chemical basis of heredity and the subsequent spectacular advances in molecular biology gave a fresh impulse to psychiatric genetics, which had been partly discredited by their misuse by the National Socialist regime. Under the name of neurosciences, these new fields of enquiry progressively acquired a dominant role in psychiatric research at the same time as the introduction of an ever-increasing number of drugs, eventually more potent, usually with less inconvenient side-effects, and sometimes with new therapeutic indications.

'Remedicalization' of psychiatry

In 1983, Melvin Sabshin, the Director of the American Psychiatric Association, summarized the overlapping chronologies of the psychodynamic, biological, and social waves as follows:[6]

> Psychoanalysis surged through the United States during the 1940s and the 1950. During the 1950s a new psychopharmacological approach emerged which had great impact on psychiatric practice generally ... The 1960s saw the dawning of a community psychiatric approach which attempted to accomplish a massive desinstitutionalization of patients from public psychiatric hospitals.

Although less radical and not strictly identical, the general picture was similar in other countries. The 1960s saw an often uneasy coexistence of three schools. 'During that decade', wrote Sabshin, 'American psychiatry enlarged its boundaries and its practices so broadly that many critics grew increasingly concerned with the "bottomless pit" of the field'. The extension of the practice of psychotherapy, frequently to cases with no clear pathological character, tended to blur the limits of the mental disease concept and to neglect the traditional diagnostic approach. Social work was also tempted to concern itself with problems with no obvious medical nature, such as those still described in 1978 in the United States by the President's Commission of Mental Health, which asserted that 'American mental health cannot be defined only in terms of disabling mental illness and identified mental disorders' and identified as a domain of concern for workers in the field 'unrelenting poverty and unemployment and the institutionalized discrimination that occurs on the basis of race, sex, class, age...'. In sharp contrast, the new biological psychiatry recognized only a strictly medical model, stressing the necessity of an accurate diagnosis for the prescription of the drugs and for the testing of their efficacy, and advocated restrictive limits in the definition of the mental diseases.

Around 1970 a profound change took place. Although the institutional modifications of the care system favoured by the generalization of drug therapy continued and expanded under its various forms everywhere, the influence of psychodynamism began to decline within the psychiatric profession. According to the Director of the National Institutes for Mental Health 'it was nearly impossible in 1945 for a non-psychoanalyst to become Chairman of a Department of Psychiatry (in the United States)' but by the mid-1970s the situation was reversed. The publication by the American Psychiatric Association of the Third Revision of the Diagnostic and Statistical Manual of Mental Disorders (DSM-III) is often considered as the symbolic expression of the change. This took place in 1980, but its origins were more than a decade previously, and it was significantly presented by its apologists, such as Klerman, as 'a decisive turning point in the history of American psychiatry... an affirmation of its medical identity'. The new nosology, which was categorical in nature and introduced diagnostic criteria borrowed from experimental psychology in the delimitation of the categories, did not allow any reference to 'unproven' aetiological factors or pathogenic mechanisms, unless 'scientifically demonstrated'. It claimed to be purely descriptive and therefore acceptable as a means of communication by all psychiatrists, whatever their individual orientation. It was in fact perceived, not only in its country of origin, as a reaction against the extreme socio-psychological positions—the deletion of the term neurosis because of its usual association with the psychoanalytic theory of intra-psychic conflicts raised violent controversies—and, despite its proclaimed 'a-theorism', as favouring the biological medical model. Although initially exclusively devised for the use of the American psychiatrists, to the surprise of its authors it was rapidly accepted in all countries and the WHO adopted finally its principles in its own nosological system, the International Classification of Diseases. Originally the result of a brutal reversal of trends in the American psychiatry, it expressed a general change of direction in the psychiatric way of thinking towards the affirmation, against the forces believed to threaten it, of the medical character of psychiatry.

Crisis in psychiatry?

At first glance the new status of psychiatry seems to have taken firm root in the last three decades. It rests on the general acceptance of the medical definition of the concept of mental disease and of the progressive realization of a diversified but co-ordinated institutional system of mental health care. The biological perspective, even if it has taken a prominent place in research and therapy, is now combined with psychological and social approaches in the bio-psychosocial model. The psychiatrist, in accordance with his medical professional responsibilities, occupies a central position in a multidisciplinary team whose members contribute their special competences to the common goal.

This idyllic picture is far from a reflection of reality, even in the developed countries, and the existence of a crisis in psychiatry is evoked with increasing frequency. An indication of the loss of prestige of psychiatry in the medical profession is the alarming decrease of the proportion of American medical students choosing a psychiatric residency; it fell to 2 per cent in 1990, a level much too low to ensure the maintenance of the present demography. Under the pressure of economic constraints, efforts are made everywhere to control the rising burden of medical care. They have taken different forms according to the country—from the managed care system in the United States to the *numerus clausus* system in France, in which the number of internships available is determined by the government—but their common aim is to limit the number of psychiatrists and the cost of their activities. Paradoxically, the recognition of the frequency of the mental disorders and the growing demand for psychiatric treatments has been associated with a reduction if the domain of action of psychiatrists, who are now often vastly outnumbered by clinical psychologists and social workers. In the United States, by 1990, 80 000 'clinical' social workers were active in the psychiatric socio-psychological domain, a quarter of them in part- or full-time private practice. The claims of these powerful professional groups are not limited to a completely autonomous status but, in the case of the clinical psychologists, extend to the demand for a legal recognition of such typical 'medical privileges' as the right to hospitalize patients and to prescribe drugs. Even within medicine, psychiatry is under attack. In Germany, a medical psychotherapeutic specialty distinct from psychiatry has been created. The most impressive change has been in the proportion of mental disorders now treated by general practitioners as a result of the availability of psychotropic drugs with fewer side-effects; in France, 60 per cent of antidepressants are now prescribed by general practitioners. These examples may not be a fair representation of the global picture, but there is undoubtedly a movement towards a limitation of the psychiatric specialty to the care of the most severe cases—in practice, the psychotic cases. However, some neuroscientists raise doubts about the usefulnesss of maintaining psychiatry as a specialty even in this field. Influential biologically oriented psychiatrists have recently proposed, on theoretical and practical grounds, that psychiatry should be absorbed into a new medical discipline, akin to the former neuropsychiatry, and all or most of its socio-psychological aspects should be left to non-medical professions.

Since psychiatry has emerged as a specialty, it has been submitted to conflicting forces. The demands of society, changes in the concept of mental disorder and of its limits, variations in the role played by different theoretical perspectives, and successive scientific discoveries have been responsible for an evolution reflected in the professional status and role of the psychiatrist. Displacements of the centre of gravity of a complex structure in which biological, psychological, and social factors interact have modified the image of psychiatry. The threat of being incorporated in other medical specialties or being deprived of its medical character is but another transitory episode in its history.

Further reading

Hunter, R. and Macalpine, I. (1963). *Three hundred years of psychiatry 1535–1860.* Oxford University Press, London.

Pichot, P. (1996). *Un siècle de psychiatrie.* Synthelabo, Le Plessis-Robinson.

Postel, J. and Questel, U. (ed.) (1994). *Nouvelle histoire de la psychiatrie.* Dunod, Paris.

Shorter, E.A. (1997). *History of psychiatry: from the era of the asylum to the age of Prozac.* Wiley, New York.

References

1. Kraepelin, E. (1918). Hundert Jahre Psychiatrie. *Zeitschrift für die gesamte Neurologie und Psychiatrie,* **38**, 161–275.
2. Leigh, D. (1961). *The historical development of British psychiatry.* Vol. I, *Eighteenth and nineteenth centuries.* Pergamon Press, Oxford.
3. Goldstein, J. (1987). *Console and classify: the French psychiatric profession in the nineteenth century.* Cambridge University Press.
4. Zilboorg, G. (1941). *A history of medical psychology.* Norton, New York.
5. Kraepelin, E. (1904). *Psychiatrie* (7th edn). Barth, Leipzig.
6. Sabshin, M. (1983). Preface. In *International perspectives on DSM-III* (ed. R.L. Spitzer, J.B.W. Williams, and A.E. Skodol). American Psychiatric Press, Washington, DC.

1.5 Psychiatric ethics: codes, concepts, and clinical practice skills

K. W. M. Fulford and Sidney Bloch

Ethical problems pervade every facet of clinical practice and research in psychiatry. Yet with occasional exceptions,[1–3] psychiatric ethics have generally been treated as an addendum to mainstream bioethics. The assumption has been that ethical 'tools' developed to deal with issues like assisted reproduction or transplant surgery can be used essentially unmodified in psychiatry.[4] These tools, as we shall see, are certainly helpful in psychiatry. But the hand-me-down approach has meant that salient features of psychiatric ethics have been widely misunderstood or even neglected altogether. We will focus on three such features: the role of ethical codes in providing a framework for good practice, the ethical significance of psychiatric diagnostic concepts, and the place of ethical reasoning as a core practice skill in psychiatry.

Codes

Codes of practice, both high-level ethical codes and practice-based guidelines, although somewhat marginalized by academic bioethics, have become a prominent feature of medical practice since the 1980s. To understand their function in contemporary practice it is helpful to set them in their historical context.[5]

The historical context

The Hippocratic Oath, devised about 400 BC, probably by Hippocrates' students, is by far the best known of early codes. It formed the basis for codes governing both early Islamic and Christian medicine and remains the inspiration for their modern counterparts. Similar codes are to be found in many of the great medical traditions. The *Caraka Samhita*, for example, written by an Indian physician in the first century AD, covers confidentiality, considerateness to patients, and keeping abreast of medical knowledge. Comparable issues are dealt with in the sixth century Hebrew *Book of Asaph Harofe* and in a text on medical ethics by the tenth century Persian physician, Haly Abbas.

The direct forerunner of modern codes, the *Code of Institutes and Precepts*, was published in 1803 by the English physician, Thomas Perceval. This was to become the foundation for both the American and British Medical Associations' early codes. The twentieth century has seen these and other national codes complemented by a series of international declarations and by derivative documents dealing with particular areas of practice. Codes specific to psychiatry were initially derived from medical codes; for example, the American Psychiatric Association's code (published in 1973) was based on that of the American Medical Association.

The functions of codes

The development of codes in the history of medicine in part reflects their importance in promoting good practice. Some codes have been a direct response to scandals: Perceval's *Principles* resulted from an unseemly battle among doctors for the control of patient referrals in the Manchester Infirmary; the Nuremberg Statement was formulated in the aftermath of Nazi medical crimes. But codes also have positive functions.

- **Protecting and promoting the profession** George Bernard Shaw famously described professions as 'conspiracies against the laity.' A professional code may be self-serving—a charter for restrictive practices, protectionist rather than protective. For a profession to function effectively, however, it must be cohesive and collegial. A code which sets out its members' obligations one to another can contribute substantially to achieving this goal. Such codes need not be wholly inward looking. Most codes have emphasized medicine's tradition of commitment and dedication; some call for 'whistle blowing' in appropriate circumstances; and the Declaration of Madrid, adopted by the World Psychiatric Association in 1996, expressly endorses a role for patient empowerment. The protective function of codes has become increasingly important in the international context. Doctors working in oppressive regimes have been supported in their resistance to abusive practices by appeals to internationally accepted codes of practice such as the Declaration of Helsinki.

- **Self-regulation** A second function of codes is to enhance high standards of practice. Professions are characterized, in part, by a corpus of specialized knowledge and skills, not readily available to others, and offered to a dependent, sometimes vulnerable clientele.[6] To the extent, therefore, that it takes an expert to judge expertise, a degree of self-regulation is essential. But this can become incestuous and must be balanced by external monitoring. In French psychiatry, for example, it took the introduction of a new law to persuade doctors to follow their own code on the requirement to obtain informed consent from their patients.[7] Similarly, where bad practice becomes the norm, self-regulation may reinforce it: the abuse of psychiatry to suppress dissent in the former USSR was promoted by leaders of the psychiatric profession.[8] The international context is again important here. As

Jim Birley, a former President of the Royal College of Psychiatrists, has put it, an 'open society' is essential if abuses arising in closed systems—whether political, cultural, or administrative—are to be prevented.[9]

- **Promoting ethical practice** It is sometimes argued that an explicit ethical code is unnecessary, implicit disciplines (such as career prospects) and a shared ethos being sufficient to maintain standards. As we have seen, history contradicts this, with codes often appearing as a direct response to a collapse in standards. What kind of codes will best promote good practice varies with circumstances, however. They have therefore differed widely in form and content, ranging from statements of aspirational principles to detailed practice guidelines. The latter are important especially in education and training. The code of the Royal Australian and New Zealand College of Psychiatrists combines general principles with detailed annotations on specific problem areas such as confidentiality and informed consent.[10] Codes also vary in ethical structure. Some are virtue-driven, emphasizing character traits which support good practice. Others are duty-based, prescribing specific responsibilities and obligations.

Codes thus have several functions in psychiatric ethics. These, furthermore, overlap and support each other. For instance, an educational quality is critical if codes are to enhance practice; without adequate standards, self-regulation can degenerate into self-protection; and self-protection ultimately damages the profession.

There are, however, important aspects of psychiatric ethics on which codes are silent. Notable among these are the ethical dimensions of diagnosis.

Concepts

The neglect of diagnosis in psychiatric ethical codes is a direct result of their derivation from medical codes. In most areas of medicine, ethical issues are confined largely to problems in management (e.g. treatment choice, resource allocation). Ethical principles of care and competence always apply to the *process* of diagnosis, of course. But in physical medicine, especially in the 'high tech' areas with which bioethics has been mainly concerned, the disease concepts on which diagnosis is grounded seem straightforwardly scientific in nature. In psychiatry, by contrast, there are a number of important *prima facie* connections between our diagnostic concepts and ethics.[11,12]

- The ethical justification for involuntary psychiatric treatment turns directly on a diagnosis of mental disorder. This is reflected in mental health law on involuntary treatment which requires, in addition to a risk element, the presence specifically of a *mental disorder* (see Chapter 1.6).

- In criminal law, similarly, the insanity defence, that someone who has committed an offence is not morally responsible for their actions, that they are 'mad not bad', is based on a diagnosis of mental disorder (usually psychotic).

- A number of differential diagnoses in psychiatry involve a moral dimension. The most notorious illustration is the distinction between psychopathic personality (a medical concept) and delinquency (a moral concept). Other medical/moral differential diagnoses include hysteria/malingering and alcoholism/drunkenness.

- Some of the worst abuses of psychiatry, in which it has been used as a means of social control, have been driven by misuses of its diagnostic concepts. In the former USSR, for example, political and other dissidents were often locked away in psychiatric institutions on the basis of 'delusions of reformism'.[8]

These *prima facie* links between diagnosis and ethics, although more obvious in the case of psychiatry, occur in all of medicine. The psychiatric 'mad not bad' as an excuse in law, for example, reflects the fact that illness in general implies loss of responsibility (an 'off work' certificate mandates sick leave, for instance). The difference between psychiatry and the rest of medicine in this respect is thus one of degree. Nonetheless, the greater prominence of the connections between diagnosis and ethics in psychiatry has led some to regard mental disorder as intrinsically different from physical disorder. In its most extreme form this view underlies antipsychiatric theory according to which mental illness should not be thought of in medical terms at all but solely in moral terms.

Medical or moral problem? A question that will not go away

Some critics of psychiatry have argued that the medical model is a relatively modern invention,[13] but as the Oxford philosopher and classicist Anthony Kenny has shown, the idea that some forms of madness might be generically linked to bodily disease dates back to ancient Greece.[14] At this time, however, and throughout history, the medical model has had to compete with a variety of spiritual or moral interpretations.[15] With the rise of modern psychiatry in the late nineteenth and early twentieth centuries it seemed that the medical model had triumphed. Yet even at the time, Karl Jaspers, one of the architects of modern scientific psychiatry, warned against naive biologism;[16] far from withering away, it was precisely when effective drugs and credible disease theories were finally coming into their own, in the 1960s and 1970s, that alternative models offered by the radical antipsychiatry movement were most influential.

Radical antipsychiatry emphasized two morally relevant features of mental disorder: agency and values.[17]

- An indirect reflection of the moral model in antipsychiatry was the importance it attached, in one form or another, to the notion of **agency**. Those suffering from mental disorder, antipsychiatry insisted, might be victims variously of labelling, of oppressive family dynamics, or of coercive societal or political forces. But they remained moral agents in their own right, capable of actively engaging with their problems, rather than patients, the passive victims of a disease process.

- A more direct reflection of the moral model in antipsychiatry was the significance it attached to the **values** by which mental disorders are (partly) defined. One prominent proponent, Thomas Szasz, based his conclusion that mental illness is a 'myth' directly on the claim that a diagnosis of mental illness is grounded on value judgements. Genuine illnesses, he argued, are defined by scientific norms derived from anatomy and physiology, whereas mental illness is defined by norms which are 'psycho-social, ethical and legal' in character.[18] Opponents of Szasz, such as R. E. Kendell,[19] counter-argued that mental illness, properly understood, can be defined by the same biological norms (of reduced life and/or reproductive expectations) as physical illness.

With major advances in neuroscience, such as neuroimaging, anti-psychotic medications, and genetics, it has again become common-place among 'biological' psychiatrists to assume that antipsychiatry is dead. Radical antipsychiatry is certainly less influential since the 1980s. Yet many of its themes have been absorbed into the mainstream. The importance of agency is evident, for example, in the widespread use of cognitive–behavioural therapies (restoring agency through the acqui-sition of self-management skills), and in the growing influence of the 'user's voice'. Similarly, far from disappearing, the value judgements involved in psychiatric diagnosis have become ever more transparent. In ICD-9[20] the relevant value judgements were largely implicit. But in DSM-IV[21] the definitions of a number of specific disorders incorpor-ate evaluative criteria. Criterion B for schizophrenia, for example, requires not just a change but a *deterioration* in social or occupational functioning; and antisocial personality disorder is defined by disregard for the '*rights* of others' and by failure to 'conform to *social norms*' (emphases added).

DSM-IV rightly emphasizes that mental disorders should not be diagnosed *solely* by reference to social norms. Besides disease, a wide range of other states, such as delinquency and despair, are defined in part (though only in part) by negative value judgements. The deterior-ation of functioning by which schizophrenia is (partly) defined under Criterion B, or the norm violations of antisocial personality disorder, must therefore be, in DSM-IV's phrase, 'clinically significant'. They must be symptoms of a 'dysfunction *in the individual*' (emphasis added—a much disputed phrase but implying a conceptual link between the medical model and loss of agency). What all this amounts to, then, is that in DSM-IV a negative value judgement, in these and similar cases, is not sufficient for a diagnosis of mental disorder. But by the same token, according to DSM-IV, a negative value judgement *is* necessary.

Value judgements in psychiatric diagnosis: an explanation from ethical theory

Diverse explanations have been offered for the prominence of overt value judgements in psychiatric diagnosis. For some it endorses the radical antipsychiatry position that psychiatry is not a part of medical science.[18] Others have argued that it reflects the primitive state of the sciences underpinning psychiatry.[22,23] Ethical theory, by contrast, the area of moral philosophy concerned with the meanings and implica-tions of value terms, offers an explanation which is fully consistent both with the status of psychiatry as a mature scientific discipline and, at the same time, with the pivotal role of value judgements in psychi-atric diagnosis.

A clear account of the relevant ethical theory has been given by a former Professor of Moral Philosophy at the University of Oxford, R. M. Hare.[24,25] We shall look briefly at his work and then apply it to the medical context. Hare pointed out that value terms have two elements of meaning:

- an **evaluative** element proper—this is the value judgement expressed by the term in question (Hare called this the term's 'prescriptive' or action-guiding meaning);

- a **factual** element—this covers the factual criteria on which the value judgement expressed by the value term is based (Hare called this the term's 'descriptive' meaning).

Thus, the value term 'good eating apple' expresses the value judgement

that an apple is good to eat (the term's evaluative meaning) based on facts about the apple in question such as that it is grub-free, clean-skinned, sweet, and so forth (the term's factual meaning).

Note, though, Hare continued, that where the use of a given value term depends on factual criteria which are widely settled or agreed upon, its factual meaning may come to eclipse its evaluative meaning. Thus, in a case like 'good eating apple' the factual criteria are widely agreed; for most people in most circumstances a good eating apple is one which is 'grub-free, clean skinned, sweet, and so forth'. By associ-ation, then, 'good eating apple' has come to mean an apple which, as a matter of fact, is grub-free, clean-skinned, sweet, and so forth. But in a case like 'good picture', by contrast, people's values differ widely; hence there are no widely agreed factual criteria available to become stuck by association to 'good picture' and the meaning of 'good picture' remains overtly evaluative.

We can now apply this to the medical case. The key point is that if 'illness' (including its cognates, such as 'disease') is a value term, then the persistence of overtly evaluative meaning in our use of '*mental* ill-ness' will reflect *diversity of values*. The details of this have been worked out by one of us elsewhere.[26] However, we can gain a general idea of the relevance of Hare's theory from the relative diversity of values in the areas with which physical medicine and psychiatry are respectively concerned.

- **Physical medicine** is concerned, by and large, with areas of human experience and behaviour over which our values are more or less *uniform*. Central chest pain and collapse, for example, are bad experiences for anyone.

- **Psychiatry**, in contrast, is concerned with areas of human experi-ence and behaviour—emotion, desire, belief, volition, and so forth—over which our values are highly *variable*. What is judged a good or bad desire, a good or bad belief, and so on, varies widely, between individuals, between cultures, and at different times.

In this respect, then, physical illness is like Hare's 'good apple' case, whereas 'mental illness' is like Hare's 'good picture' case. Hence it is by virtue of diversity of human values, rather than because of any (sup-posed) deficiency in psychiatric science, that our diagnostic concepts in psychiatry are overtly value laden. In the language of science, we can say that whereas in much of physical medicine the values relevant to diagnosis are a constant (because people's values are the same), in psychiatry they are a variable (because people's values differ).

This explanation does not imply that psychiatry is any less scientific (because more overtly value laden) than other areas of medicine. On the contrary, Hare's distinction between the factual and evaluative elements in the meanings of value terms helps to clarify what is genu-inely scientific in psychiatry. Careful examination of the mental state, the development of causal theories, and so on, remain as important here as in an exclusively scientific model of psychiatric diagnosis. This is why ethical theory is fully consistent with the status of psychiatry as a mature scientific discipline. It adds values to, rather than subtracting facts from, psychiatry. What the explanation from ethical theory *does* imply, however, is that whereas in much of physical medicine we can ignore individual values in making a diagnosis (because the relevant values are a constant), in psychiatry we cannot (because they are a variable). This conclusion has a number of important practical impli-cations for the role of ethical reasoning as a key practice skill in medicine.

Clinical practice skills

Bioethics is widely thought of as having a quasi-legal role in medicine, standing outside clinical practice, checking and curtailing the powers of doctors. An alternative model, developed for example in the medical school in Oxford, is that of ethical reasoning as a key practice skill. Practice skills are the skills required for the successful application of medical knowledge in day-to-day practice. The practice skills model combines ethics, law, and communication, as three disciplines essential to good practice skills, in a problem-solving approach to clinical training.[27]

In this section we outline three aspects of the contribution of ethical theory to clinical practice skills in psychiatry:

(1) the importance of casuistic or case-based reasoning as an aspect of the 'know-how' of medical expertise;

(2) the role of principles, standing midway in specificity between codes of practice and high-level ethical theories;

(3) the significance particularly for psychiatric ethics of balancing different value perspectives not only in treatment but also in diagnosis.

Casuistry and medical know-how

Besides knowledge, medical expertise requires a good deal of 'know-how'.[28] Knowledge can be set out explicitly, as in textbooks, in codes, and in practice guidelines. Know-how is more implicit. It is a set of skills, built on experience, which (like non-medical skills such as recognizing a face or riding a bicycle) resist definition and yet are crucial to our expertise.

Casuistry exploits the know-how of ethical reasoning by tackling ethical problems not in terms of high-level theory or general principles but from the ground up, by considering particular cases. Faced with an ethically problematic case, casuistry involves one or both of the following:

• altering the case—varying the circumstances of the case to imagine situations in which it would be more obviously right or wrong to take a particular course;

• considering related cases—comparing the given case with a series of related cases in which, again, the ethical outcomes are clearer.

These two ways of thinking help to clarify our ethical intuitions by focusing on concrete details. Casuistry has a bad name in the history of ethics in that it is associated with bending principles to suit one's purposes! We owe its rehabilitation to two philosophers working in America, Albert Jonsen and Stephen Toulmin.[29] While serving on a Presidential Commission on bioethics, they observed that its members were usually able to agree on *what* ought to be done in a given case even though they often disagreed about *why*. The way to resolve ethical problems, they concluded, is not by referring to general principles but by considering particular cases.

Casuistry is driven by shared values. Its power as a method of ethical reasoning is in allowing us to access shared ethical intuitions, which, as part of the know-how of medical expertise, are often not fully explicit. This, however, is also its weakness. As the American philosopher, Loretta Kopelman, has pointed out, where values are not shared casuistry may be at best ineffective and at worst abusive.[30] But psychiatry, as we have seen, is characterized by *diversity* of values. The importance of casuistic reasoning in psychiatry is thus not to force agreement on ethical issues but to clarify the (often legitimate) value differences underlying *dis*agreement.

Principles, codes, and ethical theory

Where casuistic reasoning is bottom-up, starting from particular cases, principles reasoning is top-down; it starts from widely held values and applies them to specific cases.

By far the best known principles in medical ethics are those pioneered in America by the philosophers Tom Beauchamp and James Childress[31] and in the United Kingdom by the doctor and philosopher Raanon Gillon.[32] They are:

• autonomy—respecting patients' wishes and freedom of choice

• beneficence—acting in patients' best interests

• non-maleficence—avoiding harm

• justice—treating equal problems equally.

Beauchamp and Childress describe these four principles as *prima facie*, i.e. likely to be pertinent in any medical ethical problem. Principles reasoning thus involves: identifying relevant ethical considerations in a given case in terms of the four principles, weighing them up appropriately, and thus reaching a conclusion on the balance of ethical considerations. For example, Beauchamp and Childress analyse the ethics of involuntary treatment in terms of the balance between beneficence and respect for autonomy, arguing that it is justified on grounds of beneficence when autonomy is undermined through a sufficient loss of rational capacity.

Principles reasoning has been widely criticized for encouraging a mechanical view of ethics, insensitive to the subtleties of real cases. This would be to misunderstand the principles approach, however. *Prima facie* principles are at an intermediate level of flexibility between the detailed prescriptions of codes and the abstractions of general ethical theory. All three levels—codes, principles, and ethical theory—are important in psychiatric ethics. The relative rigidity of codes and the specificity of their prescriptions helps to make them effective as regulators of professional conduct. General ethical theory, at the other extreme, gives us the flexibility to respond to novel problems, to adapt to changing circumstances. It also connects ethics to related disciplines. For example, deontology (the theory of rights and duties) connects ethics to law, and consequentialism, the best known example of which is utilitarianism, connects ethics to economics. Law and economics impinge importantly on psychiatry but they carry dangers which ethical theory can illuminate (see, for example, Montgomery on law[33] and Crisp on economics[34]).

The importance of principles, at an intermediate level of flexibility between codes and ethical theory, is to provide a well-structured approach to analysing the values bearing on a given case. Most of us tend to approach an ethical problem from a particular point of view: beneficence, say, may be important for one person, autonomy for another. Analysing an ethical problem in terms of *prima facie* principles helps to make us aware of aspects of the problem we had neglected, thus giving us a more balanced understanding. Again, this is crucial in psychiatry with its inherent diversity of values. But even principled reasoning cannot ensure openness to ethical perspectives other than our own.

Perspectives, concepts, and communication skills

The importance of perspectives, alongside principles and casuistry, has been emphasized by the Oxford psychiatrist and bioethicist, Tony Hope, as a key feature of the practice skills model of medical ethics.[35] Ethical reasoning, applied to clinical problem solving in everyday practice, depends on those involved understanding each other's perspectives. This in turn requires sound communication skills. However, communication skills without ethics can be used as readily for bad purposes as for good. Hence the inseparability of ethics and communication as key practice skills.

The significance of perspectives particularly in psychiatric ethics follows directly from psychiatry's inherent diversity of values. In high-tech physical medicine, where differences of values are limited mainly to issues of treatment choice, autonomy means patients 'having a say' in how they are treated. The diversity of values involved in psychiatric diagnosis means that autonomy in psychiatry must be extended to include patients having a say also in how their problems are to be understood. (We owe this clear way of making the point to Dr V. Y. Allison-Bolger.) This is no mere theoretical concern. There is growing evidence, from patients themselves and from the social sciences, of the extent to which the values of users of services—patients and carers—may be different from and conflict with those of providers[36] (see Chapters 1.1 and 2.6.2). Value differences are also important in trans-cultural psychiatry,[37] in relation to religious experience,[38] in the organization and delivery of services,[39] and, not least, in research.[40]

The practice skills model is not a consumer model of medical ethics, however, substituting patient hegemony for the traditional authority of doctors. Where values differ no one perspective should take precedence. Instead we should seek a balanced view. This is crucial in psychiatry since many of our deepest ethical questions arise in situations in which patients 'lack insight' (as in involuntary treatment). There is no easy route to achieving the required balance of perspectives. Good communication is essential. So too are the insights offered by patients' narratives and by the social sciences. There is also a key role here for the multidisciplinary team. It is true that conflicts of models within multidisciplinary teams may sometimes be highly disruptive clinically (see Chapter 1.10.1), but in the practice skills model the different perspectives represented by members of the multidisciplinary team can make a central contribution to achieving the balance of values which is essential to good practice in psychiatry.

Conclusions

We have outlined three aspects of psychiatric ethics which have been relatively neglected by mainstream bioethics: the importance of codes especially in the international context, the ethical significance of diagnostic concepts, and the value of an integrated practice skills model of ethical reasoning.

We began by suggesting that these aspects of psychiatric ethics have been neglected because, in bioethics as in biomedicine, psychiatry has been treated as an addendum to mainstream medicine. But their importance has turned out to be a consequence of the greater depth and complexity of ethical problems in psychiatry. Moreover, these three aspects of psychiatric ethics, once recognized, are seen to be important not only in psychiatry but in medicine overall. The promo-

tion of internationally recognized standards through accepted codes, the significance of patients' values in how their problems are understood as well as managed, and the full integration of ethical reasoning into clinical problem solving, are the desiderata of good practice in medicine generally. Far from being an addendum to bioethics, psychiatry thus offers a window on good practice in medicine as a whole.

References

1. Bloch, S., Chodoff, P., and Green, S.A. (ed.) (1999) *Psychiatric ethics* (3rd edn). Oxford University Press.
2. Bloch, S. (1997). Psychiatry: an impossible profession? *Australian and New Zealand Journal of Psychiatry*, **31**, 172–83.
3. Dickenson, D. and Fulford, K.W.M. (ed.) (2000). *In two minds: case studies in psychiatric ethics*. Oxford University Press.
4. Fulford, K.W.M. (1993). Bioethical blind spots: four flaws in the field of view of traditional bioethics. *Health Care Analysis*, **1**, 155–62.
5. Bloch, S. and Pargitter, R. (1996). Developing a code of ethics for psychiatry. In *Codes of ethics and the professions* (ed. M. Coady and S. Bloch), Chapter 9. Melbourne University Press.
6. Fullinwider, R. (1996). Professional codes and moral understanding. In *Codes of ethics and the professions* (ed. M. Coady and S. Bloch), pp. 72–87. Melbourne University Press.
7. Fargot-Largeault, A. (1996). National report from France. In *Informed consent in psychiatry: European perspectives on ethics, law and clinical practice* (ed. H.-G. Koch, S. Reiter-Theil, and H. Helmchen), pp. 67–96. Nomos Verlagsgesellschaft, Baden-Baden.
8. Bloch, S. and Reddaway, P. (1997). *Russia's political hospitals: the abuse of psychiatry in the Soviet Union*. Gollancz, London. (Published in the United States as *Psychiatric terror*, Basic Books, New York.)
9. Birley, J.L.T. (2000). Ethical thinking: towards an open society in health care. In *In two minds: case studies in psychiatric ethics* (ed. D. Dickenson and K.W.M. Fulford), Chapter 11. Oxford University Press.
10. Royal Australian and New Zealand College of Psychiatrists (1998). *Code of Ethics* (2nd edn). Royal Australian and New Zealand College of Psychiatrists, Melbourne.
11. Reich, W. (1999). Psychiatric ethics as an ethical problem. *Psychiatric ethics* (3rd edn) (ed. S. Bloch, P. Chodoff, and S.A. Green), Chapter 10. Oxford University Press.
12. Fulford, K.W.M. (1994). Closet logics: hidden conceptual elements in the DSM and ICD classifications of mental disorders. In *Philosophical perspectives on psychiatric diagnostic classification* (ed. J.Z. Sadler, O.P. Wiggins, and M.A. Schwartz), Chapter 9. Johns Hopkins University Press, Baltimore, MD.
13. Foucault, M. (1973). *Madness and civilization: a history of insanity in the age of reason*. Random House, New York.
14. Kenny, A.J.P. (1969). Mental health in Plato's republic. *Proceedings of the British Academy*, **5**, 229–53.
15. Robinson, D. (1996). *Wild beasts and idle humours*. Harvard University Press, Cambridge, MA.
16. Jaspers, K. (1913). Causal and meaningful connexions between life history and psychosis. Reprinted in *Themes and variations in European psychiatry* (ed. S.R. Hirsch and M. Shepherd), Chapter 5. John Wright, Bristol, 1974.
17. Fulford, K.W.M. (1998). Mental illness. In *Encylopaedia of applied ethics* (ed. R. Chadwick). Academic Press, San Diego, CA.
18. Szasz, T.S. (1960). The myth of mental illness. *American Psychologist*, **15**, 113–18.
19. Kendell, R.E. (1975). The concept of disease and its implications for psychiatry. *British Journal of Psychiatry*, **127**, 305–15.
20. World Health Organization (1978). *Mental disorders: glossary and guide to their classification in accordance with the ninth revision of the international classification of diseases*. WHO, Geneva.

21. American Psychiatric Association (1994). *Diagnostic and statistical classification of diseases and related health problems* (4th edn). American Psychiatric Association, Washington, DC.

22. Boorse, C. (1975). On the distinction between disease and illness. *Philosophy and Public Affairs*, **5**, 49–68.

23. Wakefield, J.C. (1995). Dysfunction as a value-free concept: a reply to Sadler and Agich. *Philosophy, Psychiatry, and Psychology*, **2**, 233–46.

24. Hare, R.M. (1952). *The language of morals*. Oxford University Press.

25. Hare, R.M. (1963). Descriptivism. *Proceedings of the British Academy*, **49**, 115–34. Reprinted in Hare, R.M. (1972). *Essays on the moral concepts*. Macmillan, London.

26. Fulford, K.W.M. (1989). *Moral theory and medical practice*, especially Chapters 3, 4, and 5. Cambridge University Press. (Reprinted in paperback 1995.)

27. Hope, T., Fulford, K.W.M., and Yates, A. (1996). *Manual of the Oxford Practice Skills Project*. Oxford University Press.

28. Fulford, K.W.M. (1994). Medical education: knowledge and know-how. In *Ethics and the professions* (ed. R. Chadwick), Chapter 2. Avebury Press, Aldershot.

29. Jonsen, A.R. and Toulmin, S. (1988). *The abuse of casuistry: a history of moral reasoning*. University of California Press, Berkeley, CA.

30. Kopelman, L.M. (1994). Case method and casuistry: the problem of bias. *Theoretical Medicine*, **15**, 21–38.

31. Beauchamp, T.L. and Childress, J.F. (1994). *Principles of biomedical ethics* (4th edn). Oxford University Press.

32. Gillon, R. (1986). *Philosophical medical ethics*. Wiley, Chichester.

33. Montgomery, J. (1995). Patients first: the role of rights. In *Essential practice in patient-centred care* (ed. K.W.M. Fulford, S. Ersser and T. Hope), Chapter 9. Blackwell Science, Oxford.

34. Crisp, R. (1994). Quality of life and health care. In *Medicine and moral reasoning* (ed. K.W.M. Fulford, G. Gillett, and J. Soskice), Chapter 13. Cambridge University Press.

35. Hope, R.A. and Fulford, K.W.M. (1993). Medical education: patients, principles and practice skills. In *Principles of health care ethics* (ed. R. Gillon), Chapter 59. Wiley, Chichester.

36. Campbell, P. (1996). What we want from crisis services. In *Speaking our minds: an anthology* (ed. J. Read and J. Reynolds), pp. 180–3. Macmillan, London, for The Open University.

37. Fulford, K.W.M. (1998). Philosophy and cross-cultural psychiatry. In *Studies in cross-cultural psychiatry* (ed. K. Bhui and D. Olajide), Chapter 2. W.B. Saunders, London.

38. Jackson, M. and Fulford, K.W.M. (1997). Spiritual experience and psychopathology. *Philosophy, Psychiatry, and Psychology*, **4**, 41–90.

39. Fulford, K.W.M. (1995). Concepts of disease and the meaning of patient-centred care. In *Essential practice in patient-centred care* (ed. K.W.M. Fulford, S. Ersser, and T. Hope), Chapter 1. Blackwell Science, Oxford.

40. Sadler, J.Z. (1996). Epistemic value commitments in the debate over categorical vs dimensional personality diagnosis. *Philosophy, Psychiatry, and Psychology*, **3**, 203–22.

1.6 Principles of mental health law

Alexander McCall Smith

The aims and reach of mental health law

Mental health law is concerned with the balancing of complex, and sometimes opposed, interests. Foremost amongst these is the interest that the mentally ill have in maintaining some measure of control of their lives through the making of their own decisions. This is based on the patient's right of autonomy, which is a crucial value in contemporary medical ethics. Important though the right of autonomy may be, however, the realities of mental illness mean that there are other interests to be taken into account. These include the interest that others— the patient's family and society in general—have in protecting the patient from the consequences of an illness, and the interest which the community in general has in protecting itself from potential harm caused by those suffering from mental illness.

The balancing of these interests is by no means easy. Mental health legislation may give psychiatry considerable power, including the power, normally reserved to courts of law, to deprive people of their liberty. One task of mental health law is to protect the vulnerable patient from well-intended but possibly unduly coercive intervention. Critics point out that the law has not always achieved this in the past, and that psychiatric patients have been denied many basic human rights; certainly the history of psychiatry has been marred by abuses of power over highly vulnerable people. Such criticism has been taken seriously by contemporary psychiatry, which has, in general, not attempted to defend an interventionist position but has recognized the extensive nature of the powers entrusted to it and sought to exercise them cautiously. In Britain, for example, reforms of mental health legislation in the early 1980s reflected the readiness of psychiatrists and the legislature to heed human rights concerns and to seek to achieve a balance between psychiatric power on the one hand and the rights of the patient on the other. These reforms were typical of the legislative changes made in many jurisdictions during the latter part of the twentieth century, with the result that many countries now enjoy a system of mental health law which appears transformed when compared with the previous strongly paternalistic system. This is not to say that the issue of human rights in psychiatry is no longer a live one: there continues to be a dialogue between exponents of patients' rights and those who wield compulsory treatment powers. Indeed there is also a counter-movement, which argues that legal reforms have gone too far in the direction of patient autonomy and have had the effect of denying treatment to those in need of it purely in order to avoid the use of coercive powers. Such critics hold that the case for paternalistic intervention needs to be advanced with greater conviction, and that stressing the right to resist compulsory treatment obscures the true nature of the mentally ill person's need. Joining this debate are the voices of those who argue that social protection must again be stressed as an important factor, and that concern over the right to liberty of the mentally ill has obscured the dangers inherent in premature discharge or in unsupervised presence in the community.

The legal background

Every jurisdiction has its own legal framework for mental health issues and it is impossible to provide a survey here of the wide range of legal solutions adopted. However, there is a wide range of general literature available on this topic.[1–3] The British model, which exists in English and Scottish versions, will be used here for illustrative purposes. Obviously there will be differences between the legislative arrangements in each country, but an understanding of one system will usually help to explain the rules of another system. The concerns with which mental health legislation deals are, of course, universal, and indeed there is now a strongly international flavour to the mental health law debate. This is demonstrated in the litigation on mental health matters which forms a substantial part of the business of the European Court of Human Rights. The international dimension is also underlined by a number of international codes which spell out the human rights standards to which individual countries should aspire in the promulgation of their domestic mental health legislation. Such codes do not have local force, but they are undoubtedly influential in the creation of international norms for treatment of psychiatric patients. An example of international guidelines is provided by the *Principles for the Protection of Persons with Mental Illness and the Improvement of Mental Health Care* adopted by the United Nations in 1991.[4]

At the domestic level, the common law starts from the position that every person has a right to physical integrity which must not be compromised except when there is clear legal authorization for such intervention.[5] In the medical context this means that no adult may be subjected to medical treatment of any sort unless he or she has consented to such treatment. This principle is firmly entrenched in the Anglo-American legal tradition—the legal system applicable in most English-speaking countries—and its breach may result in criminal and civil action. A person who is subjected to treatment to which he or she has not consented may have an action for civil damages against the person who treats him or her, and may also, in certain circumstances, expect criminal charges of assault to be brought in respect of the unwarranted intervention. The courts have emphasized that this right to refuse treatment may be exercised even when the treatment is necessary to save the life of the patient. In the Canadian case of *Malette* v. *Shuman*,[6] for example, substantial damages were awarded against a doctor who had administered a blood transfusion in the face of a patient's clearly-stated objection to such a procedure. English cases recognizing the right to refuse treatment include *Re T (Adult: Refusal of Treatment)*[7] and *Airedale NHS Trust* v. *Bland*.[8] It is not possible, then, to rely on an argument that the necessity of saving life justifies non-consensual treatment.

The right to reject treatment requires, however, capacity or competence to do so. A doctor is legally justified in giving emergency treatment to a person who is prevented from stating a preference by virtue of unconsciousness, and this justification extends to circumstances where the patient is, by virtue of mental disorder, unable to make a rational decision relating to treatment. The legal principle of necessity thus justifies the administration of life-saving treatment where the patient's mental condition makes it impossible to give a valid consent. It is important to note, however, that the necessity principle has strict limits. It is not possible to use it to override the preferences of patients where these are clearly expressed and where they have expressed an objection to treatment.

Mental illness raises very different legal issues. The law has developed a clear structure for the administration of treatment for persons suffering from mental disorder. This structure provides doctors with the power to treat without the consent of the patient and, as a concomitant of this, the power to deprive the patient of his or her liberty. However, the scope of this legal power is limited. Mental health powers are not intended to be used to treat other conditions, and in particular they are not intended to enable society to coerce those whose behaviour may be unconventional or antisocial but who do not suffer from a mental disorder.

Irrational behaviour and psychiatric intervention

The law in a liberal society tolerates behaviour which is irrational or socially deviant and will only intervene to prevent or punish it when a person either threatens to infringe some legal right of another or contravenes a provision of the criminal law. This tolerance includes an acceptance of self-destructive behaviour; suicide is no longer a crime in most countries even if it may be a criminal offence to assist another to commit suicide. It is therefore open to a person to embark on conduct that threatens his or her health or life, even to a significant degree. Medicine cannot force people to act in what it judges to be their own best interests, and the law will, in general, afford medicine no assistance towards the achieving of this aim. The law recognizes, then, a right to be idiosyncratic.

Legally sanctioned intervention in irrational or deviant behaviour becomes possible when the cause of the behaviour is medically identified as being a mental disorder *and where certain other criteria are met*. A psychiatric diagnosis therefore begins a process that may render the patient liable to medical intervention. It is still necessary, however, for the intervention to be directed towards the treatment of the disorder rather than towards some other, incidental goal. The legal right to impose psychiatric treatment is not a police power, nor is it a power which may be used to treat a non-psychiatric condition.

This difficult point is revealed in a number of cases involving medically inappropriate refusals of treatment on the part of pregnant women. In the case of *St George's Healthcare NHS Trust* v. *S*,[9] the Court of Appeal in England set out clear limits to the use of the Mental Health Act 1983 ('the 1983 Act') as a means of forcing a woman to submit to a Caesarean section. The patient had been admitted to hospital for assessment after she had refused to accept medical advice. The court held that no matter how unusual, irrational, or contrary to public opinion an individual's views might be, a person is nevertheless entitled to refuse medical treatment, and mental health powers should not be used to circumvent this refusal. A similar point is made in the Canadian case of *Winnipeg Child and Family Services (Northwest Area)* v. *GFG*.[10] This case involved an attempt by social service authorities to detain a pregnant women who was addicted to glue sniffing. Again, in the absence of a mental disorder of a sort which would justify detention for treatment, the court accepted the woman's right to pursue conduct that threatened the life of the fetus she was carrying.

In neither of the two cases discussed above could a legally relevant mental disorder be diagnosed; the conduct in question fell outside the boundary for intervention set out in the legislation. A different issue of boundaries arises where there has been a diagnosis of mental disorder but treatment is indicated for a non-psychiatric condition. Pregnancy was again the context for this issue in *Tameside and Glossop Acute Services NHS Trust* v. *CH (a patient)*.[11] The patient in this case suffered from acute paranoid schizophrenia and was detained for treatment under the 1983 Act. It became apparent in the 38th week of her pregnancy that she required to undergo a Caesarean section if the death of her fetus was to be avoided. She resisted this strongly, but the court ruled that she could be subjected to the procedure against her will as the birth of a healthy baby would assist in her recovery from her mental disorder, whereas the death of the fetus would have a negative effect on her mental state. The Caesarean section would therefore be considered to be part of the treatment of the mental disorder.

The mere fact that a person is suffering from a mental disorder will not prevent them from making a legally valid refusal of treatment for a condition unconnected with their mental disorder. Authority for this is found in the case of *Re C (Adult: Refusal of Medical Treatment)*.[12] The patient in this case was a chronic paranoid schizophrenic, living in an open ward of a parole house, who developed a necrotic ulcer in a grossly infected leg. He understood medical advice to the effect that without the amputation of the leg below the knee there was a strong possibility of death, but he was adamant in his refusal of an operation. The court held that this refusal should be respected on the grounds that in spite of his general capacity being impaired by schizophrenia, the patient appeared to have had the ability to understand the treatment being proposed and the implications of its refusal. In these circumstances, the court ruled, the patient was entitled to decline medical treatment. It should be noted, of course, that the patient in this case would not have been entitled to refuse treatment for schizophrenia had he wished to do so.

The effect of decisions such as *Re C* is *not* to make it impossible for medical and nursing staff to attend to the physical ills of those compulsorily detained patients. Nursing procedures are covered by the authority to detain and treat for mental disorder, and the decision in the case of *Re F*[13] suggests that there is authority to carry out day-to-day medical procedures on detained patients. More significant procedures may require more careful evaluation, and the approval of a court. Where it is clear that the mental disorder does not preclude an understanding of the condition and its treatment, careful consideration may be required as to whether the patient's refusal is attributable to the mental disorder or has some other basis.

Force feeding

Force feeding also raises the questions of determining the boundaries of intervention in mental disorder. The British courts have recognized that prisoners have the right to refuse food in the course of a hunger strike, the assumption being that they are rational persons who, if they wish to do so, may choose to decline food for political or other purposes. The force feeding of psychiatric patients raises distinct issues, and the law has tended to a rather more interventionist stance in this context.

The leading British case on this issue is B v. *Croydon Health Authority*.[14] B, who had been diagnosed as suffering from psychopathic disorder, was detained under Section 3 of the 1983 Act. She had manifested a tendency to harm herself, and this was considered symptomatic of her psychopathic condition. After a period of refusing food, during which her weight had declined to a dangerous extent, the decision was taken to feed her by nasogastric tube. A challenge to the legality of this was rejected by the court on the grounds that because the self-harming conduct was an aspect of the patient's mental disorder, resort to artificial feeding could be considered to be treatment intended to alleviate or prevent a deterioration of the disorder itself.

Courts have also considered the force feeding of patients suffering from anorexia nervosa to be part of the treatment of a mental illness. In *Riverside Mental Health Trust* v. *Fox*[15] permission was given to force feed such a patient on the grounds that the unwillingness to eat was caused by a mental disorder and was therefore a symptom which could be treated compulsorily under the terms of the 1983 Act.

Treatment or detention?

A fundamental issue facing any system of mental health law is that of determining the importance to be given to public safety considerations. One of the criteria for the exercise of compulsory psychiatric powers is that the patient poses a danger to others. This criterion emphasizes the expectation that society has of psychiatry as a guardian, a role with which psychiatrists, with good reason, tend to feel uncomfortable. The principal function of psychiatry is not to protect the public from persons who are considered dangerous, but is rather to provide treatment for those suffering from a mental disorder. In spite of this discomfort, psychiatric hospitals are nevertheless given the task of confining those whose mental condition makes them a threat to others.

The tension between custodial and therapeutic functions is particularly evident in respect of psychopathic personality disorders. Here again the issue is one of boundaries: is psychopathy properly located within the category of mental disorders, or is it a non-medical behavioural phenomenon? That is a debate for another place; what is legally significant is the fact that psychopathy is medicalized to the extent of (i) appearing in psychiatric diagnostic manuals, (ii) being acknowledged by psychiatric expert witnesses as a mental disorder, and (iii) being included by mental health legislation in the category of mental disorders. Once the condition is so recognized, medical responsibility for the psychopath becomes an issue.

The particular difficulty that psychopathy poses for mental health law is that although the condition may be acknowledged as being a mental disorder, it is also widely viewed as being untreatable. Psychiatry, having identified the condition, may then be reluctant to accept responsibility for responding to it in a therapeutic context; not an unreasonable position in circumstances of acute pressure on psychiatric resources from those suffering from conditions that are readily treatable. In one view, then, the dangerous psychopath is more appropriately housed by the prison service, although this will require that he or she first have committed an offence which will bring him or her within the purview of the criminal courts. The psychopath who has not committed an offence, or who has committed an offence but given a hospital disposal, poses a unique challenge for the mental health services. If the condition is considered as not being amenable to treatment it may be difficult to detain the person under mental health legislation, if such legislation, as is the case in Britain, makes reference to a treatability criterion for detention in hospital. It will only be if 'treatment' is interpreted sufficiently widely as to include nursing care or the provision of a structured, hospital environment that the person suffering from psychopathic personality disorder may be contained in a secure psychiatric setting. The response of the English courts to this issue is discussed by Baker and Crichton.[16]

The grounds for compulsory intervention

British legislation makes a distinction between informal and formal patients, the former being those who enter hospital voluntarily and those who are compelled to accept hospital treatment for a mental disorder. The philosophy underlying the 1983 Act was that, where possible, the treatment of patients in the former category should proceed on the same basis as the treatment of patients in non-psychiatric patients, with the patient being free to leave hospital or refuse treatment if he or she wishes. The regime governing compulsory treatment is more formal, with clear criteria being set out as to the grounds upon which such treatment may be imposed and the periods for which it may be imposed.

The 1983 Act allows for admission for assessment or removal to a place of safety if a person is suffering from, in the language of the statute, mental disorder. This is a broader criterion than is applied where a patient is admitted for treatment; in that case, he or she must suffer from one of four specifically identified forms of mental disorder, namely, mental illness, severe mental impairment, psychopathic disorder, or mental impairment. The mere fact of suffering from mental illness is not in itself grounds for admission for treatment: the illness must be 'of a nature or degree which makes it appropriate for him to receive treatment in a hospital' (Section 3 (2) (a)). This requirement should exclude from hospital those who can just as easily receive treatment in a less restrictive setting, such as the home, or the community. In practice, since medical treatment is defined in Section 145(1) of the Act as including 'nursing and care' it is legally permissible to detain a patient in hospital even if nothing more than this can be provided.

A further condition that must be satisfied before a patient may be detained in hospital for treatment is that hospital admission must be necessary 'for the health or safety of the patient or for the protection of others'. These are two separate justifications, the first being paternalistic in its inspiration, the second subordinating the therapeutic goal to that of public protection. The first of these grounds for admission—that of the health or safety of the patient—is widely accepted as justifying compulsory powers, notwithstanding the argument that the only acceptable grounds for compulsion are harm to self or others. The extent to which such criteria are open to human rights criticism depends on the interpretation of the concept of 'health' and the point at which the health of the patient is thought to be sufficiently compromised by mental disorder to justify compulsory intervention. In practice, this will be a medical decision, although appeal or review will bring lay (and judicial) examination of the medical decision. What is clear, however, is that if there is a recognized mental illness according to accepted psychiatric views as to what constitutes a mental disorder, then this may be sufficient to bring compulsory treatment of an unwilling patient. The law does not stipulate in advance how serious this illness must be and there is no requirement that there should be a severe or grave threat to the health of the patient. Any mental illness which requires hospital treatment may therefore result in compulsory hospitalization. The criterion is need, and the law entrusts the medical profession with the interpretation of need. Some countries have more restrictive legislation and focus on danger to self or others.

Consent to treatment

Adult patients who have entered hospital voluntarily or who are voluntarily receiving outpatient treatment can only be given medical treatment, including psychiatric treatment, if they consent to it (capacity is a complex issue in the law, and is discussed elsewhere[17,18]). In the absence of such consent, treatment may only be given: (1) in circumstances of necessity; (2) where the patient, by virtue of his or her mental condition, is incapable of consenting, but who has not previously stated his or her objection to treatment in such circumstances; and (3) where the patient is admitted for compulsory treatment under the legislation.

The principle of necessity justifies treatment where the patient is unable to give consent or to make a valid refusal and where the pressing nature of the circumstances makes it impossible to invoke powers under the mental health legislation. It would be legal, therefore, for a doctor to take steps to sedate a patient who requires immediate sedation in order to prevent harm to self or others. Nurses have a similar common law power to take such steps as are necessary to restrain a patient. Any necessity-based intervention, however, must involve the minimum use of force and must not persist beyond the point at which other expedients, including legislatively sanctioned compulsory measures, become feasible. It has been emphasized by a Scottish court that necessity powers should not be resorted to in the place of the procedures for non-consensual treatment which have been put in place by mental health legislation.[19]

There are certain patients who lack the capacity to give a valid consent to hospital treatment for a mental illness but who do not resist either being in hospital or receiving treatment. Such patients may be admitted to hospital as informal, voluntary patients and may therefore not be subject to the regime established for compulsorily detained patients. This means that they will also be denied some of the protection afforded to detained patients. The legality of this was questioned in the case of *R.* v. *Bournewood Community and Mental Health NHS Trust, ex parte L,*[20] in which an attempt was made to have the hospital treatment of such a patient declared illegal. On appeal to the

House of Lords it was held that the hospitalization of such patients did not constitute wrongful detention, the court clearly being concerned at the demands that would be made on the system if it became necessary formally to detain all such incompetent but compliant patients.

Patients who are involuntarily detained for treatment may, under Section 63 of the 1983 Act, be given treatment for their mental illness in the absence of consent on their part. There are restrictions, discussed below, in the period for which such treatment may be given before there must be independent medical review, and there are restrictions, also, on certain forms of hazardous or irreversible treatment.

Mental health legislation typically sets out time limits in respect of the period for which a patient may be detained involuntarily. An emergency admission under Section 4 of the 1983 Act allows a patient to be detained in hospital for up to 72 hours, but gives no powers for treatment to be imposed. It is possible, however, once the patient is admitted to hospital to resort to a longer-term admission. Only one medical opinion is needed for such an emergency admission, but it is considered desirable that the doctor furnishing the opinion should have known the patient prior to the making of the application. Longer-term admission can be made under either Section 2 (which gives authority for admission for assessment for a period of 28 days) or Section 3 (which requires two medical opinions and which requires a greater degree of specification in respect of the justification for compulsory admission). A Section 3 order lasts for 6 months, after which it may be renewed for a further period of 6 months and then for periods of 1 year at a time.

Restrictions on certain forms of treatment

British mental health legislation subjects certain treatments to special restrictions. The administration of drugs for mental disorder after the expiry of 3 months from the first administration (in the particular period of detention) requires the consent of the patient. This consent must be a real one, and there must be confirmation of the patient's understanding of the nature and effect of the treatment. If the patient does not consent, or if he or she is incapable of consenting, then there must be confirmation from an independent medical source that the drug regimen is necessary for the alleviation of the condition or for the prevention of the patient's deterioration. The doctor giving this opinion must have consulted with two other persons who have had a professional involvement in the patient's care, including a nurse but not including another doctor. The aim of this legal requirement is apparent on the face of it: the decision to follow a long-term regimen of drug therapy against the patient's will cannot be the sole decision of those responsible for the medical treatment of the patient.

Electroconvulsive therapy is subjected to the same restrictions. It may be administered with the consent of the patient, but if the patient does not consent, or is incapable of giving consent, a second medical opinion of the sort described above is required.

More demanding legal obstacles confront the use of certain hazardous, irreversible, or controversial treatments. These treatments are psychosurgery and certain hormone implantations designed to have an effect on the male libido. Psychosurgery, which involves the selective destruction of brain tissue, has a particularly controversial reputation, largely as a result of its over-enthusiastic and inappropriate use in some quarters in an earlier age when the rights of psychiatric patients were ill-protected.[21] The crudity of earlier surgery has been replaced by more refined techniques, and although there are few centres which perform it, this form of treatment of certain recalcitrant conditions has its exponents.[22]

The statutory regimen for psychosurgery in the United Kingdom is extremely restrictive. Under the 1983 Act an independent medical practitioner is required to confirm that the patient understands the procedure and its effects and has consented to it. This practitioner is also required to state that the treatment is justified as a means of preventing a deterioration in the patient's condition or promoting its alleviation. It is clear, therefore, that psychosurgery cannot be offered in those cases where the patient is incapable of giving full consent to it, thereby effectively denying it to a class of patients who might be considered for it.

Controversy over hormonal implants focuses on the issue of whether the patient in such cases can give a valid consent in circumstances in which an element of coercion may be involved. If the patient is serving a prison sentence or is facing conviction for a sexual offence, a question may be raised as to whether the treatment is wanted in itself or is merely seen as the least unattractive of two options. Again this raises the issue of paternalism: is it right to exclude a right to choose in such circumstances, even if the choice is not entirely free? In British litigation on this matter,[23] it was ruled that an injection of a hormone analogue was not covered by the Act and was therefore permissible. The recipient of the injection in this case appealed against the veto of such treatment, which he was seeking to help him avoid further sexual assaults on children.

Treatment in the community

The closure of hospital wards and the movement towards community care makes it desirable for treatment to be administered outside the hospital setting. In some countries, mental health legislation does not allow this. The powers conferred under the 1983 Act, for example, do not allow for the compulsory treatment of those who are not detained in hospital, and this led in the past to attempts to circumvent these limitations through the use of conditional leave of absence. Under such arrangements, patients were given leave of absence from hospital on the understanding that if they refused to accept treatment outside hospital their leave would be revoked. In *R. v. Hallstrom, ex parte W*[24] the court ruled that this practice was not authorized by the legislation and it was thus prevented. One solution to this problem is the possible introduction of community treatment orders, which would require patients to accept treatment in the home, clinic, or other suitable place. Community treatment orders are legally authorized in many jurisdictions in the United States[25] and in Australia and New Zealand.[26]

Arguments in favour of the extension of psychiatric supervision into the community have been reinforced by serious incidents involving discharged patients. Some of these, involving the death of the patient or fatal attacks on members of the public, attracted considerable attention and fuelled calls for closer monitoring of such patients. However, opposition to the community treatment order system has continued to be voiced from a civil libertarian perspective. Critics of community treatment orders see them as an unwarranted extension of psychiatric power outside the negotiated and closely controlled framework of compulsory hospital treatment. Indeed, their legality in terms of the European Convention on Human Rights is questionable.[27]

The Mental Health (Patients in the Community) Act 1993 introduced a compromise whereby supervised discharge is available to patients who, under former practice, may have been given leave while continuing with treatment. Under this legislation, a supervised discharge order may be made in respect of a patient suffering from mental disorder who requires to receive after-care in order to avoid a substantial risk of serious harm to his or her health or safety. Such supervision is also available if there is deemed to be a risk to the safety of other persons. A supervision order lasts for the same period as a patient's detention and may be renewed in the same way as detention may be renewed, provided that the patient is still liable for detention.

As is the case with guardianship orders, a supervision order may make broad requirements of a patient. The patient may be required, amongst other things, to live at a named place, to undergo training, and to present him- or herself for medical treatment. However, the 1993 Act does not give authority to compel the acceptance of medical treatment. Ultimately, the sanction for non-compliance with treatment directives might be the threat of detention in hospital. It is possible, however, that a supervisor might be able to exert considerable pressure within the framework of the supervision and that non-compliance with treatment recommendations could be countered with more restrictive supervision conditions.[28]

The protection of the patient's rights through review

Human rights law stresses the need for legal review of psychiatric detention. Article 5(4) of the European Convention on Human Rights, for example, requires that any person deprived of his or her liberty by detention should be entitled to have the lawfulness of his or her detention considered by a court. This right is incorporated in the 1983 Act, with provisions for appeal to a Mental Health Review Tribunal (in Scotland, appeal is to the sheriff). Appeal may be applied for by the patient (or nearest relative), but there is automatic review in the case of those who patients who do not apply for their case to go before a tribunal. This review must be initiated by the hospital manager if the patient has not applied during the first 6 months of detention, or, where there has been renewal of a detention, a patient's case has not been considered by a tribunal for a period of 3 years.

The purpose a Mental Health Review Tribunal hearing is to enable to patient, relatives, or advocate, to bring the patient's case to an independent body which can determine the justification of his or her continued detention or subjection to a regime of guardianship or supervision. A tribunal is not concerned with the legal technicalities of admission or detention, but essentially asks itself the question of whether the patient needs to be the subject of mental health compulsion, or whether he or she can be allowed to rejoin the community. Although tribunals differ from ordinary courts of law in many respects, legal representation is allowed and there is a belief that procedures have become increasingly legalistic. Unlike courts, however, where there is usually full disclosure of the evidence, a hospital may withhold from the patient matters that it considers will cause distress or lead to a deterioration in the patient's condition. This information, however, must be disclosed to a representative of the patient.

An important form of protection for the mentally ill is provided by independent bodies with broad supervisory powers over all matters affecting the welfare of this vulnerable group of people. In Britain, this function is performed by the Mental Health Act Commission (for England and Wales) and the Mental Welfare Commission (for Scotland). The Mental Health Act Commission, which is an independent body set up under the 1983 Act, is composed of both lay and professional membership appointed by the Secretary of State. It has an interest in both the treatment of individual patients and in the broader questions of treatment policy, codes of practice, and the general functioning of the 1983 Act and other mental health legislation. It is also entitled to visit hospitals and other places where patients are detained, and its members may discuss individual treatment and welfare questions with patients. Complaints may be heard by the Commission, but these may be require to be routed through hospital complaints procedures first. The Scottish Mental Welfare Commission has broader powers in some respects; it is empowered, for example, under the Mental Health (Scotland) 1984 Act to discharge patients.

The litigation rights of psychiatric patients

The fact that a person suffers from mental illness does not mean that he or she is deprived of all legal rights. There is discussion elsewhere in this work of the issue of legal capacity (such as the capacity of the mentally ill to enter into a contract or to make a will). We have seen above how the rights of the patient are protected by review arrangements and by certain restrictions placed on treatment. Another important dimension of the patient's rights is the right to litigate, which is the legal means by which the individual citizen normally protects his or her interests.

A patient in a psychiatric hospital has the same right as any other patient to pursue a claim for personal injury sustained in the course of medical treatment. Thus, a patient who is injured as a result of the negligence of the hospital or its employees may claim damages in a civil court in the normal manner. The duty of care owed by the hospital to its patients may extend to cover self-injury, including injury by suicidal patients who are not adequately supervised. The standard of care expected by the court in these circumstances will depend on the context in which the injury occurred. Clearly the constant monitoring of a patient for every minute of the day may be impossible, given limited resources and the needs of other patients, but hospitals are bound to provide a reasonably safe environment for those who are at risk of injuring themselves.

Provided that the detention of the patient is carried out in accordance with the legislative requirements, there can be no claim for deprivation of liberty. A patient may, however, be entitled to claim damages in respect of measures taken which are outside the scope of the detention, for example, in respect of the unwarranted use of force. A gratuitous assault by a nurse, for example, could be the subject of legal action. There are, however, important limitations to the patient's right of recourse to the courts. These are provided by Section 139 of the 1983 Act, which states that there will be no civil liability for anything done by a person in the course of carrying out duties under the Act provided that the act in question is not performed in bad faith or without reasonable care. This means that a doctor or nurse, for example, who acts in excess of power, will not be liable unless he or she

has done so maliciously or mischievously. It is also necessary for a patient to obtain the consent of a judge of the High Court before bringing such an action; this is a significant requirement which has the effect of curtailing the threat of litigation which would make it impossible for hospital staff and others concerned in psychiatric services to carry out their duties without the constant threat of litigation.

Psychiatric patients are entitled to confidentiality in the same way as any other patients. By the very nature of psychiatric illness, such patients are more likely than other patients to pose a threat to the safety of others, and therefore there may be occasions in psychiatric practice in which a breach of confidence in the public interest is warranted. A doctor or nurse proposing to breach confidence should nonetheless bear in mind that this should not be done for trivial reasons and should always be limited to that information which is strictly necessary. In the major English case of this point,[29] a psychiatrist commissioned by a restricted patient's solicitor to provide a report on the patient's state of health, passed on this report to the Home Office, in the belief that this was necessary to ensure that the patient should not be prematurely released. Although this was eventually held to be a justified breach of confidence, it is significant that the arguments against such a breach were not dismissed out of hand by the court.

The matter of whether a psychiatrist might be liable to a third person for damage caused by a patient for whom he or she has clinical responsibility has not been determined by a British court. There is no duty to warn of danger presented by a particular patient, although the existence of such a duty has been confirmed by American courts, most notably in the controversial Californian case of *Tarasoff v. The Regents of the University of California*.[30] In this case it was held that a psychotherapist had a duty to inform a young woman of the danger which his patient posed for her. The implications of such decisions on the exercise of clinical judgment are significant, as are the implications for discharge policies. The imposition of civil liability on hospitals for damage caused by prematurely discharged patients could have the adverse effect of encouraging detention beyond what is required. This would be a clear set-back to the right to liberty of many patients.

References

1. Hoggett, B. (1996). *Mental heath law* (4th edn). Sweet and Maxwell, London.
2. Bean, P. (1986). *Mental disorder and legal control*. Cambridge University Press.
3. Roth, M. and Bluglass, P. (1986). *Psychiatry, human rights and the law*. Cambridge University Press.
4. United Nations (1991). General Assembly, Res. 46/119.
5. Kennedy, I. and Grubb, A. (ed.) (1998) *Principles of medical law*, pp. 109–279. Oxford University Press.
6. *Malette v. Shuman* (1988), 47 Dominion Law Reports (4th) 18.
7. *Re T (Adult: Refusal of Treatment)* [1993], Law Reports Family Division 95.
8. *Airedale NHS Trust v. Bland* [1993], Appeal Cases 789.
9. *St George's Healthcare NHS Trust v. S* [1998], 3 All England Law Reports 673.
10. *Winnipeg Child and Family Services (Northwest Area) v. GFG* (1997), Dominion Law Reports (4th) 193.
11. *Tameside and Glossop Acute Services NHS Trust v. CH (a patient)* [1996], 1 Family Law Reports 762.
12. *Re C (Adult: Refusal of Medical Treatment)* [1994], 1 All England Law Reports 819.

13. *Re F* [1990], 2 Appeal Cases 1.

14. *B* v. *Croydon Health Authority* [1995], 1 All England Law Reports 683.

15. *Riverside Mental Health Trust* v. *Fox* [1994], 1 Family Law Reports 614.

16. Baker, E. and Crichton, J. (1995). *Ex parte A*: psychopathy, treatability and the law. *Journal of Forensic Psychiatry*, **6**, 101–19.

17. Gunn, M. (1994). The meaning of incapacity. *Medical Law Review*, **2**, 8–29.

18. Brabbins, C., Butler, J., and Bentall, R. (1996). Consent to neuroleptic medication for schizophrenia: clinical, legal and ethical issues. *British Journal of Psychiatry*, **168**, 540–4.

19. *Black* v. *Forsey* 1988, Scots Law Times 572.

20. *R.* v. *Bournewood Community and Mental Health NHS Trust, ex parte L* [1998], 3 Weekly Law Reports 107 (House of Lords).

21. Valenstein, E. (ed.) (1980). *The psychosurgery debate: legal and ethical perspectives*. W.H. Freeman, San Francisco, CA.

22. Sachdev, P. and Sachdev, J. (1997). Sixty years of psychosurgery: its present status and future. *Australian and New Zealand Journal of Psychiatry*, **31**, 457–64.

23. *R.* v. *Mental Health Act Commission, ex parte X* (1988), 9 Butterworths Medico-Legal Reports 77.

24. *R.* v. *Hallstrom, ex parte W* [1986], 2 All England Law Reports 306.

25. Torrey, E.F. and Kaplan, R.J. (1995). A national survey of the use of outpatient commitment. *Psychiatric Services*, **19**, 778–84.

26. McIvor, R. (1997). The community treatment order: clinical and ethical issues. *Australian and New Zealand Journal of Psychiatry*, **32**, 223–8.

27. *Winterwerp* v. *The Netherlands* [1997], 2 European Human Rights Reports 387.

28. Eastman, N. (1997). The Mental Health (Patients in the Community) Act 1995: a clinical analysis. *British Journal of Psychiatry*, **170**, 492.

29. *W.* v. *Egdell* [1990], 1 All England Law Reports 835.

30. *Tarasoff* v. *The Regents of the University of California*, 551 P 2d 334 (1976).

1.7 The education of psychiatrists

Paul R. McHugh and Phillip R. Slavney

Most successful teachers of psychiatry bring two skills to bear for the benefit of their students. The first is a clear grasp of the discipline—its concepts, information base, and practices. The second is an appreciation of the discursive methods by which knowledge is effectively transmitted. We shall examine these issues in this chapter because we believe that a lack of a conceptual structure—what to teach—and an indifference towards pedagogical methods—how to teach—thwart the education of psychiatrists. We shall conclude by describing the structure, goals, and specific components of the residency programme at the Johns Hopkins University School of Medicine to exemplify how we apply our principles.

Matters of form

Before we review these fundamental issues of psychiatric education we shall first address some perennial but less crucial matters of setting, curriculum, and 'orientation' in psychiatric education. Although we will describe our own psychiatric residency programme in some detail, we hold that excellent psychiatric education can occur wherever teachers and students meet to care for patients together in a structured fashion. The programmes may be organized around principles of thought derived from any orientation—if that orientation is acknowledged, is candidly discussed between students and faculty, and demonstrably leads to progress. Setting, curriculum, and orientation are the elements, not the essence, of an educational programme.

Setting

A diversity of settings during an apprenticeship period enhances an educational programme. Time spent on inpatient and outpatient services, in consultation in general hospital wards, and on child services leads to increased clinical competence. Local circumstances and settings can vary but do not make as crucial a difference as do the skills and commitments of teachers and students. Although some time—2 to 3 years—spent seeing a variety of patients is necessary for a thorough education, we have seen good results from centres with little diversity of settings and poor educational results from centres of great diversity. It is the people, not the places, that really count.

Curriculum

We draw the same conclusion about the curriculum. A coherent curriculum will provide a set of graded clinical experiences with progres-

sive responsibilities under supervision. These clinical experiences should be combined with didactic exercises that illuminate basic principles. In fact, licensing boards and residency review committees demand such curricula. No-one denies the value of such oversight in that it guarantees—to the student and the public alike—residency programmes that are reasonably comparable. The mistake is to confuse the satisfaction of regulations with an education. The essence of an education is supplied by neither an endorsed schedule nor a diversified setting. Excellent teaching can occur whenever committed teachers and eager students meet in the daily practice of psychiatry.

Schools of thought (orientation)

Finally, because differing schools—psychodynamic, biological, behaviourist, etc.—influence psychiatry, how can educational programmes do justice to all of them? Although much in the name of breadth of understanding can be accomplished by supervised reading of classic texts and contemporary research papers, we believe that the presentation of competing points of view is best done over particular case examples. Here explanatory theories and treatment implications can be compared without a necessary commitment of the student to any of them in a single-minded fashion. Once again excellent teaching can occur and competing viewpoints can be examined so long as well-informed teachers see patients with the students and discuss the observations and interpretations thoroughly.

Coherent discourse

Although setting, curriculum, and orientation are components of an education, the essential element is coherence. The discourse—the conversations, the observations, the lectures, and the seminars—must be interrelated and marked by a discipline of thought. What is affirmed today cannot be contradicted tomorrow without some explanation. The citizens of the educational community must share standards of observation and interpretation, so that the student moving from teacher to teacher within the community finds similar expectations and similar methods of reasoning from observations. Terms and concepts must have standard meanings and comprehensible limits. It is not just that words such as 'delusion' and 'hallucination' are to be defined; coherence must extend to reasoning, judgement, and argument.

In particular, the differences between an observation and an interpretation, between a cause and an effect, between a symptom and a syndrome must be respected and sustained in the pedagogical dialogue. Only in this way can teachers develop in their students a capacity to follow an argument and defend a position.

Conceptual structure

Conceptual structure, information, and application, in that order, are at the heart of our teaching at Johns Hopkins—structure first and foremost because we believe that a lack of understanding about the relationship of observations to explanations impedes much of the general discourse, including the teaching, of psychiatry. In fact, at Johns Hopkins we concluded that until we made *explicit* the conceptual structure of psychiatry *implicit* within the discipline, we would not progress in our teaching skills, nor for that matter in our clinical services or research.

In this century, physicians and surgeons have evolved in their practices as they came to see the disorders and treatments of their patients more coherently based on advancing knowledge of biology and biological responses to injury. Diseases came to be seen not so much as dehumanizing distinctions or harbingers of mortality but as aspects of life under altered circumstances.

Psychiatrists cannot depend upon a direct translation of information from brain mechanisms into explanations for disorders of mental life. The link between brain and mind is the least comprehended connection in the natural sciences. Psychiatrists, members of a 'top-down' discipline, recognize signs and symptoms of mental disruption but must seek their explanations either through their correlations with brain states or as meaningful reactions to life experiences. From correlation and interpretation can come 'armchair' theorizing productive of outrageous speculations and practices. These have emerged in psychiatry from time to time, have been embedded in some educational programmes, and have proved difficult to challenge and eliminate.

Before their appreciation of bodily disorders as examples of life under altered circumstances, internists and surgeons also had problems with theory gone awry. They learned to avoid these pitfalls by committing their discipline to scientifically sound reasoning and research, derived in part from laboratory investigations of bodily structure and function. Psychiatrists, because they currently lack such laboratory means for confirming or rejecting an opinion, must fight against a tendency to blur distinctions between health and disorder. They must be committed to learning a methodologically coherent structured approach to practice, one that can promote progress and eliminate error. Their education must rest upon just such an approach, their teachers exemplifying and discussing it in the process of patient care and research.

Psychiatrists have attempted to bring coherence to the amorphous character of their discipline. In the United States efforts have been made over the last two decades to bring reliability, if not validity, to psychiatric diagnoses. These efforts culminated in the third and successive editions of the American Psychiatric Association's *Diagnostic and Statistical Manual of Mental Disorders* (DSM-III, DSM-IIIR, and DSM-IV).[1] Although these classificatory manuals encourage empirical research by establishing a common nomenclature and an operationalized approach to diagnosis, they are, like their predecessors, only catalogues. They do not offer an explanatory structure for psychiatry that derives from any conception of the basic natures of the disorders they list. Indeed, the authors of DSM-IV deliberately reject an explanation-based approach to their classificatory system, opting for 'a descriptive approach that attempted to be neutral with respect to theories of etiology.' (DSM-IV, p. xviii).

When DSM-III emerged in 1980, George Engel[2] offered an encompassing theoretical approach (the 'biopsychosocial' concept) to explain the psychiatric disorders listed in that catalogue. The biopsychosocial idea, however, is so broad in its scope and so non-specific in its relation to particular mental disorders that it has proved heuristically sterile. It does not provide a foundation for teaching in that, although identifying the ingredients for explanation of mental derangements, it offers no specific recipes to validate or explain the DSM disorders. American psychiatry is committed to using DSM terminology, but it has not agreed upon a conceptual structure from which to derive its opinions, practices, and teaching.

Perspectives of psychiatry

To address these issues of diagnosis and explanation we organized our teaching at Johns Hopkins around four methods of reasoning or 'perspectives' about psychiatric disorders.[3,4] These methods bring forth an appreciation of psychiatric conditions as differing in their fundamental natures in ways critical to treatment, prevention, and research. Our views are derived in part from the methodological approach to psychiatry taken by Karl Jaspers in his classic *General Psychopathology*.[5]

We teach our students that four different classes of mental disorders exist and that an understanding of these classes—in particular, how they call for different explanatory methods with different treatment implications—offers a comprehensive conceptual structure for psychiatry. Any given patient may suffer simultaneously from disorders in several classes, even as each class of disorders is distinct in its causes, mechanisms, and apt treatments. For example, someone with a disease such as bipolar affective disorder can become entrapped in an abnormal behaviour such as the alcohol dependency syndrome and become demoralized by the disruption to his life produced by both of these conditions. These several aspects of his clinical presentation will call for different treatments co-ordinated within a comprehensive treatment plan.

We identify these methods of explanation and reasoning as 'perspectives' to emphasize, in a visual metaphor, how each method can illuminate some presentations of psychiatric disorder but obscure others. These four perspectives are the **disease perspective**, the **dimensional perspective**, the **behaviour perspective**, and the **life-story perspective**. Each generates different definitions of psychopathology and therefore what is normal and abnormal in mental life.

The disease perspective

Disease is a great word in medicine and has a long history of development as a concept. We hold that psychiatrists employ the disease perspective in the traditional medical way, which begins by clustering patients into separate groups defined by symptoms, signs, and course, and thus differentiate patients with dementia, schizophrenia, and bipolar disorder from each other and from people free of disease. The ultimate validation of any clinical disease category is the demonstration of an abnormality in structure or function of a bodily part on which the clinical phenomena depend. The correction of this abnormality—in the form of either cure or palliation—is the ultimate object of treatment.

Disease reasoning follows a standard path in medicine and psychiatry. This path logically starts with the recognition of symptoms of distress or disorder, followed by a recognition that some symptoms cluster together in patient after patient and are suitably construed as forming a clinical disease entity or syndrome. This recognition then generates a search for an abnormality in brain or body underlying this categorical disorder with the impetus to search for an aetiological agency—genes, traumas, infections, nutritional deficiencies, etc.—to explain this bodily abnormality.

For psychiatrists the brain is the major organ where injuries produce mental disorders and logically we can expect to find mental disorders afflicting any of the separate mental functions tied to brain. Thus consciousness itself is the function disordered in delirium, cognition in dementia, memory in Korsakoff's syndrome, language in aphasia, affective control in major depression, and aspects of executive control in schizophrenia. Disease reasoning opens all of these brain disorders to research and practice in palliation and cure. Careful study of those psychiatric disorders most suitably approached as diseases advances our knowledge of the forces of nature that can injure the brain and also demonstrates—through these 'experiments of nature'—just how the brain is organized so as to produce normal mental life.

The dimensional perspective

As is well known in medicine, not all disorders can be construed as diseases; some can be appreciated as derived from an aspect of human variation. The classic example is hypertension, where people are identified as being at risk for later physical illness simply because their blood pressures run at higher levels than average. Similarly in psychiatry we employ a dimensional perspective to grapple with the fact that some patients are vulnerable to mental distress because they occupy an extreme position on the 'bell curve' of human variation in cognitive capacities (the intellectually subnormal) or affective responsiveness (the emotionally unstable). These people differ psychologically from others only in degree, and treatment addresses means for strengthening and guiding them so they can manage their affairs more successfully in the future.

The Axis II categories in DSM-IV (narcissistic, histrionic, antisocial personality, etc.) fail to bring out this sense that the individuals identified as disordered are but examples of those who deviate to an extreme along human affective and cognitive dimensions. The dimensional perspective proposes that many troubling emotional responses derive from an interaction between a person's psychological potentials (cognitive or affective) colliding with specially provocative life circumstances. Treatment programmes are not aimed at a cure—as though these emotional responses were symptoms of disease—but at strengthening and guiding the individuals whose vulnerability to these responses derives from their deviation in cognitive ability and affective temperament. The purpose of treatment is to help these patients deal with difficulties in life which strike at their special weaknesses.

The behaviour perspective

Psychiatrists work to help a large and diverse group of people who are suffering not because of something they 'have', as with a disease, but rather from what they are 'doing'. A maladaptive behaviour—such as addiction, anorexia nervosa, alcoholism—has become a way of life for these people and they seek psychiatric help because of it. We employ the behaviour perspective to identify such patients and represent their problem as due to the unusual and destructive goals that they have come to seek. Some of these people have abnormal physiological drives provoking a craving, as in drug addiction. Others have disorders resting upon social circumstances provoking destructive responses, such as suicide and hysteria. Psychiatrists employ cognitive, behavioural, and pharmacological means to interrupt these behavioural activities, but, given that an aspect of choice is always found in human behaviours, the psychiatrist's task becomes the redirection of a way of life—conversion, not cure. Help in these matters depends upon persuasion and is greatly augmented if group treatment is included. Psychiatrists who treat these patients must be prepared for what is often a remitting and relapsing course of disorder. The behaviour perspective may well be the most challenging to comprehend and employ.

The life-story perspective

A distressed state of mind can be the natural, quite understandable, result of a disturbing experience in which a person's hopes and plans are thwarted by what life delivers—hence the life-story perspective. Thus grief is a universal emotional response to loss, anger or fear regularly follow a traumatic misadventure, and a dispirited sense of lost opportunities can provoke demoralization and discouragement over the future in anyone. A narrative—a chronological recounting of setting, sequence, and outcome—can make the evolution of these emotional states comprehensible to patient and physician alike. Indeed, a story is the most natural way of making sense of many of life's problems and offers the kinds of truths that can be found in histories of any type. For patients a meaningful story has a unique power to generate hope. They can easily appreciate that if the distress they are feeling is just what a story might predict from their life circumstances, then they can expect to overcome the distress if they can better understand how to manage their lives and avoid such encounters in the future. The psychotherapeutic implications of this perspective include comforting patients through a natural course of recovery, providing them with rescripted interpretations of their life circumstances that provide more optimism and a sense of control, and assisting them to avoid similar encounters in the future.

Summary

We hold that the teaching of psychiatry employs information derived from one or several of these perspectives. Each method of reasoning emphasizes a different set of theories and observations, and good teachers of psychiatry should be able to identify and explicate them. By outlining these perspectives our aim is to bring structural and conceptual coherence to psychiatric teaching and to illuminate issues that are often left vague and implicit. These methods of reasoning produce a foundation for thought over psychiatric matters and encourage collaborative efforts with disciplines ranging from molecular genetics to anthropology.

Teaching methods

A grasp of the conceptual structure of psychiatry is the first requirement of an educator, but skill in several methods of instruction is equally necessary. Teaching is a discursive exercise and with appropriate students—those with reasonably sound medical training and an attentive commitment to the subject—is best accomplished through several different methods, each of which has its own aims, purposes, and basic requirements. The three specific methods of transmitting knowledge from teacher to student are the lecture, the tutorial, and the recitation. At Johns Hopkins we have based our thinking about these methods on *The Art of Teaching* by Gilbert Highet,[6] altering them to fit into clinical settings where the teaching of psychiatrists occurs. What follows is a description of the methods as we apply them.

The lecture

The lecture, or in clinical settings the lecture–demonstration, is fundamentally a continuous and coherent talk from the teacher to the students. It may be organized around a presentation of a patient (as in a Grand Rounds) with the lecturer bringing out salient clinical facts from the examination of the patient and then expanding on what these features represent for diagnosis and treatment. Other lectures may be efforts at distilling information found in books and periodicals to make them more accessible and comprehensible.

A lecture is not a conversation to be broken into at random moments by the listeners but rather a presentation of ideas by someone who has thought them through and needs uninterrupted time to present with clarity. The time for discussion is after the lecture is finished. 'The essence of this kind of teaching, and its purpose, are a steady flow of information going from the teacher to the pupils'.[6] Indeed, a lecture is a personal presentation of a set of facts and opinions. Because any lecture must be a relatively brief presentation it cannot be encyclopaedic, but it should be a pedagogical whole resting upon the lecturer's point of view about what is most important. For psychiatrists lectures represent the best means for delivering broad-ranging facts and opinions. Lecturers can present in a brief span of time those general principles which would take a beginner much effort to gather on his or her own.

The tutorial

The second discursive teaching method is the tutorial—a term that we employ to encompass an interaction between a teacher and student over a student's presentation of material (as in ward rounds, psychotherapy supervision, seminars, or journal clubs). The tutorial differs fundamentally from the lecture in that the student brings his or her thinking about a subject to the teacher, who then criticizes and develops the ideas and points of view presented by the student.

In this form of teaching most of the work and the talking is done by the student and rests upon his or her prior preparation for the meeting. The teacher's role is that of a constructive critic who questions the student's work in a fashion that intends to correct mistakes, to provoke the student to defend his or her opinion, and to deepen the student's understanding of the matters at hand. Interaction is the essence of tutorials where student and teacher can compare what the student could do alone with what is accomplished together in the tutorial. A real appreciation by the student of how greater understanding can be achieved derives from this contrast between his or her initial efforts and the eventual opinion and knowledge arrived at after a teacher's consideration and criticism.

Tutorials, in such forms as bedside rounds, are so much a part of day-to-day running of clinical units that their structure and aims may be misaligned. They should not degenerate into mini-lectures by the leader but should rise to a meeting of the minds between an effortful prepared student and an experienced knowledgeable teacher. Thus in all forms of tutorial the student brings some work that he or she has prepared previously. That work is then the focus of constructive criti-

cism and discussion between the student and the faculty member. The tutor is the critic, not the producer of the work, even though he or she may add to the product in the discussion that follows.

The tutorial is the best forum for a consideration of subtle details and individual variations within the themes of psychiatric presentations and treatments. It can provide a sense of thorough dealing with some subject exemplified by a patient or by a research paper and ultimately can enhance the student's confidence in the subject matter.

The recitation

The third method of discursive teaching—recitation—resembles the tutorial in that there is an ongoing exchange between teacher and student, but differs in that a question-and-answer method is employed by the teacher in examining the student. Recitation is a frequently neglected form of teaching in clinical disciplines because it may seem to emphasize a paternalistic and hierarchical distinction between the questioning instructor and the responding student that is now out of pedagogical fashion. Although students are accustomed to recitation earlier in their education (as in high school or even in some college classes), they are less accustomed to its challenge after university graduation. We hold that it is most necessary in teaching a discipline such as psychiatry where the linkages between facts, observations, concepts, and opinions must be criticized as well as discursively drawn forth.

In the recitation a group of students are presented with a patient and then are questioned by the teacher one by one about what they observed and what conclusions they can draw on the basis of these observations. This enterprise, carried on as it is in a group and in a question-and-answer form, has great power in demonstrating not only what a student knows (or does not know), but also in challenging received but inaccurate opinions that have shaped the student's perceptions. It is ever an active process. The students must work for their answers. The teacher leading a recitation must sustain a coherent series of questions and develop from the answers (complete or incomplete as they may be) a fuller picture of the issues at hand. The questions that the teacher asks fit into a set of pedagogical purposes. They explore matters of evaluation and explication first, but then usually go on to explore the limits in knowledge about the subject matter.

For a successful recitation the students must bring some knowledge to the session. Efforts at questions and answers attempted with individuals who have no information quickly deteriorate into confusion and embarrassment, an agony for student and teacher alike. The exercise is to evaluate the extent of knowledge and broaden its foundations and contents. Thus the questions asked in successful recitations are seldom trivial ones that can be looked up (e.g. What is the standard dose of an antidepressant?) but rather questions that open the history of psychiatry and point to its future (e.g. What justifies the use of personality diagnoses in categorical terms?). Because all students are questioned and all listen to the answers of their peers, recitations unify a group of students in their understandings and in their conversations. Active participation in the group reassures everyone about what they know and how they know it.

Early in the course of a student's development the recitations must deal with fairly rudimentary issues of facts and theories about clinical issues—often mere restatements of the obvious are needed at the beginning, given the many ways students can be confused by the subject matter. With the gradual development of more sophistication amongst the students, recitations can evolve into discussions and explorations that go into greater depth of information and implication—all still in a question-and-answer form. The critical point about a recitation is that it should never be limited to what the pupils know but quickly move beyond the easy answers to become searching and provocative. Students often find this teaching at once challenging and exciting, particularly if it is possible to move by way of questions and answers into implications about psychiatry that have not been appreciated even though they are fundamental.

Although recitations have a fixed beginning (as with a case presentation), their course must always be improvised because the answers to initial questions determine the direction of subsequent ones and this path cannot be predicted before the first questions are asked. The recitation should conclude with some resolving consensus amongst the group. This resolution emerges as the questions ultimately move the group in a logical fashion towards a defensible proposition. The major goals of recitation are to bring—through questions asked and answers delivered, through making clear what had been vaguely presumed—a greater understanding of the subject matter to the students and a growing enthusiasm for psychiatry as a valuable, engaging, and challenging intellectual enterprise.

Recitations will always elicit many of the presumptions and pre-judgements students bring to psychiatry. The very process of composing an answer to a question reveals foundational opinions that students have and often fail to reflect upon. Presumptions and prejudgements are to be expected; prejudices (opinions maintained even after counter-evidence is provided and examined) are what are eliminated in the group encounter with fellow students. The group experience under a knowledgeable critical leader advances learning and reduces prejudices better than any other pedagogic method.

Fixing the impression

The education of psychiatrists involves all three of these means of communication with students. Still more, however, is required from a teacher. The facts and opinions that a student learns must cohere ultimately into a mature understanding of the subject matter and how that understanding translates into matters of practice. Gilbert Highet refers to this consolidation of knowledge as 'fixing the impression'. This final aspect of a psychiatric education rests on daily encounters between students and faculty in the exercise of patient care and study. The information derived from the primary teaching methods is 'fixed' by emphasis in practice and review during every clinical day. The repeated efforts at enhancing clarity of the opinions underlying practice makes the abstract ideas specific and tangible at the level of application.

As definition of the clinical problems increases so does the student's appreciation of what remains unknown and in need of future investigation for progress. The sense that there is much to discover evokes enthusiasm for the careful scrutiny of the subject. Finally, as every successful teacher will attest, the most crucial way of 'fixing the impression' offered to students is simply being with them as much as possible during their educational life. This produces a shared experience on which cross-referencing to lectures, tutorials, recitations, and simply ordinary events of the day can occur. What is taught as principle on one day can be confirmed by example on another. But only if the teachers and the students are spending days with each other and are talking together formally and informally about their common experi-

ence over patient care and research does an advanced capacity develop.

Why teach?

Given the burdens of preparation and the distractions from other enterprises that teaching an often awkward group of young people brings, why do it? The answer to this question will surely differ among individual teachers. For us, teaching psychiatry is an exercise that offers some of the greatest of professional satisfactions. It represents a real encounter with other people at a level of interaction hard to duplicate in any other way.

The teaching of students is always based on the hope that they will use this experience to advance our profession. Thus teaching is repaid by a sense of mutual commitment to the future.[7] As well though—beyond simply the experience of an encounter—teaching is a special form of creativity. This is felt in the experience of wonder and satisfaction provoked by witnessing the emergence of a new professional person from the rough beginnings—full of enthusiasm and confusion—that one first encountered. Students are most challenging and daily life with them is always a kind of 'living on the edge' of refutation and chagrin. As teachers, what do *we* know and how do *we* know it? We recommend teaching, but not to the faint-hearted!

A specific example of the application of these principles: the Johns Hopkins psychiatric residency programme

As an example of our principles in action, we now describe the goals and objectives of the psychiatric residency programme at Johns Hopkins. Because local circumstances differ, we know that our programme could not be copied everywhere. We offer it as a point of reference. Whatever the circumstances, however, programmes would do well to have their goals explicit and their objectives measurable.

Overall goal and general programmatic features

The overall goal of the Johns Hopkins psychiatric residency is to produce a well-educated broadly experienced psychiatrist who can prosper in any subsequent career. This goal is approached systematically by combining closely supervised intensive clinical experiences in multiple settings with a comprehensive didactic programme. These experiences broaden in comprehensiveness over the 4 years of the residency. The experiences are also aligned with the health-care reform demands of the contemporary era in giving residents clinical responsibilities within an integrated continuum of care system across service settings. Each year of the residency combines a clinical experience of progressive complexity on the wards and in the clinics with a didactic lecture series (1 h/week) specific to that year. In addition, an ongoing across-the-years department-wide educational programme runs concurrently and consists of weekly meetings of Departmental Grand Rounds (1.5 h), Research Seminar and Visiting Lecture Programme (1 h), Basic Science Seminar (0.5 h), Journal Club (1 h), Psychoanalytic Continuing Case Conference (1 h), and Chairman's Service Round (2 h).

All residents, juniors and seniors, participate in considering general principles of psychiatry, with an emphasis on the perspectival concepts described above, during these weekly didactic meetings. The Departmental Grand Rounds is organized as a lecture by one of the faculty. It is devoted to the consideration of a patient who exemplifies a particular psychiatric condition, what is known of its causes, and its treatment. The Journal Club is a tutorial led by a faculty member concentrating on some article from the scientific literature chosen by a resident as worthy of being carefully studied. The Research Seminar and Visiting Lecture series is a lecture directed at recent advances in psychiatry and customarily led by a visitor to the department. The Basic Science Seminar is a series organized annually around some scientific topic appropriate for detailed study by psychiatrists and led by members of the department who are expert in the topic. A year's study in this seminar has been devoted in each of the last 4 years to genetics, epidemiology, psychopharmacology, and brain imaging. The Psychoanalytic Seminar is a tutorial/seminar concentrating on a case followed over time by a resident in which the life-story perspective is closely studied in its particular exemplification. The Chairman's Service Round is a recitation based on the presentation of a patient to the residents and is led by the Chairman who directs the discussion that follows in a question-and-answer fashion.

The integration of these several didactic elements with the daily tutorial experience of ward rounds and outpatient meetings is accomplished through the more informal interactions of residents and faculty that these sessions make possible. The discourse of the departmental 'community' is a vital, but harder to delineate, element of the educational experience of everyone—student and faculty alike. Its place in student education, though, can be identified in the specific goals and objectives of each residency year that we now describe.

Year I of residency—specific goals and objectives

The goals of the first year of residency are integrative and introductory—specifically to provide a foundation, adequate for psychiatrists, in internal medicine and neurology and also to provide an initiation to the essentials of psychiatric practice through supervised responsibility for assessing and treating a diverse population of psychiatric inpatients.

Thus we expect that by the end of this year residents will have an adequate initiatory knowledge of:

- internal medicine and neurology;
- methods of patient assessment and formulation;
- different categories of psychiatric patients and the categorical implications for treatment and prognosis (e.g. DSM-IV diagnoses and the perspective concept);
- the milieu concept of inpatient psychiatric service;
- the responsibilities of the other mental health practitioners integrated in team treatment of patients—the nurse, social worker, psychologist, occupational therapist, case manager, addiction counsellor, etc.;
- the several treatment modalities—psychological, pharmacological, physical, and rehabilitative—employed with psychiatric patients.

Year II of residency—specific goals and objectives

The goals of the second year are to build on the initiatory capacities of the first year and to introduce more advanced knowledge and methods

of care. These goals are achieved by close supervision of residents on a variety of inpatient units (i.e. general psychiatry and subspecialty psychiatry) and also by introducing residents to the vertically integrated continuum of care through closely supervised experiences in specially designed day hospitals and office-based ambulatory practice. Their broad experiences with patients are amplified by a 2-year didactic programme of lectures in psychiatric assessment, treatment, and research.

We expect by the end of this year that a resident will have acquired:

- a thorough competence in the assessment and formulation of psychiatric disorders along with a clear appreciation of the corroborative methods tied to psychological testing and laboratory measurement;
- competence in treating the most seriously mentally ill patients, their frequent complicating medical and surgical problems, and the forensic issues that may affect their treatment;
- a comprehensive understanding of the psychological, pharmacological, and physical treatments involved in the care of the seriously mentally ill;
- a capacity to assume a leadership role on the treatment team in an inpatient milieu;
- experience with targeted behaviourally oriented treatment plans for the treatment of such behavioural conditions as eating disorders and addictions;
- an introductory knowledge of subspecialty psychiatry gained through experience on specialty services such as geriatric psychiatry, affective disorders, neuropsychiatry, and eating disorders;
- an introduction to both time-limited symptom-focused and long-term insight-oriented psychological treatments by delivering psychotherapy, under close supervision, to selected patients followed in an ambulatory setting;
- an initiatory experience of the vertical integration of clinical practice incorporating day hospitals and office ambulatory services in the continuum of care.

Year III of residency—specific goals and objectives

The goal of this year is to enhance the resident's acquired competencies in ambulatory care by supervised experience in more complex arenas of psychiatric service. A whole variety of new competencies are derived from this emphasis on mastering the problems of psychiatric assessment and treatment in unique domains within the health-care system. The resident continues to treat patients in an office-based practice, but, through a comprehensive outpatient service, also has closely supervised experience in the assessment and treatment of chronic schizophrenia and affective disorders, anxiety disorders, drug and alcohol disorders, and sexual disorders. Special treatment experiences—psychopharmacology for chronic disorders, couples therapy, family therapy—are provided under close supervision along with an extended series of psychodynamically oriented lecture demonstrations. A significant exposure to community-based psychiatry is provided, including rehabilitative and outreach services.

Emergency psychiatric consultation both in the emergency department and in ambulatory settings enhances the residents' confidence in methods of assessment and develops their capacity to provide crisis management and behavioural stabilization. Certain medical/psychiatric clinics—AIDS, neuropsychiatric, and chronic pain clinics—provide experience in ambulatory consultation to primary-care physicians. Such ambulatory experiences help residents learn how psychiatrists function in a large system of health care.

We expect that by the end of this year a resident will have acquired:

- mastery of skills of psychiatric assessments and treatments in complex ambulatory settings;
- diagnostic skills in recognizing the psychiatric disorders that complicate medical/surgical conditions and the capacity to provide this information in consultation to primary-care physicians in general hospital inpatient and outpatient services;
- a firm grasp of the theoretical underpinnings and the practice pitfalls of ambulatory psychotherapy both in the time-limited symptom-focused form and in long-term insight-oriented treatment;
- competence in the assessment and management of psychiatric issues seen most commonly in ambulatory settings—in particular, anxiety, family, marital, sexual, and addictive disorders;
- competence with sustaining psychopharmacology treatments for chronic schizophrenia and affective disorder;
- a knowledge of community psychiatry that rests on supervised experience in ambulatory community clinics with an outreach programme;
- a capacity to function as an effective member of a primary-care team in assessing and treating ambulatory medical patients.

Year IV of residency—specific goals and objectives

The goals of this year are those of completion and depth. The resident will add child psychiatry skills and enhance mastery of providing a continuum of care by rotating in a psychiatric day hospital. The resident, through a freely chosen elective, develops advanced experience in a psychiatric subspecialty—a 'field of concentration' with one or more faculty members to demonstrate how advancing knowledge accrues through research and close study. Finally, an appreciation of psychiatric administration is provided to residents through a weekly meeting with the Chairman of the Department where discussions review the rationales behind past and present responses of the department to the demands of health care reform, managed care, and hospital/medical school needs.

We expect that by the end of this year the resident will:

- acquire the skills of child and family assessment and gain an initiatory appreciation of the specialty of child and adolescent psychiatry;
- have an understanding of the changing health-care environment and of the competencies necessary for success in clinical practice and in other professional leadership roles;

- acquire confidence in office psychiatric practice and long-term psychotherapy given an experience with some patients extending out for years;
- have an advanced understanding of a subspecialty of psychiatry through close mentoring from a faculty member in an elective;
- have an appreciation of the rational approaches to administrative decisions within a system of psychiatric services in the contemporary challenging era for health care.

Ultimate goal of this educational programme

Our residency programme is organized according to these general and specific goals. Amplifications and modifications have occurred over time in response to the growth of knowledge in psychiatry and in response to the demands of a changing health-care system. Our ultimate goals are to open the field of psychiatry to our students and to help them become both broad- and tough-minded.

Conclusion

This chapter has emphasized the conceptual and pedagogical issues that often are lost in the details of programme construction. We hold that the best teaching of psychiatry rests not upon matters of setting, curriculum, or theoretical orientation—important as these may be for standardization—but upon teachers who can present a coherent conceptual structure that grasps the differing natures of psychiatric disorders, and who are skilled in the several discursive methods for transmitting information to students. What to teach, and how to teach, are the basic questions addressed in this chapter. Our answers—offered in a description of our residency programme and its specific goals and objectives—derive ultimately from what we have called the perspectives of psychiatry and how we believe lectures, tutorials, and recitations are best employed, within a programme of ongoing clinical services, to teach psychiatrists.

References

1. American Psychiatric Association (1994). *Diagnostic and statistical manual of mental disorders* (4th edn). American Psychiatric Association, Washington, DC.
2. Engel, G.L. (1980). The clinical application of the biopsychosocial model. *American Journal of Psychiatry*, **137**, 535–44.
3. McHugh, P.R. and Slavney, P.R. (1998). *The perspectives of psychiatry* (2nd edn). Johns Hopkins University Press, Baltimore, MD.
4. McHugh, P.R. (1992). A structure for psychiatry at the century's turn—the view from Johns Hopkins. *Journal of the Royal Society of Medicine*, **85**, 483–7.
5. Jaspers, K. (1963). *General psychopathology*. Reprinted 1997 by Johns Hopkins University Press, Baltimore, MD.
6. Highet, G. (1950). *The art of teaching*. Vintage Books, New York.
7. Lewis, A. (1967). Psychiatric education and training. In *The state of psychiatry: essays and addresses by Sir Aubrey Lewis*, pp. 138–60. Routledge and Kegan Paul, London.

1.8 The psychiatrist as manager

Dinesh Bhugra

Introduction

Management requires a number of skills. As a result of their training, most psychiatrists have a set of skills which allow them to function as good managers. They are able to manage groups and conflicts and have insight into functioning of individuals in various settings. Although in some clinical settings clinicians/psychiatrists may have a degree of autonomy which allows them to think and plan ahead for the delivery of services, this is not universal. The clinician's motivation is related to a clear sense of responsibility as well as an element of professional pride.

Clinicians who are attracted by management tasks are likely to possess some of the skills which make them respond appropriately to needs in developing and delivering services. Where services are being delivered in a hospital setting, the clinician's role is different from that in community-based services. Similarly, a different set of expectations and roles emerge if the clinician is practising in the private sector or an academic setting. The role of the psychiatrist as a manager in the United Kingdom National Health Service (**NHS**) is described in this chapter. The key functions and skills required for a clinician to function effectively as a manager are highlighted. Some of these skills are part of the clinical training (e.g. managing teams and groups, managing conflict, and negotiating), but additional training may be needed for others (e.g. time, resource, and finance management).

Historical background

In 1983, the Griffiths Report into the management of the NHS called for changes, chiefly in the form of hierarchical line management and command and control structures which reflected wider movement in both the United Kingdom and elsewhere in the world (e.g. the United States, New Zealand, and Australia). This shift from administration to management is quite an important step. Historically, the organization and delivery of government services (including health and education) in the United Kingdom had been characterized by the development of a career-based system of public service and the organization and delivery of services by established professionals. In the case of control administration, the ideal is a neutral career-based civil service that does the bidding of the government of the day.[1] In such an administrative system the politicians tend to be separated from the delivery of service by the administrative system that neutrally implements their policies and yet acts as a conduit between the politicians and the professional groups who are responsible for delivery of services. In the

1980s, public administration was gradually replaced by public management with the evolution of a top-down system of control. Whereas the administrators followed the route set by others, managers were expected to set their own targets and were expected to achieve them. The focus gradually began to shift to economy, efficiency, and effectiveness, new personal management systems, and enhancement of delegated financial management.

Providing an efficient and effective health-care system is and should be a priority of any government, as well as clinicians who are providing this care professionally. In any process of developing health-care services, clinicians are best placed to identify the needs of the population they choose to serve and also to provide a system which is effective. In addition, the professionalism has meant that clinicians themselves are responsible for self-regulation and their performance is influenced by the sanctity of the doctor–patient relationship.

Health-care management generally works as a customer service depending upon the local resources, health-care models, and socio-economic models. In private care systems there is also an intermediary between the health professional and the patient. Sometimes this is obvious but at other times it is not clear who, if anyone, is negotiating with the doctor on behalf of the patient. Clinicians have to understand their role with respect to developing services and delivering them to those most in need in a way which is effective and accessible.

In this chapter, we examine the roles and responsibilities of clinicians as managers and consider how these roles can merge in one individual. The process and content of management are described, as is the role of clinicians.

Role and responsibilities of a psychiatrist

In the United Kingdom, consultant psychiatrists in the NHS are not automatically part of a fixed line management structure although their job plans have to be agreed with the chief executive either directly or through clinical and medical directors. At present, a consultant is not answerable to a manager in a clinical situation, although this will change with new structures about to be implemented and with the introduction of clinical governance. However, the consultant psychiatrist is the essential unit of management who looks after individual named patients and working with a multi-disciplinary team. Ideally, it should be the business of all levels of management to empower individual consultants so that they can practise effectively; a group of consultants should be able to share their resources and individual consultants should be able to control their clinical resources to make their clinical services as effective as possible.[2] The psychiatrist (at a consultant or equivalent level) wears several hats—some are by virtue of his or her clinical expertise and others are due to personal interest and managerial expertise. Some of these are discussed below.

Team leader

Leadership within a multidisciplinary team is inevitably linked to the role and clinical responsibility vested in the psychiatrist. The role of consultant as a team leader depends on whether the team is based in the hospital or the community. The boundaries are amorphous in the community, where nursing staff or other professionals (e.g. occupational therapists) may be the first contact for initial clinical assessments and doctors or psychologists may be the next contact. Team leadership does not necessarily rely on personality or behavioural style but on role and clinical responsibility. Some of this may be due to comprehensive training of psychiatrists in biological, psychological, and social models of illness. Their training in diagnosis and the range of treatments that can be prescribed, their position in service planning, their effectiveness in advocacy, and the degree of contact with patients can all contribute to the possibility of the consultant taking the lead in a multidisciplinary team. In community settings the clinical responsibility for the patient may not be handed over to the multidisciplinary team at all but retained by the original referral agent. In addition to leading the team, the consultant also has to provide clinical and training leadership.

In the United Kingdom and many other countries, the psychiatrist, as a Responsible Medical Officer, is responsible for legal detention of mentally ill patients and also for overseeing their clinical care during admission aand their after-care. This responsibility is clearly associated with the resources required to provide acceptable levels of service. These responsibilities are also related to the maintenance of standards as expected by relevant training bodies such as the professional colleges and registration bodies such as the General Medical Council. In addition, being a member of a consultative body which plans and delivers appropriate services can provide an additional element of responsibility and skill. As a manager, the clinician has to be aware of local employment laws and what is expected of an employer.

Effective clinical managers need the ability to build and motivate a team, set clear and realistic targets for success, and monitor progress. To do this they must be able to relate to people—a skill that good psychiatrists must possess by virtue of their clinical training. The tasks allocated to the team member must be specific, measurable, achievable, realistic, and timed.[3]

In order to perform well, the team will need to develop a sense of responsibility and cohesiveness, where every member is pulling in the same direction. The members must be encouraged to develop a sense of self-worth, achievement, and high morale. To sustain good performance the team members must be presented with even higher goals and standards which must be achievable. Therefore the manager should monitor progress with constructive feedback and be aware of potential pitfalls. The clinician must be conscious of conflict within the team and try to resolve it as soon as possible rather than waiting for the situation to explode. Any conflicts must be resolved effectively and positively. When it is not possible to achieve this, the manager should acknowledge it and remain aware that the conflict remains unresolved.

Individual members of the team should be encouraged to take on tasks on which are within their capability, and a good manager must specify the tasks to be achieved within the limitations of experience, knowledge, and ability. The manager must not allow individuals to be overwhelmed by their tasks, and due public recognition must be given when tasks are satisfactorily completed. Clinical managers obviously need to be aware of current agreements with various professions in relation to clinical practice and also their respective legal responsibilities. An ability to delegate tasks appropriately not only enhances the motivation of others but also allows manager to prioritize their time and concentrate on other matters. Existing team members should be encouraged to retain and develop their skills, and new members must be trained and have a period of induction in order to allow them to understand the functioning of the team.

Managing people involves making decisions based on employment patterns and policies and developing new patterns of management and organizational development. A key problem arises during the management of people in changing situations, especially if the health-care system is being reorganized on a fairly regular basis.

Senior clinician

By virtue of clinical experience, the consultant is also the clinician who stays the longest in the multidisciplinary team. The clinical responsibility of the psychiatrists comes under the umbrella of professionalism which in turn is characterized by self-regulation—using one's own judgement and professional freedom or autonomy. Professional autonomy may result from intensive education or personal responsibility. On the other hand, a manager (even though a professional, highly educated, and to some degree autonomous individual) still tells other people what to do. The conflict produced within an individual between being a clinician and subsuming some degree of freedom and autonomy to be a manager is quite important. Successful managers and clinicians are able to combine these disparate skills and deal with the conflicts caused by the competing demands. The pressures related to clinical services—delivery of these services and development of new services—have to be resolved by the clinician–manager. The position of such an individual is strengthened by virtue of clinical training which enables him or her to identify the therapies which are evidence based and are likely to be successful and acceptable. The clinician is also better placed to differentiate between demands and needs, and to be able to recommend services according to needs of individual patients and their communities.

Psychiatrists often have the advantage of training in group work. Thus they are able to identify factions within such a setting and are able to identify clearer objectives and outcomes from meetings. Managing colleagues is not easy for clinicians, particularly when there is argument over the allocation of resources, but if the patients' needs are to be met then the clinician has to have the skills to fight for them.

A manager must avoid processes of demotivation which may well be related to stress within the team, manifested by absenteeism, increased sick rates, lateness, poor communications, non-participation, poor quality of work, and sudden bursts of anger. There are many reasons for demotivation including lack of recognition, boredom, lack of involvement in decisions, poor communication, lack of development, and work overload.[4] A good manager will listen, delegate appropriately, provide training, involve staff in decision-making, encourage ideas and suggestion, give praise where due, and treat people as individuals. In health-care settings the motivation of individuals is often more than simple financial self-interest and public recognition plays a very important role.

Researcher and trainer

The senior clinician, especially in university or teaching hospitals, may take the lead in developing research projects which could include empirical research or service evaluation research. Not all clinicians will have the interest or skills to carry out research—much depends upon the setting of the service, personal and past experience, and desire to carry out research. This aspect is noted here for completeness and to highlight the importance of such a process. These roles are described in more detail in Chapter 7.6.

Management processes

The process of management of health care includes the development of health strategy, its assessment and evaluation, managing finance and resources, and managing personnel and teams. Some of these processes, such as financial and strategic management, are more general tasks whereas time and stress management are more personal.

These processes are applicable to the NHS in the United Kingdom, but may not be relevant in other parts of the world and may not be appropriate in other types of health-care system. Although it is assumed here that the various management processes are discrete, in practice they often merge into one another. The implementation of these processes demands a set of specific personal skills which are described later in this chapter. A key function of the psychiatrist is that of developing strategy.

Development of strategy

Strategy development is often seen as top-down, rational, and formal. There are problems in defining and responding to strategy. Hunter[5] defines it as being contingent on both the nature of the organization (size, value system, degree of specialization) and its external environment (stable/unstable). Thus strategy is a continuum ranging from deliberate planned strategy at one extreme to emergent strategy at the other.

Strategy operates on three levels: corporate, business, and operational. Whereas corporate levels of strategy are global, operational levels have to be local. Often the strategy can be planned at the global level but with a clear indication given of how it should be implemented at the local level. A good and manageable step forward is the use of strategic management, which is a unifying concept seeking to bring together planning and management. This approach also seeks to combine the discipline of the planning and management functions with the flexibility necessary for the development and implementation of policies.

Mintzberg[6] contrasts emergent strategy with deliberate strategy, where the latter is a series of actions forming a pattern or series of patterns. Other forms of strategy combine deliberation and control with flexibility and organizational training. According to Johnson,[7] there are three views of strategy:

(1) a rational view in which strategy is seen as the outcome of a sequential planned search for optimal solutions to defined problems;

(2) an adaptive or incremental view in which strategy evolves in an additive pattern;

(3) an interpretative view in which strategy is seen as the product of individual or clinical service provision.

Policy comprises of content whereas strategy consists of content and process. Strategic management does not attempt to provide a prescription for problems but seeks to combine the deliberate and emergent approaches to strategic development and is often seen as both a process and an outcome [5]. In addition to developing strategy the clinician may be expected to have personal skills like financial, conflict, time, and stress management.

Financial management

Financial management incorporates a number of components. Wherever a clinical service is provided—in a university teaching hospital, a general hospital, or a private hospital—the cost of patient treatment will vary depending on the patient's condition, the expertise of the health professionals involved in the treatment, and additional expenses such as teaching, research overheads, etc. Costs are fixed (unchanging irrespective of the level of activity), semi-fixed (fixed for a range of activities), or variable (changing directly as activity increases or decreases). The process of consultation between the managers and the clinical service providers is crucial in financial management. Budgets have to be fixed in advance, but there is the additional responsibility of ensuring that planning variances and operational variances are taken into account. Whether the service is delivered in the private or the public sector, it must be effective, efficient, and economical.

Financial management must include a clear idea of not only all the expenses but also the costs, both fixed and flexible. Most clinicians will not be interested in the minutiae of budget management, but close collaboration with their finance directors will allow them to understand the costs and expeditures as well as incoming monies which can be used in the planning and delivery of services.

According to Bainton,[8] resource management has three components:

(1) close involvement of medical and nursing staff in management;

(2) development of information systems, particularly case mix (a method of categorizing workload by appropriate groupings);

(3) organizational development to help health-care professionals and managers to work in close collaboration.

General management

The above description of resource management recognizes the general management role of clinicians, thereby providing a clearer picture of roles and responsibilities of psychiatrists as managers.

The key tasks for managers are shown in Table 1.

The manager has to take a developmental view of organization. Each organization goes through the phases of beginning (with 'loose' organizational rules and regulations, commitment, and excitement in creating something new), expansion (when the manager's excitement and enthusiasm affects other staff who share the idealism, sense of purpose, and dreams), and consolidation and efficiency (which is characterized by quality considerations, promulgation of rules and procedures, negotiations with outside agencies, and creation of training and research programmes). Members of the team become

Table 1 Key tasks for managers

- Indicate clear directions by setting clear goals and standards, communicating goals, and clear delegation

- Encourage open communications

- Be willing to reach support staff

- Recognize the strengths of individuals and be constructive when criticizing

- Establish evaluation of service

- Encourage the staff

- Lead on innovation

- Be aware of financial implications

- Make clear decisions

- Have a high level of integrity

empowered during the final consolidation phase. Here, a good manager is able to judge when to hand over the power and in what order. In the early phases the manager may be a charismatic leader, but this may lead to jealousies and rivalries creating a disruptive state. Table 2 illustrates some of the management qualities required in a good manager.

Stress management

Managing stress at work, in oneself and others, is a key function of a good manager. Most common causes of stress have their origins outside the workplace. Some professions are stressful in themselves; for example, miners have the highest levels of stress followed by the police, and doctors are only slightly below actors.[4] Some people immerse themselves in their work in order to forget domestic problems. In addition, pressures of too much or too little work, poor supervision, isolation, frustration, and poor working conditions can all contribute to poor quality of work resulting in increased stress. Identifying the symptoms of stress at work and managing it by prioritizing, delegating, and communicating can help.

Preventive strategies can be put in place to help avoid predictable stress from life events. Once stress has developed, the individual must combat it using strategies such as relaxation and meditation. Stress can be used as a positive source of good functioning, but a good clinician

Table 2 Qualities required in a good manager

Attributes (in-born qualities)	Integrity, flexibility, decisiveness, open-mindedness, absence of bias, enthusiasm, imagination
Skills (qualities that can be learned and developed)	Listening, communicating, delegating, motivating, planning
Knowledge (information that can be learned and acquired)	Needs of staff, objectives of health-care delivery, finance, services, service development and evaluation

manager will be aware of the signs of destructive stress and burn-out.[9] Staff burn-out is considered further in Chapter 7.4.

Conflict management

Conflict can arise from time to time even in best managed teams. Conflict and disagreement are unavoidable in a team where the members are able to take positions which can become rigid and fixed. Managers are more likely to prevent the development of conflict if they avoid creating win–lose situations between team members, make clear what is expected of team members, involve the team members in decision-making processes, and develop and encourage a sense of trust within the team. Often the human response to conflict is to ignore it, to buy off one of the protagonists, and/or to work out a solution and then impose it. All these options have their advantages and disadvantages. According to Barnes,[3] in order to tackle the problem it must be seen rationally.

Managing conflict or negotiating an agreement obviously depends upon the type of conflict (see Hill[10] for further details of negotiation management). There are two kinds of conflict—integrative and distributive. In integrative conflict both parties are in some degree of agreement right from the beginning (a win–win situation). In this case they agree to negotiate and agree on the current state of affairs; this is followed by a definition of the problem which leads to the generation of solutions which are implemented and periodically reviewed. The distributive conflict is a win–lose situation, so that each party will make demands but will have to make concessions to resolve the conflict and obtain a satisfactory outcome. A good negotiator will make concessions of little value in themselves but of great importance to the other party, so that each leaves the negotiating table with feelings of success and satisfaction.[10] The stages of such a negotiation include an agreement to negotiate followed by a general discussion, an exchange of proposals, and a final bargain, with a review of the situation at a later date. A good negotiator must prepare the case thoroughly, be aware of its strengths and weaknesses, be comfortable with the best alternative to the preferred outcome, and not make concessions without obtaining something in return.

Managers must be aware of their own management styles prior to dealing with different types of conflict. Information (pre-existing data or new information obtained from logical analysis, surveys, existing services, or recognized authorities) can and should be used in resolving conflicts. Distributive conflict creates more problems for managers, who should be trained in dealing with conflicts of this kind. In this type of conflict there is less likely to be any trust or clarity, and the manager must strive to obtain both of these. Managing conflict through negotiation may involve the use of an arbitrator.

Time management

Time management is crucial for the successful manager. By prioritizing, delegating, and planning a good manager can be assertive and achieve more in a limited time. Time management is about making choices and keeping to them. Zarod[11] has illustrated some successful and pragmatic techniques for time management. The individual must identify particular time-management problems. Following processes of prioritization, a key step is to be able to delegate to others with complementary their skills. Individuals can manage time more effectively by being proactive rather than reactive.

A good manager will balance social time and working time equally

Table 3 Time management

Good time management	Bad time management
Plan	Disorganized
Prioritize	Too involved
Delegate	Welcoming interruptions
Say no	Too many meetings
Plan time for staff	Too much time on 'enjoyable' tasks
Be flexible	
Meetings only when necessary	

effectively. Allocation of time to various activities and prioritizing is an important step. Time can be managed effectively by delegating as much as possible, helping individuals to solve their problems, and managing diaries in a pragmatic manner by highlighting priorities of work for each day. Managers spend a significant period of their lives in meetings, and it is very important that the agenda and purpose of each meeting is very carefully defined. Some characteristics of good and bad time management are given in Table 3.

Managing meetings and committees

Team members often attend meetings other than clinical meetings 'because they have to'. It is important to be clear about the purpose of the meeting and to identify this in the agenda. Meetings should chaired effectively and information about decisions made should be circulated. A good chairperson will allow every individual to contribute without allowing them to dominate the meeting. The chairperson must not take sides but bring everybody into discussion. It is crucial to focus the group on the issue under discussion and to emphasize the positive. Meetings often end up as entertainment or battles, but they should be for making decisions, sharing information, and achieving agreements in public.

A good manager is able to chair committees and obtain the required results. A skilful individual will go into each committee meeting with a clear idea of their preferred outcome. Not all committees are decision-making bodies and their functions will vary depending on their structure and constitution; hence the chairperson will have to play different roles. However, preparation and planning are crucial in setting the agenda for each meeting and notifying the members of the committee. A good chairperson will control the agenda yet will give opportunity to the members to communicate their views so that they feel that their views have been heard. He or she will coax individual members to participate, clarify their views, and co-ordinate the response. By using statements and assessing verbal and non-verbal signals, the chairperson can succeed in summarizing and communicating the decisions that have been made.[12]

Management training

Good clinicians can marry managerial skills with clinical qualities. They must have a realistic appreciation of the management compon-

ent and positive attitudes towards it. There is no doubt that, although different, clinical training and management training can enhance some of these skills. The aim of training must be to increase awareness of the qualities required for management so that the service can be improved by regularly reviewing clinical practice and evaluating different components of service. Managers must foresee and attempt to eliminate barriers between different professions. They must also have the skills and ability to say no.

As discussed above, the management process includes management of resources—both financial and human—and, at a more personal level, time management, negotiation, committee management, etc. By virtue of their professional training, psychiatrists will already have the skills for negotiation and committee management, but they may need to learn other techniques and such learning can take different forms.

Management courses are one option, but significantly more can be learned by shadowing senior clinician or non-clinician managers and through practical experience. This involves management at a fairly junior level such as being involved in committee work, working parties etc. The senior clinician in private settings or in non-teaching settings in some countries may not take on these responsibilities and may not have the opportunity of doing so. The clinician manager may take the lead in establishing training programmes for nurses, psychologists, social workers, and occupational therapists as required.

Although continuing professional development has been established for some time with increased emphasis on revalidation and accreditation, the clinician has to set time aside to manage personal growth. Managers have to learn to manage emotions as well as workplace pressure in order to be able to delegate and communicate. Good verbal communication is a two-way process and, in view of their training, psychiatrists ought to be good at it. The process of communicating with people is well described by Humphries.[4] The right language, the right tone, and appropriate non-verbal communication are all important facets of good quality communication.

The medical profession continues to insist that it controls its own standards—a tradition long enjoyed and generally accepted, although pressure is increasing to change this and to make a distinction between management and clinical practice.

Conclusion

It is clear that if clinicians do not manage their own environment and resources, there are a number of others who are perfectly willing to do so. Managers must be capable of managing change by paying attention to the environment and yet have the ability to question the wisdom of the day without giving in. Managers must be aware that their role and their primary task are the same, i.e. to deliver good-quality health care for the benefit of their patients.

Successful managers achieve their aims by demonstrating enterprise and initiative, and by thinking analytically as well as influencing strategically.[3] Managers have to be aware of their own strengths and weaknesses, and must have team members around them who can complement their skills.

Leadership skills are not always hereditary, as has been demonstrated time and again in political dynasties. Some skills can be acquired but others cannot be learnt. It is vital that managers work with their teams to develop clear aims which can be achieved by co-operation and careful planning.

Some of these characteristics overlap and are present in the same individual, and individuals may change their roles as they develop and gain personal growth. The success of the team depends upon leadership qualities, which have often been described as democratic, and the team structure. Although democratic leadership may be easy when there is plenty of time to perform given tasks, a dictatorial style is vital when decisions have to be made urgently. Unfortunately, this is the style that appeals to most people if they want to demonstrate their position or power. There are problems in both approaches, and a good skilled clinician will use either or both by working within the constraints of the team.

References

1. Gray, A. and Jenkins, B. (1995). Public management and the National Health Service. In *Managing health care* (ed. J. Glynn and D. Perkins), pp. 4–32. W.B. Saunders, London.
2. Sims, A. (1995). The clinician and the clinical team in the community. In *Management for psychiatrists* (ed. D. Bhugra and A. Burns), pp. 176–82. Gaskell, London.
3. Barnes, P. (1995). Managing people. In *The clinicians management handbook* (ed. D. Hansell and B. Salter), pp. 43–68. W.B. Saunders, London.
4. Humphries, J. (1995). *How to manage people at work.* How To Do Books, Plymouth.
5. Hunter, D. (1995). Creating health services strategy. In *Managing health care* (ed. J. Glynn and D. Perkins), pp. 37–73. W.B. Saunders, London.
6. Mintzberg, H. (1990). *Mintzberg on management.* Free Press, London
7. Johnson, G. (1987). *Strategic change and the management process.* Basil Blackwell, Oxford.
8. Bainton, D. (1995) Resource management. In *Management for psychiatrists* (ed. D. Bhugra and A. Burns), pp. 75–84. Gaskell, London.
9. Waters, H. (1995). Stress management: taking the strain. In *Management for psychiatrists* (ed. D. Bhugra and A. Burns), pp. 284–308. Gaskell, London.
10. Hill, P. (1995). Negotiation. In *Management for psychiatrists* (ed. D. Bhugra and A. Burns), pp. 262–73. Gaskell, London.
11. Zarod, H. (1995). Time management. In *Management for psychiatrists* (ed. D. Bhugra and A. Burns), pp. 274–83. Gaskell, London.
12. Hill, P. (1995). Committee practice. In *Management for psychiatrists* (ed. D. Bhugra and A. Burns), pp. 248–61. Gaskell, London.

1.9 Descriptive phenomenology

Andrew Sims, Christoph Mundt, Peter Berner, and Arnd Barocka

Principles of descriptive phenomenology

Definitions and explanations

Psychopathology is the systematic study of abnormal experience, cognition, and behaviour. It includes the **explanatory psychopathologies**, where there are assumed causative factors according to theoretical constructs, and **descriptive psychopathology,** which precisely describes and categorizes abnormal experiences as recounted by the patient and observed in his behaviour.[1] Therefore the two components of descriptive psychopathology are the observation of behaviour and the empathic assessment of subjective experience. The latter is referred to by Jaspers as phenomenology,[2] and implies that the patient is able to introspect and describe what these internal experiences are, and the doctor responds by recognizing and understanding this description. Descriptive phenomenology, as described here, is synonymous with phenomenological psychopathology, and involves the observation and categorization of abnormal psychological events, the internal experiences of the patient, and its consequent behaviour. The attempt is made to observe and understand this psychological event or **phenomenon** so that the observer can, as far as possible, know what the patient's experience must feel like.

Mental phenomena in health and cultural variation

It is not surprising that the identification and classification of the phenomena of mental illness is a difficult task as there is no consensus concerning what would be acceptable as normal healthy experiences. Health has been regarded as a state of complete physical, mental, and social well-being;[3] mental illness has variously been considered as the products of a diseased brain, the symptoms that doctors treat, or a statistical variation from the norm carrying biological disadvantage, and mental illness often has legal implications. It is best to retain the use of the word 'normal' in a statistical sense; thus a phenomenon, such as hypnagogic hallucination, may be statistically abnormal but in no way an indicator of ill health or mental disease. Similarly, it is unwise to extrapolate from a population of mentally ill people and make assertions about the origins of behaviour in those who are not mentally ill.

It is important to recognize the effect of culture on subjective experience, the expression of psychological symptoms, and their manifestation in behaviour. In some cultures the very expression of subjective experience and emotion is discouraged and censored, in others feelings tend to be somatized, and in yet others the subjective experience of the individual tends to be subjugated to the sense of well being of the immediate social group. There are specific culture-bound expressions of subjective distress concerning body image in those who suffer from anxiety disorders. For delusions of passivity, although the psychopathological form remains relatively constant, the description of content will vary according to culture; for example, 'the djinn made me do it', 'my thoughts are controlled by the television'. Similarly, for possession state, although the psychopathological description remains similar, the actual cultural expression is very different for a member of a fundamentalist sect in the American Appalachian Mountains and a Buddhist girl in Sri Lanka.

Understanding the patient's symptoms

Although in internal medicine a clear distinction is made between **symptom** (the complaint which the patient makes) and **sign** (the indicator of specific disease observed or elicited on examination), in psychiatry both are contained within the speech of the patient. He complains about his unpleasant mood state, therefore identifying the symptom; he ascribes the cause of the pain in his knee to alien forces outside himself, thus revealing a sign of a psychotic illness. Because both symptoms and signs emanate from the patient's conversation, in psychiatric practice the term symptom is often used to include both. For a symptom to be used diagnostically, its occurrence must be typical of that condition and it must occur relatively frequently in the condition. Fundamental to psychiatric examination is the use of **empathic understanding** to explore and clarify the patient's subjective experiences. The method of empathy implies using the ability to 'feel oneself into' the situation of the other by proceeding through an organized series of questions, rephrasing and reiterating where necessary until one is quite sure of what is being described by the patient. The final stage is recounting back to the patient what you, the psychiatrist, believe the patient's experience to be, and the patient recognizing that as indeed an accurate representation of their own internal state. Empathy uses the psychiatrist's capacity, as a fellow human being, to experience for him- or herself what the patient's subjective state must feel like as it arises from a combination of external environmental and internal personal circumstances.

Identifying phenomena as specific indicators of defined psychopathology may be difficult. It may require recording much conversation of the patient for significant words and sentences to reveal material of diagnostic importance within the undifferentiated whole of ordinary speech. The psychiatrist, when in the role of psychopathologist, has to assume that all speech of the patient, all behaviour of the patient, and every nuance has meaning, at least to the patient at the time the speech or behaviour takes place; it is not just an epiphenomenon of brain functioning.

Jaspers has contrasted understanding (*verstehen*) with explaining (*erklären*); descriptive phenomenology is concerned with the former. Understanding is the perception of personal meaning of the patient's subjective experience and involves the human capacity for empathy. That is, I understand because I am able to put myself into my patient's situation and know for myself how he is feeling, I feel those feelings of misery myself. Explanation is concerned with observation from outside and working out causal connections as in scientific method. In psychopathology, the terms primary and secondary are based upon this important distinction between meaningful and causal connections. That which is primary can be reduced no further by understanding, i.e. by empathy. What is secondary emerges from the primary in a way which can be understood by putting oneself into the patient's situation at the time; that is, if I were as profoundly depressed as my patient, I could have such a bleak feeling that I believed the world had come to an end—a nihilistic secondary delusion.

Subjective experience and its categorization

Within certain limits subjective experience is both predictive and quantifiable. When an individual loses a close relative it can be predicted that he or she will experience misery and loss. It is possible to quantify depressive symptoms and compare the degree of depression at different times in the same individual or differences between individuals at the same time. An important distinction for psychopathology is that between form and content. The **form** of psychological experience is the description of its structure in phenomenological terms (e.g. a delusion). Its **content** is the psychosocial environmental context within which the patient describes this abnormal form: 'Nurses are coming into the house and stealing my money'. The form is dependent upon the nature of the mental illness, and ultimately upon whatever are the aetiological factors of that condition. Content is dependent upon the life situation, culture, and society within which the patient exists. The distinction is important for diagnosis and treatment; determining the psychopathological form is necessary for accurate diagnosis, whereas demonstrating the patient's current significant concerns from the content of symptoms will be helpful in constructing a well-directed treatment regime.

Whereas most science is concerned with objectivity and with trying to eliminate the observer as far as possible from being a variable within the experiment, descriptive phenomenology tries to make evaluation of the subjective both quantifiable and scientific. It is a mistake to discredit subjectivity in our clinical practice. Inevitably we use it all the time and we should learn to use it skilfully and reliably. When I make an assessment, within the Mental State Examination, that my patient is depressed, I am, at least to some extent, making a subjective judgement based upon the experienced and disciplined use of empathy: 'If I felt as my patient looks and describes himself to be, I would be feeling sad'. In psychopathology the distinction is also made between **development**, where a change of thinking or behaviour can be seen as emerging from previous patterns by understanding what the individual's subjective experience is, and **process**, where an event is imposed from outside and this cannot be understood in terms of a natural progression from the previous state. Anxiety symptoms could be seen as a development in a person with anankastic personality confronted with entirely new external circumstances; epilepsy and its psychiatric symptoms would be a process imposed upon the individual and not understandable in terms of previous life history.

Theoretical bases of descriptive phenomenology

There are important theoretical differences from dynamic psychopathology. Descriptive psychopathology does not propose explanations accounting for subjective experience or behaviour, but simply observes and describes them. Psychoanalytic psychopathology studies the roots of current behaviour and conscious experience through postulated unconscious conflicts and understands abnormalities in terms of previously described theoretical processes. The distinction between form and content and between process and development is not seen as important in psychoanalysis, but symptoms are considered to have an unconscious psychological basis. Descriptive phenomenology makes no comment upon the unconscious mind. It can only come into play when the subject is able to describe internal experiences, i.e. when material is conscious. Descriptive psychopathology is not ultimately dependent upon brain localization. It depends upon clarifying the nature of the subjective phenomenon in discussion with the patient; if links can then be shown between certain phenomena and specific brain lesions, that is, of course, highly advantageous in furthering psychiatric knowledge. Descriptive phenomenology can be a unifying factor between concepts of brain and mind. It does not ultimately depend on a particular philosophical stance on the nature of mind or brain.

Disorders of perception

Perception is a complex process which is not restricted to the screening of physical signals by sense organs but implies the processing of these data to represent reality. Ideas from structuralism, constructivism, and the philosophy of the mind have influenced psychiatric concepts of perception and the constitution of reality. Between the 1950s and 1970s Gestalt psychology highlighted the complex moulding of percepts and the disturbance of this process in psychotic phenomena. Archaic 'protopathic' Gestalt and elaborated rational 'epicritical' Gestalt processes were suggested. More recently the distinction between sensory screening and interpretative mentation has been confirmed by neurocognitive research.

Philosphical ideas have also been used. Hundert[4] used the Kantian distinction between a priori categories and a posteriori experiences as a framework for differentiating perception by the sense organs from the secondary evaluation process. Kant's emphasis on the interplay between 'distal' perception and 'proximal' conceptualization can be exemplified by the perception and recognition of faces, which are disturbed in the Capgras syndrome and to a lesser degree in schizophrenia. The processing of visual perception is organized on at least four levels of complexity: the retina, the lateral geniculate body, the occipital visual cortex, and the hippocampus. The third level (the occipital cortex), where we actually 'see', does not contain an image any more than do the preceding levels; rather, it holds a database composed of signals from specific neurones for edges, angles, curves, sudden movements, etc. Compared with the perceptual screen of the retina, these signals are 'scrambled' but even so they form a notion of what we perceive as reality. Recognition of faces needs further processing, probably in the hippocampal area where associations from other cortical fields are integrated with the visual information (e.g. the voice belonging to the face). In psychiatry we deal with very heterogeneous aetiologies and perceptual disturbances which may originate from different levels of processing, usually from a more integrated level than in neurological disease and more distant from the immediate screening of physical stimuli by the sense organs. Put in another way, psychiatric disorders of perception affect different stages of information processing—from disturbances in the sense organs to complex phenomena involving feelings and ideas.

Here we shall mainly focus on hallucinations and some related phenomena which are relevent for psychiatric illnesses.

Definitions of perceptual disturbances

Cutting[5] defines **hallucinations** as 'perception without an object (within a realistic philosophical framework) or as the appearance of an individual thing in the world without any corresponding material event (within a Kantian framework)'. There is a problem with this definition. Although some hallucinating patients mistake a hallucinatory perception for a realistic one, others can differentiate them; there is an 'as if' quality even when patients assert that they perceive real objects or events. This was demonstrated experimentally by Zucker.[6] Voices described in detail by hallucinating patients were meticulously imitated and presented to the patients without warning. The patients had no difficulty in discriminating these external voices from their hallucinations. For this reason Janzarik[7] defined hallucinations, without associating them with perception at all, as 'free running psychic contents' (using a concept similar to Jackson's disinhibition). In keeping with this idea, lack of perception may facilitate hallucinations as in sensory deprivation or in the oneiroid states of paraplegic patients.[8]

There are gradual transitions of the perceptive quality of hallucinations from similarity to sensory experiences, as in delirium, to the bizarre apprehensions of some schizophrenics. Also, the extent to which the person is affected by the hallucination varies widely from descriptions of hallucinations as film-like in amphetamine psychoses to the affectively overwhelming experiences of hallucinations associated with delusional mood.

The term **pseudohallucination** is sometimes used when the hallucinations are recognized as unreal. Jaspers[9] defined hallucinations as corporeal and tangible (*Leibhaftigkeit*); pseudohallucinations lack this quality. According to Jaspers, pseudohallucinations are not as tangible and real as hallucinatory perceptions, they appear spontaneously, they are discernible from real perception, and they are difficult, but not impossible, to overcome voluntarily. Kandinsky illustrated Jaspers' definition of pseudohallucinations with a case example. Spontaneously arising images of acquaintances arose when the patient kept his eyes closed. He was fully aware of the unrealistic character of this experience and could abandon it by opening his eyes. Thus, to Jaspers, pseudohallucinations are close to imagined images except that they arise spontaneously and are more vivid. Jaspers' definition is not used consistently in the literature. In the Anglo-American literature it is sufficient for the definition of pseudohallucination that there is subjective awareness that the percept lacks a real external equivalent and arises from the subject's mentation.

The term **imagery** describes vivid visual experiences which can be produced and manipulated voluntarily. Imagery occurs in trance states when the perceptions are produced voluntarily, but become more real and last longer than imagery occuring in a normal state of mind.

Illusions differ from hallucinations in being based on a percept of a real object or event, which is misinterpreted, usually in accordance with a mood or special theme. Illusions have to be distinguished from delusional perceptions which are percepts based on real objects to which a wrong meaning has been attached. In delusional perceptions this 'error' cannot be corrected by the patient; in illusions the true meaning can be recognized eventually.

Kurt Schneider described *Gedankenlautwerden* (also called *écho de la pensée*, or thoughts becoming aloud) as a transitional phenomenon between very vivid imagination, thoughts that are difficult to control, and auditory hallucinations. This concept is identical with that of pseudohallucinations as used in the Anglo-American literature. The patient can recognize that the words he hears are his own thoughts, but he cannot voluntarily turn them on or off. *Gedankenlautwerden* can interfere with thinking, for example disturbing concentration when talking to other people. *Gedankenlautwerden* can be differentiated from thought insertion by, for example, God or Satan, which can be distinguished from the person's own thoughts but need not be a hallucination. *Gedankenlautwerden* also differs from auditory hallucinations in that there is a lesser degree of alienation.

Klosterkötter[10] has described transitions from elementary unformed hallucinatory sensations, like a crack, bump, or hiss, through more meaningful perceptions which still can be localized 'inside' the head, to complex hallucinations which become part of a delusional cognitive structure. These transitions were related to increasing affective involvement in the themes of the hallucinations. Klosterkötter's observations support Janzarik's interpretation of hallucinations as 'free running psychic contents', as do experimental studies of model psychoses which show a regular sequence of three psychopathological states: vegetative arousal, affective change, and 'productive' phenomena like hallucinations and delusions.

Some misperceptions, found mainly in schizophrenic patients, are less complex than hallucinations, appear to be more closely related to neuropsychological disturbances, and include less systematization. They include **optical distortions** of size, colour, distance, and perspective, which can resemble experiences reported by people taking cannabis or other psychoactive drugs. These fluctuating circumscribed misperceptions are included in Huber's basic symptoms. They exemplify the way in which a more complex phenomenon of psychopathology can be built upon something more basic. Krause *et al.*[11] videotaped the non-verbal behaviour of schizophrenic patients and their healthy partners in a conversation. Very brief non-verbal cues play an important part in a dialogue, for example signalling a change of speaker or forming a non-verbal comment on the other person's words. Schizophrenic patients miss these non-verbal brief cues and are poor at judging the intentions of others; their own non-verbal communication is poorly co-ordinated. The ensuing dysfunction diminishes social competence. Schizophrenic painters who have been highly trained before the onset of their illness have been shown to misperceive perspective.[12]

Sensory modalities

Hallucinations can affect every sense modality. The most common in the idiopathic psychoses are **auditory hallucinations**, usually in the form of voices, although other kinds of sound may be associated with delusional contents. Voices talking to each other about the patient, and voices commenting about the patient's ongoing acting or thinking, are considered to be typical of but not specific to schizophrenia.[13] Voices calling the patient's name or talking without comments to the patient are considered to be nosologically non-specific.

Visual hallucinations are most frequently found in organic psychoses, particularly deliria, in which they may occur for only a couple of hours during the night if the syndrome is not full blown. Visual hallucinations, more often than those in other sensory modalities, depict animals and scenes with several persons. In alcoholic delirium in particular, optical hallucinations of fine structures (such as hairs, threads, or spider webs) occur, and are especially likely to apear if the patient stares at a white wall. A typical, although not specific, combination of hallucinations and delusions in organic psychoses is the 'siege experience', in which patients believe they are besieged by enemies and have to bar their doors and windows.

Bodily, tactile, or coenaesthetic hallucinations are associated more often with schizophrenia than with affective or organic psychoses. The phenomenology includes simple tactile sensations of the skin, sexual sensations, sensations of the contraction, expansion, or rotation of inner organs, or atypical pain. Usually these sensations are associated with delusional explanations. Tactile hallucinations localized in the skin can underlie the **delusion of parasitosis**. Elderly patients in the early stages of organic cerebral alterations are at highest risk.

Coenaesthesia is a form of misperception which may be considered as an abortive hallucination.[14] These bodily misperceptions last for minutes to days, are fluctuating (sometimes in relation to stress), and usually are not attributed to external agents or explained by delusional ideas. Patients seldom report them spontaneously. They are categorized as basic symptoms. Klosterkötter[10] suggests that when coenaesthesia is attibuted strongly to external influences, it is likely to be followed by schizophrenia.

Hallucinations may be of **gustatory or olfactory** sensations, for example a smell of gas (perhaps thought to have been infused in the flat by neighbours to kill the patient). Blunting of gustatory sensations or misperception of food as oversalted or overspiced is occasionally reported by melancholic patients.

Aetiological theories of hallucination

Aetiological theories are of three kinds:

(1) overstimulation affecting different levels of information processing;

(2) failure of inhibition of mental functions;

(3) distortion of the processing of sensory information at the interpretive level.

The work of Penfield and Perot[15] has suggested that **overstimulation** may be a pathogenetic mechanism. They stimulated the temporal regions of 500 patients, of whom 8 per cent reported scenic hallucinations, some in several modalities. Stimulation of the visual occipital cortex led to simple hallucinations like flashes, circles, stars, or lines. This phenomenon, known as *Formkonstanz*,[16] has been observed in drug-induced experimental psychosis, which is the most obvious overstimulation paradigm. It is interesting that schizophrenic patients can usually distinguish drug-induced hallucinations from those arising from their disorder. Using neural network theories, Hoffmann[17]

simulated hallucinations by using Hopfield networks; overloading the storage capacity of the network generated what can be considered as the equivalent of hallucinations.

The **disinhibition** theory originated with Hughlings Jackson, who considered that productive symptoms were caused by the disinhibition of controlling neural activities, while negative symptoms resulted from damage to the systems which generate the productive symptoms. A modern approach to disinhibition theory is sensory deprivation research using dark and sound-proofed environments, but this has yielded inconsistent results. Hallucinations, narrowly defined, seldom occur after deprivation, which may be of greater relevance to the vivid, usually visual, imaginative experiences by certain people described by Galton[18] in 1880, and later by Jaensch,[19] as 'eidetic types'. Disinhibition may also underlie the 'hypnagogic hallucinations' which can occur in healthy persons shortly before they fall asleep.

The role in the production of hallucinations of the postsensory interpretation and evaluation of stimuli is uncertain. In these terms hallucinations are a sort of deception, but this is not a sufficient description of their nature. Recent neurophysiological hypotheses and findings from neuroimaging studies have suggested that there is an 'inner censorship'[20] which deals with the ambiguities of perceptions by setting hierarchies of contingencies.

Disorders of mood

This section outlines the psychopathological elements comprising mood disorders, in particular the different varieties of depression, mania, anxiety states, and depersonalization. The account of symptoms will refer mainly to descriptive phenomenology, and only briefly to the interpretative concepts of anthropological phenomenology.

Mood can be considered as a quality of the state of mind which is more lasting than affects and feelings. Mood encompasses the whole of mentation, is not influenced by will, and is strongly related to values. The philosopher Heidegger[21] considered mood (*Stimmung, Befindlichkeit*) as the most fundamental expression of an individual's being (*Daseinsverfassung*). Kierkegaard[22] emphasized the role of existential orientation in determining mood, especially general anxiety.

The principal but not the only domain of symptoms in mood disorders is the extent and type of mood deviation. Although there are no sharp boundaries between the normal variations and pathological states of mood, the severe states are clearly abnormal and difficult to empathize. Mood can be abnormal in several ways: sad or anxious in depressive disorders; euphoric in mania; irritated in mania or agitated depression; dysphoric in depression or in mixed manic–depressive disorders; morose in chronic depressed states, often with a component of resentment; blunted (the feeling of 'having no feelings' or 'petrified' feelings) in prolonged very severe depressive disorder. Stanghellini[23] performed phenomenological analyses of depressed patients and described how a morose affect may emerge when the patient struggles against declining abilities and experiences resistance. In such cases feelings of timidity and despair may contrast with an outward appearance of hostility.

Two types of **euphoria** should be differentiated: a vital type with elation and feelings of increased spiritual, intellectual, or physical power, and a type which results from disinhibition in organic states and dementia. Other people may see this second type not as elation but as lack of interest and a negligent attitude towards the patient's actual situation.

These abnormal moods are closely related to altered **body feelings** and thinking.

Abnormal **somatic** symptoms can be divided into vegetative symptoms, such as cardiovascular dysregulation, increased sweating, and feelings of cold, and hypochondriacal symptoms, such as headaches and feelings of tightness in the chest, heavy limbs, being choked, or difficulty in swallowing. In Germany, the latter symptoms have been called 'vital' and depressive disorders which include such symptoms are known as 'vitalized'. They are considered to be related to subjective loss of energy, and are different from vegetative symptoms which represent a real somatic dysfunction.

Lopez-Ibor[24] suggested the term 'depression-equivalent' for conditions in which somatic symptoms (e.g. headaches which vary on a diurnal pattern) dominate the clinical picture. Cross-cultural research has found higher rates of such somatic symptoms in depression in Africa[25] and South America,[26] and a lower rate of guilt compared with Western industrialized countries. However, the results are not wholly consistent and reports of changing symptom profiles in American and African studies pose the question as to whether these changes are related to acculturization or to methological shortcomings in earlier studies.

A feedback loop may develop between anxiety and the **vegetative arousal**, e.g. palpitation, that accompanies it.[27,28] The prevalence of mitral valve prolapse is higher in anxiety disorder (37 per cent) than in the general population (5 per cent).[29] This finding is consistent with the idea that palpitation may lead to a conditioned anxiety response. The behaviour therapy technique of exposure aims to decondition this reflex. In social phobia and panic disorder anxiety is often complicated by anxiety-provoking situations which may lead to severe social disablement. Somatic symptoms of anxiety may be so prominent in some depressive states that patients are misdiagnosed as medically ill, with loss of weight, atypical pain, or sensory or motor disturbances. This type of depression has been called 'depressio sine depressione' or 'somatoform depression'.

Disturbances of diurnal rhythms can also be regarded as vegetative symptoms, although they influence all domains of symptomatology in mood disorders.[30] The underlying biological processes result in altered sleep architecture in the electroencephalogram with shorter REM latency (phase advance) and changes in endocrinological and cardiovascular circadian rhythms. In depression, sleep disturbance is characterized by early awakening, whereas falling asleep in the evening is often undisturbed. About 70 per cent of melancholic patients show diurnal distribution of mood, psychomotor activity, somatic symptoms, and slowed and impoverished thinking. The worst state is in the morning, with improvement in the afternoon and evening.[31]

Psychomotor retardation or acceleration is one of the most prominent symptoms of mood disorder. Often the patient's appearance and expressive movements reveal more than his or her words. The retarded patient's movements are slow, the limbs are rigid, the body is bent, and the expression is sad or anxious and does not respond to the situation. The subjective feeling may be of emptiness, weakness, and tension. If the condition is severe, it can be difficult to discriminate depressive and catatonic stupor; patients with depressive stupor seldom have increased muscular tension or rigidity. Increased psychomotor activity can appear in depression as agitation, i.e. rest-

lessness without the ability to attain goals or organize behaviour. In mania, increased psychomotor activity is also seen in sexual excesses and extravagant spending on unnecessary items.

Psychomotor retardation, and probably also acceleration, may be accompanied by a changed experience of time.[32] Depressed patients overemphasize the past, remembering guilt-connected events (*petits faux*); manic patients feel that the future is at hand. Inability to distinguish wishes from reality results in poor decision-making in both depressives and manics. Some depressives are unable even to decide how to dress in the morning. A manic patient's workroom can reflect the dissolution of his ability to distinguish between more and less important things, for example tools for immediate and frequent use and those seldom used.[33] Extreme retardation is seen in depressive stupor when patients do not move, speak, eat, or drink. Extreme acceleration occurs in mania ('the boiling over of mania') and may be accompanied by a sense of confusion.

Retardation and acceleration are closely related to depressive and manic **thought disorders**. In depression the flow of associations is reduced and slowed, and short-term memory can appear impaired (pseudodementia) (see Chapter 4.5.2). Depressed patients often ruminate about negative topics and have difficulty in terminating these thoughts. In mania, acceleration of thinking leads to a plethora of associations, 'flight of ideas', and logorrhea. Unlike patients with schizophrenic thought disorder, depressed patients retain logical connections.

The content of thoughts in mood disorders is coloured by the mood. Negative thinking about the self, the future, and the world prevails.[34] Mishaps and failures are attributed to personal faults; success is attributed to the action of other people. This depressive thinking spreads from the starting point of negative life events to more general events, and it tends to become long lasting. The fixed viewpoint that emerges is called 'cognitive schema'. After recovery from an acute episode this schema may become latent, but it can be reactivated by distressing life events. It can also prolong symptoms. Negative thinking started by minor misfortunes can become autonomous, driving down mood—which in turn intensifies negative thinking. The negative schema can prolong a depressive episode or precipitate a new one. It is uncertain whether such schemas are activated by cognitions or emotions. Probably both can do this. Guilty thoughts are closely connected with this type of thinking, and may reach the intensity of a delusion. To a degree, guilty thinking in depression is dependent on culture. In mania, the content of thought is related to the mood of elation, with diminished self-criticism and excessive self-importance. In phobic and other anxiety states, thinking centres on situations leading to anxiety. Typical contents of delusional thinking in depression concern guilt, religious failure, condemnation, personal insufficiency, impoverishment, hypochondriasis, and nihilistic ideas (e.g. the conviction of having died). In mania, delusional ideas may concern religion, with unrealistic feelings of spiritual or economic power. In contrast with schizophrenic delusions, affective delusions are synthymic, i.e. they grow out of the underlying mood exaggeration and do not appear as something new and alien to the personalilty.

Depersonalization (see later) can occur alone or as part of a depressive state. In the latter, part of the body, the self, the mind, actions, or thinking are sensed as being alienated—not belonging to the self. In mood disorders, depersonalization does not usually reach the intensity of delusion that it can in schizophrenia. Depersonalization in depression can be related to the fading of vital energy but also to anxiety, comparable with the 'emotional stupor' or 'black-out' experienced, for example, in an examination situation when a person loses memories that are normally easy to access.

Although anxiety disorders and major depression have been defined by operational criteria in the diagnostic manuals, the clinical symptoms of mood states vary considerably. Attempts have been made to define a core syndrome by using factor analyses to identify latent trait symptom profiles derived from several assessment scales and from different samples of depressives. Cross-cultural comparisons of symptom profiles can also help to identify core symptoms. Among the latent traits, retardation was found most often, together with loss of interest and alterations of diurnal rhythms. Guilt, death wishes, and affective reactivity occurred inconsistently.[25,35]

The personalities of depressive, manic, and bipolar patients have been studied before and after the onset of the disorder. There is agreement that social sensitivity, perfectionism, and dependency are very frequent features in the personality of depressives. The common features in bipolar patients are striving for autonomy, unconventional behaviour, and norm-giving behaviour. Dependency and perfectionism are probably coping attitudes to disturbed affect regulation, as well as risk factors for decompensation in response to certain life events.

Akiskal[36] has emphasized the importance of minor signs of affect dysregulation, such as temper tantrums, before the onset of affective disorders. His model of temperament (biological disposition), personality (psychological development), and character (amalgamation of both) takes into account the long-term development of the manifest syndrome, which can take a decade or more. Among the precursors to the full-blown major depression are single depressive symptoms, recurrent brief depression, and dysthymia. The viewpoint of comorbidity tries to separate personality and depression, as well as other Axis I syndromes like anxiety and alcoholism.[37]

Disorders of thinking

Types of thinking

The process resulting in a thought can vary with regard to the degree to which external reality and goal-directness are taken into account. In this perspective three types of thinking can be distinguished which represent a continuum without sharp boundaries and are intertwined in everyday life: fantasy thinking, imaginative thinking, and rational thinking.[38] Since each of these types can become dominant under some conditions, this distinction is useful to aid understanding of certain abnormal phenomena. The characterisitics of the three types can best be illustrated by considering the differences between fantasy thinking and rational thinking.

Fantasy thinking (also called dereistic or autistic thinking) produces ideas which have no external reality. This process can be completely non-goal-directed, even if the subject is to some extent aware of the mood, affect, or drive which motivates it. In other cases fantasy thinking serves to exclude reality because it requires actions that the subject does not want to accomplish. This second kind of fantasy thinking is not undirected. Its goal is not to solve a problem but to avoid it via neglect, denial, or distortion of reality. Normal subjects use fantasy thinking deliberately and sporadically. However, if its content becomes subjectively accepted as a real fact, it becomes abnormal. This pathological exclusion of reality can remain limited in extent (e.g. in

hysterical conversion and dissociation, pseudologia phantastica, and some delusions) or it may be manifested as complete autistic withdrawal from the real world.

Rational (conceptual) thinking attempts to resolve a problem through the use of logic, excluding fantasy. The accuracy of this endeavour depends on the person's intelligence, which can be affected by various disturbances of the different components involved in understanding and reasoning.

Imaginative thinking can be located between the fantasy thinking and rational thinking. It is a process of forming a representation of an object or a situation using fantasy but without going beyond the rational and possible. This thinking is goal directed but frequently leads to more general plans than the solution of immediate problems. The essential difference between imaginative and rational thinking is that the former neglects Popper's advice[39] that each theoretical assumption should be accompanied by an attempt to falsify or refute it. Imaginative thinking becomes pathological if the person attaches more weight to his representation of events than to other objectively equally possible interpretations. In overvalued ideas, the imagined interpretation surpasses other interpretations in strength; in delusions, all other possibilities are excluded.

Delusions

The term 'delusion' signifies a complex edifice of ideas in which 'delusional ideas' are linked with other ('normal') thoughts. Delusions are communicated to others in the form of judgements. In this context, the term 'delusional idea' customarily refers to pathologically falsified judgements for which three criteria have been proposed: the unrivalled conviction with which they are held, their lack of amenability to experiences or compelling counterarguments, and the impossibility of their content.[40] The last criterion must be discarded for two reasons. Firstly, collective beliefs derived from the sociocultural setting of a person can be considered, in other surroundings, as false or impossible. Taking this into account, delusion is often defined as a 'false unshakable belief which is out of keeping with the patient's social and cultural background'.[38] Secondly, in certain delusions (e.g. delusional jealousy) the content does not go beyond the possible. Thus delusions are best defined as overriding rigid convictions which create a self-evident, private, and isolating reality requiring no proof.[41]

The genesis of delusions

Delusions can occur for various reasons. Jaspers[40] introduced the distinction between primary and secondary delusions. He supposed that the first, called true delusional ideas, are characterized by their 'psychological irreducibility', whereas the second, called delusion-like ideas, emerge understandably from disturbing life experiences or from other morbid phenomena, such as pathological mood states or misperceptions. This led to the assumption that primary delusions are the direct expression of specific somatic dysfunctions which are frequently considered to be the basis of schizophrenia. Four types of primary delusions have been distinguished in this perspective.

1. **Delusional intuitions** (autochthonous delusions), occurring spontaneously, 'out of the blue'.

2. **Delusional percepts**, in which a normal perception acquires a delusional significance. Schneider[42] assumed that the 'psycho-

logical irreductibility' was clearly evident in this process, and included delusional percepts among his 'first rank symptoms' of schizophrenia.

3. **Delusional memories** can be distorted or false memories coming spontaneously into the mind like delusional intuitions. In other cases they occur, like delusional percepts, in two stages which means that normal memories are interpreted with delusional meaning.

4. **Delusional atmosphere** refers to an ensemble of minuscule and almost unnoticed experiences which impart a new and bewildering aspect to a situation. The world seems to have been subtly altered; something uncanny seems to be going on in which the subject feels personally involved, but without knowing how. From this uncertainty evolves first certainty of self-reference and then the formation of fully structured and specific delusional meanings. The apparent change in the surrounding situation is accompanied by tension, depression, or suspicion, and by anxious or even exciting expectations, so that it is often called 'delusional mood'.

The primary–secondary distinction assumes that the delusional atmosphere is part of the process underlying all primary delusional phenomena. If this preliminary perturbation is not perceived clearly or is not communicated by the patient as a general change in the situation, it may be manifested only as single delusional percepts, intuitions, or memories. In cases in which the initial change in the whole atmosphere is experienced clearly, a subsequent restriction on a perceived detail of the environment, or on a fully formed delusional idea, can lead to a release from the preceding perplexity. The origin of primary delusions is then commonly attributed to a basic cognitive anomaly perturbing information-processing, which reduces the influence of past experiences on current perception. This is considered to entail a heightened awareness of irrelevant stimuli and an ambiguous unstructured sensory input allowing the intrusion of unexpected and unintended material from long-term memory.[43]

The assumption of a purely cognitive origin for some delusional phenomena is called into question by the hypothesis that delusions only occur if they are preceded by affective disturbances. This standpoint is thrown into relief in Janzarik's concept of the 'structural-dynamic coherence'. Janzarik[7] designates as 'dynamic' a fundamental realm including affectivity and drive which he contrasts with the 'psychic structure' containing inborn recognition patterns and acquired representations. The inborn recognition patterns as well as some of the acquired representations are dynamically invested, i.e. linked with positive, negative, or ambivalent feelings. Normally, these dynamically loaded elements ('values') are kept permanently in the background by neutral representations based on learned experiences which assure a realistic critical evaluation of the situation. In addition to the feelings tied to structural elements, everybody has a certain amount of 'free floating dynamic' which may develop into a depressive, anxious, euphoric, or irritable state.

If these dynamic fluctuations reach a morbid level, reality testing becomes distorted by the exaggerated influence of values. Stable modifications of the dynamic background make the corresponding values powerful. Dynamic restriction, for example in depression, activates solely negative values which can no longer be conterbalanced by a critical evaluation of possible positive aspects of the situation. Dynamic expansion, as in mania, produces the opposite effect. In states of dynamic instability, rapid changes occur in the activation of different values, causing the puzzling uncertainty of the delusional atmosphere. In the case of schizophrenia the dynamic instability is hypothetically attributed to 'irritation' provoked by perturbed information-processing[44] or to an increased state of arousal produced by the neurochemical changes underlying the basic cognitive disturbance.[45] Similar fluctuations of affectivity and drive may occur in other conditions, for instance in temperamentally hyper-reactive personalities or rapidly alternating manic–depressive mixed states. This casts doubt on the assumption that delusional atmosphere is specific for schizophrenia.

The content of delusions

The content of delusions is determined by the mood in which they emerge and evolve, by the patient's personality and sociocultural background, and by previous life experiences. In principle, the content can embrace all kinds of presumptions which have been placed in separate categories based on certain characteristics. The following six main delusional themes are usually distinguished:

- **delusions of persecution** based on the assumption that the patient is pursued, spied upon, or harassed

- **delusional jealousy**

- **delusions of love** characterized by the patient's conviction that another person is in love with him or her

- **delusions of guilt**, unworthiness, and poverty which may sometimes reach the degree of 'nihilistic delusions' in which the patient believes that real world has disappeared completely

- **grandiose delusions** in which patients are convinced that they have great talents, are prominent in society, or possess supernatural powers

- **hypochondriacal delusions** founded on the conviction of having a serious disease.

The mood state when delusional ideas emerge favours certain themes. Delusions of guilt, or unworthiness, and hypochondriacal delusions are strongly linked with depression. Grandiose and erotic delusions generally occur in euphoric, excited, or manic states. Delusions of persecution and jealousy emerge most frequently from suspicious mood states or a delusional atmosphere, but they are occasionally observed in depressed subjects.

This broad thematic classification has been supplemented by categories taking into account specific contents:

- **religious delusions** which occur most commonly with grandiose delusions or delusions of guilt

- **delusions of infestation** which are a subtype of hypochondriacal delusions and are characterized by the conviction of infestation by small organisms

- **delusional misidentification** in which the patient believes, on the basis of a delusional percept, that a perceived person has been replaced by an imposter, or in which he is convinced that another person has been physically transformed into his own self

- **delusions of control** in which the patient experiences sensations, feelings, drives, volition, or thoughts as made or influenced by others (this type of delusion occurs in schizophrenia and is believed to result from cognitive dysfunction consisting of a failure of the system which monitors willed intentions[46].

The structure of delusions

The structure of delusions contains three criteria.

1. The alternatives 'logical' or 'paralogical' indicate whether or not the connection of ideas is consistent with logical thinking.

2. The notions 'organized' or 'unorganized' indicate whether or not the delusional ideas are integrated into a formed concept. Highly organized logical delusional edifices are known as 'systematized delusions'.

3. The third criterion concerns the relationship between delusional reality and reality:

    *   in **polarized delusions** the delusional reality is inextricably intermingled with actual facts

    *   if the delusional beliefs and reality exist side by side without influencing one another, we speak of **juxtaposition**

    *   in **autistic delusions** the patient takes no account of reality and lives wholly in a delusional world.

Overvalued ideas

An overvalued idea is a basically acceptable and comprehensible notion which preoccupies the subject to the extent of dominating his life. Overvalued ideas embrace inferences or apprehensions to which an undue probability is attributed, goals pursued beyond the bounds of reason, or overwhelming desires.

Overvalued ideas of prejudice (overvalued paranoid ideas) are characterized by an underlying self-referent interpretation of the behaviour or sayings of others; patients asume themselves to be overlooked, slighted, unfairly treated, provoked, or loved. Overvalued apprehesions become apparent as morbid jealousy, hypochondriacal phobias (e.g. parasitophobia), or dysmorphophobia in which patients assume that they attract attention because of a real or presumed bodily defect. In anorexia nervosa subjects are preoccupied by the endeavour to remain thin, and in transsexualism by the desire to change gender because they feel that they belong to the opposite sex.

Overvalued ideas generally occur in abnormal personalities whose 'psychic structure' contains representations which have become excessively dynamically invested by learning processes or previous experiences. Temperamental variants can then shape the clinical picture. Thus hyperthymic subjects may develop, on the basis of a presumed injustice, querulous or litigious paranoid overvalued ideas. Sometimes the ideas become overvalued only during abnormal mood states (of various origins) which set aside counterbalancing influences.

Phobic and anankastic disorders

Phobic and anankastic phenomena have in common that the patient experiences them as unwanted but cannot suppress them. They often occur together.

Phobic states

Phobias are inappropriate exaggerated fears which are not under voluntary control, cannot be reasoned away, and entail avoidance behaviour.[47] The fears are kindled by particular stimuli. These may either be perceived objects, such as animals (animal phobia) or pustules (in some illness phobias), or situations such as open places (agoraphobia) or confined rooms (claustrophobia).

Phobias initially triggered by a very specific stimulus can eventually generalize. Thus an elevator phobia may become extended to all kinds of closed rooms. Some phobias are linked with broader circumstances from the beginning. In social phobia, for instance, patients avoid meeting people because they fear that they will be noticed because of certain body features or personality traits. Identical types of fears can be triggered by different stimuli in different subjects. Thus illness phobia is activated in some patients by observed body changes, but in others by situations involving the risk of infection.

Phobic states are characterized by avoidance behaviour: patients avoid anxiety-provoking objects or situations. Because of stimulus generalization, this can lead to severe impairments; for instance, they cannot leave home.

Anankastic states

Anankastic phenomena are divided into two subtypes.

1. Obsessions occur as repeated thoughts, memories, images, ruminations, or impulses that patients know to be their own but are unable to prevent. The content of these ideas is often unpleasant, terrifying, obscure, or aggressive.

2. Compulsions are actions, rituals, or behaviours that the patient recognizes as part of his own behaviour, but cannot resist successfully.

Combined syndromes

In phobic–anankastic syndromes patients attempt to reduce their phobic fears by certain actions, such as handwashing in the case of an infection phobia. If obsessional thoughts or impulses induce anxiety (e.g. obscene ideas during worship, or the impulse to lean too far over a balustrade) and entail the avoidance of the situations that provoke them, the term anankastic–phobic syndrome is used.

Phobias, obsessions, and compulsions result most frequently from neurotic intrapsychic conflicts, but they also arise in functional or organic mental disorders. In all cases, conditioning processes are involved. Anankastic personalities, characterized by perfectionism, rigidity, sensitivity, and indecisiveness, are especially prone to developing obsessions and compulsions.

Disorder of the thinking process

The term 'thinking process' refers to the production of a thought. Disturbances of this process may be recognized and described by the patient himself or be deduced by an observer from the subject's speech.[48]

Impairments of thought production are conventionally named 'formal thought disorder' and contrast with abnormalities of the 'content of thought' observed in delusions. This distinction appears arbitrary, since the deviant reality-testing of deluded patients always involves a disturbance of the form of thinking.

Disorders of the flow of thinking

Association psychology indicates that the semantic memory is organized in the form of a network. This means that each representation is linked with a number of other notions, related closely as well as distantly. In rational thinking, a 'determining tendency'[40] guides the flow of ideas in the chosen direction and excludes associations which do not conform with this goal. This procedure can be disturbed in various ways which are commonly grouped together under the heading of 'formal thought disorder'.

Disturbances of the speed of thinking

In **acceleration** of thinking, associations are still formed normally but at a grossly accelerated speed. The goal is not maintained for long and the intervention of new thoughts can reach the degree of 'flight of ideas'.

Retardation refers to a slowing down of the thinking process which hampers the formation of associations and may prevent the patient from reaching the original goal of his thoughts. This results in difficulties in concentration and decision-making.

Acceleration and retardation of thinking are due to a change of affect, and are characteristic of mood disorders.

Circumstantiality

In circumstantiality the determining tendency is maintained but the patient can reach the goal only after having exhaustively explored all unnecessary associations arising in his mind. When answering a question, he relates many irrelevant details before returning to the point. This inability to exclude unimportant associations occurs in organic mental disorders and in mental retardation.

Perseveration

Perseveration is found in organic mental disorders and is defined as an inability to shift from one theme to another; a thought is retained long after it has become inappropriate in the given context. For example, a patient may give a correct answer to the first question, but repeats the same response to a subsequent completely different inquiry.

Interruptions in the flow of thinking

Thought blocking is a sudden unintended cessation in the train of thought, experienced by the patient as 'snapping off'. After this breaking off, which may even occur in the middle of a sentence, the previous idea may be taken up again or replaced by another thought. Thought blocking occurs in organic states, in depression, and frequently in schizophrenia where it is described as part of negative thought disorder.

In **loosening of associations** the flow of thinking is interrupted by deviations towards distant or unrelated thoughts, in contrast with flight of ideas in which there is only a speeding up of access to nearby associations. Since loosening of associations leads to the production of abnormal concepts, it is considered to be positive formal thought disorder. In **tangentiality** the ideas deviate towards an obliquely related theme. In **fusion**, different kinds of associations evoked by an original thought are blended to produce a word or sentence. **Derailment** is characterized by the interpolation of ideas which neither the patient nor the observer can link with the previous stream of thought. **Muddling** designates an extreme degree of derailment and fusion.

Neuropsychological research suggests that loosening of associations may be caused by a failure of inhibition in the associative network,[49] occurring as positive thought disorder in schizophrenia. In organic states, incoherent thinking, which is clinically similar to derailments, may be attributable to a primary intellectual impairment and not to an increased spread of associations.

Overinclusive thinking

This kind of thought disorder is not based on an interruption of the flow of thought but on an inability to preserve conceptual boundaries; ideas only distantly related to the concept under consideration become incorporated in it.[50] Overinclusive thinking occurs in schizophrenia, and also in other psychotic and neurotic disorders.

Concrete and abstract thinking

In organic mental disorders and subnormality of intelligence, inability to think abstractly may be attributed to a diminished capacity to structure a concept. The **concrete thinking** of schizophrenics may be caused by a dysfunction of working memory;[49] the patient cannot keep in mind the abstract use of a notion relevant in a given context and slips into more concrete meanings. This process may be enhanced by loosening of associations. The fact that schizophrenics sometimes manifest overly **abstract thinking** may also be explained by a disturbance of working memory such that the concrete meaning of the initial thought is not retained.

Disorder of control of thinking

In **obsessions** and **compulsions** the subject recognizes his thoughts as being produced by himself but is unable to control them.

In **passivity of thought**, the patient experiences his thoughts as manipulated by alien influences. The interpretations resulting from this feeling are described as 'thought withdrawal', 'thought insertion', or 'thought broadcasting' (which denotes the patient's conviction that his thoughts are diffused to other people). These 'delusions of the control of thought' were included by Schneider[42] among his 'first rank symptoms' of schizophrenia.

A particular variation of thought insertion occurring in schizophrenia is **crowding of thoughts**. In this condition, the patient experiences an excessive increase in the amount of thoughts imposed from the outside and compressed in his mind.

Language and speech disorder

'Speech disorder' refers to defects in the ability to generate and pronounce verbal statements, whereas 'language disorder' designates deficits in the use of language.[51] In view of frequent difficulties in making this distinction, the two terms are often used interchangeably.

In medical nomenclature the prefix 'a' denotes the complete loss of an ability, and the prefix 'dys' denotes a less pronounced impairment. However, this principle is not always followed strictly. Thus the terms 'aphasia' and 'dysphasia' are often used synonymously.

Disturbed generation and pronounciation of words

Aphonia designates the inability to vocalize. Thus whispering occurs in somatic illnesses (paralysis of cranial nerve IX or diseases of the vocal cords) and hysteria. **Dysphonia** is a somatic impairment with hoarseness.

Dysarthria refers to disorders of articulation occurring in various malformations or diseases which impair the mechanisms of phonation, in lesions of the brain stem, in schizophrenia, and in psychogenic disorders.

The causes of **stuttering and stammering** are still unclear, but they are often considered to be of neurotic origin. **Logoclonia** (the spastic repetition of syllables) occurs in parkinsonism (paralysis agitans).

Disturbances in talking

'Disturbances in talking' was proposed by Scharfetter[41] as a generic term for disorders of speech or language not belonging to the preceding group of disturbances.

Changes in volume of sound and in intonation occur in affective and schizophrenic states, and refer to loud excited and quiet monotonous speech.

Bradyphasia (decelerated talking) and **tachyphasia** (accelerated talking) occur in mood disorders, schizophrenia, and organic dysphasias.

Logorrhea (verbosity) is observed in various disorders, especially in manic states.

Alogia (poverty of speech) is a decrease in spontaneous talking; it occurs in depression and schizophrenia.

In **poverty of content of speech** the amount of speech is adequate but conveys little information. This is often related to schizophrenic disorganization of thinking.

Verbigeration is the monotonous repetition of syllables and words observed in organic language disorders, schizophrenia, and agitated depression.

Echolalia is the repetition of words or parts of sentences that are spoken by others. It can be observed in schizophrenia, organic states, and subnormality.

Sometimes patients give **approximate answers**, i.e. they avoid giving correct answers to questions that they have obviously understood. This occurs in organic disorders, schizophrenia, and hysteria.

Paraphasia is often used as a synonym for approximate answers. More strictly defined, it denotes the enunciation of an inappropriate sound instead of a word or phrase. This happens in organic speech disorders but may also have psychogenic causes.

Speech may be unintelligible for various reasons. **Paragrammatism** and **parasyntax** (loss of grammatical and syntactical coherence) occur in organic mental disorders and excited manic states, and in schizophrenics whose severe thought derailments become manifest as 'word salad'. **Private symbolism** can be observed in schizophrenics in three forms: use of existing words with a particular symbolic meaning, creation of 'neologisms' (new words with an idiosyncratic meaning), and production of a private incomprehensible language, which may be spoken (cryptolalia) or written (cryptographia).

Mutism (refraining from speech) may be found in various kinds of psychiatric disorder. It is a cardinal feature of stupor and also occurs as a 'hysterical' reaction to stress.

Pseudologia fantastica is characterized by excessive fluent lying which is developed into a fantastic construct. This 'mythomania' occurs in hysterical and asocial personality disorders.

Organic language disorders

This term embraces impairments of spontaneous language, naming, writing, and reading, occurring as a result of differently localized brain dysfunctions, which are sometimes combined. These disorders can be divided into 'sensory' (receptive) and 'motor' (expressive) defects containing the following principal subcategories. Dysphasic patients often present with a mixture of receptive and expressive disturbances.

Sensory language disorders

In **primary sensory dysphasia** the patient cannot understand the speech of others. His own speech remains fluent, but contains errors in the use of words, syntax, and grammar. Writing and reading are also impaired. If, in this condition, the patient's speech becomes unintelligible, the disturbance is called 'jargon aphasia'. If only the repetition of a message is disturbed, the disorder is named 'conduction dysphasia'.

In **pure word-deafness** speech, reading, and writing are fluent and correct. The patient hears words as sounds, but cannot recognize their meaning. In **pure word-blindness** (alexia) speech and writing are normal but the patient cannot read with understanding.

Motor language disorders

In **primary motor dysphasia** the verbal or written expression of words and the construction of sentences is disturbed, but the understanding of speech and writing are preserved.

In **pure word-dumbness** the disturbance is limited to an inability to produce and repeat words at will. **Pure agraphia** is an isolated inability to write. **Nominal dysphasia** is an inability to produce names and nouns.

Disorders of intellectual performance

Conceptualization of intelligence

'Intelligence' refers to the capacity to solve problems, to cope with new situations, to acquire skills through learning and experiences, to establish logical deductions, and to form abstract concepts. Several specific abilities, such as the capacity to produce spatial representations, perceptual speed, ability to calculate, comprehension of verbal meanings, memory, verbal fluency, and reasoning, have been isolated as mutually interdependent components of intelligence.[52] Some authors have suggested that there is, in addition to these specific abilities, a unitary general factor of intelligence[53] on which the capacity to recognize and establish meaningful connections is based.

Measurements of intelligence

Individual intellectual capacity is graded by reference to the intelligence quotient (**IQ**) which is defined as the ratio of a subject's intelligence to the average intelligence for his or her age. The assessment of intelligence is considered in Chapter 1.10.3.1.

In addition to the global assessment of intelligence, numerous tests have been developed to assess organic impairment, scholastic achievement, and aptitudes.

Mental retardation (learning disability)

If the development of intellectual performance does not reach an IQ level of 70, the condition is called 'mental retardation'. This condition can be subdivided according to its severity. Four levels are recognized in ICD-10:

- mild (IQ 50–69)
- moderate (IQ 35–49)
- severe (IQ 20–34)
- profound (IQ below 20).

The causes of mental retardation are considered in Part 10.

Disorders of later onset

In these disorders normally developed intellectual performance declines. This can occur as a result of organic brain disorders, and in psychotic and affective disorders.

Organic disorders may have toxic, traumatic, inflammatory, or hypoxic causes. If these conditions are treated successfully, the disturbance can be arrested or even reversed.

In dementia there is a progressive disintegration of intellectual function, which usually begins insidiously and is often first recognized through an impairment of memory.

In psychotic states the distorted testing and evaluation of reality can impair intellectual performance. In schizophrenia, formal thought disorder can contribute to this effect.

Severe affective disorder can impair perception, attention, and motivation, leading to poor intellectual performance. These disturbances are observed more often in depression, but can occur in manic mood.

Disorders of self and body image

Disorders of self

These describe the abnormal inner experiences of I-ness and my-ness which occur in psychiatric disorders. Scharfetter has added the characteristic of awareness of being or ego vitality to the four formal characteristics previously described by Jaspers: feeling of awareness of activity, awareness of unity, awareness of identity, and awareness of the boundaries of self.[2,54]

Disorder of the awareness of being

This disorder is demonstrated by **nihilistic delusions**, which frequently occur in severe depressive illness and are a feature of the eponymous Cotard's syndrome.[55] Non-psychotic abnormality is exemplified by **depersonalization** in which the sufferer experiences his mental activity, body, or surroundings as changed in quality to become unreal, remote, or automatized.

Disorder of awareness of activity

Disorder of the awareness of activity occurs with neurological lesions, such as some dyspraxias, and also in psychotic conditions in which the individual believes that no action has occurred when it has, or vice versa. This does not include action that the patient knows he has executed but with a belief it was under the influence of another. Non-psychotic disorder of activity occurs when an individual believes that he has no freedom of action and that his range of choice is limited by external circumstances, for instance a person with depressive symptoms who believes that nothing can be done to improve his state of incompetence.

Disorder of awareness of singleness

An awareness of one's essential unity implies that at any given moment 'I know that I am one person'. Disorder occurs in the rare visual perceptual experience of **autoscopy**.[56] Non-psychotic examples of disorder of singleness include both multiple personality disorder and the double phenomenon; the latter was described by Jaspers.[2] The essential feature of **multiple personality disorder** is the apparent existence of two or more distinct personalities within an individual, with only one of them being evident at any time. The **double phenomenon** is much more frequent, and describes the self-experience of those who feel that there are two different parts of themselves in conflict with each other, causing problems in all areas of life, but they are fully aware of both at the same time.

Disorder of awareness of identity

Disorder of identity is characterized by **delusion of control** or **passivity experience**, in which the sufferer believes that he has been taken over by an alien, with the belief that there is a break in continuity from 'myself' who was there before. Non-psychotic disorder of awareness of identity is exemplified by **possession disorder**, in which there is a temporary loss of the sense of personal identity and the individual may act *as if* they have been taken over by another personality, spirit, or force.

Disorder of the awareness of boundaries of self

Disorder of boundaries of self occurs in Schneiderian first-rank symptoms of schizophrenia such as thought withdrawal, control, and diffusion.[57] The patient believes that thoughts 'which I thought were under my own control are being taken out of me, influenced by an outside source'. Non-psychotic disorder of the boundaries of self occurs in ecstasy states, characteristically described as an 'as if' experience. There is disturbance of boundaries of self in that the individual may feel that there is no limit between self and the outside world.

Depersonalization

Depersonalization is the experience of one's own feelings and experiences being detached, distant, not one's own, lost or altered. Derealization is the same range of subjectivity describing awareness of the outside world. The sufferer recognizes that this is a subjective change and is not imposed by outside forces. Because the sufferer finds it difficult to describe, this experience tends to be underdiagnosed, but the misery it causes and the disturbance in functioning is considerable; it is experienced as being so subjectively unpleasant that not uncommonly deliberate self-harm results.

Disorders of awareness of the body

Bodily complaint without organic cause

Such conditions create difficulties for psychopathological understanding.

1. Aetiology is often obscure, sometimes with doubt that there may be an unrevealed physical cause.

2. The descriptive terms used come from different theoretical backgrounds and have changed their meaning over the years.

3. There is often discrepancy between the meanings attached to the symptoms by the patient and by the doctor.

ICD-10 lists a category 'Somatoform disorders' which includes both somatization and hypochondriacal disorders.[58] Somatoform disorders are characteristically repeated presentation of physical symptoms with persistent requests for medical investigation despite repeated negative findings and reassurance by doctors that the symptoms have no physical basis. The patient with **somatization** as the prominent disorder complains of multiple recurrent and often changing physical symptoms in different bodily systems over a prolonged time. However, the patient with **hypochondriasis** has a persistent preoccupation with bodily function, the possibility of illness, and the seriousness with which symptoms should be treated. Not infrequently these two groups of symptoms overlap. Comorbid anxiety and depression is quite frequent with both somatization and hypochondriasis.

The content of hypochondriasis may take the form of delusion, overvalued ideas, hallucination, anxious or depressive rumination, or anxious preoccupation.

In ICD-10 the term 'Dissociative (conversion) disorder' has replaced the confusing but graphic term hysteria. **Conversion symptoms** can be categorized as motor, sensory (including pain), or psychological. Motor symptoms include weakness or paralysis of limbs or part of a limb and abnormality of gait; sensory symptoms include glove and stocking anaesthesia. Amongst the psychological symptoms is a narrowing of the field of consciousness with selective amnesia such as may occur in fugue states. For conversion disorder, or hysteria, to be diagnosed, symptoms should appear to be psychogenic in nature, causation should be thought to be unconscious, symptoms may carry some sort of advantage to the patient, and they occur by the mediation of the processes of conversion or dissociation.

Artefactual illness includes two categories: elaboration of physical symptoms for psychological reasons, and intentional production or feigning of symptoms or disabilities, either physical or psychological. Conversion symptoms are believed to arise without the patient's conscious involvement, but artefactual illness implies that the illness, lesion, or complaint is ultimately the individual's own conscious production. **Malingering** implies feigning or producing symptoms expressly for the social advantages of being regarded as ill, while the broader category of artefactual illness includes other motivations and simply describes the behaviour.

Narcissism is not generally accepted as a disease entity but is useful to consider as a psychopathological symptom. It is an exaggerated concern with one's self-image, especially with personal appearance. This absorption with self is usually associated with marked feelings of insecurity and ambivalence concerning the self, with feelings of threat to one's integrity.

Dislike of the body and distortion of body image are subjectively different experiences but often occur together, for example in anorexia nervosa or with gross obesity. In **dysmorphophobia** the primary symptom is the patient's belief that he or she is unattractive. Sufferers believe themselves to have a physical defect, such as the size of their nose or breasts, that is noticeable to other people, but objectively their appearance lies within normal limits. The dissatisfaction with their appearance, the extent to which they feel others are aware of disfigurement, the distress this causes, and the consequences in suicidal or other self-destructive behaviour are out of proportion to the significance of the abnormality, even if such an abnormality were present. The content disorder of dysmorphophobia takes the psychopathological form of an overvalued idea in which the degree of concern and consequent distress is clearly out of proportion and comes to dominate the whole of life. The overvalued idea of dysmorphophobia may be associated with an underlying personality disorder of anankastic or dependent type or with other psychiatric disorders.

Awareness of body size and **disturbance of eating** frequently occur together; alteration of body image is associated with eating disorder. Obesity in adolescence in diet-conscious Western societies frequently results in self-loathing, more frequently in girls than boys, with overestimation of body fatness and a pathological fear of seeing themselves in mirrors. Disturbance of body image occurs in sufferers from anorexia nervosa, characteristically an overestimate of width with an accurate estimation of height or the width of inanimate objects. The more 'over-fat' an individual considers herself to be, the more dissatisfaction with herself she will experience.[59] Such disorders

of self-image, with significant overestimation of size and discrepancy between perceived and desired size, also occur in bulimia nervosa and may be associated with depression of mood and feelings of guilt and unworthiness.

Organic changes in body image

Organic change may result from either damage to the conceptualized object (e.g. following amputation, with a phantom limb) or damage to the process of conceptualization (e.g. section of the corpus callosum). Hyperschemazia or pathological accentuation of body image occurs when physical illness or neurological lesion causes enhancement of perception of an organ. Diminished or absent body image (hyposchemazia, aschemazia) may occur when innervation is lost or with parietal lobe lesions. The diminution of body image may be simple (e.g. loss or neglect of a limb) or complex. There may also be distortions of the body image (paraschemazia) in which enhancement or diminution of parts of the body may occur.

Disorder of gender and sexuality

Core gender identity is established very early in life and then retained—biologically influenced and socially reinforced. **Transsexualism** is a disorder of gender identity, much more common in biological males, in which there is discrepancy between anatomical sex and the gender that the person assigns to himself. The subjective belief is an overvalued idea, often taken to an extreme degree. (See Chapters 4.11.4 and 9.2.12.)

The more commonly occurring disorders of sexuality can be divided, psychopathologically, into disorders of sexual preference, psychological and behavioural disorders associated with sexual development and orientation, and psychosexual dysfunction—conditions which are phenomenologically distinct. Subjective experience of deviance in sexual preference is largely determined by its social context; only those exhibiting behaviour that causes difficulties in relationships with others or is overtly illegal will usually be seen by a psychiatrist. Amongst disorders of development and orientation are those where the individual has uncertainty concerning gender identity and sexual orientation. Psychosexual dysfunction implies symptoms associated with normal heterosexual intercourse, usually divided into those occurring amongst males, those occurring amongst females, or problems in the sexual relationship.

Pain as a psychopathological entity

Pain is a subjective experience which only occurs in consciousness; it is hard to describe and categorize, and it is not well charted phenomenologically. It appears to have more in common with disorder of mood than disorder of perception. Pain associated with psychiatric illness tends to be more diffuse and less well localized and to spread with non-anatomical distribution. It also tends to be complained of constantly, becoming even more severe at times but persisting without remission. It may clearly be seen to be associated with underlying disturbance of mood which appears to be primary in time and causation. It is more difficult to describe clearly the quality of psychogenic pain. Psychogenic pain tends to progress in severity and extent over time. Persistent, severe, and distressing pain which cannot be explained fully by a physiological process or physical disorder has been designated **persistent somatoform pain disorder**. (See Chapter 5.2.6.)

Insight

The clinical assessment of a patient's capacity to understand the nature, significance, and severity of his or her own illness has been called insight. Recently there has been increased interest in describing its characteristics more reliably and establishing how it correlates with other measures of illness.[60] The attitude of patients towards their illness has clear clinical implications, and the assessment of insight tries to investigate the awareness of patients about the impact that their illness has has had on their world, and their capacity to adapt to the changes brought about by illness. In clinical practice, the patient's awareness of the presence of illness and the extent to which it is interfering with function and compliance with prescribed treatment are of considerable significance. David[60] has proposed that insight is composed of three overlapping dimensions: the ability to relabel unusual mental events as pathological, the recognition that one has mental illness, and compliance with treatment. Some parallels have been drawn between the loss of insight in psychiatric patients and the denial of disease or loss of function that occurs in certain neurological conditions.

Because of its importance for clinical management of the patient there have been many attempts over recent years to measure insight, all of which depend upon a precise operational definition of the concept. McEvoy et al.[61] developed a questionnaire to measure insight based upon the definition that it was patients' awareness of the pathological nature of their experiences and also their agreement with the treating professionals about the need for treatment. The measure constructed by David et al.[62] added the ability to relabel unusual mental events as pathological to the recognition of mental illness and compliance with treatment. Other scales have included different features, but these core symptoms appear to have the most influence on clinical management.

The relationship between impairment of insight and the presence of other aspects of psychopathology is complicated; there is no clear association between impairment of insight and intellectual or neuropsychological deficit.[63] Not surprisingly, patients with unimpaired insight are found to be significantly less likely to require readmission to hospital, tend to be more compliant with treatment, and show an improved prognosis.[64] Surprisingly, and this shows how little is known about this subject, many patients are prepared to comply with treatment, even though they do not believe themselves to be ill, if the social milieu is conducive to receiving treatment.[61]

Insight is a multifaceted phenomenon with considerable clinical significance as it predicts the likelihood of patients complying with treatment. Attempts have been made to operationalize the concept and to devise scales to measure it. However, the features to be included in a definition have not yet been universally agreed. Most studies of insight have been concerned exclusively with patients suffering from schizophrenia, and it is important to extend work to other serious mental illnesses. On this topic descriptive phenomenology has implications for therapeutic practice.

Motor symptoms and signs

Motor symptoms and signs may be due to a neurological disorder causing organic brain syndrome, such as rigidity in Parkinson's disease, or may be related to emotional states such as restlessness or

Table 1 Symptoms and signs of motility disorder

Catalepsy (synonym: waxy flexibility, flexibilitas cerea)	Maintaining uncomfortable positions against resistance
Posturing	Maintaining uncomfortable positions that may have a delusional meaning
Stupor	Inability to communicate despite being awake
Akinesia	Inability to move
Mutism	Inability to speak
Echolalia	Repetition of another person's speech
Echopraxia	Repetition of another person's acts
Mannerism	Uncommon conspicuous expression by gestures, speech, or objects
Grimacing	Uncommon conspicuous facial expression
Stereotypy	Repetition of actions
Verbigeration	Repetition of speech
Tic	Rapid movements of facial or limb muscles
Akathisia	Inability to remain seated or standing
Psychomotor retardation	Slowing of mental and motor activity
Psychomotor agitation	Arousal of mental and motor activity (typically by anxiety)

tremor in anxiety. However, there is a further group of symptoms which affect voluntary movements and often occur in functional psychoses. These symptoms are neither unequivocally neurological nor clearly psychogenic in origin and are termed **motility disorder** by some authors. Table 1 gives a glossary of disordered motility. Whether patients are unable or unwilling to move normally is still a matter of debate. The origin of motility symptoms may well be a functional (rather than a morphological) abnormality of basal ganglia.

A further classification of motility disorder distinguishes psychomotor hyperphenomena (e.g. tic disorder), hypophenomena (e.g. stupor), and paraphenomena (e.g. mannerism).[65] **Tics** are rapid irregular movements involving groups of facial or limb muscles. **Stupor** is a state in which a patient does not communicate, i.e. does not speak (mutism) or move (akinesia), although he or she is alert. **Mannerisms** are uncommon; they are conspicuous expressions by gesture, speech, or objects (e.g. dress) that seem to have a particular meaning, mostly delusional.

A disorder characterized by disturbed motility is called **catatonia**. It occurs most frequently in schizophrenia, and less frequently in general medical conditions and major depression. A number of conditions, such as brain tumour, encephalitis, and endocrine and metabolic disorders, may elicit catatonic symptoms. Catatonia may take the form of hypomobility or immobility, and in extreme cases leads to catatonic stupor. Alternatively it may present as excessive motoric activity (catatonic excitement), an extreme state that might be harmful and dangerous to the patient and to others. An important symptom of catatonia is **catalepsy**, in which uncomfortable and bizarre postures are maintained against gravity or attempts to rectify them. An examiner trying to move a cataleptic limb passively will notice a 'waxy flexibility', which is quite different from rigidity or spasticity. **Echo phenomena** may occur when the patient is interacting with another person and present as echolalia (imitation of the speech of others) or echopraxia (imitation of the actions of others).

Disordered speech may also be regarded as a sign of disordered motility, as shown in the signs of mutism or verbigeration, whereas aphasia is a focal neurological symptom.

In **delirium** tremor often occurs as a vegetative sign. Anxiety is accompanied by restlessness. A particular motor pattern in delirium tremens (alcohol withdrawal delirium) makes it look as though the patient is collecting a large number of objects or brushing away dust from his blanket. Typically, the movements never seem to achieve what they are meant to and, of necessity, are therefore repetitive. Patients may show fragments of purposeful actions which, however, achieve no goal. Suggestibility in delirium may lead to movements which are based on erroneous assumptions, such as trying to take hold of a proffered, but non-existent, thread. Patients may develop panic and try to flee. Speech may be hurried and indistinct. In some cases of delirium, such as that due to hepatic failure, patients may be hypoactive before becoming drowsy and comatose. Hepatic failure may also result in catatonic disorder.

A number of conditions, such as brain tumour, encephalitis, and endocrine and metabolic disorders, may elicit catatonic symptoms. Patients with a variety of mental disorders may show abnormal movements that are of histrionic nature. They may throw themselves to the ground, seek and maintain bodily contact, or show psychomotor agitation. Alternatively, there may be psychogenic paresis.

In dementia there may be a general disturbance of psychomotor functions leading to disturbed co-ordination and clumsiness. During the further progress of dementia, lethargy and akinesia may occur.

Sequelae of encephalitis are known to include a number of motor symptoms apart from parkinsonism; a frequently mentioned example from history is the epidemic of encephalitis lethargica that occurred around 1920. **Tardive dyskinesia** is rightly regarded as a side-effect of neuroleptic therapy. However, since signs of tardive dyskinesia such as perioral hyperkinesia and dystonias were described before the introduction of neuroleptics,[66] it is also a motor symptom of mental disorder in its own right.

Disorders of memory

The following account concerns the approach to memory disorder adopted in clinical psychopathology. The psychology of memory disorder is discussed in Chapter 2.5.2.

Memory may be differentiated into short-term or recent memory and long-term or remote memory. Furthermore, ultra-short-term memory may be distinguished from short-term memory. Ultra-short-term memory encompasses immediate registration within the span of attention. Short-term memory reflects new learning. Long-term memory is usually associated with earlier data or other information that has been stored for months or years.

A variety of additional terms are used to describe memory functions; for example, the contrasting terms of declarative and procedural memory appear to be useful. Declarative memory contains facts which may be consciously recalled, whereas procedural memory contains skills and automatic activities. In dementia—both degenerative (Alz-

heimer type) and vascular (multi-infarct dementia)—recent memory is usually impaired earlier than remote memory.

Biographical memory is the recall of events in a person's past which have an emotional loading and therefore has an impact on understanding depression.

Amnesia is a period of time which cannot be recalled and it may be global or partial. With regard to time it may be retrograde—an expression derived from the idea that one is looking backwards from an event (such as brain trauma or electroconvulsive therapy) to find the period before the event to be deleted. Correspondingly, anterograde amnesia means a period of deleted memory after an event. Although it is difficult to distinguish between types of amnesia, focal lesions in the hippocampus seem to affect remote memory less than recent memory, whereas diffuse brain disease often affects both. In psychogenic amnesia it is sometimes possible to recognize specific personal meaning in the events which cannot be recalled.[67] Bonhoeffer[68] regarded amnestic disorders to be 'purely exogenous', i.e. highly specific for a cerebral disorder. Although this is not true of psychogenic amnesia, amnestic disorders should nevertheless strongly alert the examiner to the possibility of cerebral pathology.

Disorders of memory are closely connected with other disorders, such as disorders of consciousness; there is often amnesia for episodes of disturbed consciousness.

Some patients are aware of memory disorder and complain about it; others tend to neglect their memory deficits and manifest secondary signs such as confabulations. Confabulations are inventions which substitute for missing contents in gaps of memory; the patient is not aware that they are not true memories.

A disorder of short-term memory, as in Korsakoff's syndrome or transient global amnesia, is often neglected by the patient. Behaviour appears normal, and one might say that the facade of personality is intact. Apparently, such a patient is engaged in lively conversation or seemingly purposeful actions, and only after further investigation does it become obvious that these activities are not based on facts. These forms of memory disorder can be assessed directly by examining the patient. Other forms become apparent retrospectively on taking the patient's history. In these cases the patient complains about periods of global or partial amnesia. Memory of certain events may have faded or become covered by layers of other events (palimpsest), which is typical of repeated amnestic periods following bouts of drinking. In mood disorder there may be complaints about impaired memory, although no memory deficit is found in objective tests. An example of false memories (paramnesia) is *déjà vu*, an erroneous feeling of familiarity with, for example, a person or a room. *Déjà vu* may occur in temporal lobe epilepsy, although it is not specific for that disorder. Delusional memories are also examples of paramnesia.

Disorders of consciousness

Consciousness is the sum of various mental functions—in the words of Jaspers[69] 'the whole of present mental life'. Lipowski,[70] who regards the concept of consciousness to be 'completely redundant', describes what is commonly meant by clouding of consciousness on the basis of a number of behavioural features (Table 2). In contrast with Lipowski's sceptical attitude, the concept of consciousness has recently elicited fresh interest in philosophy and clinical neurology. (See Chapter 2.1.2.)

Table 2 Behavioural features indicating clouding of consciousness

The person is awake but may be drowsy

Awareness of the self and the environment is reduced

Both immediate and recent memory are impaired

Thinking is disorganized, and may be dreamlike; for instance perception
   is faulty and misperceptions may occur

The ability to learn new material is reduced

The person is unable to overcome this state by deliberate effort

Consciousness is a mode of relatedness between mind and world. Disordered consciousness may occur on a dimension of severity which ranges from lucidity to clouding and further towards unconsciousness. The latter represents a state of coma. In addition, consciousness may be assessed on a dimension of vigilance.[1] Ey[71] regards consciousness as an attribute of wakefulness. Indeed, sleepiness implies a reduction in consciousness; however, consciousness may also be reduced despite normal vigilance. This is just one example of how consciousness is connected with other mental faculties. Likewise, consciousness is impaired by a disorder of memory, orientation or coherence, as in the clouded consciousness of delirium. Some authors have suggested that disturbed consciousness could be the basis for stupor.

When consciousness is impaired there is clouding of perceptions, ideas, and images. The intensity of perceptions is diminished and there is a disintegration of order in the perceptive field. Accordingly, patients are disoriented.

The term confusional state is merely a synonym for delirium that emphasizes thought disorder and disorientation. **Disorientation** may concern time, place, or person. Temporal and geographical disorientation are very common. Remote contents are more robust then recent ones; name or date of birth are usually more available than age or name of the hospital. It is useful, after a polite excuse, to ask direct questions concerning orientation, even if they sound rather trivial, since some patients are very skilful in avoiding topics that show the degree of their disorientation.

Another aspect is described by the term **narrowing of consciousness**, which means that awareness of a person's environment is restricted, for example owing to an abnormal affective or delusional state.

In epileptic aura or after taking certain drugs, consciousness may be experienced as heightened with increased intensity of awareness.

Twilight state is a well-defined interruption of the continuity of consciousness. Consciousness is clouded and sometimes narrowed. Despite the disorder of consciousness the patient is able to perform certain actions, such as dressing, driving, or walking around. Subsequently, there is amnesia for this state. Twilight states may occur in epilepsy, alcoholism (*mania à potu* is a twilight state), brain trauma, general paresis, and dissociative disorder. *Mania à potu* describes the situation where a person reacts extremely, namely by developing twilight state, to small amounts of alcohol. Often these patients have an increased vulnerability due to pre-existing organic brain pathology. Twilight state may lead to violent behaviour and therefore needs forensic assessment.

In an **oneiroid state** the patient experiences narrowing of consciousness together with multiple scenic hallucinations. Oneiroid states may occur in schizophrenia, but are also observed in patients under intensive care who have to be totally passive and dependent on others. The atmosphere is perceived as strange and dreamlike. Accordingly patients may be aloof and behave like dreamers.[72] Unlike twilight states, the contents of oneiroid states are often remembered.

Finally, it should be noted that the subconscious of psychoanalytical theory is not open to direct clinical examination.

Disorders of attention and concentration

Attention and concentration both mean the directing of mental activities towards a particular object, with the exclusion of other objects. There is little difference between attention and concentration except that, in ordinary language, attention is associated with present alertness and concentration with longer-lasting achievement and performance. There is a distinction between selective and shared attention. Attention and concentration may be impaired by clouded consciousness or may be due to individual aspects of clouded consciousness such as sleepiness, incoherence, or memory deficits. However, there may be other reasons such as hallucinations or mood disturbances. Attention deficit is a permanent feature in the eponymous childhood disorder attention-deficit hyperactivity disorder.

Assessment of attention and concentration may consist of simple arithmetical tasks and include psychometric performance tests in addition to the clinical examination. Psychometric performance tests are also valuable tools in assessing disorder of memory and consciousness.

Disorders of sleep are described in Chapters 4.14.1 to 4.14.6.

References

1. Sims, A. (1995). *Symptoms in the mind* (2nd edn). W.B. Saunders, London.
2. Jaspers, K. (1963). *General psychopathology* (7th edn) (trans. J. Hoenig and M.W. Hamilton). Manchester University Press.
3. World Health Organization (1946). *Constitution of the World Health Organization*. WHO, Geneva.
4. Hundert, E.M. (1995). *Lessons from an optical illusion*. Harvard University Press, Cambridge, MA.
5. Cutting, J. (1997). *Principles of psychopathology*. Oxford University Press.
6. Zucker, K. (1928). Experimentelles über Sinnestäuschungen. *Archiv für Psychiatrie und Nervenkrankheiten*, **83**, 706–54.
7. Janzarik, W. (1988). *Strukturdynamische Grundlagen der Psychiatrie*. Enke, Stuttgart.
8. Schmidt-Degenhard, M. (1992). *Die oneiroide Erlebnisform*. Springer, Berlin.
9. Jaspers, K. (1965). *Allgemeine Psychopathologie*. Springer, Berlin.
10. Klosterkötter, J. (1992). The meaning of basic symptoms for the development of schizophrenic psychoses. *Neurology, Psychiatry, and Brain Research*, **1**, 30–41.
11. Krause, R., Steimer, E., Sänger-Alt, C., and Wagner, G. (1989). Facial expression of schizophrenic patients and their interactionpartners. *Psychiatry: Interpersonal and Biological Processes*, **52**, 1–12.
12. Allderidge, P. (1974). *The late Richard Dadd*, pp. 1817–86. Tate Gallery, London.
13. Huber, G. and Gross, G. (1989). The concept of basic symptoms in schizophrenia and schizoaffective psychoses. *Recenti Progressi in Medicina*, **80**, 646–52.
14. Schneider, K. (1976). *Klinische Psychopathologie*. Thieme, Stuttgart.
15. Penfield, W. and Perot, P. (1963). The brain's record of auditory and visual experience. *Brain*, **86**, 595–696.

16. Klüver, H. (1942). Mechanisms of hallucinations. In *Studies in personality* (ed. Q. McNemar and M.A. Merrill), pp. 175–207. McGraw-Hill, New York.

17. Hoffmann, R. (1987). Computer simulations of neural information processing and the schizophrenia–mania dichotomy. *Archives of General Psychiatry*, **44**, 178–85.

18. Galton, F. (1880). Statistics of mental imagery. A quarterly review of psychology and philosophy. *Mind*, **5**, 301–18.

19. Jaensch, E. (1941). *Zur Eidetik und Integrationstypologie*. Barth, Leipzig.

20. Emrich, H.M. (1989). A three-component-system hypothesis of psychosis. Impairment of binocular depth inversion as an indicator of a functional dysequilibrium. *British Journal of Psychiatry*, **155** (Supplement 5), 37–8.

21. Heidegger, M. (1963). *Sein und Zeit*. Niemeyer, Tübingen.

22. Kierkegaard, S. (1849). *Die Krankheit zum Tode*, Vol. 8. Diederichs, Jena.

23. Stanghellini, G. (1995). The interplay between personality and affective vulnerability: the case of dysphoria. Presented at World Psychiatry Association Regional Symposium, Prague.

24. Lopez-Ibor, J.J. (1969). Depressive Äquivalente. In *Das depressive Syndrom* (ed. H. Hippius and H. Selbach), pp. 403–7. Urban und Schwarzenberg, Munich.

25. Mundt, C. (1991). Endogenität von Psychosen—Anachronismus oder aktueller Wegweiser für die Pathogeneseforschung? *Nervenarzt*, **62**, 3–15.

26. Escobar, J.I., Gomez, J., and Tuason, V.B. (1983). Depressive phenomenology in North and South American patients. *American Journal of Psychiatry*, **140**, 47–51.

27. Lader, M.(1983). The psychophysiology of anxiety. *Encephale*, **9**, 205B–10B.

28. Kellner, R. (1988). Anxiety, somatic sensations, and bodily complaints. In *Handbook of anxiety* (ed. R. Noyes Jr, M. Roth, and G.D. Burrows), Vol. 2, pp. 213–37. Elsevier, Amsterdam.

29. Albus, M. (1990). Psychophysiologie der Angsterkrankungen. *Nervenarzt*, **61**, 639–46.

30. Stallone, F., Huba, G.J., Lawlor, W.G., and Fieve, R.R. (1973). Longitudical studies of diurnal variations in depression: a sample of 643 patient days. *British Journal of Psychiatry*, **123**, 311–18.

31. Kuhs, H. and Tölle, R. (1987). Symptomatik der affektiven Psychosen. In *Psychiatrie der Gegenwart* (ed. K.P. Kisker, H. Lauter, J.-E. Meyer, C. Müller, and E. Strömgren), Vol. 5, pp. 69–114. Springer, Heidelberg.

32. Mundt, C., Richter, P., van Hees, H., and Stumpf, T. (1998). Zeiterleben und Zeitschätzung depressiver Patienten. *Nervenarzt*, **69**, 38–45.

33. Meyer, J.-E. (1982). Über die Umwelt des manisch Kranken. *Nervenarzt*, **53**, 127–31.

34. Beck, A.T., Rush, A.J., Shaw, B.F., and Emery, G. (1979). *Cognitive therapy of depression*. Guilford Press, New York.

35. Philipp, M., Maier, W., and Benkert, O. (1985). Operational diagnosis of endogenous depression. II. Comparison of 8 different operational diagnoses. *Psychopathology*, **18**, 218–25.

36. Akiskal, H.S. (1996). The temperamental foundations of affective disorders. In *Interpersonal factors in the origin and course of affective disorders* (ed. C. Mundt, M.J. Goldstein, K. Hahlweg, and K. Fiedler), pp. 3–30, Gaskell, London.

37. Wittchen, H.-U. (1996) What is comorbidity—fact or artefact? *British Journal of Psychiatry*, **168** (Supplement 30), 7–8.

38. Hamilton, M. (1974). *Fish's clinical psychopathology. Signs and symptoms in psychiatry* (revised reprint). John Wright, Bristol.

39. Popper, K. (1965). *Conjectures and refutations: the growth of scientific knowledge*. Routledge and Kegan Paul, London.

40. Jaspers, K. (1975). *Allgemeine Psychopathologie* (8th edn). Springer, Berlin.

41. Scharfetter, C. (1980). *General psychopathology*. Cambridge University Press.

42. Schneider, K. (1962). *Klinische Psychopathologie* (6th edn). Thieme, Stuttgart.

43. Hemsley, D.R. (1994). An experimental psychological model for schizophrenia. In *Search for the causes of schizophrenia* (ed. H. Häfner, W.F. Gattaz, W. Janzarik), pp. 179–88. Springer, Berlin.

44. Klosterkötter, J. (1988). *Basissymptome und Endphänomene der Schizophrenie*. Springer, Berlin.

45. Grace, A.A. (1991). Phasic versus tonic dopamine release and the modulation of dopamine system responsivity: a hypothesis for the aetiology of schizophrenia. *Neurosciences*, **41**, 1–24.

46. Frith, C.D. and Done, D.J. (1989). Experiences of alien control in schizophrenia reflect a disorder in the central monitoring of action. *Psychological Medicine*, **19**, 359–63.

47. Marks, J.M. (1969). *Fears and phobias*. Heinemann, London.

48. Anderson, E.W. and Trethowan, W.H. (1973). *Psychiatry* (2nd edn). Tindall, London.

49. Spitzer, M. (1993). The psychopathology, neuropsychology and neurobiology of associative and working memory in schizophrenia. *European Archives of Psychiatry and Clinical Neuroscience*, **243**, 57–70.

50. Payne, R.W. (1996) The measurement and significance of overinclusive thinking and retardation in schizophrenic patients. In *Psychopathology of schizophrenia* (ed. P.H. Hoch and J. Zubin), pp. 77–97. Grune and Stratton, New York.

51. Rosenbaum, B. (1991). Thought and speech disorders in psychiatry. In *European handbook of psychiatry and mental health* (ed. A. Seva), pp. 541–9. Anthropos, Barcelona; Prensas Universitarias de Zaragoza.

52. Thurstone, L.L. (1938). *Primary mental abilities*. Psychometric Monograph N-1, University of Chicago Press.

53. Spearman, C.E. (1927). *The abilities of man: their nature and measurement*. Macmillan, London.

54. Scharfetter, C. (1981). Ego-psychopathology: the concept and its empirical evolution. *Psychological Medicine*, **11**, 273–90.

55. Cotard, M. (1882). Nihilistic delusions. Reprinted in *Themes and variations in European psychiatry* (ed. S.R. Hirsch and M. Shepherd). John Wright, Bristol.

56. Lukianowicz, N. (1958). Autonoscopic phenomena. *Archives of Neurology and Psychiatry*, **80**, 199–220.

57. Sims, A.C.P. (1993). Schizophrenia and permeability of self. *Neurology, Psychiatry and Brain Research*, **1**, 133–5.

58. World Health Organization (1992). *International statistical classification of diseases and related health problems, 10th revision*. WHO, Geneva

59. Slade, P.D. (1988). Body image in anorexia nervosa. *British Journal of Psychiatry*, **153** (Supplement 2), 20–2.

60. David, A.S. (1990). Insight and psychosis. *British Journal of Psychiatry*, **156**, 798–808.

61. McEvoy, J.P., Apperson, L.J., and Appelbaum, P.S. (1989) Insight in schizophrenia: its relationship to acute psychopathology. *Journal of Nervous and Mental Disease*, **177**, 43–7.

62. David, A.S., Buchanan, A., and Reed, A. (1992). The assessment of insight in psychosis. *British Journal of Psychiatry*, **161**, 599–602.

63. Kemp, R. and David, A. (1996) Insight and psychosis: a social perspective. *Psychological Medicine*, **25**, 515–20.

64. McEvoy, J.P., Freter, S., and Everett, C. (1989). Insight and the clinical outcome in schizophrenia. *Journal of Nervous and Mental Diseases*, **177**, 48–51.

65. Wernicke, C. (1894). *Grundriss der Psychiatrie in klinischen Vorlesungen*. Vol. 1, *Psycho-physiologische Einleitung*. Thieme, Leipzig.

66. Berrios, G. (1996). *The history of mental symptoms*. Cambridge University Press.

67. Lishman, W.A. (1997). *Organic psychiatry*. Blackwell Science, Oxford.

68. Bonhoeffer, K. (1917). Die exogenen Reaktionstypen. *Archiv für Psychiatrie und Nervenkrankheiten*, **58**, 58–70.

69. Jaspers, K. (1913). *Allgemeine Psychopathologie*. Springer, Heidelberg.

70. Lipowski, Z. (1990). *Delirium*. Oxford University Press, New York.

71. Ey, H. (1963). *La conscience*. Presse Universitaire de France, Paris.

72. Mayer-Gross, W., Slater, E., and Roth, M. (1955). *Clinical psychiatry*. Cassell, London.

1.10 Assessment

1.10.1 The principles of clinical assessment in general psychiatry

John E. Cooper and Margaret Oates

Introduction

This chapter is focused on the needs of the clinician in a service for general adult psychiatry, who has to carry out the initial assessment of the patient and family working either in the context of a multidisciplinary team or independently. Within this quite wide remit, the discussion is limited to general principles that guide the practice of all types of psychiatry. The chapter does not include the special procedures and techniques also needed for assessment of children and adolescents, the elderly, persons with mental retardation, persons with forensic problems, and persons requiring assessment for suitability for special types of psychotherapy.

It is assumed that the reader has already had significant experience of clinical psychiatry and has completed the first stages of a postgraduate psychiatric training programme. Therefore details of the basic methods recommended in commonly used textbooks or manuals of instruction for obtaining and recording information on essentials such as the history, personal development, mental state, and behaviour of the patient are not included in this chapter.[1-3]

Three topics have been given special attention. These are assessment by means of a **multidisciplinary team**, the trio of concepts **diseases, illness, and sickness**, and the development of **structured interviewing and rating schedules**. The first two have a special connection that justifies emphasis in view of the recent increase in multidisciplinary styles of assessment. For instance, when different members of the team appear to be in disagreement about what should be done, it is usually a good idea to ask the question: 'What is being discussed—is it the patient's possible physical disease, the patient's personal experience of symptoms and distress, or the interference of these with social activities?'. It will then often become apparent that the issues in question are legitimate differences in emphasis and priority of interest, rather than disagreements. The third topic is given prominence in order to illustrate some aspects of the background of the large number of such schedules (called 'instruments' for convenience) that are now available. They are usually given the shortest possible mention in research reports, but since most advances in clinical methods and service developments come from studies in which an assessment instrument has been used, clinicians should know something about them.

The aim of the initial clinical assessment is to allow the clinician and team to arrive at a comprehensive plan for treatment and management, that has both short-term and longer-term components. The achievement of this will be discussed under the following headings.

- Concepts underlying the procedures of assessment
- Contextual influences on assessment procedures
- Assessment as a multidisciplinary activity
- Instruments for assessment
- The condensation and recording of information
- Making a prognosis
- Reviews
- Writing reports

Concepts underlying the procedures of assessment

The separation of form from content, and from effects on activities

In psychiatric practice more than in other medical disciplines, the key items of information that allow the identification of signs and symptoms of psychiatric disorders are often embedded in a mixture of complaints about disturbed personal and social relationships, together with descriptions of problems to do with work, housing, and money. These complaints and problems may be a contributing cause or a result of the symptoms of psychiatric disorders, or they may simply exist in parallel with the symptoms. A preliminary sorting out into overall categories of information is therefore essential.

The distinction between the form and the content of the symptoms is particularly important, together with the differentiation of both of these from their effects upon the functioning of the patient (function is used here in a general sense as applying to all activities, in contrast to the specific meaning given to it in the classification of disablements). This differentiation is discussed in Chapter 1.9, so only a brief mention is needed here.

The presenting complaint of the patient is often the interference with functions, but enquiry about the reasons for this should then reveal the contents of the patient's thoughts and feelings. The form of the symptoms (i.e. the technical term, such as phobia or delusion used to identify a recurring pattern of experience or behaviour known to be important) allows the identification of the psychiatric disorder. Knowledge of the effects on functions is essential for decisions about the management of patient and family, and is an important aspect of the severity of the disorder.

This sorting into different types of information often implies a conflict of priorities during the interview. The clinician must be seen to acknowledge the concerns and distress of the patient, but also must ask questions that will allow the identification of symptoms; and the concept of a symptom (having both form and content) is probably not shared by the patient and family. Learning to balance this conflict of interest is an essential part of clinical training, and has been well recognized by previous generations of descriptive psychiatrists, including Jaspers.[4] The separation of the social effects of a symptom from the symptom itself is also a necessary part of the assessment process. Further comments on this and related issues have been made by Post[5] and, influenced to some extent by a psychodynamic background, by McHugh and Slavney.[6]

Categories of information: subjective, objective, and scientific

Is there such a thing as a truly objective account of events? If 'objective' is intended to mean absolutely true and independent of all observers, the answer must be negative. Students and trainee psychiatrists often come to psychiatric clinical work from medical and surgical disciplines where they have been encouraged to 'search for the facts' with the implication that 'true' facts exist. They may need to be reminded that the supposed facts of all medical histories, even those of clearly physical illnesses, depend upon the perceptions, opinions, and memories of individuals who may give different versions of the same events at different times.

'Objective' has several shades of meaning in ordinary usage, but in clinical assessment its most useful meaning is that an account of an event or behaviour is based on agreement between two or more persons or sources. In contrast, 'subjective' can be used to indicate that the account comes from only one person. Objective information is likely to be safer to act upon than subjective, so efforts should always be put into raising as much as possible of the information about a patient into the objective category. Nevertheless, many of the most important symptoms in psychiatry can only be subjective, since they refer to the inner experience of the one person who can describe them.

When assessing the reliability and usefulness of other types of information, such as the results of treatment or possible explanations of causes, a further useful distinction can be made between objective defined as above and 'scientific', taking this to mean that systematic efforts have been made to obtain evidence based upon comparisons (or 'controls') which demonstrate that one explanation can be preferred out of several possibilities that have been considered.

Simple definitions such as these are useful in clinical discussions, but it must be remembered that in the background are many complicated and unsolved problems of philosophy and semantics. Some of these suggestions on the status of information in clinical work are based upon the writings and clinical teaching of Kraupl Taylor.[7]

Disease, illness, and sickness

These concepts have existed in the medical and sociological literature for many years, and are best regarded as useful but inexact concepts that refer to different but related aspects of the person affected, namely pathology (disease), personal experience (illness), and social consequences (sickness), respectively.[8] They are useful as a trio because they serve as a reminder that all three levels should be considered in a clinical assessment, even though for different patients they will vary greatly in relative importance. There are no simple answers to questions about how they are best defined and how exactly they are related to each other, but time spent on these issues is not wasted because they reflect quite naturally some of the different interests and priorities of the different health professions (and are therefore often the basis of different viewpoints put forward by various members of a multidisciplinary team).

Another reason for being familiar with these concepts is that in legal and administrative settings, simple and categorical pronouncements about the presence of mental illness or mental disease and their causes and effects may be required whatever the medical viewpoint might be about the complexity of these concepts.

Clinicians of any medical discipline know from everyday experience that the disease–illness–sickness model does not always represent the simple sequence of causation that may appear to be obvious at first sight to a non-medical professional. Although disease usually causes the patient to feel ill and the state of illness then usually interferes with many personal and social activities, this sequence is by no means always present. Potentially serious physical, biochemical, or physiological abnormalities (disease) may be discovered in surveys of apparently healthy persons before any symptoms, distress, or interference with personal activities (illness) have developed, and some patients may have either or both of illness and sickness (interference with social activities) without any detectable disease.

A number of sociologists, anthropologists, and philosophers have joined psychiatrists in trying to define mental illness and mental health, but without achieving much clarification. Aubrey Lewis[9] and Barbara Wootton,[10], although writing from the different contexts of clinical psychiatry and sociology, both arrived at the conclusion that neither mental illness nor mental health could be given precise definitions, although they are useful terms in everyday language (and the same applies equally to physical health and physical illness).

More positive conclusions have resulted from attempts to define disease, in that Scadding (a general physician) has suggested that it should be defined as an abnormality of structure or function that results in 'a biological disadvantage'.[11,12] This seems reasonable if one is dealing only with conditions that have a clear physical basis, but if applied in psychiatry it implies that, for instance, behaviours such as homosexuality that reduce the likelihood of reproduction would have to be regarded as diseases alongside infections, carcinoma, and suchlike. This seems to be stretching a traditional concept too far, and different approaches clearly need to be explored.

One way forward is to accept that simple definitions and concepts encompassed by one word cannot cope with complicated ideas such as disease or health, and to take care to differentiate between definitions of these as concepts in their own right, and attempts to develop models of medical practice. The debate noted above refers to concepts of health, disease, and disorder, and it has been continued more recently with respect to psychiatry in two quite extensive reviews, in terms of the types of concepts[13] and of their possible contents.[14] What follows below is better regarded as about models of medical practice, and two points are suggested as a basis for the discussion. First, more than one dimension or aspect of the person affected always needs to be included in descriptions of health status. Second, models of medical practice and thinking do not necessarily have to start with the assumption that physical abnormalities (diseases) are the basic concept from which all others are derived.

Regarding the first point (of more than one aspect or dimension), soon after the contribution of Susser and Watson[8] noted above, Eisenberg, a psychiatrist with social and anthropological interests,[15] made a plea for all doctors, but particularly psychiatrists, to recognize the importance of appropriate illness behaviours in addition to giving the necessary attention to the diagnoses and treatment of serious and dangerous disorders.[16] He gave special emphasis to the need to minimize problems that may arise from discrepancies between disease as it is conceptualized by the physician and illness as it is experienced by the patient: 'when physicians dismiss illness because ascertainable disease is absent, they fail to meet their socially assigned responsibilities'. A similar model with a more overtly three-dimensional structure usually referred to as 'bio-psycho-social' has also been described by Engel.[17] More recently, Susser[18] has pointed out the close relationships between the disease–illness–sickness trio and the parallel classifications of impairment, disability, and handicap developed by the World Health Organization (WHO).[19] Historically, all these can be regarded as variations on and explicit developments of a theme that has been accepted implicitly by generations of psychiatrists influenced by the 'psychobiology' of Adolf Meyer and his many distinguished pupils, manifest in the importance given to the construction of the traditional clinical formulation.

The second point, to do with the disease level not being the best starting point for conceptual models of medical practice, is of more recent and specifically psychiatric origin. Both Kraupl Taylor[20] and, more recently, Fulford[21] give detailed arguments for the conclusion that the illness experience of the patient is the most satisfactory starting point from which to develop a model of medical practice. Taylor presents his case as a matter of logic, and Fulford works through lengthy philosophical and ethical justifications. This new viewpoint has the virtue of starting with the encounter between patient and doctor, which has the strength of being one of the few things that is common to all types of clinical practice. In Taylor's terms, by describing symptoms and distress the patient arouses 'therapeutic concern' in the doctor and so first establishes 'patienthood'. Whether or not a diagnosis is reached or a disease is later found to be present, and whether or not the social activities of the patient are also interfered with, are other issues of great importance, but they do not diminish the primary importance of the first interaction; in this, both patient and doctor play their appropriate roles according to their personal, social, cultural, and scientific backgrounds.

If medical training and practice are guided by this model, there is no interference with the essential obligation of the doctor to identify and treat any serious disease that may be present. However, a parallel obligation to satisfy the patient and family that the illness (comprising complaints and distress) and the sickness (interference with activities) have also been recognized and will be given attention, is equally clear.

How to answer questions by the patient and family about whether the patient has a mental illness or not, and what this implies, needs careful discussion. Within a multidisciplinary team it is usually best for the team to reach early agreement on a particular way of describing the patient's illness so that conflicting statements will not be made inadvertently by different members if asked about it. This is because the patient or family may expect this type of statement, and not because distinctions between, for instance, mental illness and physical illness, or between nervous illness and emotional upset, are regarded as fundamental from a psychiatric viewpoint. This difficult issue will be made easier if something about the patient's ideas about the nature and implications of terms such as 'mental illness' and 'nervous breakdown' is always included as part of the initial assessment information. Similarly, all members of the team need to be familiar with the concept of illness behaviour and the way this is determined by cultural influences[22] (see Chapter 2.6.2).

The diagnostic process: disorders and diagnoses

Psychiatrists learn during their general medical training that the search for a diagnosis underlying the presenting symptoms is one of the central purposes of medical assessment. This is because if an underlying cause can be found, powerful and logically based treatments may be available. But even in general medicine, as Scadding pointed out 'the diagnostic process and the meaning of the diagnosis which emerges are subject to great variation … the diagnosis which is the end-point of the process may state no more than the resemblance of the symptoms and signs to a previously recognised pattern'.[11,12] In psychiatry, 'may' becomes 'usually', and this has been recognized by the compilers of both ICD-10 and DSM-IV, in that these are presented not as classifications of diagnoses, but of disorders. These classifications use similar definitions of a disorder; the key phrases in ICD-10 are 'the existence of a clinically recognisable set of symptoms or behaviour associated in most cases with distress and with interference with personal functions', and in DSM-IV 'a clinically significant behavioral or psychological syndrome or pattern that occurs in an individual and that is associated with present distress or disability…'.

The use of such broad definitions is necessary because of the present limited knowledge of the causes of most psychiatric disorders, and a similarly limited understanding of processes that underlie their constituent symptoms. To avoid overoptimistic assumptions, there is much to be said for psychiatrists avoiding the use of the term 'diagnosis' except for the comparatively small minority of instances in which it can be used in the strict sense of indicating knowledge of something underlying the symptoms. A consequence of this viewpoint is that the currently used 'diagnostic criteria' in both these classifications should be relabelled as 'criteria for the identification of disorders'.

In spite of this, it must be accepted that the patient and family are likely to expect statements to be made about the cause of their distress and symptoms. The members of all human groups expect their healers to discover the causes of their misfortunes (i.e. to make a diagnosis), and to provide remedies. This is so whether the group is a sophisticated and scientifically oriented modern society, or a non-industrialized society that relies on ethnic healers and folk remedies. The obvious relief of a patient or family on the pronouncement of an 'official' diagnosis is often evident in any type of healing activity, even though the diagnostic terms themselves mean very little. The pronouncement of an official diagnosis is taken to show that the doctor knows what is wrong, and therefore will be able to provide successful treatment or advice. If the diagnosis is expressed in terms that the patient can understand, it will have additional power as an explanatory force.

The readiness of ethnic healers and practitioners of complementary (or alternative) medicine to provide a diagnosis and treatment in terms that have a meaning and therefore a powerful appeal to their customers is probably one of the main reasons for their continued survival and popularity alongside scientifically based medicine. This is a separate issue from the question of whether or not the treatments of complementary practitioners are successful in the sense of having effects that could be demonstrated by means of a controlled clinical trial.

Within psychiatry and clinical psychology, the medical habit of searching for a diagnosis has at times been misunderstood as an unjustified preoccupation with the presence of physical disease as a cause of mental disorders. This was most marked in the United States during the 1950s and 1960s, expressed particularly in the writings of Menninger in which the diagnostic process and attempts to classify patients were dismissed as a waste of time.[23] This viewpoint ignores two points made here and by many others; first, the choice of a diagnostic term is only one part of the overall process of assessment that leads also to a personal formulation. Second, any assessment of a person, whether made as statements about psychodynamic processes, as statements about structural and biochemical abnormalities, or as statements about interference with activities, is unavoidably an act of classification of some sort.

More detailed discussions about the importance of diagnosis have been provided by Scadding[11] as a general physician, and by Kendell[24] as a psychiatrist. A detailed analysis of the diagnostic process in psychiatry and its close relationship with classification and formulation is also given by Cooper.[25]

Concepts of disablement

Disablement will be used here as an overall term to cover any type of interference with activities by illness. This is often of more concern to the patient than the symptoms of the illness itself, since the fear of long-term dependence upon others is usually present, even though not voiced in the early stages. The question arises whether to leave the description and assessment of disablement to different members of the team as it arises in various forms, or whether in addition to encourage reference to one of the systematic descriptive schemes that are now available. Even if not used as fully as their authors intend, these have the merit of serving as checklists or reminders for the whole team, to ensure that the many different effects of the illness have been considered.

Two widely used descriptive schema are the International Classification of Impairments, Disabilities and Handicaps (**ICIDH**),[19] and a broadly similar framework described by Nagi[26] that is often used in the United States, particularly by neurologists. These are best regarded as descriptive conceptual frameworks rather than classifications, sharing a basic structure of several levels of concepts. For the ICIDH, these are **impairment**, **disability**, and **handicap**. Impairment is interference with physical or psychological functions (that is, parts of the whole person), disability is interference with activities of the whole person in relation to the immediate environment (also often figuring in other instruments as 'activities of daily living'), and handicap is the social disadvantage resulting from disability. Although the 1980 version of

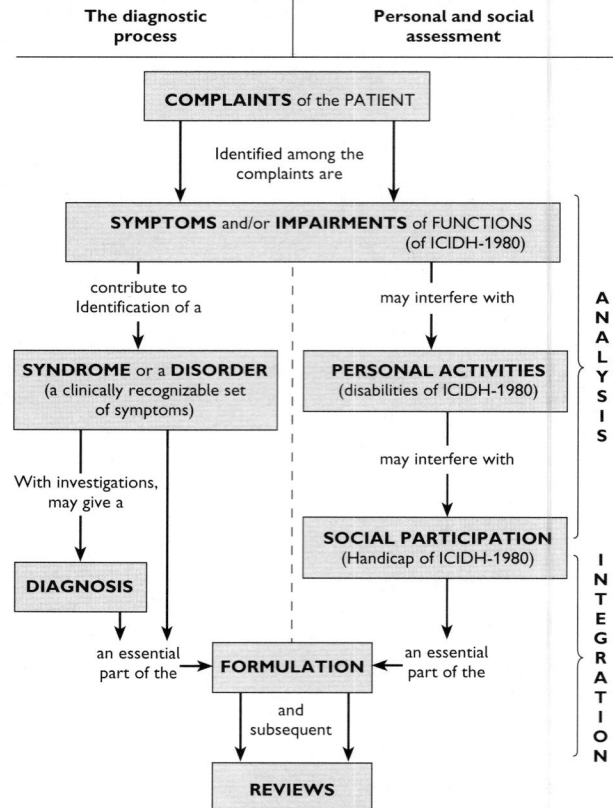

Fig. 1 Analysis and integration of information

ICIDH was not fully developed as either a classification or as a set of rating scales, the idea of thinking about interference with activities at different but related levels is very sensible.[27]

As noted in Fig. 1, these three concepts can be put alongside the sequence of ideas that leads from complaints, through symptoms to the identification of disorders or diagnoses. This may represent a causal sequence in some individuals, and this is clearest in acute physically based illnesses. But for many patients encountered in psychiatric practice, whose illnesses often have prominent social components, causal relationships may be absent or even in the opposite direction. For instance, sudden bereavement, i.e. loss of a social relationship, may be the clear cause of interference with the ability to perform daily activities (disability), and also of uncontrolled weeping (an impairment of the normal control of emotions). Social handicaps can also be imposed unjustifiably by other persons, as when a patient who is partly or fully recovered from long-standing psychiatric illness and quite able to work is refused employment due to the prejudice of a potential employer.

Many mental health workers find that to use a scheme of this sort helps to clarify how different aspects of a patient's problems fit together. Similarly, the different members of the team may be able to see more clearly how their activities with the patient and family complement one another, since the different concepts in the framework correspond approximately with the interests of different health disciplines. Social workers will focus on assessment of work and social relationships, occupational therapists will have a special expertise in the assessment of daily activities, and clinical psychologists are skilled in the assessment of cognitive and other psychological functions. Researchers in the various health disciplines have naturally devised rating scales that reflect their own interests and ideas, independently of the ICIDH or other overall schema, but it is usually found that such scales correspond quite closely with one or other of the concepts just discussed. Because of this, the ICIDH has received wide international recognition as a useful way of approaching assessment, and is now being revised.[28] The reluctance of both researchers and clinicians to adopt a standard set of terms to cover the various levels or concepts continues to be a problem; the reader needs to be aware that the terms impairment, disability, and handicap are often used synonymously by different authors.

The description of social and interpersonal relationships is in principle included in comprehensive schemas such as the ICIDH and that of Nagi, but many separate instruments that cover relationships in great detail have been devised over the years by psychotherapists, family therapists, and others.[29–31]

The sequence of assessment: collection, analysis, synthesis, and review

As information accumulates and is discussed, several different but related aspects of the patient and the illness have to be kept in mind. Good psychiatric practice is a part of what is sometimes referred to as 'whole-person medicine' in which at different times the contrasting but complementary processes of both analysis and synthesis of the information available will be needed. The patient must be seen both as an individual with a variety of attributes, abilities, problems, and experiences, and as a member of a group that is subject to family, social, and cultural influences; at different stages in the process of assessment each of these aspects will need separate consideration.

Analysis is needed to identify those attributes, experiences, and problems of the patient and the family that might require specific interventions by different members of the team. This must then be followed by several types of synthesis (or bringing together of information) to enable attempts to understand both subjective and objective relationships between the patient and the illness. First, possible interventions must be placed in order of priority for action. Second, the whole programme needs to be reviewed at intervals so as to assess progress and decide about any additional interventions that are required. At these times of review, and particularly towards the end of the whole episode of illness, global statements about 'overall improvement' or changes in 'quality of life' may be additional useful ways of summarizing and evaluating what has been happening from the viewpoint of the patient.

From complaints to formulation

Figure 1 demonstrates how the information contained in the complaints presented by the patient needs to be sorted out into different conceptual categories so that it can form the basis of actions by the various members of the multidisciplinary team.

The top box represents the complaints. Unpleasant symptoms are likely to head the list, but inability to do everyday activities or a description of problems with relationships may well come first. Symptoms that give a clue to disorders, diagnoses, and possible treatments may not be identified without close questioning by someone who knows what to ask about.

The second box indicates that the complaints need to be sorted out into symptoms and impairments (an impairment in this sense is interference with a normal physiological or psychological function, as explained below). Some complaints are both symptoms and impairments: symptoms because it is known that they can contribute towards the recognition of an underlying diagnosis or towards the identification of a disorder, and impairments because they indicate measurable interference with the function of a part of the body or of a particular organ. For instance, inability to remember the time of the day is a symptom (disorientation in time) that may contribute towards a diagnosis of some kind of dementia. It is also an impairment of cognitive functioning that is likely to interfere with the performance of everyday activities such as getting up and going to bed at the correct time, and organizing housework.

The left-hand side of Fig. 1 represents the progress towards the identification of a disorder and perhaps even an underlying diagnosis. These are important concepts because they may indicate useful treatments and likely eventual outcomes. The right-hand side shows the progression from impairment of functions of parts of the body or organs, through interference with personal and daily activities (called 'disability' in the terms of the ICIDH-1980,[19] to interference with participation in social activities ('handicap' in ICIDH-1980).

A clinical assessment is not complete until all the components of both sides of Fig. 1 have been considered. In doing this, the different components and the two pathways of concepts will need to be given widely varying emphasis for different patients, and also for the same patient at different times. For instance, if there is a physical cause for a disturbance of behaviour, an accurate diagnosis of this will lead to the best possible chance of rapid and successful treatment. In contrast, if a disturbance of social behaviour has its origin in personal relationships or has been imposed upon the patient by the social prejudices of others, the correct diagnostic category is unlikely to add much; assessments of social networks and supportive relationships will be key issues.

Life events and illness

For clarity, the right-hand side of Fig. 1 is given in a very compressed form, but in practice it is likely to need dividing into several components. The possibility of discovering relationships in time between life events and the onset of symptoms or interference with activities, particularly if repeated, should always be kept in mind, since this may be relevant to management plans and the assessment of prognosis. The best guide to this will be a lifechart. The opinions of patients and families about the causes of illness must be listened to with respect, while bearing in mind that the attribution of illness to the effects of unpleasant experiences is a more or less universal human assumption that often has no logical justification. Clinicians have to arrive at their own conclusions about such relationships by means of experience, common sense, and some acquaintance with research findings. Researchers seeking robust evidence on this topic are faced with a very difficult task, since the assessment of vulnerability to life events is a surprisingly complicated and controversial issue. The leading method in this field is the Life Events and Difficulties Schedule developed by Brown and Harris; a bulky training manual has to be mastered during a special course, and this then serves as a guide to an interview which may last for several hours. The length and detail of these procedures illustrate well the technical and conceptual problems that have to be faced.[32–34]

Psychodynamics and the life story

'Psychodynamics' refers in a general sense to the interactions between discrete life events, personal relationships, and personality attributes, in addition to its use to cover internal psychological processes (such as defence mechanisms and coping strategies). All of these need to be examined when trying to understand which of several possible causes of an illness at a particular time is the most likely.

A mixture of knowledge about local social and cultural influences and more technical psychological issues is needed for this appraisal of the patient's life story, and suggestions about different components of the overall pattern may well come from different members of the team. The different perspectives in which patients can be viewed are discussed in Chapter 1.7.

The internal psychodynamics of the patient often need to be considered in detail, and one way to do this would be to construct a subdivision of the right-hand side of Fig. 1 to show interpersonal relationships and psychodynamic processes. In some patients a major conclusion of the initial assessment will be that these aspects are paramount, indicating the need for referral to a specialist psychotherapy service. The assessment of suitability for specific forms of psychotherapy and cognitive–behavioural approaches are dealt with in Part 6.

Contextual influences on assessment

The place of assessment should not be regarded as automatically fixed in the outpatient or other clinical premises. One or more assessment interviews at home should be considered,[35] since the patient and family may feel much more at ease and therefore likely to express themselves more freely in familiar surroundings, but with the proviso that privacy may be more difficult to achieve. The assessor will often be surprised how much useful information about the home and family circumstances is gained from an interview at home, even when there appeared to be no special reason for this at first. In addition, the behaviour of both the patient and family members in the clinic or hospital is often different from that observed in familiar home surroundings. There are also obvious advantages to both assessment and care at home for mothers who have psychiatric disorders in the puerperium.[36]

Interviews on primary care premises are also often appreciated by patients who dislike going to hospitals of any sort, and the ease of consultation with the general practitioner is an additional advantage. The adoption of regular visits by a consultant psychiatrist to primary care premises as a major element in cooperation between psychiatrists and general practitioners is a style of work that seems to be spreading, with advantages to all concerned.[37]

Privacy of interviewing and confidentiality of what is discussed need careful consideration; there are few absolute rules, but the following points of procedure should be explained clearly to both patient and relatives from the start. First, the patient and any member of the family should know that if they wish they are entitled to speak to the doctor in private, and they must be able to feel that what they say will not be conveyed to any other member of the family unless they request this.

Second, in addition to the usual rules of professional secrecy, the patient must agree not to question other family members about what they said to the doctor, and vice versa. These may seem to be elementary points to trained professionals, but they are often not appreciated by patients or relatives who may be in fear of each other, or at least apprehensive about the reaction of the other on learning that statements they might construe as critical have been made about them. These are all points by which trust is established and maintained between patient and doctor, and for the same reason any attempts by relatives to seek interviews on condition that the occasion is kept secret from the patient should be firmly resisted.

An interpreter should always be sought if the patient cannot speak freely in the language of the interviewer. Mental health professionals who can also act as interpreters are increasingly available nowadays due to the presence in almost all communities of sizeable ethnic minorities. Because of the issues of confidentiality noted above, a professional of the same sex as the patient should always be preferred to family members when interpretation is needed.

Language barriers are usually, but not always, accompanied by a cultural difference. The interviewer must remember that the concept of a private interview between two strangers in which personal and often unpleasant events and experiences are discussed freely comes from 'middle-class Western' culture, and is not necessarily shared by persons from other cultures. A discussion of this point before the interview with a mental health professional familiar with the patient's background will help the interviewer to determine what to aim at in terms of intimate or possibly distressing information.

Multiple sources of information are always an advantage for those topics (mainly events) for which objective accounts are possible. Clinical experience is the best guide as to which account to use when conflicts of information arise. Serious conflicts of information arising during the initial assessment that involve the patient's account of events are best resolved by trying to obtain more information. Confrontation of the patient with important conflicts of information should be avoided since it easily leads to misunderstandings. If done at all, confrontation should be reserved for later stages in the overall management when it forms part of a planned intervention with a special purpose.

Assessment as a multidisciplinary activity

Multidisciplinary teams can take may forms, varying from the tightly organized and necessarily hierarchical surgical theatre team in which the role of each member is clearly defined and unchanging, to loosely knit groups in other types of health service in which only some of those attending meetings about patients regard what is taking place as a team event. For the purposes of discussion of the types of multidisciplinary teamwork increasingly to be found in the mental health services, it is useful to differentiate between multidisciplinary practice, familiar to many generations of mental health workers, and the more recently evolved multidisciplinary teamwork. Both of these styles of work have many variations, but they both have some key features that need to be recognized by those involved.

In multidisciplinary practice the consultant or most senior doctor present at clinical meetings or 'ward rounds' is accepted by all as the leader of the group, and listens to (and usually depends upon) the views of the senior nurses and other health professionals who may or may not be present. But the decisions about treatment and management are clearly acknowledged to be the responsibility of the doctors present. In most settings the only essential attendees at these meetings are the doctors and nurses; attendance of other health professionals is usually welcomed and valued, but they are not regarded as necessary members of the group.

Multidisciplinary teamwork has probably developed in response to a marked increase in the numbers of social workers, occupational therapists, clinical psychologists, and others, in those medical services in which patients and families with multiple needs are the rule rather than the exception. Clinical skills and techniques that were not previously available are now available, and the health professionals offering these expect quite naturally to be given increased personal and professional recognition; this can usually be found as a member of a multidisciplinary team of the sort described here. The most fully developed style of multidisciplinary teamwork involves a very significant commitment of professional time by each member so that all the team meetings can be attended, in addition to the time spent directly with the patient and family.

Some sharing of responsibilities and blurring of roles is needed, but each member also must be seen as retaining the professional skills of their parent discipline. Role blurring is most obvious in the information-gathering and information-sharing phases of assessment, and in the team discussions that lead to agreement about the content of a care programme.

Leadership

The concept of a team implies that a team leader is recognized; a leader does not have to be an obviously dominant speaker and decision maker, and many successful team leaders 'lead from behind' to great effect and to everyone's satisfaction. The main reasons for having an agreed leader are, first, to keep discussions acceptably brief and to a practical timetable; second, to facilitate decisions between reasonable alternatives; and third, to arbitrate when insoluble disagreements arise between team members.

There are a number of settings within the mental health services in which there may be no need for the leader for everyday purposes to be a doctor. This occurs most frequently in special crisis intervention and emergency units, in rehabilitation units, and in services for those with mental retardation. However, members of such teams have to acknowledge that decisions about the presence of physical illness, and the need for medication or laboratory investigations, can only be made by a medically qualified person. The team then has to accept the authority of the doctor on these occasions because of the unique ethical and legal responsibilities that accompany a medical qualification.

In teams running an inpatient unit such as an acute admission ward, there is a clear need for the whole team to accept that medical and nursing members have free access to all the patients for purposes of physical examination, laboratory investigations, the administration of medication, and a variety of nursing procedures.

Key workers and care programmes

The allocation of a team member as key worker (or case manager) for each patient being assessed is the usual method of work in teams of this sort. Which member becomes key worker for which patient depends upon the ability of the team to match the needs of each patient with the skills available amongst the team members, according to their training. Although all patients are discussed in detail at team meetings, and any team member can contribute suggestions and viewpoints, it is usually accepted that once a care programme of activities is identified and agreed upon, most if not all of the contacts with the patient and family will be made by the key worker. The key worker also has the responsibility of reporting back to the team about progress, and about problems encountered which might require new major decisions or changes in the care programme.

The terms 'case manager' and 'care programme' have been used above to refer to individual mental health professionals in direct contact with the patient, but these simple meanings must not be confused with care management, a more recently introduced concept that refers to a model of 'extended brokerage case management' recommended by, for instance, the United Kingdom Department of Health[38,39] in which care managers are not directly involved in direct service delivery. These terms are unfortunately sometimes used synonymously, and further confusion is sometimes caused by the terms and models of the Care Programme Approach, also of the United Kingdom Department of Health,[40] and the more positively evaluated Programme for Assertive Community Treatment.[41] Reviews by Burns[42] and others[41] are very helpful guides through the complexities of this topic.

In addition to the specific medical responsibilities noted above, psychiatrists as members of a multidisciplinary team have other important areas of expertise that should be recognized by the other members. Experienced psychiatrists are likely to have special skills in the assessment of dangerousness and risks of various sorts, and psychiatrists at any stage in their training should be able to show by helpful examples that they are specially trained to summarize information. Even more important is their ability to produce an overall formulation that is the key to arriving at a care programme.

For a team to be to be successful, its members have to share openly stated common goals and policies, and need to develop an indefinable but vital 'team spirit' by which they are helped both to depend upon and to support each other, even though they have marked differences in training, status, and remuneration. To be an efficient and accepted long-term member of a multidisciplinary team of this type requires personal characteristics not necessarily possessed by all mental health professionals. Tolerance of the different viewpoints of other team members is essential, in addition to the professional skills needed to carry out the work required.

The frequency of team meetings is determined by the size and nature of the workload. Special meetings to discuss topics not directly related to the patients are also usually found to be necessary, so as to deal with issues such as team policies, recruitment and appointments, relationships with outside agencies (for instance about too few, too many, or inappropriate referrals), interpersonal problems between team members, and work-related stress in the team members. This last problem is particularly important in teams dealing with crisis intervention and psychiatric emergencies because of the need to maintain a rapid turnover of patients and families who are seen over only a limited period of time.

A different type of problem that may need sensitive handling by the team leader and others in authority outside the team itself is the relationship between the team members and their immediate superiors (or 'line managers') in the hierarchy of their own discipline. Each team member has to strike a balance between personal needs for professional supervision and training, and the ability to make decisions within the team because of special skills not possessed by other team members. This type of problem will be minimized if team members are comparatively senior and experienced within their parent discipline. Student health workers are not appropriate as team members, but they can benefit greatly if attached to the team as observers. They will have the opportunity to learn something about how other disciplines operate, which is an aspect of training usually absent from the rest of their training.

Disagreements often arise within a team about the best time for patients to be discharged from care, or about the precise time for referral when it is in the patient's interests to be assessed by another service. In countries where outpatient services and inpatient services are staffed by different teams under different organizations, there will be many such breaks in care, and multidisciplinary teamwork can become frustrating. But where continuity of care between different parts of the general psychiatric services is the norm, the most frequent changes of care result from the need for the patient to be assessed for more specialized treatment such as rehabilitation, cognitive–behavioural therapy, or intensive psychotherapy. The team needs to develop agreed policies for these occasions, and these will depend largely upon the structure of the local services available.

Although no systematic information is available, there is little doubt that the style of multidisciplinary teamwork just described is spreading through the mental health services in many countries. Its popularity and success are probably due to the increased job satisfaction experienced by the non-medical team members, in addition to the recognition of multiple rather than single needs in a large proportion of psychiatric patients and families already noted. Multidisciplinary styles of working are especially important in emergency psychiatric services and crisis intervention units.[43,44]

Instruments for assessment

Reasons for the development of structured interviewing and rating instruments

The training of all mental health professionals includes instruction in some system of information gathering and recording based upon a conceptual structure that helps them to organize the large amount of information they usually need to collect. With experience, the list of headings under which this information is collected becomes incorporated in the professional's mind as an automatically available guide to the conduct of assessment interviews. For research purposes, however, it is necessary to demonstrate overtly that the essential topics have been covered in a comprehensive and systematic manner. In many types of research not only the headings covered but the detailed items also need to be recorded so that others studying the results of the research can be confident that nothing was missed, and that the information obtained was not a biased selection of the total that might have been available. It has also been generally recognized since the 1950s that for purposes of communication between researchers in different centres, conclusions must be based upon information that has been shown to have a satisfactory inter-rater reliability.

With these aims in mind, detailed and comprehensive structured interviewing and rating schedules for recording many varieties of information have been developed (nowadays these are usually called 'instruments'; for brevity this term will be used to cover any sort of published interviewing and rating schedule). The most common types cover the present mental state and behaviour. Most of these instruments are not appropriate for use in everyday clinical work because they have been designed for research studies, but nevertheless it is useful for clinicians to know something about how they originated.[45]

Since the first appearance of partly or fully structured psychiatric rating instruments in the 1950s, there has been a steady increase in their number, type, and complexity. In the discussion that follows, some of the most widely used instruments are commented upon as examples but many others are available that are not mentioned. Comprehensive lists of such instruments can be found in catalogues of instruments and reviews by the WHO and others.[46–50]

Instruments for the assessment of mental state and behaviour

The instruments now available can be grouped according to the main purposes for which they were designed.

Screening instruments such as the General Health Questionnaire[51] are needed for the identification of likely cases or high risk individuals amongst large populations. These tend to be short and economical in use, since they have to be administered to large numbers of subjects. They are designed to generate a simple score that indicates the status of the subject in relation to the populations upon which the instrument was developed and validated. This is essential for screening and for epidemiological studies, but this single score does not convey much about the details of the subject's feelings or behaviour, and so is of limited interest to the clinician.

Screening instruments are often questionnaires, defining this to mean that they are simply a means of recording the answers to a set of questions, without any further questions or enquiry about the extent to which the subject understands the question or wishes to qualify answers given. Questionnaires are usually filled in by the subject as a 'paper-and-pencil' exercise, as in the General Health Questionnaire, but one widely used questionnaire that has a very detailed content (the Composite International Diagnostic Interview[52,53]) is completed by an interviewer.

Detailed instruments may contain the following.

1. Symptoms of only one type, as in Hamilton's rating scale for depression,[54] or the Scale for Assessment of Negative Symptoms.[55]

2. A selection of symptoms for the study of the relationships between two closely related types, such as depressive and schizophrenic symptoms in the Schedule for Affective Disorders and Schizophrenia.[56]

3. A limited number of items covering different symptoms and behaviour selected as being of special importance, as in the recently developed Health of the Nation Scales of the United Kingdom.[57]

4. A more or less comprehensive array of symptoms that allows the study of the relative distribution of symptoms of many different types, such as Schedules for Clinical Assessment in Neuropsychiatry [58] and the Composite International Diagnostic Interview.[52,53] Other widely used but less tightly structured

instruments with a comprehensive content are the Brief Psychiatric Rating Scale[59] and the Composite Psychopathological Rating Scale,[60] aimed at measuring change.

The source and method for collection of information is usually specified by the designers of an instrument. These can include interviews with patients, relatives, and carers, observation of the patient, extracts from other documents, and any combination of these.

The more detailed instruments usually depend upon an interview, and the style of interviewing recommended and the training needed to achieve this depend upon both the quality of the information required and the type of research interviewer for whom the instrument is designed. These vary widely; for instance, Schedules for Clinical Assessment in Neuropsychiatry require a clinical professional training plus a special course for the instrument itself; the Comprehensive Psychopathological Rating Scale, the Brief Psychiatric Rating Scale, and the Structured Clinical Interview for DSM[61] assume a clinical professional training only. The Composite International Diagnostic Interview requires experience in interviewing such as market research plus a special course for the instrument itself, but no clinical professional training.

The time period covered varies from a cross-sectional picture of the present mental state and behaviour ('present' usually being taken to mean the immediately recent period of 2 or 4 weeks), to longer periods of follow-up, personal history, and development, and lifetime histories of psychiatric disorders. The more complicated and lengthy instruments that cover these longer periods are usually designed for particular studies, so are rarely suitable for general use.

Developments since the 1950s

A historical approach is helpful in trying to understand how and why the many instruments now available have developed. Hamilton's Rating Scale for Depression, published in 1959, is a good example of the first generation of instruments, most of which are comparatively short and simple.[54] Its contents can easily be printed on one page, and comprise the following:

(1) the names of the symptoms to be rated;

(2) a rating scale, the same for all the symptoms, by which the presence or absence and the severity of each symptom is recorded;

(3) a box in which the rating of each symptom is placed.

No special recommendations about length and style of interview are given, and no explanations or definitions of the symptoms are is given other than what is provided on the rating sheet itself. In other words, the interpretation of the ratings is based on the assumption that the raters have sufficient experience and training to know what most of their contemporaries also mean by the named symptoms. Data analysis is left to the user, other than recommendations about the likely meaning of the sum of the ratings with respect to severity of illness and 'caseness'. This and other early instruments were not tied to the use of any particular set of diagnostic categories, probably because the diagnostic classifications that were available in the 1950s and 1960s were not widely used.

The first generation of instruments made it much easier for researchers to communicate the detailed results of their clinical studies to others, mainly by facilitating the study of changes in symptoms over comparatively short periods of time. The need for this was no doubt connected with the increasing numbers of psychotropic medicines that became available around that time. Measurement of change in symptoms is more immediately useful for the study of response to treatment than reliance upon statements about overall improvement or waiting for a change in diagnosis. But in the absence of guidance about how the symptoms are defined, problems still remain in the interpretation of the results.

Improvements in more recent instruments leading to better quality and meaning of the data they collect have been of two main types, in that the structure and the associated procedures of the instruments have become more elaborate as time has passed. First, the input has been improved by the provision of written descriptions and definitions of symptoms, and by recommending particular styles of interviewing. This implies that researchers using the instrument should carry out preliminary training work so that satisfactory levels of inter-rater reliability are achieved before starting the main study (some examples of the most widely used instruments of this type are described in the next section). Second, the output has been improved by the use of computers to organize and summarize the symptom ratings, allied with the development of widely used psychiatric classifications.

Computer programs based upon decision trees (algorithms) first appeared in the 1970s, and are now commonplace. They allow the specification of sets of symptoms that identify disorders or indicate diagnoses, so that the resulting statements about symptom profiles or the presence of disorders or diagnoses are free from errors of human judgement such as carelessness, simple forgetting, and personal variations from one occasion to the next. But the biases and assumptions built into the programs by their authors still remain, and these may be a problem to others with different opinions.

Programs can also be written to assign disorders and diagnoses according to a selected classification, such as ICD-10 or DSM-IV, and some of the most recently developed instruments such as Schedules for Clinical Assessment in Neuropsychiatry and the Comprehensive International Diagnostic Interview are of this type. When used as intended, the data output from these more recent structured instruments is versatile and of high reliability, but to obtain these benefits the researcher has to pay the penalty of working hard to achieve and to maintain inter-rater reliability.

There are, of course, still plenty of uses for the simpler types of instruments; it is up to those designing and carrying out a study to decide what type of information they need and why, and to select their instruments accordingly. For the sake of those who will be interested in trying to interpret the results, a justification of the quality of the information obtained should always be included in the description of the findings.

Once an instrument (or often a related group of instruments) has demonstrated its usefulness it is likely to stay in use for many years, while at the same time being subject to extensions and improvements. Families of instruments and traditions of interviewing style therefore develop and persist in the major research centres and groups, and it is possible to identify some of these and follow them over the years.

Three such traditions of instrument development are selected for mention so as to illustrate the continuity and close relationships that sometimes exist between different instruments; these relationships may not be apparent from reports of studies in which they have been used. Three research centres that have produced particularly prominent sets of instruments are the Medical Research Council Social Psychiatry Unit at the Institute of Psychiatry in London, Biometrics

Research at the New York State Psychiatric Institute at Columbia University, New York, and the Department of Psychiatry at Washington University, St Louis, Missouri. The instruments mentioned below are only a small proportion of the many in the literature, but they are well known because of their association with some large collaborative international research studies and with widely used classifications of psychiatric disorders such as ICD-8, ICD-9, and ICD-10, and DSM-III, DSM-IIIR, and DSM-IV.

At approximately the same time in the early 1960s, but independently, research groups headed by John Wing, at the Institute of Psychiatry of the University of London (at the Maudsley Hospital), and by Robert Spitzer, at the Biometrics Research Unit at the New York State Psychiatric Institute at Columbia University, began to produce structured interviewing and rating schedules that provided extensive coverage of symptoms and were accompanied by recommendations for training procedures.

The Present State Examination

The Present State Examination (**PSE**)[62] is a semistructured procedure, based upon an interview schedule containing items that are rated as the interview proceeds. The content of the PSE has always been more or less comprehensive and it contains a number of symptoms, such as worry, muscular tension, restlessness, etc., that are not associated with particular diagnoses. These symptoms are included because they are often clinically obvious and also important to the patient (see comments below on 'bottom-up' and 'top-down' organization of interview schedules).

The ratings made by the interviewer do not depend entirely upon the immediate reply of the subject, but represent the interviewer's clinical judgement as to whether or not the subject has the symptoms as described in the glossary of definitions learned during the interview training. Questions are provided for all the symptoms and items and are used whenever possible in the order provided, but the order may be varied if the interviewer thinks fit. The interviewer is also encouraged to ask any other questions that seem relevant to determine the timing, frequency, and severity of the symptoms, as in an ordinary clinical interview. In other words, the interviewer aims to conduct a clinical interview that has been structured as much as possible so as to allow symptoms to be rated with high inter-rater reliability, but without seeming to be unpleasantly rigid to either the subject or the interviewer. Much practice and training are required before these aims can be achieved, but there is no doubt that it is possible.

The PSE was not developed with any particular diagnostic classification in mind. It was intended from the start simply to be a means of arriving at a comprehensive and defined set of symptoms described in a reliable manner, with the user being left to decide whether and how to condense the symptoms into groups and what to do with the results. This is sometimes referred to as a 'bottom-up' style of instrument organization. Versions 7 and 8 of the PSE were first used on a large scale in two studies that involved international collaboration and comparisons, namely the United States–United Kingdom Diagnostic Project between London and New York,[63,64] and the International Pilot Study of Schizophrenia co-ordinated by the WHO, Geneva.[65] Since then its content has been revised and extended as versions 9 and 10, but the techniques of interviewing and rating remain the same. PSE-10 is one of the main components of Schedules for Clinical Assessment in Neuropsychiatry.

Schedule for Affective Disorders and Schizophrenia, and the Structured Clinical Interview for DSM

The series of instruments developed by Spitzer and his colleagues at Biometrics of the New York State Psychiatric Institute have been of several different kinds and, in the early years at least, had a much more rigid structure than the PSE. Users of the Mental Status Schedule and the longer Psychiatric Status Schedule were instructed to follow the order of the questions as printed in the schedule, the only deviation from this being a repetition of the same questions if thought necessary by the interviewer. However, later instruments such as the Schedule for Affective Disorders and Schizophrenia[56] and, more recently, the Structured Clinical Interview for DSM-III and DSM-IV[61] allow more flexibility for the interviewer in both interview style and the choice of a little or a lot of training (despite its length, the Structured Clinical Interview for DSM is recommended for clinical use as well as for research). There has also been an increasing tendency for instruments from the New York group to be dedicated to a particular purpose. For instance, the content of the Schedule for Affective Disorders and Schizophrenia is keyed towards the study of relationships between schizophrenia and affective disorders, and the Structured Clinical Interview for DSM contains only those items that are necessary for identifying disorders present in the corresponding DSM. Like the Diagnostic Interview Schedule mentioned in the next section, the Schedule for Affective Disorders and Schizophrenia and the Structured Clinical Interview for DSM have a 'top-down' structure, meaning that their content is determined from the start by an already existing set of criteria or symptoms.

The instruments produced by these two centres in the 1960s and 1970s have been used widely in many countries, and their success led to the production of many similar instruments by other researchers. The adoption of the PSE for use by the WHO in a number of international collaborative studies also led to its being translated into more than 25 languages, with varying but never extensive degrees of adaptation to fit the different cultures and social settings involved.

The Diagnostic Interview Schedule

The third major research group is based at Washington University, St Louis, Missouri, and is well known as the originator of the first widely used sets of *Diagnostic Criteria for Research*.[66] Following the publication of DSM-III in 1980, there was considerable interest in discovering how the disorders it contained were distributed in the American population. Supported by the National Institute of Mental Health, Lee Robins and her colleagues designed the Diagnostic Interview Schedule (**DIS**)[67] for this purpose. This is composed of questions covering the symptoms required to identify what were considered to be the 15 most important disorders in DSM-III. The Epidemiological Catchment Area study of the National Institute of Mental Health, the very large study in which the DIS was first used, included a population sample of more than 18 000 subjects in five largely urban areas.[68]

So as to avoid the costs and other problems involved in employing trained psychiatrists or psychologists as interviewers, the DIS was designed as a highly structured questionnaire administered as an interview by lay interviewers. The interviewers, usually already experienced in interviewing for market research, had to undergo a week-long intensive training course on the DIS. The DIS questions must be given in the order printed in the schedule. Possible symptoms are not rated as present if in the opinion of the subject they may be due to physical disorders, but there is no free questioning about timing, severity, and other details of the symptoms. Questions may be repeated, but only questions provided in the schedule may be asked of the subject. This is a very different concept from that of the PSE technique, and it is based upon the assumption made by the designers of the DIS that by controlling the interviewer in this way, the DIS would 'enable the interviewer to obtain psychiatric diagnoses comparable to those a psychiatrist would obtain'.[67] Put in another way, this is an assumption that expressed complaints can be used as near equivalents of inferred symptoms for the purposes of identifying psychiatric disorders.

Schedules of Clinical Assessment for Neuropsychiatry and the Composite International Diagnostic Interview

Although originating from different groups with different traditions and purposes, the PSE and the DIS have now given rise to direct descendants, namely the Schedules of Clinical Assessment for Neuropsychiatry (**SCAN**) and the Composite International Diagnostic Interview (**CIDI**), that are closely connected. During the early 1980s, a collaborative programme of work between WHO and the National Institute of Mental Health of the United States (known as the Joint Project) resulted in the transformation of DIS into CIDI[69] by increasing its contents by adding large parts of first DSM-IIIR and then of the drafts of ICD-10 and DSM-IV. This was matched by the evolution of PSE-9 into PSE-10, the centrepiece of SCAN,[58] whose content similarly covers almost all of both ICD-10 and DSM-IV. The only sections of ICD-10 and DSM-IV not now covered by SCAN and CIDI are those dealing with disorders of adult personality, disorders of childhood and adolescence, and mental retardation.

The co-ordination by WHO of the development of the final stages of SCAN and CIDI has been aimed at the production of two instruments with different but complementary uses in epidemiological studies. CIDI can be administered to comparatively large numbers of subjects in the community since the use of lay interviewers keeps costs to a minimum. SCAN is more suitable for the professional (and therefore more expensive) assessment of subjects with obvious or severe disorders, whether these have been selected from a larger population by means of CIDI or other screening instruments, or whether they are being studied clinically for other reasons. The latest development in this long-term programme has been the establishment of WHO-sponsored training centres in a number of countries. Psychiatrists and other mental health professionals can now obtain the necessary training for both SCAN and CIDI in English, French, German, Spanish, Chinese, Japanese, and Arabic.[69]

These and other instruments will no doubt be developed further, but every new instrument and every change to an existing one carries with it problems of data interpretation. Even though the content of changed or new instruments may seem to be the same as their predecessors, quite small changes in the method or the sequence of questions may have important effects, particularly for highly structured instruments in which the ratings are not filtered through the clinical judgement of a trained mental health professional. For instance, a recent report from the United States[70] discusses the possibility that the differences in prevalence rates for some disorders found between the Epidemiological Catchment Area study[68] and the more recent

Co-morbidity Study[71] are due at least in part to changes in the 'stem questions' that introduce other specific questions rather than being due to real differences in the community subjects.

There are also unsolved problems in the study of individuals in the community, who have not sought professional help, by means of instruments originally designed for the study of psychiatric patients already in contact with services. To fulfil the criteria for a psychiatric disorder does not necessarily indicate a need for treatment, since the assessment of 'caseness' requires more than a simple count of symptoms. The debate about this problem has now stretched over 20 years, but needs to continue,[72,73] together with further examination of the closely related topic of clinical validity.[74]

Other selected issues

The importance of **negative symptoms** in the assessment of individuals with schizophrenic syndromes has led to the development of instruments devoted to these symptoms; the Scale for the Assessment of Negative Symptoms[55] is one of the most widely used, particularly in the United States. The Psychological Impairments Rating Scale (WHO/PIRS)[75] has been found to be acceptable in a variety of cultural settings, and has been used in several large international collaborative studies co-ordinated by the WHO. Both these instruments and a variety of others are useful as checklists for ordinary clinical purposes.[76] However, because of the nature of the symptoms being assessed, most of them are still beset with significant problems about inter-rater reliability and the exact meaning of their constituent items.

The **assessment of personality** poses special problems because to obtain a satisfactory account of a individual's personality, however the concept is defined, requires much more than the views of that individual; additional accounts of personal development and relationships from relatives or close friends are needed for comparison. Current concepts of personality disorders as listed in ICD-10 and DSM-IV also have serious limitations; the problems are well illustrated by a recent large international collaborative study co-ordinated by the WHO, using the International Personality Disorder Examination (IPDE).[69] Several hours of skilled interviewing are required, with at least two informants, to cover the content of the items that are needed to identify the disorders of adult personality contained in both the above classifications. This study and others with similar aims have found that if an individual fulfils the criteria for one disorder of personality, they are quite likely to fulfil the criteria for at least one more. This implies that the present categories reflect only parts of the overall personality; this may be quite useful, but a fairly drastic overhaul of the currently used categories is clearly needed if a global concept is to be retained in descriptive classifications. Whatever personality is, it does not exist in the abstract. It is one part of the complex of interacting factors that result in both past illnesses and future vulnerabilities.

Clinically, it is useful to assess three aspects of personality, according to the salience of personal characteristics and problems arising from them. First, one or more of the personality disorders described in ICD-10 or DSM-IV should be used only if there are quite clear accounts of repeated problems and behaviours as specified, and they are not due to symptoms of any other disorders that may be present. Second, for less severe but repeated problems and behaviours, the concept of 'accentuated personality type' is often useful, described simply by a short list of ordinary adjectives. These indicate recurring behaviours and attitudes likely to cause a variety of mild interpersonal or social problems, again not attributable to symptoms of other disorders. Finally, even though neither of these first two types of personality disturbance is present, it is always worthwhile describing the usual characteristics of the patient by means of a few adjectives (such as 'a worrier', somewhat shy and socially inhibited, definitely gregarious, etc.). Vaguely optimistic terms commonly offered by friends and relatives, such as 'happy-go-lucky', should be avoided.

Multiaxial descriptive systems (often optimistically called classifications) have been available for many years,[77] and now apply to both ICD-10 and DSM-IV. Multiaxial systems describe several aspects of the person in addition to the disorder, and can be regarded as providing a systematized formulation that facilitates the coded recording of several aspects of the person concerned. Most of them have been designed more for research than for everyday clinical use, but they can all serve as very useful checklists when preparing for clinical reviews. DSM-IV, like DSM-III, is presented as a multiaxial scheme covering five aspects of the subject (Axis I, clinical disorders; Axis II, personality disorders and mental retardation; Axis III, General Medical Conditions; Axis IV, Psychosocial and Environmental Problems; Axis V, Global Assessment of Functioning). Similar instruments are now available for ICD-10,[78] covering general adult psychiatry and the psychiatry of childhood and adolescence (see Chapter 9.1.1).

Quality of life has come to the fore in recent years, but in the same way as for multiaxial assessment, to use this term does no more than make explicit something that has always been implicit in a good clinical assessment. Examination of the content of the many assessment instruments that are now available with this title shows that they contain various mixtures of almost every possible attribute of the person, the illness, and the environment. There is no point in using a new term when the information collected refers only to already familiar problems such as symptoms, disablements, how the patient's time is occupied, and contacts with medical services. There is even a considerable literature on the 'quality of life' of whole communities and countries, in which indices are calculated from national or regional statistics about, for instance, standards of housing, education, transport, and consumption of material resources. Such indices are of value to economists and demographers, but are far removed from clinical assessments. There is much to be said for using the term in clinical work only when it indicates 'higher-level' value-judgements and concepts such as personal satisfaction, self-fulfilment, and freedom from distress. Most of these are subjective and difficult to measure, but in many ways they reflect the ultimate aims of all medical care. An excellent recent review of this topic from the viewpoint of psychiatry is available,[79] which illustrates well the wide range of subjects now covered by the term.

Service research into the closely related **needs assessment** has resulted in the production of some detailed instruments that, again, are of interest to clinicians largely as potential checklists. A good example from the United Kingdom is the MRC Needs for Care Assessment.[80]

Administrative pressure to provide some sort of **quantification of clinical outcome** has resulted in several comparatively brief instruments designed for clinical use. Two widely used examples are the Global Assessment of Functioning (**GAF**) scale (Axis V of DSM-IV) and, in the United Kingdom, the recently developed Health of the Nation Outcome Scale (**HONOS**).[57]

In both of these, the assessor uses whatever information is available about the patient to make judgements about the presence and severity of symptoms and troublesome behaviour, and the extent to which these interfere with activities, relationships and social performance. In the GAF scale this is expressed as a single overall score. In HONOS, 12 separate ratings are made which can be used independently, or added together to give an overall score if required. This type of instrument is likely to become increasingly important as the demand for 'evidence-based medicine' spreads, since they are designed for use by virtually any health professional in almost any setting. So long as precautions are always taken to ensure that the ratings made are as reliable and as valid as the setting permits, and likely sources of bias and error are kept in mind, their use can be a valuable aid to many forms of clinical assessment.

One further example of a **comprehensive assessment instrument** should be mentioned because it was designed for both research and clinical purposes, and it has been at times widely used in a number of European countries. The ADMP (an acronym in both German and English for the Association of Methodology and Documentation in Psychiatry) exists in English, German, French, Spanish and Japanese versions, covering virtually all the information needed for a comprehensive assessment by means of lists of items to be coded as present or absent. It is up to the user to decide the meaning of each item, and how much to train with fellow raters (or not) so as to improve inter-rater reliability.[81]

The condensation and recording of information

Summary and formulation

The skills required to produce summaries and formulations should be acquired early on in professional training, since they are central to the process of getting the information about the patient into a form which facilitates the making of decisions and the allocation of priorities for actions. Useful preliminaries to the writing of both summary and formulation are the preparation of a problem list and a lifechart; how to prepare these should also be covered in the early stages of training. The summary for an individual patient should be more or less the same whoever prepares it, since it should be a simple record of what is known, arranged under conventional headings. A 'telegram' style of writing is acceptable for the sake of brevity. In contrast, a formulation should be written as a grammatically correct narrative, and there is no necessary expectation that two different clinicians using the same summary about a patient would arrive at exactly the same conclusions in their formulations. This is because a formulation is an attempt by the writer to understand, and therefore to some extent to interpret, what has been influencing (and perhaps causing) the feelings and behaviour of the patient, and what relationships might exist between life events, illness, and contact with medical services. In other words, the writer is trying to tell the story of the patient's life and development, albeit very briefly. The complementary story of the episode of care will be clarified by clearly written **problem lists** placed in the case record at various stages. These serve both as reminders for action, and as a way of assessing progress when re-examined later.

Like the rest of the written medical records, the summary, formulation, and problem lists should be regarded as being as much for future readers as for the present carers. A clearly written summary and a well-argued formulation recorded in the case records will ensure that the reasons for treatments and decisions to do with the present illness are clear, and will be of great help to others if the patient has to be assessed in subsequent episodes of illness.

Summaries and formulations written by psychiatric members of a multidisciplinary team should be freely available to all the team, so that they can be discussed before the meetings at which a diagnosis is agreed and care programmes are set up. But it is not usually appropriate to send summaries and formulations made for hospital and team purposes to general practitioners or to consultants in other specialities. Specially written and shorter letters are best for this, taking into account the possibility that the patient or family may gain sight of, or even be shown, documents about them sent to other medical professionals.

Differential, main, subsidiary, and alternative diagnoses

A differential diagnosis should be placed in the case records in a prominent place, with a clear indication of who made it ('diagnosis' will be used in this section because of current conventions, but the difference between identifying a disorder and inferring an underlying diagnosis already noted must be kept in mind). When the patient suffers from more than one disorder it is usually possible to select one as the main diagnosis and specify the other(s) as additional or subsidiary diagnoses. The main diagnosis will usually be the one that is leading to immediate action, but the choice may depend upon the purposes for which the diagnoses are being recorded. Usually it reflects the reason for the current contact with services or admission but there are patients and occasions when, for instance, it makes more sense to record a lifetime diagnosis (such as schizophrenia or bipolar disorder) as the main diagnosis, even though something else such as anxiety or a phobic disorder is the reason for the current episode of care.

When one main diagnosis clearly applies yet does not account for some symptoms which, although a significant part of the clinical picture, still fall short of fulfilling the criteria for another disorder, it is useful to record these simply as 'additional symptoms' (for instance, depressive disorder with some obsessional symptoms; agoraphobia with some depressive symptoms, etc.). Neither ICD-10 nor DSM-IV mention this way of recording symptoms 'left over' after the main disorder has been accounted for, even though it is a useful clinical custom familiar to many generations of clinicians in a variety of countries. However, omission from formal classifications should not be allowed to inhibit clinicians from following clinical habits they find useful.

When there is reasonable debate about what is the best diagnosis out of two or more possibilities, one must be chosen provisionally as the main diagnosis as a basis for action but the other should be recorded as an alternative diagnosis. It is also good practice in quite early stages of the assessment process to record provisional diagnoses, which can then be changed as more information becomes available. About a third of psychiatric patients fulfil the criteria for more than one disorder as defined in current classifications, but as already noted, this does not carry the same implications about underlying morbid physiological, psychological, or anatomical processes as would a statement about the presence of the same number of medical or surgical diagnoses.

Making a prognosis

The final statement in the formulation should be the prognosis. This attempt to predict what will happen to the patient in the future should be expressed as clear statements about likely outcomes, avoiding vague comments such as 'the prognosis is guarded' (found all too often in case records). The patient and family usually hope to be told about the prospects for recovery and the likelihood of relapse. Efforts should be made to do this, but with due care to emphasize that a prognosis is only an estimate that may be proved wrong by events.. The ideal prognosis should contain predictions of such things as:

(1) immediate response to treatment, assuming compliance;

(2) duration of this episode of illness and/or stay in hospital;

(3) degree of recovery from this illness (i.e. partial or complete) in terms of both symptoms and return to previous activities;

(4) risk of recurrence, stated as the likely position at specific points in time, depending upon the circumstances of the case (6 months, 1 year, and 2 years from the present are often appropriate).

However difficult it may seem, attempts should be made to record a prognosis in these terms, and to sign it. To do this will fulfil the legitimate expectations of the patient and family, and the clinician will make possible a uniquely valuable learning experience when faced in the future with such statements about those patients seen in further episodes of care.

Reviews

The initial assessment should produce a list of agreed actions to be carried out in a stated order of priority by the various members of the team. Division into immediate and medium-term actions will help the whole process, and also indicate the time scale of reviews to assess progress. One of the main functions of the acknowledged team leader is to keep an eye on the progress of all the patients in the care of the team, discussing with each key worker both outside and within team meetings the best timing of the next review. Review meetings should be recorded as such in the case documents, with conclusions about progress made and any changes in plans or objectives. It is particularly important, again for future readers of the records, to write down clearly whether there was any response treatment (it is very frustrating to read in a case record of treatments given in the past, and then to find no indication of the result.)

Writing reports

Consultant psychiatrists are often asked by external agencies to provide written reports on patients for whom they have a current clinical responsibility, and requests may also be received for a report on a patient they have not seen previously. The purpose of these external reports is usually different to that of the usual clinical communications undertaken in the ordinary clinical care of the patient, in that the request is usually for an opinion about one specific issue. These requests frequently involve an opinion on the risk posed to others by the patient's inability to perform certain skills, or by the positive adverse effect of the patient's problems on others. An opinion on the capacity of the patient to understand and competently agree about important issues is also frequently requested.

The purposes of reports

Reports requested by individuals or agencies (both judicial and non-judicial) will usually fall into one of four broad groups.

1. Protection of the public or an institution:

   (a) life assurance and mortgage companies who are interested in the risk of suicide, or loss of earnings due to future illnesses;

   (b) licensing authorities and transport companies who are concerned with fitness to drive or risks due to the public, due to impairment of skills and judgement consequent upon psychiatric illness;

   (c) employment and benefit agencies who are concerned with fitness to work;

   (d) employers or occupational health physicians who are concerned about the risk posed by the patient's psychiatric disorder to an institution's clients, or about the likelihood of periods of absence because of sick leave.

2. Protection of the patient:

   (a) solicitors or courts may require reports on the competence of individual patients to conduct their financial affairs, to protect themselves from exploitation and to engage in civil contracts;

   (b) bodies concerned with the Mental Health Act (in the United Kingdom the Mental Health Act Commission and Mental Health Review Tribunals) may require reports on the competence of individuals to give informed consent to non-voluntary psychiatric treatment or inpatient care, and the risk to the safety and well being of the individual patient posed by such treatment.

3. Child protection:

   (a) Social Services Child Care Departments and others involved in the welfare of children may request reports of the supervising psychiatrist for Child Protection Case Conferences on the contribution of a psychiatric disorder to the child care problem, and on the likely impact of the psychiatric disorder on the future parenting of the patient;

   (b) solicitors acting for all parties in child care proceedings (the child, the Social Services Department, and the patient) may ask for a psychiatric report on a mentally ill parent about the likely risk to the child of suffering significant physical, developmental or emotional harm from the patient in question.

4. Medicolegal and compensation proceedings: lawyers acting for either the patient or an agency being sued may ask for a report on the impact of the event on the mental health of the patient, together with the nature of the psychiatric disorder and its prognosis. Such reports may be requested of the supervising consultant, or of another psychiatrist as an independent expert.

Reports for forensic or criminal proceedings are dealt with in Chapter 11.6.

Guiding principles

The general principles noted below apply to all reports, whether the psychiatrist knows the patient because of current or previous clinical responsibility, or whether the report is on a patient whom the psychiatrist has not seen before (this latter is known as providing an 'expert opinion').

Confidentiality

In most situations written consent must be obtained from the patient before personal information can be given to an outside agency. In almost all situations involving the writing of a report on an individual to an outside agency, that individual will gain sight of the report or will be entitled to do so. It is therefore good clinical practice for the patient to be aware of the content of the report, and particularly of any opinions or recommendations it may contain. Nevertheless, there are certain situations where the duty of care to the public or to a child overrides the duty of confidentiality, and in such circumstances the psychiatrist may write the report even without the patient's consent.

Partiality

The opinion of the psychiatrist is being sought as an expert professional. The report should not be biased in favour of one side or another and should not be influenced unduly by the interests of the commissioning agency or the psychiatrist's view of the best interests of their patient. This may cause difficulties if the patient is in the personal care of the psychiatrist because in most clinical situations psychiatrists try to be non-critical, non-judgemental, and supportive, tending to encourage rather than to prevent. But the best interests of the patient will not be served by being put in a situation where the likely outcomes are failure to do what is expected or to function at a suboptimal level.

Structure of reports

All reports should have three main sections. First, the report should begin with the patient's personal details and the reasons for which the report has been requested, together with the identity of the commissioning agency. It should also specify the relationship between the writer and the patient. If the patient is or was in the clinical care of the writer the duration of the care should be noted, and the date of the last occasion the patient was seen should be given. If a special interview had to be arranged with a patient not previously known, the duration and date of the interview should be stated. The sources of information other than the patient used to prepare the report should then be detailed, plus any other documents that have been read. Reports for civil, judicial, and child protection proceedings will also require a short paragraph on the current employment and status of the author of the report, and a note of any special experience of relevance.

The second section should describe in appropriate detail the patient's personal, social, medical, and psychiatric history, the mental state and behaviour at examination, the diagnosis and differential diagnosis, and comments upon aetiology, management, and prognosis. In almost all reports, the prognosis is the primary concern, so this should be given special attention. It is important to remember that one of the most reliable predictors of the recurrence of behaviours or episodes of illness in the future is the frequency of their occurrence in the past. Similarly, the vulnerability of the patient in the past (that is, any enduring predisposing factors and patterns of past precipitants) will tend to predict future vulnerability and the likelihood of further episodes of illness. Some mention of the past will therefore always be necessary, but in many instances this can be brief and reduced to a commentary of a few lines. But in other situations, particularly those involving civil court actions or child care proceedings, a more detailed account of the past will be necessary.

Certain aspects of the patient's past history and previous levels of functioning will need to be highlighted depending upon the purposes of the report and the nature of the questions asked of the psychiatrist. For example, if the report has been requested by an occupational physician about the fitness of a patient to return to work, then attention will need to be paid in the report to the duration of illnesses in the past and the amount of sick leave that has been taken. Detail will need to be given about the impact, if any, that the patient's ill health has had on the past to his or her capacity to work. If the report has been requested in relation to the safety of the patient to care for a child, then information will need to be given in the past history of the patient about the previous impact of the patient's illness on his or her capacity to care for children or any risks that that the patient posed to a child in the past. Life assurance and mortgage companies are likely to be particularly interested in suicidal behaviour.

The last section should contain the opinion of the psychiatrist about the specific questions posed by the commissioning agent. These questions may be unrealistically simple or there may be requests for categorical assertions of outcome that are simply not possible. The writer must avoid falling into the trap of complying with unreasonable requests about certainties. One way of avoiding this is to give opinions about risks or outcomes by stating criteria that would indicate different outcomes with different likelihoods, expressed by words such as possible, probable, and definite.

In situations where one of the variables involved in the patient's prognosis is the response of helping agencies and the availability of resources, great care must be exercised on the part of the report writer to ensure that this contingency is made clear. If possible, suggestions should be made as to how the availability of the required resources can be assured. When considering the likely impact of a future breakdown in the mental health of a patient on some other person, such as a child, consideration should be given not only to the direct impact of the illness but also to the indirect consequences and the presence or absence of other protective factors. For example, if a woman with schizophrenia lives with her parents who can safely take over the care of her child, then the impact of a further episode on that child may be much less than if she is living alone and the child needs to be removed into the care of the local authority.

An opinion is often requested on whether an accident or an act of omission such as medical negligence caused the current psychiatric disorder or disabilities of the patient. If the psychiatrist concludes that the accident or omission was definitely a contributing cause but not in itself sufficient to cause all aspects of the existing disorder and disability, then further comments will be expected on other possible contributing influences, such as predisposing personal traits, or special vulnerability to current adversities. In such circumstances, there should be an attempt to weight the contributing factors in order of their aetiological importance.

The last section of the report is usually the best place to list the sources of information used for the report, making clear distinctions between personal observations and information obtained by the writer, opinions and observations made by other team members, and written information obtained from other documents. There should always be a clear distinction between opinions based upon objective information and direct examination, and suppositions based upon interpretations, speculation, and past clinical experience. If opinions based upon research conducted by others are given, then the sources of this information should be acknowledged and referenced in the usual manner.

The language of the report should be appropriate to the commissioning agency. If the report has been requested by an occupational physician or medical officer working for a company, then it is appropriate to use accepted medical and psychiatric terminology. If the report has been requested by a civil or judicial authority, non-technical language should be used wherever possible and any medical or psychiatric terms used should be defined. At all times when writing psychiatric reports it is important to use psychiatric terms in an appropriate fashion according to a stated international classification, and to avoid idiosyncrasies.

References

1. Leff, J. and Isaacs, A.D. (1978). *Psychiatric examination in clinical practice.* Blackwell Science, Oxford.
2. Gelder, M., Gath, D., Mayou, R., and Cowen, P. (1996). *Oxford textbook of psychiatry* (3rd edn). Oxford University Press.
3. Lishman, W.A. (1998). *Organic psychiatry* (3rd edn). Blackwell Science, Oxford.
4. Jaspers, K. (1963). *General psychopathology* (7th edn) (transl. J. Hoenig and M. Hamilton), p. 825. Manchester University Press.
5. Post, F. (1983). The clinical assessment of mental disorders. In *Handbook of psychiatry*, Vol. 1 (ed. M. Shepherd and O.L. Zangwill), pp. 210–20. Cambridge University Press.
6. McHugh, P.R. and Slavney, P.R. (1986). *The perspectives of psychiatry.* Johns Hopkins University Press, Baltimore, MD.
7. Taylor, F.K. (1971). A logical analysis of the medico-psychological concept of disease: Part 1. *Psychological Medicine*, **1**, 356–64.
8. Susser, M.W. and Watson, W.B. (1971). *Sociology in medicine* (2nd edn), pp. 16–17, 216–218, 295ff. Oxford University Press.
9. Lewis, A.L. (1953). Health as a social concept. *British Journal of Sociology*, **4**, 109–204.
10. Wootton, B. (1959). Social pathology and the concepts of mental health and mental illness. *Social science and social pathology.* Allen and Unwin, London.
11. Scadding, J.G. (1967). Diagnosis, the clinician and the computer. *Lancet*, **ii**, 877–82.
12. Scadding, J.G. (1996). Essentialism and nominalism in medicine: the logic of diagnosis in disease terminology. *Lancet*, **348**, 594–6.
13. Kerr, A. and McClelland, H. (1991). *Concepts of mental disorder: a continuing debate.* Gaskell Press, London.
14. Tyrer, P. and Steinberg, D. (1993). *Models for mental disorders: conceptual models in psychiatry.* Wiley, Chichester.
15. Eisenberg, L. (1998). The social construction of mental illness (editorial). *Psychological Medicine*, **18**, 1–9.
16. Eisenberg, L. (1977). Disease and illness. Distinctions between professional and popular ideas of sickness. *Culture, Medicine and Psychiatry*, **1**, 9–24.
17. Engel, G.L. (1978). The biopsychosocial model and the education of health professionals. *Annals of the New York Academy of Sciences*, **310**, 169–81.
18. Susser, M. (1990). Disease, illness, sickness; impairment, disability and handicap (editorial). *Psychological Medicine*, **20**, 471–4.
19. World Health Organization (1980). *The international classification of impairments, disabilities and handicaps.* WHO, Geneva.
20. Taylor, F.K. (1979). *Psychopathology: its causes and symptoms.* Quartermaine House, Sunbury on Thames.
21. Fulford, K.W.M. (1989). *Moral theory and medical practice.* Cambridge University Press.

22. Mechanic, D. (1986). The concept of illness behaviour; culture, situation and personal predisposition. *Psychological Medicine*, **16**, 1–8.

23. Menninger, K. (1948). Changing concepts of disease. *Annals of Internal Medicine*, **29**, 318–25.

24. Kendell, R.E. (1975). *The role of diagnosis in psychiatry*. Blackwell Science, Oxford.

25. Cooper, J.E. (1983). Diagnosis and the diagnostic process. In *Handbook of psychiatry*, Vol. 1. *General psychopathology*, Part III (ed. M. Shepherd and O.L. Zangwill), pp. 199–209. Cambridge University Press.

26. Nagi, S.Z. (1965). Some conceptual issues in disability and rehabilitation. In *Sociology and rehabilitation* (ed. M.B. Sussman), pp. 110–13. American Sociological Association, Washington, DC.

27. Badley, E.M. (1987). The ICIDH: format, application in different settings, and distinction between disability and handicap; a critique of papers on the application of the International Classification of Impairments, Disabilities and Handicaps. *International Disability Studies*, **9**, 122–5.

28. Ustun, T.B., van Duuren-Kristen, S., and Cooper, J.E. (1995). Revision of the ICIDH: mental health aspects. *Disability and Rehabilitation*, **17**, 201–15

29. Weissman, M.M. (1975). The assessment of social adjustment: a review of techniques. *Archives of General Psychiatry*, **32**, 357–65.

30. Gurland, B.J., Yorkston, N.J., Stone, A.R., and Frank, J.D. (1972). The Structured and Scaled Interview to Assess Maladjustment (SSIAM). 1. Description, rationale and development. *Archives of General Psychiatry*, **27**, 259–64.

31. Claire, A.W. and Cairns V.E. (1978). Design, development and use of a standardised interview to assess social maladjustment and dysfunction in community studies. *Psychological Medicine*, **8**, 589–604.

32. Brown, G.W. and Harris, T.O. (1986). *Social origins of depression; a study of psychiatric disorder in women*. Tavistock Publications, London.

33. Brown, G.W. and Harris, T.O. (1986). Stressor, vulnerability and depression; a question of replication (editorial). *Psychological Medicine*, **16**, 739–44.

34. Andrews, G. and Tennant, C. (1978). Life events and psychiatric illness (editorial). *Psychological Medicine*, **8**, 545–9.

35. Jones, S.J., Turner, R.J., and Grant, J. (1987). Assessing patients in their homes. *Bulletin of the Royal College of Psychiatrists*, **11**, 117–19.

36. Oates, M.R. (1988). The development of an integrated community-oriented service for severe post-natal mental illness. In *Motherhood and mental illness*, Vol. III (ed. R. Kumar and I. Brockington), pp. 133–58. John Wright, London.

37. Tyrer, P. (1984). Psychiatric clinics in general practice: an extension of community care. *British Journal of Psychiatry*, **145**, 9–14

38. Department of Health (1990). *Caring for people: community care in the next decade and beyond. Policy guidance*. HMSO, London.

39. Department of Health (1990). *The care programme approach for people with mental illness referred to the special psychiatric services*. Department of Health, London.

40. Department of Health and Social Services Inspectorate (1991). *Care management and assessment: summary of practice guidelines*. HMSO, London.

41. Holloway, F., Oliver, N., Collins, E., *et al.* (1995). Case management: a critical review of the literature. *European Psychiatry*, **10**, 113–28.

42. Burns, T. (1997). Case management, care management and care programming (editorial). *British Journal of Psychiatry*, **170**, 393–5.

43. Katschnig, H. and Cooper, J.E. (1991). Psychiatric emergency and crisis intervention services. In *Community psychiatry: the principle* (ed. D.H. Bennet and H.L. Freeman), pp. 517–42. Churchill Livingstone, Edinburgh.

44. Cooper, J.E. (1990). Professional obstacles to implementation and diffusion of innovative approaches to mental health care. In *Mental health care delivery: innovations, impediments and implementation* (ed. I. Marks and R. Scott), pp. 233–53. Cambridge University Press.

45. Henderson, A.S. (1988). The tools of social psychiatry. In *An introduction to social psychiatry*, pp. 6–29. Oxford University Press.

46. Thompson, C. (ed.) (1989). *The instruments of psychiatric research*. Wiley, Chichester.

47. World Health Organization (1993). *Catalogue of assessment instruments used in the studies coordinated by the WHO Mental Health Programme*. WHO/MNH/92.5. Division of Mental Health, World Health Organization, Geneva.

48. Sartorius, N. and Janca, A. (1996). Psychiatric assessment instruments developed by the World Health Organization. *Social Psychiatry and Epidemiology*, **31**, 55–69.

49. Janca, A. (1997). Current trends in the development of psychiatric assessment instruments. *Current Opinion in Psychiatry*, **10**, 457–61.

50. Thornicroft, G. and Tansella, M. (ed.) (1997). *Mental health outcome measures*. Springer-Verlag, Berlin.

51. Goldberg, D.P. and Hillier, V.F. (1979). A scaled version of the General Health Questionnaire. *Psychological Medicine*, **9**, 139–45.

52. Wittchen, H.-U., Robins, L.N., Cottler, L.B., *et al.* (1991). Cross-cultural feasibility, reliability and sources of variance of the Composite International Diagnostic Interview (CIDI)—results of the multi-centre WHO/ADAMHA field trials (wave 1). *British Journal of Psychiatry*, **159**, 645–53.

53. World Health Organization (1993). *The Composite Diagnostic Interview, core version 1.1*. American Psychiatric Press, Washington, DC.

54. Hamilton, M. (1960). Rating scale for depression. *Journal of Neurology, Neurosurgery and Psychiatry*, **23**, 56–62.

55. Andreason, N.C. (1989). The Scale for Assessment of Negative Symptoms (SANS): conceptual and theoretical foundations. *British Journal of Psychiatry*, **155** (Supplement 7), 49–52.

56. Endicott, J. and Spitzer, R.L. (1978). A diagnostic interview: the Schedule for Affective Disorders and Schizophrenia. *Archives of General Psychiatry*, **35**, 837–44.

57. Wing, J.K., Curtis, R., and Beevor, A. (1994). 'Health of the Nation': measuring mental health outcomes. *Psychiatric Bulletin: Journal of Trends in Psychiatric Practice*, **18**, 690–1.

58. Wing, J.K., Babor, T., Brugha, T., *et al.* (1990). SCAN: Schedules for Clinical Assessment in Neuropsychiatry. *Archives of General Psychiatry*, **47**, 589–93.

59. Overall, J.E. and Gorham, D.R. (1962). The Brief Psychiatric Rating Scale (BPRS). *Psychological Reports*, **10**, 799–812.

60. Asberg, M., Montgomery, S.A., Perris, C., Schalling, D., and Sedvall, G. (1978). A Comprehensive Psychopathological Rating Scale (CPRS). *Acta Psychiatrica Scandinavica Supplementum*, **271**, 5–28.

61. Spitzer, R.L., Williams, J.B.W., and Gibbon M. (1987). *Structured Clinical Interview for DSM-IV (SCID)*. Biometrics Research, New York State Psychiatric Institute, New York.

62. Wing, J.K., Cooper, J.E., and Sartorius, N. (1974). *Measurement and classification of psychiatric symptoms: an instruction manual for the PSE and the CATEGO program*. Cambridge University Press, London.

63. Cooper, J.E., Kendell, R.E., Gurland, B.J., Sartorius, N., and Farkas, T. (1969). Cross-National Study of Diagnosis of Mental Disorders; some results from the first comparative investigation. *American Journal of Psychiatry*, **125** (Supplement), 21–9.

64. Cooper, J.E., Kendell, R.E., Gurland, B.J., Sharpe, L., Copeland, J.R.M., and Simon R. (1972). *Psychiatric diagnosis in New York and London: a comparative study of mental hospital admissions*. Maudsley Monograph No. 20. Oxford University Press.

65. Sartorius, N., Jablensky, A., and Shapiro, R. (1977). Two year follow-up of the patients included in the WHO International Pilot Study of Schizophrenia: preliminary communication. *Psychological Medicine*, **7**, 529–41.

66. Feighner, J.P., Robins, E., Guze, S.B., Woodruff, R.A., Winokur, G., and Munoz, R. (1972). Diagnostic criteria for use in psychiatric research. *Archives of General Psychiatry*, **26**, 57–63.

67. Robins, L.N., Helzer, J.E., Croughan, J., and Ratcliffe, K.S. (1981). National Institute of Mental Health Diagnostic Interview Schedule. Its history, characteristics and validity. *Archives of General Psychiatry*, **38**, 381–8.

68. Regier, D.A., Boyd, J.H., Burke, J.D., et al.(1988). One month prevalence of mental disorders in the United States: based on the five Epidemiological Catchment Area sites. *Archives of General Psychiatry*, **45**, 977–86.

69. Pull, C. and Wittchen, H.-U. (1991). CIDI, SCAN and IPDE: structured diagnostic interviews for ICD-10 and DSMIII-R. *European Journal of Psychiatry*, **6**, 277–85.

70. Regier, D.A., Kaelber, C.T., Rae, D.S., et al. (1998). Limitations of diagnostic criteria and assessment instruments for mental disorders. *Archives of General Psychiatry*, **55**, 9–115.

71. Kessler, R.C., McGonagle, K.A., Zhao, S., et al. (1994). Lifetime and 12 month prevalence of DSM-III-R psychiatric disorders in the United States; results from the National Co-morbidity Study. *Archives of General Psychiatry*, **51**, 8–19.

72. Wing, J.K., Bebbington, P., and Robins, L.N. (1981). *What is a case? The problem of definition in psychiatric community surveys*. Grant McIntyre, London.

73. Spitzer, R.L. (1998). Diagnosis and need for treatment are not the same (commentary). *Archives of General Psychiatry*, **55**, 120.

74. Kendell, R.E. (1989). Clinical validity.*Psychological Medicine*, **19**, 45–56.

75. Biehl, H., Maurer, K., Jablensky, A., Cooper, J.E., and Tomov, T. (1989). The WHO/PIRS : introducing a new instrument for rating observed behaviour, and the rationale of the psychological impairment concept. *British Journal of Psychiatry*, **155** (Supplement 7), 68–81.

76. Barnes, T.R.E. (ed.) (1989). Negative symptoms in schizophrenia. *British Journal of Psychiatry*, **155** (Supplement 7).

77. Mezzich, J.E. (1979). Patterns and issues in multiaxial psychiatric diagnosis *Psychological Medicine*, **9**, 125–37.

78. World Health Organization (1997). *Multiaxial presentation of ICD-10 for use in adult psychiatry*. Cambridge University Press.

79. Katschnig, H., Freeman, H., and Sartorius, N. (1997). *Quality of life in mental disorders*. Wiley, Chichester.

80. Bebbington, P., Brewin, C.R., Marsden, L., and Lesage, A. (1996). Measuring the need for psychiatric treatment in the general population: the community version of the MRC Needs for Care Assessment. *Psychological Medicine*, **26**, 229–36.

81. Woggon, B. (1986). The AMDP-III: a comprehensive instrument for recording psychiatric information. In *Assessment in depression* (ed. N. Sartorius and T. Baan), pp. 112–20. Springer-Verlag, Berlin.

1.10.2 Communication and mental health in primary care

R. M. Epstein, F. Borrell, and M. Caterina

Effective patient–physician communication is central to psychiatric diagnosis and treatment. Primary care settings offer unique challenges and opportunities to providers as compared with inpatient or outpatient mental health settings. Primary care patients often present somatic symptoms, and have somatic causal explanations for their suffering.[1–4] Many patients have one or more chronic illnesses, making 'vegetative' signs difficult to interpret. It is often difficult or undesirable to separate 'physical' from 'psychological' problems. The majority of patients with psychological distress do not have a major psychiatric disorder; many will appear to have elements of several disorders, and many will have no clear diagnosis despite adequate investigation. Primary care patients may be more reluctant to accept psychiatric referrals. Poor communication between consulting professionals is common.[5]

In the primary care setting, mental health providers need to know how to garner trust and gather information from the patient, the patient's family, friends and relevant social relations, and to involve them in an effective treatment plan. Ineffective communication is costly. Unexplored concerns lead patients to assume that the clinician is not interested, attribute the concern to a serious illness, and seek another consultation. In contrast, once a physician has responded effectively to a patient's concern, the patient is likely to be more satisfied, disclose more personal, and more accurate, information,[6,7] have improved biomedical outcomes[8,9] and may be less likely to sue.[10] Improved communication also has non-specific therapeutic effects. Often primary care patients with mental illnesses improve after discussing their concerns with their physician—without use of other psychotherapeutic interventions.

Actively inquiring into the patient's understanding of the problem, collaborating, sharing power, using language that the patient understands, seeking agreement on the nature of the problem and its treatment, and sharing emotions are skills essential to good communication.[11] In this chapter we will discuss how to overcome common communication barriers, use time effectively, set an agenda, adopt a patient-centred approach, and involve families and sociocultural networks in the care. We will also suggest methods for improving collaboration between primary care physicians and mental health professionals.

Overcoming barriers to communication

Of the many potential barriers to effective patient–physician communication (Table 1), the most important is the health professional him- or herself.[16–18] Although practising primary care is stressful because of the rapid pace and an obligation to accommodate patients' demands at inopportune moments, health professionals must meet these challenges by being empathic, assertive, and respectful. This is more easily said than done.

Being empathic is a first step in developing a patient–physician relationship. Empathy is defined as the ability to reflect accurately the inner experience of another person. It allows the clinician to open the door to patients' emotions. Despite their belief that empathy is important, physicians often are not empathic.[19] In order to express empathy, the physician must be courageous enough to tolerate and accept patients' feelings, secrets, and fears, and be willing to reveal feelings and emotions to the patient when it is appropriate and useful. Empathy requires patience. Physicians' emotions—anger, irritation, sympathy, attraction—interfere with their ability to be patient, and to listen to what their patients are trying to express. By cultivating the capacity to be aware of their own emotional reactions, physicians can fulfill their moral obligation to be respectful, that is, to put the patient's human dignity above their own values and needs. Physicians who are confident yet know their limitations can face difficult situations with flexibility and humility. An assertive positive attitude can help the professional avoid feeling aggressive, passive, or defeated, and maintain serenity. Without denying his or her emotions, or suppressing countertransference, the physician can 'recycle' feelings in a positive way.[20]

Allowing the expression of negative emotions in the patient–physician relationship has been associated with improved outcomes.[9] This 'emotional friction' is often perceived positively by patients as a

Table 1 Challenging situations in the consultation

Patient behaviours that violate physicians' personal norms

No-shows
Non-adherence
Frequent phone calls
Frequent demands for specialty referral
Seeking disability or compensation for injury
Poor hygiene
Rude foul language
Multiple sexual partners
Low motivation
Patients who do not pay bills
Emotional expression (anger, hostility)
Drug seeking

Patients with specific diagnoses[12,13]

Psychopathology—moderate to severe
Somatic distress without physical findings
Substance abuse
Hypochondriasis
Obesity
Chronic pain
Sexual behaviour-related conditions
Conditions where patient is perceived as culpable
Malignancies and other terminal illness
A complex ambiguous problem

Personality characteristics of patients that may predispose to difficulties[12,14]

Overdependency
Entitlement
Manipulativeness
Rejecting the physician's attempts to help
Self-destructive behaviour
Doctor shopping
Complaining, whining
Expressing anger
Demanding more than physician is willing to give

Personality characteristics of physicians that predispose to difficulties[12]

Like to solve problems, and like sense of closure
Like to help
Self-sacrificing, stoicism
Hard-working
Belief that science can solve human suffering
Risk aversion
Expectation that patients will share these values
Arrogance[15]

Circumstances when difficult moments are likely to surface

Diagnostic uncertainty
Deterioration of patient's functional status
Physician or hospital error
Patient dishonesty
Need for difficult decision
Conflict within the patient's family
Conflict of values between physician and patient
Secrets about, or disclosed by, patients
Patients with neurological or cognitive impairment
Cross-cultural communication
Delivering bad news
Dealing with angry or violent patients
Obtaining informed consent
Discussing advance directives
Determining competency

Table 2 Communicating by telephone

Train secretaries to recognize and triage mental health concerns, and create a simple protocol to determine whether the call is routine, urgent, or emergency. Include what information should be gathered, telephone contact, and reason for consultation

Establish telephone hours and encourage patients to use them

When the call is outside telephone hours, and is of routine nature, have the secretary indicate to the patient when the call will be returned

When interrupted by a call, try not to manifest irritation or anger, even if it comes at an inconvenient time and does not initially seem urgent. Patients usually think considerably before calling and may have undisclosed concerns

Set limits with patients who call inappropriately or frequently

marker of genuine caring. A psychiatrist can assist the primary care physician by normalizing and facilitating the patient's expression of emotions. This is especially helpful when the physician is overwhelmed or experiencing burn-out, and allows the physician to recast a positive relationship with a patient.

Using time

In general, psychiatrists working in primary care settings have more patients than time to take care of them. Effective triage of new patients, including the ability to accommodate urgent consultations, is necessary to provide good care (Table 2). Also helpful are timely and complete transfer of patient data, referral letters, and results of psychological tests that are done prior to the initial consultation. The psychiatrist must develop an interview style that can adapt to the primary care setting.

Primary care is characterized by brief but frequent patient interviews. Patient histories and family information are readily available in the primary care setting, as the physician has usually cared for several family members over time. Although it is essential to create and sustain an emotional connection with the patient during the interview, a good interview is not necessarily individual, non-directive, interpretive, or characterized by deep silences and revelations. The other interview extreme—using standardized questionnaires—allows physicians to obtain answers, but, as Balint said, only answers;[18] the most meaningful patient information may not be revealed. The 'high control' style characterized by simple yes/no responses may lead the clinician to a correct, but narrow diagnosis that does not result in understanding the patient.[21] Given the lack of time, the challenge for physicians is to find some balance between being directive versus non-directive, and listing emotions versus exploring them. Following are some guidelines to help achieve that balance.[22]

- Attend to all aspects of a patient's behaviour, appearance, speech, emotional state, thoughts, and judgement when making overall assessments of the patient's health.[23] Non-verbal cues provide valuable information from the outset of the interview. Physicians who maintain better eye contact detect more emotional distress.[24]

- Use 'windows of opportunity'.[25] Patients often do not disclose the issues that are most frightening to them in the first encounter with a clinician, and often not at the beginning of the visit. Thus,

Table 3 Basic communication skills in primary care

Greets patient and obtains patient's name
Introduces self, demonstrating interest and respect
Identifies the reason(s) for the consultation
Listens attentively, without interrupting or directing patient's response
Encourages patient to tell the story in own words
Clarifies ambiguous information
Flows from open to closed questions, eliciting information and responding to cues
Understands the patient's perspective before explaining own
Organizes delivery of information
Gives information in a way that patient understands
Checks patient understanding
Picks up verbal and non-verbal cues to patient's beliefs, reactions, and feelings
Encourages patient to take responsibility and be self-reliant
Offers future help and a follow-up plan

Data from Borrell i Carrio,[22] Kaplan *et al.*,[26] and Lipkin.[27]

probing should occur when a patient gives a clue, often indicated by a casual remark, a repeated comment, or a loaded question ('Could this be something serious?'). Often, the clinician cannot predict which topics the patient will find most difficult to discuss. A patient who speaks freely about a past history of sexual abuse, for example, may have tremendous difficulty talking about an extramarital affair (or vice versa).

- Use the words that the patient uses to describe his or her experience. Patients will often not have had experience with psychiatrists, and will not readily distinguish between problems that physicians consider somatic (e.g. fatigue) and psychiatric (e.g. depression). When describing mood, check the patient's understanding of words such as 'weak' or 'paranoid'.

- Address confidentiality. Elicit concerns from the patient, and discuss how to handle communication with other members of the team caring for the patient, as well as with the patient's family members.

- Find ways to respect the patient. This can be especially difficult when a patient discloses information that violates the physician's own personal values (such as a patient who admits to child molestation). In this instance, the physician can acknowledge the patient's courage to make such a disclosure. Let the patient know that he or she is a person with intrinsic worth and positive qualities. Actions will speak louder than words in this regard.

- Use the primary physician's long-term relationship with the patient and the family to gather historical information, especially prior adaptation to illness, and baseline level of functioning. This will provide clues to chronicity of symptoms, expectations for treatment, and underlying personality disorders. Prior psychiatric treatment, hospitalizations, and medications will give clues to previous diagnostic thinking, even if the patient is unaware of or unwilling to disclose prior psychiatric diagnoses.

Some other basic skills are summarized in Table 3.

Focusing the interview

What is the purpose of this particular clinical interview? Is it an emergency call? Am I proceeding appropriately? Do I have to change my

goals? These are questions that clinicians frequently ask themselves, sometimes unconsciously. While maintaining a focus on the patient and his or her symptoms, the physician must also maintain a more global focus to keep the interview on track. During the interview, physicians should ask: 'Have I understood fully why the patient is here now?'[28] Through active listening, the physician gathers an understanding not only of the patient's symptoms, but also of his or her beliefs, opinions, and expectations.

Aside from transference and countertransference, several factors make this task difficult: loss of perspective, inability to incorporate discordant data, and group countertransference. Sometimes, the physician can lose perspective when he or she becomes convinced of the legitimacy of the patient's beliefs, without constructing his or her own objectives and models of reality. In this way the physician can be drawn into unhelpful justifications for a patient's depression—the 'problems at home' or the 'need to convince her spouse to stop drinking'—and miss important contributing factors.

Second, the tendency to label patients as 'depressed' or 'hypochondriacal' can interfere with the clinician's ability to appreciate important diagnostic clues, and reject discordant data. This tendency may be due in part to the effort and humility required to recognize one's own mistakes, and to reclassify the patient.

Third, patients and families can stimulate issues that affect the physician's or the team's ability to provide care.[29,30] Group countertransference[31–33] is one way a health care team may respond to emotional distress. In an attempt to adapt to stressful patient situations, the team shares emotions that may result in shared attitudes toward a patient or class of patients. Teams can confuse projection, a characteristic of sympathy, with empathy, and obscure an accurate understanding of the thoughts and feelings of the patient. Teams can also idealize patients, and thus be blind to their manipulative behaviours. Inappropriate or dysfunctional attitudes on the part of the health care team occur especially when patients are viewed as intrusive, threatening, or aggressive. Group countertransference is especially common with patients who have borderline, antisocial, or addictive personality traits. Dealing with group countertransference can be difficult, as members who challenge the countertransference risk rejection and exclusion from the team. Sometimes external systems consultation is helpful.[34] The goal is for physicians and health care teams to recognize themselves as a sensitive diagnostic instrument and calibrate themselves accordingly.[18] The process of calibration involves developing self-awareness, and is one of the intangibles that distinguishes a seasoned clinician from a trainee,[17] a mature team from one that is unwilling to apply its expertise to itself.

Seeing a person rather than a patient

Human reality goes beyond DSM-IV multiaxial diagnosis. Although extremely useful, diagnostic categories do not evaluate disability, capture the patient's experience of suffering, or predict his or her capacity to heal, in part because they are pathologically driven. It is useful to view a patient's personality as his or her attempt to adapt to and remain in equilibrium with the environment rather than solely as a disorder.

Personality styles refer to 'enduring patterns of perceiving, relating to and thinking about the environment and oneself' that manifest in most or all aspects of life.[35] Understanding a patient's personality

Table 4 Personality styles

Normal trait	Potentially dysfunctional quality	Personality disorder
Cautious	Guarded/suspicious	Paranoid
Eccentric	Odd/schizoid	Schizotypal
Effusive	Dramatic	Histrionic
Self-centred	Grandiose	Narcissistic
Non-conforming	Entitled/disruptive	Antisocial
Hypersensitive	Ashamed	Avoidant
Faithful	Clinging/needy	Dependent
Attentive	Controlling/rigid	Obsessive–compulsive
Sulky	Uncooperative	Passive–aggressive
Unpredictable	Erratic	Borderline

style helps the clinician to understand the patient with the illness, as well as the illness. Patients' perceptions of their personality traits will often differ from the perceptions of others with whom they live and work. Garnering information about relationships and the perspectives of others adds rich data, whether the source of the information is the patient or family and friends.

With the stress of life circumstances, including illness, personality styles that had been very adaptive can become maladaptive; also, the patient's normal degrees of flexibility may be significantly reduced (Table 4). For example, a successful accountant with some obsessive–compulsive traits may become dysfunctionally preoccupied with his or her symptoms when confronted with the uncertainties of a chronic illness such as multiple sclerosis. A goal-directed and imaginative executive may become angry about having to wait 15 minutes to see the physician to obtain results of a 'routine' screening laboratory test. Personality styles that are maladaptive under everyday circumstances may become more maladaptive under the stress of illness. Thus, a depressive factory worker will assume that her breast lump is malignant before a biopsy is performed, and a passively dependent graduate student will schedule frequent visits for seemingly minor problems.

There are several common pitfalls in the assessment of patients' psychological profiles.

- Some personality traits may appear to be more fixed than they actually are. Defensiveness, mistrust, and anger manifested in situations of emotional distress may be state-dependent rather than traits. Clinicians may underestimate a bereaved patient's ability to cope; the deceased may have been a stabilizing force and the patient is experiencing transient disorientation.

- When there is underlying or overt turmoil in the relationship with the patient, physicians may be prone to prosecute the 'bad' patient with adjectives such as 'manipulator,' 'heartsink', or 'somatizer'.

- Physicians tend to undervalue the intelligence of illiterate, disabled, deaf, or foreign-born patients.[36,37] Physicians also tend to underestimate the level of suffering of patients from cultural groups different from their own.[38]

- Physicians are frequently misled by prior diagnoses, particularly if they are associated with legal or ethical transgressions on the part of the patient. Each patient must be given the opportunity to be different and to have a diagnosis different from that found previously.

- Hypochondriacal patients, patients who have problems with the law, and 'manipulators' can be perfect targets for physician mistakes. For these reasons, it is best to apply parsimonious and flexible adjectives when describing patients in medical records.

To overcome simplifications and facile labels (heavy, illiterate, whining, etc.), the clinician needs to maintain interest in the patient's daily life. Part of the interview should be a search for data about a previously undiscovered attribute: What are the patient's professional skills? Is he or she proud of something—a job, the family? Two biographical techniques are particularly useful for gathering such data. Pathobiography is a simple technique in which the clinician draws a time line beginning at the patient's birth and extending to the present. Important life events, including illnesses (Fig. 1), are placed to contextualize the current situation. A genogram, or family tree, can reveal important information about family structure, lifecycle developmental tasks, and family strengths as well as patterns of disharmony.[39] Both can be part of the regular medical record and updated periodically.

Interviewing children and adolescents

Children should be engaged in the interview to the degree that their development allows,[40] whether they are there for their own care or accompanying their parents. Although the parent of a preschool child undoubtedly will provide almost all of the historical information, a 3-year-old can describe where a pain is located, and can draw on a picture where he or she hurts. A 5-year-old often can provide an accurate description of his or her symptoms, and remarkably insightful descriptions of family dynamics. Intensity of symptoms, comparisons to prior experiences and temporal course can be described by an 8-year-old.

Choose a medium and style of communication that suits the child. Non-verbal communication will be more important to young children than choice of words. The clinician should be positioned to make eye contact with parent and with child. Some suggestions for engaging children are as follows:

- ask the child to draw a picture of his or her family, and then to describe what is happening in the picture

- use indirect questioning by asking the parent to ask the child a question

- be playful, but not coercive

- engage the child's interest with an object or a gift.

With the 12- to 18-year-old group, physicians frequently face a tension between maintaining the adolescent's privacy and confidentiality on the one hand and facilitating open communication within the family on the other. Although there are laws governing the care of children,

Patient: Mrs A.B.

Typhoid fever		Postpartum depression		Manic episode
1961		1982		1998
/------/----------------/---------/----------/--------- ----
1954	1974	1982	1990	2001
Birth	Marriage	First child born	Financial problems	

Fig. 1 Sample pathobiography

Table 5 Family interviewing skills

Introduce yourself to each family member, expressing interest in his or
  her perspective
Be sure that each family member has had a chance to speak
  uninterrupted
Check with each family member to make sure he or she has been heard
Do not take sides when there is a dispute
Respect confidentiality, but do not promise to keep secrets
Do not become too close or too distant from individual family members
Encourage the family to listen to and respect any opinion, regardless of
  who is talking

Adapted from McDaniel et al.[41] and Campbell and McDaniel.[43]

they are not specific enough to deal with many common situations in
practice. It is helpful to discuss with parents how important it is for the
adolescent to be able to share his or her concerns confidentially. Most
parents will agree to leave for at least part of the interview when it is
presented this way. If there is significant resistance, there may be
unspoken concerns that need to be explored further. For further information about interviews with children, see Chapter 9.1.4.

Gathering family information

The family can be an enormous asset in the care of the patient.[41] Each
family has members with a unique collection of talents, strengths, and
idiosyncrasies that have developed, in part, in response to prior life
stresses and opportunities. Most of these family patterns, as in the case
of individual personality styles, are highly adaptive. It is the clinician's
job to find out about both the adaptive and maladaptive family traits
in order to understand better how to help the patient. Most family
physicians and paediatricians, and many internists care for several
members of the same family, which provides them with a more complete picture of the family context. Home visits can also provide contextual information, and can be facilitated by the primary care
physician. When meeting with the family as a whole, developing rapport ('joining')[42] with all of those present, setting an agenda for the
meeting, eliciting each family member's perspective on the problem,
and developing a collaborative plan are crucial to a successful visit (see
Table 5).[41,43,44]

Gathering social network information

The patient's social context includes past and current affiliations with
friends, coworkers, and cultural and religious groups. Social networks
form more than a 'backdrop' for a patient's life activities; rather,
people, families, and social networks are constantly interacting with
and changing one another, and thus should be considered as part of
the patient's context.

It is helpful for the clinician to find out which social networks are
most important to the patient.

- Start with an open-ended inquiry to elicit the patient's concerns
  about the social networks he or she is describing. ('Tell me more
  about yourself—your background, work, and activities that are
  important to you.')

- Wait until the patient mentions a family member, colleague, or
  friend spontaneously, then pursue a line of questioning about

that particular relationship. ('You just mentioned your boss. How
are things going at work?' 'And, what about other people or activities that are important in your life?')

- Tie in questions about social context with observations or questions about the patient's concerns. ('You have mentioned a particularly harrowing encounter. In what ways do you think this is
  contributing to your anxiety in general?')

- Avoid premature interpretations. Although it is often tempting to
  interpret patients' reports of relationships and life events, beware
  of doing so prematurely.

The family physician often plays an important role as family counsellor, and is often central to patients' social and health care support
systems. When acting as counsellor, the family physician's knowledge
and status helps the patient and family make sense of medical information, including that from mental health professionals. Mental
health professionals can forge alliances with family physicians working
in the same community, incorporating their opinions and knowledge
of families into treatment (see Table 6).

Incorporating cultural issues

Postindustrial societies are ethnically diverse. Clinicians have the
opportunity to regard each patient as an informant from a culture that
is, in some way, foreign. The physician's curiosity about each patient's
beliefs and background will be rewarded with more information about
the patient's culturally influenced explanatory models of illness.[45] It
is a mistake to assume that all members of a culture hold the same
belief. Recent immigrants often hold beliefs different from their children. On the other hand, some generalizations may apply. In several
American studies, for example, different cultural groups had vastly
different responses to pain. Italian-Americans were most concerned
with the immediate experience of pain, Jewish-Americans were concerned more about the meaning or prognosis implied by the painful
state; both considered it dangerous not to report pain.[46] In contrast,
'old Americans' (of English descent) are expected to be more stoical in

Table 6 Guidelines for mental health professionals working with
primary care physicians

Make personal contact by letter, telephone, or e-mail with the primary
  care physician as soon as possible after the request for consultation.
  This contact will usually provide valuable information and establish a
  collaboration that will make your work easier

Be sure that the patient, family physician, and psychiatrist all understand
  the reason for consultation

Use conjoint sessions with the primary physician, psychiatrist, and the
  patient, especially for the patient who is reluctant or mistrustful

Maintain a schedule of regular communication between professionals by
  letter or e-mail for patients who have regular contact with both

At least once a year, send a treatment summary to the primary physician,
  including diagnosis, whether the patient is still in treatment, whether
  follow-up is needed, or the patient has abandoned treatment

Establish a means of contact during emergencies

Negotiate who will have responsibility for the case and for follow-up response to pain. Knowledge of Asian cultures' expectations of stoicism may be useful, for example, to the clinician caring for an 'emotionally flat' Laotian woman recovering from breast cancer surgery.

In Chinese culture, exposure to wind is thought to be harmful.[47] Disorders of a specific organ system may carry complex meanings and fear for members of a particular culture; patients fear 'heart distress' in Iranian culture,[48] and Puerto Ricans are fearful of loss of even small amounts of blood. Chinese patients will often report somatic symptoms rather than psychological ones due to the stigma that psychological distress places on the patient as well as the family.[49] Peptic ulcer disease may carry positive connotations in Japan, where it is seen as a sign of diligence and hard work. In Mediterranean cultures, it is considered healthy to express emotions, and some illnesses are attributed to 'not having cried enough' after a loss. Antidepressant or anxiolytic treatment in such cases can be counterproductive.

Patients from different ethnic groups place different emphasis on the role of the family in medical decision making. Northern European cultures value individual autonomy; many of the ethical principles are based on an individual patient–physician relationship without considering the influence of the family. Conversely, some Mediterranean,[50] Latino, and Asian[51] cultures use a family-centred model of decision making, including a preference to inform the *family*, not the patient, of his or her diagnosis and/or prognosis. These models of medical decision making are of paramount importance in mental health care, as family involvement and support of a treatment plan can make the difference between success and failure. In addition, traditional healers can play an important and adaptive role in the healing process if the clinician can maintain an open mind.

Collaborating, consulting, and referring

The success of mental health care often depends on communication between the referring primary care physician and the psychiatric consultant.[52,53] Care may be shared between the primary physician and the mental health professional according to one of several models.

A one-time psychiatric consultation with expected follow-up with the family physician might be useful to confirm a diagnosis or suggest pharmacotherapy when first-line treatments have failed. In more complex cases, the psychiatrist might assume temporary responsibility for the patient's mental health care until the patient has improved sufficiently. Long-term collaboration is necessary for patients with concurrent chronic psychiatric and medical illnesses. Shared visits with the family physician, the patient, and, sometimes, family members, can help to avoid miscommunications, and favour accurate diagnosis, appropriate treatment, and adherence. Transfer of total responsibility to a psychiatrist might be appropriate for patients with complex psychiatric illness who have no other chronic illnesses. Suggestions for effective psychiatrist–primary physician collaboration are shown in Table 6.

Conclusion

Effective communication is the core skill in mental health care in primary care settings. Communicating effectively includes gaining the patient's trust, organizing the visit so that the patient's feelings are elicited and heard, being aware of indirect cues to emotional distress, and using empathy. Inquiring about family and social issues, actively asking about topics that are difficult to discuss such as sexuality and interpersonal violence, and recognizing and adjusting to cultural differences provides the physician with more information to better understand and care for the patient. Physician self-awareness and ability to collaborate with other health care providers are also skills that will facilitate accurate inquiry into the patient's true concerns and the context in which they occur.

References

1. Schurman, R.A., Kramer, P.D., and Mitchell, J.B. (1985). The hidden mental health network. Treatment of mental illness by nonpsychiatrist physicians. *Archives of General Psychiatry*, **42**, 89–94.
2. Kroenke, K., Spitzer, R.L., Williams, J.B., *et al.* (1994). Physical symptoms in primary care. Predictors of psychiatric disorders and functional impairment. *Archives of Family Medicine*, **3**, 774–9.
3. McWhinney, I.R., Epstein, R.M., and Freeman, T.R. (1997). Rethinking somatization. *Annals of Internal Medicine*, **126**, 747–50.
4. Epstein, R.M., Quill, T.E., and McWhinney, I.R. (1999). Somatization reconsidered: incorporating the patient's experience of illness. *Archives of Internal Medicine*, **159**, 215–22.
5. Epstein, R.M. (1995). Communication between primary care physicians and consultants. *Archives of Family Medicine*, **4**, 403–9.
6. Frankel, R.M. and Beckman, H.B. (1995). Accuracy of the medical history: a review of current concepts and research. In *The medical interview* (ed. M.J. Lipkin, S.M. Putnam, and A. Lazare), pp. 511–24. Springer-Verlag, New York.
7. Roter, D.L., Hall, J.A., Kern, D.E., Barker, L.R., Cole, K.A., and Roca, R.P. (1995). Improving physicians' interviewing skills and reducing patients' emotional distress—a randomized clinical trial. *Archives of Internal Medicine*, **155**, 1877–84.
8. Bass, M.J., Buck, C., and Turner, L. (1986). The physician's actions and the outcome of illness. *Journal of Family Practice*, **23**, 43–7.
9. Kaplan, S.H., Greenfield, S., and Ware, J.E., Jr (1989). Assessing the effects of physician–patient interactions on the outcomes of chronic disease. *Medical Care*, **27**, S110–27. (Published erratum appears in *Medical Care*, **27**, 679.)
10. Beckman, H.B., Markakis, K.M., Suchman, A.L., and Frankel, R.M. (1994). The doctor–patient relationship and malpractice. Lessons from plaintiff depositions. *Archives of Internal Medicine*, **154**, 1365–70.
11. Simpson, M., Buckman, R., Stewart, M., Maguire, P., Lipkin, M., and Novack, D. (1991) Doctor–patient communication: the Toronto consensus statement. *British Medical Journal*, **303**, 1385–87.
12. Klein, D., Najman, J., Kohrman, A.F., and Munro, C. (1982). Patient characteristics that elicit negative responses from family physicians. *Journal of Family Practice*, **14**, 881–8.
13. Lin, E.H., Katon, W., Von Korff, M., *et al.* (1991). Frustrating patients: physician and patient perspectives among distressed high users of medical services. *Journal of General Internal Medicine*, **6**, 241–6.
14. Groves, J.E. (1978). Taking care of the hateful patient. *New England Journal of Medicine*, **298**, 883–7.
15. Ingelfinger, F.J. (1980). Arrogance. *New England Journal of Medicine*, **303**, 1507–11.
16. Epstein, R.M., Campbell, T.L., Cohen-Cole, S.A., McWhinney, I.R., and Smilkstein, G. (1993). Perspectives on patient–doctor communication. *Journal of Family Practice*, **37**, 377–88.
17. Novack, D.H., Suchman, A.L., Clark, W., Epstein, R.M., Najberg, E., Kaplan, C. (1997). Calibrating the physician: physician personal awareness and effective patient care. *Journal of the American Medical Association*, **278**, 502–9.
18. Balint, M. (1997). *The doctor, his patient and the illness*. International Universities Press, New York.
19. Suchman, A.L., Markakis, K., Beckman, H.B., and Frankel, R. (1997). A

model of empathic communication in the medical interview. *Journal of the American Medical Association*, **277**, 678–82.

20. Havens, L. (1986). *Making contact*. Harvard University Press, Cambridge, MA.

21. Platt, F.W. and McMath, J.C. (1979). Clinical hypocompetence: the interview. *Annals of Internal Medicine*, **91**, 898–902.

22. Borrell i Carrio, F. (1989). *Manual de entrevista clinica*. Mosby/Doyma, Barcelona.

23. Morgan, W.L. and Engel, G.L. (1969). *The clinical approach to the patient*. W.B. Saunders, Philadelphia, PA.

24. Goldberg, D., Steele, J.J., Smith, C., *et al.* (1983). *Training family practice residents to recognize psychiatric disturbances*. National Institute of Mental Health, Rockville, MD.

25. Branch, W.T. and Malik, T.K. (1993). Using 'windows of opportunities' in brief interviews to understand patients' concerns. *Journal of the American Medical Association*, **269**, 1667–8.

26. Kaplan, C.B., Siegel, B., Madill, J.M., and Epstein, R.M. (1997). Communication and the medical interview: strategies for learning and teaching. *Journal of General Internal Medicine*, **12**, S49–55.

27. Lipkin, J.M. (1994). The medical interview and related skills. In *Office practice of medicine* (ed. W.T. Branch). W.B. Saunders, Philadelphia, PA.

28. Neigbour, R. (1987). *The inner consultation: how to develop an effective and intuitive consulting style*. MTP Press, Boston, MA.

29. Mengel, M. (1987). Physician ineffectiveness due to family of origin issues. *Family Systems Medicine*, **5**, 176–90.

30. Dimsdale, J.E. (1984). Delays and slips in medical diagnosis. *Perspectives in Biology and Medicine*, **27**, 213–20.

31. Tizon, J. (1988). *Componentes psicologicos de la practica medica*. Doyma, Barcelona.

32. Tizon, J. (1992). *Atencion primaria en salud mental y salud mental en atencion primaria*. Doyma, Barcelona.

33. Bofill, P. and Folch-Mateu, P. (1999). Problemes cliniques et techniques du contre-transfert. *Revue Francaise de Psychanalyse*, **27**, 31–130.

34. Wynne, L.C., McDaniel, S.H., and Weber, T.T. (1986). *Systems consultation: a new perspective for family therapy*. Guilford Press, New York.

35. Putnam, S.M., Lipkin, M.J., Lazare, A., Kaplan, C., and Drossman, D.A. (1995). Personality styles. In *The medical interview* (ed. M.J. Lipkin, S.M. Putnam, and A. Lazare), pp. 251–74. Springer-Verlag, New York.

36. McEwen, E. and Anton-Culver, H. (1988). The medical communication of deaf patients. *The Journal of Family Practice*, **26**, 289–91.

37. Miles, S. and Davis, T. (1995). Patients who can't read. *Journal of the American Medical Association*, **274**, 1719–20.

38. Todd, K.H., Samaroo, N., and Hoffman, J.R. (1993). Ethnicity as a risk factor for inadequate emergency department analgesia. *Journal of the American Medical Association*, **269**, 1537–9.

39. McGoldrick, M. and Gerson, R. (1985). *Genograms in family assessment*. Norton, New York.

40. Dixon, S. and Stein, M.T. (1992). *Encounters with children: pediatric behavior and development*. Mosby–Year Book, St Louis, MO.

41. McDaniel, S.H., Campbell, T.L., and Seaburn, D.B. (1990). *Family-oriented primary care: a manual for medical providers*. Springer-Verlag, New York.

42. Minuchin, S. and Fishman, H.C. (1981). *Family therapy techniques*. Harvard University Press, Cambridge, MA.

43. Campbell, T.L. and McDaniel, S.H. (1995). Conducting a family interview. In *The medical interview* (ed. M.J. Lipkin, S.M. Putnam and A. Lazare), pp. 178–86. Springer-Verlag, New York.

44. Doherty, W.J. and Baird, M.A. (1983). *Family therapy and family medicine: toward the primary care of families*. Guilford Press, New York.

45. Kleinman, A. (1980). *Patients and healers in the context of culture*. University of California Press, Berkeley, CA.

46. Zborowski, M. (1952). Cultural components in response to pain. *Journal of Social Issues*, **8**, 16–30.

47. Kaptchuk, T.J. (1983). *The web that has no weaver: understanding Chinese medicine*. Congdon and Weed, New York.

48. Good, B. (1977). The heart of what's the matter: the semantics of illness in Iran. *Culture Medicine and Psychiatry*, **2**, 25–54.

49. Kleinman, A. (1982). Neurasthenia and depression: a study of somatization and culture in China. *Culture Medicine and Psychiatry*, **6**, 117.

50. Surbone, A. (1992). Truth telling to the patient. *Journal of the American Medical Association*, **268**, 1661–2.

51. Blackhall, L.J., Murphy, S.T., Frank, G., Michel, V., and Azen S. (1995). Ethnicity and attitudes toward patient autonomy. *Journal of the American Medical Association*, **274**, 820–5.

52. McDaniel, S.H., Campbell, T.L., and Seaburn, D.B. (1990). Working together: collaboration and referral to mental health professionals. In *Family oriented primary care*, pp. 343–60. Springer-Verlag, New York.

53. Seaburn, D., Lorenz, A., Gunn, B., Gawinski, B., and Mauksch, L. (1996). *Models of collaboration: a guide for mental health professionals working with health care practitioners*. Basic Books, New York.

1.10.3 Psychological assessment
1.10.3.1 Cognitive assessment

Graham E. Powell

Principles of assessment

Assessment, testing, or measurement is the evaluation of the individual in numerical or categorical terms, adhering to a range of statistical and psychometric principles. Examples of measurement are assigning people or behaviour to categories, using scales to obtain self-ratings or self-reports, using tests of ability and performance, or collecting psychophysiological readings. Even diagnosis is a form of measurement and should have various psychometric properties such as satisfactory reliability and validity. In this chapter we concentrate on cognitive or neuropsychological assessment, which typically employs standardized psychometric tests, but it is axiomatic that the basic principles are applicable to all forms of measurement without exception. For example, stating that a patient does or does not have a symptom is potentially just as much of a measurement as stating his or her IQ. It should be noted that this account is of English language tests, and readers elsewhere should note the principles but ask local psychologists what tests they use.

Psychometric tests aim to measure a real quantity—the degree to which an individual possesses or does not possess some feature or trait, such as social anxiety or spelling ability or spatial memory. This real quantity is known in classical test theory as the **true score** t, and the score that is actually obtained on the given test is the **observed score** x. It is assumed that the observed score is a function of two values, the true score plus a certain amount of **error** e, because no test is perfect. Therefore we have the most basic equation in psychometrics: $x = t + e$. The statistical aim of psychometric measurement is to keep the error term to an absolute minimum so that the observed score is equal to the true score, which happens when the error term is reduced to zero. Of course, this is never achieved, but the error term can be reduced to the minimum by making the test as reliable as possible, where reliability is simply the notion that the test gives the same answer twice.

Table 1 Types of reliability

Scorer or rater reliability	The probability that two judges will (i) give the same score to a given answer, (ii) rate a given behaviour in the same way, or (iii) add up the score properly. Scorer reliability should be near perfect.
Test–retest reliability	The degree to which a test will give the same result on two different occasions separated in time, normally expressed as a correlation coefficient. A reliability of less than 0.8 is dubious.
Parallel-form reliability	The degree to which two equivalent versions of a test give the same result (usually used when a test cannot be exactly repeated because, say, of large practice effects).
Split-half reliability	If a test cannot be repeated and there are no parallel forms, a test can be notionally split in two and the two halves correlated with each other (e.g. odd items versus even items). There is also a mathematical formula for computing the mean of all possible split halves (the Kuder–Richardson method).
Internal consistency	The degree to which one test item correlates with all other test items, i.e. an 'intraclass correlation' such as the α coefficient, which should not drop below 0.7.

In practice, of course, if a test were repeated many times, each occasion would give a slightly different result, depending on how the person felt, the precise way questions were asked, the details of how answers were scored, or whether there has been any lucky guessing. In other words, observed scores would cluster around the true score. Like the distribution of any variable, the distribution of observed scores would have a mean and a standard deviation. The mean is obviously the true score, and the standard deviation has been given a special name, the **standard error of measurement (SEM)**. Clearly the aim of a good test is to keep the SEM as near as possible to zero, and test manuals should state the actual SEM.

There is a relationship between SEM and the reliability of the test:

$$\text{SEM} = \text{SD}\sqrt{(1 - r_{11})}$$

where SD is the standard deviation of the test and r_{11} is the test–retest reliability of the test (expressed as a correlation coefficient ranging from –1 to +1). If the reliability of the test is perfect (+1), as can be seen the SEM will be zero:

$$\text{SEM} = \text{SD}\sqrt{(1 - 1)} = \text{SD}\sqrt{0} = 0.$$

Thus a test should be as reliable as possible because then the observed score will be the true score and the standard error of measurement will be zero.

An unreliable test is always useless, but if reliability can be achieved then it is worth considering the test score and, more specifically, what it measures. The degree to which a test measures what it is supposed to measure is known as **validity**. There may be various threats to validity. For example, a test of numeracy may be so stressful that scores are highly dependent upon the patient's anxiety level rather than his or her ability, or a test of social comprehension may have questions which are culturally biased and so scores may depend in part upon the person's ethnic background.

In practice, there are various types of reliability and validity, and these are summarized in Tables 1 and 2. Further discussion can be found in Kline.[1]

Having used a reliable and valid test, the next issue is how the numbers are analysed and expressed. It has to be noted first that there are three types of scale of measurement. A **nominal** scale is when numbers are assigned to various categories simply to label the categories in a manner suitable for entry onto a computer database—the categories actually bear no logical numerical relationship to each other. Examples would be marital test status or ethnic background or whether one's parents were divorced or not. Nominal scales are used to split people into groups and all statistics are based on the frequency of people in each group. The relationship or association between groups can be examined using χ^2 statistics, for example to test whether there is a relationship between being divorced and having parents who divorced. Next there is an **ordinal** scale, in which larger numbers indicate greater possession of the property in question. Rather like the order of winning a race, no assumptions are made about the magnitude of the difference between any two scale points; it does not matter whether the race is won by an inch or a mile. Ordinal scales allow people to be rank ordered and numerical scales can be subjected to non-parametric stat-

Table 2 Types of validity

Face validity	Whether a test seems sensible to the person completing it; i.e. does it appear to measure what it is meant to be measuring? This is in fact not a statistical concept, but without reasonable face validity, a patient may see little point in co-operating with a test that seems stupid.
Content validity	The degree to which the test measures all the aspects of the quality that is being assessed. Again, this is not a statistical concept but more a question of expert judgement.
Concurrent validity	Whether scores on a test discriminate between people who are differentiated on some criterion (e.g. are scores on a test of neuroticism higher in those people with a neurotic disorder than in those without such a disorder?). Also, whether scores on a test correlate with scores on a test known to measure the same or similar quality.
Predictive validity	The degree to which a test predicts whether some criterion is achieved in the future (e.g. whether a child's IQ test predicts adult occupational success; whether a test of psychological coping predicts later psychiatric breakdown). For obvious reasons, these last two types of validity are often jointly referred to as *criterion-related validity*.
Construct validity	Whether a test measures some specified hypothetical construct, i.e. the 'meaning' of test scores. For example, if a test is measuring one construct, there should not be clusters of items that seem to measure different things; the test should correlate with other measures of the construct (*convergent validity*); it should not correlate with measures that are irrelevant to the construct (*divergent validity*).
Factorial validity	If a test breaks down into various subfactors, then the number and nature of these factors should remain stable across time and different subject populations.
Incremental validity	Whether the test result improves decision-making (e.g. whether knowledge of neuropsychological test results improves the detection of brain injury).

istical analysis (which is that branch of statistics which makes minimal assumptions about intervals and distributions), including the comparison of means and distributions and the computation of certain correlation coefficients. Finally comes the **interval** scale in which each scale point is a fixed interval from the previous one, like height or speed. The types of test described in this chapter for the most part aspire to be interval scales, allowing use of the full range of parametric statistics (which assume equal intervals and normally distributed variables).

Having obtained a test score for someone, that score then has to be interpreted in the light of how the general population or various patient groups generally perform on that test. There are two general characteristics of a scale that have to be remembered. The first is the measure of central tendency. Typically one would consider the mean (the arithmetic average), but it is also sometimes useful to consider the median (the middle score) and the mode (the most frequently obtained score). This will be the first hint as to whether the score is normal or whether it is more typical of one group than another. However, in order to gauge precisely how typical a given score is, it is necessary to take into account the **standard deviation (SD)** of the test (other measures relating to the dispersion of test scores, such as the range or skew, can be considered but are not of such immediate relevance).

As long as the mean and SD of the test are known, it is possible to work out exactly what percentage of people obtain up to the observed score x. This is done by converting the observed score into a **standard score** z and converting the z-score to a **percentile**. A standard score is simply the number of SDs away from the mean m, and it will have both negative and positive values (because an observed score can be either below or above the mean respectively). In other words, $z = (x - m)/\text{SD}$. For reference, Table 3 gives some of the main values of z and what percentage of people score up to those values. It is this percentage that is known as the percentile and it is obtained from statistical tables. For example, a score at the 25th percentile means that 25 per cent of people score lower than that specific score. Obviously, the 50th percentile is the mean of the test. For illustration, the equivalent IQ scores (IQ scores have a mean of 100 and SD of 15) and broad verbal descriptors are also given in Table 3.

A knowledge of percentile scores can help to decide to which category a patient may belong. For example, if a patient completes a token test of dysphasia and scores at the 5th percentile for normal controls and the 63rd percentile for a group of dysphasics, the score is clearly more typical of the dysphasic group.

However, in clinical practice it is often not just a comparison with others that is needed, but a comparison between two of the patient's own scores. For example, verbal IQ might seem depressed in comparison with spatial IQ, or the patient's memory quotient might seem too low for his or her IQ. These are know as **difference scores**, and their analysis is a crucial part of the statistical analysis of a patient's profile. There are two key concepts: the **reliability of difference scores** and the **abnormality of difference scores**. Failure to distinguish between these two leads to all manner of erroneous conclusions. In brief, a reliable difference is one that is unlikely to be due to chance factors, so that if the person were to be retested then the difference would again be found. If the test is very reliable (see the previous discussion of reliability), even a small difference score may also be reliable. As a concrete example, the manual of the Wechsler Adult Intelligence Scale–Third Edition (**WAIS-R**)[2] indicates that a differ-

Table 3 z-scores, percentiles, IQ scores, and descriptions

z-score	Percentile	IQ	Description
−2.00	2.5th	70	Scores below the 2.5th percentile are *deficient* or in the *mentally retarded* range
−1.67	5th	75	
−1.33	10th	80	Scores between the 2.5th and 10th percentile are *borderline*
−1.00	16th	85	
−0.67	25th	90	Scores between the 10th and 25th percentile are *low average*
−0.33	37th	95	
0.00	50th	100	The mean score
+0.33	63rd	105	
+0.67	75th	110	Scores between the 25th and 75th percentile are in the *average* range
+1.00	84th	115	
1.33	90th	120	Scores between the 75th and 90th percentile are *high average*
		120+	Scores over the 90th percentile are *superior*

ence of about nine points between verbal IQ and performance IQ is statistically reliable at the 95 per cent level of certainty.

However, although a difference of this size would be reliable, this does not necessarily mean that it is abnormal and therefore indicative of pathology. The abnormality of a difference score is the percentage of the general population that have a difference score of this size or greater. Consulting published tables,[3,4] it can be seen that 18 per cent of adults and 22 per cent of children (on the children's version of the test) have a discrepancy of at least 10 points between verbal and performance IQ. Therefore a difference of 10 points is not at all unusual. In fact, to obtain an abnormal difference between verbal and performance IQ the discrepancy has to be of the order of 22 points for adults and 25 points for children (i.e. less than 5 per cent of adults or children have discrepancy scores of this size).

Having introduced the basic concepts of psychometric assessment, this is an appropriate point, prior to the description of specific tests, at which to summarize the information that can (or should) be found in a typical test manual, and this is set out in Table 4.

Tests of cognitive and neuropsychological functioning

General ability and intelligence

A very useful broad screening test, especially when it is suspected that mental functions are severely compromised, is the Mini-Mental State Examination.[5,6] It is brief, to the point, and can be repeated over time to gauge change. It measures general orientation in time and place, basic naming, language and memory functions, and basic non-verbal

Table 4 What to expect in a good test manual

Theory	The history of the development of the concept and earlier versions of the test
	The nature of the construct and the purpose of measuring it
Standardization	Characteristics of the standardization sample, how the sampling was carried out, and how well these characteristics match those of the general population
	Similar data on any criterion groups
	Similar data for each age range if the test is for children
Administration	How to administer the test in a standard fashion so as to minimize variability of administration as a factor in the error term
Scoring	How to score the test, and criteria for awarding different scores, so as to minimize scorer error
Statistical properties	Means and standard deviations of all groups
	Reliability coefficients and how they were obtained
	Validity measures and how they were derived
	Standard error of measurement
	Reliability of difference scores
	Abnormality of difference scores
	Other data on the scatter of subtest scores
	Scores of criterion groups
Special considerations	Groups for whom the test is not suitable or less suitable, i.e. the range of convenience of the tests
	Ceiling effects: at what point does the test begin to fail to discriminate between high scorers?
	Floor effects: at what point does the test begin to fail to discriminate between low scorers?

skills, and has good norms for a middle age range, especially the elderly, with appropriate adjustment for age. The maximum score is 30, and a score of 24 or less raises the possibility of dementia in older persons, especially if they have had 9 or more years of education (a score of 24 is at about the 10th percentile for people aged 65 and older).

However, the Mini-Mental State Examination is only a screening test and the presence or nature of cognitive impairment cannot be diagnosed on the basis of this test alone. A detailed cognitive assessment is provided by the Wechsler scales, i.e. the Wechsler Adult Intelligence Scale–Third Edition UK Version (**WAIS-III**^{UK}),[2] the Wechsler Intelligence Scale for Children–III UK Version (**WISC-III**^{UK}),[7] or the Wechsler Preschool and Primary Scale of Intelligence–Revised (**WPPSI-III**).[8] Outlines of the WAIS-III^{UK} and WISC-III^{UK} are given in Table 5.

IQ scores themselves are very broad measures, drawing upon a wide range of functions. This means that the scores are very stable (reliable), but also that the IQ score is relatively insensitive to anything except quite gross brain damage. Rather, a careful analysis of subtest scores is needed, always bearing in mind the concepts of reliability and abnormality of difference scores. For example, it takes a subtest range of 11 to 12 points to be considered abnormal (i.e. found in less than 5 per cent of people) on the WAIS-III^{UK}, the earlier WAIS-R,[4] and the WISC-III^{UK}.[7]

Sometimes the patient may have a language disorder or English may not be his or her first language. In such circumstances Raven's

Progressive Matrices Test,[9] which is a non-verbal test of inductive reasoning (non-verbal in the sense that it requires no verbal instructions and no verbal or written answers), can be used. The present author avoids the new norms because they were not collected in the normal fashion (i.e. not in a formal test session under the direct supervision of a psychologist), but the old norms are good. The Matrices Test has the additional advantage of having an advanced version for people in the highest range of ability.[10] No non-English versions of the WAIS-III^{UK} or the WISC-III^{UK} are available, but the non-verbal scores can be used with caution as there may be unexpected cross-cultural effects.

Speed of processing

Reasoning is not just about solving difficult problems, but also about solving them quickly; the difference between power and speed. IQ tests as above do have timed subtests sensitive to speed, but it can be useful to administer specific tests that are not quite so confounded with intellectual ability.

One example, particularly sensitive to even quite mild concussion, is the Paced Auditory Serial Addition Test (**PASAT**).[11,12] Here, the client is read a list of numbers, and as each one is read out so it has to be added to the previous number and the answer spoken aloud (Table 6). This has to be done quickly or the next number will come along. There are several trials in which the numbers are delivered at a faster and faster pace, from one number every 2.4 s down to every 1.2 s. It sounds easy but in actuality is very demanding; even at the slowest speed the average score is only about 70 per cent correct, and this falls away to only about 40 per cent at the fastest speed. Indeed, if a patient has any significant mental slowing, they often cannot do the test at all. Obviously the test cannot be used if the patient has a stammer, or is dysarthric or innumerate.

A less stressful test of mental speed is the Speed of Comprehension Test,[13] in which the person indicates as fast as possible whether simple sentences are true or false (e.g. tomato soup is a liquid, grapes are people). There are four parallel versions, and the test can be given auditorily for patients who cannot read.

Two visual tests of mental speed are Map Search (looking for target symbols on a map as fast as possible) and Telephone Search (looking for various symbols on a page from a telephone directory).[14] There are three parallel forms.

One test that tries to disentangle the relative contribution of slowed motor speed versus slowed mental speed, often a crucial issue in patients with motor deficits, is the Adult Memory and Information Processing Battery[15] which has two useful timed tests of cancelling target digits.

Attention and concentration

There are various aspects of attention and concentration: the ability to focus resources, the ability to focus on the right aspect, the ability to sustain this attention, the ability to ignore extraneous information or distracting events, and the ability to divide attention between different tasks. The tests on speed listed above are of course also measures of attention, because highly focused and selective attention has to be sustained for the duration of a pressured task. Digit span on the WAIS-III^{UK} is also a test of attention, as any lapse in attending to the incoming digits will necessarily result in a wrong answer.

However, in addition to these tests, a battery may be used, such as

Table 5 Outline of the WAIS-III[UK] and WISC-III[UK]

	WAIS-III[UK]	WISC-III[UK]
Age range	16–89 years	6.0–16.11 years
Verbal subtests	Vocabulary Similarities Arithmetic Digit span Information Comprehension Letter–number sequencing	Information Similarities Arithmetic Vocabulary Comprehension Digit Span
Non-verbal or spatial subtests	Picture completion Digit symbol Block design Matrix reasoning Picture arrangement Symbol search Object assembly	Picture completion Coding Picture arrangement Block design Object assembly Symbol search Mazes
IQ score	Verbal IQ (VIQ) Performance IQ (PIQ) Full-scale IQ (fsIQ)	Verbal IQ (VIQ) Performance IQ (PIQ) Full-scale IQ (fsIQ)
Index scores (factor scores)	Verbal comprehension Perceptual organization Working memory Processing speed	Verbal comprehension Perceptual organization Freedom from distractibility Processing speed
Mean IQ or index scores	100 (SD = 15)	100 (SD = 15)
Mean subtest scores	10 (SD = 3)	10 (SD = 3)
Test–retest reliability of IQ	0.98 for full-scale IQ	0.96 for full-scale IQ
Standard error of measurement of IQ	About 2.5, so all scores are about ±5 points[a]	About 3.2, so all scores are ±6 or 7 points
Reliable VIQ–PIQ difference	About 9 points	About 11 points
Abnormally VIQ–PIQ difference	About 22 points	About 25 points
Validity	Highly related to other tests of ability and to criteria related to ability	Highly related to other tests of ability and to criterion groups

[a] 95% of the time, true scores are the observed score ±1.96 SEM. In other words, the likely true score is within the range defined by about two SEMs either side of the score obtained.

the Test of Everyday Attention[14] which has eight different subtests. Test–retest reliability is quite good, being over 0.83 for Map Search and over 0.86 for Telephone Search, for example, both of which, in terms of validity, are also very sensitive to the effects of head injury and stroke.

Table 6 Sample from PASAT

Number on tape	(Mental process)	Patient says
7		
5	(5 + 7)	12
1	(1 + 5)	6
4	(4 + 1)	5
9	(9 + 4)	13

Memory

Memory is a complex set of processes whereby the person registers, stores, and retrieves information within different modalities (e.g. verbal memory versus spatial memory) and across different time periods (e.g. primary or shorter-term memory versus secondary or longer-term memory or learning). Therefore, as with intelligence, various batteries have evolved with subtests that tap these various aspects. Two examples of batteries are the Wechsler Memory Scale–Third Edition[16] for adults and the Children's Memory Scale,[17] which are both summarized in Table 7. Another battery, which makes a special effort to reflect real life tasks, is the Rivermead Behavioural Memory Test,[18] which also has a child's version.[19]

Sometimes inevitable time constraints make it difficult to justify giving whole memory batteries. Often, just a few key subtests are

Table 7 Summary of two memory batteries

	Wechsler Memory Scale–III	Children's Memory Scale
Age range	16–89 years	5–16 years
Subtests	Information and orientation Logical memory[a] Faces[a] Verbal paired associates[a] Family pictures[a] Word lists[a] Visual reproduction[a] Letter–number sequencing Spatial span Mental control Digit span (Means typically 10, SDs typically 3)	Dot locations[a] Stories[a] Faces[a] Word pairs[a] Family pictures[a] Word lists[a] Numbers Sequences Picture locations (Means of 10, SDs of 3)
Index Scores	Auditory immediate Visual immediate Immediate memory Auditory delayed Visual delayed Auditory recognition delayed General memory Working memory (Means of 100, SDs of 15)	Verbal immediate Verbal delayed Verbal delayed recognition Learning Visual immediate Visual delayed Attention/concentration General memory (Means of 100, SDs of 15)
Reliability	0.60–0.87 for the index scores (i.e. rather low, and note a practice effect of up to 15 points across 5 weeks)	0.76–0.91 for the index scores (note a large practice effect of about 10–15 points across a 2-month interval)
Standard error of measurement	3.88–7.40 (so true scores are at best ±8 points from the observed score)	4.5–7.4 (so true scores are at best ±9 points from the observed score)
Validity	See manual for content, criterion-related, construct, and other types of validity	See manual for content, construct, and criterion-related validity

[a] Also delayed trial.

selected, or other individual tests may be given. For example, to gauge verbal learning the Rey Auditory–Verbal Learning Test is well researched,[20] a well-researched test of visual memory is the Rey–Osterrieth Complex Figure Test;[21, 22] and a useful forced-choice recognition tests for words and faces is the Recognition Memory Test.[23] If the ability of the patient to recall details of his or her past life is an issue, the Autobiographical Memory Interview can be used.[24]

Language

Commonly used batteries for the assessment of language deficits are the Boston Diagnostic Aphasia Examination[25] and the closely related Western Aphasia Battery.[26] The Boston Examination covers auditory comprehension, oral expression, understanding written language, and writing. These tests can take a long time to give and so brief screening tests are often used, such as the Boston Naming Test[27] or the Graded Naming Test,[28] which both assess word finding, or the Token Test,[29] which assesses verbal comprehension. Finally, a good test to gauge reading and spelling ability is the Wechsler Objective Reading Dimensions Test[30] which will produce reading and spelling ages, and give the abnormality of difference scores between IQ and reading or spelling scores.

Frontal and executive functions

The term executive function derives from the theory that there is a supervisory system exerting executive control of attention.[31] Deficits of this system cause broad patterns of cognitive and behavioural change called the dysexecutive syndrome,[32] which includes changes in volition, poor planning, a disruption of purposive action, and reduced efficacy of performance. One of the most frequent causes of this syndrome is damage to the frontal lobes (frontal-lobe syndrome is a dysexecutive syndrome) but it may also be caused by other patterns of lesion. Table 8 lists some of the features of the dysexecutive syndrome, and examples of tests that are sensitive to such features.

Table 8 Features and tests of the dysexecutive syndrome

Feature	Test
Behavioural change	The Dysexecutive Questionnaire (DEX), both self-report and other-report[33]
Planning and impulsivity	Mazes subtest of the WISC-III[UK(7)]
Fluency	Of generating words: the Controlled Oral Word Association[34] Of generating spatial patterns: design fluency[35]
Concept formations and ability to shift mental set	Modified Card-Sorting Test[36] Rule Shift Cards Test[33]
Estimation	Of various amounts: the Cognitive Estimates Test[37,38] Temporal Judgement Test of time estimation[33]
Alternating plans	Switching between plans based on numbers or letters: the Trail-Making Test[39]
Screening out distracting stimuli	The Stroop Test,[40] e.g. reading the word BLUE when it is printed in red ink
Suppression of competing responses	The Hayling Test[41] which requires patients to choose connected or unconnected words to finish a sentence
Rule attainment	Brixton Test, requiring the patient to learn the rule whereby a pattern changes[41]
Planning	Action Programme Test, to use given materials to achieve a given end[33] Zoo Map Test of organizing a route[33] Modified Six-Elements Test of planning the order of tasks according to rules[33]

Some clinical issues

Sources of tests and test data

A good summary of the principles of test theory is given by Kline.[1] Information about tests and where to order them from can be found in Lezak's *Neuropsychological Assessment*[42] and Spreen and Strauss's *Compendium of Neuropsychological Tests*.[3] Slightly older, but still useful, is the *Handbook of Neuropsychological Assessment* by Crawford *et al*.[43] Many tests are 'closed', i.e. they can only be ordered by appropriately qualified people who are registered as test users within specified domains.

Understanding tests

Just because a test is published does not mean that it is a good test, any more than all published papers are good papers. The onus is upon the test user to be sufficiently knowledgeable about test theory to gauge the strengths and limitations of tests. Common problems with tests are small standardization sample sizes, unknown or unstable factor structure, poor or no theoretical adequacy, poor or no use of criterion groups, vague scoring criteria, and poor or no information on difference scores within or between tests. It is worth reading the manual of the Children's Memory Scale[17] as a good example of a psychometrically well-constructed test.

Another point to bear in mind is that even a well-normed and proven test may not actually be applicable to the particular patient at hand; tests only have a certain range of convenience. Tests have to be very carefully chosen when confounding factors are present, such as when English is not the patient's first language or when there is a sensory or motor deficit (e.g. visual problems affecting acuity or scanning, dysarthria affecting speed of verbal response, upper-limb paresis affecting manipulation of test materials).

Indeed, there are a range of potentially confounding variables even in those patients who are within the range of convenience of the test. These include effects of medication, fatigue as the testing progresses, motivation, mental state, disturbed behaviour, cultural background and beliefs, and educational background. Test manuals may provide information on such potentially confounding variables, but often it is necessary to know the primary research on the test and its sensitivity to such factors.

Assessing children

Special issues arise in the assessment of children because the neuropsychology theory and conceptual framework are different, the effects of specified lesions change with age, the pattern of recovery of function varies with age, extensive developmental norms, covering the age range, are needed, and children may be more stressed by tests or may find it harder to cooperate with test procedures. These and other issues are fully discussed in texts on developmental psychology,[44] paediatric neuropsychology,[45] and head injury in children.[46] Several children's tests have already been cited by name in preceding sections. In addition, many of the adult tests cited have also been standardized on children, often in subsequent research studies not necessarily carried out by the original test author. Examples of tests with children's norms

Table 9 Strategies for estimating premorbid IQ

Strategy	Test and/or comment
Assume that highest subtest score on the WAIS-R represents original level	Normal individuals have a profile of abilities and show quite a wide range of subtest scores.[4] It makes no sense at all to say that a person's best score is his or her 'real' potential. Anyone using this method will grossly overestimate IQ loss.
Consider scores on subtests thought to be relatively insensitive to the effects of brain injury	Vocabulary is highly correlated with IQ and also is such a deeply ingrained ability that it is relatively insensitive to the effects of brain injury. Therefore scores on the vocabulary subtest can indeed be a guide to premorbid IQ.
Gauge IQ from educational record	This is reasonable as long as the person had full access to education and the motivation to take and pass examinations. Gauging ability band is made easier now that national statistics on examination pass rates are published annually in the UK.
Gauge IQ from occupational record	Again this is reasonable as a broad approximation, but cultural and sociological constraints on choice of work or progress in work have to be taken into account.
Tests of overlearned skills such as reading	Reading ability is highly correlated with IQ, and is a very overlearned skill, not easily affected by brain injury. This is the best and safest method, as long as the patient had no history of dyslexia and is not currently dysphasic. Tests include the National Adult Reading Test, 2nd edition,[48] and the Spot the Word Test.[13]
Genetic endowment	If the patient was damaged at birth, or if the damage caused gross physical deficits adversely affecting educational and occupational potential, then the ability and educational and occupational record of natural parents and siblings may be considered.

are word fluency, design fluency, auditory verbal learning, the original Wechsler Memory Scale, the Stroop test, the token test, the trail-making test, Wisconsin card sorting, the paced serial addition test, and the progressive matrices test. There are also child norms on various memory tests not thus far mentioned, such as the Sentence Repetition Test[34] and the Benton Visual Retention Test–Revised.[47]

Assessing premorbid ability

In order to understand the effects of a brain injury, to gauge intellectual loss, to plan rehabilitation, and to advise on issues relating to personal injury compensation, it is necessary to estimate premorbid intelligence. A summary of strategies for estimating premorbid IQ is given in Table 9.

Capacity

Within the context of intellectual and cognitive functioning, a person is incapable of managing his or her own affairs if two criteria are met. First, they must have an objective deficit likely to impair problem-solving and decision-making. Second, they must be incapable of sensibly delegating responsibility to someone else. Cognitive assessment obviously bears upon both of these issues. In the first instance assessment can help gauge whether there is a deficit at all, and if so the severity of that deficit and its precise nature. For example, most people would be able to manage their own lives despite some mild reduction in intellectual efficiency or some mild memory problem—after all, this is in any case the course of natural ageing. But it is much more difficult to cope with a severe memory deficit, for example, when it may be difficult for the person to bring the relevant information to mind so as to reach a competent decision, or to hold it long enough in mind to make that decision. In the second instance, cognitive assessment can point to deficits which make it unlikely that the person can appropriately delegate certain responsibilities. For example, those with dysexecutive syndrome may be gullible or impulsive over whom to approach for advice, or may be reluctant to accept advice, may delegate only inconsistently, or may say they accept certain advice but then do the opposite. In short, they cannot plan to delegate or, if they do make such plans, the plans are poorly monitored and inconsistently implemented. All this is a question of judgement rather than pure test results. There is no psychometric test of capacity as such, but there is a growing trend for tests to reflect real life functioning, which make it easier to draw out the implications of test results for daily living. For example, Goel et al.[49] directly observed financial decision-making in analogues of planning tasks.

Malingering

There is no single test of malingering (i.e. consciously motivated deliberate underperformance on tests). Rather, a pattern builds up which gradually raises the suspicion of malingering. Features of test performance which raise the issue are as follows:

(1) a degree of deficit that is disproportionate to the severity of the injury (laboratory studies of people who are asked to feign deficits or act as if they have a certain brain injury consistently find that participants exaggerate or inflate the severity and breadth of symptoms, even when a warning about this is given[50]);

(2) bizarre errors not typically seen in patients with genuine deficits (the implication being that the person has made an uninformed guess at what the symptoms might be);

(3) patterns of test performance that do not make sense (e.g. doing as badly on easy items as hard items);

(4) not showing expected patterns (e.g. being as bad on recognition recall as on free recall, failing to show any learning whatsoever on auditory–verbal learning tasks, suppression of the first half of items on list learning tasks, discrepancies between scores on tests measuring similar processes);

(5) inconsistencies between test performance and behaviour in real life (e.g. unable to repeat short digit strings or short sentences, but in general conversation being able to respond to multistage instructions; extreme retardation, slowing, in answering test questions but converses normally and gives the history normally);

(6) inexplicable claims of remote memory loss even for important life events like weddings;[51]

(7) random responding on forced-choice tests[23] (if true this would suggest that the person had no brain at all);

(8) below random responding on forced-driven tests, i.e. suggesting that the person must know the right answer in order to give the wrong one;[52]

(9) poor performance on tests that look hard but are in fact easy, like the Rey 15- or 16-item test;[53]

(10) the absence of any sign of severe anxiety or profoundly low mood such as might cause a collapse in performance;

(11) after head injury, the absence of any improvement or indeed a worsening of performance over time;

(12) failure to report deficits following a brain injury when in retrospect those deficits are claimed to have been severe;

(13) relative absence of a history of somatization or related disorders.

Typical clinical neuropsychological assessment

Having set out the theory, tests, and issues, we can build up a picture of a typical clinical neuropsychological assessment, as given in Table 10.

Generalizability theory and ecological validity

There is a broad issue of how to make a general statement based on a test score, i.e. how to generalize from an observation made in one context to what might be observed in other contexts. As set out elsewhere,[54] one might wish to generalize from the following:

- scores obtained by one judge to those derived from other judges;

- scores on one test of, say, verbal long-term memory to scores on other test of this aspect of memory;

- scores at this particular moment to the score at some time in the future;

- scores obtained under one set of motivational conditions to those obtained under others.

In looking at these examples, it can be seen that the traditional division between reliability and validity becomes blurred; they are both expressions of the degree and nature of how a score can be generalized. This sweeps away the notion of a true score, to be replaced by the notion of a universe score, which is the mean of all possible observations under all possible conditions. Classical test theory is replaced by generalizability theory, in which variance in a test score is apportioned to various factors. An observed score becomes the product of various identifiable measurable factors, and not just a notional true score plus an entirely unpredictable error score.[55] However, in practice generalizability theory informs test construction rather than replacing classical test theory.[17]

There is one very important aspect of generalizability, and this is ecological validity or the degree to which a test score predicts real-life

Table 10 Typical protocol for a clinical neuropsychological assessment and report

Aims	The purpose of the assessment, e.g. to describe deficits, monitor improvement, inform rehabilitation planning, address certain specific issues
Background of patient	Information relevant to the interpretation of test findings, e.g. language, handedness, age, educational history, occupational history, medical and psychiatric history
Nature of the brain injury	For example, time since injury, age at injury, mechanisms of injury, retrograde amnesia, loss of consciousness, post-traumatic amnesia, results of neurological examination, results of scans
Behaviour and mental state	Motivation, co-operation with procedures, anxiety, mood, any aspect that threatens reliability or validity, a clear statement as to whether or not reliability has been compromised
Intelligence	Verbal, non-verbal, skills profile
Speed	Verbal, non-verbal, motor
Attention and concentration	Verbal/spatial tasks General behaviour and lapses on tests
Memory	Verbal/non-verbal Immediate/delayed recall Learning
Language	Reading Screening tests for dysphasia Aphasia battery if needed
Construction skills	Refer to performance subtests Copying a complex figure
Sensory deficits	Note gross deficits and subjective account Record problems noted on tests Refer to neurological examination Tests of spatial neglect Tests of visual agnosia
Motor deficits	Note gross problems and subjective accounts Record problems noted on tests Refer to neurological examination Tests of apraxia
Executive functions	Fluency Planning Estimation Personality/behaviour Record dysexecutive problems noted on other tests
Life situation	Way of life, typical day, leisure activities Nature and amount of any support Impact of deficits upon everyday living
Interview with other informant	An observer's account of deficits, changes, coping, etc.
Formulation	A coherent account of the injury and its repercussions, taking all information into account, focusing on the aims of the assessment

Table 11 Threats to the ecological validity of test results

The assessment session	Data are collected in a quiet sterile focused environment, whereas real life is noisy and full of distractions
Type of test	Cognitive tests are often constructed to measure a single pure aspect of processing, whereas real-life tasks are multidimensional
Type of interaction	The behaviour of the patient is constrained by the nature of the examiner–patient relationship, and is unlike spontaneous behaviour
Content of tests	The limited number and content of tests that can be given may not tap the real-life problems that are complained of (e.g. reduced sense of humour)
Confounding factors	Test anxiety Motivation to co-operate with the assessment or to perform in a certain way Short test sessions to avoid fatigue whereas most problems are reported when the patient *is* fatigued
Over-reliance on test data	Blinkered adherence to numbers to the exclusion of background information, general observation, information from others, and common sense
Failure to consider ecological validity	Lack of understanding of the issue Failure to follow up patients in such a way as to obtain feedback on the ecological validity of the original assessment, which is necessary to shape ecologically valid assessment procedures
Solutions	Use tests of concentration and distraction Develop new tests or new versions of tests reflecting real-life tasks Find sources of information about real-life behaviour Continue to widen the range of tests available, focusing test development on clinical need Estimate effects of confounding factors Treat numbers as only one form of data Specifically address ecological issues in the final report

trend is to make neuropsychological tests increasingly a distillation of real-life tasks so as to lessen this generalizability problem.[14,18,33]

Cognitive assessment of psychiatric disorders

It is possible to give only a summary of findings from the cognitive assessment of psychiatric and neuropsychiatric disorders. A fuller account is given by Grant and Adams.[57]

Epilepsy

There is no single cognitive profile of people with epilepsy. The relationship between epilepsy and the presence of mental retardation (learning disability) will mainly be mediated by the original brain damage causing both the epilepsy and the mental retardation. However, some patients do deteriorate intellectually if seizures are frequent or uncontrolled or if there are lapses into status epilepticus. In terms of partial seizures, the most common pattern is disturbance of verbal

functioning. Some of the various threats to ecological validity are listed in Table 11 (see Long[56] for a fuller discussion), but the recent memory if there is a left temporal (dominant) focus and of non-verbal memory if there is a right focus.[58] Anticonvulsants themselves may mildly impair performance on a wide variety of intellectual, cognitive, and speeded tasks.

Parkinsonism

The pattern of deficits in patients without overt dementia is memory disturbance and dysexecutive syndrome (e.g. reduced fluency, concept formation, ability to shift set).[59] If there is an overt (subcortical) dementia, aphasia, agnosia, and severe amnesia are relatively uncommon, but mood change is frequent.

Dementia

The most common early sign of Alzheimer's disease is poor performance on delayed verbal memory,[60] possibly with dysexecutive signs,[61] eventually joined by a deterioration is the meaningfulness of speech with a breakdown in semantic relationships and understanding; speech becomes empty of content and frontal dysexecutive deficits emerge.

Depression

In younger neurologically intact persons, depression affects attention and memory.[62,63] After head injury, the presence of above average levels of anxiety or depression can make a difference of up to about half a standard deviation in neuropsychological test scores, including IQ, mental speed, and verbal and spatial memories.[64]

Alcohol

There is a typical neurocognitive profile found in chronic detoxified alcoholics after 2 to 4 weeks abstinence: intact IQ and verbal skills, but impairment of novel problem-solving, abstract reasoning, learning and memory, visual spatial analysis, and complex perceptual–motor integration.[65] If severe thiamine deficiency arises, Wernicke–Korsakoff syndrome may ensue, with profound anterograde amnesia.

Other drugs[42]

Findings regarding the long-term neuropsychological effects of marijuana are equivocal, but if there are long-term changes they probably involve attention. Long-term cocaine use may also affect attention and memory. There are conflicting reports about the long-term use of opiates, but there may be a diffuse effect upon visuospatial and visuomotor activities. Chronic solvent abuse leads to cerebellar ataxia and also some impairment of IQ and memory.[66]

Schizophrenia

There is a growing awareness of dysexecutive deficits in the aetiology of schizophrenic symptoms,[67] relating to disorders of willed action for example. Patients with schizophrenia score poorly on the Behavioural Assessment of the Dysexecutive Syndrome[68] and show other dysexecutive features.[69]

Summary, conclusion, and future directions

Psychometric methods based on classical test theory have permitted the development of reliable and valid tests assessing a wide range of intellectual and cognitive functions. Test results assist in formulation and diagnosis, guide rehabilitation and management, provide baseline measures to detect change, and generally assist clinical decision-making regarding such issues as capacity. Tests and assessment procedures are being further developed so as to improve their ecological validity, enabling better prediction of real-life behaviour and functioning.

References

1. Kline, P. (1993). *The handbook of psychological testing.* Routledge, London.
2. Wechsler, D. (1997). *Wechsler Adult Intelligence Scale–Third Edition.* Psychological Corporation, Cleveland, OH.
3. Spreen, O. and Strauss, E. (1998). *A compendium of neuropsychological tests: administration, norms, and commentary* (2nd edn). Oxford University Press, New York.
4. Crawford, J.R. and Allan, K.M. (1996). WAIS-R subtest scatter: base-rate data from a healthy UK sample. *British Journal of Clinical Psychology,* **35**, 235–47.
5. Folstein, M.F., Folstein, S.E., and McHugh, P.R. (1975). 'Mini-Mental State'. A practical method for grading the cognitive state of patients for the clinician. *Journal of Psychiatric Research,* **12**, 189–98.
6. Tombaugh, T.N., McDowell, I., Krisjansson, B., and Hubley, A.M. (1966). Mini-Mental State Examination (MMSE) and the modified MMSE (3MS): a psychometric comparison and normative data. *Psychological Assessment,* **8**, 48–59.
7. Wechsler, D. (1992). *Wechsler Intelligence Scale for Children–Third Edition UK: manual.* Psychological Corporation, London.
8. Wechsler, D. (1989). *Manual for the Wechsler Preschool and Primary Scale of Intelligence–Revised.* Psychological Corporation, San Antonio, CA.
9. Raven, J.C. (1996). *Progressive Matrices.* Oxford Psychologists Press.
10. Raven, J.C. (1994). *Advanced Progressive Matrices, Sets I and II.* Oxford Psychologists Press.
11. Gronwall, D.M.A. (1977). Paced auditory serial addition task: a measure of recovery from concussion. *Perceptual and Motor Skills,* **44**, 367–73.
12. Stuss, D.T., Stethem, L.L. and Pelchat, G. (1988). Three tests of attention and rapid information processing: an extension. *Clinical Neuropsychologist,* **2**, 246–50.
13. Baddeley, A.D., Emslie, H., and Nimmo-Smith, I.N. (1992). *The speed and capacity of language-processing tests.* Thames Valley Test Company, Bury St Edmunds.
14. Robertson, I.H., Ward, T., Ridgeway, V., and Nimmo-Smith, I. (1994). *The test of everyday attention.* Thames Valley Test Company, Bury St Edmunds.
15. Coughlan, A.K. and Hollows, S.E. (1985). *The Adult Memory and Information Processing Battery (AMIPB): test manual.* Psychology Department, St James's University Hospital, Leeds.
16. Wechsler, D. (1997). *Wechsler Memory Scale–Third Edition.* Psychological Corporation, San Antonio, CA.
17. Cohen, M.J. (1997). *Children's Memory Scale.* Psychological Corporation, San Antonio, CA.
18. Wilson, B., Cockburn, J., and Baddeley, A. (1985). *The Rivermead Behavioural Memory Test.* Thames Valley Test Company, Bury St Edmunds.
19. Wilson, B.A., Ivani-Chalian, R., and Aldrich, F. (1991). *The Rivermead*

Behavioural Memory Test for Children Aged 5–10 Years. Thames Valley Test Company, Bury St Edmunds.

20. Schmidt, M. (1996). *Rey Auditory–Verbal Learning Test.* Western Psychological Services, Los Angeles, CA.

21. Corwin, J. and Bylsam, F.W. (1993). Translations of excerpts from André Rey's 'Psychological examination of traumatic encephalopathy' and P. A Osterrieth's 'The Complex Figure Copy Test'. *Clinical Neuropsychologist,* **7**, 3–15.

22. Meyers, J. and Meyers, K. (1995). *The Meyers scoring system for the Rey Complex Figure and the Recognition Trial: professional manual.* Psychological Assessment Resources, Odessa, TX.

23. Warrington, E.K. (1984). *Recognition Memory Test manual.* NFER-Nelson, Windsor.

24. Kopelman, M., Wilson, B., and Baddeley, A. (1990). *The Autobiographical Memory Interview.* Thames Valley Test Company, Bury St Edmunds.

25. Goodglass, H. and Kaplan, E. (1983). *The assessment of aphasia and related disorders* (2nd edn). Lea and Febiger, Philadelphia, PA.

26. Kertesz, A. (1982). *Western Aphasia Battery.* Psychological Corporation, San Antonio, CA.

27. Kaplan, E.F., Goodglass, H., and Weintraub, S. (1983). *The Boston Naming Test* (2nd edn). Lea and Febiger, Philadelphia, PA.

28. McKenna, P. and Warrington, E.K. (1983). *Graded Naming Test.* NFER-Nelson, Windsor. (New norms in 1997.)

29. McNeil, M.M. and Prescott, T.E. (1978). *Revised Token Test.* Pro-ed, Austin, TX.

30. Wechsler, D. (1993). *Wechsler Objective Reading Dimensions: manual.* Psychological Corporation, London.

31. Shallice, T. (1982). Specific impairment of planning. *Philosophical Transactions of the Royal Society of London,* **298**, 199–209.

32. Baddeley, A.D. and Wilson, B.A. (1988). Frontal amnesia and the dysexecutive syndrome. *Brain and Cognition,* **7**, 212–30.

33. Wilson, B.A., Alderman, N., Burgess, P.W., Ensie, H., and Evans, J.J. *Behavioural assessment of the dysexecutive syndrome.* Thames Valley Test Company, Bury St Edmunds.

34. Spreen, O. and Benton, A.L. (1977). *Neurosensory Center Comprehensive Examination for Aphasia (NCCEA).* University of Victoria Neuropsychology Laboratory, Victoria, BC.

35. Jones-Gotman, M. (1991). Localisation of lesions by neuropsychological testing. *Epilepsia,* **32**, 541–52.

36. Nelson, H.E. (1976). A modified card sorting test sensitive to frontal lobe defects. *Cortex,* **12**, 313–24.

37. Shallice, T. and Evans, M.E. (1978). The involvement of the frontal lobes in cognitive estimation. *Cortex,* **14**, 292–303.

38. O'Carroll, R., Egan, V., and Mackenzie, D.M. (1994). Assessing cognitive estimation. *British Journal of Clinical Psychology,* **33**, 193–7.

39. D'Esposito, M., Alexander, M.P., Fisher, R., *et al.* (1996). Recovery of memory and executive function following anterior communicating artery aneurysm. *Journal of the International Neuropsychological Society,* **2**, 565–70.

40. Sachs, T.L., Clark, C.R., Pols, R.G., and Geffen, L.B. (1991). Comparability and stability of performance of six alternate forms of the Dodrill–Stroop Color–Word Tests. *Clinical Neuropsychologist,* **5**, 220–5.

41. Burgess, P. W. and Shallice, T. (1997). *The Hayling and Brixton Tests.* Thames Valley Test Company, Bury St Edmunds.

42. Lezak, M.D. (1995). *Neuropsychological assessment* (3rd edn). Oxford University Press, New York.

43. Crawford, J.R., Parker, D.M., and McKinlay, W.W. (ed.) (1992). *A handbook of neuropsychological assessment.* Erlbaum, Hove.

44. Spreen, O., Risser, A.H., and Edgell, D. (1995). *Developmental neuropsychology.* Oxford University Press, New York.

45. Baron, I.S, Fennell, E.B., and Voeller, K.K.S. (1995). *Paediatric neuropsychology in the medical setting.* Oxford University Press, New York.

46. Broman, S.H. and Michel, M.E. (ed.) (1995). *Traumatic head injury in children.* Oxford University Press, New York.

47. Sivan, A.B. (1992). *Benton Visual Retention Test* (5th edn). Psychological Corporation, San Antonio, CA.

48. Nelson, H.E. and Willison, J. (1991). *National Adult Reading Test (NART): test manual* (2nd edn). NFER-Nelson, Windsor.

49. Goel, V., Grafman, J., Tajik, J., Gana, S., and Danto, D. (1997). A study of the performance of patients with frontal lobe lesions in a financial planning task. *Brain,* **120**, 1805–22.

50. Johnson, J.L. and Lesniak-Karpiak, K. (1997). The effect of warning on malingering on memory and motor tasks in a college sample. *Archives of Clinical Neuropsychology,* **12**, 231–8.

51. Greiffenstein, M.F., Baker, W.J., and Gola, T. (1994). Validation of malingered amnesia measure with a large clinical sample. *Psychological Assessment,* **6**, 218–24.

52. Iverson, G.L. and Franzen, M.D. (1996). Using multiple objective memory procedures to detect simulated malingering. *Journal of Clinical and Experimental Neuropsychology,* **18**, 38–51.

53. Paul, D.S., Franzen, M.D., Cohen, S.H., and Fremouw, W. (1992). An investigation into the reliability and validity of two tests used in the detection of malingering. *International Journal of Clinical Neuropsychology,* **14**, 1–9.

54. Powell, G.E. (1966). The selection and development of measures. In *Behavioural and mental health research: a handbook of skills and methods* (2nd edn) (ed. G. Parry and F. N. Watts), pp. 29–57. Erlbaum–Taylor and Francis, Hove.

55. Cronbach, L.J., Gleser, G.C., Nanda, H., and Rajaratnam, N. (1972). *The dependability of behavioural measurements.* Wiley, New York.

56. Long, C.J. (1996). Neuropsychological tests: a look at our past and the impact that ecological issues may have on our future. In *Ecological validity of neuropsychological testing* (ed. R. J. Sbordone and C.J. Long), pp. 1–41. GR Press–St Lucie Press, Delray Beach, FL.

57. Grant, I. and Adams, K.M. (ed.) (1996). *Neuropsychological assessment of neuropsychiatric disorders* (2nd edn). Oxford University Press, New York.

58. Bennett, T.L. (1992). *The neuropsychology of epilepsy.* Plenum Press, New York.

59. Levin, B.E., Tomer, R., and Rey, G.J. (1992). Cognitive impairments in Parkinson's disease. *Neurologic Clinic,* **10**, 471–85.

60. Morris, J.C., McKeel, D.W., Storandt, M., and Rubin, E.H. (1991). Very mild Alzheimer's disease: information-based clinical, psychometric, and pathological distinction from normal ageing. *Neurology,* **41**, 469–78.

61. Monsch, A.U., Bondi, M.W., Butters, N., and Paulsen, J. (1994). A comparison of category and letter fluency in Alzheimer's disease and Huntington's disease. *Neuropsychology,* **8**, 25–30.

62. Massman, P.J., Delis, D.C., Butters, N., and Dupont, R.M. (1992). The subcortical dysfunction model of memory deficits in depression: neuropsychological validation in a subgroup of patients. *Journal of Clinical and Experimental Neuropsychology,* **14**, 687–706.

63. Brand, A.N., Jolles, J., and Gipsen-deWied, C. (1992). Recall and recognition memory deficits in depression. *Journal of Affective Disorders,* **25**, 77–86.

64. Powell, G. E. (1999). Depression, anxiety and neuropsychological test performance. *Proceedings of the British Psychological Society,* **7**, 132.

65. Rourk, S.B. and Loberg, T. (1996). The neurobehavioural correlates of alcoholism. In *Neuropsychological assessment of neuropsychiatric disorders* (ed. I. Grant and K.M. Adams), pp. 423–85. Oxford University Press, New York.

66. Fornazzari, L., Wilkinson, D.A., Kapur, B.M., and Carlen, P.L. (1983). Cerebellar, cortical and functional impairment in toluene abuse. *Acta Neurologica Scandinavia,* **67**, 319–29.

67. Frith, C.D. (1992). *The cognitive neuropsychology of schizophrenia.* Erlbaum, Hove.

68. Evans, J.J., Chua, S.E., McKenna, P.J., and Wilson, B.A. (1997). Assessment of the dysexecutive syndrome in schizophrenia. *Psychological Medicine,* **27**, 635–46.

69. Shallice, T., Burgess, P.W., and Frith, C.D. (1991). Can the neuropsychological case-study approach be applied to schizophrenia? *Psychological Medicine,* **21**, 661–73.

1.10.3.2 Behavioural and observational assessment

John N. Hall

The nature of behavioural and observational assessment

One model of assessment[1] suggests that there are four main content areas for assessment, including cognition, affect (including verbal-subjective components of behaviour), physiological activity, and overt behaviour. Coverage of all these assessment domains is needed to provide both valid clinical formulations and evaluations of outcome. They also suggest that there are three main categories of assessment method, namely: self-report; the use of observation and instruments; and the use of technical equipment.

Neither cognitive tests, which offer precise and controlled information about intellectual functioning, nor responses to questioning during an interview, which tell us something of a person's thoughts and knowledge, necessarily describe how an individual behaves in detail on a day-to-day basis. It is important to know how a person will behave most of the time in either a clinical or 'normal' environment, particularly when designing treatment programmes. Behavioural and observational assessments possess high 'ecological validity' for this purpose, and are thus an essential complement to other forms of assessment.

This family of assessment methods may be used in the same way as other methods: for the initial assessment of a patient as part of a clinical formulation; for ongoing monitoring during the course of treatment; and as outcome measures. They may also be used in planning the care of groups of patients, when selecting patients from a larger population for a specific therapeutic programmes or regimes, and when planning services.

The adjective 'behavioural' then has two senses. It refers both to content—it is the overt behaviour of the patient that is being assessed, rather than some imputed or attributed inner faculty or trait—and also to a family of methods. Rating scales are the best established of the behavioural methods—the earliest such scales were developed in the 1910s, and some of those most frequently used now are over 30 years old.

A number of observational methods were refined alongside the clinical introduction of behaviour therapy procedures in the 1960s, and these continue to be associated with contemporary cognitive–behavioural interventions. An associated American term is 'functional assessment' (see ref. 2 for a detailed example), which describes the extent to which the skills possessed by an individual match those required to maintain an independent existence in the community. American managed-care companies may require a functional assessment to demonstrate how a provided treatment relates to the specific disabilities of a patient. Behavioural assessment procedures, as they have been developed in association with the growth of behavioural and cognitive–behavioural treatments, have a number of characteristics. They focus on current overt behaviour, and may seek to discern the controlling or maintaining variables in specific situations and for specific individuals.

Andrews *et al.*[3] give an excellent review of outcome measures in mental health, covering many of the most commonly used rating scales. There are a number of helpful guides to behavioural assessment, that by Bellack and Hersen[4] being one of the best established. The main members of the family of behavioural assessment procedures are given below and are summarized in Box 1.

Behavioural and observational assessment methods Box 1

Categories of behavioural and observational assessment

Behavioural observation methods
- Event sampling
- Time sampling
- Functional analysis
- Response coding

Ethological methods

Behaviour ratings and checklists

Questionnaire methods
- Self-report and self-monitoring methods

Psychophysiological methods

Behavioural observation methods

These describe methods for the immediate recording of events, usually either recording the number of times an event occurs (leading to frequency counts), or immediately coding the observed event by using a set of prescribed event categories that exhaustively and mutually exclusively cover all anticipated possibilities. The duration of an event may be of interest, or the time interval between events. As an example of event coding, any patient in a ward setting may be coded as either standing, sitting, lying, walking, or running, with supplementary codes then describing, for example, either the form of social interaction or the form of activity being concurrently undertaken.

When events of clinical interest are very complex, it may take too long to code each event fully, so then only, say, every fifth or tenth event is coded in detail—this is termed 'event sampling'. When events are happening very rapidly, or if they tend to happen at about the same rate during the day, it is time-wasting to observe all the time, so observations may then be made only every 5 or 10 min—this is termed 'time sampling'.

The term 'functional analysis' generally refers to attempts to explain and predict the functions of a phenomenon by examining any contributory relationships. Clinically, this term usually describes a special variant of behavioural observation methods, when the observation of an individual's behaviour, which is of clinical significance, is linked to the observation of those events in the immediate clinical environment that directly preceded, were concurrently associated with, and followed, the target behaviour, with the aim of uncovering any relationship between them. This sequence of antecedent environmental events, target behaviour and concurrent events, and consequent environmental events, is often called an ABC analysis. For example, incidents of aggression by a particular client in a day-setting may be a function of which other clients are near him or talking to him, so that a record of their presence or absence would be important. While a functional analysis strictly implies no particular model of behaviour, historically there has been a close association between functional and behavioural analysis.

Ethological methods

These also employ direct recording of behaviour, but they emphasize the detection of naturally occurring chains of behaviour, with an interest in the patterning, sequencing, or complexity of the behaviour, rather than the frequency or simple categorization of the behaviour.

Behaviour ratings and checklists

These are judgements about the quality or characteristics of behaviour, completed on the basis of direct observation of the behaviour in question, with the rater often being a nurse or day- or residential-care worker, or a family member or informal carer. Typically, such ratings may be completed after an observation period varying from a few hours to a few days, so that there is then a variable delay between the observation of the relevant behaviour and the rating. The British Health of the Nation Outcome Scale (**HONOS**)[5] is an example of this type. Each HONOS item consists of an item title (for example, item 1 is titled overactive, aggressive, disruptive, or agitated behaviour), followed by five response categories, ranging from 0 (no problem) to 4 (severe to very severe problem), with a verbal description of up to about 25 words of the behaviour typical of each response category. An account of the ratings completed on the basis of a clinical interview is given in Chapter 1.10.1.

Checklists are essentially the same type of method, except that by definition they simply allow a Yes/No, or Present/Absent response, without a more complex gradation of the response. Checklists may be completed by the patient as part of a behavioural programme.

Questionnaire methods

These offer the respondent a preset range of written questions covering the area of clinical interest. The questions may be completed either by ticking one of a set of provided response categories ('forced-choice' questionnaires), or by writing the patient's own response in free text. 'Self-report' and 'self-monitoring' methods are similar to the latter form of questionnaire, in that the patient is provided with, and completes, a diary or premarked sheets. However, these tend to be more open-ended, and any associated thoughts of the patient may be included. Self-report measures are often used clinically in cognitive–behavioural interventions.

Psychophysiological methods

These include the use of a range of surface sensors to measure changes in, for example, electrical conductivity (as in measuring changes in sweating), in light transmission (as in measuring changes in finger blood flow), and in volume (as in penile plethysmography). When these physical changes are found to have a close relationship with an underlying change in physiological arousal, they may then be taken as a proxy measure, which may be valuable for both the initial assessment and for monitoring therapeutic change. A major practical limitation of a number of these measures is that external environmental factors, such as changes in air temperature or humidity, may affect the reliability of the measure.

The reduction in size and cost as well as the increased sophistication and reliability of electronic, video- and audio recording equipment means that they may often be able to replace the paper-and-pencil recordings for any of the above methods. For example, hand-held electronic event recorders now allow the immediate and unobtrusive recording of events, and offer the facility of effortless data analysis. However, their use does depend on users being trained, and they are not always suitable for self-use by more disabled patients.

The formal requirements of behavioural and observational measures in clinical practice

Those psychometric principles that are applicable to all psychological measures, including the classical approaches to reliability, validity, and sensitivity to change, as well as generalizability approaches, are outlined in Chapter 1.10.3.1. Some psychometric concerns, such as those relating to speeded tests, are not applicable to behavioural measures, but on the other hand some arise primarily with behavioural measures.

Sampling procedures

A key issue with many observational methods is the adequacy of the sampling procedure used to obtain the data. Since many behaviours vary in their natural frequency during the waking day, many events should, theoretically, be observed continuously throughout the day. However, if the time needed for continual observation is unavailable, a representative sample of the whole day should be observed. Ideally, a random sample of time periods should be observed. Although only fixed observation periods may be feasible in practice, these should be distributed throughout the day—such as 9.30 to 11.00 am, 2.00 to 3.30 pm, and 7.00 to 8.30 pm. A smaller sample may be adequate if each target event or sequence of behaviour is qualitatively similar; this is in contrast to behaviour that is highly variable qualitatively, when a larger sample will be needed to obtain a stable base rate.

The effects of therapeutic learning acquired in one setting may not necessarily be displayed in another, perhaps a postdischarge, environment. This phenomenon is called 'poor generalization of learning', and is found particularly with severely mentally ill adults. Accordingly, behavioural observations, when used as an outcome measure of treatment effectiveness, should take place in both the patient's current and subsequent environments.

Interobserver reliability

Another issue is the interobserver reliability of behaviour ratings. For those standard ratings based on observation periods of more than a day, any one observer will only have been on duty for a proportion of the observation period (which may be 1 week). Therefore unless the observer, against whom reliability is being assessed, is on duty for exactly the same period, the periods of observation will not be coincident. Under these circumstances a double rating is not strictly a reliability check, but more a check of the stability of the behaviour. Patel et al.[6] discuss how the use of a simple checklist of the occurrence of key events can substantially improve the reliability of this type of scale.

Reactivity

A further issue is that of reactivity, which is the change in behaviour due to the patient's awareness of the presence of an observer. Reactivity factors may be reduced by making the observation procedure as minimally intrusiveness as possible (by, for example, careful siting of the observer). There is a debate about the ethical acceptability of completely unobtrusive measures where the patient is unaware of being assessed, since then the patient cannot give informed consent to the procedure. When a patient presents a serious risk of self-harm then some level of close observation may often be imposed without consent. Both these issues may be addressed by training the observers before the clinical use of the measure. *Any* live observer will induce some reactivity effects, and this issue is often totally ignored. However, the advent of computerized assessment procedures means that many measures, including behavioural ones, can be administered in this way, and the evidence is that they are well accepted.[7]

There are also a number of other practical factors to bear in mind. In general, shorter measures are preferred to longer ones. Coding categories should be simple enough to be entered quickly. When continuous observation is used, especially for high rates of behaviour, the observer must be allowed regular rest periods. Materials should be written at a level of vocabulary simple enough for the lowest level of educational attainment likely to be encountered by observers.

Focus of methods

Normally the assessment will focus on the presented or referred patient. However, it may be necessary to either focus on a family member (or all family members) or on formal or informal direct carers of the patient. Platt,[8] for example, reviewed five rating scales measuring the burden of psychiatric illness on the family, completed on the basis of an interview with one or more family members, and pointed out the distinction between objective and subjective burden as well as the need for such scales to be adequate psychometrically. Another example is the Camberwell Family Interview, which is a combined interview-based rating scale and observation rating, focusing on family reactions to the identified patient.

Another potential focus is the patient's environment. The range of behaviour a patient can display may be limited by the physical size or area of the environment, by the range of equipment available to the patient, and by the institutional rules of the setting (such as rules against smoking). In a small space or in a deprived environment the patient may be unable to exhibit the range of skills they possess. It may then be helpful to assess characteristics of both the physical or social environment, looking at the range of therapeutic materials available in a day room, for example. A measure of environmental restrictiveness would survey both the range of formal regulations and those informal rules followed by care staff, which might cover whether visitors can stay overnight, when lights have to be turned off, and whether residents can cook their own food.

Content of measures

Behavioural measures may include a wide range of clinically relevant content. Symptoms are most commonly elicited during clinical interviews, and their assessment is covered in Chapter 1.10.1. However, self-completed questionnaires or checklists may also supplement clinical interviews, and specific behavioural problems may be assessed by observer-completed ratings or checklists. Woo et al.[9] describe an interesting approach to symptomatic assessment, in which videotaped interactions between patients (who met research diagnostic criteria for schizophrenia, including both high and low 'expressed emotion' families) and a family member were coded for the presence of subclinical signs of pathology.

Rating scales typically cover both general social and functional behaviour. While most such measures cover a relatively limited number of functional areas, and are often designed for use with a specific subclient group, some measures are designed for wider use. An example is the Functional Performance Record,[10] comprising 600 items, that may be used not only with people with long-standing psychiatric disabilities, but also with people with enduring physical disabilities and with learning disabilities. There are 27 content topics with a number of specific questions attached to each, which enables very detailed goal-planning.

Behavioural measures have a special use in the assessment of disturbed or bizarre behaviour, where the patient commonly has little insight or knowledge of the nature or degree of their disturbance, and where the continuation of this behaviour poses either a major ongoing management problem or a barrier to their placement in the community. An example of such a measure is the Aberrant Behavior Checklist.[11] This is a 58-item behavioural rating scale completed by an informant, with the content covering five subscales: irritability, agitation, and crying; social withdrawal and lethargy; stereotyped behaviour; hyperactivity and non-compliance; inappropriate speech.

The Katz Adjustment Scales[12] are widely used self-rated questionnaires covering the pattern of everyday work and occupation, with separate scales for completion by the identified patient and the relative. The patient's scale has 134 items, covering symptoms, social adjustment, expected social activities, and performance and satisfaction with those activities (together with the discomfort experienced by the symptoms). The relative's scale comprises 205 items covering the same domains, but it only assesses the presence of symptoms and not their discomfort.

The subjective quality of life enjoyed by patients is of increasing concern, and because it is a multidimensional concept (covering physical, economic, aesthetic factors, etc.) it is often used loosely. The American Quality-of-Life scale proposed by Lehman[13] has been widely used in psychiatric studies, but British studies are increasingly using the Lancashire Scale.[14]

Most measures simply describe the current functioning of the patient, without offering a framework for translating the obtained scores into clinical priorities for treatment. The 'needs assessment' approach takes account of the views of the patient and carer as to the relative importance of different aspects of the assessment, and also takes into account the extent to which needs have been met, or remain unmet. Marshall et al.[15] derived the Cardinal Needs Schedule to measure the needs for psychiatric and social care among patients with severe psychiatric disorders. They rated 15 areas of psychiatric and social functioning (such as drug side-effects and the patient's ability to handle their own money) while considering three criteria: co-operation—the patients desire to be helped; carer stress; and severity. The 15 areas of functioning they identify (see Box 2) are a useful summary of the main areas most relevant to the rehabilitation and continuing care of severely mentally ill adults.

Box 2

Areas of functioning covered by the Cardinal Needs Schedule

Psychotic symptoms	Physical illness	Transport and amenities
Underactivity	Neurotic symptoms	ities
Side-effects	Socially embarrassing	Education
Dangerous or obstructive	Domestic skills	Occupation
	Money and own	Communication
Organic symptoms	affairs	Hygiene and dressing

In many areas of psychiatric practice the use of multiple measures, including some behavioural measures, may be helpful. Rutter,[16] in reviewing changes in child psychiatry, pays particular attention to the importance of sound measurement by contrasting standardized interviews and checklists, and points out that multiple measures involving different informants, which are repeated over time, are necessary to reduce error and minimize rater bias. Research studies may use complex multiple measures, but these are unlikely to be achievable in clinical practice. For example, Deale et al.,[17] in evaluating the outcome of a treatment trial for chronic fatigue, used ten outcome measures, namely: three functional impairment measures; two fatigue measures; two psychological distress questionnaires or inventories; and three other variables, including a global self-rating and a self-written statement of illness attributions. In clinical practice, multiple measures should be selected so that each measure is the most relevant for each category of behaviour, with care taken to consider the overall assessment load on any one individual in the light of their other clinical commitments, not forgetting the time taken to analyse the resulting data.

Standard or individualized measures?

There are many standard measures already in existence, especially ratings and questionnaires, covering most areas of clinical interest. However, the fact that a scale is well used does not necessarily mean that it is psychometrically sound,[3,18] or that the content covered is appropriate for a given clinical or research purpose. Rating scales may be widely used—such as the long-established NOSIE scale published in 1965—even when they are no longer the best scales technically, but because the volume of published research using them permits more comparisons to be made with other studies. Regier et al.[19] point out the need to standardize measures for both clinical and epidemiological work, given the 'drift' or 'mutations' that can occur with even the most carefully designed measures, with major consequences for public health and policy if prevalence estimates cannot be made reliably.

One sound solution to this dilemma is to create a totally new measure, making sure it is better than its predecessor, or systematically to improve the properties of an existing measure further. Parker et al.[20] describe a modification of the well-established Parental Bonding Instrument to include abusive parenting, which was omitted in the original version. Their article demonstrates both how to modify an original measure to improve item wording, and at the same time incorporate additional material to increase the value of the measure. An unsound solution is to change the measure in an ad hoc way—scale vandalization!—with no awareness of the principles of sound scale and item construction, this only results in an instrument that will then be of poor or unknown reliability or validity.

Direct observation methods can be used in a standardized manner for a group of patients. But they do lend themselves to flexible modification, so that the frequency of observation, and the duration of observation periods, can be chosen to suit the requirements of the task. The most common problems encountered in designing or modifying behavioural measures are as follows: choosing coding categories which cover all the most likely events and are ranked appropriately, using clear and unambiguous language, and using exact frequencies (such as 'twice a day' or 'at least every hour') rather than vague terms such as 'often' or 'frequently'.

Summary and conclusions

Behavioural and observational assessment measures constitute a clinically useful subgroup of methods. The special value of direct observation methods is that they have high validity with respect to day-to-day functioning. The value of rating and questionnaire methods is that they can be used by a variety of assessors who do not need to be qualified mental health professionals—although the need for at least some training in rating methods should not be overlooked. They can be presented in very short versions therefore making minimal demands on assessors, and so can lead to high levels of compliance. Since they can be used by patients, they can themselves be tools to increase engagement and to give patients direct feedback about their own current state. However, their very simplicity may mask the need for care in their construction, and caution in interpreting data arising from their use.

Further reading

Andrews, G., Peters, L., and Teesson, M. (1994). The measurement of consumer outcome in mental health: a report to the National Mental Health Information Strategy Committee. Clinical Research Unit for Anxiety Disorder, Sydney, Australia.

Bellack, A.S. and Hersen, M. (1988). Behavioral assessment. A practical handbook (3rd edn). Pergamon Press, Oxford.

References

1. Eifert, G.H. and Wilson, P.H. (1991). The triple response approach to assessment: a conceptual and methodological reappraisal. Behaviour Research and Therapy, 29, 283–92.

2. Farkas, M.D., O'Brien, W.F., Cohen, M.R., and Anthony, W.A. (1994). In Psychological assessment and treatment of persons with severe mental disorders (ed. J.R. Bedell), pp. 3–30. Taylor and Francis, Washington, DC.

3. Andrews, G., Peters, L., and Teesson, M. (1994). The measurement of consumer outcome in mental health: a report to the National Mental Health Information Strategy Committee. Clinical Research Unit for Anxiety Disorder, Sydney, Australia.

4. Bellack, A.S. and Hersen, M. (1988). Behavioral assessment. A practical handbook (3rd edn). Pergamon Press, Oxford.

5. Wing, J.K., Curtis, R.H., and Beevor, A.S. (1996). *HONOS: Health of the Nation Outcome Scales*. Royal College of Psychiatrists Research Unit, London.

6. Patel, V., Hope, T., Hall, J.N., and Fairburn, C.G. (1995). Three methodological issues in the development of observer-rated behaviour rating scales: experience from the development of the rating scale for aggressive behaviour in the elderly. *International Journal of Methods in Psychiatric Research*, **5**, 21–7.

7. French, C.C. and Beaumont, J.G. (1987). The reaction of psychiatric patients to computerized assessment. *British Journal of Clinical Psychology*, **26**, 267–78.

8. Platt, S. (1985). Measuring the burden of psychiatric illness on the family: an evaluation of some rating scales. *Psychological Medicine*, **15**, 383–93.

9. Woo, S.M., Goldstein, M.J., and Nuechterlein, K.H. (1997). Relatives' expressed emotion and non-verbal signs of subclinical psychopathology in schizophrenic patients. *British Journal of Psychiatry*, **170**, 58–61.

10. Mulhall, D.J. (1986). The functional performance record—an observational procedure for use with disabled people. *Behavioural Psychotherapy*, **14**, 69–80.

11. Aman, M.G., Singh, N.N., and Stewart, A.W. (1985). The aberrant behavior checklist: a behavior rating scale for the assessment of treatment effects. *American Journal of Mental Deficiency*, **89**, 485–91.

12. Katz, M.M. and Lyerly, S.B. (1963). Methods for measuring adjustment and social behaviour in the community: I rationale, description, discriminative validity and scale development. *Psychological Reports*, **13**, 503–35.

13. Lehman, A.F. (1988). A quality of life interview for the chronically mentally ill. *Evaluation and Program Planning*, **11**, 51–62.

14. Oliver, J., Huxley, P., Bridges, K., and Mohamad, H. (1996). *Quality of life and mental health services*. Routledge, London.

15. Marshall, M., Hogg, L.I., Gath, D.H., and Lockwood, A. (1995). The Cardinal Needs Schedule—modified version of the MRC Needs for Care Assessment Schedule. *Psychological Medicine*, **25**, 605–17.

16. Rutter, M. (1997). Child psychiatric disorder: measures, causal mechanisms, and interventions. *Archives of General Psychiatry*, **54**, 785–9.

17. Deale, A., Chalder, T., Marks, I., and Wessely, S. (1997). Cognitive behaviour therapy for chronic fatigue syndrome: a randomized controlled trial. *American Journal of Psychiatry*, **154**, 408–14.

18. Hall, J.N. (1980). Ward rating scales for long stay patients: a review. *Psychological Medicine*, **10**, 277–88.

19. Regier, D.A., Kaelber, C.T., Rae, D.S., *et al.* (1998). Limitations of diagnostic criteria and assessment instruments for mental disorders. *Archives of General Psychiatry*, **55**, 109–15.

20. Parker, G., Roussos, J., Hadzi-Pavlovic, D., Mitchell, P., Wilhelm, K., and Austin, M.-P. (1997). The development of a refined measure of dysfunctional parenting and assessment of its relevance in patients with affective disorders. *Psychological Medicine*, **27**, 1193–203.

1.11 Classification

H. Dilling

General issues and definitions

For thousands of years humans have tried to understand their world. Language allowed them to name all the objects pertaining to their lives, including ailments and diseases. In antiquity the question had already arisen whether things are real because humans give them a name or whether nature exists independently outside human existence. Questions of this kind can be reactivated regarding modern discussions in psychiatry concerning diagnosis. Norman Sartorius reflected that diagnosis and classification are a means of viewing the world.[1] Indeed, it is hard to imagine how it would be possible to exist without some kind of classificatory order. Classification, then, is a systematic arrangement of the world in order to master the otherwise chaotic entities and structures, and corresponds to the structure of human thinking.

In medicine, diagnosis means the description of a disease according to its symptoms and the naming of the described disease. As well as naming the disease, diagnosis can also be understood as the process of making a diagnosis. Various terms are used in general medicine: 'disease' for describing an objective pathology, 'illness' for the subjective awareness of distress, and 'sickness' for the loss of capacity to fill normal social roles. In psychiatry the term disorder is frequently used because the pathophysiology and hence the aetiology of the diagnostic category is not yet known.

Assigning a number of diagnoses a certain order with regard to their similarities and differences, within a system according to certain principles, implies building up a classification. Thus classification can be understood as a system of classes in which all described cases find a place. However, it also means the work of putting the diagnostic entities into their proper places in the system. These reflections show clearly that diagnosis and classification are connected to each other and are interdependent. There is no classification without diagnoses, and every diagnosis needs its place in a classification.

The kinds of classification used may be very different. Classification may follow a single principle (e.g. the aetiological principle), or it may be purely descriptive, or several principles may converge.

Aims of diagnosis and classification

In both general medicine and psychiatry, diagnosis is used to collect experiences concerning treatment and prognosis. Ideally, no treatment should be given without previous diagnosis. Diagnosis, treatment, and prognosis may be more standardized in general medicine than in psychiatry, but even less accurate diagnoses, such as often occur in psychiatry, are needed. Practical and scientific work performed in the clinical field cannot be communicated without a system of comparable diagnoses. Research cannot be conducted without a means of comparing groups of patients. Epidemiological data concerning different diagnoses can provide planning data for services needed in future and can enable administrative bodies to perform cost–benefit calculations. These different aims may point to different types or arrangements of diagnoses and classification according to the particular need.

Historical review

In classical antiquity physicians had already named psychiatric disorders, like depression or confusion, and the diagnoses of the Greek physician Galen were in use until a more systematical classification was devised in the eighteenth century. In Chapter 5 of *Genera Morborum*, published in 1742, Carl von Linné mentions a group of major psychiatric disorders which is complemented by minor mental disorders of neurotic nature in other chapters.[2] Only 30 years later, William Cullen published his *Synopsis Nosologiae Methodicae*, which also described psychiatric disorders.[3] In Cullen's scheme mental disorders were part of the broad class of neurosis, a term which was used very differently later on. At the same time the German philosopher Immanuel Kant described different forms of psychiatric disorders in his *Kleine Onomastik der Gebrechen des Kopfes*, providing a classical description of delusional thinking.[4] Later Heinroth from Leipzig, the first German university professor of psychiatry, built up a very complicated system of psychiatric diseases similar to the botanical system developed by von Linné. He produced many interesting diagnoses but these could not be identified reliably nor was their description reproducible.[5] In France, Pinel[6] restricted the diagnostic field to a small number of psychiatric diagnoses such as mania with and without delusions, melancholia, dementia, and idiocy. He and his pupil Esquirol[7] had a strong international influence in the nineteenth century and many psychiatrists followed their system of classification. In 1845 Wilhelm Griesinger published his textbook[8] in which he claimed that psychoses were basically only a single disorder, although he distinguished different stages and different clinical manifestations. Thus in the eighteenth and nineteenth centuries there were many different approaches to classification emerging from different backgrounds and focusing on different aspects.

In 1854 Falret[9] described *folie circulaire*, essentially the modern bipolar disorder, taking into account the course of the illness. The importance of the course of the disorders was emphasized by Kahlbaum[10] in 1863. Emil Kraepelin can be regarded as the most important nosologist at the end of the nineteenth century and in the early twentieth century. He described the symptoms and course of mental disorders and established types of disorder, consequently proposing two dominating psychotic disease entities, dementia praecox and manic–depressive disorder, in addition to several others described in his famous textbook.[11] Although his view gained worldwide recognition, Kraepelin encountered some opposition; for example, Alfred Hoche[12] demanded an alternative system of syndromes, rejecting the Kraepelinean nosological conception.

The position occupied by Eugen Bleuler[13] can be described as intermediate between those of the nosologist Kraepelin and the syndromatologist Hoche. Bleuler was not convinced that there was only one disease entity called *dementia praecox* or, as he named it, schizophrenia; thus he preferred to refer to the 'group of schizophrenias'.

In Germany, authors whose thinking was dominated by a biological view of nosology created the Würzburg neuropsychiatric diagnostic scheme,[14] which was used until ICD-8 was introduced in the 1960s. This was a rather simplistic classification and did not differentiate conditions sufficiently in either neurology or in psychiatry, let alone among psychogenic disorders.

National classifications

Although many national classifications have been developed in the twentieth century, these did not differ essentially from those which originated in central Europe. It is impossible to describe or even list the numerous classifications used in different countries; rather, only a few are noted.[15]

In France and Scandinavia, the Kraepelinean concept of psychoses was accepted only partially or rejected. Magnan and Serieux[16] developed a classification[17] which remained restricted to Francophone psychiatry. Some disturbances like acute and chronic delusional states (*bouffées délirantes* and *délires chroniques*) were recognized in France but were not really understood beyond the confines of French psychiatry. The French psychiatrists were particularly resistant to the Kraepelinean concept of schizophrenia, although they accepted the concept of manic depressive psychosis, perhaps because several French authors[9,18] had already used similar concepts. In Scandinavia the concept of psychogenic psychoses was advocated,[19] as were early concepts of multidimensional diagnosis.[20] The special classification of psychoses according to Wernicke, Kleist, and Leonhard adopted in Germany should also be noted.[21] These authors claimed that, according to the phenomenological description of psychoses, a valid prognosis including the genetic load can be given.

Outside Europe, for example in Asia, some traditional elements were related to European concepts. In Japan, traditional diagnostic thinking was abandoned after the Meiji reformation in 1868 and European influence was accepted.[22] The Kraepelinian system was very influential for a long time in Tokyo and elsewhere. Nowadays ICD-10 and DSM are widely used in Japan. In China an attempt was made to introduce modern aspects of diagnosis into the Chinese Classification of Mental Disorders, while still retaining special traditional elements.[23] Traditionally the diagnosis of neurasthenia is used frequently; this category is not found in DSM-IV but does appear in ICD-10, which offers a broader international view.

In constructing a classification which can be used worldwide, it must be remembered that many disorders like anorexia, anxiety disorders, sexual deviations, and borderline personality disorders that are prominent in the West are not important in many developing countries, where acute psychotic episodes, hysterical phenomena, and somatisation disorders are more frequent.[24] The dualism between body and mind that dominates Western psychiatry is unknown in many traditional healing systems. Thus there are fundamental differences between ayurvedic medicine in India or traditional healing in Nigeria, for example, and modern Western medicine. Nevertheless, ICD-10 satisfies a number of needs related to psychiatry in the Third World.[24]

The development of modern classifications

In the 1960s and 1970s diagnosis and classification were criticized by antipsychiatry and psychoanalysis. Many psychotherapists argued that diagnosis and classification distracted from the understanding of the individual personal problems and that they missed an acceptable goodness of fit of the diagnostic categories. On the other hand, many psychiatrists, especially those working in the field of psychopharmacological research, believed that a consistent system of diagnosis and classification was necessary.[25,26] In the United States, in reaction to the dominating psychoanalytic psychiatry, so-called 'neokraepelinianism'[27] emerged, harking back to the diagnoses and nosology of Kraepelin. The Feighner criteria[28] and later the Research Diagnostic Criteria[29] were developed for scientific purposes, and were specialized precursors of later classifications, of which DSM-III[30] should be regarded as the first large system.

The long developmental history of psychiatric classification, beginning with the diagnostic schemes of rather a few famous psychiatrists and culminating today in a consensus by many national and international experts,[31] characterizes the road to the current version of the *International Classification of Diseases* (**ICD-10**) and the American national system of psychiatric classification, the current version of the *Diagnostic and Statistical Manual of Mental Disorders* (**DSM-IV**)[32] (these classifications are reproduced at the end of this chapter). This implies that only one or two relevant classifications will survive. Nevertheless, it is hoped that certain diagnostic and classificatory tendencies or geographically determined differences in certain disorders will continue.

The first international classification of diseases in 1855 was concerned with a nomenclature of causes of death.[33] After many revisions this list was adopted by the World Health Organization (**WHO**) in 1948 and the so-called *Sixth Revision of the International Statistical Classification of Diseases, Injuries and Causes of Death* (**ICD-6**) was produced.[34] It was only after the eighth revision that the ICD[35] was accepted by psychiatrists in many countries. In this edition a glossary was published for the first time. This short description of the disorders, largely based on British views, was produced by a working group chaired by Sir Aubrey Lewis. About 10 years later the ninth revision[36] was introduced with only minor changes.

The lack of multiaxiality, the difficulties in classifying depressions and other affective disorders, the problems of diagnosing sexual disorders, and especially the insufficient description of the disorders, which in turn caused low reliability, led American psychiatrists to construct a completely new system of classification, which differed radically from that of the WHO system, in the *Third Revision of the Diagnostic and Statistical Manual of Mental Disorders* (**DSM-III**).[30]

Operationalized diagnosis

The DSM-III system of classification is characterized by operationalized diagnosis. This means that diseases are described according to their phenomenology and independent of their aetiology (the so-called atheoretical approach) using typical criteria that include the intensity and duration of the symptoms. Following a diagnostic algorithm, certain criteria (e.g. psychopathological symptoms) are obligatory while others are optional to the constitution of a diagnosis. There are 'characteristic' symptoms pertinent to the diagnosis, such as the symptom of depression which is found in many different disorders, and there are 'discriminating' symptoms, such as the delusion of thoughts being inserted into the mind, which may be of less importance to the patient but are important for diagnosis since they are not found in other disorders. Apart from characteristic and discriminating symptoms, there may be a hierarchy of symptoms, arranged in order of importance (e.g. depression over anxiety, auditory hallucinations over depression, etc.). Additionally, inclusion and exclusion criteria must be considered since diagnostic categories must be mutually exclusive without substantial overlapping.

Traditionally, psychiatrists have been used to a typologically oriented diagnosis which, although it used characteristic symptoms, was based essentially on typical cases. Thus the diagnosis was found according to maximum similarity compared with a typical case—the prototype or the leading case. There was considerable latitude concerning comparable cases which would be diagnosed by the diagnostician according to his internalized typical case.

Thus typological and operationalized diagnosis take different diagnostic pathways: the typological diagnosis starts with the typical case, whereas the operationalized diagnosis starts with symptoms and syndromes without considering aetiology. Since no nosological entities are aimed at in operationalized psychiatric diagnosis, it follows that 'disorders' not 'diseases' are diagnosed.

Categorical systems often imply a hierarchical use of diagnoses: the organic 'diseases' are located at the top, followed by psychotic 'disorders', and the hierarchy is concluded by neurotic 'disorders'. To avoid such a hierarchy in classification, the principle of comorbidity was introduced. Comorbidity lends equal weight to the diagnoses, with the current prominent disorder occupying the first place.

Disorders in a categorical classification form discrete entities, whereas dimensional diagnoses do not use discrete entities and are not clearly differentiated from either normality or other disorders. Dimensional diagnoses are widely used in clinical psychology and to some extent in the description of personality disorders.

The development of ICD-10

The psychiatric section of the *10th Revision of the International Classification of Diseases* was worked through in several conferences under the chairmanship of Norman Sartorius. After a meeting of WHO rep-resentatives and consultants, together with representatives of the American Drug and Mental Health Administration in Copenhagen in 1982, several further meetings took place (e.g. in Djakarta and in Geneva in 1984) in which a provisional psychiatric classification was designed. The first draft of the psychiatric chapter (Chapter V (F)) was written in English and distributed by the World Psychiatric Association to the national psychiatric societies for comment and criticism. Nine years later the *Clinical Descriptions and Diagnostic Guidelines*[37] were published. Following the work on the English text, the *Guidelines* were translated into many other languages including Arabic, Chinese, French, German, and Spanish; by 1995 they were available in 19 languages. Many of the translations and accompanying studies were performed by the Field Trial Coordinating Centres, later called the WHO Reference and Training Centres in Classification, Diagnosis and Assessment of Mental and Behavioural Disorders. These centres were also useful for facilitating the introduction of ICD-10 in the respective countries or language regions.

Aims of ICD-10, Chapter V (F)

The classification has to be used worldwide and therefore should be acceptable to a wide range of users in different cultures, practical, clearly understandable, and easy to translate into other languages. If possible it should serve as a reference for national and other classifications. Based on operational principles, it should be versatile and allow different versions for different users and different purposes, for example a flexible version for clinical users and a more precise version for research. Finally, it should be able to contribute to education in psychiatry.[38]

The structure and use of ICD-10, Chapter V (F)

The psychiatric classification is part of the general medical classification.[39] The earlier versions (ICD-8 and ICD-9) comprised a maximum of only 300 diagnoses. The use of an open alphanumeric system made it possible to expand ICD-10 compared with ICD-9, so that there is considerably more scope for diagnoses from all medical specialties. There are 21 chapters, each designated by a Roman numeral. The psychiatric disorders are included in Chapter V which is also identified by the letter F. The letter F is followed by Arabic numbers, the so-called second digit for the larger diagnostic groups and the third digit for more special groups. Thus the use of three digits allows a choice of 100 diagnostic possibilities. Proceeding further with a fourth digit, 1000 possible diagnoses are available, of which about one-third are used at present. This system will allow the addition of new diagnoses in future without having to change substantial parts of the classification.

Furthermore, it is possible to code the course over time or characteristic features of a disorder by using a fifth or sixth digit. By using codes from other chapters of ICD-10, such as X, Y, and Z, additional circumstances (e.g. suicide) or special symptoms (e.g. nausea) as well as psychosocial factors can be coded. Somatic comorbidity is coded from the related chapters, for example diseases of ear, nose, and throat from Chapter VIII headed by the letter H (e.g. tinnitus H93.1) or diseases of the gastrointestinal system from Chapter XI headed by the letter K (e.g. alcohol gastritis K29.2). The special difficulties encountered in diagnosing psychiatric disorders caused WHO to include short definitions plus inclusion and exclusion terms for all psychiatric disorders in Chapter V (F). In all other chapters diagnoses are named without further explanation.

The family of documents connected to Chapter V (F)

Chapter V of ICD-10 is not just a catalogue of disorders for statistical purposes, but is also a clinical manual, a textbook of diagnoses, and an instrument for research for different users. Therefore a group of texts had to be produced to serve the various purposes—the so-called 'family of documents'.[38]

The *Short Glossary of ICD-10, Chapter V (F)* is part of the basic work known as the *International Statistical Classification of Diseases and Related Health Problems*.[39] The *Short Glossary* is part of the first of three volumes, the general systematic classification, and gives short definitions which are useful not only for medical personnel but also for statisticians, health insurance clerks, and others who are not in medical or related professions.

The *Clinical Descriptions and Diagnostic Guidelines (CDDG Version)*, the so-called Blue Book, was developed first and can be regarded as the central part of the psychiatric classification[37] intended for use by psychiatric clinicians in their daily practice. An extensive description of each disorder is followed by criteria for diagnosis together with inclusion and exclusion terms.

The *Diagnostic Criteria for Research* (**DCR**), the so-called Green Book, were developed for scientific use.[40] A number of rather restrictive criteria are given for every disorder so as to facilitate the selection of groups of individuals whose symptoms resemble each other. The research criteria should be used together with the diagnostic guidelines. Compared with the Blue Book the symptom criteria are more clearly defined, the time criteria are stricter, and the inclusion and exclusion criteria are more precise. Thus many unclear cases which are unsuitable for research are excluded. However, despite its title, this book is also useful for diagnosticians in clinical practice. Its combination with the *Short Glossary*, published as the *Pocket Guide*,[41] is useful.

The *multiaxial version* of the ICD-10 classification of mental disorders allows different aspects of the patient's health and social situation to be assessed. Several attempts have been made to broaden the diagnostic view by consideration of additional aspects, for example Kretschmer's multidimensional diagnosis[42] or, much later, the multiaxial system of Essen-Möller[43] who proposed coding the clinical picture and aetiology on different axes. Introduced by Rutter *et al.*,[44] multiaxial diagnosis has been employed for many years in child and adolescent psychiatry. It contains clinical syndromes, problems of development, intelligence, somatic disorders, and psychosocial problems. In adult psychiatry many attempts were undertaken to initiate a multiaxial system. Some of these are associated with a multiaxial system of ICD-10 (**MAS**) which was developed independently after the main part of the classification was finished.

To a high degree the multiaxial version of ICD-10 is comparable with that of DSM-IV. However, in DSM-IV, axis I is for psychiatric clinical disorders, axis II is for personality disorders and mental retardation, and axis III is for general medical conditions. In ICD-10, axis I includes all three groups. Thus psychiatric disorders (F1–F5), personality disorders (F6) and mental retardation (F7), and the chapters on somatic comorbidity all use one axis.

Axis II of ICD-10 is for disability. To facilitate its use, WHO developed an instrument, the short disability assessment schedule (**WHO DAS-S**), which helps to describe and assess the consequences of axis I disorders.[45] Axis II corresponds to the widely used DSM-IV axis V, Global Assessment of Functioning (**GAF**). In connection with the disability axis, the International Classification of Impairments, Disabilities and Handicaps (**ICIDH**),[46] created by WHO for the whole of rehabilitative medicine, of which psychiatry is only a part, should be mentioned. At the time of writing, a new version of this classification (**ICIDH-II**) is being tested in field trials.[47] It uses a more positive approach, replacing disabilities by activities and handicaps by participation.

Axis III of ICD-10 covers psychosocial and other problems and corresponds to DSM-IV axis IV (psychosocial and environmental problems).

The *primary health care* (**PHC**) version of the ICD-10 classification of mental disorders[48] was constructed because of the great importance of psychiatric disorders in general practice, for example the high prevalence of depressions, anxiety disorders, and dependence on alcohol and psychotropic drugs.[48] There are 24 syndromes, including dementia, delirium, depression, etc. Each disorder is understood in a rather broad sense, and not subdivided, and the descriptions are simpler than those in the main classification. A flipcard containing symptoms, diagnostic criteria, differential diagnoses, and counselling and treatment of the patient and the family is provided for every syndrome.

Further texts in the family of documents

Reference tables ('cross-walks') are provided for valid comparison of the diagnostic categories in ICD-8, ICD-9, and ICD-10. Despite their very similar diagnoses, there is a fundamental difference between ICD-8/ICD-9 and ICD-10 in that operationalized diagnosis is used in the latter. Nevertheless, comparability has to be assured in the compilation of statistics. This is not difficult for disorders like catatonic schizophrenia or obsessive–compulsive neurosis, but it is difficult to translate the ICD-9 diagnosis of neurotic depression (300.4) into an ICD-10 diagnosis. Usually dysthymia is chosen (F34.1), but there are other diagnoses that may be even more suitable. Another problem is identifying which ICD-8/ICD-9 diagnoses correspond to the currently common diagnoses of panic disorder or somatization disorder. Therefore the reference tables produced by WHO are not an automatic translation from the old to the new system, but provide only help and guidelines. It must be emphasized that a change from one system of diagnosis to another is only possible on an individual patient basis.

Lexica for psychopathology and other terms of ICD-9, ICD-10, and transcultural psychiatry have been produced by WHO.

Casebooks have been developed to provide examples of the application of the diagnostic criteria for the individual doctor or as a help in diagnostic seminars. The English language casebook contains 100 cases, each well structured and described, systematically covering the whole of Chapter F (Üstün *et al.* 1986).[49] The German casebook[50] contains case histories whose styles differ depending on the author.

WHO has also produced **training material** for introductory lectures and seminars on diagnosis, including visual aids. This material clarifies many aspects of ICD-10; the basic set of visual aids has been translated into several other languages.

The availability of electronic data processing and the development of operational diagnoses have led to an **ICD-10 tutorial** as hypertext for use as a quick aid in demonstrations and discussions of diagnoses.[51]

Another development has been in the use of **computer diagnosis**, which can be generated from either logical decision tree programs or statistical models. Examples of decision tree program diagnosis are DIAGNO[52] and CATEGO,[53] and programs for SCAN[54] and SIDI.[55]

Operationalized psychodynamic diagnosis

ICD-10 is an open system, which means that national or traditional systems can fit into or coexist with it, and it is possible to add annexes or complementary texts to the basic classification or indicate variations. One example of a complementary text could be the operationalized psychodynamic diagnosis (**OPD**) developed by a German group comprising analytical psychotherapists and psychiatrists (Arbeitskreis OPD 1996).[56] It was felt that certain axes which could be important for diagnosis and therapy were missing from the ICD-10 texts. Therefore, as well as an ICD-10 diagnosis according to Chapter V (F), consideration is given to the subjective experience of the disorder, the conditions of treatment, relations with others, conflicts with others, and the structure of personality. The system, which requires graded ratings, could be important in many aspects of psychotherapy such as decisions about suitability for treatment and evaluation of progress and outcome.

Structure of Chapter V (F) and subchapters

At first glance, the structure of ICD-10, Chapter V (F), follows that of ICD-8 or ICD-9. The classification begins with the 'organic disorders', followed by disorders due to the abuse of psychoactive substances. The next section contains schizophrenia and other psychotic disorders. This is followed by affective disorders and then neurotic and personality disorders. The chapter ends with mental retardation and disorders of childhood and adolescence. Closer examination of the classification reveals that the traditional dualistic principle—psychoses on the one hand (in ICD-9: codes 290–299) and neuroses on the other (in ICD-9: codes 300–310)—has been abandoned. The diagnostic terms now used take a more phenomenological descriptive approach. According to the authors of ICD-10, the same psychiatric disorder may show both psychotic and non-psychotic symptoms. 'Psychotic' is defined as the manifestation of productive symptoms. The term 'neurosis' did not appear in the first drafts of ICD-10 because it is used in different and contradictory ways and is supposedly based on theories of intrapsychic processes which many of the WHO experts regarded as not generally accepted. However, after protests and objections by many clinicians worldwide, it was concluded that 'psychotic' and 'neurotic' should be used, although only as descriptive terms and not as diagnostic rubrics. Thus the term 'neurotic disorders' follows the traditional use of the word but does not imply an aetiological theory.

The subchapters are arranged in a hierarchical order, which means that the descriptions of the main diagnostic entities are also valid for the following three- and four-digit categories.

Apart from a few exceptions, the term mental disorders rather than mental diseases is used in Chapter V (F) so as to emphasize the provisional descriptive and atheoretical nature of the classification. Nevertheless, aetiological findings are considered in some subchapters, such as organic aetiology in F0, psychotropic substances in F1, and stress in F4.

Characteristics of the subchapters of Chapter V (F)

F0 Organic, including symptomatic, mental disorders

Disorders of organic aetiology are grouped in this subchapter, independent of whether they contain psychotic or non-psychotic symptoms. However, the use of the term 'organic' does not imply that conditions elsewhere in the classification are non-organic in the sense of having no cerebral substrate. Dementia may contain irreversible and reversible cases, and this term has been expanded similarly to DSM-IV, although one criterion is a duration of at least 6 months. The diagnosis of delirium is less specific than that used previously; for example, disturbances of sensory perception such as visual hallucinations are no longer obligatory.

F1 Mental and behavioural disorders due to psychoactive substance use

An improvement over ICD-9 is the compilation of all mental and behavioural disorders due to psychoactive substances within a single subchapter. The third digit indicates which substance or class of substances (e.g. F10 Alcohol) is responsible for the disorder, which is coded as a fourth digit (e.g. F10.3 Alcohol withdrawal state) or a fifth digit (e.g. F10.31 Alcohol withdrawal state with convulsions). It is possible to differentiate acute intoxication, harmful use, dependence syndrome, withdrawal state with or without delirium, different psychotic disorders, amnesic syndrome, and a number of other disorders. Thus the psychopathological syndrome can be described and related to the dominant substance class.

F2 Schizophrenia, schizotypal and delusional disorders

This subchapter covers schizophrenia, acute psychotic disorders, schizoaffective disorders, delusional disorders, and schizotypal disorders. Before schizophrenia can be diagnosed the symptoms have to be observed for at least 1 month, unlike DSM-IV where symptoms should be observed for 6 months before using this diagnosis, although only 1 month is required with florid psychotic symptoms. Special care is taken with the description of short-lasting psychoses, since acute and transient psychotic disorders are of particular interest to psychiatrists from developing countries where short-lasting acute psychoses with a good prognosis are observed quite frequently.

F3 Mood (affective) disorders

All mood disorders are combined in this subchapter, which represents a considerable change compared with ICD-9. The disorders previously known as endogenous and neurotic depressions are coded in this subchapter; the differentiation between these categories has been abandoned. The ICD-9 category of neurotic depression (300.4) is no longer found in ICD-10. Most of these cases are now coded as dysthymia (F34.1), although there is no fixed rule. Single manic episodes are coded as F30, while recurrent manic episodes are now coded as bipolar affective disorder (F31), regardless of whether or not there has been a previous depressive episode. A practical difficulty often arises concerning the differentiation between mild, moderate, and severe depressive episodes because of the number of symptoms. The structure of this chapter resembles that of DSM-IV, but unfortunately the grades of severity of the depressive disorders are based on slightly different criteria.

F4 Neurotic, stress-related, and somatoform disorders

The disorders in this subchapter are divided into a large number of categories. For instance, dissociative disorders are divided into seven subcategories, some of which represent rather rare disorders. The term hysteria is no longer used, and unfortunately there is no distinction between conversion and dissociation as in DSM-IV. In this subchapter reactions to severe stress and adjustment disorders are enumerated according to time criteria and severity. Here aetiology is generally accepted to mean exceptional mental stress or special life events. A new group of disorders in this classification are the somatoform disorders, which are of particular importance in developing countries. The traditional term neurasthenia is still maintained for a special category, in contrast with DSM-IV.

F5 Behavioural syndromes associated with physiological disturbances and physical factors

This subchapter brings together eating disorders, non-organic sleep disorders, sexual dysfunction, mental and behavioural disorders associated with the puerperium, and abuse of non-dependence-producing substances. In ICD-9 all sexual disorders were contained in one subchapter. In ICD-10 only disorders of sexual dysfunction are in F5; disorders of gender identity and sexual preference have been assigned to two different sections in subchapter F6 on personality disorders. This new classification of sexual disorders seems to be advantageous in that it accentuates the differences among the disorders. The special code F54, psychological and behavioural factors associated with disorders or diseases classified elsewhere, allows classification of psychosomatic disorders by coding an additional somatic diagnosis.

F6 Disorders of adult personality and behaviour

Specific personality disorders are coded in this subchapter. Cyclothymic personality is not included, but an equivalent appears in F3 as cyclothymia. Also, schizotypal disorders could have been assigned to this subchapter but appears instead in F2 (as F21). As in DSM-IV, the emotionally unstable personality disorder is found in this subchapter, where it is subdivided into an impulsive type (F60.30) and a borderline type (F60.31). A new entity is the factitious disorder, i.e. the intentional production or feigning of symptoms or disabilities, either physical or psychological (F68.1). If desired, narcissistic personality disorder and passive–aggressive personality disorder may be coded by using the criteria in Annex 1 of DCR.

An important aspect of this subchapter is the inclusion of enduring personality changes after catastrophic experience (F62.0) or after psychiatric illness (F62.1). Personality changes after surviving a concentration camp or torture are coded under the first of these.

Remaining subchapters

F7 Mental retardation, F8 Disorders of psychological development, and F9 Behavioural and emotional disorders with onset during childhood and adolescence are mainly used in child and adolescent psychiatry.

Empirical research associated with ICD-10

The classification in Chapter V (F) was based on the practical clinical experience of many researchers worldwide, but goodness of fit, reli-

ability, and validity had to be proved. Therefore the Mental Health Division of WHO initiated several multicentre field trials of the classification, diagnosis, and assessment of mental and behavioural disorders which were carried out by the WHO reference and training centres. Ten centres, located in China, Denmark, Egypt, Germany, India, Japan, Luxembourg, Spain, the United Kingdom, and the United States, took part so that there was a wide range of language and geographical area. Several papers describing these studies have been published.[57,58]

The first major studies were of the *Clinical Descriptions and Diagnostic Guidelines*, involving 112 centres in 39 countries, and the *Diagnostic Criteria for Research*, involving 151 centres in 32 countries. Cases were diagnosed by several clinicians in case conferences and using videotapes. The inter-rater reliability was much higher for the diagnostic criteria (0.8–1.0 κ) than for the diagnostic guidelines (0.5 κ). (Kappa (κ) values reflect the chance-corrected inter-rater reliability, with high correspondence for κ > 0.81 and low correspondence for κ < 0.20.[59]) These two studies, which formed the largest international psychiatric scientific enterprise ever conducted, showed that such large studies are possible, but that many differences and uncertainties have to be considered if a study is undertaken in so many different centres with such a large number of raters.

Another study initiated by WHO concerned the multiaxial classification. In the first part of this study 10 cases provided by WHO were rated by many centres worldwide. As the next step, the inter-rater reliability and validity of the axes was examined in cases from the centres. The inter-rater reliability of PHC has also been studied in an international research programme.

Although the inter-rater reliability of most diagnoses has been measured and is satisfactory, the same cannot be said for any measure of validity—fitting well with clinical experience (face validity), predicting the outcome (predictive validity), or satisfying associations with independent variables (construct validity).

DSM-III and DSM-IV

The separate American development of DSM began about 20 years ago when operationalized diagnosis was not offered by WHO. In 1980, shortly after the publication of ICD-9, the American Psychiatric Association published DSM-III, followed 7 years later by the revision DSM-IIIR[60] and, in 1994, by DSM-IV.[32]

The introduction of DSM-III inaugurated the use of explicit and operationally defined diagnostic criteria, multiaxiality, and, as far as possible, a classification based on neutrality rather than aetiological theories. This version of DSM was revised in the 1980s and many changes were proposed. Finally, a systematic revision process was performed for DSM-IV with reviews of the world literature and a final consensus process. WHO was involved in this process, and before it was finished representatives of the American Psychiatric Association and WHO met in several sessions. A consensus was reached on many questions, although differences persisted on others.

ICD-10 and DSM-IV

The differences between ICD-10 and DSM-IV[32] are small compared with those between ICD-9 and ICD-10. There are several reasons for this similarity; one of the most important is the involvement of American diagnosticians in designing the new ICD-10 classification. However, although the two systems have converged, they are still not fully congruent. But, despite the remaining differences, psychiatrists worldwide are converging more than ever with respect to diagnosis and classification.

The structure of DSM-IV

DSM-IV is not a general medical classification but comprises only mental disorders. The structure of DSM-IV resembles that of Chapter V of ICD-10, except that the disorders of childhood and adolescence are considered in the first chapters, followed by the chapter on organic mental disorders, which is entitled 'Delirium, dementia, amnesic and other cognitive disorders'. The title of the chapter was changed from the earlier 'Organic disorders' since research data suggest that many other mental disorders have some kind of somatic aetiology.

The difference between DSM-IV and ICD-10 in the time criterion for the diagnosis of schizophrenia has already been mentioned, as has the distinction between conversion and dissociative disorders made in DSM-IV but not in ICD-10. Furthermore, the two systems classify eating disorders differently. DSM-IV includes two distinct forms of anorexia (the restricting type and the binge eating type) and two distinct types of bulimia (the purging and the non-purging types), whereas ICD-10 only includes only anorexia, bulimia, and their (undefined) atypical forms.

Apart from these specific differences there are some structural distinctions. DSM-IV exists in one version only, so that no differences are made between diagnostic guidelines for clinical practice, for research criteria, and for use in primary health care. This may assist in the use of the DSM diagnostic criteria in research because they are primarily meant for scientific work. In some instances, however, such as in general practice, the application may be more difficult because there is no simpler version of the system. Social and occupational criteria have been avoided as far as possible in ICD-10 because of the difficulty of equating these criteria between various cultures, but they are used in DSM-IV which is a national classification. Another difference, which has been mentioned earlier, concerns the use of multiple axes.

Owing to difficulties with the registration and insurance systems, code numbers in the American edition of DSM-IV are still analogous to those of *ICD-9—Clinical Modification* (**ICD-9–CM**). However, the international edition and several translations (e.g. the German translation) have adopted ICD-10 code numbers. In about the year 2000 the United States will be ready to adopt the ICD-10 coding system and will introduce ICD-10 as a whole (i.e. for all medical disciplines). The American edition of DSM-IV will then use the same code numbers as ICD-10, Chapter V (F), but the textual differences will remain. DSM-IV provides much additional information, for example on prevalence, stress in the family or at work, and differential diagnoses. Thus it is not only a diagnostic manual but also a textbook, although without information about therapy.

Diagnostic instruments

In clinical work, typological diagnosis is based on typical cases, without the need for special instruments. In operationalized diagnosis, however, criteria and algorithms are used and can be supported by the so-called 'instruments' for use by professionals or, with certain restrictions, layworkers. Professionals often work with semistandardized interviews, which means that they have to evaluate the psychopathological picture systematically. Interviews conducted by layworkers must be standardized with questions asked exactly as written and answers recorded exactly so as to preclude any variation in the interview. For this reason certain syndromes are quite difficult to diagnose using standardized interviews, especially the acute psychotic disorders in which many of the patients' answers cannot be taken literally. To facilitate the diagnosis of mental disorders WHO has developed several instruments which are suitable for diagnosis according to both ICD-10 and DSM.

Schedule for Assessment in Neuropsychiatry (SCAN)

The Present State Examination was developed further into SCAN, a structured interview for clinicians.[61] SCAN is a semistandardized interview containing a glossary with definitions of symptoms, an item group checklist, and a questionnaire on the previous history. The interviewer has to use his or her clinical judgement about psychopathology. The interview takes about 60 to 90 minutes.

Composite International Diagnostic Interview (CIDI)

CIDI was developed on the basis of the Diagnostic Interview Schedule (**DIS**), and has been translated into a number of languages.[62] After several days of training both professionals and lay interviewers can use CIDI. In this standardized interview the answers of the interviewee are decisive. The interview takes about an hour.

International Personality Disorder Examination (IPDE)

IPDE was developed to diagnose personality disorders.[63] It should be used by experienced clinicians.

The ICD-10 International Symptom Checklists (ISCL)

ISCL enables the severity, cause, and duration of syndromes to be judged.[64,65] The Symptom Checklist (**SCL**) can be used as a screening instrument, while more exact ICD-10 diagnoses can be formulated using 32 International Diagnoses Checklists (**IDCL**). Another checklist, the IDCL-P,[66] was developed especially for personality disorders in accordance with the clinical descriptions and diagnostic guidelines. A further checklist, the ICD-10 Merkmalsliste, containing 750 criteria in 14 groups, has been developed and validated in eight German-speaking centres.[67]

Additional instruments

SIDAM, a structured interview for dementia of the Alzheimer type, multi-infarct dementia, or vascular dementia, for diagnosis of dementias according to DSM or ICD-10 was published in 1996.[68] Diagnostic instruments are considered further in Chapter 1.10.1.

Advantages of international classification

International classification makes possible future worldwide psychopharmacological studies with patients having standardized diagnoses, as well as psychotherapeutic and sociotherapeutic evaluation. In the meantime, wide use is made of standardized and structured interviews, which allow diagnoses according to ICD-10 and DSM-IV. It is expected that the use of these kinds of diagnostic instruments will be obligatory in scientific work published in future.

Internationally uniform diagnoses will enable epidemiologists to compare the prevalence and incidence of different disorders in various countries and cultures. The advantage of ICD-10 over the more regional DSM-IV may be that it satisfies both European and Third World requirements. For planning purposes it would be of great interest to compare administrative data from different countries and regions in conjunction with psychiatric diagnoses.

Risks and dangers of the international classification

Although there are major advantages of international operationalized diagnoses, there are also risks and dangers.[69] It is important to remember that most psychiatric disorders, as described in ICD-10 and DSM-IV, are conventions and not diseases based on the laws of natural science. The definition of the disorders must be flexible, so that future changes in our understanding of aetiology, epidemiology, and symptomatology can be incorporated.

There is a strong tendency in operationalized diagnosis to define categorical entities, and only in certain sections such as personality disorders are there slight dimensional tendencies. Medical categorical diagnoses are bound to aetiology, which cannot be described in the majority of mental disorders. Therefore psychiatry is forced to use conventions or constructs in many disorders. Thus, although interrater reliability of the disorders is often satisfactory, validity would require a much broader basis of knowledge.

Even if WHO encourages the maintenance of local diagnostic traditions, in the long run the uniformity of a worldwide classification will not admit different schools and local diagnoses. Nevertheless it is hoped that sensitivity and open-mindedness with respect to local cultures will not be lost; these traditions could be a source of future creativity in diagnosis.

It should not be forgotten that political correctness affects diagnosis. No terms which might offend certain individuals should be used in diagnosis. In the past, words like 'psychopath', 'sexual perversion' or 'homosexuality' were used as diagnoses without reflection. Also, some diagnoses might imply that certain criminal acts, such as arson or kleptomania, could be regarded generally as symptoms of psychiatric disorders; in ICD-10 the question is decided only after considering the individual case.

One danger inherent in current operationalized diagnosis is that only uniform international diagnoses are allowed. If a better classification were to be proposed in the future, it would have no chance to develop because scientific journals admit only the recognized systems. The same is true for research grants and scholarships.

The greatest risk attached to every codified classification is in its use in social and health insurance systems. Here, actions against the patient's interests could be taken. For instance, a health insurance company could place restrictions on inpatient treatment according to the diagnosis. The psychiatrist should defend patients against this failure to consider their individual circumstances and the individual course of the disorder. Psychiatrists should be aware of the danger that their diagnostic conventions may be misinterpreted and could be used as if they were scientific facts in both the health-care economy and the forensic field.

Another danger is that operationalized diagnosis could be used in a simplistic manner in clinical practice without applying the diagnostic criteria as demanded by ICD-10.[70] ICD-10 contains a large number of diagnoses (e.g. 50 ways of coding depression), but few are used regularly. Thus a comparison of the statistics of psychiatric diagnoses in psychiatric departments in different countries showed that only a few diagnoses were used.[71] For instance, 40 per cent of the initial diagnoses of psychiatric inpatients in Germany fall into only three categories: alcoholism, depression, and adjustment disorder.

As noted above, scientific papers that do not use international operationalized diagnoses are not accepted for publication, and there is a strong tendency to grant research funds only if one of the operationalized systems is used. However, other diagnostic concepts are often used in clinical practice and in planning treatment, and there is a need for more differentiation and additional diagnoses in some sections of the classification (e.g. psychogenic disorders).

Although ICD-10 has now been introduced, operationalized diagnosis is still not generally accepted. There are many practical difficulties, particularly in work in the community, but there is also a deep-rooted resistance. Many neurologists and psychiatrists feel that their traditional diagnostic thinking, such as the triadic system (organic, endogenous, and psychogenic mental disorders), is being destroyed by the new classification. They sense their lack of detailed knowledge of diagnosis, but are unhappy about being tied to a new system that may be imposed from outside.[70] Thus training in the new classifications should be offered not only as an introduction for beginners but also to more experienced diagnosticians. In case conferences one should try to reach a uniform and above all a high standard of diagnosis. The more the new systems are accepted, the more operationalized diagnosis will help to improve indications for therapy and the understanding of prognosis.

Future development in international classification

The development of the new global aspect of diagnosis, an expansion of many of the special sections, and the production of more diagnostic instruments can be envisaged. The descriptive diagnoses now established do not consider some traditional psychiatric and psychotherapeutic models such as the endogenous concept or the theories of neurosis. Nevertheless the influence of this type of diagnosis is increasing, even in psychodynamic psychiatry in which operationalized diagnosis would have seemed impossible some years ago. The 'reduction of psychoanalytic negligence in diagnosis and the adherence to accepted and communicable standards' has been proposed.[71] Also, a behaviour therapeutic classification of neurotic disorders has been developed and the new ICIDH-II is currently being tested in a large WHO field study. The multiaxial system may also be revised; for example, instead of axis III of ICD-10, a more comprehensive graded psychosocial diagnosis could be established.

It is to be hoped that in future a single system of classification will be used in psychiatry rather than the two current classifications. ICD-10 is used more in practice and DSM-IV more in science, a disadvantage for both!

Classification will also be developed in general practice. Diagnosis cannot be as sophisticated as that in specialist practice and many minor psychiatric disorders are treated. For these kinds of disorders general practitioners need the diagnostic help and advice on therapy which is currently offered in the primary health care version of ICD-10 (see Chapter 7.8).

However carefully the rules and criteria for the use of operationalized diagnosis are applied, some cases cannot be coded. In these cases the diagnostician needs to judge individually and to describe the patient. In any case the physician should consider the totality of the patient's suffering and his or her individuality. Diagnosis should be supplemented by an extensive biographical history of the patient.

Aetiology, diagnosis, and therapy should be interrelated. Although most current diagnoses are descriptive, it is possible that nosology may eventually have a stronger basis in aetiology. It is likely that the aetiology of the psychoses will be better understood in the future, especially if an attempt is made to study subgroups of these conditions, relating them as far as possible to somatic abnormalities. This may be achieved with bipolar affective disorders and seasonal depressions, and also with special types of schizophrena such as periodic catatonia with its high genetic load, as described by Kleist and Leonhard.[21] Future work on both psychotic and non-psychotic disorders should focus on developing a new nosology and overcoming the currently popular atheoretical approach to diagnosis.

We can expect diagnosis and classification to change faster in the next century than in the last hundred years. In the eyes of the diagnostician, the world of psychiatry will hold many surprises.

References

1. Sartorius, N. (1988). International perspectives of psychiatric classification. *British Journal of Psychiatry*, **152**, 9–14.
2. von Linné, C. (1742). *Genera morborum in auditorium usum.* Buchenroeder and Ritter, Hamburg.
3. Cullen, W. (1772). *Synopsis nosologiae methodicae.* Creech, Edinburgh.
4. Kant, I. (1983). Versuch über die Krankheiten des Kopfes. In *Vorkritische Schriften bis 1768*, Vol. 2. Wissenschaftliche Buchgesellschaft, Darmstadt.
5. Heinroth, J. (1818). *Lehrbuch der Störungen des Seelenlebens.* Vogel, Leipzig.
6. Pinel, P. (1809). *Traité médico-philosophique sur l'aliénation mentale.* Brosson, Paris.
7. Esquirol, E. (1838). *Des maladies mentales considérées sous les rapports médical, hygiénique et médico-légal.* Baillière, Paris.
8. Griesinger, W. (1845). *Die Pathologie und Therapie der psychischen Krankheiten für Aerzte und Studirende.* Krabbe, Stuttgart.
9. Falret, J.P. (1854). De la folie circulaire. *Bulletin de l'Académie de Médecine*, **19**, 382–95.
10. Kahlbaum, K. (1863). *Die Gruppierung der psychischen Krankheiten.* Kafemann, Danzig.
11. Kraepelin, E. (1896). *Lehrbuch der Psychiatrie* (5th edn). Barth, Leipzig.
12. Hoche, A.E. (1912). Die Bedeutung der Symptomkomplexe in der Psychiatrie. *Zeitschrift für die gesamte Neurologie und Psychiatrie*, **12**, 540–51.
13. Bleuler, E. (1911). *Dementia praecox oder Gruppe der Schizophrenien.* Deuticke, Leipzig.
14. Wilmanns, K. (1930). Entwurf einer für die Reichsstatistik bestimmten Diagnosentabelle für die Geisteskrankheiten. *Allgemeine Zeitschrift für Psychiatrie*, **93**, 223–34.
15. Meyer, J.E. (1961). Diagnostische Einteilungen und Diagnosenschemata in der Psychiatrie. In *Psychiatrie der Gegenwart*, Vol. 3, pp. 131–80. Springer, Berlin.
16. Magnan, V. and Serieux, P. (1893). *Le délire chronique à évolution systématique.* Gauthier Villars–Masson, Paris.
17. Pull, C.B., Pull, M.C., and Pichot, P. (1988). The French approach to psychiatric classification. In *International classification in psychiatry* (ed. J. E. Mezzich and M. von Cranach), pp. 37–47. Cambridge University Press.
18. Baillarger, J. (1854). De la folie à double forme. *Annales Medico-Psychologiques*, **6**, 369–84.
19. Wimmer, A. (1916). Psykogene sindssygdomsformer. In *Sct. Hans Mental Hospital 1816–1916, Jubilaeumsskrift*, pp. 85–216. Gad, Copenhagen.
20. Sjöbring, H. (1919). Mental constitution and mental illness. *Svenska Läkare Sällskap*, **45**, 462–93.
21. Leonhard, K. (1986). *Aufteilung der endogenen Psychosen und ihre differenzierte Ätiologie.* Akademie-Verlag, Berlin.
22. Asai, K. (1994) Psychiatric diagnosis and mental health services in Japan. In *Psychiatric diagnosis: a world perspective* (ed. J. E. Mezzich, Y. Honda, and M. C. Kastrup), pp. 228–40. Springer, New York.
23. Yu-cun, S. and Changhui, C. (1988). Principles of the Chinese Classification of Mental Disorders (CCMD). In *International classification in psychiatry* (ed. J. E. Mezzich and M. von Cranach), pp. 73–80. Cambridge University Press.
24. Wig, N.N. (1990). The Third-World perspective on psychiatric diagnosis and classification. In *Sources and traditions of classification in psychiatry* (ed. N. Sartorius, A. Jablensky, D.A. Regier, J.D. Burke, and R.M.A. Hirschfeld), pp. 181–210. Huber, Bern.
25. Kendell, R.E. (1975). *The role of diagnosis in psychiatry.* Blackwell Science, Oxford.
26. Sass, H. (1987). Die Krise der psychiatrischen Diagnostik. *Fortschritte der Neurologie-Psychiatrie*, **55**, 255–58.
27. Klerman, G.L. (1990). The contemporary American scene: diagnosis and classification of mental disorders, alcoholism and drug abuse. In *Sources and traditions of classification in psychiatry* (ed. N. Sartorius, A. Jablensky, D. A. Regier, J. D. Burke, and R.M.A. Hirschfeld), pp. 93–137. Huber, Bern.
28. Feighner, J., Robins, E., Guze, S., *et al.* (1972). Diagnostic criteria for use in psychiatric research. *Archives of General Psychiatry*, **26**, 57–63.
29. Spitzer, R.L., Endicott, J., and Robins, E. (1978). Research diagnostic criteria: rationale and reliability. *Archives of General Psychiatry*, **35**, 773–82.
30. American Psychiatric Association (1980). *Diagnostic and statistical manual of mental disorders* (3rd edn). American Psychiatric Association, Washington, DC.
31. Kendler, K.S. (1990). Toward a scientific psychiatric nosology. *Archives of General Psychiatry*, **47**, 969–73.
32. American Psychiatric Association (1994). *Diagnostic and statistical manual of mental disorders* (4th edn). American Psychiatric Association, Washington, DC.
33. Kramer, M. (1988). Historical roots and structural basis of the International Classification of Diseases. In *International classification in psychiatry* (ed. J. E. Mezzich and M. von Cranach), pp. 3–29. Cambridge University Press.
34. World Health Organization (1948). *Manual of the International Statistical Classification of Diseases, Injuries and Causes of Death (ICD-6).* World Health Organization, Geneva.
35. World Health Organization (1967). *Glossary of mental disorders and guide to their classification, for use in conjunction with the International Classification of Diseases (8th revision).* World Health Organization, Geneva.
36. World Health Organization (1978). *Mental disorders: glossary and guide to their classification, for use in conjunction with the Ninth Revision of the International Classification of Diseases.* World Health Organization, Geneva..
37. World Health Organization (1992). *The ICD-10 classification of mental and behavioural disorders—clinical descriptions and diagnostic guidelines.* World Health Organization, Geneva..
38. Sartorius, N. (1995). *Understanding the ICD-10 classification of mental disorders.* Science Press, London.
39. World Health Organization (1992). *International Statistical Classification of Diseases and Related Health Problems, 10th Revision.* World Health Organization, Geneva.
40. World Health Organization (1993). *The ICD-10 classification of mental and behavioural disorders—diagnostic criteria for research.* World Health Organization, Geneva.

41. Cooper, J.E. (ed.) (1994). *Pocket guide to the ICD-10 classification of mental and behavioural disorders with glossary and diagnostic criteria for research*. Churchill Livingstone, Edinburgh.

42. Kretschmer, E. (1919). Gedanken über die Fortentwicklung der psychiatrischen Systematik. *Zeitschrift für Neurologie*, **48**, 370–7.

43. Essen-Möller, E. (1973). Standard list for threefold classification of mental disorders. *Acta Psychiatrica Scandinavica*, **49**, 198–212.

44. Rutter, M., Shaffer, D., and Sturge, C. (1975). *A multi-axial classification of child psychiatric disorders*. World Health Organization, Geneva.

45. Janca, A., Kartrup, M., Katschnig, N., Lopez-Ibor, J.J., Mezzich, J.E., and Sartorius, N. (1996). The World Health Organization Short Disability Assessment Schedule (WHO DAS-S): a tool for the assessment of difficulties in selected areas of functioning of patients with mental disorders. *Social Psychiatry*, **31**, 349–54.

46. World Health Organization (1980). *International Classification of Impairments, Disabilities and Handicaps*. World Health Organization, Geneva.

47. World Health Organization (1998). *International Classification of Impairments, Disabilities and Handicaps (ICIDH-2)*. World Health Organization, Geneva.

48. World Health Organization (1996). *Diagnostic and management guidelines for mental disorders in primary care: ICD-10 Chapter V Primary Care Version*. WHO–Hogrefe and Huber, Göttingen.

49. Üstün, T.B., Bertelsen, A., Dilling, H., *et al*. (1996). *ICD-10 casebook. the many faces of mental disorders*. American Psychiatric Press, Washington, DC.

50. Freyberger, H.J. and Dilling, H. (ed.) (1993). *Fallbuch Psychiatrie. Kasuistiken zum Kapitel V (F) der ICD-10*. Huber, Bern.

51. Malchow, C.P., Kanitz, R.D., and Dilling (ed.) (1995). *ICD-10 computer tutorial: psychische Störungen*. Huber, Bern.

52. Spitzer, R.L. and Endicott, J. (1968). DIAGNO: a computer program for psychiatric diagnosis utilizing the differential diagnostic procedure. *Archives of General Psychiatry*, **18**, 746–56.

53. Wing, J.K., Cooper, J.E., and Sartorius, N. (1974). *Present State Examination*. Cambridge University Press.

54. Der, G., Glover, G., Brugha, T.S., and Wing, J.K. (1997). SCAN-1: algorithms and Capse-1. In *Diagnosis and clinical measurement in psychiatry: a reference manual for SCAN/PSE-10* (ed. J.K. Wing, N. Sartorius, and T.B. Üstün). Cambridge University Press.

55. Janca, A., Sartorius, N., and Üstün, T.B. (1994). New versions of World Health Organization instruments for the assessment of mental disorders. *Acta Psychiatrica Scandinavica*, **90**, 73–83.

56. Arbeitskreis OPD (ed.) (1996). *Operationalisierte psychodynamische Diagnostik—OPD*. Huber, Bern.

57. Sartorius, N., Kaelber, C.T., Cooper, J.E., *et al*. (1993). Progress toward achieving a common language in psychiatry. Results from the field trial of the clinical guidelines accompanying the WHO classification of mental and behavioural disorders in ICD-10. *Archives of General Psychiatry*, **50**, 115–24.

58. Sartorius, N., Üstün, T.B., Korten, A., Cooper, J. E., and von Drimmelen, J. (1995). Progress toward achieving a common language in psychiatry. II: Results from the international field trials of the ICD-10 diagnostic criteria for research for mental and behavioural disorders. *American Journal of Psychiatry*, **152**, 1427–37.

59. Landis, J.R. and Koch, G.G. (1977). The measurement of observer agreement for categorial data. *Biometrics*, **33**, 159–74.

60. American Psychiatric Association (1987). *Diagnostic and statistical manual of mental disorders (3rd revised edn)*. American Psychiatric Association, Washington, DC.

61. World Health Organization (1994). *Schedules for Clinical Assessment in Neuropsychiatry (SCAN), Version 2.0*. American Psychiatric Press, Washington, DC, for the World Health Organization.

62. World Health Organization (1993). *Composite International Diagnostic Interview (CIDI)*. American Psychiatric Press, Washington, DC, for the World Health Organization.

63. Loranger, A.W. (1996). *International Personality Disorder Examination (IPDE). ICD-10 Modul. Weltgesundheitsorganisation*. Huber, Bern.

64. Janca, A., Üstün, T., van Drimmelen-Krabbe, J., Dittmann, V., and Isaac, M. (1994). *The ICD-10 Symptom Checklist, Version 2.0*. World Health Organization, Geneva.

65. Janca, A., Üstün, T., Early, T., and Sartorius, N. (1993). The ICD-10 Symptom Checklist: a companion to the ICD-10 Classification of Mental and Behavioural Disorders. *Social Psychiatry*, **28**, 239–42.

66. Bronisch, T., Hiller, W., Mombour, W., and Zaudig, M. (1995). *IDCL-P internationale diagnosen Checkliste für Persönlichkeitsstörungen nach ICD-10*. Huber, Bern.

67. Dittmann, V., Dilling, H., and Freyberger, H.J. (ed.) (1992). *Psychiatrische Diagnostik nach ICD-10-klinische Erfahrungen bei der Anwendung. Ergebnisse der ICD-10-Merkmalslistenstudie*. Huber, Bern.

68. Zaudig, M. and Hiller, W. (1996). *SIDAM. Strukturiertes Interwiew für die Diagnose einer Demenz vom Alzheimer Typ, der Multiinfarkt- (oder vaskulären) Demenz und Demenzen anderer Ätiologie nach DSM-III-R, DSM-IV und ICD-10*. Huber, Bern.

69. Jablensky, A. (1991). Diagnostic criteria in psychiatry: a straitjacket or a prop? *European Psychiatry*, **6**, 323–9.

70. Arolt, V. and Dilling, H. (1994). Confounding diagnostic systems: a major risk in the use of criteria-based manuals. *Psychopathology*, **27**, 58–63.

71. Müssigbrodt, H., Michels, R., Malchow, C.P., Dilling, H., Munk-Jørgensen, P., and Bertelsen, A. (2000). Use of the ICD-10 classification in psychiatry—an international survey. *Psychopathology*, **32**, in press.

72. Hoffmann, S.O. (1996). Foreword. In *Operationalisierte psychodynamische Diagnostik—OPD* (ed. Arbeitskreis OPD). Huber, Bern.

Appendix 1

International Classification of Diseases, 10th Revision

F00–F09 Organic, including symptomatic, mental disorders

F00 Dementia in Alzheimer's disease

F00.0 Dementia in Alzheimer's disease with early onset

F00.1 Dementia in Alzheimer's disease with late onset

F00.2 Dementia in Alzheimer's disease, atypical or mixed type

F00.9 Dementia in Alzheimer's disease, unspecified

F01 Vascular dementia

F01.0 Vascular dementia of acute onset

F01.1 Multi-infarct dementia

F01.2 Subcortical vascular dementia

F01.3 Mixed cortical and subcortical vascular dementia

F01.8 Other vascular dementia

F01.9 Vascular dementia, unspecified

F02 Dementia in other diseases classified elsewhere

F02.0 Dementia in Pick's disease

F02.1 Dementia in Creutzfeldt–Jakob disease

F02.2 Dementia in Huntington's disease

F02.3 Dementia in Parkinson's disease

F02.4 Dementia in human immunodeficiency virus (HIV) disease

F02.8 Dementia in other specified diseases classified elsewhere

F03 Unspecified dementia

A fifth character may be added to specify dementia in F00–F03, as follows:

> .x0 Without additional symptoms
>
> .x1 Other symptoms, predominantly delusional
>
> .x2 Other symptoms, predominantly hallucinatory
>
> .x3 Other symptoms, predominantly depressive
>
> .x4 Other mixed symptoms

F04 Organic amnesic syndrome, not induced by alcohol and other psychoactive substances

F05 Delirium, not induced by alcohol and other psychoactive substances

F05.0 Delirium, not superimposed on dementia, so described

F05.1 Delirium, superimposed on dementia

F05.8 Other delirium

F05.9 Delirium, unspecified

F06 Other mental disorders due to brain damage and dysfunction and to physical disease

F06.0 Organic hallucinosis

F06.1 Organic catatonic disorder

F06.2 Organic delusional (schizophrenia-like) disorder

F06.3 Organic mood (affective) disorders

> .30 Organic manic disorder
>
> .31 Organic bipolar disorder
>
> .32 Organic depressive disorder
>
> .33 Organic mixed affective disorder

F06.4 Organic anxiety disorder

F06.5 Organic dissociative disorder

F06.6 Organic emotionally labile (asthenic) disorder

F06.7 Mild cognitive disorder

F06.8 Other specified mental disorders due to brain damage and dysfunction and to physical disease

F06.9 Unspecified mental disorder due to brain damage and dysfunction and to physical disease

F09 Unspecified organic or symptomatic mental disorder

F07 Personality and behavioural disorders due to brain disease, damage and dysfunction

F07.0 Organic personality disorder

F07.1 Postencephalitic syndrome

F07.2 Postconcussional syndrome

F07.8 Other organic personality and behavioural disorders due to brain disease, damage, and dysfunction

F07.9 Unspecified organic personality and behavioural disorder due to brain disease, damage, and dysfunction

F10–F19 Mental and behavioural disorders due to psychoactive substance use

F10 Mental and behavioural disorders due to use of alcohol

F11 Mental and behavioural disorders due to use of opioids

F12 Mental and behavioural disorders due to use of cannabinoids

F13 Mental and behavioural disorders due to use of sedatives or hypnotics

F14 Mental and behavioural disorders due to use of cocaine

F15 Mental and behavioural disorders due to use of other stimulants, including caffeine

F16 Mental and behavioural disorders due to use of hallucinogens

F17 Mental and behavioural disorders due to use of tobacco

F18 Mental and behavioural disorders due to use of volatile solvents

F19 Mental and behavioural disorders due to multiple drug use and use of other psychoactive substances

Four- and five-character categories may be used to specify the clinical conditions, as follows:

> F1x.0 Acute intoxication
>
> > .00 Uncomplicated
> >
> > .01 With trauma or other bodily injury
> >
> > .02 With other medical complications
> >
> > .03 With delirium
> >
> > .04 With perceptual distortions
> >
> > .05 With coma
> >
> > .06 With convulsions
> >
> > .07 Pathological intoxication
>
> F1x.1 Harmful use
>
> F1x.2 Dependence syndrome
>
> > .20 Currently abstinent
> >
> > .21 Currently abstinent, but in a protected environment
> >
> > .22 Currently on a clinically supervised maintenance or replacement regime (controlled dependence)
> >
> > .23 Currently abstinent, but receiving treatment with aversive or blocking drugs
> >
> > .24 Currently using the substance (active dependence)
> >
> > .25 Continuous use
> >
> > .26 Episodic use (dipsomania)
>
> F1x.3 Withdrawal state
>
> > .30 Uncomplicated
> >
> > .31 Convulsions
>
> F1x.4 Withdrawal state with delirium
>
> > .40 Without convulsions
> >
> > .41 With convulsions
>
> F1x.5 Psychotic disorder
>
> > .50 Schizophrenia-like
> >
> > .51 Predominantly delusional
> >
> > .52 Predominantly hallucinatory

.53 Predominantly polymorphic

.54 Predominantly depressive symptoms

.55 Predominantly manic symptoms

.56 Mixed

F1x.6 Amnesic syndrome

F1x.7 Residual and late-onset psychotic disorder

.70 Flashbacks

.71 Personality or behaviour disorder

.72 Residual affective disorder

.73 Dementia

.74 Other persisting cognitive impairment

.75 Late-onset psychotic disorder

F1x.8 Other mental and behavioural disorders

F1x.9 Unspecified mental and behavioural disorder

F20–F29 Schizophrenia, schizotypal, and delusional disorders

F20 Schizophrenia

F20.0 Paranoid schizophrenia

F20.1 Hebephrenic schizophrenia

F20.2 Catatonic schizophrenia

F20.3 Undifferentiated schizophrenia

F20.4 Post-schizophrenic depression

F20.5 Residual schizophrenia

F20.6 Simple schizophrenia

F20.8 Other schizophrenia

F20.9 Schizophrenia, unspecified

A fifth character may be used to classify course:

.x0 Continuous

.x1 Episodic with progressive deficit

.x2 Episodic with stable deficit

.x3 Episodic remittent

.x4 Incomplete remission

.x5 Complete remission

.x8 Other

.x9 Period of observation less than 1 year

F21 Schizotypal disorder

F22 Persistent delusional disorders

F22.0 Delusional disorder

F22.8 Other persistent delusional disorders

F22.9 Persistent delusional disorder, unspecified

F23 Acute and transient psychotic disorders

F23.0 Acute polymorphic psychotic disorder without symptoms of schizophrenia

F23.1 Acute polymorphic psychotic disorder with symptoms of schizophrenia

F23.2 Acute schizophrenia-like psychotic disorder

F23.3 Other acute predominantly delusional psychotic disorders

F23.8 Other acute and transient psychotic disorders

F23.9 Acute and transient psychotic disorders unspecified

A fifth character may be used to identify the presence or absence of associated acute stress:

.x0 Without associated acute stress

.x1 With associated acute stress

F24 Induced delusional disorder

F25 Schizoaffective disorders

F25.0 Schizoaffective disorder, manic type

F25.1 Schizoaffective disorder, depressive type

F25.2 Schizoaffective disorder, mixed type

F25.8 Other schizoaffective disorders

F25.9 Schizoaffective disorder, unspecified

F28 Other non-organic psychotic disorders

F29 Unspecified non-organic psychosis

F30–F39 Mood (affective) disorders

F30 Manic episode

F30.0 Hypomania

F30.1 Mania without psychotic symptoms

F30.2 Mania with psychotic symptoms

F30.8 Other manic episodes

F30.9 Manic episode, unspecified

F31 Bipolar affective disorder

F31.0 Bipolar affective disorder, current episode hypomanic

F31.1 Bipolar affective disorder, current episode manic without psychotic symptoms

F31.2 Bipolar affective disorder, current episode manic with psychotic symptoms

F31.3 Bipolar affective disorder, current episode mild or moderate depression

.30 Without somatic symptoms

.31 With somatic symptoms

F31.4 Bipolar affective disorder, current episode severe depression without psychotic symptoms

F31.5 Bipolar affective disorder, current episode severe depression with psychotic symptoms

F31.6 Bipolar affective disorder, current episode mixed

F31.7 Bipolar affective disorder, currently in remission

F31.8 Other bipolar affective disorders

F31.9 Bipolar affective disorder, unspecified

F32 Depressive episode

F32.0 Mild depressive episode

.00 Without somatic symptoms

.01 With somatic symptoms

F32.1 Moderate depressive episode

.10 Without somatic symptoms

.11 With somatic symptoms

F32.2 Severe depressive episode without psychotic symptoms

F32.3 Severe depressive episode with psychotic symptoms

F32.8 Other depressive episodes

F32.9 Depressive episode, unspecified

F33 Recurrent depressive disorder

F33.0 Recurrent depressive disorder, current episode mild

.00 Without somatic symptoms

.01 With somatic symptoms

F33.1 Recurrent depressive disorder, current episode moderate

.10 Without somatic symptoms

.11 With somatic symptoms

F33.2 Recurrent depressive disorder, current episode severe without psychotic symptoms

F33.3 Recurrent depressive disorder, current episode severe with psychotic symptoms

F33.4 Recurrent depressive disorder, currently in remission

F33.8 Other recurrent depressive disorders

F33.9 Recurrent depressive disorder, unspecified

F34 Persistent mood (affective) disorders

F34.0 Cyclothymia

F34.1 Dysthymia

F34.8 Other persistent mood (affective) disorders

F34.9 Persistent mood (affective) disorder, unspecified

F38 Other mood (affective) disorders

F38.0 Other single mood (affective) disorders

.00 Mixed affective episode

F38.1 Other recurrent mood (affective) disorders

.10 Recurrent brief depressive disorder

F38.8 Other specified mood (affective) disorders

F39 Unspecified mood (affective) disorder

F40–F48 Neurotic, stress-related, and somatoform disorders

F40 Phobic anxiety disorders

F40.0 Agoraphobia

.00 Without panic disorder

.01 With panic disorder

F40.1 Social phobias

F40.2 Specific (isolated) phobias

F40.8 Other phobic anxiety disorders

F40.9 Phobic anxiety disorder, unspecified

F41 Other anxiety disorders

F41.0 Panic disorder (episodic paroxysmal anxiety)

F41.1 Generalized anxiety disorder

F41.2 Mixed anxiety and depressive disorder

F41.3 Other mixed anxiety disorders

F41.8 Other specified anxiety disorders

F41.9 Anxiety disorder, unspecified

F42 Obsessive–compulsive disorder

F42.0 Predominantly obsessional thoughts or ruminations

F42.1 Predominantly compulsive acts (obsessional rituals)

F42.2 Mixed obsessional thoughts and acts

F42.8 Other obsessive–compulsive disorders

F42.9 Obsessive–compulsive disorder, unspecified

F43 Reaction to severe stress, and adjustment disorders

F43.0 Acute stress reaction

F43.1 Post-traumatic stress disorder

F43.2 Adjustment disorders

.20 Brief depressive reaction

.21 Prolonged depressive reaction

.22 Mixed anxiety and depressive reaction

.23 With predominant disturbance of other emotions

.24 With predominant disturbance of conduct

.25 With mixed disturbance of emotions and conduct

.28 With other specified predominant symptoms

F43.8 Other reactions to severe stress

F43.9 Reaction to severe stress, unspecified

F44 Dissociative (conversion) disorders

F44.0 Dissociative amnesia

F44.1 Dissociative fugue

F44.2 Dissociative stupor

F44.3 Trance and possession disorders

F44.4 Dissociative motor disorders

F44.5 Dissociative convulsions

F44.6 Dissociative anaesthesia and sensory loss

F44.7 Mixed dissociative (conversion) disorders

F44.8 Other dissociative (conversion) disorders

.80 Ganser's syndrome

.81 Multiple personality disorder

.82 Transient dissociate (conversion) disorders occurring in childhood and adolescence

.88 Other specified dissociative (conversion) disorders

F44.9 Dissociative (conversion) disorder, unspecified

F45 Somatoform disorders

F45.0 Somatization disorder

F45.1 Undifferentiated somatoform disorder

F45.2 Hypochondriacal disorder

F45.3 Somatoform autonomic dysfunction

.30 Heart and cardiovascular system

.31 Upper gastrointestinal tract

.32 Lower gastrointestinal tract

.33 Respiratory system

.34 Genitourinary system

.38 Other organ or system

F45.4 Persistent somatoform pain disorder

F45.8 Other somatoform disorders

F45.9 Somatoform disorder, unspecified

F48 Other neurotic disorders

F48.0 Neurasthenia

F48.1 Depersonalization–derealization syndrome

F48.8 Other specified neurotic disorders

F48.9 Neurotic disorder, unspecified

F50–F59 Behavioural syndromes associated with physiological disturbances and physical factors

F50 Eating disorders

F50.0 Anorexia nervosa

F50.1 Atypical anorexia nervosa

F50.2 Bulimia nervosa

F50.3 Atypical bulimia nervosa

F50.4 Overeating associated with other psychological disturbances

F50.5 Vomiting associated with other psychological disturbances

F50.8 Other eating disorders

F50.9 Eating disorder, unspecified

F51 Non-organic sleep disorders

F51.0 Non-organic insomnia

F51.1 Non-organic hypersomnia

F51.2 Non-organic disorder of the sleep–wake schedule

F51.3 Sleepwalking (somnambulism)

F51.4 Sleep terrors (night terrors)

F51.5 Nightmares

F51.8 Other non-organic sleep disorders

F51.9 Non-organic sleep disorder, unspecified

F52 Sexual dysfunction, not caused by organic disorder or disease

F52.0 Lack or loss of sexual desire

F52.1 Sexual aversion and lack of sexual enjoyment

.10 Sexual aversion

.11 Lack of sexual enjoyment

F52.2 Failure of genital response

F52.3 Orgasmic dysfunction

F52.4 Premature ejaculation

F52.5 Non-organic vaginismus

F52.6 Non-organic dyspareunia

F52.7 Excessive sexual drive

F52.8 Other sexual dysfunction, not caused by organic disorders or disease

F52.9 Unspecified sexual dysfunction, not caused by organic disorder or disease

F53 Mental and behavioural disorders associated with the puerperium, not elsewhere classified

F53.0 Mild mental and behavioural disorders associated with the puerperium, not elsewhere classified

F53.1 Severe mental and behavioural disorders associated with the puerperium, not elsewhere classified

F53.8 Other mental and behavioural disorders associated with the puerperium, not elsewhere classified

F53.9 Puerperal mental disorder, unspecified

F54 Psychological and behavioural factors associated with disorders or diseases classified elsewhere

F55 Abuse of non-dependence-producing substances

F55.0 Antidepressants

F55.1 Laxatives

F55.2 Analgesics

F55.3 Antacids

F55.4 Vitamins

F55.5 Steroids or hormones

F55.6 Specific herbal or folk remedies

F55.8 Other substances that do not produce dependence

F55.9 Unspecified

F59 Unspecified behavioural syndromes associated with physiological disturbances and physical factors

F60–F69 Disorders of adult personality and behaviour

F60 Specific personality disorders

F60.0 Paranoid personality disorder

F60.1 Schizoid personality disorder

F60.2 Dissocial personality disorder

F60.3 Emotionally unstable personality disorder

.30 Impulsive type

.31 Borderline type

F60.4 Histrionic personality disorder

F60.5 Anankastic personality disorder

F60.6 Anxious (avoidant) personality disorder

F60.7 Dependent personality disorder

F60.8 Other specific personality disorders

F60.9 Personality disorder, unspecified

F61 Mixed and other personality disorders

F61.0 Mixed personality disorders

F61.1 Troublesome personality changes

F62 Enduring personality changes, not attributable to brain damage and disease

F62.0 Enduring personality change after catastrophic experience

F62.1 Enduring personality change after psychiatric illness

F62.8 Other enduring personality changes

F62.9 Enduring personality change, unspecified

F63 Habit and impulse disorders

F63.0 Pathological gambling

F63.1 Pathological fire-setting (pyromania)

F63.2 Pathological stealing (kleptomania)

F63.3 Trichotillomania

F63.8 Other habit and impulse disorders

F63.9 Habit and impulse disorder, unspecified

F64 Gender identity disorders

F64.0 Transsexualism

F64.1 Dual-role transvestism

F64.2 Gender identity disorder of childhood

F64.8 Other gender identity disorders

F64.9 Gender identity disorder, unspecified

F65 Disorders of sexual preference

F65.0 Fetishism

F65.1 Fetishistic transvestism

F65.2 Exhibitionism

F65.3 Voyeurism

F65.4 Paedophilia

F65.5 Sadomasochism

F65.6 Multiple disorders of sexual preference

F65.8 Other disorders of sexual preference

F65.9 Disorder of sexual preference, unspecified

F66 Psychological and behavioural disorders associated with sexual development and orientation

F66.0 Sexual maturation disorder

F66.1 Egodystonic sexual orientation

F66.2 Sexual relationship disorder

F66.8 Other psychosexual development disorders

F66.9 Psychosexual development disorder, unspecified

A fifth character may be used to indicate association with:

.x0 Heterosexuality

.x1 Homosexuality

.x2 Bisexuality

.x8 Other, including prepubertal

F68 Other disorders of adult personality and behaviour

F68.0 Elaboration of physical symptoms for psychological reasons

F68.1 Intentional production or feigning of symptoms or disabilities, either physical or psychological (factitious disorder)

F68.8 Other specified disorders of adult personality and behaviour

F69 Unspecified disorder of adult personality and behaviour

F70–F79 Mental retardation

F70 Mild mental retardation

F71 Moderate mental retardation

F72 Severe mental retardation

F73 Profound mental retardation

F78 Other mental retardation

F79 Unspecified mental retardation

A fourth character may be used to specify the extent of associated behavioural impairment:

F7x.0 No, or minimal, impairment of behaviour

F7x.1 Significant impairment of behaviour requiring attention or treatment

F7x.8 Other impairments of behaviour

F7x.9 Without mention of impairment of behaviour

F80–F89 Disorders of psychological development

F80 specific developmental disorders of speech and language

F80.0 Specific speech articulation disorder

F80.1 Expressive language disorder

F80.2 Receptive language disorder

F80.3 Acquired aphasia with epilepsy (Landau–Kleffner syndrome)

F80.8 Other developmental disorders of speech and language

F80.9 Developmental disorder of speech and language, unspecified

F81 Specific developmental disorders of scholastic skills

F81.0 Specific reading disorder

F81.1 Specific spelling disorder

F81.2 Specific disorder of arithmetical skills

F81.3 Mixed disorder of scholastic skills

F81.8 Other developmental disorders of scholastic skills

F81.9 Developmental disorder of scholastic skills, unspecified

F82 Specific developmental disorder of motor function

F83 Mixed specific developmental disorders

F84 Pervasive developmental disorders

F84.0 Childhood autism

F84.1 Atypical autism

F84.2 Rett's syndrome

F84.3 Other childhood disintegrative disorder

F84.4 Overactive disorder associated with mental retardation and stereotyped movements

F84.5 Asperger's syndrome

F84.8 Other pervasive developmental disorders

F84.9 Pervasive developmental disorder, unspecified

F88 Other disorders of psychological development

F89 Unspecified disorder of psychological development

F90–F98 Behavioural and emotional disorders with onset usually occurring in childhood and adolescence

F90 Hyperkinetic disorders

F90.0 Disturbance of activity and attention

F90.1 Hyperkinetic conduct disorder

F90.8 Other hyperkinetic disorders

F90.9 Hyperkinetic disorder, unspecified

F91 Conduct disorders

F91.0 Conduct disorder confined to the family context

F91.1 Unsocialized conduct disorder

F91.2 Socialized conduct disorder

F91.3 Oppositional defiant disorder

F91.8 Other conduct disorders

F91.9 Conduct disorder, unspecified

F92 Mixed disorders of conduct and emotions

F92.0 Depressive conduct disorder

F92.8 Other mixed disorders of conduct and emotions

F92.9 Mixed disorder of conduct and emotions, unspecified

F93 Emotional disorders with onset specific to childhood

F93.0 Separation anxiety disorder of childhood

F93.1 Phobic anxiety disorder of childhood

F93.2 Social anxiety disorder of childhood

F93.3 Sibling rivalry disorder

F93.8 Other childhood emotional disorders

F93.9 Childhood emotional disorder, unspecified

F94 Disorders of social functioning with onset specific to childhood and adolescence

F94.0 Elective mutism

F94.1 Reactive attachment disorder of childhood

F94.2 Disinhibited attachment disorder of childhood

F94.8 Other childhood disorders of social functioning

F94.9 Childhood disorders of social functioning, unspecified

F95 Tic disorders

F95.0 Transient tic disorder

F95.1 Chronic motor or vocal tic disorder

F95.2 Combined vocal and multiple motor tic disorder (de la Tourette's syndrome)

F95.8 Other tic disorders

F95.9 Tic disorder, unspecified

F98 Other behavioural and emotional disorders with onset usually occurring in childhood and adolescence

F98.0 Non-organic enuresis

F98.1 Non-organic encopresis

F98.2 Feeding disorder of infancy and childhood

F98.3 Pica of infancy and childhood

F98.4 Stereotyped movement disorders

F98.5 Stuttering (stammering)

F98.6 Cluttering

F98.8 Other specified behavioural and emotional disorders with onset usually occurring in childhood and adolescence

F98.9 Unspecified behavioural and emotional disorders with onset usually occurring in childhood and adolescence

F99 Unspecified mental disorder

F99 Mental disorder, not otherwise specified

Appendix 2

Diagnostic and Statistical Manual of Mental Disorders (4th edition)

NOS = not otherwise specified.

An *x* appearing in a diagnostic code indicates that a specific code number is required.

An ellipsis (. . .) is used in the names of certain disorders to indicate that the name of a specific mental disorder or general medical condition should be inserted when recording the name (e.g. 293.0 Delirium due to hypothyroidism).

If criteria are currently met, one of the following severity specifiers may be noted after the diagnosis:

    mild

    moderate

    severe

If criteria are no longer met, one of the following specifiers may be noted:

    in partial remission

    in full remission

    prior history

(*Editors' note* The numerical codes used in DSM-IV follow those used in the 9th edition of the *International Classification of Diseases*. ICD-9 is no longer used internationally, having been superseded by ICD-10, but at the time of printing of this textbook the DSM system of numbering has not been changed.)

In the following list two numerical codes appear in front of each entry. The first is the code used in the DSM-IV classification. The second (in parentheses) is the corresponding ICD-10 code. The latter is provided to assist the reader who wishes to compare the entries in the two classifications.

Disorders usually first diagnosed in infancy, childhood, or adolescence

Mental retardation

Note: These are coded on Axis II.

    317 (F70.9) Mild mental retardation

    318.0 (F71.9) Moderate mental retardation

    318.1 (F72.9) Severe mental retardation

    318.2 (F73.9) Profound mental retardation

    319 (F79.9) Mental retardation, severity unspecified

Learning disorders

    315.0 (F81.0) Reading disorder

    315.1 (F81.2) Mathematics disorder

315.8 (F81.8) Disorder of written expression

315.9 (F81.9) Learning disorder NOS

Motor skills disorder

315.4 (F82) Developmental co-ordination disorder

Communication disorders

315.31 (F80.1) Expressive language disorder

315.31 (F80.2) Mixed receptive–expressive language disorder

315.39 (F80.0) Phonological disorder

307.0 (F98.5) Stuttering

307.9 (F80.9) Communication disorder NOS

Pervasive development disorders

299.00 (F84.0) Autistic disorder

299.80 (F84.2) Rett's disorder

299.10 (F84.3) Childhood disintegrative disorder

299.80 (F84.5) Asperger's disorder

299.80 (F84.9) Pervasive developmental disorder NOS

Attention-deficit and disruptive behaviour disorders

314.*xx* (—) Attention-deficit/hyperactivity disorder

.01 (F90.0) Combined type

.00 (F98.8) Predominantly inattentive type

.01 (F90.0) Predominantly hyperactive–impulsive type

314.9 (F90.9) Attention-deficit/hyperactivity disorder NOS

312.8 (F91.8) Conduct disorder

Specify type: Childhood-onset type

Adolescent-onset type

313.81 (F91.3) Oppositional defiant disorder

312.9 (F91.9) Disruptive behaviour disorder NOS

Feeding and eating disorders of infancy or early childhood

307.52 (F98.3) Pica

307.53 (F98.2) Rumination disorder

307.59 (F98.2) Feeding disorder of infancy or early childhood

Tic disorders

307.23 (F95.2) Tourette's disorder

307.22 (F95.1) Chronic motor or vocal tic disorder

307.21 (F95.0) Transient tic disorder

Specify if: Single episode/Recurrent

307.20 (F95.9) Tic disorder NOS

Elimination disorders

—.– (– –) Encopresis

787.6 (R15) With constipation and overflow incontinence

307.7 (F98.1) Without constipation and overflow incontinence

307.6 (F98.0) Enuresis (not due to a general medical condition)

Specify type: Nocturnal only

Diurnal only

Nocturnal and diurnal

Other disorders of infancy, childhood, or adolescence

309.21 (F93.0) Separation anxiety disorder

Specify if: Early onset

313.23 (F94.0) Selective mutism

313.89 (F94.*x*) Reactive attachment disorder of infancy or early childhood

(.1) *Specify type:* Inhibited type

(.2) Disinhibited type

307.3 (F98.4) Sterotypic movement disorder

Specify if: With self-injurious behaviour

313.9 (F98.9) Disorder of infancy, childhood, or adolescence NOS

Delirium, dementia, and amnestic and other cognitive disorders

Delirium

293.0 (F05.0) Delirium due to . . . *(indicate the general medical condition)*

—.– (– –) Substance intoxication delirium *(refer to substance-related disorders for substance-specific codes)*

—.– (– –) Substance withdrawal delirium *(refer to substance-related disorders for substance-specific codes)*

—.– (– –) Delirium due to multiple aetiologies *(code each of the specific aetiologies)*

780.09 (F05.9) Delirium NOS

Dementia

290.*xx* (F00.*xx*) Dementia of the Alzheimer's type, with early onset *(also code G30.0 Alzheimer's disease on Axis III)*

.10 (.00) Uncomplicated

.11 (F05.1) With delirium

.12 (.01) With delusions

.13 (.02) With depressed mood

Specify if: With behavioural disturbance

290.*xx* (F00.*xx*) Dementia of the Alzheimer's type, with late onset *(also code 331.0 Alzheimer's disease on Axis III)*

.0 (.10) Uncomplicated

.3 (F05.1) With delirium

.20 (.20) With delusions

.21 (.13) With depressed mood

Specify if: With behavioural disturbance

290.*xx* (F01.*xx*) Vascular dementia

.40 (.80) Uncomplicated

.41 (F05.1) With delirium

.42 (.81) With delusions

.43 (.83) With depressed mood

Specify if: With behavioural disturbance

294.9 (F02.4) Dementia due to HIV disease *(also code 043.1 HIV infection affecting central nervous system on Axis III)*

294.1 (F02.8) Dementia due to head trauma *(also code 854.00 Head injury on Axis III)*

294.1 (F02.3) Dementia due to Parkinson's disease *(also code 332.0 Parkinson's disease on Axis III)*

294.1 (F02.2) Dementia due to Huntington's disease *(also code 333.4 Huntington's disease on Axis III)*

290.10 (F02.0) Dementia due to Pick's disease *(also code 331.0 Pick's disease on Axis III)*

290.10 (F02.1) Dementia due to Creutzfeldt–Jakob disease *(also code 046.1 Creutzfeldt–Jakob disease on Axis III)*

294.1 (F02.8) Dementia due to ̃ . . . *(indicate the general medical condition not listed above) (also code the general medical condition on Axis III)*

—.– (– –) Substance-induced persisting dementia *(refer to substance-related disorders for substance-specific codes)*

—.– (F02.8) Dementia due to multiple aetiologies *(code each of the specific aetiologies)*

294.8 (F03) Dementia NOS

Amnestic disorders

294.0 (F04) Amnestic disorder due to . . . *(indicate the general medical condition)*

Specify if: Transient/Chronic

—.– (– –) Substance-induced persisting amnestic disorder *(refer to substance-related disorders for substance-specific codes)*

294.8 (R41.3) Amnestic disorder NOS

Other cognitive disorders

294.9 (F06.9) Cognitive disorder NOS

Mental disorders due to a general medical condition not elsewhere classified

293.89 (F06.1) Catatonic disorder due to . . . *(indicate the general medical condition)*

310.1 (F07.0) Personality change due to . . . *(indicate the general medical condition)*

Specify type: Labile type
　　　　　　Disinhibited type
　　　　　　Aggressive type
　　　　　　Apathetic type
　　　　　　Paranoid type
　　　　　　Other type
　　　　　　Combined type
　　　　　　Unspecified type

293.9 (F09) Mental disorder NOS due to . . . *(indicate the general medical condition)*

Substance-related disorders

[a]*The following specifiers may be applied to substance dependence:*

With physiological dependence/Without physiological dependence

Early full remission/Early partial remission

Sustained full remission/Sustained partial remission

On agonist therapy/In a controlled environment

The following specifiers apply to substance-induced disorders as noted:

[I]With onset during intoxication

[W]With onset during withdrawal

Alcohol-related disorders

Alcohol use disorders

303.90 (F10.2x) Alcohol dependence[a]

305.0 (F10.1) Alcohol abuse

Alcohol-induced disorders

303.00 (F10.00) Alcohol intoxication

291.8 (F10.3) Alcohol withdrawal

Specify if: With perceptual disturbances

291.0 (F10.03) Alcohol intoxication delirium

291.0 (F10.4) Alcohol withdrawal delirium

291.2 (F10.73) Alcohol-induced persisting dementia

291.1 (F10.6) Alcohol-induced persisting amnestic disorder

291.x (F10.xx) Alcohol-induced psychotic disorder

　　.5 (.51) With delusions[I,W]

　　.3 (.52) With hallucinations[I,W]

291.8 (F10.8) Alcohol-induced mood disorder[I,W]

291.8 (F10.8) Alcohol-induced anxiety disorder[I,W]

291.8 (F10.8) Alcohol-induced sexual dysfunction[I]

291.8 (F10.8) Alcohol-induced sleep disorder[I,W]

291.9 (F10.9) Alcohol-related disorder NOS

Amphetamine (or amphetamine-like) related disorders

Amphetamine use disorders

304.40 (F15.2.x) Amphetamine dependence[a]

305.70 (F15.1) Amphetamine abuse

Amphetamine-induced disorders

292.89 (F15.00) Amphetamine intoxication

(F15.04) *Specify if:* With perceptual disturbances

292.0 (F15.3) Amphetamine withdrawal

292.81 (F15.03) Amphetamine intoxication delirium

292.xx (F15.xx) Amphetamine-induced psychotic disorder

　　.11 (.51) With delusions[I]

　　.12 (.52) With hallucinations[I]

292.84 (F15.8) Amphetamine-induced mood disorder[I,W]

292.89 (F15.8) Amphetamine-induced anxiety disorder[I]

292.89 (F15.8) Amphetamine-induced sexual dysfunction[I]

292.89 (F15.8) Amphetamine-induced sleep disorder[I,W]

292.9 (F15.9) Amphetamine-related disorder NOS

Caffeine-related disorders

Caffeine-induced disorders

305.90 (F15.00) Caffeine intoxication

292.89 (F15.8) Caffeine-induced anxiety disorder[I]

292.89 (F15.8) Caffeine-induced sleep disorder[I]

292.9 (F15.9) Caffeine-related disorder NOS

Cannabis-related disorders

Cannabis use disorders

304.30 (F12.2x) Cannabis dependence[a]

305.20 (F12.1) Cannabis abuse

Cannabis-induced disorders

292.89 (F12.00) Cannabis intoxication

(F12.04) *Specify if:* With perceptual disturbances

292.81 (F12.03) Cannabis intoxication delirium

292.xx (F12.xx) Cannabis-induced psychotic disorder

    .11 (.51) With delusions[I]

    .12 (.52) With hallucinations[I]

292.89 (F12.8) Cannabis-induced anxiety disorder[I]

292.9 (F12.9) Cannabis-related disorder NOS

Cocaine-related disorders

Cocaine use disorders

304.20 (F14.2x) Cocaine dependence[a]

305.60 (F14.1) Cocaine abuse

Cocaine-induced disorders

292.89 (F14.00) Cocaine intoxication

    (F14.04) *Specify if:* With perceptual disturbances

292.0 (F14.3) Cocaine withdrawal

292.81 (F14.03) Cocaine intoxication delirium

292.xx (F14.xx) Cocaine-induced psychotic disorder

    .11 (.51) With delusions[I]

    .12 (.52) With hallucinations[I]

292.84 (F14.8) Cocaine-induced mood disorder[I,W]

292.89 (F14.8) Cocaine-induced anxiety disorder[I,W]

292.89 (F14.8) Cocaine-induced sexual dysfunction[I]

292.89 (F14.8) Cocaine-induced sleep disorder[I,W]

292.9 (F14.9) Cocaine-related disorder NOS

Hallucinogen-related disorders

Hallucinogen use disorders

304.50 (F16.2x) Hallucinogen dependence[a]

305.30 (F16.1) Hallucinogen abuse

Hallucinogen-induced disorders

292.89 (F16.00) Hallucinogen intoxication

292.89 (F16.70) Hallucinogen persisting perception disorder (flashbacks)

292.81 (F16.03) Hallucinogen intoxication delirium

292.xx (F16.xx) Hallucinogen-induced psychotic disorder

    .11 (.51) With delusions[I]

    .12 (.52) With hallucinations[I]

292.84 (F16.8) Hallucinogen-induced mood disorder[I]

292.89 (F16.8) Hallucinogen-induced anxiety disorder[I]

292.9 (F16.9) Hallucinogen-related disorder NOS

Inhalant-related disorders

Inhalant use disorders

304.60 (F18.2x) Inhalant dependence[a]

305.90 (F18.1) Inhalant abuse

Inhalant-induced disorders

292.89 (F18.00) Inhalant intoxication

292.81 (F18.03) Inhalant intoxication delirium

292.82 (F18.73) Inhalant-induced persisting dementia

292.xx (F18.xx) Inhalant-induced psychotic disorder

    .11 (.51) With delusions[I]

    .12 (.52) With hallucinations[I]

292.84 (F18.8) Inhalant-induced mood disorder[I]

292.89 (F18.8) Inhalant-induced anxiety disorder[I]

292.9 (F18.9) Inhalant-related disorder NOS

Nicotine-related disorders

Nicotine use disorder

305.10 (F17.2x) Nicotine dependence[a]

Nicotine-induced disorder

292.0 (F17.3) Nicotine withdrawal

292.9 (F17.9) Nicotine-related disorder NOS

Opioid-related disorders

Opioid use disorders

304.00 (F11.2x) Opioid dependence[a]

305.50 (F11.1) Opioid abuse

Opioid-induced disorders

292.89 (F11.0) Opioid intoxication

(F11.04) *Specify if:* With perceptual disturbances

292.00 (F11.3) Opioid withdrawal

292.81 (F11.03) Opioid intoxication delirium

292.xx (F11.xx) Opioid induced psychotic disorder

    .11 (.51) With delusions[I]

    .12 (.52) With hallucinations[I]

292.84 (F11.8) Opioid-induced mood disorder[I]

292.89 (F11.8) Opioid-induced sexual dysfunction[I]

292.89 (F11.8) Opioid-induced sleep disorder[I,W]

292.9 (F11.9) Opioid-related disorder NOS

Phencyclidine (or phencyclidine-like) related disorders

Phencyclidine use disorders

> 304.90 (F19.2*x*) Phencyclidine dependence[a]

> 305.90 (F19.1) Phencyclidine abuse

Phencyclidine-induced disorders

> 292.89 (F19.0) Phencyclidine intoxication
> (F19.04) *Specify if:* With perceptual disturbances

> 292.81 (F19.03) Phencyclidine intoxication delirium

> 292.*xx* (F19.*xx*) Phencyclidine-induced psychotic disorder

>> .11 (.51) With delusions[I]

>> .12 (.52) With hallucinations[I]

> 292.84 (F19.8) Phencyclidine-induced mood disorder[I]

> 292.89 (F19.8) Phencyclidine-induced anxiety disorder[I]

> 292.9 (F19.9) Phencyclidine-related disorder NOS

Sedative-, hypnotic-, or anxiolytic-related disorders

Sedative, hypnotic, or anxiolytic use disorders

> 304.10 (F13.2*x*) Sedative, hypnotic, or anxiolytic dependence[a]

> 305.40 (F13.1) Sedative, hypnotic, or anxiolytic abuse

Sedative-, hypnotic-, or anxiolytic-induced disorders

> 292.89 (F13.00) Sedative, hypnotic, or anxiolytic intoxication

> 292.0 (F13.3) Sedative, hypnotic, or anxiolytic withdrawal

> *Specify if:* With perceptual disturbances

> 292.81 (F13.03) Sedative, hypnotic, or anxiolytic intoxication delirium

> 292.81 (F13.4) Sedative, hypnotic, or anxiolytic withdrawal delirium

> 292.82 (F13.73) Sedative-, hypnotic-, or anxiolytic-induced persisting dementia

> 292.83 (F13.6) Sedative-, hypnotic-, or anxiolytic-induced persisting amnestic disorder

> 292.*xx* (F13.*xx*) Sedative-, hypnotic-, or anxiolytic-induced psychotic disorder

>> .11 (.51) With delusions[I,W]

>> .12 (.52) With hallucinations[I,W]

> 292.84 (F13.8) Sedative-, hypnotic-, or anxiolytic-induced mood disorder[I,W]

> 292.89 (F13.8) Sedative-, hypnotic-, or anxiolytic-induced anxiety disorder[W]

> 292.89 (F13.8) Sedative-, hypnotic-, or anxiolytic-induced sexual dysfunction[I]

> 292.89 (F13.8) Sedative-, hypnotic-, or anxiolytic-induced sleep disorder[I,W]

> 292.9 (F13.9) Sedative-, hypnotic-, or anxiolytic-related disorder NOS

Polysubstance-related disorder

> 304.80 (F19.2*x*) Polysubstance dependence[a]

Other (or unknown) substance-related disorders

Other (or unknown) substance use disorders

> 304.90 (F19.2*x*) Other (or unknown) substance dependence[a]

> 305.90 (F19.1) Other (or unknown) substance abuse

Other (or unknown) substance-induced disorders

> 292.89 (F19.00) Other (or unknown) substance intoxication
> (F19.04) *Specify if:* With perceptual disturbances

> 292.0 (F19.3) Other (or unknown) substance withdrawal

> *Specify if:* With perceptual disturbances

> 292.81 (F19.03) Other (or unknown) substance-induced delirium *(code F19.4 if onset during withdrawal)*

> 292.82 (F19.73) Other (or unknown) substance-induced persisting dementia

> 292.83 (F19.6) Other (or unknown) substance-induced persisting amnestic disorder

> 299.*xx* (F19.*xx*) Other (or unknown) subsstance-induced psychotic disorder

>> .11 (.51) With delusions[I,W]

>> .12 (.52) With hallucinations[I,W]

> 292.84 (F19.8) Other (or unknown) substance-induced mood disorder[I,W]

> 292.89 (F19.8) Other (or unknown) substance-induced anxiety disorder[I,W]

> 292.89 (F19.8) Other (or unknown) substance-induced sexual dysfunction[I]

> 292.89 (F19.8) Other (or unknown) substance-induced sleep disorder[I,W]

> 292.9 (F19.9) Other (or unknown) substance-related disorder NOS

Schizophrenia and other psychotic disorders

> 295.*xx* (F20.*xx*) Schizophrenia

The following classification of longitudinal course applies to all subtypes of schizophrenia

> Episodic with inter-episode residual symptoms

>> *Specify if:* With prominent negative symptoms

> Episodic with no inter-episode residual symptoms

> Continuous

>> *Specify if:* With prominent negative symptoms

> Single episode in partial remission

>> *Specify if:* With prominent negative symptoms

> Single episode in full remission

> Other or unspecified pattern

> .30 (.0*x*) Paranoid type

> .10 (.1*x*) Disorganized type

> .20 (.2*x*) Catatonic type

> .90 (.3*x*) Undifferentiated type

> .60 (.5*x*) Residual type

> 295.40 (F20.8) Schizophreniform disorder

Specify if: Without good prognostic features

With good prognostic features

    295.70 (F25.*x*) Schizoaffective disorder

        (.0) Bipolar type

        (.1) Depressive type

    297.1 (F22.0) Delusional disorder

Specify type: Erotomanic type

                Grandiose type

                Jealous type

                Persecutory type

                Somatic type

                Mixed type

                Unspecified type

    298.8 (F23.*xx*) Brief psychotic disorder

        (.81) With marked stressor(s)

        (.82) Without marked stressor(s)

Specify if: With postpartum onset

    297.3 (F24) Shared psychotic disorder

    293.*xx* (F06.*x*) Psychotic disorder due to . . . *(indicate the general medical condition)*

        .81 (.2) With delusions

        .82 (.0) With hallucinations

    —.– (– –) Substance-induced psychotic disorder *(refer to substance-related disorders for substance-specific codes)*

Specify if: With onset during intoxication

With onset during withdrawal

    298.9 (F29) Psychotic disorder NOS

Mood disorders

Code current state of major depressive disorder or bipolar I disorder in fifth digit:

    1 = Mild

    2 = Moderate

    3 = Severe without psychotic features

    4 = Severe with psychotic features

        Specify: Mood-congruent psychotic features

        Mood-incongruent psychotic features

    5 = In partial remission

    6 = In full remission

    0 = Unspecified

The following specifiers apply (for current or most recent episode) to mood disorders as noted:

    [a]Severity (mild, moderate, severe)

    Psychotic

    Remission specifiers (partial, full)

    [b]Chronic

    [c]With catatonic features

    [d]With melancholic features

    [e]With atypical features

    [f]With postpartum onset

The following specifiers apply to mood disorders as noted:

    [g]With or without full interepisode recovery

    [h]With seasonal pattern/With rapid cycling

Depressive disorders

    296.*xx* (– –) Major depressive disorder

        .2*x* (F32*x*) Single episode[a,b,c,d,e,f]

        .3*x* (F33*x*) Recurrent[a,b,c,d,e,f,g,h]

    300.4 (F34.1) Dysthymic disorder

Specify if: Early onset

Late onset

Specify: With atypical features

    311 (F32.9) Depressive disorder NOS

Bipolar disorders

    296.0*x* (F30.*x*) Bipolar I disorder, single manic episode[a,c,f]

Specify if: Mixed

        .40 (F31.0) Most recent episode hypomanic[g,h,i]

        .4*x* (F31.*x*) Most recent episode manic[a,c,f,g,h,i]

        .6*x* (F31.6) Most recent episode mixed[a,c,f,g,h,i]

        .5*x* (F31.*x*) Most recent episode depressed[a,b,c,d,e,f,g,h,i]

        .7 (F31.9) Most recent episode unspecified[g,h,i]

    296.89 (F31.8) Bipolar II disorder[a,b,c,d,e,f,g,h,i]

Specify (current or most recent episode): Hypomanic/Depressed

    301.13 (F34.0) Cyclothymic disorder

    296.80 (F31.9) Bipolar disorder NOS

    293.83 (F06.*xx*) Mood disorder due to . . . *(indicate the general medical condition)*

        (.32) With depressive features

        (.32) With major depressive-like episode

        (.30) With manic features

        (.33) With mixed features

    —.– (– –) Substance-induced mood disorder *(refer to substance-related disorder for substance-specific codes)*

Specify type: With depressive features

With manic features

With mixed features

Specify if: With onset during intoxication

With onset during withdrawal

    296.90 (F39) Mood disorder NOS

Anxiety disorders

    300.01 (F41.0) Panic disorder without agoraphobia

    300.21 (F40.01) Panic disorder with agoraphobia

    300.22 (F40.00) Agoraphobia without history of panic disorder

    300.29 (F40.2) Specific phobia

Specify type: Animal type

                Natural environment type

Blood–injection–injury type

Situational type

Other type

300.23 (F40.1) Social phobia

Specify if: Generalized

300.3 (F42.8) Obsessive–compulsive disorder

Specify if: With poor insight

309.81 (F43.1) Post-traumatic stress disorder

Specify if: Acute
Chronic

Specify if: With delayed onset

308.3 (F43.0) Acute stress disorder

300.02 (F41.1) Generalized anxiety disorder

293.89 (F06.4) Anxiety disorder due to . . . *(indicate the general medical condition)*

Specify if: With generalized anxiety
With panic attacks
With obsessive–compulsive symptoms

—.– (– –) Substance-induced anxiety disorder *(refer to substance-related disorders for substance-specific codes)*

Specify if: With generalized anxiety
With panic attacks
With obsessive–compulsive symptoms
With phobic symptoms

Specify if: With onset during intoxication
With onset during withdrawal

300.00 (F41.9) Anxiety disorder NOS

Somatoform disorders

300.81 (F45.0) Somatization disorder

300.81 (F45.1) Undifferentiated somatoform disorder

300.11 (F44.*x*) Conversion disorder

  (.4) *Specify if:* With motor symptom or deficit

  (.5)   With seizures or convulsions

  (.6)   With sensory symptom or deficit

  (.7)   With mixed presentation

307.*xx* (F45.4) Pain disorder

  .80 Associated with psychological factors

  .89 Associated with both psychological factors and a general medical condition

Specify if: Acute
Chronic

300.7 (F45.2) Hypochondriasis

Specify if: With poor insight

300.7 (F45.2) Body dysmorphic disorder

300.81 (F45.9) Somatoform disorder NOS

Factitious disorders

300.*xx* (F68.1) Factitious disorder

  .16 With predominantly psychological signs and symptoms

  .19 With predominantly physical signs and symptoms

  .19 With combined psychological and physical signs and symptoms

300.19 (F68.1) Factitious disorder NOS

Dissociative disorders

300.12 (F44.0) Dissociative amnesia

300.13 (F44.1) Dissociative fugue

300.14 (F44.81) Dissociative identity disorder

300.6 (F48.1) Depersonalization disorder

300.15 (F44.9) Dissociative disorder NOS

Sexual and gender identity disorders

Sexual dysfunctions

The following specifiers apply to all primary sexual dysfunctions:

Lifelong type/Acquired type

Generalized type/Situational type

Due to psychological factors/Due to combined factors

Sexual desire disorders

302.71 (F52.0) Hypoactive sexual desire disorder

302.79 (F52.10) Sexual aversion disorder

Sexual arousal disorders

302.72 (F52.2) Female sexual arousal disorder

302.72 (F52.2) Male erectile disorder

Orgasmic disorders

302.73 (F52.3) Female orgasmic disorder

302.74 (F52.3) Male orgasmic disorder

302.75 (F52.4) Premature ejaculation

Sexual pain disorders

302.76 (F52.6) Dyspareunia (not due to a general medical condition)

306.51 (F52.5) Vaginismus (not due to a general medical condition)

Sexual dysfunction due to a general medical condition

625.8 (N94.8) Female hypoactive sexual desire disorder due to . . . *(indicate the general medical condition)*

608.89 (N50.8) Male hypoactive sexual desire disorder due to . . . *(indicate the general medical condition)*

607.84 (N48.4) Male erectile disorder due to . . . *(indicate the general medical condition)*

625.0 (N94.1) Female dyspareunia due to . . . *(indicate the general medical condition)*

608.89 (N50.8) Male dyspareunia due to . . . *(indicate the general medical condition)*

625.8 (N94.8) Other female sexual dysfunction due to . . . *(indicate the general medical condition)*

608.89 (N50.8) Other male sexual dysfunction due to . . . *(indicate the general medical condition)*

—.– (– –) Substance-induced sexual dysfunction *(refer to substance-related disorders for substance-specific codes)*

Specify if: With impaired desire
With impaired arousal
With impaired orgasm
With sexual pain

Specify if: With onset during intoxication

302.70 (F52.9) Sexual dysfunction NOS

Paraphilias

302.4 (F65.2) Exhibitionism

302.81 (F65.0) Fetishism

302.89 (F65.8) Frotteurism

302.2 (F65.4) Paedophilia

Specify if: Sexually attracted to males
Sexually attracted to females
Sexually attracted to both

Specify if: Limited to incest

Specify type: Exclusive type
Non-exclusive type

302.83 (F65.5) Sexual masochism

302.84 (F65.5) Sexual sadism

302.3 (F65.1) Transvestic fetishism

Specify if: With gender dysphoria

302.82 (F65.3) Voyeurism

302.9 (F65.9) Paraphilia NOS

Gender identity disorders

302.*xx* (F64.*x*) Gender identity disorder

.6 (.2) In children

.85 (. 0) In adolescents or adults

Specify if: Sexually attracted to males
Sexually attracted to females
Sexually attracted to both
Sexually attracted to neither

302.6 (F64.9) Gender identity disorder NOS

302.9 (F52.9) Sexual disorder NOS

Eating disorders

307.1 (F50.0) Anorexia nervosa

Specify if: Restricting type
Binge eating
Purging type

307.51 (F50.2) Bulimia nervosa

Specify if: Purging type
Non-purging type

307.50 (F50.9) Eating disorder NOS

Sleep disorders

Primary sleep disorders

Dyssomnias

307.42 (F51.0) Primary insomnia

307.44 (F51.1) Primary hypersomnia

Specify if: Recurrent

347 (G47.4) Narcolepsy

780.59 (G47.3) Breathing-related sleep disorder

307.45 (F51.2) Circadian rhythm sleep disorder

Specify type: Delayed sleep phase type
Jet lag type
Shift work type
Unspecified type

307.47 (F51.9) Dyssomnia NOS

Parasomnias (579)

307.47 (F51.5) Nightmare disorder

307.46 (F51.4) Sleep terror disorder

307.46 (F51.3) Sleepwalking disorder

307.47 (F51.8) Parasomnia NOS

Sleep disorders related to another mental disorder

307.42 (F51.0) Insomnia related to . . . *(indicate the Axis I or Axis II disorder)*

307.44 (F51.1) Hypersomnia related to . . . *(indicate the Axis I or Axis II disorder)*

Other sleep disorders

780.*xx* (G47.*x*) Sleep disorder due to . . . *(indicate the general medical condition)*

.52 (.0) Insomnia type

.54 (.1) Hypersomnia type

.59 (.8) Parasomnia type

.59 (.8) Mixed type

—.– (– –) Substance-induced sleep disorder *(refer to substance-related disorders for substance-specific codes)*

Specify type: Insomnia type
Hypersomnia type
Parasomnia type
Mixed type

Specify if: With onset during intoxication
With onset during withdrawal

Impulse-control disorders not elsewhere classified

312.34 (F63.8) Intermittent explosive disorder

312.32 (F63.2) Kleptomania

312.33 (F63.1) Pyromania

312.31 (F63.0) Pathological gambling

312.39 (F63.3) Trichotillomania

312.30 (F63.9) Impulse-control disorder NOS

Adjustment disorders

309.*xx* (F43.*xx*) Adjustment disorder

.0 (.20) With depressed mood

.24 (.28) With anxiety

.28 (.22) With mixed anxiety and depressed mood

.3 (.24) With disturbance of conduct

.4 (.25) With mixed disturbance of emotions and conduct

.9 (.9) Unspecified

Specify if: Acute

           Chronic

Personality disorders

Note: These are coded on Axis II.

301.0 (F60.0) Paranoid personality disorder

301.20 (F60.1) Schizoid personality disorder

301.22 (F21) Schizotypal personality disorder

301.7 (F60.2) Antisocial personality disorder

301.83 (F60.31) Borderline personality disorder

301.50 (F60.4) Histrionic personality disorder

301.81 (F60.8) Narcissistic personality disorder

301.82 (F60.6) Avoidant personality disorder

301.6 (F60.7) Dependent personality disorder

301.4 (F60.5) Obsessive–compulsive personality disorder

301.9 (F60.9) Personality disorder NOS

Other conditions that may be a focus of clinical attention

Psychological factors affecting medical condition

316 (F54) ... *(Specified psychological factor)*

Affecting . . . *(indicate the general medical condition)*

Choose name based on nature of factors:

Mental disorder affecting medical condition

Psychological symptoms affecting medical condition

Personality traits or coping style affecting medical conditions

Maladaptive health behaviours affecting medicial condition

Stress-related physiological response affecting medical condition

Other or unspecified psychological factors affecting medical condition

Medication-induced movement disorders

332.1 (G21.0) Neuroleptic-induced parkinsonism

333.92 (G21.0) Neuroleptic malignant syndrome

333.7 (G24.0) Neuroleptic-induced acute dystonia

333.99 (G21.1) Neuroleptic-induced acute akathisia

333.82 (G24.0) Neuroleptic-induced tardive dyskinesia

333.1 (G25.1) Medication-induced postural tremor

333.90 (G25.9) Medication-induced movement disorder NOS

Other medication-induced disorder

995.2 (T88.7) Adverse effects of medication NOS

Relational problems

V61.9 (Z63.7) Relational problem related to a mental disorder or general medical condition

V61.20 (Z63.8) Parent–child relational problem *(code Z63.1 if focus of attention is on child)*

V61.1 (Z63.0) Partner relational problem

V61.8 (F93.3) Sibling relational problem

V62.81 (Z63.9) Relational problem NOS

Problems related to abuse or neglect

V61.21 (T74.1) Physical abuse of child

(code 995.5 if focus of attention is on victim)

V61.21 (T74.2) Sexual abuse of child

(code 995.5 if focus of attention is on victim)

V61.21 (T74.0) Neglect of child

(code 995.5 if focus of attention is on victim)

V61.1 (T74.1) Physical abuse of adult

(code 995.81 if focus of attention is on victim)

V61.1 (T74.2) Sexual abuse of adult

(code 995.81 if focus of attention is on victim)

Additional conditions that may be a focus of clinical attention

V15.81 (Z91.1) Non-compliance with treatment

V65.2 (Z76.5) Malingering

V71.01 (Z72.8) Adult antisocial behaviour

V71.02 (Z72.8) Child or adolescent antisocial behaviour

V62.89 (R41.8) Borderline intellectual functioning

Note: This is coded on Axis II.

780.9 (R41.8) Age-related cognitive decline

V62.82 (Z63.4) Bereavement

V62.3 (Z55.8) Academic problem

V62.2 (Z56.7) Occupational problem

313.82 (F93.8) Identity problem

V62.89 (Z71.8) Religious or spiritual problem

V62.4 (Z60.3) Acculturation problem

V62.89 (Z60.0) Phase of life problem

Additional codes

300.9 (F99) Unspecified mental disorder (non-psychotic)

V71.09 (Z03.2) No diagnosis or condition on Axis I

799.9 (R69) Diagnosis or condition deferred on Axis I

V71.09 (Z03.2) No diagnosis on Axis II

799.9 (R46.8) Diagnosis deferred on Axis II

Multiaxial system

Axis I

Clinical disorders

Other conditions that may be a focus of clinical attention

Axis II

Personality disorders

Mental retardation

Axis III

General medical conditions

Axis IV

Psychosocial and environmental problems

Axis V

Global assessment of functioning

1.12 **From science to practice**

John Geddes

The difficulties in keeping up to date

All doctors, and other health care professionals, have a considerable need for accurate and up-to-date information that often go unrecognized and unmet.[1] In psychiatry, many new treatments have been introduced over the last decade, including new antidepressants, antipsychotics, and antidementia drugs. There have also been developments in non-pharmacological treatments, such as psychotherapy and models of service organization, as well as advances in diagnosis, prognosis (including assessment of risk) and aetiology. As these clinical advances are made, it is important that doctors are informed about them in a manner that is timely, accurate, and unbiased. Ideally perhaps, every psychiatrist would have access to the original scientific articles. However, this is not often feasible. Time in clinical practice is very limited and many clinicians do not have the skills needed for an adequate systematic search, and a critical appraisal and interpretation of the findings of research studies. It has been estimated that two million papers are published in 20 000 biomedical journals every year,[2] a number clearly beyond the resources of most busy clinicians. Even restricting one's reading to those journals focusing on clinical aspects of psychiatry would mean that it would be necessary to read about 5500 papers each year—equivalent to 15 papers every day.[3] It is clear that some strategy is required for the efficient identification of research that is both methodologically sound and clinically relevant.

Traditionally, clinicians have used a number of methods of keeping up to date with research, including consulting colleagues and reading textbooks and journals. Smith[1] reviewed the research on the information needs of doctors and rated sources of information on several dimensions: their relevance to clinical practice, their scientific validity, how easy they were to use, and an overall estimate of their usefulness. Most of the sources that scored highly on all dimensions (such as regularly updated evidence-based textbooks) were of limited availability. Traditional methods of obtaining information (such as conventional textbooks and lecture-based continuing medical education) were more widely available, but of limited validity.

The difficulty of accessing reliable information means that many clinical decisions are made with a greater degree of uncertainty than is necessary, and a gap emerges between research and clinical practice. This gap is often filled by other influences including an unsystematic combination of beliefs and clinical observations. Sometimes this leads to unnecessary variations in clinical practice. These have been widely documented in psychiatry and include variations in the use of electroconvulsive therapy,[4,5] the use of antipsychotics,[6,7] and the treatment

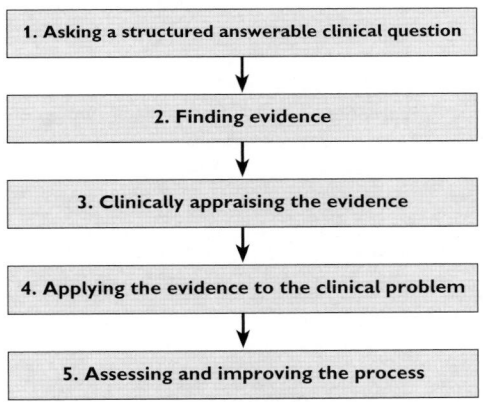

Fig. 1 The five stages of evidence-based medicine.

of depression.[8–10] The existence of these variations can only mean that some patients are not receiving the optimum treatment.

Methods of improving use of best available evidence

A set of strategies designed to assist clinicians in their attempts to base their practice on the best available evidence were first developed at McMaster University in Canada and are often referred to collectively as evidence-based medicine.[11] Evidence-based medicine is a problem-based approach and splits the process into five stages (Fig. 1). The process of evidence-based medicine also leads on to another stage—the identification of clinical questions in need of more research.

To make evidence-based practice feasible in real-life clinical practice, a number of problems need to be solved at each stage of the process.

Formulating a structured clinical question

When uncertainty arises in clinical practice, the clinician needs to formulate a structured clinical question. This step is fundamental to the process of evidence-based medicine because it allows the clinician first to classify the question, second to identify the research architecture that is most likely to yield a reliable result, and finally to determine the most efficient way of looking for the most reliable research.

Table 1 Types of clinical question and most reliable study architecture

Type of question	Form of the question	Most reliable study architecture
Diagnosis	How likely is a patient who has a particular symptom, sign, or diagnostic test result to have a specific disorder?	A cross-sectional study of patients suspected of having the disorder comparing the proportion of the patients who really have the disorder who have a positive test result with the proportion of patients who do not have the disorder who have a positive test result
Treatment	Is the treatment of interest more effective in producing a desired outcome than an alternative treatment (including no treatment)?	Randomized evidence in which the patients are randomly allocated to receive either the treatment of interest or the alternative; this is usually a systematic review of RCTs or a single high-quality RCT
Prognosis	What is the probability of a specific outcome in this patient?	A study in which an inception cohort (patients at a common stage in the development of the illness—especially first onset) are followed up for an adequate length of time
Aetiology	What has caused the disorder?	A study comparing the frequency of an exposure in a group of persons with the disease (cases) of interest with a group of persons without the disease (controls)—this may be an RCT, a case–control study, or a cohort study.

RCT, randomized controlled trial.

Example

Consider a patient who is suffering from a chronic mild depressive disorder. The clinician diagnoses dysthymic disorder but may be uncertain whether recommending an antidepressant would offer any benefit over offering non-specific support for a few sessions. The process of rapidly finding the best answer begins by formulating a clinical question:

(1) in patients with dysthymia (the **problem**)

(2) how effective are antidepressants (the **intervention**)

(3) compared with alternative treatments (including none) (the **comparison intervention**)

(4) in alleviating depressive symptoms and improving psychosocial functioning (the **outcome**)?

The next step is to classify the question. This example obviously concerns a question about therapy. Most of the questions that arise in clinical practice concern therapy, diagnosis, prognosis, or aetiology. Once the question has been formulated and classified, this suggests the most reliable research architecture (Table 1).

Finding evidence and advances in the organization of clinical knowledge

Identification of the nature of the clinical question and the most reliable study design enables the clinician to perform a focused and efficient literature search. One of the main advances of evidence-based medicine has been the development of methods of research synthesis, or the process of identifying, appraising, and summarizing primary

research studies into clinically usable knowledge. There are currently two main approaches to research synthesis—systematic reviews and clinical practice guidelines. Both these approaches are based on an explicit methodology that begins with the construction of a hierarchy of evidence in which certain forms of research architecture are considered to be reliable than others. The methodology is most clearly developed for questions about therapy and these will be the focus here.

Levels of evidence

A commonly used hierarchy of evidence for studies of treatments is as follows.

Ia. Evidence from a systematic review of randomized controlled trials

Ib. Evidence from at least one randomized controlled trial

IIa. Evidence from at least one controlled study without randomization

IIb. Evidence from at least one other type of quasi-experimental study

III. Evidence from non-experimental descriptive studies, such as comparative studies, correlation studies, and case–control studies

IV. Evidence from expert committee reports or opinions and/or clinical experience of respected authorities.

In this hierarchy, randomized evidence is considered to be more reliable than non-randomized evidence, and a systematic review of randomized evidence is considered to be the best defence against systematic bias.

Hierarchies of evidence have also been formulated for non-therapeutic studies, such as studies of aetiology, diagnosis, and prognosis. Again, the fundamental feature of these hierarchies is that the study architectures with the least susceptibility to bias are considered most reliable. The study design considered most reliable for each type of clinical question is shown in Table 1.

Systematic reviews

The need for systematic reviews and the methodology used are described in Chapter 6.1.1.2. The recognition of the need for systematic reviews of randomized controlled trials, and the development of the scientific methodology of reviews, has been one of the most striking advances in health services research over the last decade. One key development was the founding of the Cochrane Collaboration, an international organization with the objective of producing regularly updated systematic reviews of the effectiveness of all health care interventions.[12] The first Cochrane Centre was established in Oxford in 1992 as part of the information systems strategy developed to support the National Health Service Research and Development Programme; centres have since been established in several other countries.

Clinical practice guidelines

In some areas of health care there is sufficient evidence, coexisting with substantial clinical uncertainty, that it is worth developing clinical practice guidelines. Clinical practice guidelines have been defined as 'systematically developed statements to assist practitioner decisions about appropriate health care for specific clinical circumstances'.[13] Guidelines have been developed for several years, but there have been recent advances in the methodology of producing explicitly evidence-based guidelines. Evidence-based clinical practice guidelines are developed by a guideline development group consisting of key stakeholders who decide on the precise clinical questions to be answered. The evidence is then systematically reviewed and classified according to a hierarchy of evidence (see above) and presented to the guideline development group. The group then makes recommendations as appropriate. The degree to which the recommendations are directly based on the evidence is described using a second level of classification:[14]

(1) directly based on category I evidence;

(2) directly based on category II evidence *or* extrapolated recommendation from category I evidence;

(3) directly based on category III evidence *or* extrapolated recommendation from category I or II evidence;

(4) directly based on category IV evidence *or* extrapolated recommendation from category I, II. or III evidence.

Clinical practice guidelines are usually developed at a national level and need tailoring to suit local circumstances. Professional bodies such as the American Psychiatric Association and the Royal College of Psychiatrists (both of which have active guideline development programmes) usually take responsibility for developing national guidelines.

There are several limitations to clinical practice guidelines. Firstly, evidence-based clinical practice guidelines are expensive and time consuming to produce and rapidly become out of date. Secondly, to influ-ence practice, evidence-based clinical practice guidelines need to be actively disseminated and implemented. Guidelines that are developed nationally and passively sent out to doctors are often not used.[15] A number of active approaches are effective in helping change clinicians' behaviour:[16]

- outreach visits (also known as academic detailing)
- local opinion leaders
- patient-mediated interventions (including patient education)
- multifaceted interventions involving a range of techniques.

There is some evidence that guidelines can improve patient outcomes by their effect on clinical practice, especially when they are made relevant to local circumstances.[15] In one study in the United States, 217 patients with depressive disorders were randomly assigned to usual care or a mulitifaceted intervention designed to achieve the Agency for Health Care Policy and Research guidelines on management of depression.[17] Patients in the intervention group were much more likely to be treated in accordance with the guidelines, and this led to improved outcomes in patients with major depressive disorder (more than 50 per cent reduction on the Symptom Checklist-90 Depressive Symptom Scale at 4 months in 74 per cent of experimental patients compared with 44 per cent of control patients).

Understandably, clinicians also seek guidance in important clinical questions that are poorly served by high-quality, especially randomized, evidence. To assist in these clinical decisions, Frances and his colleagues have developed an innovative method of guideline development based on a systematic survey of the views of clinical experts.[18,19]

Use of electronic communication and the World Wide Web

The development of the Internet during the 1990s is closely linked to the development of evidence-based practice. The World Wide Web has become a vast information resource for doctors and patients. The improved access to information afforded to patients means that they are often very well informed about their condition. This is one of the factors contributing to the need for doctors to improve their own access to information. The Internet has several drawbacks including the disorganization of the information and the lack of quality control.[20,21] As with paper publications, resources are being developed to index critically appraised websites selectively. An example of such a site containing comprehensive links to useful information on the Web is the Centre for Evidence Based Mental Health (http://www.cebmh.com). Although in its infancy, over the next few years the Web is likely to become the main medium for transmitting and storing knowledge. Reliable electronic resources such as the Cochrane Library are already available (http://www.update-software.com/ccweb).

Improving current awareness

Another area of improvement has been the development of tools to assist doctors to maintain their current awareness of advances in research. The idea of review and abstracting journals is not new, but there has been a recognition that such journals also need a methodology to allow them to identify the most reliable and clinically important research studies.

A number of new journals have been produced with the aim improving the availability of high-quality evidence to clinicians. The first of these was *ACP Journal Club* (targeted primarily at general physicians), followed by *Evidence-Based Medicine* (targeted primarily at family doctors) and, more recently, *Evidence-Based Mental Health* (aimed at mental health clinicians of all disciplines). *Evidence-Based Mental Health* scans over 200 journals regularly and selects only those articles that both meet explicit methodological criteria (see Box 1) and are clinically important. The articles are then summarized in structured abstracts and published on one page with an accompanying commentary by a clinical expert.

A systematic approach to searching for the best available evidence

The developments in the organization of clinical knowledge make it possible for a clinician to search rapidly and efficiently for current best evidence using a standard approach (Fig. 2). This approach will change as new methods of organizing knowledge are developed.

Example (continued)

No clinical practice guideline can be found, but searching the Cochrane Library identifies the following review:

> Lima, M.S. and Moncrieff, J.A (1998). Comparison of drugs versus placebo for the treatment of dysthymia: a systematic review. In *Cochrane Database of Systematic Reviews*, Update Software.

This is a systematic review of 15 randomized controlled trials comparing a number of antidepressants (including tricyclics, selective serotonin reuptake inhibitors, monoamine oxidase inhibitors, and low-dose antipsychotics) with placebo in the treatment of dysthymia.

Critical appraisal of research articles

Once the evidence has been found, it needs to be critically appraised for its reliability and usefulness. Psychiatrists need to be able to assess the scientific value and clinical importance of a study. This requires a range of epidemiological and biostatistical skills that have not traditionally been considered to be key skills for psychiatrists. In the United Kingdom, the Royal College of Psychiatrists introduced in 1999 a new part of the main professional examination that is designed to test these skills, recognizing their fundamental importance for clinical psychiatrists.[22]

Structured critical appraisal is an active process that involves a systematic assessment of the key methodological aspects of the paper. In particular, critical appraisal focuses systematically on those aspects of the study methodology that are most likely to lead to unreliability of results. A number of checklists, designed to make the appraisal quicker and more systematic, have been produced for different research study designs.[23] For example, the critical appraisal of a systematic review involves an assessment of those aspects of methodology described in Chapter 6.1.1.2. A commonly used checklist for systematic reviews is shown in Table 2.

Example (continued)

Using the checklist, the review can be quickly critically appraised. It is a review of the effectiveness of antidepressants in dysthymia and so appears relevant to the clinical question. The authors have only

Box 1

Examples of the criteria for selection and review of articles for abstracting in *Evidence-Based Mental Health*

Articles are considered for abstracting if they meet the following criteria

Basic criteria
- Original or review articles
- In English
- About humans
- About topics that are important to the practice of clinicians in the broad field of mental health

Studies of prevention or treatment must meet these additional criteria
- Random allocation of participants to comparison groups
- Follow-up (endpoint assessment) of at least 80% of those entering the investigation
- Outcome measure of known or probable clinical importance
- Analysis consistent with study design.

Studies of diagnosis must meet these additional criteria
- Clearly identified comparison groups, at least one of which is free of the disorder or derangement of interest
- Interpretation of diagnostic standard without knowledge of test result
- Interpretation of test without knowledge of diagnostic standard result
- Diagnostic (gold) standard (e.g. diagnosis according to DSM-IV or ICD-10 criteria after assessment by clinically qualified interviewer) preferably with documentation of reproducible criteria for subjectively interpreted diagnostic standard (e.g. report of statistically significant measure of agreement among observers)
- Analysis consistent with study design

Studies of prognosis must meet these additional criteria
- Inception cohort (first onset or assembled at a uniform point in the development of the disease) of individuals, all initially free of the outcome of interest
- Follow-up of at least 80% of patients until the occurrence of a major study endpoint or to the end of the study
- Analysis consistent with study design

Studies of causation must meet these additional criteria
- Clearly identified comparison group for those at risk of, or having, the outcome of interest (i.e. randomized controlled trial, quasi-randomized controlled trial, non-randomized controlled trial, cohort analytical study with case-by-case matching or statistical adjustment to create comparable groups, case–control study)
- Masking of observers of outcomes to exposures (this criterion is assumed to be met if the outcome is objective), observers of exposures masked to outcomes for case–control studies, or masking of subjects to exposure for all other study designs
- Analysis consistent with study design

included randomized controlled trials, and this will make systematic error less likely and improve the reliability of the review. The literature search strategy is clearly documented and included electronic databases (Medline, Psyclit, Embase, Lilacs and the Cochrane Library), handsearching of journals, and correspondence with researchers active in the field. The quality of the randomized controlled trials was rated both from the description of the allocation of treatment and by assessing other methodological issues such as whether the primary analysis was done as an intention-to-treat analysis and the degree of blinding of the clinician and patient. It can be concluded that the reviewers have made a reasonable effort to identify the primary studies, although it is possible that other studies, perhaps with negative results, have not been published (publication bias, see Chapter 6.1.1.2).

The results of the primary studies are shown graphically as odds ratios (see Glossary) in Fig. 3. Odds ratios falling to the left of the vertical line indicate that the outcome (no treatment response) occurred less frequently in patients treated with the antidepressant. The smaller the odds ratio, the larger the treatment effect found in that particular study. For each study, the central diamond represents the most likely value of the odds ratio and the box around the odds ratio shows the 95 per cent confidence interval (**CI**). The larger studies (e.g. Thase *et al.*[24]) have narrower confidence intervals because they are larger and therefore have less random error and greater precision.

From the figure, it can be seen that, apart from the very small study by Stewart (1995) the odds ratios of the all the studies fall on the left-hand side of the line and therefore found approximately the same effect. There is considerable overlap in the confidence intervals from study to study. This means that there is unlikely to be significant heterogeneity between the studies (see Chapter 6.1.1.2). In the absence of heterogeneity, it was probably reasonable to combine the results of the studies to produce a pooled odds ratio which is shown as the bottom unfilled lozenge in the figure. Combining the study results produces a more precise estimate of the drug's relative effectiveness, with tighter confidence intervals. The overall pooled odds ratio for no treatment response for antidepressants compared with placebo is 0.68 (95 per cent CI (see Glossary), 0.59–0.78).

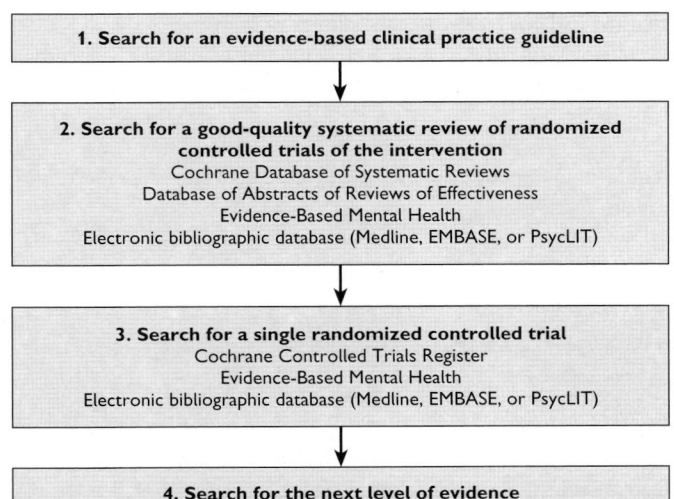

Fig. 2 A systematic approach to identifying the best evidence about a therapy.

Table 2 Checklist to assist the critical appraisal of a systematic review

Validity

1. Did the review address a clearly focused clinical question?
   Did the review describe:
       the population studied?
       the intervention given?
       the outcomes considered?

2. Did the authors select the right sort of studies for the review?
   The right studies would:
       address the review's question
       have an adequate study design (e.g. for a question re therapy, an RCT)

3. Were the important relevant studies included in the review?
       Which bibliographic databases were used?
       Personal contact with experts
       Search for unpublished as well as published studies
       Search for non-English language studies

4. Did the review's authors assess the quality of the included studies?
   Did they use:
       description of randomization?
       a rating scale?

Results

5. Were the results similar from study to study?
       Are the results of all the included studies clearly displayed?
       Are the results from different studies similar?
       If not, are the reasons for variations between studies discussed?

6. What is the overall result of the review?
       Is there a clear clinical conclusion (a clinical bottom-line)?
       What is it?
       What is the numerical result?

7. How precise are the results?
       Is there a confidence interval?

Clinical relevance of the results

8. Can I apply the results to my patient?
       Is this patient so different from those in the trial that the results do not apply?

9. Should I apply the results to my patient?
       How great would the benefit of therapy be for this particular patient?
       Is the intervention consistent with my patient's values and preferences?
       Were all the clinically important outcomes considered?
       Are the benefits worth the harms and costs?

RCT, randomized controlled trial.

Methods of using research findings at the level of individual patients

After the study has been critically appraised for its validity, the clinician needs to determine what the results are, and their importance for the patient. Patients in research studies are always different from those in real-life clinical practice in ways that may be difficult to assess. Therefore the use of results from research studies in clinical practice should be cautious and always requires a degree of extrapolation. The contribution of clinical epidemiology is in developing methods of applying research results to individual patients that are biologically

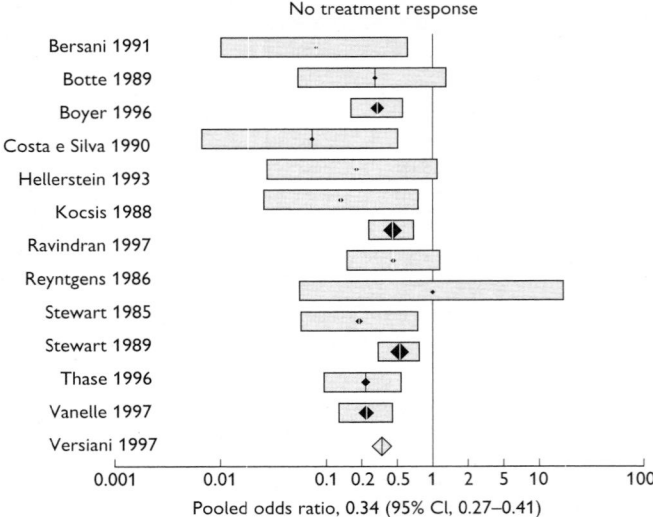

Fig. 3 Antidepressant versus placebo for the treatment of dysthymia. (Data from Lima and Moncrieff.[25])

and statistically robust and are explicit about any assumptions made. One of the most useful questions to ask when applying the results of a research study is: 'Is my patient so different from those in the study that the results cannot be used?'. The next step is to try to interpret the study results for a particular patient, in terms of his or her clinical characteristics and treatment preferences.

Odds ratios are often used in systematic reviews and meta-analyses because they have useful statistical properties. In particular, they allow treatment effects to be combined across trials with different event rates and of different durations. However, they are of limited clinical use because they are difficult to interpret clinically.[26]

A more clinically useful measure is the number needed to treat (**NNT**).[27] The NNT is an estimate of the number of patients that would need to be treated with the intervention of interest, compared with the alternative, in order to achieve one good outcome or to avoid one harmful outcome. The NNT is calculated by taking the reciprocal of the difference between the rates of the outcome of interest in the experimental and control groups.

Example (continued)

It may be considered that a selective serotonin uptake inhibitor (**SSRI**) is more appropriate then a tricyclic for patients with dysthymia because, in the review, acceptability (as measured by the overall drop-out rate from the clinical trials) was better for SSRIs than for tricyclics. A psychiatrist may want to know how effective an SSRI is likely to be in producing a full remission of symptoms rather than merely a response to treatment. The Cochrane review identifies two studies that directly answer this question. One of these[24] was a multicentre trial performed in 17 university-affiliated research clinics in the United States including 410 outpatients (mean age 42 years, 65 per cent women) who met DSM-IIIR criteria for primary dysthymia with early onset (occurring before age 21 years). One group of 134 patients were allocated to sertraline, initially 50 mg, which was increased at the physician's discretion in 50-mg increments after 3 weeks at weeks 4, 6, and 7 to a maximum dose of 200 mg/day. A second group of 136 patients were allocated to imipramine, increased weekly in 50-mg increments

from 50 to 300 mg/day unless a therapeutic response was achieved or adverse effects were dose limiting. The remaining 140 patients were allocated to matching placebo.

Appraising the validity of a randomized controlled trial

The appraisal of an individual randomized controlled trial also addresses issues of internal and external validity. The main difference compared with the appraisal of a systematic review is that the reader can appraise the trial directly, rather than relying on the author of the review to have made an adequate assessment of the quality of the studies included. The most important questions to answer during the appraisal of the article are those relating to methodological issues that have been randomly shown to affect the reliability of the results (Table 3).

This study[24] was a **randomized controlled trial**. Randomization was by a computer-generated schedule, although no details are provided about the **concealment of treatment allocation**. Concealment of allocation is one of the most important features to appraise in a randomized controlled trial, and refers to how well the treatment allocation of the next patient was concealed from the participating clinician.[28] If a clinician has definite knowledge of, or can reasonably predict, the next allocation, he may decide not to enter a patient if he favours either treatment in that specific case. This would obviously lead to a subversion of randomization and biased results. This is why methods of quasi-randomization, such as alternate allocation, are often unsatisfactory. The most satisfactory methods of random allocation are when allocation is performed by a third party following entry of the patient into the study, for example using a centralized telephone service. Concealment of allocation should be distinguished from **blinding** of treatment allocation. Blinding refers to whether the patient (**single blind**), or both the patient and the clinician (**double blind**), are kept unaware of which arm of the study the patient has been allocated to *following* randomization. Blinding protects against bias in the treatment during the trial and in the assessment of subjective outcomes, but can be difficult to maintain when the experimental treatment has characteristic side-effects (e.g. antidepressants). This study was reported to be double blind; however, it is difficult to tell how effective the blinding was and whether this affected the treatment that the patients received or the ratings of outcome.

Of the 410 patients who were randomized, 310 (75.6 per cent) completed the trial. The reasons for drop-out are clearly stated and all

Table 3 Questions that must be answered during the appraisal of an article

---

1. Was the assignment of the patients randomized?

2. Was the randomization list concealed?

3. Were all the subjects who entered the trial accounted for at its conclusion?

4. Were they analysed in the groups to which they were randomized?

5. Were subjects and clinicians 'blind' to which treatment was being received?

6. Other than the experimental treatment, were the groups treated equally?

7. Were the groups similar at the start of the trial?

---

the patients who entered the study are accounted for. Patients who drop out of a study may be different from those who complete it—this is a particular problem if there is **differential drop-out** between the arms of the study. For this reason, the most statistically reliable and clinically useful method of analysis is to include all patients who were randomized in the analysis. This is called an **intention-to-treat analysis (ITT)**. In the study by Thase *et al.*[24] the primary analysis was done on an ITT basis (with the exception of two patients who dropped out before the first follow-up assessment), and the patients were analysed in the groups to which they were randomized. However, follow-up analysis was not obtained after patients left the study and so the ITT analysis had to use the last available measure of outcome. This is a **last observation carried forward** analysis and introduces considerable uncertainty about the actual subsequent progress of the patients who left the study. The degree of this uncertainty depends on the proportion of patients who leave the study; generally, if fewer than 80 per cent of patients complete the trial, one should be cautious about the overall reliability of the results. An alternative approach to analysis that is often encountered in randomized controlled trials in psychiatry is the **endpoint** or **completers analysis**. This type of analysis includes only those patients who completed the trial and may give an idea of the comparative outcome in these patients. However, it may be misleading when there is a high drop-out rate, and when drop-out from the study is non-random, i.e. when there are systematic differences between drop-outs and completers, and perhaps also different reasons for drop-out between the comparison groups.

Lastly, although randomization will avoid bias in treatment allocation, it is possible that, by chance, the groups will be unbalanced on some key prognostic factors such as age, sex, and duration and severity of illness. Therefore it is important to assess the baseline characteristics of the patients to identify any obvious differences. In Thase *et al.*[24] the patients were reasonably similar on baseline characteristics at entry into the trial.

Are the results relevant for your patient?

To determine the relevance of the study to real-life patients, it is important to examine the inclusion and exclusion criteria of the trial. The main inclusion criteria are discussed above. Patients excluded from the trial were women who were pregnant or of child-bearing age but unwilling to use an effective contraceptive method. Exclusion criteria also included major medical conditions, bipolar disorder, psychosis, panic disorder, concurrent major depressive disorders, generalized anxiety disorder, history of alcohol or other drug dependency within the previous 12 months, serious suicidal risk, previous non-response to two or more adequate antidepressant trials, and use of psychotropic drugs within 2 weeks of enrolment. The use of the study results will have to take these inclusion and exclusion criteria into account, and the clinician needs to judge the relevance of the results for the individual patient.

What are the results?

Of the 134 patients treated with sertraline, 67 responded fully to treatment, giving a response rate, or experimental event rate (**EER**), of 50 per cent or a probability of full response of 0.5. In the placebo-treated group 39 of 140 patients fully responded, giving a control event rate (**CER**) of 28 per cent. Therefore the absolute difference between the rates was

$$EER - CER = 50 - 28 \text{ per cent} = 22 \text{ per cent}$$

and the difference between the probabilities is 0.22. This means that for every 100 patients treated with a tricyclic antidepressant, compared with placebo, 22 more responded. Therefore, to achieve one more full remission over 12 weeks, 100/22, or about five patients, would need to be treated (NNT) with sertraline.

A 95 per cent confidence interval can also be constructed for the NNT using the following formula to calculate the 95 per cent confidence interval for the absolute risk difference:

$$\text{absolute risk difference} = \pm 1.96\sqrt{\frac{CER(1 - CER)}{N(\text{control})} + \frac{EER(1 - EER)}{N(\text{experimental})}}$$

$$= \pm 1.96\sqrt{\frac{0.28(1 - 0.28)}{140} + \frac{0.50(1 - 0.50)}{134}}$$

$$= \pm 0.113.$$

This value is then added to and subtracted from absolute risk difference to produce the confidence interval for the rate, i.e. $0.22 + 0.113 = 0.333$ and $0.22 - 0.113 = 0.107$. The confidence interval for the NNT can then be calculated by taking the reciprocal of each of these values (NNTs are always rounded up to the nearest integer):

$$NNT = 5 \text{ (95 per cent CI, 3–10)}.$$

The odds ratio in this study was 0.39 (95 per cent CI, 0.24–0.64) (the odds ratio is for failure to achieve full remission).

The other study was also of 12 weeks duration and compared fluoxetine with placebo in 140 patients with dysthymia.[29] The patients in this trial were less chronic than in the study by Thase *et al.*[24], but the findings were similar. The EER was 44 per cent and the CER was 26 per cent, giving an NNT of 6 (95 per cent CI, 3 to infinity). The upper confidence interval includes infinity; this means that the result of this trial on its own is not statistically significant. The odds ratio was 0.45 (95 per cent CI, 0.20–1.01) (the odds ratio is for failure to achieve full remission).

Combining the two studies produces a pooled odds ratio of 0.41 (95 per cent CI, 0.27–0.62). The event rates and the duration of treatment in the two studies are similar and so a rough estimate of the pooled NNT can be obtained by simply pooling the results from the two studies. The EER is 48 per cent and the CER is 27 per cent. Therefore the absolute risk reduction is 21 per cent and the NNT is 5 (95 per cent CI, 4–10).

Interpretation of numbers needed to treat

The clinical interpretation of NNT depends on the seriousness of the outcome and the nature (and cost) of the intervention.

For example, if the number needed to treat with aspirin following acute stroke to avoid one death in the short-term is 100, this seems a very useful intervention because death is such a serious outcome that it is worth treating a lot of patients to save a few from dying—especially as aspirin is very cheap. Some examples of NNTs are given in Table 4.

Adjusting the NNT to the individual patient

It is often possible to calculate an NNT from a single randomized controlled trial or from a systematic review that provides the event rates. However, some meta-analyses only provide the odds ratio. There are methods for estimating the NNT by combining the odds ratio (**OR**) with the patient expected event rate (**PEER**).

Table 4 Examples of numbers needed to treat for interventions in psychiatry

Intervention	Outcome	NNT	95% CI	Reference
Cognitive therapy in bulimia nervosa	Long-term remission	2	1–4	30
Antidepressants in dysthymic disorder	Clinical response	5	3–10	25
Family therapy in schizophrenia	Relapse at 1 year	7	4–14	31
SSRIs compared with TCAs in depressive disorder	Remain in treatment at 6 weeks	39	20–426	32

SSRI, selective serotonin reuptake inhibitor; TCA, tricyclic antidepressant.

$$NNT = \frac{1 - PEER(1 - OR)}{(1 - PEER) \times PEER(1 - OR)}.$$

A psychiatrist may have evidence that in the dysthymic patients in his practice, the untreated remission rate over 12 weeks would be more likely to be around 10 per cent. Therefore the NNT would be

$$NNT = \frac{1 - [0.1 \times (1 - 0.41)]}{(1 - 0.1) \times 0.1 \times (1 - 0.41)}$$

$$= 18.$$

In other words, 18 patients would need to be treated with antidepressants to produce one full remission. This is obviously a much larger number of patients than the NNT derived from the trials and demonstrates that the NNT varies according to the expected event rate. It is usually assumed that a ratio measure of efficacy, such as the odds ratio, is more constant across different levels of baseline risk.

The NNT from a single study can also be extrapolated to an individual patient by dividing the PEER by the CER from the study. Using the values from the second study above, this would be 10/26 = 0.38. The NNT is then divided by this figure to produce a rough estimate of the NNT in this particular patient, i.e. 6/0.38 ≈ 16.

Critical appraisal of other research designs

The approach taken to the appraisal of research designs applied to other clinical questions is similar to that outlined above. Rather than passively reading the article or abstract, the clinician actively searches out the most important methodological features to determine the reliability of the study. By applying the methods developed by clinical epidemiologists, the results presented in the paper can be used to calculate more clinically meaningful measures. These can, in turn, be tailored to suit the characteristics of the individual patient. The clinician needs to develop a practical knowledge of the tools to allow him to use them routinely and quickly in clinical practice and also to develop sufficient familiarity to be able describe the results of studies to colleagues and patients.

Glossary

- **Absolute risk reduction (risk difference)** is the absolute arithmetic difference in the risk of the adverse outcome between control group (CER) and experimental group (EER). When an intervention increases the probability of a beneficial outcome it is known as the absolute benefit increase (ABI).

- **Confidence interval (CI)** is the range within which the true value of a statistical measure can be expected to lie. The CI is usually accompanied by a percentage value (usually 95 per cent) which shows the level of confidence that the true value lies within this range.

- **Event rate** is the proportion of patients in a group in whom the event is observed. In control patients, this is called the control event rate (CER) and in experimental patients it is called the experimental event rate (EER). The patient expected event rate (PEER) refers to the rate of events that would be expected in a patient who received no treatment or conventional treatment.

- **Number needed to treat (NNT)** is the reciprocal of the absolute risk reduction and is the number of patients that need to be treated to prevent one bad outcome or to achieve one beneficial outcome.

- **Odds ratio** is the odds of the outcome in the experimental group divide by the odds of the outcome in the control group. The odds ratio is often reported in meta-analyses because of its useful statistical properties.

Further reading

Sackett, D.L., Richardson, S., Rosenberg, W., and Haynes, R.B. (1997). *Evidence-based medicine: how to practise and teach EBM*. Churchill Livingstone, London.

Geddes, J.R. and Harrison, P.J. (1997). Evidence-based psychiatry: closing the gap between research and practice. *British Journal of Psychiatry*, **176**, 220–5.

References

1. Smith, R. (1996). What clinical information do doctors need? *British Medical Journal*, **313**, 1062–8.
2. Mulrow, C.D. (1994). Rationale for systematic reviews. *British Medical Journal*, **309**, 597–9.
3. Geddes, J.R., Wilczynski, N., Reynolds, S., Szatmari, P., and Streiner, D.L. (1999). Evidence-based mental health—the first year. *Evidence-Based Mental Health*, **2**, 3–5.
4. Pippard, J. (1992). Audit of electroconvulsive treatment in two national health service regions. *British Journal of Psychiatry*, **160**, 621–37.
5. Hermann, R.C., Dorwart, R.A., Hoover, C.W., and Brody, J. (1995).

Variation in ECT use in the United States. *American Journal of Psychiatry*, **152**, 869–75.

6. Meise, U., Kurz, M., and Fleischhacker, W.W. (1994). Antipsychotic maintenance treatment of schizophrenia patients: is there a consensus? *Schizophrenia Bulletin*, **20**, 215–25.

7. Lehman, A.F. and Steinwachs, D.M. (1998). Patterns of usual care for schizophrenia: initial results from the Schizophrenia Patient Outcomes Research Team (PORT) Client Survey. *Schizophrenia Bulletin*, **24**, 11–20.

8. Wells, K.B., Katon, W., Rogers, B., and Camp, P. (1994). Use of minor tranquilizers and antidepressant medications by depressed outpatients: results from the medical outcomes study. *American Journal of Psychiatry*, **151**, 694–700.

9. Hirschfeld, R.M., Keller, M.B., Panico, S., *et al.* (1997). The National Depressive and Manic–Depressive Association consensus statement on the undertreatment of depression. *Journal of the American Medical Association*, **277**, 333–40.

10. Munizza, C., Tibaldi, G., Bollini, P., Pirfo, E., Punzo, F., and Gramaglia, F. (1995). Prescription pattern of antidepressants in out-patient psychiatric practice. *Psychological Medicine*, **25**, 771–8.

11. Evidence-Based Medicine Working Group (1992). Evidence-based medicine. A new approach to teaching the practice of medicine. *Journal of the American Medical Association*, **268**, 2420–5.

12. Chalmers, I., Dickersin, K., and Chalmers, T.C. (1992). Getting to grips with Archie Cochrane's agenda. *British Medical Journal*, **305**, 786–8.

13. Field, M.J. and Lohr, K.N. (1990). *Clinical practice guidelines: direction of a new agency*. Institute of Medicine, Washington, DC.

14. Eccles, M., Freemantle, N., and Mason, J. (1988). North of England evidence based guidelines development project: methods of developing guidelines for efficient drug use in primary care. *British Medical Journal*, **316**, 1232–5.

15. Grimshaw, J.M. and Russell, I.T. (1993). Effect of clinical guidelines on medical practice: a systematic review of rigorous evaluations. *Lancet*, **342**, 1317–22.

16. Oxman, A.D., Thomson, M.A., Davis, D.A., and Haynes, R.B. (1995). No magic bullets: a systematic review of 102 trials of interventions to improve professional practice. *Canadian Medical Association Journal*, **153**, 1423–31.

17. Katon, W., Von Korff, M., Lin, E., *et al.* (1995). Collaborative management to achieve treatment guidelines. Impact on depression in primary care. *Journal of the American Medical Association*, **273**, 1026–31.

18. Kahn, D.A., Docherty, J.P., Carpenter, D., and Frances, A. (1997). Consensus methods in practice guideline development: a review and description of a new method. *Psychopharmacology Bulletin*, **33**, 631–9.

19. Frances, A.J., Docherty, J.P., and Kahn, D.A. (1998). The Expert Consensus Guideline Series: treatment of bipolar disorder. *Journal of Clinical Psychiatry*, **57**, 1–88.

20. Jadad, A.R. and Gagliardi, A. (1998). Rating health information on the Internet: navigating to knowledge or to Babel? *Journal of the American Medical Association*, **279**, 611–14.

21. Silberg, W.M., Lundberg, G.D., and Musacchio, R.A. (1997). Assessing, controlling, and assuring the quality of medical information on the Internet: caveant lector et viewor–let the reader and viewer beware. *Journal of the American Medical Association*, **277**, 1244–5.

22. Critical Review Paper Working Party (1997). MRCPsych Part II examination: proposed Critical Review Paper. *Psychiatric Bulletin*, **21**, 381–2.

23. Sackett, D.L., Richardson, S., Rosenberg, W., and Haynes, R.B. *Evidence-Based Medicine: how to practise and teach EBM*. Churchill Livingstone, London.

24. Thase, M.E., Fava, M., Halbreich, U., *et al.* (1996). A placebo-controlled, randomized clinical trial comparing sertraline and imipramine for the treatment of dysthymia. *Archives of General Psychiatry*, **53**, 777–84.

25. Lima, M.S. and Moncrieff, J. (1998). A comparison of drugs versus placebo for the treatment of dysthymia: a systematic review. In *Cochrane database of systematic reviews* (ed. M. Oakley-Brown), Update Software.

26. Sackett, D.L., Deeks, J.J., and Altman, D.G. (1996). Down with odds ratios! *Evidence-Based Medicine*, **1**, 164–6.

27. Cook, R.J. and Sackett, D.L. (1995). The number needed to treat: a clinically useful measure of treatment effect. *British Medical Journal*, **310**, 452–4.

28. Shulz, K. (2000). Assessing allocation concealment and blinding in randomised controlled trials: why bother? *Evidence-Based Mental Health*, **3**, in press.

29. Vanelle, J.M., Attar, L.D., Poirier, M.F., Bouhassira, M., Blin, P., and Olie, J.P. (1997). Controlled efficacy study of fluoxetine in dysthymia. *British Journal of Psychiatry*, **170**, 345–50.

30. Fairburn, C.G., Norman, P.A., Welch, S.L., O'Connor, M.E., Doll, H.A., and Peveler, R.C.A prospective study of outcome in bulimia nervosa and the long-term effects of three psychological treatments. *Archives of General Psychiatry*, **52**, 304–12.

31. Mari, J.J. and Streiner, D. (1998). Family intervention for schizophrenia. In *Cochrane database of systematic reviews* (ed. M. Oakley-Brown), Update Software.

32. Anderson, I.M. and Tomenson, B.M. (1995). Treatment discontinuation with selective serotonin reuptake inhibitors compared with tricyclic antidepressants: a meta-analysis. *British Medical Journal*, **310**, 1433–8.

2

The scientific basis of psychiatric aetiology

2.1 Historical development

2.1.1 Historical development of ideas about psychiatric aetiology

German E. Berrios

This chapter chronicles the 'evolution of ideas about aetiology (i.e. the concept of causality) in psychiatry' and seeks to clarify the following:

- the meaning of cause, causality, and aetiology in general
- how these ideas came to influence views on mental disorder
- whether in their current state they are helping or hindering psychiatry.

Both 'mental disorder' and 'cause' have changed their meanings throughout time. 'Cause' and 'causality' are the two ancient concepts that underlie the fancy medical term 'aetiology'. The act of explaining in psychiatry will depend on how these two terms are defined. For example, according to seventeenth century physics, 'cause' and 'effect' were ontologically stable entities (e.g. a billiard ball hitting another and causing it to move). For as long 'disease' was considered to be a stable object, the physical model worked. However, by the middle of the nineteenth century, a dynamic view of disease as a shifting state resulting from altered physiology came to the fore. This led to a major revision of the definition of causality.[1,2]

Mental disorder does not lend itself well to linear explanations of the following type: (a) a lesion causes a disorder of brain anatomy; (b) a disordered brain leads to disordered function; (c) disordered function (behaviour) dislocates psychosocial competence. Undue emphasis on (a), (b), or (c) leads to the so-called medical, psychological, and social 'models' of mental disease.[3] Apart from misusing the concept of 'model', such taxonomies fragment the causality process and render themselves sterile. It would be more useful to ask in what subtle way (a), (b), and (c) actually interact with one another to give rise to a mental illness.

Cause and aetiology: words and concepts

The *Oxford English Dictionary* (second edition) defines 'cause' as 'that which produces an effect; that which gives rise to any action, phenom-

enon, or condition', and 'aetiology' as 'that branch of medical science which investigates the causes and origin of diseases; the scientific exposition of the origin of any disease'. Through time, however, both terms (and their accompanying concepts) have undergone repeated metamorphosis.

The Latin stem *causa* meant 'reason, motive, inducement, occasion, and opportunity'. It translated the Greek αιτια and αιτιον (stems of 'aetiology'), which themselves started by meaning 'origin', 'ground', and 'the occasion of something bad' (although for the third meaning the Romans used the word *crimen*). To the Greeks, 'cause' was a relational concept, i.e. one 'without which another thing (called effect) cannot be'. In the event, *causa* came into most European languages, and up to the late medieval period all vernacular renditions shared with Aristotle[4] the recognition of four types of cause:

(1) material

(2) formal

(3) efficient

(4) final.

By the late Renaissance, however, a debate had broken out as to whether the four meanings (a) were 'really' different, (b) might work better when 'combined', or (c) were of equal importance or in fact one was more important than the others. Also, since the scientific revolution of the seventeenth century and the development of 'mechanicist' models of the world,[5] the third efficient type became the core meaning of causation.

The fourfold classification suggests the question as to which of the four senses of Aristotelian 'causation' was more influential in medicine. The view that mental illness was 'caused' by demons means something different depending on whether cause is understood as formal, material, or efficient. The received view is that it followed sense (3), i.e. that physicians believed that there were real objects called demons who could cause madness.[6] Thus understood, this aetiological view can easily be derided, but it is possible that physicians at that time (and all knew their Aristotle well) had in mind sense (2), i.e. that 'evil' was the 'formal meaning' of madness.

Aetiology, case notes, and narratives

Medical men of all periods have produced narratives to account for the 'diseases' affecting their charges. Such narratives had to be persuasive.

Hippocrates' case notes,[7] written as *aides-mémoire*, included a personal history and a history of the disease, but lacked crucial information about the cause of the disease. Causal explanations were not incorporated in medical case reports until much later. The medieval *concilia* (advice for neophytes) contained information on the causes of disease, ranging from 'constitutions' to events considered as relevant to a specific disease. The 'causal events' were more often dictated by tradition and theory than by 'observation and experience' (in the sense given to these terms by Sydenham in the seventeenth century).

The start of postmortem studies in the sixteenth century generated correlational data which led Morgagni and Bichat to place disease within the body. This interpretation of 'cause' provided the foundation for the 'anatomoclinical' model of disease and for modern medicine. By the middle of the nineteenth century, case histories had become full narratives comprising *descriptio subjecti*, *praegressa remota*, *origo morbi*, *praegressa proxima*, *status praesens*, and *cursus morbi*.[8] This narrative style, in turn, influenced the way in which medical 'causality' itself was to be conceived (see below).

Aetiological models before the nineteenth century

Hobbes and Bacon challenged the four Aristotelian definitions of cause and provided a new meaning for 'efficient cause'. Within medicine, starting with Sydenham and Willis and ending with Morgagni and Bichat, this new meaning led to a transformation of external causes into internal mechanisms. However, the old notion of antecedent, external, longitudinal, or diachronic cause did not disappear, and the two views are found side by side during the nineteenth century.

A second challenge to the old concept of cause came during the eighteenth century in the work of Hume, whose attack on the epistemological validity of 'efficient causes' set two logical requirements to future applications of the model: (1) that cause and effect were *different* entities, and (2) that the former occurred *before* the latter—'a cause is an object precedent and contiguous to another, and so united with it, that the idea of the one determines the mind to form the idea of the other, and the impression of the one to form a more lively idea of the other'.[9] This 'seriatim view' of causality governed the work of the early nineteenth-century alienists and many, such as Esquirol,[10] produced long lists of external (independent) causal events. Later, their interest shifted towards brain changes purportedly brought about by such external causes.

As neurosciences and chemistry developed during the second half of the nineteenth century, internal changes or mechanisms began to be considered as a new form of 'simultaneous', 'structural', or 'synchronic' causality. In contrast with this, and partly because no research was being done on 'external antecedents', the old causal lists became stereotyped and eventually lost most of their explanatory power (for a fuller account see Berrios[11] and Berrios and Porter[12]). However, this does not mean that they were abandoned. They were transformed into other theories and can be found surviving in psychodynamic theory, the concept of life events, and in the narrative component of case notes where they provide the rhetoric of bedside medical explanations. This is the reason why psychiatric textbooks continue listing the events preceding the onset of the disease as 'efficient causes'. Griesinger once referred to these as 'tables of physical and moral causes'.[13]

The first half of the nineteenth century

Writers on 'efficient causes' (or longitudinal, external, antecedent, or diachronic causality)

Bayle

Many consider the report by A.L.J. Bayle (1799–1858), in 1822, of six patients combining 'chronic arachnoiditis' and 'symptomatic phrenitis' as the beginning of neuropsychiatry in France,[14,15] i.e. of the view that all psychiatric disorders have an 'organic aetiology'.[16] However, Bayle did not draw this conclusion in his dissertation. But after the death of his mentor Antoine Royer-Collard he felt free to write: 'most of mental disorders are caused by a chronic, primitive inflammation of the brain membranes'.[17] At the time, Bayle had as little evidence for this statement as for the more specific claim that the 'inflammation started in the membranes and from there spread (secondarily) to the cortex'.

Bayle's views on 'causality' are historically important because of the myth that was created about his contribution, and to which he contributed. For example, in later years he believed that 'the chronic meningitis I have described is a primary disease totally different from acute arachnoiditis and of the chronic state of the latter. The term *chronic* has only been used to emphasize its duration and slow course'.[17] Chronic meningitis resulted from three types of causes: 'predisposing, occasional, and efficient (or proximal).' **Predisposing causes** were being a male, neither too young or too old, having a sanguine temperament, being in the military, having family or personal history of the disorder, being sedentary, abusing alcohol, and having suffered from sunstroke, blows about the head, venereal disease, suppression of haemorrhoidal bleeding, and disappointments and frustrations.

Amongst the **efficient causes**, Bayle listed 'cerebral congestion' which he viewed as a final common pathway. Considering a pathophysiological state as an efficient 'cause' may seem strange to a modern reader. But it is a historical fact that physiology, as a conceptual mediator between anatomy and behaviour, had not yet fully developed during the 1820s. This led Bayle, like Rostan, to conceive of 'congestion' of the brain as an independent brain state (L.L. Rostan (1791–1866) was a French physician and neuropathologist who did important work on the pathophysiology of stroke). By redefining the old efficient causes as predisposing and the internal mechanisms as the real efficient causes, Bayle paved the way for a new style of thinking about psychiatric causes that was to be taken very seriously during the second half of the nineteenth century.

Griesinger

Wilhelm Griesinger (1817–1868) was a German physician and alienist who acted as the agent of change between a psychiatry based on the concepts of *Naturphilosophie* and a new positivist science based upon the study of the brain.[18] When he wrote the second edition of his *Manual* (1861), the discussion of cause in medicine and psychiatry in Europe was beginning to be influenced by the radical ideas of Claude Bernard (1813–1878) who believed that causal information obtained from the statistical analysis of groups rarely, if ever, helped the understanding of individual cases.[19,20] Griesinger dedicated one chapter of his book to 'causes of insanity' (a conceptual introduction), a second to 'predisposing causes' (general and special), and a third to 'modes of actions of causes' (psychical, mixed and organic). Remarkable in detail, and common sense, these chapters are an excellent compendium of the state of the concept of causality in psychiatry by the middle of the nineteenth century. According to Griesinger:[13]

> under the head causes in mental as in general pathology are understood all the different classes of circumstance to which may be ascribed an influence on the development of the disease although their mode of connection may be variously exhibited. The causes comprehend, on the one hand, the external circumstances (nationality, climate, season of the year) under the influence of which insanity is generally, with more or less frequency, observed; on the other hand they signify certain external injuries (sunstroke, wounds of the head) of which insanity is frequently a consequence; finally they comprehend certain internal states depending on the organism itself (hereditary predisposition, previous disease, or other general disturbances of the organic mechanisms, such as disease of the lungs, the genital organs, etc.) which we know by experience have an influence in the development of insanity.

In other words, Griesinger believed that a complete aetiological account of a given mental disorder included a combination of 'diachronic, antecedent longitudinal or efficient causality' with knowledge of internal states of the organism itself (i.e. internal mechanisms or structural, simultaneous or synchronic explanation). Patriotically, Griesinger continued:[13]

> The German psychologists claim the merit of having always understood the etiology and pathogeny of insanity more thoroughly and correctly, and of having more successfully elaborated it, than the French school. Whilst the latter, partly even in recent times (Moreau de Jonnès (sic), Brierre, Parchappe), still adhere to abstract tables of physical and moral causes, in which drunkenness, epilepsy, ambition, prostitution, politics, loss of fortune, andc. are ranged as being of equal importance, the German psychologists (Heinroth and Ideler from the psychic side—Bergman, Flemming, Jacobi, Jensen, Nasse, Zeller, &c. partly with greater regard to bodily causes) have for long insisted on investigating the causes in each individual case; and it has been more the plan with us most carefully to consider all the circumstances, in their various connections, which can influence the development of the morbid state.

The question arises, however, as to how causes can be identified at the individual level. In this respect, Griesinger believed that:[13]

> the inquiry into the history of the case ought to embrace the whole of the bodily and mental antecedents of the individual. It must commence ab ovo, indeed from former generations—family predisposition—and minutely trace the bodily developments, the habitual state of health, the nature of the diseases to which the patient is subject, and of those which he has already has.

But such an exhaustive case-taking would leave the alienist with an enormous amount of data. One method of organizing an aetiological narrative and identifying specific factors is to be guided by theory. But there are theories and theories, and Griesinger warns against the 'French way': 'we must here endeavour by every means to keep the mind unbiased by this or that theory, and from one-sided preference

of one or of certain series of causes; for example the somatic or the mental.' Two criteria must be used instead—temporal association and reliable statistics:[13]

> An influence of causation can naturally be attributed with most certainty to those circumstances whose mode of action can be clearly traced, and whose effects therefore may be considered as physiological necessities; or, where this is not the case, to those whose influence is established by reliable statistics. A slight gastric affection, haemorrhoids, or a transient cutaneous eruption, cannot for example, be considered as causes, because no statistics warrant the opinion, no visible connection exists between these affections and insanity either as to their gravity or nature.

In other words, the alienist must resort to good old Humean causality. A realist, Griesinger concludes:[13]

> In some cases all etiological data utterly fail, and the insanity originates gradually, like many other chronic diseases, from influences wholly unknown...

With regard to causal thinking, Griesinger can thus be considered as a 'transitional' writer, i.e. one who pays attention to both 'efficient causes' and 'internal mechanisms'

Morel

Bénédict-Augustin Morel (1809–1873), who was born in Vienna, was a French alienist who, among other things, proposed the so-called 'degeneration theory'.[21] According to this theory, which had as a background the Christian myth of 'original sin', mental disorder can start at any time as a result of an environmental cause (e.g. alcoholism), the said disorder can become inheritable (by means of a Lamarckian mechanism), and when passed on from generation to generation it can become ever worse until all reproductive capacity is lost ('degeneration' theory).[22,23] Morel coined the term démence précoce, developed a model to link the neuroses with the autonomic nervous system, and wrote with much sense on epilepsy, classification, and aetiology.

A Roman Catholic, Morel's aetiological speculations are based on Aquinas's view that 'the body confers individuality on the mind [l'âme]'. The latter has a natural affinity for the former and would be incomplete without it. Without the direct intervention of God, the 'mind alone lacks in clear ideas'. Mind and body related in two ways: '(1) essential links without which the substantial unity would not be possible and which underlie normality, and (2) accidental links (in the sense of occasional) which vary according to the individual and are the domain where the will and human liberty operate'.[24] Accidental links influence essential links.

Morel believed that 'Madness develops in the wake of a change in the links between body and mind'. Because changes taking place in the body are the most common of all possible changes, madness is 'a brain disease, idiopathic or sympathetic, that deprives the individual from his physiological and psychological functions, the exercise of his moral freedom, his actions, tendencies and feelings and that affects totally or partially his intellectual function'.[24]

His views hardened in later work: 'the conventional division of the causes of mental illness between physical and moral (psychological) is no longer adequate to the current needs of science' because it is based on statistics which are too superficial to detect interactions between real events. (The influence of Claude Bernard, with whom Morel shared lodgings in Paris when a student, is evident here.) For example, 'it may be said that someone's madness was related to alcohol abuse and hence that it has a *physical* cause. However, alcohol abuse is a complex phenomenon that may result from habituation or emotional upset or from earlier mental disorder.'[25] In this case, Morel argued, it cannot even be decided whether the 'cause' of the person's current mental illness is physical or moral.

After reviewing the moral and physical causes proposed by others, Morel designed an **aetiological** classification of mental disorders: 'Three elements are needed to operate this classification: predisposition, occasional [efficient] cause, and a functional change or lesion [internal mechanism]'.[25] His classification included six groups: hereditary insanities, insanities due to intoxication, insanities caused by the transformation of certain neuroses, idiopathic insanities, sympathetic insanities, and dementia.[25]

Like Griesinger, Morel was also a transitional writer, i.e. he believed that efficient causes were incomplete, and suggested that 'internal mechanisms' also be considered as causes. One problem with 'efficient causes', when defined as 'predisposing' or 'remote' events, is that their 'truth' can only be evidenced probabilistically (i.e. by means of correlations). In other words, it is not expected that predisposition P applies to all cases. However, there is no way of telling which cases are so affected. 'Internal mechanisms', on the other hand, can be considered as 'personalized' explanations in that they are a *sine qua non* with regard to a particular individual. This creates an interesting question, namely whether the 'essence' or 'definition' of a disease should be based on the existence of its given internal mechanism (regardless of whether or not its behavioural expression is present). This was not clear during the nineteenth century, and indeed is not clear now.

An interesting dialectic play also affects the relationship between efficient causes and internal mechanisms. The former, although presenting themselves as contextualizers (i.e. as links connecting the subject to his or her environment), can only behave as probabilistic statements. The latter, although (usually) narrow biological claims, can behave as more clearly demonstrable *vis-à-vis* the individual.

In summary, the historical process described above is one of a gradual 'internalization of causes'.

The second half of the nineteenth century

The fact that during the second half of the nineteenth century 'internal mechanisms' were considered as the most important form of causal explanation requires further analysis. Both positive (i.e. contributing to the development of 'internal explanations') and negative factors (i.e. undermining the value of efficient causes) played a role in this change.

The **positive factors** included:

- the rapid increase, during the nineteenth century, of knowledge about the structure and organization of the brain[26,27]

- the development of new theories of the relationship between brain and mind[28]

- the predominance of academic psychiatry, which preferred disease-related concepts to person-related concepts.

Important **negative factors** were:

- the challenge to probabilistic causality (see the views of Claude Bernard above)

- the absence of multivariate statistical models able to handle interactions between efficient causes

- the general cultural shift from historical to structural explanations which started in linguistics[29,30] towards the end of the century and soon extended to other disciplines.

With regard to neuropsychiatric scientific dogma and accompanying social practices, the second half of the nineteenth century is similar to our own time. They also believed that only neuroscience could explain mental disorder, that descriptive psychopathology was obsolete and redundant, and that once brain lesions and patterns of inheritance were found, there would be little need for any other form of social approach to mental disorder. These beliefs were picked up by governments and university authorities alike. University hospitals were financially favoured at the expense of state hospitals, and clinical professorships (supported by funding allocated to medical education) were filled by basic scientists with scanty clinical knowledge and little interest in medical students. The Freudian backlash is only one of the historical consequences of these wrong-headed policies.

The changes noted above did not cause alienists to disown antecedent causality altogether. Rather, they led them to an increasing interest in 'internal structure or mechanisms' as shown by opinion-makers such as Meynert, Jackson, Wernicke, and von Monakow. In general, academic psychiatrists were more enthusiastic about the internal mechanisms view than asylum psychiatrists, and this was yet another reason for them to feud.[31]

To understand the idea of 'internal mechanism', the concept of 'mechanism' must be briefly discussed. Defined as 'the mode in which an act or a series of acts is performed, as the mechanism of respiration or of parturition',[32] the concept was rapidly changing, particularly in the context of biology[33] and medicine. One reason for this was the waning of 'vitalism', i.e. the view that life was assisted by the presence of some ineffable organizational force. Once this principle was abandoned, mechanisms themselves became the final object of research: 'mechanism is the view that every biological event is a pattern of non-biological occurrences'.[34] This was reinforced by the establishment of anatomy and physiology as the explanatory sciences in brain research. This is one of the reasons why, at the time, the terms 'mechanism' and 'process' became synonyms.[35] An excellent account of the 'metaphysics and epistemology of functional explanations' in biology is given by Rosenberg.[36]

We shall now briefly describe the work of those late nineteenth century writers who supported the view that 'internal mechanisms' were the true causes of disease. Little will be said about the twentieth century, because there is no evidence that later aetiological models are any better than those discussed here. For example, it is not often realized that aetiological research using techniques such as positron emission tomography or genetics is still based on nineteenth-century linear assumptions (i.e. the more of one, the more of the other, or vice versa). Thus current researchers have profited little from the lessons of history and have neglected the conceptual proposals of Meynert and von Monakow (described below) and of Jackson.

Writers on 'internal mechanisms' as causes (simultaneous, structural, or synchronic causality)

Meynert

Theodor Meynert (1833–1892), who was Professor of Psychiatry at Vienna, developed a view of mental illness based on the following assumptions.

1. All psychological processes had an organic basis (Meynert believed in a form of eliminative materialism[37]).

2. The brain was a network of innate and acquired reflex arcs (for a discussion of the relevance of reflex arc theory to nineteenth-century neurosciences, see Fearing[38]).

3. Because 'association' pathways co-ordinated and stored information and connected cortical with subcortical sites, they were crucial to mental functioning. The term 'association' in this context remains closely related to the tenets of the so-called 'association psychology' movement which, since Locke, had been the official view of philosophical empiricism. It survived well into the nineteenth century when it was supported by most alienists.[39–41]

4. Blood flow was one the central regulators of brain function (these ideas have been considered as forerunners of neuroimaging[42,43]).

These views influenced Meynert's students Freud and Wernicke.

Meynert has been seen as a precursor of current neuroscientific thinking.[42] However, claims that mental disorders are 'disorders of the brain' or that 'blood flow is relevant to brain function' mean little unless they are anchored onto a physiopathological theory. In this regard, it is sobering to remember that at the time of Meynert the full concept of 'neurone' had not yet developed. On the other hand, his neuroscientific views (like current ones) included metaphors and persuasory devices that created the mirage of 'absolute truth', achieved coherence by incorporating hidden (and in principle not testable) assumptions (this statement paraphrases a critical observation on Meynert's work by Kraepelin, quoted by Lesky[31]), and capitalized on the belief that the neurosciences alone could resolve all the problems of psychiatry.

Meynert was appointed to a chair of clinical psychiatry on the strength of his anatomical discoveries but without having had any real clinical experience. This led to a bitter struggle with the Vienna asylum psychiatrists. After Meynert's death, however, Vienna University appointed Krafft-Ebing, who believed that 'the results of research in related fields will be of value to psychiatry, but true psychiatry's progress will only result from unchangeable and unconditional observation and description of the clinical phenomena'.[44]

More than any of the other alienists mentioned in this chapter, Meynert disregarded external (predisposing or efficient) causal factors in favour of internal mechanisms. His aetiological ideas were the point of convergence of three processes, which all started at the beginning of the nineteenth century:

(1) a *reduction ad absurdum* of Cabanis's old view that the brain secreted thoughts as the liver bile;

(2) a resigned acceptance of the fact that in the field of mental illness the anatomoclinical model had to work without physiopathology and semantics;

(3) the redefinition of efficient cause in terms of internal mechanism.

With respect to the last of these processes, it has rightly been claimed that:[44]

> The explanatory system in Meynert does not really seek to establish a cause-effect relationship ... he simply states how psychological phenomena appear as the brain changes its structure and function. The crux of his doctrine was that, in opposition to Griesinger in whom there are two separate groups of phenomena, physical and psychological, Meynert considers all these phenomena and meaning exactly the same so that he does not have to explain at all how the psychological is born out of the physical.

Wernicke

Karl Wernicke (1848–1905) made three important contributions to psychiatry.[45]

1. He developed a model to encompass all brain-related diseases (both psychiatric and neurological).

2. He developed a pathophysiological model to mediate between the brain and behaviour. Until then such a model had been absent from psychiatry.

3. He introduced the first 'neuropsychological approach' to mental symptoms.

Central to Wernicke's model was the idea that the projection and (transcortical) association fibres of the brain were the organ of consciousness and of the highest intellectual functions. Hence disease of the association system generated mental illness. In this sense, Wernicke's 'organ of association' is redolent of the current concept of neural network. In current jargon, he was more of a connectionist than a conventional localizationist (for a discussion of connectionism and psychopathology, see Stein and Ludik[46]). Like his teacher Meynert, Wernicke believed that pathological changes in the association system (i.e. an internal mechanism) were the 'true' cause of mental illness.

von Monakow

Constantin von Monakow (1853–1930) was born in Russia, but at the age of 10 he emigrated with his family to Dresden. He trained as a physician in Zurich, where he later worked as a neuropathologist and neurologist. Despite making important discoveries, he had to wait until 1912 before his private research institute and clinic were incorporated into the University of Zurich.[47,48]

Together with Mourgue (a French psychiatrist), von Monakow wrote one of the most important (and neglected) books on psychopathology of the twentieth century.[49] The authors start by proposing the notion of *horme*, i.e. the 'tendency of all living beings to develop all their genetic potential. *Horme* (from the Greek ορμη, impulsion, that which sets something in motion) was a 'property of the living protoplasm'. In the human, *horme* expressed itself in the instincts that subserved the preservation of each bodily organ, development, the species, society, and culture and religion. In each individual, horme is governed by syneidesis, i.e. by a principle that regulates and balances instincts in the interest of the individual.

Based on these principles, Monakow and Mourgue developed a neuropsychiatric model of the type that Guiraud has called 'dynamo-morphological'.[50] By considering neuropsychiatry as a subfield of biology, the authors were able to adopt two crucial notions—'chronogenetic localization' and 'diaschisis'.

Chronogenetic localization

According to this concept (borrowed from Richard Semon (1859–1918), a professor of zoology at Jena University, who proposed a theory of organic memory based on the notion of the 'engram'[51,52]) 'time' is the crucial parameter of all neuropsychiatric phenomena. Functions (e.g. movement) are processes which, like music, unfold in time and according to a specific 'kinetic melody'. Hence it would be a mistake to attempt to localize processes (i.e. brain functions) in terms of specific brain sites (i.e. space alone). It would also be wrong to localize mental symptoms on specific brain addresses for, like movements, their localization was also in time. Influenced by Jackson, von Monakow and Mourgue believed that chronogenetic localization was a late acquisition in evolutionary time, and hence regarded it as a complex but unstable mechanism.

One interesting implication is that the 'chronogenetic' localization of neuropsychiatric symptoms cannot be studied by means of either cross-sectional studies or traditional longitudinal studies (i.e. as collections of cross-sectional snapshots). Neuropsychiatric symptoms unfold in time according to their own kinetic melody; for example, a hallucination can only be fully understood when the entire 'token' or hallucinatory episode has been completed, and this may take minutes or hours. This allows real longitudinal information on specific variables to be collected and integrated (e.g. modulations in intensity, changes in imagery, and accompanying emotions). Such an integrated and longitudinal knowledge is a crucial source of aetiological information.

Diaschisis

Diaschisis (from the Greek διασχιζω, I separate at a distance) refers to sudden and reversible clinical (usually negative) phenomena seen in the wake of 'shock' caused by localized lesions of the central nervous system. Its defining element is that it cannot be explained in terms of the mere extension and localization of the brain lesion. For example, a hemiplegia includes more functional deficits than the lesion can explain. Inhibition differs from diaschisis in that the former results from the activity of known nervous connection.

Two conclusions follow:

(1) some mental symptoms may result from diaschisis, i.e. have no direct anatomical localization;

(2) because chronogenetically localized functions are more unstable, their disorder is likely to give rise to more mental symptoms.

Summary and conclusions

This chapter started with a description of the historical vicissitudes of the four Aristotelian definitions of cause (formal, material, efficient, and final). The Aristotelian model was challenged by Hobbes and Bacon during the seventeenth century, and by Hume during the eighteenth century, and on both occasions the way in which doctors defined aetiology had to be adjusted.

During the nineteenth century, the concept of efficient causality (interpreted in terms of predisposing and remote causes, i.e. causes predating the onset of illness and external to the subject) was gradually found wanting and was replaced by the idea of an 'internal mechan-ism', i.e. changes that occur in the very substratum of behaviour and which are simultaneous and coexistent with the mental symptoms themselves. A host of historical reasons made this shift possible by both encouraging research into internal mechanisms and undermining the evidential value of 'efficient causes'.

By the end of the nineteenth century, 'internal mechanisms' predominated and the old lists of predisposing causes had become stereotyped and uninteresting. Nonetheless, medical doctors continued using efficient causes, particularly in the context of case-notes narrative. Interest in internal mechanisms favoured academic psychiatry and led to some progress in brain research.

Two important lessons are taught by the history of aetiological ideas in psychiatry. One is that views on causality (including current ideas) are historical events—the result of ideology and social expediency. They are not 'empirical' in any real sense, and hence it is not possible to decide on 'what is best' by empirical research alone. The second lesson is that the conventional idea of 'truth' is barely applicable in this field. It makes little sense to say that one causal model is 'truer' than another, for there is no empirical way of ascertaining this. All one can say is that, for this particular period of time, and in terms of the multiple social and cultural demands in relation to which science is performed, this or that view of causality seems acceptable, sensible, effective, profitable, attractive, etc. This is perhaps the only 'truth' that is worth remembering.

References

1. Riese, W. (1950) *La pensée causal en médecine*. Presses Universitaires de France, Paris.
2. Bunge, M. (1959). *Causality*. World Publishing, Cleveland, OH.
3. Siegler, M. and Osmond, H. (1966). Models of madness. *British Journal of Psychiatry*, **112**, 1193–1203.
4. Aristotle (1984). *Metaphysics, Book V. The complete works of Aristotle* (ed. J. Barnes), Vol. 2, p. 1600. Princeton University Press.
5. Dijksterhuis, E.J. (1961). *The mechanization of the world picture*. Oxford University Press.
6. Zilboorg, G. (1941). *A history of medical psychology*. W.W. Norton, New York.
7. Hippocrates (1923) *Epidemics I and III* (ed. trans. W.H.S. Jones), Vol. 1, pp. 139–287. Heinemann, London.
8. Laín Entralgo, P. (1961). *La historia clínica*, p. 634. Salvat, Barcelona.
9. Hume D. (1888) *A treatise of human nature* (ed. L. Selby-Bigge), p. 170. Clarendon Press, Oxford.
10. Esquirol, E. (1838). *Des maladies mentales*, Vol. I, pp. 31–3. Ballière, Paris.
11. Berrios, G.E. (2000). Aetiology. In *The great notions of psychiatry: a conceptual history*. Oxford University Press.
12. Berrios, G.E. and Porter, R. (1995) *The history of clinical psychiatry*. Athlone Press, London.
13. Griesinger, W. (1867). *Mental pathology and therapeutics* (trans. C.L. Robertson and J. Rutherford), pp. 127–31. New Sydenham Society, London. (First published in German, 1861.)
14. Coury, C. (1971). La méthode anatomo-clinique et ses promoteurs en France: Corvisart, Bayle, Laennec. *Médicine de France*, **1**, 13–22.
15. Imbault-Huart, M.J. (1981) Bayle, Laennec et la méthode anatomo-clinique. *Revue du Palais de la Découverte*, **22**, 79–90.
16. Postel, J. (1983) La paralysie générale. In *Nouvelle histoire de la psychiatrie* (ed. J. Postel and C. Quétel), pp. 322–33. Privat, Paris.
17. Bayle, A.L.J. (1826). *Traité des maladies du Cerveau et de ses membranes*, p xxiv. Gabon, Paris.
18. Wahring-Schmidt, B. (1985). *Der junge Wilhelm Griesinger in*

Spannungsfeld zwischen Philosophie und Physiologie. Gunter Narr, Tübingen.

19. Déchambre, E. (1883). Déterminisme. In *Dictionnaire encyclopédique des sciences médicales* (ed. E. Dechambre and L. Lereboullet), Vol. 28, pp. 435–49. Masson, Paris.

20. Brochin (1887) Étiologie médicale. In *Dictionnaire encyclopédique des sciences médicales* (ed. E. Dechambre and L. Lereboullet), Vol. 36, pp. 340–53. Masson, Paris.

21. Constant, F.M.C. (1970). *Introduction à la vie et à l'oeuvre de Bénédict-Augustin Morel.* Thèse de Paris.

22. Morel, B.A. (1857). *Traité des dégénérescences physiques, intellectuelles et morales de l'espèce humaine.* Baillière, Paris.

23. Friedlander, R. (1973). B.A. Morel and the development of the theory of degenerescence. PhD Dissertation, University of California.

24. Morel, B.A. (1852) *Études cliniques. Traité théorique et pratique des maladies mentales,* Vol. 1, pp. 211–12. Masson, Paris.

25. Morel, B.A. (1860). *Traité de maladies mentales,* pp. 77–8. Masson, Paris.

26. Clarke, E. and Jacyna, L.S. (1987). *Nineteenth-century origins of neuroscientific concepts.* University of California Press, Berkeley, CA.

27. Clarke, E. and O'Malley, C.D. (1996). *The human brain and spinal cord* (2nd edn). Norman, San Francisco, CA.

28. Engelhardt, H.T. (1975). J.H. Jackson and the mind–body relation. *Bulletin of the History of Medicine,* **49,** 137–51.

29. Droixhe, D. (1978). *La Linguistic et l'appel de l'histoire (1600–1800).* Droz, Geneva.

30. Aarsleff, H. (1982). *From Locke to Saussure.* Athlone Press, London.

31. Lesky, E. (1976). *The Vienna Medical School of the nineteenth century.* Johns Hopkins University Press, Baltimore, MD.

32. Power, H. and Sedgwick, L.W. (ed.) (1892). *The New Sydenham Society's lexicon of medicine and the allied sciences,* Vol. 4. New Sydenham Society, London.

33. Boirel, R. (1982). *Le mécanisme.* Presses Universitaires de France, Paris.

34. Beckner, M.O. (1966). Mechanisms in biology. In *The encyclopedia of philosophy* (ed. P. Edwards), Vol. 5, pp. 250–2. Macmillan, New York.

35. Auroux, S. (ed.) (1990). *Les notions philosophiques,* Vol. 2, p. 1582. Presses Universitaires de France, Paris.

36. Rosenberg, A. (1985). *The structure of biological science,* pp. 62–8. Cambridge University Press.

37. Churchland, P.M. (1993). Eliminative materialism and propositional attitudes. In *Folk psychology and the philosophy of mind* (ed. S.M. Christensen and D.R. Turner), pp. 42–62. Erlbaum, Hillsdale, NJ.

38. Fearing, F. (1930). *Reflex action. a study in the history of physiological psychology.* Williams and Wilkins, Baltimore, MD.

39. Claparède, E. (1903). *L'association des idées.* Doin, Paris.

40. Warren, H.C. (1921). *A history of the association psychology.* Charles Scribner's Sons, New York.

41. Rapaport, D. (1974). *The history of the concept of association of ideas.* International Universities Press, New York.

42. Whitehouse, P.J. (1985) Theodor Meynert: foreshadowing modern concepts of neuropsychiatric pathology. *Neurology,* **35,** 389–91.

43. Meynert T. (1885) *Psychiatry. a clinical treatise on diseases of the fore-brain* (transl. B. Sachs). G.P. Putnam, New York.

44. Lévy-Friesacher C. (1983). *Meynert–Freud. L'amentia.* Presses Universitaires de France, Paris.

45. Lanczik, M. (1988). *Der Breslauer Psychiater Carl Wernicke.* Jan Thorbecke, Sigmaringen.

46. Stein, D.J. and Ludik, J. (ed.) (1998). *Neural networks and psychopathology.* Cambridge University Press.

47. von Monakow, C. (1970). *Vita mea. Mein leben* (ed. A.W. Gubser and W.H. Ackerknecht). Huber, Bern.

48. Mourgue, R. (1931). L'oeuvre et la personnalité du Professeur Constantin von Monakow (1853–1930). *Encephale,* **26,** 417–28.

49. von Monakow, C. and Mourgue, R. (1928). *Introduction biologique a l'étude de la neurologie et de la psychopathologie.* Alcan, Paris.

50. Guiraud, P. (1950). *Psychiatrie générale,* p. 165. Le François, Paris.

51. Semon, R. (1908). *Die Mneme als erhaltendes Prinzip intramuscular Wechsel des organischen Geschehens* (2nd edn). Wilhelm Engelman, Leipzig

52. Schacter, D.L. (1982). *Stranger behind the engram. Theories of memory and the psychology of science.* Erlbaum, London.

2.1.2 The brain and the mind

Francisco Mora

Introduction

When thinking about the brain we have in mind an organ made up of nerve cells (the neurones), synapses (connections between neurones), chemical messengers communicating information between neurones (neurotransmitters), receptors, multiple interneuronal connections, and circuits. When we talk about the brain we use the precise specialist language of the basic sciences—mathematics, chemistry and physics, molecules, proteins, electrical potentials—the world of matter which can be manipulated, cut, separated into pieces, and analysed.[1]

But what about the mind? For perceptions, emotions, thoughts, memory, consciousness, and self-consciousness we are concerned with intimate and subjective entities that are elusive or difficult to grasp or measure. In this context we use a different language, that of psychology.

For hundreds of years we have had a clear-cut separation of these two concepts, that of the brain or matter occupying space and time, and the other of the mind or spirit occupying time and being only individually experienced and therefore unique.[2,3]

Only a few decades of research in neuroscience were necessary to start attempting to bridge the gap between brain and mind. Modern neuroscience and cognitive neuroscience are in fact trying to join the two concepts into one, that of man as a product of the Darwinian evolution, and his mind as a series of processes carried out by the brain.

Modern neuroscience and the mind

What neuroscience has provided in the attempt of unifying the two concepts is a new understanding of the brain. The brain is no longer viewed in such coarse terms of simple matter as conceived in the eighteenth century. Today we know that the brain is a continually changing organ, in its structure as well as its function. Below and inside the apparently fixed and almost universal anatomy of convolutions and sulci of the cerebral cortex, there is a constant flow of information, processing endogenous activity or sensory events (those from the environment). This flow of information is not just passive processing in which an immutable area of the brain or a distributed system in the brain has an unalterable coding to process it. The brain is a neuronal plastic organ which means that the neuronal process is constantly changing the processer. A good example is the changes of the cortical maps of somatic sensations that occur in response to learning new uses for the fingers.[4] We know now that these plastic changes are generated in neurones and pathways that release neurotransmitters and activate receptors, and this in turn activates genes, synthesis of new proteins, receptors and other membrane components, and finally morphological and physiological changes of neurones and circuit activity. It is in this dynamic way that the world of chemistry and physics of the brain is transformed into biochemistry and then into anatomy, physiology, and behaviour as a continuum. Therefore biochemistry, anatomy, and physiology are no longer conceived as discrete compartments but as a continuous dimension across space and time.

But what about the mind in this constant flow of information in the brain? Is it that the brain and its activity produce or cause what we call mind? Mind does not exist in the sense of being a real entity or global concept capturing a static or permanent thing. What does exist are mind processes, that is to say, events characterized in terms of time-varying activity of interconnected and distributed circuits in the brain. Time, not space, is the crucial dimension of the mind: 'Mind is the neural tissue sewn with the threads of time'. Needless to say, for most neuroscientists mind is not a spiritual, inmaterial entity, nor a product emerging or caused by the brain and different from the brain. Mind is the activity of the brain itself—nothing more, nothing less.

The question is then: How can it be that feelings, thoughts, and even consciousness are in fact the activity of molecules and cells in circuits of the brain? I am among those neuroscientists who believe that there is an identity between brain processes and mind processes and that it is the different descriptive language that makes them seem different. For example, when we burn a finger and describe in neurobiological terms all the events occurring in the spinal cord and brain, i.e. neurotransmitters, gene activity, electrical potentials, and activation of neuronal circuits in distributed systems of the limbic system and cerebral cortex, we are already describing the emotional reaction and the cognitive component of pain but in a different language to that of psychology. In other words, the neurobiological events are not producing something different expressed at psychological or mental level, in this example 'pain'. All events taking place in the brain are pain, first described in neurobiogical terms at one level (neurotransmitters and so on) and then when feeling it, consciously perceiving it, and verbally expressing it, described in cognitive or folk psychological common terms.

Considerable neurobiological evidence is now available concerning the activity of different sensory systems, in particular the visual system, the perception, and even the consciousness of what is visually perceived.[5–7] In this respect, vision has considerably contributed to the approximation of brain and mind. As Posner and Raichle pointed out, 'not only have scientists accumulated considerable knowledge of the visual system, but vision is a good point of entry for many forms of higher mental activity, such as pattern recognition, the construction of mental images in the absence of external stimuli and the interpretation of symbols involved in reading'.[6]

Neuroscience and the theory of the unity of knowledge

What is needed is a unified theory of knowledge.[8,9] During the last hundred years, humans have analysed the universe, included themselves, dividing it into pieces. Every group of scientists in every discipline with their available tools have analysed pieces of their field of study by dividing and subdividing it, and then, at their level of analysis, trying to understand and describe the meaning of that little piece

of reality. Today we are becoming aware that because everything is a continuum in the universe we will never reach an acceptable understanding of a single piece of reality since its full meaning only exists when linked to other fragments of that same reality, sometimes to a different level of organization.

At each level of analysis, science in general and neuroscience in particular has created its own tools of analysis which include its specific language of description and understanding. The science of man is like a Tower of Babel with many people working in it and speaking many different languages and therefore not understanding one another. The time has come for neuroscience and cognitive neuroscience to try to make a synthesis and build bridges between levels of analysis, to approximate languages for a better understanding of the unique reality which is man. This is one of the major tasks of neuroscience today.

One of the key events in such an approach is to understand that from one level of analysis to the next, there is a jump which implies the emergence of new properties in the new level that are not reducible to those of the preceding level. These new emergent properties, however, are tightly and completely dependent upon the elements of the preceding level. The most simple and classical example of this is that of water. Water is made up of oxygen and hydrogen atoms. However, we know that oxygen by itself and hydrogen by itself are not water. That particular molecule, called water, with all its peculiar characteristics and inherent properties, which are different from those of its atomic components, oxygen and hydrogen, are acquired when a particular link between the atoms of oxygen and hydrogen is formed. We know that the laws governing the molecule of water are different from those governing the atoms of oxygen and hydrogen. We also know that the properties of water are not reducible to those of hydrogen and oxygen when separated. But when oxygen and hydrogen are linked together, an emergent new thing, the molecule of water, appears, and with it the new laws governing it.

In neuroscience and cognitive neuroscience considerable effort is devoted to sewing together the different levels of analysis—from genes, molecules, organelles, microcircuits, neuronal compartments, nerve cells, specific regions, and distributed systems up to performance, mental operations, and cognitive systems. A good example of such effort is the human brain project which started in the 1980s.[10] In time, this work will provide a comparison of data obtained through different methodologies at different levels of analysis, and eventually will throw light on complex cognitive processes from their most basic building blocks—molecules, cells, and circuits.

Biological evolution, the brain, and the mind

Evolution is one of the basic elements of that continuum which constitutes man. The human brain is the result, first of several million years of evolution and then a product of a natural selection through thousands of generations. The reconstruction of how the brain has evolved with time is one of the most intriguing pieces of the integrative progress in the neurosciences. Without the reconstruction of such a history we cannot properly understand the human brain. In fact, nothing in biology can properly be understood unless it is analysed with the perspective of evolution.

Among the different biological species, man has the greatest brain volume in relation to body weight.[11] This brain volume has been acquired very rapidly during evolution of the last 2 to 3 million years, from the australopithecines (500 g) to *Homo habilis* (600–700 g), *Homo erectus* (900–1000 g), *Homo sapiens* (1.300 g), and *Homo sapiens sapiens* (1.400 g).[12–14] The brain of the present human is characterized not just by a quantitative and global increase in the number of neurones arranged in the same pre-existing pattern as in the brain of a primitive primate, but also by the reorganization of this brain with selective increases in specific areas.[12]

In this process of evolution of the human brain, the most spectacular part has been, without any doubt, the extraordinary development of those parts of the brain called the association areas. These brain areas, not directly related to sensory or motor control, seem to develop in parallel to the acquisition of mental capacities. During evolution these areas of the cerebral cortex—prefrontal and parietotemporal cortices—have selectively increased in volume and in the number of neurones (the so-called extra-neurones, damage to which does not affect sensory or motor processes). It has been estimated that in such areas, through evolution, the chimpanzee has accumulated 3.4 billion neurones, the australopithecines 4.1 billion neurones, *Homo habilis* 5.5 billion neurones, *Homo erectus* 7.0 billion neurones, and *Homo sapiens* 8.5 billion neurones.[13,14] How then can we not think that there is an intimate relationship between brain and mind?

Evolution has followed multiple and unknown routes to form the present species, including man. It is possible that many structures of the brain have changed their function throughout evolution. That is, functions of parts of the brain that first appeared with a specific survival value, determined by the environmental conditions at the time, changed their functions at later times, readapting them to new conditions of the environment. A good example is how species, including humans, evolved to perform, for instance, an apparently simple physiological function such as thermoregulation.[15]

Genes, the brain, and the mind

Today no one would challenge the idea that our brains are constructed during ontogeny through the orchestrated pattern of gene activity, and that the expression of those genes, during that early development, is also determined in part by our environment through sensory, emotional, and learning experiences. Our present knowledge of twins who have an identical genome but have different personalities and also different brain pathologies when adults argues in favour of an important role played by the environment. The external world is therefore apprehended and incorporated into the brain, not as mere functional information, but to affect the conformation of the brain itself. It is in this way that humans construct their individuality.

The most influential capacities of the environment for the development of the brain come after birth. It is interesting in this respect that humans are born with a brain weight of around 350 g, approximatively the same brain weight as a chimpanzee. However, from that time on, while the brain of the human reaches a final weight of 1400 g that of the chimpanzee will only reach 450 g. The importance of this observation is that the chimpanzee is born with 60 to 65 per cent of the final brain weight while the human is born with only 20 to 25 per cent. In other words, more than 70 per cent of the total brain weight of the

human is obtained in immediate contact with the environment, and it is this environment which shapes the final synaptology of the brain during development.

During adulthood the brain is also constantly changing its biochemistry, anatomy, and physiology. The idea that learning and memory are the activity of modified synaptic connections between neurones under the control of specific gene activity is almost fully accepted in neuroscience.[16] Training of animals in a given learning task can result in the synthesis of new neuronal proteins, and this synthesis involves first the activation of the so-called immediate early genes with the production of their protein products c-*fos* and c-*jun*. These proteins could in turn act as activators for other genes whose products may eventually change membrane structure and synapses, and hence their function. It is in this way that biochemistry becomes morphology, strenghtening in turn the synapses and therefore affecting the signal properties of neurones, circuits, and behaviour.[17]

It is also becoming clear that the learning experiences and hence memories are not confined to a single set of synapses in a defined brain locus, but as long-term memory is formed, they become widely distributed across several brain regions and therefore become a distributed property of a definite neuronal system.[18] It is in this way that a unique individual brain is constructed in continual contact with the environment.

In a recent review regarding genes, behavior, and the mind, Kandel[19] has stated:

> There can be no changes in behavior that are not reflected in the nervous system and no persistent changes in the nervous system that are not reflected in structural changes on some level of resolution. Everyday sensory experience, sensory deprivation, and learning can probably lead to a weakening of synaptic connections in some circumstances and a strengthening of connections in others.

Brain circuits and consciousness

Consciousness is, without any doubt, the central core of any neurobiological approach to processes of the mind. Many books have addressed this problem from a philosophical or cognitive point of view. Although these later approaches are of importance, many neuroscientists feel that they will never be sufficient to fully explain what consciousness is, unless other studies or theories appear to anchor them at a neurobiological level. For some, consciousness is no longer a philosophical problem but a scientific problem.[5,7] Very recently, authors have started to tackle this problem from the perspective of the brain itself.[7,20–22]

What do we mean when talking of consciousness? The definition of the term is clearly a considerable challenge and there are important difficulties in reaching a formal definition. Crick and Koch[20] admitted the difficulty in a first approach to defining conciousness and recognized that the most useful way to advance in this problem is to use the descriptions of psychologists and cognitive scientists. With such an approach, together with other series of observations, they reached the conclusion that conciousness 'is crucially dependent on some form of short-term memory and also some form of serial attentional mechanisms'. Tononi and Edelman[22] consider that 'conscious experience is a process that is unified and private, that is extremely differentiated and that evolves on a time scale of hundreds of milliseconds'. The problem of definition of consciousness is addressed more specifically by Searle.[23]

As previously mentioned, consciousness or awareness of the external world (sensory perception) has received substantial attention. For the past two decades, most work has been devoted to trying to understand how the brain could perceive a single object.[5] Today we know that a single object, say an apple, is analysed by the brain in its many single components such as form, orientation, colour, depth, movement, etc. and we also know that such varied information is distributed through the brain in different areas and circuits where it is further analysed and stored. However, we do not see the form or movement of an object separated from the perception of a unified single object. All those characteristics individually analysed by the brain should, somehow, be bound together. Therefore, the brain, when perceiving a single apple, requires a temporary unit of activity of all cells composing the different circuits relevant to the object apple—this is what is called the binding problem. It has been suggested that the activity of binding together all the properties of the object is produced by the synchronous activity (neurone firing) of all those cells relevant to the analysis of the properties of the object apple. This synchronous neural activity has been suggested to ocurr in bursts at frequencies in the 40- to 60-Hz range.[21]

Assuming that synchronous or semisynchronous activity of all these distributed circuits in the brain is activated when bringing together all the properties of that unique object called apple, how is that relevant to the neural correlates of the awareness of the apple? Both attention and re-entrant links to the areas activated have been proposed as two fundamental ingredients for consciousness to take place. Thus attention seems to play a crucial role in binding, although the exact location and mechanism of attention are unclear despite the parietal lobe mechanism that has been considered relevant in this context.[24]

The re-entrant links between the areas concerned seem to be specially significant in this regard. Zeki[5] proposed an answer to this question by suggesting that consciousness is a feature of the visual neural organization, as there are other features of the system such as movement or colour: 'It makes sense to suppose that the conscious awareness of the visual stimulus is made possible not only by the simultaneous and correlated activity of cells (in different visual areas) but also by the reentrant links between them'. As pointed out by Tononi and Edelman:[22] 'Substantial evidence indicates that the integration of distributed neuronal populations through re-entrant interactions is required for conscious experience'. Zeki[5] proposes:

> Consciousness is a feature of both types of neural organization (i.e. movement and color) and of many other, though not all, neural systems as well. There is no colour unless I see it. I cannot see it unless I am conscious. There is no conscious awareness unless certain neural organizations are intact and functioning normally and it is a feature of such neural organizations that they possess consciousness.

There have been many other different approaches to consciousness from cognitive neuroscience and neuropsychology, including studies of patients with blind sight syndrome, memory deficits, split-brain, unilateral and contralateral neglect, or patients with specific brain lesions, which allowed an understanding of some of the neurobiological bases of learning, memory, and linguistic processes in humans.[25–28] The new techniques for cognitive experimentation such as positron emission tomography, magnetic resonance imaging, and the most recent recording technique, magnetoelectroencephalography, which has a resolution capable of correlating electrical activity of specific brain areas and cognitive events measured in real time, have considerably contributed to this development.

For the most reductive neurobiological formulations of cognition and consciousness, the reader is referred to Crick and Koch,[20] Llinas and Paré,[21] and Tononi and Edelman.[22]

Crick and Koch[20] proposed that, despite the many different forms consciousness could take at any moment, this could be related to one or a few basic neurobiological mechanisms having at their core 'a particular type of activity in a transient set of neurons that use a subset of a much larger set of potential candidates'. This speculation led Crick and Koch to ask which and where these neurones are and how they are special (connections, pattern of firing, etc.).

Tononi and Edelman[22] have critized this approach after considering that 'conferring this property on neurons seems to contribute to a category error, in the sense of ascribing to things properties they cannot have'. In the light of classical lesion, stimulation, and neurophysiological studies they propose what they call the dynamic core hypothesis of conciousness:

> We propose that a large cluster of neuronal groups that together constitute, on a time scale of hundreds of milliseconds, a unified neural process of high complexity be termed the 'dynamic core', in order to emphasize both its integration and its constantly changing activity patterns. The dynamic core is a functional cluster: its participating neuronal groups are much more strongly interactive among themselves than with the rest of the brain. The dynamic core must also have high complexity: its global activity patterns must be selected within less than a second out of a very large repertoire.[22]

Perhaps one of the original formulations in this hypothesis is that the dynamic core is conceived not as an invariant set of neurones or circuits distributed along the brain, but as a set of circuits that may change over time and also that at times could underlie conscious experience while others may be involved in unconscious processes. An important component of the neuroanatomical substrates of this dynamic core would include the thalamocortical connections, both posterior and anterior regions.

Llinas and Paré[21] have proposed that, in fact, the thalamocortical system, which comprises a collection of specific thalamic regions (the ventrobasal complex and the non-specific middle-line nuclei, and a set of cortical conterparts that create resonant functional states), is a central component of the cognitive substrates of the brain. These authors maintain that the 40-Hz oscillations that can be recorded in many areas of the cerebral cortex are the resonance of neuronal oscillations in specific thalamic nuclei. These oscillations, which exhibit a 12- to 13-ms phase shift from the frontal to the posterior parts of the brain, could serve to produce a temporal binding of sensory stimuli. During that unit of time (12 ms) the brain would process a single or quantum cognitive event. Cognition, therefore, would be a collection of periods of time. Llinas and Paré concluded that 'integration of sensory events into a larger computational state that underlies cognition is a function of its temporal relation to ongoing oscillatory activities of the brain'.

Final considerations

Neuroscience is starting to be viewed as a science with scopes beyond those of aiming simply to understand the brain. In fact, in 1978, Schmitt[29] was already pointing out that 'These advances [in neuroscience] are valuable and meaningful for a significant attempt to understand the most complex known mechanism, the human brain, and to achieve the highest ultimate aim, a comprehension of human selfhood and psyche'. A recent conference on 'Neuroscience and the Human Spirit' in Washington (sponsored by the Ethics and Public Policy Center and held in Washington, DC, September 1998) and another on 'Cognitive Neuroscience and Divine Action' (sponsored by the Vatican Observatory and held in Paserbiec, Poland, June 1998) are good examples for how knowledge from neuroscience is increasingly involved in providing a new perspective on human nature. In an editorial comment in *Nature Neuroscience* entitled 'Does neuroscience threaten human values?'[30] the perspective of neuroscience being a challenge to the free will and 'a new ammunition for a materialist account of human nature and thus as an attack on traditional belief systems' was put into critical perspective.

Neuroscientists in general do not like to discuss matters of religion or morality, but certainly neuroscience provides a new perspective which embraces both brain and mind and broadens the our understanding of human nature. Implications of such a new perspective will necessarily include matters of moral values.

This new perspective in which brain and mind are viewed within the framework of identity has consequences for all fields of knowledge, mainly biology and medicine and therefore also for psychiatry. Kandel[19] has recently pointed out that not only do psycho- and neuro-pharmacological drugs alter mind processes by changing the brain machinery but also:

> We no longer think that only certain diseases, the organic diseases, affect mentation through biological changes in the brain and that others, the functional diseases do not. The basis for the new intellectual framework for psychiatry is that all mental processes are biological and therefore any alteration in those processes is necessarily organic.

As a consequence Kandel[19] points out that:

> When a therapist speaks to a patient and the patient listens, the therapist is not only making eye contact and voice contact, but the action of neuronal machinery in the therapist's brain is having an indirect and, one hopes, long-lasting effect on the neuronal machinery in the patient's brain; and quite likely, vice versa. Insofar as our words produce changes in our patient's mind, it is likely that these psychotherapeutic interventions produce changes in the patient's brain. From this perspective, the biological and sociopsychological approaches are joined.

References

1. Mora, F. and Sanguinetti, A.M. (1994). *Diccionario de neurociencias*. Alianza, Madrid.
2. Beakley, B. and Ludlow, P. (1992). *The philosophy of mind. Classical problems/contemporary issues*. MIT Press, Cambridge, MA.
3. Mora, F. (ed.) (1995). *El problema cerebro-mente*. Alianza, Madrid.
4. Jenkins, W.M., Merzenich, M.M., Ochs, M.T., and Ruiz-Robles, A.R. (1990). Functional reorganization of primary somatosensory cortex in adult owl monkeys after behaviorally controlled tactile stimulation. *Journal of Neurophysiology*, **63**, 82–104.
5. Zeki, S. (1993). *A vision of the brain*. Blackwell Science, Oxford.
6. Posner, M.I. and Raichle, M.E. (1994). *Images of mind*. Scientific American Library, New York.
7. Crick, F. (1994). *The astonishing hypothesis. The scientific search for the Soul*. Scribner's Sons, New York.
8. Mora, F. (ed.) (1996). *El cerebro intimo*. Ariel, Barcelona.
9. Wilson, E.O. (1998). *Consilience. The unity of knowledge*. Knopf, New York.
10. Shepherd, G.M., Mirsky, J.S., Healy, M.D., *et al.* (1998). The Human Brain Project: neuroinformatics tools for integrating, searching and modeling multidisciplinary neuroscience data. *Trends in Neuroscience*, **21**, 460–8.
11. Jerison, H.J. (1973). *Evolution of the brain and intelligence*. Academic Press, New York.
12. Holloway, R.L. (1995). Toward a synthetic theory of the human brain evolution. In *Origins of the human brain* (ed. J.P. Changeaux and J. Chavaillon), pp. 42–60. Clarendon Press, Oxford.
13. Tobias, P.V. (1971). *The brain in hominid evolution*. Columbia University Press, New York.
14. Tobias, P.V. (1995). The brain of the first hominids. In *Origins of the human brain* (ed. J.P. Changeaux and J. Chavaillon), pp. 61–83. Clarendon Press, Oxford.
15. Gisolfi, C.V. and Mora, F. (1999). *The hot brain: survival, temperature and the human body*. MIT Press, Cambridge, MA.
16. Kandel, E.R. (1995). Cellular mechanisms of learning and memory. In *Essentials of neural sciences and behaviour* (ed. E.R. Kandel, J.H. Schwartz, and T. M. Jessel), pp. 667–94. Appleton and Lange, East Norwalk, CT.
17. Rose, S.P.R. (1993). Synaptic plasticity, learning and memory. In *Synaptic plasticity. molecular, cellular and functional aspects* (ed. M. Baundry, R.F. Thompson, and J.L. Davis), pp. 209–29. MIT Press, Cambridge, MA.
18. Fuster, J.M. (1995). *Memory in the cerebral cortex*. MIT Press, Cambridge, MA.
19. Kandel, E.R. (1998). A new intellectual framework for Psychiatry. *American Journal of Psychiatry*, **155**, 457–69.
20. Crick, F. and Koch, D. (1990). Towards a neurobiological theory of consciousness. In *Seminars in the neurosciences 2. The neurobiology of mind* (ed. A.R. Damasio), pp. 263–75. W.B. Saunders, Philadelphia, PA.
21. Llinas, R. and Paré, D. (1996). The brain as a closed system modulated by the senses. In *The mind–brain continuum* (ed. R. Llinas and P.S. Churchland), pp. 1–18. MIT Press, Cambridge, MA.
22. Tononi, G. and Edelman, M. (1998). Consciousness and complexity. *Science*, **282**, 1846–51.
23. Searle, J.R. (1998). How to study conciousness scientifically. *Brain Research*, **26**, 379–87.
24. Crick, F. (1996). Visual perception: rivalry and consciousness. *Nature*, **379**, 485–6.
25. Damasio, A.R. (1994) *Descartes' error*. Picador, London.
26. Damasio, H. and Damasio, A. (1990). The neural basis of memory, language and behavioral guidance: advances with lesion method in humans. *Seminars in the Neuroscience 2*, pp. 277–86. W.B. Saunders, Philadelphia, PA.
27. Gazzaniga, M.S. (1995). *The cognitive neuroscience*. MIT Press, Cambridge, MA.
28. Squire, L.S., Kandel, E.R., and Kosslyn, S.M. (1966). Cognitive neuroscience. Editorial overview. *Current Opinion in Neurobiology*, **6**, 153–7.
29. Schmitt, O.F. (1978). Introduction. In *The mindful brain* (ed. G.M. Edelman and V.B. Mountcastle), pp. 1–6. MIT Press, Cambridge, MA.
30. Anonymous (1998). Does neuroscience threaten human values? (Editorial). *Nature Neuroscience*, **1**, 535–6.

2.2 Statistics and the design of experiments and surveys

Graham Dunn

Introduction

Research into mental illness uses a much wider variety of statistical methods than those familiar to a typical medical statistician. In many ways there is more similarity to the statistical toolbox of the sociologist or educationalist. It would be a pointless exercise to try to describe this variety here but, instead, we shall cover a few areas that are especially characteristic of psychiatry. The first and perhaps the most obvious is the problem of measurement. Measurement reliability and its estimation are discussed in the next section. Misclassification errors are a concern of the third section, a major part of which is concerned with the estimation of prevalence through the use of fallible screening questionnaires. This is followed by a discussion of both measurement error and misclassification error in the context of modelling patterns of risk.

The other major concern is the presence of missing data. Although this is common to all areas of medical research, it is of particular interest to the psychiatric epidemiologist because there is a long tradition (since the early 1970s) of introducing missing data by design. Here we are thinking of two-phase or double sampling (often confusingly called two-stage sampling by psychiatrists and other clinical research workers). In this design a first-phase sample are all given a screen questionnaire. They are then stratified on the basis of the results of the screen (usually, but not necessarily, using two strata—likely cases and likely non-cases) and subsampled for a second-phase diagnostic interview. This is the major topic of the third section.

At the end of this chapter pointers are given to where the interested reader might find other relevant and useful material on psychiatric statistics. One area that is not covered, however, is clinical trial methodology. This is left to others (see other chapters in this volume).

Reliability of instruments

In this section we consider two questions:

- What is meant by 'reliability'?
- How do we estimate reliabilities?

Models and definitions

Most clinicians have an intuitive idea of what the concept of reliability means, and that being able to demonstrate that one's measuring instruments have high reliability is a good thing. Reliability concerns the consistency of repeated measurements, where the repetitions might be repeated interviews by the same interviewer, alternative rat-ings of the same interview (as a video recording) by different raters, alternative forms or repeated administration of a questionnaire, or even different subscales of a single questionnaire, and so on. One learns from elementary texts that reliability is estimated by a correlation coefficient (in the case of a quantitative rating) or a kappa (κ) or weighted κ statistic (in the case of a qualitative judgement such as a diagnosis). Rarely are clinicians aware of either the formal definition of reliability or of its estimation through the use of various forms of intraclass correlation coefficient rho (ρ).

First consider a quantitative measurement X. We start with the assumption that it is fallible and that it is the sum of two components: the 'truth' T and 'error' E. If T and E are statistically independent (uncorrelated), then it can be shown that

$$\text{Var}(X) = \text{Var}(T) + \text{Var}(E) \tag{1}$$

where $\text{Var}(X)$ is the variance of X (i.e. the square of its standard deviation), and so on. The reliability ρX of X is defined as the proportion of the total variability of X (i.e. $\text{Var}(X)$) that is explained by the variability of the true scores (i.e. $\text{Var}(T)$):

$$\rho_X = \frac{\text{Var}(T)}{\text{Var}(X)} = \frac{\text{Var}(T)}{\text{Var}(T) + \text{Var}(E)}. \tag{2}$$

This ratio will approach zero as the variability of the measurement errors increases compared with that of the truth. Alternatively, it will approach 1 as the variability of the errors decreases. The standard deviation of the measurement errors (i.e. the square root of $\text{Var}(E)$) is usually know as the instrument's standard error of measurement. Note that reliability is not a fixed characteristic of an instrument, even when its standard error of measurement (i.e. its precision) is fixed. When the instrument is used on a population that is relatively homogeneous (low values of $\text{Var}(T)$), it will have a relatively low reliability. However, as $\text{Var}(T)$ increases then so does the instrument's reliability. In many ways the standard error of measurement is a much more useful summary of an instrument's performance, but one should always bear in mind that it too might vary from one population to another—a possibility that must be carefully checked by both the developers and users of the instrument.

Now let us complicate matters slightly. Suppose that a rating depends not only on the subject's so-called true score T and random measurement error E, but also on the identity R, say, of the interviewer or rater R. That is, each rater has his or her own characteristic bias (constant from assessment to another) and the biases can be thought of as varying randomly from one rater to another. Again, assuming statistical independence, we can show that, if $X = T + R + E$, then

$$\text{Var}(X) = \text{Var}(T) + \text{Var}(R) + \text{Var}(E). \tag{3}$$

But what is the instrument's reliability? It depends. If subjects in a survey or experiment, for example, are each going to be assessed by a rater randomly selected from a large pool of possible raters, then

$$\rho_{xa} = \frac{\text{Var}(T)}{\text{Var}(X)} = \frac{\text{Var}(T)}{\text{Var}(T) + \text{Var}(R) + \text{Var}(E)}. \tag{4}$$

However, if only a single rater is to be used for all subjects in the proposed study, there will be no variation due to the rater and the reliability now becomes

$$\rho_{xb} = \frac{\text{Var}(T)}{\text{Var}(T) + \text{Var}(E)}. \tag{5}$$

Of course, $\rho_{xb} > \rho_{xa}$. Again, the value of the instrument's reliability depends on the context of its use. This is the essence of generalizability theory.[1] The three versions of ρ given above are all intraclass correlation coefficients and are also examples of what generalizability theorists refer to as generalizability coefficients.

Designs

Now consider two simple designs for reliability (generalizability) studies. The first involves each subject of the study being independently assessed by two (or more) raters but that the raters for any given subject have been randomly selected from a very large pool of potential raters. The second design again involves each subject of the study being independently assessed by two (or more) raters, but in this case the raters are the same for all subjects. Equations (1) and (2) are relevant to the analysis of data arising from the first design, whilst eqns (3), (4), and (5) are relevant to the analysis of data from the second design.

Estimation of ρ and κ from ANOVA tables

When we come to analyse the data it is usually appropriate to carry out an analysis of variance (**ANOVA**). For the first design we carry out a one-way ANOVA (X by subject) and for the second we perform a two-way ANOVA (X by rater and subject). In the latter case we assume that there is no subject by rater interaction and accordingly constrain the corresponding sum of squares to be zero. We assume that readers are reasonably familiar with an analysis of variance table. Each subject has been assessed by, say, k raters. The one-way ANOVA yields a mean square for between-subjects variation (**BMS**) and a mean square for within-subjects variation (**WMS**). WMS is an estimate of $\text{Var}(E)$ in eqn (1). Therefore the square root of WMS provides an estimate of the instrument's standard error of measurement. The corresponding estimate of ρ is given by

$$r_X = \frac{\text{BMS} - \text{WMS}}{\text{BMS} + (k-1)\text{WMS}} \tag{6}$$

where rX is used to represent the estimate of ρX rather than the true, but unknown, value. In the case of $k = 2$, r becomes

$$r_X = \frac{\text{BMS} - \text{WMS}}{\text{BMS} + \text{WMS}}. \tag{7}$$

In the slightly more complex two-way ANOVA, the ANOVA table provides values of mean squares for subjects or patients (**PMS**), raters (**RMS**), and error (**EMS**). We shall not concentrate on the details of estimation of the components of eqn (3) (see Fleiss[2] or Streiner and Norman[3]) but simply note that ρ_{Xa} is estimated by

$$r_{Xa} = \frac{n(\text{PMS} - \text{EMS})}{n \times \text{PMS} + k \times \text{RMS} + (nk - n - k)\text{EMS}} \tag{8}$$

where n is the number of subjects (patients) in the study.

In reporting the results of a reliability study, it is important that investigators give some idea of the precision of their estimates of reliability, for example by giving an appropriate standard error or, even better, an appropriate confidence interval. The subject is beyond the scope of this chapter, however, and the interested reader is referred to Fleiss[2] or Dunn[4] for further illumination.

Finally, what about qualitative measures? We shall not discuss the estimation and interpretation of κ in any detail here but simply point out that for a binary (yes/no) measure one can also carry out a two-way analysis of variance (but ignore any significance tests since they are not valid for binary data) and estimate r_{Xa} as above. In large samples r_{Xa} is equivalent to κ[3]. A corollary of this is that κ is another form of reliability coefficient and, like any of the reliability coefficients described above, will vary from one population to another (i.e. it is dependent on the prevalence of the symptom or characteristic being assessed).

Prevalence estimation

Following Dunn and Everitt,[5] we ask the following questions of a survey report.

- Do the authors clearly define the sampled population?
- Do the authors discuss similarities and possible differences between their sampled population and the stated target population?
- Do the authors report what sampling mechanism has been used?
- Is the sampling mechanism random? If not, why not?
- Exactly what sort of random sampling mechanism has been used?
- Do the methods of data analysis make allowances for the sampling mechanism used?

Of course, it is vital that what counts as a case should be explained in absolute detail, including the method of eliciting symptoms (e.g. structured interview schedule), screening items, additional impairment criteria, and so on, as well as operational criteria or algorithms used in making a diagnosis. In the following we concentrate on the statistical issues. First, we consider survey design (and the associated sampling mechanisms), and then we move on to discuss the implications of design for the subsequent analysis of the results.

Survey design

Here we are concerned with the estimation of a simple proportion (or percentage). We calculate this proportion using data from the sample and use it to infer the corresponding proportion in the underlying population. One vital component of this process is to ensure that the sampled population from which we have drawn our subjects is as close as possible to that of the target population about which we want to draw conclusions. We also require the sample to be drawn from the sample population in an objective and unbiased way. The best way of achieving this is through some sort of random sampling mechanism. Random sampling implies that whether or not a subject finishes up in the sample is determined by chance. Shuffling and dealing a hand of playing cards is an example of a random selection process called simple random sampling. Here every possible hand of, say, five cards has the same probability of occurring as any other. If we can list all possible samples of a fixed size, then simple random sampling implies that they all have the same probability of finishing up in our survey. It also implies that each possible subject has the same probability of being selected. But note that the latter condition is not sufficient to define a simple random sample. In a systematic random sample, for example, we have a list of possible people to select (the sampling frame) and we simply select one of the first 10 (say) subjects at random and then systematically select every 10th subject from then on. All subjects have the same probability of selection, but there are many samples which are impossible to draw using this mechanism. For example, we can select either subject 2 or subject 3 with the same probability (1/10), but it is impossible to draw a sample which contains both.

What other forms of random sampling mechanisms might be used? Perhaps the most common is a stratified random sample. Here we divide our sampled population into mutually exclusive groups or strata (men and women, or five separate age groups, for example). Having chosen the strata, we proceed, for example, to take a separate simple random sample from each. The proportion of subjects sampled from each of the strata (i.e. the sampling fraction) might be constant across all strata (ensuring that the overall sample has the same composition as the original population), or we might decide that one or more strata (e.g. the elderly) might have a higher representation. Another commonly used sampling mechanism is multistage cluster sampling. For example, in a national prevalence survey we might chose first to sample health regions or districts, then to sample post codes within the districts, and finally to select patients randomly from each selected post code. (See Kessler[6] and Jenkins et al.[7] for discussions of complex multistage surveys of psychiatric morbidity.)

One particular design that has been used quite often in surveys designed to estimate the prevalence of psychiatric disorders is called two-phase or double sampling. Psychiatrists frequently refer to this as two-stage sampling. This is unfortunate, since it confuses the two-phase design with simple forms of cluster sampling in which the first stage involves drawing a random sample of clusters and the second stage a random sample of subjects from within each of the clusters. In two-phase sampling, however, we first draw a preliminary sample (which may be simple, stratified, and/or clustered) and then administer a first-phase screening questionnaire such as the General Health Questionnaire (see Chapter 2.7). On the basis of the screen results we then stratify the first-phase sample. Note that we are not restricted to two strata (likely cases versus the rest), although this is perhaps the most common form of the design. We then draw a second-phase sample from each of the first-phase strata and proceed to give these subjects a definitive psychiatric assessment. The point of this design is that we do not waste expensive resources interviewing large numbers of subjects who not appear (on the basis of the first-phase screen) to have any problems. Accordingly, the sampling fractions usually differ across the first-phase strata. However, it is vital that each of the first-phase strata have a reasonable representation in the second phase, and it is particularly important that all of the first-phase strata provide some second-phase subjects. The reader is referred to Pickles and Dunn[8] for further discussion of design issues in two-phase sampling (including discussion of whether it is worth the bother).

Analysis of the results

Here we are particularly concerned with the last of the questions posed at the beginning of the section. In fact, it is a question that should be asked not only of prevalence surveys but of all investigations whether they are epidemiological surveys, intervention studies, or laboratory experiments. How was the design incorporated in the analysis? Frequently the required information is missing. Either the authors are ignorant of the implications of the design, or the journal editor has insisted that technical details are stripped from the report, or both.

Consider a hypothetical sample of 100 participants who have contributed to an estimate of prevalence of, say, depression using a definitive psychiatric interview.

Seventy of the participants have been given a diagnosis of depression. What is a valid estimate of prevalence? What is the standard error of the estimate? Assuming that the data have arisen through simple random sampling, the prevalence p is estimated by 0.70 and its variance is given by

$$\text{Var}(p) = \frac{1}{Np(1-p)} \tag{9}$$

where N is the sample size. The standard error is then given by the square root of this expression.

Suppose that we are now told that the results were obtained from a two-phase survey. The size of the first-phase sample was 300. Of these, 100 were screen positive and 200 were screen negative. The second-phase sample consisted of 70 screen positives, of whom 65 were found to be depressed on interview, together with 30 screen negatives, of whom five were found to be depressed on interview. The estimate of prevalence is given by

$$p = P(\text{screen +ve}) \times P(\text{interview +ve|screen +ve}) +$$
$$P(\text{screen −ve}) \times P(\text{interview +ve|screen −ve})$$
$$= (100/300) \times (65/70) + (200/300) \times (5/30)$$
$$= 0.42 \tag{10}$$

where $P(A)$ should be read as 'probability of A' and $P(A|B)$ should be read as 'probability of A given B' or 'probability of A conditional on B having occurred'. The vertical | should not be confused with division, represented by /.

The prevalence estimate from the two-phase survey is considerably lower than if simple random sampling had been assumed. How has this arisen? Obviously the second-phase sample has been enriched for people who are likely to be depressed. The sampling fraction for the screen positives is 70/100, i.e. each second-phase participant can be thought of as representing 100/70 of screen positives from the original sample. Similarly, the sampling fraction for the screen negatives is 30/200, and each second-phase participant represents 200/30 screen-negative participants from the first-phase sample. The reciprocal of the sampling fraction is called the sampling weight. The total weighted second-phase sample size is $70 \times (100/70) + 30 \times (200/30) = 300$, the first-phase sample. Similarly, the total weighted number of cases of depression is $65 \times (100/70) + 5 \times (200/30) \approx 126$. The latter is the estimate of the number of cases in the first-phase sample. Hence the estimate of prevalence is $126/300 = 0.42$, as before. To recapitulate in a slightly more technical way, if the ith individual in the second-phase sample is assigned a sampling weight w_i, and if the interview outcome y_i has a value of 1 if the ith subject is a case and is zero otherwise, then the weighted prevalence estimate is given by

$$p = \Sigma w_i y_i / \Sigma w_i \qquad (11)$$

where Σ means 'sum over all observations in the second-phase sample' and x_i is simply an indicator that the observation is, indeed, a second-phase observation ($x_i = 1$ for everyone). This estimator is an example of the well-known Horwitz–Thompson estimator from the sampling survey literature[9] but it is not particular familiar to psychiatrists or medical statisticians. We shall discuss the use of weighting adjustments again below.

Returning to our original two-phase calculations, let $A = P(\text{screen} +ve)$ and $B = 1 - A = P(\text{screen} -ve)$. Also, let $p = P(\text{interview} +ve|\text{screen} +ve)$ and $q = P(\text{interview} +ve|\text{screen} -ve)$, so that eqn (10) becomes

$$p = Ap + Bq. \qquad (12)$$

The variance of the estimate of prevalence from the two-phase design is given by[10]

$$\text{Var}(p) = \frac{A^2 p(1-p)}{N_1} + \frac{B^2 q(1-q)}{N_2} + \frac{(p-q)^2 AB}{N} \qquad (13)$$

where N_1 is the number of first-phase screen positives and N_2 is the number of first-phase screen negatives.

Validation of screening questionnaires

It is frequently the case that data from a two-phase survey which has been designed to estimate prevalence are also used to examine the characteristics of the screen questionnaire (in particular, sensitivity and specificity). Readers who are unfamiliar with these concepts are referred to Chapter 2.7 or to Goldberg and Williams[11]. Sensitivity is the proportion of true cases who are screen positive. Specificity is the proportion of true non-cases who are screen negative. The trouble is caused because we used the screen first and then differentially subsampled to carry out the definitive diagnostic interview. Readers familiar with the use of Bayes' theorem will realize how to solve the problem, but here we use another version of the Horwitz–Thompson estimator:

$$\text{sensitivity} = \Sigma w_i y_i z_i / \Sigma w_i y_i \qquad (14)$$

and

$$1 - \text{specificity} = \Sigma w_i (1 - y_i) z_i / \Sigma w_i (1 - y_i) \qquad (15)$$

where, as before, y_i indicates whether the ith subject was a true case of depression (1=yes, 0=no). This ensures that the calculations in eqn (14) are only being carried out on the true cases and, similarly, that the calculations in (15) are only being carried out on the non-cases. Again, w_i is the second-phase sampling weight. The new variable z_i indicates whether the screen result was positive (1=yes, 0=no). An alternative, and perhaps easier, approach is to split the second-phase sample into two: cases and non-cases. Estimation of sensitivity and specificity in these two subfiles (assuming that they are being stored on a computer) is then computationally exactly the same as the weighted estimation of prevalence discussed in the previous section. In the first file, sensitivity is simply the weighted sum of the screen positives divided by the

weighted sum of the cases. Similarly, in the second file, specificity is the weighted sum of the screen negatives divided by the weighted sum of the non-cases.

Many readers will be familiar with the idea of choosing a range of cut-points for the screen questionnaire and then estimating sensitivity and specificity at each of the choices. A plot of sensitivity against $1 - \text{specificity}$ is called a receiver operating characteristic (**ROC**) curve. If the screen is of no use, then the plot will be a straight line through the origin with unit slope. A good screen will produce a convex curve (the greater the area between the observed curve and that indicated by a straight line with unit slope, the better the screen is at discriminating between cases and non-cases). It is sometimes said that one cannot investigate ROC curves using two-phase data. This view is, in fact, mistaken. One can think of the two-phase sampling design as a mechanism by which one can deliberately introduce the analogues of verification bias.[12] Note that there no necessity to restrict the first-phase stratification to just two strata (potential cases versus non-cases) to define the sampling fractions for the second phase of the survey. We start by calculating observed sampling fractions for each discrete outcome of the screening questionnaire. These define the corresponding sampling weights. We then consider all the possibilities for defining z_i in eqns (14) and (15)—there is no need for the z_i to correspond to the way that the second-phase sampling fractions were determined. We then repeatedly use eqns (14) and (15), keeping the weights constant as we change the definition of the z_i. One important point to bear in mind is that if the characteristics of the screen are not fairly well known beforehand and if one of the major aims of the survey is to carry out an ROC analysis, then this is not a particularly efficient design to use. It would be better to go back to the simple random sample—all subjects assessed by both screen and interview.

If one needs, say, confidence intervals for estimates of sensitivity and specificity, it is relatively straightforward to do this via a weighted logistic regression (see next section). The file can be split into cases and non-cases and then, using appropriate software (see below), one fits a logistic model containing a predictor variable which has the value of 1 for all subjects (i.e. just fitting a constant). One then obtains the confidence interval for the intercept term in the output. Finally, the inverse of the logistic transformation of the lower and upper confidence limits will yield the corresponding limits for the sensitivity (specificity) itself. Note that the interval will be asymmetric and will be within the permitted bounds of zero and unity.

Modelling patterns of risk

Henderson (see Chapter 2.7) has introduced the idea of an odds ratio to measure the association between a suspected risk factor and disease. In a linear logistic model the response variable is the natural logarithm of the odds (of disease). Therefore the difference between two groups on this logistic scale (i.e. $\log(a/b) - \log(c/d)$ using Henderson's notation) is equivalent to the logarithm of the odds ratio (i.e. $\log(ad/bc)$). This provides us with an easy way to calculate confidence intervals for odds ratio: $\log(\text{odds ratio})$ or $\log(ad/bc)$ is normally distributed with variance $1/a + 1/b + 1/c + 1/d$ (the corresponding standard error is the square root of this variance). The 95 per cent confidence interval for the $\log(\text{odds ratio})$, for example, is then the point estimate plus or minus 1.96 standard errors. Taking exponents (antilogarithms) of these limits provides the corresponding limits for the odds ratio itself.

The exponent of the parameter estimate in the output of the logistic regression run provides the point estimate for the corresponding odds ratio.

The great advantage of logistic regression is that it enables us to model the potential effects of several risk factors simultaneously. It allows us to adjust for the effects of suspected confounder(s) in assessing the effects of a risk factor of interest. Logistic regression can also be generalized to cope with the use of sampling weights, either to cope with data missing by design (as in a two-phase survey) or to allow for non-response and/or attrition.[13] However, one must be very wary of using weights in software packages that do not explicitly deal with sampling weights. Many packages have weighting functions but these are interpreted as frequency weights—the number of times the observation has been made instead of the number of times it might have been made (as in the case of a sampling weight). The use of frequency weights, as opposed to sampling weights, produces standard errors and confidence intervals that are far too small. This is not a subtle effect; it can make an enormous difference to a P value, giving the impression of a highly significant effect when, in reality, there is little or nothing there.[14]. We illustrate this point by reference to a two-phase survey of psychiatric morbidity in Cantabria in northern Spain.[15,16] The weighted prevalence estimate from these data is 31 per cent. The appropriate 95 per cent confidence interval (**CI**), obtained using sampling weights is (26 per cent, 40 per cent). The naive use of frequency weights produces a 95 per cent CI of (28 per cent, 35 per cent), which is much too narrow. The odds ratio indicating how much higher the prevalence of disorder is in women compared with men is 2.02 with a 95 per cent CI of (0.86, 4.74). The naive use of frequency weights gives the same point estimate (2.02), but here the 95 per cent CI is (1.45, 2.77); again, this is much too narrow. In the analysis of a similar study from Verona in northern Italy, Dunn *et al.*[14] found a corresponding odds ratio of 2.85 with a 95 per cent CI of (1.31, 6.19). The P value for this odds ratio is about 0.008. The incorrect use of frequency weights gives us a 95 per cent CI of (2.31, 3.53) and a corresponding P value of less than 0.00001—at least an 800-fold difference!

Another way in which recent theoretical developments in statistics have helped in the analysis of psychiatric surveys is in the analysis of complex survey samples containing clustered/correlated observations. There are many strands to this development. Educationalists and others have developed a comprehensive theory for hierarchical or multilevel modelling.[17] Multilevel models are also of extreme importance in the analysis and interpretation of the results from cluster-randomized intervention studies. They also allow the effects of differing explanatory variables to have an impact at different levels of the hierarchy. Generalized estimating equation approaches have also allowed the generalization of logistic regression models to cope with correlated repeated binary outcomes in longitudinal data files.[18] Finally, the increasing availability of complex survey analysis software allows us to model complex surveys involving stratification and/or clustering and/or unequal sampling fractions.[9]

Finally, what about measurement error? The 'bible' for linear modelling using explanatory models containing measurement error is Fuller.[19] Over the last few years there has been an explosion of interest in this area. Measurement error in non-linear models (e.g. logistic models) is covered in a recent monograph.[20] Path analysis or structural equation models involving latent variables have a relatively long history in psychiatric research[21–23] and they too are being developed to include logistic regression using latent predictor variables. A detailed description of structural equation modelling is beyond the scope of this chapter, but it should be stressed that regression modelling with explanatory variables acknowledged to be subject to measurement errors is an area of statistics that is particularly important in behavioural and psychiatric research, and its importance is likely to be increasingly acknowledged. The application of structural equation modelling to behaviour genetics is discussed in Chapter 2.4.1.

Conclusions

The recently published *Encyclopedia of Biostatistics*[24] comprises six large volumes of chapters such as this one, covering every area of conceivable interest to the statistically interested clinical research worker. Therefore it is inevitable that this chapter should be very restricted. Inevitably, the choice of topics might be thought to be rather idiosyncratic. Areas which might have been covered, but have been ignored, include survival modelling (particularly recent developments in so-called frailty modelling), longitudinal data analysis (with special reference to modelling patterns of attrition), genetics, and a whole range of classical multivariate methods such as principal components and factor analysis, discriminant analysis (although logistic modelling is one of the better methods of discriminant analysis), multidimensional scaling, and cluster analysis. Henderson (see Chapter 2.7) has also mentioned exciting possibilities for the development of latent trait (item response theory) and latent class models. Several years ago I was often asked to teach trainee psychiatrists all they needed to know about statistics in two 2-h sessions. The first was to cover univariate methods, and the second, multivariate analysis. It cannot be done!

So, where should the reader go from here? Which are the most useful textbooks? In terms of general medical statistics, the obvious choice is Armitage and Berry.[25] Everitt and Dunn[26] and Everitt[27] provide general introductions to multivariate methodology. Measurement error problems, including structural equation modelling, are covered by Dunn[4] and Dunn *et al.*[23] The role of statistics in genetics is well covered by Sham.[28] Although there are many texts on the use of statistics in psychology[27] and education (e.g. Plewis[17] which includes an introduction to multilevel modelling), the only specialist reference for psychiatrists appears to be that by Dunn.[22] However, there is a special issue of the review journal *Statistical Methods in Medical Research* on statistics in psychiatry (Volume 7, October 1998). Readers searching for more specialist material might find other issues of this journal useful, and there is also a mine of useful and relevant information in the *Encyclopedia of Biostatistics*.[24]

References

1. Shavelson, R.J. and Webb, N.M. (1991). *Generalizability theory: a primer*. Sage, Thousand Oaks, CA.
2. Fleiss, J.L. (1987). *The design and analysis of clinical experiments*. Wiley, New York.
3. Streiner, D.L. and Norman, G.R. (1995). *Health measurement scales: a practical guide to their development and use* (2nd edn). Oxford University Press.
4. Dunn, G. (1989). *Design and analysis of reliability studies*. Arnold, London.
5. Dunn, G. and Everitt, B.S. (1995). *Clinical biostatistics: an introduction to evidence based medicine*, Chapter 4. Arnold, London.

6. Kessler, R.C. (1994). The National Comorbidity Survey of the United States. *International Review of Psychiatry*, **6**, 365–76.

7. Jenkins, R., Bebbington, P., Brugha, T., *et al.* (1997). The National Psychiatric Morbidity Surveys of Great Britain—strategy and methods. *Psychological Medicine*, **27**, 765–74.

8. Pickles, A. and Dunn, G. (1998). Prevalence of disease, estimation from screening data. In *Encyclopedia of biostatistics* (ed. P. Armitage and T. Colton), Vol. 5, pp. 3484–90. Wiley, Chichester.

9. Lehtonen, R. and Pahkinen, E.J. (1995). *Practical methods for design and analysis of complex surveys*. Wiley, Chichester.

10. Cochran, W.G. (1977). *Sampling techniques* (3rd edn). Wiley, New York.

11. Goldberg, D.P. and Williams, P. (1988). *A user's guide to the General Health Questionnaire*. NFER–Nelson, Windsor.

12. Begg, C.B. and Greenes, R.A. (1983). Assessment of diagnostic tests when disease verification is subject to selection bias. *Biometrics*, **39**, 207–15.

13. Dunn, G. (1998). Compensating for missing data in psychiatric surveys. *Epidemiologia e Psichiatria Sociale*, **6**, 159–62.

14. Dunn, G., Pickles, A., Tansella, M., and Vázquez-Barquero, J.L. (1999). The role of two-phase epidemiological surveys in psychiatric research. *British Journal of Psychiatry*, **174**, 95–100.

15. Pickles, A., Dunn, G., and Vázquez-Barquero, J.L. (1995). Screening for stratification in two-phase ('two-stage') epidemiological surveys. *Statistical Methods in Medical Research*, **4**, 75–91.

16. Vázquez-Barquero, J.L., Garcia, J., Artal Simón, J., *et al.* (1997). Mental health in primary care: an epidemiological study of morbidity and use of health resources. *British Journal of Psychiatry*, **170**, 529–35.

17. Plewis, I. (1997). *Statistics in education*. Arnold, London.

18. Diggle, P.J., Liang, K., and Zeger, S.L. (1994). *Analysis of longitudinal data*. Oxford University Press.

19. Fuller, W.A. (1987). *Measurement error models*. Wiley, New York.

20. Carroll, R.J., Ruppert, D., and Stefanski, L.A. (1995). *Measurement error in nonlinear models*. Chapman & Hall, London.

21. Fergusson, D.M. (1998). Annotation: structural equation models in developmental research. *Journal of Child Psychology and Psychiatry*, **38**, 877–87.

22. Dunn, G. (1999). *Statistics in psychiatry*. Arnold, London.

23. Dunn, G., Everitt, B., and Pickles, A. (1993). *Modelling covariances and latent variables using equations*. Chapman & Hall, London.

24. Armitage, P. and T. Colton, T. (ed.) (1998). *Encyclopedia of biostatistics*. Wiley, Chichester.

25. Armitage, P. and Berry, G. (1994). *Statistical methods in medical research* (3rd edn). Blackwell Science, Oxford.

26. Everitt, B.S. and Dunn, G. (1993). *Applied multivariate data analysis*. Arnold, London.

27. Everitt, B.S. (1996). *Making sense of statistics in psychology*. Oxford University Press.

28. Sham, P. (1998). *Statistics in human genetics*. Arnold, London.

2.3 The contribution of neurosciences

2.3.1 Neuroanatomy

R.C.A. Pearson

Introduction

The symptoms, signs, and syndromes of psychiatry, whether organic or biological psychiatric disease or not, in the main reflect alterations in functions which reside in the cerebral cortex, including the limbic lobe, and those structures and pathways closely related to the cortex. These cortical manifestations of psychiatric disease include alterations in thought, language, perception, mood, memory, motivation, personality, behaviour and intellect. Therefore this brief account of brain structures and pathways that are important in psychiatry will concentrate on the cerebral cortex and related structures and pathways. Readers who require a fuller account of central nervous system anatomy are referred to the many standard texts, which give a more complete coverage of the subject.

Broadly speaking, neuroanatomy can be subdivided into two parts—the topographical organization of the brain and spinal cord, and the anatomical connections forming functional pathways in the central nervous system. The former is of vital importance clinically, since pathologies rarely respect the boundaries of functional systems, and knowledge of the spatial relationships of different brain structures is increasingly useful as modern imaging methods more accurately visualize detailed brain structure *in vivo*. However, it is the second subdivision of the subject which makes the greater contribution to understanding the biological basis of psychiatric disease, and it is this that will be at the centre of the present account.

The structure and organization of the cerebral cortex

The lobes of the cerebral cortex

A variable pattern of fissures (sulci) and folds (gyri), many of which have specific names, extensively groove the surface of the cerebral hemisphere. A few are relatively constant and are used to subdivide the cerebral hemisphere into lobes, named for the bones of the skull which they underlie (Fig. 1).

The deep lateral sulcus, also called the Sylvian fissure, extends from the uncus, anteriorly and medially, to the parietal lobe, posteriorly and

medially. It has a short stem, and anterior, ascending, and posterior rami. The anterior and ascending rami embrace the pars triangularis of the frontal lobe, which houses Broca's motor speech area. The much longer posterior ramus is used in defining the lobes of the hemisphere. The central sulcus is prominent approximately midway along the anteroposterior extent of the lateral surface of the hemisphere and, most commonly, extends over the medial margin, where its inferomedial tip is embraced by the U-shaped paracentral lobule. On the lateral surface, it passes from the medial margin, forwards and laterally, to reach the lateral sulcus. The line of the central sulcus closely approximates the line of the coronal suture of the adult skull, i.e. the junction between the frontal and parietal bones; consequently, the sulcus separates the frontal and parietal lobes. The demarcation of the occipital lobe is the parieto-occipital sulcus dorsally and medially, and the pre-occipital sulcus ventrally and laterally, with an imaginary line connecting the two and intersecting the posterior tip of the lateral sulcus. The temporal lobe lies anterior to this line and inferior (ventral) to the lateral sulcus. The deep lateral sulcus broadens out at its fundus, with an area of cortex forming the extensive floor of the sulcus, particularly in its anterior two-thirds. This cortex is the insula, which does not

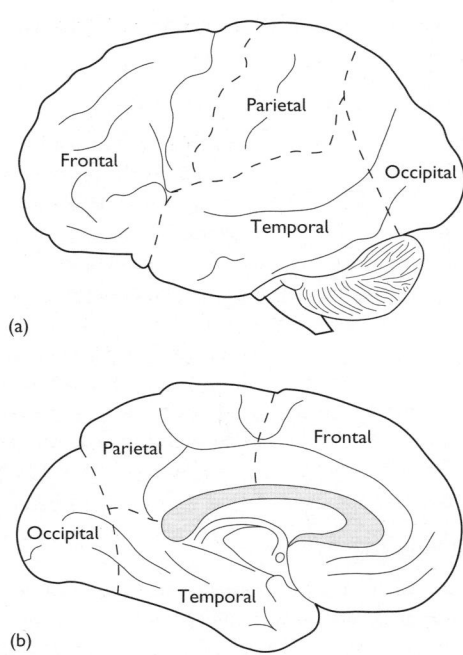

(a)

(b)

Fig. 1 The lobes of the cerebral cortex.

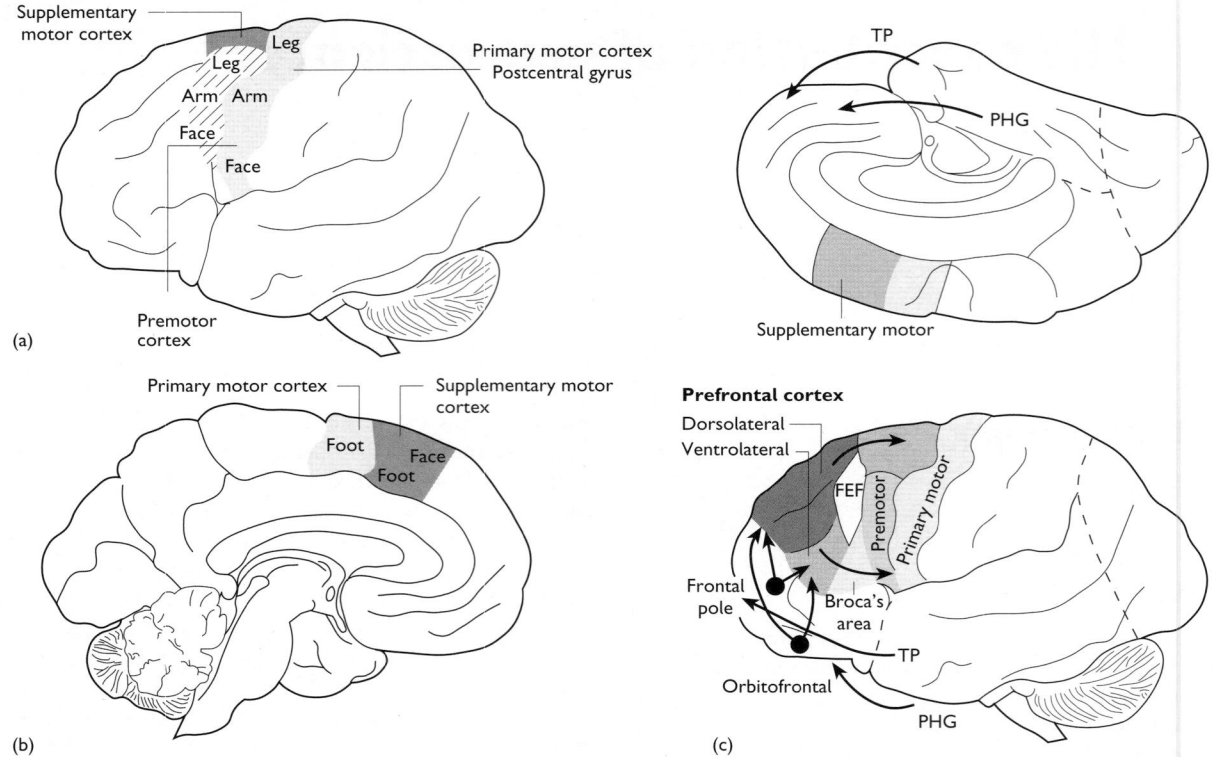

Fig. 2 Motor areas of the frontal lobe: TP, temporal pole; PHG, parahippocampal gyrus; FEF, frontal eyefields.

form part of any of the lobes mentioned above. The insula is surrounded by the circular sulcus, and is overhung by the frontal and parietal opercula superiorly, and the temporal operculum inferiorly (ventrally). The anatomical borders of the lobes of the cerebral cortex, and other sulcal and gyral landmarks, are only loosely paralleled by functional boundaries. However, lobar terminology is so firmly embedded in clinical and non-clinical neuroscience that consideration of their anatomical features is essential.

The frontal lobe (Fig. 2)

The precentral gyrus, immediately in front of the central sulcus and continuing onto the medial surface, contains the primary motor cortex. The precentral sulcus usually defines the anterior boundary, and in front of this lies the premotor cortex. The inferior margin of the sulcus runs into the pars triangularis, which includes Broca's motor speech area. On the medial margin and surface, the cortex includes the supplementary motor area. The lateral prefrontal cortex, in front of these motor and associated areas, is usually grooved by two major horizontal sulci, defining the superior, middle, and inferior frontal gyri. The cortex on the medial surface of the frontal lobe anterior to the prefrontal gyrus forms the medial prefrontal cortex. The concave inferior surface of the frontal lobe, overlying the bony orbit *in vivo*, is the orbitofrontal cortex.

The parietal lobe (Fig. 3)

Behind the central sulcus, the primary somatic sensory cortex (SI), extending onto the medial surface to occupy the posterior part of the paracentral lobule, where the sacral spinal segments are represented, occupies the postcentral gyrus. The postcentral sulcus limits the post-

central gyrus posteriorly. Behind this, the sulcal pattern is variable, but one or more horizontal intraparietal sulci divide the lobe into superior and inferior parts. The second somatic sensory cortex (SII) is located in the parietal operculum, close behind the inferolateral tip of the central sulcus. Specific sulcal patterns in the transition region between the parietal lobe and the occipital and temporal lobes (the supramarginal and angular gyri) are important landmarks for the detailed localization of language functions.

The occipital lobe (Fig. 4)

The occipital lobe is predominantly involved in vision and visual perception. The medial surface is grooved by the deep horizontal calcarine sulcus, which typically reaches the posterior pole of the hemisphere. Within its walls is the primary visual cortex. This area (area 17 of Brodmann) is often called the striate cortex; in the freshly sliced brain, a thin band of white matter, the stria of Gennari, is clearly visible running in the centre of the cortical grey ribbon. The extent of this stria precisely demarcates the primary visual cortex. Surrounding areas of the medial and lateral surface, the prestriate and peristriate cortex, contain some of the numerous separate visual association areas.

The temporal lobe (Figs 5 and 6)

Two horizontal sulci, the superior and inferior temporal sulci, divide the lateral surface of the temporal lobe into the superior, middle, and inferior gyri. The latter, extending onto the inferior surface, is also known as the inferotemporal cortex. On the medial surface, the collateral sulcus runs from close to the temporal pole to the calcarine

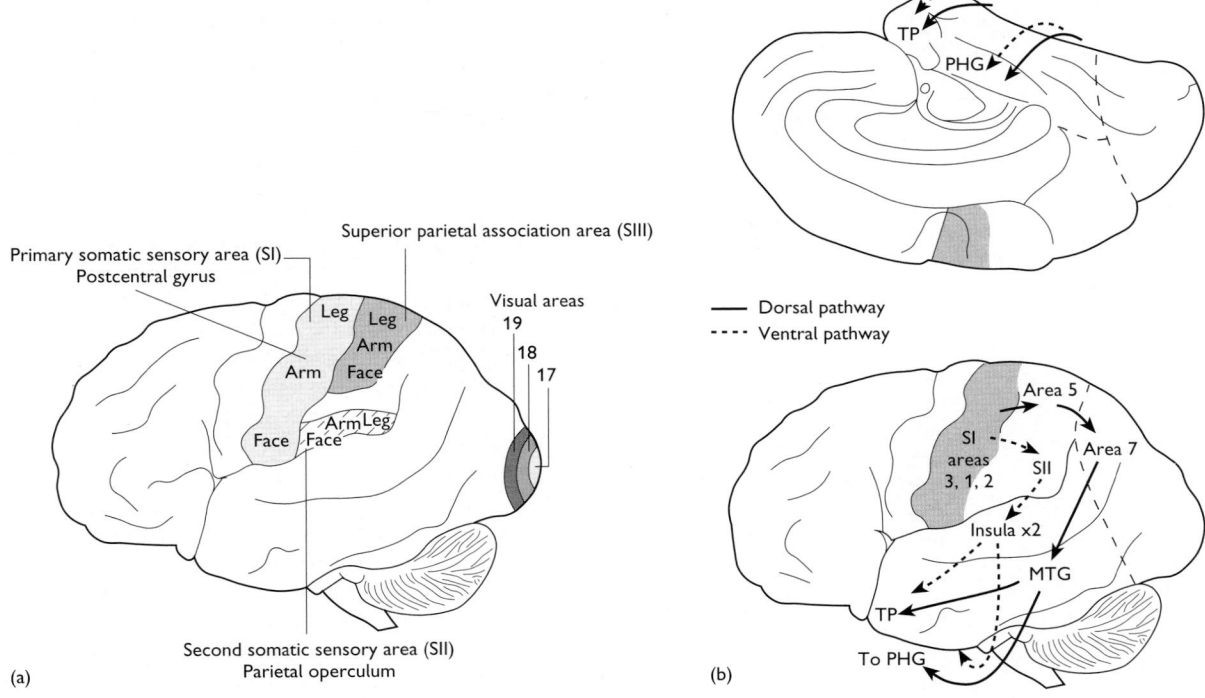

Fig. 3 (a) Areas of the parietal lobe; (b) somatic sensory association pathways. TP, temporal pole; PHG, parahippocampal gyrus; MTG, middle temporal gyrus.

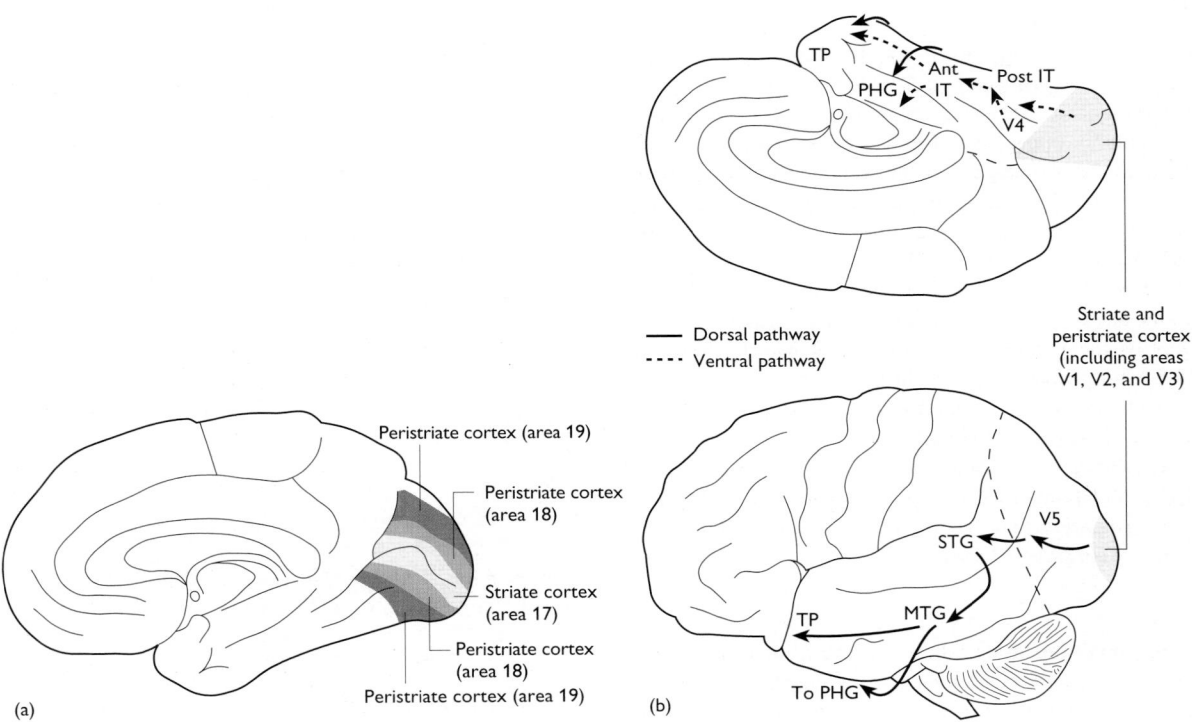

Fig. 4 The occipital lobe: (a) visual areas; (b) visual association pathways. TP, temporal pole; IT, inferotemporal cortex; PHG, parahippocampal gyrus; STG, superior temporal gyrus; MTG, middle temporal gyrus; Ant, anterior; Post, posterior.

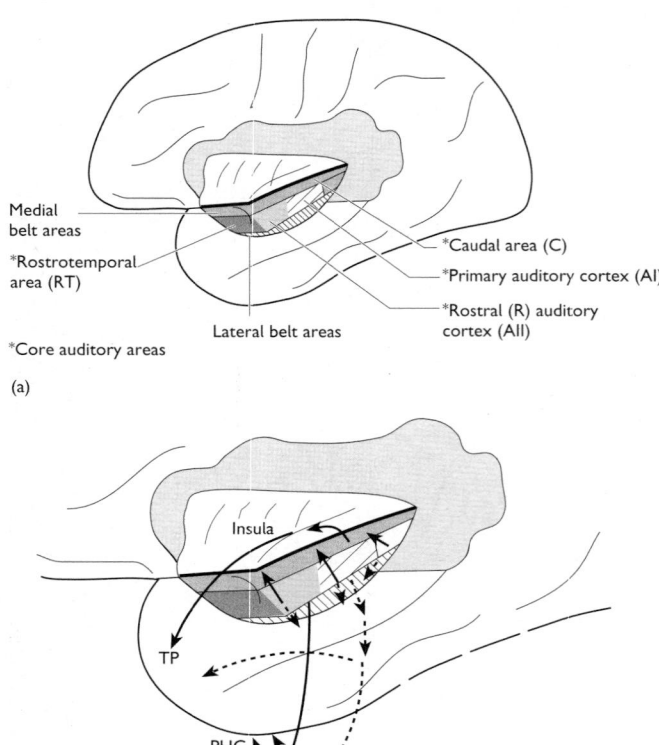

Fig. 5 Auditory association connections. TP, temporal pole; PHG, parahippocampal gyrus.

The structure of the neocortex

The neocortical grey matter is usually described as having six layers (Plate 1(a)). Wide variation in the nature of this microscopic lamination underlies the subdivision of neocortex into a multiplicity of (usually numbered) areas. At its simplest, two types of neurones make up the grey matter—pyramidal and non-pyramidal (or granular) cells. An apparent predominance of one or other type gives the extremes of granular and agranular cortex, equating with sensory areas (granular) and the motor cortex (agranular). In fact, the proportion of different cell types is constant in all areas. Indeed, with the single exception of the primary visual cortex, the numbers of neurones under a fixed surface area is also constant in all cortical areas. Variations in the size of pyramidal cells in particular lead to an apparent change in proportions. These variations probably reflect differences in the axonal volume of individual pyramidal cells, reflecting the distance and volume of projection fibres from a cortical area.

Pyramidal cells have a single main apical dendrite ascending towards the pial surface, and several horizontally spreading basal dendrites. All dendrites bear dendritic spines, which receive synapses (Plate 1(b)). All pyramidal cells use excitatory amino acids as neurotransmitters and have axons which enter the subcortical white matter; hence they are all projection neurones. They constitute approximately 60 per cent of all the neurones in the cortex. A second spiny neuronal type, the spiny stellate cells, is the next most numerous. These also use an excitatory amino acid, most probably glutamate, as their neuro-

sulcus posteriorly. Medial to this is the parahippocampal gyrus. Anteriorly, this curves dorsally and caudally to form the hook-shaped uncus. The entorhinal cortex occupies approximately the anterior third of the parahippocampal gyrus. Lateral to this, in the walls of the rhinal sulcus, lies the perirhinal cortex. The uncus closely overlies the amygdala; the primary olfactory cortex, the piriform cortex, lies immediately in front. The choroid fissure limits the parahippocampal gyrus medially. Passing into the floor of the lateral ventricle, the subicular areas of cortex lead to the hippocampus proper. A detailed consideration of the anatomy of the hippocampus is given below.

The cortex of the temporal operculum contains Heschl's gyri, within which lies the primary auditory cortex. Diverse auditory association areas surround this, extending into the superior temporal gyrus. The functions of the cortex of the middle temporal gyrus are uncertain, but include complex visual, auditory, and somatic sensory association areas. The inferotemporal cortex is largely concerned with visual perception and cognition. The anatomical pathways that underlie these functions are considered below.

The insula

The anterior margin of the insula, where the cortex becomes continuous with the anterior perforated substance, is known as the limen insulae. Above and below, where the insular cortex rolls round onto the opercula, lies the circular sulcus, the superior and inferior rami of which fuse posterosuperiorly to form the apex of the insula. Several variable sulci mark the insula, but little is known of the functional subdivisions of this cortex; gustatory, somatic sensory, and auditory areas have been described.

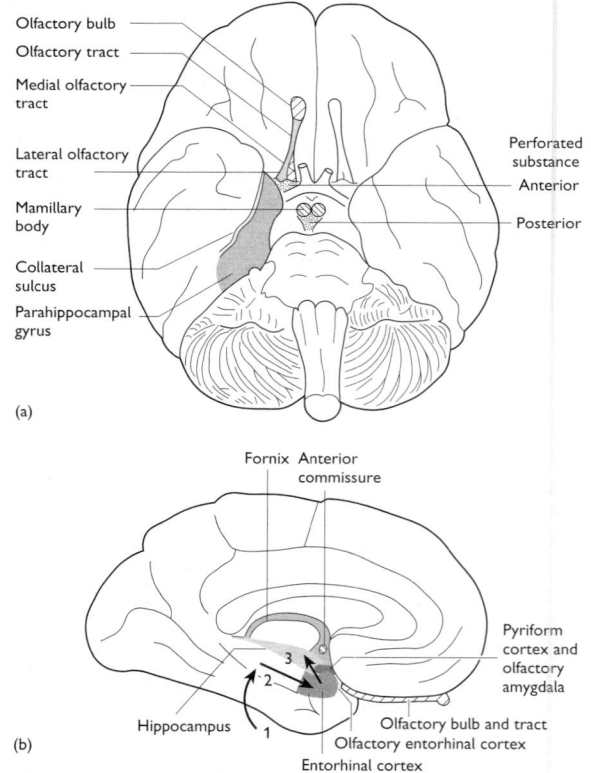

Fig. 6 Olfactory and limbic structures: (a) ventral surface of the brain; (b) medial temporal lobe. 1, Association cortex to parahippocampal gyrus; 2, parahippocampal gyrus to entorhinal cortex; 3, entorhinal cortex to hippocampus (perforant path).

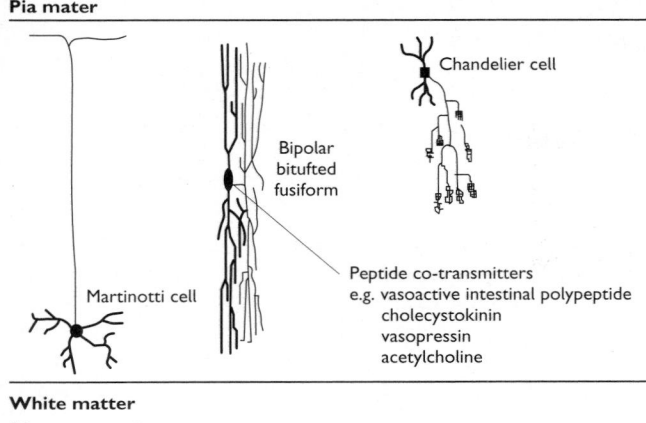

Fig. 7 Inhibitory (GABA-ergic) neurones of the neocortex: (a) vertical; (b) horizontal.

transmitter. Unlike pyramidal cells, however, their axons remain confined to the cortical grey matter; they are interneurones, accounting for a further 25 per cent of cortical neurones. All the other neurones are inhibitory interneurones, using γ-aminobutyric acid (**GABA**) as their major neurotransmitter. Many also contain one or more neuropeptides, and their content of specific calcium-binding proteins varies. They have a wide range of axonal and dendritic forms, and have been multiply classified in the past. Broadly speaking, they can be grouped into those with horizontal axonal arborizations, those whose axons ramify at right angles to the pial surface, i.e. through the depth of the cortex, and those with radial axons (Fig. 7).

The structure of the allocortex

The allocortex comprises a number of different areas, all with very different structures. They are either limbic or olfactory (or both) and are found predominantly in the medial temporal lobe. The largest of these regions is the hippocampus. Essentially this includes the three-layered cortex of the hippocampus, together with the transitional areas between it and neocortex, which are variably said to have three, four, five, or six laminae. The hippocampal formation comprises the dentate gyrus, Ammon's horn (CA fields), and the subiculum. The dentate gyrus and the CA fields each have a prominent single layer of neurones, with an overlying molecular layer and a subjacent polymorphic layer. In the dentate gyrus the cells are granule cells, whereas in the CA

fields they are predominantly large pyramidal cells—the stratum pyramidale. Both cell types are excitatory and are projection neurones. Scattered populations of GABA-ergic inhibitory interneurones are found immediately subjacent to the main cellular laminae and in the molecular layers. The CA fields are numbered 1, 2, and 3 from the subiculum to the dentate gyrus. The subiculum is the zone of transition between the three-layered hippocampus proper, and the entorhinal cortex and cortex of the parahippocampal gyrus laterally. It is sometimes further subdivided into subzones including the presubiculum, between the lateral cortex and the subiculum, and the prosubiculum, between the subiculum proper and CA1 of the hippocampus. The histological appearance of the hippocampus and adjacent areas are shown in Fig. 8, and their connections are considered in detail below.

The general pattern of connectivity of the cortex

All cortical areas share a broadly similar pattern of connections. What differs is the relative quantity of connections in each category, as well as the precise detail of origin and termination. The broad categories of connections which all cortical areas share are most easily seen in a table (Table 1). These will be dealt with in detail in subsequent sections.

A central feature of the connections of the neocortex is their organization relative to the cortical laminae (Plate 1(a)). For simplicity, it can generally be assumed that the forward-flowing stream of connections for perception and action use the central laminae, descending projections originate in deeper layers, and feedback and non-specific afferents terminate in both superficial and deep laminae. Thus, in primary sensory areas the thalamic input from the principal nuclei (e.g. the lateral geniculate nucleus in the visual cortex) terminates in layer IV. Projections to higher association areas originate from pyramidal cells immediately adjacent, in layer III. As the ipsilateral association pathway progresses from area to area, the association fibres terminate in this central region, and the thalamic afferents end in superficial and deep laminae. Projections to subcortical nuclei, such as the striatum, arise in layer V, and corticothalamic axons come from layer VI. It is as if the input of major importance, requiring detailed, focused, and faithful transmission, arrives in layer IV and is passed on from the deeper part of layer III. Inputs which moderate or modulate this pass to either side of the central layers, and outputs which are not directly part of this progression arise from deeper layers.

There is a general principle in the organization of connectivity with the cerebral cortex of overlapping connectivity of functionally related areas throughout the range of connections made. In other words, functionally related cortical areas, which are connected with each other, also tend to have overlapping or interdigitating connections with other structures. This is seen on the striatum, the thalamus, the claustrum, the cholinergic basal forebrain, and the pontine nuclei.

Subcortical afferents to the cerebral cortex

The thalamus (Plate 2)

Thalamic nuclei can be classified as specific (principal) or non-specific. In general, the specific nuclei degenerate completely when the cortex is removed, whereas the non-specific nuclei do not. This is

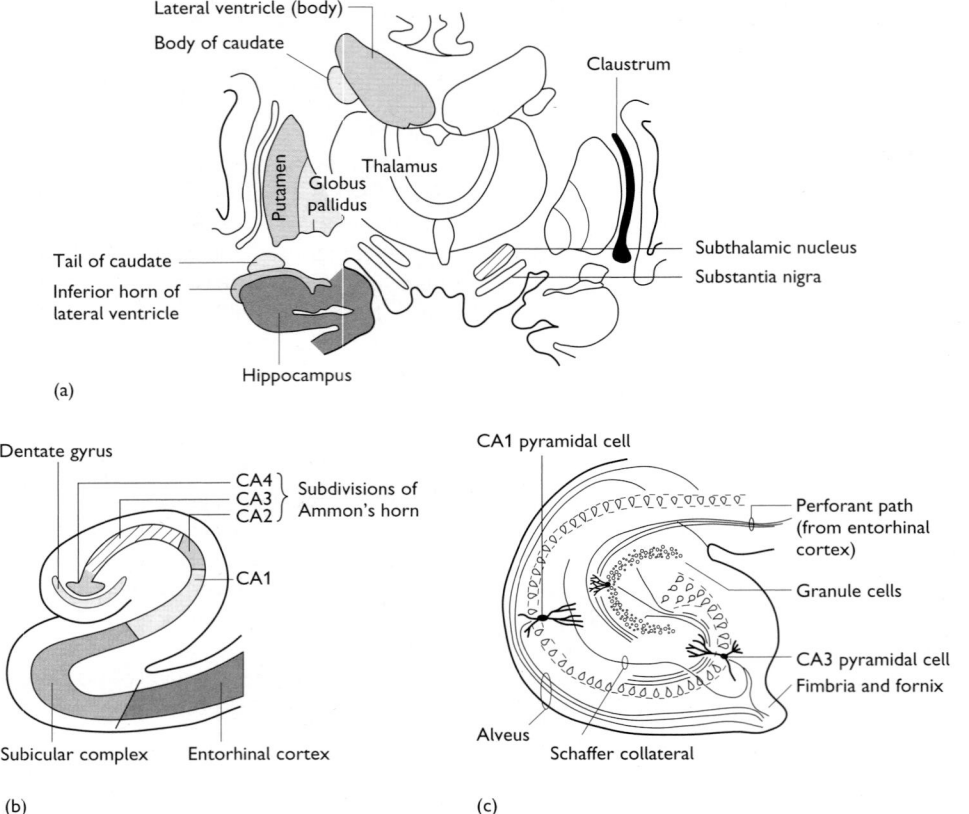

Fig. 8 (a) Hippocampal formation in the temporal lobe; (b) subdivisions of the hippocampal formation; (c) organization of the hippocampus.

because the sole major projection of the specific nuclei is to the cerebral cortex. The non-specific nuclei are the intralaminar and midline nuclei, which project to the basal ganglia as well as to cortex, and the reticular nucleus, which projects only to other thalamic nuclei.

All cortical areas receive afferents from at least one specific thalamic nucleus, and an additional input from the intralaminar/midline nuclei. Corticothalamic fibres reciprocate all thalamocortical projections, probably without exception.

Specific nuclei

The cortical projections of the specific nuclei are shown in Plate 2. Subclassification of the specific thalamic nuclei depends upon their afferent subcortical connections. The primary relay nuclei receive the major sensory pathways—the lateral and medial geniculate nuclei for the optic tract and auditory pathway respectively, and the ventral posterior nucleus for the somatic sensory pathways. The secondary relay nuclei are those which receive a known major subcortical pathway which is not sensory. These are usually taken to include the caudal subdivision of the ventral lateral nucleus, which receives the cerebellar pathway, the anterior division of the ventral lateral nucleus and the ventral anterior nucleus, which both receive fibres from the internal segment of the globus pallidus, and the anterior nuclei, which receive the mammillothalamic tract. The association nuclei are those which were not previously understood to receive a major subcortical pathway, predominantly the medial nucleus and the pulvinar. This view is no longer really tenable, since the pulvinar is now known to receive a major input from the superior colliculus, and the various subdivisions

of the medial nucleus receive fibres from the ventral pallidum and the olfactory pathway, amongst others. The subcortical afferents to the principal thalamic nuclei are shown in Plate 2(a).

The non-specific nuclei

The reticular nucleus lies lateral to the main body of the thalamus, separated from it by the external medullary lamina. Cells in the nucleus are inhibitory, using GABA as their neurotransmitter. Excitatory thalamocortical and corticothalamic fibres, passing to and from the main nuclei, traverse the reticular nucleus and give axon collaterals to the reticular nucleus cells. There is a very tight arrangement, whereby the branches of axons from the thalamus to a particular cortical area terminate in the reticular nucleus in close proximity to the corticothalamic axons from the same cortical area. The reticular nucleus cells in turn send their inhibitory axons into the thalamus, to terminate precisely in the nuclei from which they receive a collateral input.

The intralaminar and midline nuclei receive afferents from the major pathways to their adjacent principal nuclei and project to the striatum (caudate, putamen, and ventral striatum) as well as to the cortex. There is a broad topographic relationship in their projection to both areas. The midline nuclei innervate the ventral striatum (nucleus accumbens) and the limbic cortex, including the hippocampal formation. The anterior intralaminar nuclei connect with the prefrontal, parietal, occipital, and temporal cortex, and project to all parts of the caudate. The posterior intralaminar nuclei, of which the centromedian nucleus is the largest, project to the putamen and are reciprocally

Table 1 General connections of the cerebral cortex

Nucleus/area	Afferents	Efferents
Subcortical		
Thalamus		
Principal	+	+
Intralaminar	+	+
Locus coeruleus (NA)	+	–
Raphe (serotonin)	+	–
Basal nucleus (ACh)	+	–
Hypothalamus (histamine)	+	–
SN and VTA (dopamine)	+	–
Claustrum	+	+
Striatum	–	+
Pons	–	+
Superior colliculus and reticular formation	–	+
Specific (e.g. corticospinal)	–	(+/–)
Cortical		
Contralateral		
Homotopic	+	+
Heterotopic	+	+
Ipsilateral		
Short	+	+
Long	+	+

NA, noradrenaline; ACh, acetylcholine; SN, substantia nigra; VTA, ventral tegmental area.

related to the motor, premotor, and supplementary motor areas of cortex in the frontal lobe. Many axons to the cortex from the intralaminar nuclei are collateral branches of thalamostriate axons. The cortical and striatal areas to which they each project are precisely those parts of the cortex and striatum which are themselves directly connected by corticostriate fibres.

Non-thalamic subcortical afferents to the cerebral cortex

A variety of nuclei send afferents to the cerebral cortex. These fall into two categories: fibres from the so-called isodendritic core of the brainstem and basal forebrain, which are non-reciprocal and aminergic, and the two-way interconnections with the claustrum.

Acetylcholine and the basal forebrain

A system of cholinergic nuclei extend from the septum verum anteriorly, through the nuclei of the diagonal band of Broca to the basal nucleus of Meynert in the substantia innominata, ventral to the globus pallidus, most posteriorly. From these, cholinergic fibres pass to the entire cerebral cortex. Alternative nomenclature for these nuclei uses a numeric system, Ch1 to Ch4. The anterior cell groups project to the hippocampus and entorhinal cortex, and to the olfactory bulb and cortex. There is an approximate topographic relationship in the projection of the basal nucleus to the neocortex, but with considerable overlap; adjacent or overlapping regions of the nucleus project to widely separated but functionally related and interconnected areas of neocortex. Degeneration of this system is associated with the dementias of Alzheimer's disease and Lewy body disease.

Cholinergic cells in the pedunculopontine nucleus of the midbrain project to the thalamus, particularly to the midline and intralaminar nuclei.

Serotonin, noradrenaline (norepinephrine) and adrenaline (epinephrine): the raphe and associated nuclei

The median group of nuclei of the brainstem reticular formation is made up largely of the various raphe nuclei, all of which use serotonin (5-hydroxytryptamine) as their neurotransmitter. Their projections are very widespread throughout the central nervous system. Broadly speaking, there is a rostrocaudal topography to the efferent projections of these nuclei. The most rostral, notably the dorsal median raphe nucleus in the midbrain tegmentum, send projections to the entire cerebral cortex and striatum. There is a prominent projection to the thalamus, notably to the midline nuclei which in turn project in part to the hippocampal formation. The serotoninergic raphe-spinal tract, which has important functions in the gating of pain, arises from the most rostral nuclei, the raphe obscurus and the raphe magnus.

The locus coeruleus lies in the dorsolateral pons, immediately deep to the ventricular ependyma. Together with the subceruleus immediately deep to it, this nucleus supplies noradrenergic fibres to most of the central nervous system. Ascending fibres pass to the thalamus and hypothalamus, the entire cerebral cortex (neo- and allocortex), the amygdala, the septal nuclei, and the olfactory bulb. Adrenergic cells in the brainstem do not appear to send ascending projections to the cortex.

Dopamine: the substantia nigra and adjacent nuclei

The major dopaminergic cell group of the midbrain is the pars compacta of the substantia nigra, which projects to the striatum (caudate, putamen, nucleus accumbens, and olfactory tubercle). Two other adjacent nuclei, the ventral tegmental area of Tsai and the pigmented parabrachial nucleus, are also dopaminergic. Together, these three cell groups project rostrally in the medial forebrain bundle to innervate the thalamus and hypothalamus, the hippocampal formation, the entorhinal cortex and amygdala, and widespread areas of the neocortex, especially the prefrontal, orbitofrontal, and cingulate cortex.

Histamine and the posterior hypothalamus

The entire cerebral cortex, including the limbic lobe, receives a histaminergic projection from the tuberomamillary nucleus of the posterior hypothalamus. Postsynaptic receptors appear to be of two types, H1 and H2, with broadly opposing effects.

The cortex and the claustrum

The claustrum is a thin plate of grey matter lying immediately deep to the cortex of the insula, and separated from it by the white matter of the extreme capsule. Medially, the external capsule (Fig. 8(a)) separates it from the putamen. The nucleus receives fibres from and projects to the whole cortex, including the allocortex. The reciprocal connection is topographically organized, but with overlapping zones projecting to widely separated but functionally related and interconnected cortical areas. Many of the neurones of the claustrum have branching axons with collaterals going to two or more such interconnected areas. For example, the superior parietal cortex (area 5) is widely separated from the premotor cortex (area 6) but is connected to it by ipsilateral association fibres, and the two areas are functionally closely related. Both these areas project to and receive from an overlapping zone of the claustrum, and many axons of claustral cells in this zone may branch to both areas.

Modulation of cortical activation and the anatomy of the reticular activating system

Specific information to the cerebral cortex, for example relating to sensory stimuli in the periphery, is relayed via the main thalamic nuclei. The other, diffusely projecting, systems are most likely to be involved in the regulation of cortical responsivity. Such a role has been demonstrated electrophysiologically for the claustrum, and the pharmacology of the antihistamines indicates a role for this transmitter system in the regulation of cortical arousal. The cholinergic input from the basal forebrain is necessary for the proper functioning of the cortex, and its degeneration is associated with cognitive decline and memory impairment. The possible relationship of mesolimbic dopamine pathways to schizophrenia is well known. Similarly, the psychopharmacology of serotonin also implies a major role for this transmitter system in the proper functioning of the cortex. There are two routes by which these 'non-specific' pathways affect the cortex: direct projections, and an indirect pathway through the thalamus. Brainstem nuclei send fibres to the intralaminar and midline nuclei, which in turn send fibres to the entire cortex including the hippocampus. The cholinergic input from the interpeduncular nucleus to the intralaminar nuclei is prominent. Serotonin is particularly concentrated in the midline nuclei. There are other reticular formation projections to these nuclei, but the transmitters remain uncertain. This latter indirect route by which the reticular formation of the brainstem impinges on the cerebral cortex via the thalamus constitutes the reticular activating system. The role of this system in cortical arousal is well documented.

Corticocortical connections

The corpus callosum and the commissural connections of the cerebral cortex

All cortical areas both send fibres to and receive fibres from the opposite hemisphere, although the connections are not necessarily throughout the whole area. In most of the cortex, commissural fibres pass to the contralateral side in the corpus callosum. The anterior commissure carries fibres that interconnect the anterior third or so of the temporal lobe with its partner, as well as fibres that interconnect the olfactory bulbs on each side. Some fibres in the fornix cross the midline, the so-called commissure of the fornix, to interconnect the two hippocampal formations. Commissural fibres are of two types, homotopic and heterotopic. Homotopic fibres pass from one area of cortex to the same area on the other side. Heterotopic fibres pass from one area to a different, although often functionally related, area on the other side. As a generalization, the functions of the commissures can be subdivided into two categories. First, they serve to interconnect representations of the contralateral sensory surround across the midline, for example the representations of the two halves of the body, the two visual hemifields, and so on. In areas containing a lateralized sensory representation, of either the body or the visual field, the callosal fibres are confined, in both origin and termination, to the parts of the area containing a representation of midline and adjacent regions. Thus the representation of the trunk in somatic sensory areas sends and receives commissural fibres, whereas the hand and foot representations are not connected across the midline. Similarly, the vertical meridians in visuotopic representations are interconnected by callosal fibres, whereas the periphery is not. In contrast, the second function of the commissures is to connect areas in one hemisphere with areas on the other side, where the functions of each are represented on only one side, i.e. they are lateralized. Of course, this is most apparent for language areas; for example, objects held in the non-dominant hand cannot be named following callosal section because the sensory cortex of the non-dominant hemisphere cannot communicate across the midline with the language and speech areas in the dominant hemisphere.

Ipsilateral corticocortical association connections

All cortical areas interconnect with other areas in the same hemisphere. The primary sensory areas are in the parietal, occipital, and temporal lobes. From these, parallel pathways emanate in an approximately hierarchical sequence through multiple areas in the adjacent association cortex, passing towards the medial temporal lobe where all pathways converge on the parahippocampal gyrus and the cortex of the temporal pole. In general, three 'tiers' of association areas can be recognized in this sequence; the first tier receives from the core sensory areas, and the third projects into the temporal pole and the parahippocampal gyrus. Connections passing in the direction of the medial temporal cortex from the primary sensory areas have a feedforward pattern of termination, whereas the reciprocal connections have a feedback character. Although the interconnections of the multiple areas along this sequence of connections are complex, a broad pattern common to all the sensory pathways can be discerned. Essentially, each sensory modality has a core zone in the cortex, comprising three areas. Each of these is linked to the relevant main thalamic nuclei and contains a complete representation of the sensory surround. They are linked together by short association connections passing forwards from the first thalamo-recipient zone in a stepwise fashion to the other two. Two streams of connections, dealing with different aspects of sensory perception, emanate from these into the surrounding association areas. One of these, the ventral stream (the 'stimulus-relevant' or 'what' system), is primarily concerned with the detailed perception and characterization of a stimulus. The second, the dorsal stream (the 'self-relevant' or 'where' system), is concerned mainly with spatial location, particularly in extrapersonal space. Each area in this sensory hierarchy is reciprocally connected to a part of the frontal lobe, where the dual-pathway streams are represented by a dorsal and a ventral prefrontal subdivision, feeding onto the supplementary and premotor cortex, and so to the motor cortex.

Cortical association pathways for vision (Fig. 4)

The three core visual areas are V1 (the primary visual cortex, striate cortex), V2 which surrounds V1 and is contained within Brodmann's area 18, and outside this the V3 complex which is probably still within area 18. From these, feedforward projections pass to areas in the inferior parietal and superior temporal cortices, as the dorsal stream, and to V4, within Brodmann's area 19, at the junction of the occipital association cortex with the inferior temporal gyrus on the medial surface, forming the ventral pathway. Areas in the superior temporal sulcus and middle temporal gyrus form the next two tiers of association cortex for the dorsal pathway. The ventral route progresses via the posterior inferotemporal cortex on to the anterior inferotemporal cortex.

Both the anterior inferotemporal and middle temporal cortical areas at the distal end of these two visual association pathways project to the cortex of the temporal pole, and to the parahippocampal gyrus. The parahippocampal gyrus projects to the entorhinal cortex more anteriorly, and the temporal pole connects with the amygdala. The entorhinal cortex provides a major input to the dentate gyrus of the hippocampus via the perforant path (see below). Similarly, the amygdala projects into the hippocampal formation.

Cortical association pathways for somatic sensation (Fig. 3)

The three core areas for the somatic sensory cortex are Brodmann's areas 3, 1, and 2 on the postcentral gyrus, together constituting the classical primary somatic sensory cortex. Each receives a major input from the ventral posterior nucleus of the thalamus and contains a complete representation of the body. Area 3 projects forwards to areas 1 and 2, and area 1 projects similarly to area 2. All three areas project in a feedforward fashion to the second somatic sensory area in the parietal operculum. This represents the first step on the ventral association pathway. The dorsal pathway begins with the projection of all subdivisions of the primary somatic sensory cortex to Brodmann's area 5 in the superior parietal cortex. Further steps along the ventral pathway are areas in the insula. In the ventral pathway, information flows from the superior to the inferior parietal cortex, and so to the middle temporal gyrus. Areas at the ends of both these paths project on to the parahippocampal gyrus and the temporal pole.

Cortical association pathways for hearing (Fig. 5)

The association pathways from the auditory cortex are less well understood. The three core areas lie along Heschl's gyrus in the temporal operculum, with the classical primary auditory area (AI) most posterior, the rostral auditory area (AII) more anterior, and the rostrotemporal auditory area in front of that. Each of these contains a complete representation of the auditory surround, organized tonotopically, and connects with the medial geniculate nucleus. On either side of these lie multiple auditory association areas, termed the medial and lateral belt areas, representing the first steps along the two association streams of connections, although it is unclear which is 'dorsal' and which is 'ventral' in a functional sense. The medial belt areas have connections with parts of the insula, whereas the lateral belt areas project into the association cortex of the superior temporal gyrus. The first association pathway probably continues through areas of the anterior part of the superior temporal gyrus, and so to the parahippocampal gyrus and the temporal pole. The second continues from the superior to the middle temporal gyrus, and thence to the parahippocampal cortex and the temporal pole.

The olfactory pathway to the cerebral cortex (Fig. 6)

The olfactory pathway is unique among the sensory modalities in having direct access to the cerebral cortex without passing through the thalamus. The primary olfactory receptor neurones of the olfactory mucosa send their axons (the fila olfactaria) through the cribriform plate of the ethmoid bone directly into the overlying olfactory bulb, where they contact the mitral cells in synaptic glomeruli. Axons of the mitral cells pass caudally in the olfactory tract to the anterior perforated substance. Here the olfactory tract splits into medial and lateral olfactory striae. All the mitral cell axons pass in the lateral stria. The medial stria contains axons mainly from the anterior olfactory

nucleus, which are destined for the contralateral olfactory bulb by way of the anterior commissure. The lateral olfactory stria passes to the medial temporal lobe, where the axons terminate in the anterior margin of the entorhinal cortex, the pyriform cortex, and the corticomedial subdivision of the amygdala. All three termination zones interconnect. The olfactory entorhinal cortex and the olfactory amygdala both have connections with their non-olfactory partners, i.e. with the more posterior entorhinal subdivisions and the basolateral part of the amygdala respectively.

The limbic cortex and the amygdala (Figs 6 and 8)

The latter stages of the sensory association pathways all converge on the entorhinal cortex, the perirhinal cortex, and the amygdala, which are themselves interconnected. These in turn project to the hippocampus. The perirhinal cortex lies lateral to the entorhinal cortex in the banks of the rhinal fissure. It appears to receive afferents from the later stages of the sensory association pathways, notably from the temporal pole, and is extensively interconnected with the amygdala, the entorhinal cortex, and the hippocampus. The amygdala projects to the CA pyramidal cells, notably to CA1. The entorhinal input to the hippocampus arises from cell clusters in layer II and forms the perforant pathway, with axons terminating on the dendrites of granule cells of the dentate gyrus. Additional entorhinal fibres pass to the CA pyramidal cells. Axons of the dentate gyrus granule cells pass out into the molecular layer of the CA fields, notably CA3, where they synapse on the apical dendrites of pyramidal neurones. CA3 pyramidal cells project out via the fimbria, but also send collateral axons to synapse with the pyramidal cells of CA1 in particular. The activity of pyramidal neurones in the CA fields is regulated by inhibitory GABA-ergic interneurones in the molecular layer and by the basket cells, which are also GABA-ergic, sited immediately subjacent to the pyramidal layer. The latter inhibitory neurones have axons that branch around the pyramidal cell bodies, forming the baskets of terminal fibres from which they are named. CA1 sends some fibres into the fornix, but projects heavily to the subicular complex. The major output of the hippocampal formation comes from the subicular complex, and passes out into the fornix via the alveus and fimbria. The projection of fibres in the fornix to the hypothalamus, including the mamillary nuclei, is considered below. However, some hippocampal efferent fibres bypass these nuclei and enter the mamillothalamic tract without synapsing. Rather, they pass directly to the anterior thalamic nuclei, where they terminate. From the anterior thalamic nuclei, of which there are several subdivisions, axons project to the cortex of the cingulate gyrus along the whole of its length, extending into the parahippocampal gyrus inferiorly. Fibres forming the cingulum bundle interconnect these medial cortical areas, running predominantly from anterior to posterior and ending in the parahippocampal gyrus, so that they reach the entorhinal cortex. This completes Papez's circuit and defines the structures of the limbic lobe—hippocampal formation, mamillary nuclei and anterior thalamus, cingulate cortex, parahippocampal gyrus and cingulate cortex. The term 'limbic system' is often extended to include structures, such as the amygdala, which have strong connections with these components.

Association connections of the frontal lobe (Fig. 2)

The hierarchical sequence of connections in the sensory association pathways outlined above is reflected in a similar sequence passing from

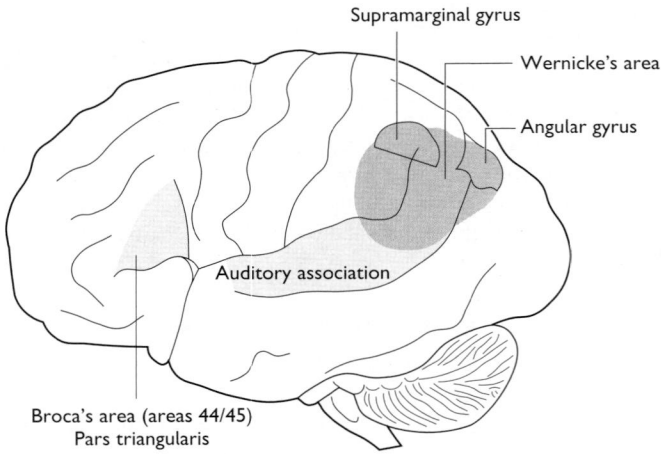

Fig. 9 Auditory association cortex and Wernicke's sensory speech area.

association areas of the prefrontal cortex back towards the primary motor cortex of the precentral gyrus. The two streams of connections are tightly linked together by long association pathways, with each tier of connections in the sensory association pathways interconnected with an area of the frontal lobe. The medial temporal areas, including the entorhinal cortex, the perirhinal cortex and the parahippocampal gyrus are closely interconnected with areas in the orbitofrontal cortex. The temporal pole is reciprocally connected with the frontal pole (Brodmann's area 10). The tiers of sensory association areas in the parietal, occipital, and temporal cortex are interconnected with the dorsolateral and ventrolateral prefrontal association cortex, occupying Brodmann's areas 9, 46, and 45. Broadly speaking, the association areas on the dorsal stream of connections for each modality interconnect with the dorsolateral prefrontal areas 9 and 46. In contrast, the ventral stream areas interconnect with the ventrolateral prefrontal cortex in areas 45 and 46. Like the sensory association areas, these regions seem to separate functionally into a dorsal hierarchy, dealing with internally generated actions, and a ventral hierarchy related to externally guided behaviours. Connections from the dorsolateral prefrontal cortex pass preferentially to the supplementary motor cortex, whereas the more ventrally placed prefrontal cortex feeds into the premotor cortex. Both the supplementary and the premotor cortex feed into the primary motor cortex of the precentral gyrus. The frontal eye-field (Brodmann's area 8), which has major ipsilateral association connections with the visual areas in the occipital lobe, is strategically placed between the prefrontal and premotor areas. It also receives ipsilateral association connections from the dorsolateral and ventrolateral prefrontal association areas.

Speech areas of the cerebral cortex

Because speech and language are not present in the subhuman primate species commonly used for neuroanatomical investigation of cortical connections, little is known about the connections of these in the human. The posterior speech area (Wernicke's area) occupies a large extent of the posterior temporal and inferior parietal cortex at the posterior limits of the superior temporal and lateral sulci, and is often taken as extending anteriorly along the superior temporal gyrus. It includes the angular and supramarginal gyri (Fig. 9). This would represent a region where the association pathways of all three

modalities—somatic sensation, vision, and hearing—lie close together. It would include many auditory association areas along the superior temporal gyrus. Within the frontal lobe, Broca's area occupies the pars triangularis between the anterior and ascending rami of the lateral sulcus. It is closely adjacent to the face area in the lateral premotor cortex. Similarly, the medial speech area lies on the medial surface immediately in front of the face representation in the supplementary motor cortex. It is, perhaps, not unreasonable to suppose that these two areas function to some extent as the premotor and supplementary motor speech areas.

Subcortical efferent pathways of the cerebral cortex

The corticostriate pathway and the basal ganglia (Fig. 10)

The anatomical definition of the basal ganglia comprises those deep grey-matter nuclei that develop from the telencephalic (cerebral) vesicle. Strictly, this would include the components of the striatum, the globus pallidus, the amygdala, and the claustrum. Because these latter two are better considered with the cortex and limbic system respectively, they are usually excluded from the term basal ganglia. Similarly, because of their close anatomical and functional relationship with the striatum and globus pallidus, the substantia nigra and subthalamic nucleus are usually included with the basal ganglia. The caudate and putamen are developmentally, anatomically, pharmacologically, and functionally a single structure, secondarily subdivided by the development of the internal capsule. The two fuse below the inferior margin of the anterior limb of the internal capsule to form the nucleus accumbens. This fusion comes to the surface of the hemisphere at the anterior perforated substance, an area sometimes called the olfactory tubercle. Together, the caudate, putamen, nucleus accumbens, and olfactory tubercle make up the striatum. The globus pallidus consists of two parts, an external segment (**GPe**) and an internal segment (**GPi**), separated by a thin white-matter lamina. Both segments extend ventrally in the region of the substantia innominata, below the anterior commissure, to form the ventral pallidum. The pars reticulata of the substantia nigra (**SNpr**) is developmentally, anatomically, pharmacologically and functionally a part of the internal segment of the globus pallidus, which has been separated off by the development of the fibres of the internal capsule passing into the crus cerebri of the midbrain. Therefore in this account the basal ganglia and related nuclei will comprise the striatum, GPe, GPi–SNpr, and the subthalamic nucleus (see Fig. 10).

The entire cerebral cortex projects to the striatum. The putamen receives predominantly from the sensorimotor cortex around the central sulcus. The caudate receives the input from most of the parietal, occipital, temporal, and frontal lobes. The limbic areas, including the entorhinal and perirhinal cortex, the hippocampus, and the amygdala, project to the ventral striatum (nucleus accumbens and olfactory tubercle) and the adjacent ventral portion of the head of the caudate. The corticostriate pathway arises from pyramidal cells predominantly in layer V of the cortex and is excitatory, using glutamate as its neurotransmitter. The termination of the pathway is broadly topographically organized, but with considerable interdigitation or overlap of the pro-

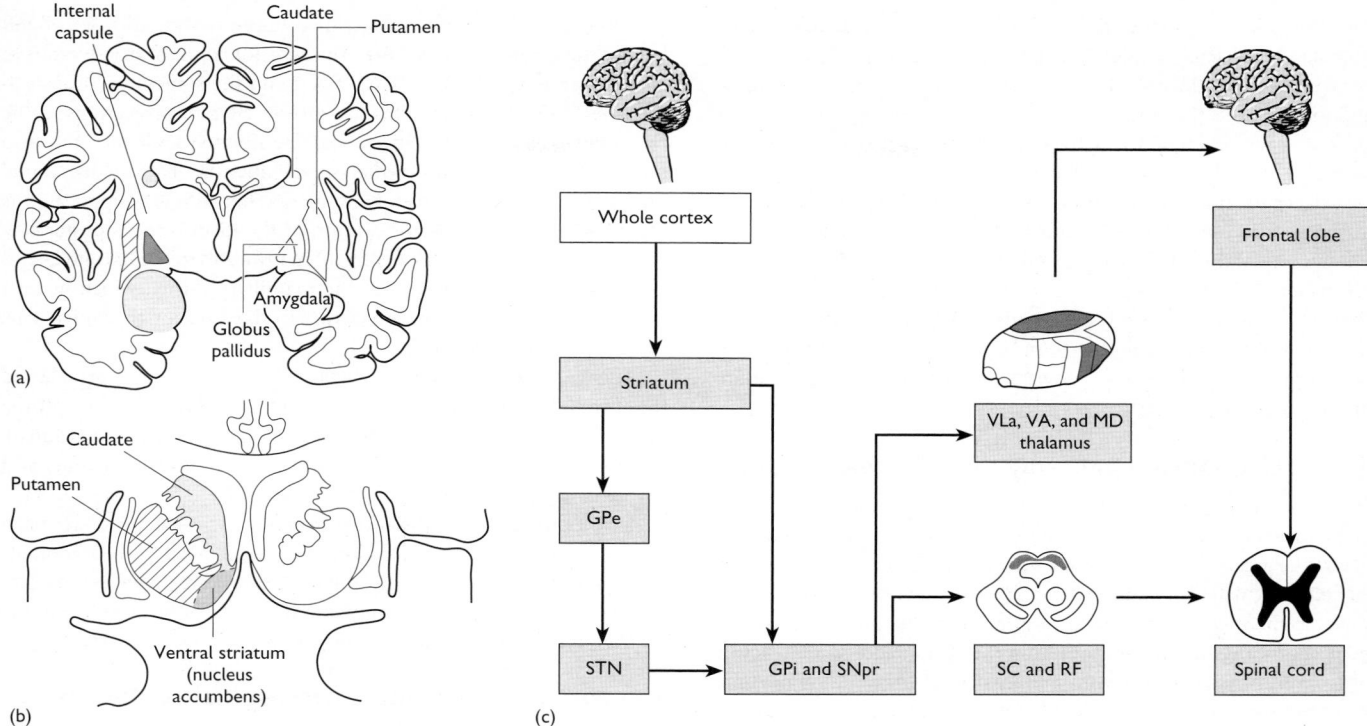

Fig. 10 The corticostriate pathway and the basal ganglia: (a) component nuclei of the basal ganglia; (b) striatum; (c) major pathways through the basal ganglia. GPe, external segment of the globus pallidus; STN, subthalamic nucleus; GPi, internal segment of the globus pallidus; SNpr, pars reticula of the substantia nigra.

jections from different cortical areas. Individual cortical areas project to a longitudinal strip of striatum orientated anteroposteriorly. The strips receiving from the frontal lobe extend more rostrally, whereas those receiving from the parietal, occipital, and temporal lobes extend more caudally. Anteriorly, zones receiving projections from interconnected areas in the frontal lobe interdigitate or overlap; centrally, zones receiving from frontal areas overlap with zones connected to areas within the parietal, temporal, or occipital cortex with which the frontal areas are connected by ipsilateral association fibres. More posteriorly, interconnected sensory association areas project to overlapping zones in the striatum. The striatum itself is compartmentalized, on the basis of acetylcholinesterase (**AChE**) histochemistry, into AChE-poor patches (striosomes) and AChE-rich matrix. The cortex projects into both compartments, but with a slightly different laminar origin. Pyramidal neurones in the deeper part of lamina V project to the patches, whereas more superficial lamina V cells and some lamina III cells project to the matrix. It is possible that apparently overlapping corticostriate projections from different cortical areas are segregated into the different compartments. The projection from a single cortical area may switch between compartments along the anteroposterior length of its zone of termination. The intralaminar nuclei of the thalamus send excitatory (glutamatergic) axons to the entire striatum. The nuclei project to those parts of the caudate or putamen which receive from the cortical areas to which the particular intralaminar nucleus projects. Many, if not all, interconnected areas in the frontal, parietal, occipital, and temporal lobes also receive a shared projection from a single intralaminar nucleus. Thus there is a tightly organized but complex topographical relationship between the connections of functionally related cortical areas with each other, with the striatum, and with the intralaminar nuclei of the thalamus. A closely similar relationship is seen in the cortical connections of the claustrum and the basal forebrain, and possibly even in the cortical projection to the pontine nuclei. Another major projection to the striatum is dopaminergic and comes from the pars compacta of the substantia nigra and adjacent nuclei. There is some topography in this projection, with the lateral and central parts of pars compacta of the substantia nigra projecting to the caudate and putamen. The medial part and the adjacent nuclei, such as the ventral tegmental area, project to the ventral striatum. The effect of dopamine on striatal neurones appears to be different in the two compartments. Additional striatal afferents come from the brainstem raphe nuclei (serotonin) and the amygdala (to the ventral striatum and the head of the caudate).

The output of the striatum passes to all parts of the globus pallidus (the ventral pallidum, GPe, and GPi–SNpr). These fibres are inhibitory, using GABA as their neurotransmitter. Here the pathway through the basal ganglia separates into a direct and an indirect route, ultimately passing to the thalamus. Fibres from the striosomes (patches) of the striatum are rich in substance P (as well as being GABA-ergic) and project to GPi. Axons from GPi go directly to the anterior part of the ventral lateral nucleus and the adjacent ventral anterior nucleus of the thalamus, forming the direct route. Neurones in the striatal matrix compartment contain enkephalin as a cotransmitter with GABA and project to GPe. Axons from GPe go to the subthalamic nucleus, which in turn projects to GPi (the indirect pathway). The ventral pallidum has equivalent pathways, but the final destination of the pallidal output is the mediodorsal nucleus of the thalamus. All efferents from the globus pallidus are GABA-ergic and inhibitory. The neurones of the subthalamic nucleus are glutamatergic and excitatory. Activation of the striatal output through the direct pathway leads to a reduced tonic inhibition of the thalamus. In contrast, activation via the indirect pathway leads to increased activation of GPi, and hence increased inhibition of the thalamus. The balance between these opposite effects is crucial in the normal functioning of the basal ganglia. Disruption of this balance is used to explain much of the pathophysiology of the extrapyramidal disorders. The ventral anterior and rostral ventral lateral nuclei of the thalamus project mainly to the premotor and supplementary motor areas of the frontal lobe. The ventral pallidal pathway through the mediodorsal thalamus feeds onto the prefrontal association areas. The major pathways through the basal ganglia are summarized in Fig. 10(c)).

The corticopontine pathway and the cerebellum

There is a major projection from the cortex to the pontine nuclei. The extent to which individual cortical areas contribute to this pathway varies. The greatest projection comes from the regions around the central sulcus, which also contribute to the pyramidal tract (see below). However, there is a substantial projection from the prefrontal cortex, and a significant number of fibres from the occipital lobe. Many fewer corticopontine axons arise from temporal neocortex, although some areas send some and it is possible that most areas send at least a few.

The pontine nuclei send their axons to the cerebellar cortex of the lateral parts of the posterior lobe. They terminate as mossy fibres, contacting granule cells. Axon collaterals pass, in addition, to the lateral dentate deep cerebellar nucleus. The anterior lobe and the midline and paramedian region of the posterior lobe are related to the spinocerebellar inputs. The flocculonodular lobe is connected to the vestibular pathway. The Purkinje cells of the cerebellar cortex send inhibitory fibres to the deep cerebellar nuclei, and it is from these that the output of the cerebellum arises. The intermediate (globose and emboliform) and medial (fastigial) deep nuclei project to the red nucleus and the vestibular nuclei and reticular formation. The dentate nucleus projects to the posterior part of the ventral lateral nucleus of the thalamus. This in turn provides the major thalamic input to the primary motor cortex of the precentral gyrus. In this way, the neocortical input to the cerebellum via the pontine nuclei is transmitted, via the thalamus, to the motor cortex.

The fornix and the cortical projection to the hypothalamus

Fibres leaving and entering the hippocampus form a thin white-matter covering on the ventricular surface, deep to the ependyma, called the alveus. These fibres pass into the fornix via the fimbria. The fornix passes initially posteriorly and superiorly, then anteriorly, curving around the outer curve of the lateral ventricle and angling towards the midline in its course. The fornices of the two sides come together at about the junction of the posterior third and anterior two-thirds of the corpus callosum. Many fibres pass across the midline, the commissure of the fornix, and turn caudally to enter the contralateral hippocampus. The two fornices, united in the midline, are suspended from the corpus callosum by the septum pellucidum as they arch over the roof of the third ventricle and the choroid fissure of the body of the lateral ventricle. They turn ventrally, immediately in front of the interventricular foramen of Monroe. The two fornices separate, and each div-

ides into an anterior and a posterior column, passing in front of and behind the anterior commissure. The anterior column carries axons to and from the septal nuclei. CA3, CA1, and the subiculum project to the lateral septal nucleus. This has diverse efferent projections to the hypothalamus, the epithalamus, and the midline thalamus, but also projects to the adjacent medial septal nucleus. The medial septal nucleus is the major source of cholinergic fibres to the hippocampus via the fornix. The posterior column of the fornix curves posteriorly through the hypothalamus, giving off many fibres to medial and lateral hypothalamic nuclei. It ends in the mamillary nuclei, which in turn project via the mamillothalamic tract to the anterior thalamus. This projection is partially bilateral.

There is a major input to the hypothalamus from the amygdala, via the stria terminalis, a white-matter tract that follows the curve of the caudate nucleus around the lateral ventricle, lying between the caudate and the thalamus. The connections between the hypothalamus and amygdala are reciprocal.

Direct projections to the cortex from the hypothalamus have been discussed earlier. Direct projections from neocortex to the hypothalamus have been described, but their extent and distribution are disputed. If they exist in the human, they probably arise from the prefrontal/orbitofrontal and insular cortex.

The corticobulbar and corticospinal pathways

The direct projection of the cortex to the brainstem and spinal cord, the pyramidal tract, arises from the cortex in front of and behind the central sulcus. About 40 per cent of fibres arise from the primary somatic sensory cortex and the adjacent superior parietal lobe. In the frontal lobe, axons arise from the primary motor, premotor, and supplementary motor areas. Apart from the direct innervation of the spinal cord and motor nuclei of the cranial nerves, direct cortical fibres innervate the red nucleus, the vestibular nuclei, the reticular formation, and the superior colliculus. In the case of the first two of these, the origin of the fibres is probably very similar to the areas of origin of the pyramidal tract. In contrast, the cortical projections to the reticular formation and superior colliculus have a much wider origin, and may include most neocortical areas to a greater or lesser degree.

The contribution of neuroanatomy to psychiatry

The above is a necessarily abbreviated account of the anatomy of the central nervous system, centring on the organization and connections of the cortex including the limbic lobe. Topographical neuroanatomy has been ignored, despite its importance in the reading of modern images of the brain in living patients. For psychiatry, the importance of the connectionist view of the brain lies in the contribution it can make to the understanding of the normal and pathological functioning of the central nervous system. Present-day neuropsychology and cognitive neuroscience are aimed towards understanding the highest levels of central nervous system processing and function. It is these areas or systems that are commonly involved in the signs and symptoms of major psychiatric disease. It is to the pathways underlying cognition, perception, memory, mood, and attention that the psychiatrist interested in the pathophysiology of mental illness must turn his or her attention, and it is this area that the above account has attempted to review.

Further reading

Gloor, P. (1977). *The temporal lobe and limbic system*. Oxford University Press.

Pearson, R.C.A. (1995). Dorsal thalamus. In *Gray's anatomy* (38th edn) (ed. P.L. Williams, L.H. Bannister, M.M. Berry, *et al.*), pp. 1080–91. Churchill Livingstone, Edinburgh.

Pearson, R.C.A. (1995). Cerebral cortex. In *Gray's anatomy* (38th edn) (ed. P.L. Williams, L.H. Bannister, M.M. Berry, *et al.*), pp. 1141–71. Churchill Livingstone, Edinburgh.

Passingham, R. (1993). *The frontal lobes and voluntary action*. Oxford University Press.

Paxinos, G. (ed.) (1990). *The human nervous system*. Academic Press, San Diego, CA.

Tovée, M.J. (1996). *An introduction to the visual system*. Cambridge University Press.

Zeki, S. (1993). *A vision of the brain*. Blackwell Science, Oxford.

2.3.2 Neurodevelopment

Karl Zilles

Neural induction

The central nervous system originates from the midline region as a specialized area of ectoderm, the neuroectoderm or neural plate. As the neuroectodermal cells proliferate an indentation, the neural groove, forms in the neural plate. The lateral folds of this groove join in the midline, forming the neural tube. The folds begin to fuse in the central part of the groove but the most rostral and caudal parts do not close, leaving rostral and caudal neuropores. A small transitional zone between the neural plate and the surrounding ectoderm provides the cells of the neural crest, which differentiate into the sensory cells of the spinal cord, the cranial ganglionic cells of the somatic and autonomic nervous systems, Schwann cells, and chromaffine cells.

Neural tube formation requires a controlled expression of cell adhesion molecules in the lateral folds of the neural groove. If the rostral neuropore fails to close, the development of the forebrain is impaired leading to anencephalus. If the caudal neuropore fails to close, the most severe result is rachischisis, a malformation with a dorsally exposed neural groove which has severe neurological consequences. The mildest result is spina bifida occulta which is a cleft of a vertebral arch covered by epidermis.

As development continues, the neural tube and crest move to a position between the ectoderm and the notochord. The rostral part of the neural tube differentiates into the brain; the caudal part differentiates into the spinal cord behind the fifth somite.

Organogenesis of the central nervous system

The embryonic brain has three vesicular enlargements: the forebrain, the midbrain and the hindbrain. Because the developing brain grows much faster than the rest of the embryo, it becomes deflected ventrally. A dorsally convex cephalic flexure marks the border between hindbrain and midbrain, and a cervical flexure marks the border between spinal cord and hindbrain (Fig. 1). The ventrally convex pontine flexure forms the hindbrain. During week 5, the forebrain differentiates further into the rostral telencephalon and the more caudal diencephalon. The telencephalon consists of two hemispheric vesicles connected by a thin lamina terminalis, the most dorsal part of which develops into the commissural plate, the *Anlage* of the corpus callosum. The ventral part of the lamina terminalis differentiates into the anterior commissure. The central cavity of the diencephalon (the third ventricle) is connected with the cavities of the hemispheric vesicles (the lateral ventricles) by the intraventricular foramen. The diencephalon develops bilateral evaginations, the eye vesicles, which differentiate into the retina and the optic nerve. Meanwhile the hindbrain becomes subdivided into a rostral metencephalon and a caudal myelencephalon.

The cerebellum starts to develop from the metencephalon during week 6 (Fig. 1). At first, the enlarged central cavity of the neural tube

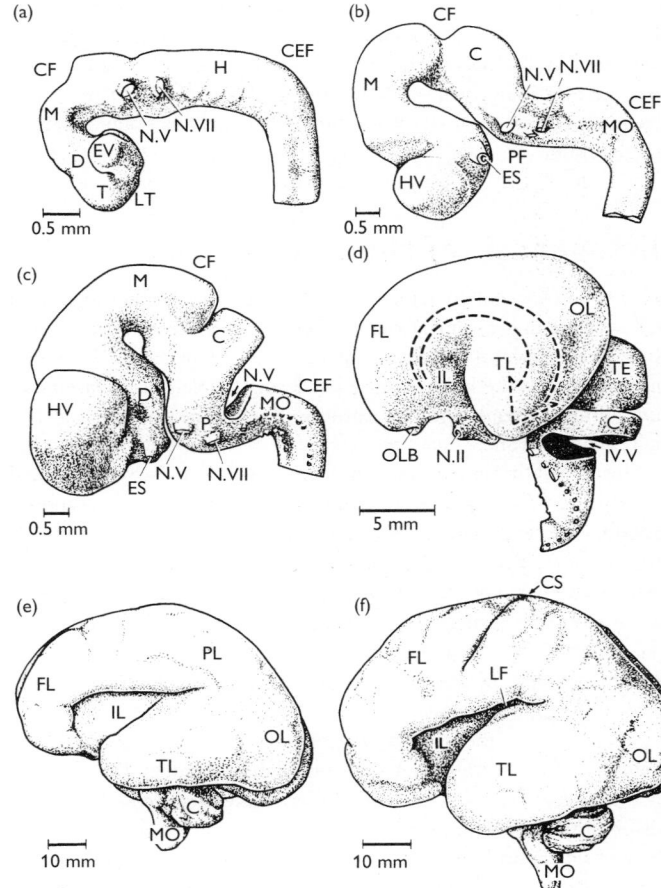

Fig. 1 Development of the human brain. Brains of (a) 4-mm (b) 10.4-mm (c), 13.8-mm, and (d) 53-mm human embryos, and (e) 21-week and (f) 24-week fetuses. C, cerebellum or cerebellar *Anlage*; CEF, cervical flexure; CF, cephalic flexure; CS, central sulcus; D, diencephalon; ES, eye stalk; EV, eye vesicle; FL, frontal lobe; H, hindbrain; HV, hemispheric vesicle; IL, insular lobe; LF, lateral fissure; LT, lamina terminalis; M, mesencephalon; MO, medulla oblongata; N.II, optic nerve; N.V, trigeminal nerve; N.VII, facial nerve; OL, occipital lobe; OLB, olfactory bulb; P, pons; PF, pontine flexure; PL, parietal lobe; T, telencephalon; TE, tectum; TL, temporal lobe; IV.V, fourth ventricle.

(the future fourth ventricle) has a thin roof plate bordered by two thickenings of the neural tube, the rhomboid lips, which merge in the midline. These thickenings develop into the cerebellar hemispheres, while the midline part develops into the vermis of the cerebellum. Fissures appear in the cerebellar hemispheres, forming the anterior and posterior lobes and the uvula. The cerebellum is connected to the hindbrain by three peduncles: the superior peduncle containing efferent fibres and the afferent ventral and rostral spinocerebellar tracts, the medial penduncle containing the afferent pontocerebellar tract; and the inferior peduncle containing other afferent tracts.

The rhombencephalon is temporarily divided into eight rhombomeres,[1] whose borders disappear during further development. Local expression of homeobox genes leads to the formation of the pallium and the ganglionic hill.

The hindbrain develops in close association with the visceral archs, which appear during week 4. It innervates these archs and the organs derived from them by a group of branchial nerves, which later become the trigeminal (V), facial (VII), glossopharyngeal (IX), vagal (X), and accessory (XI) cranial nerves. Other cranial nerves develop connections between the hindbrain and peripheral organs not derived from the visceral archs. They are the oculomotor (III), trochlear (IV), abducens (VI), vestibulocochlear (VIII), and hypoglossal (XII) nerves. The olfactory (I) and optic (II) nerves arise separately as evaginations of the forebrain.

Histogenesis of the spinal cord

The neural tube initially consists of a single layer of neuroepithelial cells surrounding a central canal filled with the cerebrospinal fluid. The outer surface of the future spinal cord has an external limiting membrane, and the inner surface bordering the central canal has an inner limiting membrane. The entire wall of the neural tube is called the ventricular zone.[2]

The cells of the neural tube proliferate, and the surface of the spinal cord enlarges. The cord then thickens as cells divide further to produce a multilayered epithelium. The daughter cells have different potentialities: one type of cell (the neuroblast) retains the capability for mitosis, whereas another type (the proneurone) is postmitotic and represents an immature neurone. The proliferation of neurones is almost complete around birth. However, there is evidence that new neurones can be formed in specific areas of the adult brain, especially in the dentate gyrus of the hippocampus.

Some neuroepithelial cells develop into precursors of glial cells, glioblasts, which differentiate into astroglial, oligodendroglial, and microglial cells. The first glioblasts differentiate into radially extended cells spanning the entire width of the spinal cord (the same occurs in the cerebral hemispheres and the cerebellar cortex as described below). During later development these cells are transformed into ependymal cells and astroglia. The adult number of glial cells is not reached until the second postnatal year.

The histogenesis of the spinal cord starts at the cervical level and progresses in a caudal direction. After week 3, a longitudinal sulcus limitans is recognizable on the inner surface of the neural tube, dividing the wall into dorsal (alar) and ventral (basal) plates. The dorsal plates of both sides are connected by a thin roof plate, and the ventral plates by a thin floor plate. The dorsal plate differentiates into the dorsal horn of the adult spinal cord, and the ventral plate differentiates into the ventral horn. The sympathetic preganglionic neurones form in the lateral horn, which is present only at thoracic levels. The subdivision into dorsal and ventral plates is important not only in the spinal cord, but also in the brainstem (see below).

During week 5, three concentrically organized zones—a cell-dense ventricular zone, a less dense intermediate or mantle zone, and a peripheral marginal zone free of neuronal cells—develop in the wall of the spinal cord. Proneurones leave the ventricular zone and migrate along radial glial cells into the intermediate zone where they become organized into nuclei. The motor neurones develop the axons of the ventral root, and the processes from spinal ganglionic cells grow into the spinal cord to form the dorsal roots. Synapses develop first in the motor zone, and later in the sensory zone, during the weeks 10 to 13.

During the third month, the ventricular zone is reduced to a small rim surrounding the central canal and is finally transformed into the ependymal cell layer. The intermediate zone becomes organized into dorsal, ventral, and (at thoracic levels) lateral horns. The ascending and descending fibre tracts of the spinal cord are increased in size in the marginal zone. During weeks 14 and 15, obligodendrocytes begin to myelinate these fibre tracts. The corticospinal, or pyramidal, tract is visible for the first time during week 14 and reaches its target neurones, mainly motor neurones of the ventral horn, between weeks 17 and 29. The myelination of the pyramidal tract is completed between the first and second postnatal years. This late myelination explains the presence of the Babinski reflex in newborns and its disappearance during the first 2 years.

Histogenesis of the brainstem and cerebellum

During histogenesis of the brainstem and spinal cord the motor, sensory, somatic, and visceral zones are organized similarly. At the level of the fourth ventricle the arrangement is different; the dorsal plate of the spinal cord is moved to a lateral position in the brainstem so that the various zones of the hindbrain are arranged in a lateral-to-medial sequence (somatosensory–viscerosensory–visceromotor–somatomotor). In the brainstem, proneurones not only migrate radially, as in the spinal cord, but also tangentially and longitudinally. This complex migration and the growth of fibre tracts lead to changes of the lateral-to-medial sequence of cranial nerve nuclei (e.g. the facial nucleus) in the adult.

In the cerebellum, between weeks 10 and 11, neuroblasts migrate from the ventricular zone through the intermediate zone into an area (the external granular layer) at the surface of the marginal zone. During weeks 12 and 13, proneurones from the ventricular zone begin to migrate along radially extended glial cells into a region below this external granular layer, where they form the Purkinje cells of the ganglionic layer of the cerebellar cortex. Other proneurones from the ventricular zone develop into the cerebellar nuclei. Proneurones from the external granular layer then migrate inwards to form the internal granular layer and the basket and star cells of the molecular layer. The migration of cerebellar proneurones is not completed until the first postnatal year. During weeks 16 and 26, synapses develop and afferent fibre systems begin to form. The external granular layer finally disappears during the first 2 years of life, leaving the three-layered organization (molecular, ganglionic, and internal granular layers) of the adult cerebellar cortex.

Histogenesis of the cerebral cortex

Initially, the wall of the hemispheric vesicle consists of a single zone. In week 5, this develops into an inner cell-dense periventricular zone and an outer cell-poor marginal zone. In week 6, postmitotic proneurones leave the inner periventricular zone and form an intermediate (mantle) zone between the other two zones. By the end of week 6, the periventricular zone is subdivided into a cell-dense ventricular zone and a less cell-dense subventricular zone.

The most important event of cortical development occurs during week 8. A cortical plate between the marginal and intermediate zones is formed by proneurones which have migrated along radial glial cells from the ventricular and subventricular zones through the intermediate zone.[2–6] A single radial glial cell can span the entire distance between the ventricular and pial surfaces. As the proneurones 'climb' to the cortical plate along the processes of the radial glial cell, they produce a vertically oriented cortical cell column. This radially guided migration is responsible for the architectonic organization of cortical layers II to VI. It is a prototype of the cortical map of the adult brain.[7] A further feature of cortical migration is the inside-to-outside layering, with the earliest proneurones being found in the deepest layers of the cortical plate and the latest in the most superficial layers. Thus layers V and VI of the adult cortex are generated before layer IV, and layer IV is generated before layers III and II. At the same time there is much tangential migration of cells.[8]

Regional differences in the development of the cortical plate subdivide the hemisphere into segments. The lateral segment, with a well-developed cortical plate and presubplate, develops into the neocortex. The mediodorsal segment, with a wide marginal zone and a thin folded cortical plate, develops into the archicortex, including the hippocampus. The mediobasal segment, with its inconspiciously developed cortical plate, is the precursor of the palaeocortex. The basolateral segment develops into the corpus striatum, the amygdala, and the septum.

During weeks 10 and 12, the axons of the serotoninergic and noradrenergic neurones contribute to the first synapses in the marginal and presubplate zones, where neurotrophin receptors (see below) are expressed. During the following 3 weeks, the subplate zone develops as axons grow in from the basal forebrain and thalamus, dendrites enlarge, and synapses form. From weeks 16 to 24, the cortical *Anlage* has a small marginal zone, a wide cell-dense cortical plate, and a very wide and less cell-dense subplate.

The transformation into the adult neocortical pattern starts between weeks 25 and 34 as the migration and proliferation of proneurones diminishes. Dendrites begin to differentiate and synapses begin to develop in the deepest cortical layers, progressing to the most superficial layer.[9] Before birth, six cortical layers can be recognized in all regions of the neocortex. In the postnatal period, layer IV (inner granular layer) disappears as part of the differentiation of the motor cortex, leaving the five-layered agranular neocortex of the motor region.[10] Shortly before birth, the subplate, the subventricular zone, and most of the ventricular zone disappear, neuronal proliferation ceases, and the intermediate zone is transformed into the white matter of the pallium. The remaining ventricular zone contributes to the ependymal layer of the ventricular surface.

Dendritic and axonal differentiation continues after birth and into adult life. Synaptogenesis reaches a maximum during the first postnatal year, but continues at a lower rate during childhood. The myelin-

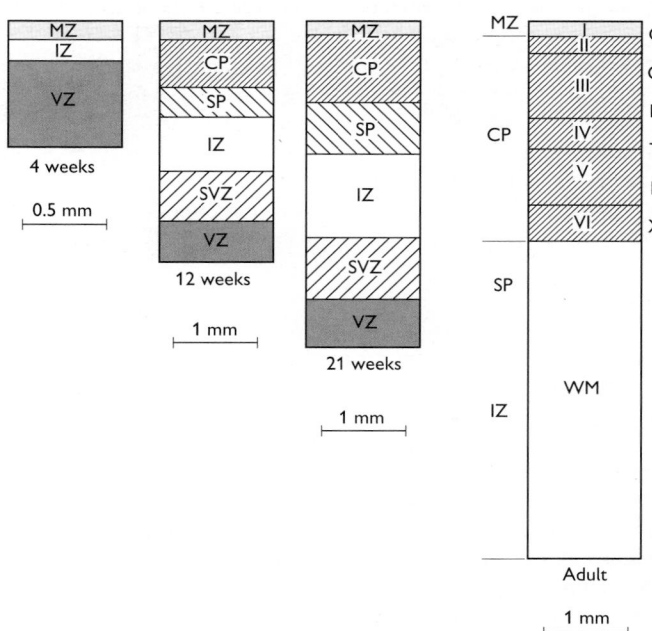

Fig. 2 Development of the neocortex between 4 weeks of gestation and adulthood. Roman numerals indicate the six cytoarchitectonically defined layers of the neocortex, which originate from the marginal zone (layer I) and the cortical plate. CP, cortical plate; IZ, intermediate zone; MZ, marginal zone; SP, subplate; SVZ, subventricular zone; VZ, ventricular zone; WM, white matter.

ation of the vestibular system is finished shortly before birth, that of the somatosensory, visual, auditory, pyramidal, and extrapyramidal fibre tracts is nearly complete by the end of the third postnatal year, and that of the associative fibre tracts in the cerebral hemispheres is continued until the second decade.[11] The key change in synapses after birth is pruning; the density of synapses in the adult brain is half that in neonates.[12]

The development of the neocortex is summarized in Fig. 2.

Hemispheric shape and the formation of gyri

The spherical shape of the early fetal hemisphere is transformed into the adult shape by differing rates of growth in the various regions of the telencephalon (Fig. 1). The future insular lobe grows less than other telencephalic regions, so that by the eighth month it is covered by the frontal, parietal, and temporal lobes. In the adult brain the insula is completely buried in the depth of the lateral fissure.

The extensive growth of the parieto-occipito-temporal association cortex leads to a bend in the temporal lobe around the lateral fissure. At the same time the temporal pole is pushed rostrally. This direction of growth (Fig. 1(d)) also affects the structures situated dorsomedially, i.e. the archicortex with the hippocampus, the corpus striatum, and the lateral ventricles. The corpus striatum is split by the ingrowing

Table 1 Important neurotrophins, their sites of synthesis in the central nervous system, receptors, and target structures

Neurotrophin	Site of synthesis	Receptors	Target structures
NGF	Hippocampus Neocortex	TrkA, p76^{NTR}	Cholinergic neurones in the basal forebrain
BDNF	Hippocampus Neocortex	TrkB, p75^{NTR}	Dopaminergic neurones in the midbrain; retinal ganglionic cells; cholinergic neurones in the basal forebrain
NT-3	Hippocampus Cerebellum	TrkC, p75^{NTR}	Dopaminergic neurones in the midbrain; neurones of the nucleus mesencephalicus nervi trigemini; neurones of origin of the pyramidal tract

NGF, NERVE GROWTH FACTOR; BDNF, BRAIN-DERIVED NEUROTROPHIC FACTOR; NT-3, NEUROTROPHIN 3.

fibres of the internal capsule into the caudate nucleus and the putamen. The head of the caudate is situated ventrolaterally to the corpus callosum in the frontal lobe, and the tail of the caudate is located in the temporal lobe dorsal to the inferior horn of the lateral ventricle. The hippocampus forms its largest extension (the retrocommisssural part) in the temporal lobe, bends around the posterior end (splenium) of the corpus callosum, and reaches a position on top of the corpus callosum (the supracommissural part). The precommissural part of the hippocampus ends in front of the genu of the corpus callosum.

After the appearance of the lateral fissure, the neocortical surface develops many sulci and gyri. The central, collateral, cingulate, parieto-occipital, superior temporal, and calcarine sulci appear between weeks 16 and 21, followed by the pre- and postcentral, frontal, temporal, and intraparietal sulci. Highly variable secondary and tertiary sulci develop between week 29 and birth, when all sulci have been formed.[13,14]

The reasons for the formation of gyri in many mammalian brains, including the human brain, are not completely understood. Since the basic organization of the cerebral cortex is vertically oriented, with cell columns positioned side by side, growth of the cortex inevitably leads to a considerable enlargement of the cortical surface. A large unfolded cortical surface would have two disadvantages: the volume of the skull would increase to such a degree during fetal development that a normal delivery would be impossible; the distance between cortical regions interconnected by intrahemispheric projection fibres would increase and with it the information transmission time. Gyri allow the maximal cortical surface in the minimal volume, and they increase the speed of neural transmission between neighbouring cortical areas. Recent measurements show that gyrification is greatest in the association cortices.[14] Although all gyri and sulci are present at birth, the depth of the sulci increases until eventually two-thirds of the cortical surface is hidden in them.[13]

Cell death and trophic factors during development

The co-ordinated expression, in space and time, of many genes underlies neurodevelopment. Mutations in these 'neurodevelopmental

genes' are increasingly being recognized as causes of developmental neurological disorders[15] such as cortical dysplasia and epilepsy; they may also be relevant to learning disability and schizophrenia. Different gene families are involved in the major component processes of neurodevelopment, such as organogenesis, neurogenesis, neuronal migration, synaptogenesis, and programmed cell death (apoptosis).[16,17] The details are beyond the scope of this book, but a few examples are given here.

Homeobox genes are important for the initial segmentation of the brain. Later, when cortical proneurones are migrating radially, their 'stop signal' is reelin, produced by specialized cells (Cajal–Retzius cells). In this way, reelin organizes the inside-to-outside layering of the cortex. Neurotrophins (growth factors) are genes which, as their name suggests, are critical for neuronal growth and survival, especially via their influence on apoptosis which is promoted by insuffiency of neurotrophins such as nerve growth factor and inhibited by enhanced nerve growth factor functioning. The effects of neurotrophins are mediated by specific tyrosine kinase (Trk) receptors (Table 1). Classical neurotransmitters and their receptors are also involved in neurodevelopment, both directly in the formation of synaptic connections and indirectly through regulation of neurotrophins and Trk receptors; particular roles have been shown for glutamate, acting via *N*-methyl-D-aspartate receptors, as well as for γ-aminobutyric acid and acetylcholine.

References

1. Lumsden, A. and Krumlauf, R. (1996). Patterning the vertebrate neuraxis. *Science*, **274**, 1109–15.
2. Kostovic, I. (1990). Zentralnervensystem. In *Humanembryologie* (ed. K.V. Hinrichsen), pp. 381–448. Springer-Verlag, Berlin.
3. Levitt, P. and Rakic, P. (1980). Immunoperoxidase localization of glial fibrillary acid protein in radial glial cells and astrocytes of the developing rhesus monkey brain. *Journal of Comparative Neurology*, **193**, 815–40.
4. Rakic, P. (1985). Limits of neurogenesis in primates. *Science*, **227**, 154–6.
5. Supèr, H., Soriano, E., and Uylings, H.B.M. (1998). The functions of the preplate in development and evolution of the neocortex and hippocampus. *Brain Research Reviews*, **26**, 40–64.

6. Schmechel, D.E. and Rakic, P. (1979). A Golgi study of radial glial cells in developing monkey telencephalon: morphogenesis and transformation into astrocytes. *Anatomy and Embryology*, **156**, 115–52.

7. Rakic, P. (1988). Specification of cerebral cortical areas. *Science*, **241**, 170–6.

8. Rakic, P. (1995). Radial versus tangential migration of neuronal clones in the developing cerebral cortex. *Proceedings of the National Academy of Sciences of the United States of America*, **92**, 11 323–7.

9. Huttenlocher, P.R. and de Courton, C. (1987). The development of synapses in striate cortex of man. *Human Neurobiology*, **6**, 1–9.

10. Brodmann, K. (1909). *Vergleichende Lokalisationslehre der Großhirnrinde in ihren Prinzipien dargestellt auf Grund des Zellenbaues*. Barth, Leipzig.

11. Yakovlev, P.I. and Lecours, A.-R. (1967). The myelogenetic cycles of regional maturation of the brain. In *Regional development of the brain in early life* (ed. A. Minkowski), pp. 3–70. Blackwell Science, Oxford.

12. Bourgeois, J.P. (1997). Synaptogenesis, heterochrony and epigenesis in the mammalian neocortex. *Acta Paediatrica Scandinavica*, **422** (Supplement), 27–33.

13. Zilles, K., Armstrong, E., Schleicher, A., and Kretschmann, H.-J. (1988). The human pattern of gyrification in the cerebral cortex. *Anatomy and Embryology*, **179**, 173–9.

14. Armstrong, E., Zilles, K., Omran, H., and Schleicher, A. (1995). The ontogeny of human gyrification. *Cerebral Cortex*, **5**, 56–63.

15. Berger-Sweeney, J. and Hohmann, C.F. (1997). Behavioral consequences of abnormal cortical development: insights into developmental disabilities. *Behavioural Brain Research*, **86**, 121–42.

16. Levitt, P., Barbe, M.F., and Eagleson, K.L. (1997) Patterning and specification of the cerebral cortex. *Annual Review of Neuroscience*, **20**, 1–24.

17. Lambert de Rouvroit, C. and Goffinet, A.M. (1998). A new view of early cortical development. *Biochemical Pharmacology*, **56**, 1403–9.

2.3.3 Neuroendocrinology

Charles B. Nemeroff

Definitions and principles

In the late 1950s a controversy arose in endocrinology and neuroscience concerning whether neurones are capable of manufacturing and secreting hormones; that is to say, is it possible that certain neurones subserve endocrine functions? Much of the ensuing debate, which persisted for approximately two decades, was centred on two major findings. First led by a husband and wife team, the Scharrers, a number of neurohistologists working with mammalian as well as with lower vertebrate and invertebrate species documented the presence—by both light and electron microscopy—of neurones that had all the characteristics of previously studied endocrine cells. They stained positive with the Gomori stain, which is claimed to be specific to endocrine tissues, and they incorporated granules or vesicles containing the endocrine substance purportedly released by these cells. The second major avenue of investigation centred around the brain's control of the secretion of the pituitary trophic hormones, which in turn were long known to control the secretion of the peripheral target endocrine hormones such as thyroid hormone, gonadal steroids, adrenal steroids, etc. A critical observation by several investigators had earlier demon-

strated the existence of a vital neuroendocrine system, namely the magnocellular cells of the paraventricular nucleus of the hypothalamus that synthesized vasopressin and oxytocin, the nonapeptides that are transported down the axon to the nerve terminals of these neurones in the posterior pituitary (neurohypophysis) and released in response to physiological stimuli. For example, the release of vasopressin, or the antidiuretic hormone as it is commonly named, acts as a critical regulator of fluid balance, and oxytocin is known to regulate the milk-letdown reflex during breast feeding.

It is now firmly established that neurones are indeed capable of functioning as true endocrine tissues, synthesizing and releasing substances, known as (neuro)hormones, that are released directly into the circulatory system and transported to distant sites of action. The release of vasopressin from the posterior pituitary gland and its action on the kidney is one often cited example; the action of the hypothalamic release and release-inhibiting factors on the anterior pituitary trophic hormone-producing cells is another.

Although it was clearly important to document the ability of neurones to function as neuroendocrine cells, particularly those in the central nervous system (**CNS**), the focus on an artificial classification system with clear demarcations of endocrine versus neuronal versus neuroendocrine, quickly lost its heuristic value. Indeed, we now recognize that the very same substances often function at one site as an endocrine substance and at another as a neurotransmitter. Thus, adrenaline (epinephrine) functions as a hormone in the adrenal medulla and as a conventional neurotransmitter substance in the mammalian CNS. Similarly corticotrophin-releasing factor (**CRF**) functions as a true hormone in its role as a hypothalamic–hypophysiotrophic factor in the hypothalamic–anterior pituitary complex, yet it is apparently a 'conventional' neurotransmitter in cortical and limbic brain areas. It may act as a paracrine substance in the adrenal medulla (see below). Thus the field has progressed to the stage where we now strive to characterize the role of a particular chemical messenger in a particular region or endocrine axis. The traditional endocrine and neurotransmitter roles for several peptides alluded to above are firmly established, but the equally important paracrine roles for such substances, namely the secretion of a substance from one cell where it acts upon nearby cells, remain largely unexplored. This is, perhaps, best illustrated in the gastrointestinal tract where several peptides that function as hormones or neurotransmitter substances in other sites, including the CNS, act to influence local cellular function. Examples would include vasoactive intestinal peptide, cholecystokinin, and somatostatin.

Neuroendocrinology thus comprises the study of the endocrine role of neuronal or glial cells as well as the neural regulation of endocrine secretion, with a major portion of the latter consisting of the biology of the various hypothalamic–pituitary–end-organ axes and the major neurohypophyseal hormones, vasopressin and oxytocin. Because of the elegant and precise regulation of peripheral endocrine hormone secretion, afforded in part by the feedback of peripherally secreted hormones at pituitary and a variety of CNS sites, the actions of such hormones on the brain has become an integral part of this discipline. The related discipline of psychoneuroendocrinology arose with the realization that there are binding sites (receptors) for peripheral hormones within the CNS that have little to do with the feedback regulation of the hypothalamic–pituitary–end-organ axes, and the further recognition of the seminal role of the CNS in regulating endocrine function, for example in the effect of stress on several such measures. Often cited as beginning with the pioneering observations of Berthold, who reported that removing roosters' testosterone-secreting gonads abolished their sexual behaviour, psychoneuroendocrinology has been expanded to include the effects of hormones on behaviour, as well as the study of endocrine alterations in psychiatric disorders and, the converse, psychiatric symptomatology in endocrine disorders. Indeed, this stepchild of neuroendocrinology and psychosomatic medicine has been one of the most rapidly growing areas of research in psychiatry, now boasting an international society (International Society of Psychoneuroendocrinology), an annual meeting, and its own journal (*Psychoneuroendocrinology*).

One of the most commonly used strategies in the 1970s and 1980s, still in occasional use today, is the so-called neuroendocrine 'window' strategy. Until the relatively recent development and availability of functional brain-imaging techniques, the brain remained relatively inaccessible for study, with the exception of cerebrospinal fluid (**CSF**) and postmortem tissue studies. With the emergence of the monoamine theories of mood disorders and schizophrenia, many investigators attempted to draw conclusions about the activity of noradrenergic, serotonergic, and dopaminergic circuits in patients with various psychiatric disorders by measuring the basal and stimulated secretion of pituitary and end-organ hormones in plasma. There is little doubt that such an approach has severe limitations, but the results, now coupled with more modern approaches, have contributed to the substantial progress made in elucidating the pathophysiology of mood and anxiety disorders and, to a considerably lesser extent, schizophrenia. One assumption of the neuroendocrine window strategy is that the monoamine-containing neurones that regulate endocrine secretion are disordered (or not disordered) to the same extent as those monoamine circuits posited to be involved in the pathophysiology of the disorder under study. Such an assumption may well be true in neural circuits in which the cells of origin are found in a circumscribed area and project to widely diffuse areas of the CNS (for example, the serotonergic and noradrenergic projections to the forebrain from the raphe and locus coeruleus cells in the brainstem, respectively). In contrast are the various dopaminergic circuits in the CNS, with their well-known topographic point-to-point distribution. Thus there is little reason to believe that the activity of the major dopamine-containing hypothalamic projection, the tuberoinfundibular system, with perikarya in the arcuate and periventricular hypothalamic nuclei and projections to the median eminence, is in any way related to the activity of the mesolimbicocortical dopamine pathway, with cell bodies in the ventral tegmentum of the midbrain and projections to the nucleus accumbens, amygdala, and cortical regions. This latter pathway has been implicated in the pathophysiology of schizophrenia. Thus study of the dopamine modulation of prolactin secretion in schizophrenia is unlikely to inform about the nature of limbic and cortical dopamine neuronal alterations in this devastating disorder.

Because a large portion of neuroendocrinology relevant to psychiatry is concerned with the hypothalamic–pituitary–end-organ axes, alterations in each of these systems in patients with a major psychiatric disorder are described later in this chapter. To avoid repetition, a generic description of the hierarchical organization of the various components of these systems is briefly outlined here. More comprehensive reviews of this subject are available.[1] In general, the hypothalamus

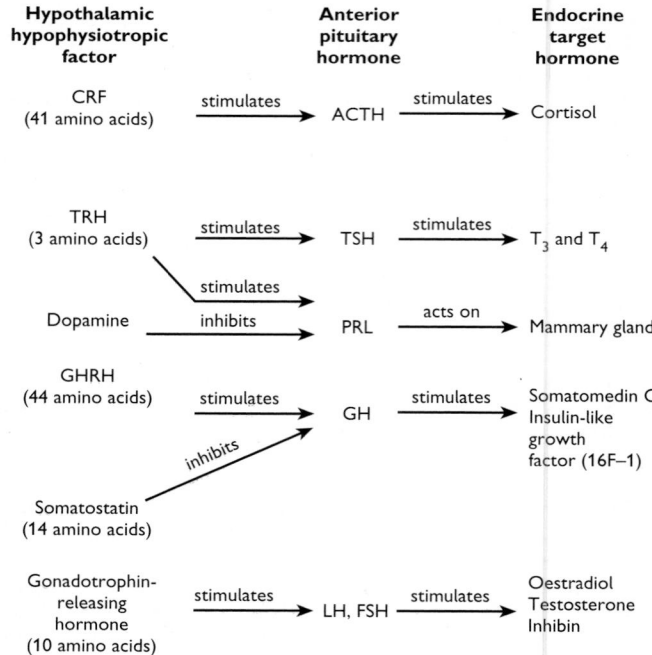

Fig. 1 Hormones of the hypothalamic–pituitary–end-organ axes: CRF, corticotrophin-releasing factor; TRH, thyrotrophin-releasing hormone; TSH, thyroid-stimulating hormone; T$_3$, tri-iodothyronine; T$_4$, thyroxine; PRL, prolactin; GHRH, growth-hormone releasing hormone; GH, growth hormone; LH, luteinizing hormone; FSH, follicle-stimulating hormone.

contains neurones that synthesize release and release-inhibiting factors. These peptide hormones, summarized in Fig. 1, are synthesized by a process beginning with transcription of the DNA sequence for the peptide prohormone. After translation in the endoplasmic reticulum and processing during axonal transport and packaging in the vesicles in the nerve terminals, the now biologically active peptide is released from nerve terminals in the median eminence and secreted into the primary plexus of the hypothalamohypophyseal portal vessels. They are transported humorally to the sinusoids of the adenohypophysis where they act on specific membrane receptors on their specific target: the pituitary trophic hormone-producing cells. Activation of their receptors results in the release or inhibition of release of the pituitary trophic hormone. The increase or decrease in pituitary trophic hormone secretion produces a corresponding increase or decrease in end-organ hormone secretion. Thus gonadotrophin-releasing hormone, a decapeptide, induces the release of the gonadotrophins, luteinizing hormone, and follicle-stimulating hormone from the anterior pituitary gland, which in turn stimulate the secretion of oestrogen and progesterone in women, and testosterone in men. The exogenous, intravenous administration of gonadotrophin-releasing hormone (GnRH), comprises the GnRH stimulation test, a very sensitive test of hypothalamic–pituitary–gonadal (HPG) axis activity. Such stimulation tests are thought to be a sensitive measure of the activity of the axis because it is influenced by GnRH secretion, gonadotrophin secretion, and feedback at the pituitary and brain by gonadal steroids. The organization of, and major feedback mechanisms thus far demonstrated in the hypothalamic–anterior pituitary–end-organ axes are illustrated in Fig. 2.

In summary, neuroendocrinology (and the related discipline psy-

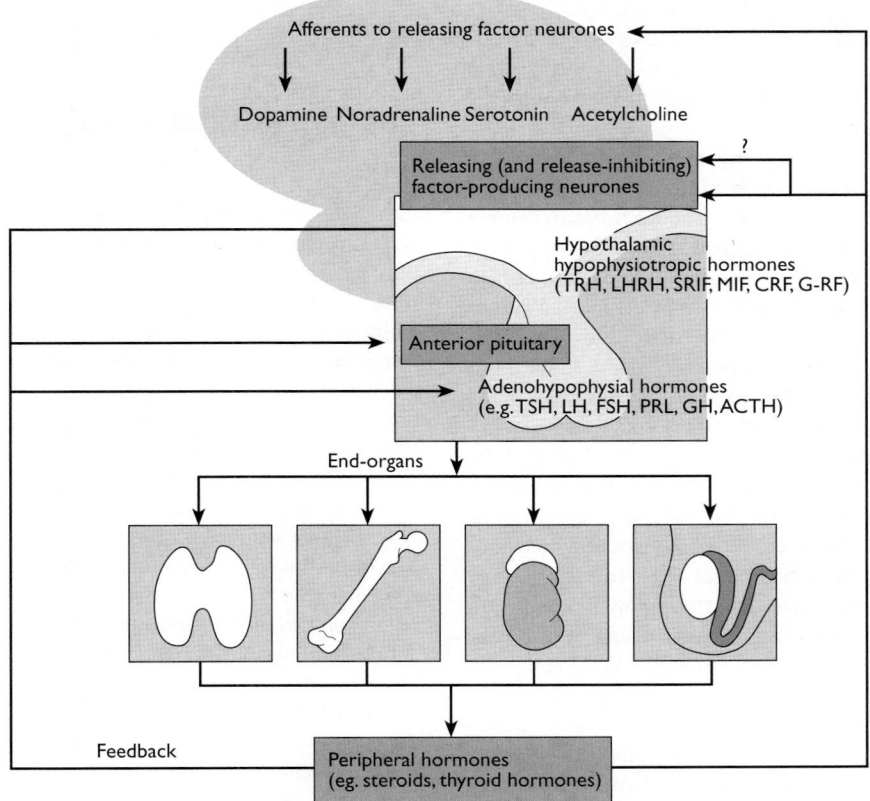

Fig. 2 Relationships between brain neurotransmitter systems, hypothalamic peptidergic (releasing-factor) neurones, anterior pituitary, and peripheral endocrine organs, illustrating established feedback loops: LHRH, luteinizing-hormone releasing hormone; SRIF, somatostatin; MIF, melanotrophin release-inhibiting factor; GHRF, growth-hormone releasing factor. Other abbreviations as in Fig. 1.

choneuroendocrinology) broadly encompasses the study of the following:

- the neural regulation of peripheral, target-organ hormone secretions, pituitary trophic hormone secretions, and secretions of the hypothalamic–hypophysiotrophic hormones;
- the role of neurotransmitter systems in the regulation of the above;
- the hormone effects of each of the endocrine axes on the CNS, alterations in the activity of the various endocrine axes in major psychiatric disorders, and conversely the behavioural consequences of endocrinopathies;
- the effects of target gland hormones on the CNS in normal individuals—for instance, the effects of synthetic glucocorticoids on memory processes.

The hypothalamic–pituitary–thyroid axis

It has been recognized for more than a century that adult patients with hypothyroidism exhibit profound disturbances in CNS function, including cognitive impairment and depression. In more recent years, attention has focused on more subtle alterations of the hypothalamic–

pituitary–thyroid (**HPT**) axis in depressed patients. Hypothyroidism is most frequently subclassified as in four grades as follows.

- Grade 1 hypothyroidism is classic primary hypothyroidism (increased thyroid-stimulating hormone (**TSH**), decreased peripheral thyroid hormone concentrations, and an increased TSH response to thyrotrophin-releasing hormone (**TRH**)).
- Grade 2 hypothyroidism is characterized by normal, basal thyroid-hormone concentrations, but an increase in basal TSH concentrations and an exaggerated TSH response to TRH.
- Grade 3 hypothyroidism can only be detected by a TRH-stimulation test; patients have a normal basal thyroid hormone and TSH concentrations, but an exaggerated TSH response to TRH.
- Grade 4 hypothyroidism is defined as normal findings on the three thyroid axis function tests noted above, but the patients have antithyroid antibodies.

Left untreated, most, if not all, patients progress from grade 4 to grade 1 hypothyroidism. Several studies have revealed an inordinately high rate of HPT axis dysfunction, largely hypothyroidism, in patients with major depression. In our pilot study, patients with comorbid depression and anxiety were especially likely to exhibit HPT axis abnormalities, especially the presence of grade 4 hypothyroidism, i.e. symptomless autoimmune thyroiditis. Patients with other major psychiatric diagnoses including schizophrenia appear to exhibit normal HPT axis function.

For patients who require thyroid-hormone replacement secondary to thyroid ablation, Bunevicius et al.[2] recently reported that treatment with a combination of tri-iodothyronine (T3) and thyroxine (T4) is optimal for mood and cognitive function, rather than the standard medication of T4 alone.

In addition, a blunted TSH response to TRH is observed in approximately 25 per cent of patients with major depression. This observation, first reported by Prange et al.[3] and Kastin et al.,[4] more than 25 years ago, has been replicated in many studies. Unfortunately, the pathophysiological underpinnings of this observation remain obscure, though there is considerable evidence that it may be due, at least in part, to chronic hypersecretion of TRH and subsequent TRH-receptor downregulation in the anterior pituitary gland. Indeed, our group[5] and others have reported elevated TRH concentrations in the cerebrospinal fluid of drug-free depressed patients.

TRH was the first of the hypothalamic-releasing factors to be chemically characterized. It is a tripeptide with the sequence pGlu–His–Pro–NH2. Once it was sequenced and antisera were raised against the peptide, immunohistochemical and radio-immunoassay methods revealed a heterogeneous brain distribution of TRH. This was the first in a series of experimental results that led to the inexorable conclusion that this peptide, and, as discussed below, other release and release-inhibiting hormones, function in extrahypothalamic brain regions as neurotransmitter substances. Thus TRH has been shown to produce direct brain effects, independent of its action on the pituitary thyrotrophs. Antidepressant effects of intravenously and intrathecally applied TRH have been reported,[3] but the results have not been confirmed in large, controlled clinical trials.[6] In contrast, several reports over the last 30 years have documented the efficacy of T3 (25–50 mg daily) in both accelerating the rate of onset of antidepressant response,[7] and in converting antidepressant non-responders to responders.[8] These studies were initiated when it became apparent that patients (and laboratory animals) with hypothyroidism do not respond to antidepressant agents. This led to the hypothesis that patients with subtle forms of hypothyroidism (grades 2–4) may not respond optimally to antidepressants unless they are adequately treated with exogenous thyroid hormone. This hypothesis is currently being tested in a large clinical trial, which seeks to determine whether the effectiveness of T3 augmentation in antidepressant non-responders is associated with subtle HPT axis dysfunction. With the cloning of the thyroid hormone receptor and its localization within the CNS, studies of its regulation in depression, as well as the regulation of TRH biosynthesis, can now be conducted in postmortem brain tissue.

A few other salient points are worth making, though a comprehensive discussion of each is beyond the scope of this review with its attendant space constraints. First is the critical role that thyroid hormones play in CNS development, and the tragic consequences of hypothyroidism early in life, namely cretinism, which is a syndrome associated with severe mental retardation.[9] The second is the reported presence within the CNS of each of the constituent hormones of the HPT axis, i.e. thyroid hormone, TSH, and TRH. The significance of this latter observation remains obscure, although TRH is considered to be a neurotransmitter in extrahypothalamic brain tissue. Third is the report by Hauser et al.[10] that an inordinately high percentage of patients with attention-deficit hyperactivity disorder exhibit thyroid hormone receptor resistance. It is likely that the development of positron emission tomographic ligands for thyroid hormone and TRH receptors will result in data that will incrementally advance the field.

The hypothalamic–pituitary–adrenal axis

Although first identified in crude form in 1955 by Saffran et al,[11] corticotrophin-releasing factor (CRF) was not chemically identified until 1981 when Vale and colleagues, working with extracts derived from 500 000 sheep hypothalami, elucidated the structure of the 41 amino acid-containing peptide.[12] This discovery finally permitted the comprehensive assessment of hypothalamic–pituitary–adrenal (HPA) axis activity, and also led to scrutiny of the role of this peptide, which is now known to co-ordinate the endocrine, immune, autonomic, and behavioural effects of stress in a variety of psychiatric disorders.

Most investigators would agree that the most important finding in all of biological psychiatry is the hyperactivity of the HPA axis observed in a significant subgroup of patients with major depression. The magnitude of HPA axis hyperactivity has been reported to be correlated to the severity of the depression.[13] Literally thousands of reports on this subject have appeared since the original and independent observations of research groups led by Board, Bunney, and Hamburg, as well as by Carroll, Sachar, Stokes, and Besser. These studies, conducted from the late 1950s to the 1980s, applied the tests largely developed for the diagnosis of Cushing's syndrome to patients with major depression and other psychiatric disorders. A panoply of such tests, ranging from urinary free-cortisol, to cerebrospinal fluid levels of cortisol, to the dexamethasone suppression test led to the inexorable conclusion that a sizeable percentage of depressed patients exhibited HPA axis hyperactivity. Our group and others, focusing on the mechanism(s) responsible for these findings, documented adrenocortical enlargement[14] and pituitary gland enlargement[15] in depressed patients, using CT and magnetic resonance imaging (MRI) respectively. The hypersecretion of cortisol is associated with hypersecretion of ACTH (and its co-secreted product of the precursor pro-opiomelanocortin), which due to its trophic properties also causes adrenocortical gland enlargement. Both direct measurements of CRF in cerebrospinal fluid,[16] and of CRF and gene expression for CRF (CRF mRNA expression) in postmortem tissue confirmed the hypothesized hypersecretion of CRF in depressed patients.[17] Like the hypersecretion of cortisol, CRF hypersecretion normalizes upon recovery from depression. Indeed, there is now considerable evidence, derived from both preclinical and clinical studies, that CRF neuronal hyperactivity is reduced by treatment with several antidepressants including paroxetine and fluoxetine, the selective serotonin-reuptake inhibitors (SSRIs), reboxetine (the noradrenaline-reuptake inhibitor), venlafaxine (the dual noradrenaline/serotonin-reuptake inhibitor), desipramine (the tricyclic antidepressant), and tranylcypromine (the monoamine oxidase inhibitor), as well as by electroconvulsive therapy.[18]

When patients who are drug free but depressed are given CRF intravenously, they exhibit, as a group, a blunted ACTH response compared with normal control subjects. This is believed to be secondary to either the downregulation of CRF receptors on the corticotrophs after long-standing CRF hypersecretion and/or intact negative feedback of the hypersecreted cortisol at anterior pituitary and higher CNS centres. As with the other measures of HPA axis function, this endocrine abnormality normalizes upon recovery from depression. Indeed, persistent alterations in HPA axis function, whether due to dexamethasone non-suppression or cerebrospinal fluid CRF hypersecretion, is the harbinger of a poor response to antidepressant treatment. In recent years Holsboer et al.[19] have pioneered the use of the combined dexamethasone–CRF test, in which patients are given the synthetic glucocorticoid and the following day receive a standardized CRF stimulation test. The results reveal that this test has a much greater sensitivity in detecting increases in HPA axis activity; it has now been used to detect axis alterations in the first-degree relatives of depressed patients who have never been symptomatic, raising for the first time the question of a trait (vulnerability) component to this measure.[20]

Space constraints preclude a more comprehensive discussion of this rich literature, but a few additional points are certainly worth interjecting. First, a robust preclinical literature has documented the depressogenic and anxiogenic effects of exogenously administered CRF in laboratory animals. When CRF was directly injected into the central nervous system it produced effects reminiscent of the cardinal symptoms of depression in patients, including decreased libido, reduced appetite and weight loss, sleep disturbances, and neophobia. Indeed, newly developed CRF1-receptor antagonists represent a novel putative class of antidepressants. Such compounds exhibit activity in virtually every preclinical screen for antidepressants and anxiolytics currently employed. A second CRF receptor, the CRF2 receptor, has now been identified. Interestingly it exhibits genetic polymorphism, i.e. it occurs in more than one naturally occurring isoform or splice variant. It is believed to utilize the recently discovered novel peptide, urocortin, as an endogenous ligand. The long-term consequences of cortisol hypersecretion in depression are just now being scrutinized. One such sequela appears to be neuronal loss in the hippocampus, one of the major feedback sites for glucocorticoids in the CNS. This has now been documented by structural brain-imaging studies that utilized MRI techniques.[21] If the degeneration of neurones that represent glucocorticoid feedback sites indeed occur in depressed patients, then this should further increase HPA axis hyperactivity, which would explain the many reports of increasing adrenocortical hyperactivity of elderly depressed patients when compared with matched younger depressed patients.

Future studies will focus on the development of positron emission tomography (**PET**) ligands for both the glucocorticoid receptor and the CRF receptor, the role of the CRF binding protein—a unique protein which binds CRF in extracellular fluid and in plasma, preventing its availability to act on its receptor—and the role of the CRF peptidase, which degrades the peptide, in normal and pathological states. Finally, are the studies from our group and others, which have documented the long-term persistent increases in the HPA axis and extrahypothalamic CRF neuronal activity after exposure to early untoward life events—for example, child abuse and neglect in both laboratory animals (rats and non-human primates) as well as in patients.[18,22] This phenomenon has been posited to underlie the now well-documented association between early abuse and neglect and increased vulnerability to mood disorders.[23–25] An early intervention strategy using CRF receptor antagonists may prevent such long-term alterations in the central nervous system.

HPA axis alterations have also been investigated in other psychiatric disorders. When depression is comorbid with a variety of other disorders such as multiple sclerosis, Alzheimer's disease, multi-infarct dementia, Huntington's disease, and others, both CRF hypersecretion and HPA axis hyperactivity are common. There is little evidence for HPA axis dysfunction in schizophrenia. In contrast, several anxiety disorders (most prominently post-traumatic stress disorder) are associated with extrahypothalamic CRF hypersecretion, as evidenced by elevated CSF concentrations of CRF,[26] but normal or reduced measures of adrenocortical activity. Finally, CRF neuronal degeneration is now well known to occur in the cerebral cortex of patients with Alzheimer's disease,[27,28] an effect which temporally occurs prior to the better-studied cholinergic neuronal involvement. With the reduction in CRF concentrations in the cerebral cortex is a reciprocal increase in CRF receptor density. Whether modification of the disease-associated effects on the CRF neuronal system in the cortex and hippocampus represents a novel strategy for the treatment of this common dementing disorder remains unclear at the present time.

The hypothalamic–growth hormone axis

Although the HPA and HPT axes have been more closely scrutinized in patients with psychiatric disorders, there is virtual universal agreement that the blunted growth-hormone response to a variety of provocative stimuli (particularly clonidine, an α_2-adrenergic agonist) in depressed patients is the most consistent finding in affective disorders research.[29] The mechanism underlying this phenomenon remains obscure, but it is of particular interest that, at least in some studies, it appears to persist upon recovery from depression, suggesting that it is a trait marker for depression vulnerability. There are reports of similar findings with other growth hormone-provocative stimuli, such as the use of apomorphine, desipramine, or levodopa. In addition, the blunted growth-hormone response to clonidine in depressed patients is particularly robust in those who have recently attempted suicide. Clearly, further work in this area is warranted, especially in the context of several reports of alterations in basal growth-hormone secretion in this disorder. The nature of this alteration is a reduction in the normal nocturnal rise in growth-hormone secretion, though this is not a universally agreed-upon finding. Alterations in growth-hormone secretion in other psychiatric disorders (particularly schizophrenia) have also been reported, though the results may have largely been due to long-term treatment of such patients with dopamine-receptor antagonists, antipsychotic drugs.

The secretion of growth hormone and the regulation of this axis are distinct from that of the other endocrine axes for several reasons. First, this is the one axis in which two hypothalamic–hypophysiotrophic hormones have unequivocally been shown to play a physiological role. The first discovered was somatostatin or growth hormone-inhibiting hormone, isolated from ovine hypothalamus in 1974. It is a tetradecapeptide, which contains a disulfide bridge linking the two cysteine residues. It is distributed in the CNS not only in cells of the periventricular nucleus of the hypothalamus, which projects to the median eminence, but in a variety of extrahypothalamic areas as well. Indeed, somatostatin is known to function as a CNS neurotransmitter and is of particular interest to psychiatrists because of its early involvement in the Alzheimer's disease process. Our group and others have documented the marked reduction in somatostatin concentrations in this dementing disorder.[28] In addition, somatostatin concentrations are markedly elevated in the basal ganglia of patients with Huntington's disease;[30] the pathological implications of this finding remain obscure. In contrast to the other peptide receptors described above in which one or at most two receptor subtypes have been identified, several distinct somatostatin receptor subtypes have now been structurally identified. Such diversity suggests the possibility of specific receptor-subtype agonists and antagonists as putative therapeutic agents.

Several years after the elucidation of the structure of somatostatin, the long-postulated growth hormone-releasing factor (**GHRF**) was found in extracts of an ectopic tumour associated with acromegaly. It is a peptide containing 44 amino acids, and it has the most limited CNS distribution of all the hypothalamic-releasing hormones thus far studied. The vast majority of the peptide is found in the arcuate nucleus of the hypothalamus from where it projects nerve terminals to the median eminence. Unlike the other axes, the growth-hormone axis is also unique in not having a single target endocrine gland. Indeed, growth hormone does stimulate the release of somatomedin C from the liver and it also exerts direct effects on a variety of targets including bone and muscle. Most, but not all, investigators have reported a blunted growth-hormone response to GHRH in depressed patients, but the total number of patients studied pales in comparison to the TRH- and CRF-stimulation test data. There are no data published on somatomedin C responses to GHRH in depressed patients. No published studies are available in which GHRH concentrations or GHRH-mRNA expression have been studied in postmortem tissue of depressed patients and matched controls, an obvious study in view of the data reviewed above.

The hypothalamic–pituitary–gonadal axis

In view of the remarkable gender differences in the prevalence rate of depression, the relatively high rates of postpartum depression, as well as the reduction in libido that is so characteristic of depression, it is plausible to posit a reduction in HPG axis activity in depressed patients. Therefore it is somewhat surprising that so little research has been conducted on HPG axis activity in depression and other psychiatric disorders. Indeed, a comprehensive database on this extraordinarily important area is simply not available, but the field has recently been reviewed.[31] A series of older studies documented no differences in basal gonadotrophin levels in depressed patients when compared to controls. The gonadotrophin-releasing hormone (**GnRH**) stimulation test has only been administered to a relatively small number of depressed patients; although the results revealed a blunted or normal response, no firm conclusions can be drawn from this limited data set. Indeed, such studies require control for menopausal status, menstrual-cycle phase, use of oral contraceptives, as well as the measurement of baseline progesterone, oestrogen, and gonadotrophin plasma concentrations. One remarkable finding relevant to these questions is the remarkable effectiveness of the GnRH agonist, leuprolide, in the treatment of the premenstrual syndrome. It is believed to act by producing a chemical ovariectomy through a marked downregulation of adenohypophyseal GnRH receptors and the expected resultant reduction in gonadotrophin and gonadal steroid secretion. Long-term treatment with this compound could theoretically result in bone-density reductions and a risk of cardiovascular disease. Therefore, supplementation with oestrogen and progesterone has been suggested in combination with leuprolide, though there are reports that such a strategy reduces the effectiveness of the treatment.

GnRH was the second of the hypothalamic–hypophysiotrophic hormones to be chemically characterized. It is a decapeptide that is relatively limited in distribution to hypothalamic regions and to the preoptic area and septum. It stimulates the secretion of both luteinizing hormone and follicle-stimulating hormone in both men and women. GnRH is known to act by stimulating GnRH receptors in the anterior pituitary gland, which results in the increased synthesis and release of the pituitary gonadotrophins, in turn causing the release of oestrogen and progesterone in women and testosterone in men. There is some evidence that oestrogens, which have receptors localized extensively throughout the CNS, may possess some antidepressant activity, though the data is far from clear.[32] There are hints from the clinical trial literature that postmenopausal women on oestrogen replacement may respond better to treatment with fluoxetine than women who are not receiving such treatment,[33] though the database is small and fraught with many confounds.

The hypothalamic–prolactin axis

This pituitary hormone, which acts on the mammary gland, plays a critical role in lactation. Unlike the other axes described, this axis is unique in having a non-peptide release-inhibiting factor, dopamine. In addition, although there is relatively strong evidence for the existence of a prolactin-releasing factor, its isolation and characterization has not yet been realized. One of the difficulties in completing this task is the presence of TRH, which is a potent prolactin-releasing factor, and may in fact function physiologically in this regard. Interestingly, although the TSH response to TRH in depressed patients is often blunted, the prolactin response is not. Although the results are not unequivocal, most studies have not observed alterations of prolactin secretion in depressed patients.[34] In contrast to this small database is a remarkably large database on the use of provocative tests of prolactin secretion in patients with psychiatric disorders. To summarize briefly, they largely use agents that increase serotonergic neurotransmission, for example L-tryptophan, 5-hydroxytryptophan (5-HTP), fenfluramine (both the racemic mixture and the (+) form). In general, the prolactin response to L-tryptophan, 5-HTP, L-(+)- and D-(+)-fenfluramine, clomipramine, and also to direct serotonin-receptor agonists, is blunted in depressed patients—as well as in patients with cluster-B personality disorder and borderline personality disorder. The available data would suggest that this blunted prolactin response is mediated by alterations in 5-HT1A-receptor responsiveness.

Discussion and summary

Although the hypothesis that the neuroendocrine window strategy would ultimately provide the long-searched for information concerning the nature of monoamine circuit alterations in patients with psychiatric disorders has never been realized, the approach has led to major advances in biological psychiatry. It has led to the CRF hypothesis of depression, which is supported by a considerable multidisciplinary database, and this in turn has directed the field towards the development of novel therapeutic approaches, namely CRF-receptor antagonists. It also apparently explains the neurobiological mechanisms responsible for the increase in depression (first postulated by

Freud in the early part of the twentieth century) in patients exposed to trauma during their early life. If CRF is indeed the 'black bile' of depression—responsible for the endocrinopathy of depression, as well as several of the other cardinal features of this disorder—then CRF-receptor antagonists should represent a novel class of antidepressants that will be a welcome addition to the armamentarium. Indeed, a number of pharmaceutical companies are now testing CRF-receptor antagonists as novel anxiolytics and antidepressants in preclinical and clinical trials.

In addition to the now widely replicated HPA axis and CRF alterations in depression, are the HPT axis abnormalities. Most depressed patients, in fact, exhibit alterations in one of these two axes. Furthermore, there is the widely replicated blunting of the growth-hormone response to clonidine and other provocative stimuli and the blunted prolactin response to serotonergic stimuli in depressed patients. It is obvious from these studies that the vast majority of studies have focused on patients with mood disorders, particularly unipolar depression. Clearly other disorders, including eating disorders, anxiety disorders, schizophrenia, and axis II diagnoses should also be critically evaluated and compared to the literature on depression. The original neuroendocrine window strategy may well have failed in terms of gleaning information about monoamine-circuit activity, but the mechanistic studies that have followed have been remarkably fruitful. As repeatedly noted above, the availability of ligands that can be utilized with positron-emission tomography to determine peptide-receptor alterations in the brain and pituitary of patients with psychiatric disorders will advance the field, as will the long-elusive ability to measure receptors for the endocrine target hormones (glucocorticoids, oestrogens, thyroid hormones, etc.) in the brains of patients with these severe mental illnesses

Finally it is important to note the increasing database suggesting that depression is a systemic disease with major implications for vulnerability to other disorders. Thus depressed patients are much more likely to develop coronary artery disease and stroke, and perhaps cancer. They have been shown to have reduced bone density, rendering them more at risk for hip fracture. Such findings may well be mediated by the described endocrine alterations in depression. This should provide a further impetus for investigating the neuroendocrinology of psychiatric disorders.

References

1. Campeau, S., Day, H.E.W., Helmreich, D.L., Kollack-Walker, S., and Watson, S.J. (1998). Principles of psychoneuroendocrinology. *Psychiatric Clinics of North America*, **21**, 259–76.
2. Bunevicius, R., Kazanavicius, G., Zalinkevicius, R., and Prange, A.J. (1999). Effects of thyroxine as compared with thyroxine plus triiodothyronine in patients with hypothyroidism. *New England Journal of Medicine*, **340**, 424–9.
3. Prange, A.J., Wilson, I.C., Lara, P.P., *et al.* (1972). Effects of thyrotropin-releasing hormone in depression. *Lancet*, **2**, 999–1002.
4. Kastin, A.J., Ehrensing, R.H., Schlach, D.S., and Anderson, M.S. (1972). Improvement in mental depression with decreased thyrotropin response after administration of thyrotropin-releasing hormone. *Lancet*, **ii**, 740–2.
5. Banki, C.M., Bissette, G., Arato, M., and Nemeroff, C.B. (1988). Elevation of immunoreactive CSF TRH in depressed patients. *American Journal of Psychiatry*, **145**, 1526–31.
6. Nemeroff, C.B. and Evans, D.L. (1989). Thyrotropin-releasing hormone (TRH), the thyroid axis and affective disorder. *Annals of the New York Academy of Sciences*, **553**, 304–10.
7. Prange, A.J., Wilson, I.C., Rabon, A.M., *et al.* (1969). Enhancement of imipramine antidepressant activity by thyroid hormone. *American Journal of Psychiatry*, **126**, 457–69.
8. Joffe, R.T., Singer, W., Levitt, A.J. *et al.* (1993). A placebo-controlled comparison of lithium and triiodothyronine augmentation of tricyclic antidepressants in unipolar refractory depression. *Archives of General Psychiatry*, **50**, 387–94.
9. Anand, K.J.S. and Nemeroff, C.B. (1996). Developmental psychoneuroendocrinology. In *Textbook of child and adolescent psychiatry* (2nd edn) (ed. M. Lewis), pp. 64–86. Williams and Wilkins, Baltimore, MD.
10. Hauser, P., Zamethlein, A.J., Martinez, R., *et al.* (1993). Attention deficit-hyper-activity disorder in people with generalized resistance to thyroid hormone. *New England Journal of Medicine*, **328**, 997–1001.
11. Saffran, M., Schally, A.V., and Benfey, B.G. (1955). Stimulation of the release of corticotropin from the adenohypophysis by a neurohypophysial factor. *Endocrinology*, **57**, 439–44.
12. Vale, W., Spiess, J., Riveir, C., *et al.* (1981). Characterization of a 41 residue ovine hypothalamic peptide that stimulates secretion of corticotropin and β-endorphin. *Science*, **213**, 1394–7.
13. Evans, D.L. and Nemeroff, C.B. (1987). The clinical use of the dexamethasone suppression test in DSM-III affective disorders: correlation with the severe depressive subtypes of melancholia and psychosis. *Journal of Psychiatric Research*, **21**, 185–94.
14. Nemeroff, C.B., Krishnan, K.R.R., Reed, D., Leder, R., Beam, C., and Dunnick, N.R. (1992). Adrenal gland enlargement in major depression: a computed tomography study. *Archives of General Psychiatry*, **49**, 384–7.
15. Krishnan, K.R.R., Doraiswamy, P.M., Lurie, S.N., *et al.* (1991). Pituitary size in depression. *Journal of Clinical Endocrinology and Metabolism*, **72**, 256–9.
16. Heit, S., Owens, M.J., Plotsky, P., and Nemeroff, C.B. (1997). Corticotropin-releasing factor, stress and depression. *Neuroscientist*, **3**, 186–94.
17. Raadsheer, F.C., Hoogendijk, W.J.G., Stam, F.C., *et al.* (1994). Increased number of corticotropin-releasing hormone neurones in the hypothalamic paraventricular nuclei of depressed patients. *Neuroendocrinology*, **60**, 436–44.
18. Nemeroff, C.B. (1999). The preeminent role of early untoward experience on vulnerability to major psychiatric disorders: the nature–nurture controversy revisited and soon to be resolved. *Molecular Psychiatry*, **4**, 106–8.
19. Holsboer, F., Von Bardeleben, U., Weidemann, K., *et al.* (1987). Serial assessment of corticotropin-releasing hormone response after dexamethasone in depression—implications for pathophysiology of DST nonsuppression. *Biological Psychiatry*, **22**, 228–34.
20. Holsboer, F., Lauer, C.J., Schreiber, W., and Krieg, J.C. (1995). Altered hypothalamic–pituitary–adrenocortical regulations in healthy subjects at high familial risk for effective disorders. *Neuroendocrinology*, **62**, 340–7.
21. Sheline, Y.I., Wang, P.W., Gado, M.H., *et al.* (1996). Hippocampal atrophy in recurrent major depression. *Proceedings of the National Academy of Sciences of the United States of America*, **93**, 3908–13.
22. Coplan, J.D., Andrews, M.W., Rosenblum, L.A., *et al.* (1996). Persistent elevations of cerebrospinal fluid concentrations of corticotropin-releasing factor in adult non-human primates exposed to early life stressors: implications for the pathophysiology of mood and anxiety disorders. *Proceedings of the National Academy of Sciences of the United States of America*, **93**, 1619–23.
23. Kendler, K.S., Neale, M.C., Kessler, R.C., Heath, A.C., and Eaves, L.J. (1992). Childhood parental loss and adult psychopathology in women. A twin-study perspective. *Archives of General Psychiatry*, **49**, 109–16.
24. McCauley, J., Kern, D., Kolodner, K., *et al.* (1997). Clinical characteristics of women with an history of childhood abuse. *Journal of the American Medical Association*, **277**, 1362–8.

25. Agid, O., Shapira, B., Zislin, J., *et al.* (1999). Environment and vulnerability to major psychiatric illness: a case control study of early parental loss in major depression, bipolar depression and schizophrenia. *Molecular Psychiatry*, **4**, 163–72.

26. Bremner, J.D., Licinio, J., Darnell, A., *et al.* (1997). Elevated CSF corticotropin-releasing factor concentrations in posttraumatic stress disorder. *American Journal of Psychiatry*, **154**, 624–9.

27. Bissette, G., Reynolds, G.P., Kilts, C.D., Widerlov, E., and Nemeroff, C.B. (1985). Corticotropin-releasing factor-like immunoreactivity in senile dementia of the Alzheimer type: reduced cortical and striatal concentrations. *Journal of the American Medical Association*, **254**, 3067–9.

28. Bissette, G., Cook, L., Smith, W., Dole, K.C., Crain, B., and Nemeroff, C.B. (1998). Regional neuropeptide pathology in Alzheimer's disease: corticotropin-releasing factor and somatostatin. *Journal of Alzheimer's Disease*, **1**, 1–15.

29. Checkley, S.A., Slade, A.P., and Shur, P. (1981). Growth hormone and other responses to clonidine in patients with endogenous depression. *British Journal of Psychiatry*, **138**, 51–5.

30. Nemeroff, C.B., Youngblood, W.W., Manberg, P.J., Prange, A.J. Jr, and Kizer, J.S. (1983). Regional brain concentrations of neuropeptides in Huntington's chorea and schizophrenia. *Science*, **221**, 972–5.

31. Young, E. and Korszun, A. (1998). Psychoneuroendocrinology of depression, hypothalamic–pituitary–gonadal axis. *Psychiatric Clinics of North America*, **21**, 309–23.

32. Schmidt, P., Rubinow, D., Neuman, L., *et al.* (1999). Estrogen replacement in perimenopause-related depression: a preliminary report. *American Journal of Obstetrics and Gynecology*, in press.

33. Schneider, L.S., Small, G.W., Hamilton, S.H., Bystritsky, A., Nemeroff, C.B., Myers, B.S., and the fluoxetine collaborative study group (1997). Estrogen replacement and response to fluoxetine in a multicenter geriatric depression trial. *American Journal of Geriatric Psychiatry*, **5**, 97–106.

34. Nicholas, L., Dawkins, K., and Golden, R. (1998). Psychoneuroendocrinology of depression—prolactin. *Psychiatric Clinics of North America*, **21**, 341–58.

2.3.4 Neurotransmitters and second messengers

Michael E. Newman and Bernard Lerer

Since the catecholamine and indoleamine hypotheses of depression and the dopamine hypothesis of schizophrenia were first proposed, the effect of psychotropic drugs on brain monoamines and their receptors has been a central focus of research in psychopharmacology and biological psychiatry. In fact, effects of psychopharmacological agents on brain monoamines were extensively studied long before these hypotheses were formulated and were cardinal tenets upon which the theories were based. As will be outlined in this chapter, there has since been an explosion of knowledge in this field. This has involved a shift in emphasis from the neurotransmitters themselves to the multitude of receptors upon which they act and to mechanisms distal to the receptor up to and including effects on target gene expression. The increasing complexity of the field places a far greater burden of understanding upon the contemporary psychiatrist than was demanded of his or her

predecessors in the more simple heyday of a few neurotransmitters and a limited number of receptors. With complexity, however, comes a far richer array of possibilities to understand the mechanism of action of antidepressant, antipsychotic, and other psychotropic drugs and a vast number of potential targets for new drug development.

Neurotransmitters in the brain, like hormones in the periphery, are located extracellularly and exert their effects by binding to receptors situated on the outer surface of the cell membrane. Transmission of the message carried by the neurotransmitter beyond the cell membrane thus depends on activation by the receptor of a signalling system which is not limited by the physical constraints of the membrane. Neurotransmitter receptors in the central nervous system have been divided into two classes.[1] The first class, known as ionotropic receptors, are directly linked to ion channels and respond to activation by a neurotransmitter within a millisecond timeframe. Each receptor consists of an oligomeric transmembrane protein containing both the ion channel and the agonist binding site(s). The molecular mass of the oligomer is 200 to 250 kDa and is composed of subunits of about 50 kDa, each subunit containing four transmembrane segments. Examples of class I receptors are the nicotinic cholinergic receptor, the γ-aminobutyric acid A (**GABAA**) receptor, and the receptors for glycine and glutamate.

The second class, known as metabotropic receptors, mediate responses over a longer time frame, with a latency of onset of at least 30 ms, and in general serve to modulate the signals generated by the class I receptors. Class II receptors have a characteristic heptahelical structure with seven hydrophobic transmembrane domains linked by hydrophilic groups (Fig. 1).[2] Attached to the N-terminal end is a large extracellular loop which contains the ligand binding domain, while the C-terminal end is cytoplasmic. These receptors are linked to effector units which are either ion channels or enzymes responsible for generating small molecules that in general are able to diffuse intracellularly. These small molecules were originally referred to as second messengers since they propagate the signal initially carried by the neurotransmitter or first messenger. It is now clear, however, that these molecules represent one step along a pathway of sequential events referred to as a signal transduction cascade. Furthermore, multiple interactions between signal cascades originally thought to be completely separate have now been documented. Although the term 'second messenger' will be retained in this chapter because of its historical importance, it should be clear that the general function of second-messenger molecules does not differ from that of other molecules that participate in the signalling cascade. A more correct terminology would therefore use the term 'intracellular messengers' for all these substances.

'Classical' second messengers

Two major second messengers are recognized. The first to be characterized, by Sutherland and Rall in the 1950s, was the compound adenosine-3′,5′-cyclic monophosphate, now referred to as cyclic AMP (**cAMP**). An early example of work involving measurement of this compound in brain tissue was the determination by Kakiuchi *et al.*[3] that electrical stimulation of isolated guinea-pig cortical slices leads to a 10-fold increase in cAMP levels. Characterization of the adenylate cyclase enzyme that forms cAMP from adenosine triphosphate, and of the phosphodiesterase enzyme that degrades cAMP to adenosine

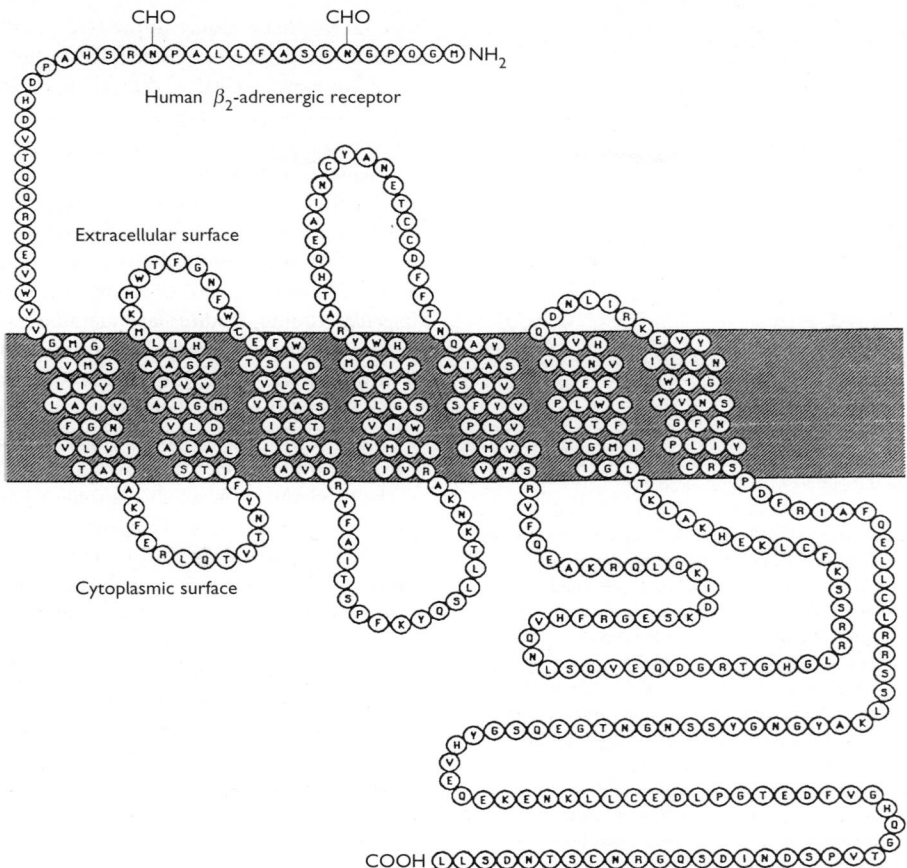

Fig. 1 The structure of a metabotropic (G-protein-coupled) receptor. The receptor illustrated is the human β₂-adrenergic receptor, but the structure is similar to that of the β₁-adrenergic receptor, the muscarinic acetylcholine receptor and to rhodopsin. The receptor possesses seven hydrophobic regions which span the plasma membrane, thus creating extracellular as well as intracellular loops. The amino terminus is extracellular while the carboxyl terminal region is cytoplasmic. (Reproduced with permission from R.J. Lefkowitz, B.K. Kobilka, and M.G. Caron (1989). The new biology of drug receptors. *Biochemical Pharmacology*, **38**, 2941–8.)

5'-monophosphate (**AMP**), in brain tissue was followed by the discovery, largely by the group led by Greengard, that adenylate cyclase can be stimulated by neurotransmitters such as noradrenaline (norepinephrine), dopamine, and histamine, thus providing a basis for the action of cAMP as a second messenger in neurones possessing receptors for these compounds.

The other major second-messenger substance is inositol-1,4,5-trisphosphate, a water-soluble compound derived from hydrolysis of the membrane phospholipid phosphatidylinositol-4,5-bisphosphate by the enzyme phospholipase C. The phosphatidylinositol cycle in which turnover of the membrane-bound phosphoinositides, which constitute about 5 per cent of membrane phospholipids, is stimulated by neurotransmitters such as acetylcholine, was first observed by Hokin and Hokin in 1953. However, the importance of this process was not recognized until Michell[4] showed that phosphoinositide hydrolysis was linked to an increase in intracellular calcium ion concentration. A further stimulus for the study of this pathway was provided by the work of Berridge *et al.*[5] who demonstrated in 1982 that lithium inhibits the phosphoinositide cycle and leads to depletion of brain inositol and accumulation of inositol phosphates. Although it was initially uncertain which of the various molecules phosphatidylinositol, phosphatidylinositol-4-phosphate, or phosphatidylinositol-

4,5-bisphosphate is hydrolysed under conditions of neurotransmitter stimulation, it is now clear that the relevant molecule is phosphatidylinositol-4,5-bisphosphate, and that inositol-1,4,5-trisphosphate is the active second messenger while inositol bisphosphate and inositol monophosphate, in their various isomeric forms, are breakdown products of inositol-1,4,5-trisphosphate (Fig. 2). Another route of metabolism involves phosphorylation of inositol-1,4,5-trisphosphate to inositol-1,3,4,5-tetrakisphosphate, which is then broken down by a phosphatase enzyme to inositol-1,3,4-trisphosphate. Inositol-1,4,5-trisphosphate acts by binding to receptors on the endoplasmic reticulum and releasing calcium ions into the cytoplasm. Calcium itself has many functions within the cell (see below) and is thus also often referred to as a second messenger. Hydrolysis of phosphatidylinositol-4,5-bisphosphate also leads to the formation of diacylglycerol, itself a second messenger which acts by stimulating the enzyme protein kinase C (see below). The cycle is completed by resynthesis of phosphatidylinositol by transfer of the phosphatidic acid moiety from cytidine diphosphate diacylglycerol to myoinositol. This process is essential to the maintenance of a sufficiently high level of phosphoinositides, since in most tissues inositol is not taken up from the bloodstream, and must therefore be provided by intracellular recycling.

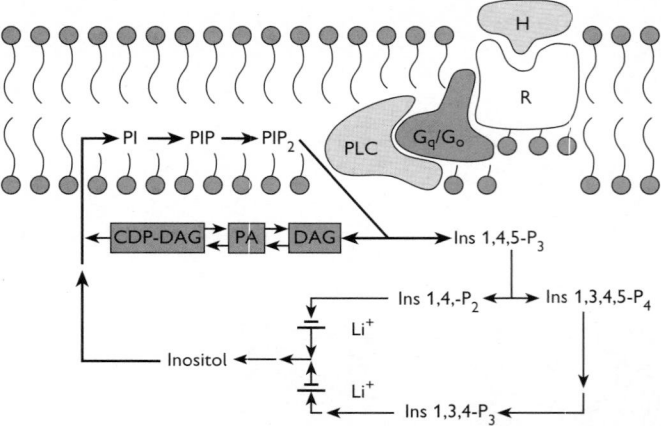

Fig. 2 The phosphoinositide cycle. Occupancy of the receptor (R) by a neurotransmitter or hormone (H) initiates the hydrolysis of phosphatidylinositol-4,5-bisphosphate (PIP₂) by phospholipase C (PLC). The signal from the receptor is conveyed to the effector (PLC) by different classes of G proteins (G_q or G_o). The hydrolysis leads to the formation of two second messengers, inositol-1,4,5-trisphosphate (Ins-1,4,5-P₃, IP₃) and diacylglycerol (DAG). IP₃ is either dephosphorylated to inositol-1,4-bisphosphate (Ins-1,4-P₂) or phosphorylated to form inositol-1,3,4,5-tetrakisphosphate (Ins-1,3,4,5-P₄), which is then itself dephosphorylated to inositol-1,3,4-trisphosphate (Ins-1,3,4-P₃). The thick horizontal lines indicate points of inhibition of the phosphatase enzymes by lithium ion (Li⁺). Resynthesis of the phosphoinositides occurs by transfer of the phosphatidic acid (PA) moiety from cytidine diphosphate glycerol (CDP-DAG) to inositol, thus generating phosphatidylinositol (PI). This is phosphorylated to phosphatidylinositol-4-phosphate (PIP) and further phosphorylated to PIP₂. (Reproduced with permission from H.K. Manji and R.H. Lenox (1994). Long-term action of lithium: a role for transcriptional and post-transcriptional factors regulated by protein kinase C. *Synapse*, **16**, 11–28.)

Transduction systems—G proteins

It was at first believed that the enzymes responsible for formation of second messengers were directly linked to the membrane-bound receptors. However, the pioneering work of Gilman and of Rodbell,[6] for which they were awarded the Nobel Prize in 1994, showed that another class of proteins exist which mediate between the receptors and effector enzymes, and are thus responsible for the phenomenon now known as 'receptor–effector coupling'. Activation of these proteins requires binding of the guanine nucleotide guanosine triphosphate, and the proteins, initially referred to as N (nucleotide binding) proteins, are now universally known as G proteins (guanyl nucleotide binding proteins).

Currently four major families of G proteins are known to exist (Table 1), defined on the basis of their sequence homologies.[7] It was initially thought that each G protein coupled to a single effector molecule only, and the G proteins were thus designated by letters specifying this action, such as G_s and G_i for stimulation and inhibition of adenylate cyclase respectively. It is now recognized that G proteins are 'promiscuous' in that they can interact with more than one effector system. G_s, for example, is capable not only of stimulating adenylate cyclase but also of opening L-type calcium channels. G_o, a member of the G_i class, is linked to calcium channels and in some systems to hydrolysis of the polyphosphoinositides via stimulation of phospho-

lipase C. Another member of the G_i class is the protein G_t, originally named transducin, which is coupled to the enzyme cyclic guanosine monophosphate (**cGMP**) phosphodiesterase. The two remaining classes of G proteins comprise G_q, which is coupled to phospholipase C-β, and G_{12}, for which the effector system is not known. Each of the G proteins consists of α-, β-, and γ-subunits, with the α-units conferring specificity. The βγ-units were originally thought to be similar or interchangeable for all G-protein heterotrimers. However, at least five β-subunits and eleven γ-subunits are now known to exist. It is not known whether certain α-subunits prefer certain βγ-complexes. Molecular cloning studies have identified at least four forms of the α-subunit of G_s, which may result from alternative splicing of a single precursor mRNA. Three forms of the α-subunit of G_i, which appear to be products of three separate genes, have been identified and named G_{i1}-α, G_{i2}-α, and G_{i3}-α. Neural tissue contains predominantly G_{i1}-α and G_{i2}-α, while platelets contain G_{i2}-α and G_{i3}-α.

The mechanism by which G proteins are activated is now understood (Fig. 3). Interaction of a ligand with a receptor results in dissociation of the α-subunit from the complex and exchange of the bound guanosine diphosphate for guanosine triphosphate. The dissociated α-units then activate the relevant intracellular effectors and also hydrolyse the bound guanosine triphosphate to guanosine diphosphate via an intrinsic guanosine triphosphatase, thus facilitating reassociation of the inactive α-β-γ heterotrimer and terminating the signal. Adenosine diphosphate ribosylation of the α-units by bacterial toxins accounts both for the diseases produced by the relevant bacteria and also enables intervention in the G-protein activation cycle. This can be used to establish the identity of the G protein involved in a particular physiological process. Cholera toxin modification of Gs inhibits guanosine triphosphatase activity and leads to constitutive stimulation of cAMP formation, while pertussis toxin modifies G_i and G_o, and blocks signal transduction by uncoupling the G protein from its receptor. Sensitivity to pertussis toxin is indeed a characteristic of the G_i group of G proteins, the one exception being G_z. It is important to note that receptors may be coupled to phosphoinositide hydrolysis by pertussis-toxin-sensitive G_i or G_o, or by pertussis-toxin-insensitive G_q.

Understanding of the roles played by the different subunits of G proteins has undergone a drastic transition in recent years. It was initially believed that messages were carried by the α-units only, and that the βγ-units served to terminate these messages by combining with and thus inactivating the α-units. βγ-units are now known to have well-defined effects on some isoforms of the classical second-messenger systems, including phospholipases C-β₂ and C-β₃ and several G-protein-responsive potassium, calcium, and perhaps also sodium ion channels. In addition, some isoforms of adenylate cyclase are activated by βγ, while others are inhibited (Table 2). While *in vitro* studies have shown that many combinations of α- and βγ-units can exist, *in vivo* a high degree of specificity may exist both for interactions between α- and βγ-units and for interactions between receptors and G proteins. This has been demonstrated using antisense oligonucleotides to suppress translation of specific G-protein subunits. Examination of subsequent impaired cellular responses indicates whether the specific subunit is involved in the signal transduction processes leading to the response. For example, it was shown that inhibition of calcium channels by somatostatin receptors in GH3 cells is mediated by the combination $\alpha_{o2}\beta_1\gamma_3$, while inhibition by M_4 muscarinic receptors is mediated by $\alpha_{o1}\beta_1\gamma_4$.[8]

Table 1 Mammalian G-protein α-subunits

Family	Subunit	Tissue distribution	Receptor agonists	Effectors
α_s	$\alpha_s(s)$ Two splice variants $\alpha_s(1)$ Two splice variants	Ubiquitous	β-Adrenergic, TSH, VIP, dopamine D_1, adenosine A_2, histamine H_2	↑Adenylate cyclase ↑Ca^{2+} channels (L-type) ↓Na^+ channels
	α_{olf}	Olfactory epithelium	Odorants	↑ Adenylate cyclase (type III)
α_i	α_{i1} α_{i2} α_{i3} α_{o1} α_{o2}	Nearly ubiquitous Ubiquitous Nearly ubiquitous Brain Brain	α_2-Adrenergic, dopamine D_2, D_4, 5-HT-la, met-enkephalin, adenosine A_1, somatostatin, muscarinic cholinergic M_2, M_4	↑K^+ channels ↓Ca^{2+} channels ↓Adenylate cyclase (types I, III, V, VI) ↑PLC ↑PLA-2
	α_{t1} α_{t2} α_g α_z	Retinal rods Retinal cones Taste buds Brain, adrenal, platelets	Rhodopsin Cone opsin Taste stimuli? Muscarinic M_2?	↑cGMP PDE ↑cGMP PDE ? ?
α_q	α_q α_{11} α_{14} $\alpha_{15/16}$	Ubiquitous Ubiquitous Kidney, lung, spleen Haematopoietic cells	α_1-Adrenergic, muscarinic M_1, M_3 histamine H_1, thromboxane A_2, neurokinin, bombesin, endothelin, vasopressin V_1, bradykinin B_2	↑Phospholipase C-β ($\beta_3 > \beta_1 >> \beta_2 = \beta_4$)
α_{12}	α_{12} α_{13}	Ubiquitous Ubiquitous	Thromboxane A_2, Thrombin	? ?

Several of the receptors and G proteins listed are not found in the central nervous system but are included for completeness.
TSH, thyroid-stimulating hormone; VIP, vasoactive intestinal peptide; 5-HT, 5-hydroxytryptamine (serotonin); PLC, phospholipase C; PLA, phospholipase A; cGMP, cyclic guanosine monophosphate; PDE, phosphodiesterase.
Modified from Hepler and Gilman[20] and Offermans and Schultz.[21]

The central role played by G proteins in the signal transduction process is illustrated by the fact that G-protein molecules vastly outnumber the receptor molecules in any given cell. G proteins thus act to amplify the relatively small chemical signals generated by transmitter and receptor molecules. The high degree of complexity generated by the interactions of G-protein-coupled receptors with G proteins may be one mechanism whereby neurons acquire the flexibility necessary to generate the wide variety of responses observed in the central nervous system.

Effector enzymes—adenylate cyclase

Eight adenylate cyclase isoenzymes have now been purified from mammalian sources (Table 2).[9] These proteins have molecular weights of approximately 120 000 and a complex topology within the membrane, consisting of a short cytoplasmic amino terminus followed by six transmembrane spans, a large cytoplasmic domain, a second set of six transmembrane spans, and a large intracellular carboxyl terminus domain (Fig. 4). This structure bears a striking resemblance to that of membrane transporter proteins. The transmembrane domains are not highly conserved between adenylate cyclases and share little or no homology with the highly conserved transmembrane domains of ion channels. The isoenzymes can be divided into three groups based on sequence similarities and shared regulatory properties. The first group, comprising types I, III, and VIII, are sensitive to stimulation by calcium ions together with its binding protein calmodulin, and to a lesser extent by G_s. Type I is inhibited by βγ-units while type III, which is found in large quantities in olfactory neurones, is insensitive to βγ. The second group, comprising types II, IV, and VII, are activated by α_s and synergistically by βγ, and have thus been proposed to act as 'coincidence detectors', i.e. molecules that integrate messages derived from different sources. This may account for the increases in cAMP formation observed in the hippocampus as a result of activation of receptors that are not coupled to G_s, such as the serotonin 5-HT_{1A} receptor. Brain tissue possesses large quantities of G_o, representing 0.5 per cent

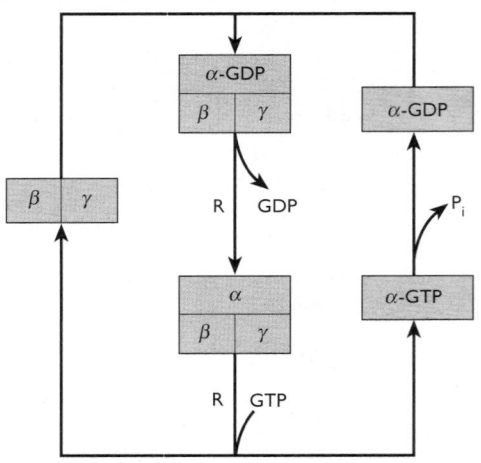

Fig. 3 The G-protein cycle of activation. During activation by a receptor (R), guanosine triphosphate (GTP) binds to the α-unit of the G-protein heterotrimer (α-β-γ) and induces its dissociation into α-GTP and $\beta\gamma$ units. GTP is then hydrolysed into guanosine diphosphate (GDP) by a guanosine triphosphatase (GTPase) enzyme intrinsic to the α-unit, and the inactive α-GDP unit then recombines with $\beta\gamma$. (Reproduced with permission from P.C. Sternweis and I.-H. Pang (1990). The G protein-channel connection. *Trends in Neurosciences*, **13**, 122–6.)

guanosine-triphosphate-containing α-subunit of G_{olf}, thus allowing substantial amplification of the odorant signal.

Further actions of second messengers—phosphorylation cascades

The earliest known action of cAMP was as a regulator of glycogen metabolism. cAMP is now known to have diverse roles in the cell. All of its actions are mediated by activation of cAMP-dependent protein kinase, an enzyme consisting of two regulatory units and two catalytic units. Binding of two molecules of cAMP to the regulatory subunits results in the release of the two catalytic subunits, which then rapidly phosphorylate membrane or cytoplasmic proteins. As well as cAMP-dependent protein kinase, cells also contain a cGMP-dependent kinase—protein kinase C—which is activated by diacylglycerol, and various calcium-dependent kinases. These can be activated by calcium ions derived either extracellularly via L-type voltage-dependent calcium channels, or from intracellular pools as a result of the action of inositol-1,4,5-trisphosphate on the endoplasmic reticulum.

Protein kinases activated by second messengers are in general referred to as serine/threonine protein kinases, since the acceptors for phosphate in the target molecules are serine or threonine residues. In protein kinase C, cGMP-dependent kinase, and Ca²⁺-calmodulin-dependent kinase, the regulatory and catalytic domains are part of the same polypeptide chain. Binding of the second messenger results in unfolding of the molecule, thus exposing and activating the catalytic region. The phosphorylation reactions mediated by these kinases may serve to integrate signals transmitted by the various second messengers. The substrates for phosphorylation in many cases include the kinase enzymes themselves. The regulatory units of cAMP-dependent protein kinase, for example, can be phosphorylated by the enzyme's catalytic units. This autophosphorylation process leads to a reduction in the rate at which the regulatory and catalytic units recombine and occurs when the cAMP concentration in the cell is low.

Protein phosphatase enzymes

Although in most instances biological activity results from kinase-mediated phosphorylation of a substrate protein, in some cases

of total brain protein, and dissociation of this G protein yields large quantities of $\beta\gamma$ which will then act synergistically with α_s to activate adenylate cyclase. The third group, comprising types V and VI, are activated by α_s and inhibited by α_i and also by calcium ions.

Figure 5 illustrates the action of adenylate cyclase type III as a coincidence detector.[10] Interaction of odorants with their receptors in the nasal epithelium leads to dissociation of the G protein G_{olf}, a member of the G_s family, into $\beta\gamma$- and α-units, which then activate adenylate cyclase. Simultaneous activation of the inositol-1,4,5-trisphosphate pathway leads to release of calcium ions, which bind to calmodulin and result in further activation of the adenylate cyclase enzyme. Calmodulin is abundant in olfactory neurones and can lead to generation of cAMP levels three to six times greater than those induced by a mixture of odorants. Activation of type III adenylate cyclase by calmodulin is most effective when the enzyme is associated with the activated

Table 2 Mammalian adenylate cyclases (grouped by structural relatedness)

Type	Stimulated by	Inhibited by	Major sources
I	α_s (slight), Ca²⁺	α_i,[a] $\beta\gamma$	Dentate gyrus, hippocampus
III	α_s, Ca²⁺		Olfactory epithelium
VIII	α_s (slight), Ca²⁺		Hippocampus
II	α_s, $\beta\gamma$, PKC		Cerebellum
IV	α_s, $\beta\gamma$		Rare
VII	α_s, PKC		Cerebellum
V	α_s	α_i, Ca²⁺	Caudate nucleus
VI	α_s	α_i, Ca²⁺	Heart

[a] Inhibition by α_i only when stimulated by Ca²⁺.
Modified from Mons and Cooper[22] and Cooper *et al.*[23]

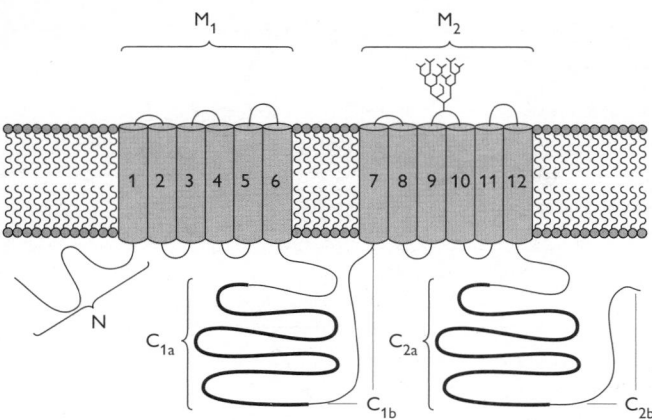

Fig. 4 The structure of adenylate cyclase. The twelve cylinders represent membrane-spanning domains divided into the two sets M$_1$ and M$_2$. The amino terminus N is cytoplasmic and there are two large cytoplasmic domains C$_1$ and C$_2$. Each of these is divided into regions of high amino acid similarity among all members of the family, indicated in bold and labelled C$_{1a}$ and C$_{2a}$; less conserved regions are labelled C$_{1b}$ and C$_{2b}$. (Reproduced with permission from R. Taussig and A.G. Gilman (1995). Mammalian membrane-bound adenylyl cyclases. *Journal of Biological Chemistry*, **270**, 1–4.)

dephosphorylation of phosphorylated proteins by phosphatase enzymes are required for signalling purposes. Eight phosphoprotein phosphatase enzymes are currently recognized, classified by whether they remove phosphate groups from phosphoserine/phosphothreonine residues or from phosphotyrosine residues. Protein phosphatase 2B is also referred to as calcineurin. Very recently, an additional molecular device for the feedback regulation of kinase signalling pathways has been described whereby a protein kinase, which is itself regulated by protein phosphorylation, becomes the substrate of a specific protein phosphatase in a self-moderating signalling complex. An example is the interaction between Ca^{2+}-calmodulin-dependent protein kinase IV and protein phosphatase 2A. Ca^{2+}-calmodulin-dependent protein kinase IV is activated in a calcium-dependent manner involving phosphorylation by the upsteam Ca^{2+}-calmodulin-depend-

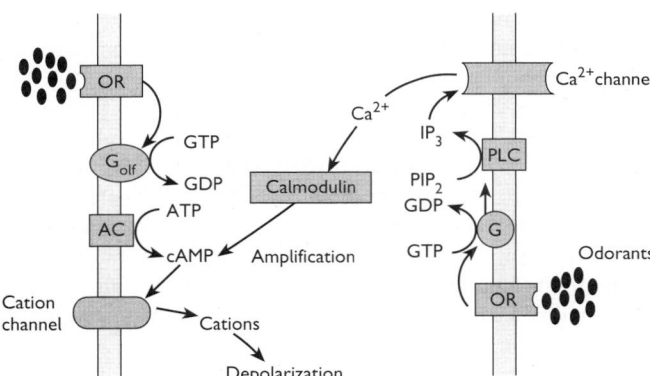

Fig. 5 Dual activation of olfactory adenylate cyclase (AC) type III by odorant-activated G$_{olf}$ and Ca^{2+}-calmodulin resulting from odorant-induced synthesis of inositol trisphosphate (IP$_3$). The odorants interact with odorant receptors (OR), which are coupled either to AC or to phospholipase C (PLC). Abbreviations as in Fig. 2. (Reproduced with permission from R.R.H. Anholt (1994). Signal integration in the nervous system: adenylate cyclases as molecular coincidence detectors. *Trends in Neuroscience*, **17**, 37–41.)

ent protein kinase kinase. Activation is transient and reversible, even in the presence of high levels of intracellular calcium ions, since protein phosphatase 2A binds to the region of Ca^{2+}-calmodulin-dependent protein kinase IV that encompasses the kinase catalytic domain. This tight regulation of Ca^{2+}-calmodulin-dependent protein kinase IV phosphorylation by the phosphatase enzyme in a constitutive signalling complex allows rapid adjustment of the signal transmitted by the kinase to achieve an appropriate cellular response.

A further level of regulation is provided by the existence of protein phosphatase inhibitors, such as DARPP-32, found in neurones which express dopamine D$_1$ receptors. DARPP-32 is a dopamine- and cAMP-regulated phosphoprotein, and by acting as a protein phosphatase inhibitor when it is phosphorylated, can regulate postsynaptic effects of dopamine in dopaminoceptive cells.

Although a variety of cellular proteins are phosphorylated by protein kinases, much attention has been given to phosphorylation of a nuclear protein known as the cAMP/calcium-responsive element binding protein. Phosphorylation of this protein requires translocation of a protein kinase from the cytoplasm to the nuclear membrane. The phosphorylated protein induces gene transcription by binding to a sequence of DNA termed the cAMP binding element. Activation of transcription requires synergism between cAMP/calcium-responsive element binding protein and the calcium-dependent protein phosphatase calcineurin. Thus the cAMP binding element acts as a coincidence detector.

Examples of genes of which transcription is activated once the cAMP binding element site is occupied include the 'immediate–early genes' such as c-*fos* and c-*jun*. The products of these genes, known as Fos or Jun proteins, are themselves transcription factors able to regulate the expression of a variety of other genes, including genes for neurotransmitter synthetic enzymes such as tyrosine hydroxylase and for neuropeptides such as dynorphin. In some cases gene transcription is controlled by a dimer of the Fos and Jun proteins, known as the AP-1 transcription factor. Thus the immediate–early genes provide a link between changes at the receptor/second-messenger level at the cell membrane and changes in gene expression in the nucleus, which then provide the basis for long-term adaptations. Induction of immediate–early gene expression always occurs in specific anatomical pathways, and neurotransmitters may have differential effects on the same target gene in different cell types or on different genes in the same cell by inducing distinct patterns of the immediate–early gene products. A corollary of this mechanism is that neurotransmitters can in some situations be thought of as growth factors, even in fully differentiated cells. This growth-factor-like action may be manifested as an ability to maintain the differentiated state of the cell by influencing the transcription of genes characteristic of the cellular phenotype.

Another function served by the phosphorylation reactions is desensitization of receptors. β-Adrenergic receptors, for example, are desensitized following phosphorylation in the cytoplasmic domain of the molecule by cAMP-dependent β-adrenergic receptor kinase, as well as by cAMP-dependent kinases or protein kinase C. Two to three molecules of phosphate are incorporated per receptor molecule, and the degree of desensitization correlates with the degree of phosphorylation. Phosphorylation slows the ability of the receptor to activate G$_s$ and also promotes binding of the inhibitory protein arrestin to the phosphorylated receptor.

Protein kinase C

Protein kinase C has a major role in regulating not only pre- and post-synaptic aspects of neurotransmission but also long-term physiological processes such as cell growth and development.[11] Activation of protein kinase C by diacylglycerol is followed by translocation of cytosolic protein kinase C to the cell membrane, where protein kinase C is further activated by extracellular calcium ions and by acidic phospholipids, in particular phosphatidylserine. It was initially thought that all the diacylglycerol present in the cell and capable of activating protein kinase C was derived from hydrolysis of phosphatidylinositol-4,5-bisphosphate. However, more recent evidence suggests that neurotransmitter-induced activation of two other phospholipase enzymes, phospholipase D and phospholipase A₂, may contribute significantly to formation of diacylglycerol and thus to activation of protein kinase C. Phospholipase D acts on the phospholipid phosphatidylcholine, and the hydrolysis of two different membrane phospholipids may lead to a biphasic increase in diacylglycerol, with an initial rapid and transient rise due to phosphatidylinositol-4,5-bisphosphate hydrolysis by phospholipase C, followed by a more sustained increase due to hydrolysis of phosphatidylcholine by phospholipase D. In addition, since activation of protein kinase C has been shown to enhance phospholipase D activity, the initial transient increase in the level of diacylglycerol arising from phosphatidylinositol-4,5-bisphosphate breakdown may act as a trigger for hydrolysis of phosphatidylcholine. This self-perpetuating cycle may be responsible for the sustained activation of protein kinase C necessary for its long-lasting biological effects.

Eight isoforms of protein kinase C have now been identified, all encoded by distinct genes. Each protein kinase C holoenzyme contains regulatory and catalytic domains in a single continuous polypeptide chain. Like cAMP-dependent protein kinase, protein kinase C can also be autophosphorylated. The major forms of protein kinase C (α, βI, βII, and γ) all have a calcium binding site and are dependent to varying extents on calcium ions, while the other 'minor' forms of protein kinase C (δ, ε, ζ, and η) lack the calcium-binding domain and therefore their activity is independent of calcium ions. In addition, protein kinase C γ is activated by low concentrations of arachidonic acid. Since arachidonic acid can also be synthesized via activation of phospholipase C (Fig. 6), it turns out that protein kinase C can be activated synergistically by at least two second messengers (diacylglycerol and calcium) and in some cases by three (diacylglycerol, calcium, and arachidonic acid).

Activation of ion channels

In addition to activation by type I receptors which are directly coupled to ion channels and by α-units derived from some G proteins such as G_s, ion channels can also be activated by phosphorylation reactions. For example, the calcium channels regulated directly by G_s are in addition phosphorylated by protein kinase A, which leads to further increases in their functional activity. Protein kinases may open channels which are closed at the resting membrane potential, an action similar to that of a transmitter on a directly gated ion channel. Kinases activated by second messengers may also close channels that are open at the resting potential, or close non-gated potassium channels which contribute to the resting potential by leakage. Closure of these channels has a depolarizing effect, increasing the excitability of the neurone and overriding its tendency to accommodate during prolonged stimu-

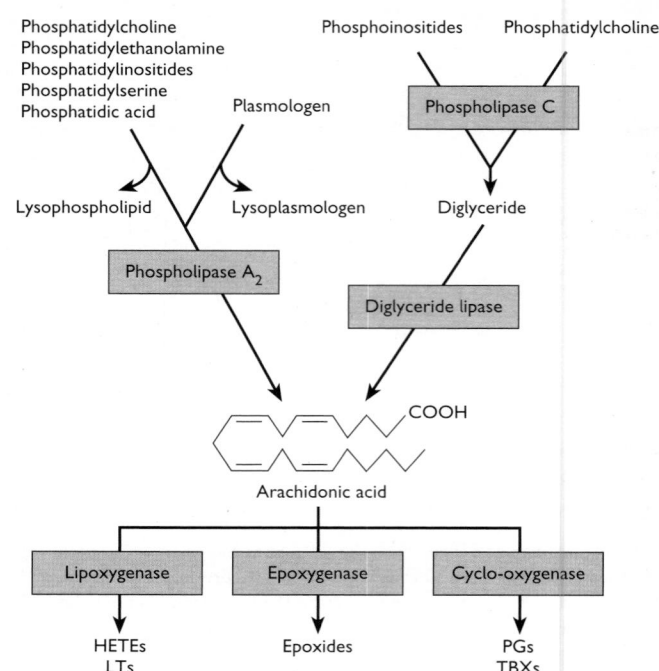

Fig. 6 Pathways for the generation and metabolism of arachidonic acid (AA). AA can arise directly from phospholipids through the action of phospholipase A₂ (PLA₂) or prior action of phospholipase C, followed by the action of diglyceride lipase. Alternatively, the diglyceride may be phosphorylated to phosphatidic acid by the action of diglyceride kinase, and AA is then released by the action of PLA₂. The released AA is metabolized by lipoxygenase, cyclo-oxygenase or epoxygenase enzymes to form leucotrienes (LTs), hydroxyeicosatetraenoic acids (HETEs), prostaglandins (PGs), thromboxanes (TXs) and epoxides. (Reproduced with permission from J. Axelrod, R.M. Burch, and C.L. Jelsema (1988). Receptor-mediated activation of phospholipase A₂ via GTP-binding proteins: arachidonic acid and its metabolites as second messengers. *Trends in Neuroscience*, **11**, 117–23.)

lation. An example of such an effect is the closure of calcium-stimulated potassium channels by noradrenaline acting through cAMP in hippocampal neurones, leading to a longer period of firing in response to glutamate. Some ion channels may be modulated directly by second messengers such as cAMP or cGMP without requiring protein phosphorylation.

Class I receptors may also be regulated by phosphorylation. An example is the nicotinic acetylcholine receptor, which is phosphorylated on its α-subunit by protein kinase C, on its β-subunit by tyrosine-specific kinases, on its γ-subunit by protein kinase A and tyrosine-specific kinases, and on its δ-subunit by all three kinases. The cAMP-dependent phosphorylation of the β- and γ-subunits increases the rate at which the receptor is desensitized. This is an example of one of the multiple feedback regulations which serve to achieve fine tuning of cellular responses.

Other second messengers

Arachidonic acid

Arachidonic acid and its metabolites, collectively known as eicosanoids, were known for a long time to be important in modulation of nervous signals, but the identification of these substances as second messengers came only in the 1980s when Axelrod's group determined that their production involved the action of a G protein.[12] Arachidonic acid can be produced directly from a variety of phospholipids by the action of phospholipase A₂, or indirectly by the action of the enzyme diglyceride lipase on diglycerides produced as a result of the hydrolytic action of phospholipase C on either phosphoinositides or phosphatidylcholine (Fig. 6). Free arachidonic acid and some of its metabolites such as prostaglandin E₂, the leucotrienes and lipoxin A can elevate cytosolic calcium concentrations independently of inositol-1,4,5-trisphosphate, and may also act as physiological regulators of guanylate cyclase. Arachidonic acid may also leave the cell and act as a first messenger for adjacent cells.

One pathway of arachidonic acid metabolism (Fig. 6) involves lipoxygenase enzymes that introduce an oxygen molecule into one of the polyunsaturated pentadiene moieties to form a hydroperoxyeicosatrienoic acid. Depolarization of brain slices with high concentrations of extracellular potassium ions, glutamate or *N*-methyl-D-aspartate has been shown to greatly increase 12-lipoxygenase activity. 12-Hydroperoxyeicosatrienoic acid and some of its metabolites act to modulate the actions of ion channels at specific synapses.

Cyclic guanosine monophosphate and nitric oxide

Cyclic guanosine-3',5'-monophosphate is a compound related to cAMP found in brain, predominantly in the cerebellum. Elucidation of the role of cGMP was delayed because initial expectations that its regulation would be similar to that exisiting for cAMP were not fulfilled. The enzyme guanylate cyclase which forms cGMP from guanosine triphosphate was found to exist in both soluble and membrane-bound forms, and no ligands that stimulated this enzyme were apparent. The first situation in which a function for cGMP was detected was in the mediation of visual signals in rod cells in the retina. The action of cGMP here differs from the conventional function of second messengers in that a decrease in its level rather than an increase stimulates the signal transduction process. In the absence of light, cGMP holds open the sodium channels in the cell membrane of the rod outer segment, allowing entry of calcium and magnesium ions to the cell. Light photons induce isomerization of the light-sensitive molecule 11-*cis*-retinal, attached to the seven-transmembrane protein rhodopsin, to all-*trans*-retinal. This process activates rhodopsin so that it interacts with the G protein transducin ($G\alpha_{t1}$), inducing its dissociation to $G\alpha$- and $\beta\gamma$-units. The $G\alpha$-unit stimulates the effector enzyme cGMP phosphodiesterase to break down cGMP, resulting in closure of the membrane sodium channels.

The soluble form of guanylate cyclase transduces the messages carried by the gaseous signalling molecules nitric oxide and carbon monoxide. These are lipid-soluble extracellular messengers which diffuse into their target cells and activate guanylate cyclase by binding to its haem moiety.[13] Nitric oxide is synthesized from arginine via the enzyme nitric oxide synthase, which is constitutively expressed in neurones and is activated by calcium and calmodulin. This enzyme can be regulated by phosphorylation by protein kinases, an increase in phosphorylation resulting in a decrease in enzyme activity. The main source of calcium ions for activation of nitric oxide synthase is the *N*-methyl-D-aspartate glutamate receptor, an ionotropic receptor pres-

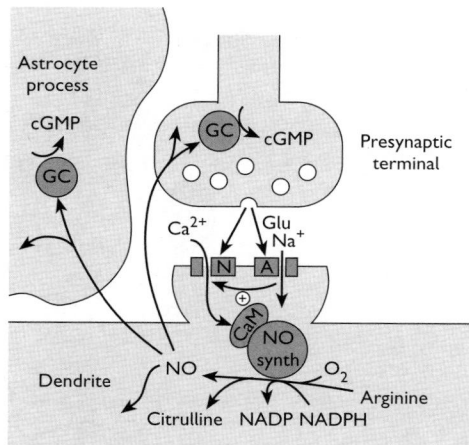

Fig. 7 Model for the operation of the nitric oxide (NO) system in the central nervous system. Glutamate (Glu) released from presynaptic terminals acts on *N*-methyl-D-aspartate (NMDA, N) and α-amino-3-hydroxy-5-methylisoxazole-4-propionic acid (AMPA, A) receptors. When the postsynaptic membrane is sufficiently depolarized, calcium ions enter and via calmodulin (CaM) activate the NO synthase. The NO formed diffuses out to neighbouring astrocyte fibres and/or to the presynaptic terminals where it activates guanylate cyclase (GC). (Reproduced with permission from J. Garthwaite (1991). Glutamate, nitric oxide and cell–cell signalling in the nervous system. *Trends in Neuroscience*, **14**, 60–67.)

ent in high concentrations on the granule cells of the cerebellum. Nitric oxide thus acts as a second messenger with respect to glutamate, but as a first messenger with respect to cGMP (Fig. 7).

Tyrosine kinases

The tyrosine kinase pathway does not strictly speaking involve second messengers in the classic sense, but is of critical importance in that it represents an alternative to the G-protein pathway for activation of effector enzymes, which themselves can be considered to be intracellular messengers. Receptors linked to tyrosine kinases, such as the receptors for epidermal growth factor, nerve growth factor, and insulin, exist either as monomers or dimers which span the membrane only once and are either situated on the same protein as the effector or in close association with it. Ligand binding to the receptor activates the effector enzyme, tyrosine kinase, at the intracellular face of the membrane without any intervening transducer protein. Elaborate signalling cascades exist to propagate the signal received by tyrosine kinase from the membrane to the nucleus, involving both autophosphorylation and phosphorylation of other substrate proteins. In a typical pathway known as the mitogen-activated protein kinase pathway, the conformational change induced by ligand binding is passed along a series of proteins known as Shc, Grb, and Sos (Fig. 8) and then activates a membrane-asssociated protein named Ras. Ras has guanosine triphosphatase activity in a manner analogous to the α-subunit of a G protein. Guanosine triphosphate-bound Ras activates a serine/threonine protein kinase known as Raf, which phosphorylates and thus activates mitogen-activated protein kinase kinase. The latter is a dual-specificity kinase which activates mitogen-activated protein kinase by phosphorylation on threonine and tyrosine residues. Mitogen-activated protein kinase is also referred to as extracellular signal-regulated kinase.

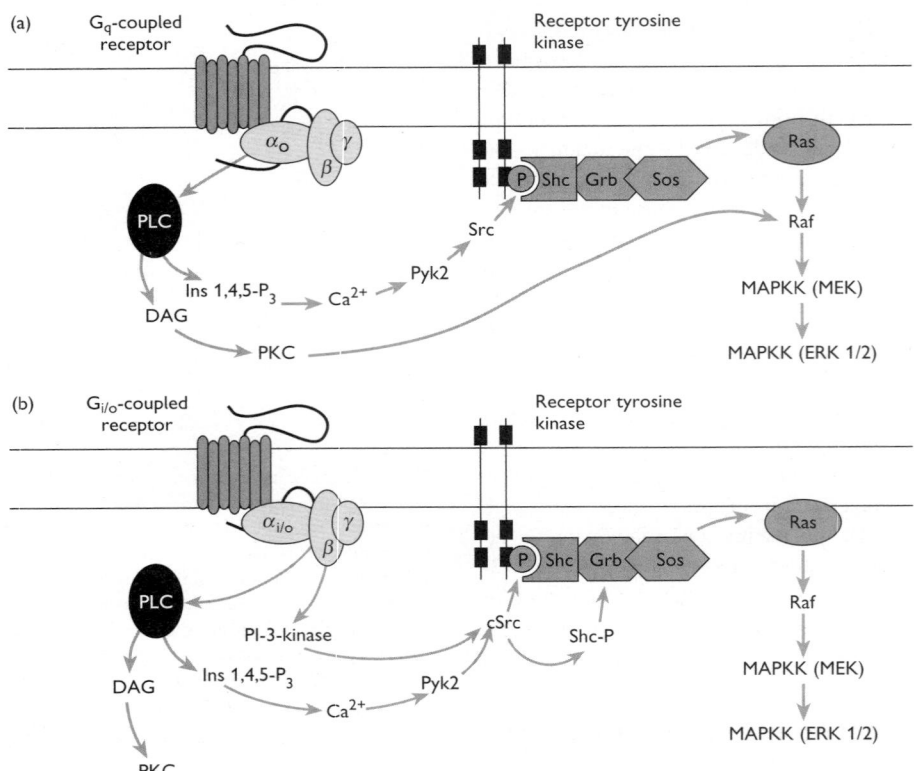

Fig. 8 Interactions between G-protein-coupled receptors and receptor tyrosine kinases. Activation of mitogen-activated protein kinase (MAPK) by (a) G_q-coupled receptors, and (b) $G_{i/o}$-coupled receptors. MAPKK is MAPK kinase, also known as MEK, PKC is protein kinase C, and ERK 1/2 is extracellular signal-regulated kinase. Other abbreviations as in Fig. 2. (Reproduced with permission from L.A. Selbie and S.J. Hill (1998). G protein-coupled-receptor cross-talk; the fine tuning of multiple receptor-signalling pathways. *Trends in Pharmacological Science*, **19**, 87–93.)

Cross-talk between this mitogen-activated protein kinase pathway and G-protein-mediated pathways may proceed via any of the second messengers cAMP, inositol-1,4,5-trisphosphate, and diacylglycerol.[14,15] Protein kinase C, activated by diacylglycerol, may activate the mitogen-activated protein kinase cascade by directly activating Raf. cAMP acting via protein kinase A can repress the activation of this pathway by inhibitory interactions either with Raf or with the receptor protein tyrosine kinase. Ca^{2+}-calmodulin-stimulated protein kinases activated by inositol-1,4,5-trisphosphate can also lead to activation of the mitogen-activated protein kinase pathway by stimulating phosphorylation of the linker protein Shc, a process involving other kinases known as Pyk2 and Src (Fig. 8). Furthermore, the reverse process by which the mitogen-activated protein kinase cascade modulates G-protein-linked receptors may also occur. Another route involves a role for G protein $\beta\gamma$-units in the activation of Ras and thus in the stimulation of mitogen-activated protein kinase. Activation proceeds via $\beta\gamma$-mediated phosphorylation of Shc, leading to an increased functional association betwen Shc, Grb, and Sos. In some cell types, the action of $\beta\gamma$ involves the enzyme phosphatidylinositol-3-kinase, which catalyses the phosphorylation of the 3 position of the inositol ring of the phosphoinositides. This route for mitogen-activated protein kinase activation is thus G-protein dependent but calcium independent.

One of the targets for convergent activation by products of the tyrosine kinase pathway and the G-protein-linked pathway is the immediate–early gene c-*fos*. This dual regulation enables c-*fos* to be activated within minutes after stimulation with diverse agents such as serum growth factors, cytokines, and neurotransmitters.

Extracellular second messengers—a contradiction in terms?

A final point of interest is that although by definition second messengers are intracellular, microdialysis and other studies have succeeded in measuring both cAMP and inositol-1,4,5-trisphosphate in the brain extracellular space. These extracellular pools of second messengers are sensitive to pharmacological manipulation, with the levels being increased by the agents that elevate their intracellular concentrations. Thus, Lazareno et al.[16] found that dopamine increased cAMP levels both in slices of rat striatum and in the incubation medium, while Egawa et al.[17] showed that the increases in extracellular cAMP produced by adding noradrenaline to rat cortical slices were equivalent to those obtained intracellularly, and furthermore that infusion of noradrenaline via a microdialysis probe implanted in the cortex produced a dose-dependent increase in cAMP. Similarly, inositol-1,4,5-trisphosphate formation in rat hippocampal microdialysate was stimulated by carbachol and inhibited by the muscarinic antagonist pirenzepine.[18]

A fascinating question concerns the role of these extracellular second messengers. The discovery by Gilman's group of the structure of the adenylate cyclase molecule and its similarity to membrane transporters suggested that adenylate cyclase itself may form a channel for cAMP efflux and that cAMP may therefore function as an intercellular signal. One possibility is that extracellular cAMP is converted to the transmitter substance adenosine, which has several important actions on neurones including inhibition of glutamate release and activation of potassium channels. Pull and McIlwain[19] found as early as 1977 that electrical stimulation of ^{14}C-adenine-labelled slices induced release of cAMP into extracellular fluid, and that extracellular adenosine derived from this cAMP.

Conclusions—implications for psychiatry

The multiple signalling systems and activation cascades described in this chapter may seem to be far removed from the problems normally encountered in psychiatry. However, it should be remembered that any drug which interacts with a receptor will of necessity either activate or inhibit at least one if not more of these second-messenger systems, and its pharmacological and therapeutic effects will thus be a direct consequence of the changes in the intracellular effector systems induced. For antidepressant drugs, the systems activated by serotonin and noradrenaline receptors may be particularly important, while for antipsychotics the intracellular effectors activated by binding to dopamine receptors are presumably involved in their actions. It is possible that drugs may attenuate some signal transduction cascades while activating others, depending on the cell type and precise combination of G proteins expressed in particular neurones. Changes in transcription of discrete sets of genes may follow, with the genes being turned on or off to yield a favourable clinical response. Furthermore, disease states such as depression or schizophrenia may themselves result from alterations in activity of distinct signal transduction cascades. Appreciation of these processes will therefore contribute in the long run to increased understanding of both the pathology of mental illness and psychopharmacology.

References

1. Strange, P.G. (1988). The structure and mechanism of neurotransmitter receptors: implications for the structure and function of the central nervous system. *Biochemical Journal*, **249**, 309–18.
2. Lefkowitz, R.J., Kobilka, B.K., and Caron, M.G. (1989). The new biology of drug receptors. *Biochemical Pharmacology*, **38**, 2941–8.
3. Kakiuchi, S., Rall, T.W., and McIlwain, H. (1969). The effect of electrical stimulation upon the accumulation of adenosine 3',5'-phosphate in isolated cerebral tissue. *Journal of Neurochemistry*, **16**, 485–91.
4. Michell, R.H. (1975). Inositol phospholipids and cell surface receptor function. *Biochimica et Biophysica Acta*, **415**, 81–147.
5. Berridge, M.J., Downes, C.P., and Hanley, M.R. (1982). Lithium amplifies agonist-dependent phosphatidylinositol responses in brain and salivary glands. *Biochemistry Journal*, **206**, 587–95.
6. Rodbell, M. (1980). The role of hormone receptors and GTP-regulatory proteins in membrane transduction. *Nature*, **284**, 17–22.
7. Simon, M.I., Strathmann, M.P., and Gautam, N. (1991). Diversity of G proteins in signal transduction. *Science*, **252**, 802–8.
8. Hamm, H.E. (1998). The many faces of G protein signalling. *Journal of Biological Chemistry*, **273**, 669–72.
9. Taussig, R. and Gilman, A.G. (1995). Mammalian membrane-bound adenylyl cyclases. *Journal of Biological Chemistry*, **270**, 1–4.
10. Anholt, R.R.H. (1994). Signal integration in the nervous system: adenylate cyclases as molecular coincidence detectors. *Trends in Neurosciences*, **17**, 37–41.
11. Nishizuka, Y. (1992). Turnover of inositol phospholipids and signal transduction. *Science*, **258**, 607–14.
12. Axelrod, J., Burch, R.M., and Jelsema, C.L. (1988). Receptor-mediated activation of phospholipase A2 via GTP-binding proteins: arachidonic acid and its metabolites as second messengers. *Trends in Neurosciences*, **11**, 117–23.
13. Garthwaite, J. (1991). Glutamate, nitric oxide and cell-cell signalling in the nervous system. *Trends in Neurosciences*, **14**, 60–67.
14. Eyster, K.M. (1998). Introduction to signal transduction: a primer for untangling the web of intracellular messengers. *Biochemical Pharmacology*, **55**, 1927–38.
15. Selbie, L.A. and Hill, S.J. (1998). G protein-coupled-receptor cross-talk; the fine tuning of multiple receptor-signalling pathways. *Trends in Pharmacological Science*, **19**, 87–93.
16. Lazareno, S., Marriott, D.B., and Nahorski, S.R. (1985). Differential effects of selective and non-selective neuroleptics on intracellular and extracellular cyclic AMP accumulation in rat striatal slices. *Brain Research*, **361**, 91–8.
17. Egawa, M., Hoebel, B.G. and Stone, E.A. (1988). Use of microdialysis to measure brain noradrenergic receptor function *in vivo*. *Brain Research*, **458**, 303–8.
18. Minisclou, C., Rouquier, L., Benavides, J., Scatton, B., and Claustre, Y. (1994). Muscarinic receptor-mediated increase in extracellular inositol 1,4,5-trisphosphate levels in the rat hippocampus: an *in vivo* microdialysis study. *Journal of Neurochemistry*, **62**, 557–62.
19. Pull, I. and McIlwain, H. (1977). Adenine mononucleotides and their metabolites liberated from and applied to isolated tissues of the mammalian brain. *Neurochemical Research*, **2**, 203–16.
20. Hepler, J.R. and Gilman, A.G. (1992). G proteins. *Trends in Biochemical Science*, **17**, 383–7.
21. Offermanns, S. and Schultz, G. (1994). Complex information processing by the transmembrane signaling system involving G proteins. *Naunyn-Schmiedebergs Archives of Pharmacology*, **350**, 329–38.
22. Mons, N. and Cooper, D.M.F. (1995). Adenylate cyclases: critical foci in neuronal signaling. *Trends in Neurosciences*, **18**, 536–542.
23. Cooper, D.M.F., Mons, N., and Karpen, J.W. (1995). Adenylyl cyclases and the interaction between calcium and cAMP signalling. *Nature*, **374**, 421–4.

2.3.5 Neuropathology

Peter Falkai and Bernhard Bogerts

Introduction

The traditional domains of neuropathology are well-defined organic brain diseases, with an obvious pathology, such as tumours, infections, vascular diseases, trauma, or toxic and hypoxemic changes, as well as degenerative brain diseases (e.g. Alzheimer's disease, Parkinson's disease, and Huntington's chorea). Neuropathological investigations of these brain disorders have been rewarding, because patients with any of these conditions can be expected to have gross morphological or more or less specific neurohistological anomalies that are related to the clinical symptoms of the disorder. Moreover, the type of brain pathology of these well-defined disease entities is quite homogenous. For example, it is highly unlikely that a patient with Parkinson's disease would not have morphological changes and Lewy bodies in the nigrostriatal system or that a person with Huntington's chorea would have a normal striatum, or that a patient with Pick's or Alzheimer's disease would not have changes in the cerebral cortex.

In contrast, the history of the neuropathology of psychiatric disorders is much more controversial, because no such obvious and homogenous types of brain pathology (as seen in neurological disorders) have yet been detected for the major psychiatric illnesses such as schizophrenia, affective disorders, substance-related disorders, or personality disorders. Furthermore it mirrors our current knowledge and beliefs concerning brain structure and function. Franz Josef Gall (1758–1828) for instance was one of the first to propose that the human brain is not a uniform mass, but different intellectual skills are localized in specific brain regions. His views were not well regarded until Paul Broca proved the connection of aphasia and lesions of the left frontal lobe.[1] With the introduction of histological methods it was possible to visualize the cytoarchitecture of the human brain. Scientists like Cajal[2] made possible a view into the complexity of brain structure and introduced the idea of a neuronal network. Based on this knowledge it was possible to unravel the neuroanatomical basis of Huntington's chorea (basal ganglia) or Parkinson's disease (substantia nigra). These findings were very encouraging and led to the belief that some psychiatric disorders like the dementias and schizophrenia had a demonstrable neuromorphological substrate. In contrast, other psychiatric disorders like depression, neurosis or personality disorders were thought to be caused by psychosocial factors or to represent variations of normal personality traits and were therefore never the subject of systematic neuropathological studies.

In 1898 Alois Alzheimer[3] described subtle abnormalities in the neocortex of patients with schizophrenia. Until 1951 about 200 pathoanatomical studies[4,5] were published describing a wealth of different findings in schizophrenia. However, at the First International Congress of Neuropathology in Rome it was concluded that there was no common neuropathological basis of schizophrenia, because no consensus was achieved on this morphological basis. Therefore schizophrenia was called a functional psychosis, in contrast with an organic psychosis where, for example, drugs or a tumour caused the symptoms. The introduction of brain imaging techniques into medicine in the mid-1970s revived the neuropathological research on psychiatric disorders. Brain imaging demonstrated *in vivo* evidence for structural changes, for example in schizophrenia an enlarged ventricle/brain ratio[6] and partly because proof was presented for brain dysfunction in disorders such as obsessive–compulsive disorder, where only psychosocial factors were thought to be central to the aetiology.

The scope of this chapter is to summarize the neuropathological findings in schizophrenia, affective disorders, and alcoholism. For this purpose the published studies are summarized in Tables 1, 2, 3, and, 4, where the significant findings are highlighted. For schizophrenia and alcoholism only the main findings are listed, as there are too many published studies to list them all. It is beyond the scope of this chapter to review the large body of literature on the senile dementias, including specifically Alzheimer's disease. The reader is referred to several comprehensive reviews.[7–9]

Table 1 Gross morphometric findings in schizophrenia

Region/parameter	Finding
General	
Brain length	($\downarrow$)
Brain weight	$\downarrow$
Ventricular area/volume	$\uparrow$
Cortex thickness	($\downarrow$)
Temporal lobe	
Lobar area/volume	—
Hippocampal area/volume	($\downarrow$)
Parahippocampal area/volume	($\downarrow$)
Parahippocampal cortical thickness	$\downarrow$
Amygdala area/volume	—
Sylvian fissure length, planum temporal volume	$\downarrow$
Sulcogyral pattern	(Abnormal)
Frontal, parietal, and occipital lobes	
Cingulate cortical thickness	—
Insula area/volume	—
Corpus callosum thickness	($\uparrow$)
Internal capsule area/volume	—
Basal ganglia	
Globus pallidum area/volume	($\downarrow$)
Nucleus accumbens area/volume	$\downarrow$
Caudate–putamen area/volume	$\uparrow$
Thalamus	
Mediodorsal nucleus area/volume	$\downarrow$
Whole and various nuclei area/volume	—
Cerebellum	
Anterior vermis area	$\downarrow$
Brainstem	
Substantia nigra volume	$\downarrow$
Locus coeruleus volume	—
Periventricular grey volume	$\downarrow$

In comparison with controls: $\downarrow$, reduced; $\uparrow$, increased; —, no difference; ( ), finding not or only partially replicated.
Adapted from Arnold and Trojanowski.[20]

Schizophrenia and other psychotic disorders

Studies between 1898 and 1975

Subsequently to Alzheimer, Southard reported cortical atrophy in schizophrenia and mentioned that association areas of the cerebral cortex were most affected in this disorder.[10] Buscaino[11] described various histopathological changes, mainly in the basal ganglia, which he assumed to be responsible for catatonia-like and stereotyped behaviour. Another approach to the neuropathology of psychiatric diseases had been made by Vogt and Vogt and their coworkers, who reported cellular alterations in the cortex, thalamus, and basal ganglia of schizophrenics.[12–19] These considerable efforts on the part of many well-known neuroanatomists and neuropathologists to prove that

Table 2 Neuronal morphometric findings in schizophrenia

Region/parameter	Finding
Temporal lobe	
Superior temporal gyrus (Tpt) neurone density	↓
Hippocampal neurone density	(↓)
Hippocampal neurone size	(↓)
Entorhinal cortex neurone density	(↓)
Entorhinal cortex neurone size	↓
Amygdala neurone density (basolateral n.)	—
Frontal lobe	
Prefrontal cortex pyramidal neurone density	(↑)
Prefrontal cortex interneurone density	(↓)
Prefrontal cortex neurone size	↓
Cingulate (anterior) pyramidal neurone density	↓
Cingulate interneurone density	↓
Cingulate neurone size	↓
Motor cortex neurone density	(↓)
Motor cortex neurone size	—
Basal ganglia and basal forebrain	
Globus pallidus neurone counts	—
Nucleus accumbens neurone counts	↓
Nucleus basalis of Meynert neurone counts	—
Thalamus	
Mediodorsal nucleus neurone counts	(↓)
Cerebellum	
Purkinje cell density	↓
Brainstem	
Substantia nigra neurone density	↓
Substantia nigra neurone size	↓
Locus coeruleus neurone density	—
Locus coeruleus neurone size	↓
Pedunculopontine nucleus neurone density	(↑)

In comparison with controls: ↓, reduced; ↑, increased; —, no difference; ( ), finding not or only partially replicated.
Adapted from Arnold and Trojanowski.[20]

schizophrenia is a primary brain disorder, ended in inconsistent and unsubstantiated findings.[4,5] To a large extent these inconsistencies can be attributed to a variety of methodological inadequacies including diagnostic uncertainties, inadequate control samples, flawed tissue-handling procedures, variable choice of brain regions for neuropathological studies, limitations in the sensitivity and specificity of classical histological stains, as well as lack of quantitative methods to delineate and analyse subtle brain abnormalities.[20]

Neuropathological findings in schizophrenia since 1975

Advances in the last 40 years have produced more reliable psychiatric diagnostic criteria, improved structural and functional neuroimaging techniques, a large array of highly sensitive and specific molecular probes and labelling procedures, suitable for use in neuropathological studies, and computer-assisted image analysis methodologies. For these and other reasons, there has been a resurgence of interest in the neurobiological substrates of schizophrenia, and contemporary neuropathological studies have enumerated many findings in the brains of patients with schizophrenia (for reviews see Bogerts and Lieberman,[21] Falkai and Bogerts,[22] Arnold and Trojanowski,[20] Roberts et al.,[23] and Harrison[24]). In addition during this period there has been extensive neurochemical and neuroreceptor research and this aspect of postmortem schizophrenia research has been the subject of several recent reviews.[23,25,26]

Diagnostic neuropathology

Stevens[27] surveyed the brains of 28 schizophrenic patients for gross and microscopic abnormalities using standard diagnostic stains, and found no abnormalities in temporal (including the amygdalohippocampal region), frontal, or parietal lobes or in the thalamus, but did find assorted abnormalites in other regions, including neuronal loss or infarction in the globus pallidus in five patients, increased cerebellar white matter gliosis in five patients, excessive Purkinje cell loss in 13, and, most notably, increased fibrillary gliosis in periventricular, periaqueductal, and basal forebrain regions bilaterally.

In another prospectively accrued series, Bruton et al.[28] found that five of 56 schizophrenics had other distinct neurological illnesses (multiple sclerosis, Friedreich's ataxia, epilepsy, stroke) and three had had prefrontal leukotomies as treatment for their schizophrenia. Of the remaining 48, there were no differences between schizophrenics and controls in the frequency of large- or small-vessel cerebrovascular disease, senile plaques, or neurofibrillary degeneration. However, there was an 'increased incidence of unexpected pathology in the schizophrenic group compared with the control group'. Of these 48 schizophrenics, 21 had some degree of focal pathology compared with 12 of 56 controls, but these abnormalites were diverse in nature and location. Holzer staining suggested a significant increase in fibrous gliosis in the cortex, white matter, and periventricular structures, but this was generally in the brains in which the other focal pathology was found. When these cases were removed, the 'purified' group showed no evidence of increased gliosis.

In a series of 101 elderly schizophrenics, Golier et al.[29] found only 10 with definite or probable Alzheimer's disease by modern neuropathological diagnostic criteria, 29 with senile plaques, 15 with vascular lesions, two with Parkinson's disease, three with unspecified tumour, and five with 'other' findings.

In summary, diagnostic neuropathological investigations find only assorted and non-specific abnormalities in the brains of schizophrenics that are likely to be representative of lesions found in age-compatible control groups.

Morphometric studies

Macroscopic findings (Table 1)

Several planimetric postmortem studies of the whole cortex have been performed, some reporting significant reduction of cortical volume (12 per cent) and central grey matter (6 per cent) and others reporting no difference in volumes of cortex, white matter and whole hemispheres between schizophrenics and controls. Other general brain parameters measured have shown reduced brain length, brain weight, and increased ventricular area/volume.

Since the first report of reduced tissue volume in temporolimbic structures of schizophrenics,[30] numerous quantitative or qualitative

Table 3 Morphometric postmortem studies in affective disorders

Study	Number of patients/ controls	Region/parameter	Finding
General			
Jellinger[43]	4/15	Entire brain	Caudate lesions
Temporal lobe			
Altshuler et al.[45]	12/27	Hippocampal area	—
		Parahippocampal area	↓
Beckmann and Jakob[47]	4/0	Cytoarchitecture of entorhinal cortex	Disturbed
		Rostroventral insula nerve cell number	↓
Casanova et al[48]	5/10	Entorhinal cortex neuronal numbers	↓
Other cortical and subcortical regions			
Brown et al.[44]	70/32	Lobar structures	—
		Callosal thickness	—
		Corpus striatum	—
		Brain weight	↑
		Lateral ventricles	↓
Diekmann et al.[49]	12/12	Cingulate cortex (interneurones in layer II)	↓
Baumann et al.[46]	8/8	Accumbens, putamen, caudate, external pallidal volumes	↓
Cerebellum			
Lohr and Jeste[50]	12/23	Cerebellum: Purkinje cells in anterior and posterior vermis and hemispheres	—
Brainstem			
Hankoff and Peress[51]	4/26	Brainstem	—
Baumann et al.[46]	12/12	Locus coeruleus neuronal number	↑
Peripheral nervous system			
Ross-Stanton and Meltzer[52]		Motor neurone branching (peripheral)	↑

In comparison with controls: ↓, reduced; ↑, increased; —, no difference; ( ), finding not or only partially replicated.

anatomical postmortem studies on limbic structures of schizophrenics were published. Of these studies the majority found subtle structural changes (15–20 per cent mean volume reduction) in at least one of the investigated areas, whereas only a few yielded entirely negative results. The findings comprise reduced volumes or cross-sectional areas of the hippocampus, amygdala, parahippocampal gyrus, which were later corroborated by morphometric magnetic resonance imaging (**MRI**) studies. Figure 1 demonstrates the subtle bilateral volume reduction of the hippocampus in schizophrenics and furthermore visualizes the kind of hypoplastic appearance of the anterior hippocampus, which can be seen in about a third of the patients (lower row of the photographs). Other findings in limbic brain regions are left temporal horn enlargement, white-matter reductions in parahippocampal gyrus or hippocampus, and an increased incidence of a cavum septi pellucidi.

Unchanged volumes of the striatum and external pallidum but a subtle volume decrease in the internal pallidal segment were found in brains from the preneuroleptic era. Pallidal volume reduction was due to a reduction in the catatonic subgroup. These initial findings have to

be pursued, as longitudinal MRI studies suggest that enlargement of basal ganglia can be seen in schizophrenia as a consequence of treatment with classical neuroleptics, which can be reversed by the use of atypical substances.

After initially finding no volumetric changes in the thalamic nuclei, subsequently the area/volume of the mediodorsal nucleus and anteroventral thalamic nucleus were found to be decreased.

Changes in area measurements of the corpus callosum were described in some studies. The findings, however, are inconsistent; there are reports of increased as well as of decreased midline areas. More consistent are reports of shape abnormalities, in that the sex difference in anterior and posterior callosal thickness in normal controls seems to be reversed in schizophrenics and the mean curvature in the corpus callosum is bent upwards.

Findings of decreased volume of the substantia nigra and the periventricular grey matter as well as no volumteric change in the locus coeruleus await replication.

In summary, macroscopic morphometric postmortem studies

Table 4 Morphometric postmortem studies in alcoholism

Region/parameter	Finding
General	
Brain weight	↓
Intracranial volume	↓
Ventricular volume	↑
White > grey matter volume	↓
Temporal lobe	
Hippocampal neuronal numbers	(↓)
Amygdala neuronal numbers	↓
Frontal, parietal, and occipital lobes	
Superior frontal cortex, neuronal numbers (BA 8)	↓
Primary motor cortex, neuronal numbers (BA 4)	—
Frontal cingulate cortex, neuronal numbers (BA 32)	—
Inferior temporal cortex, neuronal numbers (BA 20 + 36)	—
Superior frontal cortex, GABAergic pyramidal neurones	—
Thalamus	
Medial dorsal and anterior nuclei of the thalamus, volumes	(↓)
Supraoptic and paraventricular nuclei of the hypothalamus, neuronal numbers	↓
Arginine–vasopressin immunoreactive neurones	↓
Basal ganglia	
Caudate, putamen, or globus pallidus volumes	—
Cerebellum	
Cerebellar volume in general	↓
Vermal, intermediate, and lateral zone volumes	↓
Purkinje cell densities	↓
Brainstem	
Locus coeruleus noradrenergic, neuronal numbers	(↓)
Median and dorsal raphe nuclei, neuronal numbers	—
Other brain structures	
Basal nucleus, neuronal numbers	—

In comparison with controls: ↓, reduced; ↑, increased; —, no difference; ( ), finding not or only partially replicated.

demonstrate increased ventricular size and volume/area reduction of temporolimbic areas in schizophrenia. Findings on other regions such as the basal ganglia, thalamus, cerebellum, and brainstem await replication.

Microscopic findings (Table 2)

There are a number of studies of neurone number, density, and size in schizophrenia. As summarized in Table 2, the majority of these have focused on the ventromedial temporal, and frontal lobes.

In the lateral prefrontal cortex an increase in neurone density, which may relate to the observed decrease in neurone size (with decreased dendritic arborization and a decreased neuropil compartment) has been reported inconsistently. In the anterior cingulate, decreased pyramidal and local circuit neurone density accompanied by increased vertical axon density and altered dopaminergic innerv-

ation were observed. These findings have been interpreted as representing disturbed connections in the anterior cingulate.

Within the ventromedial temporal lobe reduced cell numbers or cell size and abnormal cell arrangements in the hippocampus or entorhinal cortex were described. However, some groups could not confirm cellular disarray in the hippocampus[31] and could not find significant volume and cell number reductions in the hippocampus and entorhinal cortex.[32]

Original studies demonstrating decreased neurone counts in the mediodorsal and anteriorventral nucleus of the thalamus have been supported by subsequent investigation.

The lateral (nigrostriatal) and medial (mesolimbic) parts of the mesencephalic dopaminergic systems have been evaluated and the size of the nerve cell bodies found to be significantly reduced in the medial part by 16 per cent, while the cell numbers were unchanged. The reduced cell size of the medial, mesolimbic neurones were taken to indicate dopaminergic underactivity. Two qualitative reports on degenerative changes in cholinergic cells in the basal nucleus of Meynert of schizophrenics have been published; more recent quantitative studies found normal cell numbers in the basal nucleus of schizophrenics. Volume measurements and cell counts in the noradrenergic locus coeruleus revealed a trend for decreased locus coeruleus volume without loss of neurones indicating a reduction of neuropil in the schizophrenics. These results appear comparable to those described in the substantia nigra, as mentioned above. Investigating the brainstem reticular formation, a twofold increased number of the cholinergic neurones of the pedunculopontine nucleus and the dorsal tegmental nucleus as well as a reduced cell size in the locus coeruleus were found.

In summary, morphometric microscopic studies in schizophrenia frequently find alterations in neurone density, size, shape, and positioning mainly in temporolimbic and frontal regions. Findings in other regions require replication, especially taking the small study samples into account.

Schizophrenia as a disorder of brain maturation

There is evidence from clinical research implicating aberrant neurodevelopmental processes in the pathophysiology of schizophrenia,[33] but there is also a growing literature suggestive of progressive deterioration in the disease for at least some patients.[34] It should be noted that abnormal neurodevelopmental processes are not mutually exclusive of neurodegenerative mechanisms in the pathogenesis of complex neuropsychiatric disorders. Indeed, while some genetic disorders are purely developmental (e.g. fragile X syndrome) and others purely neurodegenerative (e.g. Huntington's disease), some have both developmental and degenerative pathologies (e.g. Down syndrome). Based on the neuropathological literature of the last 30 years some suggestions can be made concerning the pathophysiology of schizophrenia.

Gliosis

Glial cells, mainly astrocytes (Figs 2 and 3), show changes in response to almost every type of injury or disease in the central nervous system. Therefore in typical degenerative brain disorders such as Alzheimer's disease or Huntington's chorea increased glial cell densities are found. Studies using glial cell counts, neurone-to-glial ratios and glial cell nuclear volumes found no difference between schizophrenics and controls in temporolimbic structures, the thalamus, and cingulate cortex.

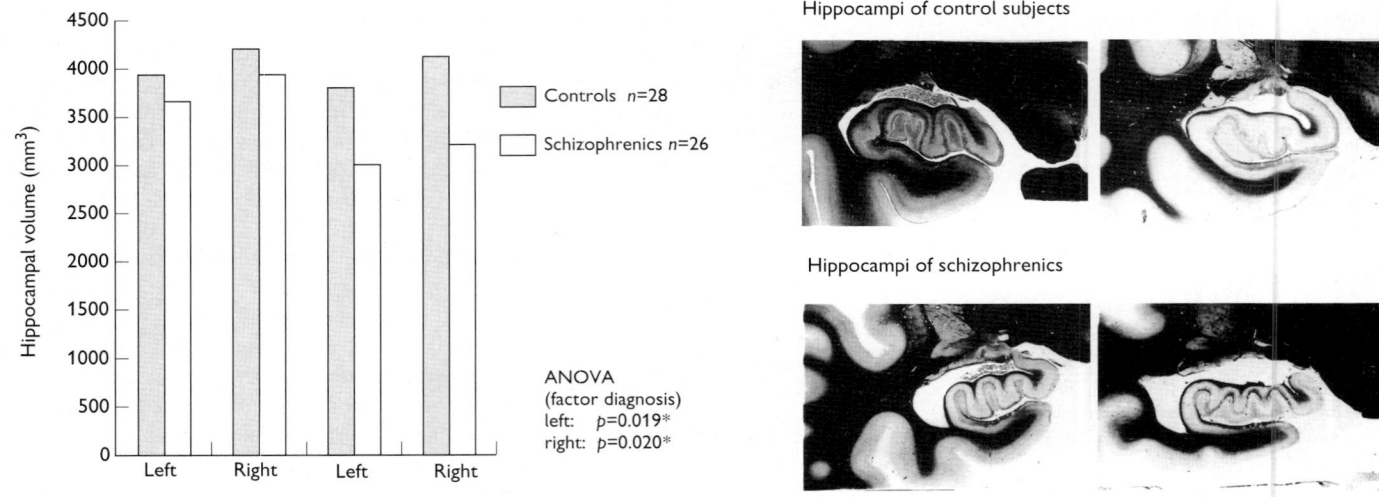

Fig. 1 Hippocampal volumes (left) and representative photographs at the level of the mamillary body (right) in schizophrenics and controls.

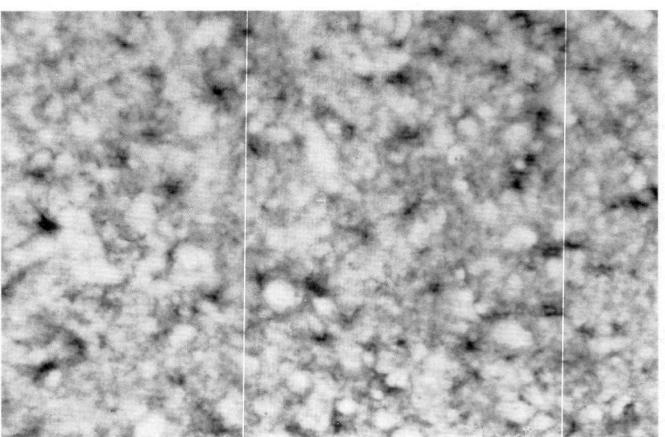

Fig. 2 Glial fibrillary acidic protein (GFAP) positive astrocytes in the human cortex.

In our own large-scale study we counted the number of astrocytes in several key regions such as the area surrounding the temporal horn and found no evidence for astrogliosis in schizophrenia (Fig. 3).[35] Although the question of fibrous gliosis (i.e. increase in glial cell fibres) remains more controversial, the well-controlled study by Bruton *et*

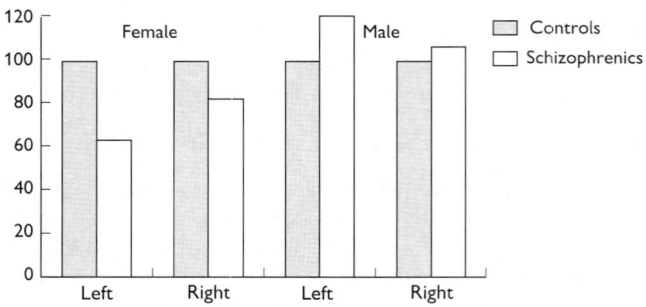

p-values from ANOVA (diagnosis by sex): *p*=0.40 (left), *p*=0.59 (right)

Fig. 3 Astrocyte counts (cells per field of vision) around the temporal horns.

al.[28] also rejects fibrous gliosis in schizophrenia. Therefore it seems unlikely that the majority of schizophrenic patients show a considerable degree of gliosis.

Neurohistological indications of disturbed brain development

Subtle cytoarchitectural anomalies were described in the hippocampal formation, frontal cortex, cingulate gyrus, and entorhinal cortex in patients suffering from schizophrenia compared with control subjects. For example, a significant cellular disarray in the CA3–CA4 interface was described in the left and replicated in the right hippocampus.[36] This was interpreted as a bilateral migrational abnormality and broadly correlated with the degree of disease severity. One subsequent study was not able to fully replicate this findings, but did confirm a within-case correlation with severity; whereas another examination did not find any significant disarray distinguishing schizophrenics from controls. Another prominent finding was of an abnormal sulco-gyral pattern or abnormal gross configuration of the temporal lobe and cytoarchitectonic abnormalities of the rostral entorhinal region as well as of the ventral insular cortex of schizophrenics.[37,38] The cytoarchitectonic abnormalities of the rostral entorhinal region consisted of heterotopic pre-α-cells in the pre-β-layer (layer III), which would normally belong to the pre-α-layer (layer II). This observation stimulated considerable research, with some studies supporting these findings, while others did not.

In conclusion, cytoarchitectonic abnormalities recently described in different limbic structures in schizophrenia are very subtle and can easily be missed using classical neuropathological methods. Quantifying them often needs sophisticated staining methods, for example immunohistochemistry, serial sections and a matched control group and even than replicating original findings seems difficult, as outlined above. These findings can be interpreted as a sign for disturbed late neuronal migration or could mirror disturbed programmed cell death as heterotopias are frequently found in the temporal cortex of autopsied children, which seem to dissapear in adults.

Investigations of connectivity

There is some evidence from postmortem studies for disturbed cerebral asymmetry in schizophrenia, for example the planum temporale (for overview see Falkai and Bogerts[22]). Changes in the asymmetry pattern of the human brain in closely linked to connectivity. Recently, quantitative studies of axons, dendrites, synapses and synapse-related proteins, and mRNAs have begun to explore the hypothesis of disturbed connectivity in schizophrenia. Although the results reported to date have been somewhat inconsistent, the preliminary data look promising. Benes et al.[39] have focused on the anterior cingulate cortex describing decreased neurone density and abnormally spaced aggregates of neurones in this region. Subsequently they found decreased density of interneurones[40] and increased numbers of vertical axons (glutamatergic in origin) in cortical layers in which the altered cytoarchitecture had been found.[41] Together these findings have been interpreted as representing a miswiring of the anterior cingulate. More specific investigations of connectivity are at an early stage but describe abnormal dendritic spine densities in the cortex, various changes in synaptic vesicle protein expression in limbic, temporal, and frontal cortices, and alterations in glutamatergic, catecholaminergic, and intrinsic innervation in anterior cingulate cortex. These findings suggest a 'miswiring' in the brain of schizophrenic patients.

In summary there is growing evidence for pathomorphological abnormalities in the postmortem brains from patients suffering from schizophrenia. The changes are focused on the frontal lobe and temporolimbic regions. They are subtle, lacking the typical signs of degeneration, and point to problems in prenatal (cell migration) and postnatal (connectivity) periods of brain development. Currently, underlying causes are unclear, but the interaction between genetic and non-genetic factors (e.g. birth complications) has to be discussed.

Mood disorders (Table 3)

The number of published pathoanatomical studies in schizophrenia contrasts sharply with the scant number of neuropathological examinations in affective disorders. In reviewing the world literature of the last 60 years, Jeste et al.[42] found 15 neuropathological studies on affective disorders. Seven of them were published between 1949 and 1969, had fewer than four cases, and utilized qualitative tissue evaluation. Using Medline Research between 1970 and 1999 we found 11 morphometric postmortem studies, where patients with affective disorders were included (Table 3). However, they were usually included as control cases searching for abnormalities in schizophrenic brains.

Macroscopic findings

Four studies examined macroscopic measures such as the gross brain morphology,[43] brain weight and ventricular volume,[44] and the area or volume of specific regions such as the hippocampus, parahippocampal gyrus,[45] striatum, globus pallidus, and corpus callosum.[44,46] In comparison to schizophrenic patients and/or non-psychiatric control subjects, patients with affective disorders revealed caudate lesions,[43] reduced area of the right parahippocampal gyrus,[45] increased brain and reduced ventricular volume.[44]

Microscopic findings

Seven studies examined the cytoarchitecture and nerve cell or interneuronal numbers of the entorhinal and insular cortex,[47,48] cingulate,[49] cerebellum,[50] and brainstem[46,51] and in the peripheral nervous system.[52] Findings in patients with affective disorders

included overall reduced neuronal numbers, together with disturbed cytoarchitecture of entorhinal cortex, reduced neuronal numbers in the rostroventral insula, reduced Purkinje cells in anterior and posterior vermis and hemispheres of the cerebellum, reduced interneuronal numbers in layer II of the cingulate, but increased neuronal numbers of the locus coeruleus and peripheral motor neurone branching.

Summary and pathophysiological conclusions

In summary, the number of postmortem studies on mood disorders is still very limited, but there is some evidence for changes in the basal ganglia and brainstem. Structural brain imaging studies support the notion that mood disorders are associated with regional structural brain abnormalities, in particular regions involved in mood regulation, such as the limbic portion of the basal ganglia and brainstem structures. Because small numbers of subjects were studied, only some postmortem studies distinguished between unipolar and bipolar depression.[46] Nevertheless, a recent review of the structural imaging studies[53] found this distinction worthwhile. The main abnormalities found in unipolar depression were smaller basal ganglia, cerebellum, and possibly frontal lobe, which may reflect local atrophy. Bipolar disorder appeared to be associated with larger third ventricle, smaller cerebellum, possibly smaller temporal lobe, and perhaps changes in the hippocampus. In both groups there seems to be an increased rate of subcortical white-matter lesions and periventricular hyperintensities. Further studies are needed, combining endocrine/biochemical parameters with structural parameters,[54] to identify the key regions involved in processes central to mood disorders such as changes in the regulation of the hypothalamic–pituitary–adrenal axis.[55] This would allow a focus on these regions in future postmortem-studies, which should yield promising results.

Alcoholism (Table 4)

The best known neuropathological feature of alcoholism is Wernicke's encephalopathy, which is characterized by degenerative changes including gliosis and small hemorrhages in structures surrounding the third ventricle and aqueduct (i.e. the mamillary bodies, hypothalamus, mediodorsal thalamic nucleus, colliculi, and midbrain tegmentum), as well as cerebellar atrophy. Most of the clinical features associated with the Wernicke–Korsakoff syndrome including ophthalmoplegia, nystagmus, ataxia, and mental symptoms such as confusion, disorientation, and even coma can be related to damaged functional systems in the hypothalamus, midbrain, and cerebellum.[56] Other important neuropathological manifestations of chronic alcoholism are central pontine myelinolysis, Marchiafava syndrome, and fetal alcohol syndrome (see Chapter 4.2.2.3).

Studies on alcohol-specific brain damage

Most of the changes mentioned above occur in association with thiamin deficiency, which is frequently, but not always, correlated with the long-term use of excessive amounts of alcohol. One major challenge is to identify those lesions caused by alcohol itself (uncomplicated alcoholism[57]) and those caused by other common alcohol-related factors, principally thiamin deficiency. The following summarizes recent results in this field, which has been reviewed in detail by others.[57,58]

Brain shrinkage can be found in uncomplicated alcoholism, which can largely be accounted for by loss of white matter. Some of this damage appears to be reversible. However, alcohol-related neuronal loss has been documented in specific regions of the cerebral cortex (superior frontal association cortex), hypothalamus (supraoptic and para-ventricular nuclei), and cerebellum. The data are conflicting for the hippocampus, amygdala, and locus coeruleus. No changes are found in the basal ganglia, nucleus basalis, or serotonergic raphe nuclei. As pointed out above, many of the regions that are normal in uncompli-cated alcoholics are damaged in those with Wernicke–Korsakoff syn-drome. Dendritic and synaptic changes have been documented in uncomplicated alcoholics, and these, together with receptor and trans-mitter changes, may explain functional changes and cognitive deficits that precede the more severe structural neuronal changes.

Summary and pathophysiological considerations

In summary, there is neuropathological evidence showing that alcohol *per se* causes damage to both grey and white matter. White-matter damage is predominant and results in a reduction in brain volume. A component of the white-matter loss appears to be reversible in some cases, given a significant period of abstinence. The grey-matter dam-age appears to be regionally selective, but many areas of the brain appear to be resistant to damage.

Thiamin deficiency accounts for a major component of the brain damage in alcoholics. Animal models suggest that the distribution and extent of neuronal loss seems to depend on the duration of alcohol exposure, the magnitude and mode of exposure (ingestion, inhalation, etc.), the genetic susceptibility of the species, and the strain of animals studied.[57] It has been suggested that alcohol withdrawal may play a role in brain damage, evidenced by the fact that a number of workers have shown loss of granule cells in the dentate gyrus of the hippo-campus continues even after alcohol exposure stops.[59] It was further-more suggested that up-regulation of N-methyl-D-aspartate receptors may lead to withdrawal seizures and enhanced susceptibility to excito-toxicity, which may explain the continuing damage described.[60]

Further reading

Arnold, S.E. and Trojanowski, J.Q. (1996). Recent advances in defining the neuropathology of schizophrenia. *Acta Neuropathologica* 92, 217–31.

Bogerts, B. and Lieberman, J. (1993). Neuropathology in the study of psychiatric disease. In *International review of psychiatry*, Vol. 1 (ed. N.C. Andreasen and M. Sato), pp. 515–55. American Psychiatric Press, Washington, DC.

David, G.B. (1957). The pathological anatomy of the schizophrenias. In *Schizophrenia: somatic aspects* (ed. D. Richter), pp. 93–130. Pergamon Press, Oxford.

Falkai, P. and Bogerts, B. (1995). The neuropathology of schizophrenia. In *Schizophrenia* (ed. S.R. Hirsch and D.R. Weinberger), pp. 275–93. Blackwell Science, Oxford.

Harper, C.G. (1998). The neuropathology of alcohol-specific brain damage, or does alcohol damage the brain? *Journal of Neuropathology and Experimental Neurology*, 57, 101–10.

Harper, C.G. and Kril, J.J. (1990). Neuropathology of alcoholism. *Alcohol and Alcoholism*, 25, 207–16.

Harrison, P.J. (1999). The neuropathology of schizophrenia. A critical review of the data and their interpretation. *Brain*, 122, 593–624.

Jellinger, K.A. and Bancher, C. (1998). Neuropathology of Alzheimer's disease: a critical update. *Journal of Neural Transmission Supplementum*, 54, 77–95.

Jeste, D.V., Lohr, J.B., and Goodwin, F.K. (1988). Neuroanatomical studies of major affective disorders. A review and suggestions for further research. *British Journal of Psychiatry*, 153, 444–59.

Ohuoha, D.C., Hyde, T.M., and Kleinman, J.E. (1993). The role of serotonin in schizophrenia: an overview of the nomenclature, distribution and alterations of serotonin receptors in the central nervous system. *Psychopharmacology*, 112 (Supplement 1), S5–15.

Peters, G. (1967). Die symptomatischen Schizophrenien. In *Psychiatrie der Gegenwart*, Vol. I (ed. H.W. Gruhle, R. Jung, W. Mayer-Gross, and M. Müller), pp. 298–305. Springer-Verlag, Berlin.

Price, D.L., Tanzi, R.E., Borchelt, D.R., and Sisodia, S.S. (1998). Alzheimer's disease: genetic studies and transgenic models. *Annual Review of Genetics* 32, 461–93.

Roberts, G.W., Royston, M.C., and Weinberger, D.R. (1997). Schizophrenia. In *Greenfield's neuropathology* (6th edn) (ed. D.I. Graham and P.L. Lantos), pp. 897–931. Arnold, London.

Rosenblum, W.I. (1999). The presence, origin, and significance of A beta peptide in the cell bodies of neurons. *Journal of Neuropathology and Experimental Neurology*, 58, 575–81.

Shapiro, R.M. (1993). Regional neuropathology in schizophrenia: where are we? Where are we going? *Schizophrenia Research*, 10, 187–239.

Soares, J.C. and Mann, J.J. (1997). The anatomy of mood disorders—review of structural neuroimaging studies. *Biological Psychiatry*, 41, 86–106.

Weinberger, D.R. (1996). On the plausibility of 'the neurodevelopmental hypothesis' of schizophrenia. *Neuropsychopharmacology*, 14, 1S–11S.

Woods, B.T., Yurgelun-Todd, D., Goldstein, J.M., Seidman, L.J., and Tsuang, M.T. (1996). MRI brain abnormalities in chronic schizophrenia: one process or more? *Biological Psychiatry*, 40, 585–96.

References

1. Broca, P. (1865). Sur la faculté du langage articulé. *Bulletins de la Societé d'Anthropologie*, 6, 377–93.

2. Cajal, S.R. (1911). *Histologie du systeme nerveux de l'homme de des vertebres*, Vol. II. Instituto Ramon y Cajal, Madrid.

3. Alzheimer, A. (1898). Beiträge zur pathologischen Anatomie der Hirnrinde und zur anatomischen Grundlage der Psychosen. *Monatsschrift Psychiatrie und Neurologie*, 2, 82–120.

4. David, G.B. (1957). The pathological anatomy of the schizophrenias. In *Schizophrenia: somatic aspects* (ed. D. Richter), pp. 93–130. Pergamon Press, Oxford.

5. Peters, G. (1967). Die symptomatischen Schizophrenien. In *Psychiatrie der Gegenwart*, Vol. I. (ed. H.W. Gruhle, R. Jung, W. Mayer-Gross, and M. Müller), pp. 298–305. Springer-Verlag, Berlin.

6. Johnstone, E.C., Crow, T.J., Frith, C.D., Husband, J., and Kreel, L. (1976). Cerebral ventricular size and cognitive impairment in chronic schizophrenia. *Lancet*, ii, 924–6.

7. Jellinger, K.A. and Bancher, C. (1998). Neuropathology of Alzheimer's disease: a critical update. *Journal of Neural Transmisson Supplementum*, 54, 77–95.

8. Rosenblum, W.I. (1999). The presence, origin, and significance of A beta peptide in the cell bodies of neurons. *Journal of Neuropathology and Experimental Neurology*, 58, 575–81.

9. Price, D.L., Tanzi, R.E., Borchelt, D.R., and Sisodia, S.S. (1998). Alzheimer's disease: genetic studies and transgenic models. *Annual Review of Genetics*, 32, 461–93.

10. Southard, E.E. (1915). On the topographic distribution of cortex lesions and anomalies in dementia praecox with some account of their functional significance. *American Journal of Insanity*, 71, 603–71.

11. Buscaino, V.M. (1920). Le cause anatoma-pathologiche della manifestatione schizophrenica della demenza precoce. *Rivista di Patologia Nervosa e Mentale*, **25**, 197–226.

12. Fünfgeld, E. (1925). Pathologisch-anatomische Untersuchungen bei Dementia praecox mit besonderer Berücksichtigung des Thalamus opticus. *Zeitschrift der Gesellschaft für Neurologie und Psychiatrie*, **95**, 411–63.

13. Fünfgeld, E.W. (1952). Der Nucleus anterior thalami bei Schizophrenie. *Journal für Hirnforschung*, **1**, 147–55.

14. Vogt, C. and Vogt, O. (1948). Über anatomische Substrate. Bemerkungen zu pathoanatomischen Befunden bei Schizophrenie. *Ärztliche Forschritte*, **3**, 1–7.

15. Vogt, C. and Vogt, O. (1952). Resultats de l'etude anatomique de la schizophrenie et d'autres psychoses dites fontionelles faite a l'institut du cerveau de Neustadt, Schwarzwald. In *First International Congress of Neuropathology*, Vol. 1, pp. 515–32. Rosenberg and Sellier, Turin.

16. Bäumer, H. (1954). Veränderungen des Thalamus bei Schizophrenie. *Journal für Hirnforschung*, **1**, 157–72.

17. Hopf, A. (1954). Orientierende Untersuchung zur Fraged pathoanatomischer Veränderungen intramuscular Pallidum und Striatum bei Schizophrenie. *Journal für Hirnforschung*, **1**, 97–145.

18. Buttlar-Brentano, K. (1956). Zur weiteren Kenntnis der Veränderungen des Basalkerns bei Schizophrenen. *Journal für Hirnforschung*, **2**, 271–91.

19. Treff, W.M. and Hempel, K.J. (1958). Die Zelldichte bei Schizophrenen und klinisch Gesunden. *Journal für Hirnforschung*, **4**, 314–69.

20. Arnold, S.E. and Trojanowski, J.Q. (1996). Recent advances in defining the neuropathology of schizophrenia. *Acta Neuropathologica*, **92**, 217–31.

21. Bogerts, B. and Lieberman, J. (1993). Neuropathology in the study of psychiatric disease. In *International review of psychiatry*, Vol. 1 (ed. N.C. Andreasen and M. Sato), pp. 515–55. American Psychiatric Press, Washington, DC.

22. Falkai, P. and Bogerts, B. (1995). The neuropathology of schizophrenia. In *Schizophrenia* (ed. S.R. Hirsch and D.R. Weinberger), pp. 275–93. Blackwell Science, Oxford.

23. Roberts, G.W., Royston, M.C., and Weinberger, D.R. (1997). Schizophrenia. In *Greenfield's neuropathology* (6th edn) (ed. D.I. Graham and P.L. Lantos), pp. 897–931. Arnold, London.

24. Harrison, P. J. (1999). The neuropathology of schizophrenia. A critical review of the data and their interpretation. *Brain*, **122**, 593–624.

25. Ohuoha, D.C., Hyde, T.M., and Kleinman, J.E. (1993). The role of serotonin in schizophrenia: an overview of the nomenclature, distribution and alterations of serotonin receptors in the central nervous system. *Psychopharmacology*, **112** (Supplement 1), S5–15.

26. Shapiro, R.M. (1993). Regional neuropathology in schizophrenia: where are we? Where are we going? *Schizophrenia Research*, **10**, 187–239.

27. Stevens, J.R. (1982). Neuropathology of schizophrenia. *Archives of General Psychiatry*, **39**, 1131–9.

28. Bruton, C.J., Crow, T.J., Frith, C.D., Johnstone, E.C., Owens, D.G.C., and Roberts, G.W. (1990). Schizophrenia and the brain: a prospective clinico-neuropathological study. *Psychological Medicine*, **20**, 285–304.

29. Golier, J.A., Davidson, M., Haroutunian, V., *et al.* (1995). Neuropathological study of 101 elderly schizophrenics: preliminary findings. *Schizophrenia Research*, **15**, 120.

30. Bogerts, B., Meertz, E., and Schönfeldt-Bausch, R. (1983). Limbic system pathology in schizophrenia: a controlled post mortem study. *7th World Congress of Psychiatry*, Vienna, 1983, Vortrag, Abstract F6.

31. Christison, G.W., Casanova, M.F., Weinberger, D.R., Rawlings, R., and Kleinman, J.E. (1989). A quantitative investigation of hippocampal pyramidal cell size, shape and variability of orientation in schizophrenia. *Archives of General Psychiatry*, **46**, 1027–32.

32. Heckers, S., Heinsen, H., Heinsen, Y.C., and Beckmann, H. (1990). Limbic structures and lateral ventricle in schizophrenia. *Archives of General Psychiatry*, **47**, 1016–22.

33. Weinberger, D.R. (1996). On the plausibility of 'the neurodevelopmental hypothesis' of schizophrenia. *Neuropsychopharmacology*, **14**, 1S–11S.

34. Woods, B.T., Yurgelun-Todd, D., Goldstein, J.M., Seidman, L.J., and Tsuang, M.T. (1996). MRI brain abnormalities in chronic schizophrenia: one process or more? *Biological Psychiatry*, **40**, 585–96.

35. Falkai, P., Honer, W.G., David, S., Bogerts, B., Majtenyi, C., and Bayer, T.A. (1999). No evidence for astrogliosis in brains of schizophrenic patients. A post-mortem study. *Neuropathology and Applied Neurobiology*, **25**, 48–53.

36. Kovelman, J.A. and Scheibel, A.B. (1984). A neurohistological correlate of schizophrenia. *Biological Psychiatry*, **19**, 1601–21.

37. Jakob, J. and Beckmann, H. (1986). Prenatal developmental disturbances in the limbic allocortex in schizophrenics. *Journal of Neural Transmission*, **65**, 303–26.

38. Jakob, H. and Beckmann, H. (1989). Gross and histological criteria for developmental disorders in brains of schizophrenics. *Journal of the Royal Society of Medicine*, **82**, 466–9.

39. Benes, F.M., Davidson, B., and Bird, E.D. (1986). Quantitative cytoarchitectural studies of the cerebral cortex of schizophrenics. *Archives of General Psychiatry*, **43**, 31–5.

40. Benes, F.M., McSparren, J., Bird, E.D., San Giovanni, J.P., and Vincent, S.L. (1991). Deficits in small interneurons in prefrontal and cingulate cortices of schizophrenic and schizoaffective patients. *Archives of General Psychiatry*, **48**, 996–1001.

41. Benes, F.M., Sorensen, I., Vincent, S.L., Alsterberg, G., Bird, E.D., and SanGiovanni, J.P. (1992). Increased GABAa receptor binding in superficial layers of cingulate cortex in schizophrenics. *Journal of Neuroscience*, **12**, 924–9.

42. Jeste, D.V., Lohr, J.B., and Goodwin, F.K. (1988). Neuroanatomical studies of major affective disorders. A review and suggestions for further research. *British Journal of Psychiatry*, **153**, 444–59.

43. Jellinger, K.A. (1977). Neuropathologic findings after neuroleptic long term therapy. In *Neurotoxicology* (ed. L. Roizin, H. Shiraki, and N. Grcevic), pp. 25–42. Raven Press, New York.

44. Brown, R., Colter, N., Corsellis, J.A.N., *et al.* (1986). Postmortem evidence of structural brain changes in schizophrenia. Differences in brain weight, temporal horn area and parahippocampal gyrus compared with affective disorder. *Archives of General Psychiatry*, **43**, 36–42.

45. Altshuler, L.L., Casanova, M.F., Goldberg, T.E., and Kleinman, J.E. (1990). The hippocampus and parahippocampus in schizophrenic, suicide, and control brains. *Archives of General Psychiatry*, **47**, 1029–34.

46. Baumann, B., Danos, P., Krell, D., *et al.* (1999). Unipolar–bipolar dichotomy of mood disorders is supported by noradrenergic brainstem system morphology. *Journal of Affective Disorders*, **54**, 217–24.

47. Beckmann, H. and Jakob, H. (1991). Prenatal disturbances of nerve cell migration in the entorhinal region: a common vulnerability factor in functional psychoses? *Journal of Neural Transmission. General Section*, **84** (1–2), 155–64.

48. Casanova, M.F., Saunder, R., Altshuler, L., *et al.* (1991). Entorhinal cortex pathology in schizophrenia and affective disorders. In *Biological psychiatry* (ed. G. Racagni *et al.*), pp. 504–6. Elsevier, Amsterdam.

49. Diekmann, S., Baumann, B., Schmidt, U., and Bogerts, B. (1998). Significant decrease in calretinin immunoreactive neurons in layer II in the cingulate cortex in schizophrenics. *Pharmacopsychiatry*, **31**, 12.

50. Lohr, J.B. and Jeste, D.V. (1986). Studies of cerebellum and hippocampus in major psychiatric disorders. In *Biological psychiatry* (ed. C. Shagass , R. Josiassen, S. Bridger, K. Weiss, D. Stoff, and G.M. Simpson), pp. 1024–6. Elsevier, New York.

51. Hankoff, L.D. and Peress, N.S. (1981). Neuropathology of the brain stem in psychiatric disorders. *Biological Psychiatry*, **16**, 945–52.

52. Ross-Stanton, J. and Meltzer, F.A. (1981). Motor neuron branching patterns in psychotic patients. *Archives of General Psychiatry*, **38**, 1097–103.

53. Soares, J.C. and Mann, J.J. (1997). The anatomy of mood disorders— review of structural neuroimaging studies. *Biological Psychiatry*, **41**, 86–106.

54. Sheline, Y.I., Wang Po, W., Gado, M.H., Csernansky, J.G., and Vannier, M.W. (1996). Hippocampal atrophy in recurrent major depression. *Proceedings of the National Academy of Sciences*, **93**, 3908–13.

55. Duman, R.S., Heninger, G.R., and Nestler, E.J. (1997). A molecular and cellular theory of depression. *Archives of General Psychiatry*, **54**, 597–606.

56. Victor, M., Adams, R.D., and Collins, G. (1989). *The Wernicke–Korsakow syndrome and related neurologic disorders due to alcoholism and malnutrition*. Davis, Philadelphia, PA.

57. Harper, C.G. and Kril, J.J. (1990). Neuropathology of alcoholism. *Alcohol and Alcoholism*, **25**, 207–16.

58. Harper, C.G. (1998). The neuropathology of alcohol-specific brain damage, or does alcohol damage the brain? *Journal of Neuropathology and Experimental Neurology*, **57**, 101–10.

59. Cavazos, J.E., Das, I., and Sutula, T.P. (1994). Neuronal loss induced in limbic pathways by kindling: evidence for induction of hippocampal sclerosis by repeated brief seizures. *Journal of Neuroscience*, **14**, 3106–21.

60. Hoffmann, P.L., Iorio, K.R., Snell, L.D., and Tabakoff, B. (1995). Attenuation of glutamate-induced neurotoxicity in chronically ethanol-exposed cerebellar granule cells by NMDA receptor antagonists and ganglioside GM1. *Alcoholism, Clinical and Experimental Research*, **19**, 721–6.

2.3.6 Functional positron emission tomography in psychiatry

P. M. Grasby

Introduction

Positron emission tomography (**PET**) and single-photon emission tomography (**SPET**) are tools for investigating the pathophysiology of psychiatric illnesses and the action of psychotropic drugs. With these techniques monoaminergic, cholinergic, opioid and benzodiazepine receptors, regional cerebral blood flow, glucose and oxygen metabolism can be measured in the living brain (Table 1). Thus, neural function of direct relevance to neurochemical and anatomical theories of psychiatric illnesses can be sampled.

Methodology of PET and SPET[1,2]

In brief, PET and SPET comprise the following.

1. The production and incorporation of a gamma-emitting radio-isotope into a molecule of biological interest to form a radiotracer administered to humans (Plate 3).

2. Imaging of the distribution of the radiotracer, over minutes or hours, in living human brain. PET or SPET cameras are used to detect the emitted gamma radiation from the decaying radio-isotope (Plate 4).

3. Quantification of a physiological parameter of interest, such as total number of receptors (B_{max}) or regional cerebral blood flow,

from the measurement of radio-activity in the brain over time (Plates 5 and 6).

Production of isotopes

Common PET radio-isotopes, produced by a cyclotron, are oxygen-15 (^{15}O), carbon-11 (^{11}C), and fluorine-18 (^{18}F) (with half-lives of 2.03 min, 20.4 min and 109.8 min respectively) whilst SPET radio-isotopes include technetium (^{99m}Tc) and iodine-123 (^{123}I) (with half-lives of 6.02 h and 13.2 h respectively). SPET isotopes are less versatile than PET isotopes because the atoms are not normal constituents of many organic molecules (unlike carbon and oxygen) and because the large molecular size alters the properties of the molecule to which they are attached. However, SPET is cheaper than PET and less technically demanding, making it more readily available in hospitals and research centres.

Radiochemistry

To produce, for example, the radio-isotope [^{11}C]raclopride (used to study striatal dopamine D_2 receptors), protons are accelerated by a cyclotron to hit a target of nitrogen gas. The nuclear reaction produces [^{11}C]carbon dioxide (^{11}CO$_2$). ^{11}CO$_2$ is converted to [^{11}C]iodomethane which is then used to label a raclopride precursor to form [^{11}C]raclopride. This radiosynthesis procedure requires rapid automated synthetic chemistry facilities. Following quality control procedures, to estimate specific activity and chemical purity, [^{11}C]raclopride is injected intravenously into subjects lying in the PET camera (Plate 3). Importantly, the total mass of radiotracer injected is very small (typically less than 5 μg) and therefore the radiotracer has no pharmacological effect itself.

Imaging of radiotracer, data collection, and analysis

PET involves the disintegration of positrons emitted from unstable nuclei such as ^{11}C (Plate 4). Emitted positrons travel a short distance in tissue before annihilation by collision with an electron.[1] On annihilation, two high-energy gamma rays are generated with a separation angle of 180° (Plate 4). Radiation detectors (e.g. bismuth germanate), 180° apart and linked in electronic coincidence circuits, detect the resulting gamma radiation and therefore localize the source of radiation to a volume between any two detectors (Plate 3). By arranging rings of detectors around the subject's head and using computer-based back-projection techniques, the distribution of radiotracer within tomographic slices of the brain can be obtained.[1,2] SPET radio-isotopes, in contrast, decay by emitting a single gamma ray and therefore the radiation detectors are not linked in coincidence circuits. State-of-the-art PET and SPET cameras have transaxial spatial resolutions of the order of 4 to 5 mm (full-width half maximum—a standard measure of spatial resolution) and can detect subnanomolar concentrations of receptors.[1,2]

Table 1 Established and novel radiotracers for psychiatry

Radiotracer	Application	Comments
PET radiotracers		
$C^{15}O_2/H_2^{15}O$	Blood flow	Used to map dysfunctional brain areas involved in psychiatric illnesses. May be replaced by functional MRI techniques
[18F]deoxyglucose	Glucose metabolism	Used for many resting-state studies and to define antipsychotic drug effects
[11C]SCH 23390	Dopamine D_1 receptor	Receptor occupancy studies with many neuroleptics. Recent report of reduced cortical D_1 receptors in drug-naive schizophrenics
[11C]raclopride	Dopamine D_2 receptor	Robust demonstration of no elevation of striatal D_2 receptors in drug-naive schizophrenics. Striatal D_2 receptor occupancy studies with many neuroleptics
[11C]FLB-457	Dopamine D_2 receptor	High-affinity ligand; may enable extrastriatal D_2 populations to be measured
[11C]RTI 121 and 32	Dopamine reuptake site markers	Studies in Parkinson's disease in progress
[18F]dopa and [18F]metatyrosine	Dopaminergic neurone density and integrity	Radiotracer predominantly imageable in basal ganglia. Cortical signal weak. Some application to psychosis studies
[11C]flumazenil	Central benzodiazepine receptors	Labels all subtypes of central receptor. Studies in anxiety disorders in progress
[18F]altanserin	5-HT$_2$ receptor	Low specific signal in human brain. Studies in depressed patients in progress
[18F]setoperone	5-HT$_2$ receptor	Low specific signal in human brain. Studies in depressed patients in progress
[11C]methylspiperone	Cortical 5-HT$_2$ receptors and striatal D_2 receptors	Neuroleptic occupancy studies
[11C]MDL-100907	5-HT$_{2A}$ receptors	May be most suitable ligand for imaging 5-HT$_2$ receptors
[11C]WAY 100635	5-HT$_{1A}$ receptors	Studies in major depressive disorder in progress
[11C]McN 5652	Serotonin transporter	Studies in ecstasy abusers in progress
[11C]methyltryptophan	Possible measure of serotonin synthesis rate	A potentially important tracer for psychiatry. Validity of measure being investigated
[11C]diprenorphine	μ, κ, and δ receptors	Potential for studies in depressive disorder
[11C]carfentanil	μ opiate receptors	
SPET radiotracers		
[99mTc]HMPAO	Blood flow	Many resting state and two-scan activation studies in psychosis
[123I]iodobenzamide	Dopamine D_2 receptors	Occupancy and displacement studies
[123I]epidepride	Dopamine D_2/D_3 receptors	Studies of schizophrenia in progress. Can measure extrastriatal dopamine receptors
[123I]iomazenil	Benzodiazepine receptors	Studies in alcoholism
[123I]nor-β-CIT	Dopamine and serototonin transporter	Studies in ecstasy abusers in progress

Positron-emitting isotopes can be incorporated into molecules associated with diverse biochemical processes in the brain. For example, the positron emitter ^{11}C can be incorporated into a molecule WAY 100635, which selectively binds to 5-HT$_{1A}$ receptors, and injected intravenously in tracer amounts; the resulting gamma radiation is detected with a positron camera. Brain regions will show different profiles of radio-activity accumulation over time as the radiotracer binds in areas with a high density of 5-HT$_{1A}$ receptors (medial temporal cortex) whilst in regions with no or sparse receptors (cerebellum), it will be washed out (Plate 5). By this means, specific and non-specific binding can be distinguished. With an appropriate model of the radiotracer's history in tissue over time, a quantitative measurement of 5-HT$_{1A}$ receptor number in tomographic slices of the human brain can be obtained.[2] With some radiotracers (e.g. [11C]diprenorphine to label opiate receptors) it may be necessary to undertake radial artery cannulation to obtain an 'input function'[2] that describes the time course of presentation of radiotracer to the brain used in the quantitative modelling of the radiotracer (Plate 6).

Technical and practical limitations of PET and SPET compared with other imaging modalities

PET and SPET excel in the measurement of neurochemical parameters *in vivo* at very low (subnanomolar) concentration.[1,2] Such sensitivity cannot be matched by other *in vivo* methods such as proton magnetic resonance spectroscopy (millimolar range). However, radiation dosimetry limits the number of scans that subjects may receive. Full quantitation can often be achieved with PET, unlike SPET. However, for imaging blood flow change, functional magnetic resonance imaging (**MRI**) now offers the possibility of repeated measures (without radiation exposure) that far exceed that possible with PET- and SPET-based methods of flow mapping. However, full quantitation of blood flow is not yet readily achievable with functional MRI without injection of contrast agents. One disadvantage of functional MRI over PET, for some subjects, is the noisy claustrophobic environment of the scanner, but generally subjects and paradigms studied with PET flow mapping can be readily investigated with functional MRI (see Chapter 2.3.8), although all test materials in the vicinity of the scanner have to be non-magnetic.

Structural MRI scanning is often used in conjunction with PET activation and ligand binding techniques. The high-resolution anatomical information contained in MRI images can be used to precisely define areas of activation or radiotracer binding observed in PET studies from single subjects.[2]

PET and SPET, and even functional MRI, have relatively poor temporal resolution (seconds) compared with electrophysiological methods such as EEG, event-related potentials, and magnetoencephalography (milliseconds), but these methods in turn suffer from poor spatial resolution. Attempts to integrate information from these different modalities are now a major focus of methodological research in many imaging centres.

Standard brain spaces, statistical parametric mapping, and databases

A challenge for functional brain imaging is to maximize the detection of small signal changes whilst maintaining precision in the description of where signal change has occured.[2–4] Many centres have approached these tasks, particularly for flow studies, by using one or more of the following: smoothing image data; stereotactic transformation of PET images, from individual subjects, into a standard brain space; and voxel by voxel analysis of signal change using statistical tests that account for the multiple comparisons made.

A standard brain space commonly used is that of Talairch and Tournoux. In this brain space, images are orientated in planes parallel to a transverse plane that passes through the anterior and posterior commisures. Thus, for example, images of regional cerebral blood flow from different subjects in an activation experiment can be transformed to match a template blood flow image in this space. The co-ordinates of signal change for the group can then be specified by co-ordinates in the *x*, *y* and *z* axes of the Talairch space allowing comparisons with other studies in other centres.

Voxel-by-voxel-based methods of image analysis, which reduce

Table 2 Summary of PET functional brain imaging approaches

Functional brain mapping: rCBF or metabolism is measured as an index of local neural activity

(a) Studies in normal volunteers in which 'activation' paradigms are used to identify functional anatomy that is relevant to psychiatric disorders

(b) Activation studies in patients who are compared with matched control subjects

(c) Studies in which the biological variable (e.g. rCBF) is correlated with a relevant clinical variable (e.g. hallucinations) within the patient group

(d) The longitudinal comparison of patients before and after various treatments and into clinical recovery

(e) Cross-sectional studies of resting-state brain activity in patient groups in comparison with appropriate controls

Radioligand imaging: the specific uptake and binding of radiolabelled tracer compounds is measured

(a) To estimate baseline radioligand uptake at rest in patient groups in comparison with controls

(b) Within-patient group correlations between radioligand uptake and particular symptoms/signs

(c) Longitudinal comparison of radioligand uptake in patients before and after various treatments and into clinical recovery

(d) 'Displacement' or radioligand activation studies designed to detect changes in the levels of intrasynaptic neurotransmitters in response to a pharmacological or cognitive challenge

(e) Investigation of the receptor binding and occupancy characteristics of psychotropic drugs

rCBF, regional cerebral blood flow.

error variance and are devoid of observer bias, are now widespread. One such technique is statistical parametric mapping[3,4] which comprises realignment of images, spatial normalization, spatial smoothing, and voxel-wise statistical analysis. In the near future it is envisaged that a generic brain atlas database will be readily available in which PET, SPET, and functional MRI study results will be entered as standard co-ordinates allowing meta-analysis and easy comparison of results from different imaging centres.[4]

PET and SPET imaging strategies in psychiatry

These techniques (see Table 2) are used to either measure brain receptors and neurochemistry, or map functional brain activity via the indices of regional blood flow and glucose utilization. Each approach attempts to define trait and state abnormalities of psychiatric illnesses or the effect of psychotropic drug action.

Because of the technical complexities of brain imaging, it is important to bear in mind the following questions when judging experimental results. What assumptions are made about the behaviour of the radiotracer *in vivo*? Has the radiotracer been well validated for the physiological parameter measured? Is the spatial resolution of the PET camera sufficient for the regions measured? What is the test–test reliability for the PET measure? How have the raw PET images been treated in the data analysis? How have regions of interest been defined?

What statistical techniques have been used, and are the statistical thresholds appropriate?

Measuring brain receptors and neurochemistry[5]

Many neurochemical hypotheses, generated by post-mortem and animal data, can be rigorously tested with PET and SPET in the living brain whilst avoiding many of the confounding variables inherent in other techniques. Many receptor systems can be studied (Table 1). However, the rate of discovery of new radiotracers, suitable for use in humans, is relatively slow. Many conditions have to be satisfied to produce a suitable radiotracer for human use including blood–brain barrier permeability, high specific binding, receptor selectivity, absence of radioactive metabolites, and adequate modelling of tracer kinetics (Plate 6).

Mapping brain activity by imaging blood flow and glucose metabolism

Regional cerebral blood flow and glucose metabolism are indicators of regional neuronal synaptic activity.[6] Radiotracers for these processes, such as $H_2^{(15)}O$ to index blood flow, are used to image brain activity in psychiatric illness. Glucose metabolic mapping using $[^{(18)}F]$deoxyglucose has some disadvantages over flow mapping. Radiation dosimetry limits for $[^{(18)}F]$deoxyglucose and the long half-life of the tracer restrict repeated measurement in a subject over a short time-scale. In contrast $^{(15)}O$-based methods allow, for example, 12 measurements of regional blood flow over a 3-h period in a single subject.

The rapid development of PET cameras and automated data analysis techniques in the last decade has established flow-based functional imaging as a large and active research activity.[4] Early studies examined patients and normal controls while they were at rest in the scanner. Because of the unconstrained nature of subjects' cognitive states at rest some investigators have asked patients to rate certain mental experiences, such as presence of hallucinations whilst being scanned.

As the techniques of regional cerebral blood flow mapping have advanced there has been an equivalent sophistication of experimental design with rest state studies being overshadowed by activation paradigms.[4] In an activation design, subjects are engaged in a specific cognitive task whilst being scanned, for instance generating words, and the blood flow pattern is compared with flow present in a baseline condition such as repeating words. PET activation experiments may involve categorical, correlational, and factorial designs.[4]

Categorical comparisons: cognitive subtraction

The majority of PET activation studies have used the categorical comparison of cognitive subtraction[4–6] to isolate the neural correlates of cognitive processes. The cardinal assumption of cognitive subtraction is that the regional cerebral blood flow difference between two sets of PET scans (in each of which subjects perform different psychological tasks) isolates the neural correlates of the difference in cognitive components between tasks. The validity of cognitive subtraction rests on assumptions about the componential nature of the psychological processes underlying a particular task (perhaps not always valid). Specifically, it is assumed psychological tasks can be resolved into unique components that can be added or subtracted from one another to isolate a psychological component of interest.

Correlational designs: graded response

An alternative approach, resting on fewer assumptions about the componential nature of the psychological processes under investigation, is that of a correlational design or so-called 'graded response' paradigm. Here a parameter of psychological/physiological interest is systematically varied across PET scans and correlations are obtained between regional cerebral blood flow and the parameter manipulated. Such an approach may identify brain systems that respond over a range, or above a threshold, of the manipulated variable.[4]

Factorial designs

PET $^{(15)}O$ techniques allowing for multiple measures of blood flow in single subjects (typically six to 12 scans) has enabled factorial designs to be implemented. In such a design two or more experimental variables are examined for effects on flow, alone and in combination. An example of this design would be a study where the influence of task A on flow activations induced by task B is examined. These factorial designs can be used to examine the modulatory influence of a psychotropic drug on psychological processes.[4,5]

Novel data analysis methods for PET

Developments in this area are very rapid.[2,4] Recent examples would include the use of principal components technique to analyse PET activation data sets and attempts to determine measures of functional and effective connectivity between brain regions activated by a given task. For PET receptor studies, the use of cluster analysis, parametric approaches and simplified reference region models are of considerable interest.

Imaging pathophysiology: examples from schizophrenia research

Imaging dopamine receptors

Much research effort has focused on in vivo PET/SPET measurement of striatal dopamine D_2-receptor number in schizophrenia following the initial post-mortem reports of increased striatal dopamine receptor number. Initially, using $[^{(11)}C]N$-methylspiperone as a radiotracer, a two- to threefold raised striatal D_2-receptor number in drug-naive schizophrenics was reported.[7] However, subsequently other investigators using $[^{(11)}C]$raclopride, $[^{(11)}C]N$-methylspiperone, $[^{(123)}I]$iodobenzamide, $[^{(76)}Br]$bromolisuride failed to detect such elevations of striatal dopamine D_2-receptor number.[8,9] The different radiotracer methodologies used, the selectivity of radiotracers for dopamine D_2, D_3, and D_4 receptor subtypes, and the clinical characteristics of the patients studied have been advanced as possible explanations for the failure to replicate raised striatal dopamine D_2-receptor number. However, given these conflicting but essentially negative results, attention has shifted in recent years to reports of increased presynaptic dopaminergic function measured with $[^{(18)}F]$dopa[10] and decreased cortical dopamine D_1 receptors measured with $[^{(11)}C]$SCH 23390[11] in schizophrenia. These studies await further replication.

A novel extension to studies utilizing PET/SPET radiotracers for imaging dopamine D_2 receptors has been to index dopamine release during a pharmacological challenge in schizophrenia. Theoretically,

PET/SPET has the potential to detect neurotransmitter release associated with behavioural and pharmacological challenges if sufficient endogenous neurotransmitter is released to cause appreciable change (via receptor occupancy) in the number of 'available' receptors that can be 'seen' by a radioligand.[5] For example, pre-dosing animals and human subjects with D-amphetamine, which releases dopamine, results in decreased [^{11}C]raclopride and [^{123}I]iodobenzamide binding to dopamine D_2 receptors.[12] Recently enhanced release of striatal dopamine in acutely symptomatic patients with schizophrenia following pharmacological challenge has been reported by Laruelle *et al.*[13] In these studies the displacement of radiotracer (presumably reflecting increased release of dopamine) correlated with worsening of positive symptoms. Whether this important finding of increased dopaminergic responsivity will be prove to be reliable state or trait marker for schizophrenia remains to be fully established.

Imaging blood flow change and hypofrontality

From the outset of the functional neuroimaging of schizophrenia there has been discussion as to whether the frontal lobes of patients are 'less active' than those of normal subjects. The term 'hypofrontality' has indicated either reduced activity 'at rest' or a failure of activation (relative to a baseline condition) when the subject performs a given cognitive task.[14] Studies by Weinberger's group, using the Wisconsin Card Sorting Task whilst scanning, demonstrated that schizophrenic cohorts performing this task exhibit relative hypofrontality.[14] This hypofrontality was replicated in other schizophrenic cohorts, on and off medication, and task performance was positively correlated with prefrontal blood flow.

However, hypofrontality, whether at rest or during cognitive challenge, has not been a universal finding in all studies, making it a somewhat unreliable trait marker of schizophrenia. It has been found in about 50 per cent of resting-state studies but more often in activation paradigms.[15] Discrepant results might be attributable to the nature and demands of the task used, task performance, and the symptom profiles of patients studied. For example, Frith and Fletcher used PET to study paced verbal fluency activations in chronic and acute schizophrenic patients, on and off neuroleptic medication, respectively, and failed to find hypofrontality.[16] But pacing tasks could be criticized on the grounds that slowing the task so that patients and normal subjects perform equally fails to address a dysfunction that may be expressed when patients are required to produce 'normal' levels of performance. This is a difficult issue to resolve. Pacing patients and controls means that performance levels may be matched, and therefore differences of brain activation are not confounded by the patients' failure to do the task. Yet it may be instructive to image patients attempting to perform a task that stresses (dysfunctional) cognitive processes, produces altered brain activity and hence impaired performance.

Many authors have suggested hypofrontality may be most pronounced in schizophrenic patients who have predominantly 'negative' symptoms. This view has received support from a large cross-sectional study of chronically symptomatic patients where resting blood flow was measured in 30 patients.[17] Within this group of schizophrenic patients, greater hypofrontality was seen among those with the most pronounced negative symptoms as assessed by factor analysis. That symptoms and not the diagnosis of schizophrenia *per se* may be an important factor in hypofrontality is apparent in one study where poverty of speech (a sign of psychomotor retardation or poverty) was

associated with reduced regional cerebral blood flow in the left dorsolateral prefrontal cortex, irrespective of diagnosis of depression or schizophrenia.[18] Some SPET and PET studies also suggest a relationship between hypofrontality and the presence of positive symptoms,[19,20] and hypofrontality (at rest or on activation) may resolve when symptoms improve.[21]

In conclusion, hypofrontality may not be a stable trait, but rather a state-related abnormality in schizophrenic psychoses (and possibly other diagnoses), perhaps related to the presence and/or severity of particular symptom clusters.

Imaging pathophysiology: examples from depressive disorders

Imaging 5-hydroxytryptamine receptors

Recent progress has seen the development of new radiotracers for the 5-hydroxytryptamine (5-HT) system; hypothesized to be dysfunctional in affective illness and to be the prime target for many antidepressant treatments.[5] In particular, radioligands for 5-HT$_{1A}$ and 5-HT$_{2A}$ receptors, the 5-HT transporter, and radiotracers of 5-HT synthesis are being developed (Table 1).

One recent success is the radioligand [^{11}C]WAY 100635 for imaging 5-HT$_{1A}$ receptors in the human brain.[22] As many different antidepressant treatments alter 5-HT$_{1A}$ receptor function in rodents, this ligand will be useful investigating 5-HT$_{1A}$ receptor populations in depressed patients before and after treatment especially.

[^{11}C]N-methylspiperone, [^{18}F]altanserin, [^{18}F]ethylspiperone, [^{18}F]setoperone or [^{18}F]altanserin, and the SPET tracer [^{123}I]ketanserin have been used to measure 5-HT$_2$ receptor number; a receptor implicated in depressive illness, suicidal behaviour, and psychosis. Many of these 5-HT$_2$ ligands have been hampered by either the lack of selectivity, or the relatively low ratio of specific to non-specific signal obtained in the human brain,[23] although a few reports have appeared reporting reduced 5-HT$_2$ receptor number in drug-free depressed patients. Further studies are needed using more selective ligands with higher signal to noise ratios, such as [^{11}C]MDL 100907, a promising selective ligand for 5-HT$_{2A}$ receptors (Table 1).

Imaging blood-flow change in depressive disorder

Similarly to brain-mapping studies of patients with schizophrenia, regional deficits of neural activity (indexed by cerebral blood flow or glucose utilization) can be detected in the 'resting' brains of depressed patients.[24,25] Many resting-state studies have shown a reduction of regional brain functional activity, most frequently reported in the prefrontal cortex, compared with normal controls. However, the exact location of prefrontal change (dorsolateral, ventrolateral, orbitofrontal, and medial frontal areas) has been variably emphasized by different authors.[24–26]

As demonstrated in schizophrenia, significant associations between cortical activity and cognitive function, symptom clusters, including mood, and response to treatments are apparent.[25] Similarly to schizophrenia, the resting-state functional brain abnormalities may represent the physiological correlates of aspects of the depressed state such as depressed mood, retardation, or cognitive impairment rather than trait markers of the illness itself.

Psychological challenge paradigms have been applied in a few studies in depressed cohorts to test whether specific brain regions, subserving select cognitive processes, are impaired in depressed patients. For example, the Tower of London planning task has been used to investigate a 'planning network' in depressed patients.[27] Patients in this study showed reduced activity throughout the network with complete loss of functional activity in the anterior cingulate cortex; a cortical region involved in attentional processing and highly connected with other prefrontal areas. Using a different activation strategy, mood induction paradigms have mapped the neural correlates of subjective mood. In one of the first of these studies, recall of sad situations resulted in increased activity in inferior orbitofrontal cortex. In more recent studies, increased flow in limbic and paralimbic structures including the left prefrontal, bilateral anterior cingulate, hypothalamus, and inferomedial prefrontal cortex have been observed.[27]

Imaging psychotropic drug action

Of direct clinical relevance are imaging studies of antipsychotic drug action where clinical efficacy and side-effects are related to receptor occupancy.[9,28]

Many studies have investigated the occupancy of striatal dopamine D_1 and D_2 and cortical serotonin 5-HT$_2$ receptors by neuroleptic drugs. Farde's group first demonstrated that clinically efficacious doses of a variety of classical antipsychotics cause between 65 per cent and 89 per cent occupancy of central dopamine D_2 receptors.[9,28] Higher receptor occupancy ({gt}85 per cent) is associated with an increased incidence of extrapyramidal side effects. Thus, there may be a therapeutic window for occupancy of between 65 per cent and 85 per cent, which is antipsychotic and yet less likely to cause extrapyramidal side effects. In contrast, treatment with classical antipsychotics produces variable levels of occupancy of striatal D_1 receptors. Interestingly, efficacious doses of the atypical antipsychotic clozapine are associated with a relatively low D_2 receptor occupancy (38–63 per cent) and a D_1 occupancy of 38 to 52 per cent.[9,28] This unexpected finding of low D_2 receptor occupancy, reproduced in different patient groups with both PET and SPET techniques, has challenged theories of a simple relationship between D_2 occupancy per se and clinical efficacy. Further evidence for this view comes from studies showing that schizophrenic antipsychotic non-responders have the same levels of dopamine D_2 occupancy as responders and that occupancy occurs as rapidly as 2 h after acute administration of the antipsychotic yet efficacy takes weeks to appear.

PET/SPET is also proving useful in the characterization of atypical antipsychotics. The binding of antipsychotic drugs to central 5-HT$_2$ receptors is a possible candidate for the mechanism of 'atypicality' and studies suggest high cortical 5-HT$_2$ occupancy with risperidone (80 per cent) and clozapine (84–90 per cent).[9,28,29]

Conclusions

So far, the PET and SPET radiotracer techniques and applications described have not yielded a diagnostic test, or an exact guide to outcome in the major psychiatric illnesses. However, they have been immediately valuable in assessing the receptor occupancy effects of antipsychotic drugs and of mapping the neural correlates of dysfunctional cognitive processes and psychiatric symptoms. The definition of an endophenotype of a major psychiatric illness is perhaps some way off but in the long term the techniques will almost certainly provide essential information about the pathophysiology of psychiatric illnesses.

References

1. Myers, R., Spinks, T.J., Luthra, S.K., et al. (1992). Positron emission tomography. In Quantitative methods in neuroanatomy (ed. M.G. Stewart), pp. 117–61. Wiley, New York.
2. Myers, R., Cunningham, V., Bailey, D., and Jones, T. (1996). Quantification of brain function using PET. Academic Press, London.
3. Friston, K.J., Holmes, A.P., Worsley, K.J., et al. (1995). Statistical parametric maps in functional imaging: a general linear approach. Human Brain Mapping, 2, 189–210.
4. Frackowiak, R.S.J., Friston, K.J., Frith, C.D., Dolan, R.J., and Mazziotta, J.C. (1997). Human brain function. Academic Press, San Diego, CA.
5. Grasby, P., Malizia, A., and Bench, C. (1996). Psychopharmacology—in vivo neurochemistry and pharmacology. British Medical Bulletin, 52, 513–26.
6. Raichle, M.E. (1987). Circulatory and metabolic correlations of brain function in normal humans. In Handbook of physiology. Section 1, The nervous system. Vol. 5, Higher functions of the brain (ed. F. Plum), pp. 643–74. Oxford University Press, New York.
7. Wong, D.F., Wagner, H.N., Tune, L.E., et al. (1986). Positron emission tomography reveals elevated D2-dopamine receptors in drug-naive schizophrenia. Science, 234, 1558–63.
8. Farde, L., Wiesel, F.-A., Stone-Elander, S., et al. (1990). D2 dopamine receptors in neuroleptic naive schizophrenic patients. Archives of General Psychiatry, 47, 213–19.
9. Sedvall, G. and Farde, L. (1995). Chemical brain anatomy in schizophrenia. Lancet, 346, 743–9.
10. Hietala, J., Syvalahti, E., and Vuorio, K., et al. (1995). Presynaptic dopamine function in striatum of neuroleptic naive schizophrenic patients. Lancet, 346, 1130–1.
11. Okubo, Y., Suhara, T., Suzuku, K., et al. (1997). Decreased prefrontal dopamine D1 receptors in schizophreia revealed by PET. Nature, 385, 634–6.
12. Volkow, N.D, Wang, G.-J., Fowler, J.S., et al. (1994). Imaging endogenous dopamine competition with 11C-raclopride in the human brain. Synapse, 16, 255–62
13. Laruelle, M., Abi-Dargham, A., van Dyck, C.H., et al. (1996). Single photon emission computerized tomography imaging of amphetamine-induced dopamine release in drug-free schizophrenia subjects. Proceedings of the National Academy of Sciences of the United States of America, 93, 9235–40.
14. Weinberger, D.R. and Berman, K.F. (1996). Prefrontal function in schizophrenia: confounds and controversies. Philosophical Transactions of the Royal Society of London. Series B: Biological Sciences, 351, 1495–503.
15. Chuam, S.E. and McKenna, P.J. (1996). Schizophrenia—a brain disease? A critical review of structural and functional cerebral abnormality in the disorder. British Journal of Psychiatry, 166, 563–82.
16. Frith, C.D., Friston, K.J., Herold, S., et al. (1995). Regional brain activity in chronic schizophrenic patients during the performance of a verbal fluency task. British Journal of Psychiatry, 167, 343–9.
17. Liddle, P.F., Friston, K.J., Frith, C.D., Hirsch, S.R., Jones, T., and Frackowiak, R.S.J. (1992). Patterns of cerebral blood flow in schizophrenia. British Journal of Psychiatry, 160, 179–86.
18. Dolan, R.J., Bench, C.J., Liddle, P.F., et al. (1993). Dorsolateral prefrontal cortex dysfunction in the major psychoses; symptom or disease specificity? Journal of Neurology, Neurosurgery and Psychiatry, 56, 1290–4.

19. Andreasen, N.C., O'Leary, D.S., Flaum, M., *et al.* (1997). Hypofrontality in schizophrenia: distributed dysfunctional circuits in neuroleptic-naive patients. *Lancet*, **349**, 1730–4.

20. Sabri, O., Erkwoh, R., Schreckenberger, M., *et al.* (1997). Correlation of positive symptoms exclusively to hyperperfusion or hypoperfusion of cerebral cortex in never-treated schizophrenics. *Lancet*, **349**, 1735–9.

21. Spence, S.A., Hirsch, S.R., Brooks, D.J., and Grasby, P.M. (1998). Prefrontal cortex activity in people with schizophrenia and control subjects. Evidence from positron emission tomography for remission of 'hypofrontality' with recovery from acute schizophrenia. *British Journal of Psychiatry*, **172**, 316–23.

22. Pike, V., McCarron, J.A., Lammerstma, A.A., *et al.* (1995). First delineation of 5-HT$_{1A}$ receptors in the living human brain using $^{(11)}$C-WAY-100635. *European Journal of Pharmacology*, **283**, R1–R3.

23. Pike, V. (1993). Positron emitting radioligands for studies *in vivo*—probes for human psychopharmacology. *Journal of Psychopharmacology*, **7**, 139–58.

24. Goodwin, G. (1996). Functional imaging, affective disorder and dementia. *British Medical Bulletin*, **52**, 495–512.

25. Bench, C.J., Friston, K.J., Brown, R.G., *et al.* (1993). Regional cerebral blood flow in depression measured by positron emission tomography: the relationship with clinical dimensions. *Psychological Medicine*, **23**, 579–90.

26. Drevets, W.C., Price, J.L., Simpson, J.R., *et al.* (1997). Subgenual prefrontal cortex abnormalities in mood disorders. *Nature*, **386**, 824–7.

27. Grasby, P.M. and Bench, C.J. (1997). Neuroimaging of mood disorders. *Current Opinion in Psychiatry*, **10**, 73–8.

28. Farde, L., Nordstrom, A.-L., Wiesel, F.A., Pauli, S., Halldin, C., and Sedvall, G. (1992). Positron emission tomographic analysis of central D1 and D2 dopamine receptor occupancy in patients treated with classical neuroleptics and clozapine. Relation to extrapyramidal side effects. *Archives of General Psychiatry*, **49**, 538–54.

29. Nyberg, S., Farde, L., and Erikson, L. (1993). 5-HT2 and D2 dopamine receptor occupancy in the living human brain: a PET study with risperidone. *Psychopharmacology*, **110**, 265–72.

2.3.7 Structural magnetic resonance imaging

J. Suckling and E. T. Bullmore

Introduction

Magnetic resonance imaging (**MRI**) is a versatile and evolving technology for visualizing the structure, function, and metabolism of the living human brain. All kinds of MRI data can be acquired without exposing subjects to ionizing radiation or radioactive isotopes. Installing the hardware for MRI represents a major capital investment, of approximately £1.5 million, but this is considerably less than the costs of setting up a positron emission tomography unit. For these three reasons of versatility, safety, and (relative) affordability, MRI is likely to be the dominant brain-imaging technique in psychiatric practice and research for at least the next 15 years.

In this chapter, we introduce the principles and practicalities of MRI and describe common methods of structural MRI data acquisition and analysis. Chapter 2.3.8 on functional MRI provides greater detail on statistical issues arising in image analysis.

Historical background

Naturally occurring magnets or lodestones were considered magical by the early inhabitants of Magnesia in modern Turkey—hence the word magnetism. Physical principles were formulated by Karl Friedrich Gauss in the eighteenth century. James Clerk Maxwell discovered the fundamental laws of electromagnetism in the nineteenth century. In 1946, Felix Bloch and Edward Mills Purcell independently reported the phenomenon of nuclear magnetic resonance (**NMR**). For this discovery they were jointly awarded the Nobel Prize for Physics in 1952. The technique was quickly taken up and magnetic resonance spectroscopy *in vitro* was developed over the following decades. In the late 1960s other technologies converged: superconducting magnets, computers, and image reconstruction techniques developed by Sir Godfrey Hounsfield for X-ray tomography were combined to produce the first *in vivo* magnetic resonance images in the early 1970s. Technological and engineering developments have continued apace, as have ideas for new imaging perspectives. The limits of MRI remain unreached.

Magnetization

If iron filings are scattered on a piece of paper they will be oriented at random. If a bar magnet is then placed under the paper the iron filings will align themselves so that each filing lies parallel to the magnetic field produced by the magnet. More technically, we can say that iron filings have a susceptibility to be magnetized by a static magnetic field.

Susceptibility refers both to the effect of a magnetic field on an object, and the effect of that object on the field. Paramagnetic materials, like some metals, tend to be attracted by magnets and cause a local increase in magnetic field strength. Diamagnetic materials, like carbon and many organic compounds, tend to be repulsed by magnets and cause a local decrease in field strength.

The brain also has a susceptibility to be magnetized. It is largely composed of water and each molecule of water comprises, of course, two hydrogen atoms and one oxygen atom. The hydrogen nucleus is a single positively charged proton, which has a dynamic property called spin. Like all moving charged particles, spinning protons generate a magnetic field. The axis of the magnetic dipole generated by a spinning proton is sometimes called its magnetic moment, and is drawn as a vector.

When the brain is placed in a strong magnetic field, the spinning protons align themselves with the external field, just as iron filings align themselves to the field of a bar magnet. The angle of alignment between each proton's moment and the (longitudinal) axis of the external magnetic field is α. Protons obey the laws of quantum mechanics, and so two modes of alignment or spin states are possible, one with the magnetic moment in the direction of the field ($\alpha = 0°$) and one with the moment in the opposite direction ($\alpha = 180°$). Depending on the strength of the applied field, the spin states have slightly different probabilities, with those protons aligned in the direction of the field in excess by about 5 ppm at an external field strength of 1.5 T. (Magnetic field strength is measured in units of gauss (**G**) or tesla (**T**): 1 T = 10 000 G. The Earth's magnetic field is approximately 0.5 G; a child's toy magnet has a field of around 10 G.)

Thus, if the magnetic moments for all spinning protons are averaged, the net, or bulk, magnetization vector for the brain as a whole

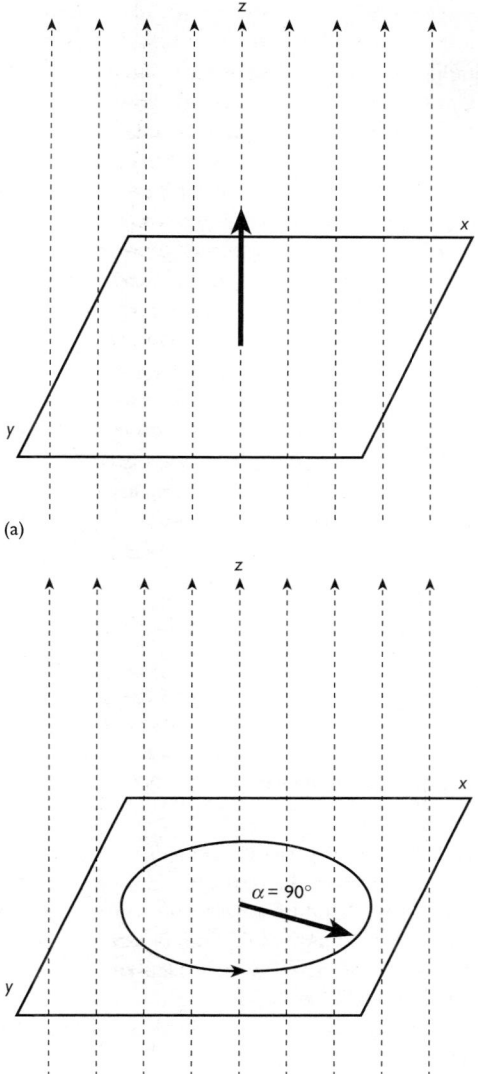

Fig. 1 Net magnetization vector. (a) In a static magnetic field, the vector is aligned parallel to the longitudinal z axis of the field and α = 0. (b) Immediately after a 90° excitation pulse of radiofrequency energy at Larmor frequency, the angle of alignment α is increased (transverse magnetization) and the phase of precession in the x–y plane is coherent over all protons in the brain. As protons relax following excitation, the angle of the net vector becomes smaller (return of longitudinal magnetization) and the phase of precession becomes more variable from one proton to another (dephasing).

Nuclear magnetic resonance

When a wineglass is tapped by a knife, it produces a high-pitched sound of characteristic frequency. If a singer can exactly match that frequency with her voice then the glass will resonate and may break. The basic idea is that if an object has a characteristic frequency of oscillation, exposing it to energy precisely at that frequency will cause a change in physical state.

Analogously, if we supply a pulse of radiofrequency energy at (and only at) the Larmor frequency to a brain located in a magnetic field, the protons within the brain will absorb the energy and resonate. Their angle of alignment α with the external field increases. If sufficient energy is supplied to cause α = 90°, the radiofrequency pulse is called a '90° pulse'. If the net magnetization vector is flipped to an angle α = 180°, the radiofrequency pulse is called a '180° pulse'. At the same time as the angle of alignment is increased by radiofrequency irradiation, the phase of precession becomes coherent over all protons. In other words, in place of the random variation in the phase of precession that existed before the radiofrequency pulse, protons are now 'marching in step' with each other around the axis of the external field.

After the radiofrequency pulse has ceased, the resonating nuclei gradually relax back to the equilibrium state of random precession in alignment with the external field. The two components of this relaxation process are characterized by relaxation times. The first relaxation time (T_1), also called the spin–lattice relaxation time, describes the time taken for the strength of longitudinal magnetization to return to 63 per cent of its value before radiofrequency irradiation. This is a measure of the time taken for α to return to zero having been flipped to 90° or 180°. T_1 is determined by interactions between protons and their long-range (molecular) environment or lattice. The second relaxation time (T_2), also called the spin–spin relaxation time, describes the time taken for the flipped nuclei to stop 'marching in step' around the axis of the field. This process of dephasing begins as soon as the radiofrequency pulse stops, but its rate is determined by the immediate (atomic) environment of the protons. Small variations in the applied magnetic field accentuate spin–spin relaxation, resulting in an observed relaxation time T_2^* which is somewhat faster than the 'true' relaxation time T_2 that would have been observed in an ideally homogeneous field.

As protons relax, they release the energy absorbed from the radiofrequency pulse in the form of a weak radiofrequency signal, which decays at a rate normally determined by T_2^*. This process is called free induction decay, and the emitted signal forms the data from which magnetic resonance images are ultimately constructed.

Magnetic resonance imaging

Spin echo sequence

The basic principles of NMR can be exploited to generate magnetic resonance images of the brain. One widely used MRI technique is the spin echo sequence. A 90° radiofrequency pulse is repetitively applied to the brain with a constant repetition time (TR ms) between consecutive pulses. Following each 90° pulse, protons are excited and then relax. The dephasing component of relaxation can be reversed by applying a second 180° pulse some time (TE/2 ms) after the 90° pulse. We can imagine that following the first 90° pulse, protons immediately

will have α = 0°. The length of the net magnetization vector then represents the strength of longitudinal magnetization (Fig. 1).

Protons aligned with a static magnetic field are not static themselves. They rotate or precess at very high frequency around the axis of the external field. The precession frequency, or Larmor frequency, is constant for a given type of atomic nucleus and external field strength. For protons, the Larmor frequency at 1.5 T is 63.9 MHz. However, although all hydrogen nuclei in the brain precess at the same frequency in the same field, they will not all precess with the same phase. At any given time, different nuclei have reached a different point in their rotation around the external field axis.

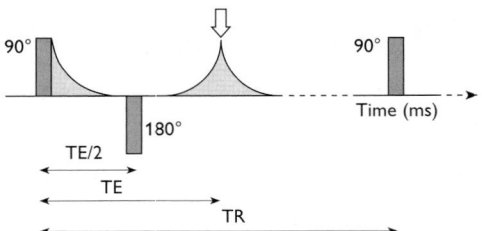

Fig. 2 Spin echo pulse sequence. A 90° excitation pulse of radiofrequency energy is immediately followed by exponential decay of the T_2-weighted signal. A 180° pulse TE/2 ms later causes rephasing of proton spins and an exponential increase in T_2-weighted signal with maximum (echo) TE ms after the 90° pulse. Images are acquired at TE (thick arrow). The protons are allowed to relax completely before the next 90° pulse, TR ms after the previous excitation.

begin to precess idiosyncratically and the emitted signal decays. By reversing this process, the 180° pulse causes rephasing and an increase in emitted signal which has a maximum or echo at TE ms (time to echo) after the initial 90° pulse (Fig. 2).

The spatial location of the radiofrequency signal emitted by free induction decay in a given volume of the brain is encoded in three spatial dimensions by slice-selective radiofrequency irradiation combined with frequency- and phase-encoding gradients. To improve scan time, multiple slices can be excited in an interleaved fashion (multi-slice acquisition). This means that after the output signal is detected from one slice, and while the net magnetization vector is relaxing back to its equilibrium state, other slices can be excited. The in-plane resolution (voxel size) of the image is determined by the field of view and the number of voxels in the image. Typically, in-plane resolution at 1.5 T is in the order of 0.5 to 2 mm, and slice thickness is 2 mm or more.

Tissue contrast

The outstanding advantage of MRI for the anatomical examination of the brain is the easily visible contrast in the images between grey matter, white matter, and cerebrospinal fluid. In particular, contrast between parenchymal tissues (grey and white matter) has made MRI the imaging research tool of choice for identifying subtle cortical abnormalities in a wide variety of psychiatric disorders.

Tissue contrast in magnetic resonance images is determined by differences in the density of protons, and their physical and chemical environment. A tissue that is largely composed of air, like the lungs, will have a lower proton density than a tissue, such as the cerebrospinal fluid, that is composed largely of water, which in turn will have a lower proton density than parenchymal brain tissues. The physicochemical environment of protons has a marked effect on spin–lattice relaxation. If protons are mainly in freely diffusing water molecules, as they are in cerebrospinal fluid, T_1 will be prolonged, whereas if they are mainly bound to large macromolecules, as they are in fat, T_1 will be short (Table 1). Since grey matter contains proportionally less fat than myelinated white matter, T_1 is longer for grey matter. Spin–spin relaxation is likewise determined, in part, by the immediate physical environment of protons in the tissue; liquid tissues will have prolonged T_2 times compared with solid tissues. Other effects on apparent relaxation times (T_2^*) include minute fluctuations or inhomogeneities in the strength of the external magnetic field, which may be due to the

local paramagnetic effects of iron-containing compounds such as haemoglobin.

The parameters of the spin echo pulse sequence, repetition time (TR), and time to echo (TE), can be judiciously adjusted to acquire images that are sensitive to or weighted by one or other of these possible sources of tissue contrast.

If TR is long (> 1000 ms) and TE is short (< 20 ms), contrast in the images will be weighted by differences between tissues in proton density. Proton-density-weighted images show good contrast between relatively hyperintense parenchymal tissue and hypointense cerebrospinal fluid (Plate 7).

If TR is short (< 1000 ms) and TE is short (< 20 ms), contrast in the images will be weighted by tissue differences in spin–lattice relaxation. T_1-weighted images show excellent contrast between hyperintense white matter and relatively hypointense grey matter (Plate 7) (Plate 7). For this reason, T_1-weighted images are widely used to measure quantitative abnormalities in size or shape of the cerebral cortex.

If TR is long (> 1000 ms) and TE is long (> 20 ms), contrast in the images will be weighted by tissue differences in spin–spin relaxation. T_2-weighted images show strong contrast between hyperintense cerebrospinal fluid and parenchymal tissues (Plate 7), unless there is congestion or oedema of the parenchyma, in which case the T_2-weighted signal will be increased. For this reason, T_2-weighted images are widely used to identify acute, inflammatory, and ischaemic lesions.

Fast spin echo sequence

Fast spin echo imaging involves a refinement of the basic spin echo sequence. Instead of eliciting a single signal echo after a 180° rephasing pulse in each cycle of length TR, fast spin echo imaging elicits several signals, an echo-train, by multiple 180° pulses after a single 90° pulse. Earlier echoes (TE < 20 ms) are used to form a proton-density-weighted image and those arriving later (TE > 80 ms) are used to form a T_2-weighted image. This pair of dual-echo images provides complementary tissue contrast for no increase in scan time, making fast spin echo a favoured sequence.

Diffusion-weighted imaging

Diffusion-weighted imaging is another refinement of the spin echo sequence. It can provide information about the organization of white matter tracts in the brain that cannot be obtained by other MRI methods.

The basic idea is that protons move within and between cells by random motion. Typically, a proton may travel around 20 μm in 100 ms by this Brownian motion or diffusion. The rate of diffusion

Table 1 Relaxation times at 1.5 T for different tissue types

Tissue type	T_1 (ms)	T_2 (ms)
Grey matter	980–1040	64–71
White matter	740–770	64–70
CSF	> 2000	> 300
Fat (at 1 T)	180	90

CSF, cerebrospinal fluid.

will be greatest for protons that are moving freely through the cerebrospinal fluid and less for protons constrained by physical barriers such as myelinated cell membranes. The rate of diffusion affects the spin–spin relaxation time, with rapidly diffusing protons tending to relax more quickly. To acquire images that are weighted by differences in diffusion, two extra gradients are briefly applied during a spin echo sequence.[1]

White matter is generally hyperintense in diffusion-weighted imaging because closely packed axonal tracts provide the greatest barrier to the free diffusion of water in the brain. Furthermore, it is possible to deduce from diffusion-weighted imaging data how compactly organized the white matter is, and even to estimate in what direction the fibre tracts are oriented (Plate 8). This information is of considerable interest to psychiatry, since the pathology of many psychiatric disorders may involve the axonal connections between multiple cortical areas.[2]

Safety

MRI is absolutely contraindicated in patients who have any strongly magnetized metal object in their heads. This includes aneurysm clips, reconstructive metal plates, or traumatically embedded metal fragments. MRI is also contraindicated in patients who have implanted electronic devices, such as cardiac pacemakers. It is advisable to screen all subjects undergoing MRI by questionnaire for possible contraindications. A skull radiograph is a useful preliminary examination if there is any doubt about the presence of intracranial metal. All subjects need to provide informed consent in writing.

Static magnetic fields as strong as 2 T cause no harmful effects to biological tissue. Rapid switching of field gradients can induce electrical currents in tissue, but at the switching speeds used in MRI these induced currents are several times less than needed for muscle contraction. Since radiofrequency energy can cause heating, limits to the amounts of energy absorbed are set by national standards.

Artefacts

Quality assurance protocols and diligent hardware servicing are necessary to maintain high standards in MRI. Image artefacts refer to loss of image quality (i.e. spatial resolution or tissue contrast) owing to a specific cause. It is often possible to effect a remedy and an awareness of their causes can often pre-empt the problem.

Movement

Subject motion is the most common artefact and has two components: voluntary and involuntary (physiological). The result of voluntary motion during acquisition may be an obvious blurring (Plate 7). The co-operation of subjects is vital and special regard is required for children, the elderly, and those with neurological or psychiatric disorders who may find the MRI environment disconcerting. The subject's head is physically restrained by additional padding and by Velcro straps placed across the forehead. Involuntary motion arises primarily from the cardiorespiratory cycle causing pulsation of the blood vessels and cerebrospinal fluid. This is most apparent in structural images showing major arteries.

Susceptibility

Where two materials with very different susceptibilities are closely adjacent, there may be severe distortion of the magnetic field, causing artefactual loss or exaggeration of the magnetic resonance signal. This is clearly seen in an image acquired with a metallic clip placed close to the scalp (Plate 7). Ferromagnetic (highly paramagnetic) materials that may cause artefacts include metallic dental fillings and plates, hairgrips, ear or nose rings, and even some cosmetics. A less obvious form of susceptibility artefact arises if more (diamagnetic) tissue is situated at one end of the image field of view than the other. A field gradient is set up across the image resulting in signal loss. This is termed bulk susceptibility artefact and is often seen in images of both the head and neck (Plate 7).

Partial volume

Voxel sizes are larger than some scales of anatomical organization in the brain. A voxel may represent a heterogeneous mixture of tissue classes, or be only partially occupied by tissue of a single type. This partial-volume artefact is particularly evident at the interface between cortical grey matter and sulcal cerebrospinal fluid, and at the interface between cortical grey matter and central white matter. It causes error in the estimation of tissue class volumes.

MRI hardware

Superconducting magnet

Magnetic fields greater than 0.5 T can only be generated by extremely heavy electromagnets or by much lighter superconducting magnets. Superconducting magnets are almost universally preferred. Ancillary equipment includes the liquid-helium cooling systems required to keep the temperature low enough (4 K) for superconduction. Cooling consumes the majority of the supplied power. Only a small current is initially required to generate the field, which is then self-sustaining.

Small variations in the homogeneity of the magnetic field give rise to distortions and artefacts. The field is minutely adjusted to improve homogeneity using additional magnets in an automated procedure known as shimming.

Magnetic field gradients are essential to MRI. Rapid switching of gradient coils produces the loud 'knocking' sound associated with magnetic resonance scanners. However, three orthogonal gradients are available which are coupled to generate gradients in any direction.

Radiofrequency coil

The function of the radiofrequency coil is twofold—to transmit the radiofrequency pulses of the imaging sequences and to receive the emitted output signal. Head coils used for neuroimaging fit snugly over the subject's head, and are often of a three-dimensional bird-cage design with good sensitivity throughout the volume they enclose. Surface coil designs are used to image small regions with high spatial resolution, and phased-array coils combine several surface coils for more extensive coverage.

Computers

MRI produces large quantities of data, which require rapid processing and storage so that images may be viewed and other sequences prescribed during the same appointment. The computer system is integral to the machine and contains specialized hardware and software for data acquisition and image reconstruction, as well as control of the magnet, gradient and radiofrequency coils, and other components of the scanner.

The scanner room

The room housing the scanner must be specially designed. It must have a reinforced floor and be environmentally controlled to maintain a constant temperature and humidity. The walls and ceiling contain a magnetic shield, which both prevents leakage of the field outside the room and stops FM radio broadcasts from being picked up by the radiofrequency coil.

Case–control design

Structural MRI studies in psychiatry have most commonly adopted a cross-sectional or case–control design. This involves scanning two groups of subjects, patients and matched controls, on a single occasion. The objective is generally to identify anatomical differences in brain structure between cases and controls. In evaluating or planning such a study, it is important to pay attention to several design issues, some of which are summarized below.

Power

What is the power of the study to refute the null hypothesis (zero anatomical difference between the case and control populations) when it is not true? Unfortunately, few published imaging studies consider this question explicitly. In general, the power of a study is proportional to the sample size (the number of subjects scanned), the effect size (the anatomical difference between populations), and the probability threshold or p value adopted for hypothesis testing. The p value will often be decided in relation to the number of tests conducted—the greater the number of tests, the smaller is the appropriate p value. Therefore the risk of low power and associated type 2 error is likely to be greatest when differences between two small groups have been multiply tested on the basis of many anatomical variables. In general, it is reasonable to be sceptical about negative findings reported in samples comprising less than 30 or 40 individuals per group.

Representativeness

What population is represented by the sample of patients studied, and is this the population of interest? If the ambition of the study is to make inferences about the population of patients with, say, manic–depressive disorder, then it is important that the diagnosis is made according to standard and reliable criteria and that the sampling procedure is such that any patient in that population has an equal chance of being included in the study. This means that the authors of the study will need to sample cases from general practice and the community as well as from hospital clinics and wards. Sampling hospital patients is generally much easier; the patients are already well characterized and hospital treatment facilities are likely to be relatively few in number and close to the scanning unit. However, if only hospital patients are sampled, it follows that inference can only be made about the population of hospital patients, rather than the larger and more general population of individuals with the disorder.

Heterogeneity

Diagnostic categories in psychiatry may subsume considerable heterogeneity in terms of phenomenology and aetiology. For example, patients with a diagnosis of schizophrenia may differ profoundly in terms of positive or negative symptom profiles, cognitive deficit, and genetic or environmental risk factors. These natural sources of heterogeneity may be compounded by differences in treatment. Any or all of these factors may affect brain structure. Studies which simply ignore heterogeneity, or attempt to deal with it by *post hoc* statistical correction, may have less power to detect a group difference than studies which define cases according to refined or subdiagnostic criteria. Thus studying a sample of schizophrenic patients with high negative symptom scores and marked working memory deficits may be more likely to reveal anatomical abnormalities of frontal cortex than studying an unrefined sample of patients with schizophrenia. However, there are disadvantages to refined sampling. It is likely to be more time consuming to ascertain a sample of adequate size, and the scope of inference is reduced to the diagnostic subgroup in question.

Matching

Ideally, the control or comparison subjects should be indistinguishable from the patients in every characteristic apart from features of the disorder. For example, it is important that cases and controls should be matched for age, handedness, and sex, since all of these factors may affect brain structure, and a spurious difference between cases and controls might well arise if, say, the patients were on average 20 years older than the controls. Unfortunately, there are a number of other possible confounding factors which are not so obviously unrelated to presence of the disorder. For example, an unrefined sample of patients with schizophrenia will generally have lower IQ and smaller head size than an age- and sex-matched group of comparison subjects. Should we try to correct these differences as if they were spurious (by either refined sampling or *post hoc* statistical modelling), or should we accept that they represent real features of the disorder? In practice, most published studies tend to correct group differences on global variables by statistical modelling in order to focus attention on regional differences which may be more interesting. A comparable problem arises in relation to medication. Cases are likely to have been treated, often for many years, by drugs that can cause structural change to the brain; control subjects, by definition, will not have had this treatment. Because exposure to drug treatment is systematically confounded with diagnostic status, it cannot be well corrected by statistical modelling after the data have been acquired. The only way to be sure that group differences are uncontaminated by medication effects is to sample selectively those patients who have never been treated. However, sampling such a naive group of patients is likely to be time consuming and will also limit the scope of inference.

Other designs

A probable future trend in psychiatric MRI research over the next few years is that the hypotheses under investigation will become more concerned with aetiological mechanisms and pathogenetic models and less concerned with the basic question of whether a given group of patients has abnormal brain structure. This shift in hypothetical interest will dictate a shift in design away from case–control or cross-sectional studies.

Longitudinal designs, in which a cohort of patients are scanned repeatedly over a period of months or years, are a powerful way of demonstrating degenerative or developmental changes in brain structure.[3] They have the obvious disadvantage that they are time consuming to complete and subjects may not attend for multiply repeated examination. Mixed longitudinal designs, in which each subject is scanned just a few times but the sample as a whole includes subjects over a wide range of ages, are a pragmatic alternative for studies of normal and abnormal brain development.

Genetic designs involve subjects that are defined genotypically, rather than phenotypically as in the standard case–control design. Imaging studies of monozygotic twins discordant for a disorder,[4] and of families multiply affected by a disorder, are examples of genetic designs in which there may be complete knowledge about the proportion of genetic information that is shared between subjects but incomplete knowledge about the genetic constitution of each subject. As the human genome becomes better characterized and genetic risk factors for psychiatric disorder are more precisely identified, it is likely that genetic imaging designs will increasingly be focused on the anatomical expression of one or more specific genes.

Overall, there is no single perfect design for an imaging study. Often designing a study will entail finding pragmatic and arguably justifiable solutions to problems for which there is not an absolutely correct answer. Furthermore, the 'goodness' of a design can really only be judged in relation to the hypothesis under investigation and the methods of analysis applied to the data. The best imaging studies will convey a sense that the design is both ingenious and inevitable, given the hypothesis and available methods, and will probably also include a frank discussion of the limitations or implications of the particular design adopted.

Data analysis

Clinical analysis

Structural MRI is most often used in clinical practice to exclude non-psychiatric causes for psychopathology. For example, it is routine in many centres to obtain an MRI examination in all first episodes of psychotic illness to exclude tumours, arteriovenous malformations, or other rare (but surgically treatable) causes of psychosis. Clinical examination of these cases may also sometimes reveal abnormalities such as hippocampal sclerosis or callosal agenesis which suggest that psychopathology has been determined by birth injury or abnormal development. In assessment of a patient with dementia, MRI may usefully demonstrate signs of vascular disease (such as infarcts or periventricular white matter changes), or a focal pattern of grey matter atrophy suggestive of Pick's disease (frontal cortex) or Huntington's disease (caudate nucleus and frontal cortex). All of these abnormalities may be detected simply by skilled visual examination of the data. However, clinical diagnosis of the subtler abnormalities associated with, say, schizophrenia, obsessive–compulsive disorder, or autism would require quantitative analysis of the patient's data and access to a data-

base of normative MRI measurements on appropriately matched samples of the general population. Neither quantitative analysis nor normative databases are widely used in current radiological practice, thus limiting the value of MRI to clinical psychiatry, but this may be expected to change in the future.

Quantitative analysis

There are broadly two requirements for quantitative analysis of structural MRI data. The first is to measure the anatomical structure of the brain (this is often called morphometry). The second is to test hypotheses of interest on the basis of these morphometric variables.[5] Here we shall focus on morphometry.

Morphometry

The most widely used method of measuring brain structure from magnetic resonance images is based on the hypothetical expectation that one or more anatomically defined regions of the brain are particularly relevant to the disorder.[6] The area or volume of each of these regions of interest (**ROIs**) can then be measured directly by drawing a line around the region on a computerized display of the data and counting the number of voxels enclosed by the line. Measurements of several ROIs may be combined to produce summary measures of asymmetry[7] or of spatially distributed anatomical systems such as heteromodal association cortex. The advantages of ROI morphometry are that it is conceptually simple and that it allows measurement of structures (e.g. the hippocampus) or parts of structures (e.g. segments of the corpus callosum) which may be difficult to measure otherwise. Some familiar disadvantages are that it is time consuming and imperfectly reliable. More fundamentally, ROI morphometry is of limited use if it is not obvious in advance what the region of interest is, or there are several possible regions of abnormality (as is likely if the disorder is determined by an insult early in the course of brain development). For these reasons, and although most psychiatric imaging research published to date has used ROI morphometry, it is expected that future studies will preferentially use alternative techniques which are computationally more intensive.

Such techniques are currently an active focus for research and different research groups have adopted somewhat different approaches; the approach adopted by our own group is summarized in Plate 9. In this scheme, the first step in image processing is removal of extracerebral tissues like skull and scalp leaving an image of the brain alone. The brain image is then segmented into the three main tissue classes. There are a variety of techniques for segmentation or brain tissue classification,[8] but generally the quality of segmentation is improved if a dual-echo (fast spin echo) image is available. One method, based on discriminant analysis, requires the operator to select a subset of voxels in the image that are representative of each tissue class; these training data are then used to make a probabilistic assignment of each voxel to one of the three possible classes. Other methods have been developed to avoid even this minimal requirement for human operator intervention, thereby improving speed and reliability.

Once the brain image has been divided into its component classes, or even prior to segmentation in some laboratories, it can be registered in a standard anatomical space.[9] This can be done by finding the mathematical transformation which minimizes the difference between the image and a template image already registered in standard space. The value of making this transformation is potentially twofold. First, it then becomes possible to compare brain structure between individuals at the spatial resolution of the image, i.e. in terms of the percentage occupancy of each voxel by each tissue class. This means that one is able ultimately to test anatomical differences between groups over the whole brain in detail, without having to assume *a priori* that pathological change is located in a particular region.[10] The second major advantage of image registration is that the parameters of the transformation used to align the image with the template may themselves be used as measures of brain structure. Thus, if an image represents a brain that is structurally abnormal in some way, the mathematical deformation which must be applied to align it with a standard template may be abnormally great.[11]

Statistical testing

Morphometric variables of any description can be used to test hypotheses by a variety of statistical analyses. For example, the null hypothesis of zero difference in brain structure between two groups can be addressed by a *t*-test of a single ROI or by many thousands of *t*-tests of, say, grey matter occupancy measured at each and every voxel. Similarly hypotheses concerning the relationship between brain structure and psychological function can be addressed by testing the correlation between a morphometric variable and the subjects' scores on a psychometric instrument.[12] Alternatively, the relationships between several morphometric variables may be explored by multivariate methods such as principal component or factor analysis.[13]

Further reading

1. Pierpaoli, C., Jezzard, P., Basser, P.J., Barnett, A., and Di Chiro, G. (1996). Diffusion tensor MR imaging of the human brain. *Radiology*, **201**, 637–48.
2. Buchsbaum, M.S., Tang, C.Y., Peled, S., *et al.* (1998). Fronto-striatal circuitry, MRI white matter diffusion anisotropy, and PET metabolic rate in schizophrenia. *NeuroReport*, **9**, 425–30.
3. Weinberger, D.R., Berman, K.F., Suddath, R., and Fuller Torrey, E. (1992). Evidence of dysfunction of a prefrontal-limbic network in schizophrenia: a magnetic resonance imaging study and regional cerebral blood flow study of discordant monozygotic twins. *American Journal of Psychiatry*, **149**, 890–7.
4. Saeed, N., Puri, B.K., Oatridge, A., Hajnal, J.V., and Young, I.R. (1998). Two methods for semi-automated quantification of changes in ventricular volume and their use in schizophrenia. *Magnetic Resonance Imaging*, **16**, 1237–47.
5. Bullmore, E.T., Suckling, J., Overmeyer, S., Rabe-Hesketh, S., Taylor, E., and Brammer, M.J. (1999). Global, voxel and cluster tests, by theory and permutation, for a difference between two groups of structural MR images. *IEEE Transactions on Medical Imaging*, **18**, 32–42.
6. Lawrie, S.M. and Abukmeil, S.S. (1998). Brain abnormality in schizophrenia. A systematic and quantitative review of volumetric magnetic resonance imaging studies. *British Journal of Psychiatry*, **172**, 110–20.
7. Bilder, R.M., Wu, H., Bogerts, B., *et al.* (1994). Absence of regional volume asymmetries in first episode schizophrenia. *American Journal of Psychiatry*, **151**, 1437–47.
8. Clarke, L.P., Velthuizen, R.P., Camacho, M.A., *et al.* (1995). MRI segmentation: methods and applications. *Magnetic Resonance Imaging*, **13**, 343–68.
9. Andreasen, N.C., Arndt, S., Swayze, V., *et al.* (1994). Thalamic abnormalities in schizophrenia visualised through magnetic resonance image averaging. *Science*, **266**, 294–8.
10. Wright, I.C., Ellison, Z.R., Sharma, T., Friston, K.J., Murray, R.M., and
McGuire, P.K. (1999). Mapping of grey matter changes in schizophrenia. *Schizophrenia Research*, **35**, 1–14.
11. Csernansky, J.G., Joshi, S., Wang, L., *et al.* (1998). Hippocampal morphometry in schizophrenia by high dimensional brain mapping. *Proceedings of the National Academy of Sciences of the United States of America*, **95**, 11406–11.
12. Barta, P.E., Pearlson, G.D., Powers, R.E., Richards, S.S., and Tune, L.E. (1990). Auditory hallucinations and smaller superior temporal gyral volume in schizophrenia. *American Journal of Psychiatry*, **147**, 1457–62.
13. Tien, A.Y., Eaton, W.W., Schlaepfer, T.E., *et al.* (1996). Exploratory factor analysis of MRI brain structure measures in schizophrenia. *Schizophrenia Research*, **19**, 93–101.

2.3.8 Functional magnetic resonance imaging

E. T. Bullmore and J. Suckling

Introduction

Functional magnetic resonance imaging (**fMRI**) is a relatively new technique for measuring changes in cerebral blood flow. The first fMRI studies, showing functional activation of the occipital cortex by visual stimulation and activation of the motor cortex by finger movement, were published in the early 1990s[1–3]. In the few years since then, fMRI has been used to investigate the physiological response to a wide variety of experimental procedures in both normal human subjects and diverse patient groups. By 1997, there were approximately 500 sites worldwide with the capacity to perform functional MRI research. This number can be expected to increase considerably over the next 15 years. Over the same time, fMRI will probably establish a role for itself in radiological and psychiatric practice; currently the clinical role of fMRI is limited to specialized applications such as assessment of hemispheric dominance prior to neurosurgery.[4]

The outstanding advantage of fMRI over alternative methods of imaging cerebral blood flow, such as positron emission tomography (**PET**) and single-photon emission computed tomography (**SPECT**), is that it does not involve exposure to radioactivity. This means that a single subject can safely be examined by fMRI on many occasions, and that the ethical problems of examining patients are minimized. Functional MRI also has superior spatial resolution (of the order of millimetres) and temporal resolution (of the order of seconds) compared with PET and SPECT.

In this chapter, we provide an introduction to technical issues relevant to fMRI data acquisition, study design, and analysis. An introduction to the basic physical principles of magnetization and nuclear magnetic resonance, and the technology, is given in Chapter 2.3.7.

Cerebral activation and blood-flow changes

Try closing your eyes and then opening them again. At the moment that you open your eyes, neurones in the occipital cortex that are specialized for the perception of visual stimuli will show a sudden and dramatic increase in their rate of discharge. There is a short delay (approximately 100 ms) between the stimulus and neural response owing to the propagation of electrical activity from the retina via the optic nerves and tracts to the visual cortex. Later, some 3 to 8 s after stimulus onset, there will be an accompanying change in the local blood supply to the stimulated area of cortex. Blood flow increases without a commensurate increase in oxygen uptake by the visual cortex, leading to a local increase in the ratio of oxygenated to deoxygenated forms of haemoglobin.

The linkage between neural activity and regional cerebral blood flow, sometimes called neurovascular coupling, has been known since Roy and Sherrington first reported 'changes in blood supply in accordance with local variations of functional activity' in 1894. However, the molecular mechanisms for neurovascular coupling are still uncertain. Neuronal activity causes a local accumulation of vasodilating metabolites, such as hydrogen ions, which might mediate a vascular response. There may also be a neurogenic mechanism whereby groups of neurones control their own perfusion by innervating the smooth muscular walls of the arterioles supplying them with blood.

Exogenous and endogenous contrast agents

The fact that neural activity is linked to local blood flow provides the opportunity for functional MRI. Broadly, there are two ways in which altered blood flow can produce measurable change in magnetic resonance signals.

The first involves the administration of an exogenous contrast agent, such as gadolinium diethylenetriaminepentaacetic acid (**Gd-DTPA**). Gd-DTPA has marked paramagnetic properties causing a local change in the effective magnetic field. When given intravenously as a bolus while the subject is exposed to experimental stimulation, Gd-DTPA causes locally increased field strength in those regions (and only those regions) that are neurally activated by the stimulus. This effect on the field alters the magnetic resonance properties of protons, namely the spin–spin relaxation time, creating tissue contrast between brain regions activated by the stimulus and regions that are not activated.

The second approach involves exploiting the existence of an endogenous contrast agent. Iron in deoxygenated haemoglobin has paramagnetic properties similar to Gd-DTPA. It also does not diffuse out of the vascular compartment. Neural activity causes a local reduction in the ratio of deoxygenated to oxygenated haemoglobin, so that the paramagnetic effects of deoxyhaemoglobin are 'diluted'. Since apparent spin–spin relaxation or dephasing is accelerated by microscopic inhomogeneities in the magnetic field due to the presence of paramagnetic contrast agents, the net effect of diluting deoxyhaemoglobin will be to prolong T_2^* times in areas of the brain that receive an increased blood flow as a consequence of neural activity. The haemodynamic effect on spin–spin relaxation can be measured by a T_2^*-weighted signal which is blood oxygen level dependent (**BOLD**).

Note that gadolinium infusion causes a somewhat larger signal decrease (about 5 per cent) than the signal increase (about 3 per cent) associated with the activity-dependent dilution of deoxyhaemoglobin. However, endogenous contrast is generally preferable on the grounds that it does not require an intravenous infusion.

Imaging sequences for fMRI

Several different pulse sequences can be used to collect MRI data which are sensitive to functionally determined changes in signal strength. Here we will concentrate on gradient echo sequences which, combined with special techniques for very rapid data acquisition, have been most widely used to date for fMRI. However, note that spin echo sequences can also be used for functional MRI data acquisition, and that gradient echo sequences can be used for structural MRI.

Gradient echo sequence

The basic principle is similar to spin echo imaging. An initial excitation pulse of radiofrequency energy is supplied at the Larmor frequency to the brain in the presence of a powerful static magnetic field. Protons are excited to a state characterized by increased transverse magnetization and a coherent phase of precession around the axis of the external field. Immediately the radiofrequency pulse has ceased, protons begin to relax back to their equilibrium state of maximum longitudinal magnetization and random phase of precession, emitting a radiofrequency signal by free induction decay.

In gradient echo imaging, the process of spin–spin relaxation (dephasing) is first accelerated by briefly applying a gradient to the magnetic field shortly after the excitation pulse. Then, at some time (TE/2) after the excitation pulse, a second gradient is applied to reverse the process of dephasing, causing rephasing and a signal maximum or echo some time (TE) after excitation. The sequence is repetitively applied with a constant time interval between consecutive excitations (TR).

The objective is to manipulate spin–spin relaxation by brief perturbations of the external magnetic field rather than by supplying additional pulses of radiofrequency energy as in spin echo imaging. Frequency- and phase-encoding gradients are applied to locate the sources of signal in three-dimensional space (see Chapter 2.3.7).

One advantage of gradient echo imaging is that TE and TR can both be shorter than in spin echo imaging, allowing an overall reduction in scanning time. However, if TR is short, spoiler gradients or radiofrequency pulses may be needed to ensure that the protons have returned to equilibrium before the next excitation pulse is supplied. The flip angle α induced by radiofrequency excitation can be adjusted to generate images weighted by different sources of tissue contrast. T_1-weighted images are generated by radiofrequency pulses causing flip angles of the order of 10° to 20°. For functionally sensitive T_2-weighted images, more radiofrequency energy must be supplied in the excitation pulse to give a flip angle approaching 90°.

Echo-planar imaging

The gradient echo sequence equivalent to a fast spin echo sequence is obtained by rapidly applying, or blipping, a series of rephasing gradients following the excitation pulse and dephasing gradient. Gradient blipping is done extremely rapidly (< 1 ms), and up to 128 echoes can be generated from a single excitation. Clearly, the advantage of such echoplanar imaging is the speed of acquisition. Multislice images of the entire cortex, with slice thickness of only a few millimetres, can be acquired in 3 s or less. Such high-speed imaging is highly desirable for functional MRI, where we wish to detect physiologically determined changes in magnetic resonance signal with the best possible temporal resolution. However, the hardware required for rapid gradient blipping has only become available on clinical machines in the last few years.

Artefacts

The main sources of artefact in functional MRI are the same as for structural MRI (see Chapter 2.3.7).

Movement

Movement of the subject's head during fMRI data acquisition is inevitable, and attempts to eliminate it by fixing the head in the scanner may paradoxically exacerbate the problem. The best approach to minimizing movement is to ensure that the subjects are not unduly anxious about the scanning procedure, that they understand clearly what they are being asked to do, and that they are comfortable in the scanner before data acquisition begins. Experiments should be designed so that they do not require the subject to move extensively; small finger movements required for button pressing do not generally cause severe head movement. However, even very small movements of the head (less than 1 mm) can cause significant artefacts in fMRI data.

Involuntary or physiological movements are mostly due to the cardiorespiratory cycle causing pulsation of the cerebrospinal fluid and vascular spaces. Therefore these movements often occur at a higher frequency than the frequency of image volume acquisition, and are aliased into the signal as a low-frequency confound. The problem can be minimized by cardiac gating, which means timing the acquisition of images relative to the cardiac cycle measured by ECG.

Susceptibility

The susceptibility artefact is exaggerated by gradient echoplanar imaging, typically causing signal loss in inferior temporal and orbitofrontal brain regions close to bone or sinuses. The problem is further compounded if subjects are asked to speak during scanning, since slight deformations of the sinuses associated with overt articulation can cause changes in susceptibility artefact which can mimic signal changes due to speech-related neural activity. If overt articulation is necessary to monitor the subject's performance on the experimental task, then it is advisable to design the sequence so that images are not acquired while the subject is speaking.

Hardware

The hardware requirements for functional MRI include a superconducting magnet, a radiofrequency coil, computers, and a purpose-built room, as described in Chapter 2.3.7.

Gradient coils

The essential extra prerequisite is gradient coils capable of very rapidly blipping the external magnetic field for echoplanar imaging. The gradients required are small compared with the external field (1 to 10 mT/m) but may need to be applied for less than 1 ms. The speed with which the gradient is switched on, the slew rate, is necessarily fast (up to 200 mT/m/s). Such rapidly changing gradients can cause eddy currents in the gradient coils, adversely affecting the homogeneity of the field. This problem is minimized by actively shielding the coils, which requires yet another set of coils.

Audiovisual equipment

It must be possible to present visual and auditory stimuli to subjects while they are lying with their heads in the bore of the magnet. Headphones are required to clearly present auditory stimuli in the presence of the loud background noise of gradient switching. Visual stimuli can be projected on to a screen which is viewed through a system of mirrors. The subject should have access to an alert button. In addition, it is generally useful for subjects to use a button-press device to indicate their response to cognitively demanding experimental tasks. These behavioural data will need to be monitored during scanning.

Experimental design

The basic principle of experimental design in fMRI is to manipulate the subject's experience or behaviour in some way that is likely to produce a functionally specific neurovascular response. It is usually important that the experiment should be designed to allow some other measure of response, for instance a button press, to be monitored simultaneously. We shall illustrate these and other principles by considering how one might design an experiment to identify the regions of the brain that are important in making a (semantic) decision about the meaning of words. As will become clear, no single design is ideal; each has its strengths and weaknesses, and the choice between them should be considered carefully in the light of the particular hypothesis one is using fMRI to test.

Blocked periodic design

This is the most common experimental design and is adaptable to a wide range of investigations. The simplest form involves alternately presenting the subject with two conditions: an activation (A) condition and a baseline (B) condition. Each condition is presented for an identical epoch of time. During each epoch, several stimuli are sequentially presented with an interstimulus interval (**ISI**) that is less than the epoch length. The cycle of alternation between A and B conditions is repeated a number of times over the course of each experiment.

For example, during each 30-s epoch of the A condition, we could visually present subjects with a series of 12 common concrete nouns (ISI = 2.5 s) and ask them to decide for each word whether it refers to an animate object (e.g. 'goat') or an inanimate object (e.g. 'bucket'). The subjects could be asked to indicate their decision by pressing one of two buttons: left for living objects and right for non-living objects. During each 30-s epoch of the B condition, we could present words at the same rate, but ask subjects to decide whether they are written in upper- or lower-case letters. This decision could be monitored by button press as in the A condition. The two epochs could be presented alternately, beginning with the B condition, in five cycles for a total experimental time of 5 min. Functional MRI data would be acquired continuously throughout the experiment (Fig. 1).

The rationale for this design is that the two conditions are matched in all respects apart from semantic analysis; words are visually presented at an identical rate, and subjects are asked to signal their decision by an identical device. But while condition A demands semantic

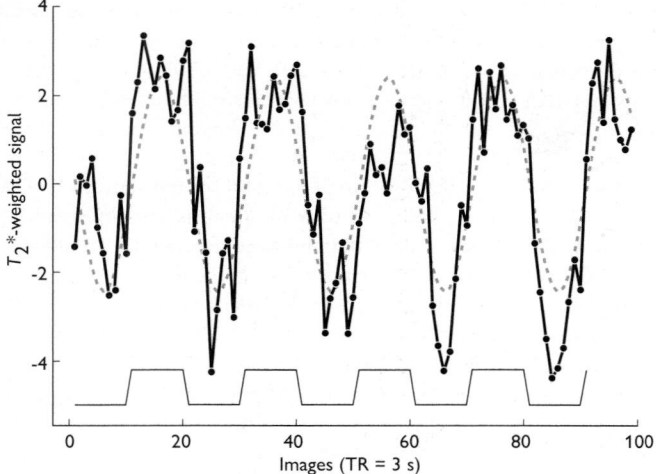

Fig. 1 Design, response, and modelled response for a blocked periodic experiment. The experimental design or input function is represented by a square wave (solid line), which alternates periodically between a baseline (B) and an activation (A) condition. The B condition is presented first, and the BA cycle is repeated five times in the course of the experiment. Images are acquired every 3 s during the experiment, and the T_2*-weighted signal observed at an activated voxel is shown by points joined by a solid line. There is clearly a signal increase during the A condition. The modelled response, a phase-shifted sine wave, is shown by the broken line. In these data the estimated haemodynamic delay is 3.6 s.

analysis of the words (what do they mean?), condition B demands only orthographic analysis (what do they look like?). We assume that only those regions of the brain that are specifically responsible for semantic analysis will show an increased magnetic resonance signal during condition A; those regions responsible for visual perception and motor output will be activated identically under both conditions, and so will not demonstrate a periodic signal change at the frequency of AB alternation. This set of assumptions is sometimes referred to as cognitive subtraction.[5]

Blocked periodic designs can generate robust signal changes in fMRI, as long as the two conditions are not too closely matched. The drawbacks are that it is impossible to assess the response to a single stimulus and the critical assumption of cognitive subtraction may not always be valid. Sometimes two experimental tasks that appear to differ only in terms of one component process may actually invoke entirely different cognitive strategies and so cause activation of entirely different neurocognitive networks.

Parametric design

Parametric designs are so called because the same task is presented throughout the experiment but some continuously variable parameter of the task is experimentally manipulated.[6,7] For example, we could ask subjects to perform the semantic analysis task for 5 min, but continuously vary the interval between consecutive stimuli (words) from 10 s at the start of the experiment to 1 s at the end. Here we are assuming that as the task becomes more difficult, i.e. the interstimulus interval becomes shorter, blood flow to the regions specialized for semantic analysis will increase. The main advantage of this design is that it avoids the assumption of cognitive subtraction; the main disadvantage is that it may lack specificity. Motor and visual cortex, as well as brain

regions specialized for semantic analysis, will probably show an increased blood flow as the rate of stimulus presentation is increased.

Single-trial design

Single-trial designs are sometimes called event-related designs.[8,9] A series of stimuli are presented and the magnetic resonance signal response to each individual stimulus is measured. Single-trial designs may be coupled with sequences for very rapid image acquisition so that the temporal pattern of response to a single event can be resolved in detail. A single-trial design would be advantageous for our semantic analysis experiment if we were particularly interested in correlating some aspect of the behavioural response to each stimulus, for instance accuracy of decision or reaction time, with the neurovascular response measured using fMRI. A disadvantage of such designs is that signal changes induced by a single trial are generally weak compared with the 2 to 5 per cent signal changes that are typical in blocked periodic experiments.

Beyond a single experiment

If the hypothesis in question demands the investigation of more than a few subjects and/or more than one experimental condition, it is advisable to seek expert statistical advice at the outset. In general, it is important that randomization should be used appropriately to eliminate confounding effects of the order in which experiments are conducted, and of the order in which different subjects are scanned. Practice on a task may substantially alter the neurovascular response, and so all subjects should receive preliminary training on the task according to a standard protocol. If there is considerable variability between subjects in their ability to perform a task, consider adjusting the difficulty of the task presented in the scanner so that each subject is performing at the same level in terms of accuracy or reaction time. The use of functional MRI to study longitudinal changes by repeated examination of the same subject(s), for instance before and after the administration of a drug, will generally improve the statistical power to detect the effect of interest by controlling for idiosyncratic variability of functional response between subjects.

Data analysis

General principles of data analysis are reviewed here; for more detailed coverage of the issues and the methods implemented in a variety of software packages, see the reviews by Lange[9] and Rabe-Hesketh *et al.*[10]

Movement estimation and correction

The first step in fMRI data analysis is to estimate the extent of head motion during data acquisition and to correct it.[11] Gross head movement (of several millimetres) can be detected simply by viewing the images acquired over time at a given slice. However, because of the multislice acquisition protocols generally used for fMRI, the magnetic field to which the brain is exposed will change dramatically within the space of a few micrometres at the superior and inferior edges of a selectively irradiated slice. This means that minute head movements

(< 1 mm) can have disproportionately large effects on magnetic resonance signal emission.

Head movement occurring at the same time as experimental stimuli are presented, namely stimulus correlated motion, can artefactually exaggerate the neurovascular response. Head movement occurring randomly with respect to the experimental design is more likely to cause the opposite problem of artefactually attenuating the measured response. Therefore it is essential to supplement visual inspection of the data by computerized methods for movement estimation and its correction.

Statistical models for the neurovascular response

The next step in analysis is to estimate the strength of the experimentally determined signal change in the time series of magnetic resonance signal measurements at each voxel in the image. This requires some sort of statistical model for the response. The simplest model, for a blocked periodic design, is a square wave at the same frequency as the experimental input function. This model assumes that a brain region activated specifically by condition A will show an immediate increase in signal intensity, which is sustained throughout the epoch until the onset of condition B. The problem with this model is that the increase in magnetic resonance signal during condition A is due to changes in blood flow and oxygenation, which are delayed by several seconds relative to the onset of condition A. Furthermore, this haemodynamic delay between stimulus onset and measurable response will be variable from one fMRI time series to another. Therefore it is important that the experimental effect should be modelled as an increase in signal intensity that is arbitrarily delayed relative to the onset of the activating stimulus. Various suitable models have been proposed for periodic designs, including a phase-shifted sine wave at the frequency of AB alternation (Fig. 1). Failure to allow for a variable haemodynamic delay may cause underestimation of the experimental effect, and subsequent loss of statistical power to detect activated voxels.

No model is perfect and, whatever model is chosen for the neurovascular response in fMRI, there will probably be some mismatch with the data. For example, both square-wave and sine-wave models for the response to a periodically designed experiment assume that the amplitude of response is exactly the same for each epoch of the activation condition. In fact, it is not unusual for the amplitude of response to vary from one epoch to another. Mismatch between the data and the model means that the residuals obtained by fitting the model to the data may not be pure noise. In turn, this can lead to voxels being incorrectly identified as activated. Another source of this problem is high-frequency physiological movements due to the cardiorespiratory cycle.

Activation mapping

The next step in analysis is often to decide which of the several thousand voxels in the image have demonstrated such a strong response to the experiment that it is unlikely to be due to chance. In other words, we want to identify the significantly activated voxels. Let us assume that we have estimated the neurovascular response by the amplitude of a sine wave at each and every voxel, and refer to this as our test statistic. The problem is then to assign a probability to each estimated amplitude under the null hypothesis that the experiment had no effect on the brain. To do this we need to know the probability distribution of our test statistic under the null hypothesis. There are broadly two ways

we can know this distribution: we can work it out from mathematical theory, or we can sample it by randomly permuting the data. Theoretical distributions are quicker to evaluate than permutation distributions, but permutation entails many fewer assumptions and is the gold standard against which the validity of theoretical approximations should be checked.

Once we have a probability distribution for the test statistic, we still have to decide what p value we wish to adopt as our threshold for activation. If we choose a small (conservative) p value (i.e. < 0.00001), only those voxels that demonstrate a very powerful response will be identified as activated. There will be few false-positive or type 1 errors, i.e. almost all the voxels we identify as activated will truly be activated. But there will probably be a large number of false-negative or type 2 errors, i.e. many voxels that are truly activated will not be identified as such. Conversely, if we choose a large (lenient) p value (i.e. 0.01), there will be a larger number of false-positive errors but a smaller number of false-negative errors. The choice of p value should be informed by the search volume, or the number of voxels tested for significance. The larger the search volume, the smaller the p value will need to be for an acceptable degree of type 1 error control. A rule of thumb is that the p value should be approximately the reciprocal of the search volume. More elaborate methods have been advocated for correcting p values for large numbers of tests on imaging data.

An alternative approach to testing tens of thousands of voxels against a suitably small probability threshold, with an associated risk of major type 2 error, is to combine information about the experimental response over several voxels. For example, we can initially apply a lenient threshold ($p = 0.05$) to the test statistics estimated at each voxel, and set to zero any voxel that does not have a test statistic greater than the corresponding critical value. The result will be a map of several spatially contiguous clusters, ranging in size from a single voxel to several hundred voxels (Plate 10). We can ascertain the probability distribution for cluster size under the null hypothesis either by theory or permutation. Then we can proceed to identify significantly activated clusters instead of voxels. The advantage of hypothesis testing at cluster level is a greater power to detect significant foci of activation, partly because there will be many fewer clusters than voxels to test, so the p value can be legitimately increased. The disadvantage is the loss of spatial resolution of activation.

Multivariate approaches

Many of the 'higher-order' cognitive tasks that are likely to be of greatest interest to psychiatric research do not activate a single modular region of the brain. Instead, they typically activate several spatially distinct or distributed regions that together comprise a large-scale neurocognitive network for performance of the task. It may then be of interest to investigate functional integration between different regions or nodes of the network. The simplest way to do this is by estimating the correlation between a pair of fMRI time series observed at different voxels or regions. Large correlations, whether negative or positive, may be described as evidence for functional connectivity. Psychiatric disorders may be characterized by abnormal functional relationships between coactivated regions, or functional dysconnectivity.

More sophisticated techniques for investigating functional relationships between large numbers of voxels or regions include multivariate methods such as principal component analysis, discriminant analysis, and path analysis. These methods are equally applicable to structural MRI data, where they may provide indirect evidence for anatomical connectivity between regions.

Within- and between-group analysis

Once a measure or parameter of experimental response has been estimated in each fMRI time series, the resulting parameter maps can be registered in standard space. There are many possible computational algorithms for spatial registration. The most commonly used at present is an affine transformation, which applies a global and linear rescaling in three dimensions to each individual image. The most commonly adopted standard space is that represented in a stereotactic atlas of the brain originally written by Talairach and Tournoux to assist neurosurgeons in locating subcortical structures.[12] In both systems, each voxel is assigned a set of $\{x,y,z\}$ coordinates which define its position. In Talairach–Tournoux space, the coordinates are defined relative to the cerebral midline and a line is drawn between the anterior and posterior commissures (intercommissural or AC–PC line). After registration, parameter maps are usually smoothed by applying a two- or three-dimensional Gaussian filter to accommodate variability in sulcogyral anatomy between subjects and error in spatial registration.

It is then possible to test a wide variety of hypotheses about the response parameters measured over several subjects at each voxel in standard space. For example, one can test the null hypothesis that there is zero mean or median power of experimental response within a group, or the null hypothesis that there is zero difference in the power of response between two groups. It is also possible to test for correlations between the power of functional response and some behavioural or symptom measure within a group. All these statistical tests can be conducted by permutation as well as by theory, and at cluster level as well as voxel level (see above).

Visualization

The final result of fMRI data analysis will often be visualized as a map in standard space. The background for the map will generally be a grey-scale image of cerebral anatomy. This image could be simply the fMRI data averaged over time at each slice. Alternatively, one might wish to use a structural MRI dataset with superior spatial resolution or tissue contrast between grey and white matter. In this case, one should beware of the potential discrepancy in geometric distortion between images of the same brain acquired using different sequences.

The background image will often be combined with, or substituted by, a rectangular grid allowing any feature of interest to be referred directly to the appropriate atlas of standard anatomical space. If the image is displayed as a series of two-dimensional slices, the z co-ordinate for each slice in standard space should also be displayed. Images are often rendered so that the right side of the brain is represented by the left side of each slice.

Voxels or clusters that demonstrate a significant effect are generally coloured against the grey-scale background image (Plate 11). A range of colours can be used to encode additional information. For example, the haemodynamic delay of response at each generically activated voxel may be colour coded by a continuous spectrum. Other strategies for visualization include use of three-dimensional rendering to show foci of activation in the context of the sulcogyral anatomy of a whole hemisphere, and 'flat mapping' whereby the template image is deformed to a smooth sphere and then mapped to a plane before activation foci are superimposed on it.[13]

Further reading

1. Kwong, K.K., Belliveau, J.W., Chesler, D.A., *et al.* (1992). Dynamic magnetic resonance imaging of human brain activity during primary sensory stimulation. *Proceedings of the National Academy of Sciences of the United States of America*, **89**, 5675–9.
2. Stehling, M.K., Turner, R., and Mansfield, P. (1991). Echo-planar imaging: magnetic resonance imaging in a fraction of a second. *Science*, **254**, 43–50.
3. Le Bihan, D. and Karni, A. (1995). Applications of magnetic resonance imaging to the study of human brain function. *Current Biology*, **5**, 231–7.
4. Desmond, J.E., Sum, J.M., Wagner, A.D., *et al.* (1995). Functional MRI measurement of language lateralisation in Wada-tested patients. *Brain*, **118**, 1411–19.
5. Friston, K.J., Price, C.J., Fletcher, P., Moore, C., Frackowiak, R.S.J., and Dolan, R.J. (1996). The trouble with cognitive subtraction. *NeuroImage*, **4**, 97–104.
6. Braver, T.S., Cohen, J.D., Nystrom, L.E., Jonides, J., Smith, E.E., and Noll, D.C. (1997). A parametric study of prefrontal cortex involvement in human working memory. *NeuroImage*, **5**, 49–62.
7. Buckner, R.L., Bandettini, P.A., O'Craven, K.M., *et al.* (1996). Detection of cortical activation during averaged single trials of a cognitive task using functional magnetic resonance imaging. *Proceedings of the National Academy of Sciences of the United States of America*, **89**, 11069–73.
8. Zarahn, E., Aguirre, G., and D'Esposito, M. (1997). A trial-based experimental design for fMRI. *NeuroImage*, **6**, 122–38.
9. Lange, N. (1996). Statistical approaches to human brain mapping by functional magnetic resonance imaging. *Statistics in Medicine*, **15**, 389–428.
10. Rabe-Hesketh, S., Bullmore, E.T., and Brammer, M.J. (1997). The analysis of functional magnetic resonance images. *Statistical Methods in Medical Research*, **6**, 215–37.
11. Bullmore, E. T., Brammer, M.J., Rabe-Hesketh, S., *et al.* (1999). Methods for diagnosis and treatment of stimulus correlated motion in generic brain activation studies using fMRI. *Human Brain Mapping*, **7**, 38–48.
12. Talairach, J. and Tournoux, P. (1988). *Co-planar stereotaxic atlas of the human brain*. Thieme, Stuttgart.
13. Sereno, M.I., Dale, A.M., Reppas, J.B., *et al.* (1995). Borders of multiple visual areas in human brain revealed by functional magnetic resonance imaging. *Science*, **268**, 889–93.

2.3.9 Neuronal networks, epilepsy, and other brain dysfunctions

John G. R. Jefferys

Aims

The hippocampal formation is implicated in several important psychiatric and neurological problems. The hippocampus and amygdala are often the site of epileptic foci which can lead to problems in learning and memory, emotion, anxiety, and other problems. This kind of epilepsy is variously known as temporal lobe epilepsy, complex partial seizures, or limbic epilepsy. The hippocampus, with associated limbic areas, has been linked both to affective disorders and to psychoses including schizophrenia. This chapter will consider the cellular organization of the hippocampus and then outline aspects of the emergent

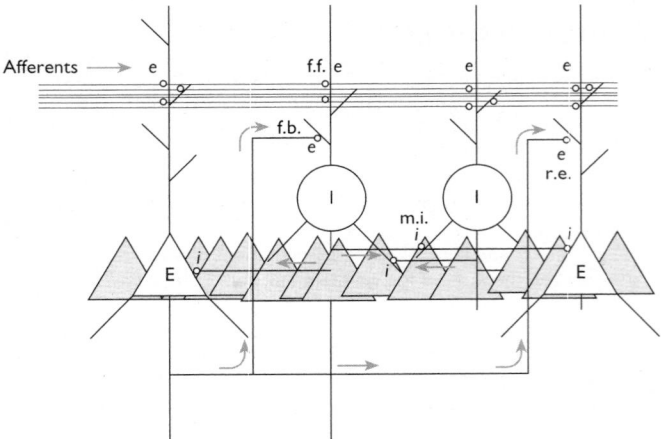

Fig. 1 Schematic illustration of hippocampal neuronal network. There are many more excitatory pyramidal cells (E and triangles) than inhibitory interneurones (I and circles). As with most neurones, they receive inputs onto their dendrites and somata (the latter contain the nucleus and are represented by a triangle or circle). The level of simplification is clear from the observation that each pyramidal cell receives tens of thousands of synapses. Axons from other regions, known as afferents, make excitatory synapses (e) with both pyramidal cells and interneurones. Most of the interneurones make inhibitory synapses (i) onto pyramidal cells. The inhibition of the pyramidal cell is called 'feed-forward' (f.f.) when the interneurones were excited by afferent axons and 'feed-back' (f.b.) when they were excited by pyramidal cells. Interneurones also inhibit each other forming a mutually inhibitory network (m.i.); this network is important in some kinds of physiological network oscillation (see text). Finally, pyramidal cells make excitatory synapses onto each other (r.e.) which can lead to epileptic discharges if not held in check by inhibitory mechanisms.

properties of neuronal networks in the hippocampus and speculative role in psychiatric disorders. Cellular and network mechanisms of focal epilepsy, and learning impairments associated with limbic epilepsy will be reviewed.

A central element in this chapter is the idea that the functional organization of neuronal networks plays a key role in the normal and pathological operation of the brain. For brevity (and for the author's convenience) the examples concern the hippocampus, but similar principles apply in the neocortex and other parts of the brain.

Hippocampal organization

Anatomy

The hippocampus resembles the neocortex in containing a majority of excitatory neurones, the pyramidal cells and granule cells, which use glutamate as their neurotransmitter (E in Fig. 1).[1,2] Most of the remaining neurones in the hippocampus are inhibitory, and use γ-aminobutyric acid (GABA) as their neurotransmitter (I in Fig. 1). The inhibitory neurones fall into several distinct subtypes according to where their axons go (and hence which cells they inhibit), where their cell bodies are, the shapes of their dendrites, whether they contain more than one transmitter, and whether they contain particular calcium-binding proteins. This chapter will ignore most of the diversity of interneurones.

Evoked responses

Each hippocampal (or cortical) area receives 'afferent' synaptic inputs from other areas. Most afferents are excitatory; stimulating them provides a convenient tool to study the operation of the neuronal circuits involved. The responses evoked in hippocampal neurones typically start with an excitatory postsynaptic potential. If the excitatory postsynaptic potential is strong enough, it will result in an action potential triggered at a low-threshold zone near the cell body, probably a short distance down the axon. The excitatory postsynaptic potential is followed by a fast and a slow inhibitory postsynaptic potential. Both the fast inhibitory and the excitatory postsynaptic potentials are due to ligand-gated channels where the transmitter receptor (GABA$_A$ and glutamate α-amino-3-hydroxy-5-methyl-4-isoxazolepropionic acid (AMPA)/kainic acid or N-methyl-D-aspartate respectively) is part of the same molecular structure as the ion channel (chloride and partially selective cationic respectively). The slow inhibitory postsynaptic potential is due to GABA$_B$ receptors which are G protein coupled and use second messengers to open separate potassium channels.

Inhibitory neurones can be triggered both by activity in the principal cells (pyramidal or granule), resulting in recurrent or feedback inhibition, and directly by the incoming afferents, resulting in feedforward inhibition. The synchrony of the stimulation of the afferent input imposes synchrony on the response with the useful consequence that the extracellular currents generated by the activity of individual pyramidal or granule cells can summate (because the cells are located in tight layers) and produce large 'field potentials' comprising a population excitatory postsynaptic potential, followed by a population spike.

Evoked field potentials are over in 10 to 20 ms and the slowest intracellular components end within a few hundred milliseconds to a second. However, stimulation can elicit much more prolonged responses in the hippocampus. The best known of these is long-term potentiation, in which a brief train of stimuli can result in an increase, lasting hours or days, in the response to a fixed test stimulus. The modest conditioning event and the enduring consequence make long-term potentiation an attractive model of learning and memory, although the evidence that it really is the direct cellular substrate for learning remains circumstantial.[3] It is perhaps more likely that long-term potentiation provides an artificial experimental tool that depends on cellular and molecular mechanisms that may also be involved in learning and/or other plastic changes in synaptic strength.

Local circuits

Hippocampal neurones are not just arranged as a simple synaptic relay where afferents excite target cells to produce an output depending on the size of the input and the state of inhibition at that time. Instead there exists a complex synaptic network, or local circuit, interlinking neurones of all kinds (Fig. 1 gives a very much simplified illustration of some of the salient features of hippocampal local circuits). This chapter considers two kinds of emergent network activity that arise from this organization: focal epilepsy and gamma rhythms.

Experimental approaches

Unravelling the cellular and network mechanisms of emergent network phenomena depends on a combination of electrophysiology, pharmacology, anatomy, and realistic computer simulations. Two practical issues may need a brief introduction

Brain slices

Brain slices have played a pivotal role in developing theories on the operation of neuronal networks. Slices about 0.4 mm thick are cut from the brains of deeply anaesthetised or recently killed experimental animals, or sometimes from humans undergoing neurosurgery. Brain slices can survive many hours *in vitro* in an artificial cerebrospinal fluid, usually equilibrated with 95 per cent oxygen and 5 per cent carbon dioxide (with bicarbonate providing a pH buffer). If the slices are prepared under sterile conditions, they can survive for weeks as 'organotypic slice cultures'. In both cases the visualization of the anatomy of the living slice helps locate electrodes, the mechanical stability greatly simplifies recordings from inside neurones, and the lack of a blood–brain barrier facilitates drug applications and changes in ion concentrations. Brain slices have proved immensely popular and successful, but it is important to remember that they are only one tool in the armoury needed to study brain function, and that ultimately results from them must be put in the context of the whole organism.

Realistic computer simulations

Computer simulations provide the means to determine whether what we know at one level, for instance of the properties of individual neurones and their interconnections, are necessary and sufficient to explain the emergent properties at the next level, here of circuits of a few thousand neurones. The most useful models for this purpose are tightly constrained by experimental data, and ideally are used to make experimentally testable predictions. Mostly they consist of several 'compartments' to represent the anatomy of the neurone's dendrites and soma. Each compartment consists of several differential equations representing specific ion channels which may be gated by membrane potential, extracellular neurotransmitters, or intracellular calcium. Large numbers of neurones can then be wired together in larger-scale simulations, using biologically realistic anatomical connectivity and synaptic properties.[4,5]

Emergent properties of hippocampal networks

Hippocampal rhythms

The organization of hippocampal networks (Fig. 1) leads to several distinct kinds of oscillation, which can be considered as 'emergent' properties of the network.[2] Perhaps the most prominent rhythm in the hippocampus is theta (3–7 Hz) which, at least in rats, is associated with locomotion. Theta results from interactions of the hippocampus with two other limbic structures, the septum and the entorhinal cortex. Often superimposed on theta is a faster rhythm known as gamma (30–100 Hz). The best evidence we have now is that gamma is generated by local circuits in the hippocampus and that inhibitory neurones play a crucial role.[4] The role of gamma in the hippocampus remains unclear; in the neocortex it has been implicated in higher cognitive processes such as the 'binding' of individual sensory features into coherent perceived objects.

Networks for gamma rhythms[4]

The first strong clue that inhibitory neurones played a central role in gamma rhythms came from hippocampal and neocortical slices in which fast excitatory postsynaptic potentials had been blocked by drugs. Excitation by pulses of glutamate or agonist drugs acting at metabotropic (i.e. G-protein-coupled) glutamate receptors resulted in rhythmic inhibitory postsynaptic potentials in the gamma frequency band. A series of experimental tests of predictions from realistic computer simulations showed that this gamma rhythm was generated by the mutual inhibition of inhibitory neurones which produced a synchronous interruption of the fast discharge the metabotropic glutamate receptor activation would otherwise have evoked. These interruptions lasted for a time, of the order of 25 ms, that depended on the time course of the inhibitory postsynaptic potentials in interneurones. We named this phenomenon 'interneuronal network gamma'.

During interneuronal network gamma pyramidal cells generate rhythmic inhibitory postsynaptic potentials, but do not reach threshold unless they are driven by some other input. If pyramidal cells are brought close to threshold at the same time as the inhibitory neurones, the properties of gamma change. This happens when slices are subject to short trains of electrical stimuli (typically 20 shocks over a period of 200 ms), in the absence of drugs to block excitatory postsynaptic potentials. An intermediate kind of gamma rhythm occurs when slices are exposed to cholinergic drugs such as carbachol, or to non-desensitizing glutamate agonist drugs such as kainic acid. Here each pyramidal cell fires on some cycles of the rhythm, so that on average some fluctuating fraction of pyramidal cells fires on each cycle.

New properties appear in tetanic gamma, including the ability to synchronize rhythms at pairs of sites separated by long distances (several millimetres) with phase lags shorter than predicted by conduction delays. The details are complex, but one theory argues that the long-range synaptic connections from pyramidal cells to interneurones at the remote site result in action potential doublets which play an error-correction role. A second intriguing aspect of this theory concerns the slowing of gamma to beta (15–30 Hz) frequencies, which is attributed partly to the recovery of the after-hyperpolarization and partly to potentiation of synapses between the pyramidal cells (this differs from long-term potentiation, which mainly affects incoming 'afferent' synapses rather than local associational synapses). These ideas on tetanic gamma are controversial, with recent evidence pointing to an alternative non-synaptic model, which may be more closely related to epileptic seizures than to cognition. Whatever the outcome of this debate, the concepts developed for tetanic gamma are proving very valuable in understanding the carbachol/kainate gamma mentioned above, and in time will play a major role in unravelling the mechanisms of gamma rhythms *in vivo*.

Significance of gamma

Gamma rhythms have been linked with sensory processing and with perception and other cognitive functions. Gamma rhythms may play roles in other psychiatric conditions. For instance, a recent study reveals increased beta and decreased gamma band signals in patients with schizophrenia. It is tempting to speculate that rather subtle changes in the networks responsible for gamma and beta rhythms could be at fault.

Gamma rhythms are intimately linked with epilepsy. Coherent neural activity at gamma frequencies is associated with some kinds of epileptic activity. Gamma rhythms are disrupted in at least one chronic model of epilepsy associated with learning impairments. Finally, the ideas behind the synaptic network mechanisms of the two kinds of phenomena have much in common.

Epilepsy—an emergent property of neuronal networks

Epileptic discharges typically involve excessively synchronous activity in principal neurones. In experimental focal epilepsy this excessive synchronization is due to the mutual excitation of pyramidal cells in the hippocampus, neocortex, or related areas. The essential idea is of a chain reaction. Areas that are especially prone to epileptic discharges have strong synaptic interconnections between their principal cells (e.g. the pyramidal cells of the CA3 region of the hippocampus or layers 3 and 5 of the neocortex). Activity in a few pyramidal cells can propagate through the synaptic network to recruit the whole population of neurones. Normally this propagation is held in check by inhibitory neurones; if the control mechanism is ineffective then epileptic discharges result. In experimental models the balance of synchronization versus control is compromised by treatments that weaken inhibition (usually by drugs such as bicuculline or picrotoxin), strengthen excitation (incubating brain slices in solutions lacking magnesium ions) or strengthen synaptic potentials in general (4-aminopyridine). Combined experimental and theoretical studies of such models have led to some general principals.[5] Synchronous epileptic discharges will result under the following conditions.

1. Connections between excitatory neurones are divergent, i.e. each connects to more than one postsynaptic excitatory neurone.

2. Connections between excitatory neurones are powerful enough to make their postsynaptic cells fire with a high probability. Precisely how high a probability depends on factors such as the connectivity and size of the network. The 'intrinsic' electrical properties of the neurones are important. Many epilepsy-prone areas have cells with prominent voltage-sensitive calcium currents, which are more prolonged than the classical voltage-sensitive sodium currents of the axonal action potential, and which cause neurones to fire bursts of fast sodium action potentials. Such intrinsic bursts greatly amplify transmission between pyramidal cells.

3. The network is large enough to allow all the neurones to link together. The critical mass for a network where the probability of any two cells being directly connected is 1 per cent, and the probability of one cell exciting its target cells is approximately 50 per cent, works out at about 1000 to 2000 neurones.

These features explain experimental brief epileptic discharges very effectively. The brain contains inhibitory mechanisms, both synaptic (inhibitory postsynaptic potentials, presynaptic inhibition) and intrinsic (voltage- and calcium-sensitive potassium channels), to terminate hypersynchronous discharges. Other mechanisms are needed to overcome the burst-termination mechanisms for the crucial transition to full-blown seizures lasting tens of seconds to minutes. These include slower synaptic mechanisms (both N-methyl-D-aspartate and metabotropic glutamate receptors, GABA, which paradoxically can become depolarizing if present in excess), non-synaptic mechanisms (potassium accumulation, electric fields[6]), and abnormal activity arising in axons (ectopic spikes, gap junctions).[5]

Convulsant drugs can trigger seizures in normal brains, including those of humans. People with epilepsy have a reduced seizure threshold. The reasons are far from clear, but may include abnormalities in intrinsic properties of neurones or in the connectivity of the neurones.

Improvements in non-invasive imaging and in neuropathology increasingly reveal misplaced neurones and other more or less subtle anatomical malformations in many focal epilepsies, which suggests that the local circuitry is disturbed.

Other kinds of epilepsy have very different mechanisms. Absence epilepsy is the other major class where cellular mechanisms are relatively well understood. They involve the interaction of the thalamus and neocortex, although the received wisdom on the underlying mechanism has recently been challenged by experiments on one of the key animal models of absence epilepsy.[7]

Epilepsy—learning and memory

Patients with temporal lobe epilepsy can have problems with learning and memory. Antiepileptic drugs can have marked side-effects, but the observation that chronic animal models of temporal lobe epilepsy also have impairments in learning and memory suggests that this is not the only cause. Memory impairments could result from gross damage, such as hippocampal sclerosis. Gross hippocampal pathology will have effects similar to experimental lesions of the hippocampus, but the observation that at least some of the chronic animal models lack gross hippocampal pathology does not support neuronal death as being the sole cause of impaired learning and memory.

At least two chronic experimental epilepsies have either limited or no cell loss during their induction. These are kindling and stereotaxic injection of a minute dose of tetanus toxin. The tetanus toxin model results in a well-characterized and enduring impairment of learning and memory, which outlasts the active epileptic syndrome in all but a few rats that show relapse. The absence of medication and of cell loss suggest that the psychological impairments in this model have some functional cause. Long-term potentiation remains intact, at least over a period of up to an hour. There is an association of learning impairment with the size of population spikes recorded from the same rats *in vivo* and under anaesthesia. Inhibition remains impaired in rats at a stage (>3 months after injection) when they had recovered from the active epileptic stage, but retained learning impairments. Abnormalities of the cellular electrophysiology of the postepileptic phase can lead to disruption of network properties, including gamma rhythms, which may, in time, provide a link to the behavioural problem.

Humans with limbic epilepsy often do have substantial hippocampal damage, and this will contribute to learning impairments. The experimental evidence suggests that even in the absence of gross hippocampal damage learning impairments can arise as a result of functional disruption of the hippocampal network.

Conclusions

Understanding the operation of networks of neurones provides valuable insight into a range of neurological and psychiatric diseases. The role of synaptic networks of excitatory neurones in focal epilepsies is now well established. The ways in which brief epileptic discharges transform into events lasting as long as full seizures are starting to be clarified, and may offer new avenues for developing rational therapies. New ideas on the generation of physiological rhythms suggest novel models of psychiatric and neurological problems ranging from impairments in learning and memory in limbic epilepsies to (more speculatively) the disruption of sensory perception in psychoses. Real clinical cases will inevitably be much more complex, but the ideas and models outlined above will aid the understanding of the underlying mechanisms.

References

1. Somogyi, P., Tamás, G., Lujan, R., and Buhl, E.H. (1998). Salient features of synaptic organisation in the cerebral cortex. *Brain Research Reviews*, **26**, 113–35.
2. Traub, R.D. and Miles, R. (1991). *Neuronal networks in the hippocampus*. Cambridge University Press.
3. Bliss, T.V.P. and Collingridge, G.L. (1993). A synaptic model of memory: long-term potentiation in the hippocampus. *Nature*, **361**, 31–9.
4. Traub, R.D., Jefferys, J.G.R., and Whittington, M.A. (1999). *Fast oscillations in cortical circuits*. MIT Press, Cambridge, MA
5. Traub, R.D. and Jefferys, J.G.R. (1996). Epilepsy *in vitro*: electrophysiology and computer modeling. In *Epilepsy. A comprehensive textbook* (ed. J. Engel Jr and T.A. Pedley), pp. 405–18. Raven Press, New York.
6. Jefferys, J.G.R. (1995). Non-synaptic modulation of neuronal activity in the brain: electric currents and extracellular ions. *Physiological Reviews*, **75**, 689–723.
7. Pinault, D., Leresche, N., Charpier, S., *et al*. (1998). Intracellular recordings in thalamic neurones during spontaneous spike and wave discharges in rats with absence epilepsy. *Journal of Physiology*, **509**, 449–56.

2.3.10 Psychoneuroimmunology

George Freeman Solomon

Definition

Psychoneuroimmunology is the transdisciplinary scientific field concerned with interactions between brain (mind/behaviour) and the immune system and their clinical implications.[1] Psychoneuroimmunology, or PNI, is the term coined by Robert Ader in the latter 1970s, but the field is also known by the equally ponderous terms neuroimmunomodualtion and, less commonly, neuroendocrinimmunology or behavioural immunology. Its clinical aspects range from an understanding of the biological mechanisms underlying the influence of psychosocial factors on the onset and course of immunologically resisted and mediated diseases to an understanding of immunologically generated psychiatric symptoms. Its basic science aspects involve understanding the complex interaction of neuroendocrine and immunologically generated networks in maintaining health and combating disease. Psychoneuroimmunology may provide a basis for understanding the biological basis of humanistic medicine and of alternative or complimentary medical techniques, and offers the hope of developing new non-linear models of health and disease.

By its very nature, psychoneuroimmunology bridges the traditional disciplines of psychiatry, psychology, neurology, endocrinology, immunology, neuroscience, internal medicine, and even surgery (wound healing). Interdisciplinary collaboration is generally essential and intrinsic to its research. The field is rapidly growing, as evidenced by the 14 chapters of the first edition of the major textbook *Psycho-neuroimmunology*, the 46 chapters of the second edition in 1991,[2] and the anticipated 80 chapters of the three-volume third edition in preparation at the time of writing.

History

Ancient and pre-modern wisdom reflected awareness of body–mind bidirectional interaction. Aristotle said: 'Psyche and body react sympathetically to each other, it seems to me. A change in the state of the psyche produces a change in the structure of the body, and conversely, a change in the structure of the body produces a change in the state of the psyche'. Sir Francis Bacon similarly suggested: 'Let us enquire how and how far the humours and affects of the body do alter and work upon the mind, or again, how and how far the passions or apprehensions of the mind do alter or work on the body'.

Wise physicians have long been aware of the role of emotions in the onset and course of immunologically resisted and mediated diseases. Sir William Osler is reported to have said that it is just has important to know what is going on in a man's head as in his chest in order to predict the outcome of pulmonary tuberculosis. The British phthisiologist George Day noted 'increasing difficulty in adjustment' in the 18 to 24 months prior to the onset of the disease and said: 'that psychological factors can and do influence the course of tuberculosis, once its is established, can be witnessed by anyone who has the opportunity of watching a patient's progress over a reasonably long period'.[3] During the years since the 1940s many 'psychosomatic' observations have been made regarding emotional factors in the onset and course of autoimmune diseases, mainly rheumatoid arthritis, but including systemic lupus erythematosis, Graves' disease/thyroiditis, and others.[4] In perhaps the most intriguing observation of this period, it was found that physically healthy relatives of patients with rheumatoid arthritis who had in their sera the autoantibody characteristic of that disease, rheumatoid factor (anti-immunoglobulin G), were better adjusted psychologically, on average, than those lacking the factor, suggesting that psychological well being might have a protective influence in the face of a genetic vulnerability.[5] Conversely, at least one autoimmune disease, systemic lupus erythematosis, can produce psychiatric symptoms, even as an initial clinical feature.[6] The relatively voluminous literature, of highly varied quality, on personality factors predisposing to cancer and psychological factors predictive of outcome are harder to interpret psychoneuroimmunologically, since only some cancers (such as malignant melanoma, non-Hodgkin's lymphoma, and some breast cancers) clearly are resisted immunologically, although the case for immunological resistance to metastatic dissemination (via natural killer (**NK**) cell cytotoxicity) is impressive.[7,8]

The scientific foundations of psychoneuroimmunology are the subject of a compilation of historical papers, a few of which will be cited.[9] By the late 1950s and early 1960s, animal experiments implied that stress could affect both humoral and cellular immunity. Rasmussen, Marsh, and Brill found that mice subjected to avoidance learning stress were more susceptible to herpes simplex virus infection. Wistar and Haldemann found that the same stress prolonged the retention of homografts. The first direct experimental evidence of stress effects on immunity was the observation of a reduction of antibody response to antigen as a result of group-housing stress in rodents by Vessey and by Solomon in the 1960s. At about the same time, Solomon, Levine, and

Kraft demonstrated that early life experience (infantile handling) might affect antibody response in adult life. Investigation of the larger area of immunological abnormalities that occur in conjunction with mental illnesses began with work of Solomon and Fessel on abnormal immunoglobulin levels and brain-reactive antibodies in some patients with schizophrenia.

The most definitive early research in psychoneuroimmunology, largely overlooked in the West, was that of Korneva and Khai working in Leningrad (St Petersburg). In 1963, they reported that destructive electrolytic lesions in the dorsal hypothalamus of rabbits led to a suppression of the development of complement-fixing antibodies and prolonged retention of antigen in the blood. Thus they had proved that the brain was involved in immunoregulation, a subject of speculation in the 1964 paper 'Emotions, immunity, and disease' by Solomon and Moos,[4] sometimes referred to as a 'marker' of the beginning of the field. A number of prescient papers were published in the 1960s and 1970s by the Yugoslav immunologist B.D. Jankovic. For example, he pointed out antigenic similarities between brain and immunological proteins. However, the most critical paper establishing the credibility and significance of brain–immune system communication was that of Ader and Cohen in 1975 on taste-aversion-conditioned immunosuppression. If a conditioned stimulus (saccharin) could produce the immunosuppression of an unconditioned stimulus (the drug cyclophosphamide), the brain and learning must relate to immunological responses. Subsequently, Ader and Cohen discovered, relevantly both clinically and with regard to the nature of the placebo response, the ability to utilize this type of conditioning to prolong the life of mice with an autoimmune disease (systemic lupus erythematosus) by treatment mainly with saccharin.[10] Remarkably, only after a general acceptance of the phenomenon of conditioning of immunity (which was subsequently shown to be able to be accomplished in upregulatory as well as downregulatory directions) was it realized that the phenomenon had been demonstrated in peritoneal inflammation by Metal'nikov and Chorine in 1926—science truly before its time. The critical immune system to brain limb of the neuroendocrine–immune axis was convincingly demonstrated by Besedovsky and Sorkin in the late 1970s. They showed that immune activation (antigenic stimulation) triggers the hypothalamic–pituitary–adrenal axis in an immunoregulatory role. The next milestone was the then controversial finding by Blalock[11] that immunologically competent cells (lymphocytes) can synthesize hormones (ACTH) and neuropeptides (β-endorphin), formerly thought only to be produced by neuroendocrine cells.

Classes of evidence of central nervous system–immune system interactions

There are a variety of categories of evidence—experimental and naturalistic, basic and clinical, animal and human, *in vitro* and *in vivo*, medical and psychiatric—for bidirectional communication between the central nervous system and various components of the immune system. Teleologically, it makes sense that these two systems should be linked. Both relate the organism to the outside world and assess its components as harmless or dangerous, both serve functions of defence and adaptation, both possesses memory and learn by experience, both contribute to homeostasis, and errors of defence by each can produce

illness, for example autoimmunity or allergies on the one hand and phobias or panic on the other. Blalock[11] has referred to the immune system as a 'sixth sense', forwarding information to the brain about molecular and cellular aspects of the environment not accessible by the five senses, and, more recently, as a 'mirror on the mind'.

The classes of evidence for central nervous system–immune system interaction, some of which have been mentioned, include the following:

- direct (lesion) evidence of brain region control of immunity and of innervation of immune organs;

- psychological (trait and state) factors in the onset and course of immunologically resisted (infectious and neoplastic) and mediated (autoimmune and allergic) diseases;

- influences of stress-response hormones on immunity;

- effects of neurotransmitters and neuropeptides on immunity;

- effects of experimental stress on immunity in animals;

- effects of experimental and naturalistic life stress and exercise on immunity in humans;

- behavioural modifiers of stress effects on immunity in animals and humans;

- effects of psychoactive drugs on immunity;

- correlation of individual psychological differences with immunity in animals and man;

- occurrence of immunological abnormalities in conjunction with mental illnesses (depression and schizophrenia);

- influence of products of the immune system on the central nervous system, including immunologically induced behaviours;

- alteration by psychological intervention and exercise of immunity and the course of immunologically related diseases.

Direct evidence

Pioneering work on the hypothalamus has been noted as providing direct evidence of neural modulation of immunity.[12] Hypothalamic neurones fire in spatial and sequential ways after antigen administration, and the hypothalamic–pituitary–adrenal axis is activated by antigen and proinflammatory cytokines in a stress-like way. Immune organs, including thymus, spleen, and bone marrow, receive sympathetic innervation with synapse-like junctions between nerve endings and immunocytes. Immunity is regulated in a cerebrocortical laterally specific way, with the left cortex influencing T-cell maturation and function.

Psychological factors

Emotional factors in the onset and course of autoimmune diseases include claims of personality trait/coping style predisposing factors such as tension and insecurity, shyness, difficulty in expressing feelings and in being assertive, 'martyr' type and masochistic characteristics, and sensitivity to the anger of others. Psychological state factors include loss/bereavement and depression and situational factors such as loss of a previously successful mode of adaptation.[13] Negative affect and failure of coping have been related to rate of progression, degree of incapacitation, and poorer response to medical treatment, particularly of rheumatoid arthritis. With regard to the less well-studied area of allergies, stress, anxiety, and depression have been related to both delayed (T-cell) and immediate (B-cell) hypersensitivities and to atopic dermatitis and asthma.[14–16] There is a somewhat controversial literature suggesting that hypnosis can alter immediate and delayed hypersensitivity.[17]

The psychoneuroimmunology of cancer is an area of increasing attention.[18] The antigenicities of neoplasms, and thus the ability of the immune system to resist specific cancers, vary. Immunotherapies are gaining attention, particularly for treatment of melanoma, lymphomas, and breast cancer. 'Cooley's toxins', which had some efficacy before the advent of chemotherapy, are now known to have been powerful immune stimulants. The NK cell, a non-B non-T lymphocyte, has cytotoxic activity that is non-specific and non-HLA-restricted. Many experimental and clinical studies in humans and animals have shown the numbers and activity of this cell type to be sensitive to stressors and psychosocial factors. The NK cell may play a role in immune surveillance against newly emerged neoplastic cells, and is clearly known to play an important role in prevention of metastatic spread of cancer. Stress increases metastatic spread of mammary carcinoma in the rat via suppression of NK cell cytotoxicity.[19] Psycho-oncology, which is discussed in Chapter 5.3.7, is concerned with quality as well as duration of life in cancer patients. Psychoneuroimmunology suggests that these are linked. To date, only one psychotherapeutic intervention study has included immunological as well as clinical outcome variables.[20] Compared with controls, patients with malignant melanoma undergoing a structured psychiatric group intervention at 6-month follow-up showed more effective coping, less distress, and greater stimulability of NK cells. Intervention patients showed less recurrence and greater survival 6 years later.

Psychoneuroimmunology, stress, and infection—the topic of old observations and early experimental work—is now the focus of rigorous research.[21] Subjects given a variety of cold-causing viruses intranasally developed both antibody evidence of infection and clinical colds in a dose-response manner with increases in degree of perceived psychological stress.[22] There is much confirmation of earlier work on stress effects on viral and bacterial (including mycobacterial) infections in experimental animals.

Stress-responsive hormones

Stress-responsive hormones, including but not limited to adrenal corticosteroids and catecholamines, have a myriad of effects on various aspects of the immune response in both down- and upregulatory fashion.[23] Often hormones affect immunity in an 'inverted U-shaped' way, being suppressive at either abnormally high or abnormally low levels. As mentioned above, the hypothalamic–pituitary–adrenal axis, itself triggered by immunological as well as psychological events, is immunoregulatory, and both corticotrophin-releasing factor and ACTH have direct effects on immunity in addition to those via induction of release of cortisol. Growth hormone increases T- and NK-cell functions in aged animals. Prolactin antagonizes glucocorticoid-induced immune suppression. Gonadal hormones affect immunity. NK cell activity is higher in the luteal phase of the menstrual cycle (which should influence surgeons in the timing of cancer surgery in premenopausal women). Cellular immunity is depressed during pregnancy. Thyroid hormones may stimulate NK activity and affect T-cell

development, and may modulate the affect of cytokines on immune cells.[24]

Neuropeptides

Neuropeptides, which are stress responsive,[25] have multiple immunological effects[26] and have even been referred to as 'conductors of the immune orchestra'.[27] β-Endorphin is a stimulant of NK cell activity. Substance P, co-released with noradrenaline (norepinephrine) at sympathetic nerve endings, may be particularly important in local immunity (and psychological influences thereon). Vasoactive intestinal peptide modulates immunoglobulin production. The sympathetic neurotransmitter noradrenaline (also a hormone) mobilizes NK cells into the circulation and is probably responsible for their increase during acute stress. Cerebral catecholamines and indolamines (e.g. serotonin) are released by immune activation and proinflammatory cytokines like interleukin 1 (**IL-1**), which, in turn, probably influence neuroimmunomodulation.[24]

Experimental stress and immunity

Animals

Experimental stress and immunity in animals, already mentioned in pioneering studies, is the subject of a very large literature.[28] Type, duration, intensity, timing (in relation to antigen administration), and controllability of the stressor are all relevant to its immunological impact. In primates, social support is a modifier of stress effects.[29] Behavioural response to the stressor, such as defeat posture, may be critical to the immunological outcome.

Humans

Acute experimental stress in humans (akin to the fight-or-flight reaction), such as mental arithmetic, generally results in a transient increase in 'first-line-of-defence' immunity, such as NK cell numbers and activity, and such effects have psychophysiological correlates.[30]

Naturally occurring human life stresses, both acute (e.g. examinations) and chronic (e.g. caring for patients with Alzheimer's disease), adversely affect a wide array of immune measures.[31] These include T-cell function, NK cell activity, antibody response to immunization, macrophage function, and activation of latent viruses like herpes simplex (controlled by cellular not humoral immunity). Such effects are increasingly being shown to have health implications. Social support can ameliorate stress effects. Natural disasters can have prolonged effects on immunity.[32]

Behaviour modifiers of stress effects

Exercise can affect immunity positively or negatively.[33] Acute aerobic exercise transiently increases NK cell numbers and activity. Overtraining without adequate periods of rest and recovery can diminish NK- and T-cell functions and increase incidence of infectious diseases. Several studies have reported an association between physical inactivity and risk of colon cancer, and animal tumorigenesis experiments tend to show that regular exercise reduces tumour burden. Even moderate exercise in very frail elderly people can reduce both NK- and T-cell functions, quite contrary to the effects of moderate endurance exercise on increasing resistance to infectious disease in normal subjects. Exercise increases lifespan in rats fed *ad libitum*. The combination of exercise and severe food restriction found in patients with anorexia nervosa leads (as in experimental animals) to morbid immuno-suppression.

Effects of psychoactive drugs

Drugs of abuse, particularly alcohol, have adverse effects on various aspects of immunity and susceptibility to infectious diseases.[34,35] Fetal alcohol exposure can permanently affect endocrine and immune responses. Alcohol inhibits production of proinflammatory cytokines, reduces NK cell activity and suppresses B- and T-cell immunity. Alcoholics are infection prone. Although HIV-seronegative heroin addicts generally have reduced immune functions, persons maintained on methadone in a state of steady tolerance have normal immunity. Marijuana suppresses production of α- and β-interferon and the cytolytic activity of macrophages. Other psychoative drugs often have immune effects. Benzodiazepines antagonize suppression of NK cell activity by corticotrophin-releasing factor and thus may modify stress effects on immunity.[36]

Individual differences

Individual differences in behaviour, coping styles, and psychological traits may be accompanied by differences in immunological characteristics. Inbred female mice with spontaneous fighting behaviour showed greater immunological resistance to a virus-induced tumour.[37] A pessimistic explanatory style correlated with lower measures of cell-mediated immunity.[38]

Immunological abnormalities in mental illness

The topic of immunological abnormalities that occur in conjunction with major mental illnesses needs to be separated into those associated with depression (affective disorders) and those associated with schizophrenia, a much more muddled area of research. Given that the central nervous system and the immune system have intimate linkages, which are being ever more fully elucidated by psychoneuroimmunology, it would seem to follow that major functional perturbations in one system would be reflected in the other. Some of these may have implications for physical health, implying the inseparability of mental and physical health. However, the contribution of immunological processes to the aetiology of mental illness is highly problematic, unlike their contribution to some neurological disorders, particularly multiple sclerosis which is an autoimmune disease.

Important decrements in immunological functions have been well documented in depression, particularly major depressive disorder[39] in which T-cell function declines in an age-dependent way. Thus persons in their twenties or thirties with a significantly elevated score on a psychological test of depression might have no T-cell functional decrement, whereas an elderly person with the same depression score would be likely to suffer a clinically significant decline. Intensity and duration of depressive symptoms are relevant. In contrast, depression-associated declines in NK cell cytotoxicity are age independent. Latent virus activation occurs in depression. It is noteworthy that depression is associated not only with immunosuppression but also with signs of immune activation (such as lymphocyte cell surface activation markers like HLA-DR). Depression has even been referred to as an 'inflammatory disease'. Effective treatment of depression by whatever modality is accompanied by gradual return of immune functions to

normal. (Tricyclic antidepressant drugs are somewhat immunosuppressive *in vitro*, whereas lithium may have some immunostimulatory properties.)

It is beyond the scope of this chapter to discuss the many immunological abnormalities that have been found in some patients with schizophrenia, particularly the long-standing claims that schizophrenia itself might be an autoimmune disease.[40] There have been a number of claims, largely based on epidemiological evidence, that schizophrenia has a viral or postviral aetiology.[41] A variety of abnormalities of levels of different classes of immunoglobulins in serum and cerebrospinal fluid has been inconsistently reported in conjunction with schizophrenia. It does appear that, relative to normal controls, there is a higher incidence of a variety of autoantibodies, including rheumatoid factor (anti-IgG) and anti-nuclear factor, in schizophrenia. Much more controversial has been the concept of schizophrenia as an autoimmune disease based on a considerable number of reports of antibrain antibodies (usually heterologous) in the sera of schizophrenic patients, studies begun by Fessel and particularly promoted by Heath, whose claims of producing schizophrenic-like symptoms by injection of patients' immunoglobulins into monkeys and humans were never replicated. An autoimmune theory of schizophrenia remains attractive because of evidence that other autoimmune diseases have both genetic and psychological predisposing and exacerbating factors. More modern work has suggested immunopathology of neurotransmitter receptors, both serotonergic and dopaminergic. (Autoantibodies can act as blockers or stimulants of neurotransmitter receptors, as in myasthenia gravis and Graves' disease respectively. It has been postulated that an autoantibody could act as a dopamine agonist in schizophrenia.) Abnormalities in cytokine production, particularly IL-2, have been found. An early observation by Hirata-Hibi of morphological abnormalities in lymphocytes of many patients with schizophrenia (particularly those with 'negative' symptoms) and some of their family members seems to have been supported by replication studies. The probable cell is an activated T cell. These many, varied, and generally inconsistent findings, possibly reflective of subtypes of schizophrenia, are hard to interpret. The linked neuropsychological–immunological perturbation hypothesis seems the most conservative.

Influence of products of the immune system on the central nervous system

The immune system affects brain and behaviour, especially via the effects of immune cytokines on the central nervous system.[42] Although cytokines are relatively large molecules, some, particularly IL-1, can cross the blood–brain barrier via active transport. IL-1 is also produced in the brain by both microglia, which are macrophages resident in the central nervous system, and astrocytes. Peripheral IL-1 can affect the brain, including its production of cytokines, via stimulation of the vagus afferent fibres. There are cytokine receptors in the brain, including those for IL-1, IL-8, and interferon, on both glial cells and neurones. Cytokines play a role in the development and regeneration of myelin-producing oligodendrocytes. Brain cytokines play a role in immune effector mechanisms as regulated by the brain, including a role in brain infection and inflammation. Cytokines are relevant to the progression of multiple sclerosis, gliomas, HIV-associated dementia, brain injury, and probably Alzheimer's disease. Proinflammatory cytokines, particularly IL-1 and tumour necrosis factor, are responsible for sickness behaviour that includes fever, sleepiness, anorexia, and fatigue. Sickness behaviour is adaptive. Microbes grow less well at high body temperature, which also is immunostimulatory. Production of IL-1 is facilitated by slow-wave sleep. Low blood sugar 'starves' bacteria. Fatigue conserves energy for battling infection. Not 'listening to the body', ignoring sensory messages that are immunologically induced, and not modifying behaviour appropriately for illness can adversely affect the course of infection. There is some evidence that chronic fatigue syndrome, which may occur following a viral infection, physical exhaustion, or psychological stress, and which may be accompanied by depression, is related to inappropriate cytokine signalling, as if there were infection, and elevated levels of IL-1 have been reported.[43] Chronic fatigue syndrome is associated with low levels of cortisol, unlike depression where the cortisol level is usually elevated. Evidence of immunosuppression and activation occur in both chronic fatigue syndrome and depression. IL-1 can produce both cognitive defects and lowered pain threshold in animals. Cognitive defects, myalgias, and headaches are often prominent symptoms of chronic fatigue syndrome. Therapeutic use of cytokines, particularly interferon, can produce psychiatric symptoms—psychotic, affective, or anxious.

Effects of psychosocial factors on the course of disease

Links between brain and behaviour and between psychiatry and medicine are well illustrated by the substantial research on the influence of psychosocial factors on the course of HIV infection and AIDS.[44] Sustained depressed mood and negative expectancies, especially when complicated by bereavement, are associated with more rapid decline of CD4+ helper T cells and an increase in other markers of progression (such as the activation marker β_2-microglobulin), as is lack of open acknowledgment of sexual orientation (being 'in the closet'). Passive coping (including denial and disengagement) is inversely related to long-term CD4 cell count. Long-term survivors with clinical AIDS and those who remain asymptomatic for prolonged periods of time in the face of very low CD4 counts seem to be those who have good coping skills, lead meaningful lives, find new meanings as a result of illness, are relatively not distressed, and are emotionally expressive and assertive. HIV-associated dementia, which is reversible in its early stages, appears to be closely related to the action of proinflammatory cytokines, particularly tumour necrosis factor, on neurones. Psychiatric symptoms, as well as cognitive defects, probably also cytokine induced, also occur in conjunction with HIV infection (primarily of microglia) of the brain; they include apathy, withdrawal, psychosis, and regressive behaviours.

Towards new models of health and illness

Health can be viewed as the capacity of the organism to regulate its own behaviour and physiology and produce co-ordinated response patterns to challenges. The two systems mediating interaction with the environment, the central nervous and immune systems, communicate with each other and can be thought of as a single integrated system for adaptation and defence. Psychoneuroimmunology is dissolving the dualisms of mind–body, body–environment, and individual–population. In realizing that the states of the medical body are correlated with individual's bodily experience, the philosopher David Levin and the present author have expressed the hope that patients will experience their bodies and themselves in new ways.[45] Somatic awareness is akin to psychological insight, and each has a role in maintenance of physical and mental health. A patient may realize that the body he or she presents for treatment is a body of integrated mental and somatic awareness and of meaningful experience, and is influenced by his or her own sensitivity. Psychoneuroimmunology should help us not only to understand the pathophysiology and psychophysiology of disease in a more systems-theory-oriented way, but also to value the doctor–patient relationship and the patient's own role in recovery from disease and maintenance of health. Thus, psychoneuroimmunology provides a scientific basis for the practice of humanistic medicine.

References

1. Solomon, G.F. (1998). *Immune and nervous system interactions*. Fund for Psychoneuroimmunolgy, Malibu, CA.
2. Ader, R.A., Felten, D.L., and Cohen, N. (ed.) (1991). *Psychoneuroimmunology* (2nd edn). Academic Press, San Diego, CA.
3. Day, G. (1951). The psychosomatic approach to pulmonary tuberculosis. *Lancet*, 12 May, 1025–8.
4. Solomon, G.F. and Moos, R.H. (1964). Emotions, immunity, and disease: a speculative theoretical integration. *Archives of General Psychiatry*, 11, 657–74.
5. Solomon, G.F and Moos, R.H. (1965). The relationship of personality to the presence of rheumatoid factor in asymptomatic relatives of patients with rheumatoid arthritis. *Psychosomatic Medicine*, 27, 350–60.
6. Fessel, W.J. and Solomon, G.F. (1960). Psychosis and systemic lupus erythematosus: a review of the literature and case reports. *California Medicine*, 92, 266–70.
7. Fox, B.H and Newberry, B.H. (ed.) (1984). *Impact of psychoendocrine system in cancer and immunity*. C.J. Hogrefe, Lewiston, NY.
8. Cooper, C.L. and Watson, M. (1991). *Cancer and stress. Psychological, biological, and coping studies*. John Wiley, Chichester.
9. Locke, S., Ader, R., Besedovsky, H., Hall, N., Solomon, G., and Strom, T. (1985). *Foundations of psychoneuroimmunology*. Aldine, New York.
10. Ader, R. and Cohen, N. (1983). Behaviorally conditioned immunosuppression and murine systemic lupus erythematosus. *Science*, 214, 1534–6.
11. Blalock, J.D. (1984). The immune system as a sensory organ. *Journal of Immunology*, 132, 1070–7.
12. Guillemin, R., Cohn, M., and Melnechuk, T. (ed.) (1985). *Neural modulation of immunity*. Raven Press, New York.
13. Solomon, G.F. (1981). Emotional and personality factors in the onset and course of autoimmune disease, particularly rheumatoid arthritis. In *Psychoneuroimmunology* (ed. R.A. Ader, D.L. Felten, and N. Cohen), pp. 159–82. Academic Press, San Diego, CA.
14. Paciante, C.M., Carpihiello, B., Rudas, N., Pilodu, G., and Del Giacco, G.S. (1997). Anxious symptoms influence delayed-type hypersensitivity skin test in subjects devoid of any psychiatric morbidity. *International Journal of Neuroscience*, 79, 275–83.
15. Gil, K.G., Keefe, F.J., Sampson, H.A., McCaskill, C.C., Rodin, J., and Crisson, J.E. (1987). The relation of stress and family environment to atopic dermatitis symptoms in children. *Journal of Psychosomatic Research*, 31, 673–84.
16. Djuric, V.J., Overstreeet, D.H., Bienenstock, J., and Perdue, M.H. (1995). Immediate hypersensitivity in the Flinders rat: evidence for a possible link between susceptibility to allergies and depression. *Brain, Behavior, and Immunity*, 9, 196–206.

17. Zochariae, R., Bjerring, P., and Arendt-Nielsen, L. (1989). Modulation of type I immediate and type IV delayed immunoreactivity using direct suggestion and guided imagery during hypnosis. *Allergy*, **44**, 537–42.

18. Lewis, C.E., O'Sullivan, C., and Barraclough, J. (ed.) (1994). *The psychoneuroimmunology of cancer*. Oxford University Press.

19. Ben-Eliyahu, S., Yirmiya, R., Liebeskind, J.D., Taylor, A.N., and Gale, R.P. (1991). Stress increases metastatic spread of mammary tumor in rats: evidence for medication by the immune system. *Brain, Behavior, and Immunity*, **5**, 193–205.

20. Fawzy, F.I., Hyan, C.S., Elashoff, R., Guthrie, D., Fahey, J.L., and Morton, D.L. (1993). Malignant melanoma. Effects of an early structured psychiatric intervention, coping, and affective state on recurrence and survival 6 years later. *Archives of General Psychiatry*, **50**, 681–9.

21. Friedman, H., Kein, T.W., and Friedman, A.L. (ed.) (1996). *Psychoneuroimmunology, stress and infection*. CRC Press, Boca Raton, FL.

22. Cohen, S., Tyrell, D.A.J., and Smith, A.P. (1991). Psychological stress and susceptibility to the common cold. *New England Journal of Medicine*, **325**, 606–12.

23. Buckingham, J.C., Gillies, G.E., and Cowell, A.M. (ed.) (1997). *Stress, stress hormones and the immune system*. Wiley, Chichester.

24. Marsh, J.A. and Kendall, M.D. (ed.) (1996). *The physiology of immunity*. CRC Press, Boca Raton, FL.

25. Taché, Y., Morley, J.E., and Brown, M.R. (ed.) (1989). *Neuropeptides and stress*. Springer-Verlag, New York.

26. O'Dorisio, M.S. and Panerai, A. (ed.) (1989). Neuropeptides and immunopeptides: messengers in a neuroimmune axis. *Annals of the New York Academy of Sciences*, **594**.

27. Morley, J.E., Kay, N.E., and Solomon, G.F. (1987). Neuropeptides: conductors of the immune orchestra. *Life Sciences*, **41**, 526–44.

28. Koolhas, J.M. and Bohus, B. (1995). Animal models of stress and immunity. In *Stress, the immune system and psychiatry* (ed. B.E. Leonard and K. Miller), pp. 69–83. Wiley, Chichester.

29. Coe., C.L., Rosenberg, L.T., Fischer, M., and Levine, S. (1987). Psychological factors capable of preventing the inhibition of the antibody response in separated infant monkeys. *Child Development*, **58**, 1420–8.

30. Naliboff, B.D., Benton, D., Solomon, G.F., *et al.* (1991). Psychological, psychophysiological, and immunological changes in young and old subjects during brief laboratory stress. *Psychosomatic Medicine*, **53**, 121–32.

31. Glaser, R. and Kiecolt-Glaser, J. (ed.) (1994). *Handbook of human stress and immunity*. Academic Press, San Diego, CA.

32. Solomon, G.F., Segerstrom, S.G., Grohr, P., Kemeny, M., and Fahey, J. (1997). Shaking up immunity: psychological and immunologic changes following a natural disaster. *Psychosomatic Medicine*, **59**, 114–27.

33. Hoffman-Goetz, L. (ed.) (1996). *Exercise and immune function*. CRC Press, Boca Raton, FL.

34. Watson, R.R. (ed.) (1995). *Alcohol, drugs of abuse, and immune function*. CRC Press, Boca Raton, FL.

35. Friedman, H., Klein, T.W., and Specter, S. (ed.) (1996). *Drugs of abuse, immunity, and infections*. CRC Press, Boca Raton, FL.

36. Irwin, M., Hauger, R., and Braitton, K. (1993). Benzodiazepines antagonize central corticotropin releasing hormone-induced suppression of natural killer cell activity. *Brain Research*, **631**, 114–18.

37. Amkraut, A. and Solomon, G.F. (1972). Stress and murine sarcoma virus (Maloney)-induced tumors. *Cancer Research*, **32**, 1428–33.

38. Kamen-Siegel, L., Rodin, J., Seligman, M.E., and Dwyer, J. (1991). Explanatory style and cell-mediated immunity in elderly men and women. *Health Psychology*, **90**, 229–35.

39. Miller, A.H. (ed.) (1989). *Depressive disorders and immunity*. American Psychiatric Press, Washington, DC.

40. Henneberg, A.E. and Kaschka, W.P. (ed.) (1995). *Immunological alterations in psychiatric diseases*. Karger, Basel.

41. Kurstak, E., Lipowski, A.J., and Morozov, P.V. (ed.) (1987). *Viruses, immunity, and mental disorders*. Plenum, New York.

42. Ransohoff, R.M. and Beneviste, E.N. (ed.) (1996). *Cytokines and the CNS*. CRC Press, Boca Raton, FL.

43. Goodnick, P.J. and Klimas, N.G. (ed.) (1993). *Chronic fatigue and related immune deficiency syndromes*. American Psychiatric Press, Washington, DC.

44. Nott, K. and Vedhara K. (ed.) (2000). *Psychosocial and biomedical interactions in HIV infections*. Harwood Academic, Chur, Switzerland.

45. Levin, D.M. and Solomon, G.F. (1990). The discursive formation of the body in the history of medicine. *Journal of Medicine and Philosophy*, **15**, 515–37.

2.4 The contribution of genetics

2.4.1 Quantitative genetics

Anita Thapar and Peter McGuffin

Patterns of inheritance

Our understanding of how traits and disorders are passed from one generation to the next began with the work carried out by an Augustinian monk, Gregor Mendel. Although Mendel's published work in 1866 was initially ignored, its rediscovery at the beginning of the twentieth century heralded the beginning of modern genetics. Mendel's experiments on pea plants and his observations of the patterns of inheritance of certain characteristics led to the development of his particulate theory of inheritance. It was only later in 1909 that the units of inheritance that he had described were named genes and alternative forms of a gene were termed alleles. It was also at this time that the terms phenotype, used to describe the observed characteristic, and genotype, used to refer to the genetic endowment, were introduced.

Mendel's laws

Mendel examined clear-cut dichotomous characteristics such as smooth versus wrinkled coats in peas. He first noted that when parents of different types were crossed, the first generation (F1) offspring displayed **uniformity** of that characteristic. He inferred that this uniformity was due to one phenotype being dominant and the other being recessive. Thus, when homozygous parents AA and aa produced heterozygote Aa offspring, these offspring displayed the phenotype of the AA parent rather than manifesting a phenotype intermediate to those of both parents.

Mendel then demonstrated that when the F1 heterozygotes (Aa) were intercrossed (Aa × Aa), **segregation** resulted in the second F2 generation showing recessive and dominant phenotypes in the ratio of 1 to 3. He then inferred that this F2 generation consisted of three types (AA, Aa, and aA, aa) occurring with a probability of 1 : 2 : 1.

Finally, Mendel showed that when the transmission of two different phenotypic traits was studied, they showed **independent assortment**. We now know that independent assortment occurs when the genes coding for these traits are either located far apart on the same chromosome or are on different chromosomes (see linkage).

Single-gene disorders

Although disorders showing a simple Mendelian pattern of inheritance are rare, they tend to be clinically severe and collectively impose a significant burden.

For **autosomal dominant** disorders to manifest themselves, only one disease allele is necessary, i.e. both heterozygotes as well as homozygotes (those who carry both disease genes) will be affected. In most instances, where there is one affected parent who is a heterozygote for the disease, approximately 50 per cent of the offspring will show the disorder. Autosomal disorders tend to be severe and manifest themselves in every generation. Huntington's disease and acute intermittent porphyria are examples of autosomal dominant conditions that often present with psychiatric symptoms.

Autosomal recessive conditions such as phenylketonuria require the presence of two disease alleles to show clinical manifestations of the disorder. Thus, they often appear to skip generations. These disorders usually occur in the offspring of two 'carrier' heterozygote parents and are more common where there is a high rate of consanguinity (e.g. marriages between cousins) as these inbred populations will show greater homozygosity at all loci.

The other group of single gene disorders consists of **sex-linked** conditions such as fragile X syndrome. Normal females have two X chromosomes whereas normal males have one X chromosome and one Y chromosome. Thus, for recessive disorders on the X chromosome, if the mother is a carrier (X*X) and assuming that the father is unaffected (XY), half of her sons will manifest the disorder (X*Y) and half of her daughters will be carriers (X*X). Where the father is affected by an X-linked recessive condition, all the daughters will be carriers. As sons have to inherit their X chromosome from their mother, there will be an absence of father to son transmission. X-linked dominant conditions are extremely rare.

Continuous traits

Mendel's laws are based on the transmission of dichotomous characteristics, yet many important human phenotypes such as height, weight, and blood pressure are continuously distributed. However, we are able to show that Mendelian principles can also be applied for these types of quantitative traits.

Let us first consider a phenotype measured on a continuous scale which results from the influence of a single gene with two alleles A_1 and A_2 (see Fig. 1). We can now describe the phenotypes of the three possible genotypes in terms of a quantitative value on the continuous scale. A_1A_1 has a value of $-a$; A_2A_2 has a value of $+a$; and A_1A_2, the

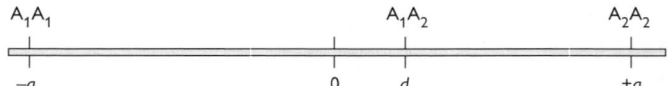

Fig. 1 A phenotype, measured on a continuous scale, resulting from a single gene with two alleles A_1 and A_2.

heterozygote, has a value of d. When $d = 0$, A_1A_2 lies exactly half way between A_1A_1 and A_2A_2, that is the genetic contribution is entirely additive. When $d = -a$, A_2 is recessive to A_1 and when $d = +a$, A_2 is dominant to A_1.

At the simplest level, we assume that there are no dominance effects and that there is no mutation, selection, migration, or inbreeding in the population. If p is the frequency of allele A_1 and q is the frequency of A_2 in the population where $p + q = 1$ then the frequency of genotypes can be expressed as follows:

$$A_1A_1 \quad A_1A_2 \quad A_2A_2$$
$$p^2 \quad 2pq \quad q^2$$

This is known as the Hardy–Weinberg equilibrium. If we now simplify further and state allelic frequencies where $p = q = 0.5$, then the phenotypic values of A_1A_1, A_1A_2, and A_2A_2 would be distributed in the population with relative frequencies of $1 : 2 : 1$.

Now if we consider a trait which results from two genes each of which has two alleles of equal frequency and additive effect, there would be five possible phenotypic values with relative frequencies of $1 : 4 : 6 : 4 : 1$. Overall as the number of genetic loci (n) increases, the number of phenotypic values increases ($2n + 1$) and the distribution of phenotypic values more closely approximates a normal distribution. It is thought that most quantitative or continuous traits result from the additive action of genes at many loci which is otherwise known as **polygenic** inheritance. Where familial transmission is explained by environmental factors as well as by multiple genes, we then call this a **multifactorial** mode of inheritance.

Complex disorders and irregular phenotypes

Polygenic/multifactorial threshold models

Most common human psychiatric and medical disorders such as schizophrenia, diabetes, and heart disease do not show a Mendelian pattern of inheritance. Neither can they be considered as continuous traits in that people are described as being affected or unaffected. However, these conditions could be regarded as quasi-continuous in that those who are affected can be graded along a continuum of severity. It is possible to extend this to assume that there is an underlying liability to develop the disorder which is continuously distributed in the population. Those who pass a certain threshold manifest the condition. If the underlying liability to develop the disorder is inherited in a polygenic or multifactorial fashion, then we can assume that the distribution will be approximately normally distributed (Fig. 2). The genetic liability of relatives of affected individuals will be increased and their liability distribution will be shifted to the right (Fig. 2). Thus, the proportion of relatives above the disease threshold will be greater compared with the general population. If we know the proportion of affected relatives of probands and the proportion of those affected in the general population, it is possible to calculate the correlation in liability between pairs of relatives using this type of model.

Single major locus model and atypical patterns of Mendelian inheritance

An alternative to a polygenic model of complex disease is a single major locus model. Single gene disorders do not always show typical Mendelian patterns of inheritance. For example familial transmission can be modified by variable **expression** and **penetrance**. Some conditions can show great variability in terms of clinical expression. For example neurofibromatosis, an autosomal dominant disorder can express itself as the full blown disorder or merely as a few café-au-lait spots. Penetrance is defined as the probability of manifesting the disorder given a particular genotype. For Mendelian disorders this is always 1 or 0, but irregular patterns of inheritance may occur because of incomplete penetrance where the probability of manifesting the disorder is greater than 0 but less than 1.

Finally, there are now molecular explanations for other types of unusual patterns of inheritance for single genes. Anticipation where disorders show a progressively earlier onset and greater severity with subsequent generations is now known to be explained by heritable unstable nucleotide repeat sequences (see later). Huntington's chorea and fragile X syndrome are examples of disorders caused by heritable unstable repeats. For some conditions such as the Angelman syndrome and the Prader–Willi syndrome, manifestation of the disorder depends on the parental origin of the gene. This is known as imprinting.

Other models

Alternative explanations of how complex conditions such as psychiatric disorders are inherited include mixed and oligogenic patterns of transmission. A mixed model includes a major gene and a polygenic/multifactorial contribution. However, for many of these disorders, genes of major effect may not exist. It may be that these irregular phenotypes are best explained by oligogenic models where the co-action or interaction of a small number of genes contributes to the disorder. These issues remain to be resolved by molecular genetic studies (see later).

Components of phenotypic variation

We will now consider the different influences that contribute to phenotypic variation in a population. The total observed variation in an observed trait (phenotype v_p) at the simplest level (ignoring non-additive effects) can be partitioned into a proportion due to genetic

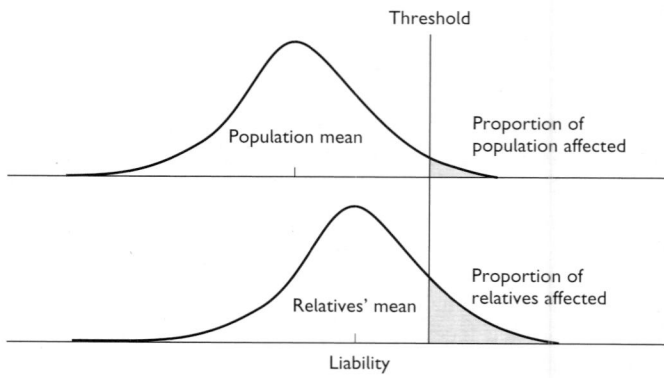

Fig. 2 A polygenic or multifactorial threshold model of disease transmission.

influences (v_g), a component explained by shared environmental factors (v_c) and a remainder accounted by non-shared environmental factors which includes error (v_e):

$$v_p = v_g + v_c + v_e$$

Shared or common environmental influences are aspects of the environment, such as poverty, that are shared by family members. Non-shared environmental factors refer to environmental influences that are specific to individuals (e.g. a head injury) and not common to family members.

Although we have so far only considered one type of genetic contribution, the genetic variance v_g can be further subdivided into variance due to additive genetic influences (v_a) and dominance effects (v_d).

The relative influence of genetic factors is expressed as **heritability** and when defined as the proportion of the total phenotypic variance attributable to additive genetic variance, is known as **narrow-sense heritability**:

$$h^2_n = v_a/v_p.$$

Heritability is also sometimes used to describe the proportion of variance explained by the *total* genetic variance (additive and non-additive genetic variance) and it is then known as **broad-sense heritability**:

$$h^2_b = v_a/v_g.$$

Similarly we can estimate the proportion of the total phenotypic variance explained by shared environment where $c^2 = v_c/v_p$ and the remaining proportion attributable to non-shared environmental factors and error (e^2).

It is important to remember that the estimate of heritability and the contribution of shared environment and non-shared environment are proportions of total variation within a given population, i.e. these parameters tell us about sources of difference between individuals in a population and have no meaning at an individual level. For example, if an individual was selected from a population where IQ had been shown to have a heritability of 50 per cent, it could not be said that 50 per cent of that individual's IQ was determined by genes. Another important point is that these estimates are specific to the population studied and may differ for other populations.

Non-additive genetic effects

So far we have simplistically assumed that phenotypic variation is influenced in an additive fashion. However, the contribution of genes and environment is likely to be more complex than this. We have already referred to genetic **dominance** effects where there is non-additive interaction of alleles within a locus. Another potential source of influence is the non-additive interaction between alleles at different loci which is known as gene–gene interaction or **epistasis**.

Similarly, it is possible that genes and environment also interact non-additively. For example, it has been shown that although the performance of mice on certain tasks improves when they are reared in an enriched environment, the degree of response to this environment depends on the genotype of the mouse. However, so far it has been difficult to show these types of **gene–environment** effects for human behaviour and psychopathology.

Gene–environment correlation

Gene–environment correlation further adds to the complexity of interplay between genes and environment. Gene–environment correlation arises when a person's genotype is correlated with the environment that they are exposed to. For example, sociable parents not only endow their children with genes but also provide an environment that encourages greater sociability in their children (passive gene–environment correlation). Moreover, positive gene–environment correlation would result where a sociable child actively seeks out more situations where socializing occurs (active gene–environment correlation) or where he or she evokes friendly responses in others (evocative gene–environment correlation).

Family, twin, and adoption studies

So far we have considered the theoretical basis of inheritance and possible sources of phenotypic variation and familial resemblance. Clearly, the investigation of the genetic basis of psychiatric disorders first requires us to examine whether genes contribute to a given disorder or trait. Secondly, we need to examine the role of both genes and environmental influences and finally to investigate the genetic basis of disorders at a molecular level.

Traditional methods in psychiatric genetics research include family, twin, and adoption studies. Family studies enable us to examine to what extent a disorder or trait aggregates in families. Familiality of a disorder can of course by explained by shared environmental influences as well as by shared genes. Twin and adoption studies allow us to disentangle the effects of genes and shared environment.

Family studies

Methods

Family studies allow us to determine whether a disorder aggregates in families by examining the rate of disorder in the relatives of affected individuals (probands) and comparing this with the rate of disorder in the general population or in a control group. Alternatively we can compare the frequency of disorder in the relatives of probands with the frequency among relatives of a control group of normal individuals or those with another disorder.

There are two types of family studies. The **family history** method is more economical in that the psychiatric history is taken from the proband. However, given that most individuals are unlikely to know as much about family members as about themselves, this method results in an underestimate of diagnoses in relatives. A more thorough but more time-consuming approach is the **family study** method where all available relatives are directly interviewed.

Ascertainment

An important issue is how a family study sample is ascertained. Ideally, probands should be ascertained independently from each other. This is unlikely to pose a problem for rare disorders. However, for more common conditions where a series of cases is collected, for example, by consecutive referrals of the disorder to a particular hospital, it is possible that families included in a family study contain more than one proband. This is known as multiple incomplete ascertainment. Complete ascertainment, where all affected individuals in a given population are included is rarely possible and in most instances probands are identified after some selection process (e.g. referrals to a particular hospital). Thus, factors influencing selection, such as comorbidity and help seeking may also influence observed patterns of familial aggregation.

Age correction

For genetic studies, we are interested in the proportion of individuals who have ever had the disorder (lifetime prevalence) rather than the proportion who show the disorder at one point in time (point prevalence). However, a difficulty encountered when carrying out family studies is that the observed rates of disorder will also depend on the age of the individual, the risk period for the disorder, and whether or not the individual has lived through that risk period. Thus, some members may not yet have reached the age of risk for the disorder, some are currently unaffected but will become affected at some later point, and others may have died whilst still unaffected. The most appropriate method is to correct for age and express the rate of disorder in relatives as the **morbid risk** or lifetime expectancy.

There are many methods of age correction, of which Weinberg's shorter method is the most straightforward. The uncorrected frequency of affected relatives $F = A/(A + U)$ where A = the number of affected relatives and U = the number of unaffected relatives. However, there are three types of unaffected relatives (U): those who have yet to pass through the age of risk (u_1), those within the period of risk (u_2), and those who are older than the age of risk (u_3). The frequency of affected relatives is then corrected by assigning weights to the three groups of affected relatives, namely 0 for u_1, 0.5 for u_2, and 1 for u_3.

The corrected frequency of affected relatives, i.e. morbid risk, is then given as

$$F = \frac{A}{A + 0.5u_2 + u_3}.$$

Twin studies

Identical or monozygotic twins, by virtue of arising from the fertilization of one egg, share 100 per cent of their genes. Non-identical or dizygotic twins are from two fertilized eggs and like full biological siblings share on average 50 per cent of their genes. Thus, assuming that monozygotic twins and dizygotic twins share environment to the same extent, monozygotic twins would share greater similarity than dizygotic twins for a disorder that is genetically influenced. Twin studies are an important method for disentangling the effects of genes and shared environment and can be used to estimate the contribution of genetic influences, shared environmental factors and non-shared environmental factors to the total variation for a given trait or disorder.

For continuous traits, twin similarity is expressed as an intraclass correlation coefficient where:

$$r_{mz} = h^2 + c^2$$
$$r_{dz} = 0.5h^2 + c^2$$

Thus, from observed monozygotic and dizygotic correlations for a given trait we can calculate heritability from the above equations where $h^2 = 2(r_{mz} - r_{dz})$, $c^2 = 2r_{dz} - r_{mz}$, and e^2 is the remaining variance $= 1 - h^2 - c^2$ (see path analysis below).

For dichotomous characteristics (e.g. affected with a disorder and unaffected), twin similarity is expressed as concordance rates. A **pairwise concordance rate** is estimated as the number of twin pairs who both have the disorder divided by the total number of pairs. However, where there has been systematic ascertainment, for example a twin register, it is preferable to report a **probandwise concordance rate** which is calculated as the number of affected twins divided by the total number of cotwins.

Ascertainment

One potential source of bias in twin studies stems from ascertainment procedures. For example, affected twins referred to a specific study or volunteer samples are likely to include more twin pairs who are monozygotic and who are concordant. Ascertainment of twin pairs through hospital registers overcomes this problem to some extent, but for some disorders may be biased by the process of referral. Population-based samples overcome these biases, although when examining disorders rather than traits extremely large sample sizes are required to obtain an adequate number of affected individuals.

Zygosity

A further potential source of error is in the assignment of zygosity. Ideally zygosity should be determined by DNA typing. However, it may be more practical to use a twin similarity questionnaire which includes questions such as whether the twins share the same hair/eye colour, and whether they look alike as two peas in a pod. This method of assigning zygosity is simple and inexpensive with a reported accuracy of over 90 per cent.

Equal environments assumption

It is sometimes argued that a major drawback to the twin study method is that monozygotic twins may experience a more similar environment and may be treated more similarly than dizygotic twins. However, where there is evidence that monozygotic twins share greater environmental similarity than dizygotic twins it is difficult to infer whether this contributes to their similarity for the disorder or whether this is the consequence of greater genetic similarity. There have been several approaches adopted to further explore this issue.

In some studies questionnaire measures of environmental sharing (e.g. being dressed alike as children, sharing friends) have been used. These suggest that environmental sharing is indeed greater for monozygotic twins than for dizygotic twins. However, it appears that for many traits and disorders such as cognitive ability, personality, depressive symptoms and depressive disorder this degree of similarity for childhood environment does not account for monozygotic twin similarity for the trait. One way of disentangling cause and effect is to use direct observational studies. Although this method has not been much used, one study of young twins suggested that the greater similarity of parental responses to monozygotic twins compared to dizygotic twins appeared to be elicited by the twins themselves.

An alternative method of examining the effects of environmental sharing is to study twins who are mistaken about their zygosity. However, most studies which have used this method suggest that perceived zygosity is a less important influence on twin similarity than true zygosity.

Finally, the most powerful means of examining the effects of environmental sharing is to look at monozygotic twins who have been reared apart. However, such twin pairs are rare and have mostly been ascertained in a biased fashion. Nevertheless, studies of reared-apart twins have informed us that there is a substantial genetic contribution to cognition, personality, and psychosis.

Comparability of twins

The final potential criticism of the twin method is whether twins can be regarded as representative of the general population given some important differences. Twin births are relatively common (1 in 80 births), although the number of dizygotic twins varies in different countries and is influenced by factors such as maternal age and multi-parity, a family history of twins and increasingly, the use of fertility drugs. Twins are more likely to experience greater intrauterine and perinatal adversity and the experience of being brought up as a twin is unusual in itself. There is also some evidence that depression is more common in mothers of young twins than among mothers of single-tons. However, these differences are only important if they result in different rates of disorder or symptoms in twins compared to single-tons. So far there is little evidence to suggest that the rate of psychiatric disorder in twins is any higher than amongst singletons.

Adoption studies

Adoption studies provide another means of teasing apart the effects of genes and environment. The basic method of the adoption study lies in comparing the rates of disorder in biological relatives and adoptive relatives There are three main types of adoption study.

1. **The adoptee study**: here the rate of disorder in the adopted-away offspring of affected individuals is compared with the rate of dis-order in control adoptees whose biological parents are unaffected.

2. **The adoptee's family study**: in this design, the rate of disorder in the biological relatives of affected adoptees is compared with that among the adopted relatives.

3. **The cross-fostering study**: this allows us to examine gene–envir-onment interaction by comparing the rate of disorder in adoptees who have well biological parents and affected adoptive parents with the rate of disorder in adoptees who have affected biological parents and normal adoptive parents.

Although adoption studies allow us to examine the effects of both genes and environment, there are several potential drawbacks to the method. First, adoption is in itself an unusual event and there is a tendency for higher rates of some psychiatric difficulties such as anti-social personality traits amongst adoptees. Second, adoptive place-ments are not random in that adoption agencies are likely to attempt to match adoptive and biological parents for physical, social, and other characteristics. Nevertheless, despite these difficulties, adoption evi-dence has given much support to the role of both genes and environ-ment for traits and behaviours such as cognitive ability and criminality.

Methods of analysis

Although the statistical methods used in quantitative genetics may seem complex, the principles are straightforward. We will now con-sider the methods of analyses that are most commonly used for exam-ining the contribution of genetic and environmental factors to psychiatric disorders and traits.

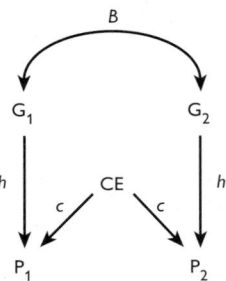

Fig. 3 A single path model of the sources of resemblance between twins or pairs of siblings. G_1 and G_2 are genotypes with correlation B, CE is common environment, P_1 and P_2 are phenotypes, and h and c are path coefficients.

Path analysis

Path analysis provides a simple diagrammatic method of estimating the contribution of genetic and environmental factors. The basic path diagram in Fig. 3 shows the sources of resemblance for phenotypes (P_1 and P_2) in a pair of siblings. Using the rules of path analysis, the correl-ation between the siblings (r_{sib}) is derived by multiplying the path coefficients for each connecting path and then summing these coef-ficients. Thus

$$r_{sib} = h \times r_g \times h + c \times c.$$

The genetic correlation r_g is 1 for monozygotic twins who share 100 per cent of their genes in common and is 0.5 for full siblings or di-zygotic twins. Thus, using path analysis we obtain the equations described earlier where

$$r_{mz} = h^2 + c^2$$
$$r_{dz} = \tfrac{1}{2}h^2 + c^2.$$

Model fitting

Although we can simply estimate h^2, c^2, and e^2 from the equations above for more complex data, solving multiple linear equations becomes difficult. We may also wish to test alternative models, for example one where there is no genetic contribution or one where shared environmental influences are dropped. Model fitting allows us to first statistically test how well a given model explains the observed data and to then compare different models.

Computer packages such as Mx[1] are all based on the same prin-ciples. The raw data are read into the program and the researcher sup-plies the initial starting values for the unknown parameters (h, c, and e for a full genetic model). The program then iterates with different par-ameter estimates until values are found which give an optimum fit (usually this involves maximizing a likelihood function or minimizing a χ^2). The goodness of fit of the model is then assessed by examining the χ^2 goodness of fit where a smaller value indicates a better fit.

The fit of a reduced model (R) can then be compared against the full model (F) by subtracting the χ^2 values ($R - F$). Alternatively the fit of models can be compared by using the likelihood ratio test where twice the difference between the log likelihoods for each model (this approximates a χ^2 distribution) is calculated.

An example of model fitting is shown in Table 1.

A full ACE model (additive genes, common/shared environment, and non-shared environment) gives a good fit ($\chi^2 = 0.6$, df = 3, $P = 0.90$) with estimates of 0.59 for h^2, 0.15 for c^2, and 0.26 for e^2. When we compare the fit of the reduced AE model where we have dropped

Table 1 Data on depressive symptoms for school-aged twins: example of model fitting

	h^2	c^2	e^2	χ^2	df	P
ACE	0.59	0.15	0.26	0.60	3	0.90
AE	0.75	[0]	0.25	1.36	4	0.85
CE	[0]	0.61	0.39	15.18	4	0.004
E	[0]	[0]	1	102.3	5	0.000

Reproduced with permission from A. Thapar and P. McGuffin (1996). The genetic aetiology of childhood depressive symptoms—a developmental perspective. *Development and Psychopathology*, **8**, 751–60.

shared environmental effects, there is no significant difference in the fit of the model ($\chi^2 = 1.36 - 0.6 = 0.76$, df = 1, $P < 0.001$). However, there is a significant worsening of fit for the CE model ($\chi^2 = 15.18$) and a very poor fit for a model of no familial transmission E ($\chi^2 = 102.3$). Thus, on the grounds of goodness of fit and parsimony (accepting the simplest model), an AE model provides the most satisfactory explanation of the data.

Multivariate model fitting

So far we have considered the influence of genes and environment on variation in a single phenotype. This type of analysis is known as univariate genetic analysis. Increasingly we have become more interested in the contribution of genes and environment to the covariation or correlation of two or more phenotypes (multivariate genetic analysis). This strategy allows us to examine to what extent the covariation or correlation between two phenotypes, for example depression and anxiety, is due to genetic factors that influence both phenotypes and how much can be explained by an environmental aetiology common to both disorders. Thus, multivariate genetic analysis can be used to examine the co-occurrence or comorbidity of different psychiatric disorders. This method, for example, has shown that the same set of genes, but different non-shared environmental factors influence anxiety and depressive disorders (and symptoms). Similarly this method is increasingly being utilized to examine the relationship between environmental risk factors and psychopathology and the role of genetic and environmental mediating factors.

Multiple regression analysis

Another commonly used method of analysing twin data is multiple regression analyses.[3] Here the score of the co-twin C is predicted by the score of the proband twin P, the coefficient of the relationship or zygosity R and an interaction term PR. The partial regression coefficients provide direct estimates of heritability and shared environment. The advantage of this method is that it can then also be used to test whether the genetic aetiology of extreme scores for a continuous trait differs from scores within the normal range.

Segregation analysis

We began the chapter by considering simple Mendelian inheritance. Segregation analysis was originally developed to test the hypothesis of a trait segregating in families according to either a dominant, recessive, or X-linked pattern. As such, the statistical procedures are straightforward, most commonly involving a χ^2 goodness-of-fit test. The com-

plications that arise largely result from differing methods of ascertainment. We have already mentioned this briefly in the earlier section discussing family studies. When a disorder is rare in a given population, such that the probability of ascertainment is low and no family contains more than one proband, this is called **single ascertainment**. The opposite is complete ascertainment when all probands are identified with certainty. In practice, with moderately common disorders there will be multiple-incomplete ascertainment with some families containing more than one proband (and hence being including in the sample more than once). The different methods of ascertainment affect the expected segregation ratios and hence they are important to specify. A detailed account is provided by Sham.[4]

The principles of segregation analysis have been extended to common disorders that do not show an obvious straightforward Mendelian pattern of transmission within pedigrees and where other evidence (for example less than 100 per cent concordance in monozygotic twins) indicate that there are environmental as well as genetic influences.[5] The details of such methods are beyond our scope but in essence they can applied either to continuous traits or to present/absent traits (such as being affected or unaffected by disease) by assuming that there is a continuum of liability to the trait with only those beyond a certain threshold value manifesting it (see the discussion of threshold models earlier in this chapter). Probably the most commonly applied and the most rigorous approach is embodied in the so called 'unified' model of Lalouel *et al.*[6] This allows the investigator to test how well a set of family data is explained by a combination of a major locus plus a multifactorial background and to compare this (as described earlier in the section on model fitting) with reduced models using a likelihood ratio test. The reduced models consist either of single gene alone or multifactorial transmission alone. If there is evidence for a single gene it is then possible to apply a further test of whether the transmission probabilities[7] conform to Mendelian expectation.

In practice, complex segregation analysis of this type has proved to be disappointing in psychiatric genetics. For example, in schizophrenia the findings have been inconclusive with the ability to distinguish between competing models being poor.[8] Furthermore, segregation analysis has produced misleading results such as suggesting an autosomal locus for the enzyme, platelet monoamine oxidase, which is now known to be encoded at two distinct X-linked loci.[9] Attempting to apply the approach to traits that are familial but not necessarily genetic can also be a pitfall for the unwary so that one study suggested that attendance at medical school among the relatives of medical students could best be explained by the segregation of a recessive gene.[10]

Gene mapping

A more direct approach to locating and identifying genes involved in psychiatric disorders is to attempt to map them. Gene mapping technology has advanced at an astonishing pace over the past 20 years. Early studies in psychiatric disorders such as schizophrenia[11] had to rely purely on 'classical' genetic markers such as HLA antigens blood groups and various protein polymorphisms. Capabilities in systematic gene mapping, which involves mounting a search throughout the whole genome (i.e. the 22 pairs of autosomes and the sex chromosomes), only became possible after the discovery of markers based on variation in DNA length. The first of these were the restriction frag-

Table 2 Double back-cross mating

	Parent 1		x	Parent 2
	AB/ab			ab/ab
Offspring	AB/ab	Ab/ab	aB/ab	ab/ab
	Non-recombinant	Recombinant	Recombinant	Non-recombinant
No linkage	¼	¼	¼	¼
Linkage	$(1-\theta)/2$	$\theta/2$	$\theta/2$	$(1-\theta)/2$

ment length polymorphisms and these have largely been supplanted by simple sequence repeat polymorphisms such as dinucleotide repeat polymorphisms. There is now a very detailed 'reference map' of the genome based on several thousand, more or less evenly spaced dinucleotide repeats. We can look forward to an even better map within the next few years, with the Human Genome Project on course to sequence the human genome before its target date of 2003 and the introduction of tens of thousands of new marker maps based upon single nucleotide polymorphisms. Such marker maps allow the genes contributing to traits or diseases to be located which is the first stage in positional cloning in which the genes themselves are then identified. The methods for mapping are linkage and association. Gene mapping is discussed further in Chapter 2.4.2.

Linkage

In linkage studies, rather than just studying the segregation of a disease in families, the co-segregation of the disease and a set of genetic markers is investigated. The aims are, first, to detect linkage, indicated by the disorder and the marker co-occurring more often than would be expected by chance (i.e. not showing Mendelian independent assortment) and, second, to estimate the distance between a linked marker and the gene conferring to susceptibility to the disorder.

It is possible to detect linkage only in families containing at least one parent who is a double heterozygote (i.e. heterozygous at both the marker and the disease loci). Technically such families are referred to as double back-cross or intercross/intercross matings but, for simplicity, we will just focus on the double back-cross type (Table 2). The table shows a double hetrozygote parent where the alleles *A* and *B* are on one chromosome with *a* and *b* on the other. Consequently offspring of the types *aaBb* or *Aabb* result from recombination or crossing over between the homologous pair of chromosomes during meiosis. These types of offspring are called **recombinants**. Offspring of the same type as the parents (i.e. *AaBb aabb* are non-recombinant. We can then simply define the recombination fraction, θ, as the number of recombinants divided by total number of offspring.

For two loci that are very widely separated on the same chromosome (and all pairs of loci carried on to two different chromosomes) independent assortment occurs and $\theta = 1/2$. When the two loci are close together dependent assortment may be observed indicated by a recombination fraction of less than a half. The size of the recombination fraction depends on the physical distance between the two loci and (within certain limits) is proportional to it, so that for loci that are very close together recombination rarely occurs and θ tends to zero. Genetic distances estimated by linkage studies are measured in centimorgans (cM) with 1 cM the equivalent of a recombination fraction of

0.01. For reasons that are not fully understood, recombination occurs more frequently in female than in male meioses. Hence, the size of the female human genome expressed in centimorgans is larger than the male genome. The sex-averaged size of the human genome is about 3700 cM. With reasonable sample sizes major gene effects can be confidently detected over distances of around 10 to 15 cM. Hence, a whole genome search can be carried out using 200 to 300 polymorphic markers, provided they are approximately evenly spaced. A **polymorphism** can be defined as a gene or sequence of DNA that occurs in two or more common forms. Classically, 'common' means an allele frequence of at least 1 per cent. However, modern markers such as simple sequence repeat polymorphisms are generally highly polymorphic having multiple very common alleles. Since, as we have noted, heterozygosity in the parental generation is a prerequisite for linkage analysis, simple sequence repeat polymorphisms are much more often informative than earlier less polymorphic types of marker.

Linkage analysis

The standard method of carrying out linkage analysis in humans is the lod score approach devised by Morton.[12] Essentially, for a given set of data, lod scores are calculated over a range of values of θ between 0 and 0.5. Where the lod score reaches a maximum, provides the best (or maximum likelihood) estimate of θ. The lod score is so called because it is the common **log** of the **od**ds that θ has a certain value θ' rather than a value of 0.5, i.e.

$$\text{lod} = \log_{10}\frac{\text{probability } (\theta = \theta')}{\text{probability } (\theta = 0.5)}.$$

By convention, a lod of 3 or more is accepted indicating that linkage has been detected, while a lod of −2 or less indicates that linkage can be excluded at that particular value of θ. A lod of 3 corresponds to odds on linkage of 1000 : 1 and to a nominal *P* value of 0.0001. This therefore seems at first sight to be a very stringent criterion. However, linkage between two loci taken at random is inherently unlikely[13] and Morton's[12] original argument took into account the low prior probability of linkage to arrive at a criterion that gave a posterior probability, or reliability, of 95 per cent. More recently workers have been concerned about the effects of carrying out many statistical tests in a genome-wide search for linkage and have sought to set an appropriate level of lod score to compensate for this. In fact, as it turns out, the original suggestion of a lod of about 3 is close to recent calculations of what lod is required to conclude in favour of genome-wide significance.[14]

As originally devised, the lod method deals purely with regular Mendelian traits. However, it can be readily adapted for detection of single genes that have incomplete penetrance by applying the general single major locus model discussed earlier.[15] The main drawback is that the model (as specified by the penetrance values, and less critically the gene frequency) must be known accurately. Where the model is mis-specified there is a high risk that linkage will fail to be detected.[16]

A further difficulty is that diseases may show locus heterogeneity, i.e. there may be two or more different (and unlinked) loci where mutations result in similar phenotypes. There are many instances of this among rare Mendelian diseases. A good example is Usher's syndrome causing deafness and retinitis pigmentosa, which can result from mutations in any one of six different genes.[17] Subforms of common diseases can also show locus heterogeneity, the most relevant to psychiatry being early onset familial Alzheimer's disease where autosomal dominant forms can result from mutations in three different genes, called presenilin 1, presenilin 2, and amyloid precursor protein. Although methods exist for detecting linkage in the presence of heterogeneity[12,15] these have not so far in practice been of great help in psychiatric or other common disorders. Rather, the most frequent general strategy has been to focus on multiplex families (i.e. those containing multiple members with the disorder under study) and to make the following simplifying assumptions.

1. There are major gene subforms of the disorder in at least some families.

2. Although the mode of transmission is unknown, a reasonable guess at the defining parameters can be made.

3. Although there may be locus heterogeneity in the disorder as a whole, within any given family there is likely to be homogeneity.

This has worked very well for several disorders, including, as we have just mentioned, Alzheimer's disease, but has so far produced a rather confusing set of results from a large number of different centres for schizophrenia[18] and manic–depressive disorder.[19] The most likely cause of this is that assumption 1 is incorrect and that subforms of these conditions resulting from major genes are very rare or perhaps non-existent. Consequently there has been a shift towards other methods of tackling linkage studies in psychiatry which do not rely on any assumptions about the mode of transmission. These concentrate on affected siblings or other pairs of relatives both affected by the disorder.

Methods based on relative pairs

The underlying principle of the affected sib-pair approach is simple. For any given locus the probabilities that siblings share 0, 1, or 2 alleles that are identical by descent from their parents is respectively $\frac{1}{4}$, $\frac{1}{2}$, $\frac{1}{4}$. On the other hand, if both members of a sib pair are affected by the same disease and we are studying a locus close to a gene that confers susceptibility to that disease, there will be increased allele sharing. This will occur irrespective of the mode of transmission of the susceptibility gene and hence simple non-parametric statistics can be used to test whether there is any perturbation of the expected identical-by-descent proportions. Affected sib-pair methods are therefore robust and are now generally considered to be the method of choice in detecting linkage in oligogenic or polygenic disorders. In order to be certain that a pair of siblings share alleles identical by descent, one needs to know their parents' genotypes. Otherwise it could be that a shared allele identical by state results from one of the pair having inherited it from the father and the other from the mother. However, an advantage of using highly polymorphic single sequence repeat polymorphisms is that it may not always be necessary to genotype parents, i.e. where the population is reasonably homogenous and where gene frequencies can be estimated, it is possible to compute the likelihood that a pair who share one or two alleles identical by state are truly identical by descent. This means that in return for a fairly modest reduction in power (because one is now dealing with a probability rather than a certainty of counting alleles that are identical by descent) there is a halving in the amount of genotyping that needs to be done.[20] In our own experience, the other advantage of being able to make do without parental genotypes is that they are often difficult to obtain in adult-onset disorders such as schizophrenia.

Another use of sib-pair methods is in studying continuous traits

Table 3 Case–control allelic association

Marker	N affected	N unaffected
Present	a	b
Absent	c	d

(e.g. height, weight, personality test scores) to attempt to detect the quantitative trait loci that contribute to their heritability.[21] One approach is to select probands who have extreme scores on some quantitative measure and investigate the extent to which marker allele sharing by siblings predicts the regression to the population mean of the siblings' scores.[22] This has been successfully used in mapping a quantitative trait locus contributing to reading ability in children. Unfortunately the drawback of such methods and of sib-pair linkage approaches generally is that they are only capable of detecting moderately large effects. This means that a quantitative trait locus contributing less than about 10 per cent of the variance or a disease susceptibility locus conferring a relative risk of less than 2 will probably require very large samples running into several hundreds, perhaps thousands, of pairs. If we assume that most common diseases and complex behaviours involve the combined action of many genes of small effect, complementary strategies based on allelic association are required.

Association

In their classic form, allelic association studies are more straightforward to carry out than linkage studies. A sample of cases affected by a disorder (or subjects who have scores higher than a given threshold on a quantitative measure) is compared with controls who do not have the disorder (or subject whose scores are near average). The frequency of alleles at the marker locus is then compared in the two groups. The significance of the difference can then be compared in the usual way for contingency table analysis using a χ^2 test (or Fisher's exact test if expected frequencies are small). In addition to significance it is useful to have a measure of the strength of association. A variety of statistics can provide this but probably the most useful and intuitively appealing is the **relative risk**, i.e. the proportion of cases among those carrying the marker allele or risk factor, P_1, divided by the proportion of cases, P_2, among those not carrying the factor. As we can calculate from Table 3, $RR = P_1/P_2 = (a/(a + b))/(c/(c + d))$. If the disorder is uncommon, i.e. a and c are small relative to b and d, RR can be approximated by another, easier-to-obtain statistic, the odds ratio, $OR = a \times d/(b \times c)$. If a positive marker disease association has been found the odds ratio will be significantly greater than 1.

Before the current era of molecular genetics many association studies of disease with classical markers were carried out most notably with blood groups and with the HLA system. One of the earliest well-replicated findings was an association between blood group O and duodenal ulcer. The odds ratio was less than 2 in most studies and Edwards[23] pointed out that the proportion of variance in liability to the disorder explained by the association was only about 1 per cent. Even though later disease association studies on HLA, with other diseases such as type I diabetes and various auto immune disorders, were stronger, it has been pointed out that here too only a small proportion of variance is accounted for. Although this could in one respect be considered disappointing, it demonstrates that allelic association can

Table 4 Transmission disequilibrium test: affected subjects with at least one parent heterozygous for allele A

Transmitted	Non-transmitted	
	A$_1$	A$_2$
A$_1$	a	b
A$_2$	c	d

χ^2, 1 df = $(b - c)^2/(b + c)$

detect small gene effects in polygenic or multifactorial traits and may therefore prove to be more useful than linkage.

How does allelic association arise and what does its detection tell us? There are three principal mechanisms of association. The first is linkage disequilibrium. Normally pairs of alleles at two different loci occur together no more often than would be expected by chance (i.e. they are in 'equilibrium'). In most cases this is the result of independent assortment. However, even if loci are linked they will usually approach equilibrium very rapidly with the proportion of associated alleles decreasing by $1 - \theta$ each generation. Only where the two loci are very close together does disequilibrium tend to persist. For example, where the distance is 1 cM corresponding to a recombination rate of one meiosis in 100, the time taken for an association to go half way to equilibrium is 69 generations. For a distance of 0.1 cM the time taken is 693 generations, or about 20 000 years. The second cause of association is when a polymorphism within a gene itself has a functional effect which results in susceptibility to a disease. The third, and in most cases least interesting, phenomenon is population stratification. This occurs where there has been recent admixture of populations or two or more ethnically distinct populations living side by side with little interbreeding. If the populations differ in terms of the frequency of alleles of the genetic markers and in the frequency of the disease being studied, marker disease associations can arise if there is not careful ethnic matching of patients and controls.

Another way of overcoming stratification is not to study unrelated cases and controls but to study families and derive the controls 'internally'. The most familiar method in current use is the transmission disequilibrium test.[24] This requires affected individuals to have at least one parent who is heterozygous at the test locus. The affecteds can therefore each receive one of two alleles from such parents. A 2 × 2 contingency table can then be constructed of whether a particular allele is the transmitted or the non-transmitted allele. This is illustrated in Table 4 for a marker with two alleles, A1 and A2 . The entries in each cell of the table, *a*, *b*, *c*, and *d* are counts of the number of parents transmitting or not transmitting each allele to their affected offspring. The significance of the transmission disequilibrium test is simply assessed by a McNemar χ^2 test.

Assuming that stratification can be overcome there are broadly two ways to proceed with association studies. The first is to concentrate on polymorphisms in or near candidate genes, i.e. genes that encode for proteins that are likely to be involved in the disorder. This has so far been the commonest type of association study in psychiatry as in most other common diseases, and there are some interesting early results relating to, for example, polymorphisms at the serotonin 5-HT$_{2a}$ receptor in schizophrenia, the serotonin transporter in affective disorders, and the dopamine (DAT$_1$) transporter in attention-deficit–

hyperactivity disorder. The second is to attempt a systematic search through a chromosomal region or, more ambitiously, the entire genome with the aim of detecting linkage disequilibrium. It follows from what we have discussed earlier that a genome-wide search for linkage disequilibrium has a particular attraction in the study of polygenic disorders in that it should be capable of detecting genes of small effect. The disadvantages are twofold. There are problems to do with multiple statistical testing and there are feasibility issues to do with the amount of genotyping necessary to scan the entire genome. This has led some authorities to conclude that systematic genome scans for genes involved in complex disorders are not practicable.[17]

Let us deal with the second problem first. It follows from our discussion of the mechanisms underlying association that it will require a very large number of markers to scan the entire genome. This is because linkage disequilibrium is usually only detectable over very short distances of a centimorgan or less. This means that thousands of evenly spaced markers will be needed. If we add to this the problem that small effects require large samples of subjects to provide adequate power of detection, the task becomes daunting. Let us suppose that we wish to test 3000 markers on 1000 subjects (500 patients and the same number of controls). This would mean 3 million genotypings—a huge amount of work. Fortunately two recent developments make this more achievable. DNA pooling methods[25] allow the initial screening to be carried out on combined samples such that all of the controls can be processed as one batch and all of the patients as the other. Positive findings can then be followed up by doing individual genotyping. This means that the initial screen involves 6000 rather than 3 million genotypings. The other innovative development in very high throughput genetic analysis involves hybridizing DNA to microarrays of hundreds of oligonucleotides bound to 'chips' which means that a very large number of biallelic single nucleotide polymorphisms can be tested for very rapidly.

The problem of multiple testing can be overcome either, as in the DNA pooling approach, by carrying out a two-stage analysis with fairly liberal test criteria in the first stage followed by stringent criteria in the second stage, or by simply setting a very stringent criterion at the beginning. It has recently been shown that, even with an alpha level set at 1×10^{-6}, detection of linkage disequilibrium with genes of small effect is feasible with realistic sample sizes.[26] In short, the linkage disequilibrium mapping approach using either DNA pooling or single nucleotide polymorphisms on chips is likely to greatly advance the discovery of susceptibility loci and quantitative trait loci over the next few years.

References

1. Neale, M. C. and Cardon, L. R. (1991). *Methodology of genetic studies of twins and families*. Kluwer, Dordrecht.
2. Thapar, A. and McGuffin, P. (1996). The genetic aetiology of childhood depressive symptoms—a developmental perspective. *Development and Psychopathology*, **8**, 751–60.
3. De Fries, J.C. and Fulker, D.W. (1988). Multiple regression analysis of twin data: etiology of deviant scores versus individual differences. *Acta Geneticae Medicae et Gemellolologiae*, **37**, 205–16.
4. Sham, P. (1998). *Statistics in human genetics*. Arnold, London.
5. Morton, N.E. (1982). *Outline of genetic epidemiology*. Karger, Basel.
6. Lalouel, J.M., Rao, D.L., Morton, N.E., and Elson, R.C. (1983). A unified model for complex segregation analysis. *American Journal of Human Genetics*, **35**, 816–26.

7. Elston, R.C. and Yelverton, K.C. (1975). General models for segregation analysis. *American Journal of Human Genetics*, **27**, 31–45.

8. Vogler, G.P., Gottesman, I.I., McGue, M.K., and Rao, D. C. (1990). Mixed model segregation analysis of schizophrenia in the Lindelius Swedish pedigrees. *Behavior Genetics*, **20**, 461–72.

9. Rice, J.P., Endicott, J., Knesevich, M.A., and Rochberg, N. (1987). The estimation of diagnostic sensitivity using stability data: an application to major depressive disorder. *Journal of Psychiatric Research*, **21**, 337–45.

10. McGuffin, P. and Huckle, P. (1990). Simulation of Mendelism revisited: the recessive gene for attending medical school. *American Journal of Human Genetics*, **46**, 994–9.

11. McGuffin, P. and Sturt, E. (1986). Genetic markers in schizophrenia. *Human Heredity*, **16**, 461–5.

12. Morton, N.E. (1955). Sequential tests for the detection of linkage. *American Journal of Human Genetics*, **7**, 277–318.

13. Edwards, N.H. (1991). The formal problems of linkage. In *The new genetics of mental illness* (ed. P. McGuffin and R. Murray), pp. 58–70. Butterworth Heinemann, Oxford.

14. Lander, E. and Kruglyak, L. (1995) Genetic dissection of complex traits: guidelines for interpreting and reporting linkage results. *Nature Genetics*.

15. Ott, J. (1991). *Analysis of human genetic linkage.* Johns Hopkins University Press, Baltimore, MD.

16. Clerget-Darpoux, F. (1991). The uses and abuses of linkage analysis in neuropsychiatric disorder. In *The new genetics of mental illness* (ed. P. McGuffin and R. Murray), pp. 44–57. Butterworth Heinemann, Oxford.

17. Strachan, T. and Read, A.P. (1996). *Human molecular genetics*. BIOS, Oxford.

18. Moldin, S.O. (1997). The maddening hunt for madness genes. *Nature Genetics*, **17**, 127–9.

19. Risch, N. and Botstein, D. (1996). A manic depressive history. *Nature Genetics*, **12**, 351–3.

20. Holmans, P. (1993). Asymptotic properties of affected-sib-pair linkage analysis. *American Journal of Human Genetics*, **52**, 362–74.

21. Plomin, R.G., McClearn, G.E., Smith, D.L., *et al.* (1995). Allelic associations between 100 DNA markers and high versus low IQ. *Intelligence*, **21**, 31–48.

22. Fulker, D.W. and Cardon, L.R. (1994). A sib-pair approach to interval mapping of quantitative trait loci. *American Journal of Human Genetics*, **54**, 1092–103.

23. Edwards, T.H. (1965). The meaning of the associations between blood groups and disease. *Annals of Human Genetics*, **29**, 77–83.

24. Spielman, R.S., McGinnis, R.E., and Ewenst, W.J. (1993). Transmission test for linkage disequilibrium: the insulin gene region and insulin-dependent diabetes mellitus (IDDM). *American Journal of Human Genetics*, **52**, 506–16.

25. Daniels, J.P., Holmans, P., Williams, N., *et al.* (1998). A simple method for analysing microsatellite allele image patterns generated from DNA pools and its application to allelic association studies. *American Journal of Human Genetics*, **62**, 1189–97.

26. Risch, N. and Merikangas, K.(1996). The future of genetic studies of complex human diseases. *Science*, **273**, 1516–17.

2.4.2 **Molecular genetics**

Jonathan Flint

Introduction

The considerable impact of molecular genetics on medicine, most visibly in terms of diagnosis,[1] has raised expectations of similar advances in psychiatric aetiology and nosology, hopes that have been partly realized with the successful identification of genetic mutations in the dementias and some forms of mental retardation. Moreover, even if the mixed success in applying molecular approaches to common psychiatric conditions might be taken as an indication that genetics will remain a peripheral subject for psychiatry, it is at the very least likely that the genetic bases of psychosis and depression will soon be unravelled.[2,3] Once this has been worked out, psychiatrists will need to have a grasp of sufficient molecular genetics to communicate diagnostic advances to their patients.

But there is another reason why molecular genetics will soon be a basic tool for psychiatrists. Mental states emerge from activity in neural systems, which are being delineated with increasing sophistication by neuroscientists down to the level of anatomical, cellular, and now molecular components. Changes in mental states, whether environmentally or genetically determined, have biological correlates, which in some circumstances can be observed (for instance by functional magnetic resonance imaging). We now know that persistent changes in mental function involve alterations in gene expression, as research into memory has demonstrated; animal studies show that learned behaviour results in molecular changes in synaptic connections.

We are close to a point at which it is possible to correlate changes in gene expression with changes in behaviour. Thus genetic approaches to psychiatry are not limited to understanding inherited disease. They have become central to a biological understanding of psychiatric disorders, and all psychiatrists will need to have some familiarity with molecular biology.[4]

Expositions of molecular genetics are hampered by the rapid pace of change in the field and an associated proliferation of jargon. In this chapter the background essential for appreciating the issues currently reported in the research literature is outlined and an attempt is made to cover areas of molecular genetics that are likely to become relevant with the completion of the Human Genome Project and the ability to screen every gene for sequence differences that may be disease related. The chapter starts with a basic introduction to DNA structure and function, which is followed by an outline of the ways in which disease genes are identified.

The second part of the chapter reviews the molecular pathology of psychiatric disorders (still limited to rare single-gene disorders). Research that is likely to have an impact on clinical practice in the near future is covered in the last two sections, which deal with the biological basis of mental processes and the genetic effects on common psychiatric disorders. Work in both areas is still in its infancy, but is progressing fast.

The section on the neurobiology of learning and memory shows how genetic influences on cognitive processes can be interpreted as acting at the level of a neural system (spatial memory), the first time such a feat has been achieved and no doubt a paradigm for further developments. In the last part of this chapter, the scant data on the molecular basis of complex genetic disorders and their implications for psychiatric disorders are reviewed. Despite a huge amount or work, we still do not have good candidates for susceptibility genes, except in the case of diabetes. The complexities encountered in that disorder are again paradigmatic and indicate that we will need a sophisticated knowledge of genetics to make sense of the coming results of mapping susceptibility genes for common psychiatric disorders.

Nucleic acid structure and function

The chemical constituents of genetic information are deoxyribo-nucleic acid (**DNA**) and ribonucleic acid (**RNA**). Both molecules consist of linear chains of nitrogenous bases bound to a sugar (ribose) and a phosphate backbone. Because of the way the sugars are joined together, one end of each nucleic acid strand will have a terminal sugar residue in which the carbon atom at position number 5 of the ribose molecule is not linked; the other end has a free carbon atom at position 3. These two ends are termed the 5′ (5 prime) and 3′ (3 prime) ends respectively. It is usual to describe a DNA or RNA sequence by writing the order of bases in a single strand, in the 5′ to 3′ direction. DNA contains four nitrogenous bases: adenine (A), guanine (G), cytosine (C), and thymine (T). RNA differs in that it contains uracil instead of thymine.

Two structural differences between DNA and RNA are important for understanding nucleic acid function. First, DNA has a hydroxyl group on part of its sugar constituent whereas RNA has a hydrogen atom. The result is that, in most biological environments, RNA is much more unstable. Second, RNA normally exists as a single molecule, whereas DNA is a double helix in which two strands are held together by weak hydrogen bonds between opposed base pairs (**bp**), C joined to G and A to T. The sequence of one strand can therefore be inferred from the other. The two strands are said to be complementary to each other, and this property is exploited whenever DNA is copied (during meiosis, mitosis, or *in vitro* processes such as amplification of DNA using a polymerase chain reaction).

As befits an unstable molecule, RNA mediates the expression of genetic information; its production, and degradation, are under tight regulation. RNA is translated into a linear order of amino acids in proteins according to a three-letter code (e.g. GAA encodes the amino acid glutamine). DNA acts as a template for the production of RNA in a process termed transcription. But DNA is more than a stable repository of encoded protein sequence information; it also contains information that controls the transcription of RNA.

Disorders of the template function of DNA are the molecular basis of inherited dispositions and illness, and are the subject matter of genetics. By contrast, gene expression (the transcription and translation of RNA) is not entirely genetically predetermined. It is tightly regulated, but in response to changes in the cellular environment which in turn reflect changes in the state of the organism. Unfortunately we do not know much about how gene expression is regulated in eukaryotes, although this subject is rapidly progressing and will certainly have a major impact on the understanding and treatment of human disease. An introduction to this important subject is given below. For further details the reader is recommended to consult the textbook by Strachan and Read.[5]

Gene expression and regulation

A gene is a section of DNA that is transcribed into RNA which in turn encodes a protein (although a small number of unusual genes are not translated and indeed cannot be translated into protein). For reasons that are still unclear, large portions of transcribed RNA are excised (by RNA splicing enzymes) and additional modifications are made to the ends of the RNA molecule (capping of one end and polyadenylation of the other). The final product, messenger RNA (**mRNA**), contains a central section, translated into protein, and flanking non-coding

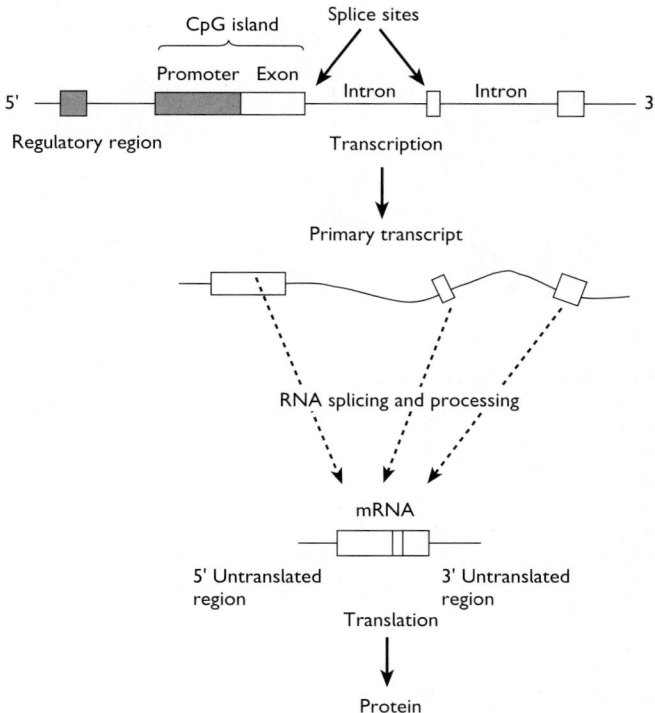

Fig. 1 The figure shows the process of transcription by which mRNA is produced from DNA. At the top of the figure the organization of a gene in genomic DNA is shown. Unshaded boxes correspond to coding regions (exons) and the two shaded boxes correspond to control regions. The control region immediately 5′ of the first exon, where transcription is initiated, is known as the promoter and often has a characteristic sequence composition. In almost all ubiquitously expressed genes (and in many tissue-specific genes) it is unmethylated, GC rich, and has a relative excess of the dinucleotide CpG. The region, which typically contains the first exon as well as the promoter, is called a CpG island. The boundaries between exons and introns are called splice sites and are conserved; introns virtually always start with the sequence GT and end with the sequence AG. The entire genomic region is transcribed into a primary transcript (bold arrow) which is then processed to excise the introns. Many human genes undergo alternative splicing to yield a number of different mRNA products. Mature mRNA is then translated into a protein product.

regions. The consequence of these manipulations is that DNA and mRNA are not coterminous; sections of DNA that encode mRNA (termed exons) are interrupted by often very large stretches of DNA that are not translated (termed introns) (Fig. 1).

We know of a number of ways in which gene expression is controlled. Predominantly it occurs at the level of transcription (but post-transcriptional processing and translational control are important for some genes). Transcriptional control involves at least three mechanisms, which are illustrated in Fig. 2.

First, transcription factors exercise control over gene expression. Transcription occurs when RNA polymerases manufacture RNA from the template DNA, a process that requires the help of transcription factors, proteins that recognize and bind to specific DNA sequences (note that transcription factors can also *repress* transcription). Although transcription factor binding sites are found close to a gene, at a 5′ region known as the promoter (see Fig. 1), they may also be situated far away, sometimes within other genes. Transcription factors

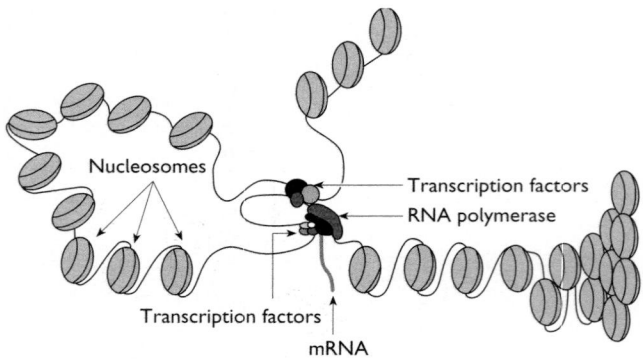

Fig. 2 Factors involved in regulating the transcription of DNA. Gene expression requires an RNA polymerase which initially binds to the 5′ end of the gene at the promoter. The figure shows polymerization occurring once transcription factors have bound to DNA and to the polymerase. Note that the transcription factors are binding not only close to the gene, but also at a distance. Transcription occurs in the centre of the figure, in a region of DNA devoid of chromatin. Shaded ovals indicate nucleosomes, one level at which chromatin packages DNA. The higher-order structure of chromatin is unknown, but is indicated on the right of the figure by tightly packed nucleosomes.

are themselves the products of genes, so that they may control their own expression or be part of more complex sets of interacting regulatory pathways.

Second, transcription can be controlled by the extent to which the DNA is made accessible to the transcriptional machinery. DNA does not exist in a free state in the cell; it is closely associated with a complex of proteins called chromatin. For a long time chromatin was considered to be merely a way of packing DNA into the nucleus, but it is now clear that it is intricately involved in DNA metabolism. Figure 2 shows how DNA is wrapped around nucleosomes, which are composed of chromatin proteins. On the right the nucleosomes are packed together and, although the higher-order structure is not known, tightly packed nucleosomes mean that DNA cannot be transcribed. DNA has to be free of nucleosomes for it to be accessible to transcription factors and the large complex of proteins that constitutes RNA polymerase. Actively transcribed DNA lies in regions of relatively open chromatin, which can be experimentally identified by their accessibility to enzymes that digest DNA (nucleases). Therefore understanding what controls chromatin packaging will reveal one way of controlling gene expression. For this reason there has been much interest in characterizing proteins that remodel chromatin and consequently influence many biochemical pathways, including the control of genes involved in the development and activity of the central nervous system. For example, the mental retardation syndrome ATRX (discussed below) is due to a mutation in a transcriptional regulator that probably acts by remodelling chromatin.[6]

Gene expression can also be altered by the addition of methyl groups to cytosine bases. Methylation of DNA does not change the DNA sequence but, when it affects control regions, is associated with gene inactivation. It is not clear whether methylation is an independent mechanism for regulating gene expression, since methylation directs chromatin into an inactive conformation, mediated by methylated DNA binding proteins. Changes in methylation are involved in at least two mental retardation syndromes (the Prader–Willi and Angelman syndromes, discussed below).

Genome organization

Few disciplines are more burdened with jargon than molecular genetics. This is partly due to a proliferation of molecular techniques, but it is also partly intrinsic to the subject; the only unifying principle is evolution, which often operates in a very *ad hoc* fashion. Biological solutions to the problems posed by selection result in the adaptation of existing structures to new uses, rather than to the invention of purpose-built systems. Nowhere is this more true than at the level of the genome which, rather than being an efficiently organized plan of the organism consisting of precise drawings, resembles a working copy written over countless rough drafts and discarded versions, among which there are literally thousands of jottings and scribbles, mostly irrelevant to the final structure.

DNA within cells is packaged into chromosomes in the cell nucleus, with a tiny amount (16 569 bases containing 37 genes) in the mitochondria. Since mitochondria in the fertilized egg are maternally derived, mitochondrial inheritance is through the female lineage. Although small, mitochondrial disorders contribute substantially to degenerative disorders including ageing.[7] More important is nuclear DNA. The total size of the nuclear genome is approximately 3000 million bp (megabases) and codes for between 65 000 and 100 000 genes. Only 3 per cent of the genome codes for protein. Perhaps 90 per cent of nuclear DNA has no function, consisting primarily of repetitive sequences.

Nuclear DNA is contained in the 22 pairs of chromosomes (the autosomes), one inherited from the mother and one from the father, and the two sex chromosomes, X and Y. Each chromosome pair exchanges stretches of DNA during sexual division (meiosis) in a process called recombination (without which genetic mapping, the basic method of finding disease genes, would be impossible).

Chromosomes have three functional elements: origins of replication, centromeres, and telomeres. Replication origins are required to initiate DNA replication and maintain chromosome copy number. Their molecular structure is unknown. Centromeres are responsible for the segregation of chromosomes during cell division. Their molecular nature is also not understood, but they are visible in light microscopy as a constriction where the duplicated chromosomes (called chromatids) are held together. Chromosomes are said to have two arms, separated by the centromere which, despite its name, is not always at the centre. Short arms are termed p (petit) and long arms q (queue). Telomeres are the ends of chromosomes and their molecular nature is well understood. They consist of long stretches of the sequence TTAGGG without which the chromosome is unstable, tending to break apart and fuse with itself or to other chromosomes.

No one has found any general principles that organize genetic material within chromosomes. While there are examples of gene families clustered in the same chromosomal location (for instance genes involved in immune regulation are clustered on chromosome 6p), more commonly the position of genes on chromosomes does not reflect functional similarity. For example, the most complete structural and functional analysis to date of a large region of human genomic sequence (the terminal region of chromosome 16p) shows that genes expressed only in erythroid tissue are immediately adjacent to widely expressed housekeeping genes.[8]

Figure 3 shows the organization of genes at the end of chromosome 16p and summarizes many of the points made here. It highlights our

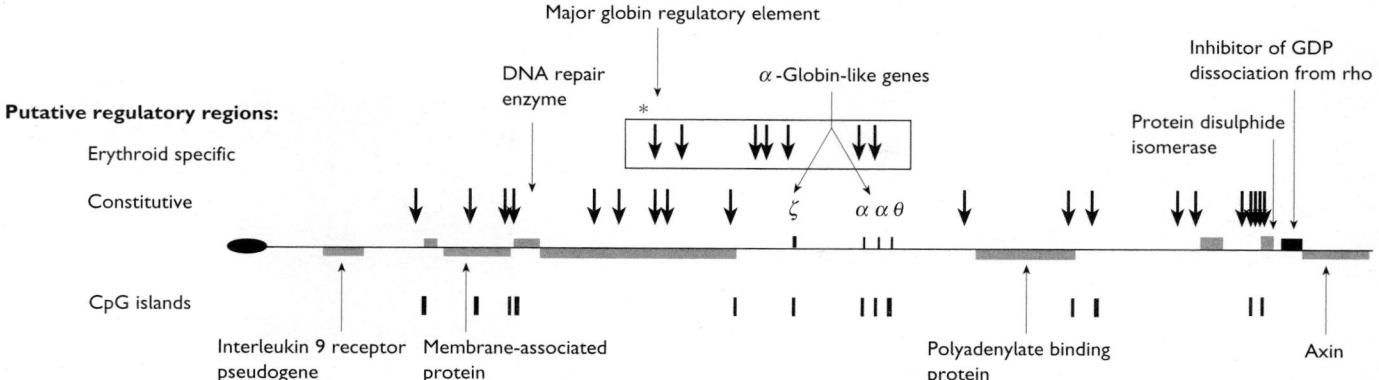

Fig. 3 The relationship between chromosome structure and function at the end of chromosome 16p. The oval on the left of the figure indicates the telomere (the end of the chromosome). Boxes above the line indicate genes transcribed towards the centromere and boxes under the line indicate genes transcribed towards the telomere. Black boxes are tissue-specific genes: the four α-globin-like genes (one ζ, two α, and one θ gene) and a liver-specific gene (an inhibitor of the dissociation of guanine diphosphate from rho). Grey boxes are ubiquitously expressed genes. The distinction between introns and exons is not shown. The function of only some genes is known, as indicated on the figure. Apart from the globins, we are confident of the function of only four genes (the DNA repair enzyme, protein disulphide isomerase, the inhibitor of guanine diphosphate dissociation, and axin). The function of a few others is inferred from sequence analysis, but for the remainder we have no clue at all. Two sorts of putative control regions are indicated. Above the line, arrows indicate regions devoid of nucleosomes where regulatory proteins may bind. They fall into two classes, those present in every tissue (constitutive) and those present only in erythroid tissues (erythroid specific). Note that the latter extend well beyond the region containing the α-globin genes. Underneath the line are shown the position of CpG islands (as defined in Fig. 1).

poor understanding of the relationship between genome structure and function, for, despite extensive characterization of the region, we know the function of only a few of the genes shown. Potential binding sites for regulatory proteins are scattered across the region, with no apparent logic. The major regulatory element for the α-globin genes (which encode one half of the oxygen-transporting protein haemoglobin) lies within an intron of another gene (of unknown function). Similar pictures of genome organization are emerging from analysis of other regions of the genome.

Genetic and physical mapping

Molecular characterization of genetic disease is based on the supposition that it is possible to identify an alteration in gene expression that causes the disease. In single-gene disorders the task is conceptually straightforward (although often technically demanding); the aim is to establish that all those with the disorder have DNA sequence changes (mutations) affecting the same gene and that such changes are not found in unaffected individuals. Enough is known about sequence codes to recognize a mutation that will disrupt gene expression, and this can be experimentally verified by looking at the production and structure of mRNA. The technical challenge is to find the one mutation in 3000 million bases which is responsible for the change in gene expression.

Genetic mapping is still the basic method for locating a disease gene to a small region of a chromosome. Before explaining what gene mapping entails, some terminology needs to be explained. A position on a chromosome is termed a locus, a general term which can refer to a gene or a segment of DNA with no known function. DNA sequences that differ at the same locus are termed allelic variants. Since we have two copies of each chromosome, by definition we have two alleles at each

locus. If these alleles are identical the individual is said to be a homozygote at that locus; if they are different, the individual is a heterozygote. The number of alleles at any locus varies remarkably; at the most polymorphic loci, hundreds of alleles may be found. Polymorphism in the human genome is important in a practical sense because it permits gene mapping, and hence disease gene identification.

The basic idea of gene mapping is to track genetic recombinants in pedigrees. Recombination can occur almost anywhere on a chromosome and will break up the association of alleles between different loci along that chromosome (such an association is called a haplotype). Alleles, like most single-gene disorders, follow Mendelian laws of segregation so that it is possible to ask whether one is segregating with a disease and test the result statistically using methods described in Chapter 2.4.1. The expected result is an estimate of the probability that an allele and a disease locus will recombine; the lower the probability, the closer together the two loci are on the chromosome.

The statistical test tells us the likelihood that the estimate of recombination distance is correct. If the likelihood is acceptably high, then the next task is further genetic mapping to reduce the genetic interval as much as possible, at which point physical mapping and characterization of the region takes over as the principal tool of disease gene identification. The latter process is currently the most time consuming and expensive, but will become easier with the completion of the Human Genome Project.

Genetic mapping of disease genes is a powerful method because it does not require any knowledge of a gene's function to find the chromosomal location and then the identity of the disease gene. It is a successful method because the genome is replete with DNA sequence polymorphisms whose only known use is to enable geneticists to map disease genes. On average, every 1000 bp will contain 1.4 bases that differ between two randomly chosen individuals (although the full extent of variation is not known), almost all of which have no phenotypic consequence. In addition, there are small runs of repeated

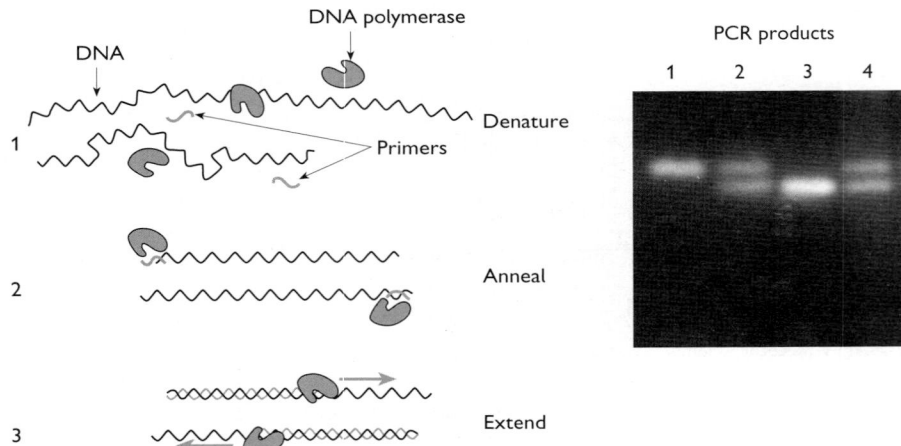

Fig. 4 The polymerase chain reaction. The essential ingredients for *in vitro* DNA amplification are as follows: a DNA polymerase (shaded shape); a pair of oligonucleotides (referred to as primers in the figure and shown as short grey wavy lines), which are synthetic single-stranded DNA, usually between 15 and 25 bases long, complementary to two sequences on opposite strands of the target DNA; the target DNA itself; all four nucleotides, usually present in excess; appropriate buffer and cofactors for the reaction. The reaction proceeds in a cycle of three steps: (1) the mixture is heated to over 90°C for 1 min to separate the complementary strands of target DNA; (2) the mixture is cooled, to about 50°C, so that the oligonucleotides anneal to their complementary sequence in the target DNA and allow the DNA polymerase to bind (oligonucleotides are required to prime the polymerase); (3) the temperature is adjusted to allow the polymerase to function in the extension component of the reaction. Typically the polymerase is from a thermophilic bacterium with a permissive temperature of 72°C. Products from the first cycle can serve as targets for a second round of amplification and the cycle can be repeated, usually up to about 40 times. One way of visualizing the products of a PCR reaction is shown on the right of the figure. The DNA has been electrophoresed through an agarose gel, which resolves the PCR products by size so that smaller fragments are lower down the gel. The PCR products in the gel are stained with a dye that fluoresces under ultraviolet light and appear as white bands in the photograph. The gel shows samples from four individuals at a polymorphic locus. Lanes 2 and 4 are heterozygotes and lanes 1 and 3 are homozygotes.

sequence (most commonly CA) which differ in length between individuals. At least one of these short tandem repeats (**STRs**), or **microsatellites**, is found every 50 kilobases (**kb**) and they also have no known phenotypic consequences. There are other more complex sequence polymorphisms, but single-nucleotide polymorphisms (**SNPs**) and microsatellites are the most useful for identifying disease genes. The process of defining which alleles a person has at a polymorphic locus is termed genotyping.

Microsatellites are currently preferred as genetic markers in disease mapping because they can be detected using the polymerase chain reaction (**PCR**) (see Fig. 4). Many thousands have already been placed on a genetic map which provides the basic cartographic resource for molecular cloning, and eventually sequencing, of the human genome. However, recent technical innovations promise to make genotyping SNPs the favoured way to map genetic disease.

A number of approaches are now available for genotyping many thousands of SNPs in a few hours. One method uses mass spectrometry to measure size differences between DNA fragments; another uses hybridization to a minute glass slide (smaller than a postage stamp and called a DNA chip) containing tens of thousands of small stretches of DNA (oligonucleotides). Hybridization is the process whereby two strands of genomic DNA, separated chemically or by heat (the DNA is said to be denatured), will pair to their complementary sequences, which can be either their original partner or any other DNA with the same complementary sequence. The chip technology involves hybridizing DNA labelled with a fluorescent nucleotide to oligonucleotides that have been synthesized directly onto glass.

The advantage of the new techniques is the high throughput they permit, so that it is possible to genotype very large numbers of individuals with very large numbers of markers.[9] For statistical reasons, successful genetic analysis of common psychiatric disorders may only be possible with the massive genotyping provided by SNP analysis.

How to find a disease gene

Cloning a disease gene on the basis of positional information is still an extremely labour-intensive and technically demanding process, made very much easier if additional information is available. One of the most helpful things to know is what genes are present in the region thought to contain the disease gene, permitting the researcher to test each candidate.[10] Once an enormous undertaking, finding genes at a locus can now be done by anyone with access to the Internet, making positional candidate approaches to disease gene identification a very effective strategy. Genes, and more besides, are identified every day as part of the Human Genome Project and made publicly available at the websites of the participating laboratories (e.g. http://www.sanger.ac.uk and http://www. genome.wi.mit.edu.) Procedures for the identification of disease genes are so inextricably tied up with the progress of the Human Genome Project that molecular genetic approaches to human health and illness cannot be discussed without considering the Project's aims and scope.

Ever since its inception there has been discussion as to whether resources should be focused on sequencing only coding DNA. The biological interest of the human genome lies primarily in the genes, which could be sequenced at a fraction of the cost and effort required to sequence the entire genome. Genes can be identified by isolating mRNA, using an enzyme (reverse transcriptase) to copy RNA into

DNA, and then sequencing the DNA. Making RNA from many different tissues and from different developmental stages increases the chances of obtaining a representative collection of expressed sequences, and this project has been undertaken by a number of academic and industrial research groups.[11] Small fragments of DNA complementary to the mRNA (termed **cDNA**) are sequenced to generate a set of expressed sequence tags (**ESTs**) that are then placed on the existing physical and genetic maps of the human genome.[12] These advances mean that disease gene identification can be achieved by searching a database of ESTs and other sequence information within the region known to contain the disease locus. The size of the databases is enormous; at the time of writing publicly available databases include 1.7 million EST entries.

However, sequencing cDNA is now only a small portion of the effort that is being put into the Human Genome Project. A number of laboratories are devoted entirely to cloning, and then sequencing, human chromosomes, so that once a disease gene has been localized, the most efficient method to identify the abnormal transcript is to contact the appropriate laboratory. Much basic biology can then be done with a computer and a telephone. Indeed, bio-informatics is likely to take over from bench work as the major tool for disease gene identification.

Molecular techniques have been most successful in identifying genetic mutations in disorders with a simple genetic basis—one mutated gene segregating according to Mendelian genetics causing disease in a recessive or dominant fashion. Such single-gene mutations make a small contribution to psychiatric disorders, with the exception of syndromes associated with mental retardation. Can the same strategy work for common psychiatric disorders? There are three reasons to be cautious.

First, not all genetic conditions that have a simple genetic basis have yielded to positional cloning strategies. A good example is fascio-scapulo-humeral muscular dystrophy (FSHD) which has been mapped to the end of 4q and associated with the presence of an unusual series of repeats. Despite extensive characterization and sequencing of the region, no mutated genes have been found. The suspicion is that the repetitive region is involved in controlling a set of distant, as yet uncharacterized genes.[13,14] Similar complexities have beset attempts to clone genes implicated in some chromosomal deletion syndromes (see below). Thus our knowledge of gene regulation is not sufficiently advanced to permit us to recognize all mutations.

Second, it is known that the same phenotype can arise from mutations at different loci (genetic heterogeneity); conversely, mutations in a single gene can result in a set of different phenotypes (an allelic series). Perhaps the best example of an allelic series is the mutations in one of the fibroblast growth factor receptor genes (FGFR2) which are responsible for four different craniofacial syndromes.[15] No examples of allelic series are recorded (yet) in psychiatric genetics. However, genetic heterogeneity is already documented for Alzheimer's disease, which can be due to mutations in presenilin genes on chromosomes 1 and 14, and to mutations in the amyloid precursor protein gene on chromosome 21.[16–19] Genetic heterogeneity is almost certainly an important feature of the genetic architecture of schizophrenia and manic–depressive psychosis. Both allelic series and genetic heterogeneity seriously complicate the task of associating genotypes with phenotypes, the basis of disease gene mapping and identification.

Third, the genetic contribution to many common psychiatric disorders may not be a mutation that disrupts gene expression but one that has a more subtle effect and is considerably harder to detect. Traits such as anxiety and depression are normally distributed *quantitative* traits for which the distinction between clinical disorder and normality is conventional. It is hard to believe that the molecular basis of allelic differences underlying quantitative traits is due to the type of mutation mentioned above. While the genetic basis for some extreme phenotypes might be due to the deletion of a gene or to an inactivating mutation, it is much more likely that extremes of traits such as anxiety and depression are due to subtle changes in gene expression, perhaps affecting developmental genes early in life and possibly arising from allelic differences in unexpressed regions of the genome that contain sequences controlling gene expression. Consequently it will be very hard to devise a way of proving that a candidate gene really does underlie the phenotype. There may be no discernible sequence differences or expression differences to identify the gene and even if there are, their presence does not prove that they are of aetiological significance.

While association studies can go some way to implicating a particular sequence, they can never be proof of a causal relation. A functional assay is needed—a way to alter the sequence and see whether that change results in an altered phenotype. Such experiments are currently only possible in animals and may be the only way to understand how genetic differences result in individual variation in susceptibility to common psychiatric disorders.

Genetic manipulation of animals

The molecular techniques described above are used in attempts to find genetic alterations that either cause or increase susceptibility to psychiatric disease. Because so little is assumed about the pathogenesis of the condition (other than it has a genetic component), the methodology is extremely useful when we have little or no aetiological information. The drawback is that once the gene is identified we may have no idea what it does. One of the great surprises of the genome sequencing projects is that there are so many genes with unknown functions (more than 80 per cent of identified expressed sequenced genes in the human genome, and 70 per cent of genes in yeast,[20] have no known function). A whole discipline, functional genomics, is now developing to find out what genes do. With the completion of the Human Genome Project, functional genomics will become the cynosure of biology.

One of the most fruitful ways of investigating gene function is by genetic manipulation of animals, generally either introducing a copy of the gene into a mouse or mutating the mouse version of the gene. Both approaches work because exogenous DNA can integrate into chromosomes. If the site of integration can be targeted, rather than being random, the exogenous DNA can be used to create mutations in specific genes.

Transgenic mice are made by injecting human DNA into fertilized mouse oocytes. Integration is a rare and random event, but almost always involves multiple copies entering at a single site, making interpretation of some transgenic experiments difficult. More specific genetic manipulation is achieved by exploiting homologous recombination in embryonic stem (**ES**) cells, although the technique is very technically demanding. DNA containing a mutated copy of the gene of interest in tandem with a selectable marker (e.g. an antibiotic resistance gene) is introduced into ES cells where in a small number of cases it recombines with, and consequently replaces, the cell's copy of the gene. ES cells are isolated from embryos and can be grown in flasks while retaining the potential to develop into any tissue. Once they have been genetically manipulated and reinjected back into the pregnant mouse, the resulting embryo is a mixture of mutant and normal cells. If some of the ES cells contribute to the germ line of the embryo, then its offspring will be full heterozygote mutants, from which homozygotes can be bred.

Two improvements in knockout technology are already making an impact on neuroscience research.[21] Inducible gene knockouts use homologous recombination to replace the gene of interest, but in addition to the mutant gene and selectable marker, the replacement DNA contains a sequence that puts expression of the gene under exogenous control; gene expression from the construct can then be altered by feeding the animal tetracycline, for instance. A slightly different technology is involved in the creation of cell-type restricted knockouts. Sequences recognized by an enzyme that excises DNA are introduced either side of the gene of interest and mice are crossed with a strain that contains the gene for the excision enzyme, which is itself under exogenous control (generally in a tissue- or cell-type-specific fashion). In progeny with the gene flanked by recognition sites, the gene is excised only in those cells in which the enzyme is activated.

The power of genetic engineering technology is impressive but, as with all new technologies, its limitations are still unclear. At least two reservations should be borne in mind. First, the effects of any knockout experiment will be present in all tissues and throughout development. Consequently, effects observed in the adult could be the result of developmental abnormalities. The newer tissue-specific knockouts, or those where gene expression is said to be regulated by a tissue-specific promoter, are improvements but they are not perfect models. As explained above, understanding of tissue-specific gene regulation is still rudimentary and we do not know exactly which sequences are required for controlling gene expression.

Second, the genetic background of a mutant can have an effect on the mutant.[22] Most targeting experiments use the ES stem cells derived from substrain 129 mice, which are crossed with another inbred line. The choice of inbred line into which the mutation is bred can be critical because many inbred lines have specific behavioural phenotypes; for instance, the inbred strain DBA shows poor hippocampal-dependent learning[23] and C57BL/6 mice are poor avoidance learners.[24]

Neither reservation should obscure the fact that genetic manipulation of animals has already made considerable inroads into problems of neurobiology, as described later in this chapter. The technique is an invaluable way of exploring gene function, and will undoubtedly be necessary to work out the pathogenesis of common psychiatric disorders.

Molecular pathology

Almost all molecular analyses of human disease end in the characterization of DNA sequence variants that produce the disease. The experimental approaches described at the end of this chapter give an alternative approach to understanding the relationship between gene and behaviour, but at present, at least in humans, we are limited to documenting the mutation and observing the phenotype. The following section documents what we know about this relationship in naturally occurring mutants that cause psychiatric disease.

Mutational mechanisms

The complexity of both the patterns of inheritance and phenotypes of psychiatric disorders suggests that the underlying genetic abnormalities are equally complex. In fact there is probably nothing unique about the molecular defects, although it has to be admitted that we know next to nothing about the molecular basis of common psychiatric conditions. Where mutations have been described in single genes that give rise to behavioural disorders, they are typical of other human genetic disorders; changes in a single base pair (e.g. from C to T) of the coding sequence of the gene may alter the function of the protein (**mis-sense mutations**), result in premature termination of the protein product (**non-sense mutations**), or create or destroy a splice site. In addition, deletions (of a single base pair or many megabases of DNA) and insertions (again of any size) disrupt transcription and translation of a gene. Deletions or insertions that do not affect a multiple of three bases alter the way that the message is translated and are known as frame-shift mutations. None of these mechanisms is special to psychiatric genetics and by themselves tells us nothing about how the mutation produces the disorder.

One mutational mechanism that does deserve special comment is expansion of trinucleotide repeats.[25] Its importance in psychiatry is that it occurs in neurological disorders, some with behavioural phenotypes, and in two mental retardation syndromes (Table 1). No one knows why trinucleotide repeat expansions tend to be found in disorders of the central nervous system, and the unusual mutational mechanism has not so far explained the pathogenesis of any of the disorders in which it occurs. The mechanism was first discovered in 1991 as the cause of fragile X syndrome, a common form of inherited X-linked mental retardation.[26]

The most common repeat types are AGC and CGG (Table 1) which can expand dramatically from a small array in unaffected individuals to many hundreds of copies. At each locus there is a normal range of copy numbers above which the repeat array becomes unstable—the larger the number of copies, the more unstable is the allele. Furthermore, larger alleles result in more severe disease with earlier onset. The consequence is that the age of onset of a disorder may become progressively earlier with each new generation of affected individuals in a pedigree, a phenomenon called anticipation. The association between trinucleotide repeat expansions and central nervous system disorders, together with claims that anticipation occurs in manic–depressive psychosis and, less credibly, in schizophrenia, prompted a search for expanded trinucleotide repeats in the psychoses. The results, although preliminary, suggest that schizophrenics may have an excess of expanded trinucleotide repeats compared with controls.[27-29] However, it should again be stressed that molecular mechanisms have not yet told us anything about pathogenesis.

Mutational spectrum

Describing the mutational basis of a genetic disorder is an initial step in understanding how the disorder arises; what the DNA sequence change does to the protein gives a clue to the protein's function (if unknown) and to the pathogenesis of the condition. Analysis of

Table 1 Triplet repeat diseases

Disease	Normal	Premutation	Affected	Repeat
Fragile X syndrome (FraxA)	6–54	43–200	>200	CCG
FRAXE	6–30		>200	CCG
Huntington's disease	4–36	36–41	42–121	AGC
Spinocerebellar ataxia 1	6–39		39–83	AGC
Spinocerebellar ataxia 2	14–32	32–34	35–77	AGC
Spinocerebellar ataxia 3	12–40	41–62	63–86	AGC
Spinocerebellar ataxia 6	4–18	19–21	22–30	AGC
Dentatorubral pallidolyusian atrophy	3–36	37–38	39–62	AGC
Spinobulbar muscular atrophy	9–36	37–41	42–121	AGC
Myotonic dystrophy	5–50	50–100	>100	AGC
Friedrich's ataxia	7–32		>100	AAG

mutants causing dementia, isolated by positional molecular cloning, are an example.

The presenilins are ubiquitously expressed transmembrane proteins of unknown function, in which mutations give rise to rare forms of inherited Alzheimer's disease.[16–18,30] All but one of the many mutations that have been described are mis-sense mutations. Why are there no frame-shift or non-sense mutants? Recall that mis-sense mutants alter an amino acid in the protein and therefore can alter its function. Presumably therefore the mutations in presenilin result in a gain of function, although what that may be is unknown. One clue comes from looking at where the mutations occur within the protein, to discern whether some parts of the molecule are more frequently involved than others. The distribution of mutations in the presenilins is indeed non-random; they occur at residues which are the same in both presenilin genes, lying on one side of the α helix in transmembrane domains, predominantly in exon 8. Thus the mutational spectrum highlights key residues for understanding the protein's functions.[31,32]

Where a gene's function is known, the distribution of mutations may point out the likely pathogenesis. For example, mutations in the tau gene are now known to cause frontotemporal dementia with parkinsonism (Pick's disease).[33,34] The most common mutation occurs in the 5′ splice site of exon 10, resulting in overproduction and accumulation of one form of tau; mutations in other regions of the gene lead to accumulation of a different form of the protein. The position of the mutations in tau indicate that they cause disruption of tau microtubule binding, which may cause cell death by the degeneration of microtubules or through an increase in unbound tau.

Molecular pathogenesis

The immense efforts involved in positional cloning of a disease gene are rarely rewarded with as much insight into the biology of the condition as has been the case with the dementias. Indeed, stages subsequent to cloning are often even more arduous. Tables 2 and 3 give a list of disorders with a behavioural phenotype (excluding metabolic conditions), due either to abnormalities of a single gene or of a small chromosomal region, analysed at the molecular level. For some conditions, mutant genes have been identified; for others, the cause remains obscure despite immense amounts of genetic analysis. Often, even where a gene has been found, its function is unknown.

We can interpret the tables in two ways: either they suggest that molecular approaches are not an efficient way of understanding the pathogenesis of genetic conditions, or the pathogenesis is extremely

Table 2 Cloned genes responsible for mental retardation

Disorder	Phenotype	Location	Gene	Function
Angelman syndrome	Syndromal mental retardation	15q11–q13	UBE3A	E6–Ap ubiquitin protein ligase
Fragile X syndrome	Syndromal mental retardation	Xq27	FMR1	Unknown
X-linked hydrocephalus/spastic paraplegia/MASA	Syndromal mental retardation	Xq28	L1 CAM	Neural cell adhesion molecule
Kallman syndrome	Syndromal mental retardation	Xp22	NCAM	Neural cell adhesion molecule
Rubinstein–Taybi syndrome	Syndromal mental retardation	16p13	CBP	cAMP-responsive element binding protein
Tuberous sclerosis	Syndromal mental retardation	16p13	Tuberin	
ATRX	Syndromal mental retardation	Xq13	ATRX	Regulator of gene expression
Optiz G/BBB	Syndromal mental retardation	Xp22	MID1	Regulates midline development
FRAXE	Non-specific mental retardation	Xq27	FMR2	Unknown
X-linked mental retardation	Non-specific mental retardation	Xp11	MAOA	Monoamine metabolism
X-linked mental retardation	Non-specific mental retardation	Xq12	Oligophrenin	Rho GTP activating protein
X-linked mental retardation	Non-specific mental retardation	Xq28	GDI 1	Rab3a GDP dissociation inhibitor
X-linked mental retardation	Non-specific mental retardation	Xq22	PAK3	Links Rac and Cdc42 to the actin cytoskeleton

MASA, mental retardation–adducted thumbs–spastic paralysis–aphasia.

Table 3 Segmental aneusomy syndromes

Disorder	Phenotype	Location	Mechanism	MR gene	Function
Williams syndrome	Syndromal mental retardation	7q11.23	Haploinsufficiency	LIM 1 kinase	Unknown
Angelman syndrome	Syndromal mental retardation	15a11–q13	Deletion/imprinting disorder	UBE3A	Ubiquitin-mediated protein degradation
Prader–Willi syndrome	Syndromal mental retardation	15q11–q13	Deletion/imprinting disorder	Many candidates	
Langer–Giedion syndrome	Syndromal mental retardation	8q24.1	Haploinsufficiency	Unknown	
Miller–Dieker syndrome	Syndromal mental retardation	17p13.3	Haploinsufficiency	LIS1	Platelet-activating factor–neurotransmitter
Smith–Magenis syndrome	Syndromal mental retardation	17p11.2	Haploinsufficiency	Unknown	
DiGeorge/velocardiofacial syndrome	Syndromal mental retardation	22q11.2	Haploinsufficiency?	Many candidates	
Wolf–Hirschhorn syndrome	Syndromal mental retardation	4p16.3	Haploinsufficiency	Unknown	
Cri-du-chat	Syndromal mental retardation	5p13–5pter	Haploinsufficiency	Unknown	
ATR-16	Syndromal mental retardation	16p13.3	Haploinsufficiency	Unknown	
Turner syndrome	Syndromal mental retardation	X	Haploinsufficiency	Unknown	
WAGR	Syndromal mental retardation	11p13	Haploinsufficiency	Unknown	

complex. Unfortunately the latter may well be the case. A description of what is known about the relevant conditions is given below.

Mental retardation

It is useful to divide mental retardation into two categories: syndromal and non-syndromal (see Table 2). The distinction is based on the observation that many of the more than 800 genetic and chromosomal disorders associated with mental retardation have a complex phenotype including, for example, facial dysmorphism, minor congenital anomalies of the hands and feet, cardiac defects, genitourinary abnormalities, short stature, and microcephaly. In non-syndromal mental retardation the only known abnormality is cognitive, and a number of families have been found in which the disorder segregates as a single Mendelian gene. Since affected individuals are less likely to reproduce, it is not surprising that known pedigrees show linkage to the X chromosome (X-linked mental retardation (XLMR)).[35]

Non-syndromal mental retardation

The genetic basis of four non-syndromal XLMR conditions has been identified and, remarkably, three of the four genes are related. They are GDI1, oligophrenin, and PAK3.[36–38] GDI1 is a guanine diphosphate (**GDP**) dissociation inhibitor of the protein Rab3a, a small guanosine triphosphate (**GTP**) binding protein that plays a role in the recruitment of synaptic vesicles for exocytosis.[39] Oligophrenin encodes a rhoGAP protein that stimulates the intrinsic GTPase activity of small G proteins. PAK3 links Rac and Cdc42 to the actin cytoskeleton and to transcriptional activation. Thus GDI1, oligophrenin, and PAK3 are all involved in Rho GTPase signalling networks. What does this tell us about the pathogenesis of mental retardation?

At present, there are two possibilities. The first is that normal development of axonal connections is disrupted in patients with mutations in these genes. As yet that hypothesis is unproved, but it fits with what is known about the cell biology of the Rho GTPases.[40] Axons and neurites find their way through the developing brain by sampling

molecular signals, helped by GTPases, and dendritic formation (like other cellular extensions, filopodia, and lamellae) is reduced by inhibiting Rho GTPases. Furthermore, the pattern of GDI1 expression in the developing brain is consistent with a developmental role.[37] The second possibility is that synaptic function is compromised. The main evidence here comes from our understanding of the function of Rab3a, a protein that is only expressed in neurones and neuroendocrine cells and localizes to secretory vesicles. A decrease in intracellular Rab3a concentrations, due to the GDI1 mutation, could reduce neurotransmitter release.

The fourth gene implicated in non-syndromal mental retardation is FMR2.[41,42] We know next to nothing about what the gene does, other than that it encodes a nuclear protein that may regulate transcription.[43,44] The dearth of information about its function is more typical of our knowledge of genes involved in mental retardation than is suggested by the success with Rho GTPase family of genes.

Syndromal mental retardation

Single genes

Molecular analysis of syndromal mental retardation has identified numerous genes, but has not cast much light on the pathogenesis of the condition. A division into conditions due to mutations in a single gene and those due to chromosomal rearrangements is helpful for descriptive purposes, but this probably does not reflect a major distinction in pathogenesis.

Perhaps the most disappointing result comes from the cloning of the FMR1 gene, mutations in which give rise to the fragile X syndrome, a common heritable cause of mental retardation (see Chapter 10.4). The mechanism of gene inactivation has turned out to be extremely interesting (amplification of a CGG repeat in the first exon of the gene), but although the gene was cloned in 1991, its function is still a mystery.[26,45,46] In normal brain, the protein is found in nearly all neurones but is absent from non-neuronal cells. The protein can bind RNA, including its own transcript, and it has been postulated that FMR protein has a role in the machinery of translation.[47–51]

FMR1 knockout mice have macro-orchidism and impaired spatial learning abilities, but nothing more to tell us what the gene does.[52]

We know more about a gene for a much rarer mental retardation syndrome, ATRX.[6] The disorder is X linked and patients have an anaemia (α-thalassaemia), a characteristic facial appearance, profound developmental delay, neonatal hypotonia, and genital abnormalities. The gene contains sequence motifs indicating that it belongs to a group of proteins that bind to chromatin. ATRX may be involved in chromatin remodelling (see Fig. 2). Possibly it regulates expression of a restricted class of genes, accounting for the pleiotropic effects of the mutant.

The final example is Optiz G/BBB syndrome, an X-linked multiple-organ disorder which includes developmental delay. Mutations have been found in a gene called MID1 whose features suggest that it is involved in developmental regulation by protein–protein interactions.[53] Again, this has not (yet) been helpful in advancing our understanding of pathogenesis of mental retardation.

Segmental aneusomy syndromes

A number of syndromes associated with mental retardation have been found to be due to chromosomal rearrangements among which Down syndrome (trisomy 21) is by far the most common (accounting for about a third of all cases with moderate to severe retardation). Chromosomal rearrangements can be extremely complex, as can the nomenclature used to describe them. Abnormalities of the number of chromosomes result in aneuploidy. Deletion of part or an entire chromosome is termed monosomy (or haploinsufficiency); an extra copy of either part of or an entire chromosome is called trisomy. A general term to describe either loss or excess of chromosomal material is aneusomy.

The phenotypes of chromosomal rearrangements are thought to arise because of the loss, in the case of monosomy, or addition, in the case of trisomy, of dosage-sensitive genes, of unrelated function, that happen to lie next to each other on the chromosome. Most chromosomal abnormalities involve small regions of aneusomy and consequently are known as segmental aneusomy syndromes[54] (see Table 3). The small size of some of the aneusomic regions has enabled a search for dosage-sensitive genes, and there are currently two examples where this approach appears to have been successful. Unfortunately, in neither case can it be said that the discovery has led to an understanding of the pathogenesis of mental retardation.

In Williams syndrome (see Chapter 10.4) it has been possible to identify genes that contribute to different components of the syndrome, one of which is cognitive impairment. Families have been found with a mutation affecting the elastin gene and presenting with supravalvular aortic stenosis and facial features typical of Williams syndrome, but normal intelligence. Other, very rare, families have some facial features, supravalvular aortic stenosis, verbal ability, and short-term memory similar to unaffected members, but marked impairment of visuoconstructive skills. Molecular characterization of these individuals showed that the chromosomal deletion was small (only 84 kb, compared with more than 500 kb found in the majority of Williams syndrome patients) which permitted the researchers to isolate a candidate gene, LIMK1 kinase.[55] The LIM domain, first identified in three homeodomain (developmental) proteins, is a zinc finger motif believed to function as protein–protein binding module in neural development.[56] LIMK1 binds to several isoforms of protein kinase C and to neuregulin.[57] Transmembrane neuregulins interact with LIMK1 and co-localize at the neuromuscular synapse, suggesting that the two proteins have a role in synapse formation and maintenance, although how this explains the defect in visuospatial cognition in Williams syndrome patients is a mystery.

Rubinstein–Taybi syndrome is characterized by abnormal craniofacial features, broad thumbs, and mental retardation. It arises from monosomy of a small region on 16p13.3, where mutations have been documented in the Cbp gene.[58] The protein product of the Cbp gene binds to the cyclic adenosine monophosphate (**cAMP**) response element binding protein, and to several elements of the basal transcriptional machinery, suggesting that mutations will disturb the transcription of numerous genes. Thus, as is the case with the ATRX syndrome, the molecular basis of Rubinstein–Taybi syndrome lies in a gene with effects on many different systems.

Non-Mendelian disorders

Two clinically distinct disorders, Prader–Willi syndrome (**PWS**) and Angelman syndrome (**AS**), arise from abnormalities of a small region of 15q11-q13.[59] The two syndromes have characteristic and distinct neurobehavioural profiles. In AS the retardation is severe (very few affected individuals can talk) and there is ataxia, seizures, an abnormal electroencephalogram, microcephaly, facial dysmorphism, hyperactivity, and paroxysmal laughter. In contrast, in PWS the mental retardation may be only mild. There is a characteristic facial appearance and a specific behavioural abnormality: hyperphagia resulting in severe obesity.

Despite the phenotypic differences, the basic defect is the same in both disorders—a failure of parent-of-origin-specific gene expression. Normally one chromosome 15 is inherited from the mother and the other from the father. If both derive from the mother, the individual will have PWS; if both derive from the father, the phenotype is AS. In both cases the DNA sequence is the same as in a normal individual, yet the phenotype is abnormal, showing that the chromosomes bear an additional molecular signal that affects gene expression and indicates their parent of origin. The signal is termed an imprint and is believed to be DNA methylation.

The majority (about 70 per cent) of cases of AS and PWS arise because there is a deletion within a 1.5-Mb region of 15q11-q13. A deletion on the maternal chromosome leaves only paternally expressed genes, resulting in AS, and conversely a deletion on the paternal chromosome leads to PWS. About a quarter of cases of PWS and 2 per cent of AS are due to uniparental disomy, i.e. inheritance of both chromosome 15s from one parent.

Mutations in a ubiquitin protein ligase gene (UBE3A) have been found in a few rare families with AS[60] and it has been proposed that the UBE3A gene is maternally expressed. If the mutations are the cause of AS, then it is unlikely to tell us much about the origin of the phenotype. The gene product is part of a widely used ubiquitin-mediated protein degradation pathway. The deletion almost certainly has pleiotropic effects that will be difficult, if not impossible, to disentangle.

PWS is probably not the result of a defect in a single gene. Seven genes (and candidate genes) have been identified in the PWS region, all of which appear to be brain specific. The function of these genes is not known; one, IPW, does not even code for a protein. Potentially, therefore, the phenotype arises from deficits in all these genes. Again, it is not known how the specific behavioural abnormalities can be explained by the genetic defect.

Similar problems beset attempts to understand how deletions of 22q11 give rise to cognitive disabilities. DiGeorge, velocardiofacial, and conotruncal anomaly face syndromes are different manifestations of deletions of 22q11.[61] DiGeorge and velocardiofacial syndromes are associated with mental retardation; additionally psychosis is found in some patients with 22q11 deletions.[62] The region most consistently deleted is large (> 1.5 megabases), containing at least 14 genes. Cloning and sequencing of the entire region has not identified any obvious candidates for the cognitive defect and it now seems likely that the syndromes arise from combined monosomy of more than one gene.[54] For example, one gene in this region, HIRA, encodes a protein similar to yeast transcriptional repressors. Potentially HIRA, like ATRX, remodels chromatin locally, altering the expression of many genes.[63]

Aneuploidy

Both Down syndrome and Turner syndrome are due to an abnormal number of chromosomes, an extra chromosome 21 in the case of Down syndrome and a single X (without a Y) in the case of Turner syndrome. Epstein has argued that the phenotypes of the aneuploid syndromes (of which these are just two examples) cannot be due to non-specific effects of chromosome imbalance because the phenotypic features are distinct.[64] This view is not without its critics,[65] and there certainly are some common phenotypic features of chromosome abnormalities, for instance small stature, microcephaly, and mental retardation. Nevertheless Turner and Down syndrome have sufficient specific features to encourage a search for dosage-sensitive genes that determine the syndromal phenotype.

Candidate genes for some of the somatic features of Turner syndrome have been proposed: SHOX/PHOG encodes a homeodomain protein that may explain the short stature; RPS4Y (which encodes an isoform of a ribosomal small subunit protein) and ZFY (which encodes a transcription factor of unknown function) may have pleiotropic effects.[66] There are no candidates for the unusual cognitive profile. However, there is one report that Turner syndrome patients with a paternally derived X chromosome have superior verbal abilities and skills involved in social interactions.[67] Therefore there may be an imprinted gene on the X chromosome that mediates some cognitive abilities.

Attempts have been made in Down syndrome to correlate regions of trisomy with different phenotypic abnormalities and hence infer the location of specific genes. While no genes have been identified solely on this basis, the information has been crucial in driving attempts to make a mouse model of Down syndrome. First, mice with three copies of chromosome 16 (the mouse homologue of human chromosome 21) show many of the features of Down syndrome.[68] Astrocytosis, craniofacial abnormalities, and seizures in trisomy 16 mice mimic the phenotype of Down syndrome. Second, attention has been focused on 21q22.2 as a potential site for dosage-sensitive genes that affect learning and behaviour. By putting pieces of human DNA from 21q22.2 into mice, and testing the mice for deficits in memory, one gene has been identified.[69] It is a human homologue of the *Drosophila minibrain* gene, a tyrosine/serine kinase expressed in developing neuroblasts. The use of transgenic mice to isolate *minibrain* demonstrates how complex phenotypes may be dissected down to their molecular basis, but there is as yet no proof that *minibrain* in humans is either dosage sensitive or a critical determinant of mental retardation in Down syndrome.

Neurobiology of learning and memory

The final section of this chapter deals with molecular genetic approaches to the neurobiology of learning. In so far as changes in behaviour are learnt (a proposition that applies as much to therapeutic interventions as to the development of disordered behaviour), understanding the neurobiology of learning encompasses almost all psychiatric practice.[4] In the future, a neurobiological understanding of the relationship between brain and mind will be possible, using the sort of approaches described below. While they are still far from making an impact on clinical practice, the potential for them to do so is very great indeed.

Animal studies of memory indicate that learning induces gene expression, which in turn leads to the growth of new synaptic connections, as explored most fully in the snail *Aplysia*.[70] In a typical experiment the snail is given a noxious stimulus and then develops a vigorous withdrawal response to a previously neutral or indifferent stimulus. The key finding here is that the animal's memory has at least two forms; while a single noxious stimulus gives rise to sensitization lasting minutes to hours, repetitive stimulation produces sensitization that can last days to weeks. The short- and long-term changes have different properties; long-term, but not short-term, sensitization is blocked by inhibitors of RNA and protein synthesis, and long-term sensitization involves synaptogenesis. Thus long-term changes require gene induction, which is essential for the development of new neuronal connections.

At least part of the molecular pathway involved has now been identified: cell surface receptors activate protein kinase A (**PKA**) via an increase in cAMP. PKA acts in the nucleus to activate cAMP response element binding protein 1 (CREB1) and to relieve CREB2-mediated repression. One consequence is downregulation of cell adhesion molecules (in *Aplysia* these are termed apCAMs), decreasing the interaction of neurites and resulting in the generation of new synaptic connections.

It is now clear that the same pathway is used by other organisms; mutations in PKA or its subunits disrupt olfactory learning in the fruitfly *Drosophila*.[71] Two forms of CREB have been identified that have complementary effects on olfactory learning in *Drosophila*, just as they do in *Aplysia*. The situation in mammals is more complex, but CREB has been identified as a key molecule in learning. Mice with a targeted mutation in the CREB gene have spatial memory deficits.[72] The animals could be conditioned to a tone and could learn to find a hidden platform in a water bath, but both skills were lost after 30 min. In other words, the deficit specifically affected long-term memory. Successful short-term training ruled out motivational sensory or motor deficits as an explanation.

The involvement of CREB in long-term memory in molluscs, flies, and mice indicates the existence of an evolutionary conserved pathway that operates in neurones. There seems little doubt that what applies at the neuronal level in molluscs, flies, and mice will apply to humans. While this is consoling, it also suggests that genetic approaches may not tell us what we would really like to know. Molecular neurobiology is very good at revealing the commonalities between species, but most psychiatrists are concerned with the behavioural repertoire that makes humans distinct. From a strictly biological point of view, that means asking what is distinctive about neural connections and activity in humans.

An answer requires that we know first how genetic effects determine neural activity, and that is now possible. The best example comes again from the study of memory, this time in the hippocampus. Pyramidal cells in the hippocampus fire when a rodent is in a restricted region, and information about the location of an animal can be estimated from the simultaneous firing patterns of many hippocampal neurones.[73,74] Genetic knockouts have been used to investigate the molecular basis of this phenomenon.

A modification of gene-knockout technology was used to ablate the N-methyl-D-aspartate receptors specifically from hippocampal pyramidal neurones,[75,76] resulting in impaired spatial memory. How is this genetic effect mediated? A miniaturized multi-electrode recording device was used to examine the firing patterns of hippocampal neurones. Fairly normal place cell activity was observed, but there were significant alterations in the size and quality of place fields. Cells with overlapping fields tend not to fire at the same time, giving incorrect signals about the animal's position and impairing its spatial memory. Thus genetically determined changes in synaptic plasticity are linked to both electrophysiological and behavioural impairments. This experiment demonstrates for the first time how genetic influences on cognitive processes can be interpreted as acting at the level of a neural system (spatial memory) and not just on its cellular components (neurones).

Thus, while molecular neurobiology has not yet progressed to the point of explaining how neural activity determines behaviour, it has begun to give us a molecular description of a neural system. Does this mean that we can expect similar advances in our understanding of other neural systems? A moment's reflection will show that successful application of genetic approaches requires that the neurobiology of the system is already well worked out. Consider again the example of the CREB gene in long-term memory.[72]

CREB proteins are not specific to the hippocampus. Indeed, they are widely distributed throughout the tissues of the body and involved in so many fundamental cellular processes that it is surprising that the CREB knockout mouse is viable. Thus the knockout experiments, while strongly supporting the view that CREB is required for long-term memory, raise another question. Why, contrary to our expectations, are the effects of the knockout apparently so specific?

The answer probably lies in the fact that specific effects arise because there is considerable redundancy in most genetic systems; another gene can at least partly take over the role of a missing or abnormal gene. However, such an answer raises new problems. If phenotypes arise due to the partial rescue of mutant, to what do we attribute the effect? Is it simply a reduced effect from a single gene acting in many different brain systems, is it complete absence of gene effect in one brain system (where isoforms cannot compensate), or is it the accumulated, and presumably unpredictable, result of compensatory mechanisms? As yet, we do not have definitive answers to these questions.

The important observation here is that genetic approaches on their own do not tell us how genes shape behaviour. In fact they often raise more questions than they answer, and this has implications for the hopes placed in positional cloning as a method of unravelling the biology of the mind. Accessing the neural correlates of mood disorders and psychosis or normal behavioural and cognitive traits appears possible by using the positional candidate cloning strategies described above. But, even with the genes in our hand, we may be no wiser about what they do. The detailed functional assays described above for memory have only been possible because so much was already known about its anatomical, cellular, and molecular basis.

The molecular basis of complex disorders

We do not know the molecular basis of any common psychiatric disorder, but it is almost certain that we will before long. Loci that determine susceptibility to psychosis, mood disorders, and personality disorders are being mapped, despite fluctuating levels of agreement between research groups. Once genes are identified, there is every reason to expect that subsequent genetic investigations will be equally daunting, as has been explained in the context of the neurobiology of learning and memory. The complex genetic basis of disorders with simple patterns of inheritance suggests that understanding complex inheritance will be, quite simply, very difficult.

The complexity of the subject does not diminish its clinical relevance; many patients and their families will want to know what the new genetic analyses mean, both in general, for our understanding of the disorder, and in particular, for the management of affected individuals and their relatives. What issues are psychiatrists likely to have to deal with?

In addition to the complexities of understanding gene action, it will be necessary to know how a phenotype arises from a combination of genes, and what predisposition means at a molecular level. Our understanding of the former issue is only in its infancy, but one concept is essential.

Soon after the discovery of Mendelian genetics it became clear that it was not always possible to predict a phenotype by a simple combination of the known effects of each gene. Thus if an allele (a) on chromosome 1 contributed 10 cm to height and an allele (b) on chromosome 2 contributed 5 cm, it was not always the case that an individual with both alleles (a) and (b) would be 15 cm taller than an individual without either allele. Epistasis is the term frequently used to describe the phenomenon where the effect of one locus masks the effects of another (thus in the example above the individual would be 5 cm taller because of the epistatic effect of (a) on (b)).[77] More complex interactions are possible, and often epistasis is used in a general way to describe all gene interactions. We do not even know how common a phenomenon epistasis is, and some have argued that it may be more extreme in disease states.[78] We certainly know nothing about its molecular mechanisms.

What is genetic predisposition likely to mean for a complex genetic disorder? In the simple case, we will identify a predisposing allele that will increase the chance that an individual develops the disorder. The presence of epistasis would certainly complicate this simple relationship, but unfortunately much more complex scenarios are possible, as the following example demonstrates. Insulin-dependent diabetes (**IDDM**), or type 1 diabetes, is a paradigm for genetically complex diseases[79] and an exemplar of the difficulties we can expect to find in the interpretation of genetic data. A number of studies have looked throughout the entire genome (without identifying the same loci [80,81]) and the insulin gene is now recognized as a susceptibility gene.[82] The interest of this locus is the immense complexity of the inheritance of susceptibility.

Just 5′ of the gene is a short stretch of tandemly repeated sequence which, like many other repeats, is polymorphic. In Caucasians, the alleles divide into two classes. Class I alleles predispose to IDDM in a recessive fashion, while the other class (confusingly called class III) are dominantly protective. This simple situation hides a parent-of-origin effect. Paternally inherited class I alleles are protective, but (here is the next level of difficulty) not in every case. What could be determining whether class I alleles predispose or protect? The answer appears to be the other paternal allele.[83] Class I alleles are protective if the father is heterozygous and has a class III allele. In other words the protective effect of class III alleles is transmitted to the class I allele when the two alleles are together in the father, in a way that suggests an unusual form of parental imprinting.

Discussion of the molecular basis of complex disorders is necessarily brief because of our limited knowledge. However, it is probably very relevant to understanding genetic disorders in psychiatry. Within the next few years it is likely that the situation will be very different, and much more information will be available about gene interaction and the inheritance of complex genetic disorders. The indications are that the subject will very complex.

References

1. Weatherall, D.J. (1991). *The new genetics and clinical practice*. Oxford University Press.
2. McGuffin, P. and Owen, M.J. (1996). Molecular genetic studies of schizophrenia. *Cold Spring Harbor Symposia on Quantitative Biology*, **61**, 815–22.
3. Karayiorgou, M. and Gogos, J.A. (1997). A turning point in schizophrenia genetics. *Neuron*, **19**, 967–79.
4. Kandel, E.R. (1998). A new intellectual framework for psychiatry. *American Journal of Psychiatry*, **155**, 457–69.
5. Strachan, T. and Read, A.P. (1996). *Human molecular genetics*. Bios Scientific, Oxford.
6. Gibbons, R.J., Picketts, D.J., Villard, L., and Higgs, D.R. (1995). Mutations in a putative global transcriptional regulator cause X-linked mental retardation with α-thalassemia (ATR-X syndrome). *Cell*, **80**, 837–45.
7. Wallace, D.C. (1997). Mitochondrial DNA in aging and disease. *Scientific American*, **277**, 40–7.
8. Flint, J., Thomas, K., Micklem, G., *et al.* (1997). The relationship between chromosome structure and function at a human telomeric region. *Nature Genetics*, **15**, 252–7.
9. Wang, D.G., Fan, J.B., Siao, C.J., *et al.* (1998). Large-scale identification, mapping, and genotyping of single-nucleotide polymorphisms in the human genome. *Science*, **280**, 1077–82.
10. Collins, F. (1995). Positional cloning moves from perditional to traditional. *Nature Genetics*, **9**, 347–50.
11. Adams, M.D., Kerlavage, A.R., Fleischmann, R.D., *et al.* (1995). Initial assessment of human gene diversity and expression patterns based upon 83-million nucleotides of cDNA sequence. *Nature*, **377**, 3–17.
12. Schuler, G.D., Boguski, M.S., Stewart, E.A., *et al.* (1996). A gene map of the human genome. *Science*, **274**, 540–6.
13. Tupler, R., Berardinelli, A., Barbierato, L., *et al.* (1996). Monosomy of distal 4q does not cause facioscapulohumeral muscular-dystrophy. *Journal of Medical Genetics*, **33**, 366–70.
14. Lemmers, R., van der Maarel, S.M., van Deutekom, J.C.T., *et al.* (1998). Inter- and intrachromosomal sub-telomeric rearrangements on 4q35: implications for facioscapulohumeral muscular dystrophy (FSHD) aetiology and diagnosis. *Human Molecular Genetics*, **7**, 1207–14.
15. Wilkie, A.O.M. (1997). Craniosynostosis: genes and mechanisms. *Human Molecular Genetics*, **6**, 1647–56.
16. Levy-Lahad, E., Wijsman, E.M., Nemens, E., *et al.* (1995). A familial Alzheimer's-disease locus on chromosome-1. *Science*, **269**, 970–3.
17. Levy-Lahad, E., Wasco, W., Poorkaj, P., *et al.* (1995). Candidate gene for the chromosome-1 familial Alzheimer's-disease locus. *Science*, **269**, 973–7.
18. Sherrington, R., Rogaev, E.I., Liang, Y., *et al.* (1995). Cloning of a gene bearing missense mutations in early-onset familial Alzheimer's-disease. *Nature*, **375**, 754–60.
19. Goate, A., Chartierharlin, M.C., Mullan, M., *et al.* (1991). Segregation of a missense mutation in the amyloid precursor protein gene with familial Alzheimer's-disease. *Nature*, **349**, 704–6.
20. Mewes, H.W., Albermann, K., Bahr, M., *et al.* (1997). Overview of the yeast genome. *Nature*, **387**, 7–8.
21. Tonegawa, S., Li, Y., Erzurumlu, R.S., *et al.* (1995). The gene knockout technology for the analysis of learning and memory, and neural development. *Progress in Brain Research*, **105**, 3–14.
22. Threadgill, D.W., Dlugosz, A.A., Hansen, L.A., *et al.* (1995). Targeted disruption of mouse Egf receptor—effect of genetic background on mutant phenotype. *Science*, **269**, 230–4.
23. Upchurch, M. and Wehner, J. (1988). Differences between inbred strains of mice in the Morris water maze performance. *Behavior Genetics*, **18**, 55–68.
24. Schwegler, H. and Lipp, H.-P. (1983). Hereditary covariations of neuronal circuitry and behaviour: correlations between the proportions of hippocampal synaptic fields in the regio inferior and two-way avoidance in mice and rats. *Behaviour and Brain Research*, **7**, 1–39.
25. Gusella, J. F. and MacDonald, M. E. (1996). Trinucleotide instability: a repeating theme in human inherited disorders. *Annual Review of Medicine*, **47**, 201–9.
26. Verkerk, A.J.M.H., Pieretti, M., Sutcliffe, J.S., *et al.* (1991). Identification of a gene (FMR-1) containing a CGG repeat coincident with a breakpoint cluster region exhibiting length variation in fragile X syndrome. *Cell*, **65**, 905–14.
27. Bowen, T., Guy, C.A., Craddock, N., *et al.* (1998). Further support for an association between a polymorphic CAG repeat in the hKCa3 gene and schizophrenia. *Molecular Psychiatry*, **3**, 266–9.
28. Odonovan, M.C., Guy, C., Craddock, N., *et al.* (1995). Expanded CAG repeats in schizophrenia and bipolar disorder. *Nature Genetics*, **10**, 380–1.
29. Odonovan, M.C., Guy, C., Craddock, N., *et al.* (1996). Confirmation of association between expanded CAG/CTG repeats and both schizophrenia and bipolar disorder. *Psychological Medicine*, **26**, 1145–53.
30. Rogaev, E.I., Sherrington, R., Rogaeva, E.A., *et al.* (1995). Familial Alzheimer's-disease in kindreds with missense mutations in a gene on chromosome-1 related to the Alzheimer's-disease type-3 gene. *Nature*, **376**, 775–8.
31. Hardy, J. (1997). Amyloid, the presenilins and Alzheimer's disease. *Trends in Neuroscience*, **20**, 154–9.
32. Hardy, J., Duf, K., Hardy, K.G., Perez-Tur, J., and Hutton, M. (1998). Genetic dissection of Alzheimer's disease and related dementias: amyloid and its relationship to tau. *Nature Neuroscience*, **1**, 355–8.
33. Hutton, M., Lendon, C. L., Rizzu, P., *et al.* (1998). Association of missense and 5′-splice-site mutations in tau with the inherited dementia FTDP-17. *Nature*, **393**, 702–5.
34. Spillantini, M.G., Murrell, J.R., Goedert, M., Farlow, M.R., Klug, A., and Ghetti, B. (1998). Mutation in the tau gene in familial multiple system tauopathy with presenile dementia. *Proceedings of the National Academy of Sciences of the United States of America*, **95**, 7737–41.
35. Glass, I. (1991). X linked mental retardation. *Journal of Medical Genetics*, **28**, 361–71.
36. Billuart, P., Bienvenu, T., Ronce, N., *et al.* (1998). Oligophrenin-1 encodes a rhoGAP protein involved in X-linked mental retardation. *Nature*, **392**, 923–6.
37. Dadamo, P., Menegon, A., LoNigro, C., *et al.* (1998). Mutations in GDI1 are responsible for X-linked non-specific mental retardation. *Nature Genetics*, **19**, 134–9.
38. Allen, K.M., Gleeson, J.G., Bagrodia, S., *et al.* (1998). PAK3 mutation in nonsyndromic X-linked mental retardation. *Nature Genetics*, **20**, 25–30.

39. Geppert, M., Bolshakov, V.Y., Siegelbaum, S.A., *et al.* (1994). The role of Rab3a in neurotransmitter release. *Nature*, **369**, 493–7.

40. Van Aelst, L. and D'Souza-Schorey, C. (1997). Rho GTPases and signaling networks. *Genes and Development*, **11**, 2295–322.

41. Gu, Y., Shen, Y., Biggs, R.A., and Nelson, D.L. (1996). Identification of FMR2, a novel gene associated with the FRAXE CCG repeat and CpG island. *Nature Genetics*, **13**, 109–13.

42. Gecz, J., Gedeon, A.K., Sutherland, G.R., and Mulley, J.C. (1996). Identification of the gene FMR2, associated with FRAXE mental retardation. *Nature Genetics*, **13**, 105–8.

43. Gecz, J., Bielby, S., Sutherland, G.R., and Mulley, J.C. (1997). Gene structure and subcellular localization of FMR2, a member of a new family of putative transcription activators. *Genomics*, **44**, 201–13.

44. Gecz, J., Oostra, B.A., Hockey, A., *et al.* (1997). FMR2 expression in families with FRAXE mental retardation. *Human Molecular Genetics*, **6**, 435–41.

45. Yu, S., Pritchard, M., Kremer, E., *et al.* (1991). Fragile X genotype characterized by an unstable region of DNA. *Science*, **252**, 1179–81.

46. Oberle, I., Rousseau, F., Heitz, D., *et al.* (1991). Instability of a 550 base pair DNA segment and abnormal methylation in fragile X-syndrome. *Science*, **252**, 1097–1102.

47. Verheij, C., Bakker, C.E., de Graaff, E., *et al.* (1993). Characterisation and localisation of the FMR-1 gene product associated with fragile X syndrome. *Nature*, **363**, 722–4.

48. Siomi, H., Siomi, M.C., Nussbaum, R.L., and Dreyfuss, G. (1993). The protein product of the fragile X gene, FMR1, has characteristics of an RNA-binding protein. *Cell*, **74**, 291–8.

49. Devys, D., Lutz, Y., Rouyer, N., Bellocq, J.-P., and Mandel, J.-L. (1993). The FMR-1 protein is cytoplasmic, most abundant in neurons and appears normal in carriers of fragile X premutation. *Nature Genetics*, **4**, 335–40.

50. Siomi, H., Choi, M., Siomi, M.C., Nussbaum, R.L., and Dreyfuss, G. (1994). Essential role for KH domains in RNA binding: impaired RNA binding by a mutation in the KH domain of FMR1 that causes fragile X syndrome. *Cell*, **77**, 33–9.

51. Feng, Y., Zhang, Z., Lokey, L.K., *et al.* (1995). Translational suppression by trinucleotide repeat expansion at FMR1. *Science*, **268**, 731–4.

52. Dutch–Belgian Fragile X Consortium. (1994). Fmr1 knockout mice: a model to study fragile X mental retardation. *Cell*, **78**, 23–33.

53. Quaderi, N.A., Schweiger, S., Gaudenz, K., *et al.* (1997). Opitz G/BBB syndrome, a defect of midline development, is due to mutations in a new RING finger gene on Xp22. *Nature Genetics*, **17**, 285–91.

54. Budarf, M.L. and Emanuel, B.S. (1997). Progress in the autosomal segmental aneusomy syndromes (SASs): single or multi-locus disorders. *Human Molecular Genetics*, **6**, 1657–65.

55. Frangiskakis, J.M., Ewart, A., Morris, C.A., *et al.* (1996). LIM-kinase 1 hemizygosity implicated in impaired visuospatial constructive cognition. *Cell*, **86**, 59–69.

56. Wanaka, A., Matsumoto, K., Kashihara, Y., *et al.* (1997). LIM-homeodomain gene family in neural development. *Developmental Neuroscience*, **19**, 97–100.

57. Wang, J.Y., Frenzel, K.E., Wen, D.Z., and Falls, D.L. (1998). Transmembrane neuregulins interact with LIM kinase 1, a cytoplasmic protein kinase implicated in development of visuospatial cognition. *Journal of Biological Chemistry*, **273**, 20 525–34.

58. Petrij, F., Giles, H.R., Dauwerse, H.G., *et al.* (1995). Rubinstein–Taybi syndrome caused by mutations in the transcriptional co-activator CNP. *Nature*, **376**, 348–351.

59. Nicholls, R.D., Saitoh, S., and Horsthemke, B. (1998). Imprinting in Prader–Willi and Angelman syndromes. *Trends in Genetics*, **14**, 194–200.

60. Kishino, T., Lalande, M., and Wagstaff, J. (1997). UBE3A/E6-AP mutations cause Angelman syndrome. *Nature Genetics*, **15**, 70–3.

61. Scambler, P.J. (1993). Deletions of human chromosome 22 and associated birth defects. *Current Opinion in Genetics and Development*, **3**, 432–7.

62. Karayiorgou, P., Morris, M.A., Morrow, B., *et al.* (1995). Schizophrenia susceptibility associated with interstitial deletions of chromosome 22q11. *Proceedings of the National Academy of Sciences of the United States of America*, **17**, 7612–16.

63. Magnaghi, P., Roberts, C., Lorain, S., Lipinski, M. and Scambler, P. (1998). HIRA, a mammalian homologue of *Saccharomyces cerevisiae* transcriptional co-repressors, interacts with Pax3. *Nature Genetics*, **20**, 74–77.

64. Epstein, C.J. (1988). Mechanisms of the effects of aneuploidy in mammals. *Annual Review of Genetics*, **22**, 51–75.

65. Shapiro, B.L. (1997). Whither Down syndrome critical region? *Human Genetics*, **99**, 421–3.

66. Zinn, A.R. and Ross, J.L. (1998). Turner syndrome and haploinsufficiency. *Currrent Opinion in Genetics and Development*, **8**, 322–7.

67. Skuse, D.H., James, R.S., Bishop, D.V.M., *et al.* (1997). Evidence from Turner's syndrome of an imprinted X-linked locus affecting cognitive function. *Nature*, **387**, 705–8.

68. Reeves, R.H., Irving, N.G., Moran, T.H., *et al.* (1995). A mouse model for Down-syndrome exhibits learning and behavior deficits. *Nature Genetics*, **11**, 177–84.

69. Smith, D.J., Stevens, M.E., Sudangunta, S.P., *et al.* (1997). Functional screening of 2 Mb of human chromosome 21q22.2 in transgenic mice implicates *minibrain* in learning defects associated with Down syndrome. *Nature Genetics*, **16**, 28–36.

70. Bailey, C.H. and Kandel, E.R. (1993). Structural changes accompanying memory storage. *Annual Review of Physiology*, **55**, 397–426.

71. Tully, T. (1996). Discovery of genes involved with learning and memory: an experimental synthesis of Hirschian and Benzerian perspectives. *Proceedings of the National Academy of Sciences of the United States of America*, **93**, 13 460–7.

72. Bourtchuladze, R., Frenguelli, B., Blendy, J., Cioffi, D., Schutz, G., and Silva, A.J. (1994). Deficient long-term memory in mice with a targeted mutation of the cAMP-responsive element-binding protein. *Cell*, **79**, 59–68.

73. Wilson, M.M. and McNaughton, B.L. (1993). Dynamics of the hippocampal ensemble code for space. *Science*, **261**, 1055–8.

74. O'Keefe, J. (1993). Hippocampus, theta, and spatial memory. *Current Opinion in Neurobiology*, **3**, 917–24.

75. Tsien, J.Z., Huerta, P.T., and Tonegawa, S. (1996). The essential role of hippocampal CA1 NMDA receptor-dependent synaptic plasticity in spatial memory. *Cell*, **87**, 1327–38.

76. Tsien, J.Z., Chen, D.F., Gerber, D., *et al.* (1996). Subregion- and cell type-restricted gene knockout in mouse brain. *Cell*, **87**, 1317–26.

77. Phillips, P.C. (1998). The language of gene interaction. *Genetics*, **149**, 1167–71.

78. Crow, J.F. (1990). How important is detecting interaction? *Behavioural and Brain Sciences*, **13**, 126–7.

79. Bennett, S.T. and Todd, J.A. (1996). Human type 1 diabetes and the insulin gene: principles of mapping polygenes. *Annual Review of Genetics*, **30**, 343–70.

80. Concannon, P., Gogolin-Ewens, K.J., Hinds, D.A., *et al.* (1998). A second generation screen of the human genome for susceptibility to insulin-dependent diabetes mellitus. *Nature Genetics*, **19**, 292–6.

81. Mein, C.A., Esposito, L., Dunn, M.G., *et al.* (1998). A search for type 1 diabetes susceptibility genes in families from the United Kingdom. *Nature Genetics*, **19**, 297–300.

82. Todd, J.A. and Farrall, M. (1996). Panning for gold: genome-wide scanning for linkage in type 1 diabetes. *Human Molecular Genetics*, **5**, 1443–8.

83. Bennett, S.T., Wilson, A.J., Esposito, L., *et al.* (1997). Insulin VNTR allele-specific effect in type 1 diabetes depends on identity of untransmitted paternal allele. *Nature Genetics*, **17**, 350–2.

2.5 The contribution of psychological science

2.5.1 Developmental psychology throughout life
2.5.1.1 Developmental psychology through infancy, childhood, and adolescence
William Yule

Introduction

'The child is father to the man.' This saying seems so obviously true that it may surprise some people that it needs to be analysed and certain assumptions inherent in it need to be challenged if psychiatric practice across the lifespan is to be properly informed by findings from developmental psychology. This chapter examines different conceptualizations of children and childhood through the ages and the ideas and theoretical models that have shaped popular, as well as professional, views on how children develop. It notes that there are no overarching theories of child development, but rather a potpourri of smaller models, most of which address disparate aspects of development.

Developmental psychology is not just about charting the norms of development, although knowledge of such is essential in all clinical practice. Rather, there are many issues that need to be critically examined in trying to understand how individuals develop. Taking a 'developmental perspective' is about integrating this knowledge and understanding the patient's presenting problems within such a framework.

The significance that the clinician will place on a particular piece of behaviour will depend not only on the child's sociocultural background, but also on the child's developmental age. Cox and Rutter[1] note four reasons for taking a developmental perspective.

1. Children behave differently at different ages. The clinician must be familiar with the range of behaviours and their age-appropriateness in separating the normal from the abnormal. For instance, simple consonant substitutions are widespread in the speech of preschool children, but indicate some delay or deviation in the speech of teenagers.

2. Many aspects of behaviour can be viewed as progressing through a normal sequence. Admittedly, discrete stages are overemphasized by stage theorists such as Freud, Piaget, and Bowlby, whereas the continuities in development are more emphasized by social learning theorists such as Staats, Bijou, and Baer. Either way, an understanding of the normal sequences and ages permits a judgement as to whether the child has deviated in his or her development.

3. Different stages of development are associated with different stresses and different developmental tasks. Bladder and bowel training are normally achieved between the ages of 2 and 4 years. Major stresses on the child or the family at the time may interfere with the achievement of proper bladder and bowel control. Mood swings are very common in adolescence, making it difficult to diagnose the severity of depression at this stage.[2,3]

4. An understanding of the processes that underlie both normal and abnormal development will help in the understanding of how the problems have arisen.[4] Such an historical perspective can help explain to the parents why a particular problem developed, as well as give possible clues for future programmes for prevention. A major implication of this for clinical practice is that it is always necessary to obtain a good account of the child's developmental history.

5. A better understanding of the processes underlying a child's development will lead to far better interventions and prevention. Once we have a better understanding of the distal and proximal causes of behaviour, better targeted interventions will follow.

Developmental theories and views

There is a bewildering set of mini-models and mini-theories of developmental processes, each trying to deal with changes in children's functioning either at different periods in their lives or in different psychological functions such as perception, language, and memory. By and large, the different theorists seem to ignore each other's work—and many also seem keener on theories than on data that might test the theories.

For example, Piaget's theories predominantly address how children develop a cognitive understanding of their world. His was a biological view of development, and his cross-sectional methodology emphasized the separation between the stages he posited. Staats[5] argued that most of the phenomena described by Piaget and his followers could be interpreted within a social learning theory framework that instead emphasized the continuity of development across stages.

Kohlberg's theory of moral judgement is a stage theory that differs radically from Piaget's in that the different forms of reasoning said to typify different stages can coexist. However, the way in which children (or adults for that matter) judge an ethical dilemma does not necessarily determine how they behave. Most financiers would have little difficulty in providing sophisticated moral judgements on Kohlberg-type tasks, but many financiers also present the 'unacceptable face of capitalism' in their ruthless dealings. It is not the case that the older we are, the wiser we behave.

In Freud's theory of psychosexual development, children are seen as passively passing through stages, their development being impeded by obstacles or even regressing in the face of trauma. This view owes more to literature than to science, and the evidence on children's psychosexual development clearly shows that whatever Freud was unaware of during the 'latency' period, children are certainly far from inactive.[6]

Apart from being 'stage' theories, these three sets of influential theories really have very little in common. The psychological mechanisms determining growth of cognitive understanding bear little relationship to any that supposedly underlie socio-emotional behaviour. None of the theories takes into account all of the work done in perceptual development, language development, development of memory, development of peer relationships, development during adolescence, and so on. They pay little attention to the work on individual differences in personality or temperament, or to biological development generally.

A totally biological determinist view of development was anathema to the new theorists of behaviour modification and behaviour therapy in the 1960s. It was seen as too pessimistic, offering little hope of change. By ignoring the biological basis of behaviour and seeking explanations solely in the here-and-now (proximal) influences on behaviour, they undoubtedly broke through to a much more optimistic era of interventions.

Simultaneously, child developmentalists were recognizing the contributions the child brought to all aspects of development. The child has increasingly been seen as an active participant in development. The direction of influence was not all one way: the child helped shape the environment. Thus, parents react to individual differences in children. Different children 'call out' different responses from their social environment. As parents have known all along, children do have different temperaments from birth, and these shape their development.[7,8]

The implications of this for child psychiatry are many. For example, it implies that clinicians must take into account a child's temperament when planning treatment.[7,9] Children who are extremely introverted react differently to praise and punishment than children who are extremely extroverted.[9,10] They also respond to different teaching styles in the classroom. Such differences need to be accommodated in setting up individualized treatment programmes.

With young infants, it can be very reassuring to a parent to be told that anyone would find their unpredictable child difficult to rear. It can boost parental self-confidence to be told (when true) that their parenting style is perfectly adequate for most children—just not effective with this particular one. This reassurance should greatly alter the way such a parent participates in parent training programmes that are increasingly part of primary and secondary level child mental health services.

All this is not to say that stage theories carry no implications for child mental health services. Far from it. It is very helpful to remember that young children think and reason about their worlds differently from older children. This has to be borne in mind when interviewing children, when trying to elicit their own understanding of their problem, and, equally, when giving them instructions, feedback, or explanations. However, it must again be emphasized that the 'stages' should only ever be regarded as rough guidelines. We know that there are such wide individual differences in the rate at which children develop that we should never make assumptions about the individual child knowing only his or her chronological age.

Let us take one example that increasingly confronts clinicians—the issue of helping children deal with bereavement (see also Chapter 9.3.5). It is not until around the age of 10 or 11 that most children appreciate that death is both universal and irreversible.[11–13] This helps to explain why some younger children show an almost casual matter-of-fact interest in death of a loved one and are less upset by it than adults are.[13] But it would be wrong to assume that all younger children fail to have an adult appreciation of the significance of death, and indeed some children as young as 4 years old have been found to have a mature understanding. Knowledge of the broad outline of the development of the conceptualization of death helps clinicians formulate their questions, but the onus must always be on the clinician to check whether or not the individual child conforms to the average. The adult's task may not be finished when they have helped a young child to understand a bereavement at the level the child can cope with. That same child will probably want to revisit the issue when he or she is older and can understand it in a more mature way. What is true of bereavement also holds true for understanding any other major life event and its effects on the child.

Critical issues in development

When one takes a closer look at how children develop, one cannot help but be amazed at the complexities of the process. Children the world over start using words around their first birthday, and within a couple of years more they are talking in complex sentences using complicated ideas. The contrast between the language development of most children and the minority who suffer a severe mental handicap is devastating. Likewise, blind children start to smile at the same time as sighted children; deaf children start to use a similar range of phonemes; children in Japan, France, and the United Kingdom all start uttering the same range of sounds only to have them narrowed down to those they need in their native language—with the later consequence that they may not even be able to discriminate some of the unused sounds, let alone incorporate them when learning a foreign language. The broad developmental trajectory seems very similar across cultural groups, but particular children do not always follow the average in a smooth, predictable way.

Rutter and Rutter[14] drew attention to a number of issues that need to be considered when trying to understand developmental processes. Clinicians are understandably focused on trying to make sense of cases where something has gone wrong in development. Mostly in child psychiatry, abnormal behaviours of children are quantitatively rather than qualitatively different from normal. Disorders following brain damage or genetic/chromosomal abnormalities and many involving very severe degrees of mental handicap, including infantile autism, are increasingly recognized as being qualitatively different. Most of the other disorders seen in child and adolescent mental health services are probably best viewed as deviations lying at the extreme of a continuum. But why do some children break down under stress while others do not? Why are some more resilient than others? What factors protect children against environmental and social stressors? Is it really the case that severe depression in late adolescence is just the extreme end of a continuum ranging from happiness through sadness to suicidality? In order to tackle these issues, it is necessary to clarify some of the concepts of development.

1. One should not assume that the same mechanisms underlie both normal and abnormal development.

2. A biological perspective is necessary to understand human development fully. The brain is clearly the most important organ concerned—the genetic inheritance, insults during critical periods of brain growth, and hormonal changes all have considerable influence on how children develop.

3. One has to expect both continuities and discontinuities in development. At times, continuities are intrinsic to the particular process as in language development; at other times, continuities—as in academic attainment—are in large part influenced by continuities imposed by the social environment. Parents concerned about education influence the choice of schools and provide support for learning.

4. The timing of an experience is as important as its nature. The brain is most vulnerable to insult when it is developing most rapidly, at and shortly after birth. Severe disruptions in caretaking have their greatest effects from around 9 months to 2 or 3 years. Before then, the infant does not show the same quality of selective attachments; after language is well established, the child can better hold the memory of a loved one, and that may act as a protection against the separation.

5. Children are active creatures. Not only do they call out responses from others, but as they develop cognitively and linguistically, they actively seek to make sense of their world. They appraise threat from others, even if they do not always get it right. When they are involved in a major catastrophe, their 'assumptive world'[15] can be literally turned upside down and they take a long time to reconstruct the world as a safe place. The way the child interprets experience will come to determine in part how similar experiences are responded to in the future.

6. 'Continuity may be heterotypic as well as homotypic.'[14] The brilliant idea developed in the New York Longitudinal Study[16] of temperament was that rather than seeking evidence for predictability and continuity in particular infant behaviours across times when behaviour was developing rapidly, the investigators looked instead at how a variety of topographically different behaviours were expressed, and found considerable continuities in such aspects as regularity of functions, strength of response, and predominant reaction to new stimuli. Thus, they adduced evidence of temperamental characteristics that were independent of the specific behaviours shown, and, moreover, these temperamental characteristics proved to be predictive of later behaviour and adjustment.[16]

7. Both risk and protective factors, and the interactions between them, must be considered. Not all apparently adverse experiences are necessarily wholly bad for healthy development. In the same way that exposure to a virus or infection can boost resistance to infection, so exposure to mild stressors may boost resistance to other stressful experiences later. In part, this is the basis for stress inoculation therapy.[17] Some would argue that young children should have practice in separating from parents under enjoyable conditions so that in the event of a sudden, unexpected, or traumatic separation being necessary, the effects of experience will be mitigated.

8. As noted earlier, continuities may arise indirectly in that the way parents or society in general support attainment and in turn entry to the job market. The moderately high correlations between early attainment and later earning power are thereby in part determined and supported environmentally.

9. Similarly, the achievement of a particular behaviour may set in motion a chain of events. It is important to understand the processes underlying such a sequence. Too often studies are short-term and cross-sectional in nature and despite being aware of the pitfall of confusing correlation with causality, investigators remain prone to identifying a correlate as being a causal agent. For example, in the early days of studies of reading difficulties, it was noted that poor readers did badly on tests of visual perception. It was assumed that they therefore had a visual perceptual deficit and generations of poor readers were subjected to hours of mindless tracing of lines and walking along benches. The end result was that they performed better on the particular visual–perceptual test but they were no better at reading! A different experimental design was needed to demonstrate causal relationships between psychological processes and poor reading,[18] and when that was understood, the way was open for better remedial work based on a proper understanding of causal mechanisms.

This can also be viewed as an error in confusing a risk indicator with a risk process. Thirty years ago, studies of the dehumanizing effects of institutionalization on adults and children[19] found that poor living conditions and 'block treatment' of residents were related to a greater risk of behavioural and emotional problems. In one set of studies, a good indicator of block treatment was whether patients had their own toothbrushes. Clearly, providing individual toothbrushes to all would not make much difference if all the other aspects of institutionalization remained in force. A fuller understanding of the process of institutionalization is needed in order to be able to develop more humane care that improves development.

These critical issues demonstrate just how complicated the relationship between nature, experience, and development can be. But human beings are indeed very complicated, and so a proper appreciation of all these factors is needed in order to be able to understand how a particular child reached a particular point in development, to be able to predict what the future may hold for a child, and to be able to develop rational interventions that have a hope of making a real difference to children's lives.

Developmental psychopathology

Developmental psychopathology emerged in the 1980s to bridge the rift between academic and clinical child psychology.[20,21] 'The developmental psychopathologist is concerned with the time course of a given disorder, its varying manifestations with development, its precursors and sequelae, and its relation to non-disordered patterns of behaviour.'[21] Developmental psychopathologists, like social learning theorists, look to normal development to illuminate pathological development. They are interested in continuities and changes in behaviour across time. This fits in well with the tradition of risk research[22] and attempts to answer questions not only about why some children are more vulnerable than others, but also about what protective factors operate to lessen the impact of stressors.

Sroufe and Rutter,[21] following Santostefano,[23] articulated several propositions that are broadly agreed across the many different theories alluded to above.

- **Holism**: '...the meaning of behaviour can only be determined within the total psychological context'.[21] Thus, a behaviour such as crying can only be evaluated according to the age of the child and the circumstances in which it occurs. Crying on separation would be seen as usual for a 3-year-old, but unusual in a 15-year-old. One cannot simply judge the significance of a behaviour simply on the basis of its physical, stimulus properties, but one has to evaluate it within the broader social context.

- **Directedness**: children are not passive reactors to the demands of the environment. Development consists of a reorganization of previous elements, skills, and behaviour, not just a linear addition of skills.

- **Differentiation of modes and goals**: over time, children's reactions to their environment become both more flexible and increasingly complex in organization. Thus, one sign of pathology is for children to get stuck in a particular way of trying to solve a problem.

- **Mobility of behavioural functions**: earlier behaviour becomes integrated into later patterns, and '...the individual does not operate only in terms of behaviours that define a single stage. Especially in periods of stress, early modes of functioning may become manifest'.[21] In other words, under stress, those patterns of behaviour that have most recently become integrated into the child's repertoire are most susceptible of disruption. This is very different from the unsatisfactory concept of 'regression' in that all skills achieved remain available in the child's repertoire; some earlier ones also manifest at times of stress.

- **The problem of continuity and change**: above all, development is seen as lawful, even though we are still far from understanding the processes involved in these laws. Sroufe and Rutter[21] emphasize: 'The continuity lies not in isomorphic behaviours over time but in lawful relations to later behaviour, however complex the links'. As noted, Thomas et al.[16] were among the first to demonstrate continuities in the style of behaviour (temperament) rather than continuities of behaviour per se.

It is now recognized that there are many complex ways in which child behaviour is related to later and even adult adjustment.[24] One of the most powerful predictors of later adult psychopathology is inadequate peer relations. The mechanism by which these work may be due to two interacting processes: poor peer relations are signs of failure to adapt during childhood, and that failure persists; social support later acts as a buffer against adult stressors.[21]

Clearly, this view of development, with its implications for psychopathology, is far removed from the lessons learned from the Skinner box. And yet what has been learned from the paradigms of classical and operant conditioning must also be integrated into ways that child therapists assess children's problems if we are to provide better treatments. This holistic view manages to incorporate ideas on the biological basis for behaviour and the notion of the child as an active participant interacting with his or her effective social environment within a broad social learning framework.[25,26] Understanding how a problem has arisen may provide useful guidance on what aspects to focus on, but the treatment will still focus on the present. There will be implications for maintaining treatment gains and preventing future problems, as well as implications for preventing such problems arising in other children.

For clinicians more used to working with adult patients, it is worth pointing out children differ in many ways from their grown-up counterparts. This has implications for improving diagnostic classificatory systems in that both DSM and ICD are still too adult oriented and pay insufficient attention to developmental aspects of disorders.[27–29]

Garber[30] makes the point that children differ from adults in cognition, language, physiology, and emotions: 'Such maturational differences may impact children's abilities to experience or express certain affects, cognitions, or behaviours, and thus the manner in which symptoms are expressed may differ over the course of development'. In the author's recent work on the effects of major disasters and acute stress on children's adjustment, it became evident that children as young as 8 years old showed most of the symptoms of post-traumatic stress disorder (**PTSD**), with unpleasant thoughts, poor concentration, and sleep disorders predominating.[31,32] Parents and teachers were often unaware of the nature and extent of the children's subjective distress, and only sympathetic but direct questioning elicited the full spectrum of symptomatology.

The criteria for PTSD are less appropriate for children under 8 years of age. Preschool children often react with more repetitive play and drawing than older ones. Even the youngest children will report very disturbing intrusive thoughts about the disaster. Almqvist and Brandell-Forsberg[33] report on one way of eliciting developmentally appropriate symptoms of stress reactions using standard play material, while Scheeringa et al.[34] suggest varying criteria for making the diagnosis of PTSD in young children. Leaving aside the logical problem of altering criteria but keeping the same name for the supposed underlying condition, this clearly is one aspect of the isomorphism mentioned earlier. It is also interesting to speculate whether the repetitive play seen in 6-year-olds is functionally equivalent to the intrusive thoughts seen in 10-year-olds, and when the one changes into the other.

Garber[30] also notes that some disorders, such as mental handicap and autism, first manifest in childhood and persist into adulthood. Others, such as encopresis and enuresis manifest in childhood, but rarely persist into adulthood unless part of a more global developmental delay. Some, such as anorexia and bulimia, are more typical of adolescence. Suicide, although rare before puberty, is rapidly becoming the major cause of death in adolescence, but peaks in old age. Major depression and schizophrenia are rare in childhood, although precursors are being more firmly established. While the wish to treat disorders in childhood so as to prevent them continuing to adulthood is laudable, treating them to improve adjustment during childhood is equally valid.

Plates for Chapter 2.3.1

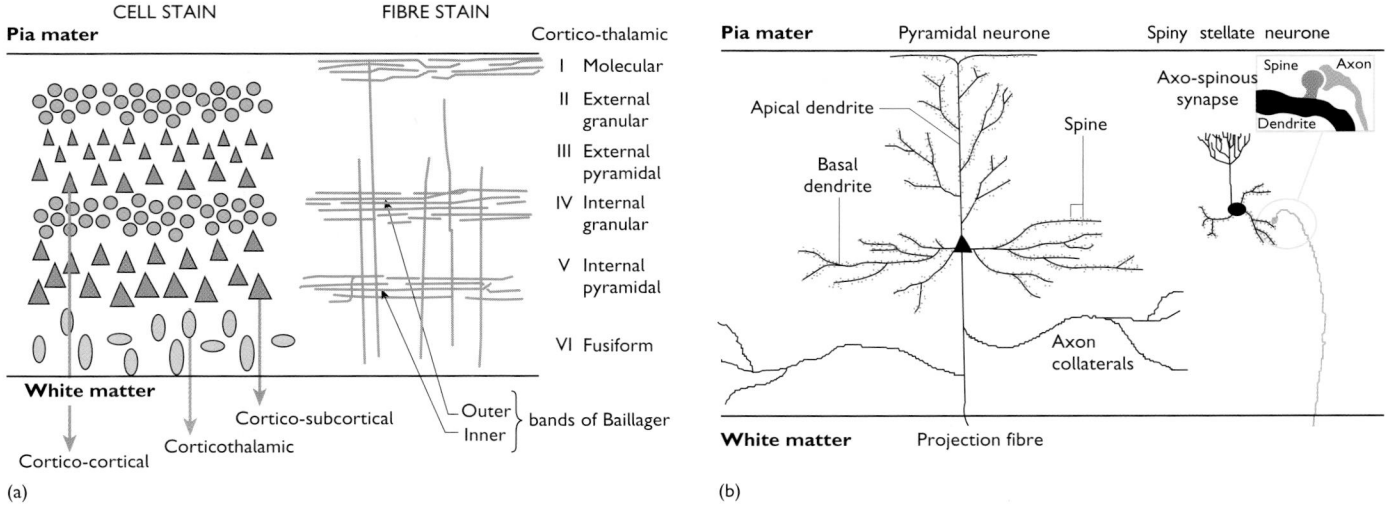

Plate 1 (a) Laminar structure of the cerebral neocortex; (b) excitatory amino acid using spiny neurones of the neocortex.

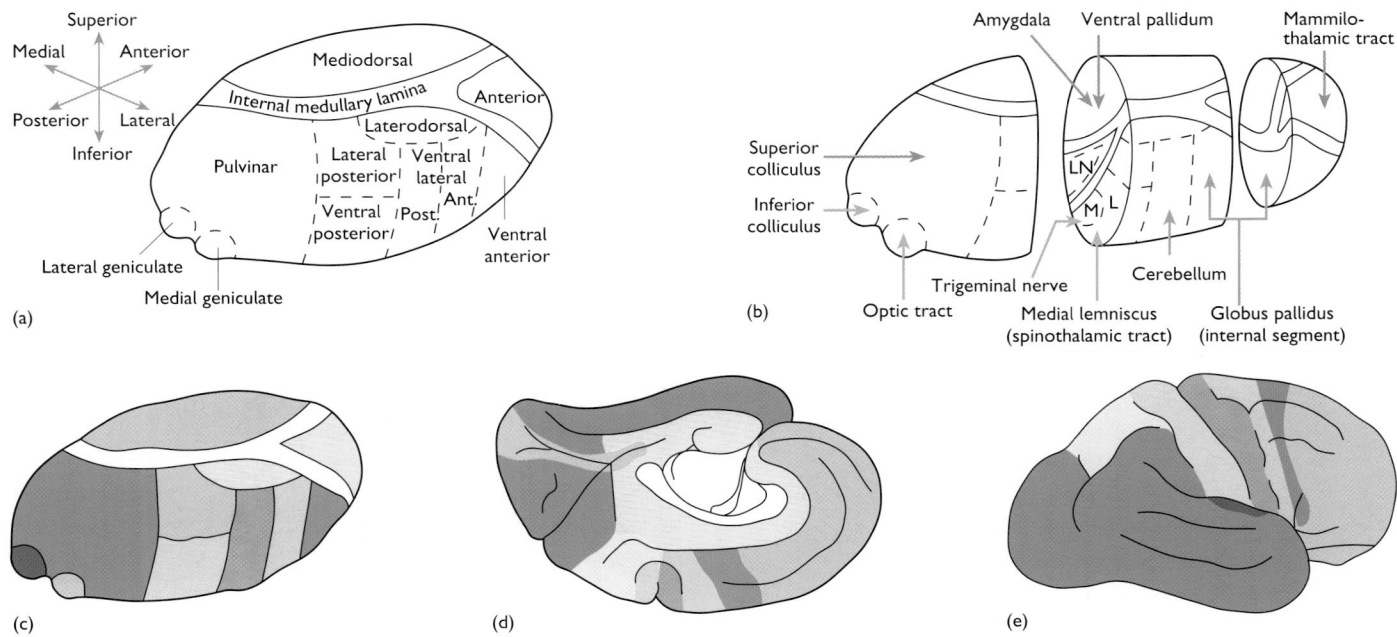

Plate 2 (a) The thalamus is shown as if removed from the brain at the top, with the individual major nuclei indicated. (b) Schematic diagram showing the isolated thalamus divided approximately at the middle of its anteroposterior extent; the arrows indicate known sources of major subcortical afferents to the individual named nuclei. (c) The diagram of the isolated thalamus shown in (a) with the individual main nuclei colour coded. (d), (e) Schematic diagrams of the cerebral surfaces (medial and lateral) showing the regions of cortex colour coded to correspond to the main thalamic nuclei with which they have major connections.

Plates for Chapter 2.3.6

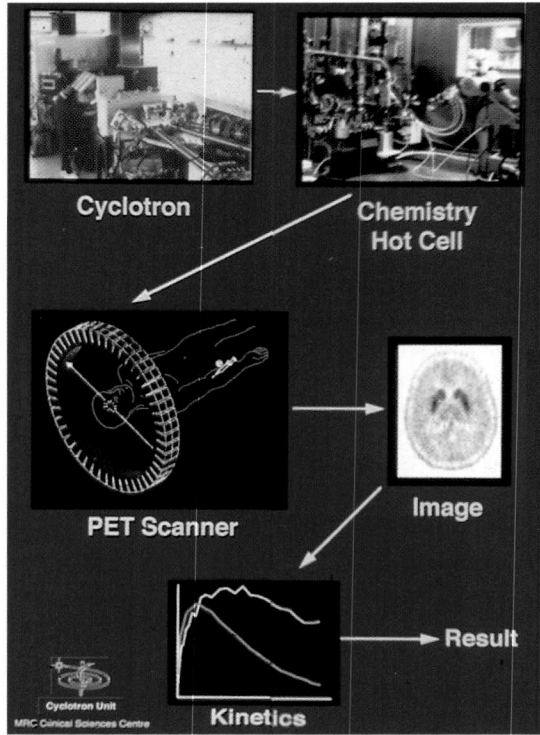

Plate 3 Steps in the production and use of PET radio-isotopes.

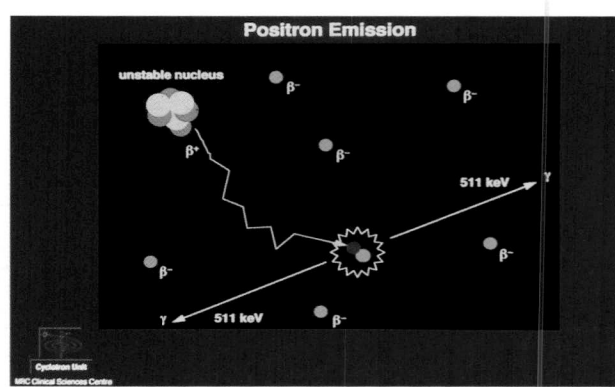

Plate 4 Principles of positron emission: β^- is an electron and β^+ is a positron. Two high-energy gamma rays (γ) are produced on annihilation of a positron by an electron.

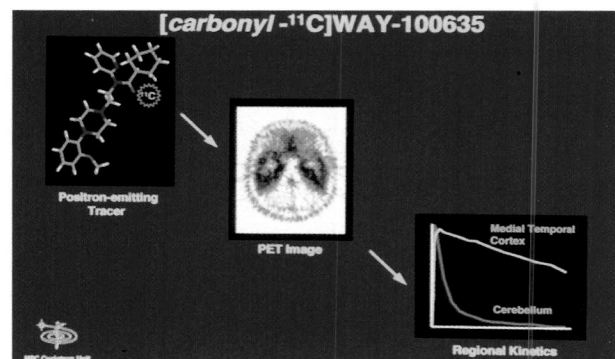

Plate 5 Use of a PET radiotracer to image 5-HT$_{1A}$ receptors in the human brain.

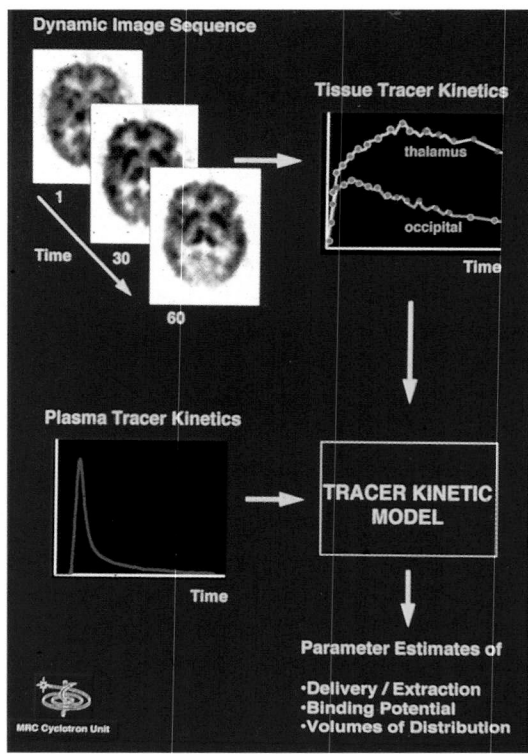

Plate 6 Steps in the data analysis of a PET radiotracer.

Plate for Chapter 2.3.7

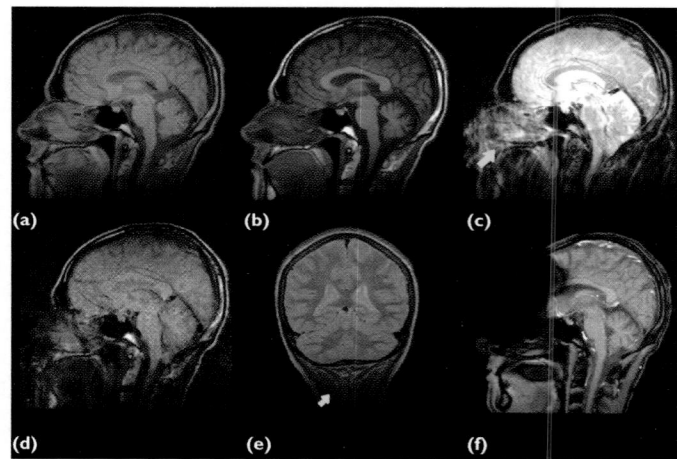

Plate 7 Spin echo MR images and artefacts. Top row, spin echo images: left, proton density image (TR = 2000 ms, TE = 20 ms); middle, T_1-weighted image (TR = 350 ms, TE = 20 ms); right, T_2-weighted image (TR = 2000 ms, TE = 90 ms). The arrow on the T_2-weighted image indicates blurring caused by movement (swallowing) during acquisition. Bottom row, examples of poor tissue contrast and susceptibility artefact: left, spin echo image showing poor contrast due to injudicious prescription of pulse sequence (TR = 350 ms, TE = 90 ms); middle, bulk susceptibility artefact; right, ferromagnetic susceptibility artefact caused by a metallic hairgrip.

Plate for Chapter 2.3.7 *(continued)*

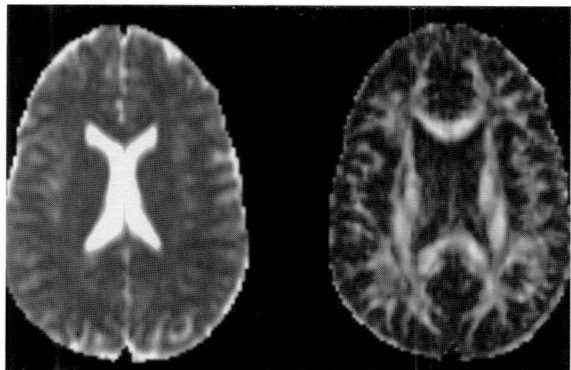

Plate 8 Diffusion-weighted MRI data can be used to generate maps of (left) the apparent diffusion coefficient (**ADC**) and (right) the anisotropy of diffusion. Diffusion of protons is most rapid and isotropic in cerebrospinal fluid, and least rapid and most anisotropic in white matter. White matter is clearly defined by relative hyperintensity in the anisotropy map.

Plates for Chapter 2.3.8

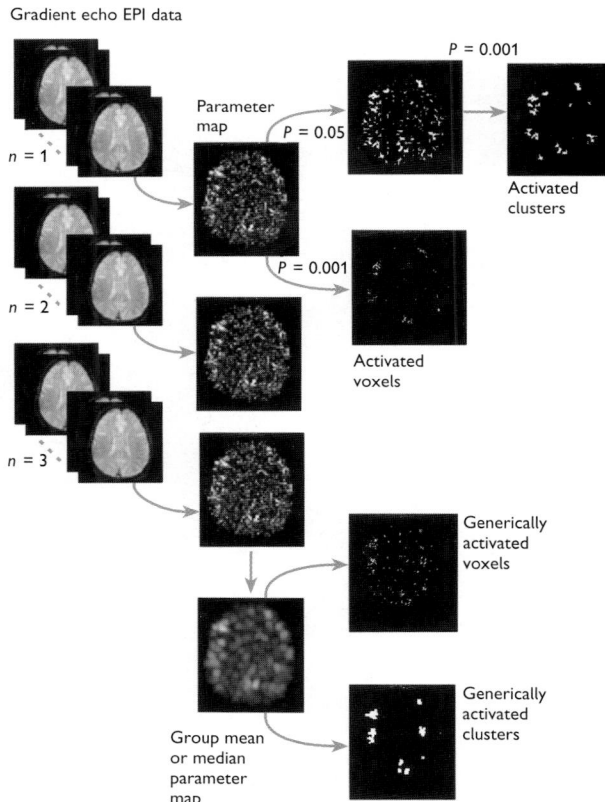

Plate 10 Steps in computerized data analysis. Gradient echoplanar imaging data have been acquired from three subjects under identical conditions. The time series at each voxel is analysed to estimate a measure or parameter of the experimental effect, which is represented as a parameter map. Significantly activated voxels or clusters can be identified in each individual image. Parameter maps can be averaged over individuals and generically activated voxels or clusters identified over the group of subjects. The power to detect activation is enhanced by cluster-level analysis and by combining data from several subjects.

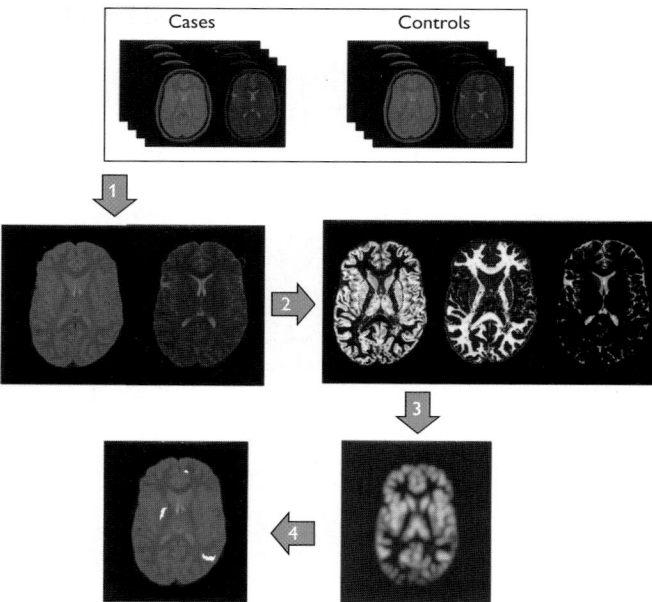

Plate 9 Steps in computerized image analysis. Dual-echo (fast spin echo) data are acquired from several cases and controls in a cross-sectionally designed study. Extracerebral tissue is removed (1) from each image before segmentation or tissue classification (2). Tissue-classified images are registered with a template image in standard space (3) before hypothesis testing (4). Voxels or clusters, which demonstrate a significant difference in tissue class volume between groups, are colour coded.

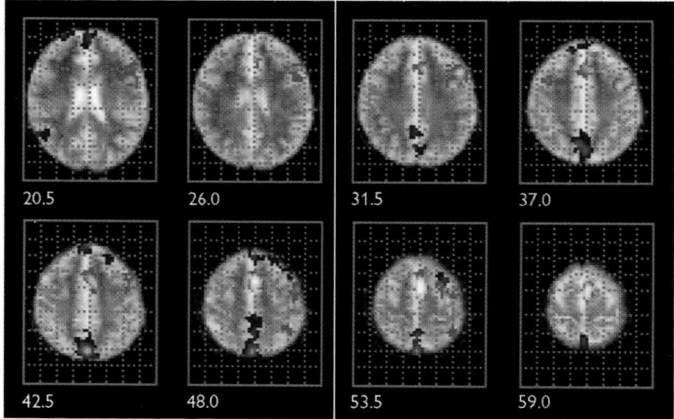

Plate 11 Activation map. Generically activated voxels are colour coded against a grey-scale background of gradient echoplanar imaging data. The grid represents the standard Talairach–Tournoux space;[12] z-coordinates for each slice are shown at the bottom left. Colour codes the timing and power of a periodic response to a covert verbal-fluency experiment. Blue voxels show increased magnetic resonance signal during condition B (repeat a word covertly); light blue represents a greater power of response than dark blue. Red voxels show increased magnetic resonance signal during condition A (generate a word beginning with a cue letter); yellow and orange represent a greater power of response than dark red. The voxel-wise probability of a false-positive error is $p = 0.0001$. The main areas activated during condition A are the dorsolateral prefrontal cortex, inferior frontal gyrus, and supplementary motor area; the main areas activated during condition B are the medial parietal cortex and posterior cingulate gyrus.

Plate for Chapter 4.1.4

Plate 12 Regional cerebral blood flow (rCBF) measured using SPECT with exametazine (left) and the xenon-133 inhalation method (right) in a 54-year-old female with clinical signs of FTD. The variation of regional cerebral blood flow is measured with xenon-133, above (red) or below (green) the average flow level, as indicated by the colour code. The patient showed the first signs of personality change, and stereotypy of speech and behaviour at the age of 48 years. EEG was normal, and CT and MRI showed slight frontal cortical atrophy. The regional cerebral blood flow measurement with xenon-133 showed a normal average flow level and marked bilateral, frontal flow decreases. The SPECT scan showed a severe perfusion deficit in the frontal and anterior cingulate cortex. (Courtesy of Department of Neurophysiology, University Hospital, Lund, Sweden.)

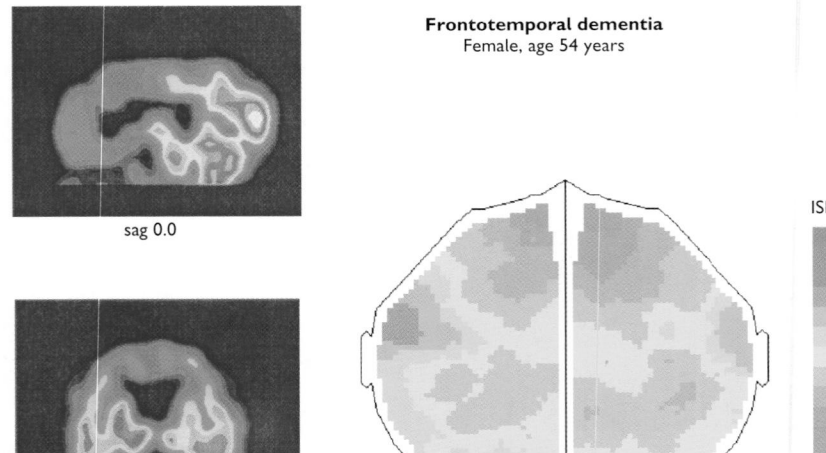

sag 0.0

Rt   om4   Lt

Frontotemporal dementia
Female, age 54 years

ISI (2–3)%

24
20
16
12
8
4
0
–4
–8
–12
–16
–20
–24

Lt 46.1   Rt45.3

Plate for Chapter 4.2.1

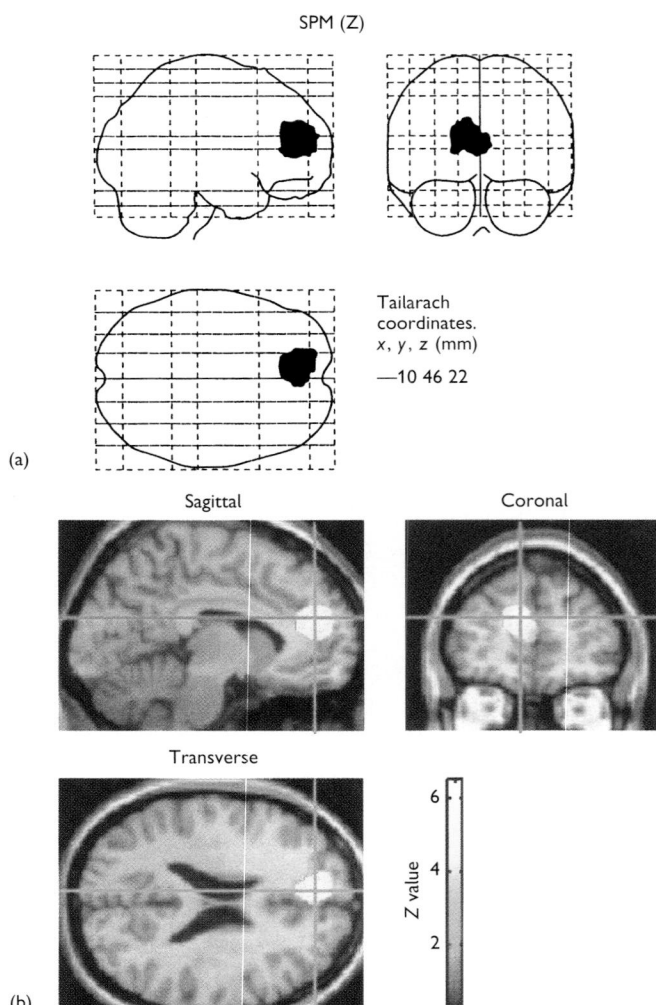

SPM (Z)

Tailarach coordinates.
x, y, z (mm)

—10 46 22

(a)

Sagittal   Coronal

Transverse

Z value

(b)

Plate 13 Area of activation during opiate craving: (a) $[^{15}O]H_2O$ PET SPM image; (b) area of activation superimposed on magnetic resonance image.

Plate for Chapter 4.5.5.2

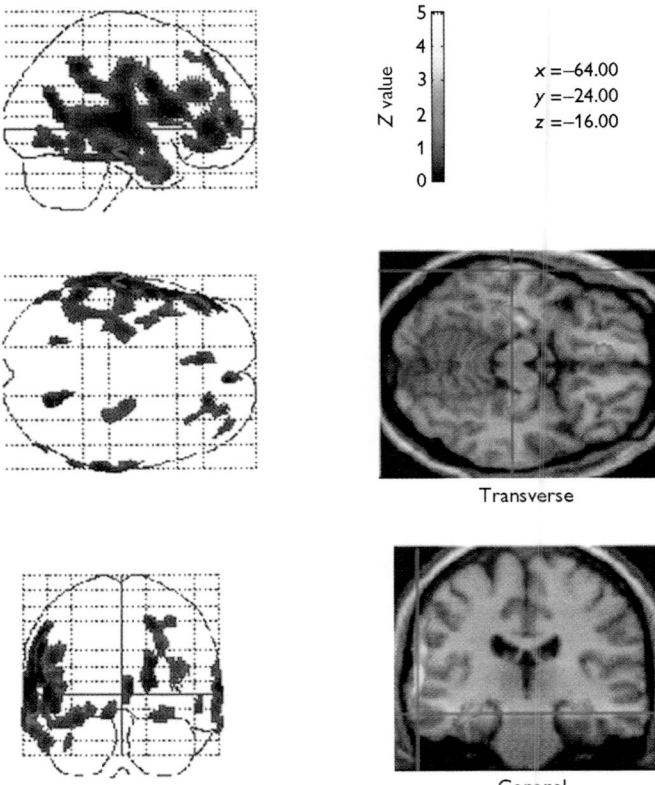

Z value

x = –64.00
y = –24.00
z = –16.00

Transverse

Coronal

Plate 14 Statistical parametric maps ($p < 0.001$) for reductions in grey matter densities in subjects with chronic refractory depression compared with controls. Effects are controlled for age. (Reproduced with permission from P.J. Shah *et al.* (1998). Cortical grey matter reductions associated with treatment-resistant chronic unipolar depression: controlled MRI study. *British Journal of Psychiatry*, **72**, 527–32.)

Table 1 Temperamental characteristics

Mainly:	Mainly:
1. Active	1. Passive
2. Regular (e.g. in feeding and sleeping habits)	2. Irregular
3. Reacts intensely (strongly)	3. Reacts mildly
4. Shows 'approach' behaviour to new people, places, toys, foods, etc.	4. Shows withdrawal behaviour
5. Adaptive—adapts fairly easily to change	5. Non-adaptive
6. Reacts easily to small changes	6. Reactions slow
7. Predominantly 'good' moods—happy contented disposition	7. Predominantly 'bad' disposition—fretful, hard to please
8. Persistent in what he or she is doing as regards time and in the face of difficulties	8. Non-persistent
9. Not easily distracted	9. Easily distracted from whatever he or she is doing

Linking developmental psychopathology to developing children

These exciting ideas need to be brought out of experimental settings and into clinics—the aim of developmental psychopathology theorists. In this second half of the chapter, some of the key aspects of child development relevant to clinical practice will be highlighted in this framework.

Individual differences

Children differ in their personality, character, or temperament. European psychologists have always emphasized these individual differences and adduced evidence that many were based on biologically determined ways of responding to the world. While the three-factor structure of personality developed by Eysenck evolved into the 'big five' structure of today, an issue remained as to how one could demonstrate continuity in personality from a very early age. The same issue bedevilled studies seeking to establish continuity in differences in intellectual functioning—simply put, little babies show such a different repertoire of behaviour from mobile talking preschool children that it was impossible to test the same behaviours at different ages.

In part, the problem was solved in the New York Longitudinal Study[16] by looking at differences in style of behaviour rather than differences in content or topography. By avoiding talking of biologically based personality, the findings reawakened interest in the genetics of individual differences. Through a mixture of observation and exhaustive interviews with mothers, they originally developed nine different categories of behavioural style or temperament (Table 1).

In the original sample of 78 babies, the investigators were able to demonstrate considerable individual differences in temperament.

There was good inter-rater reliability in making these judgements, and direct observations agreed well with reports from parents. The temperamental characteristics were found to be stable over both the short (2-year) and medium term, and even predicted reasonably well into late childhood.

Three broad types of temperament were characterized: children who were regular, predictable, and showed generally positive reactions—the easy babies, those who were almost the opposite, whom Chess called the 'mother killers', and a sizeable minority who were 'slow to warm up' to new situations but who adjusted eventually. The difficult children were over-represented in those who developed behavioural problems in later childhood.

Cognitive development

One of the major aspects of development that exercises parents and teachers alike is how best to improve the intellectual functioning of children, be that in language, reading, memory, or general intelligence. To what extent individual differences in these areas are predominantly related to heredity or to environment continues to be a popular, if sterile, source of argument. Clearly, the end result comes from an interaction between genetic predisposition and experience, but there remain issues of how best to manipulate the environment so as to help children gain their maximum potential. To that end, an understanding of modern behavioural genetics is essential (see Chapters 2.4.1 and 2.4.2). Here, some of the methodological issues involved in assessing babies' cognitive processes and findings in cognitive development, language, and memory are considered.

Getting inside the baby's head

Until babies start to speak, it is difficult to know what they are thinking. Fond parents interpret wind-driven grimaces as smiling; every child is seen as recognizing people and being smart from a young age. But how can one tell what really goes on inside a baby's head?

Fantz[35] developed an experimental method based on earlier work with chicks. Soon after hatching, chicks start pecking at things to eat. Presented with a variety of different-shaped objects, chicks preferred round to angular objects, and solid rather than two-dimensional objects. These preferences emerged even in chicks deprived of early experience, and so this innate preference was seen as having survival value as round solid objects the size of seeds are most likely to be edible.

Fantz decided to look at infants' eye movements and use fixation time as a measure of preference for different stimuli. Film recordings were made of light reflected off the baby's eyes. In a study of 30 infants tested weekly from 1 to 15 weeks of age, it was shown that the infants spent longer looking at complex than simple patterns. This demonstration of a clear perceptual preference in the first few weeks after birth gave the lie to the view that all begins as a 'big booming confusion'. Infants as young as 1 week show clear preference for human faces over other shapes presented to them some 10 inches (25 cm) away.

Fantz took advantage of the technology of the day. Since then, others have utilized measures of changes in temperature, galvanic skin response, and heartbeat to provide behavioural indices of preferences. In addition, not only have crude indices of time spent gazing at an object been utilized, but also investigators have used various indices from learning and conditioning paradigms. Shaffer and Parry[36] compared the performance of 6-month-old and 12-month-old children on a test where novel stimuli were presented within their reach. For the first seven presentations, the same 'nonsense' object was presented and both groups of children rapidly lost interest (or habituated). When a novel toy was shown on the eighth trial, both groups showed renewed interest, but only the older children were able to act on the information and be cautious in reaching out for the toy. One explanation of this finding is that knowledge and action are out of step in the second half of the first year. Visual recognition exerts no control over behaviour. But by 12 months, the infant can act on the information. This ability to tell known from unknown, to tell friend from foe, but also to be able to take appropriate action has obvious survival value.

Similar studies have shown that new-born babies recognize their mothers' voices, and also recognize the signature tunes of 'soap operas' that the mothers watched during the latter stages of pregnancy! Fagan[37] tested visual preference in 7-month-old babies and later measured their intelligence when they were 3 and 5 years old. The time spent looking at the novel stimulus when a baby had a correlation of 0.42 with performance on the later Picture Vocabulary Test. Thus it is becoming easier to measure various indices of baby's reactions, and some of these are found to be usefully predictive of later development and adjustment.

Piaget and cognitive development

Piaget was a biologist who studied amoebas in his doctoral research. Biological models found useful for that purpose clearly influenced the way he regarded cognitive development. He held to a sort of moving homeostasis—children develop a model of the world. New information that challenges that model is gradually assimilated and eventually the model accommodates the new ways of thinking—somewhat similar to an amoeba reaching out to a piece of food, surrounding it, and assimilating it.

According to his theory, children pass through three broad stages of thinking (see Box 1): a sensorimotor stage, a long stage where they think in terms of what he called concrete operations, and finally a stage where they can think logically.

Piaget's stage theory has been very influential, and helpfully sparked off a great deal of research which has led to a much better understanding of how children develop cognitively. However, his original models were somewhat simplistic, and to have seen only three major stages covering a period of such rapid development appears to be inadequate. Moreover, for the clinician, the question one often wants to raise is how this understanding can be used to bolster the reasoning of a child who is developmentally delayed—what Piaget witheringly dismissed as 'the American question'. Piaget tended to argue that children could not be hurried through the stages. However, critics soon argued that some of the regularities that were apparently replicated in his work owed more to the manner in which the tasks were presented to the child than to any necessary underlying cohesion in types of thinking.

A typical experiment is to give a child two pieces of clay that are identical. Then one is rolled out into a sausage and the child is asked if they remain the same. Alternatively, the child is shown two test tubes of differing diameters. The same amount of liquid is poured into each but, of course, reaches different heights. Which test tube has more liquid? Not surprisingly, younger children make more errors than older ones, and it has been shown that an understanding of conser-

Box 1

Piaget's stages of cognitive development

Birth to 18 months: sensorimotor stage

Cognition is based mainly on the child's actions and six substages were described. A key concept at this stage is that of 'object permanence'—the ability to understand that an object continues to exist even when it is out of sight. Infants of 12 months will continue to look for an object where an experimenter hides it, even when they watch the experimenter move it. It is as if the object 'belongs' only in a particular place.

18 months to 12 years: concrete operations

This is the stage of concrete operations. At the early stage, language develops rapidly. Children begin to demonstrate symbolic play, showing that they have memories and internal representations. Many ingenious little experiments were developed to illustrate how children's thinking about their worlds develops. Various other conservation tasks—of length, mass, and number for instance—convince teachers that children think differently about the world than adults and this has had a major, if not always beneficial, effect on ways of teaching.

12 years and over: formal operations

From around puberty onwards, the child is able to formulate and test hypotheses about the world. The child realizes that mass and volume can be altered in many ways, but they remain essentially unchanged. Children can examine their own thought processes and can begin to reason more logically.

vation of mass (seeing that the quantity of material remains the same despite of changes in shape) is acquired around 7 to 8 years, while conservation of weight is not understood until 9 or 10 years. It is not until the age of 11 or 12 that the child typically thinks that each shape also occupies the same amount of space (i.e. understands conservation of volume).

Bruner was one of the earliest to demonstrate that children's judgements could be radically manipulated by small changes in the ways the tasks were presented. For example, in the studies of conservation of volume, a screen was placed between the child and the test tubes so that only the tops showed but not the levels reached by the liquid. This simple change meant that many younger children now understood that by pouring liquid from one container to another—perhaps something done daily in the bath—nothing had changed. Some children as young as 4 years were able to perform the revised task, but once they had to make the judgement again without the screen, they reverted to the more primitive form of reasoning. In other words, young children are more at the mercy of their perceptual impressions—a finding that needs to be taken into consideration in many circumstances.

Language development

Children communicate from the beginning. They signal their basic needs, often by crying. Parents soon learn to respond to the differing signals. Their own child's crying can be very aversive to most parents and so they quickly learn how to switch the noise off! Autistic and brain-damaged children produce grossly abnormal cries, but often parents with little experience do not recognize the unusual nature of the cry. Whilst lower primates and other animals can communicate, none uses language in the flexible way that human infants come to do. Language, both spoken and written, is truly the most human of attributes.

However, it was not the subject of serious study until 40 years ago. Beginning with simple descriptive studies of the acquisition of words, the complexities of grammar and cross-cultural comparisons, studies of language development now encompass many other dimensions from neuropsychological, brain imaging, and genetics. What stands out is just how difficult it is to affect the onset of language by manipulating the environment. It takes extraordinary environmental deprivation to interfere with language development and even then, when the environment is normalized, considerable catch-up occurs.

The grunts and single syllables of the first couple of months soon give way to the production of the full range of phonemes and babbling between 2 and 4 months. States of feelings are communicated clearly by 3 to 7 months. From 6 months, the baby begins to imitate simple sounds and unreinforced phonemes disappear from the vocabulary. By 8 months, the baby begins to utter two-syllable combinations such as 'ma-ma' and 'da-da'—among the easiest to produce physically and, perhaps not coincidentally, the most emotionally evocative words parents want to hear. At around 12 months, the first true word appears, usually as the infant takes his or her first step—girls reaching the milestone slightly ahead of boys.

Studies in the 1960s and 1970s established that language development followed complicated underlying rules. The idea that children learned language by successive approximations to adult speech being differentially reinforced was quickly laid to rest. Such techniques have an important place in remedial intervention for children with deviant language development, but for ordinary children the sheer inevitability, speed, and beauty of acquisition is overwhelming. This led many to postulate that there is a genetically encoded language acquisition device that guides communication, although not the particular form of language that a particular child will develop. That still depends on what language they are exposed to.

Early sentences are telegraphic with some words acting as pivots on which other words hang to form flexible sentences. Thus, the pivot 'all-gone' can have 'sock', 'milk' or 'daddy' added to create a whole range of meaningful simple sentences. Children develop rules for expression. A common error is for them to extract a rule and then overgeneralize it to a situation that is an exception in their particular language. For example, the present tense is used before the past tense. Instead of saying 'I went' children often form past participles by adding '-ed' to a stem and come up with the often heard 'I goed'. This shows they are learning a rule, even though they make some mistakes on the way.

Different ways of describing and classifying language disorders have been proposed in the past few years.[38] The findings of Bishop's[39] twin study that when language disorder is defined as a discrepancy between non-verbal IQ and language score the heritability is far less than when language delay and disorder are considered without reference to IQ is important for clinicians in identifying children with such difficulties (see Chapter 9.2.11).

Vocabulary grows astronomically from 1 to 3 years and beyond. Children's sentences become longer and more complex.[40] A good working approximation is that the average length of sentence is in keeping with the number of years of age (Table 2).

Table 2 Average length of sentences: 2 to 5 years

Age (months)	24	42	30	36	48	54	60
Average number of words per sentence	1.7	4.0	2.4	3.3	4.3	4.7	4.6

Memory

One of the most intriguing observations in the current child development literature is the contrast between the ever-increasing evidence of just how complicated children's cognitive development is and the phenomenon known as 'infantile amnesia'. Basically, people have very few memories before the age of 3 years. Clearly from all that has been described earlier about the differential reactions of babies to specific stimuli, to their recognizing their mother's voice or holding out their arms to their father rather than to a stranger, children increasingly have some form of central representations that they can work on. However, these early memories are not accessible in later life. It is really not until language is well established that people have what is ordinarily termed memory for past events.

Clearly, infantile amnesia poses a major challenge to any theory of child development or personality that tries to link very early experiences with later adjustment. But early experience does affect the way in which relationships are formed, so what are the mechanisms? As the different types of memory are better understood, so better assessment of these functions is possible.

Some very recent work has looked at implicit and explicit memory as well as attentional processes in children with generalized anxiety disorder, PTSD, and depression. Broadly speaking, the preliminary findings are in accord with the voluminous findings with adult patients, namely that depressed children tend to have biases in memory for sad things, while anxious children do not. In contrast, children with anxiety disorders (including PTSD) have biases in attention that make them attend more to threatening cues in their environment, or at least to threatening words projected on computer screens. Studies using these adult-generated paradigms but utilized within a developmental framework should greatly increase our understanding of why some children break down under stress and others do not. Biases in cognitive processing of emotional reactions are implicated and can now be studied more readily.

Goswami[41] summarizes many ingenious experiments that establish the parameters of children's memory. While parents and teachers often talk about children having problems with memory and even 'short-term memory', developmental psychologists have worked on much more complex paradigms and identified a number of different memory systems:

- **Recognition memory** is simply the ability to realize that a particular stimulus has been encountered before. Recognition is always easier than recall, as those learning a foreign language can testify. Once established in the first year of life, recognition memory does not change much.

- **Implicit memory** is another term for 'memory without awareness'. Although not able to put it in to words, people can act differently to previously exposed stimuli than to novel ones. This seems to be fully developed by around 4 years of age.

- **Episodic memory** involves awareness. It is this memory system that organizes memories into stories or scripts concerning similar activities. These scripts contain both temporal and causal information. The ability to learn sequences in a particular chain of events does develop with age. It is now that one realizes that there needs to be some mechanism to get rid of many of the memories for everyday activities, otherwise the whole memory will get clogged up with non-essential information. In other words, memory processes are seen as being very active with some memory traces remaining in (technically) short-term memory for only a few seconds unless operated upon and stored in long-term store.

- **Eye-witness memory** has taken on a special importance as children are expected to testify in court on things they have witnessed happening to themselves or to others. Children can recall things fairly accurately, as long as deliberate leading questions are not put to them.[42] Three-year-olds are more suggestible than 5-year-olds. Bruck *et al.*[42] found that experienced adults, such as psychiatrists or judges, evaluated children's responses to questioning about a real event using the child's behaviour while giving their answer. Where children gave firm answers with lots of supporting details, they were judged to have clear and accurate memories. Where children were uncertain and hesitant, they were seen as fabricating whereas they were hesitating because the questioner was asking the wrong questions—ones that were in conflict with what had actually happened: they were the ones who were actually telling the truth. The younger confident children were often telling adults what they wanted to hear! A great deal more needs to be done in relation to helping children recall what has happened to them without using leading questions. (Children's ability to testify as witnesses is considered further in Chapter 9.4.2.)

- **Working memory** was seen by Baddeley and coworkers as consisting of a central executive linked to two separate subsystems: a phonological loop and a visuospatial sketchpad. Information decays in the phonological loop in 1 or 2 s, unless it is actively rehearsed. It is thought that children predominantly use a visuospatial encoding until they switch to the phonological–verbal system around the age of 5 years. Deaf children continue to rely on the visual encoding for much longer.

Social and emotional development

Alongside cognitive development, children are developing both socially and emotionally. It has been recognized for years that children brought up in institutions, away from their natural parents, often develop serious and subtle problems in social interactions and emotional development.

Arising in part from his studies of infants in institutions and his collaborative studies of children's reactions to being in hospital, as well as his dissatisfaction with contemporary psychoanalytic theory, Bowlby turned to ethology for an understanding of early infant relationships. He came to view the intense relationship between the infant and the caretaker, usually but not always the biological mother, as serving a biological survival value and having been produced by natural selection.

As memory develops in the first year of life, and as the infant becomes more able to express emotion and to move independently, so there is evidence for selective attachment. This is shown round about 6 to 8 months onwards by the upset at leaving the attachment figure, by seeking his or her comfort when feeling threatened, and by a general wariness of strangers.

The idea that attachments were simply associative learning—the baby comes to love the person who feeds him or her—was quickly dismissed by the evidence from Harlow's studies of infant monkeys. They attached to the cuddly terry-towelling surrogate rather than the wire surrogate where they were fed. Rather, selective attachments in the human served to protect the infant during the prolonged period of helplessness. The function of attachment changes over the years, with children using an attachment figure as a secure base from which to explore. Thus, almost paradoxically, the well-attached toddler may move away from the attachment figure more than the insecurely attached counterpart. Attachment is not the same as clinginess.

By the age of 3 to 4 years, most children show good evidence of having multiple attachment figures. By this age, their memories are so much greater that they are less dependent on the physical presence of the attachment figure to provide security and comfort. Bowlby saw good attachments in infancy as laying the basis for future social and intimate relationships and there is currently an explosion of work re-examining psychiatric conditions from an 'attachment perspective'.

Bowlby's theory places considerable emphasis on the child's real experience. As Belsky and Cassidy[43] put it:

> Central to Bowlby's theory of the working model of the self and of the attachment figure is the idea that, over time, there is an inextricable intertwining of the working model of the self and of the attachment figure. Thus, a child whose attachment needs are rebuffed not only comes to develop a model of the mother as rejecting, but of himself as unworthy of love and attention … working models become so deeply ingrained that they influence feelings, thoughts and behaviour unconsciously and automatically.

Thus, Bowlby saw the child as developing a cognitive model of his or her effective social world, in keeping with the views of other cognitive theorists such as George Kelly, Aaron Beck, and Ronnie Janoff-Bulmann.

It needs to be emphasized that the pattern of attachment characterizes a particular dyadic relationship and children can show different types of attachment to different caretakers. Even so, the characterization of such attachment behaviour in the 12- to 18-month period has been shown to predict reasonably to patterns of social behaviour 4 years later. A major problem for workers in this area has been to develop measures to characterize social attachments after infancy. As Belsky and Cassidy[43] conclude, '…the notion of internal working models as the causal process explaining the associations between attachment security and developmental sequelae remains a useful interpretive heuristic in need of empirical evaluation'.

A negative aspect of the focus on attachments has been the emergence of an ill-defined disorder described as 'reactive attachment disorder' which seems to be diagnosable by the presence of any or all of a long list of symptoms and signs that haunted previous generations under such labels as minimal brain dysfunction and the like. This has been associated in some countries with the use of assaultative 'holding therapies' intended to break the child's resistance to forming attachments. Clearly, more careful studies need to be undertaken to try to pinpoint the subtle social difficulties presented by children whose early lives have been disrupted as in fostering and adoption, but care also needs to be taken to adduce evidence for appropriate interventions.

Ainsworth *et al.*[44] developed the theory and a method for detecting individual differences in attachment. They introduced the 'strange situation' test in which an infant is left in the care of a stranger for a few minutes. The observer then notes how the infant copes both with the separation and with the reunion with the attachment figure. These observations led to a tripartite classification of attachments.

- **Secure attachment**: the infant tends to seek proximity and contact with the attachment figure, shows a preference for the attachment figure over a stranger, and shows very little distress before and after separation. Any distress is easily soothed by the comfort of the attachment figure.

- **Avoidant insecure**: the baby does not cling when held, avoids the mother (or caretaker) during the reunion, and does not differentiate greatly between the caretaker and a stranger.

- **Resistant insecurity**: the infant resists contact and interaction with the mother. There is great distress at reunion.

- **Disorganized or avoidant insecurity**: this category had to be introduced when it was found that infants of severely depressed and abusive mothers showed a mixed pattern of attachments. The child shows contradictory patterns and unusual patterns of negative emotions.

Having good supportive social relationships has been shown to be a major protective factor in the aetiology and maintenance of many psychiatric disorders. The ability to make and maintain friends—initially of the same age and later of any age—is often related to the existence of disorders such as personality disorders, social anxiety disorders, depression, and even PTSD. The emphasis on social skills training for socially inadequate persons points to the early basis for such deficits even though they may have their greatest impact in adulthood. Some children are less sensitive to social cues than others, and some misinterpret the intentions of other people. Both lead to difficulties, albeit of different sorts.

Boys and girls tend to develop different types of social relationships. Children tend to prefer playing with others of the same gender when freed from adult influence. Boys tend to play in larger, looser groups in which issues of dominance and play fighting predominate; girls relate in smaller groups of more intense relationships, with best friends often changing.

Young children show an interest in each other from a very early age:

- 2 months—infants will orient to other babies

- 3 months—will reach out and try to touch other babies

- 6 months—additionally will smile and vocalize to the other baby

- 6 to 12 months—increase in attempted interactions, but low rate of response

- 12 to 24 months—more varied interactions, with negative ones increasing.

Altruism and empathy are present in normal children from early on with positive interactions increasing. But competitiveness and rivalry also increase in the preschool years. Indeed, Patterson's early observational studies of children in nurseries showed how these were all too effective in training children to be more assertive.[45]

Psychosexual development

While sexual activity is often the focus of parental concern when a child reaches adolescence, psychosexual development arises from birth, if not before. In the second half of the first year of life, infants can tell genders apart and by the second year they are aware of their own gender. As noted earlier, they then prefer to play with children of their own gender. In the preschool years, they are increasingly aware of their own bodies. Far from confirming the stereotype of fatness equalling jollity, fat children are more likely than physically disabled children to be rejected by other children and to become depressed. Concern with size and image currently predominate in many Western cultures, and even elementary school children show concerns about being too fat.

Empirical studies have moved us far on from the primitive and misleading 'stage theories' of psychosexual development popularized in the 1920s. Children's interest in bodily functions continues throughout childhood and there is no latency period. Masturbation and sexual play are common well before puberty. Sexual behaviour in young children is common, and should only be regarded as a sign of sexual abuse when it is out of context and is inappropriate.

With puberty, things change and sexual identity and behaviour, as well as fertility management, take on a new importance. Despite the rise of unwanted teenage pregancies in many Western countries, there are still too many uninformed debates about the role and importance of sex education and contraception.[6,14,46] The emergence of HIV is beginning slowly to focus people's minds on the issues.

While physical gender is mainly determined by chromosmes, hormonal activity *in utero* can also influence physical and psychosexual development to some extent. Problems associated with gender identity ('tomboy girls' and 'sissy boys') arise in the toddler and preschool years. Follow-up studies of feminine boys find that they show an increased rate of homosexual behaviour later, but there is still considerable debate as to the mechanisms underlying the development of homosexuality. As more societies develop less discriminatory practices, so more homosexual behaviour is shown. Even so, homosexual boys—often clear about their sexual orientation before puberty—still experience discrimination and show higher rates of exclusion and even suicidal behaviour than others.

A better empirically based understanding of psychosexual development would help underpin an enhanced understanding of the formation and maintenance of happy healthy relationships throughout the lifespan. Failed relationships can greatly harm the children caught up in divorcing families.

Concluding comments

Taking a developmental perspective to mental health issues should apply across the lifespan. Psychiatrists working with adults need to understand where their clients are coming from and where they are going to. They need to understand the pleasures and pressures that children bring to their parents, and where appropriate they should be considering the impact of parental illness on the children. The institutionalized separation of child and adult psychiatry (in terms of service delivery) should not lead to a separation in ways of considering the developmental context of presenting problems.

This chapter has shown that there are many small focused models of development that deal with discrete areas. Stage theories emphasize differences at different stages; social learning theories emphasize continuities on processes of development. As long as practitioners are aware that when they say a child is 'at a particular stage', this is but a rough guide to describing the child, that may be acceptable. It is when such models are taken literally that oversimplification leads to poor practice. There is no single overarching theory of child development, and while this may be inconvenient for examiners, it truly reflects the rich diversity of human development. By paying more attention to the interactions between biological, social, and psychological factors, a better understanding of healthy normal development will emerge. Empirical studies will help identify risk and protective factors which in turn will lead to better mental health promotion and more effective interventions when mental disorders manifest.

References

1. Cox, A. and Rutter, M. (1985). Diagnostic appraisal and interviewing. In *Child psychiatry: modern approaches* (2nd edn) (ed. M. Rutter and L. Hersov), pp. 233–48. Blackwell Science, Oxford.

2. Rutter, M., Graham, P., Chadwick, O., and Yule, W. (1975). Adolescent turmoil: fact or fiction? *Journal of Child Psychology and Psychiatry*, **17**, 35–56.

3. Harrington, R. (1993). *Depressive disorder in childhood and adolescence.* Wiley, Chichester.

4. Rutter, M. (1975). *Helping troubled children.* Penguin Books, Harmondsworth.

5. Staats, A.W. (1971). *Child learning, intelligence and personality: principles of a behavioral interaction approach.* Harper and Row, New York.

6. Rutter, M. (1980). Psychosexual development. In *Scientific foundations of developmental psychiatry,* (ed. M. Rutter), pp. 322–39. Heinemann Medical, London.

7. Berger, M. (1985). Temperament and individual differences. In *Child psychiatry: modern approaches* (2nd edn) (ed. M. Rutter and L. Hersov), pp. 3–16. Blackwell Science, Oxford.

8. Kagan, J. (1997). Temperament. In *Handbook of child and adolescent psychiatry,* Vol. 1: *Infants and preschoolers* (ed. J.D. Noshpitz), pp. 268–75. Wiley, New York.

9. Keogh, B.K. (1982). Children's temperament and teachers' decisions. In *Temperamental differences in infants and young children* (ed. R. Porter and G.M. Collins), pp. 269–78. Pitman, London.

10. Eysenck, H.J. and Eysenck, S.B.G. (1969). *Personality structures and measurement.* Routledge and Kegan Paul, London.

11. Childers, P. and Wimmer, M. (1971). The concept of death in early childhood. *Child Development*, **42**, 1299–301.

12. Koocher, G.P. (1974). Talking with children about death. *American Journal of Orthopsychiatry*, **44**, 404–11.

13. Wolff, S. (1969). *Children under stress.* Penguin Books, Harmondsworth.

14. Rutter, M. and Rutter, M. (1993). *Developing minds: challenge and continuity across the life span.* Basic Books, New York.

15. Janoff-Bulman, R. (1985). The aftermath of victimization: rebuilding shattered assumptions. In *Trauma and its wake* (ed. C.R. Figley), Vol. 1, pp. 15–35. Brunner–Mazel, New York.

16. Thomas, A., Chess, S., and Birch, H.G. (1968). *Temperament and behavior disorders in children.* University of London Press.

17. Meichenbaum, D. (1993). Stress inoculation training: a 20-year update. In *Principles and practice of stress management* (2nd edn) (ed. P.M. Lehrer and R.L. Woolfolk). Guilford Press, New York.

18. Bradley, L. and Bryant, P.E. (1983). Categorizing sounds and learning to read—a causal connection. *Nature*, **301**, 419–21.

19. King, R.D., Raynes, N.V., and Tizard, J. (1971). *Patterns of residential care: sociological studies in institutions for handicapped children.* Routledge and Kegan Paul, London.

20. Cicchetti, D. (1984). The emergence of developmental psychopathology. *Child Development*, **55**, 1–7.

21. Sroufe, L.A. and Rutter, M. (1984). The domain of developmental psychopathology. *Child Development*, **55**, 17–29.

22. Garmezy, N. (1974). Children at risk: the search for the antecedents of schizophrenia. I: Conceptual models and research methods. *Schizophrenia Bulletin*, **8**, 14–90.

23. Santostefano, S. (1978). *A biodevelopmental approach to clinical child psychology.* Wiley, New York.

24. Rutter, M. (1983). Continuities and discontinuities in socioemotional development: empirical and conceptual perspectives. In *Continuities and discontinuities in development* (ed. R. Harmon and R. Emde), pp. 41–68. Plenum Press, New York.

25. Bandura, A. (1973). *Aggression: a social learning analysis.* Prentice-Hall, London.

26. Yule, W. (1978). Behavioural treatment of children and adolescents with conduct disorders. In *Aggression and anti-social behaviour in childhood and adolescence* (ed. L. Hersov, M. Berger, and D. Shaffer), pp. 115–41. Pergamon Press, Oxford.

27. Cantwell, D.P. (1988). DSM-III studies. In *Assessment and diagnosis in child psychopathology* (ed. M. Rutter, A.H.Tuma, and I.S. Lann), pp. 3–36. David Fulton, London.

28. Rutter, M. and Shaffer, D. (1980). A step forward or back in terms of the classification of child psychiatric disorders? *Journal of the American Academy of Child Psychiatry*, **19**, 371–94.

29. Yule, W. (1981). The epidemiology of child psychopathology. In *Advances in clinical child psychology,* Vol. 4 (ed. B.B. Lahey and A.E. Kazdin), pp. 1–51. Plenum Press, New York.

30. Garber, J. (1984). Classification of childhood psychopathology: a developmental perspective. *Child Development*, **55**, 30–48.

31. Yule, W. and Williams, R. (1990). Post traumatic stress reactions in children. *Journal of Traumatic Stress*, **3**, 279–95.

32. Yule, W., Perrin, S., and Smith, P. (1999). Post-traumatic stress disorders in children and adolescents. In *Post-traumatic stress disorders: concepts and therapy* (ed. W. Yule), pp. 25–50. Wiley, Chichester.

33. Almqvist, K. and Brandell-Forsberg, M. (1997). Refugee children in Sweden: post-traumatic stress disorder in Iranian preschool children exposed to organized violence. *Child Abuse and Neglect*, **21**, 351–66.

34. Scheeringa, M.S., Zeanah, C.H., Drell, M.J., and Larrieu, J.A. (1995). Two approaches to the diagnosis of posttraumatic stress disorder in infancy and early childhood. *Journal of the American Academy of Child and Adolescent Psychiatry*, **34**, 191–200.

35. Fantz, R.L. (1961). The origin of form perception. *Scientific American*, Reprint 459.

36. Shaffer, H.R. and Parry, M.H. (1969). Perceptual motor behaviour in infancy as a function of age and stimulus familiarity. *British Journal of Psychology*, **60**, 1–9.

37. Fagan, J.F. (1984). The relationship of novelty preferences during infancy to later intelligence and later recognition memory. *Intelligence*, **8**, 339–46.

38. Yule, W. and Rutter, M. (ed.) (1987). *Language development and disorders.* MacKeith Press, London.

39. Bishop, D.V.M. (1998). Is specific language impairment a valid diagnostic category? Genetic and psycholinguistic evidence. In *Perspectives on the classification of specific developmental disorders* (ed. J. Rispens, T. van Yperen, and W. Yule), pp. 139–53. Kluwer, Dordrecht.

40. Smith, M.E. (1926). An investigation of the development of the sentence and extent of vocabulary in young children. *University of Iowa Studies in Child Welfare*, **3** (no. 5).

41. Goswami, U. (1998). *Cognition in children.* Psychology Press, Hove.

42. Bruck, M., Ceci, S., and Hembrooke, H. (1998). Reliability and credibility of young children's reports. *American Psychologist*, **53**, 136–51.

43. Belsky, J. and Cassidy, J. (1994). Attachment: theory and evidence. In

Development through life: a handbook for clinicians (ed. M. Rutter and D.F. Hay), pp. 373–402. Blackwell Science, Oxford.

44. Ainsworth, M.D.S., Blehar, M.C., Waters, E., and Wall, S. (1978). *Patterns of attachment*. Erlbaum, Hillsdale, NJ.

45. Patterson, G.R., Littman, R.A., and Bricker, W. (1967). Assertive behavior in children: a step towards a theory of aggression. *Monographs of the Society for Research in Child Development*, **32** (5), Series 113.

46. Paikoff, R. and Brooks-Gunn, J. (1994). Psychosexual development across the lifespan. In *Development through life: a handbook for clinicians* (ed. M. Rutter and D.F. Hay), pp. 403–55. Blackwell Science, Oxford.

2.5.1.2 Lifespan psychology: illustrations from adulthood and old age

Alexandra M. Freund and Ursula M. Staudinger

Lifespan psychology defines development as selective age-related change in adaptive capacity.[1] Inasmuch as mental health can be considered one important indicator of adaptation, lifespan psychology is of relevance to researchers and practitioners in the field of psychiatry. Lifespan psychology specifies conditions and constraints on development across the whole life. We start this chapter by outlining three of the propositions of lifespan psychology which address the effects of biological and cultural processes on human development. Next, we present a model that identifies three processes regulating the interplay of biological and cultural influences in individual development, namely selection, optimization, and compensation. We then illustrate the application of these theoretical conceptss in one area of psychological functioning—self and personality. Finally, we outline the specific characteristics of very old age and some of their consequences for research and practice in psychiatry. This late period of the lifespan, sometimes called the 'fourth age', poses specific challenges for science and society.

Lifespan development: the dynamic between biology and culture

Unlike traditional conceptions of development, lifespan psychology proposes that development is not completed when entering adulthood but continues throughout mid-life into old and very old age.[2] Lifespan psychology holds that development is best described as the dynamic interplay between biological and cultural factors, resulting in multiple trajectories comprising growth and decline, gains and losses.[3]

Although some resources may increase throughout the lifespan (e.g. life experience), internal and external resources are finite. Resources can be defined as personal or environmental characteristics that support or facilitate a person's transaction with the environment. Resources include biological–genetic characteristics (e.g. temperament), psychological characteristics (e.g. conscientiousness), and social–cultural characteristics (e.g. health system). Although these resources are limited throughout the lifespan, their availability and

efficiency change with age.[3,4] Childhood is primarily characterized by an increase of resources (e.g. the acquisition of new skills), although children's developmental trajectories also include some losses. Starting out highly positive, the ratio of gains to losses becomes progressively less positive with age. Resources are replenished less as the individual grows old, and are drawn upon more exhaustively. There are three reasons for this:[3]

(1) the advantages of evolutionary selection decline with increasing age;

(2) the need for culture increases across the lifespan;

(3) the efficacy of culture decreases across the lifespan and particularly in old age.

Life expectancy has only fairly recently extended into old age. As argued in more detail elsewhere,[1,3] the benefits of evolutionary selection decrease with age leading to less effective genetic material, mechanisms, and expressions for developing and maintaining high levels of functioning. In addition, our culture has not had enough time to evolve into one that provides the same richness of opportunity for the elderly as for children.[3] In old age, when culture most needs to compensate for biologically based decreases in functioning, it provides the least support. Moreover, owing to reduced resources, old people make less use of supportive environmental conditions. It takes more cultural investment to reach comparable goals and some goals cannot be attained any more. Overall, the three developmental trajectories result in a less favourable balance of growth (gains) and decline (losses) with increasing age. Thus, with increasing age individuals have to allocate more resources to maintenance of functioning and resilience against losses rather than processes of growth.[5]

An important assumption underlying our notion of resilience is that development is a dynamic process of both reacting to and proactively shaping one's environment as well as oneself. People not only react to environmental demands but also shape their environment.[6] Indeed, shaping one's environment so that it better suits one's needs is an important source of resilience when confronted with adverse conditions (e.g. a move to a ground-floor apartment in which a wheelchair can be used when mobility decreases).

One important way in which individuals play an active role in their development is by choosing, committing to, and pursuing a set of (life) goals such as having a child or pursuing a certain career. A person's goals are constrained by sociocultural, biological, and phylogenetic factors. The less the influence of these factors, the more freedom a person has to develop and choose his or her goals and ways of pursuing them. During childhood, adolescence, and young adulthood there are relatively strong biological constraints and social expectations with regard to the kinds of goals that ought to be pursued.[7] There are also social opportunity structures[8] such as financial or institutional incentives for entering the workforce or for founding a family.

In late adulthood and old age, there are fewer normative age-related expectations about the goals a person ought to pursue.[9] This greater social freedom in older age gives more weight to goal selection and goal pursuit as processes of developmental regulation. On the other hand, old age is characterized by diminishing resources that limit the degree to which a person is able to shape the environment according to his or her goals.[10,11] When resources tend to be more limited than in earlier life, it is crucial to make a wise selection of goals on which to focus.[12]

Thus, it is not surprising that goal selection and goal pursuit have a prominent place in models of successful development in general and successful aging.[3,10–12] In the next section, we shall describe the selection, optimization, and compensation (**SOC**) model,[1,12–14] which is particularly useful for conceptualizing adult development.

Selection, optimization, and compensation as processes of adaptive mastery in adulthood

The SOC metamodel conceptualizes general processes of adaptive mastery across the lifespan.[12–14] Here, we provide only a brief definition of these three processes of developmental regulation; for a more detailed description see Freund and Baltes.[13]

The limitation of resources (e.g. time, energy, social support, money) present throughout the lifespan necessitates the careful selection of domains of functioning on which to focus resources, as not all opportunities can be pursued. **Selection** refers to delineating the range of alternative domains of functioning by developing, elaborating, and committing to a set of goals. Selection gives development a direction because goals organize behaviour into meaningful action sequences which may motivate and guide behaviour across situations and over time. Moreover, to be committed to a set of goals allows a person to focus his or her resources on the domains he or she considers to be most important and that best match his or her values, opportunity structures, and environmental demands.

Selection refers either to developing goals or preferences, building a goal hierarchy, and committing oneself to these goals (i.e. elective selection), or to restructuring one's goal hierarchy, adapting goal standards, or selecting new goals as a response to loss or decline in goal-relevant means (i.e. loss-based selection). The distinction between elective and loss-based selection is based on the assumption that development involves both gains and losses. Whereas elective selection addresses goal-setting processes that are associated with trajectories of gains/growth, loss-based selection addresses the mastery of loss or decline in goal-relevant means. Loss-based selection encompasses such strategies as disengaging from a goal that can no longer be achieved due to decline or loss of resources, reconstructing one's goal hierarchy or searching for new goals that better match the resources available to the person.

To reach optimal levels of functioning in the selected domains (goals), one needs to acquire, allocate, and refine internal or external resources (optimization). In other words, the SOC model posits that people need to invest goal-relevant resources into optimizing their level of functioning. **Optimization** refers to the acquisition, application, and orchestration of means (resources) aimed at achieving optimal functioning or desired outcomes. The adaptiveness of a specific means for achieving a goal depends on such factors as the content of the goal, the characteristics of the person (e.g. age, skills), and the given opportunity structure. On a more abstract level, a number of strategies contributing to goal attainment can be identified:[13] planning and forming specific intentions,[15] the investment of time and energy, the acquisition of new skills or resources, the practice of skills,[16] persistence,[17] modelling successful others,[18] and control beliefs.[19]

Optimization addresses processes related to goal attainment and growth, i.e. means are invested in fostering developmental gains. Loss of the means of attaining goals is managed by compensatory processes,[12,20] i.e. means are invested avoiding a loss in functioning.[5,13] Compensation involves substitution of means or use of external accessories, for example hearing aids.[21]

Compensation may be of particular importance in old age when losses are prevalent in health,[22] sensory functioning,[23] size of social network,[24] and cognitive functioning.[25] Functioning in these domains is a resource when pursuing goals. For instance, if taking regular walks is threatened when mobility is severely impaired, a good compensatory strategy would be to use an external aid such as a wheelchair. Another example of compensation is the use of external memory aids such as calendar entries when memory declines. As losses of this kind are more frequent in old age, the maintenance of functions in the face of loss becomes more important than the achievement of new goals[11] and the need for compensation may be greater.[5]

There is some evidence supporting the usefulness of the SOC model for conceptualizing life mastery in adulthood. For instance, in young adulthood self-reported selection, optimization, and compensation are positively related to subjective indicators of life mastery in the domains of work and family.[26] In late adulthood, selection, optimization, and compensation are correlated with subjective indicators of successful aging (satisfaction with aging, lack of agitation, positive emotions, and absence of loneliness).[27] In the next section, we shall present more specific illustrations of resilience in two areas of self and personality, namely self-definition and personal life investment in old age.

Two illustrations of resilience in old age

Old people, particularly the very old, experience losses more frequently than younger people. Most old people are excluded from productive employment, and experience a decline in physical capacity and health.[28] Old people are also likely to lose same-aged acquaintances, friends, or social partners, i.e. their social network and support patterns change.[24] However, most old people do not feel depressed or dissatisfied. Indeed, they are at least as happy and satisfied with their lives as their young and middle-aged counterparts.[29] The maintenance of subjective well being in the face of loss and decline has been called a paradox.[5,10] The capacity for recovery and maintenance of the status quo in response to stressful events or adverse conditions has been called resilience.[30] Psychological resilience is a concept originally used in research on childhood and adolescence but more recently has been applied to adults.[5,31] What are the processes that help older people to maintain a sense of well being when confronted with stressful events?

Increasing health-related problems are one cause of the constraints and losses of old age.[22,28,32] A moderate association between physical symptoms and subjective well being has been found in numerous cross-sectional studies. In one of the few longitudinal studies investigating the relationship between objective health and subjective well being, Feist *et al.*[33], found that health predicts subjective well being. In general, however, the association between objective measures of health (e.g. number of medical diagnoses) and subjective well being is rather low.[34,35] This is consistent with the general finding that subjective well being is more strongly associated with subjective perceptions and evaluations than with objective factors of a person's life circumstances.[29] Self and personality seem to moderate the relation between objective life circumstances and subjective well being. In very old age, however, high multimorbidity might expose the limits of such compensatory power.

In our own research,[36–39] we found that self-related characteristics contributed to resilience and buffered the negative effect of health-related impairment in old age. More specifically, we found that selectivity regarding personal life investment is adaptive when resources (e.g. energy) are limited by health-related losses. Also, a multifaceted self-definition helps to prevent depression in the face of health-related risks.

Self-definition

Self-definition, i.e. what a person considers central to who he or she is, organizes and structures experience, guides behaviour, provides orientation for interaction with the environment, and offers a sense of identity.[40] To fulfil this function, self-definition must have some degree of temporal stability. Without continuity the person's sense of identity would be threatened.[41]

Because of the losses in various domains of functioning in old age,[22] the maintenance of self-definition may be particularly at risk in this age group.[10] For instance, constraints in mobility might prohibit sports activities that are important for self-definition. In late adulthood, the number of self-defining domains declines with increasing age because of health-related constraints.[36]

According to the SOC model, an older person's self-definition should be better maintained if it comprises a variety of domains of functioning. A self-definition that consists of different domains provides a back-up supply of self-defining domains that can help to compensate the loss of one.[36,42] Consistent with this hypothesis, a multifaceted self-definition contributes to resilience against depression when faced with health-related risks.[39] However, it does not provide positive emotional well being in such situations.[36] This suggests that there may be limitations to resilience in very old age. In a situation of a wide-ranging limitation of resources, it may be more adaptive to disengage from self-relevant domains or goals that are subject to loss. When resources are so diminished, a multifaceted self-definition may overwhelm rather than stabilize the person. If this happens, it may be more adaptive to abandon those domains of functioning that are not of central importance for the self-definition. This interpretation is supported by findings from the area of personal life investment.

Personal life investment

Personal life investment is one facet of the goal system. It refers to the amount of thought and effort people report in investing in life domains such as family, work, leisure, or health.[37,38,]

The content and priorities of personal life investments are not arbitrary. They are embedded in subjective conceptions of the life course, and also reflect the changing developmental tasks and themes of life. Across the adult lifespan people report most investment (in terms of time and effort) in domains that reflect the developmental tasks and themes of their particular life period.[43] From 25 to 35 years, work, friends, family, and independence are ranked highest in personal investment. From 35 to 45 years, family, work, friends, and cognitive fitness figure centrally. From 55 to 65, the top four ranks of personal life investment are occupied by family, health, friends, and cognitive fitness. For 70- to 85-year-olds, the only change is that friends and cognitive fitness reverse position. Finally, in very old age (85 to 105), health becomes the most important investment theme, followed by family, thinking about life, and cognitive fitness. Towards the end of life (70–105 years) the overall amount of psychological energy that people invest in central domains of life decreases slightly, but much less than biological markers of vitality would suggest[37]

Teleological theories of well being have claimed, and empirical evidence has demonstrated, that both involvement in the pursuit and selection of goals contribute to subjective well being.[44] The relationship between life investment ratings in central life domains, such as work, health, or family, and indicators of subjective well being is rather weak as investment in such domains seems to be a necessity of life and does not differentiate between people.[37] However, when such necessities of life cannot be taken for granted or become threatened, the protective power of personal life investment emerges. For example, in bad health, reduced levels of overall life investment (averaged across 10 domains) and selective increase in investment in health is related to higher levels of well being both cross-sectionally[38] and longitudinally.[39]

This result is consistent with the SOC model,[12,13] which predicts that the selection of goals on which to focus time and energy becomes particularly important for successful life-mastery when resources are limited. Focusing on a small set of the most important goals when confronted with bad health appears to have an adaptive value.

Limits of resilience: the 'fourth age'

The two illustrations of resilience outlined above lead to two important conclusions: throughout adulthood, people possess resources that allow them to master constraints and losses successfully; advanced old age—the 'fourth age'[3]—might be a period when people are more likely to experience the limits of resilience. The three conditions outlined at the beginning of the chapter (decreased biological functioning, less cultural support, and decreased efficiency of cultural support) may together have a cumulative effect that seriously challenges the resilience of very old people by depleting their (internal and external) resources.[45]

As many of the processes contributing to resilience draw on resources (e.g. energy), the depletion of internal or external resources can reach a point at which efforts relevant to resilience are themselves restricted. When losses occur in a variety of domains, means that can be invested into selection, optimization, and compensation are scarce. In a sample of old and very old people aged 70 to 103, it was found that self-reported selection-, optimization-, and compensation-related behaviours declined with increasing age.[27] The engagement in selection, optimization, and compensation might have exceeded the elderly person's resources.

Reaching the limits of resilience in advanced old age might also have important implications for mental health. The relatively high frequency of depression and dementia in advanced old age[46] may reflect such a breakdown associated with the depletion of internal and external resources. For instance, whereas it is possible to compensate for the losses in the early phases of Alzheimer's disease (e.g. through social support or the use of memory aids), compensatory means lose their efficiency with the progression of the disease. Cognitive training research provides some evidence for this decreasing efficiency and eventual breakdown of compensation.[47]

The 'fourth age' poses challenges for science and society. We do not yet possess enough knowledge about the various processes contributing to resilience in old age. Moreover, society is not yet sufficiently supportive of the particular needs in very old age. More work will have to be done in both areas to make the 'fourth age' a time of life that people look forward to.

References

1. Baltes, P.B., Lindenberger, U., and Staudinger, U.M. (1998). Life-span theory in developmental psychology. In *Handbook of child psychology*, Vol. 1, *Theoretical models of human development* (ed. R.M. Lerner), pp. 1029–143. Wiley, New York.

2. Baltes, P.B., Reese, H.W., and Lipsitt, L.P. (1980). Life-span developmental psychology. *Annual Review of Psychology*, **31**, 65–110.

3. Baltes, P.B. (1997). On the incomplete architecture of human ontogeny. Selection, optimization, and compensation as foundation of developmental theory. *American Psychologist*, **52**, 366–80.

4. Lerner, R.M. (1986). *Concepts and theories of human development* (2nd edn). Random House, New York.

5. Staudinger, U.M., Marsiske, M., and Baltes, P.B. (1995). Resilience and reserve capacity in later adulthood: potentials and limits of development across the life-span. In *Developmental psychopathology*, Vol. 2, *Risk, disorder, and adaptation* (ed. D. Cicchetti and D. Cohen), pp. 801–47. Wiley, New York.

6. Lerner, R.M. and Busch-Rossnagel, N.A. (1981). Individuals as producers of their development: conceptual and empirical bases. In *Individuals as producers of their development: a life-span perspective* (ed. R.M. Lerner and N.A. Busch-Rossnagel), pp. 1–36. Academic Press, New York.

7. Neugarten, B.L., Moore, J.W., and Lowe, J.C. (1965). Age norms, age constraints, and adult socialization. *American Journal of Sociology*, **70**, 710–17.

8. Riley, M.W. (1987). On the significance of age in sociology. *American Sociological Review*, **52**, 1–14.

9. Atchley, R.C. (1982). The aging self. *Psychological Theory, Research, and Practice*, **19**, 338–96.

10. Brandtstädter, J. and Greve, W. (1994). The aging self: stabilizing and protective processes. *Developmental Review*, **14**, 52–80.

11. Heckhausen, J. and Schulz, R. (1995). A life-span theory of control. *Psychological Review*, **102**, 284–304.

12. Baltes, P.B. and Baltes, M.M. (1990). Psychological perspectives on successful aging: the model of selective optimization with compensation. In *Successful aging: perspectives from the behavioral sciences* (ed. P.B. Baltes and M.M. Baltes), pp. 1–34. Cambridge University Press, New York.

13. Freund, A.M. and Baltes, P.B. (in press). The orchestration of selection, optimization, and compensation: an action-theoretical conceptualization of a theory of developmental regulation. In *Control of human behavior, mental processes, and consciousness* (ed. W.J. Perrig and A. Grob). Erlbaum, Mahwah, NJ.

14. Marsiske, M., Lang, F.R., Baltes, M.M., and Baltes, P.B. (1995). Selective optimization with compensation: life-span perspectives on successful human development. In *Compensation for psychological defects and declines: managing losses and promoting gains* (ed. R.A. Dixon and L. Bäckman), pp. 35–79. Erlbaum, Hillsdale, NJ.

15. Gollwitzer, P.M. (1996). The volitional benefits of planning. In *The psychology of action* (ed. P.M. Gollwitzer and J.A. Bargh), pp. 287–312. Guilford Press, New York.

16. Ericsson, K.A. (1996). *The road to excellence: the acquisition of expert performance in the arts and sciences, sports, and games.* Erlbaum, Mahwah, NJ.

17. Mischel, W. (1996). From good intentions to willpower. In *The psychology of action* (ed. P.M. Gollwitzer and J.A. Bargh), pp. 197–218. Guilford Press, New York.

18. Bandura, A. (1977). Self-efficacy: toward a unifying theory of behavioral change. *Psychological Review*, **84**, 191–215.

19. Skinner, E.A., Chapman, M., and Baltes, P.B. (1988). Children's beliefs about control, means–ends, and agency: developmental differences during middle childhood. *International Journal of Behavioral Development*, **11**, 369–88.

20. Carstensen, L.L., Hanson, K.A., and Freund, A.M. (1995). Selection and compensation in adulthood. In *Compensating for psychological deficits and declines: managing losses and promoting gains* (ed. R.A. Dixon and L. Bäckman), pp. 107–26. Erlbaum, Hillsdale, NJ.

21. Dixon, R.A. and Bäckman, L. (ed.) (1995). *Psychological compensation: managing losses and promoting gains.* Erlbaum, Hillsdale, NJ.

22. Manton, K.G., Stallard, E., and Corder, L. (1995). Changes in morbidity and chronic disability in the U.S. elderly population: evidence from the 1982, 1984, and 1989 National Long Term Care Surveys. *Journal of Gerontology*, **50B**, S194–204.

23. Marsiske, M., Delius, J., Maas, I., Lindenberger, U., Scherer, H., and Tesch-Römer, C. (1999). Sensory systems in old age. In *The Berlin Aging Study: aging from 70 to 100* (ed. P.B. Baltes and K.U. Mayer), pp. 360–83. Cambridge University Press, New York.

24. Lang, F.R. and Carstensen, L.L. (1998). Social relationships and adaptation in late life. In *Comprehensive clinical psychology*, Vol. 7 (ed. A.S. Bellack and M. Hersen M), pp. 55–72. Pergamon Press, Oxford.

25. Lindenberger, U., Mayr, U., and Kliegl, R. (1993). Speed and intelligence in old age. *Psychology and Aging*, **8**, 207–20.

26. Wiese, B.S., Freund, A.M., and Baltes, P.B. (1999). Selection, optimization, and compensation in day-to-day life: consequences for general, work-related, and partnership-related well-being. Unpublished report, Max Planck Institute for Human Development, Berlin.

27. Freund, A.M. and Baltes, P.B. (1998). Selection, optimization, and compensation as strategies of life-management: correlations with subjective indicators of successful aging. *Psychology and Aging*, **13**, 531–43.

28. Steinhagen-Thiessen, E. and Borchelt, M. (1999). Morbidity, medication, and functional limitations in very old age. In *The Berlin Aging Study: aging from 70 to 100* (ed. P.B. Baltes and K.U. Mayer), pp. 131–66. Cambridge University Press, New York.

29. Diener, E. and Suh, E. (1998). Subjective well-being and age: an international analysis. *Annual Review of Gerontology and Geriatrics*, **17**, 304–24.

30. Rutter, M. (1987). Resilience in the face of adversity: protective factors and resistance to psychiatric disorder. *British Journal of Psychiatry*, **147**, 598–611.

31. Ryff, C.D., Singer, B., Love, G.D., and Essex, M.J. (1998). Resilience in adulthood and later life. In *Handbook of aging and mental health: an integrative approach* (ed. J. Lomranz), pp. 69–96. Plenum Press, New York.

32. Baltes, M.M., Maas, I., Wilms, H.-U., Borchelt, M., and Little, T.D. (1999). Everyday competence in old and very old age: theoretical considerations and empirical findings. In *The Berlin Aging Study: aging from 70 to 100* (ed. P.B. Baltes and K.U. Mayer), pp. 384–402. Cambridge University Press, New York.

33. Feist, G.J., Bodner, T.E., Jacobs, J.F., Miles, M., and Tan, V. (1995). Integrating top-down and bottom-up structural models of subjective well-being: a longitudinal investigation. *Journal of Personality and Social Psychology*, **68**, 138–50.

34. Smith, J., Fleeson, W., Geiselmann, B., Settersten, R.A. Jr, and Kunzmann, U. (1999). Well-being in very old age: predictions from objective life conditions and subjective experience. In *The Berlin Aging Study: aging from 70 to 100* (ed. P.B. Baltes and K.U. Mayer), pp. 450–71. Cambridge University Press, New York.

35. Watson, D. and Pennebaker, J.W. (1989). Health complaints, stress, and distress: exploring the central role of negative affectivity. *Psychological Review*, **96**, 234–54.

36. Freund, A.M. and Smith, J. (1999). Content and function of self-definition in old and very old age. *Journals of Gerontology: Psychological Science*, **54**, P55–67.

37. Staudinger, U.M., Freund, A., Linden, M., and Maas, I. (1999). Self, personality, and life regulation: facets of psychological resilience in old age. In *The Berlin Aging Study: aging from 70 to 100* (ed. P.B. Baltes and K.U. Mayer), pp. 302–428. Cambridge University Press, New York.

38. Staudinger, U.M. and Fleeson, W. (1996). Self and personality in old and very old age: a sample case of resilience? *Development and Psychopathology*, **8**, 867–85.

39. Staudinger, U.M. and Freund, A.M. (1998). Krank und arm intramuscular hohen Alter und trotzdem guten Mutes? *Zeitschrift für Klinische Psychologie*, **27**, 78–85.

40. Swann, W.B., Jr (1990). To be adored or to be known; The interplay of self-enhancement and self-verification. In *Motivation and cognition*, Vol. 2 (ed. R.M. Sorrentino and E.T. Higgins), pp. 408–48. Erlbaum, Hillsdale, NJ.

41. Epstein, S. (1973). The self-concept revisited. Or a theory of a theory. *American Psychologist*, **28**, 404–16.

42. Rosenberg, S. and Gara, M.A. (1985). The multiplicity of personal identity. In *Review of personality and social psychology*, Vol. 6 (ed. P. Shaver), pp. 87–113. Sage, Beverly Hills, CA.

43. Staudinger, U.M. (1996). Psychologische Produktivität und Selbstentfaltung intramuscular Alter. In *Produktivität und Altern* (ed. M.M. Baltes and L. Montada), pp. 344–73. Campus Verlag, Frankfurt.

44. Emmons, R.A. (1996). Striving and feeling: personal goals and subjective well-being. In *The psychology of action: linking cognition and motivation to behavior* (ed. P.M. Gollwitzer and J.A. Bargh), pp. 313–37. Guilford Press, New York.

45. Baltes, P.B. and Smith, J. (1998). Multilevel and systemic analyses of old age: theoretical and empirical evidence for a fourth age. In *Handbook of theories of aging* (ed. V.L. Bengtson and K.W. Schaie), pp. 153–73. Springer, New York.

46. Helmchen, H., Baltes, M.M., Geiselmann, B. *et al.* (1999). Psychiatric illnesses in old age. In *The Berlin Aging Study: aging from 70 to 100* (ed. P.B. Baltes and K.U. Mayer), pp. 167–96. Cambridge University Press, New York.

47. Baltes, M.M., Kühl, K.-P., and Sowarka, D. (1992). Testing the limits of cognitive reserve capacity: a promising strategy for early diagnosis of dementia? *Journal of Gerontology: Psychological Sciences*, **47**, 165–67.

2.5.2 **Memory and memory disorders**

Barbara A. Wilson

Introduction

A young man with head injuries described his memory functioning in the following words: 'My memory is like a tape on a tape recorder with large chunks erased or of poor quality'. Like this young man, people often talk about memory as though it were one particular skill or single function. We might hear someone say, 'He has a photographic memory' or 'My memory is dreadful'. In fact, memory comprises a number of subskills, subsystems, or subfunctions working together. The number of these subdivisions, and their roles, depend on the model or classification system used to interpret or explain memory functioning. One influential model proposed by Baddeley and Hitch[1] subdivides memory into three main categories depending on the

length of time information is stored. We can also divide memory into a number of systems for remembering different types of information that can be labelled as semantic, episodic, or procedural. Yet another way to conceptualize memory is by considering the different stages involved in remembering: namely encoding, storing, and retrieving. Other ways of regarding memory include subdividing the kinds of remembering required into recall or recognition; or by demonstrating that something has been remembered in terms of whether it is explicit or implicit; or, in the case of lost memories, whether they date from before or after a neuropsychological insult, that is whether there is retrograde or anterograde amnesia. We shall consider all these subsystems and categories in more detail in this chapter.

Although dementia is probably the biggest cause of organic memory impairment, memory problems are common after many other neurological insults including traumatic head injury, encephalitis, vascular disorders, chronic alcohol abuse, temporal lobe epilepsy, cerebral tumour, and anoxia. Whatever the cause, memory-impaired people tend to share certain characteristics in that they do not lose personal identity, their immediate memory functioning is normal or nearly normal, they have problems remembering after a delay or distraction, they have difficulty learning new information, they usually recall things that happened some time before the insult better than things that happened a short time before, and they typically do not forget how to do things they learned well before the insult such as reading, swimming, or riding a bicycle. Of course, there are exceptions to this general pattern particularly with certain syndromes such as semantic dementia. We shall discuss typical amnesic patients together with some of the less common memory disorders as this chapter progresses.

Although few people working in memory rehabilitation would claim to be able to restore memory functioning in someone whose problems result from an organic cause, there is nevertheless a considerable amount that can be done to help memory-impaired people and their families or carers. We can organize the environment to make it easier for people to cope without adequate memory functioning; we can help memory-impaired people to learn more efficiently; we can teach them to compensate for their impairments; and we can reduce the anxiety or other emotional sequelae resulting from impaired cognition. Again, these rehabilitative approaches will be discussed more fully later in this chapter.

Ways of understanding memory

Length of storage

The working memory model of Baddeley and Hitch[1] subdivides memory into three main types depending both on time-based and conceptual differences. The first system, **sensory memory**, is a brief and rather literal trace that results from a visual, auditory, or other sensory event, probably lasting no longer than a quarter of a second. This is the system we use to make sense of moving pictures (visual sensory memory) or language (auditory sensory memory). Most people with damage to this system would present with perceptual or language disorders and we would not normally think of them as having memory problems.

The second system, **working memory**, is considered to have two main components or functions. The first of these is short-term or immediate memory, which lasts for several seconds. This period of time can be extended to several minutes if the person is rehearsing or concentrating on the particular information. Unlike sensory memory, information in working memory has already undergone substantial cognitive analysis, so it is typically represented in meaningful chunks such as words or numbers. We use this system when looking up a new telephone number and holding on to it long enough to dial.

The second component of working memory is a central executive that can be conceived of as an organizer, controller, or allocator of resources. This component enables us to both drive a car and talk to our passenger at the same time. Sufficient resources are allocated to each of these tasks, and if a demanding or unusual situation occurs on the road we stop talking while all our resources are required to deal with the unexpected situation.

The third system in the Baddeley and Hitch model[1] is **long-term memory**, which encodes information in a reasonably robust form and can last for decades. Although there are differences in memory for things that happened 10 minutes ago and things that happened 10 years ago, the differences are less clear-cut than those between sensory (quarter of a second) and immediate (a few seconds) memory systems. Nevertheless, because long-term memory means different things to different people, the following terms can be used to reduce ambiguity:

1. Delayed memory refers to memory for information presented in the last few minutes.

2. Recent memory refers to knowledge accumulated in the last few days or weeks.

3. Remote memory refers to knowledge accumulated over several years.

All the systems described so far are connected with retrospective memory, that is remembering information or events that have already occurred. Frequently, however, we want to remember to do something in the future, such as take our medicine, water the plants, or make a telephone call. The system activated for remembering to do something is known as prospective memory. It is significant that many of the complaints of memory-impaired people refer to failures in prospective memory.

Type of information to be remembered

In 1972 Tulving[2] produced an influential paper distinguishing two types of memory: semantic and episodic. Semantic memory is memory for our knowledge about the world, for example remembering that Dublin is the capital of Eire, or that a fox has a bushy tail. Semantic memory is also concerned with our knowledge of social customs, the meanings of words, the colours and textures of objects, and how things smell. Most memory-impaired patients do not forget this kind of information, although they may have difficulty adding to their store of semantic knowledge. Amnesic patients are often unable, for example, to learn new words that enter the vocabulary after their neurological insult. Thus CW, an ex-patient of mine, cannot understand the terms 'AIDS' or 'e-mail', or 'mad cow disease', all of which came into widespread usage after 1985 when CW developed herpes simplex encephalitis.

Episodic memory, on the other hand, represents what most of us would think of as memory, in that it refers to a specific episode that has been experienced and can be recalled. Thus remembering what you ate for dinner last night, when you last phoned your mother, or what you read a few minutes ago are all examples of episodic memory. This system is frequently damaged in people with organic memory impairment and episodic memory deficits are perhaps the most noticeable characteristic of the amnesic syndrome.

A third system that operates differently from either semantic or episodic memory is procedural memory, the system used for learning skills such as riding a bicycle or learning to type. People get better with practice and can demonstrate the skill even though they may not remember how they learned to ride a bicycle or type. JC, a young amnesic patient of mine, successfully learned to type even though he had no conscious recollection of learning. In his words, 'Practical skills developed without me being aware of how this came about. I could do things without being able to explain how.' Procedural memory is typically normal or nearly normal in amnesic patients.

The stages involved in remembering

Typically there are three stages involved in remembering: encoding, storage, and retrieval. Encoding refers to the registration stage or getting the information into memory. Storage refers to the maintenance of information in the memory store, and retrieval refers to the stage of extracting or recalling the information when it is required. After a neurological insult to the brain each of these stages can be affected.

The following are some suggestions for improving encoding, storage, and retrieval:

1. Simplify the information you give to a memory-impaired person.

2. Reduce the amount of information supplied at any one time.

3. Ensure that there is minimal distraction.

4. Make sure the information is understood—by asking the person to repeat it in his/her own words.

5. Encourage the person to link or associate information with material that is already known.

6. Try to ensure processing at a deeper level—by encouraging the person to ask questions.

7. Use the 'little and often' rule.

8. Make sure learning occurs in different contexts to avoid context specificity and enhance generalization.

Recall and recognition

Recall and recognition are two of the main ways we remember information. Recall involves actively finding the information to be remembered. If I asked someone to summarize what they had read in this chapter so far they would demonstrate this by recalling the information. In some situations, however, we do not need to recall the information but to recognize it. Most of us at some time have been unable to tell someone how to find a particular street but can nevertheless take ourselves there with no trouble. We recognize which turns to make and when but cannot actively recall the route. Most memory-impaired people find recall harder than recognition, although both systems are usually affected. Some people might have difficulty with both verbal and visual information, while others might have problems in only one of these modalities.

Explicit and implicit memory

In many situations we need to consciously recall information we have received. For example, if I asked someone where they went for their summer holidays last year, and they could tell me, they would be using explicit memory as they could consciously recall the information wanted. If, on the other hand, I asked someone when and where they learned to ride a bicycle, and the steps by which they gained expertise, they would probably find this difficult. They might demonstrate how to ride a bicycle without much trouble, that is they would have implicit memory of this skill, they would remember how to do it even if they were unable to explain it with any great ease or remember when and how they learned the skill. Like procedural memory, implicit memory is usually intact or relatively intact in people with organic memory impairment.

Retrograde and anterograde memory

One of the questions frequently asked by relatives of memory-impaired people is, 'Why can she/he remember what happened several years ago but not what happened yesterday?' The short answer is that old memories are stored differently in the brain from new memories. Although information acquired before a neurological insult may be forgotten, this is usually for a specific time period—ranging from a few minutes for some head-injured people to several decades for some people with Korsakoff's syndrome or herpes simplex viral encephalitis. Memory loss dating from before the insult is known as **retrograde amnesia**. This form of amnesia is usually less of a problem and less handicapping for the memory-impaired person than **anterograde amnesia**, which refers to memory difficulties dating from the time of the neurological insult (although see Kapur[3] for a review of retrograde amnesia).

Conditions that give rise to memory problems, and typical presentations

A variety of brain pathologies can give rise to severe memory impairment, the most common being the following:

(1) degenerative disorders (particularly Alzheimer's disease and Huntington's disease);

(2) chronic alcohol abuse giving rise to Korsakoff's syndrome;

(3) traumatic head injury;

(4) temporal lobe surgery;

(5) encephalitis;

(6) cerebral vascular disorders (including subarachnoid haemorrhage resulting from ruptured aneurysms);

(7) anoxic brain damage (following, for example, myocardial infarction, carbon monoxide poisoning, or respiratory arrest);

(8) cerebral tumours.

These conditions are described in the chapters in Section 4.1 of this book and in more detail in a number of publications: Kapur[4] and Lishman[5] both provide good accounts of all these pathologies as well as less common ones.

Clients referred to rehabilitation centres for memory-therapy rehabilitation are most likely to have sustained a severe traumatic head injury, a cerebral vascular accident (**CVA**), herpes simplex encephalitis, or anoxic brain damage. It should also be remembered that these conditions are not mutually exclusive. I once saw a man who had a CVA while driving, thus sustaining some brain damage from the stroke; he then crashed his car because of the CVA and sustained further brain damage from a head injury caused by the crash; following this he stopped breathing for a while and appeared to sustain further damage from the anoxia; then on top of everything else a haematoma developed and the man required surgery to remove the blood clot. Thus he sustained damage from four separate causes. He went on to respond reasonably well to rehabilitation and, although never able to return to work as a university lecturer, he became a secretary of his local Headway Group (The National Head Injuries Association).

Whatever the cause of the organic memory impairment, certain characteristics tend to be seen in survivors. People with a classic amnesic syndrome show an anterograde amnesia, that is they have great difficulty learning and remembering most kinds of new information. Immediate memory, however, is normal when this is assessed by forward digit span or the recency effect in free recall. There is usually a period of retrograde amnesia. This gap or period of retrograde amnesia is very variable in length and may range from a few minutes to decades. Previously acquired semantic knowledge and implicit memory (remembering without awareness or conscious recollection) are typically intact in amnesic subjects. Other cognitive skills, apart from memory, are normal or nearly normal. As the majority of patients with severe memory disorders present with additional cognitive problems such as attention deficits, word-finding problems, or slowed information processing, those with a classic amnesic syndrome are relatively rare.

Nevertheless, people with a 'pure' amnesic syndrome and people with more widespread cognitive deficits tend to share certain characteristics. In both cases immediate memory is reasonably normal; there is difficulty remembering after a delay or distraction; new learning is difficult, and there is a tendency to remember things that happened a long time before the accident or illness better than things that happened a short time before. People with organic amnesia never seem to lose memory for personal identity, unlike those with a functional amnesia following, say, an emotional trauma. Despite the rather exaggerated interest in functional amnesia by the media, organic amnesia is far more commonly encountered in clinical practice. In some cases it is not easy to distinguish between the two, and indeed some people have memory problems resulting from both brain injury and from an overlying or functional memory disorder, possibly caused by a need for sympathy or some other secondary gain. Kopelman[6] believes there is a continuum between totally organic amnesia and totally functional problems rather than two orthogonal dimensions.

Less common manifestations of memory disorders

Despite the typical picture of organic memory impairment described above, other manifestations are possible and are encountered every now and again. Returning for a moment to the working memory model of Baddeley and Hitch[1] referred to earlier, one can find patients with deficits in the short-term or immediate (that is to say a few seconds) memory system. Baddeley and Hitch subdivide this system into several 'slave' systems that aid the central executive in its role as co-ordinator of temporary storage systems. Two of these slave systems have been studied in detail. One is the phonological loop that utilizes subvocal speech and is involved in many short-term verbal memory tasks. The second system is the visuospatial sketchpad—a temporary system used in creating and manipulating visual images. Patients with phonological loop or verbal short-term memory difficulties have been reported,[7] and visuospatial sketchpad or visual short-term memory deficits have also been reported.[8] Wilson et al.[9] describe a sculptress with an autoimmune disorder, systemic lupus erythematosus, that caused her to have an impaired visual short-term memory (**VSTM**) together with image generation problems. This dramatically affected her sculpting style; prior to the episode causing the VSTM difficulties she produced sculptures that were full of detail, while afterwards the sculptures were abstract and completely lacking in detail. Her style changed because she could not hold images in her mind to see where the details should go. If she tried looking in a mirror or using a model she 'lost' the visual memory in the brief period between looking at the model and looking at the material with which she was working.

Patients with semantic memory impairments are another group of people who show yet another different pattern of characteristics. Semantic memory is the system we use to store knowledge about the world. Not only knowledge such as the meaning of the word 'happy' or the name of the world's largest ocean, but knowledge about what things look like, sound like, smell like, or feel like and knowledge about social customs such as when to shake hands. Damage to the semantic memory store (or impaired access to this store) may be caused by brain injury. Warrington,[10] for example, suggests that visual object agnosia (the failure to recognize objects despite adequate eyesight, language, and naming) is due to a deficit of the visual semantic memory system. Furthermore, Warrington and Shallice[11] demonstrated that there are category-specific deficits so that some patients lose the ability to recognize living things but are still able to recognize non-living things. Hillis and Caramazza[12] describe the reverse, that is subjects who show greater knowledge of living things than of manufactured objects. Patients with semantic memory deficits are likely to have problems recognizing objects in the real world, problems expressing themselves, and may be considered intellectually disabled because of the errors they make.

In recent years there has been considerable interest in the syndrome known as semantic dementia, a term coined by Snowden et al.,[13] and studied in some detail by Hodges and Patterson.[14] The essential characteristics of semantic dementia are as follows:

(1) selective impairment of semantic memory causing severe anomia, impaired single-word comprehension (both spoken and written), reduced generation of exemplars on category-fluency tests, and an impoverished fund of general knowledge;

(2) relative sparing of other components of speech production, notably syntax and phonology;

(3) unimpaired perceptual skills and non-verbal problem-solving abilities;

(4) relatively well-preserved episodic memory.

Patients with semantic dementia show a progressive deterioration of the semantic memory store associated with damage to the temporal neocortex. However, semantic memory impairments may also be seen in patients with non-progressive conditions. Wilson[15] describes four patients, two of whom had sustained a severe head injury and two with herpes simplex viral encephalitis (**HSVE**). In many ways Wilson's patients were similar to those reported by Hodges and Patterson,[14] although younger and with more serious episodic memory deficits (particularly the two patients with HSVE).

In this section we have looked at a few of the more atypical memory disorders. For those readers interested in retrograde without anterograde amnesia see Kapur,[3] and for those wanting to know how post-traumatic amnesia differs from the amnesic syndrome and from chronic memory impairment see Wilson et al.[16]

Management and remediation of memory difficulties

Although there is no known cure for memory impairment there are a number of ways we can help memory-impaired people and their families or carers. The main methods are: environmental adaptations, improving learning, compensating for memory problems, and managing anxiety or other emotional sequelae resulting from impaired cognition.

Environmental adaptations

One of the simplest ways to help people with memory impairment is to arrange the environment so that they rely less on memory. Examples include using written labels or drawings for cupboards in the kitchen or bedroom as reminders of where things are kept; positioning objects so that they cannot be missed or forgotten (for instance tying a front-door key to a belt); or painting the toilet door a distinctive colour so that it is easier to find. Sometimes changing the wording of our questions or comments can reduce problems. For example, CW, a former musician, became very densely amnesic following encephalitis. He frequently thinks he has just woken up and says, 'This is the first time I've been awake. I don't remember you coming into this room but now I'm awake' (or words to that effect). Sympathizing with him, or offering explanations, seems to increase his agitation and causes escalation of the number of repetitions he makes about awakening. One partial solution is to distract him by introducing another topic of conversation or asking him a question about music. Such a ploy can also be viewed as an environmental adaptation, although in this case it is the verbal rather than the physical environment that is being modified.

For people with severe intellectual deficits, or progressive deterioration, or extremely dense amnesia, environmental adaptations may be the best we can offer to enable them and their families or carers to cope, and to reduce some of the frustration and confusion associated with their conditions.

Improving learning in memory-impaired people

One of the greatest handicaps for memory-impaired people is their inability to learn new information. In recent years a number of studies have been carried out to investigate errorless learning in memory rehabilitation. Errorless learning is a teaching strategy whereby people are prevented, as far as possible, from making mistakes while they are learning a new skill or acquiring new information. Instead of teaching by demonstration, which may involve the learner in trial and error, the experimenter or teacher presents the correct information or procedure in ways that minimize the possibility of erroneous responses.

There are two theoretical backgrounds influencing errorless learning work with cognitively impaired people. The first is errorless discrimination learning from behavioural psychology, first developed by Terrace[17] in his work with pigeons, and later used with mentally retarded (learning disabled) people.[18] The second influence is from studies of implicit learning in amnesic subjects,[19] showing that people with amnesia can learn some information normally although they may have no conscious recollection (explicit recall) that they have previously engaged in the task.

Building on these two strands of research we posed the question, 'Do amnesic subjects learn better when prevented from making errors during the learning process?' In one group study and several single-case studies[20] it was demonstrated that people with severe memory disorders learn more successfully with an errorless learning strategy. Others have adapted this strategy with non-progressive amnesic patients,[21] and recently we have used errorless learning procedures with patients who have Alzheimer's disease.[22] All patients benefited to a greater or lesser degree and were able to learn some useful everyday information.

Compensating for memory loss

Much of the work in memory rehabilitation involves teaching people to compensate for their impairments by employing aids such as diaries, tape recorders, organizers, computers, and other similar items. These external memory aids are probably the most useful devices for helping memory-impaired people and they are likely to be used more by them in the long run.[23] Despite their value, it is not always easy to persuade patients to use compensatory strategies. Some feel it is cheating and believe they should not rely on such aids, others feel such devices will reduce their chances of natural recovery occurring, and others simply forget to use them or may use them in a disorganized manner. After all, remembering to use a compensation is in itself a memory task. Despite these difficulties, some memory-impaired people use compensatory aids and strategies very efficiently. Kime *et al.*[24] describe a young amnesic woman who was able to get back to paid employment once she had been taught to use a comprehensive system of external aids. Wilson *et al.*[25] describe the 10-year natural history of a compensatory memory system devised by a young man who became amnesic following the rupture of a posterior cerebral artery aneurysm. Using results from a long-term follow-up study, Wilson and Watson[23] made some predictions as to which people are more likely to use compensatory aids effectively and which are not. Age, absence of additional cognitive deficits, and scoring above floor level on a test of everyday memory were all predictors of independence and the use of aids.

Other work looking at how to help memory-impaired people compensate involves the use or modification of new technology.[26] One fairly recent development that appears to help people with a wide range of conditions and degrees of memory impairment is Neuro-Page®,[27] which is a simple and portable paging system with a screen that can be attached to a belt. It utilizes an arrangement of microcomputers linked to a conventional computer memory and, by telephone, to a paging company to produce a programmable messaging system. The scheduling of reminders or cues for each individual is entered into the computer and from then on no further human inter-

facing is required. On the appropriate date and time NeuroPage® accesses the user's data files and transmits the appropriate information by modem to a terminal where the reminder is converted and transmitted to the receiver corresponding to the particular user. The reminder is graphically displayed on the screen of the receiver. NeuroPage® is easy to use and avoids many of the problems inherent in other external aids. It is highly portable, has an audible alarm that can be adapted to vibrate if required, together with an accompanying explanatory message, and, rather than being embarrassing to use, it conveys a certain amount of prestige. In a pilot study,[28] the average number of target behaviours achieved by 15 people during a 2- to 6-week baseline was 37 per cent. Once the pager was provided (for a 12-week period) the average number of targets achieved rose to over 85 per cent. Preliminary analysis of the first 38 clients in a larger study of 200 people, many of whom have very severe impairments, suggests similar (if less dramatic) results, ranging from 50 per cent of targets achieved in the baseline to 77 per cent in the treatment stage.

Managing anxiety and other emotional sequelae resulting from impaired cognition

Anxiety and depression are frequently seen in memory-impaired people. Kopelman and Crawford[29] found depression in over 40 per cent of 200 consecutive referrals to a memory clinic. Evans and Wilson[30] found anxiety to be common in attenders of a weekly memory group. Dealing with these emotional problems should be an integral part of memory rehabilitation. Obviously, listening, trying to understand, and providing information are key factors in encouraging families to cope with their difficulties. Wearing[31] provides a helpful reference on the problems faced by families of memory-impaired people, and makes suggestions as to what can be done to help. Providing information or explanations is one very simple and therapeutic strategy that can help reduce the fear and anxiety accompanying memory impairment. Written information is best, as most people, whether memory impaired or not, are unlikely to have good recall of information at times of stress. *Memory Problems After Head Injury*,[32] written for the National Head Injuries Association; *Managing Your Memory*,[33] and *Coping With Memory Problem*[34] are all useful publications to have available for patients and their relatives.

In addition to providing information, it may be necessary to offer therapy for anxiety and depression. Relaxation therapy can be helpful in reducing anxiety, even if memory problems are severe enough to prevent a participant from remembering the actual therapy sessions. Depression, too, may exacerbate difficulties in people with organic memory impairment. It is possible that cognitive behavioural therapy approaches such as those employed by Beck[35] might be appropriate for those with depression associated with organic memory impairment, although no studies appear to have been reported. Psychotherapy, on the other hand, is a well-established intervention for patients with neurological damage. Prigatano *et al.*[36] firmly believe in group and individual psychotherapy with brain-injured clients. Jackson and Gouvier[37] provide descriptions and guidelines for group psychotherapy with brain-injured adults and their families.

Other groups for memory-impaired people can be useful in reducing social isolation, which is also common in people with memory problems.[31] Wilson and Moffat[38] describe several kinds of groups for patients. Moffat[39] reports on a relatives' memory group for people with dementia, and Wearing[31] offers suggestions for setting up self-help groups. Evans and Wilson[30] point out the social value of memory groups as well as their effect in reducing anxiety.

Conclusions

This chapter has emphasized that memory should be regarded as a multifunctional cognitive system that can be understood in a number of ways. We can consider the length of time information is stored, the type of information being stored, the stages involved in remembering, whether information is recalled or recognized, or whether memories date from before or after neurological insult.

The chapter has described a number of conditions that can give rise to organic memory impairment, the most common of which are degenerative conditions, Korsakoff's syndrome, traumatic head injury, temporal lobe surgery, encephalitis, anoxic brain damage, and cerebral tumours.

Most memory-impaired people have difficulty in learning and remembering new information; they have a normal or nearly normal immediate memory span but have problems remembering after a delay or distraction, and they usually have a period of retrograde amnesia that may range from minutes to decades. Less common memory disorders include semantic memory impairment and immediate verbal or visuospatial deficits.

Although restoration of memory functioning is unlikely to occur in the majority of people whose memory impairments follow neurological insult, there is, nevertheless, much that can be done to reduce the impact of disabling and handicapping memory problems and foster understanding of the issues involved. These include environmental modifications that can enable very severely impaired people to cope in their daily lives despite the lack of adequate memory functioning, the employment of errorless learning principles to improve the learning ability of memory-impaired people, teaching how to use external memory aids to help compensate for memory difficulties, and dealing with emotional sequelae such as anxiety and depression, which are often associated with organic memory impairment.

References

1. Baddeley, A.D. and Hitch, G. (1974). Working memory. In *The psychology of learning and motivation*, Vol. 8 (ed. G.H. Bower), pp. 47–89. Academic Press, New York.
2. Tulving, E. (1972). Episodic and semantic memory. In *Organization of memory* (ed. E. Tulving and W. Donaldson), pp. 381–403. Academic Press, New York.
3. Kapur, N. (1993). Focal retrograde amnesia in neurological disease: a critical review. *Cortex*, **29**, 217–34.
4. Kapur, N. (1988). *Memory disorders in clinical practice*. Butterworths, London.
5. Lishman, W.A. (1998). *Organic psychiatry: the psychological consequences of cerebral disorder* (3rd edn). Blackwell Science, Oxford.
6. Kopelman, M.D. (1995). The assessment of psychogenic amnesia. In *Handbook of memory disorders* (ed. A.D. Baddeley, B.A. Wilson, and F.N. Watts), pp. 427–48. Wiley, Chichester.
7. Vallar, G. and Baddeley, A.D. (1984). Fractionation of working memory. Neuropsychological evidence for a phonological short-term store. *Journal of Verbal Learning and Verbal Behavior*, **23**, 151–61.
8. Farah, M.J. (1984). The neurological basis of mental imagery: a componential analysis. *Cognition*, **18**, 245–72.
9. Wilson, B.A., Baddeley, A.D., and Young, A.W. (1999). LE, a person who lost her 'mind's eye'. *Neurocase*, **5**, 119–27.
10. Warrington, E.K. (1975) The selective impairment of semantic memory. *Quarterly Journal of Experimental Psychology*, **27**, 635–57.
11. Warrington, E.K. and Shallice, T. (1984) Category specific semantic impairments. *Brain*, **107**, 829–54.
12. Hillis, A.E. and Caramazza, A. (1991). Category-specific naming and comprehension impairment: a double dissociation. *Brain*, **114**, 2081–94.
13. Snowden, J.S., Goulding, P.J., and Neary, D. (1989). Semantic dementia: a form of circumscribed cerebral atrophy. *Behavioural Neurology*, **2**, 167–82.
14. Hodges, J.R. and Patterson, K. (1997). Semantic memory disorders. *Trends in Cognitive Sciences*, **1**, 68–72.
15. Wilson, B.A. (1997). Semantic memory impairments following non-progressive brain damage: a study of four cases. *Brain Injury*, **11**, 259–69.
16. Wilson, B.A., Baddeley, A.D., Shiel, A., and Patton, G. (1992). How does post traumatic amnesia differ from the amnesic syndrome and from chronic memory impairment? *Neuropsychological Rehabilitation*, **2**, 231–43.
17. Terrace, H.S. (1963). Discrimination learning with and without 'errors'. *Journal of Experimental Analysis of Behavior*, **6**, 1–27.
18. Sidman, M. and Stoddard, L.T. (1967). The effectiveness of fading in programming simultaneous form discrimination for retarded children. *Journal of Experimental Analysis of Behavior*, **10**, 3–15.
19. Graf, P. and Schacter, D.L. (1985). Implicit and explicit memory for new associations in normal and amnesic subjects. *Journal of Experimental Psychology: Learning, Memory and Cognition*, **11**, 501–18.
20. Wilson, B.A., Baddeley, A.D., Evans, J.J., and Shiel, A. (1994). Errorless learning in the rehabilitation of memory impaired people. *Neuropsychological Rehabilitation*, **4**, 307–26.
21. Squires, E.J., Hunkin, N.M., and Parkin, A.J. (1997). Errorless learning of novel associations in amnesia. *Neuropsychologia*, **35**, 1103–37.
22. Clare, L., Wilson, B.A., Carter, G., Breen, E.K., Gosses, A., and Hodges, J.R. Intervening with memory problems in dementia of Alzheimer type: an errorless learning approach. *Journal of Clinical and Experimental Psychology*, in press.
23. Wilson, B.A. and Watson, P.C. (1996). A practical framework for understanding compensatory behaviour in people with organic memory impairment. *Memory*, **4**, 465–86.
24. Kime, S.K., Lamb, D.G., and Wilson, B.A. (1996). Use of a comprehensive program of external cuing to enhance procedural memory in a patient with dense amnesia. *Brain Injury*, **10**, 17–25.
25. Wilson, B.A., and Hughes, E. (1997). Coping with amnesia: the natural history of a compensatory memory system. *Neuropsychological Rehabilitation*, **7**, 43–56.
26. Kapur, N. (1995). Memory aids in the rehabilitation of memory disordered patients. In *Handbook of memory disorders* (ed. A.D. Baddeley, B.A. Wilson, and F.N. Watts), pp. 533–56. Wiley, Chichester.
27. Hersh, N. and Treadgold, L. (1994). NeuroPage: the rehabilitation of memory dysfunction by prosthetic memory and cueing. *NeuroRehabilitation*, **4**, 187–97.
28. Wilson, B.A., Evans, J.J., Emslie, H., and Malinek, V. (1997). Evaluation of NeuroPage: a new memory aid. *Journal of Neurology, Neurosurgery, and Psychiatry*, **63**, 113–15.
29. Kopelman, M. and Crawford, S. (1996). Not all memory clinics are dementia clinics. *Neuropsychological Rehabilitation*, **6**, 187–202.
30. Evans, J.J. and Wilson, B.A. (1992). A memory group for individuals with brain injury. *Clinical Rehabilitation*, **6**, 75–81.
31. Wearing, D. (1992). Self help groups. In *Clinical management of memory problems* (2nd edn) (ed. B.A. Wilson and N. Moffat), pp. 271–301. Chapman & Hall, London.
32. Wilson, B. A. (1989). *Memory problems after head injury*. National Head Injuries Association, Nottingham.
33. Kapur, N. (1991). *Managing your memory. A self help memory manual for improving everyday memory skills*. Available from the author at the

Wessex Neurological Centre, Southampton General Hospital, Southampton.

34. Clare, L. and Wilson, B.A. (1997). *Coping with memory problems: a practical guide for people with memory impairments, relatives, friends and carers.* Thames Valley Test Co., Bury St Edmunds.

35. Beck, A.T. (1976). *Cognitive therapy and emotional disorders.* International Universities Press, New York.

36. Prigatano, G.P., Fordyce, D.J., Zeiner, H.K., Roueche, J.R., Pepping, M., and Wood, B. C. (ed.) (1986). *Neuropsychological rehabilitation after brain injury.* Johns Hopkins University Press, Baltimore, MD.

37. Jackson, W.T. and Gouvier, W.D. (1992). Group psychotherapy with brain-damaged adults and their families. In *Handbook of head trauma: acute care to recovery* (ed. C.J. Long and L.K. Ross), pp. 309–27. Plenum Press, New York.

38. Wilson, B.A. and Moffat, N. (1992). The development of group memory therapy. In *Clinical management of memory problems* (2nd edn) (ed. B.A. Wilson and N. Moffat), pp. 243–73. Chapman & Hall, London.

39. Moffat, N. (1989). Home based cognitive rehabilitation with the elderly. In *Everyday cognition in adulthood and late life* (ed. L.W. Poon, D.C. Rubin, and B.A. Wilson), pp. 659–80. Cambridge University Press.

2.5.3 Contributions of psychology to the understanding of psychiatric disorders

Marcel van den Hout, Arnoud Arntz, and Harald Merckelbach

Introduction

The contribution of psychology to psychiatry dates back to the early days of experimental psychology. Indeed, Kraepelin performed his pioneering work on psychopharmacology in Wundt's laboratory,[1] and Jung studied the electrodermal reactions of schizophrenic patients during word associations tasks that he derived from the British associanist doctrine.[2] Since that time, the impact of psychology on psychiatry has steadily grown. A quick glance at the most influential journals in the field of psychiatry shows that many authors have their roots in experimental psychology.

Psychiatric problems are as numerous as the psychological contributions to their understanding, with contributions ranging from developmental psychology to psychopharmacology. It is not possible to cover even the essentials of the theoretical and empirical work that has been carried out in this field in this chapter. Therefore, rather than trying to summarize the theoretical or empirical contributions, we focus on three lines of research that we believe have been the most important contributions of psychology to psychiatry. The types of contributions that are addressed originate from biological psychology, from information processing frameworks, and from theories about schemas, beliefs, and intentions. The aim is to give a critical, yet balanced and non-technical, overview of the relative merits of these three approaches. In doing so, the emphasis will be on anxiety disorders and affective disorders. The justification for this is both epidemiological

and theoretical; anxiety and affective disorders are the most prevalent mental health problems in modern industrial societies, with lifetime prevalences of about 25 per cent for anxiety disorders and 20 per cent for affective disorders.[3] Accordingly, psychological analyses of these disorders have been extensive and have yielded results that are clinically relevant.

People try to make sense of their environment and the behaviour of fellow humans, and to the extent that this is successful, it allows for some prediction and control. When trying to understand how others behave in daily life, people tend to follow a rather specific explanatory strategy. Behaviour and emotional expressions are reduced to beliefs and intentions that are attributed to the person whose behaviour or emotions are to be explained. Consider a simple but straightforward example: if we want to explain why X is carrying an umbrella, this piece of behaviour is reduced to a combination of belief (it might rain) and intention (X does not want to become wet). This combination of belief and intention is thought to provide an adequate explanation. Thus knowledge about beliefs concerning the weather enables us to predict the behaviour of others and to change their behaviour by changing their beliefs.

Almost from its onset, academic psychology has been profoundly discontented with this type of 'intentional explanation' of behaviour. The problems that arise with such explanations are numerous, but in the present context it will suffice to mention the following points. To begin with, knowledge about beliefs and intentions critically depends on the individual's ability to give a reliable and valid introspective account. However, there is a large body of knowledge from experimental psychology indicating an asymmetry between people's readiness to verbalize their cognitive activity and their inaccuracy in this domain. Intriguing examples can be found in Nisbett and Wilson's classical paper 'Telling more than we can know'.[4] Another case in point is provided by all sorts of memory illusions which may occur in children and adults, and which often take the form of grossly inaccurate autobiographical recollections that are described with strong subjective confidence.[5]

A second problem with intentional explanations is perhaps even more fundamental. No doubt, beliefs and intentions can be associated with behaviour or emotions. But the type of feelings and thoughts that enter consciousness and are accessible to verbalization may be 'end-products' of deeper processes.[6] In daily life, people may have access to these end-products and may understandably rely on them when they try to predict behaviour of others. Meanwhile, many researchers believe it to be the task of scientific psychology to move beyond end-products and to treat beliefs and intentions as phenomena to be explained rather than as explanatory constructs.

A final objection to intentional explanations is especially relevant for psychopathology. Intentional explanations assume that subjects are rational in the sense that, given their intentions and beliefs, they are thought to act in their best interests. Yet, in this sense of the word, psychiatric patients almost by definition behave irrationally. Thus, even if one would accept a role for intentional explanation in the psychology of healthy individuals, one could argue that, certainly in psychiatry, intentional explanations are doomed to fail.

If psychology has a contribution to make to the understanding of psychiatric problems, it should be able to pinpoint psychiatric problems to 'underlying' psychological processes. The success of this explanatory endeavour should be apparent from its fruits; it should produce powerful predictions of clinical phenomena and effective interventions, preferably successful not only in psychological laboratories but also in treatment settings. The three categories of psychological contributions to psychiatry that are the focus of the present chapter will be introduced below.

In the first category, clinical phenomena to be explained and treated are reduced to biopsychological phenomena. Cognition, emotion, and behaviour are all organized by the brain, and some authors take this to indicate that mental disorders are, in fact, disorders of the brain. This approach stands in the tradition of the 'mental diseases are brain diseases' doctrine that was successfully launched by Wilhelm Griesinger in his *Mental Pathology and Therapeutics* (for a detailed appreciation, see Arens[7]) and is still influential. In the words of one of the pioneers of modern biological psychiatry, 'abnormal behaviour presupposes disturbed cerebral functioning'.[8] Prominent illustrations of this approach are theories and data about the neuropsychology of anxiety and its disorders.[9,10] Obviously, notions like beliefs and intentions have no place in biopsychological contributions to psychiatry. If anything, these concepts deserve explanation.

A second category of contributions circumvents intentional explanation not by focusing on central nervous system dysfunctions, but rather by emphasizing aberrations in the way psychiatric patients process information. When relating information processing approaches to biopsychology, it is tempting to draw parallels with computer technology. Whereas biopsychology focuses on the neuronal 'hardware' of patients, information processing research concentrates on the 'software'. Disturbances in the filtering of stimuli, the regulation of attention, the functioning of memory, and so on are investigated as possible antecedents or maintaining factors of psychopathology. In the same way as aberrations of computer software can be analysed without assuming 'intentions' of the machine, psychiatric problems should be explicable without invoking beliefs and intentions as explanatory notions.

Finally, there are psychological approaches that explicitly and deliberately challenge the widely held assumption, referred to above, that beliefs are but epiphenomena with little or no explanatory power. The central idea here is that many psychiatric problems can be fruitfully and validly reduced to erroneous beliefs held by patients. Like normal people's beliefs about the weather, such beliefs are assumed to be accessible to introspection and open to verbalization. Futhermore, these beliefs are thought to be far more than end-products; they are held to contribute to the origin and maintenance of the disorder.

The remainder of this chapter will be devoted to illustrations of these three types of contributions to the understanding of psychiatric disorders. To the degree that the knowledge is valid and relevant, it should enable one to predict and change psychiatric phenomena. When discussing the various contributions, we shall focus on these two criteria of validity and relevance; what insights allow for predictions and interventions that are relevant to the pragmatic science that psychiatry is by its very nature.

Biological psychology

To a large extent, psychiatric symptoms can be interpreted in terms of radicalized temperaments and extreme emotions.[11] For example, the shyness implicated in social phobia is connected to neuroticism or, as some researchers prefer to call it, negative affectivity. Likewise, the impulsive behaviour of a psychopathic criminal is the extreme manifestation of a trait known as sensation-seeking. Phobic reactions represent exaggerations of normal fear, while the blunted affect of a schizophrenic patient indicates the breakdown of normal emotion regulation. Thus it is obvious that the study of temperament and emotions is relevant to psychiatry.

Emotion, mood, psychopathology, and temperament all refer to what Oatley and Jenkins[11] have termed the 'affective realm'. The primary difference between these constructs has to do with the time course of the affective phenomena involved, with emotional states lasting for a few seconds and temperaments lasting for years. Although it is tempting to view affective phenomena as subjective inner experiences, research shows that they can fruitfully be conceptualized as biologically based action tendencies. Indeed, the function of affective phenomena is to guide and manage our thoughts and actions in a complex world that is difficult to predict. Accordingly, severe emotional disorders undermine real-life planning. This is exactly what the work of, for instance, Damasio[12] demonstrates. Consider the following experiment. Normal subjects and patients with bilateral frontal-lobe damage are instructed to play a gambling game that involves several card decks. Some of the decks are advantageous in that they result in overall gain in the long run, while other decks are disadvantageous because they cost money in the long run. Meanwhile, it is not possible for subjects to make an exact calculation of the gains and losses associated with each deck. Therefore subjects have to sample all decks and, on the basis of this information, they gradually have to adopt a strategy in which bad decks are avoided. Normal subjects are able to develop such a strategy, but patients with bilateral frontal damage are not. They continue to sample the bad decks and consequently lose all their money. This is associated with the insensitivity of these patients to repeated losses and punishment. In more general terms, the results of this experiment accord well with the observation that, owing to their blunted affect, patients with bilateral frontal-lobe damage have great difficulties in planning ordinary life. Thus affective phenomena provide us with heuristics that guide our decisions.[11]

Emotions and affective style

The idea that the two cerebral hemispheres make different contributions to the development of dysphoric emotions (e.g. depression, anxiety) has attracted considerable attention in the past few years. Evidence for this idea comes from two separate research lines. The first is exemplified by the experimental work of Hugdahl,[13] who directly manipulated hemisphere information processing (e.g. by confining visual stimuli to one visual field/hemisphere) in order to examine the differential involvement of the two hemispheres in emotional reactions. His studies indicate that fear-relevant stimuli (e.g. pictures of snakes) evoke a cardiac defence reaction when they are flashed to the right hemisphere (i.e. left visual field) of healthy subjects, but not when they are flashed to the left hemisphere (i.e. right visual field) of these subjects. Also, the two hemispheres of normal subjects apparently differ in their conditionability. That is, when visual stimuli flashed to either the right or the left side of the brain are followed by electric shocks, only the stimuli presented to the right hemisphere eventually elicit conditioned fear reactions. Similarly, studies by Wittling[14] indicate that emotionally provocative film clips presented to the right hemisphere of normal subjects produce a higher increase in cortisol secretion than do left-hemisphere presentations of the same film clips. This suggests that cortisol reaction to emotional stimuli is under the primary control of the right hemisphere. Taken together, these findings seem to imply that the right hemisphere is more sensitive to emotional information.

A second line of research relies on direct measures of brain activity. A good example is provided by the electroencephalography (**EEG**) studies of Davidson,[15] who demonstrated that, in normal subjects, negative emotions (e.g. disgust, fear) are accompanied by a stronger right-hemisphere than left-hemisphere activation. Research findings such as these have led many authors to conclude that the right frontal areas sustain negative emotions and avoidance behaviour, while the left frontal areas are more involved in pleasant emotions and approach behaviour (for a more refined version of this theory, see Heller and Nitschke[16]). There are good reasons to take this argument one step further and to assume that right- and left-frontal overactivation are trait-like characteristics that reflect susceptibility to avoidance-related and approach-related behaviour respectively. That is, habitual overactivation of one frontal area or underactivation of the other frontal area corresponds to certain affective styles. Germane to this issue is a study which found that young infants with a strongly activated right frontal hemisphere tend to react with crying to subsequent maternal separation.[17] The idea that asymmetries in frontal activation are linked to affective styles is further buttressed by the finding that heightened right-hemisphere activation during rest predicts the extent to which healthy adults react with fear and disgust to emotional film clips.[18]

Research on frontal asymmetry and affective phenomena is important because it may shed light on certain psychiatric conditions, such as poststroke depression. Depression is considered to be the most common emotional consequence of stroke, occurring in 20 to 50 per cent of stroke patients. There are robust indications that poststroke depression has a negative impact on the rehabilitation of stroke patients.[19] Additionally, damage to the left-frontal area is more likely than damage to any other cortical region to be associated with depression. A plausible interpretation of this association is that left-frontal lesions result in a decreased activity in this region which, in turn, would lead to a deficit of the positively valenced approach system sustained by the left-frontal areas. Such an interpretation accords well with the finding that neurologically intact patients with current unipolar depression or a history of unipolar depression exhibit reduced left-frontal EEG activity.[20]

Some authors have argued that left-frontal underactivation represents a risk factor for depression because it biases individuals in favour of a negatively valenced avoidance system. Interestingly, there is tentative evidence that left-frontal underactivation is accompanied by cognitive biases (see below) that are known to play a role in the aetiology of depression. Future research on affective brain asymmetry may clarify the neuropsychological basis of these cognitive biases.[21] In addition, research in this domain may provide us with clinical tools for predicting treatment outcome. A study by Bruder et al.[22] nicely illustrates this point. These authors measured hemisphere activation by means of a dichotic listening task before depressive patients underwent cognitive-behavioural treatment. Cognitive therapy responders exhibited higher left-hemisphere activity (as indexed by larger right-ear advantages for verbal material) than non-responders. In fact, left-

hemisphere activation was the best predictor of a favourable response to cognitive therapy.

Temperament

Although the details are still a matter of debate, most researchers agree that only a few dimensions are needed to classify a wide variety of personality types.[23] Students of personality accept that neuroticism (or negative affectivity, behavioural inhibition, or avoidance) corresponds to one core dimension, while extraversion (or positive affectivity or approach) refers to another core dimension. Furthermore, most researchers consider psychoticism (or impulsive sensation-seeking) to be a basic trait. The widely used Big Five taxonomy[24] lists agreeableness and openness to experience as two additional basic traits.

As Gray[25] and Zuckerman[23] have pointed out, there is no one-to-one relationship between basic traits and neurohormone systems. For example, the enzyme monoamine oxidase, which has an important function in dopamine breakdown, is negatively correlated with sensation-seeking.[26] This is in line with the observation that disinhibitory forms of psychopathology (e.g. borderline personality disorder, bipolar disorder, positive schizophrenic symptoms) are accompanied by low levels of monoamine oxidase. However, sensation-seeking also correlates strongly with testosterone. Likewise, the arousal component of neurotic anxiety is thought to be mediated by high levels of noradrenaline (norepinephrine), while the avoidance component has been related to low levels of γ-aminobutyric acid. The important point to note is that personality dimensions can be decomposed in more basal behavioural tendencies which probably do correspond to discrete neurohormone systems. For example, the trait of impulsive sensation-seeking involves strong approach behaviour which is a function of dopamine and testosterone, weak inhibition which is a function of serotonin, and low arousal which is a function of noradrenaline. Thus, a high score on sensation-seeking is brought about by several neurohormone systems interacting with each other.[23,26]

Clarifying the precise linkages between personality, behavioural tendencies, and neurohormones will lead to a better appreciation of studies concerned with the genetics of psychopathology. For example, in their twin study, Andrews et al.[27] found evidence for a genetic transmission of depression and anxiety disorders, but they also concluded that this genetic component involves the general vulnerability factor of neuroticism rather than specific symptoms or diagnostic categories. However, it should be noted that, in the final analysis, it is not personality traits such as neuroticism that are inherited, but genes that code for proteins which, in turn, regulate neurohormones.

The concept of behavioural inhibition is closely linked to neuroticism and negative affectivity.[28] It refers to the tendency of some children to interrupt ongoing behaviour and to react with vocal restraint and withdrawal when confronted with unfamiliar people or settings. Behavioural inhibition is thought to be a stable and inherited response disposition that characterizes approximately 10 to 15 per cent of children.[29] Cross-sectional and longitudinal data collected by Biederman et al.[30] indicate that behavioural inhibition is a vulnerability factor for a broad range of anxiety disorders. As to the biological underpinnings of behavioural inhibition, relevant parameters have been identified by Schmidt et al.,[31] who noted that behaviourally inhibited children exhibit relatively high morning levels of the stress hormone cortisol. They speculated that these high cortisol levels may sensitize subcortical arousal circuits (e.g. the amygdala) and this would make children more prone to developing serious anxiety symptoms. Interestingly, work on psychophysiological parameters that tap subcortical fear responsivity (e.g. the eye-blink startle reflex[32]) supports this interpretation. For example, Grillon et al.[33] measured startle reflexes in children with a parental history of an anxiety disorder (such children often meet the criteria for behavioural inhibition). They noted that these children displayed a heightened startle reflex magnitude. This is in agreement with the notion that anxiety-prone (i.e. behaviourally inhibited) children have hyperexcitable subcortical circuits that may promote fear behaviour and avoidance.

People high in positive affectivity or extraversion frequently feel joyful, optimistic, and assertive, while those low in positive affectivity are disinterested and pessimistic. Positive affectivity is a stable temperamental dimension with a substantial genetic component. There is also evidence that it is specifically linked to depression. However, the details of this link are far from clear. Some studies indicate that low positive affectivity reflects a predisposition to developing depressive symptoms, while other studies suggest that it modulates the course of depressive symptoms.[34] Another unresolved issue concerns the precise cognitive variables that mediate the connection between positive affectivity and depression. It is well established that individuals who rely on a pessimistic explanatory style (i.e. who habitually ascribe bad life events to their own faults) run a greater risk of becoming depressed than those who rely on an optimistic explanatory style. It is also clear that explanatory style has a genetic component[35] and is a good predictor of the long-term outcome of cognitive treatment for depression.[36] However, solid evidence for the idea that a pessimistic explanatory style functions as a specific cognitive mediator between low positive affectivity and depression is lacking. It may well be the case that such a style predisposes individuals to both anxiety and depression.[34]

Psychophysiological parameters

In general, the search for unique biological markers of psychiatric diagnoses has produced disappointing results. A good diagnostic marker is one that possesses sufficient sensitivity (i.e. high detection rate of a specific disease) and specificity (i.e. strong discrimination between a specific disease and other diseases). Although psychophysiological research has discovered a variety of deviations in psychiatric populations, ranging from an excess of fast EEG activity in alcoholism to abnormal eye-tracking movements in schizophrenia,[37,38] none of these deviations satisfy the criteria for being good markers. Apparently, the organizing principle behind these deviations is quite different from that of the Diagnostic and Statistical Manual of Mental Disorders (DSM). This has led some authors to conclude that we should stop looking for biological markers of the nosological categories listed in the DSM. After all, there is no reason to treat the taxonomy provided by the DSM as the gold standard.[39]

This is not to say that the psychophysiological abnormalities that have been revealed in various psychiatric populations are meaningless. Space limitations preclude a systematic review of this issue, and therefore we shall focus on a few arbitrarily chosen examples.

About 40 to 60 per cent of schizophrenic patients fail to show an electrodermal orienting response to simple sensory stimuli (e.g.

sounds). This electrodermal non-response is not due to hospitalization or medication effects, but reflects a profound attentional disturbance. Electrodermal non-response in schizophrenia has a number of interesting clinical correlates. For instance, electrodermal non-response has been found to be related to poor premorbid adjustment, negative and/or more severe schizophrenic symptoms (e.g. blunted affect), poor response to neuroleptics, CT scan abnormalities (e.g. increased ventricular brain ratios), and poor long-term social functioning.[40,41] Thus, even though electrodermal non-response is neither a sensitive (i.e. only a subgroup of schizophrenic patients exhibit the phenomenon) nor a specific (there are other conditions such as autism and schizotypical personality disorder in which the phenomenon occurs) marker of schizophrenia, it is a clinically relevant phenomenon.

One hypothesis about the origins of hallucinations is that patients misinterpret their own subvocal speech about emotionally charged topics as voices. This idea has been tested in a number of studies where electromyographic data on vocal muscle activity were collected together with reports of hallucinations.[42] The results of these studies were generally negative in that no clear temporal association was found between increased vocal activity and the onset of hallucinations. Although the subvocalization theory of hallucinations proved to be incorrect, it inspired a whole new avenue of research that focused on what has been termed inner speech.[43] Indeed, neuroimaging studies of activity in the language areas of the brain (e.g. Broca's area) during hallucinations did find evidence to suggest that hallucinations are linked to inner speech.[44] Findings such as these have been a major impetus to cognitive theories about schizophrenia. A good example is provided by Frith[45] who argued that most schizophrenic symptoms can be interpreted in terms of self-monitoring deficits. According to this view, hallucinations occur when people attribute their own inner speech to an external source.

Some decades ago, Chapman and Chapman[46] concluded in their classic monograph on schizophrenia that 'most clinical psychologists and psychiatrists believe, almost as an article of faith, that thought disorders and the other symptoms of schizophrenia are a response by the patient to his emotional problems'. This situation has drastically changed due to the extensive biopsychological work in this field. This work has revealed systematic relationships between schizophrenic symptoms and cognitive deficits.[47] Although it is not clear which of these deficits are primary and central to the disorder and which are secondary reactions to the symptoms, some authors have concluded that the time is ripe for small-scale cognitive remediation programmes for schizophrenia.[48]

Psychophysiological parameters such as electrodermal response or electromyographic activity are traditionally viewed as the peripheral ends of a chain. They may reflect central dysfunctions, but do not themselves serve as determinants of these dysfunctions. A further example of such a peripheral parameter is the eye-blink startle reflex. The central antecedents of startle reflex have been well studied because this reflex provides an objective index of defensive action tendencies. For example, patients with phobias, panic disorder, or post-traumatic stress disorder all exhibit exaggerated startle potentiation when startle reflexes are probed in the context of threatening stimuli (e.g. pictures of phobic objects). In contrast, psychopathic individuals fail to show any startle potentiation in the presence of threatening stimuli. Precisely because startle reflexes do not depend on introspection, startle probe analysis may be useful in assessing the effects of behavioural or pharmacological interventions.[49]

Recent animal studies suggest that there are conditions in which peripheral parameters may act as the determinants of central dysfunctions. An interesting example is provided by cortisol. Exposure to aversive events mobilizes the hypothamalamic–pituitary–adrenal axis, which results in an increased secretion of cortisol. High levels of cortisol may have neurotoxic effects on hippocampal circuits, thereby producing memory impairments. These findings may elucidate some clinical features of depression and post-traumatic stress disorder. Both conditions are associated with stress and memory disturbances, and there are some preliminary indications that at least some patients with these disorders have a reduced hippocampal volume.[50]

Conclusions

Many of the findings summarized above invite a diathesis–stress view of psychopathology. According to this view, psychiatric symptoms are the end-product of a biologically based predisposition (e.g. neuroticism) interacting with aversive life experiences. While this approach has proved to be a fruitful framework for many disorders,[51] it should not limit our thinking about the aetiology of psychiatric symptoms. For example, the diathesis–stress framework has often been taken to imply that biological abnormalities of symptomatic individuals are somehow more fundamental than the symptoms and therefore must precede these symptoms. In their excellent review, Harrop et al.[52] demonstrate that this line of reasoning is problematic. Even in the case of ventricular enlargements or dopamine disruptions in schizophrenia, there is the possibility that the pertinent central nervous system abnormalities are produced by schizophrenic symptoms or certain environmental factors that operate in the aetiology of schizophrenia.[53] Note that there are well-researched examples of psychological conditions resulting in biological abnormalities. Consider the learned helplessness paradigm. When animals are made helpless by inescapable shocks, they not only become passive, but also exhibit noradrenaline and serotonin depletion.[54] This implies that a certain learning history may give rise to neurotransmitter abnormalities that have traditionally been conceptualized as the causes of depression. Likewise, while positron-emission tomography scanning revealed profound brain abnormalities in obsessive–compulsive patients, these cerebral differences between patients and controls were abolished after successful behavioural treatment.[55]

Even when it is plausible to assume that a biological abnormality precedes the onset of symptoms, it is not self-evident that this abnormality plays a significant aetiological role. For example, a biologically based dysfunction (e.g. scoring low on positive affectivity) may affect the course rather than the onset of a disorder. This type of causation is known as the pathoplasty model and, compared with the widespread diathesis–stress approach, it has received too little consideration.

Perhaps, then, the benefit of psychobiology to psychiatry does not consist of grand theories about causation, but of reliable measurements of basic concepts. That is, psychobiology can inform psychiatry about fundamental personality traits, the nature of emotions, and how they relate to the brain. It can also contribute good psychophysiological and neuropsychological tools that possess diagnostic and prognostic value. In doing so, it may help to define the limits within which good theorizing must occur.

Information processing

In the first half of the twentieth century academic psychology was predominantly behaviouristic in its orientation, concentrating on relations between stimuli (input) and responses (output) and largely ignoring the processes that take place between input and output. Given the ambition to develop a true science of behaviour, this reluctance to dwell upon non-observables in the 'black box' is understandable, but the approach had serious limitations.[56,57] For example, early century behaviourists, especially in the United States, were largely silent about individual differences as it was assumed that all behavioural manifestations result from stimulus configurations. Evidently, however, people differ very much from each other, and these individual differences are to a large extent linked to biologically based temperaments. A psychological science that ignores individual differences would be of little use to psychiatry.[58]

Another serious shortcoming of behaviouristic psychology was that it ignored the important issue of how the organism manages to produce a response after a stimulus has been perceived. It is clear that stimulus perception and response preparation must be involved, but some stimulus–response relations (e.g. fear conditioning) are acquired through learning processes. Does not learning involve memory? And does not the notion of memory implicate certain qualities of the black box? Likewise, intelligent behaviour requires attention, self-monitoring of motor acts, emotion, and speech, and again all these functions imply a highly specific cognitive architecture of the black box.

In the 1960s, computer sciences began to offer a powerful metaphor for conceptualizing this cognitive architecture. Within a decade, studying the black box became an appealing and scientifically respectable challenge, dramatically changing the landscape of psychology. This shift has sometimes been referred to as the 'cognitive revolution' in psychology.[59] Whereas the behavioural tradition concentrated on how organisms learn, the central issue for cognitive psychology became how intelligent systems process information. The relevance to psychiatry is straightforward. Given a specific disorder, say depression, the question arises as to whether it is associated with peculiarities in processing information and whether these peculiarities play a role in the genesis or maintenance of the disorder. Before discussing some of the main findings from this research, two preliminary remarks are in order.

First, possibly because of its association with computer sciences, much of the early information processing research in psychiatry concentrated on emotionally neutral information. In memory tests, patients were asked to memorize emotionally neutral or even nonsense words. The self-relevance and 'emotional valence' of information was regarded as reflecting irrelevant 'noise'. It is now clear that this is incorrect; the valence or meaning of the information to be processed is highly relevant to the cognitive psychology of emotional disorders. Depressive patients, for instance, perform poorly on tests measuring memory for emotional neutral information. Interestingly, the memory performance of depressives is better for emotionally negative material (e.g. words like dead, guilty, suffering) than for neutral information. This indicates that, apart from a general memory dysfunction, depressive patients exhibit a domain-specific memory bias. Another illustration is provided by patients suffering from obsessive–compulsive disorder who are sometimes extremely uncertain about their own memory performance (Did I turn the gas off or didn't I?) This uncertainty may contribute to checking behaviour and suggests a failure of metamemory, i.e. the ability to judge whether or not a retrieved piece of memory relates to events that really took place. However, given the clinical picture of obsessive–compulsive disorder, it does not make sense to assume a general deficit in metamemory. Patients do trust their memory when it relates to whether or not they went to the grocery store. What these examples illustrate is that aberrations in information processing do occur in psychopathology, but that such aberrations are often domain specific and confined to the processing of information with a specific emotional valence.

A second preliminary issue is concerned with the fact that information processing takes place at separate stages that are hierarchically organized. These stages involve attention to the information to be processed, sensory registration of the information, comparison of incoming stimuli with information stored in memory, interpretation, decision about action, motor preparation and execution, etc. There is some debate about the precise number of stages that need to be distinguished and their exact sequence. We shall not enter this debate here, but will concentrate on those aspects and information processing stages that are both best studied and most relevant to psychiatry, i.e. attention, memory, and interpretation.

Attention

We cannot possibly process all the information that is available. By allocating the limited attentional resources that we have to specific stimuli, some information is selected for further processing at the expense of other information. Aberrations in the regulation of attention occur in a wide range of psychiatric disorders.

First, severe disorders like schizophrenia or attention-deficit hyperactivity disorder are accompanied by a general deficit in attentional selection. Patients display attentional deficits that are largely independent of the semantic content of the information to be processed. A good illustration is provided by the systematic work of Shakow and colleagues who sought to identify the earliest stage at which cognitive deficits occur in schizophrenics. This work revealed that schizophrenic patients perform at a normal level on repetitive motor tasks and tasks measuring visual acuity, but display a slowing of speed when they have to react to a signalled target stimulus.[60] This accords well with Kraepelin's clinical observation that a general attentional dysfunction is one of the core disturbances in schizophrenia.

In many other conditions, however, attentional disruptions are not general but domain specific, because they depend on the content (or 'valence' or 'meaning') of the information to be processed. As there is no reason to suppose that such an 'attentional bias' is accessible to introspection, researchers adopted paradigms from experimental psychology for documenting and unravelling the phenomenon. Typically, several groups of patients and healthy controls are asked to perform a task during which distractors, which vary in content (e.g. emotionally neutral versus emotionally negative), are presented. To the degree that attention is selectively allocated to emotionally negative material, for example, performance on the primary task will deteriorate more when negative distractors are presented than when the distractors are neutral. When certain patients are more distracted by, for example, specific negative distractors than by neutral distractors, relative to healthy or psychiatric controls, it is inferred that they display a domain-specific 'attentional bias'. While a wide variety of such tasks is available, by far the best studied is the so-called emotional Stroop test.

Patients are seated before a computer screen and are presented with a sequence of words varying in colour. Words are sometimes emotionally neutral and sometimes emotionally valent (e.g. related to threat). The subject's task is to ignore the word's meaning and to name its colour. Findings with this paradigm rank among the most robust data in the cognitive psychology of emotional disorders. Anxious patients typically slow down when colour naming emotionally provocative words relative to neutral words. Healthy controls typically do not. Attentional bias, measured with this approach, has been documented in addiction and eating disorders, but most notably in anxiety disorders, i.e. phobias, panic disorder, social phobia, generalized anxiety disorder, post-traumatic stress disorder, and obsessive–compulsive disorder.[61–63] The most intriguing aspect of this phenomenon is not that patients selectively attend to issues of personal concern, but that they are apparently unable to abstain voluntarily from selective attention to threat. After all, they do try to ignore the meaning of the distracting word content. In psychology, such involuntariness is seen as a feature of 'automatic processing', which is contrasted with 'controlled processing' which does require willful effort.[64]

Another psychological feature distinguishing controlled from automatic processing is awareness. Whereas controlled processing (e.g. driving a car by a novice driver) requires awareness of the information to be processed and of the operations to be carried out, automatic or automatized processing (e.g. driving a car by an experienced driver) does not require such awareness. Thus the question arises as to whether anxiety-related non-volitional selective attention to threat requires consciousness of the material that is processed. The answer to this is negative. There are good reasons to believe that even when anxiety patients cannot possibly be aware of the information that is presented to them, they preferentially process information with a negative content. Evidence comes mainly from a modification of the Stroop test. Words to be colour named are presented for an ultrashort period of time, say 20 ms, after which they are replaced by a coloured mask that effectively blocks the after-image of the word, preventing conscious recognition. These masked words are emotionally neutral or negative, and the subject is asked to name the colour of the mask as quickly as possible. Again, anxious patients selectively slow down when a mask is preceded by a threat word as opposed to neutral words. This selective attention to cues that are not consciously identified has been observed with high-trait anxious subjects,[65–67] with phobics,[68] and with patients suffering from generalized anxiety disorder.[69] Selective attending to preconscious threat cues in anxiety not only affects ongoing low-level cognitive operations, but also seems to activate the sympathetic branch of the autonomic nervous system; fearful subjects display increased electrodermal activity when confronted with masked presentations of threat pictures, whereas controls do not.[70]

While attentional bias has been observed in several disorders, a curious exception to this rule is depression. Depressed patients tend to selectively remember negatively valenced information ('memory bias'), but they typically do not selectively attend to threat.[71] This may be because depressed people are preoccupied with (perceived) loss in the past and not, like anxious people, with (perceived) future harm. From a functionalist position, it seems that selective attention is to be expected for those cues that are relevant for immediate action, like approach or avoidance. In line with this implication from general emotion theory, it was found that attentional bias also occurs for emotionally positive cues, given that the cues relate to highly desirable immediate action. For example, subjects who fast for 24 h selectively attend to positively valenced cues related to eating.[72]

Theoretically and clinically, a crucial question is the causal status of attentional bias: is it related to the genesis and/or maintenance of disorders or is it a result of these disorders? The empirical evidence that has accumulated favours both interpretations. Thus several studies have found that attentional bias disappears or is reduced after successful cognitive behaviour therapy.[73–75] The finding that cognitive behaviour therapy affects not only behaviour and self-reported complaints but also objective manifestations of information processing, while encouraging for cognitive behaviour therapy, suggests that attentional bias results from anxiety. Obviously, the relevance of attentional bias would be rather limited if there were an epiphenomenal and superficial feature of the disorder, appearing and disappearing with the waxing and waning of the syndrome. Still, there is more to attentional bias than this. MacLeod and Hagan,[65] using the preconsciously operating 'masked' Stroop test in a prospective study, observed that future distress could be predicted from a currently present tendency to selectively attend to threat. This was replicated in a cross-sectional study.[67] Of particular interest is that the prediction of distress from current attentional bias was unrelated to current anxiety levels. Independent of current anxiety, attentional bias was a predictor of subsequent symptoms. This suggests that anxiety and attentional bias are reciprocally related; anxiety may foster attentional bias, but in and of itself attentional bias may be a vulnerability factor. A therapeutic implication would be that reducing attentional bias may help in reducing anxiety disorders or preventing relapse after successful treatment. While promising observations have been reported,[76] no controlled data are yet available.

Memory

Memory is not what lay people often think it is. It is not a hard disk from which information can be easily retrieved by a simple command. Information represented in memory can sometimes be temporarily inaccessible and can pop up unexpectedly at other times. Not all information is stored in the memory in the same way. Sometimes memories are so vivid that it seems as if one experiences the event again, but other memories are only global abstract ways of knowing what has happened. In some mood states things are remembered that would not easily be remembered in other mood states. Since memory-related disturbances often accompany psychiatric problems, even if there is no direct organic cause for these disturbances, and since memory seems to essential for our daily functioning, the study of memory processes in different forms of psychopathology has become a major topic in psychological research.

One important issue is the influence of mood on the accessibility of specific memories. Numerous experiments indicate that a person's mood influences what memories are reported when the person is asked to retrieved a memory related to a specific cue; the cue word can be neutral (e.g. street) or highly affect laden (e.g. disappointment). Memories of negative events of unhappy life periods, and even of negative self-descriptors recently learned, are more accessible in a negative mood than in a happy mood, while the reverse is true for memories of positive events of happy periods in life and positive self-descriptors. This seems to hold for naturally fluctuating mood and experimentally induced mood, as well as for psychopathological mood states, notably clinical depression.[62,63,77]

This phenomenon of mood-congruent memory seems to be rather specific for depressive patients or patients with concomitant depressive mood. Accordingly, researchers have focused on the role that it might play in the origins or maintenance of depressive disorders. Teasdale's model is probably the best known and has been very influential. This model states that depressive patients are caught in a vicious circle, such that their negative memories lead to negative interpretations of current events, which in turn maintain the depressive mood, while the depressed mood maintains the increased accessibility of negative memories and the reduced accessibility of positive memories.[78] The precise status of the influence of mood on memory has not been fully elucidated[79] and the findings in this field do not lead to direct therapeutic interventions, other than the type of cognitive therapeutic methods which seemed to be more related to schema theories (see section below on schemas and beliefs) than to memory theories. However, it is clear that the recall of autobiographical memories is influenced by the current mood of the individual. Thus memory functioning in depression is not disturbed in a general way, but is biased towards the emotionally laden content of the memories. As with attentional bias, memory bias is related to the content of the information that is to be processed.

Why do anxious patients display a clear attentional bias, whereas depressed patients do not display attentional bias but are characterized by a mood-congruent memory bias? One speculation is that this has to do with the original functions of the patient's emotional state. It is helpful to view anxiety disorders as dysfunctional variants of normal anxiety and depressive disorders as dysfunctional variants of normal states of grief. In 'normal' or 'functional' anxiety, there is a (potential) danger and the resulting anxious state is directed at immediate survival. Thus the attentional system aims at a quick (although perhaps somewhat 'dirty') signalling of danger, thereby facilitating sufficiently early fight or flight. By definition, the perspective is on the future. In conditions of grief, however, the focus is on what has been lost, and the information processing aims at integrating the new fact (e.g. the death of a loved one) with memories of the lost object. Thus the perspective is on the past, until the new fact has been sufficiently assimilated. It seems that in dysfunctional anxiety and in depressive disorders, the information processing system displays biases directly related to the processes that have priority in the functional variants.

Research on memory functioning in depressed patients has recently focused more on the degree to which memories are specific. Williams[80] observed that suicidal and depressed patients find it more difficult than somatic patients and healthy people to report memories of specific events, i.e. depressive patients tend to react with very global memories to cue words. For example, a depressed patient might react to the cue word 'party' with 'I've never liked parties', rather than 'I did not like the party my neighbour organized last Sunday afternoon; there was almost nobody I know, and the music was very loud so that you couldn't talk to each other'. Although it is unclear how specific this phenomenon of 'overgeneral memory' is for depression, Williams[80] has speculated that this deficit may play a crucial role in maintaining depressive disorders. One way in which overgeneral memory might be problematic is that if one cannot find memories of specific events, problem solving becomes very difficult. Memories of specific events can help us to find effective solutions for present problems and to avoid ineffective ways of coping with life. For example, Evans et al.[81] reported that the failure of depressed patients to react with detailed memories to cue words is related to their poor problem-solving capacity, and a longitudinal study by Brittlebank *et al.*[82] showed that overgeneral recall of autobiographical memories predicts a failure to recover from depression following psychopharmacological intervention.

Again, one could speculate about the original function of overgeneral memories in depression. One possibility, related to our speculation about the mood-congruent memory bias in depressed mood, is that in grief the major task for the individual is to integrate the loss into general schematic representations of the self and the world. It does not seem helpful to integrate the loss of a child, for example, into every separate memory of the thousands of specific events one has shared with the child. Thus the observed bias again seems to be closely related to the content of the disorder. However, there are other speculations about the original functions of overgeneral memories.[83] For example, it has been proposed that overgeneral memories result from overlearned strategies to avoid painful traumatic memories. Yet another speculation is that the inability to produce specific memories results from a sort of cognitive stagnation in early childhood; young children have more difficulties in producing specific memories than adults, and traumatic experiences during these periods might lead to such a stagnation.

Most recently, attention has been drawn to traumatic memories. In psychopathological conditions directly related to traumas, such as post-traumatic stress disorder, efforts to remember fully what happened seem to be less successful than expected, given the fact that emotional events are usually better memorized than neutral events.[84] However, extremely vivid memories seem to pop up and can have an almost real quality; the patient sometimes smells, sees, hears, etc. what has happened during the trauma. It seems as if verbally stored memory, i.e. the conceptual meaning of the traumatic event, is poorly developed, whereas memory on a sensory level is highly developed. Apparently, these 'sensory-coded' memories are poorly accessible for voluntary attempts to remember. According to one psychological memory theory[85] this may be related to how the experience was encoded; experiences encoded on the level of sensory data are poorly accessible to explicit attempts to remember, but easily accessible when cues resembling the original data are used (implicit memory). However, when people process an experience by giving it a conceptual meaning, the opposite seems to occur—explicit memory is relatively good, but implicit memory is relatively poor. What may happen during highly traumatic experiences is that the often unexpected experience, which is difficult to understand conceptually, is processed on a low level (i.e. on the sensory data level) and not at a conceptual level. High stress levels and uncontrollability may also play a role in paralysing higher cognitive functions, so that there is poor conceptual processing of the trauma. This hypothesis explains how lively intrusions and poor explicit memory are both parts of psychopathological conditions that can follow a traumatic experience. Moreover, there is a direct therapeutic implication; by helping patients to give better organized conceptual meanings to the traumatic experience, the memories on the sensory data level are transformed to a conceptual level and memory-related complaints should reduce. In the coming decades, psychological studies of memory will undoubtedly further clarify how memory-related problems following a traumatic experience can be understood and how treatment could help patients recover from its aftermath.

Interpretation

Research on attention and memory emphasizes biased processing of relatively isolated pieces of emotionally charged information. At a level of processing that is typically characterized as 'higher', such pieces of information from memory and the outside world are integrated to create a more or less coherent representation of what is going on. For convenience, we refer to this integration of information by the generic term 'interpretation'. Meanwhile, it should be acknowledged that interpretation, thus defined, covers cognitive activity that ranges from the immediate effortless imposition of a Gestalt on an ambiguous visual stimulus configuration (e.g. the famous Rubin illusion that can be seen as either a vase or two faces) to the rather effortful logical deduction of a valid conclusion from a set of premises.

The present focus will be on three related types of interpretation biases: disambiguation bias, the inference of correlations that are illusory, and using emotional responses as a source of information about the safety or danger of the immediate environment.

The degree to which situations are positive or negative, dangerous or safe, and so on is often quite ambiguous, and assessing the meaning of such situations requires interpretation or 'disambiguation'. Psychologists have studied how affect is related to the interpretation of ambiguous material. In such studies, anxious or depressed people and normal subjects are invited to disambiguate inherently ambiguous stimuli. For instance, subjects are asked to write down orally presented homophones like 'killed' and 'kilt', or 'dye' and 'die'. Relative to non-anxious people, anxious subjects tend to favour the negative version of an ambiguous word over the neutral version.[86] Likewise, clinically anxious patients, unlike recovered patients and non-patients, tend to negatively disambiguate sentences like 'They discussed the priests' convictions' or 'The doctor examined little Emma's growth'.[87] Similarly, anxious people tend to overestimate the chances that unfortunate events will happen to them,[88] and they take less time to understand negative turns in narratives but are slower to understand positive turns of the story.[89]

The fact that disambiguation bias in anxiety disappears after successful treatment[87] suggests that the bias follows from anxiety. This idea is strengthened by the observation that experimentally lowering the mood in healthy subjects is attended by the emergence of a negativistic interpretation bias.[63] On the other hand, it seems obvious that disambiguating the world in a negative way may contribute to the maintenance of negative affect. Thus it appears that interpretation bias and negative affect are reciprocally related—negative affect fosters interpretation bias and vice versa.

Research on disambiguation biases has at least two limitations. First, the stimulus configurations to be interpreted are presented simultaneously rather than sequentially. It cannot be established whether the interpretations relate to causal sequences that are assumed by patients but not by normal subjects. Furthermore, the validity of the interpretations given by patients and normal subjects cannot be independently established; patients may be more negativistic than normal controls, but there is no gold standard which can be used to decide whether patients are overly negativistic or whether non-patients are unduly optimistic.

Research on interpretation bias that does not suffer from these problems was instigated by Tomarken *et al.*[90] In the first study, subjects with high and low anxiety were presented a series of slides from three categories, two neutral and one fear-relevant. Each slide was immediately followed by one of three outcomes: a tone, nothing, or shock. The conditional probability of any outcome given any preceding slide was exactly one-third. After exposure to dozens of slide–outcome combinations, subjects were asked to rate the probability of a given outcome provided that it was preceded by a given slide. Highly anxious subjects systematically overestimated the covariation between fear-relevant slides and shock. In an extended replication, de Jong et al.[91] showed spider slides, weapon slides, and neutral slides to severe spider phobics. Slides were randomly paired with shock, tone, or nothing. Again, spider phobics tended to overestimate highly the association between spider slides and shock. This suggests that anxiety is associated with a tendency to overestimate the association between a feared cue and personal harm.

Selective processing of spider–shock combinations was manifest not only from 'illusory correlations', as reported by the subjects, but also from electrodermal response. Subjects not only reacted with stronger electrodermal responses to spider slides, but also reacted with stronger electrodermal responses to shocks that were preceded by spider slides rather than control slides.[91,92]

As to the question of causality, the reasoning of de Jong and coworkers was similar to that employed in the above studies of selective attention. If illusory correlations between cue and harm result from anxiety, reductions in anxiety should be followed by reductions in illusory correlations. However, if illusory correlations act as an antecedent anxiety, they should predict future anxiety, independent of present anxiety, and inducing fearful expectation in normal subjects should make them confirmation biased and suffer from an illusionary correlation.

In line with the notion that anxiety causes illusory correlations, it was reported that, using the paradigm of Tomarken et al.,[90] untreated phobics show larger illusory correlations than treated phobics not previously tested.[91,92] It should be noted that, although illusory correlations after therapy tend to be low, there is substantial interindividual variation. Likewise, although long-term follow-up of behaviour therapy for spider phobias tends to be good, here too the variance is considerable. By testing whether residual illusory correlation after therapy predicts relapse, one may obtain a first impression of an anxiogenic role of illusory correlation. The correlation between residual illusory correlation after therapy and the increase in phobia severity from post-test to follow-up after 2 years was found to be 0.61. This correlation remained unchanged, even when post-treatment severity of complaints was partialled out.[93] This indicates that the tendency to overestimate the association between phobic cue and harm, in and by itself, independent of anxiety, may contribute to the (re)occurrence of fear.

If illusory correlations in and by themselves contribute to the maintenance of anxiety, normal subjects should become resistant to disconfirmation after an illusory correlation between cue and harm is induced. In an experiment that specifically addressed this issue,[94] normal subjects were shown a random series of two neutral slides (circles and crosses), each of which was sometimes paired with shock and sometimes not. During the initial trials, suggestive combinations were given with the target slide being paired with shock in 70 per cent of the presentations and the control slide in 30 per cent of the presentations. During the remainder of the trials, target slides were gradually paired less frequently with shock whereas control slides were paired more frequently with shock so that, finally, both target and control slides had been paired with shock in exactly 50 per cent of the trials. Throughout the experiment, probability estimates of the connection between slides

and shocks were obtained after each slide. In the suggestive phase, subjects reported that they expected the target slide to be specifically related to shock. After the suggestive series, even though the true target–shock association dropped below 50 per cent and below the association of control slide and shock, subjects remained convinced of the target–shock association and there was no sign that the disconfirmatory evidence resulted in extinction of this belief. Thus it is quite easy to induce an illusory correlation between cue and harm in healthy subjects. The striking observation was that, once established, the illusory correlation remained unchanged, even in the face of disconfirming evidence.

Anxious subjects report that they think fear cues are predictive of harm. The present experiments indicate that, if such an association is established, it becomes self-supporting. Confirmatory evidence is overvalued, disconfirmatory evidence is ignored, and fearful expectations remain intact.

Research on illusory correlations is interesting but seems to suffer from a lack of clinical or 'ecological' validity. Under laboratory conditions, patients may see unrealistic associations between cues and feared consequences, but outside the laboratory the association between feared cues and anticipated disasters is virtually absent; touching door knobs does not result in HIV infection, palpitations do not predict cardiac arrest, and so on. Although feared and avoided cues do not predict objective harm, they reliably predict something else—the occurrence of an anxiety response. Could the very occurrence of an output phenomenon like an emotional response influence the interpretation of the stimulus that served as the input? There is strong evidence that it can. To a large extent, people derive the meaning and valence of a situation from their responses to that situation. This is illustrated by the social psychology work of Valins[95] who showed, for example, that when male students received false feedback about cardio-acceleration when seeing a particular erotic picture, the subjective attractiveness of the picture increased. There is a wealth of data from psychopathology indicating that panic patients in particular take the 'output phenomenon' of anxiety responses as predictors of serious harm.[96] In line with this, Ehlers et al.,[97] using set-ups not unlike the one mentioned above, showed that once panic patients are provided with false feedback about cardio-acceleration, subjective fear increases just like heart rate and blood pressure.

The tendency to interpret fear responses as indicators of danger has been labelled 'emotional reasoning'. In the realm of anxiety and threat, such emotional reasoning appears to be a prominent characteristic not only of panic patients, but of anxious patients in general. Groups of 41 panic patients, 20 spider phobics, 58 social phobics, other anxiety patients, and normal subjects were given written scenarios that related to panic, social interaction, confrontation with a spider, and a non-disorder relevant situation. Four subtypes were constructed and administered for each scenario: information about objective danger was either given or not given; similarly, information about the occurrence of a fear response was given or not given. Subjects were asked to rate each of the four subtypes of the scenarios in terms of objective danger.

Normal subjects were barely influenced by response information. Their danger ratings simply followed danger information provided by the scenarios, but scores were not affected by fear information. The pattern in the patient groups was strikingly different. Compared with controls, patients generally gave higher danger ratings, even when object safety information was provided. More important was that patients, but not normal controls, engaged in 'emotional reasoning'; the dangerousness of a situation was inferred from the fact that anxious responses were included in the scenarios. Remarkably, this 'emotional reasoning' of patients was not specific, i.e. all groups of patients displayed the reasoning pattern to the same degree in all domains that were studied (panic relevant, socially relevant, and spider relevant).[98]

Schemas and beliefs

Reducing emotions and behaviour to a person's beliefs and goals appears to be closely associated with the idea of the human as rational actor. This notion may have some explanatory virtue in non-clinical areas, but it may be hard to see how beliefs and intentions may account for psychiatric problems.

An initial solution was proposed by psychoanalytic theory, which stated that intentions (wishes, desires) unknown to rational consciousness direct the emotions and behaviour of people with emotional problems. The main problem with this view is that there is no corpus of scientific data to support it.[99] That is, many psychological processes like memory or attention do not require consciousness (see the discussion of attention above), but these 'unconscious' or 'preconscious' processes are typically rather diffuse and non-specific, or 'quick and dirty',[100] and far less elaborate than beliefs.

A second way of applying intentional explanations to psychopathology is bluntly to assume that the emotions and behaviour of patients and healthy people are guided to the same degree by beliefs. The crucial difference between clinical and non-clinical groups may be the content of their beliefs. In cognitive theories of the type discussed here, it is assumed that various forms of psychopathology are associated with specific beliefs about the self, others, or the outside world. According to cognitive psychology, such basic beliefs are organized in schemas. Schema is a highly theoretical term denoting a hypothetical knowledge structure in memory. Schemas are assumed to organize selective attention, interpretation of events, and strategies for survival. In other words, schemas underlie information processing, conscious thoughts, emotions, and behaviour. Although much of the content of the knowledge represented in these schemas is not necessarily accessible to direct introspection, it is possible to reconstruct it in verbal terms. Such reconstructions are usually called assumptions or beliefs, and it is assumed that, in psychiatric patients, such 'pathogenic' beliefs are unrealistic or dysfunctional, resistant to disconfirmation by corrective information, and play a crucial role in the genesis and/or maintenance of the disorder.[63] In the remainder of this section, we first discuss evidence relating to the existence and nature of such unrealistic ideas, and then consider the rather important issue of the causal status of unrealistic/dysfunctional beliefs in psychiatric disorders.

Presence and subjective credibility of 'pathogenic' beliefs

Traditionally, it has been believed that 'neurotic' symptoms are experienced by the patient as egodystonic and that patients recognize the irrational character of their emotions or behaviour. Recent data show that this widely held idea needs to be qualified. The common way of gaining access to someone's beliefs is to ask the person. A number of studies have followed this approach and yielded findings that do not support the hypothesis of egodystonicity of neurotic problems. One could counter that when, for example, an obsessive–compulsive patient claims that she really believes that not washing her hands after turning a doorknob will result in catching a disease, this may be a rationalization. That is, confronted with her own irrational washing behaviour, the formulated belief may be a *post hoc* explanation intended to justify the behaviour to herself and/or to others.[101] However, it is far from obvious that it is socially more desirable to express beliefs that others regard as highly irrational (touching doorknobs results in disease) than to 'admit' that one endorses the view that the behaviour is irrational.[102] Widely held impressions about egodystony, obtained in the consulting room, may be caused by patients denying beliefs that they expect the clinician to find untenable.

Irrational beliefs about the outside world are common in anxiety disorders. Especially interesting are people with monosymptomatic phobia who tend, in contrast to other anxiety patients, not to suffer from comorbid pathology and who present the clearest case of irrational emotions and behaviour in otherwise healthy people. While egodystony in specific phobias is even a diagnostic criterion of DSM-IV ('The person recognizes that the fear is excessive or unreasonable'), systematic questioning using a paper-and-pencil task, without the social pressure of an interviewer, reveals that spider phobics tend to endorse highly irrational beliefs about the dangerousness of spiders. The credibility of these frightening ideas is especially high in the presence of the phobic cue.[102] Social phobics appear to have negative beliefs about their own social performance and about others, whom they believe to be more critical and rejecting than they actually are.[103–105] Furthermore, prominent other-centred problem-related convictions are found in patients suffering from borderline personality disorder who tend to believe that other people are malevolent, and will abuse, punish, or abandon the patient when the relationship becomes intimate.[106]

Apart from beliefs about the outside world and others, a number of psychiatric disorders appear to be characterized by problematic beliefs about the self in general or about specific internal events. Generalized beliefs about the self being worthless and vulnerable are found in depression[107] and borderline personality disorder.[106] Panic patients firmly belief that specific benign bodily sensations such as palpitations predict imminent catastrophes (e.g. cardiac infarction).[108] Interestingly, the paroxysmal occurrence of the sensations feared by panic patients is highly prevalent in the general population.[109] The crucial difference between such non-clinical and clinical panic is that non-clinical panickers are far less inclined to believe, during the attacks, that they may die from suffocation, have a cardial arrest, lose consciousness, and so on.[110] Remarkably, phobics appear to expect similar catastrophic consequences of experiencing fear and related bodily sensations during confrontation with the phobic object.[102]

Other internal events that can be subject to distorted beliefs are cognitive processes. Examples are the belief, found in many elderly people, that one's memory is failing although objective memory performance is, by all standards, normal.[111] Just as the bodily sensations that panic patients fear are quite common, so are the types of intrusions that obsessive patients report. The content of the clinical intrusions is no different from that of non-clinical intrusions. The latter also circle around themes like sex, aggression, blasphemy, and illness.[112] What is different, however, is the appraisal of the intrusions. While obsessive–compulsive patients regard them as highly aversive and try to resist them,[112,113] healthy people do not. Relatedly, negative intrusions are common after loss and trauma. Post-trauma intrusions can be interpreted as normal and adaptive responses to extremely aversive events or, alternatively, as indications that one is losing control, that one can never concentrate or enjoy life anymore, etc. Victims suffering from post-traumatic stress disorder report far more negative ideas about intrusions than do victims without post-traumatic stress disorder.[114] Worry is a hallmark of generalized anxiety disorder, in which patients appear to hold a wide range of beliefs about the pros and cons of worrying (so called 'meta-cognitions') which are hypothesized to fuel the worry process.[115] Hearing voices, curious as it may sound, is not a pathognomic sign of schizophrenia This phenomenon occurs in approximately 10 per cent of the general population and is related to conditions like sensory deprivation, sleep difficulties, intense imagery, and so on. How people cope with voices might be relevant when considering to what extent hallucinations might develop into pathological phenomena.[116]

Thus there is good evidence that patients with a variety of disorders maintain problem-related beliefs that are highly unrealistic or dysfunctional. Two questions arise. First, given that there are no formal thought disorders, why do patients not give up such beliefs in the light of disconfirming evidence? Second, are there arguments that these beliefs are causally related to the problems? If so, what are the clinical implications?

Immunity against disconfirmation

It is perfectly possible that a large number of people develop irrational beliefs of the types discussed above, but the vast majority are quick to reject them and do not present for mental health care. However, that would make the question even more compelling for those who do seek help. Why do these patients fail to reject problem-related beliefs that are logically and/or empirically untenable or extremely dysfunctional?

Behavioural processes seem to be involved in irrational fear. The conviction that a particular situation predicts harm motivates avoidance and escape of that situation. This deprives the patient of the opportunity to experience the fact that the feared situation is innocuous. In traditional behavioural accounts of fears and phobias, avoidance and escape were also seen as maintaining factors. Escape and avoidance were held to reduce anxiety immediately, and this anxiety reduction was thought to reinforce avoidance. From the present cognitive stance, this view appears not to be entirely correct. Patients do not avoid because otherwise they will become anxious, but because they believe that harm will be inflicted if they do not avoid. Thus avoidance maintains anxiety disorders because it prevents disconfirmation of fear-related beliefs. Likewise, depressed patients seem to behave in ways that tend to confirm their dysfunctional beliefs and they do not engage in activities that might yield disconfirming information. Depressed patients who believe that they are unlovable tend to isolate themselves, and the lack of social interaction is likely to be interpreted as further evidence for their belief.

Feared situations can be avoided but, as indicated above, some beliefs relate to internal events. Some patients fear internal events like bodily sensations (e.g. panic patients or hypochondriacs) or intrusions (e.g. obsessive–compulsive patients), and such internal events cannot be avoided. Panic patients have experienced hundreds of attacks attended by feared sensations but not followed by the catastrophe that they believe to be predicted by these sensations. Likewise, obsessive patients have typically experienced hundreds or thousands of intrusions without the feared outcome materializing. Why do these patients not give up their beliefs in the light of such clear and personally experienced contradicting evidences?

The phenomenon of safety behaviour, which appears to be functionally equivalent to avoidance and escape, may be relevant here. Once the feared situation is encountered and the patient believes harm is about to occur, he or she may try to prevent this. For instance, panic patients may sit down and try to relax in order to prevent cardiac failure. The non-occurrence of a heart problem may then be attributed not to the harmlessness of palpitations, but to the effectiveness of sitting down and relaxing. The rituals by which obsessive–compulsive patients respond to intrusions seem to serve the same function; predicted harm is prevented by some safety operation.

Apart from avoidance, escape, or safety behaviours that immunize against disconfirmation, the cognitive biases discussed earlier may, of course, be relevant here. The phenomenon of emotional reasoning appears to be especially relevant to our understanding of hypochondriasis. The feared sensations are not followed by any catastrophe, but they are followed by intense anxiety. Given that anxious patients take the occurrence of anxiety as evidence for the presence of danger, beliefs may be strengthened by the very fear to which the beliefs give rise.[98] Other cognitive biases may also serve to maintain the disorder.[90] Selective attention to threat reinforces the experience of living in a threatening environment and selectively remembering negative experiences may foster hopelessness. Interpretation biases may provide subjective evidence that the disturbing beliefs are valid.

Causality and clinical relevance

The issue of causality of beliefs to behaviour and emotions can be treated not only as a philosophical topic, but also as a straightforward empirical issue. If beliefs are causal to pathology, normal subjects should show pathology-related behaviour and emotions once they are experimentally made to endorse the beliefs held by patients. In contrast, reducing the credibility of irrational beliefs in patients should result in a reduction of symptomatology. If the beliefs are rejected altogether, pathology should disappear. There is some evidence that allows for an evaluation of the causal status and (hence) clinical relevance of problem-related beliefs in neurotic disorders.

When healthy subjects are made to believe, as panic patients do, that particular bodily sensations predict harm, they immediately become anxious upon experiencing these sensations.[117] Likewise, normal subjects tend not to become anxious during lactate infusion, whereas panic patients do so. But once normal subjects are made to believe that lactate infusion is a highly aversive experience, they become extremely upset during the infusion.[118] Some authors[119] have pointed out that a certain type of appraisal bias known as thought–action fusion underlies the aetiology of pathological obsessions. Briefly, thought–action fusion refers to an overevaluation of intrusive thoughts, such that unwanted thoughts are appraised as equivalents of unwanted actions. An example would be the belief that unacceptable thoughts are as bad as the actual actions they describe. It is easy to see how thought–action fusion could contribute to an inflated sense of responsibility and, eventually, to suppression and neutralization attempts. A recent study explored the effects of experimentally induced thought–action fusion. Students underwent a bogus

EEG recording session. The experimental group were informed that the apparatus was able to pick up the word 'apple' and that thinking of that word could result in the administration of electrical shocks to a person in an adjacent room. The control group were only told that the EEG equipment was sensitive to 'reading' simple words such as 'apple'. After having spent 15 min in the EEG laboratory, students completed a short questionnaire about the characteristics (e.g. frequency, aversiveness) of the target word (i.e. apple). Results showed that students in the experimental group reported a higher frequency of target thoughts, more discomfort, and a greater urge to suppress compared with control students. These findings are consistent with the idea that thought–action fusion promotes intrusive thinking.[120]

Even more relevant may be the numerous experiments indicating that reducing the credibility of catastrophic misconceptions greatly reduces the panicogenic effects of so-called pharmacological challenge tests in panic disorder. Pharmacological interventions such as lactate infusion or CO_2 inhalation induce salient bodily sensations in both normal subjects and panic patients. Panic patients believe that these sensations predict harm, while normal subjects do not. If, prior to the challenge, panic patients are reassured about the procedure by a careful explanation of the nature of the sensations to be experienced, by giving them the illusion that there are in control, or by greatly increasing the predictability of what will happen, the challenge become far less frightening and panic attacks are blocked.[121,122]

Yet another demonstration of the causal role of beliefs in psychopathology is provided by an experiment by Lopatka and Rachman.[123] Obsessive–compulsive patients are known to believe that they are excessively responsible for the catastrophes that may happen if they make a mistake in a specific area, which varies from patient to patient. They feel uncomfortable if they are not very sure that they undertook every possible action to reduce their responsibility and compulsively check, wash, or perform other rituals to ensure that they did not play a role in bringing about any misfortune to others or to themselves. Lopatka and Rachman[123] asked obsessive–compulsive patients to sign contracts that stated that the experimenter took all responsibility for possible harmful consequences following a specific action of the patients which usually elicited discomfort and compulsive behaviours. Compared with those who had signed neutral contracts, not only the feelings of responsibility, but also the urge to check, discomfort, and related variables, were significantly lower when the patient had signed the contract in which the experimenter took all responsibility. When the contract stated that all responsibility was given to the patient, perceived responsibility increased compared with those who had signed neutral contracts, and obsessive–compulsive complaints also tended to increase. This experiment demonstrated that obsessive–compulsive complaints can be increased or decreased by experimentally manipulating responsibility beliefs,.

If reducing the credibility of negative beliefs results in a reduction of pathology-related phenomena in the laboratory, the theoretical relevance may be clear: apparently, the manipulated beliefs play some role in the origin or maintenance of the pathology. Clinically much more interesting are the effects of reducing catastrophic beliefs outside the laboratory and in treatment settings. These efforts typically take the form of cognitive therapy for specific disorders. These interventions target specific beliefs assumed to be the cognitive nucleus of a certain disorder. The therapist identifies the specific content that the supposed pathogenic belief has for a certain patient, while the tactical aim of the therapist is to have these beliefs replaced by less irrational and less invalidating ones. From the assumed causal status of such beliefs it follows that cognitive therapy should be uniquely effective.

Of course it would be incorrect to infer aetiology from treatment effects. However positive, it can never be ruled out that the effectiveness of cognitive therapy, or any other biological or psychological treatment, may result from other processes than the ones that were intended to target. What can be said however, is that failures of cognitive therapy would have posed huge problems for the underlying theory. So far, the literature shows that cognitive theories rank among the most effective treatment for psychopathological problems.[124–128]

Summary

This chapter has been organized around three psychological perspectives on psychiatric problems: biological psychology, information processing approaches, and the cognitive psychology of beliefs. These perspectives reflect three hierarchically related levels on which psychiatric problems can be studied. Human information processing presupposes neural hardware, and beliefs presuppose information processing. When psychiatric phenomena are to be explained in psychological terms, they should be reduced to underlying psychological processes. It is often assumed that the further this reduction is taken, the more respectable and fundamental theories become. On this view, theories focusing on beliefs would be relatively superficial, while theories about neural hardware would be relatively fundamental, if not 'the real thing'. We shall not enter the somewhat philosophical discussion about the merits and necessity of reduction, but reiterate that we do not share the view that the quality of explanations critically depend on the degree of reduction. Rather, it is suggested that the optimal degree of reduction is pragmatic, i.e. the degree of reduction should be dictated by what scientific stance offers the best opportunities for prediction and experimental manipulation of psychopathological phenomena. After all, it would be hard to defend that a certain psychological perspective is superficial when it allows for effective prediction and intervention. The other way round, it would be problematic to claim that perspectives that do not result in precise prediction and intervention nevertheless offer profound understanding.

The merits of neuroscientific contributions to psychiatry are extensively discussed elsewhere in this volume. Technological developments in the field of neuroimaging offer tantalizing prospects of relating disordered behaviour to its neural hardware. It will be particularly interesting to find out what neurophysiological patient–control differences reflect emotions and cognitions of patients, and what brain characteristics represent true pathophysiology. In obsessive–compulsive disorder, for instance, positron emission tomography (**PET**) scans reveal distinctive brain changes. These changes disapear after successful treatment of obsessive–compulsive disorder, no matter whether the treatment is pharmacological or behavioural.[55] Of course, this suggests that the observed PET scan deviations reflect, rather than cause, obsessive–compulsive pathology. The implication is that normal subjects who are, experimentally, made to feel, think, and act like obsessive–compulsive patients will display the same abnormalities found in patients. Studies like these will no doubt be undertaken and most probably a differentiated picture will occur: just as differences between patients and controls in beliefs may or may not be epiphenomena, visualized differences in brain function may or may not be a mere reflection, rather than a biological cause, of the disorder. Happily, these issues are empirical and can and will be solved by obtaining controlled data.

Theories and paradigms from information-processing approaches have been applied to a wide range of psychopathological phenomena. The emphasis in this chapter was on the selective processing of emotionally valent information. Distinguishing between processing of neutral and negatively valenced information proved to be fruitful; a number of robust processing biases, related to the emotional valence of the information, were identified. There are some indications that such processing biases serve to maintain psychiatric disorders. For instance, relapse after behaviour therapy could be predicted from the tendency of successfully treated patients to see illusory correlations between phobic cues and harm.[93] Also, the occurrence of anxious and depressive problems after severe life stress could be predicted from a tendency to attend selectively to threatening material that was unconsciously perceived.[65]

While explanation of neurotic disorders in terms of beliefs is at odds with popular views about egodystony, the unreliability of introspection, and the epiphenomenal status of beliefs, such 'intentional' explanations have proved remarkably successful. Not only did they generate successful laboratory research, but their clinical implications are straightforward and have made effective treatments available for bulimia, anxiety disorders, and depression, for example.[124–126] Cognitive therapies have recently been developed even for notoriously difficult disorders such as schizophrenia,and results from controlled trials are quite encouraging.[129,130]

In clinical psychology, a distinction is commonly made between causal processes in the origin of disorders (aetiology and pathogenesis) and causal factors involved in their maintenance. As to the aetiology, progress in behavioural genetics and in the identification and measurement of stable individual differences in temperament have indicated traits that act as vulnerability factors for the development of psychopathology. In the area of anxiety and affective disorders, so-called 'negative affectivity' is of particular relevance. Meanwhile, although negative affectivity, or 'neuroticism' contributes to the develoment of pathology and while patients with anxiety or affective disorders almost invariably score in the extremes of negative affectivity, the vast majority of people high in negative affectivity do not suffer from Axis I disorders. There is very little data to indicate under what conditions some people at risk develop maladaptive and negative schemas about the self, others, and the outside world. Far more is known about how such schemas or beliefs, once established, are maintained. Processing biases and avoidance, escape, and safety behaviour may act in concert to maintain neurotic disorders. No doubt this picture is very incomplete, but it covers much of the existing data, it has a good record when it comes to experimental validation, and it has therapeutic implications that are encouragingly effective.

References

1. Shepherd, M. (1993). The placebo: from specificity to the non-specific and back. *Psychological Medicine*, **23**, 569–78.
2. Peterson, F. and Jung, C.G. (1970). Psychophysical investigations with the galvanometer and pneumograph in normal and insane individuals. *Brain*, **30**, 153–218.
3. Kessler, R.C., McGonagle, K.A., Shanyang, Z., *et al.*(1994). Lifetime and 12-month prevalence of DSM-II-R psychiatric disorders in the United States. *Archives of General Psychiatry*, **51**, 8–13.
4. Nisbett, R.E. and Wilson, T.D. (1977). Telling more than we can know: verbal reports on mental processes. *Psychological Review*, **84**, 231–59.
5. Schacter, D.L., Kagan, J., and Leichtman, M.D. (1995). True and false memories in children and adults: a cognitive science perspective. *Psychology, Public Policy and Law*, **1**, 411–28.
6. Neisser, U. (1967). *Cognitive psychology*. Appleton-Century-Crofts, New York.
7. Arens, K. (1996). Wilhelm Griesinger: psychiatry between philosophy and praxis. *Philosophy, Psychiatry and Psychology*, **3**, 148–52.
8. van Praag, H. (1993). *Make believes in psychiatry or the perils of progress*, p. 7. Bruner-Mazel, New York.
9. Gray, J.A. (1982). *The neuropsychology of anxiety. An enquiry into the functions of the septo-hippocampal system*. Clarendon Press, Oxford.
10. LeDoux, J.E. (1996). *The emotional brain.* Simon and Schuster, New York.
11. Oatley, K. and Jenkins, J.M. (1996). *Understanding emotions*. Blackwell, Cambridge, MA.
12. Damasio, A.R. (1994). *Descartes' error*. Putnam, New York.
13. Hugdahl, K. (1989). Human Pavlovian aversive conditioning: effects of brain asymmetry and stimulus lateralization. In *Aversion, avoidance, and anxiety: perspectives on aversively motivated behavior* (ed. T. Archer and L.G. Nilsson), pp. 145–7. Erlbaum, Hillsdale, NJ.
14. Wittling, W. (1996). Brain asymmetry in the control of autonomic–physiological activity. In *Brain asymmetry* (ed. R.J. Davidson and K. Hugdahl), pp. 305–57. MIT Press, Cambridge, MA.
15. Davidson, R.J. (1992). Anterior cerebral asymmetry and the nature of emotion. *Brain and Cognition*, **20**, 125–51.
16. Heller, W. and Nitschke, J.B. (1998). The puzzle of regional brain activity in depression and anxiety: the importance of subtypes and comorbidity. *Cognition and Emotion*, **12**, 421–47.
17. Davidson, R.J. and Fox, N. (1989). Frontal brain asymmetry predicts infants'response to maternal separation. *Journal of Abnormal Psychology*, **98**, 127–31.
18. Tomarken, A.J., Davidson, R.J., and Henriques, J.B. (1990). Resting frontal brain asymmetry predicts affective responses to films. *Journal of Personality and Social Psychology*, **59**, 791–801.
19. Hosking, S.G., Marsh, N.V., and Friedman, P.J. (1996). Poststroke depression: prevalence, course, and associated factors. *Neuropsychology Review*, **6**, 107–33.
20. Davidson, R.J. (1998). Affective style and affective disorders: perspectives from affective neuroscience. *Cognition and Emotion*, **12**, 307–30.
21. Tomarken, A.J. and Keener, A.D. (1988). Frontal brain asymmetry and depression: a self-regulatory perspective. *Cognition and Emotion*, **12**, 387–420.
22. Bruder, G.E., Stewart, J.W., Mercier, M.A., *et al.* (1997). Outcome of cognitive-behavioral therapy for depression: relation to hemispheric dominance for verbal processing. *Journal of Abnormal Psychology*, **106**, 138–44.
23. Zuckerman, M. (1995). Good and bad humors: biochemical bases of personality and its disorders. *Psychological Science*, **6**, 325–32.
24. Costa, P.T. and McCrae, R.R. (1992). *Neo-PI-R: revised personality inventory*. Psychological Assessment Resources, Odessa, FL.
25. Gray, J.A. (1987). Discussions arising from Cloninger, C.R. A unified biosocial theory of personality and its role in the development of anxiety states. *Psychiatric Developments*, **4**, 377–94.
26. Zuckerman, M. (1994). *Behavioral expressions and biosocial bases of sensation seeking*. Cambridge University Press, New York.
27. Andrews, G., Stewart, G., Allen, R., and Henderson, A.S. (1990). The genetics of six neurotic disorders: a twin study. *Journal of Affective Disorder*, **19**, 23–9.
28. Craske, M.G. (1997). Fear and anxiety in children and adolescents. *Bulletin of the Menninger Clinic*, **61**, 4–36.

29. Kagan, J., Reznick, J.S., Clarke, C., Snidman, N., and Garcia-Coll, C. (1984). Behavioral inhibition to the unfamiliar. *Child Development*, **55**, 2212–25.

30. Biederman, J., Rosenbaum, J.F., Chaloff, J., and Kagan, J. (1995). Behavioural inhibition as a risk factor for anxiety disorders. In *Anxiety disorders in children and adolescents* (ed. J.S. March), pp. 61–81. Guilford Press, New York.

31. Schmidt, L.A., Fox, N.A., Sternberg, E.M., Gold, P.W., Smith, C.C., and Schulkin, J. (1997). Behavioral and neuroendocrine responses in shy children. *Developmental Psychobiology*, **30**, 127–40.

32. Vrana, R.J., Spence, E.L., and Lang, P.J. (1988). The startle probe response: a new measure of emotion? *Journal of Abnormal Psychology*, **97**, 487–91.

33. Grillon, C., Dierker, L., and Merikangas, K.R. (1997). Startle modulation in children at risk for anxiety disorders and/or alcoholism. *Journal of the American Academy of Child and Adolescent Psychiatry*, **36**, 925–32.

34. Clark, L.A., Watson, D., and Mineka, S. (1994). Temperament, personality, and the mood and the anxiety disorders. *Journal of Abnormal Psychology*, **103**, 103–16.

35. Schulman, P., Keith, D., and Seligman, M.P. (1993). Is optimism heritable? A study of twins. *Behaviour Research and Therapy*, **31**, 569–74.

36. Hollon, S., Evans, M., and DeRubeis, R. (1990). Cognitive mediation of relapse prevention following treatment for depression: implications for differential risk. In *Psychological aspects of depression* (ed. R. Ingram), pp. 117–36. Plenum Press, New York.

37. Iacono, W.G. and Ficken, J.W. (1989). Research strategies employing psychophysiological measures: identifying and using psychophysiological markers. In *Handbook of clinical psychophysiology* (ed. G. Turpin), pp. 45–70. Wiley, Chichester.

38. Turpin, G. (1989). An overview of clinical psychophysiological techniques: tools or theories? In *Handbook of clinical psychophysiology* (ed. G. Turpin), pp. 3–44. Wiley, Chichester.

39. van Praag, H.M., Kahn, R., Asnis, G.M., *et al.* (1987). Denosologization of biological psychiatry or the specificity of 5-HT disturbances in psychiatric disorders. *Journal of Affective Disorders*, **13**, 1–8.

40. Hultman, C.M., Öhman, A., Ohlund, L.S., Wieselgren, I.-M., and Lindstrom, L.H. (1996). Electrodermal activity and social network as predictors of outcome of episodes in schizophrenia. *Journal of Abnormal Psychology*, **105**, 626–36.

41. Katsanis, J. and Iacono, W.G. (1994). Electrodermal activity and clinical status in chronic schizophrenia. *Journal of Abnormal Psychology*, **103**, 777–83.

42. Junginger, J. and Rauscher, F.P. (1987). Vocal activity in verbal hallucinations. *Journal of Psychiatric Research*, **21**, 101–9.

43. Bentall, R.P. (1990). The illusion of reality: a review and integration of psychological research on hallucinations. *Psychological Bulletin*, **107**, 82–95.

44. David, A.S. (1994). The neuropsychological origins of auditory hallucinations. In *The neuropsychology of schizophrenia* (ed. A.S. David and J.C. Cutting), pp. 269–313. Erlbaum, Hove.

45. Frith, C.D. (1992). *The cognitive neuropsychology of schizophrenia*. Erlbaum, Hillsdale, NJ.

46. Chapman, L.J. and Chapman, J.P. (1973). *Disordered thought in schizophrenia*, p. 224. Appleton-Century-Crofts, New York.

47. Strauss, M.E. (1993). Relations of symptoms to cognitive deficits in schizophrenia. *Schizophrenia Bulletin*, **19**, 215–31.

48. Foster Green, M. (1993). Cognitive remediation in schizophrenia: is it time yet? *American Journal of Psychiatry*, **150**, 178–87.

49. Lang, P.J., Bradley, M.M., and Cuthbert, B.N. (1992). A motivational analysis of emotion: reflex–cortex connections. *Psychological Science*, **3**, 44–9.

50. O'Brien, J.T. (1997). The glucocorticoid cascade hypothesis in man. *British Journal of Psychiatry*, **170**, 199–201.

51. Magnusson, D. and Öhman, A. (1987). *Psychopathology: an interactional perspective*. Academic Press, Orlando, FL.

52. Harrop, C.E., Trower, P., and Mitchell, I.J. (1996). Does the biology go around the symptoms? A Copernican shift in schizophrenia paradigms. *Clinical Psychology Review*, **16**, 641–54.

53. Miller, G.A. (1995). How we think about cognition, emotion, and biology in psychopathology. *Psychophysiology*, **33**, 615–28.

54. Weiss, J.M., Simson, P.G., Ambrose, M.J., Webster, A., and Hoffman, L.J. (1985). Neurochemical basis of behavioral depression. *Advances in Behavioral Medicine*, **1**, 253–75.

55. Baxter, L., Schwartz, J.M., Bergman, K.S., *et al.* (1992). Caudate glucose metabolic rate changes with both drug and behaviour therapy for obsessive–compulsive disorders. *Archives of General Psychiatry*, **49**, 681–9.

56. Hornstein, G.A. (1992). The return of the repressed: psychology's problematic relations with psychoanalysis. *American Psychologist*, **47**, 254–63.

57. Mandler, G. (1996). The situation of psychology: landmarks and choicepoints. *American Journal of Psychology*, **109**, 1–35.

58. Eysenck, H.J. (1987). Behavior therapy. In *Theoretical foundations of behavior therapy* (ed. H.J. Eysenck and I. Martin), pp. 3–35. Plenum Press, New York.

59. Dember, W.N. (1974). Motivation and the cognitive revolution. *American Psychologist*, **29**, 161–8.

60. Shakow, D. (1977). *Schizophrenia: selected papers*. International Universities Press, New York.

61. Brewin, C. (1988). *Cognitive foundations of clinical psychology*. Erlbaum, Hove.

62. Mineka, S. and Sutton, S.K. (1992). Cognitive biases and the emotional disorders. *Psychological Science*, **3**, 65–9.

63. Williams, J.M.G., Watts, F.N., MacLeod, C., and Mathews, A. (1997). *Cognitive psychology and emotional disorders*. Wiley, Chichester.

64. McNally, J.M. (1995). Automaticity and the anxiety disorders. *Behaviour Research and Therapy*, **33**, 747–54.

65. MacLeod, C. and Hagan, R. (1992). Individual differences in the selective processing of threatening information and emotional responses to a stressful life event. *Behaviour Research and Therapy*, **30**, 151–61.

66. MacLeod, C. and Rutherford, E. (1992). Anxiety and the selective processing of emotional information. Mediating roles of awareness, trait and state variables and personal relevance of stimulus materials. *Behaviour Research and Therapy*, **30**, 479–91.

67. van den Hout, M.A., Tenney, N., Huygens, K., Merckelbach, H., and Kindt, M. (1995). Responding to subliminal threat cues is related to trait anxiety and emotional vulnerability: a successful replication of MacLeod and Hagan (1992). *Behaviour Research and Therapy*, **33**, 451–4.

68. van den Hout, M.A., Tenney, N., Huygens, K., and de Jong, P.J. (1997). Preconscious processing bias in specific phobia. *Behaviour Research and Therapy*, **35**, 29–34.

69. Mogg, K., Bradley, B.P., Williams, R. and Mathews, A. (1993). Subliminal processing of emotional information in anxiety and depression. *Journal of Abnormal Psychology*, **102**, 304–11.

70. Öhman, A. and Soares, J.J.F. (1994). 'Unconscious anxiety': phobic responses to masked stimuli. *Journal of Abnormal Psychology*, **103**, 304–11.

71. Mineka, S. and Gilboa, E. (1998). Cognitive biases in anxiety and depression. In *Emotions in psychopathology: theory and research* (ed. W.F. Flack Jr and J.D. Laird), pp. 216–29. Oxford University Press, New York.

72. Lavy, E.H. and van den Hout, M.A. (1993). Attentional bias for appetitive cues: effects of fasting in normal subjects. *Behavioural and Cognitive Psychotherapy*, **21**, 297–310.

73. Lavy, E.H., van den Hout, M.A., and Arntz, A. (1993). Attentional bias and facilitated escape: a pictorial test. *Advances in Behaviour Research Therapy*, **15**, 279–89.

74. Mattia, J.I., Heimberg, R.G., and Hope, D.A. (1993). The revised Stroop color-naming task in social phobics. *Behaviour Research and Therapy*, **31**, 305–15.

75. Mathews, A.M., Mogg, K., Kentish, J., and Eysenck, M. (1995). Effects of

psychological treatment on cognitive bias in generalised anxiety disorder. *Behaviour Research and Therapy*, **33**, 293–303.

76. Wells, A., White, J., and Carter, K. (1997). Attention training: effects on anxiety and beliefs in panic and social phobia. *Clinical Psychology and Psychotherapy*, **4**, 226–32.

77. Blaney, P.H. (1986). Affect and memory: a review. *Psychological Bulletin*, **99**, 229–46.

78. Teasdale, J.D. (1983). Negative thinking in depression: cause, effect, or reciprocal relationship. *Advances in Behaviour Research and Therapy*, **5**, 3–25.

79. Bower, G.H. (1987). Commentary on mood and memory. *Behaviour Research and Therapy*, **25**, 443–55.

80. Williams, J.M.G. (1992). Autobiographical memory and emotional disorders. In *The handbook of emotion and memory. Research and theory* (ed. S.A. Christianson), pp. 451–77. Erlbaum, Hillsdale, NJ.

81. Evans, J., Williams, J.M.G., O'Loughlin, S., and Howless, K. (1992). Autobiographical memory and problem solving strategies of parasuicide patients. *Psychological Medicine*, **22**, 399–405.

82. Brittlebank, A.D., Scott, J., Williams, J.M., and Ferrier, I.N. (1993). Autobiographical memory in depression: state or trait marker? *British Journal of Psychiatry*, **162**, 118–21.

83. Kuyken, W. and Brewin, C.R. (1995). Autobiographical memory functioning in depression and reports of early abuse. *Journal of Abnormal Psychology*, **104**, 585–91.

84. Cahill, L., Prins, B., Weber, M., and McCaugh, J.L. (1994). Beta-adrenergic activation and memory for emotional events. *Nature*, **371**, 702–4.

85. Roediger, H.L. (1990). Implicit memory. Retention without remembering. *American Psychologist*, **45**, 1043–56.

86. Mathews, A., Richards, A., and Eysenck, M.W. (1989). Interpretations of homophones related to threat in anxiety states. *Journal of Abnormal Psychology*, **98**, 31–4.

87. Eysenck, M.W., Mogg, K., May, J., Richards, A., and Mathews, A. (1991). Bias in interpretation of ambiguous sentences related to threat in anxiety. *Journal of Abnormal Psychology*, **100**, 144–50.

88. Butler, G. and Mathews, A. (1987). Anticipatory anxiety and risk perception. *Cognitive Therapy and Research*, **11**, 551–65.

89. Da Calvo, M.G., Eysenck, M.W., and Castillo, M.D. (1997). Interpretation bias in test anxiety: the time course of predictive inferences. *Cognition and Emotion*, **11**, 43–63.

90. Tomarken, A.J., Mineka, S., and Cook, M. (1989). Fear relevant selective associations and covariation bias. *Journal of Abnormal Psychology*, **98**, 381–94.

91. de Jong, P.J., Merckelbach, H., and Arntz, A. (1993). Covariation detection in treated and untreated spider phobics. *Journal of Abnormal Psychology*, **101**, 724–7.

92. de Jong, P.J., Merckelbach, H., and Arntz, A. (1995). Covariation bias in phobic women: the relationship between a priori expectancy, on-line expectancy, autonomic responding, and a posteriori contingency judgement. *Journal of Abnormal Psychology*, **104**, 55–62.

93. de Jong, P.J., van den Hout, M.A., and Merckelbach, H. (1995). Covariation bias and the return of fear. *Behaviour Research and Therapy*, **33**, 211–13.

94. de Jong, P.J., Merckelbach, H., and Arntz, A. (1991). Illusory correlation, on-line problability estimates, and electrodermal responding in a quasi-conditioning paradigm. *Biological Psychology*, **31**, 201–12.

95. Valins, S. (1974). Cognitive effects of false heart-rate feedback. *Journal of Personality and Social Psychology*, **4**, 400–8.

96. Clark, D.M. (1996). A cognitive approach to panic. *Behaviour Research and Therapy*, **34**, 461–70.

97. Ehlers, A., Margraf, J., Roth, W.T., Taylor, B., and Birbaumer, N. (1988). Anxiety induction by false heart rate feedback in patients with panic disorder. *Behaviour Research and Therapy*, **26**, 2–11.

98. Arntz, A., Rauner, M., and van den Hout, M.A. (1995). 'If I feel anxious, there must be danger': *ex-consequentia* reasoning in inferring danger in anxiety disorders. *Behaviour Research and Therapy*, **33**, 917–25.

99. Loftus, E.F. and Klinger, M.R. (1992). Is the unconscious smart of dumb? *American Psychologist*, **47**, 761–5.

100. Greenwald, A.G. (1992). New look 3. Unconscious cognition reclaimed. *American Psychologist*, **47**, 766–79.

101. Enright, S.J. (1996). Forwards, backwards, and sideways: progress in OCD research. In *Current controversies in the anxiety disorders* (ed. R.M. Rapee), pp. 206–13. Guilford Press, New York.

102. Arntz, A., Lavy, E., van den Berg, G., and van Rijsoort, S. (1993). Negative beliefs of spider phobics: a psychometric evaluation of the spider phobia beliefs questionnaire. *Advances in Behaviour Research and Therapy*, **15**, 257–77.

103. Clark, D.M. and Wells, A. (1995). A cognitive model of social phobia. In *Social phobia—diagnosis, assessment and treatment* (ed. R. Heimberg, M. Liebowitz, D.A. Hope, and F.R. Schneier), pp. 69–93. Guilford Press, New York.

104. Rapee, R.M. and Lim, L. (1992). Discrepancy between self- and observer ratings of performance in social phobics. *Journal of Abnormal Psychology*, **101**, 728–31.

105. Stopa, L. and Clark, D.M. (1993). Cognitive processes in social phobia. *Behaviour Research and Therapy*, **31**, 255–67.

106. Arntz, A., Dietzel, R., and Dreessen, L. (1999). Specificity and stability of cognitive assumptions in borderline personality disorder and their relationship with childhood traumas. *Behaviour Research and Therapy*, **37**, 545–57.

107. Beck, A.T., Brown, G., Steer, R.A., Eidelson, J.I., and Riskind, J.H. (1987). Differentiating anxiety and depression: a test of cognitive content-specificity hypothesis. *Journal of Abnormal Psychology*, **96**, 179–83.

108. Chambless, D.L., Caputo, G.C., Bright, P., and Gallagher, R. (1984). Assessment of fear in agoraphobics: the body sensations questionnaire and the agoraphobic cognitions questionnaire. *Journal of Consulting and Clinical Psychology*, **52**, 1090–7.

109. Norton, G.R., Harison, B., Hauch, D., and Rhodes, L. (1985). Characteristics of people with infrequent panic attacks. *Journal of Abnormal Psychology*, **94**, 216–21.

110. McNally, R.M. (1994). *Panic disorder. A critical analysis*. Guilford Press, New York.

111. Ponds, R.W.H.M. and Jolles, J. (1996). Memory complaints in elderly people: the role of memory abilities, metamemory, depression, and personality. *Educational Gerontology*, **22**, 341–57.

112. Rachman, S. and DeSilva, P. (1978). Abnormal and normal obsessions. *Behaviour Research and Therapy*, **16**, 233–48.

113. Salkovskis, P.M. and Harrison, J. (1984). Abnormal and normal obsessions: a replication. *Behaviour Research and Therapy*, **22**, 549–52.

114. Ehlers, A. and Skil, R. (1995). Maintenance of intrusive memories in posttraumatic stress disorder: a cognitive approach. *Behavioural and Cognitive Psychotherapy*, **13**, 217–49.

115. Wells, A. (1995). Meta-cognition and worry: a cognitive model of generalized anxiety disorder. *Behavioural and Cognitive Psychotherapy*, **23**, 301–20.

116. Romme, M.A.J. and Escher, A.D. (1988). Hearing voices. *Schizophrenia Bulletin*, **15**, 209–15.

117. Salkovskis, P.M. and Clark, D.M. (1990). Affective responses to hyperventilation: a test of the cognitive model of panic. *Behaviour Research and Therapy*, **28**, 15–28.

118. van der Molen, G.M., van den Hout, M.A., Vroemen, J., Lousberg, H., and Griez, E. (1986). Cognitive derminants of lactate induced anxiety. *Behaviour Research and Therapy*, **24**, 677–80.

119. Rachman, S. (1997). A cognitive theory of obsessions. *Behavioural Research and Therapy*, **35**, 793–802.

120. Rassin, E., Merckelbach, H., Muris, P. and Spaan (1999). Thought–action fusion as a causal factor in the development of intrusions. *Behaviour Research and Therapy*, **37**, 231–7.

121. van den Hout, M.A. (1988). The explanation of experimental panic. In *Panic: psychological perspectives* (ed. S. Rachman and J.D. Maser), pp. 237–58. Erlbaum, Hillsdale, NJ.

122. Clark, D.M. (1993). Cognitive mediation of panic attacks induced by biological challenge tests. *Advances in Behaviour Research and Therapy,* **15,** 75–84.

123. Lopatka, C. and Rachman, S. (1995). Perceived responsibility and compulsive checking: an experimental analysis. *Behaviour Research and Therapy,* **33,** 673–84.

124. Chambless, D.L. and Gillis, M.M. (1993). Cognitive therapy of anxiety disorders. *Journal of Consulting and Clinical Psychology,* **61,** 248–60.

125. DeRubeis, R.J. and Crits-Christoph, P. (1998). Empirically supported individual and group psychological treatments for adult mental disorders. *Journal of Consulting and Clinical Psychology,* **66,** 37–52.

126. Gloaguen, V., Cottraux, J., Cuchedrat, M., and Blackburn, I.M. (1998). A meta-analysis of the effects of cognitive therapy in depressed patients. *Journal of Affective Disorders,* **49,** 59–72.

127. Roth, A. and Fonagy, P. (1996). *What works for whom? A critical review of psychotherapy.* Guilford Press, New York.

128. Smith, M.L., Glass, G.V., and Miller, T.I. (1980). *The benefits of psychotherapy.* Johns Hopkins University Press, Baltimore, MD.

129. Fowler, D., Garety, P., and Kuipers, E. (1998). Cognitive therapy for psychosis: formulation, treatment, effects and service implications. *Journal of Mental Health UK,* **7,** 123–33.

130. Haddock, G., Morrison, A.P., Hopkins, R., Lewis, S., and Tarrier, N. (1998). Individual cognitive-behavioural interventions in early psychosis. *British Journal of Psychiatry,* **173,** 101–6.

2.6 The contribution of social sciences

2.6.1 Medical sociology and issues of aetiology

George W. Brown

Introduction

David Mechanic, in his pioneering textbook, *Medical Sociology,*[1] views human activity within an adaptive framework—as a struggle of human beings to control their environment and life situation. Whilst this view informs the research to be outlined, there are a number of ways it differs in emphasis from much medical sociology. First, by its concern with particular disorders defined in medical terms. Second, by its emphasis on the use of the investigator rather than respondent to characterize phenomena—to decide, for example, whether an incident should be classified as a life event or whether a person's account of sadness and tearfulness is sufficient to be classed as 'depressed mood'. Third, by its recognition that emotion needs to be taken into account if meaning of environmental happenings are to be assessed, since it is emotion that makes things matter for us: 'A world experienced without any affect would be a pallid, meaningless world. We would know that things happened, but we would not care whether they did or not'.[2] It is emotions that give us feedback about what is important and meaningful in our lives; about what is good or bad.[3,4] And finally by its emphasis on the need to take account of context. In order to grasp, for example, the likely meaning of an event such as a loss of a job it is essential to know whether it cast the person in a bad or humiliating light; its impact on the person's family; his or her chances of getting another job, and so on. It is such surrounding circumstances to an event such as loss of a job or a marital separation.that usually give it meaning via the emotion they help to create.

Context and measurement

Concern with context in the social sciences was central to the *Geisteswissenschaften* and the problem of meaning was discussed widely in Germany in the late nineteenth century.[5] The ideas were introduced into sociology by Max Weber[6] and into psychiatry by Karl Jaspers,[7] although none of these early writers showed how to apply the methods systematically to concrete examples.[8] Jaspers, in his *Allegemeine Psychopathologie*, emphasized the way in which *Verstehen*, or understanding, on the part of an investigator 'depends primarily on the tangible facts' (i.e. verbal contents, cultural factors, people's acts, ways of life

and expressive gestures) in terms of which the connection is understood, and which provides the objective data.[7] While this view influenced the approach to meaning in what follows, there is one major difference. No attempt has been made to extend the method to make a link between a particular set of circumstances so defined and the development of a particular psychiatric episode. The method is restricted to making a judgement about the likely meaning of a set of circumstances in the light of whatever 'tangible factors' about past and present appear relevant. Once this has been established, any link with disorder is explored using established scientific procedures.

As noted by Jaspers, it has been possible to take note of cultural factors; for example, when rating the likely implications of a birth, as part of research among women in a black township in Zimbabwe, we took into account the importance placed on a wife producing a male child for her husband and his family.[9]

A second, more limited, use of context deals with the actual observation of emotion.[10,11] The Camberwell Family Interview, by taking account of verbal and vocal aspects of speech, for example, considers how far a parent's talk about a son or daughter conveys 'criticism' rather than 'non-critical' dissatisfaction.[12,13] The relevant context is here limited to the interview itself and what this conveys about a person's emotional style.[14,15] In everyday life we automatically make allowances for the fact, say, that some people show warmth in a more open way and even expressed in an extroverted fashion, and, by taking this into account in the rating of expressed emotion, it is possible for quite disparate expressive styles to be counted as equivalent, for example in rating 'warmth'.

Such use of context makes it possible to take account of individual differences even when dealing with core sociological concepts. For example, working-class mothers in North London have been shown to differ substantially in commitment to roles such as 'mother' or 'wife'. This is judged by how enthusiastically activities typical of the roles are spoken about in an interview encouraging them to talk at length about their lives.

Some methodological considerations

These developments have enabled what are often seen as 'soft' variables to be quantified, and this in turn has allowed a reasonably persuasive case to be made that significant bias has not followed the use of the investigator as the primary measuring instrument. For example, Creed,[16] in a study of stressful life events and appendectomy, documented a relationship between severely threatening events rated contextually and the onset of non-inflamed but not inflamed conditions. The research was persuasive for two reasons. First, on the basis of a detailed description of the event and surrounding circumstances a consensus rating team reached agreement about the likely degree of threat of each life event, blind to the person's reported response and whether or not he or she was a patient. Second, the interviewer, who provided the team with this edited account was blind to clinical details. (He only consulted the medical records after the ratings had been made.) Such flexibility is difficult, if not impossible, with a questionnaire-based instrument which hands over the task of measurement to the respondent and because of this is in a much weaker position to deal with possible bias.

There are now a number of investigator-based instruments covering areas ranging from 'expressed emotion' (e.g. critical comments, warmth, etc.), attitudes to self (e.g. self-esteem), plans and concerns (e.g. commitment to various roles), behavioural systems (e.g. styles of attachment), experience of adversity in childhood (e.g. sexual and physical abuse), and characteristics of non-family groups (e.g. restrictiveness of a psychiatric ward regimen). Each of the instruments with their component scales can be used with some confidence because of the kind of methodological safeguards already noted and because a fair amount of replicable and theoretically relevant findings have emerged. Particularly important was the development in the 1960s of the clinically informed interview-based Present State Examination (**PSE**) by Wing et al.,[17] later amended to deal with a 12-month period,[18] and psychosocial measures such as that of 'expressed emotion'[12,13,15,19] and the Life Events and Difficulties Schedule.[20] Part of the strength of the resulting research has been due to the levels of inter-rater reliability achieved and the ability of the approach to deal with time order. It is frequently overlooked that even with longitudinal designs it is important to be able to establish time order about what has happened between interviews, for example whether a 'stressor' occurred before or after an onset of a disorder, and this is only possible by asking in detail about what has occurred.

Life events and building aetiological models

The characteristic features of the aetiological studies that have emerged with the development of such instruments can be illustrated by those dealing with life events (and to a lesser extent ongoing difficulties). While the Life Events and Difficulties Schedule is the most detailed and comprehensive instrument, it is only one of a variety that have been utilized. The significance of findings concerning depression is enhanced by the fact that most studies have produced broadly consistent findings about the role of events.[21–27] Indeed, for some years the challenge has been not so much to establish the presence of an effect due to life events, but to learn more about the nature of the events involved and to integrate findings into a more comprehensive aetiological model.[28]

In what follows, four questions concerning life events are discussed.

- Meaning: what makes them so critical?

- Vulnerability: what is the role of other current psychosocial factors?

- Lifespan: do experiences in childhood and adult life contribute to risk?

- A population perspective: what social factors are implicated when differences are found in rates of depression across populations?

The role of life events in the aetiology of depression

Measurement and meanings

The original version of the Life Events and Difficulties Schedule was developed to study schizophrenic episodes[29,30] and there has since been a large amount of research dealing with psychotic patients.[31] An early achievement was to make clear that the amount of change in activity as such brought about by a life event appears to be irrelevant and that the impact of events results from their meaning.[32] It has also been clear that some attention needs also to be given to ongoing difficulties that can either be brought about by an event (e.g. the death of husband leading to financial problems), or lead to an event (e.g. a marital difficulty eventually ending in a separation).

In dealing with meaning, two perspectives have proved productive. The first is summed up by the statement that we cannot fully know the meaning of an event or set of circumstances until we relate it in some manner to our concerns. One way of conceiving of such concerns is in terms of the impact of a particular event on plans and purposes that stem from role activity caught up in the crisis: how, for example, being turned down for rehousing by a local authority thwarts a woman's wish to move from an overcrowded and damp flat to give her children 'a better start in life'.

A second perspective assumes that evolutionary-based response patterns that help to guide us in terms of what to want or to avoid are often involved, and that such behavioural systems are sensitive to a particular range of stimuli. The attachment system and fear responses are obvious examples.[33] Of course, such responses will be influenced by individual differences of various kinds and by cultural display rules concerning emotions, but there is good reason to believe that such behavioural systems are often involved in the development of psychiatric disorders. For example, the central importance in a number of cultures of 'critical comments' rather than 'dissatisfaction' in a schizophrenic relapse probably reflects an evolutionary-based sensitivity to emotionally toned criticism interacting with some constitutional predisposition to the disorder.[34]

The Life Events and Difficulties Schedule deals with both kinds of meaning. Blind consensus ratings usually based on 4-point scales, made by several investigators are employed to rule out reporting artifacts using 'edited' accounts supplied by the person who carried out the interview. General as well as specific kinds of threat are rated in this way. They are contextual in the sense of taking into account a person's likely concerns of relevance for the event in so far as these can be assessed from a person's current circumstances and biography. In making such ratings no account is taken of reported feelings or whether or not a disorder followed the event. As already noted, it has been possible in this way to deal with possible bias on the part of raters. It also deals with the problem that the cognitive processes involved in the appraisal of an event are not necessarily ones a person is willing or able to report.[35] General guidelines for rating severity of threat are given in an extensive manual containing thousands of examples listed in terms of a number of event categories (such as

Table 1 Onset of depression within 6 months of a severe event or a severe difficulty among 303 women in Islington

	Percentage onset
Severe event	22 (29/130)
Severe difficulty and no severe event	5 (1/20)
Neither	1 (2/153)
Total	11 (32/303)

'demotion at work' and 'unplanned pregnancy'). A similar procedure is followed for difficulties.

Some findings

The first use of the Life Events and Difficulties Schedule to study depressive conditions took place in the early 1970s and involved a patient series seen at the Maudsley Hospital together with a random series of women from the local Camberwell population. All were aged between 18 and 65. A threshold of 'caseness' developed at that time reflected what an outpatient psychiatrist would accept as a 'case'.[18] This enquiry, and a number of subsequent ones, have established that the majority of episodes of clinical relevance are preceded by a severely threatening event.[20] Only events having long-term threat some 10 to 14 days later are considered for a severe rating. The presence of a severe ongoing difficulty has turned out to be of less significance. Nothing has so far emerged to suggest that events with only short-term threat play a role.

Table 1 gives a typical result from a prospective enquiry of 400 women living in Islington in North London with at least one child at home. The table shows the women who at the time of first contact did not qualify as cases of depression; 29 of the 32 onsets in the first follow-up year were preceded by at least one severe event in the prior 6 months with most occurring within a matter of weeks.[36] For example, a woman experiencing a second miscarriage after persistent attempts to have her first child would probably have the event rated severe, but a first miscarriage shortly after marriage would most likely be rated upsetting but not severely so.

This set of results emerged despite the use of contextual ratings of events that, as already made clear, are based on a limited amount of information and deliberately designed to be approximate and probabilistic. Moreover, it was possible to obtain more direct evidence about the relevance of plans and purposes. Their importance was confirmed by the use of a measure of commitment to a number of core roles made at the time of the first interview based on how they and the activities associated with them were talked about. Where a severe event (e.g. a child's delinquency) in the subsequent follow-up year 'matched' an area of high emotional commitment (e.g. to motherhood), risk of an onset was considerably increased when compared with a non-matching severe event.[36]

Specific meaning

The original contextual ratings of severity of threat have been used as a basis for taking account of more specific aspects of meaning. Severe events preceding an onset of depression generally involve loss, if this is defined broadly not only in terms of loss of a person but loss of a role or a cherished idea—the latter about oneself or someone close.[37] (In contrast, events preceding the onset of anxiety tend to involve 'danger'—the threat of future loss.) However, although loss is typically present it may not be the factor of central aetiological importance. Table 2 illustrates this by the development of a more comprehensive rating scheme—again carried out by the investigator. Four overall types of meaning are considered, covering in all nine categories. The ratings are hierarchical. Where more than one rating is possible the highest on the scale is taken. The first three categories concern possible types of **humiliation,** i.e. the likelihood of the event provoking a sense of being put down or a marked devaluation of self. The first category, for example, covers separating from a partner or a lover where they either took the initiative or the respondent was 'forced' to leave or break off a relationship because of violence or the discovery of infidelity.

Events associated with **entrapment,** the second main type, had to have failed to meet criteria for one of the three humiliation categories. Such events emphasized the fact of being imprisoned in a punishing situation that had gone on for some time. The third type deals with four kinds of **loss** (in the absence of humiliation or entrapment) with the final type, **danger,** involving threat of a future loss.[37]

The table shows whether a particular severe event (or sequence of closely related events) was followed by an onset, taking the event (or sequence) nearest the onset when there was more than one event within 6 months of onset. Using a 2-year period for the Islington women, it shows that there were large differences in risk by event type. If events involving humiliation are combined with those of entrapment, risk was increased threefold.[38] The relatively low risk associated with loss alone, except following a severe event involving a death, suggests that while the majority of depressogenic events involve loss,

Table 2 Onset by type of severe event over 2-year period in the Islington community series

Hierarchical event classification	No. of onsets	Percentage onset rate
(a) All 'humiliation' events	31/102	30
Humiliation: separation	12/34	35
Humiliation: other's delinquency	7/36	19
Humiliation: put down	12/32	38
(b) All 'trapped' alone events (i.e. not (a))	10/29	34
(c) All 'loss' alone events (i.e. not (a) or (b))	14/157	9
Death	7/24	29
Separation: subject initiated	2/18	11
Other key loss	4/58	7
Lesser loss	1/57	2
(d) All 'danger' alone events (i.e. not (a), (b), or (c))	3/89	3
All severe events	58/377	15

something more than this is usually involved and that the experience of humiliation or entrapment associated with the loss is often critical.

Diagnostic issues

So far only depressive onsets in the general population, almost entirely of a 'neurotic' kind, have been considered. In the Camberwell patient enquiry, while events were rather less frequent before 'melancholic' depression than before 'neurotic' depression, there was considerable overlap between the types of depression. This lack of a clear link between the presence of a provoking life event and diagnosis had been reported earlier[39] and also in several subsequent studies.[40,41]

A recent study of North London psychiatric patients has thrown possible light on this somewhat unexpected picture. When episode number was taken into account, those patients with both a melancholic/psychotic diagnosis and a prior episode of depression had a much smaller chance of experiencing a severe event before onset.[42] A patient series from Pittsburgh produced consistent findings.[43] These results, if confirmed, may also help to explain inconsistencies in published results since the proportion with a melancholic/psychotic picture and a prior episode is bound to vary by type of treatment centre.

It is of interest that the smaller number with provoking events as episode number rises has also been found to relate to the course of bipolar conditions where there is some evidence for a sensitization or kindling mechanism.[44] It is also of note that this same London study concluded that, despite detailed questioning, as many as one-tenth of patients with a 'neurotic' depressive disorder gave no hint of being provoked by social adversity of any kind.[42]

Course and remission

Life-event research has also thrown some light on the processes involved in remission or recovery from depression. Evidence has begun to emerge that these often involve the reverse of the process leading to onset. A positive event or the reduction in the level of a severe difficulty (with or without an event) is commonly found to have been present in the 20-week period before any remission (or marked improvement). However, it is of interest that although the events involved were rated contextually as likely to have given renewed hope about the future, one-third were at the same time judged as severely threatening.[45]

In the Islington general population series somewhat over half of the remissions of episodes that had lasted 20 weeks or more were preceded by such an event. There was no such link with episodes lasting less than this. In the patient series the result was much the same, although the chances of a positive event or difficulty reduction for those on antidepressant medication was somewhat less.[46]

A different approach to the issue of outcome concerns determinants of the length of a particular episode. Here the presence of severe interpersonal difficulty at the point of onset (but no other difficulty) was an important predictor of whether a depressive episode would go on to last for at least 1 year, and this held for both series.[47,48] (Much the same result in terms of chronicity held if the predictor was the presence of the difficulty throughout the episode.) Ongoing difficulties therefore need to be taken into account in terms both remission and in terms of whether an episode takes a chronic course.

Psychosocial vulnerability

The part played by severe events in depression has proved to be a particularly effective platform for exploring psychosocial vulnerability. The importance of this question was, in fact, illustrated in Table 1 where, despite the fact that the majority of onsets were preceded by a severe event, only one-fifth of those who experienced a severe event developed depression. While, as already discussed, taking account of event type somewhat reduces this ratio, it is still necessary to ask why only a minority go on to develop clinically relevant depression following a severe event.

In the Islington series, two background factors present at the time of the first interview proved highly predictive of onset during the following year: a negative psychological factor (negative evaluation of self or chronic anxiety or subclinical depressive symptoms) and a negative environmental factor (negative interaction with others in the home and in addition, for single mothers, lack of a close confidant seen fairly often).

Their predictive power can be judged by the fact that, while only 23 per cent of the women without depression at the time of first contact had both, three-quarters of onsets in the follow-up period occurred among these women.[49] The result has recently been broadly confirmed in a second prospective enquiry.[50]

In terms of an overall aetiological model, the predictive power of the two indices appears to be largely because they relate to a greater chance of both a severe event occurring and to a lack of effective emotional support from a close confidant once the event has occurred.[51–53] Consideration of social support, of course, links the research, with social science concepts such as 'social integration', 'social bond', and 'social alienation'.[54] The topic is too complex to pursue in any detail in the present brief review. Research has so far underlined the need to recognize that support at one point in time does not necessarily predict what will occur in a subsequent crisis and, indeed, that a significant aspect of a number of severe events is the fact they involve the withdrawal of social support that up to that point had largely been taken for granted.[55] There is also some indication that the ability of a woman to make supportive ties that can be used in a future crisis, and also to go on actually to use them in such circumstances, is adversely influenced by the early experience of childhood abuse and neglect.[56–58] Finally, the predictive power of these two 'negative' vulnerability factors is partly due to their link with lack of core support with a severe event in the follow-up year.

Figure 1, dealing with the Islington series, sums up research on the issue of vulnerability. It takes into account both event type and vulnerability and it shows that a severe event, however threatening, was not enough to provoke depression without the presence of at least one vulnerability factor. Subsequent research has confirmed this general picture, although it does indicate that on occasions it is possible for a severe event to provoke a depressive onset without the presence of one of the vulnerability factors.[53]

Gender differences

One issue not considered so far concerns gender. Most research on depression using the Life Events and Difficulties Schedule has dealt with women, although in the original Camberwell enquiry a small series of men gave similar results, as did a subsequent population enquiry.[59] However, recent research has gone further to suggest that the well-recognized greater risk of a depressive onset among women may well relate to their greater sensitivity to severe events involving their role as mothers. In a study of couples experiencing a severe event in common, women were twice as likely to develop a depressive episode following events involving procreation, children, and housing; for other events, risk was much the same.[60] While this research requires replication, it does support the increasingly held opinion that the large gender difference in the experience of 'neurotic' depression is likely to have an essentially psychosocial explanation.[61]

A lifespan perspective

So far only current environmental circumstances have been taken into account. The Camberwell research had also identified loss of a mother before the age of 11 as a risk factor.[62] While there has been a good deal of controversy about this finding,[57,62–65] two further population studies produced equally clear evidence with the added suggestion that such a loss between 11 and 17 may also increase risk.[57,62,66,67] The mode of the impact of such an early loss of mother for women is undoubtedly complex, but several studies have now established the critical importance of untoward experiences *after* the loss and have downplayed the role of loss as such.[57,62,66,67] It has been necessary to trace the history of a woman from the loss itself to any later experience of depression in a way that makes it possible to gain some sense of a life trajectory. Certain early experiences are particularly associated with the chance of experiencing one or another of the two risk factors already discussed.[57,66]

More important than the loss of the mother itself was the quality of replacement parental care after the loss (in terms of an index of parental indifference or lax control). Risk of adult depression was doubled for those positive on the index.

A factor playing a critical mediating role was the experience of a premarital pregnancy, and, like the care index itself, this was found to be associated with the subsequent experience of severe events.[32] What seemed to be crucial about these premarital pregnancies was that they often trapped women in relationships which they might well not otherwise have chosen and which became a source of ongoing problems—such as severe housing and financial difficulties consequent upon a couple starting a family too young to have built up adequate savings, or marital difficulties with undependable partners. These women also emerged as less upwardly mobile, in terms of social class, than their peers without such pregnancies. In interpreting this

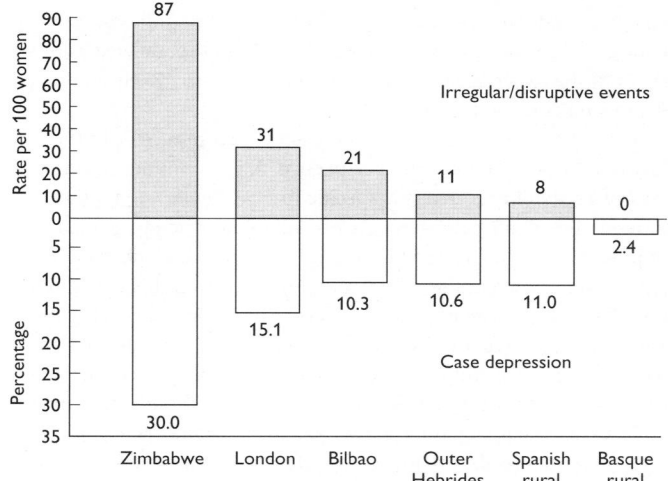

Fig. 2 Yearly rate of irregular or disruptive severe events per 100 women in six populations and prevalence of caseness of depression in year.

complex of experiences, a conveyor belt of adversities was outlined, on which some women often appeared to move inexorably from one crisis to another, starting with lack of care in childhood and passing via premarital pregnancy to current working-class status, lack of social support and high rates of severe events.[68]

Although it was often hard to see from the women's accounts of their lives how they could have left this conveyor belt once their childhood had located them on it, a more personal element is likely to have played a role in many instances. Here the work of Quinton and Rutter[69,70] has been particularly significant in developing a lifespan perspective in this regard, and over this issue the results of the two research programmes have largely complemented each other.[71,72]

The kind of early adverse experience just outlined was subsequently incorporated into a broader index of childhood adversity that included severe physical abuse within the family and also severe sexual abuse in any setting.[73] This index not only relates to a doubling of the risk of a depressive onset in adult life, but also to a number of other adverse outcomes, for example to the risk of an episode taking a chronic course (over and above risk, noted earlier, from a current severe interpersonal difficulty) and also to the risk of a depressive condition comorbid with anxiety disorder defined by DSM-IIIR criteria (excluding simple phobias and mild agoraphobia).[74]

A population perspective

In terms of the final of the four questions about events listed earlier, 'neurotic' conditions that form the bulk of depressive disorders, even in patient series, need to be considered in terms of a population perspective. Figure 2 summarizes the findings of six population studies of women aged between 18 and 65 carried out in a comparable manner, using the same semistructured interview-based measures as in the Islington survey, including the Present State Examination. The bottom half of Fig. 2 shows the rate of depressive caseness in a 12-month period. Between the two extreme populations there is a 10-fold difference—3 per cent in a rural Basque-speaking population in

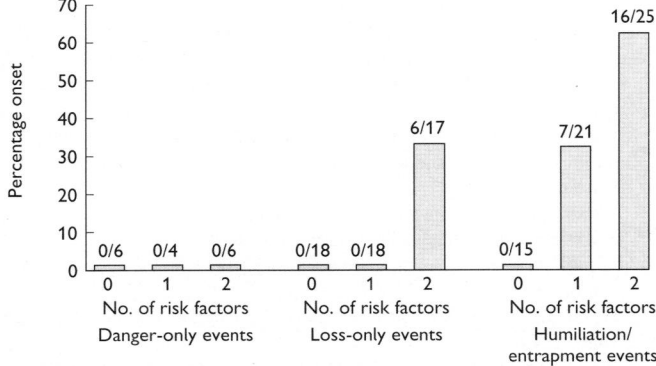

Fig. 1 Onset rate among 130 Islington women with a severe event by type of event and number of background risk factors.

Spain[75] and 30 per cent in a black urban population in Zimbabwe.[8,76] In addition these rates are fairly closely paralleled by differences in the experience of severe events particularly likely to provoke depression (see top half of Fig. 2).

One of the implications of these results becomes clear in the context of a behavioural genetic perspective. A key point about the concept of heritability is that it is specific to a particular population. The index is based on consideration of individual discrepancies from a population mean. While it is certainly possible that heritability for depression in each of the six populations is positive, this would reflect only the contribution of genetic factors to individual variability in risk within each population. Even if large, they would be unlikely to be of relevance for explaining the actual population differences in rates of depression. The most plausible interpretation of these is that the differences are essentially the result of psychosocial factors.

Differences in the frequency of relevant genes would need to be extremely large to explain such differences and in addition it now seems likely that significant secular changes in rates of depression are possible.[77–79] There is, however, no inherent conflict between the two perspectives—they refer to different ways of looking at the 'variance' of a condition.[80] The general point is that the study of individual variability within particular populations cannot rule out the possibility that the mean level of disorder is largely under environmental control; that it can be increased or decreased markedly by external changes quite uninfluenced by the genetic make-up of a population.

A population perspective is also concerned with variability in rates of disorder within populations in terms of social categories such as socio-economic status. Thus, the survey in Camberwell in South London in the early 1970s found that, while the rate of severe events was related to social class position, this explained comparatively little of the large class difference in prevalence of depression; of greater importance were background vulnerability factors such as an unsupportive marriage.[19] However, the picture has recently become more complex with the finding that severe events involving humiliation and entrapment are not only especially depressogenic but particularly common in high-risk populations (such as Harare) and within populations in high-risk subgroups (such as working-class women in London). In Islington such events were common among single mothers, a social category that has expanded dramatically in most Western populations in recent years and among whom there is a high risk of depression.[81]

Final comments

There are two ways of looking at the findings that have been reviewed. First, that the study of life events has been an effective way of opening up wider issues concerning the aetiology of depression—and, it can be added, other psychiatric conditions that have not been reviewed.[82–86] This has been possible because, given the presence of a substantial causal link, a platform is provided for the study of a whole range of other experiences. As research has progressed it has pushed back in time to consider the aetiological role of early experiences of neglect and abuse which can have event-like characteristics. In more general terms the study of events has led to consideration of issues of vulnerability and protection, event production, chronicity and course of particular episodes, and also issues not covered in this account such as coping and social support.

So far this kind of extension of life-event research has remained largely within the psychosocial realm, but potential ramifications are broader (for an exception concerning biological research see Calloway and Dolan[87]). In diagnostic terms, for example, it has raised issues concerning the role of kindling in explaining the lessening of the importance of stress in terms of episode number in onsets of melancholic/psychotic depressive conditions.

It has also been possible to isolate a small group of 'endogenous' neurotic depressive episodes. Such findings call out for collaborative research and hint at the possible advantage of taking into account of the aetiological models that have been developed around the event–onset link. Further, while this review has largely restricted itself to work on depression, the approach has been successfully employed with a number of other psychiatric and physical conditions and may prove of relevance for a wider range of issues in medical research such as 'illness behaviour' and the doctor–patient relationship.

The second contribution concerns insight about the depression–event link itself. This is a complex issue because depressogenic life events correlate with a whole range of factors ranging from genetic/personality[88] to macrolevel/societal.[89] However, the findings concerning events involving humiliation and entrapment may need to be viewed from an evolutionary perspective, i.e. that in some way a response pattern which has developed in group-living animals, closely linked to issues surrounding defeat and exclusion, may often be involved.[90] It is possible that clinically relevant depressive conditions are often a complication of essentially non-pathological submission and appeasement responses to defeat in group-living mammals.[81] Therefore the high rates of clinically relevant depression that appear to be possible in some populations may well be a result of the more highly developed cognitive developments of *Homo sapiens* together with the event-creating potential of many societies experiencing periods of marked social change due to factors such as war, industrialization, technological development, urbanization, changing sexual mores.

References

1. Mechanic, D. (1978). *Medical sociology* (2nd edn). Free Press, New York.
2. Tomkins, S.S. (1979). Script theory: differential magnification of affects. In *Nebraska symposium on motivations*, Vol. 26 (ed. H.E. Howe and R.A. Dienstbier), pp. 201–36. University of Nebraska Press, Lincoln, NE.
3. Gilbert, P. (1997). The biopsychosociology of meaning. In *The transformation of meaning in psychological therapies* (ed. M. Power and C.R. Brewin), pp. 33–56. Wiley, Chichester.
4. Greenberg, L.S. and Pascual-Leone (1997). Emotion in the creation of personal meaning. In *The transformation of meaning in psychological therapies* (ed. M. Power and C.R. Brewin), pp. 193–208. Wiley, Chichester.
5. Bolton, D. and Hill, J. (1996). Mind, meaning and mental disorder. *The nature of causal explanation in psychology and psychiatry.* Oxford University Press.
6. Weber, M. (1964). *The theory of social and economic organisation* (ed. and trans. T. Parsons). Collier-Macmillan, London.
7. Jaspers, K. (1962). *General psychopathology* (trans. J. Hoenig and M.W. Hamilton). Manchester University Press.
8. Scheff, T.J. (1990). *Microsociology: discourse, emotion and social structure.* University of Chicago.
9. Broadhead, J.C. and Abas, M.A. (1998). Life events, difficulties and depression among women in an urban setting in Zimbabwe. *Psychological Medicine*, **28**, 29–38.

10. Boulton, M.G. (1983). *On being a mother*. Tavistock Publications, London.

11. O'Connor, P. and Brown, G.W. (1984). Supportive relationships: fact or fancy? *Journal of Social and Personal Relationships*, **1**, 159–75.

12. Brown, G.W. and Rutter, M. (1966). The measurement of family activities and relationships: a methodical study. *Human Relations*, **19**, 241–63.

13. Rutter, M. and Brown, G.W. (1966). The reliability and validity of measures of family life and relationships in families containing a psychiatric patient. *Social Psychiatry*, **1**, 38–53.

14. Brown, G. W. (1985). The discovery of 'expressed emotion': induction or deduction? In *Expressed emotion in families: its significance for mental illness* (ed. J. Leff and C. Vaughn), pp. 7–25. Guilford Press, New York.

15. Leff, J. and Vaughn, C. (ed.) (1985). *Expressed emotion in families: its significance for mental illness*. Guilford Press, New York.

16. Creed, F. (1981). Life events and appendectomy. *Lancet*, **i**, 1381–5.

17. Wing, J.K., Cooper, J.E., and Sartorious, N. (1974). *The measurement and classification of psychiatric symptoms: an instruction for the Present State Examination and CATEGO Programme*. Cambridge University Press.

18. Finlay-Jones, R., Brown, G.W., Duncan-Jones, P., Harris, T., Murphy, E., and Prudo, R. (1980). Depression and anxiety in the community. *Psychological Medicine*, **10**, 445–54.

19. Brown, G.W., Birley, J.L.T., and Wing, J.K. (1972). The influence of family life on the course of schizophrenia. *Journal of Health and Social Behavior*, **9**, 203–14.

20. Brown, G.W. and Harris, T.O. (1978). *Social origins of depression: a study of psychiatric disorder in women*. Tavistock Publications, London; Free Press, New York.

21. Paykel, E.S., Myers, J.K., Dienelt M.N., Klerman, G.L., Lindenthal, J.J., and Pepper, M.P. (1969). Life events and depression. A controlled study. *Archives of General Psychiatry*, **21**, 753–60.

22. Jenaway, A. and Paykel, E.S. (1997). Life events and depression. In *Depression: neurobiological psycho-pathological and theraputic advances* (ed. A. Honig and H.M. van Praag), pp. 279–96. Wiley, Chichester.

23. Bebbington, P., Hurry, J. Tennant, C., Sturt, E., and Wing, J.K. (1981) Epidemiology of mental disorders in Camberwell. *Psychological Medicine*, **11**, 561–79.

24. Dohrenwend, B.P., Shrout, P.E., Link, B.P., Martin, J.L., and Skodol, A.E. (1986). Overview and initial results from a risk-factor study of depression and schizophrenia. *Mental Disorders in the Community*, **10**, 184–215.

25. Henderson, A.S., Byrne, D.G., and Duncan-Jones, P. (1981). *Neurosis and the social environment*. Academic Press, Sydney.

26. Surtees, P. G., Miller, P.M., Ingham, J.G., Kreitmann, B., Rennie, D., and Sashi Dharan, S.P. (1986). Life events and the onset of affective disorders: a longitudinal general population study. *Journal of Affective Disorders*, **10**, 37–50.

27. Surtees, P.G. and Rennie, D. (1983). Adversity and the onset of psychiatric disorder in women. *Social Psychiatry*, **18**, 37–44.

28. Harris, T.O. (1998). A psychosocial model of depression: implications for management. In *The management of depression* (ed. S. Checkley), pp.70–93. Blackwell Science, Oxford.

29. Brown, G.W. and Birley, J.L.T. (1968). Crises and life changes and the onset of schizophrenia. *Journal of Health and Social Behaviour*, **9**, 203–14.

30. Birley, J.L.T. and Brown, G.W. (1970). Crises and life changes preceding the onset and relapse of schizophrenia: clinical aspects. *British Journal of Psychiatry*, **116**, 327–33.

31. Bebbington, P., Wilkins, S., Sham, P.I., *et al.* (1996). Life events before pysochotic episodes: do clinical and social variables affect the relationship? *Social Psychiatry and Psychiatric Epidemiology*, **31**, 122–8.

32. Brown, G.W. and Harris, T.O. (1989). *Life events and illness*. Guilford Press, New York; Unwin and Hyman, London.

33. Gilbert, P. (1989). *Human nature and suffering*. Erlbaum, Hove.

34. Ohman, A. (1986). Face the beast and fear the face: animal social fears as prototypes for evolutionary analysis of emotion. *Psychophysiology*, **23**, 123–45.

35. Frijda, N.H. (1993). The place of appraisal in emotion. *Cognition and Emotion*, **7**, 357–87.

36. Brown, G.W., Bifulco, A., and Harris, T.O. (1987). Life events, vulnerability and onset of depression: some refinements. *British Journal of Psychiatry*, **150**, 30–42.

37. Finlay-Jones, R. and Brown, G.W. (1981). Types of stressful life event and the onset of anxiety and depressive disorders. *Psychological Medicine*, **11**, 803–15.

38. Brown, G.W., Harris, T.O., and Hepworth, C. (1995). Loss, humiliation and entrapment among women developing depression. A patient and non-patient comparison. *Psychological Medicine*, **25**, 7–21.

39. Paykel, E.S., Prusoff, B.A., and Klerman, G.L. (1971). The endogenous-neurotic continuum in depression, rater independence and factor distributions. *Journal of Psychiatric Research*, **8**, 73–90.

40. Katschnig, H., Pakesch, G., and Egger-Zeidner, E. (1986). Life stress and depressive subtypes: a review of present diagnostic criteria and recent research results. In *Life events and psychiatric disorders: controversial issues* (ed. H. Katschnig), pp. 201–45. Cambridge University Press.

41. Bebbington, P. and McGuffin, P. (1989). Interactive models of depression. In *Depression, an integrative approach* (ed. E. Paykel and K. Herbst), pp. 65–80. Heinemann Medical Books, London.

42. Brown, G.W., Harris, T.O., and Hepworth, C. (1994*a*). Life events and endogenous depression: a puzzle re-examined. *Archives of General Psychiatry*, **51**, 525–34.

43. Frank, E., Anderson, B., Reynolds, C.F., Ritenour, A., and Kupfer, D.J. (1994). Life events and research diagnostic criteria endogenous subtype. *Archives of General Psychiatry*, **51**, 519–24.

44. Post, R.M., Rubinow, D.R., Ballenger. J.C. (1986). Conditioning and sensitisation in the longitudinal course of affective illness. *British Journal of Psychiatry*, **149**, 191–201.

45. Brown, G.W., Lemyre, L., and Bifulco. A. (1992). Social factors and recovery from anxiety and depressive disorders: a test of the specificity hypothesis. *British Journal of Psychiatry*, **161**, 44–54.

46. Brown, G.W. (1993). Life events and affective disorder: replications and limitations. *Psychosomatic Medicine*, **55**, 248–59.

47. Brown, G.W. and Moran, P. (1994). Clinical and psychosocial origins of chronic depressive episodes. I: a community survey. *British Journal of Psychiatry*, **165**, 447–56.

48. Brown, G.W., Harris, T.O., Hepworth, C., and Robinson, R. (1994). Clinical and psychosocial origins of chronic depressive episodes. II. A patient enquiry. *British Journal of Psychiatry*, **165**, 457–65.

49. Brown, G.W., Bifulco, A., and Andrews, B. (1990). Self-esteem and depression: 3. Aetiological issues. *Social Psychiatry and Psychiatric Epidemiology*, **25**, 235–43.

50. Bifulco, A., Brown, G.W. Moran, P., Ball, C., and Campbell, C. (1998). Predicting depression in women. The role of past and present vulnerability. *Psychological Medicine*, **28**, 39–50.

51. Brown, G.W. (1992). Social support: an investigator-based approach. In *The meaning and measurement of social support* (ed. H.O.F. Veiel and U. Baumann), pp. 235–57. Hemisphere, Washington, DC.

52. Harris, T.O. (1992). Some reflections of the process of social support: and nature of unsupportive behaviors. In *The meaning and measurement of social support* (ed. H.O.F. Veiel and U. Baumann), pp. 171–89. Hemisphere, Washington.

53. Edwards, A.C., Nazroo, J., and Brown, G.W. (1998). Gender difference in marital support following a shared life event. *Social Science and Medicine*, **46**, 1077–85.

54. Veiel, H.O.F. and Baumann, U. (ed.) (1992). *The meaning and measurement of social support*. Hemisphere, Washington, DC.

55. Brown, G.W., Andrews, B., Harris, T.O., Alder, Z., and Bridge, L. (1986). Social support, self esteem and depression. *Psychological Medicine*, **16**, 813–31.

56. Andrews, B. and Brown, G.W. (1998). Marital violence in the community. A biographical approach. *British Journal of Psychiatry*, **153**, 305–12.

57. Harris, T.O., Brown, G.W., and Bifulco, A. (1986). Loss of parent in childhood and adult psychiatric disorder. The role of lack of adequate parental care. *Psychological Medicine*, **16**, 641–59.

58. Harris, T.O., Brown, G.W., and Bifulco, A. (1990). Loss of parent in childhood and adult psychiatric disorder: a tentative overall model. *Development and Psychopathology*, **2**, 311–28.

59. Bebbington, P.E., Brugha, T., MacCarthy, B., *et al.* (1988). The Camberwell Collaborative Depression Study 1. Depressed probands: adversity and the form of depression. *British Journal of Psychiatry*, **152**, 754–65.

60. Nazroo, J.Y., Edwards, A.C., and Brown, G.W. (1997). Gender differences in the onset of depression: a study of couples. *Psychological Medicine*, **27**, 9–19.

61. Bebbington, P. (1996). The origins of sex differences in depressive disorder: bridging the gap. *International Review of Psychiatry*, **8**, 295–332.

62. Brown, G.W., Harris, T.O., and Bifulco, C. (1986). Long-term effect of early loss of parent. In *Depression in childhood: developmental perspectives* (ed. M. Rutter, C. Izard, and P. Read), pp. 251–96. Guilford Press, New York.

63. Crook, T. and Eliot, J. (1980). Parental death during childhood and adult depression. *Psychological Bulletin*, **87**, 252–9.

64. Tennant, C., Bebbington, P., and Hurry, J. (1980). Parental death in childhood and risk of adult depressive disorders; a review. *Psychological Medicine*, **10**, 289–99.

65. Harris, T.O. and Brown, G.W. (1985). Interpreting data from aetioloical studies: pitfalls and ambiguities. *British Journal of Psychiatry*, **147**, 5–15.

66. Harris, T.O., Brown, G.W., and Bifulco, A. (1987). Loss of parent in childhood and adult psychiatric disorder: the role of social class position and premarital pregnancy. *Psychological Medicine*, **17**, 163–83.

67. Bifulco, A., Brown, G.W., and Harris, T.O. (1987). Childhood loss of parent, lack of adequate parental care and adult depression: a replication. *Journal of Affective Disorders*, **12**, 115–28.

68. Harris, T.O. (1988). Psycho-social vulnerability to depression: the biographical perspective of the Bedford College Studies. In *Handbook of social psychiatry* (ed. A.S. Henderson and G.D. Burrows), pp. 55–71. Elsevier, Amsterdam.

69. Quinton, D. and Rutter, M. (1984). Parents with children in care: 1. Current circumstances and parenting skills. *Journal of Child Psychology and Psychiatry*, **25**, 211–29.

70. Quinton, D. and Rutter, M. (1984). Parents with children in care: 2. Intergenerational continuities. *Journal of Child Psychology and Psychiatry*, **25**, 231–50.

71. Pawlby, S.J., Mills, A., and Quinton, D. (1997). Vulnerable adolescent girls: opposite-sex relationships. *Journal of Child Psychology*, **38**, 909–20.

72. Quinton, D., Pickle, A., Maughan, B., and Rutter, M. (1993). Partners, peers and pathways: assertive pairing and continuities in conduct disorder. *Development and Psychopathology*, **5**, 763–83.

73. Bifulco, A., Brown, G.W., and Harris, T.O. (1994). Childhood experience of care and abuse (CECA): a retrospective interview measure. *Child Psychology and Psychiatry*, **35**, 1419–35.

74. Brown, G.W. and Harris, T.O. (1993). Aetiology of anxiety and depressive disorders in an inner-city population. 1. Early adversity. *Psychological Medicine*, **23**, 143–54.

75. Gaminde, I., Uria, M., Padro, D., Querejete, I., and Ozamiz, A. (1993). Depression in three populations in the Basque country—a comparison with Britain. *Social Psychiatry and Psychiatric Epidemiology*, **28**, 243–51.

76. Abas, M.A. and Broadhead, J.C. (1997). Depression and anxiety among women in an urban setting in Zimbabwe. *Psychological Medicine*, **27**, 59–71.

77. Klerman, G.L. and Weissman, M.M. (1989). Increasing rates of depression. *Journal of the American Medical Association*, **261**, 2229–35.

78. Hagnell, O., Lanke, J., Rorsman, B., and Ojesjo, L. (1982). Are we entering an age of melancholy? Depressive illnesses in a prospective epidemiological study over 25 years: the Lundy Study, Sweden. *Psychological Medicine*, **12**, 279–89.

79. Fombonne, E. (1995). Depressive disorders: time trends and possible explanatory mechanisms. In *Psychosocial disorders in young people: time trends and their causes* (ed. M. Rutter and D.J. Smith), pp. 616–85. Wiley, Chichester.

80. Weizmann, F. (1971). Correlational statistics and the nature–nurture problem. *Science*, **171**, 589.

81. Brown, G.W. (1998). Genetic and population perspectives in life events and depression. *Social Psychiatry and Psychiatric Epidemiology*, **33**, 363–72.

82. Craig, T.K.J. (1989). Abdominal pain. In *Life events and illness* (ed.G.W. Brown and T.O. Harris), pp. 233–57. Guilford Press, New York.

83. Craig, T.K.J., Boardman, A.P., Mills, K., Daly-Jones, O., and Drake, H. (1993). The South London Somatisation Study. I: Longitudinal course and the influence of early life experiences. *British Journal of Psychiatry*, **163**, 579–88.

84. Craig, T.K.J., Drake, H., Mills, K., and Boardman, A.P. (1994). The South London Somatisation Study. II: Influence of stressful life events, and secondary gain. *British Journal of Psychiatry*, **165**, 248–58.

85. Harris, T.O. (1989). Disorders of menstruation. *Life events and illness* (ed. G.W. Brown and T.O. Harris), pp. 261–94. Guilford Press, New York.

86. Creed, F.H., Craig, T., and Farmer, R. (1988). Functional abdominal pain, psychiatric illness and life events. *Gut*, **29**, 235–42.

87. Calloway, P. and Dolan, R. (1989). Endocrine changes and clinical profiles. In *Life events and illness* (ed. G.W. Brown and T.O. Harris), pp. 139–57. Guilford Press, New York.

88. Owens, M.J. and McGuffin, P. (1997). Genetics and psychiatry. *British Journal of Psychiatry*, **171**, 201–2.

89. Brown, G.W. (1996). Genetics of depression: a social science perspective. *International Review of Psychiatry*, **8**, 387–401.

90. Gilbert, P. (1992). *Depression: the evolution of powerlessness*. Erlbaum, Hove.

2.6.2 Social and cultural anthropology: salience for psychiatry

Arthur Kleinman

Social and cultural anthropology

One of the social sciences (together with history, economics, political science, sociology, and social psychology), social and cultural anthropology is principally concerned with the study of society, in almost all of its aspects. Together with linguistics, archaeology, and biological anthropology, social and cultural anthropology formed the classic (and now considered overly ambitious) four-field base of anthropology, the science of man. Yet still, in many universities, anthropology departments bridge the traditional divisions of the humanities, social sciences, and natural sciences. From the outset, anthropologists defined their subject in holistic terms meant to contextualize men and women in a nested hierarchy of influential environments that ran from the human body to the social body, and that assumed that these levels were related to each other, so that individual and collective processes (biological, psychological, social relational, and cultural) intersected in some way. Social and cultural anthropology, in particular, took as its subject matter studies of communities, ranging from small-scale preliterate groups to neighbourhoods or institutions in megacities. Comparison of different societies, or different structures and processes in those societies, is still seen as a defining approach, as is the analysis of cultural symbol systems (from languages to aesthetics), history of kinship, and other systems of social relationship, as well as research on large-scale social changes such as our decade's globalization, ethnonationalism, and resurgence of religious fundamentalism.

Anthropology's chief research methodology is ethnography, the close study of a local world—a village, an urban neighbourhood, an institution, a network. Ethnography privileges local language, conceptual categories, values, and practices. Its procedure is to begin with local definitions and perceptions of reality (sometimes called 'emics', from phonemics), and only when these experience-near patterns are understood in a particular context of everyday life (with the larger political, economic, and cultural forces that influence it) are comparisons made with other local worlds in the framework of experience-distant scientific definitions of reality (referred to as 'etics', from phonetics). Knowledge is generated by participant observation, informal interviews, and the use of more formal procedures from structured interviews to questionnaires. While some ethnographers use statistically oriented quantitative methods, most gather qualitative data that is closer in type to the findings of social history, scholarship in the humanities, and the writing of biography. But in many instances ethnographers combine narratives and numbers. Cross-cultural comparison is another core mode of knowledge production. Both ethnography and cross-cultural comparisons draw on empirical data to engage larger questions in social theory, which itself is constantly being reorganized in this dialectical engagement. Social theory, which conceptualizes how societies are organized and work, is based in classical formulations by Karl Marx, Emil Durkheim, Max Weber, Franz Boas, E.E. Evans-Pritchard, and others, but over the past half-century has proliferated in various directions, among them structuralism (Claude Lévi-Strauss), meaning-centred analysis (Clifford Geertz), postmodernism (Michel Foucault, George Marcus, David Harvey, and others), and interactionism (George Herbert Mead, Pierre Bourdieu), to mention a few examples.

In this century, social and cultural anthropology's division of labour has spun off at least two subfields that are of particular relevance for psychiatry: psychological anthropology and medical anthropology. The former grew out of the culture and personality school (c. 1930–1950), when psychoanalysts and anthropologists sought to collaborate to understand how mental processes differed or were similar across greatly different societies. Margaret Mead, Ruth Benedict, and Irving Hallowell are those anthropologists most often associated with this school. But in a broader sense psychological concerns were influential throughout American anthropology and even among such leading figures in British social anthropology as Bronislaw Malinowskii and Meyer Fortes. However, social and cultural anthropologists in both countries became increasingly critical of psychoanalytical assumptions, the orientation to individuals, and the dubious correlation of individuals with entire cultures which, among other things, had the unfortunate side-effect of legitimating ethnic stereotypes. A small group of social and cultural anthropologists continue, none the less, to pursue this direction, and over time they have developed broader ties with psychology, as can be readily seen by their leading research interests in cognition, lifecycle development, and ethno-

psychological categories. Anthropologists working in this tradition have studied self-concepts and self-images, emotion terms, interpersonal processes and their relation to personhood, as well as experiences of childhood, child rearing, adolescence, midlife, and ageing. Memory, affects, especially depression, anger, and guilt, sexual meanings and practices, and experiences of trance/possession and other altered mental states have all received considerable research attention. Other processes, notably bereavement, have received far less attention. (A strange irony given all the attention anthropologists have devoted to the study of funeral practices.) Psychological anthropology has been influential in recent years in psychology, where a sister subdiscipline called cultural psychology has started up in close connection to it.

Medical anthropology, the other relevant subfield, has had a different history. Physicians were among the founders of anthropology, and some, like the British polymath W.H.R. Rivers, combined medicine and anthropology. Rivers wrote about illness meanings and healing practices, and, during the First World War, practised a form of psychotherapy that was informed by ethnography. Another source of medical anthropology was social medicine and public health; indeed the great German pathologist and social medicine advocate, Rudolph Virchow, was one of the first to use the term 'medical anthropology'. Thus, medical anthropology's early roots were applied. After the Second World War, the field took off as anthropologists developed an interest in the theoretical and empirical aspects of non-Western medical traditions, religious healing and its relation to medicine, and increasingly in experiences of suffering. In more recent years, medical anthropologists, of whom there are several thousand worldwide, have developed special interests in infectious diseases (especially diarrhoeal disease, malaria, tuberculosis, and AIDS), female reproductive lifecycle problems, the health problems of children and the aged, substance abuse, cancer, diabetes, disabilities, medical ethics, and the economic and social transformation of health care. One of the earliest and abiding interests has been in psychiatric diagnosis, disorders, and treatments. While the term psychiatric anthropology is not as frequently used as medical anthropology, there are hundreds of medical anthropologists worldwide who conduct research and teach courses on mental illnesses and psychiatry as a profession. An increasing number of these are themselves psychiatrists with training in anthropology. This subfield of social and cultural anthropology has many ongoing relationships to cultural psychiatry (see Chapter 4.16) and has been active in recent years in the effort to introduce mental health concerns into international health (see Chapter 1.3.1). Indeed, the cultural sections of the DSM-IV were contributed by a taskforce that included both medical anthropologists and cultural psychiatrists, in equal numbers.

Major contributions of anthropology to psychiatry

Cultural critique of biomedicine

Theory is downplayed in academic psychiatry, although there is much more of it than the naïve positivist view of atheoretical psychiatric diagnosis portrayed in DSM-IV allows. Yet, one of the crucial contributions of anthropology is theoretical, namely a critique of the theoretical biases inherent in psychiatric science and clinical practice. And how could this not be? For unlike any other branch of medicine, there is no blood test, biopsy, or radiograph to diagnose psychiatric disorder (leaving aside Alzheimer's disease, which is after all a neurological disorder). That means that psychiatric diagnosis is based on the establishment of symptom and syndromal criteria, which are based in turn in language, lay categories, and everyday social experience. In other words, there is no biological validity but only psychosocial reliability in psychiatric assessment. Cultural bias can enter this process in several ways. Anthropologists have shown that this can happen when diagnostic criteria which have been developed in one society are applied to another where they lack validity. This is called a 'category fallacy,' a term introduced by Kleinman.[1] Classic examples include trance and possession states in many non-Western societies, which are frequently normative and normal experiences. Failure to recognize this phenomenon, and therefore the diagnosis of persons in religious trance as psychotic, creates a category fallacy in the application of the diagnostic criteria of psychosis to normal people. In a related manner, anthropologists have faulted international diagnostic criteria for failing to take into account indigenous syndromes (such as *ataques* and *nervios* among Puerto Ricans), and thereby either underdiagnosing indigenously defined psychopathology that may (or may not) have a family resemblance to established professional categories, or overdiagnosing (ICD- or DSM-defined) psychopathology. What they are hearing are collective idioms of distress that are culturally patterned and socially shared ways of complaining about social or personal problems in an idiom of bodily and psychological terms, which do not necessarily signify psychiatric disease. The cultural critique has been applied to personality disorders as well, because this category of disorder models self-processes on a decidedly Euro-American, middle-class, and usually male behavioural type and lifestyle. Anthropologists argue for a much more flexible and interactive understanding of subjectivity that changes in basic ways in response to different social circumstances. Extremely high rates of sociopathy among adolescents from ethnic minorities in the inner city, they argue, is the result of such cultural bias in diagnosis. The anthropological framework for understanding personality and pathology sets the conditions in the conjunction of changing cultural representations, collective processes, and individual experience. Anthropologists are divided on the issue of human nature. Some see human conditions as a continuous process of change without a fixed 'nature'; others deem human nature only one element in the process. Yet, on the whole, even anthropologists who draw on the idea of human nature regard it as historically and cross-culturally malleable. They try to avoid naturalizing or essentializing human nature by emphasizing its inseparability from particular contexts.

In the 1990s, cultural critique has been deployed by anthropologists and ethnic psychiatrists to examine the influence of institutional racism in psychiatric diagnosis, referral, and treatment. Leading examples are the overdiagnosis of African-Americans and African-Caribbean Britons with schizophrenia, the tendency to perceive them as more dangerous and less amenable to psychotherapy, and differences in the way their discharge and aftercare are organized. Anthropologists have examined how racism is unwittingly built into psychiatric categories and infiltrates the model cases used to illustrate diagnostic criteria, and also the way that psychiatrists are trained to replicate such patterns in the practice of triage.

Cultural critique, informed by the cross-cultural and international data, is the basis for anthropologists' doubts about the validity of many of the psychiatric conditions detailed in DSM-IV and ICD-10. The idea that there are no stable psychiatric syndromes cross-culturally is an idea few psychiatric anthropologists would advance, although in an

earlier era of the most radical cultural relativism in the field, this idea had more than a few supporters. But the ethnographic database strongly suggests that, apart from brain tumours and infections, Alzheimer's disease, metabolic encephalopathy, substance abuse, and other well-documented brain-based disorders such as certain sleep disorders, only five psychiatric syndromes of adults can be found cross-culturally; i.e. only these have stability as syndromes outside the cultural mainstream of Euro-American societies. The conditions are schizophrenia, brief reactive psychoses, major depression, bipolar disease, and a range of anxiety disorders from panic states through phobias to obsessive–compulsive disorder. Most of the other hundreds of conditions described in DSM-IV, for example, are culture bound to Euro-America. This point has also led many medical anthropologists to be suspicious about the idea of culture-bound disorders generally. Why should railway psychosis, *shenjing shuairuo* (neurasthenia as diagnosed by Chinese psychiatrists), and pathological trance and possession states in China be listed as culture-bound syndromes, when at the very least they are stable syndromes among one-fifth of the world's population? These anthropologists also ask: When many conditions listed in the DSM and ICD systems that are found in Europe and America are not to be found in China, or in most of the rest of the non-Western world, why should they not be regarded as culture bound?

Related to these contributions of cultural critique, anthropologists have also contributed to the development of culturally informed diagnostic criteria, questionnaires, structured interviews, and guidelines for working with translators. Globalizing and indigenizing psychiatric approaches is an even more general emphasis in anthropology. Largely because of the politics of ethnicity and the worldwide movement of globalization, psychiatric researchers and practitioners must pay attention to the international database and to the concerns of ethnic communities and individual patients. Yet, few seem to be serious readers of relevant anthropological literature, which after all is the basic science in this field. Anthropology contains numerous concepts and methods that might be tried out, but relatively few have been experimented with or adopted. Besides those described below, several examples of the concepts, methods, and findings from anthropology that await trial in psychiatry are listed in Table 1.

Local moral worlds: interpersonal basis of illness experience

Ethnographies—hundreds of them, including many on psychiatric topics—demonstrate, with great consistency, that most people and most patients are not isolated individuals but rather live their lives as active members of local worlds. By local worlds, ethnographers mean villages, neighbourhoods, networks, and families, as well as particular social institutions, including hospitals and outpatient systems. Ethnographic research illustrates the interpersonal processes of communication, negotiation, and contestation that make up everyday experience in local worlds everywhere. Rarely are communities or even networks homogeneous, as was erroneously thought to be the case earlier. Rather, local worlds are differentiated by class, ethnicity, gender, age cohort, political faction, religious ties, and still other social differences. That is why one must be extremely cautious about characterizing a local world as if it were one distinct thing. But what does hold for each and every local world is that there are crucial things at stake that orient the attention and actions of participants. What is at

Table 1 Anthropological concepts, methods, and findings that await trial in psychiatry

Ethnography

Ethnography as a research strategy in clinical and epidemiological research. For example, as a means of studying the clustering of psychiatric conditions with social problems. Ethnography also has uses in evaluation research, in generating categories and questions in epidemiological studies, and in sociosomatic research. It is also a means of training researchers

Ethnographic database

Ethnographic database as a routine source of knowledge about communities (foreign and domestic) for clinicians, mental health planners, and researchers

Cross-cultural comparisons

Cross-cultural comparisons as a routine form of knowledge production. For example, cross-cultural comparisons of psychotherapy might help (a) to clarify what is common among religious, moral, and medical healing, (b) to determine how culture influences psychotherapeutic practice, and (c) to develop psychotherapeutic techniques for use with patients and families from different minority, ethnic, and international populations

Social theory

Systematic reading of social theory as a source of hypotheses for research in social psychiatry and as a means of preparing clinicians to practise community psychiatry. Concepts such as social and symbolic capital, globalization, marginalization, ethnic identity, and institutional racism, among many others, can be used to frame psychiatric research and clinical intervention

stake, most at stake, may be shared (status, resources, survival, transcendence), but it also can be as distinctive as the different meanings of ultimacy that make religions distinguishable from each other.

Illness experience and experiences of treatment are as much caught up in these transpersonal processes of agonistic and antagonistic engagement over what is at stake in experience as are experiences of normality. Thus, for anthropology how a person's illness is encountered, coped with, understood, and lived is simply crucial for understanding the illness and the treatment. It is for this reason that anthropologists write about the social course of illness: meaning that local worlds shape the course of illness so thoroughly that the same disease process (diabetes, AIDS, depression, schizophrenia) can take different trajectories. When sick people go for treatment, who they first seek out, whether they comply with the therapeutic regime, how they assess their experience of treatment—all are in one way or another influenced by what is most at stake for communities, families, networks, and individuals. The anthropological contribution here is to highlight the processes through which individuals relate to collectives. Thus, Estroff[2] shows that collective and individual definitions of identity affect how schizophrenic patients live their schizophrenia as an illness identity, which in turn affects their careers as patients and their experiences in other domains (family, workplace, etc.).

Another example of the difference between anthropological and psychiatric approaches to human conditions is the way the two disciplines understand suicide. In American psychiatry, at least, it is widely accepted that most of the time suicide occurs in the context of depressive disorder, and that that disorder as well as individual impulsivity are the principal determinants of suicide. Anthropological understandings are derived from the study of suicide as a collective experience. Hence, anthropologists note that suicide rates index a variety of social changes, most notably economic depression and political vio-

lence. In China today, the rate of suicide is at least twice that of the United States, and possibly may be three times as high. Yet rates of depressive disorder in China are very low by international standards; indeed the most recent epidemiological data from China suggests the rates of depressive disorder may be as much as five to 200 times less than in North America. Hence it is highly unlikely that depression can be the major determinant of China's enormous rate of suicide. Moreover, suicide in China is unlike suicide in the rest of the world because it is more common in women than men. Of all suicides in the world, 40 per cent occur in China (which accounts for 20 per cent of the world's population) and an astonishing 50 per cent of all reported female suicides occur there. Rural women from 15 to 25 years of age and men and women over 55 years of age are most at risk for suicide.[3] Recent research (psychological autopsies in the context of village-based epidemiological studies) suggests that in most instances there was no evidence of serious depression. Rather, family conflicts and other well-documented interpersonal problems were found to be present. Furthermore, analysis of suicide notes suggests that in many instances suicide was an act of social resistance against oppressive patriarchal conditions such as forced marriage, pressures following failure to produce sons, infanticide, abusive husbands, husbands who took second wives or mistresses, and so forth. Marginalization and relative powerlessness as social positions correlate better with suicide than does psychological status. Here societal and individual perspectives lead to vastly different interpretations of the determinants of suicide. The Chinese concept of 'loss of face' (loss of embodied moral status, *lianmian*) points to interpersonal connections between the moral and the emotional levels of experience that seem particularly important for understanding suicide (for the reason that many suicides in China follow serious loss of face and can be viewed as a desperate but still acceptable means of regaining face), and perhaps not only in China. Altruistic suicide is also valued.

Practical clinical relevance

Immigration processes have so altered national demographic patterns that most nation states today have plural populations representing distinctive ethnic backgrounds. In 1900, the population of the United States, for example, included only 13 per cent categorized as ethnic minority members. By 1990 that figure was greater than 25 per cent. The percentage is projected to be one-third in 2010, and by mid-century to reach an astonishing 50 per cent. In California, the largest American state, non-Hispanic white Americans are already in a minority.

Ethnic background has been shown empirically to influence epidemiological rates of disease, patterns of access to health care, help-seeking, and patient–doctor interactions, often with negative outcomes such as delayed treatment, misdiagnosis, non-compliance, and treatment failure. Taking ethnicity into account in the provision of services means a variety of things, such as making translators available, putting up signs in several languages, holding clinics at times when working-class patients can attend, and paying attention to differences in cultural meanings and practices. The now popular idea of providing culturally informed and sensitive care is premised on anthropological concepts and methods. Several of these have been elaborated in the literature.

1. The distinctions between illness and disease: for medical anthropologists illness is the patient's experience of symptoms in the

context of family, work, and community; disease is the practitioner's model of the pathological process. Help-seeking is usually orientated around the illness experience with respect to what is most at stake for the patient and significant others. Care can founder when the patient's primary concerns with the illness experience conflicts with or is entirely different from the physician's focus on disease. Thus, many patients with chronic pain experience interrogation of the disease process by the sceptical physician as delegitimizing their illness experience. This leads to high rates of dissatisfaction with care among this group of patients. Many so-called 'orphan diseases'—chronic pain, chronic fatigue syndrome, etc.—produce this result. When patients and families are from ethnic minority backgrounds, differences in cultural meanings and practices intensify conflicts between patient and physician models.

2. Medical anthropology sponsors a method to reduce this explanatory gap and thereby to improve clinical relationships. Called the explanatory models' methodology, it involves three steps.

   (a) Elicitation of patient and family explanatory models of the illness experience and treatment, which can be accomplished by asking the following questions.

   - What do you call your problem?
   - What do you think caused it?
   - Why did it start when it did?
   - What course will it take from here on?
   - How does it work in your body?
   - What do you most fear about the illness?
   - What kind of treatment do you desire for this illness?
   - What do you most fear about the treatment?

   (b) Presentation of the clinician's explanatory model of the disease process.

   (c) Negotiation of a mutually acceptable understanding of the clinical problem across patient, family, and physician models.[4]

Closely related to this technique is the development of a mini-ethnography. This is a brief description, based on interviewing the key parties about the impact of family and work context on the illness experience and vice versa. The mini-ethnography and the explanatory models' elicitation generally give rise to patient stories of the illness experience. These illness narratives can be assessed with respect to the chief meanings and practices associated with the condition and its treatment. The illness narrative can be interpreted with respect to core metaphors, culturally particular content, as well as biographical issues with which psychiatrists are more familiar. The influence of cultural categories, values and practices on the illness and treatment can be assessed from this standpoint.[5]

Cultural formulation

Appendix I to DSM-IV contains an outline of how psychiatric cases can be culturally formulated. The outline includes:

- the cultural identity of the individual
- cultural explanations of the individual's illness
- cultural factors related to the psychosocial environment and levels of functioning

- cultural elements of the relationship between the individual and the clinician.

This is a feasible approach to routine patient care with members of ethnic minorities and recent immigrants and refugees that has a high likelihood of making that care culturally informed and culturally sensitive. Key to it, as it is to anthropology's core methodology, ethnography, is the display of genuine respect for patients, families, and their meanings and practices. That respect for the person and his or her illness experience is the indispensable condition of anthropologically informed care. It includes, as its first step, the ethical act of acknowledging the suffering of the other in his or her own terms as the basis for diagnosis and treatment. In this sense, it reverses the cultural preoccupation of the biomedical practitioner with the disease process, and establishes the interpersonal relationship as the grounds of knowledge as well as caregiving.

Conclusions

Anthropology's chief contribution to psychiatry is to emphasize the importance of the social world in diagnosis, prognosis, and treatment, and to provide concepts and methods that psychiatrists can apply (the appropriate cross-disciplinary translation first being made, however). But that is not the only contribution that anthropology offers. Ethnographers are aware that knowledge is positioned, facts and values are inseparable, and experience is simply too complex and robust to be easily boxed into tight analytical categories. Hence a sense of the fallibility of understanding, the limitation of practice, and irony and paradox in human conditions is the consequence of ethnography as a method of knowledge production. Of course this is not very different from the 'humanistic' insight provided by the experience of 'doing' psychotherapy. Both forms of knowledge are transpersonal and incomplete and, for those very reasons, deeply human. They both disclose that just as patients are caught up in the moral processes of everyday life so too are clinicians absorbed by what is at stake in professional institutions and careers (which after all is also a moral process). They both require that these moral processes of everyday life be engaged by ethical (and epistemological and ontological) self-reflection, so that practitioners and patients are able to open a space of self-awareness in the milieu of psychobiological and sociocultural affairs which are so very influential (although not determinative) in most of experience. This self-awareness and the space required for it, as well as its uses in assisting others, is why ethnography has attracted generations of physicians and why anthropology, like psychotherapy, will always have a role in psychiatry.

Anthropology also complements the idea of psychosomatic relationships with evidence and theorizing about sociosomatic relationships. Here moral processes—namely what is at stake in local worlds—are shown to be closely linked with emotional processes, which are frequently about experiences of loss, fear, vexation, and betrayal of what is collectively and individually at stake in interpersonal relationships. Change in the former can change the latter, and this can at times work in reverse as well. Examples include the way symptoms intensify or even arise in response to fear and vexation concerning threats perceived as serious dangers to what is most at stake.

The relationship of poverty to morbidity and mortality is a different example of sociosomatic processes. Poverty correlates with increased morbidity and mortality. Psychiatrists have often had trouble getting the point that public health and infectious disease experts have long understood. But it is not just diarrhoeal disease, tuberculosis, AIDS, heart disease, and cancer that demonstrate this powerful social epidemiological correlation—so do psychiatric conditions. Depression, substance abuse, violence, and their traumatic consequences not only occur at higher rates in the poorest local worlds, but also cluster together (much as do infectious diseases), and those vicious clusters define a local place, usually a disintegrating inner-city community. Hence the findings of the National Co-Morbidity Study in the United States of America that most psychiatric conditions occur as comorbidity is a step toward this ethnographic knowledge—that in the most vulnerable, dangerous, and broken local worlds, psychiatric diseases are not encountered as separate problems but as part of these sociosomatic clusters.

Finally, anthropology is also salient for policy and programme development in psychiatry. Against an overly narrow neurobiological framing of psychiatric conditions as brain disorders, anthropology in psychiatry draws on cross-national, cross-ethnic, and disintegrating community data to emphasize the relationship of increasing rates of mental health problems, especially among underserved, impoverished populations worldwide, and increasing problems in the organization and delivery of mental health services to fundamental transformations in political economy, institutions, and culture that are remaking our epoch. In so doing, anthropology projects a vision of psychiatry as a discipline central to social welfare and health policy. It argues as well against the profession's ethnocentrism and for the field as a larger component of international health. Anthropology (together with economics, sociology, and political science) also provides the tools for psychiatry to develop policies and programmes that address the close ties between social conditions and mental health conditions, social policies, and mental health policies. In this sense, anthropology urges psychiatry in a global direction, one in which psychiatric knowledge

and practice, once altered to fit in more culturally salient ways in local worlds around the globe, have a more important place at the policy table.[6]

Further reading

Barrett, R. (1996). *The psychiatric team and the social definition of schizophrenia: an anthropological study of person and illness.* Cambridge University Press.

Kleinman, A. and Good, B. (ed.) (1985). *Culture and depression.* University of California Press, Berkeley, CA.

Littlewood, R. (1995). *The butterfly and the serpent: essays in psychiatry, race and religion.* Free Association Books, London.

Young, A. (1995). *The harmony of illusions: inventing post-traumatic stress disorder.* Princeton University Press.

References

1. Kleinman, A. (1977). Depression, somatization and the new cross-cultural psychiatry. *Social Science and Medicine*, **11**, 3–10.
2. Estroff, S.E. (1993). Disability and schizophrenia. In *Knowledge, power and practice: the anthropology of medicine and everyday life* (ed. S. Lindenbaum and M. Lock), pp. 247–86. University of California Press, Berkeley, CA.
3. Lee, S. and Kleinman, A. (1997). Mental illness and social change in China. *Harvard Review of Psychiatry*, **5**, 43–5.
4. Kleinman, A. (1988). *The illness narratives.* Basic Books, New York.
5. Kleinman, A. (1988). *Rethinking psychiatry: from cultural category to personal experience.* Free Press, New York.
6. Desjarlais, R., Eisenberg, L., Good, B., and Kleinman, A. (ed.) (1995). *World mental health: problems and priorities in low-income countries.* Oxford University Press, New York.

2.7 The contribution of epidemiology to psychiatric aetiology

Scott Henderson

Introduction

Epidemiology deals with overall patterns. On the one hand, people are unique with their own genetic endowment and life experiences. This idiographic paradigm is balanced by the nomothetic in which recurrent and predictable patterns are sought in the whole of humankind. It is the business of psychiatric epidemiology to determine the distribution of mental disorders in populations, the factors determining that distribution, and measures that may help in their prevention.

From their undergraduate years onward, clinicians are accustomed to patients who have a disorder and who at the same time give a history of certain experiences dating from birth to their present. It may be tempting for both patient and doctor to make causal links. But if the principles of epidemiology are brought into play, some questions need to be asked first. What proportion of the general population have had the same experiences but not developed the disorder? What proportion have the same disorder but have not had these experiences? What proportion have the same disorder but are not known to health services? And could having the exposure itself be linked in some way with being known, or not known, to health services? These are the questions that are prompted by a simple two-by-two table (Table 1).

The rows are made up of persons in a population who have or do not have a particular disorder. The columns are the numbers who have or have not had a certain exposure. That exposure is being considered as a putative risk factor. It may be biological or psychosocial and may have taken place at any time from conception to the present. In every one of these questions, the clinician's traditional perspective is expanded to consider the whole population and not only the sick who have reached clinics or hospitals.

To establish a causal link between some phenomenon and a disorder is a demanding but most engaging exercise. It is well worth reading the classic expositions by Bradford Hill[1] and Mervyn Susser[2,3] on how a cause can reasonably be inferred from the data.

Table 1 Cases and exposure: a two-by-two table

		Case	
		Yes	No
Exposed	Yes	a	b
	No	c	d

Letters refer to numbers of persons.

The uses of epidemiology

In his celebrated monograph bearing this title, J.N. Morris[4] described seven uses of epidemiology. It continues to give us a framework for assessing the state of psychiatric epidemiology in relation to the biological and psychosocial conditions of the contemporary world. Morris's list can be reinterpreted for our use as follows in the next sections.

Completing the clinical picture

This means knowing about all the ways in which a disorder may present and what is its usual course. But it also means relating subclinical cases to fully developed ones. An excellent example here would be the anxiety, depressive, or somatization states seen in general practice or field surveys compared to the more severe syndromes specified in the international criteria and encountered by psychiatrists.

Community diagnosis

Here one obtains estimates of morbidity as it occurs at the general population level, not just in persons who have reached primary care or mental health services. Examples are the National Comorbidity Study in the United States,[5] the Survey of Psychiatric Morbidity in the United Kingdom,[6] and the National Survey of Mental Health and Wellbeing in Australia.[7] Only by having such estimates of prevalence or incidence for whole populations can the size of their disease burden be determined. This is because community-based measures of morbidity include not only persons with treated conditions but also those who are symptomatic yet have not reached services.

Secular changes in incidence

This refers to the rise and fall of diseases in populations, with the possibility of making projections into the future. For example, there is some evidence that schizophrenia has been dropping in incidence and becoming more benign in its clinical course,[8] it is possible that depressive disorder has become more frequent in persons born since the Second World War[9,10] (the suicide rate of young persons has indisputably increased in many industrialized countries), it is likely that eating disorders have increased in frequency in some industrialized countries, and it is certain that the use of heroin and the AIDS epidemic with its neuropsychiatric sequelae are new arrivals and will be a continuing burden.

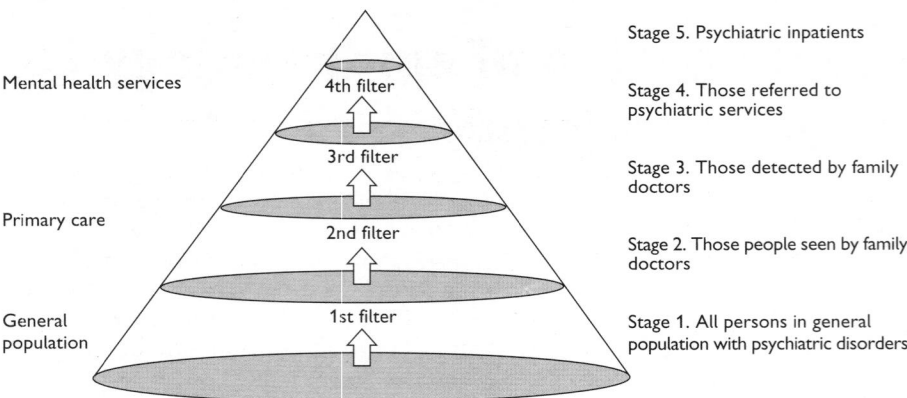

Fig. 1 Pathways to care. (Adapted from Goldberg and Huxley.[14])

The search for causes

Here, epidemiology is looking for aetiological clues both within groups of individuals and within the communities they live in. It is the substance of this chapter.

Applying population data to individual risk

In this, the focus moves from the population back to the individual. For example, if the annual incidence rate for schizophrenia is known in a population and if this information is age-specific, it is possible to estimate the probability that a person of a given age will develop this disorder within the next year. This is the base rate, before one starts to consider risk factors such as family history. Next, by aggregating data on the course of schizophrenia, it is possible to estimate the chances of recovery for persons who are currently having their first episode. The common principle is that data based on large numbers of persons are used to make probability estimates for individuals.

Delineation of syndromes

This is done by examining the distribution of clinical phenomena as they occur in the population. It fits well with recent experience of repetitive strain injury, chronic fatigue syndrome, and post-traumatic stress disorder or its congeners.

Health services research

This begins with a determination of needs and of resources, then an analysis of services currently in action, and ends with attempts to evaluate them. Research activity in this area has expanded greatly in recent years, driven by the forces of economic rationalism.

Prevention

To Morris's seven uses of epidemiology should be added prevention, which Ernest Gruenberg[11] said was its 'ultimate service'. All other uses are subsidiary to this. Examples are the current activity in the prevention of suicide in young persons and of alcohol or drug abuse. In these, the traditional medical approach of targeting high-risk groups should be contrasted with the epidemiological and population-based approach described by Rose.[12,13] (Prevention is discussed further in Chapter 7.4.)

Research on aetiology: three levels and three designs

Epidemiological methods can be applied at any of three levels: to disorders as these present in hospitals and specialist health services, in primary care, or in the general population. These three levels are represented diagrammatically in Fig. 1 as a three-dimensional cone, derived from the seminal volume on pathways to care by Goldberg and Huxley.[14] The base of the cone consists of those in the general population who have clinically significant psychological symptoms (Stage 1). When these symptoms become unmanageable to self or to others, people seek help from their doctor or other health practitioners (Stage 2). But only some of them are recognized by the professional to have significant mental health problems (Stage 3). A small proportion may be referred to mental health services (Stage 4), of whom an even smaller fraction are admitted to inpatient care (Stage 5). Note that undergraduate teaching and the diagnostic criteria in international use are largely based on Stages 4 and 5!

Commonly used designs

At any of these levels, research directed at aetiology uses one of three designs: cross-sectional, prospective longitudinal, or case–control. A cross-sectional study is often an excellent start, because it provides a picture of how much morbidity is present at one point in time and the variables most closely associated with this. But because it is only a 'snapshot', the cross-sectional study can rarely allow much to be said about causes. For example, suppose that in a community sample of several thousand adults one has a measure of the psychiatric symptoms each has experienced in the previous month and their self-reported exposure to adverse life events in the previous year. The data will show that persons who have had many adversities also tend to have more symptoms of anxiety or depression than those not so exposed. But it would be unwise to conclude from these findings alone that adversity contributes to the onset of symptoms. First, persons with anxiety or depression may be more likely to report that they have had many troubles. This may be through selective recall of unpleasant events, because it is known that depressed people are more likely to remember bad times than good times.[15,16] Another mechanism is effort after meaning, whereby people try to account for feeling psychologically unwell. Second, symptomatic persons may be more likely to have unpleasant things happen to them, secondary to their mental state. Third, persons with anxiety or depression may have certain personality traits or lifestyles that make them more likely to have troubled lives and also be vulnerable to common mental disorders.

Such problems in methodology can be resolved to some extent by graduating to a prospective longitudinal design or cohort study. In this, a population sample is assessed at the start when most persons are psychologically well. In one type of cohort study, the sample may deliberately include a group who have had a particular exposure, such as a head injury or natural disaster. The information in a prospective study is less likely to be biased by mood state or selective recall. At the start, data are obtained on personality, lifestyle, recent or past exposure to adversity, past health, and family history. The cohort is then re-examined at least once after an appropriate interval. Some will have developed symptoms. The research question to be asked is whether the putative risk factors that were assessed at the start were more frequently present in those who later developed symptoms. A design of this type yields considerably more information about the causal processes likely to be at work, either those leading to mental disorders or protecting against them. It also overcomes the problem of a putative risk factor really being a consequence rather than an antecedent of a disorder. But it is obviously very demanding in resources—human, administrative, and financial. It also takes a long time. For these reasons, epidemiologists often use the case–control method as a more practicable alternative.

Case–control designs have been underused in psychiatric research, but they can be a powerful strategy for identifying risk factors for a specified disorder.[17,18] The essence of the case–control design lies in obtaining data to complete the cells in Table 1. The aim is to find a sample of all persons in a population who have reached case level for a particular disorder and an equivalent number of persons who are similar in age, gender, and other variables, but who do not have the disorder—at least not yet. The cases should ideally be 'incident' or recent in onset. If instead, the study has to have recourse to all the cases of the disorder known to the service, some of these will be long-standing and some more recent. This could lead to misleading results because a putative risk factor may show up as 'positive' not because it is a cause or true risk factor, but because it is associated with chronicity, either through prolonging the duration of the disorder, or prolonging the life of the sufferer. This problem can be avoided only by recruiting recent-onset or incident cases for case–control studies. The cases and controls are then asked about the various possible exposures. If the cases are unable to give information because they are cognitively impaired (as in dementia), at least one informant has to be found for each case, usually a partner or close family member.

In Table 1, the important question is whether there are more persons in cell a than would occur by chance. We do not know the incidence of the disorder in all persons in the population who were exposed to each risk factor, nor do we know the number not exposed. Likewise, we do not know how many people in the population have recently developed the disorder. As a consequence, we cannot compare the incidence in those exposed and not exposed for the whole population. All we have are the data from the cases examined, who are necessarily only a fraction of all incident cases in the population; and data from a fraction of all healthy persons. But we can proceed as follows. First, the relative risk is calculated from Table 1. The relative risk is

$$\frac{a/(a + b)}{c/(c + d)}.$$

By simple algebra this becomes

$$\frac{a(c + d)}{c(a + b)}.$$

Then something very helpful can be done. Where a disorder is fairly uncommon in the general population, a will be very small compared with b, and c will be small compared with d. If we assume a negligible contribution by a in the term $a+b$, and by c in the term $c+d$, the relative risk will be nearly equal to

$$\frac{ad}{bc}.$$

This is the odds ratio, which is an expression of the strength of a risk factor.

Who to study: principles of sampling

Whichever the design, there are few occasions when it is practicable to examine a total population. In studies at the general population level, it would mean carrying out an assessment of every individual in an entire city or region. In a primary healthcare setting, it would mean assessing every person who consults staff in every general practice or health centre during a specified period. In clinics or hospitals, it would mean examining all individuals who present with a particular disorder across a whole country, in both public and private sectors. The solution is to sample the group under investigation.

The essential principle is that everyone in the true denominator (usually the total population within a defined geographical or administrative area) must have an equal probability of being included in that sample. If this is not achieved, there is the likelihood of bias whereby the achieved sample may be systematically different in ways that could be important in the analysis. For example, the sample of cases should not differ from all the incident cases in that population in attributes such as level of education, age, or likelihood of having been exposed to a candidate exposure or risk factor. So in a study of the association between, say, sexual abuse in childhood and depressive disorder in adult life, the cases of depression should be representative of all those with depressive disorder in that community and not just those reaching a particular service. This applies especially if that service is known to have a special interest in childhood abuse.

Non-ignorable non-response

In field surveys, it has long been accepted that not everyone who is in the 'target sample' will agree to be interviewed or will be available at the time the interviewer calls. It is common to find that only 70 to 90 per cent are actually assessed. Furthermore, those who refuse or are repeatedly not available are known to be more likely to have the mental disorder under investigation. For this reason, the prevalence that is found will often be an underestimate. A putative risk factor may itself increase the chances of a person's not being in a sample in the first place, of dropping out, or of dying during the study. Statistical methods have been available for many years for estimating how much error may have occurred due to refusals and how to correct for this in the conclusions drawn.

The other occasion when non-response is a problem is in longitudinal studies, where a sample is followed over several years. If a disorder with an increased mortality is the topic, such as dementia or schizophrenia, it is recognized that some cases will be lost at follow-up. This means that those who are successfully re-examined are a survival élite and are different in important ways from the original cohort. These distortions could lead to mistaken conclusions if the losses are not allowed for. Various techniques have been developed to handle these difficulties, including Bayesian methods which adjust final estimates on the basis of prior knowledge.[19]

Specifying the disorders

Diagnostic categories

The epidemiology of mental disorders could have made no real progress without methods for specifying the disorders to be investigated, then measuring these, so that research on, say, depression or schizophrenia can be comparable between sites, within and between countries. Whether the study is at the level of the community, primary healthcare or mental health services, it is essential to specify which symptoms or which diagnoses are to be studied. Having consistency in diagnosis has been made much easier through the development of the diagnostic criteria now in wide international use.

The first of these is the *International Classification of Diseases (10th Revision)* (**ICD-10**) with its *Classification of Mental and Behavioural Disorders*. This comes in two mutually complementary presentations: the *Clinical Descriptions and Diagnostic Guidelines*;[20] and the *Diagnostic Criteria for Research*.[21] These sets of diagnostic criteria have been prepared after wide consultation with expert psychiatrists in some 40 countries. They therefore represent an international consensus. Furthermore, the *Diagnostic Criteria for Research* have been used as the basis for diagnostic instruments that have computer algorithms to apply these criteria, precisely and invariably, to the information obtained at interview (see below).

Another system is the *Diagnostic and Statistical Manual, 4th edition* (**DSM-IV**) of the American Psychiatric Association.[22] This is a national system that is used throughout the United States and quite widely elsewhere. Through a process of extensive consultation between the World Health Organization and the architects of DSM-IV, it is closely similar to ICD-10. These two sets of diagnostic criteria have brought a common language to clinical practice and to research. When authors now submit a paper to a reputable scientific journal, it is virtually mandatory that the disorders investigated be according to one or both systems.

These classifications are described further in Chapter 1.11.

Continuous measures of morbidity

Case ascertainment might be assumed to be the *sine qua non* for any progress in the epidemiology of mental disorders. But to use the traditional expression 'case ascertainment' nicely illustrates the very problem that has to be re-thought, because it implies a categorical structure in the morbidity that we wish to study. In a population, there are trad-itionally cases and non-cases. As expressed by Pickering,[23] 'Medicine in its present state can count up to two, but not beyond'. He was referring to hypertension, but others have argued that most mental disorders have dimensional properties.[12,13] The frequency distribution of their component symptoms such as anxiety, depression, or cognitive impairment is usually a reversed J-shape, with most people having none or only a few symptoms and progressively fewer persons having higher counts. A committee of clinicians in Geneva or Washington, whose experience is largely derived from teaching hospitals, has decided by consensus where the cut-point should be placed for persons to be 'cases'. While this is entirely appropriate for some purposes, it may not always be a true representation of the underlying pathology. In statistical terms, it may lose information.

It is not disputed that mental disorders exist in categorical states and that these have some utilitarian value: a depressive episode, Alzheimer's disease, anorexia nervosa, or alcohol dependency are clinically realistic entities. What is proposed here is that, in epidemiological studies at the general population level, hypotheses about the aetiology of case-level conditions are not well served unless large numbers of respondents are interviewed, solely because the base rates for such conditions are not large. But it is possible to identify persons with some symptoms of depression, of cognitive impairment, of abnormal eating, or of alcohol misuse, and the score on a scale of these symptoms can become the dependent variable in an analysis of candidate risk factors. So it is usually more powerful statistically to look for associations between a putative risk factor and morbidity expressed as a continuous variable, rather than as a dichotomy of cases and non-cases.

When a continuous measure of common psychological symptoms such as the General Health Questionnaire (**GHQ**)[24] is applied to a population, a unimodal distribution curve is found, with no break between so-called cases and so-called normals. Rose[12,13] argued that there are three important consequences from this approach to studying morbidity. First, a characteristic of the community as a whole emerges. This is the mean and standard deviation of its GHQ scores. Second, this collective characteristic may show large differences between men and women, geographical regions, social strata, and income groups. These differences are based on shifts of the entire distribution. The third consequence is that differences between these groups in the prevalence of probable cases (those with a score above a threshold) are related to different average scores in these groups. As Rose[12] concisely put it, 'The visible part of the iceberg (prevalence) is a function of its total mass (the population average)'.

He suggested[13] that '*Psychiatrists, unlike sociologists, seem generally unaware of the existence and importance of mental health attributes of whole populations, their concern being only with sick individuals*' (emphasis added). It is an appealing notion that populations, while they are undeniably made up of individuals and, as far as we know, no other component, take on properties of their own, much as molecules acquire attributes not found in their constituent atoms. The concept of populations having different frequency distributions of morbidity, not just different prevalence rates for clinical cases, carries with it the implication that some factors are shifting the overall distribution in some populations but not in others. The idea is that there is some pervasive force active in the biological or social environment and which promotes the onset or persistence of a disorder. This is a highly attractive hypothesis—but not a new one. It is not far removed from Galen's atmospheric factor, the katastasis or miasma, or the societal forces that Durkheim[25] proposed were related to national suicide rates.

Disablement

There is yet a further advantage in considering morbidity as a continuum in a population. Morbidity refers to symptoms, syndromes, or disorders. But there is a universe of discourse closely linked to this, namely disablement. This is the collective noun now used to refer to the impairment, disability, and social role handicap in daily life that disorders bring with them. It is self-evident that the main categories of mental disorder, especially the psychoses, affective disorders, and dementias, are almost always associated with substantial disablement. But subclinical levels of mental disorders also carry with them a certain amount of disablement. From the point of view of a whole population, the amount of disablement from subclinical or milder conditions is cumulatively substantial. This is because such conditions have a high point prevalence. Therefore, from a public health perspective, the significance of milder mental disorders is not trivial because of the disablement they bring in daily life. Disablement has recently come to carry new significance in the interpretation of prevalence estimates from large community surveys. These typically produce 12-month prevalence rates of 15 per cent or more for all types of mental disorder taken together. But it is most unlikely that 15 per cent of the population require professional treatment. Only a proportion of the 15 per cent may find their symptoms disabling. The interpretation and administrative significance of prevalence estimates are therefore likely to command much more attention in the future. This is necessary if such epidemiological information is to inform us about the burden of mental disorders in the community.[26–28]

The measurement of psychiatric symptoms

Instruments for epidemiological research fall into two types: questionnaires and psychiatric examinations.

Questionnaires

The more simple type is a symptom scale, which can be completed by respondents themselves or administered by an interviewer. The best-known instrument is the GHQ used in its 60, 30, 28, or 12-item versions.[24] The GHQ detects symptoms of anxiety and depression. The briefest version, the GHQ-12, is a highly efficient screening tool. A score of 2 or more indicates that the person is likely to have one of what Goldberg and Huxley[29] have usefully termed common mental disorders. Another screening instrument is the Hopkins Symptom Checklist,[30] while a good general measure is the 14-item Anxiety and Depression module in the Delusions–Symptoms–States Inventory (**DSSI**) by Bedford and Foulds.[31] For depressive states specifically, examples are the Center for Epidemiologic Studies Depression Scale (**CES-D**)[32] and the Beck Depression Inventory.[33]

The Alcohol Use Disorders Identification Test (**AUDIT**) was developed by the World Health Organization for population screening. This 10-item test has been shown to have satisfactory psychometric and predictive properties. The total score is 40 and a score of 8 or more (7 for women) is recommended for a range of adverse consequences of drinking.[34]

Table 2 Screening a population sample

		Criterion (cases by full psychiatric assessment)	
		Yes	No
Cases by screening test	Yes	a	b	a+b
	No	c	d	c+d
		a+c	b+d	

Letters refer to numbers of persons.

For cognitive impairment, the Mini-Mental State Examination (**MMSE**)[35] gives a score for a person's current cognitive function, or by applying a cut-point to that score, it can be used to identify persons who are likely to have a dementia.[36,37] The MMSE has been used in many community studies of older persons and has proved to be a valuable screening tool for moderate and severe dementia, though not for milder cases. Like any other cognitive test, it cannot itself make a diagnosis of dementia. It detects cognitive impairment, not cognitive decline, which requires a history. The MMSE is known to be sensitive to education, in that persons with limited intelligence or education may have low scores without their having had any cognitive decline.

All these instruments can be used in two ways: by applying a cut-point to identify persons who are likely to be clinically significant cases; and by using the score as a continuous variable. When a questionnaire or self-rated instrument is used in research, its psychometric properties should be known beforehand and these are often specific to the population being studied. Two important properties are the sensitivity and specificity of the instrument. These refer to its performance when compared with a criterion or 'gold standard', such as a comprehensive psychiatric examination or a consensus diagnosis amongst experts. In Table 2, a sample of persons has been examined with both the screening instrument and a full examination. We consider the number of persons who are 'cases' according to both assessments (a), according to one but not the other (b or c) and according to neither (d).

Sensitivity is the proportion who screen positive and who are indeed cases by the criterion; that is: $a/a + c$, while specificity is the number who screen negative and who are indeed not cases: $d/b + d$.

The sensitivity and specificity of a test are expressed as a percentage and vary according to where the cut-point is placed on the scores. As sensitivity increases, specificity tends to decrease, so that an appropriate balance between the two has to be determined. For some purposes, such as in screening for depression, it is more important to identify as many as possible of the true cases, but it does not matter if there are quite a few false-positives because these can be corrected by a more extensive second-stage examination. Under these conditions, one would want a highly sensitive screening test that placed most of the true cases in cell a and few in c. It matters rather less if quite a few of the true non-cases are incorrectly placed in b.

Standardized psychiatric interviews

Even the best-designed questionnaires with the best psychometric properties cannot be a substitute for a psychiatric interview. Only the latter can obtain the information that leads to a diagnosis, reached according to the international criteria. But for many years, psychiatric assessments were entirely in the hands of the individual clinician. As a consequence, different psychiatrists obtained different information; and different psychiatrists assembled the information in different ways to reach a diagnosis. Not unexpectedly, agreement between interviewers was poor even within one centre, as shown by Kreitman.[38] Progress of fundamental significance for all of psychiatry has been made since the late 1960s with the development of standardized assessments. These are standardized in two mutually complementary ways. First, neither the questions asked nor the ratings of behaviour are left to the idiosyncrasies of the interviewer. Instead, this information variance is reduced by having interviewers ask about symptoms in the same way. Second is the reduction of criterion variance, where the symptoms or signs elicited are, like building bricks, assembled in exactly the same way, both within and across studies. This is achieved by applying to the data an algorithm that is a precise expression of the diagnostic criteria in ICD-10 or DSM-IV. The algorithm can be computerized so that the responses to each item in the interview are assembled automatically. This determines if the person's symptoms and behaviour fulfil the diagnostic criteria. By appropriate programming, a symptom score can also be obtained in addition to the categorical diagnosis.

There are two types of standardized psychiatric examination. This is for the good reason that, although full clinical interviews in the field by experienced clinicians may be the ideal, such resources are often not available. The first type of instrument is designed for use by experienced clinicians after some training. These instruments allow some flexibility in questioning, and enable the clinicians to use their judgement when making a rating about the presence or absence of each symptom or behaviour. The second type of instrument is for use by lay interviewers. These interviews are 'fully scripted', where the questions asked are invariable and must be strictly adhered to, with only very few of the items calling for any judgement. Such instruments can now be computerized for use on a laptop. The scoring of responses is then both error-free and available immediately the interview is completed.

The Schedule for Clinical Assessment in Neuropsychiatry (SCAN) belongs to the first type. It is the successor to the groundbreaking Present State Examination (PSE) developed by Wing et al.[39] and now revised[40] for the World Health Organization. SCAN is a clinician's instrument because it requires familiarity with the phenomenology of mental disorders. It assumes that the interviewer is comfortable in examining persons with a mental disorder. In complete contrast to interviews for use by laypersons, the clinician asks the main question, but is allowed to probe with further questions if necessary, before deciding if a symptom is present or not. The correct use of SCAN requires formal training in one of the designated centres around the world. SCAN has a number of modules, each dealing with a group of disorders such as anxiety states, affective disorders, substance abuse, or psychoses. It is available from the World Health Organization.

The Clinical Interview Schedule—Revised (CIS-R)

This instrument was developed from an earlier version for clinicians so that it could be used by lay interviewers.[41] It was used in the National Survey of Psychiatric Morbidity in the United Kingdom.[6,42] CIS-R generates diagnoses by ICD-10 and DSM-IV, but is also able to give scores for symptoms. It is known to have been well received by respondents and to have been user-friendly for interviewers in the British survey.

The Composite International Diagnostic Interview (CIDI)

CIDI was developed by Robins et al.[43] for the World Health Organization and the United States Alcohol, Drug Abuse and Mental Health Administration. It combines questions from its predecessor, the Diagnostic Interview Schedule, with items from PSE and SCAN. However, CIDI is constructed in such a way that it can be administered by laypersons after only a few days' training. Its performance, including reliability and validity has been described.[44,45] CIDI is fully scripted and has been automated for administration on laptop computers by Peters and Andrews.[46] Its modules cover the main categories of mental disorder, generating both ICD-10 and DSM-IV diagnoses as well as symptom scores.

Validity issues

The quality of information these instruments obtain is clearly of central importance. We know that they do not obtain the same information as each other, nor do they identify the same persons as cases of a particular diagnostic category. Their validity is therefore a matter of considerable concern for administrators using the data obtained in large surveys to guide planning. But it is also a matter of concern for aetiological research. A general tendency is for the lay interviews to obtain higher case rates than an instrument such as SCAN. An important study by Brugha et al.[47] compared SCAN, CIS-R, and CIDI on a sample of the general population, finding that agreement was generally poor, with kappa values between 0.1 and 0.4. Their recommendation is that SCAN now be assessed for its performance when it is in the hands of thoroughly trained lay interviewers. Meanwhile, it is not possible to say which of the available instruments is superior. Further technical developments are urgently needed in this demanding area.

Instruments for assessing dementia and depression in the elderly

Epidemiological research on mental disorders in late life calls for specially built instruments to detect cognitive impairment, cognitive decline, depressive states, psychotic symptoms, and performance in the activities of daily living. All of the following have a section for assessing the elderly person and a separate section for an informant, who is usually a relative or close friend. The first to be developed was the Geriatric Mental State Examination (GMS),[48] which has now been widely used. The second is CAMDEX,[49] which was intended as a clinician's instrument but can be used by laypersons after some training. A combination of parts of GMS and CAMDEX was used in a large United Kingdom study of cognitive impairment and dementia.[50] The third instrument is the Canberra Interview for the Elderly (CIE),[51] which is available in English, German, and French versions.[52] From CIE, Jorm and Mackinnon[53] developed the highly parsimonious Psychogeriatric Assessment Scales (PAS) to enable non-clinicians working with elderly persons to detect depression, cognitive decline, and stroke in a standardized manner.[54,55] PAS is now in wide use internationally.

Typical prevalence estimates

The above instruments have been used in a large number of surveys of the prevalence of the main mental disorders in the general population.

Table 3 Some community prevalence estimates (per cent)

	Depressive disorders		Anxiety disorders		Alcohol abuse or dependence		Schizophrenia or non-affective psychosis		Instrument used
	M	F	M	F	M	F	M	F	
Henderson et al., [100] Canberra (1 month)	2.6	6.7	4.1	3.0	—	—	—	—	GHQ/PSE
Bebbington et al., [101] London (1 month)	4.8	9.0	1.0	4.5	—	—	—	—	PSE
Von Korff et al.,[102] USA (lifetime)	—	—	—	—	—	—	0.4	0.8	DIS
Mavreas et al.,[103] Athens (1 month)	3.0	7.4	3.9	12.1	—	—	—	—	PSE
Lehtinen et al.,[104] Finland (1 month)	3.6	5.5	4.6	7.5	—	—	—	—	PSE
Regier et al.,[105] USA (1 month)	3.5	6.6	4.7	9.7	5.0	0.9	0.7	0.7	DIS
Kessler et al.,[5] USA (12 months)	8.5	14.1	11.8	22.6	14.1	5.3	0.5	0.6	CIDI
Jenkins et al.,[6] UK (1 week)	1.7	2.5	2.8	3.4	7.5	2.1	0.4	0.4	CIS-R
Australian Bureau of Statistics,[7] Australia (12 months)	4.2	7.4	7.1	12.1	9.4	3.7	—	—	CIDI-A

Examples are shown in Table 3. What is important about these is that they provide an estimate of the prevalence in the community of those syndromes that are familiar to psychiatrists working in clinics and hospitals. This puts the public health significance of these syndromes into perspective both for clinicians and for health service administrators.

Disablement

The most comprehensive measure is the Disability Assessment Schedule (**DAS**)[56] that assesses an individual's functioning in daily life. Its short form[57] is suitable for survey use. Self-completion instruments are the Brief Disability Questionnaire (**BDQ**)[58] and the SF-36[59] or its briefer version, the SF-12.

Possible causes of mental disorders: the domains

Having specified the psychiatric disorder or class of symptom and having developed methods to measure it, the next task is to measure whatever factors are suspected to contribute to its onset or course. These lie in the traditional three domains: the biological, social, and psychological. But in epidemiology, any variable used to tap these is rarely specific to one domain. Some biological, some social, and some psychological factors are often conflated. For example, gender expresses biological differences but may also carry different social experiences in the past, different social contexts in the present, and different psychological or intrapersonal differences in personality traits and behaviour.

Likewise, age-group can also reflect social role, educational opportunities in the past, marital status, and physical health. It is therefore important not to be misled into thinking that a variable is tapping only what one is primarily interested in. Confounding is ever present—and often unexpected.

Sociodemographic variables

When data on a population sample is divided by age, gender, marital status, ethnic background, and socioeconomic or educational level, the average level of psychiatric morbidity may differ significantly. Depressive disorders are consistently more prevalent in women[60] and dementia has a higher prevalence in groups with low education.[61,62] Furthermore, there may be important interaction effects between variables in their relation to morbidity. For example, the average age of onset in schizophrenia is different in men and in women (see Chapter 4.3.4).

The social environment

This can be considered in two parts: first is the individual's immediate social environment—what the sociologist Cooley[63] called the primary group—consisting of those around a person with whom there is both interaction and commitment. There is then the wider community with its standard of living, lifestyle, and cultural values. Plausibly, both may have some influence on the incidence of mental disorders and on their course. Instruments to measure the individual's immediate social environment and the support it may afford have been usefully reviewed by Turner.[64] Most instruments are interviews taking about 30 min.[65,66] The hypothesis that social support protects against depression and other common mental disorders has proved hard to investigate.[67] This is because social support is probably influenced by some intrapersonal factors rather than being a product solely of the individual's environment. Here is a good example of confounding: a major variable concerning the social environment of individuals turns out to be determined not solely by environmental factors, but partly by their own personality attributes. The evidence suggests that social support, stripped of these confounding factors, is not a powerful factor in aetiology.[68] A separate issue is whether social support influences the outcome of psychiatric disorders once these have developed.

Societal (macrosocial) variables have long been suspected of playing an important role in aetiology. It was such a hypothesis that was investigated in the celebrated Stirling County Study in Canada by Dorothea and Alexander Leighton[69,70] with their concept of sociocultural disintegration. The current increase in depression and suicide in the young is also attributed to a macrosocial variable. The problem is that satisfactory indicators are elusive.

Experiential variables

'Experiential' is a useful term to refer inclusively to all that individuals are exposed to, from conception to death. In epidemiological research, it includes intrauterine exposures—such as maternal influenza or malnutrition—and perinatal events. In infancy and childhood, social and interpersonal experiences have been the main focus of research. Maternal deprivation was intensively studied in both clinical and community samples for two decades. The expectation from Bowlby's attachment theory was that loss or separation from the mother would be pathogenic for depression and possibly personality disorders.[71] This hypothesis has proved very hard to test because of confounding by other factors. Where people have lost their mother through death or separation, a number of other disadvantageous experiences are also likely to have been present. Maternal deprivation promised to be an important topic both for psychiatric theory and for social policy. The evidence has been assembled by Rutter[72] who concluded that '…the residual effects of early experiences on adult behaviour tend to be quite slight because of both the maturational changes that take place during middle and later childhood and also the effects of beneficial and adverse experiences during all the years after infancy…'.

More recently, promising findings have been obtained on the association between parenting style and depressive disorders in adulthood. Parker[73,74] developed the Parental Bonding Instrument (**PBI**) to measure two fundamental dimensions of the manner in which parents behave towards their children: care and affection as one dimension and protectiveness as the other. Studies of clinical samples using PBI have suggested that low parental care and parental overprotection, separately or together, are associated with some psychiatric disorders in adult life. The 'toxic' exposure was found to be affectionless control: that is, parents who had been highly controlling but not affectionate or caring. Parker[75] has reviewed the evidence for inadequate parental care as a risk factor to adult depression, integrating this with the evidence on parental loss and, importantly, on compensating or mitigating factors. The PBI is too lengthy for epidemiological research on community samples where the interview is often already extensive.

Parker and his colleagues have subsequently developed a briefer instrument, the Measure of Parenting Style (**MOPS**), which includes the experience of physical and sexual abuse.[76] MOPS is likely to prove useful in case–control and prospective studies of psychiatric disorders for systematically obtaining information on exposures of theoretical relevance.

Childhood abuse

It seems intuitively likely that children who have been physically or sexually abused have an increased risk of having anxiety, depression, or other psychiatric disorders in adulthood. The findings from epidemiological studies on unreferred samples point to the many other adverse experiences that accompany childhood sexual abuse, including physical violence, unstable and untrustworthy relationships with parents, and emotional deprivation.[77] Knutson[78] has given a review of the psychological consequences of physical abuse in childhood. Valuable reviews on the consequences of sexual abuse can be found in Browne and Finkelhor[79] and Beitchman et al.[80]

Recent exposure to adversity

Adverse experiences have been very extensively studied for their contribution to the onset and course of psychiatric disorders. In epidemiological research, much attention has been accorded to issues that arise in the measurement of adversity. Some of these issues are equally relevant in clinical practice. They include the following.

- The duration of the stressor: acute or long-standing.

- Its magnitude and how to determine this independently of the person's reaction to it.

- The independence of the event from the individual: some events are entirely independent while others may have come about because of the individual's own behaviour or psychiatric state.

- Interaction with sociodemographic variables: the same experience may have markedly different significance according to these.

- The personal context of the experience may augment or reduce its psychological impact.

- Confounding by personality traits that may be independently associated with psychiatric morbidity.

- The additive effect of multiple events, some of which may be causally linked in a chain.

- The quality of the event: a loss or a threat.

- Effort after meaning, whereby patients and doctors may attribute symptoms to a particular experience as a way to explain the onset of illness.

These issues have been comprehensively described in Katschnig[81] and in Brown and Harris.[82] A valuable conspectus of the issues and the evidence is in the volume edited by Dohrenwend.[83] Instruments for measuring life events are of two types. The most simple are brief inventories, usually for self-completion. An example is the measure by Brugha et al.[84] A radically different approach is to make the assessment interviewer based. First the adverse experiences are identified at interview from a very full list, then the overall context for that person is determined. But the rating of severity is made by the external judgement of a research team. This method, the Life Events and Difficulties

Schedule, was developed by Brown and his colleagues and is recognized to obtain high-quality information.[85] Dohrenwend et al.[86] have also developed a comprehensive assessment for administration by interview. (Life events are discussed further in Chapter 2.6.1.)

Personality variables

Although personality traits may contribute to how vulnerable individuals are to adverse experiences, it has not often been possible to measure personality traits in general populations, then follow the sample prospectively to demonstrate if the incidence of specific disorders is indeed higher in some types. Many measures of personality are too lengthy to be used in surveys. One exception is the Eysenck Personality Questionnaire (**EPQ-R**)[87] in which the trait of neuroticism has consistently been found to confer increased risk of anxiety and depression.[64,88,89]

Molecular genetics and epidemiology

In its search for aetiological factors, psychiatric epidemiology has worked mainly with psychosocial variables. The dominant paradigm has been that the causes of most mental disorders are likely to be found in the social environment and the experiences it imposes. A major contribution towards correcting this has come from Kendler and his collaborators. Instead of the general population, they used a large sample of adult twins from the Virginia Twin Registry. This enabled them to estimate how much of a disorder is attributable to genetic inheritance; how much to a common environment that both twins shared; and how much to each twins' unique environment. This method has generated findings of fundamental importance for aetiology.[90–92] It is in this context that the technical advances described below become highly attractive.

It has long been recognized by psychiatric epidemiologists that the addition of biological measures would be theoretically desirable, but these have not been highly practicable for administration to large numbers of persons in field surveys. The situation has recently changed and exciting new opportunities have become available. These lie in the unprecedented advances being made in molecular genetics. What has become available is a new set of predictor variables in the form of genotypes. It is not a matter of psychiatric epidemiology turning its back on psychosocial variables. Instead, genes can be assessed in their interaction with a full range of experiential and social factors. Two complementary strategies are being followed. The first is a continuing search for genes associated with discrete diseases such as bipolar affective disorder or schizophrenia. The second strategy is quite different: to search not for genes that may cause or be directly related to disorders, but for genes that confer vulnerability to them. Such an approach is well suited to epidemiological methods.

Cloninger et al.[93] have commented on the difficulties of replicating genetic associations with complex psychiatric disorders, and have argued that it may be more fruitful to map genes contributing to temperament, not symptoms. Within populations, personality traits are distributed as continua and probably involve many genes, each of which is neither necessary nor sufficient for the trait. In recent years, there has been increasing interest in genes that contribute to variation in quantitative traits. These quantitative trait loci (**QTLs**) may vary in the size of their effect on a trait from small to modest. The aim of current QTL research is to find the loci that have the largest effect. There are a number of techniques available for the study of QTLs,

including linkage analysis in families, allele-sharing methods between relatives, and association studies in population samples. It is argued that allelic association studies are at present the strategy of choice for detecting QTLs.Table 4 Because a large number of candidate markers are being investigated, there is a high risk of type I errors.

In the next few years, it can be expected that some personality traits will be found to occur more often in people with particular alleles in genes related to brain function. Amongst these, a preferred group of candidates are genes with known polymorphisms that alter the function of neurotransmitter systems, either by affecting the metabolism of a transmitter or some aspect of its function such as transport, receptor binding, or signal transduction. The attraction for psychiatric epidemiology is twofold: the promise of introducing to population studies a biological variable of fundamental significance; and the possibility of looking for interaction between biologically based vulnerability and life experiences. Although several studies reporting associations between personality traits and polymorphisms related to serotonin and dopamine metabolism have already been published, it would be premature to accept any association as established until replications have been achieved in sizeable samples across different populations.[94]

Other strategies for finding quantitative trait loci are emerging. One is to obtain general population samples not of individuals but of sib pairs or triads of first-degree relatives. Genomic scanning and gene expression technology are also now practicable. The prospects have been critically assessed by Henderson and Blackwood,[95] but the field is moving so rapidly that interested readers will need to maintain close vigilance on the literature.

How epidemiologists think

We can now look back on the strategies used to find causes of mental disorders and how epidemiologists go about the task. To find aetiological clues, they looks for links. This is best done by working not with individual patients, nor even with series of patients in one clinic. Instead it is better to have data that represent all cases of a disorder in a defined population. Anything short of that could well be biased, in that the data would fail to represent all occurrences. Then one can start to ask questions that may throw light on aetiology.

1. Is there a gender difference in prevalence, or if the data are available, in incidence? If there is, one gender may carry greater biological susceptibility; or may be exposed to more of some environmental factor.

2. Does incidence vary regionally, or between contrasted environments, or between different socioeconomic groups? If there is little variation, it suggests that environmental factors may play little part in the aetiology.

3. If persons who have the disorder are compared with those who do not, have the cases been exposed to some environmental factor more often than the controls?

Each of these questions leads to a testable hypothesis.

The way in which a candidate risk factor comes to be proposed is itself very interesting. There are three types.

1. **The inspired hypothesis** A sharp-eyed clinician develops the idea that some factor—in any of the three domains—is present more often than by chance in a certain disorder; and that that factor

Table 4 The search for cause: a matrix for epidemiological studies

		Child psychiatric disorders	Anxiety disorders	Affective disorders	Schizophrenia	Dementias	Personality disorders	Eating disorders	Alcohol and substance abuse	Suicide	Parasuicide	Intellectual disability	Psychological well being
Sociodemographic factors	Gender												
	Age												
	Marital status												
	Social class												
	Education												
	Employment status												
	Urban/rural												
	World region												
Experiential factors	Season of birth												
	Parental age												
	Childhood separation												
	Parental style												
	Cultural or subcultural beliefs and attitudes												
	Adverse experiences												
	Extreme experiences												
	Bereavement												
	Expressed emotion (for relapse)												
	Social support												
	Secular changes in society												
	Other macrosocial factors (economic depression, war, social cohesion)												
	Migration												
	Climate and daylight												
	Noise												
	Environmental toxins												
	Diet												
	Alcohol and drugs												
	Medication												
	Infections												
	Physical illness												
	Interaction of two or more factors												
	Comorbidity												
	Genetics: major genes												
	quantitative trait loci												

No attempt has been made to be exhaustive in either the classes of morbodity or the putative causal factors.

may contribute to the onset of the disorder. This is exactly what happened to the ophthalmologist Sir Norman Gregg in Sydney when he noticed that many disabled children had mothers who had contracted rubella during the pregnancy. The association was later confirmed and shown to be causal. So here a hypothesis arising in the course of clinical work was taken out of the clinic and tested by epidemiological methods, then the knowledge applied in prevention.

2. **A coarse observation** A second pathway to a hypothesis starts with a coarse observation of a link between a disorder and, say, some demographic variable. In the aetiology of schizophrenia, a slight excess in winter birthdates was noticed in persons who later developed schizophrenia. This has led to others over the years, such as the possible excess of schizophrenia in the offspring of women who had influenza during the second trimester of their pregnancy. One study reported an increased risk in the female offspring of women who were pregnant during the Dutch Famine of 1944 to 1945.[96] Work on the 1946 birth cohort in Britain has yielded the important finding that persons who later developed schizophrenia had been recorded as children to have had more speech and educational problems, more social anxiety, and a preference for solitary play.[97] From the simple observation of a slight excess of winter births in schizophrenia, a series of other studies have followed, all based on a neurodevelopmental hypothesis. These are far removed from the hypothesis about 'schizophrenogenic' families so seriously espoused only three decades ago.

3. **The enquiry is theory driven** A good example is what came from attachment theory. The hypothesis was that if a close affectional relationship were not experienced in childhood, the individual would be vulnerable to depression and anxiety in adult life. In epidemiological research on Alzheimer's disease, it was theory that led to a search for putative risk factors such as a family history of Down syndrome, aluminium in drinking water, maternal age at the patient's birth, and a history of previous head injury. It was also theory that led Jenkinson et al.[98] to find an inverse association between Alzheimer's disease and rheumatoid arthritis. This subsequently led to studies of people who had been treated with long-term anti-inflammatory drugs. Breitner's conclusion is that they probably have a lower probability of developing Alzheimer's disease.[99]

4. **A matrix** All these three approaches can be brought together, then used as the building material to construct a matrix. This can then drive a systematic search. In Table 4, the main categories of mental disorders are listed across the top to form the columns, while the rows are made up of those variables that may contribute to the onset or course of morbidity. The matrix proves to be a tidy way of organizing what information is already available; but it also acts heuristically by proposing associations that call for investigation but might not otherwise have been considered. The variables can be placed in categories: sociodemographic, experiential, intrapersonal (psychological), and biological. The alert observer will notice that the matrix has one limitation: it is in only two dimensions and therefore does not display the interactions between two or more variables, yet these can be of the greatest importance. Basic examples are the indisputable interaction between age and gender in the onset of schizophrenia; or the possible interaction between head injury and having the apo-

lipoproteinE ε4 allele. To think about such interactions, users of the matrix need to select their own combinations in, or expand it by adding other disorders or putative risk factors.

Conclusion

Research on the epidemiology of psychiatric disorders becomes more and more exciting. There is an abundance of testable hypotheses on aetiology and on factors influencing the course of mental disorders. Of particular significance is the emergent capability to advance our understanding of the contribution made to aetiology by specific genes in interaction with environmental exposures.

Useful information

- Copies of the Schedule for Clinical Assessment in Neuropsychiatry can be obtained from Publications, World Health Organization, Avenue Appia, 1221 Geneva-27, Switzerland.

- The Composite International Diagnostic Interview (CIDI) and its automated version (CIDI-A) can be obtained from the WHO Collaborating Centre for Mental Health and Substance Abuse, St Vincent's Hospital, 299 Forbes Street, Darlinghurst, NSW 2010, Australia. Order forms are available at http://www.crufad.unsw.edu.au

- The Canberra Interview for the Elderly (CIE) and the Psychogeriatric Assessment Scales (PAS) are available free from the Secretary, NHMRC Psychiatric Epidemiology Research Centre, The Australian National University, Canberra, ACT 0200, Australia.

References

1. Hill, A.B. (1965). The environment and disease: association or causation? *Proceedings of the Royal Society for Medicine*, **58**, 295–300.
2. Susser, M. (1973). *Causal thinking in the health sciences*. Oxford University Press, New York.
3. Susser, M. (1991). What is a cause and how do we know one? A grammar for pragmatic epidemiology. *American Journal of Epidemiology*, **7**, 635–48.
4. Morris, J.N. (1964). *Uses of epidemiology*. Williams and Wilkins, Baltimore, MD.
5. Kessler, R.C., McGonagle, K.A., Zhao, S., *et al.* (1994). Lifetime and 12-month prevalence of DSM-III-R psychiatric disorder in the United States: results from the National Comorbidity Survey. *Archives of General Psychiatry*, **51**, 8–19.
6. Jenkins, R., Bebbington, P., Farrell, M., *et al.* (1997). The National Psychiatric Morbidity Surveys of Great Britain—initial findings from the Household Survey. *Psychological Medicine*, **27**, 775–89.
7. Henderson, S., Andrews, G., and Hall, W. Australia's mental health: an overview of the general population survey. *Australian & New Zealand Journal of Psychiatry*, in press.
8. Jablensky, A. (1995). Schizophrenia: recent epidemiologic issues. *Epidemiologic Reviews*, **17**, 10–20.
9. Hagnell, O., Lanke, J., Rorsman, B., and Öjesjö, L. (1982). Are we entering an age of melancholy? Depressive illnesses in a prospective epidemiological study over 25 years: the Lundby Study, Sweden. *Psychological Medicine*, **12**, 279–89.
10. Klerman, G.L. (1988). The current age of youthful melancholia: evidence for increase in depression among adolescents and young adults. *British Journal of Psychiatry*, **152**, 4–14.

11. Gruenberg, E.M. (1966). Epidemiology of mental illness. *International Journal of Psychiatry*, **2**, 78–134.
12. Rose, G. (1992). *The strategy of preventive medicine*. Oxford University Press.
13. Rose, G. (1993). Mental disorder and the strategies of prevention. *Psychological Medicine*, **23**, 553–5.
14. Goldberg, D.P. and Huxley, P. (1980). *Mental illness in the community: the pathway to psychiatric care*. Tavistock Publications, London.
15. Neugebauer, R. and Ng, S. (1990). Differential recall as a source of bias in epidemiologic research. *Journal of Clinical Epidemiology*, **43**, 1337–41.
16. Jorm, A.F. and Henderson, A.S. (1992). Memory bias in depression: implications for risk factor studies relying on self-reports of exposure. *International Journal of Methods in Psychiatric Research*, **2**, 31–8.
17. Schlesselman, J.L. (1982). *Case–control studies: design, conduct, analysis*. Oxford University Press, New York.
18. Anthony, J.C. (1988). The epidemiologic case–control strategy, with applications in psychiatric research. In *Handbook of social psychiatry* (ed. A.S. Henderson and G.D. Burrows), pp. 157–71. Elsevier, Amsterdam.
19. Best, N.G., Spiegelhalter, D.J., Thomas, A., and Brayne, C.E.G. (1996). Bayesian analysis of realistically complex models. *Journal of the Royal Statistical Society*, **159**, 323–42.
20. World Health Organization (1992). *The ICD-10 classification of mental and behavioural disorders. Clinical descriptions and diagnostic guidelines*. World Health Organization, Geneva.
21. World Health Organization (1993). *The ICD-10 classification of mental and behavioural disorders. Diagnostic criteria for research*. World Health Organization, Geneva.
22. American Psychiatric Association (1994). *Diagnostic and statistical manual. Fourth edition (DSM-IV)*. American Psychiatric Association, Washington, DC.
23. Pickering, G.W. (1968). *High blood pressure*. Churchill, London.
24. Goldberg, D.P. and Williams, P. (1988). *A user's guide to the GHQ*. NFER/Nelson, London.
25. Durkheim, E. (1897). *Le Suicide: Etude de Sociologie*. Felix Alcan, Paris.
26. Regier, D.A., Kaelber, C.T., Rae, D.S., *et al.* (1998). Limitations of diagnostic criteria and assessment instruments for mental disorders. *Archives of General Psychiatry*, **55**, 109–15.
27. Frances, A. (1998). Problems in defining clinical significance in epidemiological studies. *Archives of General Psychiatry*, **55**, 119.
28. Spitzer, R.L. (1998). Diagnosis and need for treatment are not the same. *Archives of General Psychiatry*, **55**, 120.
29. Goldberg, D. and Huxley, P. (1992). *Common mental disorders*. Tavistock Publications/Routledge, London.
30. Derogatis, L.R., Lipman, R.S., Rickels, K., Uhlenhuth, E.H., and Covi, L. (1974). The Hopkins Symptom Checklist (HSCL): a self-report symptom inventory. *Behavioral Science*, **19**, 1–15.
31. Bedford, A. and Foulds, G.A. (1978). *Manual of the Delusions–Symptoms States Inventory (state of anxiety-depression)*. NFER, Windsor.
32. Radloff, L.S. (1977). The CES-D scale: a self-report depression scale for research in the general population. *Applied Psychological Measurement*, **1**, 385–401.
33. Beck, A.T. (1967). *Depression: clinical, experimental and theoretical aspects*. Harper and Row, New York.
34. Conigrave, K.M., Hall, W.D., and Saunders, J.B. (1995). The AUDIT questionnaire: choosing a cut-off score. *Addiction*, **90**, 1349–56.
35. Folstein, M.F., Folstein, S.E., and McHugh, P.R. (1975). 'Mini-Mental State': a practical method for grading the cognitive state of patients for the clinician. *Journal of Psychiatric Research*, **12**, 189–98.
36. Brayne, C. and Calloway, P. (1990). The association of education and socioeconomic status with the Mini-Mental State Examination and the clinical diagnosis of dementia in the elderly. *Age and Ageing*, **19**, 91–6.
37. Henderson, A.S., Jorm, A., Mackinnon, A., *et al.* (1994). A survey of dementia in the Canberra population: experience with ICD-10 and DSM-III-R criteria. *Psychological Medicine*, **24**, 473–82
38. Kreitman, N. (1961). The reliability of psychiatric diagnosis. *Journal of Mental Science*, **7**, 876–86.
39. Wing, J.K., Cooper, J.E., and Sartorius, N. (1974). *The measurement and classification of psychiatric symptoms*. Cambridge University Press.
40. Wing, J.K., Babor, T., Brugha, T., *et al.* (1990). SCAN. Schedules for Clinical Assessment in Neuropsychiatry. *Archives of General Psychiatry*, **47**, 589–93.
41. Lewis, G., Pelosi, A.J., Araya, R., and Dunn, G. (1992). Measuring psychiatric disorder in the community: a standardized assessment for use by lay interviewers. *Psychological Medicine*, **22**, 465–86.
42. Jenkins, R., Bebbington, P., Farrell, M., *et al.* (1997). The National Psychiatric Morbidity Surveys of Great Britain—strategy and methods. *Psychological Medicine*, **27**, 765–74.
43. Robins, L.N., *et al.* (1988). The Composite International Diagnostic Interview. *Archives of General Psychiatry*, **45**, 1069–77.
44. Wittchen, H.-Ü. (1994). Reliability and validity studies of the WHO Composite International Diagnostic Interview (CIDI): a critical review. *Journal of Psychiatric Reviews*, **28**, 57–84.
45. Andrews, G. and Peters, L. (1998). The psychometric properties of the Composite International Diagnostic Interview. *Social Psychiatry and Psychiatric Epidemiology*, **33**, 80–8.
46. Peters, L. and Andrews, G. (1995). Procedural validity of the computerized version of the Composite International Diagnostic Interview (CIDI-auto) in the anxiety disorders. *Psychological Medicine*, **25**, 1269–80.
47. Brugha, T.S., Bebbington, P.E., Jenkins, R., *et al.* (1999). Cross validation of a general population survey diagnostic interview: a comparison of CIS-R with SCAN ICD-10 diagnostic categories. *Psychological Medicine*, **29**, 1029–42.
48. Copeland, J.R.M., Kelleher, M.J., Kellett, J.M., *et al.* (1976). A semi-structured clinical interview for the assessment of diagnosis and mental state in the elderly: the Geriatric Mental State Schedule. I. Development and reliability. *Psychological Medicine*, **6**, 439–49.
49. Roth, M., Tym, E., Mountjoy, C.Q., *et al.* (1986). CAMDEX. A standardised instrument for the diagnosis of mental disorder in the elderly with special reference to the early detection of dementia. *British Journal of Psychiatry*, **149**, 698–709.
50. Medical Research Council Cognitive Function and Ageing Study (1998). Cognitive function and dementia in six areas of England and Wales: the distribution of MMSE and prevalence of GMS organicity level in the MRC CFA study. *Psychological Medicine*, **28**, 319–35.
51. Social Psychiatry Research Unit (1992). The Canberra Interview for the Elderly: a new field instrument for the diagnosis of dementia and depression by ICD-10 and DSM-III-R. *Acta Psychiatrica Scandinavica*, **85**, 105–13.
52. Mulligan, R., Mackinnon, A., Berney, P., and Giannakopoulos, P. (1994). The reliability and validity of the French version of the Canberra Interview for the Elderly. *Acta Psychiatrica Scandinavica*, **89**, 268–73.
53. Jorm, A. and Mackinnon, A. (1995). *The Psychogeriatric Assessment Scale*. ANUTECH, Canberra.
54. Jorm, A., Mackinnon, A., Henderson, A.S., *et al.* (1995). The Psychogeriatric Assessment Scales: a multi-dimensional alternative to categorical diagnoses of dementia and depression in the elderly. *Psychological Medicine*, **25**, 447–60.
55. Jorm, A., Mackinnon, A.J., Christensen, H., Henderson, A.S., Jacomb, P.A., and Korten, A.E. (1997). The Psychogeriatric Assessment Scales (PAS): further data on psychometric properties and validity from a longitudinal study of the elderly. *International Journal of Geriatric Psychiatry*, **12**, 93–100.
56. World Health Organization (1988). *Psychiatric disability assessment schedule (WHO/DAS)*. World Health Organization, Geneva.
57. Janca, A., Kastrup, M., Katschnig, H., López-Ibor, J.J., Mezzich, J.E., and Sartorius, N. (1996). The World Health Organization Short Disability Assessment Schedule (WHO DAS-S): a tool for the assessment of difficulties in selected areas of functioning of patients with mental disorders. *Social Psychiatry and Psychiatric Epidemiology*, **31**, 349–54.
58. Von Korff, M., Üstün, T.B., Ormel, J., Kaplan, I., and Simon, G.E.

(1996). Self-report disability in an international primary care study of psychological illness. *Journal of Clinical Epidemiology*, **49**, 297–303.

59. Brazier, J.E., Harper, R., Jones, N.M.B., *et al.* (1992). Validating the SF-36 health survey questionnaire, new outcome measure for primary care. *British Medical Journal*, **305**, 160–4.

60. Bebbington, P. (1998). Sex and depression. *Psychological Medicine*, **28**, 1–8.

61. White, L., Katzman, R., Losonczy, K., *et al.* (1994). Association of education with incidence of cognitive impairment in three established populations for epidemiologic studies of the elderly. *Journal of Clinical Epidemiology*, **47**, 363–74.

62. Orrell, M. and Sahakian, B. (1995). Education and dementia. *British Medical Journal*, **310**, 951–2.

63. Cooley, C.H. (1909). *Social organization: a study of the larger mind*. Scribner, New York.

64. Turner, R.J. (1992). Measuring social support: issues of concept and method. In *The meaning and measurement of social support* (ed. H.O.F. Veiel and U. Baumann), pp. 217–33. Hemisphere, New York.

65. Henderson, S., Byrne, D.G., and Duncan-Jones, P. (1981). *Neurosis and the social environment*. Academic Press, Sydney.

66. Brugha, T.S., Sturt, E., and MacCarthy, B.E.A. (1987). The interview measure of social relationships: the description and evaluation of a survey instrument for assessing personal social resources. *Social Psychiatry*, **22**, 123–8.

67. Henderson, A.S. and Brown, G.W. (1988). Social support: the hypothesis and the evidence. In *Handbook of social psychiatry* (ed. A.S. Henderson and G.D. Burrows), pp. 73–85. Elsevier, Amsterdam.

68. Henderson, A.S. (1998). Social support: its present significance for psychiatric epidemiology. In *Adversity, stress and psychopathology* (ed. B.P. Dohrenwend), pp. 390–7. Oxford University Press, New York.

69. Leighton, D.C., Harding, J.S., Macklin, D.B., Hughes, C.C., and Leighton, A.H. (1963). Psychiatric findings of the Stirling County study. *American Journal Psychiatry*, **119**, 1021–6.

70. Leighton, D.C., Harding, J.S., Macklin, D.B., Macmillan, A.M., and Leighton, A. (1963). *The character of danger*. Basic Books, New York.

71. Bowlby, J. (1977). The making and breaking of affectional bonds. I. Aetiology and psychopathology in the light of attachment theory. *British Journal of Psychiatry*, **130**, 201–10.

72. Rutter, M. (1981). *Maternal deprivation reassessed*, p. 197. Penguin, Harmondsworth.

73. Parker, G., Tupling, H., and Brown, L.B. (1979). A parental bonding instrument. *British Journal of Medical Psychology*, **52**, 1–10.

74. Parker, G. (1983). *Overprotection: a risk factor in psychosocial development*. Grune and Stratton, New York.

75. Parker, G. (1992). Early environment. In *Handbook of affective disorders* (2nd edn) (ed. E.S. Paykel), pp. 171–83. Guilford Press, New York.

76. Parker, G., Roussos, J., Hadzi-Pavlovic, D., Mitchell, P., Wilhelm, K., and Austin, M.-P. (1997). The development of a refined measure of dysfunctional parenting and assessment of its relevance in patients with affective disorders. *Psychological Medicine*, **27**, 1193–203.

77. Mullen, P.E., Martin, J.L., Anderson, J.C., Romans, S.E., and Herbison, G.P. (1993). Childhood sexual abuse and mental health in adult life. *British Journal of Psychiatry*, **163**, 721–32.

78. Knutson, J.F. (1995). Psychological characteristics of maltreated children: putative risk factors and consequences. *Annual Review of Psychology*, **46**, 401–31.

79. Browne, A. and Finkelhor, D. (1986). Impact of child sexual abuse: a review of the research. *Psychological Bulletin*, **99**, 66–77.

80. Beitchman, J.H., Zucker, K.J., Hood, J.E., *et al.* (1992). A review of the long term effects of child sexual abuse. *Child Abuse and Neglect*, **16**, 101–18.

81. Katschnig, H. (ed.) (1986). *Life events and psychiatric disorders*. Cambridge University Press.

82. Brown, G.W. and Harris, T.O. (1989). *Life events and illness*. Guilford Press, London.

83. Dohrenwend, B.P. (ed.) (1998). *Adversity, stress and psychopathology*. Oxford University Press, New York.

84. Brugha, T., Bebbington, P., Tennant, C., and Hurry, J. (1985). The list of threatening experiences: a subset of 12 life event categories with considerable long-term contextual threat. *Psychological Medicine*, **15**, 1–6.

85. Brown, G.W. and Harris, T.O. (1978). *Social origins of depression: a study of psychiatric disorder in women*. Tavistock Publications, London.

86. Dohrenwend, B.P., Raphael, K.G., Schwartz, S., Stueve, A., and Skodol, A. (1993). The structured event probe and narrative rating method for measuring stressful life events. In *Handbook of stress* (ed. L. Goldberger and S. Breznitz), pp. 174–99. Free Press, New York.

87. Eysenck, S.B.G., Eysenck, H.J., and Barrett, P. (1985). A revised version of the psychoticism scale. *Personality and Individual Differences*, **6**, 21–9.

88. Fergusson, D.M., Horwood, L.J., and Lawton, J.M. (1989). The relationships between neuroticism and depressive symptoms. *Social Psychiatry and Psychiatric Epidemiology*, **24**, 275–81.

89. Surtees, P.G. and Wainwright, N.W.J. (1996). Fragile states of mind: neuroticism, vulnerability and the long-term outcome of depression. *British Journal of Psychiatry*, **169**, 338–47.

90. Kendler, K.S., Neale, M.C., Kessler, R.C., Heath, A.C., and Eaves, L.J. (1993). Childhood parental loss and adult psychopathology in women. *Archives of General Psychiatry*, **49**, 109–16.

91. Kendler, K.S. (1995). Adversity, stress and psychopathology: a psychiatric genetic perspective. *International Journal of Methods in Psychiatric Research*, **5**, 163–70.

92. Kendler, K.S. and Karkowski-Shuman, L. (1997). Stressful life events and genetic liability to major depression: genetic control of exposure to the environment? *Psychological Medicine*, **27**, 539–47.

93. Cloninger, C.R., Adolfsson, R., and Svrakic, N.M. (1996). Mapping genes for human personality. *Nature Genetics*, **12**, 3–4.

94. Baron, M. (1998). Mapping genes for personality: is the sagga sagging? *Molecular Psychiatry*, **3**, 106–8.

95. Henderson, S. and Blackwood, D. Molecular genetics in psychiatric epidemiology. *Psychological Medicine*, in press.

96. Susser, E. and Lin, S.P. (1994). Schizophrenia after prenatal exposure to the Dutch hunger winter of 1944–1945. *Archives of General Psychiatry*, **51**, 333–6.

97. Jones, P., Rodgers, B., Murray, R., and Marmot, M. (1994). Child developmental risk factors for adult schizophrenia in the British 1946 birth cohort. *Lancet*, **344**, 1398–402.

98. Jenkinson, M.L., Bliss, M.R., Brain, A.T., and Scott, D.L. (1989). Rheumatoid arthritis and senile dementia of the Alzheimer's type. *British Journal of Rheumatology*, **28**, 86–8.

99. Breitner, J.C.S. (1996). Inflammatory processes and anti-inflammatory drugs in Alzheimer's disease: a current appraisal. *Neurobiology of Aging*, **17**, 789–94.

100. Henderson, S., Duncan-Jones, P., Byrne, D.G., Scott, R., and Adcock, S. (1979). Psychiatric disorders in Canberra: a standardised study of prevalence. *Acta Psychiatrica Scandinavica*, **60**, 355–74.

101. Bebbington, P., Hurry, J., Tennant, C., Sturt, E., and Wing, J.K. (1981). Epidemiology of mental disorders in Camberwell. *Psychological Medicine*, **11**, 561–79.

102. Von Korff, M., Nestadt, G., Romanoski, A., *et al.* (1985). Prevalence of treated and untreated DSM-III schizophrenia. *Journal of Nervous and Mental Disease*, **173**, 577–81.

103. Mavreas, V.G., Beis, A., Mouyias, A., Rigoni, F., and Lyketsos, G.C. (1986). Prevalence of psychiatric disorders in Athens. A community study. *Social Psychiatry*, **21**, 172–81.

104. Lehtinen, V., Joukamaa, M., Lahtela, K., *et al.* (1990). Prevalence of mental disorders among adults in Finland: basic results from the Mini Finland Health Survey. *Acta Psychiatrica Scandinavica*, **81**, 418–25.

105. Regier, D.A., Farmer, M.E., Rae, D.S., *et al.* (1993). One-month prevalence of mental disorders in the United States and sociodemographic characteristics: the Epidemiologic Catchment Area Study. *Acta Psychiatrica Scandinavica*, **88**, 35–47.

3

Psychodynamic contributions to psychiatry

3.1 The historical development of dynamic psychiatry

Anthony Storr

The adjective 'psychodynamic' is variously defined by different authorities. In this chapter, it will be taken as applying to psychological systems and theories which describe persons as changing and developing rather than as static entities, and which assume that individuals are motivated by drives of which they may or may not be consciously aware.

Nineteenth century psychiatry

Until the end of the nineteenth century, psychiatry was chiefly concerned with the custodial care of the insane in asylums. Insanity was believed to be caused by disease of the brain, although it was recognized that the brain displayed no obvious signs of abnormality at postmortem in some common forms of insanity. Mental illness was considered to be a sign of degeneration, perhaps caused by factors like alcoholism in one or other parent.

Kraepelin's important differentiation of manic–depressive illness from dementia praecox (schizophrenia) did not begin to be defined until 1896. Asylums contained patients suffering from many varieties of psychiatric illness who had nothing in common with one another except their inability to comply with the standards of behaviour demanded by society.

Patients suffering from mental illness were subjected to a variety of medical treatments ranging from the application of electricity and the wet pack to the prescription of purges and emetics, bromides, chloral hydrate, paraldehyde, and even injections of morphine. Since none of these treatments were effective, asylums became depressing institutions in which chronic cases accumulated and from which very few inmates were or could be discharged as cured. The consequence was that no doctor aiming at professional distinction chose to work in an asylum, and the doctors who did so were despised by their medical colleagues.

Neurosis as 'incipient lunacy'

This deplorable state of affairs was gradually modified when a few leading figures like Henry Maudsley began to build private practices. The affluent insane were directed toward small private asylums; but an increasing proportion of patients seeking advice from alienists did not require certification or confinement, but were described as suffering from 'neurasthenia' or 'incipient lunacy' rather than full-blown insanity. These patients, whom we should now deem neurotic, were thought to be carriers of some form of hereditary taint, or suffering from 'latent brain disease'.[1] Because the assumption was that neurosis, as well as insanity, was constitutional, it followed that not much could be expected from treatment other than minimal alleviation. Neurology became established as a medical speciality in the 1870s and 1880s, and many neurotic patients preferred to seek the advice of neurologists who were recognized as 'nerve-specialists', but who lacked any stigma of association with asylums. Because of the comparative rarity of organic neurological disease, many neurologists continued to make their living by treating neurotics with sedatives until the 1940s or later.

The first dynamic psychiatry

Alongside this depressing static picture of mental illness, another conception of mental disorder was developing outside the asylum. In his book *The Discovery of the Unconscious*, Henri Ellenberger refers to the *first dynamic psychiatry* which he dates as lasting from 1775 to 1900; that is, from the time of Mesmer to the time of Charcot. Throughout this period, students of the mind's vagaries were predominantly concerned with the phenomena allied to, or brought about by, hypnosis. Hypnotic subjects, when aroused from the hypnotic state, commonly had no recollection of what had transpired during the period of trance. This demonstrated that the mind could not necessarily be regarded as a single entity, and might sometimes be divided against itself. Somnambulism, fugue states, multiple personality, and automatic writing all confirmed this conception of mind as a playground or battlefield of interacting or conflicting forces; and where there is conflict, there is also the possibility of resolution of conflict.

Mesmer and his successors had shown that suggestion could alter mental states and rid some subjects of disturbing symptoms. Mesmer believed that a mysterious fluid resembling the 'ether' of the physicists permeated the body, and that disease was caused by unequal distribution of this fluid. By means of what he called 'animal magnetism', equilibrium could be restored. In other words, at least some forms of mental disturbance could be modified or cured, which threw doubt on their origin being wholly genetic or degenerative.

The idea of the unconscious

Lancelot Law Whyte, in *The Unconscious Before Freud*, describes the *Transition from Static towards Process Concepts*, which he dates as beginning around 1750. Many thinkers contributed to this change in how men regarded themselves and the mind, including Vico, Herder,

Goethe, Schopenhauer, and Nietzsche. Whyte wrote: 'I have given enough evidence to show that the general conception of unconscious mental processes was *conceivable* (in post-Cartesian Europe) around 1700, *topical* around 1800, and *fashionable* around 1870–1880'.[2]

The rise of individualism

So the pessimistic static concept of mental illness current within the asylum became opposed by a more optimistic dynamic concept in which change and development within the mind could lead to better balance or even complete cure. Psychodynamic theories are primarily concerned with the psychology of the individual, and could not have been developed in pre-industrial societies, which have little perception of a person as a separate entity rather than a member of a tribe or family. The growth of individualism and self-consciousness can be traced by studying the dictionary. For example, most of the compound words which combine the word *self* with other words, like *self-sufficient*, *self-knowledge*, *self-determination*, *self- conscious*, entered the language during the seventeenth century. A quotation from Southey dated 1809 is the first example of the use of the word *autobiography* given by the *Oxford English Dictionary*. The modern psychoanalyst is concerned with making coherent sense out of his patient's life history by encouraging him to produce a detailed verbal autobiography. This procedure could only be undertaken or thought worthwhile in a society which valued individualism.

The change from static to process concepts could also be perceived in ideas about society. In 1848, Mrs Alexander had written in the hymn *All Things Bright and Beautiful*:

> The rich man in his castle,
> The poor man at his gate,
> God made them, high or lowly,
> And order'd their estate.

Modern congregations find that singing this hymn is embarrassing unless this verse is omitted.

The dynamic view of society can be illustrated by Karl Marx's famous sentence, written in 1888:

> Philosophers have previously offered various interpretations of the world. Our business is to change it.[3]

Although Marx was not introspective, whilst Freud was intensely so, the two men shared certain characteristics. Both were dogmatically certain that their discoveries were right, and both regarded ordinary people with distaste or even contempt. Marx dismissed the majority of the people he met as either fools or sycophants; Freud wrote that most human beings were trash.

Static versus dynamic

Psychiatrists adopting the static concept were likely to be objective detached observers who were principally concerned with diagnostic classification, and who emphasized nature rather than nurture. Psychiatrists adopting the dynamic concept were less interested in exact description and diagnosis, more interested in empathizing with the patient's emotional inner life, and emphasized nurture rather than nature.

Both attitudes are limiting when carried to extremes. It is possible for a psychiatrist to be so objectively scientific that he only perceives his patient as an example of one or other mental abnormality, and fails to understand him as a person. It is equally possible for a psychiatrist so to empathize with his patient that he cannot perceive the latter diagnostically or critically, and is likely to see progress and improvement where none exists. The nature versus nurture controversy has also been evident in the dispute about the inheritance of IQ and educability. It is clear that temperamental prejudice influences which stance a psychiatrist or a psychologist chooses to adopt.

Freud's early theories

The rise of modern psychodynamic theory, led by Freud, began around the end of the nineteenth century, and was directly derived from Freud's period of study with Charcot during the winter of 1885–1886. Charcot had been studying hypnosis for some years in the hope of discovering a diagnostic technique which would enable him to distinguish between paralyses which were the consequence of organic disease and those which were hysterical. When a patient developed a hysterical paralysis, the form which it took could not be explained in terms of a lesion of a particular peripheral nerve, but was determined by the patient's idea of where his leg or arm began and ended. Such paralyses could often be both cured and later reinstated by hypnotic suggestion, whereas paralyses caused by organic disease of the nervous system remained unaffected.

Freud learned two main lessons from Charcot's demonstrations. The first was that, since subjects who had been hypnotized could not recall what had happened during the hypnotic trance, it must be the case that mental processes influencing behaviour took place unconsciously. The second lesson was that ideas could be causal agents in the production of hysterical symptoms.

Freud at first treated his neurotic patients with hypnosis. In addition to suggesting ideas of positive health, Freud used hypnosis as a means of enabling the patient to recall the forgotten origin of particular symptoms. This technique derived from Freud's colleague and friend, Josef Breuer, who had been treating his famous case 'Anna O.' with hypnosis. Breuer discovered that if 'Anna O.' could recall the exact moment at which a particular symptom started and could also recover and express the emotion which she felt at the time, the symptom disappeared. Breuer named this form of treatment *catharsis*. Breuer and Freud proclaimed, in a famous sentence: *Hysterics suffer mainly from reminiscences.*[4]

Sexuality and repression

Freud discovered that most of these reminiscences were painful or shameful, and not easily accessible to conscious recall. This led him to postulate a mental mechanism which he called **repression**, which tended to banish unpleasant memories from consciousness. Freud, therefore, was postulating a state of **conflict** within the mind in which a painful emotion was seeking to be discharged, while another part of the mind was refusing to allow this to happen. According to Freud, nearly all these reminiscences were concerned with sexual experience.

Freud remained convinced that sexual satisfaction was the key to happiness, and that what was wrong with the neurotic was failure to achieve a normal sex life. This central conviction had two roots. In his autobiographical study, Freud acknowledges his debt to the ideas of G.T. Fechner, a professor of physics and then philosophy at Leipzig

University. During the course of a manic–depressive illness, Fechner introduced the idea of a universal 'pleasure principle', which Freud adopted. Freud also took from Fechner the notion of a 'principle of constancy', the idea that the main function of the mental apparatus was to bring about the discharge of instinctual tension in order to maintain stability. Freud thought that one dominating principle governing human behaviour was the need to reach a state of tensionless tranquillity (he called it the Nirvana principle). Freud treated powerful emotions as disturbances to be abolished rather than as pleasures to be sought. He seems to have been unaware of 'stimulus hunger'. Human beings in a restricted boring environment are far from being contented with tranquillity: in reality they yearn for intellectual and emotional stimuli, but Freud does not consider this.

Second, Freud hoped that neurosis would ultimately be shown to be physical in origin. In 1895, he used his neurological knowledge to represent psychological processes in terms of what little was then known about neuronal function within the brain. This 'project for a scientific psychology', as Freud's English translators named it, continued to influence Freud's later work, but it was never published during his lifetime. It is an attempt to link psychology and neurology which still awaits fulfilment.

However, sex goes some way toward bridging the gap between physical and mental. It is obviously physical and hormonal in origin, but it also gives rise to purely psychological phenomena like thoughts, phantasies, and dreams. As Freud wrote to Jung:

> In the sexual processes we have the indispensable 'organic foundation' without which a medical man can only feel ill at ease in the life of the psyche.[5]

Healing the Cartesian split

In the seventeenth century, Descartes had claimed a sharp division between mind and body.

> While it is possible (or rather, it is certain, as I shall say further on) that I have a body, which is very closely joined to me; nevertheless, since on the one hand I have a clear and distinct idea of myself, as purely a thing that thinks and is not extended, and, on the other hand, I have a distinct idea of the body as a thing that is extended and does not think, it is certain that this *I*, that is to say my soul, which makes me what I am, is entirely and truly distinct from my body, and can be or exist without it.[6]

L.L. Whyte considers this claim to be one of the fundamental blunders made by the human mind, and suggests that one reason why Freud's ideas became so appealing was that, by linking mind indissolubly with body, he was repairing Descartes's dualistic error. Whyte might also have pointed out, although he does not do so, that Freud was an agnostic who had no need to postulate a soul, since he did not believe in the soul's immortality. Freud thought that all mental activity was ultimately driven by unconscious, 'instinctual', physical drives, and thus came close to affirming that the body itself 'thinks', in sharp contrast with Descartes's conception.

The original idea that neurosis was caused by specific traumas occurring in early childhood which had been repressed, was gradually replaced by the idea that neurosis in adult life came about because the child's sexual development had been partly arrested at an immature stage, which made adult sexual fulfilment difficult or impossible.

Freud's account of infantile development does not take account of cognition, perception, or conventional ideas of learning, but is exclusively concerned with sex, which, in the widest sense, includes all types of physical pleasure.

Infantile sexuality

Freud's stages of development were based upon which bodily organ he considered predominant. During the first year of life, the infant's capacity for physical gratification is centred upon the mouth, so this stage is labelled 'oral.' From the ages of 1 to 3, the anus gains pride of place. The anal stage is succeeded by the phallic stage, in which libidinal interest focuses upon the genitals and masturbation, although the child is still incapable of sexual fulfilment through intercourse with another person. After puberty, the 'normal' individual reaches the genital stage, in which satisfying sexual relations with a person of the opposite sex become possible; but traces from all the previous stages persist into adult life in even the most mature characters. If a patient could overcome the blocks imposed by repression and recall the earliest infantile sexual impulses, these could be brought into consciousness and abreacted, thus opening the previously impeded path towards sexual maturity.

Breuer and Freud published *Studies on Hysteria* as joint authors in 1895. This is generally reckoned to be the first psychoanalytic book. The second was *The Interpretation of Dreams* which appeared in November 1899. The term 'psychotherapy' was introduced by the followers of the leader of the so-called Nancy school of hypnosis, Hippolyte Bernheim (1840–1919), and became widely popular. Bernheim, for a time, rivalled the fame of Charcot. Freud visited him in the summer of 1889. One of the facts Freud learned from Bernheim was that hypnosis was much more successful with the lower classes, who tended to comply with the suggestions of their social superiors. The time was ripe for the introduction of a form of psychotherapy suitable for the 'carriage trade', who might respond better to a less authoritarian approach. Freud discovered that traumatic memories could be recovered without the dubious aid of hypnosis. If the patient lay supine on the couch and was honest enough to reveal everything which was passing through his mind, he would inevitably come upon disturbing material relevant to his neurotic problems. This technique was named free association. From 1892 onwards, Freud gradually abandoned the use of hypnosis in favour of this new procedure. This was an important innovation, because the employment of free association demanded that the patient took the lead, while the analyst remained a passive listener who issued interpretations rather than behaving like a conventional physician who gave orders or advice. Freud's clientèle, who were mostly upper class, may have welcomed an approach which allowed the patient to take the initiative rather than obey orders.

The ways in which the 'medical model' of the cause and treatment of neurosis was progressively modified is dealt with in greater detail in Chapter 3.2. Freud's discovery of transference eventually led to psychoanalysis and its derivatives becoming more concerned with the development and maldevelopment of the patient's relationships with significant others from infancy onward than with his or her infantile sexuality. Psychoanalysis became a technique of emotional re-education in which investigation, interpretation, and consequent modification of the patient's attitudes toward the analyst, rather than exploration of infantile sexuality, became the principal vehicle of change.

Psychoanalysis and psychosis

Although Freud had practically no experience of psychotic patients, and specifically stated that psychotic patients were not suitable subjects for psychoanalysis, this did not deter him from writing about their presumed psychopathology in psychoanalytic terms. For example, he wrote a penetrating account of severe depressive illness in *Mourning and Melancholia*[7] and a less convincing interpretation of paranoia in *Psycho-Analytic Notes on an Autobiographical Account of a Case of Paranoia*[8] and *A Case of Paranoia Running Counter to the Psycho-Analytic Theory of the Disease.*[9] Psychoanalytic ideas were eagerly discussed in psychiatric hospitals because they offered a new interpretation of mental illness in terms of psychopathology even when there was no prospect of cure. Psychoanalysis was gradually establishing itself throughout Europe.

Two 'heretics'

Alfred Adler

Alfred Adler (1870–1937) joined Freud's discussion group in 1902, and was made President of the Vienna Psycho-Analytic Society in 1910. However, Adler's ideas became increasingly at variance with those of Freud, and, in 1911, together with six adherents, he parted company with Freud, later founding his own Society for Individual Psychology. Adler, who had himself suffered from rickets in childhood, studied the ways in which individuals compensated, or overcompensated, for physical defects. In his view, 'aggression,' in the wide sense of self-assertion and the will to power, took precedence over sex as the prime mover of human conduct. Freud's approach was historical; Adler's was teleological. That is, Freud attempted to reconstruct the patient's infancy, while Adler strove to determine the patient's goals. Adler pictured the child as feeling itself to be weak and inferior to adults, but as striving to overcome such feelings of inferiority in a variety of ways which were dictated by genetic endowment, position within the family, and type of upbringing. Thus, the clever child strives to achieve superiority through his intellect, while his physically more agile brother develops his muscles. Adler believed that the individual adopted a characteristic 'style of life' at an early age which dictated his further development. Individuals were pictured as striving toward a variety of hidden goals of which they were only partially aware. The fully mature individual should, ideally, replace striving for superiority over his fellows by *Gemeinschaftsgefühl*, that is, 'social interest' within a co-operating community.

Adler, a socialist by conviction, a Protestant by conversion, and, through his Russian wife, an acquaintance of Trotsky and other revolutionaries, was passionately concerned with social problems, and was influenced by both Nietzsche and Marx. Freud regarded society as a limitation on the individual, restraining him from uninhibited instinctual fulfilment. Adler, true to his socialist convictions, believed that social interaction and co-operation were essential to mental health.

Adler's *Individual Psychology* reached its peak of popularity during the 1920s and early 1930s. At one time there were 34 local associations

promoting Adlerian ideas. The majority of these were in Central Europe, but there were also associations in Great Britain and the United States, and there were Adlerian journals in English on both sides of the Atlantic. The advent of Hitler put an end to most Adlerian associations in Europe, and the majority of Adler's associates were compelled to emigrate. For a time, Adler's name faded from sight. He was essentially a teacher and a publicist rather than a theoretician. Unlike Freud and Jung, he left no large corpus of scholarly work. His books are written in a popular style because they nearly all took origin from lectures. Many of his ideas were appropriated by others, often without acknowledgment; but he did make important and original contributions to psychiatry.

Adler's interest in psychological reactions to physical defects, 'organ inferiority' and its consequences, provided a springboard for the development of psychosomatic medicine. In addition, he was a pioneer in the development of child guidance clinics. These were attached to schools in Vienna, where psychiatrists and teachers collaborated in treating educational and emotional problems in children. These clinics were abolished by the Nazis, presumably because Alfred Adler was a Jew.

Freud did not fully acknowledge the importance of aggression until 1920. Adler emphasized aggression, the will to power, and the wish for dominance over others from the beginning. Adler's conviction that every mature individual needed to contribute to, and be a part of, society, contrasted sharply with Freud's negative view of society as a brake upon instinctual expression, and with Jung's concentration upon the development of the individual in isolation.

C. G. Jung

In December 1900, Jung obtained a post as an assistant in the Burghölzli mental hospital in Zürich, then directed by Eugen Bleuler, the psychiatrist who introduced the term 'schizophrenia'. In 1905, he was appointed a lecturer in psychiatry at the University of Zürich and was also promoted to Senior Staff Physician at the Psychiatric Clinic. During these first years in psychiatry, Jung wrote his MD dissertation *On the Psychology and Pathology of So-called Occult Phenomena*, and began his studies based on word-association tests. At this date, associationist theories of mental functioning were paramount. Jung transformed the word-association test from a way of investigating similarity, contrast, and contiguity into a technique for uncovering emotional preoccupations. A list of 100 words is read out, and the subject is asked to respond to each with the first word that occurs to him. By timing the interval between stimulus and response, it was possible to show that, unknown to themselves, subjects are influenced by words which arouse emotion, because such words slow down their responses. This was an important piece of research, because it demonstrated experimentally that unconscious mental contents could influence behaviour.

Freud's ideas were eagerly discussed at the Burghölzli. Eugen Bleuler lists five references to Freud in his famous monograph *Dementia Praecox oder die Gruppe der Schizophrenien*. Bleuler wrote to Freud and told him that his writings were being studied there. In 1907, Jung published a pioneering book on schizophrenia, *The Psychology of Dementia Praecox*[10], which was the first notable attempt to interpret the phenomena of insanity from a psychoanalytic viewpoint. Jung demonstrated that even the fragmented utterances of the insane can have a personal meaning. Jung sent the book to Freud, which prompted Freud to invite him to Vienna. Their first meeting took place in March 1907. Jung (see Chapter 3.3.1) continued to write dynamically orientated papers on schizophrenia until a few years before his death, but he also thought it probable that a chemical factor was involved in the disease. In a lecture *On the Problem of Psychogenesis in Mental Disease*,[11] given at the Royal Society of Medicine in July 1919, Jung gives examples of psychotic behaviour precipitated by emotionally charged events, and insists that psychological factors must be considered along with disease of the brain if mental disease is to be fully comprehended.

From 1907 to 1913, Freud and Jung collaborated, albeit mostly at a distance, since Freud lived in Vienna and Jung lived in Zürich. Jung was a particularly welcome recruit to the psychoanalytic cause for two reasons. First, he was already a distinguished psychiatrist from another country; second, unlike the majority of Freud's close associates, he was not a Jew. However, temperamental and theoretical differences between the two men became more and more evident. Jung finally parted from Freud in 1913; that is, some 2 years after Adler, and 6 years after he first met Freud in 1907. Finally, Jung resigned from the Presidency of the International Psychoanalytic Association in 1914.

Adler and Jung were not the only 'heretics' who defected from the Vienna Psycho-Analytic Society, but they were the most important and original members to do so.

The spread of psychoanalysis

In 1909, Freud, Jung, and Ferenczi visited the United States and lectured at Clark University, Worcester, Massachusetts. By 1911, Havelock Ellis was able to report that psychoanalysis was being practised in Austria, Switzerland, and the United States, and also in England, India, and Canada. Before the outbreak of the First World War, psychoanalysis had already begun to assume the character of a worldwide movement.

'Shell-shock'

The First World War prompted increasing interest in psychodynamic explanations of neurosis because of the large number of serving soldiers who suffered from 'shell-shock.' Some exhibited deaf-mutism, blindness, amnesia, or other hysterical symptoms. Many complained of recurrent nightmares, or had waking visions of the horrors of the trenches which were of hallucinatory intensity. The devastating effects of prolonged lack of sleep were not fully appreciated. The term 'shell-shock', introduced in 1915, indicated the current belief that proximity to exploding shells, even without physical injury, could damage the nervous system. But the British Army was slow to accept the actuality of what we should now call post-traumatic stress disorder, and the diagnosis of shell-shock was no defence in cases where men had deserted:

> Even as late as May 1916, said Colonel Myers, who was then the Consulting Psychologist to the Army, 'From a military standpoint, a deserter was either "insane" and destined for the "mad house", or responsible and should be shot'.[12]

Shell-shock became such a problem that special hospitals had to be set up for its treatment. The official casualty figures show that there were 28 533 cases of shell-shock reported in France up to the end of 1917.[13] It was gradually realized that even the bravest of men break down if the stress imposed upon them is sufficient. Some years later, study of Communist methods of interrogation reinforced the realization that no-one can indefinitely withstand intense stress accompanied by sleep deprivation . Study of what would now be called 'war neurosis' contributed to the general perception that psychological conflict was an important determinant of illness, and that the sufferer might be unaware, or only partially aware, of the opposing forces within his psyche.

During the 1920s, psychoanalysis began to interest English intellectuals. James Strachey, whose translation of Freud's writings was published as *The Standard Edition of the Complete Psychological Works of Sigmund Freud* between 1953 and 1974, had undergone analysis with Freud in Vienna in 1920. Interest in psychoanalysis permeated Bloomsbury to the extent of influencing Lytton Strachey's book *Elizabeth and Essex*. On Christmas Day 1928, Freud himself wrote a cautious letter to Lytton Strachey about the book. Lionel S. Penrose, who later became famous for his work on the genetics of mental handicap, was another intellectual who studied with Freud.

Hitler's promotion of psychoanalysis

The Second World War also promoted the spread of pychodynamic ideas, for an entirely different reason. A very high proportion of European psychoanalysts were, like their founder, Jews. Hitler's persecution led to their emigration. Some came to England, but the majority found refuge in the United States and profoundly influenced the development of psychiatry in that country. It has been argued that psychoanalysis was likely to make an especially strong impact upon a society based upon immigrants who were cut off from the network of stable social relationships, family ties, and religion which characterized older cultures. Whereas members of traditional societies make sense out of their experience in terms of these relationships, immigrant cultures have fewer reference points, and people therefore look for ways of understanding themselves which are based upon the psychological development of the isolated individual.

As psychoanalysis spread beyond the consulting room to make incursions into anthropology, sociology, religion, literature, art, and the occult, it became what Ernest Gellner called 'the dominant idiom for the discussion of the human personality and of human relations'.[14] Gradually, more and more psychoanalytic training institutes were established. By the 1970s, such institutes existed in every continent except Africa.

Even in England, where there was always less enthusiasm for psychoanalysis and its variants than in the United States, the principal training school for psychiatrists at the Maudsley Hospital and Institute of Psychiatry found it advisable to recruit dynamically orientated psychotherapists to its teaching staff. In the late 1940s, a Kleinian, a Jungian, and an eclectic psychoanalyst rubbed shoulders without generating too much friction.

The Tavistock Clinic became established as a centre where psychoanalytic psychotherapy was available for selected out-patients and where the staff were predominantly trained in Freudian methods. The Cassel Hospital was another institution staffed by psychoanalysts which offered psychoanalytic treatment to in-patients.

In the United States, psychoanalysis became so essential a part of the psychiatrist's training that, from the 1930s to the 1960s, it was virtually impossible to be appointed to a leading position in psychiatry without proffering as a qualification membership of one or other of the psychoanalytic institutes. Since the introduction of effective drugs, the pendulum has swung so violently in the opposite direction in the United States that young psychiatrists in training have barely heard of Freud and have certainly never read his writings.

The influence of psychodynamic theories

Research has shown that psychoanalysis, in the form originally promulgated by Freud and his followers, is no more effective in relieving neurotic symptoms than other less demanding and less expensive forms of psychotherapy. Freud's theory of dreams, which he himself considered to embody his deepest insight, has not stood the test of time. Nor have his views on religion, anthropology, and art. Although many of his psychopathological interpretations are open to question, he was a great clinical observer and a great writer whose descriptions of obsessional neurosis and melancholia remain unsurpassed. In spite of the comparative failure of psychoanalysis as either a system of psychopathology or a technique of treatment, psychoanalytic ideas have caused a revolution in the way Western man thinks about himself, and have also had a major effect upon twentieth-century art and literature. Psychoanalysis has entered the language we use, and it would be difficult to discard from our writing and speaking such words as 'repression', 'sublimation', 'ego', 'id', superego', 'unconscious', 'projection', and 'defence mechanisms'. Freud's uncompromising reductive stance tended to explain human behaviour in terms of the lowest common instinctual denominator. One result has been to make us less inclined to take what were considered virtues at their face values. So altruism and self-sacrifice are interpreted as masochistic, and celibacy is considered a flight from sex or as masking perversion.

Although psychodynamic theories have made us more aware of the human tendency to self-deception, they have also made us more tolerant. Because Freud laid it down that neurosis has its roots in early childhood, psychiatrists and others working in child guidance clinics have studied the child's development within the family and based their treatment of the child's difficulties upon understanding family dynamics. Psychiatrists, hospital administrators, and others have become aware of the young child's need for secure attachment, and of the dire consequences which are likely to follow if such attachment is suddenly disrupted. For example, mothers and infants are kept together rather than separated whenever possible, even if one or the other has to be admitted to hospital.

Although we are no better at preventing crime or treating criminals than before the advent of psychodynamic theories, there is a greater appreciation among forensic psychiatrists that crime reflects alienation from society rather than innate wickedness, and a greater realization that savage penalties are ineffective.

Sexual diversity is no longer attributed to moral degeneration. Freud attempted to account for homosexuality and other forms of sexual deviance in terms of the vicissitudes of infantile emotional development. Although it is now believed that some varieties of sexual deviance are due to variations in the development of the brain in infancy, Freud's frank discussion of infantile sexuality did much to dispel the cloud of moral disapproval which had hitherto hindered our understanding of these phenomena.

Freud's employment of free association instead of hypnosis was referred to above. Freud's technique of listening to distressed people over long periods has had a profound and beneficial influence upon all techniques of psychotherapy derived from psychoanalysis. Psychoanalysis and its derivatives have in common that they are techniques of helping the patient to understand and help himself rather than obeying doctor's orders or carrying out instructions. In spite of this, Freud discovered that his patients tended to put him in the position of a father figure, an idealized lover, or even a saviour. Freud's discovery of what he called 'transference' has affected every subsequent type of analytical psychotherapy. Today, exploration and interpretation of the patient's changing attitude to the analyst is a major tool in enabling the patient to understand and improve his relationships with others in the world outside the consulting room.

Although psychoanalysis and its derivatives have not led us into the promised land for which Freud had hoped, the impact of psychodynamic theories has been considerable. Freud did cause a revolution in the way we think about ourselves. As Karl Popper claimed, our understanding of the world and of ourselves progresses by the refutation of existing hypotheses. Even if every theory which Freud put forward could be proved wrong, we should still be greatly indebted to him.

References

1. Scull, A. (1993). *The most solitary of afflictions: madness and society in Britain 1700–1900*, p. 255. Yale University Press, New Haven, CT.
2. Whyte, L.L. (1962). *The unconscious before Freud*, pp. 168–9. Tavistock Publications, London.
3. Marx, K., quoted in Berlin, I. (1978) *Karl Marx* (4th edn), p. 107. Oxford University Press.
4. Breuer, J. and Freud, S. (1893). *The standard edition of the complete psychological works of Sigmund Freud* (translated by James Strachey in collaboration with Anna Freud, assisted by Alix Strachey and Alan Tyson). Vol. 2, *Studies on hysteria*, p. 7. Hogarth Press and Institute of Psycho-Analysis, London, 1955.
5. McGuire, W. (ed.) (1974). *The Freud/Jung letters* (translated by Ralph Manheim and R.F.C. Hull), pp. 140–1. Hogarth Press and Routledge & Kegan Paul, London.
6. Quoted in Williams, B. (1978). *Descartes: the project of pure enquiry*, pp. 104–5. Penguin, Harmondsworth.
7. Freud, S. (1917). Mourning and melancholia. In *The standard edition of the complete psychological works of Sigmund Freud* (translated by James Strachey in collaboration with Anna Freud, assisted by Alix Strachey and Alan Tyson), Vol. 14, pp. 239–58. Hogarth Press and Institute of Psycho-Analysis, London, 1957.
8. Freud, S. (1911). Psycho-analytic notes on an autobiographical account of a case of paranoia. In *The standard edition of the complete psychological works of Sigmund Freud* (translated by James Strachey in collaboration with Anna Freud, assisted by Alix Strachey and Alan Tyson), Vol. 12, pp. 3–82. Hogarth Press and Institute of Psycho-Analysis, London, 1958.
9. Freud, S. (1915). A case of paranoia running counter to the psychoanalytic theory of the disease. In *The standard edition of the complete psychological works of Sigmund Freud* (translated by James Strachey in collaboration with Anna Freud, assisted by Alix Strachey and Alan Tyson), Vol. 14, pp. 261–72. Hogarth Press and Institute of Psycho-Analysis, London, 1957.
10. Jung, C.G. (1900). The psychology of dementia praecox. In *The collected works of C.G. Jung* (translated by R.F.C. Hull) (ed. Sir Herbert Read, Michael Fordham, and Gerhard Adler), Vol. 3, pp. 3–151. Routledge and Kegan Paul, London, 1960.
11. Jung, C.G. (1907). On the problem of psychogenesis in mental disease.

In *The collected works of C.G. Jung* (translated by R.F.C. Hull) (ed. Sir Herbert Read, Michael Fordham, and Gerhard Adler), Vol. 3, pp. 211–25. Routledge & Kegan Paul, London, 1960.

12. Babington, A. (1997). *Shell-shock*, p. 57. Leo Cooper, London.
13. Babington, A. (1997). *Shell-shock*, p. 104. Leo Cooper, London.
14. Gellner, E. (1985). *The psychoanalytic movement*, p. 5. Paladin, London.

3.2 Psychoanalysis: Freud's theories and their contemporary development

Otto F. Kernberg

Psychoanalysis is:

(1) a personality theory, and, more generally, a theory of psychological functioning that focuses particularly on unconscious mental processes;

(2) a method for the investigation of psychological functions based on the exploration of free associations within a special therapeutic setting;

(3) a method for treatment of a broad spectrum of psychopathological conditions, including the symptomatic neuroses (anxiety states, characterological depression, obsessive–compulsive disorder, conversion hysteria, and dissociative hysterical pathology), sexual inhibitions and perversions ('paraphilias'), and the personality disorders.

Psychoanalysis has also been applied, mostly in modified versions, i.e. in psychoanalytic psychotherapies, to the treatment of severe personality disorders, psychosomatic conditions, and certain psychotic conditions, particularly a subgroup of patients with chronic schizophrenic illness.

All three aspects of psychoanalysis were originally developed by Sigmund Freud,[1–3] whose theories of the dynamic unconscious, personality development, personality structure, psychopathology, methodology of psychoanalytic investigation, and method of treatment still largely influence the field, both in the sense that many of his central ideas continue as the basis of contemporary psychoanalytic thinking, and in that corresponding divergencies, controversies, and radical innovations still can be better understood in the light of the overall frame of his contributions. Freud's concepts of dream analysis, mechanisms of defence, and transference have become central aspects of many contemporary psychotherapeutic procedures.

Freud's ideas about personality development and psychopathology, the method of psychoanalytic investigation, and the analytic approach to treatment gradually changed in the course of his dramatically creative lifespan. Moreover, the theory of the structure of the mind that he assumed must underly the events that he observed clinically changed in major respects, so that an overall summary of his views can hardly be undertaken without tracing the history of his thinking. The present overview will lead up to summaries of his final conclusions as to the structure of the mind and how this is reflected in personality development and psychopathology. Psychoanalysis will then be described as a method of treatment, as seen from the point of view of resolution of conflict between impulse and defence, and from that of object-relations theory. We shall explore significant changes that have occurred in all these domains, and conclude with an overview of con-

temporary psychoanalysis, with particular emphasis upon the presently converging tendencies of contemporary psychoanalytic approaches, and new developments that remain controversial.

Freud's theory of the mental apparatus: motivation, structure, and functioning

Unconscious mental processes: the topographic theory; defence mechanisms

Freud's starting point[4] was his study of hysterical patients and the discovery that, when he found a way to help these patients piece together a coherent account of the antecedents of their conversion symptoms, dissociative phenomena, and pathological affective dispositions, all these psychopathological phenomena could be traced to traumatic experiences in their past that had become unconscious. That is, these traumatic experiences continued to influence the patients' functioning despite an active defensive mechanism of 'repression' that excluded them from the patient's conscious awareness. In the course of a few years Freud abandoned his early efforts to recover repressed material by means of hypnosis, and replaced hypnosis with the technique of 'free association', an essential aspect of psychoanalytic technique until the present time. Freud instructed his patients to eliminate as much as possible all 'prepared agendas', and to try to express whatever came to mind, while attempting to exert as little censorship over this material as they could. He provided them with a non-judgemental and stable setting in which to carry out their task, inviting them to recline on a couch while he sat behind it. The sessions lasted for an hour and were conducted five to six times a week. There has been little change in the essentials of this format, except that sessions have been shortened to 45 to 50 min and are carried out three to five times a week. The method of free association led to the gradual recovery of repressed memories of traumatic events. Originally, Freud thought that the recovery of such events into consciousness would permit their abreaction and elaboration, and thus resolve the patients' symptoms.

Practising this method led Freud to several lines of discovery. To begin, he conceptualized unconscious mechanisms of defence that opposed the recovery of memories by free association. He described these mechanisms, namely repression, negation, isolation, projection, introjection, transformation into the opposite, rationalization, intellectualization, and, most important, reaction formation. The last of these involves overt chronic patterns of thought and behaviour that serve to disguise and disavow opposite tendencies linked to unconscious traumatic events and the intrapsychic conflicts derived from them. The discovery of reaction formations led Freud to the psychoanalytic study of character pathology and normal character formation, and still constitutes an important aspect of the contemporary psychoanalytic understanding and treatment of personality disorders (for practical purposes, character pathology and personality disorders are synonymous concepts).

A related line of development in Freud's theories was the discovery of the differential characteristics of conscious and unconscious thinking. Freud differentiated conscious thinking, the 'secondary process', invested by 'attention cathexis' and dominated by sensory perception and ordinary logic in relating to the psychosocial environment, from the 'primary process' of the 'dynamic unconscious'. That part of the unconscious mind he referred to as 'dynamic' exerted constant pressure or influence on conscious processes, against the active barrier constituted by the various defensive operations, particularly repression. The dynamic unconscious, Freud proposed, presented a general mobility of affective investments, and was ruled by the 'pleasure principle' in contrast to the 'reality principle' of consciousness. The 'primary process' thinking of the dynamic unconscious was characterized by the absence of the principle of contradiction and of ordinary logical thinking, the absence of negation and of the ordinary sense of time and space, the treatment of a part as if it were equivalent to the whole, and a general tendency towards condensation of thoughts and the displacement of affective investments from one to another mental content.

Finally, Freud proposed a 'preconscious', an intermediate zone between the dynamic unconscious and consciousness. It represented the storehouse for retrievable memories and knowledge and for affective investments in general, and it was the seat of daydreaming, in which the reality principle of consciousness was loosened, and derivatives of the dynamic unconscious might emerge. Free association, in fact, primarily tapped the preconscious as well as the layer of unconscious defensive operations opposing the emergence of material from the dynamic unconscious.

This model of the mind as a 'place' with unconscious, preconscious, and conscious 'regions' constituted Freud's 'topographic theory'.[1] He eventually replaced it with the 'structural theory', namely, the concept of three interacting psychic structures, the ego, the superego, and the id.[5] This tripartite structural theory is still the model of the mind that dominates psychoanalytic thinking. A major determinant of the shift from the topographic to the structural model was Freud's recognition that the 'regions' of conscious, preconscious, and unconscious were fluid, and that the defence mechanisms directed against the emergence in consciousness of the dynamic unconscious were themselves unconscious. Another consideration was Freud's[6] discovery of a specialized unconscious system of infantile morality, the superego. What follows is a summary of the characteristics and contents of these structures, an analysis that will lead us directly into contemporary psychoanalytic formulations.

The structural theory, the dual-drive theory, and the Oedipus complex

The id: infantile sexuality and the Oedipus complex

The id is the mental structure that contains the mental representatives of the 'drives', i.e. the ultimate intrapsychic motivations that Freud[7]

described in his final 'dual-drive theory' of libido and aggression, or metaphorically, the sexual or life drive and the destruction or death drive to be examined below. Behind this categorical formulation lies a complex set of discoveries regarding the patients' unconscious experiences that Freud came across in the course of the application of the psychoanalytic method to the treatment of neurotic and characterological symptoms. In exploring unconscious mental processes, what at first appeared to be specific traumatic life experiences turned out to reflect surprisingly consistent, repetitive intrapsychic experiences of a sexual and aggressive nature.

Freud[4] was particularly impressed by the regularity with which his patients reported the emergence of childhood memories reflecting seductive and traumatic sexual experiences on the one hand, and intense sexual desires and related guilt feelings on the other. He discovered a continuity between the earliest wishes for dependency and being taken care of (the psychology, as he saw it, of the baby at the mother's breast) during what he described as the 'oral phase' of development; the pleasure in exercising control and struggles around autonomy in the subsequent 'anal phase' of development (the psychology of toilet training); and, particularly, the sexual desire towards the parent of the opposite gender and the ambivalent rivalry for that parent's exclusive love with the parent of the same gender. He described this latter state as characteristic of the 'infantile genital stage' (from the third or fourth to the sixth year of life) and called its characteristic constellation of wishes and conflicts the positive Oedipus complex. He differentiated it from the negative Oedipus complex, i.e. the love for the parent of the same gender, and the corresponding ambivalent rivalry with the parent of the other gender. Freud proposed that Oedipal wishes came to dominate the infantile hierarchy of oral and anal wishes, becoming the fundamental unconscious realm of desire.

Powerful fears motivated the repression of awareness of infantile desire: the fear of loss of the object, and later of the loss of the object's love was the basic fear of the oral phase, directed against libidinal wishes to possess the breast; the fear of destructive control and annihilation of the self or the object was the dominant fear of the anal phase directed against libidinal wishes of anal expulsion and retentiveness; and the fear of castration, 'castration anxiety', the dominant fear of the Oedipal phase of development, directed against libidinal desire of the Oedipal object. Unconscious guilt was a dominant later fear, originating in the superego and generally directed against drive gratification (see under superego). Unconscious guilt over sexual impulses unconsciously equated with Oedipal desires constitute a major source of many types of pathology, such as sexual inhibition and related character pathology.

Prototypical intrapsychic infantile experiences linked to the Oedipus complex were phantasies and perceptions around the sexual intimacy of the parents (the 'primal scene'), and unconscious phantasies derived from experiences with primary caregivers ('primal seduction'). In all these phases of infantile development of drive motivated wishes and fears, powerful aggressive strivings accompanied the libidinal ones, such as cannibalistic impulses during the oral phase of physical dependency on the breast and psychological dependency on mother, sadistic phantasies linked to the anal phase, and parricidal wishes and phantasies in the Oedipal stage of development.

Freud described the oral phase as essentially coinciding with the infantile stage of breast feeding, the anal phase as coinciding with struggles around sphincter control, and the Oedipal stage as developing gradually during the second and through the fourth years, and culminating in the fourth and the fifth years of life. This last phase would then be followed by more general repressive processes under the dominance of the installation of the superego, leading to a 'latency phase' roughly corresponding to the school years, and finally, to a transitory reactivation of all unconscious childhood conflicts under the dominance of Oedipal issues during puberty and early adolescence.

The id: drives

The drives represent for human behaviour what the instincts constitute for the animal kingdom, i.e. the ultimate biological motivational system. The drives are constant, highly individualized, and developmentally shaped motivational systems. Under the dominance of the drives and guided by the primary process, the id exerts an ongoing pressure towards gratification, operating in accordance with the pleasure principle. Freud initially equated the drives with primitive affects. After discarding various other models of unconscious motivation, he ended up with the dual-drive theory of libido and aggression.

He described the libido or the sexual drive as having an 'origin' in the erotogenic nature of the leading oral, anal, and genital bodily zones; an 'impulse' expressing the quantitative intensity of the drive by the intensity of the corresponding affects; an 'aim' reflected in the particular act of concrete gratification of the drive; and an 'object' consisting of displacements from the dominant parental objects of desire.

The introduction of the idea of an aggressive or 'death' drive, arrived at later in Freud's writing,[7,8] stemmed from his observations of the profound self-destructive urges particularly manifest in the psychopathology of major depression and suicide, and of the 'repetition compulsion' of impulse-driven behaviour that frequently seemed to run counter to the pleasure principle that supposedly governed unconscious drives. He never spelt out the details of the aggressive drive as to its origins. This issue was taken up later by Melanie Klein,[9] Fairbairn,[10] Winnicott,[11] Edith Jacobson,[12] and Margaret Mahler and her colleagues.[13] Freud described drives as intermediate between the body and the mind; the only thing we knew about them, Freud suggested,[14] were 'representations and affects'.

The structure and functions of the ego

While the id is the seat of the unconscious drives, and functions according to the 'primary process' of the dynamic unconscious, the ego, Freud proposed,[5] is the seat of consciousness as well as of unconscious defence mechanisms that, in the psychoanalytic treatment, appear as 'resistances' to free association. The ego functions according to the logical and reality-based principles of 'secondary process', negotiating the relations between internal and external reality. Guided by the reality principle, it exerts control over perception and motility; it draws on preconscious material, controls 'attention cathexes', and permits motor delay as well as selection of imagery and perception. The ego is also the seat of basic affects, particularly anxiety as an alarm signal against the danger of emergence of unconscious, repressed impulses. This alarm signal may turn into a disorganized state of panic when the ego is flooded with external perceptions that activate unconscious desire and conflicts, or with overwhelming, traumatic experiences in reality that resonate with such repressed unconscious conflicts, and overwhelm the particularly sensitized ego in the process. The fact that the ego was seen by Freud as the seat of affects, and that affects had previously been described by him as discharge phenomena reflecting drives (together with their mental representations) tended to dissociate affects from drives in psychoanalytic theory, in contrast to

their originally being equated in Freud's early formulations. As we shall see, this issue, the centrality of affects in psychic reality and interactions, has gradually re-emerged as a major aspect of contemporary psychoanalytic thinking.

Freud originally equated the 'I', i.e. the categorical self of the philosophers, with consciousness; later, once he established the theory of the ego as an organization of both conscious and unconscious functions, he at times treated the ego as if it were the subjective self, and at other times, as an impersonal organization of functions. Out of this ambiguity evolved the contemporary concept of the self within modern ego psychology as well as in British and American object relations and cultural psychoanalytic contributions.[15] An alternative theory of the self was proposed by Kohut,[16] the originator of the self-psychology approach within contemporary psychoanalysis.

Nowadays, an integrated concept of the self as the seat of subjectivity is considered an essential structure of the ego, and the concept of 'ego identity' refers to the integration of the concept of the self: because of developmental processes in early infancy and childhood better understood today, an integrated self concept usually goes hand in hand with the capacity for an integrated concept of significant others. An unconscious tendency towards primitive dissociation or 'splitting' of the self concept and of the concepts of significant objects runs counter to such integration: we shall return to this process later. Already Freud,[17] in one of his last contributions, described a process of splitting in the ego as a way of dealing with intolerable intrapsychic conflict, thus opening up the road for considering splitting processes of the ego as an alternative, pathological defence against intolerable intrapsychic conflict (alternative, that is, to the repression of that conflict and to drawing important related ego functions into repression as well).

Character, from a psychoanalytic perspective, may be defined as constituting the behavioural aspects of ego identity (the self concept) and the internal relations with significant others (the internalized world of 'object relations'). The sense of personal identity and of an internal world of object relations, in turn, reflect the subjective side of character. It was particularly the ego-psychological approach—one of the dominant contemporary psychoanalytic schools—that developed the analysis of defensive operations of the ego, and of pathological character formation as a stable defensive organization that needed to be explored and resolved in the psychoanalytic treatment. In the process, ego psychology contributed importantly to the psychoanalytic treatment of personality disorders.

Personality disorders reflect typical constellations of pathological character traits derived from abnormal developmental processes under the influence of unconscious intrapsychic conflicts. The description of 'reaction formation' as one of the defences of the ego led Freud to the description of the 'oral', 'anal', and 'genital' characters, particularly to the description of the obsessive–compulsive personality as a typical manifestation of reaction formations against anal drive derivatives. This was followed by the description by Abraham[18] of the hysterical personality as a consequence of multiple reaction formations against the female castration complex. Over the years, psychoanalytic explorations led to the description of a broad spectrum of pathological character constellations, which today are a part of the spectrum of personality disorders.

Perhaps the most important psychoanalytic contribution to character pathology and the personality disorders is the clinical description of the narcissistic personality disorder. While Freud provided the basic elements that led to its eventual description, psychoanalytic understanding, and treatment, it was not he who crystallized the concepts of normal and pathological narcissism. Freud[19] conceptualized narcissism as the libidinal investment of the ego or self, in contrast to the libidinal investment of significant others ('objects'). In proposing the possibility of a withdrawal of libidinal investment from others with an excessive investment in the self as the basic feature of narcissistic pathology, he pointed to a broad spectrum of psychopathology, and thus first stimulated the contribution of Abraham,[20] and later those of Melanie Klein,[21] Herbert Rosenfeld,[22] Grunberger,[23] Kohut,[16] Jacobson,[12] and Kernberg.[24] Thus crystallized the description of the narcissistic personality as a disorder derived from a pathological integration of a grandiose self as a defence against unbearable aggressive conflicts, particularly around primitive envy.

The superego in normality and pathology

In his analysis of unconscious intrapsychic conflicts between drive and defence, Freud regularly encountered unconscious feelings of guilt in his patients, reflecting an extremely strict, unconscious infantile morality which he called the superego. This unconscious morality could lead to severe self-blame and self-attacks, and particularly, to abnormal depressive reactions, which he came to regard as expressing the superego's attacks on the ego. It was particularly in studying normal and pathological mourning that Freud[6] arrived at the idea of excessive mourning and depression as reflecting the unconscious internalization of the representation of an ambivalently loved and hated lost object. In unconsciously identifying the self with that object introjected into the ego, the individual now attacked his or her own self in replacement of the previous unconscious hatred of the object; and the internalization of aspects of that object into the superego reinforced the strictness of the individual's pre-existing unconscious infantile morality.

Freud traced the origins of the superego to the overcoming of the Oedipus complex via unconscious identification with the parent of the same gender; in internalizing the Oedipal parent's prohibition against the rivalry with him or her and the unconscious death wishes regularly connected with such a rivalry, and against the incestuous desire for the parent of the other gender, this internalization crystallized an unconscious infantile morality. The superego, thus based upon prohibitions against incest and parricide, and a demand for submission to, and identification with, the Oedipal rival, became the guarantor of the capacity for identification with moral and ethical values in general. In simple terms, the little boy renounces mother out of fear and love of father, takes father's phantasized prohibition against the little boy's sexuality into the superego as a fundamental prohibition, and establishes an identification with his father in the consolidation of his character structure. The little boy thus enacts the unconscious phantasy that, in identifying with father, he will gradually grow into his role, and satisfy his sexual desire in the distant future by choosing another woman who, unconsciously and symbolically, will represent mother. The superego thus introduces a new time perspective into the functioning of the psychic apparatus.

Freud also described the internalization of the idealized representations of both parents into the superego in the form of the 'ego ideal'. He suggested that the earliest sources of self-esteem, derived from mother's love, gradually fixated by the baby's and small child's internalizations of the representations of the loving mother into the ego ideal, led to the parental demands becoming internalized as well. In

other words, normally self-esteem is maintained both by living up to the expectations of the internalized idealized parental objects, and by submitting to their internalized prohibitions. This consideration of self-esteem regulation leads to the clinical concept of narcissism as normal or pathological self-esteem regulation, in contrast to the theoretical concept of narcissism as the libidinal investment of the self.

The superego, in summary, is a mental structure constituted by the internalized demands and prohibitions from the parental objects of childhood, the 'heir to the Oedipal complex'. This unconscious structure is of fundamental importance in determining unconscious 'fixations' to infantile prohibitions against drive derivatives and the corresponding unconscious motivation for the activation of a broad spectrum of ego defences against them, thus preventing the ego from re-examining and reintegrating unresolved pathogenic conflicts from early childhood. In health, this internal sense of unconscious morality is the underpinning of moral and ethical systems. Excessive superego severity, usually derived from excessive parental strictness, determines excessive repressive mechanisms and ego inhibitions, irrational moralistic behaviour, or pathological activation of depression and loss of self-esteem.

Having thus summarized the basic psychoanalytic theory of motivation (drives), of development (the stages of development from the early oral phase to the dominance of the Oedipal complex), of structure (the tripartite model), and their implications for psychopathology, I shall now describe more specifically the contemporary psychoanalytic theory of psychopathology and of psychoanalytic treatment.

Psychoanalytic treatment

The psychoanalytic theory of psychopathology

The psychoanalytic theory of psychopathology proposes that the clinical manifestations of the symptomatic neuroses, character pathology, perversions, sexual inhibitions, and selected types of psychosomatic and psychotic illness reflect unconscious intrapsychic conflicts between drive derivatives following the pleasure principle, defensive operations reflecting the reality principle, and the unconscious motivations of the superego. Unconscious conflicts between impulse and defence are expressed in the form of structured conflicts between the agencies of the tripartite structure: there are ego defences against impulses of the id; the superego motivates inhibitions and restrictions in the ego; at times the repetitive, dissociated expression of id impulses ('repetition compulsion') constitutes an effective id defence against superego pressures. The resolution of unconscious conflicts implies the analysis of all these intersystemic conflicts.

All these conflicts are expressed clinically by three types of phenomena:

(1) inhibitions of normal ego functions regarding sexuality, intimacy, social relations, and affect activation;

(2) compromise formations between repressed impulses and the defences directed against them;

(3) dissociative expression of impulse and defence.

The last category implies a dominance of the splitting mechanisms referred to before; these have acquired central importance in the understanding of severe character pathology as reflected in contemporary psychoanalytic thinking.

The structural formulation of the psychoanalytic method

Psychoanalytic treatment consists, in essence, in facilitating the reactivation of the pathogenic unconscious conflicts in the treatment situation by means of a systematic analysis of the defensive operations directed against them. This leads to the gradual emergence of repressed impulses, with the possibility of elaborating them in relation to the analyst, and their eventual adaptive integration into the adult ego. Freud[25] had described the concept of 'sublimation' as an adaptive transformation of unconscious drives; drive derivatives, converted into a consciously tolerable form, are permitted gratification in a symbolic way while their origin remains unconscious. The result of this process is an adaptive non-defensive compromise formation between impulse and defence. In analysis, the gradual integration into the patient's conscious ego of unconscious wishes and desires from the past and the understanding of the phantasized threats and dangers connected with them, facilitates their gradual elaboration and sublimatory expression in the consulting room and in everyday life as well.

The object-relations theory formulation of psychoanalytic treatment

In the light of contemporary object-relations theory, the formulation based upon the structural theory (resolution of unconscious conflicts between impulse and defence) has changed, in the sense that all unconscious conflicts are considered to be embedded in unconscious internalized object relations. Such internalized object relations determine both the nature of the defensive operations and of the impulses against which they are directed. These internalized object relations constitute, at the same time, the 'building blocks' of the tripartite structure of id, ego, and superego. Object-relations theory proposes that the gradual analysis of intersystemic conflicts between impulse and defence (structured into conflicts between ego, superego, and id) decomposes the tripartite structure into the constituent conflicting internalized object relations. These object relations are reactivated in the treatment situation in the form of an unconscious relation between self and significant others replicated in the relation between patient and analyst, i.e. the 'transference'.

The transference is the unconscious repetition in the 'here and now' of unconscious, conflicting pathogenic relationships from the past. The transference reflects the reactivation of the past conflict not in the form of a memory, but in the form of a repetition. This repetition provides essential information about the past, but constitutes, at the same time, a defence in the sense that the patient repeats instead of remembering. Therefore transference has important informative features that need to be facilitated in their development, and defensive features that need to be therapeutically resolved once their nature has been clarified. Transference analysis is the fundamental ingredient of psychoanalytic treatment.

The psychoanalytic treatment process

Psychoanalytic treatment consists of the creation of an atmosphere of safety in which a patient is willing to try to express whatever comes to mind. In 45- to 50-min sessions, three to five times per week, the patient usually reclines on a couch while the analyst, generally sitting behind the patient, helps the patient become aware of his or her defensive operations ('resistances') by means of interpretations. The systematic interpretation of resistances gradually permits an ever-growing freedom of free association, and helps the patient to become aware of his or her unconscious desires and fears, phantasies and terrors, traumatic situations, and unresolved mourning. Defensive operations are usually classified as ego defences (in the form of the mechanisms listed earlier), superego defences in the form of excessive guilt feelings activated during the treatment, id resistances in the form of repetition compulsion, the development of secondary gain from symptoms as a powerful resistance, and, last and most importantly, the transference as the dominant resistance and source of information.

Merton Gill,[26] in a classical definition that is still relevant today, proposed the definition of psychoanalysis as a treatment that facilitates the development of a 'regressive transference neurosis' and its resolution by means of interpretation alone, carried out by the analyst from a position of technical neutrality. Let us define these concepts.

'Regression' refers to the patient's return to earlier experiences (temporal regression), and modes of functioning (structural and formal regression) under the effect of the analysis of resistances, and is an expression of the reactivation of his or her unconscious conflicts from the past in the transference. In essence, the patient activates or enacts earlier object relations in the transference. Certain past stages of development where particular traumatic experiences occurred act as gathering points ('fixations') that foster regression towards them. The concept of a regressive transference neurosis refers to the gradual gathering into the relationship with the analyst of the patient's most important past pathogenic experiences and unconscious conflicts. The concept of a regressive transference neurosis has been largely abandoned in practice because, particularly in patients with severe character pathology, transference regression occurs so early and consistently that the gradual development of a regressive transference neurosis is no longer a useful concept.

Merton Gill's proposal that the resolution of the transference be achieved 'by interpretation alone', refers to 'interpretation' as a set of the psychoanalyst's interventions that starts with 'clarification' of the patient's subjective experiences communicated by means of free association, expands with the tactful 'confrontation' of aspects of the patient's patterns of behaviour that are expressed in a dissociated or split-off manner from his or her subjective awareness, and thus complements the total expression of the patient's intrapsychic life in the treatment situation, and finally evolves into 'interpretation *per se*'. Interpretation *per se* implies the formulation of hypotheses regarding the unconscious meanings in the 'here and now' of the patient's material, and the relation of these unconscious meanings with the 'there and then' of the patient's unconscious, past pathogenic experiences. The analysis of the transference is 'systematic', in the sense that all emerging transference dispositions are interpreted, ideally, in the natural sequence of their emergence in the analytic situation. Gill's phrase, 'by interpretation alone', implies that the psychoanalyst abstains from measures other than helping the patient to fully understand the unconscious conflicts activated in the here and now. Thus, providing guidance about life decisions, or attempting to modify the patient's behaviour or state by means of praise, prohibition, or reward is not part of the psychoanalytic method of treatment.

The concept of 'technical neutrality' refers to the analyst's impartiality regarding both impulse and defence, with a concerned objectivity that provides a helpful collaboration with the patient's efforts to come to grips with his or her intrapsychic conflicts.

This definition of the nature of psychoanalytic treatment needs to be complemented with the contemporary concepts of 'transference', 'countertransference', 'acting out', and 'working through'.

An object-relations theory model of the transference and countertransference

Modern object-relations theory, further explored below, and presented in more detail in terms of particular schools in Chapter 3.3.2, proposes that, in the case of any particular conflict around sexual or aggressive impulses, the conflict is embedded in an internalized object relation, i.e. in a repressed or dissociated representation of the self ('self representation') linked with a particular representation of another who is a significant object of desire or hatred ('object representation'). Such units of self-representation, object representation, and the dominant sexual, dependent or aggressive affect linking them are the basic 'dyadic units', whose consolidation will give rise to the tripartite structure. Internalized dyadic relations dominated by sexual and aggressive impulses will constitute the id; internalized dyadic relations of an idealized or prohibitive nature the superego; and those related to developing psychosocial functioning and the preconscious and conscious experience, together with their unconscious, defensive organization against unconscious impulses, the ego. These internalized object relations are activated in the **transference** with an alternating role distribution, i.e. the patient enacts a self representation while projecting the corresponding object representation onto the analyst at times, while at other times projecting his or her self representation onto the analyst and identifying with the corresponding object representation. The impulse or drive derivative is reflected by a dominant, usually primitive affect disposition linking a particular dyadic object relation; the associated defensive operation is also represented unconsciously by a corresponding dyadic relation between a self representation and an object representation under the dominance of a certain affect state.

For example, a conflict between unconscious aggression and unconscious guilt feelings, respectively located in id and superego, is clinically represented by manifestations of a guilt-provoking object representation relating to a guilty self (the superego defence), and an enraged self representation attempting to attack a threatening or frustrating object representation (the id impulse). The development of the transference, therefore, consists of a sequence of activation of such impulsively determined and defensively determined internalized object relations and their systematic clarification, confrontation, and interpretation by the analyst.

The concept of **countertransference**, originally coined by Freud as the unresolved, reactivated transference dispositions of the analyst, is currently defined as the total affective disposition of the analyst in response to the patient and his or her transference, shifting from moment to moment, and providing important data of information to the analyst. The countertransference, thus defined, may be partially derived from unresolved problems of the analyst, but stems as well from the impact of the dominant transference reactions of the patient, from reality aspects of the patient's life, and sometimes from aspects of the analyst's life situation, that are emotionally activated in the context of the transference developments. In general, the stronger the transference regression, the more the transference determines the countertransference; thus the countertransference becomes an important diagnostic tool. The countertransference includes both the analyst's

empathic identification with a patient's central subjective experience ('concordant identification') and the analyst's identification with the reciprocal object or self representation ('complementary identification') unconsciously activated in the patient as part of a certain dyadic unit, and projected onto the analyst.[27] In other words, the analyst's countertransference implies an identification with what the patient cannot tolerate in him- or herself, and must dissociate, project, or repress.

At this point, it is important to refer to certain primitive defensive operations that were described by Melanie Klein[9] and her school in the context of the analysis of severe character pathology. Primitive defensive operations are characteristic of patients with severe personality disorders, and emerge in other cases during periods of regression. They include splitting, projective identification, denial, omnipotence, omnipotent control, primitive idealization, and devaluation (contempt). All these primitive defences centre around splitting, i.e. an active dissociation of contradictory ego (or self) experiences as a defence against unconscious intrapsychic conflict. They represent a regression to the phase of development (the first 2 to 3 years of life) before repression and its related mechanisms mentioned are established.

Primitive defensive operations present important behavioural components that tend to induce behaviours or emotional reactions in the analyst, which, if the analyst manages to 'contain' them, permit the analyst to diagnose in him- or herself projected aspects of the patient's experience. Particularly 'projective identification' is a process in which:

(1) the patient unconsciously projects an intolerable aspect of self-experience onto (or 'into') the analyst;

(2) the analyst unconsciously enacts the corresponding experience ('complementary identification');

(3) the patient tries to control the analyst, who now is under the effect of this projected behaviour;

(4) the patient meanwhile maintains empathy with what is projected.

This scenario is in contrast to the more mature mechanism of 'projection', secondary to repression, where there is no longer any conscious emotional contact with what is projected. Such complementary identification in the countertransference permits the analyst to identify him- or herself through his or her own experience with the aspects of the patient's experience communicated by means of projective identification. This information complements what the analyst has discovered about the patient by means of clarification and confrontation, and permits the analyst to integrate all this information in the form of a 'selected fact' that constitutes the object of interpretation. Interpretation is thus a complex technique that is very much concerned with the systematic analysis of both transference and countertransference.

Contemporary trends of the psychoanalytic method

Contemporary psychoanalytic technique can be seen as having evolved from a 'one-person psychology' into a 'two-person psychology' and then into a 'three-person psychology'. The concept of 'one-person psychology' refers to Freud's original analysis of the patient's unconscious intrapsychic conflicts by analysing the intrapsychic defensive operations that oppose free association. The 'two-person psychology' refers to the central focus on the analysis of transference and counter-transference. In the views of the contemporary intersubjective, inter-personal, and self-psychology psychoanalytic schools, the relationship between transference and countertransference is mutual, in the sense that the transference is at least in part a reaction to reality aspects of the analyst, who therefore must be acutely mindful of his or her contribution to the activation of the transference. The so-called 'constructivist' position regarding transference analysis assumes that it is impossible for the analyst to achieve a totally objective position outside the transference–countertransference bind.

In contrast, the contemporary 'objectivist' position, represented by the 'three-person psychology' approaches of the Kleinian school, the French psychoanalytic mainstream, and significant segments of contemporary ego psychology proposes that the analyst has to divide him- or herself between one part influenced by transference and counter-transference developments, and another part that, by means of self-reflection, maintains him- or herself outside this process, as an 'excluded third party', who, symbolically, provides an early triangulation to the dyadic regression that dominates transference developments. This triangulation in the treatment situation becomes particularly important in the treatment of severe personality disorders.

The 'enactment' of pathogenic past internalized object relations in the form of both transference and countertransference developments needs to be differentiated from **acting out**, the replacement of self-awareness by often dramatic, and at times, violent action. It is characteristic of patients with severe character pathology, and may occur in both patient and analyst under the influence of regression. Acting out may occur both during and outside the sessions. While it reflects an intense defensive operation and resistance, it also offers the opportunity for a very fundamental exploration of a primitive conflict, if dealt with by consistent interpretations in as much depth as possible. Acting out may also be considered an extreme, behavioural manifestation of 'enactment' as the usual experience of transference/countertransference manifestations.

The **repetition compulsion** as a resistance of the id is most probably a form of acting out as a defence against emotional containment of an extremely painful or traumatic set of experiences. **Working through** refers to the repeated elaboration of an unconscious conflict in the psychoanalytic situation. It is a major task for the analyst, who has to be alert to the subtle variation in meanings and implications of what on the surface may be appear to be an endless repetition of the same conflict in the transference. The patient elaboration of the conflict that presents itself with these repetitive characteristics also implies the function of 'holding' originally described by Winnicott.[11] It consists of the analyst's capacity to withstand the onslaught of primitive transferences without retaliation, abandonment of the patient, or a self-devaluing giving up, and the maintenance of a working relationship (or 'therapeutic alliance') that addresses itself consistently to the healthy part of the patient, even when the latter is under the control of his or her most conflicting behaviours. Bion's concept[28] of 'containing' is complementary to 'holding', in the sense that holding deals mostly with the affective disposition of the analyst, and containing with his or her cognitive capacity to maintain a concerned objectivity and focus on the 'selected fact', permitting the integration in the analyst's mind what the patient can only express in violently dispersed or split-off behaviour patterns.

Dream analysis developed in the context of the method of free association, and constituted, in Freud's view,[29] a 'royal road to the unconscious'. Freud's discovery of primary process thinking derived from his method of dream analysis. By now, psychoanalytic thinking has evolved into the view that there are many 'royal roads' to the unconscious. The analysis of character defences, for example, or of particular transference complications, may be equally important avenues of entry into the patient's unconscious mind.

The technique of dream analysis consists, in essence, in asking the patient to free associate to elements of the 'manifest content' of the dream, in order to arrive at its 'latent' content, the unconscious wish defended against and distorted by the unconscious defensive mechanisms that constitute the 'dream work', and have transformed the latent content into the manifest dream. The latent content is revealed with the help of the simultaneous analysis of the way in which the dream is being communicated to the analyst, the 'day residuals' that may have triggered the dream, the unconscious conflicts revealed in it, and the dominant transference dispositions in the context of which the dream evolved. Dreams also provide some residual, universal symbolic meanings that may facilitate the total understanding of the latent content.

The **analysis of character** may be the single most important element of the psychoanalytic method in bringing about fundamental characterological change. Character analysis is facilitated by the patient's use of reaction formations, i.e. his or her defensively motivated character traits, as transference resistances. Thus, the activation of defensive behaviours in the transference, reflecting the patient's characterological patterns in all interpersonal interactions, facilitates both the analysis of the underlying unconscious conflicts, and in the process, the resolution of pathological character patterns. The result is an increase in the patient's autonomy, flexibility, and capacity for adaptation. Character analysis was originally developed by Wilhelm Reich[30] within an ego-psychology perspective, but has re-emerged in the work of Herbert Rosenfeld[31] and John Steiner[32] in the analysis of 'pathological organizations' in the transference, within the Kleinian school.

Character analysis, although not always referred to under this specific heading, constitutes a major focus of contemporary psychoanalytic treatment. In essence, its technique addresses repetitive, ego-syntonic behaviour patterns in the transference, raising the patient's curiosity about their function in the relationship with the analyst, and inviting the patient to associate about this behaviour. Gradually, their explorations makes character resistances ego-dystonic, and facilitates the discovery of the underlying internalized object relations condensed in these pathological character traits, both in their defensive and impulsive meanings. The question, to what extent such rigid behaviours should be analysed first, in order to free the patient's capacity for analytic work, or to what extent they should be left for later, until more fluid conflicts have been resolved, has been settled in favour of the general psychoanalytic technical principle of focusing interpretations upon what is affectively dominant in each hour.[33] Affective dominance refers once more to the 'selected fact',[28] to be interpreted. All interpretations are usually carried out from surface to depth, which in practice means first analysing the object relation activated by the need for defence before analysing the corresponding object relation activated by impulse.

The overall objective of psychoanalytic treatment is not only the resolution of symptoms and pathological behaviour patterns or characteristics, but fundamental structural change, i.e. the expansion and enrichment of ego functions as the consequence of resolution of unconscious conflict and the integration of previously repressed and dynamically active id and superego pressures into ego potentialities. Such change is reflected in the increasing capacity for both adaptation to and autonomy from psychosocial demands and expectations, and an increased capacity for gratifying and successful functioning in love and work.

Derived modalities of treatment

One of the most important contributions of psychoanalytic theory and technique to the contemporary treatment of a broad spectrum of patients with severe psychopathology who, for various reasons, cannot benefit from psychoanalytic treatment proper, is the development of psychoanalytic psychotherapy, also called expressive or exploratory psychotherapy, and of supportive psychotherapy based on psychoanalytic principles. These treatment are explored below.

Psychoanalytic psychotherapy

Psychoanalytic psychotherapy may be characterized by the same basic techniques as psychoanalysis, but with quantitative modifications that, in combination, result in a qualitative shift in the nature of the treatment. Any given session of psychoanalytic psychotherapy may be indistinguishable from a psychoanalytic session, but over time, the differences emerge quite clearly. Psychoanalytic psychotherapy utilizes interpretation, but with patients with severe psychopathology, a good deal of time must be devoted to clarification and confrontation before interpretation can be effective; and interpretations of unconscious meanings in the 'here and now' occupy the foreground until late in the treatment, when genetic interpretations in the 'there and then' become useful.[15,34]

In the treatment of patients with severe character pathology, transference analysis is the essential focus of psychoanalytic psychotherapy from the very beginning; it must be modified, however, by active interpretive connection of transference analysis with exploration in depth of the patient's daily life situation, an approach made necessary by the predominance of primitive defence operations in these patients. Splitting operations in particular tend to dissociate the therapeutic situation from the patient's external life, and may lead to severe, dissociated acting out either in the sessions or outside the sessions. Therefore, interpretive linkage between the patient's external reality and transference developments in the hour becomes central.

In order to enable the therapist to analyse transference developments in sufficient depth, psychoanalytic psychotherapy requires a minimum frequency of two sessions per week. It is usually carried out in 'face-to-face' sessions.

Technical neutrality is an essential feature of analysis in general, but in the treatment of patients with severe character pathology the need to set limits may necessitate repeatedly abandoning neutrality, in order to control life-threatening or treatment-threatening acting out. The self-perpetuating nature of acting out in these cases may prove impossible to resolve interpretively without such structuring or setting limits. Whenever the analyst has to abandon technical neutrality to protect the patient or the treatment, it is essential to explore the episode immediately. The transference implications of the therapist's structuring behaviour must be laid out, followed by the analysis of the transference implications of the patient's behaviour that necessitated the imposition of limits or the initiation of a new structure in the treatment; this in turn is followed by the gradual resolution of the structure or limit setting by interpretive means, thus restoring technical neutrality. In short, technical neutrality in psychoanalytic psychotherapy is an ideal working state that is again and again preventively abandoned and interpretively reinstated.[15,35,36]

Supportive psychotherapy

Supportive psychotherapy based on psychoanalytic theory may also be defined in terms of the three major techniques of interpretation, transference analysis, and technical neutrality. Supportive psychotherapy utilizes the preliminary steps of interpretive technique, i.e. clarification and confrontation, but rarely uses interpretation *per se*. It seeks to strengthen the ego by bolstering adaptive compromises between impulse and defence through the provision of cognitive support in the form of information, persuasion, and advice, and emotional support via suggestion, reassurance, encouragement, and praise. Supportive psychotherapy may call upon direct environmental intervention by the therapist, relatives, or other mental health personnel engaged in auxiliary therapeutic functions.[37]

While the transference is seldom interpreted in supportive psychotherapy, it is not ignored either. Careful attention to transference developments helps the therapist to analyse any maladaptive transference developments, to call the patient's attention to the reproduction with the therapist of pathological interactions the patient generally engages in with significant others, and to encourage the patient to reduce such pathological behaviours. Pointing out the distorted, unproductive, destructive, or confusing nature of the patient's behaviour is accompanied by clarifying the patient's conscious reasons for his or her behaviour, followed by the transfer or 'export' of the knowledge thus achieved to the patient's relationships outside the treatment. In short, supportive psychotherapy includes the clarification, reduction, and 'export' of the transference, thus contributing to the re-educative functions of supportive psychotherapy together with the direct cognitive and affective support of adaptive combinations of impulse and defence, and direct supportive environmental interventions.

Technical neutrality is systematically abandoned in supportive psychotherapy, with the therapist taking a stance alternatively on the side of the ego, superego, id, or external reality, according to which agency represents, at a certain point, the more adaptive potential for the patient. The main dangers, of course, in supportive psychotherapy are, on the one hand, infantilizing the patient by an excessively supportive stance, and, on the other, countertransference acting out as a consequence of the abandonment of the position of technical neutrality. The therapist carrying out supportive psychotherapy, therefore, needs a heightened awareness of the risk of these complications. Like psychoanalytic psychotherapy, supportive psychotherapy is carried out in 'face-to-face' sessions. It has the advantage of considerable flexibility regarding its frequency, from several sessions a week, to one session a week, or one or two sessions per month, according to the urgency of the patient's present difficulties, the long-range objectives of the treatment, and the patient's ability to tolerate and use the relationship with the therapist.

Indications and contraindications for psychoanalysis and derived psychotherapies

The **indications** for these three modalities of treatment remain controversial. With the recognition of the limitations of psychoanalysis in many cases with severe, chronic, life-threatening, self-destructive behaviour, such as chronic suicidal behaviour, severe eating disorders, dependence upon drugs or alcohol, and severely antisocial behaviour, psychoanalytic psychotherapy has proven to be a highly effective treatment for many but by no means all patients with these conditions. The differential diagnosis of a spectrum of severity of antisocial behaviour and those cases of severe self-destructive and antisocial behaviour who are amenable to treatment with psychoanalytic psychotherapy has been one of the important side-products of the psychoanalytic exploration of these cases.[35]

Supportive psychotherapy, originally conceived as the treatment of choice for patients with severe personality disorders, now may be considered the alternative treatment for those patients with severe personality disorders who are unable to participate in psychoanalytic psychotherapy. The Menninger Foundation Psychotherapy Research Project showed that patients with the least severe psychopathological disturbances tend to respond very positively to all three modalities derived from psychoanalytic theory, although best to standard psychoanalysis.[38]

Standard psychoanalysis is the treatment of choice for patients with neurotic personality organization, i.e. with good identity integration and a repertoire of defences centring on repression along with sufficient severity of illness to warrant such a major therapeutic intervention. Psychoanalysis has also expanded its scope to some of the severe personality disorders, particularly a broad spectrum of patients with narcissistic personality disorders, patients with mixed hysterical–histrionic features, and selected cases of patients with severe paranoid, schizoid, and sado-masochistic features.

We are still lacking systematic studies of the relationship between particular types of psychopathology and outcome with the various psychotherapeutic treatments derived from psychoanalytic theory. As a tentative generalization it may be stated that there is a definite relationship between outcome and the severity of illness in any diagnostic category. The least severe cases will respond favourably to either brief psychoanalytic psychotherapy, supportive psychotherapy, or psychoanalysis. Psychoanalysis represents the opportunity for most improvement if the severity of the case warrants psychoanalytic treatment. For cases of neurotic personality organization of moderate severity, psychoanalysis is the treatment of choice; definitely less can be expected in these cases from psychoanalytic psychotherapy. For the most severely ill patients (those with severe identity diffusion, predominance of primitive defences centring on splitting, and general 'ego weakness') psychoanalytic psychotherapy is the treatment of choice, with supportive psychotherapy a second choice if psychoanalytic psychotherapy is contraindicated. A few such cases may be able to participate in psychoanalysis and benefit from it.

In all cases, individualized **contraindications** for the respective treatment are important: in the case of psychoanalysis, individual contraindications depend on the questions of ego strength, motivation, introspection or insight, secondary gain of illness, intelligence, and age. In the case of psychoanalytic psychotherapy, secondary gain, the impossibility of control of life- or treatment-threatening acting out, limited intelligence, significant antisocial features, and a desperate life situation may constitute individual contraindications, particularly when they occur in combination. When psychoanalytic psychotherapy is contraindicated for such reasons, supportive psychotherapy becomes the treatment of choice. Participation in supportive psychotherapy requires a sufficient capacity for commitment to an on-going treatment arrangement, and the absence of severe antisocial features as minimal individual requirements. This is not meant to be a complete list, but an illustration of the kind of criteria that become dominant in the individual decisions regarding the selection of the treatment and its contraindications.

Psychoanalytic object-relations theories: overview and critique

Given the centrality of object-relations theory in practically all contemporary psychoanalytic formulations and treatment approaches, the following summary is included. It should help the reader to clarify further the references made earlier to this theory.

Psychoanalytic object-relations theories may be defined as those that place the internalization, structuralization, and reactivation in the transference and countertransference of the earliest dyadic object relations at the centre of their clinical formulations, and of their thinking about motivation, pathogenesis, development, and psychic structure. Internalization of object relations refers to the concept that, in all interactions of the infant and child with the significant parental figures, what the infant internalizes is not merely an image or representation of the other ('the object' of fear, hatred or desire), but the relationship between the self and the other, in the form of a self-image or self representation linked to an object image or object representation by the affect that dominates their interaction. This internal structure replicates in the intrapsychic world both real and phantasied relationships with significant others.

Several major issues separate different object-relations theories, the most important of which is the extent to which the theory is perceived as harmonious with or in opposition to Freud's traditional drive theory: i.e. whether object relations are seen as replacing drives as the motivational system for human behaviour. From this perspective, Klein,[9,21] Mahler et al.,[13] and Jacobson[12] occupy one pole. They combine Freud's dual-drive theory with an object-relations theory. For Fairbairn[10] and Sullivan,[39] on the other hand, object relations themselves replace Freud's drives as the major motivational system. Here, the establishment of gratifying object relations in itself constitutes the major motivational system. Contemporary interpersonal psychoanalysis as represented by Greenberg and Mitchell,[40] based upon an integration of principally Fairbairnian and Sullivanian concepts, asserts the essential incompatibility between drive-based and object-relations-based models of psychic motivational systems. Winnicott,[11] Loewald,[41] Sandler,[42] and Sandler and Sandler[43] (each for different reasons) maintain an intermediate posture; they perceive the affective frame of the infant–mother relationship as a crucial determinant in shaping the development of drives. While adhering to Freud's dual-drive theory, Kernberg[15] considers drives supraordinate motivational systems, while affects are their constituent components.

A related controversy has to do with the origin and role of aggression as motivator of behaviour. Those theoreticians who reject the idea of inborn drives,[39] or equate libido with the search for object relations,[10] conceptualize aggression as secondary to the frustration of libidinal needs, particularly traumatic experiences in the early mother–infant dyad. Theoreticians who adhere to Freud's dual-drive theory, in contrast, believe aggression is inborn and plays an important part in shaping early interactions: this group includes Klein in particular, and to some extent Winnicott, and ego psychology object-relations theoreticians such as Kernberg.[35]

Finally, contrast may be made between object-relations theories and French approaches, both Lacanian and (non-Lacanian) mainstream psychoanalysis. The French psychoanalytic mainstream[44,45] has maintained close links with traditional psychoanalysis, including the British object-relations theories. Insofar as Lacan[46] conceptualizes the unconscious as a natural language and focuses on the cognitive aspects of unconscious development, he underemphasizes affect—a dominant element of object-relations theories. At the same time, however, in postulating a very early Oedipal structuralization of all infant–mother interactions, Lacan emphasizes archaic Oedipal developments, which implicitly links his formulations with those of Kleinian object-relations theory in general. French mainstream analysis also focuses on archaic aspects of Oedipal developments, but places a traditional emphasis on Freud's dual-drive theory and on the affective nature of the early ego–id. As neither French mainstream nor Lacanian psychoanalysis spells out specific structural consequences of dyadic internalized object relations, however, neither would fit the definition that frames the field of object-relations theory as proposed in this chapter.

All object-relations theories focus heavily on the enactment of internalized object relations in the transference, and on the analysis of countertransference in the development of interpretive strategies. They are particularly concerned with severe psychopathologies, including those psychotic patients who are approachable with psychoanalytic techniques; borderline conditions; severe narcissistic character pathology; and the perversions ('paraphilias'). Object-relations theories explore primitive defensive operations and object relations both in cases of severe psychopathology and at points of severe regression with all patients, regarding such exploration as essential in facilitating transference analysis and conflict resolution.

The contemporary re-evaluation of Freud's dual-drive theory that has occurred mostly in France is relevant to the relationship between object-relations theory and drive theory. Perhaps particularly the work of Laplanche[47] and Green[44] has emphasized the central importance of unconscious destructive and self-destructive drive manifestations in the form of attacks on object relations, and the central role of unconscious erotization in the mother–infant relationship in libidinal development, all of which tends to link drive theory and object-relations theory in intimate ways.

Another important development within psychoanalytic theory has been the growing emphasis on affects as primary motivators, and the centrality of the communicative functions of affects in early development, particularly the infant–mother relationship.[48] This emphasis has linked affect theory and object-relations theory quite closely, despite the persistent controversy between those who see affect, particularly peak affect states, as essential representatives of the drives,[48] and those who stress the psychophysiological nature of the affective response, and attempt to replace drive theory with an affect theory.[49]

The basic (self representation–object representation) units of internalized object relations include the representative affects, or else the constituent affective components of the drives. One might say that the affect of sexual excitement is the central affect of libido, in the same way as the affect of primitive hatred constitutes the central affect of the aggressive or death drive. The id is conceptualized in this object-relations theory model as the sum total of repressed, desired, and feared primitive object relations. The gradual integration of successive layers of persecutory and idealized, prohibitive and demanding, internalized object relations become part of the primitive superego, while internalized object relations activated in the service of defence consolidate as part of an integrated self-structure surrounded by integrated representations of significant others. In short, the id or dynamic unconscious, the superego, and the ego are constituted by different constellations of internalized object relations, so that the development of the drives and the development of the psychic apparatus—the tripartite structure—occur hand in hand.

Perhaps the most important practical implication of object-relations theory is the conception of identification as a series of internalization processes of dyadic units of self representation and object representation linked by a dominant affect state, ranging from earliest introjections to identifications per se, to the development of complex identity formation. Each step includes the internalizing of both self and object representations and their affective interactions under the conditions that prevail at different developmental levels.

In the transference of healthier patients, with a well-consolidated ego identity, the diverse self-representations are relatively stable in their coherent mutual linkage. This fosters the relatively consistent projection onto the analyst of the object representation aspect of the enacted object relationship. In contrast, patients with severe identity diffusion lack such linkage of self representations into an integrated self. They tend to alternate rapidly between projection of self and object representations in the transference, so that the analytic situation seems chaotic. Systematic interpretation of how the same internalized object relation is enacted again and again with rapid role reversals between patient and analyst makes it possible to clarify the nature of the unconscious object relation, and the double splitting of self representation from object representation and idealized from persecutory object relations. This process of interpretation promotes integration of the split representations which characterize severe psychopathology and account for the marked instability of the emotions, behaviour, and interpersonal relationships of these patients.

Kernberg[35] proposes that affects are the primary motivational system and that, internalized or fixated as the very frame of internalized 'good' and 'bad' object relations, affects are gradually integrated into libidinal and aggressive drives to form hierarchically supraordinate motivational systems. In other words, primitive affects are the 'building blocks' of the drives. He sees unconscious intrapsychic conflicts as always between the following:

(1) certain units of self and object representations under the impact of a particular drive derivative (clinically, a certain affect disposition reflecting the drive derivative side of the conflict);

(2) contradictory or opposing units of self and object representations and their respective affect dispositions reflecting the defensive structure.

Unconscious intrapsychic conflicts are never simply between impulse and defence; rather, both impulse and defence find expression, respectively, through certain internalized object relations.

In patients with borderline personality organization and severe conflicts around early aggression, splitting mechanisms stabilize such dynamic structures within an ego–id matrix and permit the contradictory aspects of these conflicts to remain at least partially conscious, in the form of primitive, mutually split-off, idealized and persecutory transferences. In contrast, patients with neurotic personality organization present impulse–defence configurations that contain specific unconscious wishes of an integrated though infantile self, reflecting sexual and aggressive drive derivatives embedded in unconscious phantasies relating to the Oedipal objects. Repressed unconscious wishes, however, always come in the form of corresponding units composed of self representation and object representation and affect linking them.

Patients with neurotic personality organization present well-integrated superego, ego, and id structures; within the psychoanalytic situation, the analysis of resistances brings about the activation, in the transference, first of relatively global characteristics of these structures, and later, the internalized object relations of which they are composed. Oedipal conflicts dominate the dynamic unconscious of these patients. The analysis of drive derivatives occurs in the context of the analysis of the relation of the patient's infantile self to significant parental objects as projected onto the analyst.

Patients with severe personality disorders or borderline personality organization, in contrast, show a predominance of psychic representations of pre-Oedipal conflicts, with pre-Oedipal aggression, in particular, condensed with representations of the Oedipal phase. Conflicts are not predominantly repressed and therefore unconsciously dynamic; rather, they are avoided by being represented in mutually dissociated ego states reflecting the defence of primitive dissociation or splitting. The activation of primitive object relations that predate the consolidation of ego, superego, and id is manifest in the transference as apparently chaotic affect states, which have to be analysed in sequential steps as follows:

(1) the clarification of a dominant primitive object relation in the transference, with its corresponding self and object representation, and the dominant affect linking them;

(2) the analysis of the alternative projection of self and object representation onto the therapist, while the patient identifies with a reciprocal self or object representation of this object relationship, leading to the patient's gradual capacity to become aware of his or her identification with an object in that relationship;

(3) the interpretive integration of mutually split-off, idealized, and persecutory 'part object' relations with the characteristics mentioned.

This analysis may gradually bring about a transformation of mutually split, idealized, and persecutory ('part object') relations into 'total object' relations, or of primitive transferences (largely reflecting Mahler's stages of development that predate object constancy) into the advanced transferences of the Oedipal phase. In other words, a gradual integration of self representations into an integrated self-concept, and a parallel integration of significant object representations into integrated concepts of significant others develop first in the transference, and later generalize in the patient's relations with significant others. The analyst's exploration of his or her countertransference, including concordant and complementary identifications in the countertransference,[27] facilitates transference analysis, and the analysis of primitive defensive operations, particularly splitting and projective identification, in the transference also contributes to strengthening the patient's ego.

Treatment results: research on outcome

The psychoanalytic profession has been slow in developing systematic research on treatment process and results, let alone controlled randomized comparison of treatment methods evaluating efficacy and efficiency. The reasons are multiple: the complexity of the psychoanalytic treatment, and the changes in its technique; the long duration of treatment, making systematic research and controlled comparison with other treatment methods difficult; the private nature of psychoanalytic exploration in the context of patients' regression, and the related concerns over disturbing the therapeutic relationship by recording or direct observation. In addition, the general methodology of psychotherapy research evolved to a degree of sophistication applicable to the evaluation of psychoanalytic treatment only in recent decades. With all these reservations, significant progress has been made, and outcome studies are beginning to be available.

The Menninger Psychotherapy Research Project, a naturalistic study comparing psychoanalysis, psychoanalytic psychotherapy, and supportive psychotherapy, showed psychoanalysis to be the most effective of these approaches with patients presenting relatively good ego strength, while patients with severe ego weakness—what nowadays would be described as presenting severe personality disorders or borderline personality organization—improved most with psychoanalytic psychotherapy.[38] This research also showed how important supportive elements were throughout all modalities of treatment.[50] A comprehensive review of outcome studies on psychoanalytic psychotherapy and psychoanalysis by Bachrach et al.[51] concluded that the improvement rates are in the range from 60 to 90 per cent, but it also pointed to limitations and problems in the methodology utilized.

Recently, studies regarding the treatment process and outcome of psychoanalysis and psychoanalytic psychotherapy have become more precise in defining the specific treatment variables of psychotherapeutic and psychoanalytic treatments, and several systematic studies on psychoanalytic psychotherapies and psychoanalysis are in progress.[52] A recent study by the Stockholm Outcome of Psychoanalysis and Psychotherapy Project has found, on the basis of a relatively large patient population, that psychoanalytic treatment, in comparison with psychoanalytic psychotherapy, obtained a significantly higher degree long-range symptomatic improvement.[53] The extent to which the psychotherapist had years of experience linked with appropriate long-term supervisory experiences, i.e. an 'experiential learning cluster', was related to treatment outcome, in the sense that those therapists with long experiences in doing teaching or supervision of psychotherapy had a significantly better outcome than therapists who only had been in supervision or personal therapy for long periods. It also appeared that the maintenance of a rigid 'psychoanalytic' attitude as part of a psychoanalytic psychotherapy was not as effective as a more flexible shift in techniques in psychotherapy, but not in analysis proper.[54] A manualized psychoanalytic psychotherapy for a specific patient population, namely the psychotherapy research project of the Cornell Personality Disorders Institute's manualized treatment for borderline patients, is presently under way.[36] It has provided evidence for the efficacy of the treatment with severely ill patients, although comparative studies with other treatment modalities, or with 'treatment as usual' still remains to be done.

In summary, process research has predated outcome research on psychoanalysis and derived psychotherapies; major efforts at outcome research are being made, and should contribute to clarify the effects, not only of psychoanalysis proper, but also of the derived psychotherapeutic approaches now being carried out in clinical practice.

References

1. Freud, S. (1963). Introductory lectures on psycho-analysis. In *Standard edition of the complete psychological works of Sigmund Freud*, Vol. 16 (ed. J. Strachey), pp. 243–463. Hogarth Press, London.
2. Freud, S. (1964). An outline of psycho-analysis. In *Standard edition of the complete psychological works of Sigmund Freud*, Vol. 23 (ed. J. Strachey), pp. 141–207. Hogarth Press, London.
3. Breuer, J. and Freud, S. (1955). Studies on hysteria. In *Standard edition of the complete psychological works of Sigmund Freud*, Vol. 2 (ed. J. Strachey), pp. 3–311. Hogarth Press, London.
4. Freud, S. (1953). Three essays on the theory of sexuality. In *Standard edition of the complete psychological works of Sigmund Freud*, Vol. 7 (ed. J. Strachey), pp. 125–245. Hogarth Press, London.
5. Freud, S. (1961). The ego and the id. In *Standard edition of the complete psychological works of Sigmund Freud*, Vol. 19 (ed. J. Strachey), pp. 3–66. Hogarth Press, London.
6. Freud, S. (1957). Mourning and melancholia. In *Standard edition of the complete psychological works of Sigmund Freud*, Vol. 14 (ed. J. Strachey), pp. 237–58. Hogarth Press, London.
7. Freud, S. (1955). Beyond the pleasure principle. In *Standard edition of the complete psychological works of Sigmund Freud*, Vol. 18 (ed. J. Strachey), pp. 3–64. Hogarth Press, London.
8. Freud, S. (1961). Civilization and its discontents. In *Standard edition of the complete psychological works of Sigmund Freud*, Vol. 21 (ed. J. Strachey), pp. 57–145. Hogarth Press, London.
9. Klein, M. (1952). Notes on some schizoid mechanisms. In *Developments in psycho-analysis* (ed. J. Riviere), pp. 292–320. Hogarth Press, London.
10. Fairbairn, W.R.D. (1954). *An object-relations theory of the personality.* Basic Books, New York.
11. Winnicott, D. (1965). *The maturational processes and the facilitating environment.* International Universities Press, New York.
12. Jacobson, E. (1964). *The self and the object world.* International Universities Press, New York.
13. Mahler, M., Pine, F., and Bergman, A. (1975). *The psychological birth of the human infant.* Basic Books, New York.
14. Freud, S. (1957). Instincts and their vicissitudes. In *Standard edition of the complete psychological works of Sigmund Freud*, Vol. 14 (ed. J. Strachey), pp. 109–40. Hogarth Press, London.
15. Kernberg, O. (1984). *Severe personality disorders. Psychotherapeutic strategies.* Yale University Press, New Haven, CT.
16. Kohut, H. (1971). *The analysis of the self.* International Universities Press, New York.
17. Freud, S. (1964). Splitting of the ego in the process of defence. In *Standard edition of the complete psychological works of Sigmund Freud*, Vol. 23 (ed. J. Strachey), pp. 273–4. Hogarth Press, London.
18. Abraham, K. (1920). Manifestations of the female castration complex. Reprinted in *Selected papers on psycho-analysis*, pp. 338–69. Brunner–Mazel, New York, 1979.
19. Freud, S. (1957). On narcissism. In *Standard edition of the complete psychological works of Sigmund Freud*, Vol. 14 (ed. J. Strachey), pp. 69–102. Hogarth Press, London.
20. Abraham, K. (1919). A particular form of neurotic resistance against the psychoanalytic method. Reprinted in *Selected papers on psycho-analysis*, pp. 303–11. Brunner–Mazel, New York, 1979.
21. Klein, M. (1957). *Envy and gratitude.* Basic Books, New York.
22. Rosenfeld, H. (1964). On the psychopathology of narcissism: a clinical approach. *International Journal of Psycho-Analysis*, **45**, 332–7.
23. Grunberger, B. (1979). *Narcissism: psychoanalytic essays.* International Universities Press, New York.
24. Kernberg, O.F. (1975). *Borderline conditions and pathological narcissism.* Jason Aronson, New York.
25. Freud, S. (1953). Fragment of an analysis of a case of hysteria. In *Standard edition of the complete psychological works of Sigmund Freud*, Vol. 7 (ed. J. Strachey), pp. 3–122. Hogarth Press, London.
26. Gill, M. (1954). Psychoanalysis and exploratory psychotherapy. *Journal of the American Psychoanalytic Association*, **2**, 771–97.
27. Racker, H. (1957). The meaning and uses of countertransference. *Psychoanalytic Quarterly*, **26**, 303–57.
28. Bion, W.R. (1967). Second thoughts. *Selected papers on psychoanalysis.* Basic Books, New York.
29. Freud, S. (1953). The interpretation of dreams. In *Standard edition of the complete psychological works of Sigmund Freud*, Vol. 4 (ed. J. Strachey), pp. 1–338; Vol. 5 (ed. J. Strachey), pp. 339–625. Hogarth Press, London.
30. Reich, W. (1972). *Character analysis.* Farrar, Straus, and Giroux, New York.
31. Rosenfeld, H. (1987). *Impasse and interpretation.* Tavistock Press, New York.
32. Steiner, J. (1993). *Psychic retreats.* Routledge, London.
33. Fenichel, O. (1941). *Problems of psychoanalytic technique.* Psychoanalytic Quarterly, Albany, NY.
34. Kernberg, O.F., Selzer, M.A., Koenigsberg, H.W., Carr, A.C., and Appelbaum, A.H. (1989). *Psychodynamic psychotherapy of borderline patients.* Basic Books, New York.
35. Kernberg, O.F. (1992). *Aggression in personality disorders and perversion.* Yale University Press, New Haven, CT.
36. Clarkin, J.F., Yeomans, F., and Kernberg, O.F. (1999). *Psychotherapy for borderline personality.* Wiley, New York.
37. Rockland, L.H. (1989). *Supportive therapy: a psychodynamic approach.* Basic Books, New York.
38. Kernberg, O.F., Burnstein, E., Coyne, L., Appelbaum, A., Horwitz, L., and Voth, H. (1972). Psychotherapy and psychoanalysis: final report of the Menninger Foundation's Psychotherapy Research Project. *Bulletin of the Menninger Clinic*, **36**, 1–275.
39. Sullivan, H. (1953). *The interpersonal theory of psychiatry.* Norton, New York.
40. Greenberg, J.R. and Mitchell, S.A. (1983). *Object relations in psychoanalytic theory.* Harvard University Press, Cambridge, MA.
41. Loewald, H.W. (1960). On the therapeutic action of psycho-analysis. *International Journal of Psycho-Analysis*, **41**, 16–33.
42. Sandler, J. (1987). *From safety to superego: selected papers of Joseph Sandler.* Guilford Press, New York.
43. Sandler, J. and Sandler, A.M. (1998). *Internal objects revisited.* Karnac Books, London.
44. Green, A. (1993). *Le travail du négatif.* Les Editions de Minuit, Paris.
45. Laplanche, J. (1987). *Nouveaux fondements pour la psychanalyse.* Presses Universitaires de France, Paris.
46. Lacan, J. (1966). *Ecrits.* Editions du Seuil, Paris.
47. Laplanche, J. (1992). *Seduction, translation, drives.* Psychoanalytic Forum, Institute of Contemporary Arts, London.
48. Krause, R. (1998). *Allgemeine Psychoanalytische Krankheitslehre*, Vols 1 and 2. Kohlhammer, Stuttgart.
49. Mitchell, S. (1988). *Relational concepts in psychoanalysis.* Harvard University Press, Cambridge, MA.

50. Wallerstein, R. (1986). *Forty-two lives in treatment: a study of psycho-analysis and psychotherapy*. Guilford Press, New York.

51. Bachrach, H.M., Weber, J.J., and Murray, S. (1985). Factors associated with the outcome of psychoanalysis. Report of the Columbia Psychoanalytic Research Center (IV). *International Review of Psychoanalysis*, **12**, 379–89.

52. Fonagy, P. (1998). *An open door review of outcome studies in psychoanalysis*. International Psychoanalytic Association, London.

53. Sandell, R., Blomberg, J., and Lazar, A. (1997). When reality doesn't fit the blueprint: doing research on psychoanalysis and long-term psychotherapy in a public health service program. *Psychotherapy Research*, **7**, 333–44.

54. Sandell, R., Schubert, J., Blomberg, J., Carlsson, J., Lazar, A., and Bromberg, J. (1997). The influence of therapist factors on outcomes of psychotherapy and psychoanalysis in the Stockholm Outcome of Psychotherapy and Psychoanalysis Project (STOPP). Paper presented at the Annual Meeting of the Society for Psychotherapy Research, Geilo, Norway.

3.3 Other psychodynamic schools

3.3.1 Analytical psychology (Jung)

Anthony Storr

'Analytical Psychology' was the name given by C.G. Jung to his variety of psychodynamic theory in order to distinguish it from Freud's 'Psychoanalysis'.

Jung's background and early work

Jung was born on 26 July 1875, the son of a pastor in the Swiss Reformed Church who was also an Oriental and classical scholar. He was an only child for his first 9 years and, since he was more intelligent than most of his rural schoolfellows, remained somewhat isolated. He became a medical student at the University of Basel. On completing his medical degree, he had almost decided to become a surgeon, when he came across a textbook of psychiatry by Krafft-Ebing which persuaded him to specialize in this neglected branch of medicine. From 1900 to 1909, he was a psychiatrist at the Burghölzli mental hospital in Zürich, where he became particularly interested in schizophrenia and carried out original research which is reported in the first two volumes of *The Collected Works of C.G. Jung*.[1,2]

Archetypes and the collective unconscious

Jung's research into schizophrenia led him to conclude that there was a myth-making substratum of mind common to all men: a 'collective unconscious' which lay beneath the merely personal, and which was responsible for the spontaneous production of myths, visions, religious ideas, and certain types of dream which were common to various cultures and different periods of history. Jung was widely read in history and comparative religion. He referred to the images of the collective unconscious as 'archetypes'.

Hero myths

For example, many cultures have 'hero myths' in which the hero has to go through various trials and tribulations and prove his courage before gaining a mate and possibly a throne. This is an exposition, in fairy-tale language, of a child's progress from infancy to maturity. Every child has to leave the mother, grow up, face the dangers associated with becoming independent, win a sexual partner, and achieve a position in society. Different cultures have different ideas of what a hero should be like. Galahad, the perfect knight, exemplifies one English idea of a hero; Odysseus, the wily trickster, personifies a Greek ideal. The two ideas of the heroic are very different, but each is an expression of the heroic archetype. It is as if there was some kind of a flexible mould underlying the idea of the hero which could not be clearly defined until a culture had filled it with a myth, but which was itself indefinable.

Anima, animus, and shadow

In the course of analysis of their dreams, patients would encounter various typical 'primordial images' or archetypes which are experienced as being of profound significance. For example, the primordial image of the opposite sex, which in men is named the 'anima', may be someone resembling Rider Haggard's 'She'. The aptly named 'She' is not only spectacularly beautiful, but also an immortal priestess with access to divine wisdom. 'She' is not an actual woman, but an image of the eternal feminine. The phenomenon of being in love, which Freud referred to as 'the normal prototype of the psychoses',[3] consists in projecting an anima image upon the beloved, who may in reality be unremarkable in the eyes of everyone except those of the deluded lover. Film stars and princesses are often similarly perceived. The primordial image of the opposite sex in women is named 'animus', and is projected in similar fashion upon film stars from Valentino to Cary Grant. The image is often at odds with the actual character of the idealized person.

Another archetypal image is the 'shadow', that is, a personification of least acceptable aspects of human nature, often symbolized by a sinister dark 'other' who is felt to be terrifying or alien. Coming to terms with the shadow is one way of expressing the need to accept the worst in oneself.

Jung found that the myths and religious beliefs of primitive peoples had much in common with the bizarre delusions of the insane. Delusional systems and religious beliefs both had the function of making sense out of the individual's experience and giving meaning to his existence. For example, a paranoid delusional system which explains an individual's failure in life by alleging that he is the victim of malicious persecution preserves the subject's self-esteem and prevents him from perceiving his own life as futile. So does a belief that one is a child of God. Regarded from the cold standpoint of reason, most human lives are of little lasting significance. Perhaps ordinary people, as well as psychotics, need a religious faith or myth to persuade them that their lives are not entirely trivial.

Jung's concept of the collective unconscious has often been criticized, but the existence of a mythological substratum to human experience is recognized by psychoanalysts of an entirely different theoretical orientation. Analysts who refer to 'internal objects' are delineating the same phenomena. The Kleinian stage of infantile development known as the 'paranoid–schizoid' position postulates that the infant perceives the mother as wholly 'good' or wholly 'bad' in accordance with whether she fulfils or fails to fulfil the infant's needs. The mother is perceived as an evil witch on the one hand, or as the Virgin Mary on the other. In Jung's terminology, these are typical archetypal images. The concept of the collective unconscious simply postulates that, just as human beings share a similar anatomy, so they also share a common tendency to enshrine their deepest experiences in similar myths, phantasies, and images.

Jung's contributions to psychotherapy

Jung's contributions to psychiatry and psychotherapy were both practical and theoretical. Unlike Freud, he preferred a face-to-face encounter with the patient, and did not employ a couch. He did not insist on seeing his patients five times a week, and, after an initial period of perhaps four meetings a week, reduced the frequency to two or three. In addition, he thought that there should be 'holidays' from analysis in which patients could work on their problems alone.

Jung introduced a technique which became known as 'active imagination,' in which the patient was instructed to suspend judgement and enter a state of reverie. Whatever phantasies then occurred were to be written down, painted, sculpted, or recorded in any fashion preferred by the patient. Whereas Freud regarded phantasy as an escape from reality, Jung held it in high regard, and referred to his technique as 'developing the creative possibilities latent in the patient himself'.[4] Although Jung specifically forbade his patients to regard their phantasy productions as works of art, he was in fact inducing the state of mind which most writers and composers describe as the one in which new creative ideas occur to them. Jung's initiative is largely responsible for the widespread development of departments of art therapy in mental hospitals.

Dreams and the self-regulating psyche

Jungian analysis always made considerable use of dreams, but Jung's view of the dream differed sharply from that of Freud. Freud regarded the majority of dreams as disguised hallucinatory fulfilments of repressed unacceptable sexual wishes deriving from early childhood. Jung thought this view too narrow. Dreams might be expressed in a symbolic language which was difficult to understand, but there was no reason to assume that they were invariably concealing the unacceptable. Dreams often seemed to be compensatory; that is, expressing the opposite to a one-sided conscious attitude.

This view of dreams derives from Jung's conception of the mind as a self-regulating system. As a medical student, Jung had learned that human physiology is governed by a system of checks and balances which ensure that any tendency to go too far in one direction is compensated by an opposing swing in the other. Thus, if if the blood becomes too alkaline, various mechanisms are set in operation which

ensure that the kidney excretes more alkali and retains acid. This physiological tendency to seek equilibrium is known as 'homeostasis', and is dependent on the cybernetic mechanism known as negative feedback.

Jung applied this physiological concept to the mind. He believed that there was a reciprocal relationship between conscious and unconscious which ensured that, if a person's conscious attitude became exaggerated or distortedly one-sided, unconscious mechanisms would be set in operation which, through dreams, neurotic symptoms, or even mental breakdown, might force the individual to reconsider himself and his attitude to life. Jung therefore regarded neurosis in an entirely different way from Freud. Instead of trying to reconstruct the patient's infantile past, Jung asked why he or she had become neurotic at a particular time in the present.

Psychological types

In his book *Psychological Types* (1921), Jung had introduced the terms **extraversion** and **introversion**, concepts which would be taken over by experimental psychologists. Jung believed that people approached the study of the mind and life in general from bascially different attitudes. The extravert was primarily interested in the world of external objects; the introvert in what went on within his own mind. Both attitudes were necessary for a full comprehension of reality, but men were usually one-sided and tended to one or other extreme. A typical example would be the extraverted businessman who pursued the accumulation of wealth to the exclusion of all other aspects of life, but who was brought to his knees by a mid-life depression. Neurotic symptoms were not always residues of childhood experience, as Freud supposed, but were often attempts on the part of the mind to correct its own lack of equilibrium, and therefore pointers to a new and more satisfactory synthesis. Jung sometimes said of a patient, 'Thank God he became neurotic'.

The process of individuation

The idea that the psyche, like the body, is self-regulating implicitly assumes that there is something within both body and mind which 'knows better' than the conscious self. We are accustomed to the fact that fatigue, hunger, or lack of sleep are physical messages to which we have to listen, and which constitute restraints upon what we might wish to accomplish. We are less attuned to the signals coming from within our minds. Jung pioneered the analysis of middle-aged patients whom Freudian analysts rejected as too old to benefit. Many of these patients, having achieved conventional success, were not suffering from a clinically definable neurosis, but complained that life seemed senseless and aimless. Through the analysis of dreams and phantasies, Jung started such people on a journey of personal psychological development which he named the process of individuation. This might be described as a kind of Pilgrim's Progress without a creed, aiming not at heaven, but at integration and wholeness.

Most of Jung's later work is concerned with the process of individuation. Jung became more a guru than a doctor or scientist. As he himself acknowledged, the concept of individuation has subjective origins. Early in childhood, Jung began to have doubts about the Christian faith which his father taught; in adolescence, he finally abandoned it.

But, like others who have been brought up in a strongly religious atmosphere, Jung found it hard to live without a faith.

After his break with Freud, Jung passed through a psychotic episode, which lasted throughout the First World War. He was nearly overwhelmed; but his illness taught him that, at the same time at which his mind appeared to be disintegrating, a healing process was proceeding which was striving to make sense out of chaos and achieve a new integration. He himself wrote: 'The years when I was pursuing my inner images were the most important in my life—in them everything essential was decided.'[5] He found that he had to submit to being guided by something within himself which was independent of his conscious intention. Could this be the psychological equivalent of God—a kind of 'God within' rather than a 'God out there'? Jung wrote:

Among all my patients in the second half of life—that is to say, over thirty-five—there has not been one whose problem in the last resort was not that of finding a religious outlook on life. It is safe to say that every one of them fell ill because he had lost what the living religions of every age have given to their followers, and none of them has really been healed who did not regain his religious outlook. This of course has nothing to do with a particular creed or membership of a church.[6]

Summary

Today, when psychiatry is dominated by biochemistry and genetics, Jung's ideas are likely to be disregarded. But research has shown that properly conducted psychotherapy by trained professionals still has an important role in psychiatry. Jung made original contributions to psychotherapy. He demonstrated that the middle-aged and elderly were not beyond the reach of help. His main contribution was in the field of adult development. By exhorting his patients to record and portray their psychological conflicts, he demonstrated the value of self-exploration and promoted the patient's independence from the analyst. He drew attention to a phenomenon which has not been sufficiently investigated: the need which those who have lost their faith feel for something to replace it, and the dangers which threaten us all when whole populations worship Hitler or Stalin or Mao rather than a god beyond the skies.

Every psychotherapist has seen patients who have not been cured of all their neurotic symptoms, but who nevertheless claim that psychotherapy has transformed their lives. Jung describes such people as achieving peace of mind after 'long and fruitless struggles'.

If you sum up what people tell you about their experiences, you can formulate it this way: They came to themselves, they could accept themselves, they were able to become reconciled to themselves, and thus were reconciled to adverse circumstances and events. This is almost like what used to be expressed by saying: He has made his peace with God, he has sacrificed his own will, he has submitted himself to the will of God.[7]

This change in attitude to life and its problems could be expressed in other terms more in accord with modern thought. But Jung is describing a phenomenon which undoubtedly takes place during the course of analytical psychotherapy more often than has been generally recognized. Perhaps changes in attitude to life are actually more important factors in healing than the cure of symptoms.

References

1. Jung, C.G. (1902–1905). *The collected works of C.G. Jung* (translated by R.F.C. Hull) (ed. Sir Herbert Read, Michael Fordham, and Gerhard Adler). Vol. 1, *Psychiatric studies*. Routledge & Kegan Paul, London, 1957.
2. Jung, C.G. (1904–1911). *The collected works of C.G. Jung* (translated by R.F.C. Hull) (ed. Sir Herbert Read, Michael Fordham, and Gerhard Adler). Vol. 2, *Experimental researches*. Routledge & Kegan Paul, London, 1973.
3. Freud, S. (1913). Totem and taboo. In *The standard edition of the complete psychological works of Sigmund Freud* (translated by James Strachey in collaboration with Anna Freud, assisted by Alix Strachey and Alan Tyson), Vol. 13, p. 89. Hogarth Press and Institute of Psycho-Analysis, London, 1958.
4. Jung, C.G. (1931). The aims of psychotherapy. In *The collected works of C.G. Jung* (translated by R.F.C. Hull) (ed. Sir Herbert Read, Michael Fordham, and Gerhard Adler). Vol. 16, *The practice of psychotherapy*, p. 41. Routledge & Kegan Paul, London, 1954.
5. Jung, C.G. (1932). *Memories, dreams, reflections* (recorded and edited by Aniela Jaffé) (translated by Richard and Clara Winston), p. 191. Collins and Routledge & Kegan Paul, London, 1958.
6. Jung, C.G. (1932). Psychotherapists or the clergy. In *The collected works of C.G. Jung* (translated by R.F.C. Hull) (ed. Sir Herbert Read, Michael Fordham, and Gerhard Adler). Vol. 11, *Psychology and religion: West and East*, p. 334. Routledge & Kegan Paul, London, 1958.
7. Jung, C.G. (1932). The history and psychology of a natural symbol. The third of the Terry Lectures published as *Psychology and religion*. In *The collected works of C.G. Jung* (translated by R.F.C. Hull) (ed. Sir Herbert Read, Michael Fordham, and Gerhard Adler). Vol. 11, *Psychology and religion: West and East*, pp. 81–2. Routledge & Kegan Paul, London, 1958.

3.3.2 Object relations, attachment theory, self-psychology, and interpersonal psychoanalysis

Jeremy Holmes

Despite many splits and schisms, dating back to Adler and Jung's early break with Freud, there has been an enduring attempt within psychoanalysis to hold to a central psychodynamic vision and to find common ground between differing theoretical and clinical approaches. The aim of this chapter is to describe the work of some of the major figures who have extended and developed Freud's ideas, pointing to areas of both conflict and convergence, and, wherever possible, to relate their concepts to the everyday practice of psychiatry.

From drive theory to object relations

Psychoanalysis started its life as a drive theory. By what means, Freud asked, did the instinctual life of the infant become tamed in the process of development so that the end result was the civilized man and woman of adult society? To this he had two sets of answers. The first, roughly, was repression and sublimation. In the Oedipal situation the child experiences sexual desire for the opposite-sex parent. These feelings arouse anxiety ('castration anxiety'), and so are repressed, or diverted into harmless exploratory and creative sublimatory activities. If, however, the process of repression is excessive the consequence in adult life is emotional inhibition. When repression is insufficient, anxiety-based or psychosomatic disorders result, or, ultimately, psychosis. A second answer, coming later, and forged in the face of the horrors of the First World War, was to suggest that 'civilization' was only skin deep. Here Freud invoked the death instinct and regression. Eros, the love instinct, is balanced by thanatos, the death instinct. Humans can all too easily regress to a state in which the death instinct is unleashed, producing, at an individual level the self-defeatingness and perversity of personality disorder, and at a group level social disruption and war.

As Freud's thought evolved, so a new paradigm began to emerge. Drive theory had little to say about relationships: other people appear merely as satisfiers or thwarters of an individual's instinctual needs. Freud began to ask how children as they developed, and later adults, reconciled their own wishes and desires—their drives or instincts—with those of their caregivers and peers. Struggling with this problem, while remaining within the confines of drive theory, he now differentiated between self-love, or narcissism, and other, or 'anaclitic', love, directed outwards. In this model, the individual gradually emerges from egg-like self-absorption and healthy narcissism into the world of relationships.

A further push towards a more relational theory came from Abraham, later to become Melanie Klein's analyst, who noticed the parallels between the phenomena of grief and depression. The intense psychic pain and disruption associated with a loss suggested a much more intimate connection between relationships and the architecture of the psyche than drive theory would allow. 'The unconscious' is not so much a repository of drives and desires, but an inner world populated by significant others or 'objects'. The self is forged out of these 'objects' with whom the individual has or has had important relationships: 'the shadow of the object falls on the ego'.[1] A further theoretical move arose from considering the origins of conscience and ideals. It is a matter of observation that much of development depends on processes of imitation and identification. The developing child internalizes, or in psychoanalytic terms 'introjects', his or her parent's values and standards. How, and where in the psyche, does this process take place? In Freud's 'tripartite model', the 'superego', alongside the ego and the id, is the focus for these internalized parental values and aspirations. The inner world now contained not just 'objects', but value-based relations between them: prohibitions, encouragements, injunctions, and gratifications. Much of post-Freudian theory consists of attempts to develop and elaborate these ideas.

Object relations 1: Klein, Fairbairn, and their successors

This was the state of theoretical play in psychoanalysis when Melanie Klein first burst on to the scene in the late 1920s. Like Freud, her work can be divided into a number of phases.[2,3]

Psychoanalysis is concerned with early mental life, which it sees as the basis for much adult disturbance. But how do we gain access to the thought processes of small children, whose verbal and introspective capacities are limited or non-existent? Klein's great technical innovation was the introduction of play therapy. She provided her little patients with play materials—paper and pencils, a doll's house with

figures, a sandpit, and farmyard animals—and observed the pictures and games which the children set up, making her interpretations around them. Here she used the methods of dream interpretation to formulate her ideas. What she observed in play—movement of figures in and out; bringing things together, often violently; separation and disruption—she took to represent the workings of the child's mind. Still deeply influenced by drive theory, and by Freud's insistence on the pre-eminence of sexuality and castration anxiety, she found sexual and aggressive meanings in all that was presented to her. Every vertical line or orifice-shaped circle drawn had a sexual significance; every conjoining or emitted sound stood for parental intercourse, by which the child was both fascinated and frightened. Exploration and the drive to know were seen as an expression of the desire to possess the mother's body, and inhibitions of learning as manifestations of castration anxiety.

Here Klein began to depart from Freud. For him the Oedipus complex arose around the age of three, when the child begins to observe his or her parents' relationship and to feel such emotions as passionate love, envy, fear, and jealous vengefulness. Klein, by contrast, saw Oedipal phenomena as arising much earlier in development. For example, the infant may experience weaning as a punishment or symbolic castration, and believe that his mother's breast in his mouth has been displaced by the paternal penis in her vagina. Two other aspects of Kleinian thought emerge from this. First, in Klein's schema the infant has an instinctual knowledge of the body and its relationships. There appears to be a reservoir of unconscious phantasy, which she saw as the mental accompaniment of bodily function: phantasies about the breast, the mouth, the penis, the vagina, and their relationships that could not have arisen from direct observation, and therefore must be present from within, as correlates of the child's bodily sensations, which Klein saw as dominating the early years of life. Unconscious phantasies are akin to Jungian archetypes: preformed mental constructs unconsciously shaping experience and patterns of relationship.

Second, and closely related to unconscious phantasy, is the idea of internal objects—initially body parts, and later 'whole objects' that are salient to emotional life—the mother and her breast, the father and his penis, bellies and their contents such as unborn babies, faeces, and sphincters. These objects are endowed with motivational properties reflecting the infant's emotional life, which Klein saw as dominated by persecutory fears. The 'death instinct' ensures that the child reacts to frustration with overwhelming feelings of hatred and destructiveness. These feelings are then projected outwards on to the objects in the child's emotional environment, which are in turn reintrojected to populate the inner world. To preserve good feelings from these terrifying bad objects, the child also projects goodness outwards. Thus a radical split arises between good and bad experiences, which are attributed to good and bad objects: 'in the very earliest stage every unpleasant stimulus is related to the 'bad', denying, persecuting breasts, every 'good' experience to the 'good' gratifying breasts'.[2]

Klein depicts early emotional life as dominated by the infant's fears of annihilation from without, and the use of the mechanisms of splitting and projection to reduce these fears. She postulated the onset of a new type of anxiety towards the end of the first year of life. Here the infant is beginning to bring the image of the 'good' and the 'bad' breast together, and to realize that they are one and the same. With weaning, the child experiences his first major loss. Now 'depressive' anxiety comes into the picture. The child believes that he is responsible for the loss, and that he has destroyed the good object with his aggression and sadism. He begins to feel guilt and remorse, and wants to repair the damage he believes he has inflicted on his objects. His attempts at creation, the gifts he offers, and the charm with which he approaches his caregivers are all motivated by this sense of depressive despair and the wish to make reparation.

Klein thus described a developmental sequence: inherent aggression, annihilation anxiety, projection and splitting of the object into good and bad, loss, bringing together the split objects, depressive despair, concern for the object, and finally reparation. For her this was a description of normal development, and she saw pathological states as resulting from developmental arrest along this line. The fulcrum of this sequence is the movement from what, drawing on Fairbairn's term (see below) Klein now called the 'paranoid–schizoid' position (**PSP**) to the 'depressive' position (**DP**), a movement from splitting, blaming, and avoidance, to integration, responsibility, and concern for the object (see Hobson et al.[4] for objective evidence of the validity of the PSP–DP distinction). Klein saw the struggle between PSP and DP as a lifelong process, an equilibrium driven one way or the other depending on life experience and constitutional endowment.

Klein was generally rather unconcerned about the impact of external reality on psychological development (a point which, as we shall see, stimulated Bowlby's divergence from her ideas). To the extent that she did consider the real as opposed to the phantasized role of the parents, it was as benign figures whose job it is to mitigate the strength of the infant's need to hate, project, and split. An important late theoretical contribution, however, concerned the role of envy in psychic life (one of her students complained: 'I was just nearing the end of my long analysis when Mrs Klein discovered envy—that meant another five years!'). One of the great strengths of a psychoanalytical approach to psychotherapy is that it takes seriously the phenomenon of resistance, and the fact that psychic growth is usually hard-won, often with much backsliding and self-defeatingness. With her emphasis on the dark side of human nature, Klein realized that the infant may feel persecuted not just by frustration and separation, but also by the very capacity of the caregiver to satisfy his needs. The breast upon which the baby depends for satisfaction and pleasure can also be a source of envy and hatred in its plenitude and ability to create dependency. This envy then becomes a basis for destructiveness within psychotherapy, and more generally: an explanation, perhaps, for the graffiti which inevitably appear on beautiful buildings, or, at times, the fact that patients attack and seem to want to destroy the very help that is offered to them.

Envy links the inner world, which in the Kleinian as opposed to the original Freudian schema has become a world of phantasy rather than drives, with caregivers and other significant people in the environment—with objects and their relations. Kleinians increasingly use the phrase projective identification (**PI**) as a general term to describe this relationship between the inner and outer worlds. Projective identification is an important but difficult and perhaps misnamed concept, coined almost casually by Klein in an attempt to describe how parts of the ego may be split off and projected not just on to objects in the environment as visualized in Freud's notion of projection, but into them.

The phrase projective identification is used in a number of different ways. As originally conceived by Klein it referred to the solipsistic world of the infant described above, in which unbearable feelings of rage and hatred are split off, projected into the breast, which is then perceived by the child as 'having' properties that in fact originated in the self. Projective identification here is a form of misperception or delusional perception, which can be used both to explain the fact that normal adults' experience of the world is inevitably coloured by their emotional state (the gloomy or rose-tinted spectacles with which we view the world), and to account for delusional ideas in psychosis, such as paranoid feelings of persecution which, it is hypothesized, originate in the subject's own aggressive phantasies but are attributed, via projective identification, to persecutors.

Projective identification differs from simple projection in that the objects of PI are induced or controlled by the projection in such a way that they then enact the phantasy which has been transferred into them. Paranoid people have the capacity to make those around them behave in suspicious or hostile ways, and thus projective identification can be thought of as a form of communication in which the recipient of the projection is induced to think or feel in ways that properly 'belong' to the projector. Post-Kleinian authors, notably Bion,[5] Heimann,[6] and later Grotstein[7] and Ogden,[8] have extended the concept of projective identification, with an emphasis on this communicative aspect, in that PI requires a recipient as well as a projector.

As a 'primitive' mode of communication projective identification is widespread, for example in 'tit-for-tat' relationships. Thus if one member of a couple has an affair, the other, unable to show directly their hurt, may retaliate by themselves sleeping with someone else. Here the initially injured party communicates pain, humiliation, and rage not by direct expression of anger, but by inducing those feelings in the other via PI. While such everyday use of PI is common, excessive reliance on it is usually a sign of pathology and is a frequent feature of people with borderline personality disorder.

Bion, an analysand of Klein, realized that projective identification also underlies normal empathy and fellow feeling. PI is primitive in the sense perhaps that preverbal children rely on it almost exclusively to communicate their feelings, but this denotes immaturity rather than pathology. Bion went on to develop his container–contained theory of early emotional communication. Here the mother, or 'breast', acts, via PI, as a recipient or container for the infant's unmanageable feelings of fear, hatred, annihilation, etc. These feelings are contained or held by the mother, and 'detoxified' before they are 'returned' to the infant through her understanding and empathic handling. She knows intuitively—through projective identification—when her child cries whether it is hungry or cold, or bored or wet, etc., and responds appropriately, often putting those feelings into words as she does so. In this way the infant begins to build up a sense of himself through the reflective awareness of the mother. Disruptions of this process, for example through maternal depression or the violent use by the parent of the infant as a container (role reversal) as occurs in child abuse, may sow the seeds of disorders of identity found in borderline personality disorder in later life.

PI is important in psychotherapy in the contemporary understanding of countertransference. Paula Heimann pointed out that the therapist's reactions to the patient, while no doubt coloured to some extent by her own conflicts (Freud's classical conceptualization of countertransference), also represent feelings induced by contact with the patient, that is to say they are a manifestation of projective identification. By attending to these thoughts and feelings the therapist gains clues about the patient's state of mind, which can then be put into words as interpretations. Here the therapist's mind is the container for the patient's split-off feelings. Sometimes this container–contained relationship fails, and the therapist is induced to enact some aspect of the patient's inner world, for instance by forgetting an appointment with a patient who has felt neglected and overlooked as a child, or by expressing anger or boredom in his tone of voice, being himself moved by feelings which properly belong to the patient.

The firm boundaries of psychotherapy are, in part, designed to minimize these occurrences (although they are unavoidable, and often, if thought about, can be put to good use in the form of deepened understanding), but in the much more uncontained setting of general psychiatric wards or community mental health centres such enactments are widespread. A common example would be the polarization which disturbed people with borderline personality disorder can induce in their carers, some seeing the patient as manipulative and demanding, others feeling intense sympathy and the wish to repair past hurts on the patient's behalf. Each perspective represents a split-off aspect of the patient's inner world that has been picked up via PI by different staff members. This is an essentially interactive process, since, no doubt, what determines which aspect depends on the carers' own developmental history and defensive strategies.

Working in the relative isolation of Scotland, and coming to essentially similar conclusions to Klein about the importance of splitting, W.R.D. Fairbairn[9] further developed this interpersonal perspective. For him drives were 'a signpost to the object', the glue that held human beings together. Sex is what gets us close to those who matter, rather than vice versa, as originally conceived by Freud. Like Bion later, Fairbairn also placed great emphasis on the role of the mother and of environmental failure as a source of psychopathology. Frustration plays a central part in his schema. With a perfectly responsive mother, the child has no need to think or develop an inner world. When separation and frustration come into play, the child then builds up an image of the object, which is split into three parts: the ideal object (one that would never cause frustration), the libidinal object (one that could satisfy the child's drive-related needs), and the antilibidinal object (the one that frustrates). This in turn sets up a split of the self into three corresponding parts—ideal self, libidinal self, and antilibidinal self. The Fairbairnian model provides clarity in understanding some typical phenomena found in severe personality disturbance: the swing between idealization and denigration of therapists and partners (who become the antilibidinal withholding object at that point), the self-destructiveness of the antilibidinal self, or 'internal saboteur', and the split-off search for pure libidinal satisfaction unrelated to persons represented by substance abuse and promiscuity.

Fairbairn's notion of schizoid withdrawal was conceptualized as a typical interpersonal strategy in the face of frustration. John Steiner[10] has developed a similar idea in his notion of the psychic retreat, an inner place to which individuals with borderline personality may repair in the face of environmental trauma, and which may make them relatively inaccessible in therapy. Another important neo-Kleinian development has been Ronald Britton's[11] attempt to link the Oedipus complex with the tolerance of separateness and loss implicit in the depressive position. Britton sees the ability, at times, to let go of the mother as the Oedipal stage is successfully negotiated—in which the child comes to see that his mother and father are sexually involved with one another and he is necessarily excluded—as an important developmental step towards the establishment of an inner world and the ability to see things from varying perspectives. This can be linked with Bion's idea of creative thought in which ideas are brought together to create 'conceptions', in contrast to the destructiveness of schizoid thinking in which, as a way of reducing anxiety, the links

between things and ideas are attacked, and the world emptied of meaning. The restoration of meaning is a central task of psychotherapy. The dialectic of close involvement and repeated separation inherent in the therapeutic relationship fosters this capacity, enabling disturbed or even psychotic patients first to find their experience mirrored by the responsive therapist, then gradually to tolerate loss and envy, and so to gain the capacity to think and to feel more autonomously.

Object relations 2: Balint and Winnicott

'Object relations' is a broad church containing disparate thinkers, united mainly by their common membership of the British Psychoanalytic Society, which managed to avoid the splits typical of some psychoanalytic societies by its 'gentleman's agreement' that created a structure in which different theoretical tendencies could coexist within the one society—a good example, perhaps, of 'depressive position thinking' outlined above.

Klein's view of the mind and of psychopathology was essentially a conflictual model: defensiveness and difficulty arise out of the inherent conflict in an immature mind between love and hate, and attempts to avoid the inevitability of loss. For her, such conflict was characteristic of normal development, and pathology merely an exaggeration of normal conflict in which the environment has failed to mitigate its potentially destructive effects (thus Kleinian psychoanalysis might be seen as a secularized version of the doctrine of original sin). By contrast, the non-Kleinian members of the 'object relations' school tend to espouse some variety of a deficit model, in which normal and abnormal development are more sharply differentiated, and the basis for psychopathology is a failure of the environment to provide the conditions needed for healthy psychic growth.

Michael Balint[12] is perhaps best known for his work in raising psychological awareness among general practitioners through the use of 'Balint groups', but he was also a significant figure in psychoanalysis, introducing a number of key terms and concepts. In contrast to Klein, who saw the newborn infant as wracked with fear and conflict, Balint proposed a state of primary love characterizing the early mother–infant relationship—which he described as a 'harmonious interpenetrative mixup'. Where parenting was inadequate, due to neglect, over-intrusiveness, aggression, or abuse he claimed that the child would be permanently scarred at the level of the 'basic fault'. He emphasized the importance of regression in the therapy of such cases, and argued that therapy could only be effective if it reached the level of the basic fault. His model of therapy implied a remedial, rather than purely interpretative, experience with the therapist, including both quiet acceptance, and on occasion therapeutic 'acting in': Balint would sometimes gently hold the patient's hand, and, famously, once encouraged a patient who stated that she had never had the courage to do a somersault to try one out in the consulting room then and there (behaviour therapy meets psychoanalysis!). Freud originally identified two fundamental defences against anxiety: schizoid withdrawal, seen in obsessive–compulsive disorders and psychosis, and the dependent clinging characteristic of hysteria. Balint developed this theme, dividing patients into those who are frightened of the spaces between people, and so tend to cling to their objects, while others find close contact with people threatening and use avoidance as a way of controlling anxiety. Attachment theory (see below) has provided some experimental evidence to support this dichotomy.

Donald Winnicott,[13] after Klein perhaps the best known of the British psychoanalysts, was a maverick figure combining exceptional clinical sensitivity with great theoretical originality. His work bridges Klein and the independent group, and like Bowlby (see below) reached a wide audience through his writings and broadcasts on child development. A number of his phrases and concepts have passed into the vernacular, especially that of the good-enough mother and transitional object. Winnicott's central focus was on the interaction between mother and baby, like most of the object relations school; unlike Freud, he had relatively little to say about fathers, whose main role he saw as protecting the mother–baby couple from outside interference, including their own.

Winnicott visualized an intermediate zone in the early years of life that was neither the realm of pure phantasy (as described by Klein), nor that of reality (to which adaptation by the ego was required, as described by Freud), although it partakes of both. In this intermediate, or transitional, zone the infant learns, with the help of the mother, to play (another key Winnicottian theme). Here phantasies can become reality, at least for the duration of the interactive play. In this transitional space Winnicott saw the origins of creativity and culture generally, and of a nascent sense of self. He suggested that the mother's face is a kind of mirror in which the child sees his own feelings reflected, and through this recognition begins to gain a sense of who he is. This process is disrupted if the mother is depressed or abusive, and here perhaps are the germs of borderline personality disorder, characterized by a deficient sense of self, and feelings of inner emptiness and sterility. Winnicott saw 'learning to play' as a key task in therapy in helping patients to regain their sense of self.

A related phenomenon is that of the transitional object—the special handkerchiefs, teddy bears, and precious playthings that toddlers often need for comfort and to help them sleep. Winnicott saw these as buffers against loss, objects that are invested with the properties of the primary object (the mother and her breast) but remain under the control of the child. They are 'transitional' in the sense that they lie between the ideal object of phantasy and the real, but potentially unreliable, objects of external reality.

The subtlety of Winnicott's thought is exemplified by his notion of the good-enough mother. Unlike some psychoanalytical writers he did not attribute all the evils of mankind to parental failure. Just as Freud saw phantasy as a reaction to loss (there is no need to imagine/phantasize a breast if you are in proximity to one), so Winnicott realized that a 'perfect' mother, who is always and intrusively in tune with her infant's needs could inhibit rather than foster the development of a sense of oneself as a separate and autonomous being. Mothers (and presumably fathers) should be 'good enough', not perfect, not least because through healthy protest about parental failure the child learns his own strength and finds limits which reassure him that his parents can withstand his aggression and still love him. Transitional objects can help children negotiate such conflict, as representatives of an intact inner world of loving objects, while external relationships are stormy.

Winnicott realized that developmental deficit does not always take the form of neglect or overt violence. He was particularly concerned with the ways that parents, driven by their own unconscious needs, may subtly impose their will on a compliant child, thereby inhibiting the growth of a robust and distinct sense of self. The false-self–real-self distinction tries to capture the ways in which children, and later personality disordered adults, may present an acceptable face to the world that is radically at variance with inner feelings of terror, emptiness, or rage. In his seminal, but today largely forgotten, classic *The Divided Self*, R.D. Laing[14] took Winnicott's false-self–real-self distinction as a central theme in his psychodynamic account of schizophrenia, seeing delusions as representing a way of holding together, albeit 'falsely', a disintegrating 'real' self and its inner world.

John Bowlby and attachment theory

Winnicott's contemporary John Bowlby[15] was considered for many years as a psychoanalytical renegade, despite (or perhaps because of) the fact that his life's work was essentially an attempt to bring logical and scientific rigour to psychoanalytical thought. Attachment theory, which can be thought of as an empirically validated version of object relations theory, starts from Freud's[16] revised theory of anxiety, in which, rather than viewing it as the result of incomplete repression of incestual wishes, anxiety is conceptualized in interpersonal terms as a response to the threat of the loss of a loved one. Based on his observations of delinquent youths, many of whom had suffered the loss of a parent during early childhood, and the depressive reactions of small children to separation from their parents on entering hospital, Bowlby saw that protection from danger was a key component of the parent–child relationship, and that there were built-in psychological mechanisms to ensure the maintenance of attachment bonds.

Attachment theory postulates that, when faced with threat, illness, or exhaustion, children will seek proximity to their caregivers. A protective response from the caregiver assuages the child's attachment needs, who can then return to play or exploratory behaviour, secure in the knowledge that help will once more be at hand if needed. This provides the conditions for secure attachment, and the child builds up an internal working model (Bowlby's preferred term for the inner world) of a secure robust self and responsive others. This formulation is very similar to Winnicott's notion of 'alone in the presence of the mother', a typically Winnicottian paradox depicting a child absorbed in play but with an overseeing protective but non-intrusive mother, his attempt to capture the conditions under which a strong sense of self can develop, and the capacity to withstand or even enjoy being alone.

Secure attachment arises out of responsive and sensitive parenting and is contrasted with insecure attachment which Bowlby saw as a factor predisposing to adult neurosis. Bowlby's collaborator, Mary Ainsworth, and her students, have researched different patterns of insecure attachment and the conditions under which they arise.[17] They delineate three main types of insecure attachment: insecure-avoidant, insecure-ambivalent, and insecure-disorganized. The avoidant child has experienced brusque or aggressive parenting, and tends to avoid close contact with people, hovering near caregivers rather than going directly to them when faced with threat. The ambivalent child clings to his inconsistent parents, and finds exploratory play difficult, even when the danger has past. Disorganized children behave in bizarre ways when threatened, and seem to have parents who are emotionally absent, often in the context of a parental history of abuse in their childhood. Disorganization is thought to be a severe form of insecure attachment and a possible precursor of severe personality disorder and dissociative phenomena in adolescence and early adulthood.

Mary Main[18] has developed a psychodynamic interview schedule, the Adult Attachment Interview (**AAI**), which is rated for the interviewee's narrative style, and, in long-term follow-up studies of children whose attachment patterns have been classified in infancy, yields interesting links with these earlier patterns of attachment. As with response to threat in childhood, adults ways of talking about themselves and their lives vary enormously. Some, in the secure-autonomous style, talk freely about themselves and their past pain in a coherent and apposite way. The insecure-dismissive style minimizes problems and is characterized by unelaborated speech lacking in metaphor or vividness. The insecure-enmeshed style is rambling and emotionally laden, while an insecure-disorganized pattern has evident breaks in continuity and logical flow. These insecure speech patterns, typical of those found in psychotherapeutic interviews with the psychologically disturbed, are manifestations of the underlying psychobiological relational dispositions which the various theories of object relations attempt to capture. The way we speak about ourselves reveals the state of our inner world. Peter Fonagy[19] has suggested that the capacity to represent experience, which he calls reflexive function, especially if problematic or traumatic (a contemporary version of the classical psychoanalytic notion of 'insight'), is a buffer against psychiatric disturbance. Once pain is thus represented the sufferer can distance himself from it, and consider alternative ways of responding. Enhancement of reflexive function is a generic psychotherapeutic strategy and applies as much to cognitive therapy (becoming aware of negative cognitions and automatic thoughts) as in psychodynamic therapies.

Bowlby objected to what he saw as the hijacking of the term 'biological' by organic psychiatry, since he believed the attachment relationship and its vicissitudes, adaptively shaped by evolutionary pressures, was no less 'biological' than the neurochemistry which presumably mediates it. For him human psychology was fundamentally relational, and he also resisted the idea that dependency was in some way a mark of psychological immaturity, or conversely, that the splendid isolation of autonomy was a good measure of maturity. He saw attachment needs as existing throughout the lifecycle, and thus put separation and loss as central to his view of the origins of psychiatric disturbance. In the attachment model, separation from a caregiver is a threat: we are biologically programmed to respond with shock, denial, anger, and searching behaviours when separated from a loved person or object. Loss is an irrevocable separation, and the early phases of the bereavement response are all vain attempts to restore the *status quo*. Despair and depression come with the recognition that separation is final, and, beyond that, reorganization of internal working models, sustained, perhaps, by what Klein called 'reinstatement of the lost object'—the recognition that although the loved one is lost in reality, good memories live on in the inner world.

Thus, ironically, Bowlby and Klein, despite radically different views especially on the role of the environment in mental ill health, agree on the importance of the ability to cope with loss, and see the capacity to become appropriately sad, as opposed to depressed, as a sign of mental health. Research on psychosocial factors in depression have tended to confirm these views. The attachment perspective also has implications for the day-to-day practice of psychiatry. One function of the psychiatric hospital and of the psychiatrist is to provide the patient with a 'secure base', which in itself goes some way to reducing anxiety. Appropriate dependency is integral to the supportive psychotherapeutic relationship which is such a key part of the psychotherapeutic dimension of psychiatry. Short-term training rotations, and unresponsive or rejecting relationships with psychiatrists and other mental health workers reinforce insecure attachment and may lead patients to redouble their efforts to cling on to the psychiatric institution—an all too familiar vicious circle.

The ego and its defences: Anna Freud, Hartmann, and Lacan

The interpersonal focus of object relations meant that Freud's abiding interest, psychic structure, received little attention from its theorists. The role of the ego and of defence mechanisms was, however, a particular concern of Anna Freud,[20] who represented a parallel tendency to the object relations school. She elaborated a taxonomy of defences used by the ego to maintain its integrity in the face of both internal threat from the id, and the demands and impingements of external reality. Valliant[21] groups Anna Freud's defences into those that are immature (like projective identification and splitting), neurotic defences (which include intellectualization, reaction formation, and identification with the aggressor), and mature ones (such as humour and sublimation).

Reaction formation describes the ways in which the ego counteracts unconscious desires or impulses that threaten its equilibrium by consciously held views directly contrary to these: the militant pacifist who is out of touch with any feelings of aggression for example, or the self-effacing secret narcissist. Identification with the aggressor, first described by Anna Freud, is frequently invoked in discussions of the psychological effects of childhood abuse. One way of dealing with the horror of abuse is to 'dis-identify' with oneself (a form of dissociation), and to put oneself in the place of the person who is attacking, thereby reducing feelings of pain and helplessness. This idea helps to explain how those who have been abused in childhood may become abusers themselves in adult life. A frequent experience in working with severely disturbed patients, many of whom are abuse survivors, is that healthcare workers may themselves feel attacked or symbolically 'abused' by these patients—seeing how the patient may have unconsciously identified with their aggressor can help carers to a greater understanding of their patients' problems and to respond less defensively to these attacks.

Valliant has found that men who use more mature defence mechanisms are less vulnerable to physical and psychological illness, and an important aim of psychotherapy would be to help the patient move from the use of more- to less-primitive defence mechanisms. Defences are therefore legitimately seen as adaptive, and, from a developmental perspective, the earlier the presumed psychic trauma, the more likely are primitive defence mechanisms to be employed. Heinz Hartmann,[22] the founder of the ego psychology school, emphasized the adaptive aspect of ego-function and a positive view of defences. For Freud the ego is a relatively weak structure, doing its best to moderate the overweening demands of the id, and the strictures of the superego, and so help the individual to survive in the face of environmental trauma. Hartmann proposed a more benign model. For him there was a 'conflict-free sphere of the ego' in which the ego can, if circumstances are reasonably favourable, deal smoothly with the external world. The basic psychological functions of thinking, perception, memory, planning, and even the experience of pleasure and satisfaction are manifestations of this conflict-free aspect of the ego. An advantage of

Hartmann's formulation, and one that is consistent with psychiatric thinking, is that it makes a clear distinction between normal and abnormal mental functioning, unlike, for example, the Freud–Klein model in which normality is built on an infrastructure of universal infantile disturbance and unintegration.

David Malan's[23] triangular model of anxiety, defence, and 'hidden impulse' is another variety of ego psychology which has found favour in psychiatric circles. It provides a clear formula for thinking about neurotic difficulties: for example people suffering from agoraphobia commonly defend against anxiety by avoidance and dependency; underlying this there may be hidden feelings of dissatisfaction and aggression, immediately towards a spouse, and in the past towards a controlling but unaffectionate mother. There are interesting links between Malan's formulation and non-psychodynamic schools of therapy, and with integrative therapies such as cognitive analytic therapy and interpersonal therapy (see Chapter 6.3.3). Behaviour therapy helps the ego to tolerate anxiety and thus face the feared situation. For Malan, the task of therapy is to allow the ego to tolerate and express the hidden feelings; cognitive therapy similarly would help the patient to become aware of and then counteract the automatic thoughts (equivalent to hidden feelings) that undermine the ego's attempts to achieve conflict-free functioning.

Ego psychology has been strongly criticized by Lacan, the French psychoanalyst, and his followers, who claim that it undermines the radical component of Freud's message. Lacan claims that Hartmann's view encourages the subject to adapt to, and therefore accept, the social *status quo*. Lacan advocates a 'return to Freud', which means emphasizing the importance of the inescapable conflict between the wishes and desires of an infant or small child, especially for possession of the mother, and the power relationships of the adult world, embodied in the father's capacity to say 'no', and to impose his reality on the child, including that of language. The anxiety generated by this conflict was seen by Freud as 'castration anxiety'. Feminist psychoanalysts have adopted Lacan's critique to demonstrate how patriarchy, rather than being a biological given, is a social construct deeply embedded in our psychology. The 'alternative reality' of psychosis can be understood in Lacanian terms as an attempt to evade this built-in collision between infantile desire and social conditioning.

The self, meaning, and interpersonal psychoanalysis: Sullivan, Horney, and Kohut

Freud's models of the mind were essentially intrapsychic, and couched in quasi-scientific language. Object relations, in varying degrees, retained this perspective but introduced a relational dimension never fully developed by Freud. Interpersonal psychoanalysis in the United States was even more radically interpersonal than object relations, and also critical of Freudian orthodoxy, which it saw as neglecting the human domain with its use of jargon and rigid intellectual dogmatism. Harry Stack Sullivan[24] was a free thinker who emphasized this existential aspect of psychotherapy, while remaining within the psychoanalytical tradition. He worked particularly with people suffering from schizophrenia, of whom Freud had little experience. Sullivan puts The Self at the centre of his psychology, in the sense of 'what one takes oneself to be'—equivalent to the contemporary notion of 'self-representation'. Patients suffering from schizophrenia suffer from low self-esteem and overwhelming anxiety, which Sullivan saw as the product of neglectful parenting, anxiety being equated in his schema, as for Klein, with a 'bad mother' representation. Humans have two sets of needs: the need for satisfaction and the need for security. 'Good mother', as in attachment theory, arises out of a sense of security and the absence of anxiety.

Sullivan believed in close involvement with his psychotic patients. His mission was always to find meaning in their experience, rather than dismiss it as an unintelligible manifestation of organic illness. He was a major influence on a generation of psychoanalytically informed psychiatrists including Harold Searles, Freida Fromm-Reichman, and Karen Horney.[25] The latter, like Sullivan, was critical of the pseudo-biological aspects of psychoanalysis, especially in relation to female psychology. For her, castration complex and penis envy were social rather than biological phenomena, manifestations of social relations that subjugated women, and from which by appropriate action, including psychotherapy, they could be liberated. Horney's contemporary, Eric Fromm, brought a Marxist influence into psychoanalysis, emphasizing the part played by capitalist production methods in contributing to isolation and anomie of modern men and women and their psychological troubles.

Although conventional psychoanalytical treatment for schizophrenia is now largely discredited, there is increasing interest in the role of psychosocial interventions in psychosis. Here the Sullivanian principles of respect for the patient's experience and its meaning, the need for a long-term supportive psychotherapeutic relationship, attention to the social precipitants of psychosis, and a focus on the ways in which the therapist may, through countertransference, foster recovery or reinforce pathology, are all highly relevant to contemporary psychiatry.

Heinz Kohut[26] was concerned not so much with schizophrenia, but with that intermediate world between neurosis and psychosis which psychoanalysts call 'borderline' pathology. The link with Sullivan is that for Kohut borderline and narcissistic disorders are analysed in terms of deficiencies of the self. Like Sullivan, Kohut puts self-esteem and its disorders at the centre of his psychology. Like Balint, Bowlby, and Winnicott (with whom his thought is most closely allied), he sees the origins of self-esteem in the empathic responsiveness of caregivers in the early years of life. For him there is a core of healthy narcissism which is based on the grandiosity and omnipotence of the young child ('his majesty the baby', as Freud put it) which is both accepted and fostered by effective parenting. Parents at this stage are 'self-objects', a concept akin to Winnicott's transitional objects, who partake both of the self and of the responsive environment, and which the infant believes, in his state of healthy delusion, to be there exclusively for his benefit.

Like Winnicott, Kohut emphasizes 'mirroring' as a key interpersonal theme. For Winnicott parental mirroring helps the child to own his emotions and begin to know who he is. Kohut, by contrast, takes up the narcissistic aspect of the mirror: the child sees his reflected glory in the eyes of his admiring parents, and this contributes towards his own positive self-regard. As development proceeds there is a process of 'optimal disillusionment', similar to the resolution of the Oedipus complex, in which the child gradually learns that his objects have a life of their own. By this time, however, his sense of a valued and effective self will be sufficiently developed, and residual narcissism will serve the useful functions of ambition, aspiration to success and admiration, or a sense of duty and concern for others.

Where the environment is unempathic, mirroring is deficient, fragile grandiosity squashed, or disillusionment traumatic, the stage is set for borderline pathology, in which self-absorption, and the use of others as self-objects, appropriate to the infantile years, persists into adult life (although in normal psychology self-object needs are never fully outgrown). Self-injurious behaviour such as drug abuse, eating disorders, and deliberate self-harm are 'breakdown products' of a disintegrated self, trying to use the environment as a self-object that will provide momentary and illusory satisfaction and self-affirmation.

A therapeutic implication of Kohut's approach is that the therapist is more supportive than in classical analysis, tolerant of the patient's grandiose designs, especially in the early stages of treatment. This contrasts with the approach of Otto Kernberg[27] who synthesizes classical and Kleinian concepts, and advocates rigorous interpretation, especially of destructive and self-defeating behaviour in borderline patients. Kohut's and Kernberg's theories reflect the typical polarization that such patients evoke in clinical settings, perhaps mirroring an inner world rigidly split into good and bad objects. Effective treatment requires a synthesis: empathy and tolerance is needed to form a working alliance, but firm limit-setting and confrontation of destructiveness is also essential. Another interpersonal synthesis is to be found in the work of Stephen Mitchell[28] whose approach reminds the therapist of the reciprocity of the therapeutic relationship in what Robert Lang calls the 'bipersonal field': patient and therapist form a system of mutual influence, the job of the therapist being both to participate in this, and at the same time to be sufficiently detached to be able to reflect upon it.

The shift in interpersonal psychoanalysis away from the analyst as an objective and privileged observer to a co-participant has given rise to a contemporary interest in narrative or hermeneutic explanations in psychotherapy,[29] in contrast to the scientific psychology which Freud originally hoped to establish. These authors argue the case for psychoanalysis as a hermeneutic discipline whose aim is to explore meaning rather than objective truth. If Freud is one of the intellectual founding fathers of modernism, their approach is 'post-modern' in the sense that it stresses the relativism of values and meanings, and the importance of power in determining one's view of the world. Here is a link—albeit so far rather distant—with the emerging 'user' movement in psychiatry, and the importance of giving as much weight to the client's voice as to that of the professional. Psychological truths are inherently contextual, and without awareness of the social context they can be obfuscatory.

Conclusions

Many new perspectives have emerged in the century since psychoanalysis was conceived. Emphasis has shifted from the intrapsychic to the interpsychic and interpersonal. Kleinian psychoanalysis offers a unique vision of the ways in which interpersonal reality is inescapably coloured by the emotional state of the participants. Attachment theory has begun to provide an account of human psychological development that both takes account of meaning and is empirically based. Psychoanalysis is emerging from its isolation and bridges have begun to be built with cognitive science: the inner world of phantasy is not unlike the world of schemata and assumptions that are the focus of cognitive therapy. There are, through modern neuroimaging techniques, even links being forged with neurobiology: we can now see the impact of effective therapeutic interventions on brain architecture. Progress will depend on further theoretical syntheses and technological advances, while holding firm to the humanistic emphasis on personal meaning and inner experience that is the fundamental contribution of psychoanalysis to contemporary psychiatry.

Further reading

Bateman, A. and Holmes, J. (1995). *Introduction to psychoanalysis: contemporary theory and practice*. Routledge, London.

Greenberg, J. and Mitchell, S. (1982). *Object relations in psychoanalytic theory*. Harvard University Press, Cambridge, MA.

Kohon, G. (1986). *The British school of psychoanalysis—the independent tradition*. Free Association, London.

Sandler, J., Holder, A., and Dare, C. (1992). *The patient and the analyst* (2nd edn). Karnac, London.

Symington, N. (1986). *The analytic experience: lectures from the Tavistock*. Free Association Books, London.

Wallerstein, R. (1992). *The common ground of psychoanalysis*. Jason Aronson, New York.

References

1. Freud, S. (1917). Mourning and melancholia. In *Standard edition of the complete psychological works of Sigmund Freud* (ed. J. Strachey), Vol. 14, pp. 239–58. Hogarth Press, London, 1957.
2. Klein, M. (1986). *The selected Melanie Klein* (ed. J. Mitchell). Penguin, Harmondsworth.
3. Spillius, E. (1988). *Melanie Klein today*. Routledge, London.
4. Hobson, R.P., Patrick, M., and Valentine, J. (1998). Objectivity in psychoanalytic judgements. *British Journal of Psychiatry*, **173**, 172–7.
5. Bion, W. (1988). In *Melanie Klein today* (ed. E. Spillius), pp. 178–86. Routledge, London.
6. Heimann, P. (1950). On countertransference. *International Journal of Psychoanalysis*, **31**, 81–4.
7. Grotstein, J. (1981). *Splitting and projective identification*. Basic Books, New York.
8. Ogden, T. (1979). On projective identification. *International Journal of Psychoanalysis*, **60**, 357–73.
9. Fairbairn, W.R. (1952). *Psychoanalytic studies of the personality*. Routledge, London.
10. Steiner, J. (1993). *Psychic retreats*. Routledge, London.
11. Britton, R., Feldman, M., and O'Shaughnessy, E. (1989). *The Oedipus complex today*. Karnac Press, London.
12. Balint, M. (1968). *The basic fault*. Tavistock Press, London.
13. Winnicott, D. (1971). *Playing and reality*. Penguin, Harmondsworth.
14. Laing, R. (1961). *The divided self*. Penguin, Harmondsworth.
15. Bowlby, J. (1988). *A secure base: clinical applications of attachment theory*. Routledge, London.
16. Freud, S. (1926). Inhibitions, symptoms, and anxiety. In *Standard edition of the complete psychological works of Sigmund Freud* (ed. J. Strachey), Vol. 20. Hogarth Press, London.
17. Holmes, J. (1996). *Attachment, intimacy, autonomy: using attachment theory in adult psychotherapy*. Jason Aronson, New York.
18. Main, M. (1995). In *Attachment theory: social, development and clinical perspectives* (ed. S. Goldberg, R. Muir, and J. Kerr), pp. 407–74. Analytic Press, New York.

19. Fonagy, P. (1995). In *Attachment theory: social, development and clinical perspectives* (ed. S. Goldberg, R. Muir, and J. Kerr), pp. 233–78. Analytic Press, New York.

20. Freud, A. (1936). *The ego and the mechanisms of defense.* Hogarth Press, London.

21. Valliant, G. (1992). *Ego mechanisms of defense: a guide for clinicians and researchers.* American Psychiatric Press, Washington, DC.

22. Hartmann, H. (1964). *Essays in ego psychology.* International Universities Press, New York.

23. Malan, D. (1996). *Individual psychotherapy and the science of psychodynamics* (2nd edn). Butterworth, London.

24. Sullivan, H.S. (1962). *Schizophrenia as a human process.* Norton, New York.

25. Horney, K. (1939). *New ways in psychoanalysis.* Norton, New York.

26. Kohut, H. (1977). *The restoration of the self.* International Universities Press, New York.

27. Kernberg, O. (1975). *Borderline conditions and pathological narcissism.* Jason Aronson, New York.

28. Mitchell, S. (1988). *Relational concepts in psychoanalysis: an integration.* Harvard Universities Press, Cambridge, MA.

29. Roberts, G. and Holmes, J. (ed.) (1998). *Healing stories: narrative in psychiatry and psychotherapy.* Oxford University Press.

3.4 Existential and phenomenological approach to psychiatry

Otto Doerr-Zegers

Introduction

It is a practical impossibility to give a brief summary of the principles and methods of phenomenology and their enormous influence on the human sciences, as well as the basic features of one of its derivations—existential psychiatry. We can only highlight the elements which seem to be fundamental to our understanding of their role in the history of psychiatry.

Phenomenology and the phenomenological movement are considered to have been founded by the German philosopher Edmund Husserl at the beginning of the twentieth century. Husserl first studied mathematics and later philosophy with Franz Brentano, from whom he adopted the concept of the *intentionality* of consciousness: 'And thus we can define psychic phenomena by saying that they are those phenomena which, precisely as intention, contain an object in themselves'.[1] Husserl later expresses the same idea in his own words: 'In simple acts of perceiving we are directed to the things perceived, in remembering, to the remembered ones, in thinking, to thoughts, in evaluating, to values, in willing, to objectives and perspectives . . .'.[2] Reality is, in the first place, experienced as the 'noema' of a 'noesis', as the content of our conscious acts.

Philosophy has to develop a direct and immediate approach to objects and to avoid the many prejudices which characterize history and human knowledge. Husserl's command 'To the things themselves' does not simply mean withdrawing from all traditional dogmas; rather, it is an invitation to become fully immersed in things. Eugen Fink, Husserl's follower, wrote: '[it is a matter of] an immersion in the authentic problems as such . . . [without] keeping up with ingenuous evidences'.[3] A return to things as they are in themselves does not mean that one takes concrete facts at face value, as one does in realism for example. On the contrary, one should reach *beyond* the realm of *that which shows itself*. Furthermore, phenomenology does not restrict its investigational data to sense experiences, but accepts on equal terms non-sensory data (such as relations and values) which present themselves intuitively. Phenomenology obtains its knowledge from a full and direct 'givenness' (the intuition) of the object.

Phenomenological experience is certainly not a natural experience, although it stems from this. In everyday life one finds oneself in a natural attitude ingenuously directed towards the world of objects. However, this directs us neither to *knowledge* nor, even less, to *scientific knowledge*. In order to transform this natural attitude to scientific knowledge we reduce the living object to only one of its aspects. For example, when chemists consider water, they reduce all meanings of the subject to its mere molecular composition: two hydrogen atoms and one oxygen atom. In essence, the natural scientist projects the chemical–physical theory of reality upon the entirety of the phenomenon, disregarding all other elements constituting the real object 'water'. Chemists do not consider the capacity of water to quench thirst or to make fields bear fruit, nor do they invoke the symbolisms of the depth of the sea, the importance of clouds, or the beauty of a lake. In contrast, when phenomenologists adopt a reflexive attitude, they direct their attention to the totality of the many ways in which an object is perceived in consciousness. Broekman, an outstanding Husserl scholar, states in this context: 'This fundamental division into two attitudes (natural and phenomenological) and their respective fields is a leitmotive which can be found in all of phenomenology'.[4]

According to Blankenburg, the phenomenological attitude tries:

> . . . to be as open as possible to the different ways of being of the object, that is to say, it tries to be (even) 'more natural' than natural experience itself. But on the other hand, it also tries to be 'more scientific' than scientific experience, as it does not limit itself to one particular project, but transforms in its subject [the totality of] the ways of being of what faces us.[5]

In other words: in every real experience we experience more than that which is given by perception of the mere object. This was brilliantly formulated almost 100 years before Husserl by Goethe, who stated in one of his aphorisms: 'The experience is always only half of the experience'.[6] We always live more than we live, and experience more than we experience, and to explore this other part is the great task of phenomenology. The Goethean principle, itself so parallel to Husserl's, leads us directly to the *oeuvre* of the French author Marcel Proust. The deep meaning of his novel *Remembrance of Things Past* lies in the recovery of everything that he experienced in the past and lived at that moment almost without becoming aware of it. The major features of his work parallel the founding phases of the phenomenological method: a total openness to reality, a reflexive attitude which perceives reality as given to a consciousness, and a progressive elimination of all presuppositions, prejudices, and accidental elements as an instrument to achieve insight into the essence of what is experienced.

The approach of Jaspers

The German physician and philosopher Karl Jaspers was the first to apply the phenomenological method to psychiatry.[7,8] According to Jaspers, phenomenology is a 'descriptive psychology'. It is strongly related to facts and delivers a unbiased description of patients' experiences. Jaspers combined an appeal to empathy (*Einfühlen*) with immediate understanding (*Verstehen*) of the other person, without exploiting phenomenological techniques of self-reduction, free variation in imagination, and intuition of essential features. However, the present author does not share the opinion of Berríos,[9] who strongly contrasted Husserl and Jaspers. The differences between them are not so extreme as claimed by Berríos, at least not as far as the application of their phenomenological approaches to psychiatry are concerned. Some of Jaspers' statements illustrate this opinion: 'Phenomenology relates to what is experienced as real; it observes the psyche "from inside" through immediate representation (*Vergegenwärtigung*)', or '[He] who has no eyes cannot practice histology; [he] who repudiates himself or is unable to image the psyche and to perceive it as a living entity, can never understand phenomenology'.[7] Thus Jaspers' points of departure were in fact the same as those of Husserl: the return to things, the intentionality of psychic phenomena, and the change from a natural to a phenomenological attitude. A scrupulous search of the writings of Jaspers eventually also leads us to Husserl's intuition of essences, as when Jaspers call for 'an ordering which puts the phenomena of the psyche together, in accordance with their phenomenological kinship, not unlike that which occurs with the infinitely manifold colours in the rainbow'.[7] Significant American authors, such as Wiggins and Schwartz,[10,11] have recently expressed a similar opinion regarding Jaspers' link with Husserl.

The approach of Binswanger

The second psychiatrist to apply the phenomenological method to psychiatry was the Swiss–German Ludwig Binswanger. In his paper 'On phenomenology'[12] he is already suggesting that 'the intuition of essences is the fundamental process of the phenomenological method (in psychiatry)'. Later, he was strongly influenced by Heidegger's *Being and Time*[13] and was converted to existentialism. Through this conversion, Binswanger placed the way of being and the biography of psychiatric patients within the realm of Heidegger's description of human existence as 'being-in-the-world'. Thus, according to Binswanger, 'We do not say "mental illnesses are brain diseases" but in mental illnesses we encounter modifications of the essential structure and structural elements of the being-in-the-world as transcendence'.[14]

This approach has at least two advantages. First, analyses of various forms of psychotic worlds showed how these deviations lead to the understanding of new forms of being-in-the-world. Examples include the feeling that the world is full of light in mania[15] or the eccentricity in schizophrenia.[16] Secondly, the use of language is of great importance. The biological psychiatrist studies the alterations of language within the boundaries of the clinical picture and the psychoanalyst investigates its biographical content, whereas the existential analyst directs his attention to 'the world projects in which the speaker lives or has lived'.[14] Thus, existential analysis enquires into ways in which *Dasein* 'discovers' and 'projects' worlds.[15] We shall now try to summarize Binswanger's findings pertaining to the life-history and the world of schizophrenic patients.

1. First, the unfolding of a schizophrenic existence is characterized by 'the breaking of the coherence of natural experience'. Binswanger regarded this pattern of 'incoherence' as a major tendency

even in the childhood of these patients. For this reason, their lives are painful and difficult; they are permanently searching for forms and means to re-establish a lost order.

2. Another essential element of schizophrenic existence is its splitting into alternatives which are not reconcilable. One dominant alternative is usually an eccentric ideal. This tendency to split often appears in the period preceding the illness and in different realms of life, such as work, social relations, or the relationship with one's own body.

3. The third constitutive feature is the concealment of the rejected side of the alternative in favour of the absolute supremacy of the eccentric ideal. This perspective allows one to understand the relationship between schizophrenia and the search for original forms of expression found in the Mannerist movement in the arts, because concealment of the feared alternative is often achieved by means of arbitrary, twisted, and unnecessarily detailed modes of expression (language, writing, movement, and drawing).

4. The final characteristic is the drive to 'annihilation' which becomes manifest as the culmination of conflicting tensions and withdrawal from the world. This is the 'longing for the end', which can be reached as passive autism, chronic delusion, or suicide.

At the end of his life, Binswanger abandoned these biographical analyses, so closely linked to Heidegger's work, and returned to Husserl's transcendental phenomenology. In his last two books, *Melancholie und Manie*[17] and *Wahn*,[18] he tried to describe the constitution of pathological worlds as alterations of transcendental consciousness. In understanding time in terms of his concept of intentionality (see above), Husserl differentiates between *protentio* (future), *retentio* (past), and *prasentatio* (present). In the case of endogenous depression, Binswanger described a profound alteration in the constitution of the experience of time. The *protentio* is invaded by elements of the past (in a depressive delusion a mere possibility, for example that I may become ruined, is transformed into a fact that has already occurred). The *retentio* is invaded by elements of the future (as in the frequent self-reproaches, where events in the past are experienced as if they are still active in the present).

In mania, Binswanger found a loosening of the links between the three elements of the experience of time. The future is not anchored in the present or the past, and the past is no longer needed to sustain the present or the future. Thus a person who is manic does not need to have studied medicine to consider himself a great physician. Binswanger also found a failure in the experience of other beings. This is the result of a very complex process, which begins with the perception of the other's body and continues with the 'aperception' of that body as different from one's own. From there, one proceeds to what Husserl called *Appräsentation* ('appresentation') of the other in his entirety and *Alterität* (the conviction of being another person). Our common shared world stems from the reciprocity of these representations. This is made clear in the example of a teacher and his students given by Szilasi.[19] The ways in which the teacher sees the students as being present and they see him are different. However, both share the 'appresentation' that he is the teacher and they are the students. Binswanger observed how the manic patient demonstrates a lack of respect towards the other person and constantly evaluates the other by his weak points. He formulated this attitude as a failure in 'the continuity of appresentation'.[17] The loss of this shared 'appresentation' is devastating, as it forms the basis of mutual experience of the other person.

Binswanger's return to Husserl's pure transcendental phenomenology has been criticized by some of his followers, including Kisker[20] and Tellenbach.[21] They doubt whether this return to the study of transcendental consciousness and its different constitutions is real progress towards a scientific foundation for psychiatry. They regret that Binswanger abandoned existential analysis with its accent on historicity, and proceeded to the study of the ahistoric structures of transcendental consciousness.

However, one cannot deny that the application of Husserl's truly transcendental phenomenology can be fruitful for psychiatry. Blankenburg has demonstrated this,[5,22] and it has been underlined by recent efforts to construct a link between phenomenology and psychopathology in the light of emerging trends in both neurobiology and the philosophy of consciousness.[23]

Other European authors contemporary with Binswanger, for example von Gebsattel, Straus, and Zutt in Germany, Minkowski in France, and López-Ibor in Spain, were influenced equally by Husserl and Heidegger. von Gebsattel[24] developed a new understanding of the world of phobia and obsession. His descriptions of the hypersensitivity of phobics to space, and of decomposition, dirtiness, and impurity as constitutive elements of the world of the obsessed contributed to the understanding of both diseases. Straus[25] made important contributions to understanding of the experience of space, and his studies were equally relevant to the experience of time in depression. Equally noteworthy is Minkowski's book *Le Temps Vécu*[26] which, on the basis of the philosophy of Bergson, is not only a profound study of the experience of time in psychosis but also a conclusive contribution to our understanding of 'autism'. López-Ibor's work, which strongly influenced the Spanish-speaking world, is a good example of how phenomenological intuition runs ahead of the results of empirical research. In 1950, López-Ibor[27] had already defined the 'endogenous' character of states then termed 'neurotic'. The disappearance of the concept of 'neurosis' since the publication of DSM-III in 1980 and the broadening of the concept of depression in recent decades have vindicated his phenomenological insights.

The work of Zutt

Another author who has made a major contribution to the phenomenological orientation in psychiatry is Jürg Zutt. His analysis of hallucination[28] is one of the best examples of how a phenomenological approach can disclose the essence of a psychpathological phenomenon. Many patients hear voices, and this has traditionally been interpreted as 'false perceptions by the ear'. If the 'deceived' sensorial organ is the ear, then the alteration in function should be the acoustic tract. According to Zutt, empirical research to find such alterations was carried out during the first half of the twentieth century without any obvious result. In addition, classical authors had been puzzled by the fact that schizophrenic patients *listen to voices*, but *do not see visions*. Why does this discrepancy exist? This approach to hallucination and its discrepancy relates to the theory that the human organism is based on anatomy and physiology. However, there are other theories, like psychoanalysis, where hallucination is not interpreted as an alteration in auditory perception but rather as the result of a 'weak ego' con-

fronted with threatening contents of the consciousness. However, the symptom 'to hear voices' as such was not investigated in either the organic or the psychoanalytic theory. Such theories tend to 'conceal' the phenomenon; they do not let it speak for itself. What remains constant in the schizophrenic patient's 'hearing voices' when we set it free from all the contingent factors, both anecdotal and specific? The present author has contributed to Zutt's analysis, in so far as he compared schizophrenic hallucinations with those associated with alcoholic psychosis.[29] Alcoholic patients listen to non-existent persons who suddenly appear in real space and talk to them ('behind the door', 'in the street') while schizophrenics feel perplexed and overwhelmed by the voices and generally do not act in accordance with what they hear. The alcoholic hallucination is an active perception, which implies an identification ('it's the police'), a localization ('they've already entered the door'), and an action (the patient hides away under the bed), whereas, as Zutt pointed out, the schizophrenic hallucination is characterized by passivity and defencelessness because the patient *does not truly hear voices* (as the alcoholic patient does) but is the person to whom the voices speak—he *is talked to*. However, this formulation leads us to realize that the discrepancy mentioned above has disappeared, because the schizophrenic patient, as he *is talked to*, is also *looked at*. Consequently, the contextual relation is not voice–vision, but voice–look. Therefore in this clinical picture the fundamental disorder is not of perception but rather of the more complex phenomenon of interpersonal relationships.

The appointment of first von Baeyer (in 1955), and later Janzarik (in 1973), to the chair of psychiatry in Heidelberg initiated a new era in phenomenological and existential psychiatry, also associated with Blankenburg, Braeutigam, Haefner, Kisker, and Tellenbach. Many psychiatrists from Germany and elsewhere were trained at the Heidelberg Clinic, or were influenced by this school, and the majority of them remained attached to phenomenology. These psychiatrists include Kraus (an outstanding follower of Tellenbach), Lang, Schmidt-Degenhard, and Spitzer in Germany, Bin Kimura in Japan, Ballbé in Argentina, and Figueroa, Lolas, Parada, and Doerr-Zegers in Chile. Since it is not possible to comment here on the work of each author, we will focus only on Tellenbach and Blankenburg, whose work had the greatest impact outside Germany.

The work of Tellenbach and Blankenburg

Tellenbach's work is prodigious; it shows not only the power of phenomenology for understanding the essence of mental illnesses, but also the many possibilities for applying that approach in clinical practice. His major field of investigation was depression,[30] but he also contributed to the understanding of delusion, 'the atmospheric', by which he meant the aura associated with a person or place. He was also interested in the importance of the father's role in psychopathology, and in the different ways in which this has been conceived in the course of history. He also carried out numerous hermeneutic analyses of literary and religious characters such as King Oedipus, Hamlet, Othello, King Lear, and Prince Myshkin,[31] investigating what these characters can teach us about psychopathological phenomena such as delusion, melancholy, jealousy, dementia, and epilepsy. Tellenbach also describes a specific human type, the 'typus melancholicus', who carries a predisposition for unipolar depression. The fundamental characteristic of this type is what he terms 'orderliness'. This is a manner of remaining fixated to life's natural orders, such as home, marriage, maternity, work, etc., so that hazards of human life and the impossibility of maintaining the usual order can become an existential threat and trigger the change towards depression ('endokinesis'). Perhaps the most interesting point in Tellenbach's conceptualization is that he succeeded in demonstrating a perfect coherence between the predepressive personality, the triggering situation, and the symptoms of depression. His comprehensive and visionary insight allowed him to show, as early as 1961, the existence of only one 'endoreactive' unipolar depressive syndrome, whereas at that time approximately 20 types of depression were distinguished. Tellenbach's description was some 20 years ahead of the DSM-III concept of 'major depression'. Later, von Zerssen[32] empirically demonstrated the validity of Tellenbach's intuitions.

Earlier, Blankenburg attempted a strict application of Husserl's transcendental phenomenology to a case of delusional mood (*Wahnstimmung*). A young student standing in front of the display of a bookstore had the extraordinary feeling that all the books were exposed *for him*: 'It was like a reproach. Perhaps that meant that I had to study more at the university'.[5] Blankenburg's point of departure is the analysis of the perplexity that he himself experiences when confronted with the episode lived by the patient, and he discovers how his own capacity for astonishment had been surpassed, somehow overwhelmed. Therefore he tries to probe more deeply into the meanings of 'astonishment' and 'being overwhelmed'. In 'astonishment', 'what emanates from the world [*Zuwurf*] will be contained in an even wider plan [*Entwurf*] of human existence',[5] while in 'being overwhelmed' the same emanation, or 'stream' (*Zustrom*), surpasses the limits of what human existence can contain. This is the case with the young student. The books had lost their neutral character and something is released from them which urges and presses upon the patient, leaving him feeling exposed, without any protection, and finally leading to a loss of the coherence of his natural experience. This is the seed of what we know in more serious cases as 'constraint of thought' (*Gedankenbeeinflussung*).

A further important contribution by Blankenburg is his conceptualization of 'the loss of natural evidence' (*der Verlust der natürlichen Selbstverständlichkeit*) in schizophrenia.[22] His observations about this phenomenon were made on a series of patients with a high intellectual level and a large capacity for self-reflection. One patient expressed this by saying: 'I lack something, something small . . . but so important that I can not live without it'.[22] Another said that health and happiness were only possible because there was 'something' that one is usually not aware of. The same patient ended up in saying that 'this mysterious "something" seems to stubbornly resist awareness'.[22] Healthy people do not think about the natural evidence which schizophrenic patients sometimes reflect upon compulsively because they have lost it to a certain extent. The only situation in which healthy people come very near to what occurs in schizophrenic patients is in the phenomenological reduction or *epoché*. This consists 'in releasing the everyday existence from the simple naive ways of forming opinions in which we are rooted in our personal world'.[22] In doing so, we adopt a reflexive attitude and distance ourselves from the everyday world. The resistance which phenomenologists experience, when they adopt this attitude, is absent in the case of the schizophrenic patient who, in contrast, lives in a more or less permanent *epoché*.

The French phenomenologists

Phenomenological psychiatry also developed in France, paralleling its development in Germany, particularly in Paris, under the leadership of Pelicier, and in Marseilles, where it was associated with Sutter, Tatossian, Azorin, Giudicelli, and Naudin. France is one of the most important centres of phenomenological research today, as can be seen in the periodical *L'Art de Comprendre*, edited by Philippe Forget and Georges Charbonneau. Pelicier's work is far reaching and characterized by a clinical point of view combined with important ethical concerns. He has touched on almost all themes in psychiatry, with contributions on anxiety, depression, addictions, dementia, and psychosomatic illnesses.[33] His method could be described as being between Jaspers and Husserl. Like Jaspers, he remains close to the subjective experience of the concrete patient, but like Husserl he searches for the essential characteristics and invariant elements within the complexity of psychopathological facts. However, he does not pretend to reach the very constitution of the acts of consciousness in the Husserlian sense. Tatossian's book *Phénoménologie des Psychoses*[34] provided the first systematic review of knowledge in the field of psychoses, including an introduction, for French readers, to the work of German authors from Binswanger to Blankenburg. One cannot conclude this brief overview of French phenomenology without mentioning Naudin's extraordinary book *Phénoménologie et Psychiatrie: Les Voix et la Chose*,[35] which is the most complete phenomenological analysis of hallucination in the Husserlian sense. For Naudin, as earlier for Zutt, hallucination is not a disturbance of perception but of intentionality itself: 'It is an insoluble dehumanization which lays bare the very "phenomenality" of intentional processes'. Later he adds:[35]

> Transparent and with a single voice, the hallucinated other is characterized by its lack of reciprocity. This other is not an *alter ego*, since it is lived [by the patient] in the immediate present. Everything occurs as if the processes of perception, which put things in perspective through a succession of schemas, were inverted: here, the idea appears as a whole, all of a sudden.

Other approaches

France is not the only country where psychiatric phenomenology is being developed. The journal *Philosophy, Psychiatry and Psychology* brings together important authors from the United Kingdom and the United States, including Fulford from the former and Schwartz from the latter. In addition, the major journal *Current Opinion in Psychiatry*, edited by the World Psychiatric Association, is publishing an increasing number of phenomenological contributions.

Future developments

As for the future, we are in agreement with the ideas recently expressed by Wiggins and Schwartz.[36] Phenomenology can contribute to psychiatry firstly by allowing an understanding of mental illnesses beyond the mind–body dualism, and secondly by enforcing a rigorous scientific method. In doing this, it can highlight aspects of psychopathology which differentiate, for example, delusions in schizophrenia, mania, and exogenous psychosis.[37]

Finally we suggest a critique of psychiatric phenomenology and at the same time offer some solutions. The application of the phenomenological method in psychiatry always results in the determination of a 'loss' of something owned by the healthy person, a problem also identified by Broekman.[38] For example, we talk of the 'loss of natural evidence' (Blankenburg) or the 'loss of the coherence of natural experience' (Binswanger). The search for the mere deficiency can mean that phenomenology appears to be only the translation of psychopathological concepts into another language; for example, instead of schizophrenic 'devastation' (*Verblödung*) one speaks of 'existential withdrawal' (*Rückzug*). We see only one way of overcoming this difficulty, and that is to develop a *positive* phenomenological understanding of psychopathological deviations. This means that they should be understood not as mere deficiencies, 'but as the emancipation of particular aspects of human reality, which in the healthy person remain integrated'.[39] In the case of delusions (phenomena pertaining to the realm of intentional acts which fixate reality and solidify themselves in judgements), Blankenburg has demonstrated how the normal constitution of a judgement about reality appears itself as a delusional formation *in statu nascendi* which is permanently being corrected or abolished. In delusion there is an emancipation and radicalization of human possibilities, for instance the capacity to proceed from the particular to the general or the imagination of things that are beyond reality or the zealous search for truth. Doerr-Zegers and Tellenbach[37] have shown how delusion and truth are closely related. Strictly speaking, delusion possesses almost all the attributes of truth, even its capacity to illuminate (in the sense of the Greek *aletheia*); however, its radicalizing character leads to blinding and isolation of the patient.

This phenomenological–dialectic perspective is of interest for psychopathology in two ways. The first is that it allows one to understand those styles of experience and behaviour which appear in our daily clinical practice not as a pure deviation from a presupposed norm, but as behaviours which exist in their own right. The second is the positive view of the negative, originally developed by Hegel and applied to psychiatry by Blankenburg[40] and later by Doerr-Zegers.[41] This approach directs attention not only to the deficiencies of schizophrenic patients (what is negative), but also to the many positive aspects, such as their metaphysical sense, their capacity to perceive nuances of reality which are bewildering to average people, and their search for an uncompromising truth.[37] The same approach could be adopted for depressive, hysteric, or obsessive patients. The depressive personality displays loyalty to social norms, a high work performance, and self-oblivion. The hysterical personality adapts to any context, possesses a great capacity for emotional warmth, and is an outstanding entertainer. The obsessive patient displays a strong capacity to carry out projects, a sober appearance, and scrupulous care in relations with other persons.

This way of thinking is not only of theoretical but also of practical importance. When psychiatrists do not simply take the negative view, they will be forced to widen their horizons of understanding, change their frames of reference, and question the traditional concept of illness. Furthermore, from this perspective psychopathological states appear as polarities (e.g. schizophrenia versus depression or hysteria versus obsession) with multiple transitions which correspond to clinical experience rather than fixed nosological categories. The observation of the positive aspects of psychopathological states leads to improved methods of therapeutic action. Thus the doctor should avoid merely adapting the patient to a norm which in reality does not exist. Instead, the patient is made aware of the positive values of features that are often defined as abnormal and helped to develop in the opposite direction, towards the other pole, for example from the schizophrenic to the depressive pole and vice versa. In doing this, the existential–phenomenological attitude helps the patient to approach what the Ancient Greeks called 'measure' which, according to Aristotle, is the perfect position between two imperfect extremes. As Heraclitus stated, '[In the end] what is cold gets warm, what is warm gets cold, what is humid gets dry, and what is dry gets humid' (Fragment 126).

References

1. Brentano, F. (1925). *Psychologie vom empirischen Standpunkt.* Meiner, Leipzig.
2. Husserl, E. (1962). *Husserliana*, Vol. IX, *Phänomenologische Psychologie.* Nijhoff, The Hague.
3. Fink, E. (1958). *Studien zur Phänomenologie.* Nijhoff, The Hague.
4. Broekman, J.M. (1965). Phänomenologisches Denken in Philosophie und Psychiatrie. *Confinia Psychiatrica*, **8**, 165–87.
5. Blankenburg, W. (1962). Aus dem phänomenologischen Erfahrungsfeld innerhalb der Psychiatrie. *Schweizer Archiv für Neurologie, Neurochirurgie und Psychiatrie*, **90**, 412–21.
6. Goethe, W. (1966). *Naturwissenschafte Schriften II, Sprüche in Prosa*, No. 172. Artemis, Zürich.
7. Jaspers, K. (1963). Die phänomenologische Forschungsrichtung in der Psychopathologie. In *Gesammelte Schriften zur Psychopathologie*, pp. 314–28. Springer, Berlin.
8. Jaspers, K. (1963). *Allgemeine Psychopathologie.* Springer, Berlin
9. Berrios, G.E. (1989). What is phenomenology? *Journal of the Royal Society of Medicine*, **82**, 425–8.
10. Wiggins, O.P., Schwartz, M.A., and Spitzer, M. (1992). Phenomenological/descriptive psychiatry: the methods of Edmund Husserl and Karl Jaspers. In *Phenomenology, Language and Schizophrenia* (ed. C. Mundt), pp. 1–25. Springer, New York.
11. Wiggins, O.P. and Schwartz, M.A. (1997). Edmund Husserl's influence on Karl Jaspers' phenomenology. *Philosophy, Psychiatry, and Psychology*, **4**, 15–36.
12. Binswanger, L. (1947). Über Phänomenologie. In *Ausgewählte Vorträge und Aufsätze*, Vol. I, pp. 13–49. Francke, Bern.
13. Heidegger, M. (1963). *Sein und Zeit* (10th edn). Niemayer, Tübingen.
14. Binswanger, L. (1947). Über die dasesinsanalytische Forschungsrichtung in der Psychiatrie. In *Ausgewählte Vorträge und Aufsätze*, Vol. I, pp. 190–217. Francke, Bern.
15. Binswanger, L. (1945). Über die manische Lebensform. In *Ausgewählte Vorträge und Aufsätze*, Vol. II, pp. 252–63. Francke, Bern.
16. Binswanger, L.(1957). *Schizophrenie.* Neske, Pfullingen.
17. Binswanger, L. (1960). *Melancholie und Manie.* Neske, Pfullingen.
18. Binswanger, L. (1965). *Wahn.* Neske, Pfullingen.
19. Szilasi, W. (1959). *Einführung in die Phänomenologie Edmund Husserls.* Niemayer, Tübingen.
20. Kisker, K.P. (1961). Die phänomenologische Wendung Ludwig Binswanger's. *Jahrbuch für Psychologie, Psychotherapie und Medizinische Anthropologie*, **8**, 143–153.
21. Tellenbach, H. (1962). Abbreviatur und Epikritisches zu Ludwig Binswanger's Buch 'Melancholie und Manie'. *Nervenarzt*, **33**, 515–20.
22. Blankenburg, W. (1971). *Der Verlust der natürlichen Selbstverständlichkeit.* Enke, Stuttgart.
23. Mishara, A. and Schwartz, M.A. (1997). Psychopathology in the light of emergent trends in the philosophy of consciousness, neuropsychiatry and phenomenology. *Current Opinion in Psychiatry*, **10**, 383–9.
24. von Gebsattel, V.E. (1954). *Prolegomena einer medizinischen Anthropologie.* Springer, Berlin.

25. Straus, E. (1960). *Psychologie der menschlichen Welt*. Springer, Berlin.

26. Minkowski, E. (1933). *Le temps vécu*. Collection de L'Évolution Psychiatrique, Paris.

27. López-Ibor, J.J. (1950). *La angustia vital*. Paz Montalvo, Madrid.

28. Zutt, J. (1963). *Auf dem Wege zu einer anthropologischen Psychiatrie*. Springer, Berlin.

29. Doerr-Zegers, O. (1997). *Psiquiatría antropológica* (2nd edn). Universitaria, Santiago.

30. Tellenbach, H. (1983). *Melancholie* (4th edn). Springer, Berlin.

31. Tellenbach, H. (1992). *Schwermut, Wahn und Fallsucht in der abendländischen Dichtung*. Pressler, Hürtgenwald.

32. von Zerssen, D. (1982). Personality and affective disorders. In *Handbook of affective disorders*, pp. 213–28. Churchill Livingstone, New York.

33. Pelicier, Y. (1987). Asthme, souffle et culture. *Psychologie Médicale*, **19**, 1849–50.

34. Tatossian, A. (1979). *Phénoménologie des psychoses*. Masson, Paris.

35. Naudin, J. (1997). *Phénoménologie et psychiatrie*. Presses Universitaires du Mirail, Toulouse.

36. Wiggins, O. and Schwartz, M. (1997). Psychiatry. In *Encyclopaedia of phenomenology* (ed. L. Embree), Vol. 18. Kluwer, Boston, MA.

37. Doerr-Zegers, O. and Tellenbach, H. (1980). Differential-phänomenologia des depressiven Syndroms. *Nervenarzt*, **51**, 113–18.

38. Broekman, J. (1998). Schizophrenie als Erkenntnisproblem. *Fundamenta Psychiatrica*, **12**, 47–52.

39. Blankenburg, W. (1985). Perspectiva antropológica y analítico-existencial del delirio. *Revista Chilena de Neuropsiquiatría*, **23**, 165–78.

40. Blankenburg, W. (1981). Wie weit reicht die dialektische Betrachtungsweise in der Psychiatrie? *Zeitschrift für Psychiatrie und Psychotherapie*, **29**, 45–66.

41. Doerr-Zegers, O. (1990). Hacia una concepción dialéctica en psiquiatría. *Actas Luso-Españolas de Neurología y Psiquiatría* **18**, 244–57.

3.5 Current psychodynamic approaches to psychiatry

Glen O. Gabbard

Psychodynamic psychiatry is broadly defined today. In fact, the term psychodynamic is now used almost synonymously with psychoanalytical. Freud originally used the term psychodynamic to emphasize the conflict between opposing intrapsychic forces: a wish was opposed by a defence, and different intrapsychic agencies, such as ego, id, and superego, were in conflict with one another. Indeed, for much of the twentieth century psychoanalytical theory was dominated by the drive-defence model, often referred to as ego psychology.

In the last decades of the twentieth century, however, the hegemony of ego psychology waned, and other models of the mind gained wide acceptance. Through the influence of Melanie Klein and the British School of object relations, psychoanalytical theory expanded beyond the notion of conflict among intrapsychic agencies. Internal object relations became paramount in models deriving from these sources. In addition, a deficit model of symptomatology arose from the work of the British object-relation theorists, such as Balint and Winnicott. In the United States, Kohut's self-psychology also developed a model based on developmental deficits. In other words, disturbed patients who came to treatment were seen as suffering from absent or weakened psychic structures based on developmental failures by parents or caretakers in the early childhood environment. (See Chapter 3.2 for an account of the development and modern practice of psychoanalysis.)

As a result of these innovations in psychoanalytical theory, psychodynamic psychiatry is practised today in an era of pluralism. The typical psychodynamic psychiatrist then uses multiple models to assist in the understanding of a particular patient. Moreover, the diagnostic and treatment approach to an individual patient is psychodynamically informed even when a decision has been made to forego psychodynamic psychotherapy. Psychodynamic thinking provides a conceptual framework within which all treatments are prescribed, including pharmacotherapy, psychotherapy, inpatient or partial hospital treatment, and group or family modalities. Psychodynamic psychiatry is not synonymous with psychodynamic psychotherapy.

A comprehensive definition of current psychodynamic psychiatry is the following:[1]

> Psychodynamic psychiatry is an approach to diagnosis and treatment characterized by a way of thinking about both patient and clinician that includes unconscious conflict, deficits and distortions of intrapsychic structures, and internal object relations.

In this definition emphasis is placed on the presence of two individual psychologies or subjectivities that interact in the field of treatment. Clinicians must recognize that their own unconscious beliefs, biases, and feelings will inevitably influence the way they view the patient.

Basic principles

A set of time-honoured basic principles, all derived from psychoanalytical technique and theory, define the overall approach of the dynamic psychiatrists (Table 1).

The unconscious

A fundamental premise of psychodynamic psychiatry is that mental activity going on outside our awareness can be profoundly influential. Freud saw signs of the unconscious in two major types of clinical evidence: parapraxes and dreams. Parapraxes, commonly referred to as slips of the tongue or 'Freudian slips,' involve substituting one word for another. For example, a patient who intends to say 'Protestant,' may unwittingly say 'prostitute'. Parapraxes may also involve actions, such as forgetting, or executing one action when intending to do another.

Freud regarded dreams as the 'Royal Road' to the understanding of the unconscious. Although dreams are no longer regarded as the exclusive avenue to the patient's unconscious conflicts, fears, and wishes, they are still of considerable value in helping the clinician gain a greater grasp of the patient's difficulties. The dream work typically disguises an unconscious childhood wish, so there can be no facile analysis of a dream based on the assumption that one symbol always means the same thing. Rather, there needs to be a psychotherapeutic collaboration in which the patient talks about the connection of the dream to past experiences, current concerns, and current conflicts.

Another primary way that the unconscious manifests itself in the clinical setting is the patient's behaviour toward the clinician. Certain characteristic patterns of relatedness to others set in childhood become

Table 1 Basic principles of psychodynamic psychiatry

The unconscious
Psychic determinism
Developmental orientation
Emphasis on the uniqueness of the individual rather than how the individual is like others
Transference
Countertransference
Resistance

internalized and are manifested automatically and unconsciously as part of the patient's character. Hence certain patients may consistently act deferentially toward the clinician, while others will behave in a highly rebellious way. This type of procedural memory is closely linked to Squire's[2] notion of implicit memory, which occurs outside the realm of verbal narrative memory.

While declarative or autobiographical memory involves remembered events and narratives of one's life, procedural memory stores the 'how' of executing sequences of actions, such as motor skills. Once guitar-playing or bicycle-riding has been mastered, no conscious recall is necessary when one sits down with a guitar or jumps on a bicycle. The schema referred to as unconscious internal-object relations are to some extent procedural memories repeated again and again in a variety of interpersonal situations. They are non-conscious, but not dynamically unconscious, in the sense of being defensively banished from conscious awareness.

The notion that much of mental life is unconscious is one that is most challenged by psychoanalytical critics, but it is also one that is extensively validated by literature from experimental psychology.[3] Research subjects who have bilateral lesions to the hippocampus have great difficulty learning that two discrete events are connected, but their emotional responses suggest that they have made an unconscious connection between the two events.[4] Subliminal presentation of stimuli that have emotional or psychodynamic meanings to research subjects have been shown to influence a wide range of behaviour, even though the subjects have no conscious awareness of the stimuli.[5] Studies of brain-evoked related potentials found that emotional words evoke more electroencephalograph alpha waves than neutral words, even before they are consciously recognized.[6] In another study, a team of clinicians assessed which conflicts were relevant to identified patient symptoms. Words reflecting those conflicts were selected and presented both subliminally and superliminally.[7] A different pattern of response was documented for those words consciously related to the patient's symptoms and those hypothesized to be unconsciously related.

Psychic determinism

The notion of psychic determinism is intimately linked with the construct of the unconscious. Freud felt that behaviour and mental life were related to multiple and complex causation.[8] The term over-determination implies that a variety of intrapsychic and unconscious factors come together to produce specific symptoms or behaviours. The notion of multiple causation implies that there can be alternate sets of sufficient conditions, some involving primarily unconscious conflicting forces, others stemming from biological and environmental influences, that ultimately produce similar symptoms or behaviours.

While unconscious factors powerfully influence much of human experience, we must also recognize that there are powerful biological factors at work as well. A patient who has a brain injury may forget the name of someone important to him, but it does not necessarily reflect a parapraxis based on unconscious conflict. Similarly, to say that unconscious factors are relevant does not rule out the possibility that conscious intent can override the unconscious forces. Psychodynamic clinicians must avoid colluding with patients who say they cannot change because they are a passive victim of unconscious forces beyond their control.

Developmental orientation

Regardless of which psychoanalytical theory seems to fit best with a particular patient, the dynamic psychiatrist always thinks in terms of developmental models. Patterns of relatedness established in childhood are repeated in adult relationships. Modern dynamic psychiatrists avoid the early psychoanalytical reductionism that attempted to link an adult psychopathological syndrome to a specific developmental arrest or fixation in childhood. Today, full account is taken of genetic contributions to personality and to psychiatric disorders. Environmental influences and genetic factors interact with one another reciprocally to shape the human being in health and illness. Still, the wisdom of the psychodynamic approach is that within each of us is a child yearning to complete some unfinished business from earlier in life.

Emphasis on the uniqueness of the individual

In much of descriptive psychiatry the major focus is on taxonomy—specifically: How do groups of patients fit together under one classification? In psychodynamic psychiatry, by contrast, there is great interest in how a particular patient is unique, in other words different from others. The subjective experience of the individual has been forged through an idiosyncratic narrative that is different from all other life stories and involves a specific interaction between genetic predisposition, intrapsychic factors, and environmental influence.

Transference

Intrinsic to the developmental model of mental organization is that adults are constantly repeating childhood patterns in the present. Transference is the best-known example of this phenomenon. The patient unconsciously experiences the doctor as a significant figure from the past and reacts to the doctor based on a set of unconscious attributions based on those past experiences. Transference has undergone considerable revision in more recent writings, so that today much more emphasis is placed on the clinician's contributions to the patient's transference. In other words, if a clinician is silent and remote, the patient may experience that clinician as disengaged and cold. While an internal template of past experiences with authority figures may correlate with that perception, we would also recognize that the clinician's real behaviour contributes to that precise transference paradigm. In that regard, a more contemporary view of transference would be that every treatment relationship is a mixture of new features based on real characteristics of the clinician and old experiences from the patient's past. Psychodynamic clinicians also recognize a bidimensional quality to transference: while one dimension involves repetition of the past, another dimension is seeking an experience with a new object to facilitate further emotional growth.

Countertransference

Central to the psychodynamic viewpoint is that the clinician and the patient bring their own separate subjectivities to an encounter, and mutually influence one another. Countertransference, in this respect, is the counterpart of transference. In other words, as Freud originally used the term, it referred to the analyst's attribution of certain qualities to the patient based on the analyst's past experiences with similar figures. This perspective, often referred to as the narrow view of countertransference, regarded the phenomenon as an obstacle to be removed because it interfered with the analyst's objectivity.

Subsequent contributors to the literature on countertransference[9,10] noted that countertransference with severely disturbed patients often involves an objective component. The patient behaves in such a provocative manner that virtually anyone would respond with a certain set of emotional reactions to that patient. This way of looking at countertransference is often regarded as the broad or totalistic view. Inherent in this perspective is that the clinician's reaction has much less to do with his or her own individual past than with the specific characteristics of the patient and that patient's capacity to induce strong reactions in others.

As the definition has continued to evolve, countertransference is now generally regarded as involving both the narrow and the broad characteristics. In other words, most theoretical perspectives view countertransference as entailing a jointly created reaction in the clinician that stems, in part, from contributions of the clinician's past and, in part, from feelings induced by the patient's behaviour.[11] In some cases the emphasis may be more on the contributions of the clinician than the patient, while in other cases the reverse may be true. This model also regards countertransference as something of a unique construction that varies depending on the two subjectivities involved (see Box 1). In this contemporary perspective, countertransference is both a source of valuable information about the patient's internal world and something of an interference with the treatment.

Resistance

In 1912 Freud[12] wrote, 'The resistance accompanies the treatment step by step. Every single association, every act of the person under treatment must reckon with the resistance and represents a compromise between the forces that are striving towards recovery and the opposing ones'. The patient's resistance defends the patient's illness from the clinician's attempt to treat it and change it. Resistance may be conscious, preconscious, or unconscious. It may take many forms, including not taking medication as prescribed, forgetting appointments with the psychiatrist, changing the subject in the middle of an appointment to something trivial, and discounting every insight the psychiatrist offers. The patient's characteristic defence mechanisms are often transformed into resistances in the treatment situation. If a patient sexualizes relationships as a way of avoiding abandonment,

Box 1

Changing views of countertransference

Narrow The original Freudian view connoting the analyst's transference to the patient: an obstacle to be removed through careful analysis of the clinician.

Broad or totalistic *All* the feelings experienced towards the patient, some of which are *induced* by the patient's behaviour.

Joint creation The contemporary perspective that emphasizes mutual contributions from the patient's behaviour toward the clinician and the clinician's past experiences with similar figures. This perspective emphasizes countertransference as a source of valuable information in addition to being an interference

that same patient may sexualize the treatment relationship to assure the therapist's continued interest and allay the fear that the therapist may stop the treatment. The dynamic psychiatrist knows that all progress will be accompanied by some degree of resistance, and the exploration of resistance is a major part of therapeutic work. Resistance is intimately related to transference because the patient often rebels against the doctor resulting from unconscious transference configurations that lead the patient to oppose the doctor's help.

The mind–brain interface

The psychodynamic psychiatrist eschews reductionism. Recognizing that mental life and psychiatric symptoms are both overdetermined and multiply caused, psychodynamic clinicians are always interested in the interface between the biological and the psychosocial. Psychodynamic psychiatry is not antibiological. The psychodynamic psychiatrist is the integrator *par excellence*. Avoiding Cartesian dualism, the mind is seen as the expression of the activity of the brain.[13] Subjective experience affects the brain just as mental phenomena arise from the brain. Every treatment intervention is seen as being biopsychosocial in nature. Medications have psychological effects. Psychotherapeutic interpretations affect the brain. Moreover, psychodynamic psychotherapy and medications may work synergistically to provide better outcomes for patients. For example, a patient with a bipolar disorder who is denying that he has an illness and refusing to take lithium may ultimately have better compliance with the medication if the clinician explores the meaning of his denial and his reluctance to consider himself as someone requiring treatment.

The comprehensive mind–brain strategy of the contemporary psychodynamic psychiatrist fits well with our growing knowledge of the interaction between genes and the environment. In an inspired series of experiments with the marine snail *Aplysia*, Kandel[14,15] has demonstrated that synaptic connections are strengthened and permanently altered through regulation of gene expression connected with learning from the environment. In *Aplysia* the number of synapses actually double or triple as a result of learning. Kandel has suggested that psychotherapy might make similar neuroanatomical changes in the synapses. He argues that just as representations of self and others are malleable, the brain itself is a dynamic and plastic structure. He postulates that psychotherapy is a form of learning that produces alteration of gene expression and thereby alters the strength of synaptic connections. While the template function or the sequence of the gene is not affected by environmental experience, the transcriptional function of the gene (namely the ability of a given gene to direct the manufacture of specific proteins) is highly regulated and responsive to environmental factors.

There is also evidence in mammalian species that the brain is plastic and influenced by environmental factors. Rats raised in a social environment that requires complex learning to survive have significantly greater numbers of synapses per neurone compared to rats raised in isolation.[16] Environmentally derived activity appears to drive the development of dendrites so that they conform to cognitive schemes for the construction of mental representations. The brain is not a blank screen, and the individual's genetic endowment will constrain the impact of environmental factors. Nevertheless, neural connections between the limbic system, the cortex, and the autonomic nervous system become connected into circuits in accordance with specific experiences of the developing organism. This developmental pattern may be summarized as follows: 'Neurons that fire together, wire together'.[17]

Primate research suggests that specific types of relatedness may serve to overcome genetic vulnerability. For example, Suomi[18] identified a cohort of infants comprising about 20 per cent of the Rhesus monkey colony in his laboratory who appeared to have an inborn vulnerability on a genetic basis. These infant monkeys reacted to brief separations with depressive reactions, increased cortisol and ACTH levels, and exaggerated noradrenaline turnover. He then placed these infants with unusually nurturant mothers within the monkey colony that he referred to as 'supermothers'. He observed that inborn vulnerability to separation anxiety and depressive reactions was overcome when the infants were allowed to have round-the-clock access to these extraordinarily nurturing mothers. Indeed, the interaction led these infant monkeys to become leaders in the social hierarchy. One can speculate that with a special type of nurturing relationship, the heightened sensitivity characteristic of these monkeys on a genetic basis was transformed into a highly adaptive means of relating to their peers in the social context.

Primate research is also serving to confirm certain psychoanalytical developmental notions. In a study of milder trauma,[19] infant monkeys were randomly assigned either to normal mothers or to mothers temporarily made anxious by an unpredictable feeding schedule. Those with anxious mothers became socially subordinate and showed diminished capacity for normal social interaction. However, these social changes did not appear until adolescence, confirming the psychoanalytical notion that disturbances at early phases of development can produce delayed psychopathological changes in adolescence and adulthood. These behavioural changes were accompanied by serotonergic and noradrenergic alterations, indicating that the mild trauma of having a mother made anxious about how she will obtain sufficient food also produces brain changes.

The research summarized here points to the dynamic interplay between genetic expression and the environment. Gene expression cannot be considered static. It is a dynamic phenomenon that interacts with and reacts to environmental experiences. Heritable characteristics of children actually shape their relationships with their parents and siblings.[20] In turn, the response of family members to the child affect the genetic expression. Hence genetic influences on some types of psychopathology may be dependent on the mediation of social processes. A child's genetic endowment will influence the way parents relate to a child, and the way the parents treat the child will then influence that child's developing brain. Biological and psychosocial processes are constantly intertwined, and neither is prior.

In many major psychiatric disorders, such as depression, genetic factors appear to influence whether a stressor produces an episode of illness.[21] From a psychodynamic perspective, the meaning of stressors must also be incorporated. Some stressors that may seem mild to one individual are overwhelming to another because of their idiosyncratic conscious or unconscious meaning. In addition, the presence of biologically generated symptoms in no way diminishes the importance of meaning. Pre-existing psychodynamic conflicts may attach themselves to biologically driven symptoms, and the symptoms then function as a vehicle for the expression of the conflicts.[22] Auditory hallucinations are generated by alterations in neurotransmitters in persons with schizophrenia, but the content of the hallucination often has specific meanings based on the patient's psychodynamic conflicts.

Hence a patient who is being told that he is a failure and should kill himself by a hallucinated voice may be tormented by a sense that his life is shattered by his illness and that he no longer has any purpose in living.

The impact of psychotherapy on the brain

In the past, psychotherapy was often regarded as the treatment for 'psychologically based' disorders, while pharmacotherapy was prescribed for disorders that were considered to be 'biologically based.' This distinction is rapidly becoming obsolete with advances in imaging techniques that demonstrate how psychotherapy alters the brain.[23,24]

Both behaviour therapy and fluoxetine appear to produce similar decreases in cerebral metabolic rates in the head of the right caudate nucleus when used in the treatment of obsessive–compulsive disorder.[25] The local cerebral metabolic rates for glucose can be measured using positron emission tomography methodology, and they are found to have the same response in reaction to the two different treatments.

A Finnish study[26] suggested that psychodynamic therapy may have a significant impact on the neurotransmitter serotonin. At the beginning of a 1-year psychotherapy process, single-photon emission CT (SPECT) imaging was undertaken with a 25-year-old man suffering from personality disorder and depression. Another man with similar problems also underwent imaging but did not receive psychotherapy or any other treatment.

Initial SPECT imaging showed that both patients had markedly reduced serotonin uptake in the medial prefrontal area and the thalamus compared with 10 healthy control subjects. After 1 year of psychodynamic therapy, repeat SPECT imaging showed that the patient who received the psychotherapy had normal serotonin uptake, while the control patient who did not receive psychotherapy continued to have markedly reduced serotonin uptake. Since the patient who received psychotherapy did not take medication in conjunction with the therapy, the findings suggest that the dynamic therapy itself may have normalized the serotonin metabolism. These preliminary data, as well as many other studies that do not use imaging techniques but nevertheless show results with psychotherapy that are comparable to medication, make a case for psychotherapy as an intervention that is just as 'medical' as pharmacotherapy. The brain responds to words as well as to chemicals.

Development of personality

Another key component of the psychodynamic approach is that the clinician treats the person and not just the illness. In practice, that perspective means taking the personality into account in every case. The interface of the biological and the psychosocial is particularly apparent in the area of personality. The psychobiological model of personality developed by Cloninger et al.[27] recognizes an equal contribution of biological and environmental factors (see Table 2). The four dimensions of temperament are roughly 50 to 60 per cent heritable independently of one another. They all manifest themselves early in life, and they involve preconceptual biases, habit formation, and perceptual memory. They include the following:

(1) novelty-seeking, characterized by active avoidance of frustration,

Table 2 Development of personality

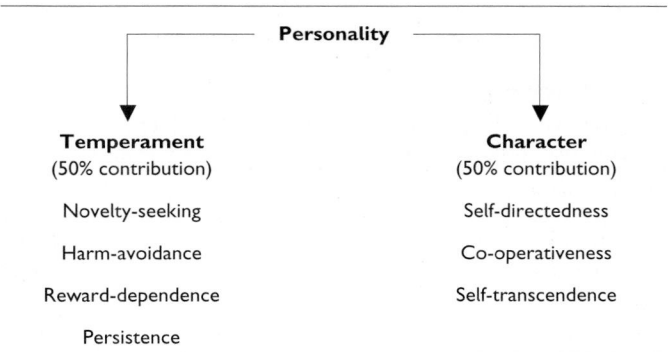

	Personality	
Temperament (50% contribution)		**Character** (50% contribution)
Novelty-seeking		Self-directedness
Harm-avoidance		Co-operativeness
Reward-dependence		Self-transcendence
Persistence		

Data from Cloninger *et al.*[27]

quick loss of temper, impulsive decision-making, frequent exploratory activity in response to novelty, and extravagance in the approach to cues and rewards;

(2) harm-avoidance, which involves pessimistic worry about the future, passive avoidant behaviour such as fear of uncertainty, shyness regarding strangers, and rapid fatiguability;

(3) reward-dependence, characterized by sentimentality, social attachment, and dependence on the approval of others;

(4) persistence, which refers to the capacity to persevere despite fatigue and frustration.

Certain of these temperament dimensions appear to correlate with specific types of personality disorders. The cluster A personalities in DSM-IV, for example, are strongly associated with low reward-dependence. Cluster B personality disorders have been shown to be high in novelty-seeking, while cluster C personality disorder patients tend to rate high in harm-avoidance.

The other component of personality in this model is character. While temperament is genetically based, character is shaped by environmental experiences, such as family relationships, peer relationships, trauma, and neglect. These dimensions appear to make up about 50 per cent of personality. There have been three dimensions of character identified that appear to mature in adulthood. These dimensions influence social and personal effectiveness by insight-learning about self-concepts. The three character dimensions are self-directedness, co-operativeness, and self-transcendence.

Self-directedness is a developmental process with several aspects:

(1) acceptance of self-responsibility for the choices one makes instead of externalizing or blaming others;

(2) identification of personally valued goals and purposes versus a lack of direction or goalessness;

(3) development of confidence and skills in problem-solving (resourcefulness versus apathy);

(4) self-acceptance versus self-striving;

(5) congruent second nature versus personality distrust.

The second dimension of character, co-operativeness, refers to the extent to which a person is agreeable, on the one hand, or hostile and self-centred, on the other. It, too, has several aspects associated with it:

(1) social acceptance versus intolerance;

(2) empathy versus social disinterest;

(3) helpfulness versus unhelpfulness;

(4) compassion versus vengefulness;

(5) pure-hearted principles versus those based on self-advantage.

Individuals who are uncooperative regard the world as adversarial and hostile, while those who are high in co-operativeness view themselves as involved in compassionate and mutually supportive social networks.

The third dimension of character, self-transcendence, also has several aspects:

(1) the capacity to lose or forget oneself versus self-conscious experience;

(2) identification with transpersonal values or goals versus self-differentiation;

(3) spiritual acceptance versus rational materialism.

Low self-directedness and low co-operativeness are associated with all categories of personality disorder in the DSM-IV system.[27] Self-transcendence, on the other hand, does not differentiate patients with personality disorders from those without personality disorders.

Self-directedness and co-operativeness reflect two fundamental tasks in personality development as defined by Blatt *et al.*[28]: the achievement of a stable, differential, realistic, and positive identity, and the establishment of enduring, mutually gratifying relationships with others. These two dimensions evolve in a dialectical and synergistic relationship to one another throughout the lifecycle. Patients with character pathology tend to divide into two groups: introjective types, who are primarily focused on self-definition; and anaclitic types, who are more concerned about relatedness.

The character dimensions readily lend themselves to typical psychodynamic constructs. The self-directedness dimension is closely linked to what are often called ego functions or self-structures. The dimension of co-operativeness is a direct measure of a person's characteristic pattern of internal object relations as they are externalized in relationships with others. In one's assessment of a patient's personality, the transference–countertransference dimensions of the clinical interaction provide a privileged glimpse of the typical patterns of relatedness that cause difficulties in the patient's outside relationships.[29] The patient is involved in an ongoing attempt to actualize certain patterns of relatedness that reflect various wishes in the patient's unconscious. Through the patient's behaviour, he or she subtly tries to impose on the clinician a certain way of responding and experiencing.[30]

An individual internalizes a self-representation in interaction with an object representation connected by an affect through a series of repetitive interactions in childhood. This pattern ultimately leads to an internalized set of self- and object representations in interaction with one another. The adult individual repeats these patterns again and again as an effort to fulfil an unconscious wish. Even abusive or painful relationships involving a 'bad' or tormenting object may be wished for because of the safety and affirmation such relationships provide. In other words, a child who has been abused has internalized a highly conflictual abusive relationship as a predictable and familiar pattern. Having an abusive object may be preferable to having no object at all or being abandoned. Many patients with histories of an abusive childhood become convinced that the only way to remain connected to a significant person is to maintain an abuser–victim relationship.

The repetitive interactions seen in patients with personality disorder may reflect actual relationships with real objects in the past, but they may also involve wished-for relationships, such as those often seen in patients with childhood trauma who seek a rescuer. Clinicians who are influenced by the patient's interpersonal pressure to respond in a particular way may unconsciously accept the role in which they have been cast. When this phenomenon occurs, it is often referred to as projective identification.[11] In other words, the patient may 'nudge' the therapist into assuming the role of an abuser in response to the patient's 'victim' role, and the therapist may feel countertransference hate or anger and begin to make sarcastic or demeaning comments to the patient.

In addition to this pattern of object relations, the other major component of character, from a psychodynamic perspective, is the particular constellation of defence mechanisms that characterizes the individual patient.[31] While defences were traditionally regarded as intrapsychic mechanisms designed to prevent awareness of unconscious aggressive or sexual wishes, the current understanding of defence mechanisms has been expanded far beyond Freud's dual-drive theory. We now understand that defences also preserve a sense of self-esteem in the face of narcissistic vulnerability, assure safety when one feels dangerously threatened by abandonment, and serve to insulate one from external dangers through, for example, denial or minimization.

Different personality types or disorders use characteristic sets of defence mechanisms. For example, the paranoid personality may typically use projection as a way of disavowing unacknowledged feelings and attributing them to others. Patients with obsessive–compulsive personality disorder may use defensive operations such as isolation of affect, intellectualization, and reaction formation to control affective states that are highly threatening. In the relationship with the clinician, as noted previously, these defences will manifest themselves as resistances. Hence, if a patient with an obsessive–compulsive personality disorder uses intellectualization as a defence against painful affects, when the patient comes to treatment, intellectualization will be used as a resistance to avoid getting at feelings in psychotherapy.

Applications of psychodynamic thinking to diagnosis and treatment

Dynamic pharmacotherapy

The commonly used psychodynamic constructs, such as therapeutic alliance, transference, countertransference, and resistance apply to all modalities of psychiatric treatment, even though their usage is generally associated with psychodynamic psychotherapy. In a study of the relationship between the therapeutic alliance and the outcome of 250 depressed outpatients in the National Institute of Mental Health Treatment of Depression Study,[32] the therapeutic alliance was found to be of extraordinary importance. The patients had been randomly assigned to one of four conditions: brief interpersonal therapy, brief cognitive–behavioural therapy, imipramine plus clinical management, or placebo plus clinical management. The researchers found that the therapeutic alliance was just as important for drug therapy as for psychotherapy. In all four treatment cells, the therapeutic alliance counted for more of the variance of treatment outcome than the treatment method itself! This was the first empirical study to show the importance of the therapeutic alliance in psychotherapy, pharmacotherapy, and placebo outcome.

Non-compliance is one of the most challenging problems facing psychiatric practitioners. After 12 weeks of antidepressant prescription, only 40 per cent of patients were complying with the medication as prescribed.[33] In patients with bipolar illness, up to 60 per cent of patients may be non-compliant with lithium carbonate.[34] In one study of schizophrenia, Weiden et al.[35] found that 74 per cent of schizophrenic outpatients became non-compliant with their neuroleptic regimen within 2 years of discharge from the hospital. Overall, only about one-third of patients comply adequately with medications, one-third comply somewhat, and one-third are non-compliant.[36]

Many factors go into compliance. Although many patients blame side-effects, they often unconsciously undermine the treatment plan. The patient may have a negative transference to the prescribing clinician related to attitudes toward parents and other authority figures that lead the patient to rebel and defy the doctor's orders. Some clinicians may have countertransference reactions to specific patients that lead them to prescribe in a highly authoritarian manner or a tentative and ambivalent manner, giving unconscious messages to the patient that reflect the doctor's attitude about the medication. Patients who feel the doctor is bullying them to take the medication may not comply. Similarly, patients who sense their doctor is ambivalent about the value of the medication may also choose not to fill the prescription.

Unconscious resistance is frequently a major factor in non-compliance. Medications may have idiosyncratic meanings to patients based on unconscious identifications with family members who have taken the same medication, views of psychiatric illness as moral weakness, or fears about the effects of the medication. In Jamison's[37] autobiographical account of her struggles with bipolar illness, she made a strong argument for the combination of psychotherapy and medication in the treatment of bipolar illness. Working psychotherapeutically with her psychiatrist, she came to realize that one of her reasons for non-compliance with lithium was a secret fear that it might not work, leaving her with a sense of despair associated with an untreatable illness.

Multiple-treater settings

In inpatient units and partial hospital settings, psychodynamic concepts are of considerable value in understanding the patient's psychopathology as it unfolds in a group setting. Patients re-create their internal object relations in the inpatient or partial hospital milieu.[38] The conflicts that occur in their family context will re-emerge in their relationships with hospital staff members. Through projective identification the patient subtly pressures various staff members to play the roles that are in keeping with the patient's internal world. Hence a patient who has been physically and/or sexually abused by a parent will behave in such a way toward a certain nurse, for example, that the nurse begins to feel abusive toward the patient. The same patient may treat another nurse as an idealized rescuer figure, eliciting loving and protective feelings from that nurse. This form of splitting[38] may create extraordinary conflicts between staff members over the best treatment approach to the patient. Therefore failure to attend to the transference–countertransference dimensions of the milieu treatment may lead to a total disruption of the staff members' capacity to be effective with certain patients.

Moreover, individual patients often act out covert staff conflicts.[39]

Psychodynamically informed hospital treatment may help to identify these conflicts and allow staff to process them in such a way that the patients no longer need to enact them. When covert conflicts between staff members become overt and open to discussion, the patient's disruptive behaviour often settles down.[39] This observation reflects how the dynamics of the patient group and staff group often parallel each other. The psychodynamic clinician also understands that individuals behave differently in groups than they do alone or in a one-to-one context. Powerful group forces, such as scapegoating, can be recognized and processed so they do not become destructive to treatment. Similarly, the patient's recurrent problems in groups can be diagnosed, in part, by a careful study of the transference and countertransference responses.

Two-person context of treatment

One of the major shifts in psychodynamic thinking in recent years has been a greater acknowledgement of the influence of the clinician's perspective on the observations about the patient. Postmodern contributions from intersubjectivity and social constructivism have challenged the view that the clinician assesses the patient from a detached and objective frame of reference. Fundamental to this perspective is that clinicians can never transcend their irreducible subjectivity.[40] The psychiatrist in this context can never fully know how his or her subjectivity is influencing the diagnostic assessment or the treatment process. Countertransference is viewed as both unconscious and continuous, so that a therapist cannot possibly be capable of keeping up with every emotional reaction to the patient.[41]

This two-person model of the treatment situation has contributed to the demise of the classical psychoanalytical view of the therapist or analyst as a blank screen or a dispassionate observer. The influence of the clinician's biases and unconscious feelings toward the patient may have far-reaching implications for a variety of situations in psychiatry. Frustration about a patient's non-responsiveness to treatment, for example, can lead a clinician to recommend electroconvulsive therapy as a reaction to despair, rather than as a result of systematic decision trees or algorithms about refractory depression. Even in the case of physician-assisted suicide, countertransference may play a major, though hidden, role.[42] Within this context the patient's wish to die may stem from a self-concept as worthless and a burden to others that is, in part, a reflection of what the physician brings to the encounter. Similarly, the doctor's death-anxiety might underlie an omnipotent need to triumph over death through the prescription of physician-assisted suicide that strives to preserve an illusion of control and mastery. In the worst scenario, a clinician's intense countertransference hate toward a patient may lead to a wish to kill that is transposed into a recommendation for physician-assisted suicide.

Psychodynamic approaches to specific disorders

A psychodynamic approach is relevant to the treatment of the vast majority of psychiatric disorders encountered in clinical practice. Depending on the nature of the illness, the setting in which the illness is treated, and the psychological mindedness of the patient, psychodynamic strategies may be the major emphasis in the treatment plan

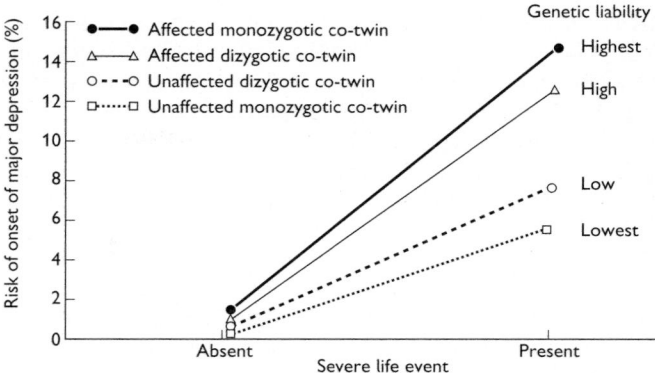

Fig. 1 Risk of onset of major depression per person-month as a function of genetic liability and the presence or absence of a severe stressful life event in that month among 2060 female twins. (Data from Kendler et al.[21])

or a relatively minor contribution. Space considerations preclude a comprehensive discussion of psychodynamic approaches to all the major disorders, but a sampling of three major entities may provide a general guide to the approach to other disorders.

Major depression

Few disorders illustrate the interaction between genetics and environment more clearly than major depression. In Kendler's study of twins[21] he followed 2164 members of female–female twin pairs. Recent stressful events were the single most powerful risk factor for an episode of major depression. Genetic factors were substantial, but not overwhelming. He followed this cohort of subjects for 17.3 months. During that time 14 per cent of them had major depressive episodes. He found that the four most powerful predictors of a major depression in the month of the occurrence were death of a close relative, serious marital problems, assault, and divorce or separation within a marriage. Genetic factors appeared to alter the sensitivity of individuals to the depression-inducing effect of stressful life events (Fig. 1). In other words, those with the highest genetic risk had only a 1.1 per cent probability of having a depressive episode without a life stressor, but the risk rose to 14.6 per cent if they were exposed to a severe life event. On the other hand, those subjects with the lowest genetic risk had only a 0.5 per cent probability of depression onset per month if they were unexposed to a life stressor. The probability of a depression episode increased to 6.2 per cent with a stressor.

As noted earlier, the meaning of the stressor to the individual patient has a great deal to do with whether or not a depressive episode results. Research has shown that a stressor is more likely to produce depression if its content matches the area of the patient's self-definition.[43] Events that are interpreted to mean depletion of self-worth and the expectation of inability to replenish needed supplies are more likely to cause depression. A relatively minor insult to one's self-esteem, then, can result in a major depressive episode because it is attached to a more profound sense of worthlessness.

In the treatment of major depression, brief dynamic therapy has been shown to be as effective as cognitive–behavioural therapy.[44] However, even when the primary treatment is antidepressant medication, a dynamic approach to the pharmacotherapy can be very helpful, particularly because some depressed patients feel they do not deserve to get better because they have 'sinned'. Hence these compliance problems can be explored dynamically. Moreover, an examination of the stressors and their meaning may be critical as part of an ongoing maintenance approach to prevent future episodes.

A subgroup of depressed patients requires more extended and intensive psychodynamic therapy. In a reanalysis of the NIMH Treatment of Depression Collaborative Research Program data, Blatt *et al.*[45] found that perfectionism had consistently negative relationships with all outcome measures in all four treatment conditions. They noted that the profile of highly perfectionistic depressed patients is one associated with a high risk of suicide, and the investigators recognized that a substantial period of time is required to alter deeply entrenched, negative mental representations of self and others. Uncontrolled studies have suggested that patients fitting this profile may improve with extended psychodynamic therapy.[28]

Anxiety disorders

The atheoretical categorizations of anxiety disorders in the official nomenclature and the associated research on the biological underpinnings of anxiety tend to categorize anxiety as only an illness, rather than an overdetermined symptom of unconscious conflict.[1] In this conceptual framework, anxiety is to be eliminated, or at the very least, minimized primarily through pharmacotherapeutic interventions. An important psychodynamic perspective that is in danger of disappearing is that anxiety has value as a signal of internal conflict and distress that may require reflection and understanding.

Eradication of all anxiety is not necessarily desirable. In the Menninger Foundation Psychotherapy Research Project, 18 out of 35 patients showed increased anxiety at the termination of psychoanalysis or long-term psychoanalytical psychotherapy, even though 13 of these 18 cases were judged by independent raters to have undergone substantial improvement.[46,47]

The findings in this study were consistent with the clinical observation that an increase in anxiety tolerance, defined as the capacity to experience anxiety without having to discharge it, may be one of the results of long-term psychoanalytical psychotherapy or psychoanalysis, reflecting an expansion of the ego's capacity to deal with anxiety. The investigators differentiated anxiety that is used as a signal from primary or disorganizing anxiety, such as that associated with panic disorder. Many of the patients with good outcomes in this follow-up study had greatly enhanced their capacity to use ideational activity more effectively in the service of understanding anxiety.

The psychodynamic clinician also wants to understand the developmental correlates of the anxiety as a way of gaining a greater grasp of what the patient fears. Based on psychoanalytical theory, a developmental hierarchy of anxiety can be constructed (Table 3).

This developmental hierarchy can be used to understand the danger situations implied by the patient's anxiety. The most primitive form of anxiety involves a fear of disintegrating or falling apart and was called by Kohut[48] disintegration anxiety. One can also feel that he or she will disintegrate through merger or fusion with another person. Persecutory anxiety is a paranoid fear based on the conviction that malevolent forces from outside will invade and destroy the patient from within. Separation anxiety involves a fear of being abandoned and losing a significant object. This is related to the notion of Kleinian depressive anxiety, where the individual fears that his or her aggression will destroy the loved object.

Table 3 A developmental hierarchy of anxiety

| Superego anxiety |
| Castration anxiety |
| Fear of loss of love |
| Fear of loss of the object (separation anxiety) |
| Persecutory anxiety |
| Disintegration anxiety |

Data from Gabbard.[1]

Moving up the developmental ladder, fear of the loss of love is more associated with neurotically organized individuals, and is characterized by a fear that one must behave in a specific manner because the love and attention of another is tenuously balanced. Castration anxiety is connected to the Oedipal fear that a powerful same-sex parent will respond with violent attack if the individual is too competitive or in a rivalrous situation for the opposite-sex parent. Finally, superego anxiety involves concern that one will disappoint one's own internal ideals and values, that stem from the internalization of parental values.

Medication and dynamic psychotherapy may work synergistically in some anxiety disorders. In one randomized controlled investigation involving the treatment of panic disorder, patients were assigned to treatment with either clomipramine for 9 months or clomipramine for 9 months combined with 15 weekly sessions of brief dynamic therapy.[49] While all patients in both groups were free of panic attacks within 20 weeks of the beginning of treatment, the relapse rate was significantly higher in the group that received only clomipramine when the pharmacotherapy was terminated. The investigators concluded that brief dynamic therapy may reduce the psychosocial vulnerability associated with panic disorder.

Borderline personality disorder

The psychobiological model of personality proposed by Cloninger *et al.*[27] suggests a treatment strategy that combines medication and psychotherapy. Certain medications appear to improve target symptoms associated with temperament, such as impulsivity and affective lability, while psychotherapy may address the character problems such as self-directedness and co-operativeness. At least three studies using a double-blind placebo-controlled design have demonstrated that impulsivity and anger in patients with borderline personality disorder are significantly improved with the use of serotonin-selective reuptake inhibitors.[50–52] These agents do not cure borderline personality disorder, but they do facilitate the psychotherapy process. When the affect and the impulsivity is toned down by the use of medication, patients often find it easier to reflect on internal states and process what is happening between them and others.

The improvement of temperament through the use of medications is only a partial treatment strategy because, as previously noted, the character variables determine whether or not an individual has a personality disorder. Psychodynamic therapy may address the chaotic pattern of object relations and the deficiencies in self-esteem and self-cohesiveness. Although no systematic study has been conducted with the combined use of dynamic psychotherapy and medication, one follow-along study using a pre–post design with twice-weekly dynamic therapy appeared to produce substantial and durable changes after 12 months of treatment.[53] While the conceptual model of temperament and character provides a basis for the combination of medication and psychotherapy, further research is necessary to demonstrate the efficacy of the two-pronged approach.

Future directions

The evidence regarding the impact of psychotherapy on the brain opens up new lines of investigation to enhance our understanding of psychopathology and treatment. These include the following:

(1) the mechanisms of action of psychotherapy;

(2) the interrelationships between the mechanisms of action of psychotherapy and medication;

(3) a clearer understanding of pathogenesis itself and the malleability of some components of the pathogenetic mechanisms of major psychiatric disorder.

Research is sorely needed on psychodynamic treatments because there is only a modest empirical base for psychodynamic therapy. Many more studies are needed, especially those with a randomized controlled design targeted at specific disorders. Studies investigating extended dynamic therapy of a year or more are needed to demonstrate which patients benefit from the additional investment of time and money. In the current climate of cost containment, practitioners of psychodynamic therapy must take cost-effectiveness into account.

The optimal treatment for many psychiatric patients involves a combination of medication and psychotherapy, but research support for this view is also rather modest. Controlled studies of combined treatment versus single modalities are needed for personality disorders and anxiety disorders. In addition, the role of psychodynamic thinking in compliance problems needs rigorous investigation.

In the meantime, the psychodynamic model continues to enrich the patient's understanding and the psychiatrist's practice. The time-honoured principles elaborated here serve as windows into the murky recesses of the unconscious and illuminate human motivation. They also provide the clinician with a 'second sight' that helps make sense out of bewildering and complex clinical situations.

References

1. Gabbard, G.O. (1994). *Psychodynamic psychiatry in clinical practice: the DSM-IV edition*. American Psychiatric Press, Washington, DC.

2. Squire, L.R. (1987). *Memory and brain*. Oxford University Press, NY.

3. Westen, D. The scientific status of unconscious processes: is Freud really dead? *Journal of the American Psychoanalytic Association*, in press.

4. Bechara, A., Tranel, D., Damasio, H., Adolphs, R., Rockland, C., and Damasio, A. (1995). Double association of conditioning and declarative knowledge relative to the amygdala and hippocampus in humans. *Science*, **269**, 1115–18.

5. Bowers, J.S. and Schachter, D.L. (1990). Implicit memory and test awareness. *Journal of Experimental Psychology: Learning, Memory, and Cognition*, **16**, 404–16.

6. Heinemann, L.G. and Emrich, H. (1971). Alpha activity during inhibitory brain processes. *Psychophysiology*, **7**, 442–50.

7. Shevrin, H., Bond, J., Brakel, L.A., Hertel, R.K., and Williams, W.J. (1996). *Conscious and unconscious processes: psychodynamic, cognitive, and neurophysiological convergences*. Guilford Press, New York.

8. Sherwood, M. (1969). *The logic of explanation in psychoanalysis*. Academic Press, New York.

9. Winnicott, D.W. (1949). Hate in the countertransference. *International Journal of Psycho-Analysis*, **30**, 69–74.

10. Kernberg. O.F. (1965). Notes on countertransference. *Journal of the American Psychoanalytic Association*, **13**, 38–56.

11. Gabbard, G.O. (1995). Countertransference: the emerging common ground. *International Journal of Psycho-Analysis*, **76**, 475–85.

12. Freud, S. (1912). The dynamics of transference. In the *Standard edition of the complete works of Sigmund Freud*, Vol. 12 (ed. J. Strachey), pp. 97–108. Hogarth Press, London, 1958.

13. Andreasen, N.C. (1997). Linking mind and brain in the study of mental illness: a project for a scientific psychopathology. *Science*, **275**, 1587–93.

14. Kandel, E.R. (1983). From metapsychology to molecular biology: explorations into the nature of anxiety. *American Journal of Psychiatry*, **140**, 1277–93.

15. Kandel, E.R. (1998). A new intellectual framework for psychiatry. *American Journal of Psychiatry*, **155**, 457–69.

16. Greenough, W.T., Black, J.E., and Wallace, C.S. (1987). Experience and brain development. *Child Development*, **58**, 539–59.

17. Schatz, C.J. (1992). The developing brain. *Scientific American*, **267**, 60–7.

18. Suomi, S.J. (1991). Early stress and adult emotional reactivity in rhesus monkeys. In *Childhood environmental and adult disease: Symposium 156* (ed. CIBA Foundation Symposium Staff), pp. 171–88. Wiley, Chichester.

19. Rosenblum, L.A. and Anderson, M.W. (1994). Influences of environmental demand on maternal behavior and infant development. *Acta Paediatrica Supplement*, **397**, 57–63.

20. Reiss, D., Plomin, R., and Hetherington, E.M. (1991). Genetics and psychiatry: an unheralded window on the environment. *American Journal of Psychiatry*, **148**, 283–91.

21. Kendler, K.S., Kessler, R.C., Walters, E.E., *et al.* (1995). Stressful life events, genetic liability, and onset of an episode of major depression in women. *American Journal of Psychiatry*, **152**, 833–42.

22. Gabbard, G.O. (1992). Psychodynamic psychiatry in the decade of the brain. *American Journal of Psychiatry*, **149**, 991–8.

23. Gabbard, G.O. (1994). Mind and brain in psychiatric treatment. *Bulletin of the Menninger Clinic*, **58**, 427–46.

24. Gabbard, G.O. and Goodwin, F. (1996). Clinical psychiatry in transition: integrating biological and psychosocial perspectives. In *Review of psychiatry*, Vol. 15 (ed. L.J. Dickstein, M.B. Riba, and J.M. Oldham), pp. 527–48. American Psychiatric Press, Washington, DC.

25. Baxter, L.R., Schwartz, J.M., Bergman, K.S., *et al.* (1992). Caudate glucose metabolic rate changes with both drug and behavior therapy for obsessive–compulsive disorder. *Archives of General Psychiatry*, **49**, 681–9.

26. Viinamäki, H., Kuikka, J., Tiihonen, J., and Lehtonen, J.L. (1998). Change in monoamine transporter density related to clinical recovery: a case–control study. *Nordic Journal of Psychiatry*, **52**, 39–44.

27. Cloninger, C.R., Svrakic, D.M., and Pryzbeck, T.R. (1993). A psychobiological model of temperament and character. *Archives of General Psychiatry*, **50**, 975–90.

28. Blatt, S.J., Ford, R.Q., Berman, W.H. Jr, *et al.* (1994). *Therapeutic change: an object relations perspective*. Plenum Press, New York.

29. Gabbard, G.O. (1997). Finding the 'person' in personality disorders. *American Journal of Psychiatry*, **154**, 891–3.

30. Sandler, J. (1981). Character traits and object relationships. *Psychoanalytic Quarterly*, **50**, 694–708.

31. Gabbard, G.O. (1999). Psychoanalysis and psychoanalytic therapy. In *The DSM-IV personality disorders* (ed. W.J. Livesley). Guilford Press, New York.

32. Krupnick, J.L., Sotsky, S.M., Simmens, S., *et al.* (1996). The role of the therapeutic alliance in psychotherapy and pharmacotherapy outcome: findings in the National Institute of Mental Health Treatment of Depression Collaborative Research Program. *Journal of Consulting and Clinical Psychology*, **64**, 532–9.

33. Myers, E.D. and Branthwaite, A. (1992). Outpatient compliance with antidepressant medication. *British Journal of Psychiatry*, **160**, 83–6.

34. Keck, P.E., McElroy, S.L., Strakowski, S.M., *et al.* (1996). Factors associated with pharmacologic noncompliance in patient with mania. *Journal of Clinical Psychiatry*, **57**, 292–7.

35. Weiden, P.J., Dixon, L., Frances, A., *et al.* (1991). Neuroleptic noncompliance in schizophrenia. In *Schizophrenia research*. Vol 1. *Advances in neuropsychiatry and psychopharmacology* (ed. C.A. Tamminga and C.S. Schulz), pp. 285–96. Raven Press, New York.

36. Wright, E.C. (1993). Noncompliance—or how many aunts has Matilda? *Lancet*, **342**, 909–12.

37. Jamison, K.R. (1995). *An unquiet mind*. Vintage Books, New York.

38. Gabbard, G.O. (1989). Splitting in hospital treatment. *American Journal of Psychiatry*, **146**, 444–51.

39. Stanton, A. and Schwartz, M. (1954). Pathological excitement and hidden staff disagreement. In *The mental hospital*, pp. 342–65. Basic Books, New York.

40. Renik, O. (1993). Analytic interaction: conceptualizing technique in light of the analyst's irreducible subjectivity. *Psychoanalytic Quarterly*, **62**, 553–71.

41. Hoffman, I.Z. (1998). *Ritual and spontaneity in the psychoanalytic process: the dialectical constructivist view*. Analytic Press, Hillsdale, NJ.

42. Varghese, F.T. and Kelly, B. (1999). Countertransference and assisted suicide. In *Review of psychiatry* (ed. J. Oldham and M. Riba). Vol. 18, *Countertransference in psychiatric treatment* (ed. G. Gabbard), pp. 85–118. American Psychiatric Press, Washington, DC.

43. Hammen, C., Marks, T., Mayol, A., *et al.* (1985). Depressive self-schemas, life stress, and vulnerability to depression. *Journal of Abnormal Psychology*, **94**, 308–19.

44. Gallagher-Thompson, D. and Steffen, A.M. (1994). Comparative effects of cognitive-behavioral and brief psychodynamic therapies for depressed family caregivers. *Journal of Consulting and Clinical Psychology*, **62**, 543–9.

45. Blatt, S.J., Quinlan, D.M., Pilkonis, P.A., and Shae, M.T. (1995). Impact of perfectionism and need for approval on the brief treatment of depression: the National Institute of Mental Health Treatment of Depression Collaborative Research Program revisited. *Journal of Consulting and Clinical Psychology*, **63**, 125–32.

46. Siegel, R.S. and Rosen, I.C. (1962). Character style and anxiety tolerance: a study of intrapsychic change. In *Research in psychotherapy*, Vol. 2 (ed. H. Strupp and L. Luborsky), pp. 206–17. French-Bray, Baltimore, MD.

47. Appelbaum, S.A. (1997). *The anatomy of change: a Menninger report on testing the effects of psychotherapy*. Plenum Press, New York.

48. Kohut, H. (1977). *The restoration of the self*. International Universities Press, New York.

49. Wiborg, I.M. and Dahl, A.A. (1996). Does brief dynamic psychotherapy reduce the relapse rate of panic disorder? *Archives of General Psychiatry*, **53**, 689–94.

50. Coccaro, E.F. and Kavoussi, R.J. (1997). Fluoxetine and impulsive aggressive behavior in personality disordered subjects. *Archives of General Psychiatry*, **54**, 1081–8.

51. Markovitz, P. (1995). Pharmacotherapy of impulsivity, aggression, and related disorders. In *Impulsivity and aggression* (ed. E. Hollander and D.J. Stein), pp. 263–87. Wiley, New York.

52. Salzman, C., Wolfson, A.N., Schatzberg, A., *et al.* (1995). Effect of fluoxetine on anger in symptomatic volunteers with borderline personality disorder. *Journal of Clinical Psychopharmacology*, **15**, 23–9.

53. Stevenson, J. and Meares, R. (1992). An outcome study of psychotherapy for patients with borderline personality disorder. *American Journal of Psychiatry*, **149**, 358–62.

4

Clinical syndromes of adult psychiatry

4.1 Delirium, dementia, and amnesic and other cognitive disorders

4.1.1 Introduction to cognitive disorders

Demetrio Barcia

Introduction

The three terms delirium, dementia, and amnesic syndrome appear together in the classification manuals because they share a common, but not exclusive, organic aetiology. However, these conditions have little in common from a historical, clinical, and psychopathological perspective. Because the notion of 'organicity' is imprecise, it would perhaps be preferable to use Schneider's term 'corporeally based manifestations' (*körperlich begründbaren Psychosen*). In this chapter, delirium, dementia, and the amnesic syndrome will be discussed separately from historical and psychopathological perspectives.

Delirium

Georget introduced the term *stupidité* (stupor) to replace Esquirol's term acute dementia to indicate a state in which a person appears to have no ideas or cannot express them. The term was adopted by German as well as French authors. Baillarger[1] suggested that patients with this syndrome were melancholic, and the term 'melancholy with stupor' became widely accepted despite problems with differential diagnoses. According to Griesinger:[2]

> Melancholy with stupor has not only a great theoretical importance due to the strongly marked psychic symptoms and characteristic brain injuries existing in some cases, but also due to the fact that they are easily and frequently mixed up with dementia, which can lead to great errors in relation to the prognosis and treatment; for this they have also a great practical interest.

This controversy resembles that surrounding the term 'depressive pseudodementia' today. Other authors, while accepting that melancholy with stupor existed, thought that most cases of stupor were independent.

Chaslin[3] included *stupidité* under the term mental confusion. Both the concept and many of the clinical features correspond to Bon-

hoeffer's exogenous reaction type (*die exogenen Reaktionstypus*),[4] which he classified into three groups:

(1) characteristic forms, which comprised amentia, delirium, twilight states, and hallucinosis;

(2) homonymous forms, i.e those with manifestations similar to schizophrenia, mania, and depression;

(3) a residual group including hyperaesthetic, sensory, or neurastheniform disorders together with Korsakoff's syndrome.

Two properties are essential: the manifestations lack specificity, and they share a disturbance of consciousness (*Bewusstsein*). Kraepelin[5] attempted to study organic or exogenous psychoses using the medical aetiological model, believing that each aetiology corresponded to a specific aetiopathogenic mechanism and a characteristic symptomatology. This view was contradicted by Bonhoeffer,[4] who pointed out that in the characteristic forms each aetiology could give rise to any syndrome, and each syndrome could be caused by any aetiological factor.

Characteristic forms are characterized by a disorder of the consciousness; amentia, delirium, and twilight states are due to a decrease of consciousness, whereas hallucinosis is due to an increased clarity of consciousness.[6]

All Bonhoeffer's characteristic forms are included in the current classifications under the term delirium, but this is an error. Firstly, the disturbance of consciousness is not sufficiently emphasized and, secondly, syndromes which should be separated because of their different psychopathological characteristics appear together. In amentia, there is little decrease in consciousness; indeed, it may even go unnoticed although it is always present. Amentia is characterized by incoherent thought and severe motor disorder, whereas delirium is characterized by a more severe disturbance of consciousness with oneirism, hallucinations, and delusions (frequently occupational). In a twilight state, the level of consiousness is intense but fluctuating. It may occur with a decrease of the 'awake' consciousness (*Bewustsein*), but without any alteration in 'reflexive' consciousness' (Ey's *conscience de soi*[7]). Finally, in hallucinosis increased clarity of consciousness is accompanied by anxiety, auditory hallucinations, and a tendency to paranoid ideas.

Some consider that all four syndromes described by Bonhoeffer should be mantained mainly to avoid diagnostic errors. Amentia, with little change of consciousness, is sometimes mistaken for schizophrenia or, in older people, dementia. The patient is perplexed, makes false identification, and is depersonalized. These manifestations of amentia may also be present in acute endogenous disorders such as the cycloid psychoses. Sometimes these subconfusional manifestations are chronic, with a long evolution when it is easy to mistake them with dementia. The possibility that enhanced amentia in the old may be of psychogenic origin (psychogenic unresponsiveness) has to keep in mind.

Dementia

The term 'dementia' refers to patients with chronic brain damage and severe deterioration of intellectual processes. Frequently, psychotic symptoms (hallucinations and delusions) and affective symptoms are also present. This syndrome has a long history; in antiquity it had a meaning similar to that understood today when used in a medical context (Celsus, 150 BC). The term 'dementia' was recognized by Pinel,[8] and Esquirol[9] distinguished acute dementia (later called mental confusion) and chronic dementia. Georget[10] subdivided the latter into primary dementias, so called because the intellectual disorder appeared first, and secondary dementias, in which other mental manifestations (e.g. mania and *dementia praecox*) preceded the intellectual disorder.

There are two periods in the subsequent history of dementia. In the first and longest, from the beginning of psychiatry to the 1970s, dementia was considered as an illness. Since then, dementia has been considered to be a syndrome.

The concept of dementia as an illness was based on an anatomical and clinical approach. Three illnesses were characterized:

(1) general paresis of the insane, identified by Bayle[11] and later attributed to syphilis;[12]

(2) vascular dementias as described by Klippel,[13] i.e. dementias that were exclusively vascular in origin;

(3) parenchymatous dementias.

In 1898 precise knowledge of the structure of the brain became available using the silver impregnation technique developed by Ramón y Cajal. When analysing the dementias, Alzheimer[14] pointed out that not all are due to a vascular aetiology, and in 1911 he described parenchymatous dementias with neurofibrillar degeneration and senile plaques.[15] This finding was soon confirmed by other authors. Kraepelin[5] called this condition senile dementia, and included in it Kahlbaum's presbyophrenia as a form of dementia arising at an earlier age.

In 1906 Alzheimer[16] described a 52-year-old female patient who presented a severe dementia, with neurological symptoms, aphasia, apraxia, and agnosia, initiated with delusions of jealousy, and whose brain showed the histopathology described in senile dementia. He published this case without being able to ascribe a cause. Similar observations were reported by other authors between 1908 and 1910.[17–19] Kraepelin[5] called the condition the presenile dementia of Alzheimer.

Between 1892 and 1904 Pick carried studied lesions in the brains of aphasic patients and published several cases including two of persons aged over 50 with clinical features similar to the presenile dementia of Alzheimer but without its characteristic lesions. Subsequently, Ornari and Spatz[20] coined the term presenile dementia of Pick and described the histopathological characteristics of the disorder and the topography of the lesions. They suggested a hereditary-degenerative aetiology.

Some other forms were subsequently added to the four main

Table 1 Pathological conditions associated with Alzheimer's anatomopathological types

Primary degenerative polioencephalitis of Alzheimer type
Alzheimer's disease (presenile and of late onset)
Alzheimer-like senile dementia
Alzheimer-like juvenile dementia

Secondary Alzheimer's disease
Down syndrome and possibly other forms of mental retardation
Post-traumatic syndromes (e.g. dementia pugilistica)
Endocrine dysfunction

Atypical Alzheimer's disease (i.e. congophilic angiopathy)

Alzheimer neuropathy
Normal senescence
Senilis simplex and presbyophrenic dementia
Postencephalic Parkinson syndrome
Guam–Parkinson complex dementia
Chronic sclerosing panencephalitis
Other rare organic encephalopathies

dementing illnesses, including the spastic pseudosclerosis described by Creutzfeldt and Jakob in 1927. In the 20 years following the Second World War research raised new questions, including the importance and frequency of mixed vascular and parenchymatous forms,[21] the correlation between the amount of anatomical damage and the seriousness of the dementia,[22] and the identification of new clinical manifestations such as 'mild dysfunction of the memory'.[23] In general, however, the dementias were still thought of as illnesses, each with specific histopathological findings.

Changes in the concept of dementia

In the 1950s two important events occurred which led to new approaches to the concept of dementia.

1. Forms intermediate between senile dementia and the presenile dementia of Alzheimer were identified. Sjögren[24] described cases of dementia appearing at older ages than those reported for the presenile dementia of Alzheimer, without extrapyramidal signs, strokes, or signs of aphasia, agnosia, and apraxia, but with similar histopathology although the senile plaques and neurofibrillar tangles were less dense. Sjögren called this condition 'atrophia senilis cerebri'. During these years the Geneva School showed that patients with senile dementia could present, during the evolution of their disorder, with focal manifestations and lesions analogous to the those found in presenile dementia, in what they called 'Alzheimerized senile dementia'. This finding lead to a unifying thesis, so that parenchymatous dementias were usually referred to as 'senile dementia of Alzheimer type'.

(2) Studies of lesions of senile dementia and non-age-associated illnesses led to the abandonment of the idea that senile dementia was a severe form of normal ageing[25] and to the view that the lesions of parenchymatous dementias were not due to ageing. In 1970, Sourander and Sjögren[26] described a series of cases in which characteristic lesions of senile dementia were present (Table 1). Their findings led to the idea of dementia as a syndrome produced by more than one underlying condition. As a

Table 2 Classification of primary degenerative dementias

Frontotemporal predominance
Pick's disease
Non-Alzheimer frontal-lobe degeneration
Atypical Alzheimer's disease
Unusual familial forms

Temporoparietal predominance
Early-onset Alzheimer's disease
Late-onset Alzheimer's disease
Down syndrome with dementia
Alzheimer-type traumatic dementia

Subcortical predominance
Huntington's disease
Progressive supranuclear paralysis
Shy–Drager syndrome
Multisystemic degeneration with dementia
Progressive subcortical gliosis
Hallervorden–Spatz disease
Other forms

Other types of dementia
Parkinson's disease
Lewy body dementia

consequence, the terms reversible and irreversible dementias appeared, together with tables of conditions that could produce chronic brain disorder.

Gradually another approach, based on understanding of the functioning of the nervous system, was considered, which made the study of dementia as a syndrome more comprehensible. Barcia[27] suggested that the concept of dementia should be based on the organization of the nervous system and that two concepts are important: the functional levels of the nervous system, as proposed by Jackson,[28] and the idea of specialization of the nervous system.

The first of these ideas led to the differentiation of cortical and subcortical dementias. However, a description which better coincides with Jackson's concepts differentiates three types of dementias: cortical, axial, and dementias due to diseases of the basal ganglia and extrapyramidal diseases.

The concept of the specialization of the nervous system leads to the distinction between 'left brain and right brain', 'anterior brain' responsible for mental processes, and 'posterior brain' responsible for perception of the external and internal worlds.

An alternative scheme proposed by the Swedish Consensus[29] refers to three types of degenerative disease of the nervous system: frontotemporal, temporoparietal, and subcortical dementias (Table 2).

Subcortical dementia was described by Albert *et al.*[30] and McHugh and Folstein[31] in relation to progressive supranuclear paralysis and Huntington's disease. In fact the term had already been used by von Stocker[32] in 1932 (*subcortical Demenz*). The clinical features correspond closely to those described by Wilson[33] in his account of hepatolenticular degeneration, and to those of the 'bradyphrenia' of Naville[34] and of the dementia of the cerebral trunk (*Hirnstammdemenz*) reported by Sterz.[35] Sterz probably carried out the best study

of this condition prior to 1974 when American authors introduced the term 'subcortical dementia' and encouraged research to differentiate it from cortical dementia.

Cortical and subcortical dementias can be distinguished satisfactorily on anatomical grounds, but it is interesting that they are characterized by different clinical syndromes. The most characteristic differences are listed in Table 3.[36] Subcortical dementia can be subdivided into an axial syndrome, of which the main model is Korsakoff's syndrome, and a syndrome arising from lesions of the basal ganglia.

Cortical dementias

Cortical dementias are classified into frontotemporal dementias, temporoparietal dementias, and occipital dementias.

Frontotemporal dementias

Frontotemporal dementias are characterized not by a loss of function but by an inability to act. There is apathy, indifference, or in contrast lack of inhibition, and the patient fails to make plans to change from one activity to another, and to select the actions needed to solve a problem. This syndrome is not necessarily due to lesions of the frontal lobe, but may arise from lesions in the frontal projection system and from other subcortical diseases, including Korsakoff's syndrome.

Cummings[37] recognized three complex syndromes of the frontal lobe which he ascribed to prefrontal circuits:

(1) **prefrontal dorsolateral syndrome** which is characterized by neuropsychological deficits, including decreased verbal fluency, decreased ability to plan, anomalous motor programming, failures of learning and recovery of memories, and inability to solve problems;

(2) **orbitofrontal syndrome** which is characterized by lack of inhibition, irritability, and alterations of initiative and introspection depending on environmental cues;[38]

(3) **anterior cingulate syndrome** which is characterized by apathy and reduction of initiative, which in extreme cases manifests as akinetic mutism.

Temporoparietal dementia

Temporoparietal dementia includes Alzheimer's disease. In a series of studies, the Geneva School[39,40] have found that this disease is characterized by a disintegration of psychological functions which occurs in the opposite order to that in which they are acquired in Piaget's scheme. Disintegration starts with abstract functions and extends to concrete functions and finally to a 'preoperative' level.

When patients are examined with a test battery proposed by these authors, it is possible to diagnose which psychopathological functions are damaged. For example, in a test using different-sized cubes, in which the smaller ones are heavier, patients with Alzheimer's disease generally identify the larger cubes as heavier, indicating a loss in the ability to differentiate volume and weight. In another test an object is brought closer to the patient from behind so that it can be seen in a mirror in front of the patient. When Alzheimer's patients are asked to takethe object, they are unable to do so because they have lost spatial representation. Findings such as these are of interest not only because they increase understanding of cerebral organization but also because

Table 3 Differences between cortical and subcortical dementia

Characteristic	Subcortical dementia	Cortical dementia
Language	No aphasia (if dementia is severe, difficulties in comprehension and anomy)	Early aphasia
	Dysarthria	No dysarthria
Memory	Damage to memory	Damage to memory and remembrance
	Normal memory	
Visuospatial disorders	Damaged	Damaged
Calculation	Preserved until the end	Damaged from the beginning
Frontal abilities	Disproportionately affected compared with other functions	Severely damaged together with other functions
Speed of cognitive processes	Slowed down at the beginning	Normal until the end
Personality	Apathetic, inert	Indifferent
Mood	Depressed	Euthymic
Posture	Stooped	Upright
Co-ordination	Damaged	Normal
Abnormal movements	Chorea, trembling, tics	Not present (sometimes myoclonus)
Motor speed	Slowed	Normal

they allow Alzheimer's dementia to be differentiated from pseudo-dementia.

Occipital dementia

Occipital dementia was first reported in 1902 by Dide and Bocazzo,[41] who described a Korsakoff syndrome produced by bilateral occipital injuries. In 1912, Dide and Perzet[42] described the occipital syndrome as characterized by oblivion, fantasizing, temporospatial disorientation, reduction of the visual field, and psychic blindness. This condition is present in a large proportion of patients with occipital tumours: 24 per cent according to Delay[43] and up to 60 per cent according to Allen.[44] The condition is superimposed on the Korsakoff syndrome (see below) and is produced by symmetrical focal lesions in the middle of occipital lobe and lingual gyri. There is destruction of grey and white matter, although not beyond the tapetum and the occipital horn of the ventricles. Although it is a cortical dementia, this condition is related to the diencephalic syndromes.[45]

Axial and diencephalic dementias

The **Korsakoff syndrome** is the prototype of the axial or diencephalic dementias. It is characterized by anterograde and retrograde amnesia, temporospatial disorientation, confabulation, false recognition, and occasionally euphoria. The main lesions are localized to the structures of the Papez system, especially the mamillary bodies, although there is always some frontal involvement. The amnesia is anterograde as well as retrograde, and it is reported that patients lack insight into it.[46] However, Shimamura and Squire[47] have reported that most patients with Korsakoff syndrome are aware of their amnesia and of their failures on tests. There is dissociation between explicit and implicit memories. The Korsakoff patient can learn, but is unable to remember the learning process, a fact described by Calparede in 1911.[48] For example, if a Korsakoff patient is pricked while shaking hands, he learns not to shake hands again although he is unable to explain why. The Korsakoff syndrome is described in Chapter 4.1.13.

Another diencephalic syndrome is **diencephalic vascular demen-**tia, a condition recognized recently as a result of the study of cerebral lesions using modern radiological techniques.[49,50]

There are other subcortical **dementias associated with extrapyramidal syndromes**. Although most of their characteristics had been known for a long time, the studies of progressive supranuclear paralysis by Albert *et al.*[30] and of Huntington's disease by McHugh and Folstein[31] led to increased interest in these disorders and to recognition of the need to differentiate subcortical from cortical dementias.

In general, instrumental processes are preserved, and cognitive failures are generally referred to disturbances of their onset. In Parkinson's disease the motor or visospatial perception is disturbed and there is difficulty in changing attitude or orientation.[51] Dementia in Parkinson's disease is described further in Chapter 4.1.7.

These forms of subcortical dementia are mainly related to abnormalities in the striate nuclei and the structures commonly involved with them, including the substantia nigra, the subthalamic nuclei, the septal area, the locus coeruleus, and the deep hemispheric tracts of the white matter. These structures have important connections with the limbic system and with the cerebral cortex, especially the frontal lobes.[37,52,53] These circuits are the motor circuit, the oculomotor circuit, the dorsolateral prefrontal circuit, the lateral orbitofrontal circuit, and the anterior angled circuit. The main neurotransmitters involved are dopamine, noradrenaline (norepinephrine), serotonin, acetylcholine, and γ-aminobutyric acid (GABA), which are the mediators for alterations of mood, motivation, movement, and intellectual function in subcortical dementias.

Conclusion

The term 'dementia' refers to a large number of conditions, specific symptom patterns, and psychopathological changes. To simplify, there is disorganization of functions in senile dementia of the Alzheimer type, an alteration in the programming of tasks in frontal dementia, an alteration in the temporal organization of experiences in Korsakoff's syndrome, an alteration of perceptive and psychomotor tasks in diencephalic dementia, and an alteration in spatial structures in extrapyramidal subcortical dementia.

References

1. Baillarger, J. (1843). De l'état désigné chez les aliènes sous le nom de stupidité. *Annales Médico-psychologiques*, **1**, 76–256.

2. Greisinger, W. (1861). *Die Pathologie und Therapie der psychischen Krankheit* (2nd edn). Krabe, Stuttgart.

3. Chaslin, P. (1895). *La confusion mentale primitive*. Asselin et Houreau, Paris.

4. Bonhoeffer, K. (1917). Die exogene reaktion Typen. *Archiv für Psychiatrie und Krankheiten*, **58**, 58–70.

5. Kraepelin, E. (1899). *Psychiatrie. Ein Lehrbuch für Studirende und Ärzte* (6th edn). Barth, Leipzig.

6. Zutt, J. (1943). Über die polare Struktur der Bewussteins. *Nervenartz*, **16**, 145–63.

7. Ey, H. (1963). *La conscience*. Presses Universitaires de France, Paris.

8. Pinel, P. (1801). *Traité médico-philosophique sur l'aliénation mentale ou la manie*. Richard, Caille et Ravier, Paris.

9. Esquirol, J.E.D. (1814). Démence. In *Dictionnaire des sciences médicales par une societé de medecins et chirurgiens*, Vol. 8, pp. 280–93. Pankouke, Paris.

10. Georget, E.J. (1820). *De la folie: considerations sur cette maladie*. Chero, Paris.

11. Bayle, A.L.J. (1922). *Recherche sur les maladies mentales*. Thèses de Médecine, Paris.

12. Nogouchi, H. and Moore, J.W. (1913). A demonstration of treponema pallidum in the brain in cases of general paralysis. *Journal of Experimental Medicine*, **17**, 232–8.

13. Klippel, M. (1891). Caractères histologiques différentiels de la paralysie générale. Classification histologique des paralysies générales. *Archives de Médecine Experimental*, **3**, 660–76.

14. Alzheimer, A. (1898). Neuere Arbeiten über die Dementia senilis und die atheromatoser Gefasserkrankung bassirenden Gehirnkrankheiten. *Monatsschrift für Psychiatrie und Neurologie*, **3**, 101–15.

15. Alzheimer, A. (1910-1911). Über eigenartige Krankheitsfalle des späteren Alters. *Zeitschrift für die Gesamte Neurologie und Psychiatrie*, **4**, 356–85.

16. Alzheimer, A. (1907). Über eigenartige Erkrankung der Hirnrinde. *Allgemeine Zeitschrift für Psychiatrie*, **64**, 146–8.

17. Bonfiglio, F. (1908). Di speziali riperti in un caso di probabile sifilide cerebrale. *Rev. Sper. Feniat.*, **34**, 196–206.

18. Perusini, G. (1909). Über klinisch und histologisch eigenartige psychische Erkrankungen des späteren Lebensalter. *Histologie und Pathologie Arbeit*, **3**, 297–302.

19. Rodríguez Lafora, G. (1910). Beitrag zur Kenntnis der Alzheimer'schen oder presenilen Demenz mit Herdsymptomen. *Zeitschrift für die Gesamte Neurologie und Psychiatrie*, **6**, 211–50.

20. Ornari, K. and Spatz, H. (1926). Anatomische Beiträge zur lehre von der Pickschen umschriebene Grosshirnrindatrophie (Picksche Krankheit). *Zeitschrift für die Gesämte Neurologie und Psychiatrie*, **101**, 470–511.

21. Raskin, N. and Ehrenberg, R. (1956). Senescence, senility and Alzheimer's disease. *American Journal of Psychiatry*, **113**, 133–7.

22. Tomlinson, B., Blessed, G., and Roth M. (1968). The association between quantitative measures of dementia and of degenerative changes in the cerebral grey matter of elderly subjects. *British Journal of Psychiatry*, **114**, 797–801.

23. Kral, V.A. (1962). Senescent forgetfulness: benign and malignant. *Canadian Medical Association Journal*, **86**, 257–60.

24. Sjögren, H. (1956). Twenty-four cases of Alzheimer's disease. A clinical analysis. *Acta Medica Scandinavica*, **246** (Supplement), 225–33.

25. Simkowitz, T. (1924). Sur la signification des plaques séniles et sur la formule sénile de l'écorce cérébrale. *Revue de Neurologie*, **31**, 221–7.

26. Sourander, P. and Sjögren, H. (1970). The concept of Alzheimer's disease and clinical implications. In *Alzheimer's disease and related conditions* (ed. G.E. Wolstenholme and M. O'Connor). Churchill, London.

27. Barcia, D. (1988). *Demencias*. Jarpyo, Madrid.

28. Jackson, J.H. (1884). Evolution and dissolution of the nervous system (Firts Croonian Lecture). *British Medical Journal*, **1**, 591. Reprinted in *Selected writings of John Hughlings Jackson* (ed. J. Taylor). Hodder and Stoughton, London, 1932.

29. Guftanson, L. (1992). Clinical classification of dementia conditions. *Acta Neurologica Scandinavica*, **139** (Supplement), 16–20.

30. Albert, M., Feldman, R., and Willis, A.L. (1974). 'The 'subcortical dementia' of progressive supranuclear palsy. *Journal of Neurology, Neurosurgery and Psychiatry*, **37**, 121–30.

31. McHugh, P.R. and Folstein, M.F. (1975). Psychiatric symptoms of Huntington's chorea: a clinical and phenomenologic study. In *Psychiatric aspects of neurological disease* (ed. D.F. Benson and D. Blume), pp. 267–85. Raven Press, New York.

32. von Stocker, A. (1932). Subcorticale Demenz. *Archiv für Psychiatrie*, **37**, 77–100.

33. Wilson, S.A.K. (1912). Progressive lenticular degeneration: a familial nervous disease associated with cirrhosis of the liver. *Brain*, **34**, 296–508.

34. Naville, F. (1922). Etudes sur les complications et les secuelles mentales de l'encephalites epidemiques: la bradifrenie. *Encephale*, **17**, 369–75.

35. Sterz, G. (1933). Probleme der Swischenhirns. *Archiv für Psychiatrie*, **38**, 441–4.

36. Cummings, J.L. (1990). Introduction. In *Subcortical dementia* (ed. J.L. Cummings), pp. 3–16. Oxford University Press, New York.

37. Cummings, J.L. (1990). Frontal-subcortical circuits and human behaviour. *Archives of Neurology*, **50**, 873–80.

38. Lhermite, F. (1968). Human autonomy and the frontal lobes. Part II. Patients' behaviour in complex and social situations: the environmental dependency syndrome. *Annals of Neurology*, **19**, 35–43.

39. Ajuriaguerra, J. and Tissot, R. (1967). Aspects de la desintegration psychoneurologique dans les démences du grand age. Presented at the International Symposium on Senile Dementias, Lausanne.

40. Ajuriaguerra, J., Rey, M., and Tissot, R. (1986). Desintegración operativa en el envejecimiento. Presented at Envejecimiento Patológico y Salud, Instituto de Ciencias del Hombre, Madrid.

41. Dide, M. and Bocazzo, A. (1902). Amnesia continue, cecite verbale pure, perte du sens topographique, Ramollissement double du lobe linguale. *Revue Neurologique*, **10**, 676–80.

42. Dide, M. and Perzet, C. (1912). Syndrome occipital avec dyspraxie compléte surajoutée. *Bulletin de la Societé des Cliniciens Médicales et Mentales*, 279–91.

43. Delay, J. (1969). *Les maladies de la memoire*. Presses Universitaires de France, Paris.

44. Allen, I.M. (1930). A clinical study of tumors involving the occipital lobe. *Brain*, **53**, 196–213.

45. Benson, D.F., Davis, R.J., and Snyder, B.D. (1988). Posterior cortical atrophy. *Archives of Neurology*, **45**, 789–93.

46. Schachter, D. (1991). Unawareness of deficit and unawareness of knowledge in patients with memory disorders. In *Awareness of deficit after brain injury. Clinical and theoretical issues* (ed. G. Prigtano and D. Schachter). Oxford University Press, New York.

47. Shimamura, A. and Squire, L. (1986). Memory and metamemory: a study of the feeling-of-knowing phenomenon in amnestic patients. *Journal of Experimental Psychology*, **12**, 452–60.

48. Calparede, E.D. (1911). Recognition et moi. *Archives de Physiologie, Gévève*, **11**, 79–90.

49. Graf-Redford, R., Tranel, D., van Hoesen, G., *et al.* (1990). Diencephalic amnesia. *Brain*, **54**, 633–8.

50. Markowitsch, H.J. (1991). Memory disorders after diencephalic damage: heterogeneity of findings. In *memory mechanisms: a tribute to G.V. Goddard* (ed. W.C. Corbalis and K.G. White). Erlbaum, Hillsdale, NJ.

51. Leiva. C. and Gimeno, A. (1985). Affectación psíquica en la enfermedad de Parkinson. In *Síndromes extrapirimidale. Parkinson y Parkinsonosmos.* Chapter 3. Médica Internacional, Madrid.

52. Alexander, G.E., DeLong, M.R., and Strok, L.P. (1986). Parallel organization of functionally segregated circuits linking basal ganglia and cortex. *Annual Review of Neuroscience*, **9**, 356–81.

53. Alexander, G.E., Crutcha, M.D., and DeLong, M.R. (1990). Basal ganglia–thalamocortical circuits: parallel substrates for motor, oculomotor, 'prefrontal' and 'limbic' functions. *Progress in Brain Research*, **85**, 119–46.

4.1.2 Delirium

David Gill and Richard Mayou

The term delirium has a very long history, and has been used with many different meanings, lay and medical. In modern psychiatry it means a clinical syndrome comprising a diminished level of consciousness, cognitive impairment, perceptual abnormalities including both hallucinations and illusions, typically visual though in any modality, and disturbance of behaviour, typically agitation. The disorder tends to present over a short period, from hours to a few days. Severity typically fluctuates, being worse at night when darkness makes visual misperceptions more likely and behaviour disturbance consequently greater.

History

Until the nineteenth century delirium was used to indicate a disorder of thinking, but later there was considerable international confusion about overlapping terminologies. In the English literature it was applied to an organic brain syndrome with impaired consciousness. In contrast, in France *délire* was originally used to describe a primary disturbance of perception. In 1909 Bonhoeffer defined delirium as a clinical pattern of acute brain failure. Whilst the complexities of his classification have been abandoned, the central concept of an acute organic syndrome has been retained. It has often been seen as having several subtypes according to the degree of behavioural disturbance and psychotic symptoms. In clinical practice, during most of this century, the word delirium has generally been reserved for patients exhibiting disturbed overactive behaviour, often with pronounced visual hallucinations.[1]

An important change was introduced in DSM-III, in which delirium was used to cover all types of acute disturbance of consciousness with general impairment of cognition, whether or not the patient was overactive and disturbed. This is in line with clinical experience that a delirious patient who is disturbed and hallucinating at one moment is often drowsy and inactive shortly later. This change of definition has gained general acceptance, so that both DSM-IV and ICD-10 use delirium in this wider sense. Nevertheless, other misunderstandings and confusions about terminology are common throughout medicine. It is important to emphasize that delirium is the preferred term and that it includes acute organic brain syndrome, acute organic mental disorder, and confusional state. 'Confusion' is best not used to denote delirium since in its lay meaning it may also be applied to patients with dementia, anxiety, severe depression, and other conditions.

Clinical features

- **Impairment of consciousness** is the key feature that separates delirium from most other psychiatric disorders. There is a continuum between mild impairment of consciousness and near unconsciousness. There is fluctuation in intensity, and symptoms are often worse at night. The patient may be unmistakably drowsy, but milder states are easy to miss, especially by those who are unfamiliar with the patient's normal intellectual performance. They may be apparent only in reduced or slowed performance on bedside cognitive testing. There is disorientation in time, place, and the identity of other people (Table 1).

- **Appearance and behaviour**: the patient looks unwell and behaviour may be marked by agitation or hypoactivity, by a fluctuation between these states, or by a mixture of them—for example, a drowsy patient plucking aimlessly at the bedclothes.

- **Mood** is frequently labile, with perplexity, intermittent periods of anxiety or depression, or occasionally of other mood states such as elation and irritability. Usually, the mood states have an empty and transitory quality.

- **Speech**: the patient may mumble and be incoherent.

- **Perception**: visual perception is the modality most often affected. Illusions and misinterpretations are frequent. For example, a patient may become agitated and fearful, believing that a shadow in a dark room is actually an attacker. Visual hallucinations also

Table 1 Clinical features of delirium

Appearance and behaviour
Overactive and agitated/underactive and drowsy/mixed
Fluctuates, worse at night
Features of underlying medical cause

Mood
Anxious/irritable/depressed/perplexed; tends to vary

Thought
Speed reduced
Form muddled
Content— ideas of reference, delusions

Speech
Mumbling, incoherent

Perception
Visual illusions/misinterpretations/hallucinations; less common in other modalities

Cognition
Abnormalities in all areas
Memory registration, retention, and recall all impaired
Orientation disturbed
Concentration impaired; mild cases may only have slow task performance or wandering of attention

Insight
Impaired

occur. The small living creatures which may be seen in delirium tremens are the best-known example. Auditory and tactile hallucinations also occur. Complex sensory distortions, such as colours being experienced as tastes, would suggest intoxication with hallucinogens.

- **Cognition**: there are abnormalities in all areas of cognitive function. Memory registration, retention, and recall are all affected. Mild cases may show their most pronounced abnormalities in slow performance on tasks or in the wandering of attention away from the task at hand.

- **Orientation**: in obvious cases, orientation in person, time, and place will all be disturbed. Milder degrees of disorientation will need to be interpreted in the context of the individual patient. For example, it may be considered not abnormal for a person who has been seriously ill in hospital for a long time to be unaware of the day of the month.

- **Concentration** is impaired, for example, on tests such as 'serial sevens' or 'days of the week backwards'.

- **Memory** disturbances are seen, with impaired registration (e.g. digit span), short-term recall (e.g. name and address), and long-term recall (e.g. current news items). After recovery from the illness there is usually (but not always) amnesia for the illness.

- **Insight** is usually impaired. The patient will have no understanding of why a psychiatric assessment has been requested.

Epidemiology

Delirium is a very common disorder, accepted as an inevitable concomitant of serious acute illness in children or adults. The probable lifetime risk is 100 per cent, in that everyone has the potential to suffer delirium symptoms with severe physical illness. It is more frequent among people with brain damage and in conditions of low sensory input (such as poor lighting and isolation).

Therefore medical attention is focused on those cases where there is no obvious cause, where there are troublesome features such as disturbed behaviour or psychotic symptoms, or where the diagnosis is uncertain. Less conspicuous cases are usually not recognized as suffering from a diagnosable psychiatric disorder. Surveys also find many patients with transient, subthreshold cognitive disturbances on neuropsychological testing that do not satisfy the full criteria for delirium. For example, it has been reported that six of 70 patients had DSM-III delirium on the second or third day after coronary artery bypass grafting; a larger number had milder disturbances, which did not meet full DSM criteria. Patients who developed delirium had worse cognitive function and worse cardiac function preoperatively.[2]

Delirium in children

Children are more susceptible to delirium than adults. They may develop delirium with any severe acute illness, most commonly with pyrexia due to an acute infection. Such cases are frequently seen by general practitioners in the community. The underlying cause may be a simple upper respiratory infection, or a serious disorder such as pneumonia. Febrile convulsions may supervene. Any child with severe delirium, or where the cause is unclear, requires urgent specialist referral for diagnosis and management.

Delirium in the elderly

Delirium in this population, alone or superimposed on dementia, is described in Chapter 8.5.1. The elderly are considerably more susceptible than younger adults. They may become delirious due to otherwise minor physical problems such as constipation or urinary tract infection, or to combinations thereof. Prescription of multiple medicines (including psychotropics, especially hypnotics), dehydration, and chronic medical conditions are frequently contributing factors. Those with pre-existing dementia are especially vulnerable to developing delirium; indeed, an episode of delirium is frequently the first presentation of patients with dementia to medical services.

Delirium in the general hospital

Delirium may be seen in any hospital department. It occurs in about 15 per cent of all general medical and surgical inpatients and a substantially higher proportion of those who are elderly. It is common in those with severe illnesses, postoperatively,[3] in intensive care and in other settings where patients are severely ill. It is readily diagnosed in those medical settings where it is reasonably common, such as in alcohol or substance misuse services, or in inpatient wards with many elderly patients. However, it may be missed in other settings, where it occurs more sporadically, such as in the accident and emergency department. Delirium should be part of the differential diagnosis for any acute change in behaviour or reduced conscious level, including those patients who are intoxicated with alcohol. Drowsiness and disturbed behaviour may be ascribed to alcohol, and delirium due to another cause (e.g. head injury, diabetes) may be missed, with potentially disastrous clinical (and medicolegal) consequences.

Delirium in psychiatric patients

It is important not to miss uncommon presentations of delirium in psychiatric patients, especially in the elderly. Prevalence is high amongst older psychiatric inpatients. occasionally, neurological causes of delirium, such as epilepsy and problems with anticonvulsant medication, may need to be dealt with, especially by child and learning disability psychiatrists; management should be in collaboration with physicians.

In adult psychiatry, delirium tremens is probably the most common form of delirium seen. The full syndrome of delirium tremens includes florid hallucinations and illusions (both auditory and visual), delusions, marked impairment of consciousness, tremor, agitation, and autonomic overactivity. Anxiety, even terror, is conspicuous. Less dramatic presentations of confusion, hallucinations, and tremor are much more frequent. In severe cases signs and symptoms of cardiovascular collapse and hyperthermia may occur. It must not be missed, as it may proceed to convulsions, with an appreciable morbidity and mortality. Usually the diagnosis will be obvious, with a known history of alcohol abuse, and/or clinical signs. It is essential to remember that the patient does not crave alcohol during the acute episode.

The neuroleptic malignant syndrome (see Chapter 6.2.5) is an uncommon but important cause of delirium. Patients develop agitation and hyperpyrexia, usually whilst on high doses of antipsychotics.

Delirium and death may follow if the condition goes unrecognized. It requires general hospital referral.

Delirium due to infections may also be seen by psychiatrists. HIV-related delirium and dementia may be seen not uncommonly in some groups in some countries. Tuberculosis and syphilis should not be forgotten. Neuropsychiatrists may see a variety of other causes of delirium, including head injury.

Classification

Until recently, delirium was classified as part of a group of 'organic brain disorders' in both the main international classifications. However, differences between them have emerged with the advent of ICD-10 and DSM-IV. DSM-IV dropped the section on 'Organic mental syndromes and disorders', which had appeared in previous editions, because 'the term organic mental disorders ... incorrectly implies that 'non-organic' mental disorders do not have a biological basis'. DSM-IV introduced a new general category of 'Delirium, dementia, amnestic and other cognitive disorders' grouped into three sections.

1. Dementia, delirium and amnestic and other cognitive disorders.

2. Mental disorders due to a general medical condition.

3. Substance-related disorders.

Relevant DSM-IV codings of subcategories include:

- 291.0 delirium due to alcohol (intoxication or withdrawal)

- 292.0 delirium due to other substances (intoxication or withdrawal)

- 293.0 delirium due to a general metabolic condition, delirium due to multiple aetiologies

- 780.09: delirium not otherwise specified.

The category 'delirium due to multiple aetiologies' is useful, as it reflects clinical experience that delirium often results from several factors (e.g. dehydration, fever, and polypharmacy).

In contrast, ICD-10 retains the general term 'Organic mental disorders'. ICD diagnostic criteria for the presence of delirium are somewhat more restrictive than those of DSM. Symptoms have to be present in all the following areas:

- impairment of consciousness

- global disturbance of cognition

- psychomotor disturbances

- disturbance of sleep–wake cycle

- emotional disturbance.

Like DSM, ICD-10 also has subcategories for the various causes and types of delirium. Delirium due to substance use is coded F1x.0 (intoxication) or F1x.3 (withdrawal), where x denotes a numerical code for the particular substance concerned. There are further subcodings to denote the presence or absence of convulsions and of dependence. ICD-10's other main category of delirium is defined by exclusion: 'F05, Delirium, not induced by alcohol and other psychoactive substances'. There is also a subcategory 'F05.1 Delirium, superimposed on dementia'. Other categories are described very generally only ('F05.0 Delirium, not superimposed on dementia'; 'F05.8 Other delirium', 'F05.9 Delirium, unspecified').

Table 2 Causes of delirium

I	**I**nfection: intracerebral (meningitis, encephalitis), extracerebral
W	**W**ithdrawal: alcohol, sedatives
A	**A**cute metabolic: hypoglycaemia, renal or hepatic failure
T	**T**rauma: head injury, burns, heatstroke
C	**C**NS pathology: space-occupying lesion, infection, epilepsy (status and postictal states), Wernicke's and other encephalopathies
H	**H**ypoxia
D	**D**eficiency: thiamine, vitamin B$_{12}$, folate, etc.
E	**E**ndocrine: over- or underactivity of thyroid, parathyroid, adrenal
A	**A**cute vascular: TIA, stroke, hypertensive encephalopathy, shock
T	**T**oxins or drugs (legal or illicit)
H	**H**eavy metals, e.g. lead, mercury

Modified from Wise and Trzepacz.[4]

Aetiology

Table 2 lists the many possible causes of delirium, using the well-known I WATCH DEATH mnemonic.[4,5] However, the links between these insults and the neuropathogenesis of delirium are poorly understood. Electrophysiological, brain imaging, and neurotransmitter studies all show a generalized disturbance of cortical and subcortical function. It is unclear whether there are subtypes associated with different mechanisms, though delirium tremens is said to have a different electroencephalographic pattern of fast activity, from the slow activity seen in other forms of delirium.[4] There is limited evidence[6] regarding mechanisms after cardiac surgery (the possible role of microemboli) and some other types of disorder, including renal failure, and following trauma.

There is evidence of increased susceptibility to delirium with increasing age. This is generally ascribed to reduced 'cerebral reserve', which may be related to reduced acetylcholinesterase activity, and to cerebrovascular changes. Pre-existing brain pathology of any kind (e.g. degenerative conditions such as Parkinson's disease, cerebrovascular disease, dementia, chronic infections such as HIV) is likewise a risk factor. The more severe the precipitating illness and the more acute its onset, the more likely it is to be followed by delirium.[4,5] A reduced serum albumin level is an important contributory factor in many cases of chronic disease. Decreased protein binding of psychoactive and other drugs leads to higher concentrations of the free drug, and hence to greater toxicity at a given dose level.

Psychoactive drugs of all types are especially prone to cause, or contribute to, delirium. This includes antipsychotics (especially those with anticholinergic actions, notably thioridazine), antidepressants, and hypnotics.

There has been considerable research on some neuropsychiatric consequences (including delirium) of some disorders (such as liver and renal failure) and treatments. An example of the latter is the now considerable evidence of the acute neuropsychological deficits following cardiac surgery, some of which are transient but which may also be permanent. Clinical and psychometric features have been related to perfusion procedures, the relationship to postoperative microembolic damage, and the role of various protective procedures.[6]

A further particularly important example is intoxication by alcohol, which may cause delirium. This also applies to other psychoactive substances, licit or otherwise, such as LSD (lysergic acid diethylamide) and MDMA ('ecstasy', methylenedioxymethamphetamine). Most such episodes occur in the community, however, and do not present to doctors. Delirium tremens (delirium due to sudden withdrawal of alcohol in a person chemically dependent on alcohol) is a common cause of referral in liaison psychiatric practice. It is important because it carries a significant morbidity and mortality, yet it is largely preventable and treatable. (See also Chapter 4.2.2.3.)

Course and prognosis

Evidence is limited.[4,5] The usual clinical experience is that delirium is a disorder which is seen as appropriate to acute illness, is not specifically diagnosed, and usually has a good outcome. Those who have recovered from delirium often have little memory of what happened, but a small minority may have distressing memories of being frightened and of being unable to understand what was happening to them.

In the elderly, research confirms clinical experience that delirium may proceed not only to death or to recovery, but that it is frequently followed by survival with impairment. A systematic review and meta-analysis examined the prognosis of delirium in the elderly:[7] eight reports involved 573 patients with delirium. At 1 month after admission 46.5 per cent were in institutions, and 14.2 per cent had died; only 54.9 per cent had improved mentally. At 6 months after admission 43.2 per cent were in institutions. Compared with unmatched control subjects they had longer hospital stays, higher mortality rates at 1 month, and higher rates of institutional care at 1 and 6 months. The presence of severe physical illness or dementia may have been related to some outcomes. The authors concluded that delirium in the elderly appears to have a poor prognosis, although this finding may have been confounded by the presence of concomitant dementia or severe physical illness.

Treloar and MacDonald[5] confirmed that the clinical diagnosis of delirium in geriatric medical inpatients did not necessarily indicate that survivors would have normal cognitive function, as judged by the Mini-Mental State Examination.

Diagnosis and differential diagnosis

It is important to consider delirium in any psychiatrically disturbed patient who has evidence of physical disorder. The diagnosis is mainly clinical. It consists of two components. First, the diagnosis of delirium itself, and second, the diagnosis of the cause. Cognitive testing must be carried out if the diagnosis is not readily apparent. It is essential that assessing psychiatrists are able quickly and accurately to assess cognitive function at the bedside, using clinical methods (see below). Otherwise, many cases of delirium may be missed or the diagnosis delayed. Atypical clinical patterns are frequent.

It is unusual for patients with delirium to seek medical attention themselves; the main exception being the alcoholic who notices the emergence of visual hallucinations whilst withdrawing. Rather, drowsiness or disturbed behaviour will alert others. Disturbed behaviour may include agitation at the presence of delusions or hallucinations, or the expression of false ideas, for example that a carer or family member is trying to harm them. The presence of a diminished level of consciousness may be obvious in some cases, but can easily be missed if it is mild and not associated with overactive behaviour disturbance. A common presentation to liaison psychiatry is for general hospital ward staff to refer a patient as '?psychotic', on the basis of apparent delusions or hallucinations. The task here includes distinguishing a new episode of functional psychosis (uncommon) from delirium (common in this situation).

Diagnosis of delirium

Information from other informants can be very helpful, but bedside clinical testing is the mainstay. Tests such as the Mini-Mental State Examination are extremely useful, but the psychiatrist must not be in the position of being unable to proceed if they are unavailable. If there is suspicion of cognitive impairment, cognitive testing should tactfully be introduced near the start of the assessment, lest time be wasted attempting to take an incoherent history from a patient who turns out to have gross cognitive abnormalities when tested at the end of the interview. Formal testing is also useful for monitoring progress.

There are numerous assessment scales, some intended for routine clinical testing by non-specialists.[8] An example of a brief assessment is the Cognitive Test for Delirium.[9] However, only two of the scale's attributes (visual attention span and recognition memory for pictures) were able to distinguish delirium from dementia, schizophrenia, and depression ($p < 0.0001$) and delirium from moderate to severe dementia ($p < 0.0002$). This confirms the importance of testing attention and short-term memory in this group. Special investigations (such as electroencephalography[10]) have little role in the diagnosis of delirium itself. Their main role is in identifying the underlying cause of delirium (see above), especially in making sure that treatable causes have been excluded.

Differential diagnosis of delirium

- **Functional psychotic disorders** can mimic the positive features of delirium, such as hallucinations. However, functional psychosis occurs in clear consciousness, and delirium's usual predominance of visual hallucinations would not be typical.

- **Stupor** due to severe depression or mania can be mistaken for a diminished level of consciousness. However, these states are now rare in developed countries; a gradual onset with worsening symptoms would differentiate from delirium.

- **Dementia** occurs, except in the terminal stages, in clear consciousness. Marked hallucinations would be unusual in early dementia. The combination of dementia and delirium is frequent in the elderly. Assessment of the relative importance of delirium and dementia may be difficult in the acute situation. However, the position usually declares itself with time.

- **Amnestic disorders**, such as Korsakov's syndrome, also occur in clear consciousness, but the cognitive deficits are concentrated in short-term memory. Immediate recall (e.g. digit span) is normal in amnestic disorders, and long-term memory is relatively preserved: both are impaired in delirium.

- **Sleep disorders** (e.g. narcolepsy) and various forms of epilepsy (e.g. the rare petit mal status epilepticus in children) may also need to be excluded.

Treatment

A search of the Cochrane Library[11] identified only one systematic review of the effects of treatment, by Cole and colleagues.[12] This examined prevention strategies, and is discussed below. A large number of individual randomized trials were also identified, all but two were evaluations of drug treatments of delirium tremens. For example, Breitbart et al.[13] performed a double-blind trial of haloperidol, chlorpromazine, and lorazepam in the treatment of delirium in 30 hospitalized patients with AIDS. They found that delirium symptoms could be effectively treated with low doses of either of the antipsychotics with few unwanted effects. They terminated the lorazepam arm of the study early due to side-effects. However, this represented only six patients, so it is probably unsafe to conclude that antipsychotics are superior to benzodiazepines in delirium generally. Another recent study found no difference between alprazolam and low-dose haloperidol in older, cognitively impaired patients (who were resident in nursing homes) with disruptive behavioural episodes associated with delirium, dementia, and amnesic and other cognitive disorders.[14] Therefore it appears that there is little randomized evidence on the relative effectiveness of various medications for delirium except in delirium tremens.

The treatment of delirium tremens follows general principles and also combines management of physical problems, such as cardiovascular collapse, infection, and hypothermia, with multivitamin replacement and psychotropic medication. Benzodiazepines are the treatment of choice, beginning with an adequate regular dose to control withdrawal symptoms. Drugs are then gradually reduced over several days. An alternative medication which is widely used is chlormethiazole, but its use should be restricted to inpatient treatment as there are risks of dependency and abuse.

Practice guidelines for the treatment of patients with delirium have recently been published.[15]

Clinical management

Caring for delirious patients on the busy general wards of over-stretched hospitals often presents problems. In most situations in developed countries, the initial assessment and treatment is the responsibility of physicians.

The role of the liaison psychiatrist is to help where the diagnosis is unclear and to advise on treatment, including the organization of consistent nursing care. It is often necessary to explain the diagnosis and likely prognosis to ward staff, who may believe the patient is 'going mad' or 'becoming psychotic', and seek their inappropriate removal to psychiatric care.[4]

Doctors are often asked to assess delirium as an urgent clinical problem. Although it is essential to treat immediate problems effectively, it is also necessary to establish a continuing, but flexible, regime of management over a period of days. This requires regular medical and nursing review. The main principles are summarized in Table 3.

In all patients, good general medical and nursing care is required. This includes adequate hydration, and measures to control fever if present. Bowel and pressure area care are important.

- Special one-to-one nursing is often needed, sometimes in a side-room. The use of bright light may help patients with prominent visual hallucinations.

Table 3 Management of delirium

Obtain information from other informants and medical notes
Assess patient's mental state
Confirm the diagnosis of delirium
Determine the physical cause
Treat the physical cause if possible
Reduce disorientation; reorientate repeatedly; consistent routine
Reduce anxiety; reassurance
Avoid over- or understimulation
Inform and support relatives
If calm monitor progress
If agitated, disturbed or distressed: • consider hypnotic at night   • consider regular medication   • monitor progress, review medication

- Patients need reassurance and reorientation to reduce anxiety and disorientation; this should be repeated frequently.

- Relatives find delirium upsetting and they require a clear explanation for the disorder so as to relieve their own anxiety and to help them to join in reassuring and reorienting the patient.

- In hospital, a predicable and consistent routine should be planned. It may be that this is best provided by nursing the patient in a quiet single room. Relatives and friends should be encouraged to visit frequently and help to reassure the patient. There should be enough light throughout the night to enable the patient to know easily where he is but not so much that sleep is disturbed.

- It is important to give as few drugs as possible, since these may worsen the delirium.

Sedation should not be used merely because the patient has delirium. If he is drowsy and underactive, or if he merely has muddled thinking or perceptual disturbance, medication should be avoided as the drugs themselves will tend to make the patient drowsy and therefore militate against recovery from the delirium itself.

However, medication may be necessary if the patient is severely distressed or in danger of injuring himself or others.[4] In acute situations, it may be necessary to start with injected medication or with relatively large oral doses in liquid form, but the aim should be to move towards regular oral doses, which are reviewed daily. The drug of choice depends on patient characteristics. Response is unpredictable and the prescriber should be prepared to modify the type of drug and dosage as necessary.

Major tranquillizers may be the first choice. Haloperidol is the preferred drug of some authorities,[3] although this does not seem to be based on randomized trial evidence of superiority. Delirious patients are very susceptible to parkinsonian side-effects, and so starting doses should be low, especially in the elderly. Among the phenothiazines, promazine is a useful sedative with less anticholinergic action than chlorpromazine and so is less prone to add to cognitive problems.

Benzodiazepines are an alternative; they may be also be helpful in re-establishing the sleep–wake cycle, but often at the cost of increased daytime drowsiness. Therefore a short-acting agent should usually be chosen.

Medicolegal issues

Physical restraint can usually be avoided with adequate nursing care and medication. The psychiatrist should not become party to dubious practices in this area, such as the use of *de facto* restraint with tight blankets or deliberately induced parkinsonism with major tranquillizers. If continued physical restraint is necessary in rare cases, it should be as an explicit part of the treatment plan after medicolegal advice.

Informed consent to treatment also involves important medicolegal issues.[16] Patients with delirium are often very ill, and frequently require surgery or other invasive procedures that they are incapable of understanding and consenting to. The legal position is complex, and will vary in different jurisdictions. However, legal capacity should certainly be assessed before seeking consent. It is almost always wise to involve relatives in decisions in these circumstances. It may be necessary to consult medicolegal advisers, including the hospital authorities.

Prevention

A variety of methods for delirium prevention in hospitalized patients have been subjected to controlled evaluations. Cole and coworkers identified ten studies, of which three were randomized, in a systematic review;[12] patients were middle-aged or elderly medical and surgical cases. Interventions included preintervention psychiatric assessment, and pre- and postoperative nursing assessments. Of these studies, only one showed a significant reduction of delirium in the treated group, but this was a non-randomized study. Therefore it appears that there is little evidence to support the introduction of special measures, over and above routine care, to prevent delirium.

Good general medical and nursing care must be the key to prevention as well as to early recognition and effective treatment. Screening for alcohol dependence is important, for example with the CAGE questions. Elderly patients who are very unwell physically or who are having a major procedure, who have pre-existing cognitive problems, and who are receiving polypharmacy (especially psychoactive drugs) are the most likely to develop delirium, and should be monitored clinically for this condition. Hypnotics are associated with an increased risk of delirium; routine use should be avoided, especially in such vulnerable patients.

References

1. Berrios, G. and Porter, R. (1995). *A history of clinical psychiatry. The origin and history of psychiatric disorders.* Athlone, London.
2. Walzer, T., Herrmann, M., and Wallesch, C.W. (1997). Neuropsychological disorders after coronary bypass surgery. *Journal of Neurology, Neurosurgery and Psychiatry*, **62**, 644–8.
3. Dyer, C.B., Ashton, C.M., and Teasdale, T.A. (1995). Postoperative delirium. *Archives of Internal Medicine*, **155**, 461–5.
4. Wise, M.G. and Trzepacz, P. (1994). Delirium. In *Textbook of consultation–liaison psychiatry* (ed. J.R. Rundell and M.G. Wise). American Psychiatric Press, Washington, DC.
5. Treloar, A.J. and Macdonald, A.J. (1997). Outcome of delirium: Part 1. Outcome of delirium diagnosed by DSM-III-R, ICD-10 and CAMDEX and derivation of the Reversible Cognitive Dysfunction Scale among acute geriatric inpatients. *International Journal of Geriatric Psychiatry*, **12**, 609–13.
6. Newman, S. and Stygall, J. (2000). Changes in cognition following cardiac surgery (Editorial). *Heart*, in press.
7. Cole, M.G. and Primeau, F.J. (1993). Prognosis of delirium in elderly hospital patients. *Canadian Medical Association Journal*, **149**, 41–6.
8. Trzepacz, P.T. (1994). A review of delirium assessment instruments. *General Hospital Psychiatry*, **16**, 397–405.
9. Hart, R.P., Best, A.M., Sessler, C.N., and Levenson, J.L. (1997). Abbreviated cognitive test for delirium. *Journal of Psychosomatic Research*, **43**, 417–23.
10. Hughes, J.R. (1996). A review of the usefulness of the standard EEG in psychiatry. *Clinical Electroencephalography*, **27**, 35–9.
11. Cochrane Library, Issue 3 on CD-ROM. Update Software/BMJ Publishing, London.
12. Cole, M.G., Primeau, F., and McCusker, J. (1996). Effectiveness of interventions to prevent delirium in hospitalized patients: a systematic review. *Canadian Medical Association Journal*, **155**, 1263–8.
13. Breitbart, W., Marotta, R., Platt, M.M., *et al.* (1996). A double-blind trial of haloperidol, chlorpromazine and lorazepam in the treatment of delirium in hospitalized AIDS patients. *American Journal of Psychiatry*, **153**, 231–7.
14. Christensen, D.B. and Benfield, W.R. (1998). Alprazolam as an alternative to low-dose haloperidol in older, cognitively impaired nursing facility patients. *Journal of the American Geriatrics Society*, **46**, 620–5.
15. American Psychiatric Association (1999). Practice guidelines for the treatment of patients with delirium. *American Journal of Psychiatry*, **156**, Supplement to Issue 5.
16. Auerswald, K.B., Charpentier, P.A., and Inouye, S.K. (1997). The informed consent process in older patients who developed delirium: a clinical epidemiologic study. *American Journal of Medicine*, **103**, 410–18.

4.1.3 Dementia: Alzheimer's disease

Simon Lovestone

Introduction

Alzheimer's disease (**AD**) and other dementias incur huge costs to society, to the families of those affected, and to the individuals themselves. Costs to society include both direct costs to health and social services and indirect economic costs in terms of lost productivity, as carers are taken out of the workplace, and the economic costs to those families caring for or funding the care of their relative. Increasingly, as treatments become available, these costs are targets for change and are part of the cost–benefit analysis of new compounds, especially the largest single direct cost, that of the provision of nursing and other forms of continuing care. Apart from the financial cost to families there is the emotional impact resulting in distress and psychiatric morbidity.

As the population ages, these costs pose substantial social and economic problems. Although lifespan itself has remained static, the numbers of elderly in both developed and developing societies is increasing rapidly. In the developed world the sharpest projected growth is in the very elderly cohort—precisely the one that is at most risk of AD. Within the developing world the total number of elderly people is projected to rise substantially, reflecting to a large part better child health and nutrition. For countries in South America and Asia, with large and growing populations, the costs involved in caring for people with dementia in the future will become an increasing burden on health and social services budgets. In the absence of such services families will inevitably shoulder the main part of providing care, although the very process of development is associated with increasing urbanization and, to some degree, a diminution of the security provided by extended family structures.

From discovery towards understanding

In the early part of the twentieth century, Alois Alzheimer described his eponymous disorder in a middle-aged woman who suffered not only cognitive deterioration and functional decline but psychotic experiences, including delusions and auditory hallucinations. Neuropathology included gross atrophy and plaques and tangles on microscopy. Although all the important features of AD were described at this stage, two important developments came much later. First, in the 1960s with the studies of Roth and colleagues in Newcastle[1] and others elsewhere, it was appreciated that much dementia in the elderly has an identical neuropathological appearance to that of AD in younger people. The other development was the rediscovery that AD has a rich phenomenology. The non-cognitive symptomatology of AD is integral to the clinical manifestation of this disease, and is a major cause of carer burden and medical intervention. This second phase of research—the recognition that both the neuropathology and clinical phenomenology described by Alzheimer occur in what had previously been though of as senile dementia or, worse, just ageing, was accompanied by a growing understanding of the neurotransmitter deficits in AD. The cholinergic hypothesis provided the first glimpse of possible interventions, and remains the most important finding from this period of AD investigations. The third phase of AD research encompasses the use of molecular approaches to understanding pathogenesis. The techniques of molecular biology have been applied to understanding the formation of plaques and tangles, to a growing understanding of the genetic aetiology of much of AD, and, through the use of transgenic approaches, to developing animal and cellular models of pathogenesis.

Just as research can broadly be seen to have three phases—discovery, neuropathology, and molecular aspects—so too does the clinical response to AD. For many years cognitive impairment in the elderly was perceived as senility. As a process thought to be an inevitable consequence of ageing it was difficulty to establish medical-care models. Hence the needs of the elderly with AD were not seen as requiring specialist intervention, carers needs were not realized, and public appreciation of the impact of dementia on the elderly themselves or on the family was negligible. The change in perception of AD from 'just ageing' to a disease was accompanied, and to some degree led, by the development of 'old age psychiatry' as a specialism on the one hand and by the rapid growth of the Alzheimer disease societies on the other. During this second phase of AD treatment, the goals have been to ensure that the care needs of patients are met, that families'

concerns are addressed, and that behavioural disturbance is minimized. The third phase of AD treatment began with the arrival of specifically designed interventions. Compounds have been introduced that were designed to ameliorate some of the deficits incurred by the disease process, and other approaches are being developed to treat those disease processes themselves.

Clinical features

Cognitive impairment

Dementia is an acquired and progressive cognitive decline in multiple areas; AD is one cause of dementia and the core clinical symptom of AD is cognitive impairment. However, as noted above, AD is clinically heterogeneous and includes diverse non-cognitive symptoms and inevitable functional impairment. Cognitive decline is manifested as amnesia, aphasia, agnosia, and apraxia (the 4As).

Amnesia

Memory loss in AD is early and inevitable. Characteristically, recent memories are lost before remote memories. However, there is considerable individual variation, with some patients able to recall specific and detailed events of childhood and others apparently having few distant memories accessible. With disease progression, even remote and emotionally charged memories are lost. The discrepancy between recent and remote memory loss suggests that the primary problem is of acquisition or retrieval of memory rather than a destruction of memory, and this is confirmed in early AD,[2] although as the disease progresses it is likely that all memory processes are impaired. Retrieval of remote memory is assumed to be preserved for longer because of rehearsal over life.

Aphasia

Language problems are found in many patients at presentation, although the language deficits in AD are not as severe as those of the frontotemporal degenerations[3] and may only be apparent on detailed examination. Word-finding difficulties (nominal dysphasia) are the earliest phenomena observed and are accompanied by circumlocutions and other responses, for example repetitions and alternative wordings. As the disorder progresses, syntax is affected and speech becomes increasingly paraphasic. Although harder to assess, receptive aphasia, or comprehension of speech, is almost certainly affected. In the final stages of the disorder, speech is grossly deteriorated with decreased fluency, preservation, echolalia, and abnormal non-speech utterances.

Agnosia

Patients with AD may have difficulty in recognizing as well as naming objects. This can have implications for care needs and safety if the unrecognized objects are important for daily functioning. One particular agnosia encountered in AD is the loss of recognition of one's own face (autoprosopagnosia). This distressing symptom is the underlying cause of perhaps the only clinical sign in AD—the mirror sign. Patients exhibiting this will interpret the face in the mirror as some other individual and respond by talking to it or by apparent fearfulness. Autoprosopagnosia can present as an apparent hallucinatory experience, until it is realized that the 'hallucination' is fixed in both content and space, occurring only when self-reflection can be seen.

Apraxia

Difficulties with complex tasks that are not due to motor impairment become apparent in the moderate stages of AD. Typically, difficulties with dressing or tasks in the kitchen are noticed first, but these are inevitably preceded by loss of ability for more difficult tasks. Strategies to avoid such tasks are often acquired as the disease progresses, and it is only when these fail that the dyspraxia becomes apparent.

Other cognitive impairments

There appear to be no cognitive functions that are truly preserved in AD. Visuospatial difficulties commonly occur in the middle stages of the disorder and may result in topographical disorientation, wandering, and becoming lost. Difficulties with calculation, attention, and cognitive planning all occur.

Functional impairment

Although the cognitive decline in AD is the core symptom, it is the functional deterioration that has the most impact on the person themselves and it is the functional loss that necessitates most of the care needs of patients with AD, including nursing-home residency.[4] Increasingly, abilities to function in ordinary life (activities of daily living (**ADLs**)) are lost, starting with the most subtle and easily avoided and progressing to the most basic and essential. In general, functional abilities decline alongside cognitive abilities. However, the precise correlation between these functions is not perfect, suggesting that factors other than disease severity account for part of the variance between patients.[5] Functional abilities are related to gender; for example, cooking abilities are rehearsed more frequently in women, and home-improvement skills in men. However, the overall pattern shows some similarities between groups of patients with similar disease severity. This is exploited in the Functional Assessment Staging (**FAST**) scale;[6] in the original form, this is a seven-point scale of functional impairment, with stage 1 as no impairment and stage 7 as severe AD. A sequential decline is mapped by descriptions of the abilities that are lost: stage 2, difficulties with language and finding objects; stage 4, difficulties with finances; stage 6, incontinence and inability to dress or wash oneself.

ADLs are divided into those that relate to self-care and those that concern instrumental activities. Instrumental ADLs, those related to the use of objects or the outside world, are lost first and can be subtle.[7] A change in the ability to use the telephone properly or to handle finances accurately may not be apparent. Self-care ADLs include dressing and personal hygiene and are also lost gradually; for example, untidiness in clothing progresses to difficulties in dressing. Personal hygiene becomes poor as dentures are not cleaned and baths taken less often, before finally assistance is required with all self-care tasks.

Neuropsychiatric symptoms

Mood

The relationship between AD and depression is complex. Depression is a risk factor for AD, depression can be confused with dementia (pseudodementia), depression occurs as part of dementia, and cognitive impairments are found in depression. Depression occurring as a symptom of dementia will be considered here. Assessing the mood of a person with dementia is difficult for obvious reasons. However, psychomotor retardation, apathy, crying, poor appetite, disturbed sleep, and expressions of unhappiness all occur frequently. The rates of depression found in cohorts of patients with AD vary widely, reflecting changes in prevalence at different levels of severity and difficulties in the classification of symptoms suggestive of depression in those with cognitive loss. A major depressive episode is found in approximately 10 per cent of patients, minor depressive episode in 25 per cent, some features of depression in 50 per cent, and an assessment of depression by a carer in up to 85 per cent.[8–10] It is commonly believed that depression is more common in the early than in the later stages of AD, although this may reflect the difficulties of assessing depression in the more severely affected and least communicative patients. Indeed, severely affected patients in nursing homes may be particularly prone to depression.[11] Elation, disinhibition, and hypomania all occur in AD but are relatively infrequent, elevated mood being found in only 3.5 per cent of patients by Burns et al.[10]

The underlying cause of mood change in AD is not known. However, loss of serotonergic and noradrenergic markers accompanies cholinergic loss; some studies have found a greater loss of these markers at postmortem in AD patients with depression than in non-depressed patients.[12,13]

Psychosis

Psychotic symptoms occur in many patients, although, as with depression, the difficulty in determining the presence of delusions or hallucinatory experiences in the moderately to severely demented gives rise to a very wide range of frequency rates. Few studies have been able to determine the rates of psychosis in community-dwelling, fully representative samples of patients with AD. However, of those known to, largely, psychiatric services, between 10 and 50 per cent suffer from delusions and between 10 and 25 per cent experience hallucinations.[14–16] Delusions are frequently paranoid and the most common delusion is one of theft. In the context of the confusion and amnesia of dementia, it is easy to appreciate how the experience of mislaying an object becomes translated into conviction of a theft. Other patients become convinced that someone, often a family member, is trying to harm them.

Hallucinations are only somewhat less frequent than delusions—the median of one series of studies being 28 per cent.[17] Visual hallucinations are reported more commonly than auditory ones, and other modalities are rare.[16] Most studies of the non-cognitive symptomatology of AD precede the wide recognition and accepted criteria of dementia with Lewy bodies, one of the cardinal symptoms of which is visual hallucinations.[18] It is probable that a large number of those AD patients experiencing visual hallucinations reported in the studies would now be classified as having dementia with Lewy bodies.

Phenomena falling short of delusions or hallucinations, such as persecutory ideas or intrusive illusionary experiences, are common in AD as are misidentification syndromes. Capgras' syndrome may occur, but frequently the symptom is less fully evolved with the patient mistaking one person for another. Failure to recognize one's own face may be due to visuospatial difficulties or to a true misidentification syndrome—distinguishing between the two is difficult.

Various factors have been associated with psychosis in AD, but few have been substantiated in multiple studies. Burns et al.[16] found that more men than women suffered delusions of theft, although others find that psychosis occurs more often or earlier in women. An association with polymorphic variation in serotonin receptors has been reported.[19] Patients with psychotic symptoms show regional metabolic differences on functional neuroimaging.[20] The relationship between psychosis and dementia severity is not as clear cut as that between functional ability and dementia severity. Psychosis can occur at any stage of the disease process, although most studies find the maximal rate of psychosis in those with at least moderate dementia.[16,17]

Although the biological basis of psychosis within AD is not fully understood, it is probable that psychosis symptoms impact upon carers causing increased distress,[21] and that underlying psychosis accounts for much of the behavioural disturbance and aggression encountered in AD.[22]

Personality

Changes in personality are an almost inevitable concomitant of AD. Indeed, it is difficult to envisage how profound cognitive impairment resulting in the loss of recognition of loved ones, and an understanding of and ability to react with the outside world, could not result in a change in personality. Family members have described the loss of personality as a 'living bereavement'—the person remains, but the person once known has gone. Personality change is most frequently one of loss of awareness and normal responsiveness to the environment. Individuals may become more anxious or fearful, there is a flattening of affect, and a withdrawal from challenging situations. Catastrophic reactions are short-lived emotional reactions that occur when the patient is confronted, and cannot avoid, such a challenging situation. Less commonly, personality changes may be of disinhibition with inappropriate sexual behaviours or inappropriate affect. Aggressiveness is, as noted above, often accompanied by psychosis, but it may be part of a more general personality change.

Other behavioural manifestations

Behavioural complications in AD have become a target of therapy. However, the term encompasses a wide rage of behaviours, some of which include neuropsychiatric syndromes, some caused by neuropsychiatric syndromes, and some of which have little apparent relationship to mood or to thought content. Behavioural complication is itself a largely subjective term that relies to a great extent on informer evaluation: but a behaviour may be a complication in one context, although not in another.

Behaviours exhibited in AD include wandering, changes in eating habit, altered sleep or circadian rhythms, and incontinence. These behaviours are closely linked to disease severity and occur to some extent in the majority of patients with AD. Wandering may be a manifestation of topographical confusion, a need for the toilet, or it may reflect hunger, boredom, or anxiety. Sleep is frequently disturbed, with many patients exhibiting altered sleep–wake cycles and others experiencing increased confusion towards evening ('sundowning').[23] A central defect in the regulation of circadian rhythms underlying these phenomena is postulated.[24] Excessive or inappropriate vocalizations (grunting and screaming) occur in the late stages.

Classification

AD is classified, as with all other disorders, by DSM-IV and by ICD-10. In addition, it also has a specialized classification system resulting from the National Institute of Neurological and Communicative Disorders and Stroke–Alzheimer's Disease and Related Disorders Association

(**NINCDS–ADRDA**).[25] This clinical diagnostic system is internationally accepted and widely observed. There are other classification systems for neuropathological diagnosis, most notably the Consortium to Establish a Registry for Alzheimer's Disease (**CERAD**) criteria.[26]

DSM-IV stipulates that a dementia syndrome is characterized by a decline in multiple cognitive deficits, including amnesia, resulting in impairment. A gradual onset and decline in the absence of other conditions sufficient to cause dementia indicates AD. ICD-10 shares with DSM-IV the definition of a dementia syndrome as a deterioration in more than one area of cognition, but including memory that is sufficient to impair function. Again an emphasis on insidious onset and slow decline in the absence of other disorders sufficient to cause dementia indicates AD. The NINCDS-ADRDA criteria defines possible, probable, and definite categories; the latter being restricted to neuropathological confirmation of a clinical diagnosis.[25] It is important to note that both clinical and neuropathological data are required—no single neuropathological lesion is pathognomonic of AD, and it is still uncertain how often or to what extent the neuropathological lesions of AD also occur in normal ageing. Probable AD, according to NINCDS–ADRDA, requires a dementia with progressive decline in memory and other cognitive areas, cognitive impairment established by formal testing, no disturbance of consciousness, and absence of other disorders sufficient to cause dementia. Supporting features include decline in function, change in behaviour, positive family history, and decline in specific cognitive areas including aphasia, apraxia, and agnosia. Non-specific change on electroencephalography (**EEG**) and progressive changes on CT are supporting, but not necessary, features. Possible AD should be diagnosed if there are variations in the clinical presentation, another disorder sufficient to cause a dementia (even if it is not thought to do so in this case), or a restricted cognitive decline.

A number of studies have attempted to determine the accuracy of diagnostic criteria against postmortem diagnosis. One of the difficulties in these studies is that because AD is the most common dementia (by some way), such studies are very likely to find a high-positive predicative value. Kukull et al.[27] found the specificity of DSM-III to be higher than NINCDS–ADRDA (0.8 versus 0.65), but NINCDS–ADRDA had a higher sensitivity (0.92 versus 0.76); others find an even lower specificity.[28]

Diagnosis

AD is the most common of the dementias, occurring in some 60 to 70 per cent of cases. However, this oft-stated figure must be treated with some caution for two reasons. First, cases that come to postmortem represent a biased sample, and the proportion of pathologically confirmed AD in community-dwelling representative samples is unknown. Second, even at postmortem the distinction between different dementias is not clear cut—many AD brains show the presence of Lewy bodies and others have considerable evidence of vascular damage. The proportion of mixed pathologies is actually rather high, between 15 and 30 per cent of all dementias.

History

Making a clinical diagnosis of AD is a positive process and not one of exclusion. The most valuable diagnostic assessment is a careful informant history, paying attention to the pattern and timing of onset and progression. In the research context, a family history interview conducted by telephone provides a degree of accuracy compatible with a full clinical assessment.[29,30] Detailed semistructured family informant diagnostic schedules are available, such as CAMDEX.[31] A history should be taken for the presence of risk factors for AD (e.g. a positive family history) and vascular and other risk factors (e.g. hypertension and head injury). Taking a family history for late-onset disorders such as AD requires special attention. Because of attrition due to other illness, many elderly people have had too few relatives reach the age of onset of dementia to make a pedigree analysis informative. The ages at death of all relatives should be established, together with cause of death and the presence or absence of dementia or memory problems in late life. The term 'sporadic' dementia should be avoided, and is misleading when applied to an individual with a dementia where one parent died young and where no sibling reached the age of 65 to 70 years. The history should also screen for the presence of other illnesses sufficient to cause a dementia, and for systemic health in general. The presence of any significant physical illness, from chronic pain to delirium, may significantly alter cognitive abilities in the elderly, and especially so in those with AD.

A careful history should also establish the presence of any behavioural disturbance that has occurred. The relationship of aggression, wandering, agitation, or other behaviours to care tasks and other recent changes in the provision of the care package should be established. As the mainstay of the management of behavioural disturbance in all dementias is behavioural, establishing the antecedents to behaviour is an absolute prerequisite to effective management.

Examination

In addition to an examination of the mental state to establish the presence of disorders of mood and thought content, the examination will establish the specific pattern of cognitive impairment and the degree of impairment. Screening tests used to establish the presence of cognitive impairments include the Mini Mental State Examination;[32] this is a 30-point scale routinely used in all clinical trials of drugs for the treatment of AD, which is also a useful proxy measure for severity. It should be accompanied by other cognitive testing, including supplementary examination for aphasia and apraxias. Other cognitive and physical examinations will be necessary where the differential diagnosis is between a lobar dementia (e.g. frontotemporal dementia) or a subcortical dementia (e.g. that accompanying Huntington's disease).

In addition to the cognitive examination, a physical examination should be conducted in all patients with AD, although this might not be most effectively and conveniently performed at the initial assessment. Physical illness, including chronic pain, infection, cardiac insufficiency, or anaemia are all common in the elderly and can both complicate the diagnosis of AD and increase confusion in those known to have AD.

Assessment of function

Clinical assessment of function can be performed by informant history and by direct observation. The occupational therapist fulfils an invaluable role in establishing the detailed functional ability of those with AD, in addition to implementing changes in the home designed to maximize function. The FAST scale[6] is based on the premise that the pattern of decline in function is relatively uniform in AD, and hence establishes a staging of severity on function rather than cognition. As

in most instances functional severity is of more relevance for the provision of services, there is much to recommend such an approach.

Global assessment

Driven largely by the United States Food and Drugs Administration, global assessment has become part of the assessment of all patients with AD in clinical trials and is finding its way into clinical practice. The underlying premise is that an assessment by a clinician, often supplemented by an informant history, provides information on severity that neither a cognitive assessment nor a functional assessment alone can provide. One scale, the Clinicians Interview of Change, has become widely used in this context and is an interesting attempt to semiformalize the routine clinical impression without operationalized criteria.

Investigations

At the initial assessment, patients with dementia should be investigated for other disorders that could complicate, exacerbate, or be confused with AD. A dementia screen might include routine biochemistry, thyroid function tests, vitamin B_{12} and folate estimations, and a full blood count; many would also include syphilis serology, although the frequency of abnormal findings is low. A CT brain scan is not necessary in many cases and is not a required investigation in the NINCDS–ADRDA classification, although worsening atrophy on CT is supportive evidence. Functional scanning (single-photon emission CT (SPECT) in particular) can be useful where regional dementias are suspected, and magnetic resonance imaging can provide supportive evidence where vascular dementia is a possibility. An EEG is nearly always non-specifically abnormal even in the early stages of AD, in contrast with frontotemporal degenerations where an EEG remains unaffected at a broadly equivalent severity. This can help to distinguish the conditions, particularly where there is neuroimaging evidence of regional insufficiency.

Aetiology and molecular neurobiology

AD is the most common dementia, affecting more than 20 per cent of the population over the age of 85 years. Epidemiological evidence has suggested risk factors and putative protective factors, but the greatest advances in understanding its pathogenesis have come from the combination of molecular and epidemiological approaches.

Neuropathology

At postmortem, the brain in AD is lighter than aged-unaffected controls with more prominent sulci and a larger ventricular volume. Microscopic examination reveals the most prominent lesions described by Alzheimer—the extracellular plaque and intracellular neurofibrillary tangle.[26] No consensus has developed regarding which of these lesions is responsible for the cognitive impairment of AD. Plaques, or more precisely amyloid load, might correlate with the degree of cognitive impairment,[33] although a significant amyloid deposition is also found in normal, unimpaired, aged individuals.[34] However, there is a high degree of correlation between dementia severity and neurofibrillary tangle formation,[35] although it is possible that some of the features of AD are more stable than others; for example, extracellular neurofibrillary tangles persist after the neurone has died, whereas extracellular Lewy bodies are not found.

The plaque consists of an amyloid core surrounded by dystrophic neurites, which are themselves filled with highly phosphorylated tau protein. Studies of Down syndrome brains have suggested a temporal course to plaque formation. First, peptides derived from the amyloid precursor protein (**APP**) are deposited in a diffuse plaque.[36] Over time this becomes organized as the amyloid peptides become fibrillar and form the amyloid deposit, neuritic change then occurs, and the plaque becomes fully mature.

Neurofibrillary tangles are composed of paired helical filaments, structures which are also found in the dystrophic neurites around mature plaques, and together with straight filaments, in neuropil threads. These filaments are themselves composed of the microtubule-associated protein, tau, which is present in a stably and highly phosphorylated state.[37] Tau is a neuronal-specific protein, found predominantly in the axon, that functions to stabilize microtubules, a property that is regulated by phosphorylation. Phosphorylated tau is less effective in promoting tubulin polymerization into microtubules, and in cells highly phosphorylated tau does not stabilize microtubules.[38] In normal adult brain a proportion of tau is highly phosphorylated, but this proportion is considerably greater in AD. Tau deposits are a feature of other disorders, such as progressive supranuclear palsy and some frontotemporal degenerations. Mutations have been found in frontotemporal degenerations with parkinsonism (FTDP-17),[39] and progressive supranuclear palsy has also been associated with changes in the tau gene[40] thereby emphasizing the importance of this molecule to neurodegeneration.

Braak and Braak[41] studied large numbers of brains from individuals who died at various ages and at different stages of dementia severity, which has resulted in the wide acceptance of the neuropathological staging of AD. The very earliest stages, before the clinical manifestation of dementia, are characterized by the appearance of highly phosphorylated tau in the hippocampus. In later stages, neurofibrillary tangles appear in the same brain regions and then become more widely distributed.

The cholinergic hypothesis

The pathological changes in AD are localized both structurally and functionally. Plaques and tangles first occur in the hippocampus before spreading to involve other regions. Some areas of the brain are relatively preserved—the occipital lobe is affected relatively late and the cerebellum appears to be spared from neuritic change (neurofibrillary tangles and the fully matured plaques, although diffuse amyloid deposits do occur). Functional localization was demonstrated by evidence of the relatively greater and earlier loss of cholinergic neurotransmission. At postmortem there is evidence of significantly greater neuronal loss in the cholinergic nucleus basalis of Meynert and loss of cholinergic markers.[42–44] These observations led to the cholinergic hypothesis, which stated that the cognitive impairment of AD was due to a disorder predominantly affecting cholinergic neurones. It was this hypothesis that led to the development of pharmacological strategies to rectify cholinergic loss and the introduction of the first compounds specifically designed for and efficacious in AD. However, the cholinergic hypothesis was something of a simplification as other neurotransmitter systems (e.g. serotonergic and noradrenergic) are also affected in AD.

The amyloid cascade hypothesis

In 1984, the protein deposited in blood vessels (congophilic angiopathy) in AD was shown to be a 4-kDa peptide known as β-amyloid.[45] This peptide, which is identical to the amyloid in plaques, is derived from a larger peptide, APP, the gene for which is coded on chromosome 21. After a series of misleading linkage studies, mutations in the APP gene were found in a family with autosomal dominant early-onset AD.[46] These two discoveries—the identification of β-amyloid and the discovery of mutations in the parent APP gene—led the way to the amyloid cascade hypothesis, which has remained the dominant molecular model of the disorder.[47] Many subsequent molecular observations have been consistent with this model, which posits the formation of β-amyloid as the initiating, or at least early event, leading to all the other changes observed including tau aggregation and phosphorylation, neuronal loss, cholinergic deficits, and clinical symptoms. Perhaps the most convincing evidence that there is such a unidirectional cascade comes from the observation that mutations in the APP gene give rise to plaque formation and also to neurofibrillary tangle pathology, whereas mutations in the tau gene give rise to tangle formation but not to plaque formation in FTDP-17.

Much subsequent research has concentrated upon understanding the metabolism of APP and the formation of β-amyloid peptide.[48,49] APP is a ubiquitous single-pass cell-membrane protein expressed in many cell lines with a high degree of evolutionary conservation. At least three putative secretases cleave APP and the metabolic products can be detected in individuals unaffected by AD; the processing is not pathological in AD, but the balance between different metabolic routes may be shifted in the disease state. α-Secretase cleaves APP at the outer cell-membrane surface at a site within the β-amyloid moiety itself. Clearly, α-secretase cannot therefore yield intact β-amyloid, and this metabolic route, resulting in a secreted product, APPs, and other fragments, is termed non-amyloidogenic. α-Secretase activity is increased following stimulation of protein kinase C.[50] This might have some clinical relevance as certain neuronal receptors are coupled to protein kinase C and, indeed, muscarinic agonists do increase non-amyloidogenic metabolism. These studies predict that therapies designed to correct the cholinergic deficit in AD might have a disease modification effect.[51]

Amyloidogenic metabolism is the result of β-secretase cleaving APP beyond the amino terminus of β-amyloid and of γ-secretase cleaving the resulting peptides at the carboxy terminus in the cell. The β-amyloid products vary in length, with predominant species having a length of 40 or 43 amino acids. The longer peptides are somewhat more prone to forming fibrils *in vitro*. It is probable that the proportion of β-amyloid[42–43] peptides relative to β-amyloid[40] peptides is critical in pathogenesis,[49] and that mutations in the APP gene increase these longer amyloid peptides.[52,53] Transgenic mice overexpressing the mutated APP gene also produce more β-amyloid peptide and have amyloid deposits in brain.[54] Interestingly, these animals do not develop other aspects of AD pathology.

The presenilin genes

Mutations in presenilin-1 (PS-1) and presenilin-2 (PS-2), two very similar genes on chromosome 14 and chromosome 1 respectively, also cause early-onset autosomal dominant AD.[55] The function of these genes is not fully understood, but homology with genes in flies and worms suggests that the presenilins participate in NOTCH signalling—a complex signal-transduction cascade critical, amongst other things, in determining neuronal cell fate. Mutations in the presenilin genes, and hence their role in AD pathogenesis, may result in an interference with the normal functioning of the protein or may induce a gain in a novel pathogenic function. Whatever the mechanism, it is clear that mutations in the presenilins result in an increase in the production of β-amyloid.[49] Therefore the finding of mutations in these genes adds to, rather than detracting from, the amyloid cascade hypothesis although, as with any hypothesis, the complexity of an originally simple idea increases.

Tangle formation and tau phosphorylation

Tangles are composed of paired helical filaments, themselves composed of hyperphosphorylated tau. It is not fully determined whether tau phosphorylation precedes tau aggregation, but tau is highly phosphorylated in fetal brain and, albeit to a lesser extent, in normal adult brain.[37] However, neuropathological evidence suggests that highly phosphorylated tau does begin to accumulate in the brain before the formation of tangles, and before the clinical manifestation of AD.[56] It seems as though, if not the only event in paired helical-filament formation, increased tau phosphorylation is at least an early event.

Protein phosphorylation is a product of kinase and phosphatase activity. It is likely that many such enzymes may participate in the regulation of tau phosphorylation in the brain, but two have been shown to be predominant. In cells, and *in vitro*, glycogen synthase kinase-3 is the main tau-kinase and protein phosphatase 2A is the predominant tau phosphatase.[57,58]

Molecular genetics

Mutations in three genes have been found to cause early-onset familial AD, which is inherited in an autosomal dominant fashion.[59] Mutations in the *APP* gene (on chromosome 21) are the least common, only affecting perhaps 20 families worldwide. Mutations in PS-1 (on chromosome 14) are somewhat more frequent, although are still a rare cause of AD. Mutations in PS-2 (on chromosome 1) appear to be largely restricted to an ethnic German people residing in the United States, suggesting an individual founder effect. Mutations in these genes have not been identified in true late-onset AD. Individuals with Down's syndrome are at extremely high risk of AD, with neuropathological evidence being present in virtually all individuals living to middle age, probably because of trisomy APP.

The genetic component of late-onset AD has been demonstrated by epidemiological studies, showing that a family history of dementia is the largest single risk factor for AD.[60] However many, perhaps most, patients with AD do not have a positive family history, thus giving rise to the idea of 'sporadic' AD with a separate aetiology to 'familial' AD. For late-onset AD this concept is outmoded and redundant. Many patients with AD do not have a family history because of attrition of family members due to death by other causes. For the cohort currently suffering from AD their parents were born in the latter part of the nineteenth century or early years of the twentieth, lived through two major world wars, and reached adulthood before the discovery of antibiotics. It is not surprising that few patients with late-onset AD have two parents and more than one sibling living to the age of onset of AD, and if one parent died young and there are no elderly siblings then the family history is non-informative. Well-designed studies examining the rate of AD in first-degree relatives by age find a cumulative incidence reaching 50 per cent or higher by the age of 90 years.[61,62]

One gene has been unequivocally associated with late-onset AD, although even this gene accounts for only something like 50 per cent of the genetic variance.[63] The apolipoprotein E gene (*APOE*, gene; apoE, protein) on chromosome 19 has three common alleles, coding for three protein isoforms that differ by the substitution of an amino acid at just two positions. Of the three alleles ε3 is the most frequent and ε2 the least; following linkage to chromosome 18 it was demonstrated that the ε4 allele confers risk, whilst the ε2 may be protective.[64] This finding has been replicated in a huge number of studies and in many different populations, although there are some, as yet, unexplained differences as black African-Americans apparently do not show an increased risk with the ε4 allele.[65]

The mechanism of action of the *APOE* gene in increasing the risk of AD is not known. As *APOE* variation is a major genetic influence on serum cholesterol (people with the *APOE* ε4/* genotype have higher serum cholesterol levels), it is possible that an altered lipid metabolism—either peripherally or locally—might affect the pathogenesis of AD.[66] Alternative theories arise from *in vitro* studies, which show a differential binding of APOE protein isoforms both to amyloid protein and to tau protein.[64] Certainly it does seem as though APOE isoforms affect neurones in culture in different ways, with apoE4 isoforms inducing shorter neurites and microtubule collapse.[67]

Other genes have been associated with AD, but none have been replicated in as many studies as *APOE*. It is likely that a combination of linkage and association studies using large populations will identify the other genes that influence AD, either alone or in interactions with other genes or the environment.

Treatment

For many conditions the goals of treatment or intervention are self-evident—cure, prevention of relapse, and resolution of symptoms. For AD, however, the goals of treatment can be less obvious and differ between patients and for individual patients over time. Ultimately, the quality of life of the patient should be improved, but assessing quality of life is difficult in those with dementia, and given the early loss of insight who is to judge such issues?[68] Quality of life may appear poor—patients may have diminished emotional repertoires, few pleasurable activities, and considerable handicap—but they may share none of the negative cognitions experienced by others with a similarly questionable quality of life induced by different illnesses. Other patients may appear content or happy, despite the loss of the autonomy and self-awareness normally considered an essential component of a good quality life. Equally, the treatment unit in AD includes carers, and there are times when the patient's quality of life is in conflict with the quality of life for other members of the family. Resolving such conflicts of interest and other moral and ethical issues is part of the treatment process in AD. With the arrival of specific treatments for AD and the prospect of disease-modifying therapies, an even harder question arises regarding prolonging life for those with dementia: if quality of life appears poor to observers, is it right to prolong the process, can quality of life in those with dementia truly be assessed, or should carers and families be allowed to assess for themselves the benefits and costs of treatment?[69]

There is no single model of management of patients with AD. In many countries management is the role of the gerontologist or neurologist. In others, as in the United Kingdom, the old-age psychiatry team provide the core specialist services. Many, perhaps even the majority, of those with AD are managed within primary care with the support of social services. Referral from primary care to specialist services will be according to local agreements, but most would concur that behavioural disturbance or the use of specific drugs to treat AD warrant referral to secondary care. Interventions for AD, whether provided in primary or secondary care, can be thought of as directed towards the patient, the patient's family, and the patient's environment. Guidelines on the identification and management of patients with dementia have been produced and may be a constructive approach to ensuring best clinical practice.[70–72]

Managing the patient

Management of the patient with dementia is discussed in greater detail in Chapter 4.1.14. Management starts with the assessment and diagnosis, and perhaps the difficult dilemma is how much of the diagnosis and prognosis to discuss with the patient.[73] Most practitioners do not discuss the diagnosis with the patient themselves, although especially in the early stages a frank consultation can be beneficial. For most patients, however, cognitive impairment renders an appreciation of the diagnosis and prognosis difficult.

A large part of managing the patient is directed towards managing mood and behavioural disturbance. Accurate assessment of the disturbance is critical, and includes determining the antecedents and responses to the behaviour as well as a full description of the behaviour and any associated abnormalities in the mental state. Treatments of behavioural disturbance in AD are most often behavioural and sometimes restricted to giving information to careers. However, pharmacological interventions are an important part of the management of behavioural disturbance, even though caution regarding the use of psychotropic medications in those with dementia is necessary.

Specific treatments for AD have been developed, concentrating in clinical trials on ameliorating the core symptom of cognitive impairment. The cholinomimetic approaches are the most advanced, but other therapies are receiving extensive evaluation. Although designed for the large part as strategies to enhance cognition, these compounds also favourably appear to affect function and may reduce behavioural disturbance. Further evaluation is being conducted to determine whether there are disease-modifying effects. Drug treatments for AD are described in Chapter 6.2.7.

Managing the family

Although patients may not appreciate or be able to follow a detailed discussion of the diagnosis and prognosis, their relatives, spouses, and other carers will. This is an important part of the treatment process; as the carer provides the main interventions for much of the period of the disease process, care should be taken to ensure that appropriate and sufficiently complete information is given.

Caring for a patient with AD can be difficult and stressful and some carers suffer accordingly.[74] The characteristics of both carers and patients influence the impact that this 'burden' of caring has on the carers themselves. Men in general, and husbands in particular, seem to be less vulnerable to the adverse effects of caring, possibly because of the response seen in many male carers of rapidly and effectively recruiting outside help.[75] Women may be socialized into accepting more caring roles themselves and therefore seek less help. Non-white carers appear to suffer from less adverse consequences of caring, perhaps because of cultural differences in the perception of family bonds.[76] Patient characteristics that increase the burden of caring include behavioural disturbances,[77,78] depression,[79] and unawareness of cognitive impairment,[80] but not the cognitive impairment itself. Although the core outcome variable in clinical trials of AD drugs is the severity of cognitive impairment, it is not the variable that induces most stress in relatives nor is it the variable that predicts entry to residential care. Other variables are almost certainly protective, and caring for a loved one with dementia is not a universally negative experience. Much caring is done willingly, effectively, with love, and without complaint.

Carer support groups offer much to a person with a relative afflicted by AD. Through support groups, and especially through the national AD societies and the umbrella group—Alzheimer's Disease International—carers can obtain up-to-date and useful information regarding all aspects of AD. A support group can help individuals practically and emotionally through difficult times. Many carers talk of the support group as a life-line, although little empirical evidence exists as to the impact on carer well being.

One particular intervention for the family is that of genetic counselling. Many relatives are worried about inheriting AD. This concern might arise from two sources—the frequent discussion of genes 'for' AD in the media and the observation of familial occurrence of AD in many individual families. For families with clinically apparent familial AD, advice, information, and where appropriate, genetic testing can be arranged through a genetics centre. Where predictive testing is contemplated for genes causing autosomal dominant, early-onset AD this will adhere to guidelines established for Huntington's disease. It is unlikely that true predictive testing will become available for late-onset AD.[81]

Managing the environment

The mainstay of interventions for AD are provided by social services. The goal of the provision of social care in people with AD is to provide an environment that is comfortable, stimulating, and, above all, safe. For most patients, and for all patients in the early stages, this means care at home, perhaps with the support of home-meal delivery and home-helps to provide shopping and cleaning assistance. Further home care may become necessary as the patient requires assistance with basic self-care tasks such as washing and dressing. The carer may require a sitting service, either for periods during the day to allow them time to themselves or in the evening to allow them to attend a carers group or for socializing. Safety issues are especially important for those with dementia living alone. There are inherent risks to the patient themselves if they wander out of the home and risks to others if the gas can be left on or fires started.

Day care is appropriate for many patients, ideally in a specialist unit. In a generic facility for elderly people those with early dementia can receive little input and those with moderate or advanced dementia can necessitate too much input from the day-centre staff. A good dementia specialist day-care facility will provide the staffing ratio appropriate to patients with a range of severities, in addition to providing a varied programme of group and recreational facilities to maintain interest and stimulation. Day centres, where patients are arrayed around the edge of the room with a television as a focal point, are, or should be, consigned to history. Day care provides essential respite to many carers, and longer periods of occasional or regular respite can prolong the period a patient can remain in their own home.

The multidisciplinary team consisting of care workers, social services, community psychiatric nurse occupational therapist, and psychologist can maintain patients at home more effectively and for longer periods than can clinicians alone. However, long-term care becomes a necessity for many patients at some point. The costs of providing nursing-home care are huge and far outweigh the costs of providing relatively intensive community care or relatively costly drugs. If treatments were shown to reduce the total length of stay in nursing homes then this would affect the cost–benefit ratio of these compounds considerably.

Preventing AD and future treatments

A number of factors such as non-steroidal anti-inflammatory drugs, hormone replacement therapy, and the antioxidant vitamin E, might be of some use in strategies to prevent AD. Prevention could be primary before any signs of the disease or secondary after some manifestation of the process. Primary preventive measures would have to be directed at either the entire population or to groups at risk (identified by family history or genotype, for example), and therefore would have to be entirely benign and almost cost-free to be acceptable. Secondary prevention, possibly in those with memory impairments not amounting to dementia (minimal cognitive impairment), is a more realistic prospect rendering the determination of the very earliest signs of disease or evidence of a prodromal state a high priority. A biological marker for AD would have immense utility in both clinical practice and in clinical trials. Markers suggested have included platelet membrane fluidity and measurement of amyloid, apoE, and tau in cerebrospinal fluid, as well as genetic markers.[82] Of these only cerebrospinal fluid tau appears to have any possible value as a biomarker.

Tertiary prevention or disease modification refers to treatments to arrest or slow down the disease process after it has become clinically evident. Some evidence exists that drugs already available might have a disease-modifying effect, and other compounds designed to reduce amyloid formation or aggregation or tau phosphorylation are in development. Other approaches have been developed to reduce the inflammatory component of pathogenesis, or to enhance function and provide support for the remaining neurones using nerve growth factor. This latter promising approach is made problematic by the fact that oral or parenteral administration of a peptide would result in its rapid degradation.

Given that AD is a chronically deteriorating condition, determining efficacy of disease modification is difficult. Two approaches have been suggested.[83] The randomized start trial assigns patients to drug or placebo at random, and at some predetermined point those on placebo are switched to treatment. If the treatment is symptomatic only it would be expected that on switching to treatment these individuals would 'catch-up' with those treated from the outset. However, if the treatment has slowed the disease, those treated from the outset would remain relatively improved compared to the switched group. The randomized withdrawal trial is a reverse of this, with patients withdrawn from active treatment failing to fall to the placebo group results if the compound had affected the disease process.

Conclusions

For the foreseeable future, AD will remain a disorder afflicting a large proportion of the world's elderly. The impact on developing countries especially will be considerable. Care for these patients will continue to be provided from many sources, with specialist services being necessary to compliment primary and generic services, particularly for those patients exhibiting the complex psychiatric phenomenology described by Alzheimer and for those patients where specific drugs are indicated. As the molecular pathogenesis of AD is increasingly understood it is to be hoped that this is translated into treatments ever more effective in modifying or preventing the disease process itself.

References

1. Tomlinson, B.E., Blessed, G., and Roth, M. (1970). Observation on the brains of demented old people. *Journal of Neurological Science*, **11**, 205–42.
2. Petersen, R.C., Smith, G.E., Ivnik, R.J., Kokmen, E., and Tangalos, E.G. (1994). Memory function in very early Alzheimer's disease. *Neurology*, **44**, 867–72.
3. Neary, D., Snowden, J.S., Northen, B., and Goulding, P. (1988). Dementia of frontal lobe type. *Journal of Neurology, Neurosurgery and Psychiatry*, **51**, 353–61.
4. Riter, R.N. and Fries, B.E. (1992). Predictors of the placement of cognitively impaired residents on special care units. *Gerontologist*, **32**, 184–90.
5. Reed, B.R., Jagust, W.J., and Seab, J.P. (1989). Mental status as a predictor of daily function in progressive dementia. *Gerontologist*, **29**, 804–7.
6. Reisberg, B. (1988). Functional assessment staging (FAST). *Psychopharmacology Bulletin*, **24**, 653–9.
7. Green, C.R., Mohs, R.C., Schmeidler, J., Aryan, M., and Davis, K.L. (1993). Functional decline in Alzheimer's disease: a longitudinal study. *Journal of the American Geriatrics Society*, **41**, 654–61.
8. Levy, M.L., Cummings, J.L., Fairbanks, L.A., Bravi, D., Calvani, M., and Carta, A. (1996). Longitudinal assessment of symptoms of depression, agitation, and psychosis in 181 patients with Alzheimer's disease. *American Journal of Psychiatry*, **153**, 1438–43.
9. Rovner, B.W., Broadhead, J., Spencer, M., Carson, K., and Folstein, M.F. (1989). Depression and Alzheimer's disease. *American Journal of Psychiatry*, **146**, 350–3.
10. Burns, A., Jacoby, R., and Levy, R. (1990). Psychiatric phenomena in Alzheimer's disease. III: Disorders of mood. *British Journal of Psychiatry*, **157**, 81–6.
11. Rovner, B.W., German, P.S., Broadhead, J., *et al.* (1990). The prevalence and management of dementia and other psychiatric disorders in nursing homes. *International Psychogeriatrics*, **2**, 13–24.
12. Zubenko, G.S., Moossy, J., and Kopp, U. (1990). Neurochemical correlates of major depression in primary dementia. *Archives of Neurology*, **47**, 209–14.
13. Förstl, H., Burns, A., Luthert, P., Cairns, N., Lantos, P., and Levy, R. (1992). Clinical and neuropathological correlates of depression in Alzheimer's disease. *Psychological Medicine*, **22**, 877–84.
14. Deutsch, L.H., Bylsma, F.W., Rovner, B.W., Steele, C., and Folstein, M.F. (1991). Psychosis and physical aggression in probable Alzheimer's disease. *American Journal of Psychiatry*, **148**, 1159–63.

15. Drevets, W.C. and Rubin, E.H. (1989). Psychotic symptoms and the longitudinal course of senile dementia of the Alzheimer type. *Biological Psychiatry*, **25**, 39–48.

16. Burns, A., Jacoby, R., and Levy, R. (1990). Psychiatric phenomena in Alzheimer's disease. I: Disorders of thought content. *British Journal of Psychiatry*, **157**, 72–6.

17. Wragg, R.E. and Jeste, D.V. (1989). Overview of depression and psychosis in Alzheimer's disease. *American Journal of Psychiatry*, **146**, 577–87.

18. McKeith, I.G., Galasko, D., Kosaka, K., *et al.* (1996). Consensus guidelines for the clinical and pathologic diagnosis of dementia with Lewy bodies (DLB): report of the consortium on DLB international workshop. *Neurology*, **47**, 1113–24.

19. Holmes, C., Arranz, M.J., Powell, J.F., Collier, D.A., and Lovestone, S. (1998). 5-HT$_{2A}$ and 5-HT$_{2C}$ receptor polymorphisms and psychopathology in late onset Alzheimer's disease. *Human Molecular Genetics*, **7**, 1507–9.

20. Kotrla, K.J., Chacko, R.C., Harper, R.G., Jhingran, S., and Doody, R. (1995). SPECT findings on psychosis in Alzheimer's disease. *American Journal of Psychiatry*, **152**, 1470–5.

21. Victoroff, J., Mack, W.J., and Nielson, K.A. (1998). Psychiatric complications of dementia: impact on caregivers. *Dementia*, **9**, 50–5.

22. Gormley, N., Rizwan, M.R., and Lovestone, S. (1998). Clinical predictors of aggressive behaviour in Alzheimer's disease. *International Journal of Geriatric Psychiatry*, **13**, 109–15.

23. Evans, L.K. (1987). Sundown syndrome in institutionalized elderly. *Journal of the American Geriatrics Society*, **35**, 101–8.

24. Satlin, A., Volicer, L., Stopa, E.G., and Harper, D. (1995). Circadian locomotor activity and core-body temperature rhythms in Alzheimer's disease. *Neurobiology of Aging*, **16**, 765–71.

25. McKhann, G., Drachman, D., Folstein, M., Katzman, R., Price, D., and Stadlan, E.M. (1984). Clinical diagnosis of Alzheimer's disease: report of the NINCDS–ADRDA Work Group under the auspices of Department of Health and Human Services Task Force on Alzheimer's Disease. *Neurology*, **34**, 939–44.

26. Gearing, M., Mirra, S.S., Hedreen, J.C., Sumi, S.M., Hansen, L.A., and Heyman, A. (1995). The Consortium to Establish a Registry for Alzheimer's Disease (CERAD). Part X. Neuropathology confirmation of the clinical diagnosis of Alzheimer's disease. *Neurology*, **45**, 461–6.

27. Kukull, W.A., Larson, E.B., Reifler, B.V., Lampe, T.H., Yerby, M.S., and Hughes, J.P. (1990). The validity of 3 clinical diagnostic criteria for Alzheimer's disease. *Neurology*, **40**, 1364–9.

28. Nagy, Z., Esiri, M.M., Hindley, N.J., *et al.* (1998). Accuracy of clinical operational diagnostic criteria for Alzheimer's disease in relation to different pathological diagnostic protocols. *Dementia*, **9**, 219–26.

29. Shimomura, T. and Mori, E. (1998). Obstinate imitation behaviour in differentiation of frontotemporal dementia from Alzheimer's disease. *Lancet*, **352**, 623–4.

30. Devi, G., Marder, K., Schofield, P.W., Tang, M.X., Stern, Y., and Mayeux, R. (1998). Validity of family history for the diagnosis of dementia among siblings of patients with late-onset Alzheimer's disease. *Genetic Epidemiology*, **15**, 215–23.

31. Roth, M., Tym, E., Mountjoy, C.Q., *et al.* (1986). CAMDEX. A standardised instrument for the diagnosis of mental disorder in the elderly with special reference to the early detection of dementia. *British Journal of Psychiatry*, **149**, 698–709.

32. Folstein, M.F., Folstein, S.E., and McHugh, P.R. (1975). Mini-Mental State, a practical method of grading the cognitive state of patients for the clinician. *Journal of Psychiatric Research*, **12**, 189–98.

33. Cummings, B.J. and Cotman, C.W. (1995). Image analysis of β-amyloid load in Alzheimer's disease and relation to dementia severity. *Lancet*, **346**, 1524–8.

34. Haroutunian, V., Perl, D.P., Purohit, D.P., *et al.* (1998). Regional distribution of neuritic plaques in the nondemented elderly and subjects with very mild Alzheimer disease. *Archives of Neurology*, **55**, 1185–91.

35. Nagy, Z., Esiri, M.M., Jobst, K.A., *et al.* (1995). Relative roles of plaques and tangles in the dementia of Alzheimer's disease: correlations using three sets of neuropathological criteria. *Dementia*, **6**, 21–31.

36. Mann, D.M., Brown, A., Prinja, D., *et al.* (1989). An analysis of the morphology of senile plaques in Down's syndrome patients of different ages using immunocytochemical and lectin histochemical techniques. *Neuropathology and Applied Neurobiology*, **15**, 317–29.

37. Lovestone, S. and Reynolds, C.H. (1997). The phosphorylation of tau: a critical stage in neurodevelopmental and neurodegenerative processes. *Neuroscience*, **78**, 309–24.

38. Lovestone, S., Hartley, C.L., Pearce, J., and Anderton, B.H. (1996). Phosphorylation of tau by glycogen synthase kinase-3β in intact mammalian cells: the effects on organisation and stability of microtubules. *Neuroscience*, **73**, 1145–57.

39. Spillantini, M.G., Murrell, J.R., Goedert, M., Farlow, M.R., Klug, A., and Ghetti, B. (1998). Mutation in the tau gene in familial multiple system tauopathy with presenile dementia. *Proceedings of the National Academy of Sciences of the United States of America*, **95**, 7737–41.

40. Higgins, J.J., Litvan, I., Pho, L.T., Li, W., and Nee, L.E. (1998). Progressive supranuclear gaze palsy is in linkage disequilibrium with the τ and not the α-synuclein gene. *Neurology*, **50**, 270–3.

41. Braak, H. and Braak, E. (1991). Neuropathological stageing of Alzheimer-related changes. *Acta Neuropathologica (Berlin)*, **82**, 239–59.

42. Davies, P. and Maloney, A.J.F. (1976). Selective loss of central cholinergic neurones in Alzheimer's disease. *Lancet*, **2**, 1403–6.

43. Wilcock, G.K., Esiri, M.M., Bowen D.M., and Smith, C.C. (1983). The nucleus basalis in Alzheimer's disease: cell counts and cortical biochemistry. *Neuropathology and Applied Neurobiology*, **9**, 175–9.

44. Francis, P.T., Palmer, A.M., Sims, N.R., *et al.* (1985). Neurochemical studies of early-onset Alzheimer's disease. Possible influence on treatment. *New England Journal of Medicine*, **313**, 7–11.

45. Glenner, G.G. and Wong, C.W. (1984). Alzheimer's disease: initial report of the purification and characterization of a novel cerebrovascular amyloid protein. *Biochemical and Biophysical Research Communications*, **120**, 885–90.

46. Chartier Harlin, M.C., Crawford, F., Houlden, H., *et al.* (1991). Early-onset Alzheimer's disease caused by mutations at codon 717 of the beta-amyloid precursor protein gene. *Nature*, **353**, 844–6.

47. Hardy, J.A. and Higgins, G.A. (1992). Alzheimer's disease: the amyloid cascade hypothesis. *Science*, **256**, 184–5.

48. Selkoe, D.J. (1994). Alzheimer's disease: a central role for amyloid. *Journal of Neuropathology and Experimental Neurology*, **53**, 438–47.

49. Hardy, J. (1997). Amyloid, the presenilins and Alzheimer's disease. *Trends in Neuroscience*, **20**, 154–9.

50. Hung, A.Y., Haass, C., Nitsch, R.M., *et al.* (1993). Activation of protein kinase C inhibits cellular production of the amyloid β-protein. *Journal of Biological Chemistry*, **268**, 22 959–62.

51. Lovestone, S. (1997). Muscarinic therapies in Alzheimer's disease: from palliative therapies to disease modification. *International Journal of Psychiatry in Clinical Practice*, **1**, 15–20.

52. Kosaka, T., Imagawa, M., Seki, K., *et al.* (1997). The βAPP717 Alzheimer mutation increases the percentage of plasma amyloid-β protein ending at Aβ42(43). *Neurology*, **48**, 741–5.

53. Citron, M., Vigo-Pelfrey, C., Teplow, D.B., *et al.* (1994). Excessive production of amyloid β-protein by peripheral cells of symptomatic and presymptomatic patients carrying the Swedish familial Alzheimer disease mutation. *Proceedings of the National Academy of Sciences of the United States of America*, **91**, 11993–7.

54. Price, D.L. and Sisodia, S.S. (1994). Cellular and molecular biology of Alzheimer's disease and animal models. *Annual Review of Medicine*, **45**, 435–46.

55. Da Silva, H.A.R. and Patel, A.J. (1997). Presenilins and early-onset familial Alzheimer's disease. *Neuroreport*, **8**, 1–12.

56. Braak, E., Braak, H., and Mandelkow, E.-M. (1994). A sequence of cytoskeleton changes related to the formation of neurofibrillary tangles and neuropil threads. *Acta Neuropathologica (Berlin)*, **87**, 554–67.

57. Lovestone, S., Reynolds, C.H., Latimer, D., *et al.* (1994). Alzheimer's

disease-like phosphorylation of the microtubule-associated protein tau by glycogen synthase kinase-3 in transfected mammalian cells. *Current Biology*, **4**, 1077–86.

58. Goedert, M. (1996). Tau protein and the neurofibrillary pathology of Alzheimer's disease. *Annals of the New York Academy of Sciences*, **777**, 121–31.

59. Blacker, D. and Tanzi, R.E. (1998). The genetics of Alzheimer disease— current status and future prospects. *Archives of Neurology*, **55**, 294–6.

60. van Duijn, C.M., Clayton, D.G., Chandra, V., *et al.* (1994). Interaction between genetic and environmental risk factors for Alzheimer's disease: a reanalysis of case–control studies. *Genetic Epidemiology*, **11**, 539–51.

61. Korten, A.E., Jorm, A.F., Henderson, A.S., Broe, G.A., Creasey, H., and McCusker, E. (1993). Assessing the risk of Alzheimer's disease in first-degree relatives of Alzheimer's disease cases. *Psychological Medicine*, **23**, 915–23.

62. Huff, F.J., Auerbach, J., Chakravarti, A., and Boller, F. (1988). Risk of dementia in relatives of patients with Alzheimer's disease. *Neurology*, **38**, 786–90.

63. Owen, M., Liddell, M., and McGuffin, P. (1994). Alzheimer's disease. *British Medical Journal*, **308**, 672–3.

64. Higgins, G.A., Large, C.H., Rupniak, H.T., and Barnes, J.C. (1997). Apolipoprotein E and Alzheimer's disease: a review of recent studies. *Pharmacology, Biochemistry and Behavior*, **56**, 675–85.

65. Maestre, G., Ottman, R., Stern, Y., *et al.* (1995). Apolipoprotein E and Alzheimer's disease: ethnic variation in genotypic risks. *Annals of Neurology*, **37**, 254–9.

66. Sparks, D.L. (1997). Coronary artery disease, hypertension, ApoE, and cholesterol: a link to Alzheimer's disease. *Annals of the New York Academy of Sciences*, **826**, 128–46.

67. Nathan, B.P., Chang, K.C., Bellosta, S., *et al.* (1995). The inhibitory effect of apolipoprotein E4 on neurite outgrowth is associated with microtubule depolymerization. *Journal of Biological Chemistry*, **270**, 19 791–9.

68. Howard, K. and Rockwood, K. (1995). Quality of life in Alzheimer's disease. *Dementia*, **6**, 113–16.

69. Hollister, L. and Gruber, N. (1996). Drug treatment of Alzheimer's disease. Effects on caregiver burden and patient quality of life. *Drugs and Aging*, **8**, 47–55.

70. Lovestone, S., Graham, N., and Howard, R. (1997). Guidelines on drug treatments for Alzheimer's disease. *Lancet*, **350**, 232–3.

71. Whitehouse, P.J. and Reidenbach, F. (1997). Guidelines for early identification of Alzheimer disease. *Alzheimer Disease and Associated Disorders*, **11**, 61–2.

72. Fisk, J.D., Sadovnick, A.D., Cohen, C.A., *et al.* (1998). Ethical guidelines of the Alzheimer Society of Canada. *Canadian Journal of Neurological Science*, **25**, 242–8.

73. Meyers, B.S. (1997). Telling patients they have Alzheimer's disease— important for planning their future, and no evidence of ill effects. *British Medical Journal*, **314**, 321–2.

74. Dunkin, J.J. and Anderson Hanley, C. (1998). Dementia caregiver burden: a review of the literature and guidelines for assessment and intervention. *Neurology*, **51**, S53–60.

75. Bedard, M., Molloy, D.W., Pedlar, D., Lever, J.A., and Stones, M.J. (1997). Associations between dysfunctional behaviors, gender, and burden in spousal caregivers of cognitively impaired older adults. *International Psychogeriatrics*, **9**, 277–90.

76. Connell, C.M. and Gibson, G.D. (1997). Racial, ethnic, and cultural differences in dementia caregiving: review and analysis. *Gerontologist*, **37**, 355–64.

77. Coen, R.F., Swanwick, G.R., O'Boyle, C.A., and Coakley, D. (1997). Behaviour disturbance and other predictors of carer burden in Alzheimer's disease. *International Journal of Geriatric Psychiatry*, **12**, 331–6.

78. Donaldson, C., Tarrier, N., and Burns, A. (1998). Determinants of carer stress in Alzheimer's disease. *International Journal of Geriatric Psychiatry*, **13**, 248–56.

79. Teri, L. (1997). Behavior and caregiver burden: behavioral problems in patients with Alzheimer disease and its association with caregiver distress. *Alzheimer Disease and Associated Disorders*, **11** (Supplement 4), S35–8.

80. Seltzer, B., Vasterling, J.J., Yoder, J.A., and Thompson, K.A. (1997). Awareness of deficit in Alzheimer's disease: relation to caregiver burden. *Gerontologist*, **37**, 20–4.

81. Lovestone, S. (1998). Genetics consortiums can offer views facilitating best practice in Alzheimer's disease. *British Medical Journal*, **317**, 471.

82. Foster, N.L. (1998). The development of biological markers for the diagnosis of Alzheimer's disease. *Neurobiology of Aging*, **19**, 127–9.

83. Leber, P. (1997). Slowing the progression of Alzheimer disease: methodologic issues. *Alzheimer Disease and Associated Disorders*, **11** (Supplement 5), S10–20.

4.1.4 Frontotemporal dementias

Lars Gustafson

Nosological classification of organic dementia is based on current knowledge and theories of aetiology, clinical picture, the pathological substrate, and the predominant location of brain damage. This chapter is concerned with dementia caused by a degenerative disease primarily affecting the frontal and temporal lobes called frontal-lobe dementia[1] or frontotemporal dementia (**FTD**).[2] The terminology should be viewed from a historical perspective. The relationship between localized cortical atrophy within the frontal and temporal lobes in dementia and symptoms of aphasia was first reported by Pick in a series of publications, starting in 1892.[3] The pathological account of this lobar degeneration by Alzheimer in 1911 described inflated, 'ballooned' neurones (Pick cells) and argentophilic globes (Pick bodies),[4] and in the 1920s this clinicopathological entity was named Pick's disease.[5]

However, 'pure' Pick's disease is rare, and in recent decades attention has been drawn to a much larger group of frontal-lobe dementias clinically similar to Pick's disease but lacking the pathological characteristics of Pick's disease and Alzheimer's disease.[6–8] The disease was named frontal-lobe degeneration of non-Alzheimer type (**FLD**)[6] to mark its dissimilarity to Alzheimer's disease. Alternative designations are 'dementia lacking distinctive histology'[9] and 'primary degenerative dementia without Alzheimer pathology'.[10] In 1994 the Lund–Manchester consensus delineated the clinical and neuropathological criteria for FTD, with Pick's disease, FLD, and motor neurone disease with dementia as the main constituents.[2] Other diseases, such as progressive non-fluent aphasia,[11] and FTD with parkinsonism linked to chromosome 17 (**FTDP-17**) are considered as belonging to the same clinicopathological spectrum.[12]

Neuropathology

The neuropathological characteristics of Pick's disease, FLD, motor neurone disease with dementia, and Alzheimer's disease are summarized in Table 1.

The cortical atrophy in Pick's disease is severe, circumscribed with knife-blade appearance, often asymmetrical, and involves the striatum and hippocampus. The degeneration involves all cortical laminae, with

Table 1 Pathological features in frontotemporal dementia and Alzheimer's disease

Feature	Pick's disease	FLD	Motor neurone disease dementia	Early-onset Alzheimer's disease
Circumscribed frontal atrophy	+	–	–	–
Principal cortical topography	Frontotemporal	Frontotemporal	Frontal	Parietotemporal
Laminar involvement	I–VI	I–III	I–III	I–VI
Neuronal inclusions	Tau and ubiquitine positive	–	Ubiquitine positive	–
Plaques, tangles, and amyloid	–	–	–	+

inflated neurones and Pick bodies, which are tau and ubiquitin positive.[13] The white-matter degeneration and atrophy are quite pronounced. FLD is characterized by mild to moderate atrophy which is most marked in the frontal convexity cortex, the anterior cingulate gyrus, and in about a third of the cases also in the anterior temporal cortex. Degenerative changes are restricted to the cortical layers 1, 2, and 3, and the histopathological changes are non-specific with neuronal loss and atrophy, microvacuolation, and astrocytic gliosis. The posterior cingulate gyrus, hippocampus, and striatum are unremarkable but the substantia nigra sometimes shows moderate degeneration, although never as severe as in Parkinson's disease.[14] The frontal white matter often shows mild loss of myelin.[15] The parietal cortex and the posterior cingulate gyrus are comparatively spared in contrast with the pattern of degeneration in Alzheimer's disease with similar age at onset.[6] There are no neuronal inclusions or prions, plaques, tangles, or Lewy bodies and no amyloid in FLD. The brain pathology in motor neurone disease with dementia is similar to that described in FLD, but in addition there are ubiquitin-positive neuronal inclusions in the superficial laminae, for example in the frontotemporal cortex, in addition to anterior horn cell loss.[13,16]

Prevalence and age characteristics

Pick's disease as defined above is rare, with a prevalence of 1 to 2 per cent in post-mortem studies of dementia,[17] compared to a prevalence of 7.5 per cent of FLD and 40 to 50 per cent of Alzheimer's disease.[18] Little is known about the true prevalence and incidence of FTD. It might be responsible for as much as 20 per cent of all early onset dementia.[19] Most demographic data concern the grouping of FTD, not separating FLD and Pick's disease. The overall frequency of Pick's disease in a wider sense has been estimated at 24 to 60 per 100 000 in Minnesota and 30 to 60 in Switzerland.[20] The estimated prevalence of FTD in the Netherlands is 10.7 per million between 50 and 60 years of age, and 28 between 60 and 70 years.[21] Pasquier et al.[22] diagnosed FTD in 4.8 per cent, and probable or possible Alzheimer's disease in 71.4 per cent of 1015 consecutive cases examined at the Memory Clinic in Lille, France. The marked geographic variation of the prevalence of FTD might be due to genetic and environmental factors, but it might also be influenced by differences in the diagnostic process. The prevalence of dementia with a mainly presenile clinical onset in motor neurone disease has been estimated at 2 to 6 per cent.[23]

Clinical features

The first clinical manifestations of FTD usually appear in the presenium, in some cases as early as 35 and seldom after 70 years of age. The mean age at onset in postmortem-verified FLD cases is 56 ± 7.6 years with a mean duration of 8 ± 3.4 years (range 3–17 years).[18] The mean age of onset in Pick's disease is similar, 62 years, with a range of 45 to 80 years, and a mean survival of 9.8 years with a range of 4.8 to 21.2 years.[20] This large variation of the duration of FLD and Pick's disease is similar to that of early-onset Alzheimer's disease, which is 10.6 ± 3 years, with a range of 5 to 16 years.[18] The clinical onset of dementia in motor neurone disease is usually in the sixth decade and the mean duration is about 30 months.[24]

Disordered behaviour

The Lund–Manchester consensus on clinical criteria for FTD is summarized in Table 2. The early stage of FLD and Pick's disease is characterized by changes of personality and behaviour, affective symptoms, and a progressive reduction of expressive speech, revealing the dysfunction of frontotemporal brain structures. The clinical onset is insidious with slow progression without ictal events. Therefore the duration of the disease may easily be underestimated. The changes of personality and behaviour are mainly non-specific and easily misinterpreted as expressions of non-organic mental disease such as mood disorder, hypochondriasis, schizophrenia, or other psychotic reaction. Other explanations of the patient's behaviour such as a reaction to problems in the family may also be suggested, especially by people lacking previous knowledge of the patient. Loss of insight concerning the mental changes and their consequences is an early and alarming manifestation of the disease. Although most patients deny any awareness of mental change or illness, several patients ask for medical examination referring to symptoms such as anxiety, tiredness, and strange somatic complaints combined with bizarre hypochondriacal ideas. The hypochondriasis may sometimes be secondary to hallucinations or sensory distortion.

The early loss of personal and social awareness is seen as neglect of personal hygiene and grooming, and tactlessness and antisocial behaviour. The impaired control and modulation of emotions are seen as increased sentimentality, inadequate smiling, inappropriate joking, irritability, and acts of aggressiveness, leading to conflicts at home and at work. Craving for affection and sexual contact may be easily provoked, but usually expressions of sexual disinhibition are rather childish and innocent, and possible to divert. Impulse buying, shoplifting,

Table 2 The Lund–Manchester consensus on clinical criteria for frontotemporal dementia

Core features
Behavioural disorder
    Insidious onset and slow progression
    Early loss of insight
    Early loss of personal and social awareness
    Early signs of disinhibition and lack of judgement
    Mental rigidity and inflexibility
    Stereotyped, repetitive, and imitating behaviour
    Hyperorality, oral/dietary changes
    Utilization behaviour
    Distractibility, impulsivity, and impersistence

Affective symptoms
    Depression, anxiety, excessive sentimentality
    Hypochondriasis, bizarre somatic complaints
    Emotional bluntness, apathy, and lack of empathy
    Amimia

Speech disorders
    Progressive reduction of speech output
    Stereotypy of speech, perseveration
    Echolalia
    Late mutism

Spatial orientation, receptive speech, and praxis comparatively spared

Physical signs
    Early primitive reflexes
    Early incontinence
    Late akinesia, rigidity and tremor
    Low and labile blood pressure

Investigations
    Normal EEG despite clinically evident dementia
    Brain imaging (structural and/or functional): predominant frontal
        and/or anterior temporal abnormality
    Neuropsychology: profound failure on 'frontal-lobe' tests in the
        absence of severe amnesia, or perceptual spatial disorder

Supportive diagnostic features
    Onset before 65 years of age
    Positive family history or similar disorder in a first-degree relative
    Bulbar palsy, muscular weakness and wasting, fasciculations (motor
        neurone disease)

indecency, and other disinhibited behaviour may, however, lead to rejection by the family and society. Such unpredictable and pseudo-psychopathic behaviour imposes severe strain on the patient's family, leading in some cases to economic problems, divorce, and even suicide in the family. Complications of this type are uncommon in families with an Alzheimer patient. Traffic accidents may also result from the patient's impaired regulation of conduct. FTD patients tend to become inattentive and careless; although using the correct traffic lane they may neglect traffic lights, speed limits, and other regulations. The typical Alzheimer patient is more self-critical and anxiously aware of the difficulties in driving. Changes in drinking behaviour are sometimes reported. Patients with previous restricted alcohol consumption start to drink more frequently and in larger quantities than before. The alcohol is probably sometimes used to reduce anxiety and depressed mood. The pathological drinking behaviour, which may lead to mis-

diagnosis of alcohol-induced dementia, can often be controlled by a firm attitude from relatives.

Affective symptoms

The FTD patient becomes emotionally shallow and blunt, showing less concern about family and friends. The patient is described as egocentric, rigid, and lacking empathy. The early emotional changes may be difficult to differentiate from non-organic personality disorders and affective disorder. Mood changes towards euphoria, especially when associated with increased talkativeness and restlessness, may at first be mistaken for a hypomanic or manic state. Slowly developing apathy, in combination with sparse mimical movements and verbal aspontaneity, may be misdiagnosed as depression. During the depressive reactions, which are mostly of short duration, the patient may become agitated or dysphoric, and may dwell on suicidal thoughts. FTD patients are often diagnosed as depressed and treated with antidepressant medication during the early stage of the disease.

Early symptoms of dementia must be judged against information about the patient's premorbid personality, education, and social background. The vast majority of cases show normal premorbid personality although a few have previously manifested anxiety and restlessness. The emotional features in FTD do not seem primarily related to premorbid personality traits but rather to the distribution of brain pathology as shown at autopsy and brain imaging.[25]

Other symptoms

A striking feature of FTD is the **stereotyped and perseverative behaviour** seen as wandering, clapping, humming, dancing, and hoarding of objects, as well as complex rituals involving washing and dressing. The intensity of such behaviour sometimes reaches psychotic intensity. Imitative behaviour seen as repetition of other people's gestures and utterances is frequent in FTD and occurs more often than in Alzheimer's disease.

Hallucinations and delusions are reported in about 20 per cent of FTD and early-onset Alzheimer's disease cases and even more frequently when the patients are followed closely from the easily stage of the disease. The psychotic symptoms in FTD are often bizarre and the combination with loss of insight, emotional blunting, restlessness, and stereotypy of speech and behaviour gives the impression of functional psychosis with schizophrenia as an early tentative diagnosis.[7–9] The psychotic symptoms in early-onset Alzheimer's disease seem more strongly related to the cognitive failure with memory failure, impaired recognition, and disorientation, and the degeneration of the temporo-parietal association cortex.

The **human counterpart of the Klüver–Bucy syndrome** with elements such as blunted affect, hyperorality, and unrestrained sexuality has been reported in FLD and in Pick's disease. The hyperorality and changes of oral/dietary behaviour are seen as overeating, food fads, excessive smoking and alcohol consumption, and oral exploration of inanimate objects. Utilization behaviour, defined as an irresistible impulse to explore and use objects in the visual environmental, shows important similarity to the hypermetamorphosis and distractibility of the Klüver–Bucy syndrome especially when oral exploration is present.[26] The Klüver–Bucy syndrome in Alzheimer's disease is usually less complete than in FTD with less hypersexuality and utilization behaviour, supporting the suggestion that frontal as well as temporal lobe involvement is needed to produce the syndrome in humans.

Dissolution of language

A core feature of FTD is progressive impairment of expressive speech described as *dissolution du langage* or *Sprachverödung*.[27] Speech becomes aspontaneous with word-finding difficulties and frequent use of stereotyped comments and set phrases. During the early stage there may be a period of increased pressure of speech. The FTD patient may also loose his or her normal pitch of voice and speaks in an unmodulated inappropriately high tone. The language dysfunction is dominated by dynamic expressive failure rather than by a semantic receptive one, which is in agreement with damage in the frontal cortex especially premotor areas. Echolalia is observed in about 50 per cent of FTD and Pick cases.[18] Finally the patients become mute which in combination with the amimia makes communication extremely difficult. The ability to understand information and instructions usually remains until comparatively late in the course of the disease, as does the ability to write. The handwriting may, however, change in magnitude, spelling, and speed of writing. These disturbances are unlike the temporoparietal type of dysgraphia and global dysphasia observed in Alzheimer's disease. The symptom constellation of palilalia (stereotypy of speech), echolalia, mutism, and amimia (PEMA syndrome of Guiraud) is typical of FTD and seldom found in Alzheimer's disease.

There are important similarities between the speech disorder of early FTD and the clinical spectrum of progressive non-fluent aphasia,[11] characterized by effortful speech production and relative preservation of memory and practical abilities. Dementia often develops later in the course, and the underlying degenerative process may be similar to that of FLD, with a predominant and early involvement of the speech-dominant hemisphere.

Physical signs

Few pathological somatic findings including neurological symptom are reported in FTD. Primitive reflexes such as grasp, snout, and sucking reflexes may appear comparatively early, while akinesia, rigidity, and tremor are late phenomena. Increased muscular tension is significantly more common in Alzheimer's disease, although it also occurs in FTD.[7] Recently the spectrum of dementing frontotemporal disorder has expanded to include the syndrome of the disinhibition–dementia –parkinsonism–amyotrophy complex,[28] also named FTDP-17.[29]

Generalized epileptic seizures may appear in FTD although less prevalent than in Alzheimer's disease, and myoclonic twitchings which are present in 50 per cent of early-onset Alzheimer's cases are uncommon in FTD. Urinary incontinence, which is reported early in about 50 per cent of FTD cases, is a comparatively late feature in uncomplicated early-onset Alzheimer's disease. This feature is also common in vascular dementia and late-onset Alzheimer's disease and seems related to frontobasal and anterior cingulate gyral damage.

FTD patients in general have low and labile blood pressure with a high prevalence (50 per cent) of orthostatic blood pressure drops and syncopal attacks. These symptoms are, however, also reported in early-onset Alzheimer's disease (40 per cent) and late in the course of vascular dementia (50 per cent).[30] The relationship between blood pressure changes and brain damage especially the white-matter changes in FTD are still unclear.[14]

Comparison between FLD and Pick's disease

The clinical similarities between FLD and Pick's disease are important, in spite of differences in histopathology and distribution of brain pathology. Deterioration of personality and behaviour, expressive speech disorder, and gradual loss of mimical expression are found in both diseases as are an early normal EEG, incontinence, and low and labile blood pressure. Severe memory failure and confabulation are probably more prevalent in Pick's disease, while affective symptoms, especially depression, are more often reported in FLD. The analysis of larger patient materials and the use of functional brain imaging, and genetic and other biological markers will further elucidate the relationship between FLD and Pick's disease.

Dementia in motor neurone disease

The clinical picture of the dementia in motor neurone disease is similar to that in FLD with early changes of personality and behaviour, lack of insight, and signs of disinhibition such as restlessness, irritability, unrestrained sexuality, and hyperorality.[16,31] Speech becomes stereotyped and perseverative, later developing into mutism. Receptive speech function, orientation and practicable abilities remain relatively untouched by the degenerative process. Emotional changes such as euphoria and apathy may appear and the face becomes expressionless. The mental changes may appear early in motor neurone disease and even precede development of typical neurological features.

Investigations

EEG

The EEG may be normal or only slightly pathological in FTD at a stage when dementia is strongly suspected or clinically evident, but it is usually pathological late in the course. This has been shown in FLD, Pick's disease, and motor neurone disease with dementia.[32] By contrast, EEG is almost always pathological in Alzheimer's disease even at an early stage. Quantitative EEG mapping and repeated recordings may strongly improve the differential diagnosis between FTD and Alzheimer's disease.[32]

Brain imaging

Structural and functional brain imaging has strongly improved the recognition of frontal and frontotemporal degeneration in FTD. Cortical atrophy with more or less frontal focal accentuation is shown with CT and magnetic resonance imaging (**MRI**).[9,33] MRI may show significantly more prevalent and severe periventricular hyperintense deep white-matter lesions in FTD patients than in matched normal controls.[34] The differential diagnosis from vascular dementia with frontal subcortical lesions, but lacking large cortical infarctions, may be difficult.

Brain imaging of metabolism and regional cerebral blood flow has radically improved recognition and differential diagnosis of dementing diseases. The frontotemporal regional cerebral blood flow abnormalities in FTD shown with xenon clearance technique, single-photon emission CT (**SPECT**) (Plate 12), and positron emission tomography

(PET) contrast with the temporoparietal pathology in Alzheimer's disease.[35–37] The findings are not disease specific, but are also found in vascular brain damage, in Alzheimer's disease with marked frontal-lobe involvement,[38] and in progressive supranuclear palsy. The regional cerebral blood flow pathology in progressive aphasia is most pronounced in the left hemisphere.[11]

Assessment of cognitive impairment

The cognitive symptoms, which appear early in FTD, may be difficult to evaluate due to the patient's emotional and behavioural changes. Distractibility and slightly reduced recent memory are common findings and remote memory is also impaired although to a lesser extent than in Alzheimer's didease. The patients show significant impairment on 'frontal-lobe' tests such as the Wisconsin card sorting test, word fluency test, and the Stroop and trail-making tests. The early test profile is characterized by slow verbal production and relatively intact visuospatial ability, reasoning, and memory, while intellectual and motor speed are reduced.[39] Early Alzheimer's disease usually shows a relatively preserved verbal ability and simultaneous impairment of reasoning ability, verbal and spatial memory dysfunction, dysphasia, and dyspraxia.[39,40] Difficulties in understanding instructions are found early only in a minority of FTD cases. Misspelling and dyscalculia are sometimes reported early in FTD.

Discrimination between FTD and Alzheimer's disease can be based on a short test-battery (verbal ability, visuospatial ability, and verbal memory), when used in the context of a neuropsychological evaluation of qualitative as well as quantitative aspects of test performance.[39,41] Using a screening instrument based on frontal release signs, awareness of social/ethical dilemma in a short story, and the number of preservation errors, FTD was classified correctly in 83 per cent, validated against clinical diagnosis.[42] The Mini-Mental State Examination[43] does not reflect the FTD patient's true competence because of influence of motivational and behavioural factors.[44]

The deterioration of personality and behaviour in FTD contrasts with the comparatively spared spatial orientation, receptive speech, and practical ability.

Differential diagnosis

Differential diagnosis between FTD and Alzheimer's disease and other dementias is often possible using well-defined clinical criteria, neuropsychological testing, and brain imaging. Organic dementias with frontal features are listed in Table 3.

The clinical differences between FTD and Alzheimer's disease are often obvious at an early stage (Table 4). The initial stages of FTD are dominated by emotional and personality changes, and consequently severe dyspraxia, memory failure, and spatial disorientation develop comparatively late with the relative sparing of the temporoparietal occipital cortical areas. In contrast, early-onset Alzheimer's disease is characterized by memory failure, dyspraxia, dysgnosia, and impaired sense of locality, whereas habitual personality traits, social competence, and insight are better preserved in agreement with the consistent pattern of cortical involvement. A minority of Alzheimer's cases, about 5 per cent, show a marked frontal-lobe involvement at an early stage and consequently also present a frontal-lobe clinical pattern in addition to the temporoparietal symptoms.[38] The PEMA syndrome with stereotypy of speech (palilalia), echolalia, late mutism, and ami-

Table 3 Organic dementia with frontal features

Frontotemporal dementia and closely allied conditions
Frontal-lobe degeneration of non-Alzheimer type (FLD)
Pick's disease
Motor neurone disease with frontal dementia
Dementia lacking distinctive histological features
Frontotemporal dementia with parkinsonism (FTDP-17)
Progressive language disorder due to lobar atrophy, primary progressive aphasia, semantic dementia, etc.

Other clinically similar disorders
Alzheimer's disease with frontal emphasis
Vascular dementia with frontal emphasis
   Selective incomplete white-matter infarction
   Binswanger's disease
   Multi-infarct dementia with frontal emphasis
   Bilateral thalamic infarctions
Huntington's disease
Progressive supranuclear palsy
Corticobasal degeneration
Creutzfeldt–Jakob disease with frontal emphasis
General paresis

mia is typical of FTD and rare in Alzheimer's disease. Certain neurological features may also contribute to the differentiation between the two, for example generalized epileptic seizures, myoclonus, and logoclonia are more prevalent in Alzheimer's disease. Moreover, EEG may remain normal in FTD cases with evident signs of dementia while EEG

Table 4 Clinical characteristics in frontotemporal dementia (FTD) and early-onset Alzheimer's disease (AD)

	FTD	AD
Early features		
Loss of insight	++	–
Loss of social awareness	++	–
Disinhibition	++	–
Memory impairment	+	++
Dyspraxia	+	++
Incontinence	+	–
Low and labile blood pressure	++	+(+)
Speech disorder		
Stereotypy	++	–
Echolalia	+	–
Mutistic but receptive	++	–
Logoclonia	–	+
Hypomimia/amimia	++	+
Extrapyramidal signs	(+)	++
Grand mal	–	+
Myoclonia	–	++
Normal EEG	++	–
Klüver–Bucy-like syndrome		
Hyperorality	++	+
Utilization behaviour	+	–
Hypersexuality	+	–

in Alzheimer's disease is almost always pathological. The Klüver–Bucy syndrome in Alzheimer's disease is usually less complete than in FTD with less hypersexuality and utilization behaviour, supporting the suggestion that frontal as well as temporal lobe involvement is needed to produce the syndrome in humans. Imitating behaviour, seen as echolalia and repetition of other people's gestures, is more prevalent in FTD than in Alzheimer's disease.

Vascular dementia with frontal emphasis may be caused by selective incomplete white-matter infarction, Binswanger's disease, and frontal and strategic thalamic infarctions. The frontal-lobe dysfunction caused by vascular lesions may closely mimic the course of FTD, when developing gradually without dramatic onset on fluctuations.[38,45]

The clinical distinction between FTD and Huntington's disease may be difficult when personality changes and psychotic features dominate, and when the neurological characteristics of Huntington's disease are less obvious or appear late in the course. Brain imaging showing striatal involvement and genetic analysis may contribute to the diagnosis.

Progressive supranuclear palsy and the rare progressive subcortical gliosis may also show a frontal-lobe clinical and imaging pathology.[46,47] Corticobasal degeneration may also present with a dementia of frontal-lobe type in addition to the typical asymmetric akinetic–rigid dystonic syndrome. These three diseases have grown increasingly important because of studies suggesting a linkage to chromosome 17.[12]

Dementia of the frontal and frontal subcortical type is also found in Creutzfeldt–Jakob disease,[38] in the AIDS dementia complex, and in general paresis.

Classification

The Lund–Manchester consensus (Table 2) is recommended as guidelines for clinical recognition of FTD. Guidelines for diagnosis of dementia, such as the NINCDS-ADRDA criteria for diagnosis of Alzheimer's disease,[48] may easily lead to the inclusion of FTD and Pick cases in the Alzheimer's group. DSM-IV presents Pick's disease as 'One of the pathologically distinct etiologies among the heterogeneous group of dementing processes that are associated with frontotemporal brain atrophy. The specific diagnosis of a frontal-lobe dementia such as Pick's disease is usually established at autopsy with a pathological finding of characteristic intraneuronal argentophilic Pick inclusion bodies'. Moreover, the frontal-lobe dementias are 'characterized clinically by changes in personality early in course, deterioration of social skills, emotional blunting, behavioural inhibition, and prominent language abnormalities. Difficulties with memory, apraxia and other features of dementia usually follow later in the course.'[1]

ICD-10[49] describes 'Dementia in Pick's disease' as 'a progressive dementia, commencing in middle life (usually between 50 to 60 years) characterized by slowly progressive changes of character and social deterioration, followed by impairment of intellect memory and language functions with apathy, euphoria and (occasionally) extrapyramidal phenomena. The social and behavioural manifestations often precede frank memory impairment.' ICD-10 points out that Pick's disease is a non-Alzheimer degenerative brain disease, but it does not introduce the concepts of frontal-lobe dementia or FTD.

Aetiology and pathogenesis

The aetiology and pathogenesis of FLD and Pick's disease and the relationship between the diseases are unknown. About 40 to 50 per cent of patients with FLD have a history of similar disorder in a first-degree relative.[18,21] A Swedish pedigree with FTD in 10 out of 21 family members in three generations has been described.[50] Typical FLD was confirmed post-mortem in three cases. There is at present no solid proof of an autosomal dominant inheritance in the majority of studies of Pick's disease. A linkage to chromosome 17q21–22 has been found in 13 families with an autosomal dominantly inherited FTDP-17.[12] The FTDP-17 locus has been mapped to a region where the tau gene also lies. Pathological tau proteins may therefore be of pathophysiological significance in FTD, Alzheimer's disease, and other degenerative dementias.[29] Another possible gene has been indicated by mapping to chromosome 3 in a Danish family with dementia of frontal-lobe type.[51] Conflicting results exist concerning the relation of FLD to chromosome 19 and the ApoE allele pattern has been reported.[52] A prion aetiology has been excluded in FLD and also in FTDP-17.[29] The pattern of degeneration in FTD may be related to selective vulnerability of different brain regions to factors such as oxidative stress, environmental toxins, neurotransmittor dysfunction, and certain mutations.

FTD patients tend to develop low and orthostatic blood pressure, but the pathological changes do not indicate an association with anoxic or ischaemic damage.

There are few systematic neurochemical studies of FTD. No alternations in cholinergic markers have been found in Pick's disease, FLD, or motor neurone disease with dementia.[9,10,20] Nigrostriatal dopamine decrease and reduction of serotonin receptors and substance P levels in substantia nigra and frontal cortex have been found in Pick's disease.[53,54] Cerebrospinal fluid analysis has shown reduced somatostatin levels both in FTD and Alzheimer's disease, while delta-sleep-inducing peptide was significantly reduced in Alzheimer's disease but not in FTD, and the corticotrophin-releasing factor was significantly reduced in FTD but not in Alzheimer's disease.[55] Pathological tau proteins have been found in the frontotemporal cortex in FTD despite the absence of neurofibrillary lesions.[56]

Treatment and care

FTD is a heterogeneous group, but with important clinical features and probably also aetiological factors in common. Early diagnosis is a prerequisite for adequate treatment and care of the patient and for information and support for the family and other carers involved.

There is presently no specific pharmacological treatment for the underlying degenerative disease, but symptomatic treatment may be effective for the patient's anxiety, depressed mood, restlessness, aggressiveness, hallucinations, and delusions. However, the FTD patient may be extremely sensitive to psychotropic medication with disturbing side-effects and paradoxical reactions. The important consequence of the diagnostic process is the possibility of understanding and explaining the patient's strange behaviour, and to differentiate from early-onset Alzheimer's disease for which pharmacological treatment is now available. FTD patients are often restless and show stereotyped movements with a strong need for physical activity, which, as well as the comparatively preserved memory, and spatial and practicable abilities, should be channelled in a meaningful way, rather than restricted. A well-structured programme for daily activities, considering the patient's premorbid personality and interests, may be rewarding and minimize the need for pharmacological treatment. Daily activities should be carried out together with someone well aware of the patient's difficulties to plan, initiate, and control emotions and behaviour. The long duration of the dementing process and the awareness of hereditary factors have a strong impact on family members, who need information, support, and training through many critical years. Prevailing psychotic features and unpredictable aggressive behaviour should managed by special psychiatric or psychogeriatric services for diagnosis, treatment, living, and care.

References

1. American Psychiatric Association (1994). *Diagnostic and statistical manual of mental disorders* (4th edn). American Psychiatric Association, Washington, DC.

2. Brun, A., Englund, E., Gustafson, L., *et al.* (1994). Consensus statement—clinical and neuropathological criteria for frontotemporal dementia. *Journal of Neurology, Neurosurgery and Psychiatry* 57, 416–18.

3. Pick, A. (1892). Über die Beziehungen der senilen Hirnatrophie zur Aphasie. *Prager Medizinische Wochenschrift*, 17, 165–7.

4. Alzheimer, A. (1911). Über eigenartige Krankheitsfälle des späteren Alters. *Zeitschrift für die Gesamte Neurologie und Psychiatrie* 4, 356–85.

5. Schneider, C. (1927). Über Picksche Krankheit. *Monatschrift für Psychiatrie und Neurologie*, 65, 230–75.

6. Brun, A. (1987). Frontal lobe degeneration of non-Alzheimer type. I. Neuropathology. *Archives of Gerontology and Geriatrics*, 6, 193–207.

7. Gustafson, L. (1987). Frontal lobe degeneration of non-Alzheimer type. II. Clinical picture and differential diagnosis. *Archives of Gerontology and Geriatrics*, 6, 209–23.

8. Neary, D., Snowden, J.S., Northern, B., and Goulding, P.J. (1988). Dementia of frontal lobe type. *Journal of Neurology, Neurosurgery and Psychiatry*, 51, 353–61.

9. Knopman, D.S., Mastri, A.R., Frey, W.H., Sung, J.H., and Rustan, T. (1990). Dementia lacking distinctive histologic features. A common non-Alzheimer degenerative dementia. *Neurology*, 40, 251–6.

10. Clark, A.W., White, C.L. III, and Manz, J.H. (1986). Primary degenerative dementia without Alzheimer pathology. *Canadian Journal of Neurological Sciences*, 13, 462–70.

11. Neary, D., Snowden, J.S., and Mann, D.M.A. (1993). The clinical pathological correlates of lobar atrophy. *Dementia*, 4, 154–9.

12. Hutton, M., Lendon, C.L., Rizzu, P., *et al.* (1998). Association of missence and 5′-splice-site mutation in tau with the inherited dementia FTDP-17. *Nature*, 393, 702–5.

13. Delacourte, A., Robitaille, Y., Sergeant, N., *et al.* (1996). Specific pathological tau protein varaints characterize Pick's disease. *Journal of Neuropathology and Experimental Neurology*, 55, 159–68.

14. Brun, A. (1993). Frontal lobe degeneration of non-Alzheimer type, revisited. I. Neuropathology. *Archives of Gerontology and Geriatrics*, 4, 126–31.

15. Englund, E. and Brun, A. (1987). Frontal lobe degeneration of non-Alzheimer type. II. White matter changes. *Archives of Gerontology and Geriatrics*, 6, 235–43.

16. Mitsuyama, Y. (1993). Presenile dementia with motor neuron disease. *Dementia*, 4, 137–42.

17. Jellinger, K., Danielczyk, W., Fischer, P., and Gabriel, E. (1990). Clinicopathological analysis of dementia disorders in the elderly. *Journal of the Neurological Sciences*, 95, 239–58.

18. Gustafson, L. (1993). Clinical picture of frontal lobe degeneration of non-Alzheimer type. *Dementia*, 4, 143–8.

19. Neary, D. (1990). Dementia of frontal lobe type. *Journal of the American Geriatrics Society*. 38, 71–2.

20. Markesbery, W.R. (1998). Pick's disease. In *Neuropathology of dementing disorders* (ed. W.R. Markesbery), pp. 142–57. Arnold, London.

21. Stevens, M., Van Duijn, C.M., Kamphorts, W., *et al.* (1998). Familial aggregation in fronto-temporal dementia, *Neurology*, 50, 1541–5.

22. Pasquier, F., Lebert, F., and Amouyel, P. (1995). In *Les démences frontotemporales, épidémiologie* (ed F. Pasquier and F. Lebert), pp. 23–9. Masson, Paris.

23. Lopez, O.L., Becker, J.T., and De Kosky, S.T. (1994). Dementia accompanying motor neuron disease. *Dementia*, 5, 42–7.

24. Salazar, A.M., Masters, C.L., Gajdusek, D.C., and Gibbs, C.J. (1983). Syndromes of amyotrophic lateral sclerosis and dementia: relation to transmissible Creutzfeldt–Jakob's disease. *Annual Neurology*, 14, 17–26.

25. Lebert, F., Pasquier, F., and Petit, H. (1995). Personality traits and frontal lobe dementia. *International Journal of Geriatric Psychiatry*, 10, 1046–9.

26. Cummings, J.L. and Duchen, L.W. (1981). Klüver–Bucy syndrome in Pick's disease: clinical and pathological correlations. *Neurology*, 31, 1415–22.

27. Van Mansfelt, J. (1954). Pick's disease. A syndrome of lobar, cerebral atrophy; its clinico-anatomical and histopathological types. Unpublished Thesis, Enschede, Utrecht.

28. Lynch, T., Sano, M., Marder, K.S., *et al.* (1994). Clinical characteristics of a family with chromosome 17-linked disinhibition–dementia–parkinsonism–amyotrophy complex. *Neurology*, 44, 1878–84.

29. Foster, N.L., Wilhelmsen, K., Sima, A.A.F., Jones, M.Z., D'Amato, C., and Gildman, S. (1997). Frontotemporal dementia and parkinsonism linked to chromosome 17: a consensus. *Annals of Neurology*, 41, 706–15.

30. Passant, U., Warkentin, S., and Gustafson, L. (1997). Orthostatic hypotension and low blood pressure in organic dementia: a study of prevalence and related clinical characteristics. *International Journal of Geriatric Psychiatry*, 12, 395–403.

31. Neary, D., Snowden, J.S., and Mann, D.M.A. (1990). Frontal lobe dementia and motor neuron disease. *Journal of Neurology, Neurosurgery and Psychiatry*, 53, 23–32.

32. Rosén, I., Gustafson, L., and Risberg, J. (1993). Multichannel EEG frequency analysis and somatosensory-evoked potentials in patients with different types of organic dementia. *Dementia*, 4, 43–9.

33. Förstl, H., Hentschel, F., Besthorn, C., *et al.* (1994). Frontal und temporal beginnende Hirnatrophie. *Nervenarzt*, 65, 611–18.

34. Larsson, E.-M., Passant, U., Sundgren, P.C., *et al.* Magnetic resonance imaging and histopathology in dementia, clinically of frontotemporal type. *Dementia and Geriatric Cognitive Disorders*, in press.

35. Risberg, J. and Gustafson, L. (1997). Regional cerebral blood flow measurements in the clinical evaluation of demented patients. *Dementia and Geriatric Cognitive Disorders*, 8, 92–7.

36. Miller, B.L., Laurent, I., Li, J., *et al.* (1995). Atrophy-corrected cerebral blood flow in frontotemporal dementia. In *Facts and research in geriatrics* (ed. A. Bruno, F. Chollet, and B.J. Vellas), pp. 93–103. Springer, New York.

37. Ludolph, A.C., Langen, K.J., Regard, M., *et al.* (1992). Frontal lobe function in amyotrophic lateral sclerosis: an neuropatholgoical and positron emission tomography study. *Acta Neurologica Scandinavica*, 82, 81–9.

38. Brun, A. and Gustafson, L. (1991). Psychopathology and frontal lobe involvement in organic dementia. In *Alzheimer's disease: basic mechanisms, diagnosis and therapeutic strategies* (ed. K. Iqbal, D.R.C. McLachlan, B. Winblad, and H.M. Wisnewski), pp. 27–33. Wiley, Chichester.

39. Johanson, A. and Hagberg, B. (1989). Psychometric characteristics in patients with frontal lobe degeneration of non-Alzheimer type. *Archives of Gerontology and Geriatrics*, 8, 29–137.

40. Frisoni, G.B., Pizzolato, G., Geroldi, C., Rossato, A., Bianchetti, A., and Trabuceti, M. (1995). Dementia of the frontal type: neuropsychological

and (99Tc)-HMPAO SPET features. *Journal of Geriatric Psychiatry and Neurology*, **8**, 42–8.

41. Elfgren, C., Brun, A., Gustafson, L., *et al.* (1994). Neuropsychological tests as discriminators between dementia of Alzheimer type and frontotemporal dementia. *International Journal of Geriatric Psychiatry*, **9**, 635–42.

42. Gregory, C.A., Orrell, M., Sahakian, B., and Hodges, J.R. (1997). Can frontotemporal dementia and Alzheimer's disease be differentiated using a brief battery of tests? *International Journal of Geriatric Psychiatry*, **12**, 375–83.

43. Folstein, M.F., Folstein, S.E., and McHugh, P.R. (1975). 'Mini-Mental State'. A practical method for grading the cognitive state of patients for the clinician. *Journal of Psychiatric Research*, **12**, 189–98.

44. Pasquier, F. (1996). Neuropsychological features and cognitive assessment in frontotemporal dementia. In *Frontotemporal dementia* (ed. D. Pasquier, F. Lebert, and P. Scheltens), pp. 46–69. ICG, The Netherlands.

45. Benson, D.F. (1993). Progressive frontal dysfunction. *Dementia*, **4**, 149–53.

46. Esmonde, T., Giles, E., Xuereb, J., and Hodges, J. (1996). Progressive supranuclear palsy presenting with dynamic aphasia. *Journal of Neurology, Neurosurgery and Psychiatry*, **60**, 403–10.

47. d'Antona, R., Baron, J.C., Samson, Y., *et al.* (1985). Subcortical dementia. *Brain*, **108**, 785–99.

48. McKhann, G., Drachmann, D.A., Folstein, M., Katzmann, R., Price, D., and Stadlan, E.M. (1984). Clinical diagnosis of Alzheimer's disease: report of the NINCDS-ADRDA Work Group. *Neurology*, **34**, 939–44.

49. World Health Organization (1992). *The ICD-10 classification of mental and behavioural disorders. Clinical descriptions and diagnostic guidelines.* World Health Organization, Geneva.

50. Passant, U., Gustafson, L., and Brun, A. (1993). Spectrum of frontal lobe dementia in a Swedish Family. *Dementia*, **4**, 160–2.

51. Brown, J., Asworth, A., Gydesen, S., *et al.* (1995). Familial non-specific dementia maps to chromosome 3. *Human Molecular Genetics*, **4**, 1625–8.

52. Pickering-Brown, S.M., Siddons, M., Mann, D.M.A., Owen, F., Neary, D., and Snowden, J.S. (1995). Apolipoprotein E allelic frequencies in patients with lobar atrophy. *Neuroscience Letters*, **188**, 205–7.

53. Kanazawa, I., Kwak, S., Sasaki, H., *et al.* (1988). Studies on neurotransmitter markers of the basal ganglia in Pick's disease, with special reference to dopamine reduction. *Journal of the Neurological Sciences*, **83**, 63–74.

54. Francis, P.T., Holmes, C., Webster, M-T., Stratmann, G.C., Procter, A.W., and Bowen, D.M. (1993). Preliminary neurochemical findings in non-Alzheimer dementia due to lobar atrophy. *Dementia*, **4**, 172–7.

55. Edvinsson, L., Minthon, L., Ekman, R., and Gustafson, L. (1993). Neuropeptides in cerebrospinal fluid of patients with Alzheimer's disease and dementia in frontotemporal lobe degeneration. *Dementia*, **4**, 167–71.

56. Vermersch, P., David, J.P., Frigard, B., *et al.* (1995). Cortical mapping of Alzheimer pathology in brains of aged non-demented subjects. *Neuropsychopharmacology and Biological Psychiatry*, **19**, 1035–47.

4.1.5 Prion disease

John Collinge

Introduction

The human prion diseases, also known as the subacute spongiform encephalopathies, have been traditionally classified into Creutzfeldt–Jakob disease (**CJD**), Gerstmann–Sträussler syndrome (**GSS**) (also known as Gerstmann–Sträussler–Scheinker disease), and kuru. Although rare, affecting about one person per million worldwide per annum, remarkable attention has been recently focused on these diseases. This is because of the unique biology of the transmissible agent or prion, and also because bovine spongiform encephalopathy (**BSE**), an epidemic bovine prion disease, appears to have transmitted to humans as 'new variant' CJD (**vCJD**), opening the possibility of a significant threat to public health through dietary exposure to infected tissues.

The transmissibility of the human diseases was demonstrated with the transmission, by intracerebral inoculation with brain homogenates into chimpanzees, of first kuru and then CJD in 1966 and 1968 respectively.[1,2] Transmission of GSS followed in 1981. The prototypic prion disease is scrapie, a naturally occurring disease of sheep and goats, which has been recognized in Europe for over 200 years[3] and which is present in the sheep flocks of many countries. Scrapie was demonstrated to be transmissible by inoculation in 1936[4] and the recognition that kuru, and then CJD, resembled scrapie in its histopathological appearances led to the suggestion that these diseases may also be transmissible.[5] Kuru reached epidemic proportions amongst the Fore linguistic group in the Eastern Highlands of Papua New Guinea and was transmitted by ritual cannibalism. Since the cessation of cannibalism in the 1950s the disease has declined but a few cases still occur as a result of the long incubation periods in this condition. The term Creutzfeldt–Jakob disease was introduced by Spielmeyer in 1922 bringing together the case reports published by Creutzfeldt and Jakob. Several of these cases would not meet modern diagnostic criteria for CJD and indeed it was not until the demonstration of transmissibility allowed diagnostic criteria to be reassessed and refined that a clear diagnostic entity developed. All these diseases share common histopathological features; the classical triad of spongiform vacuolation (affecting any part of the cerebral grey matter), astrocytic proliferation, and neuronal loss may be accompanied by the deposition of amyloid plaques.[6]

Aetiology

Prion diseases of both humans and animals are associated with the accumulation in the brain of an abnormal, partially protease-resistant, isoform of a host-encoded glycoprotein known as prion protein (PrP). The disease-related isoform, PrP^{Sc}, is derived from its normal cellular precursor, PrP^{C}, by a post-translational process that involves a conformational change. PrP^{C} is rich in α-helical structure while PrP^{Sc} appears to be predominantly composed of β-sheet structure. According to the 'protein-only' hypothesis,[7] an abnormal PrP isoform[8] is the principal, and possibly the sole, constituent of the transmissible agent or prion. PrP^{Sc} is hypothesized to act as a conformational template, promoting the conversion of PrP^{C} to further PrP^{Sc}. PrP^{C} appears to be poised between two radically different folding states, and α and β forms of PrP can be interconverted in suitable conditions.[9] Soluble β-PrP aggregates in physiological salt concentrations to form fibrils with morphological and biochemical characteristics closely similar to PrP^{Sc}. A molecular mechanism for prion propagation can now be proposed.[9] Prion replication, with recruitment of PrP^{C} into the aggregated PrP^{Sc} isoform, may be initiated by a pathogenic mutation (resulting in a PrP^{C} predisposed to form β-PrP) in inherited prion diseases, by exposure to a 'seed' of PrP^{Sc} in acquired cases, or as a result of the spontaneous conversion of PrP^C to β-PrP (and subsequent formation of aggregated material) as a rare stochastic event in sporadic prion disease.

The human PrP gene (*PRNP*) is a single-copy gene located on the short arm of chromosome 20 and was an obvious candidate for genetic linkage studies in the familial forms of CJD and GSS, which both showed an autosomal dominant pattern of disease segregation. A turning point in understanding the human prion diseases was the identification of mutations in the prion protein gene in familial CJD and GSS in 1989. The first mutation to be identified in *PRNP* was in a family with CJD and constituted a 144-bp insertion into the coding sequence.[10] A second mutation was reported in two families with GSS and genetic linkage was confirmed between this missense variant at codon 102 and GSS, confirming that GSS was an autosomal dominant Mendelian disorder.[11] Uniquely, these diseases are therefore both inherited and transmissible. Current evidence suggests that around 15 per cent of prion diseases are inherited and at least 20 coding mutations in *PRNP* are now recognized.[12]

With the exception of the rare iatrogenic CJD cases mentioned above, most prion disease occurs as sporadic CJD. While, by definition, there will not be a family history in sporadic cases, mutations are seen in occasional apparently sporadic cases, as with a late-onset disease the family history may not be apparent or non-paternity may occur. However, in the majority of sporadic CJD cases there is neither a coding mutation nor a history of iatrogenic exposure. Human prion diseases can therefore be subdivided into inherited, sporadic, and acquired forms. However, a common PrP polymorphism at residue 129, where either methionine or valine can be encoded, is a key determinant of genetic susceptibility to acquired and sporadic prion diseases, the large majority of which occur in homozygous individuals.[13,14] This protective effect of *PRNP* codon 129 heterozygosity is also seen in some of the inherited prion diseases.[15,16]

The aetiology of sporadic CJD remains unclear. It has been speculated that these cases might arise from somatic mutation of *PRNP* or spontaneous conversion of PrP^C to PrP^Sc as a rare stochastic event. The alternative hypothesis, that such cases arise as a result of exposure to an environmental source of either human or animal prions, is not supported by epidemiological evidence.[17]

A major problem for the 'protein-only' hypothesis of prion propagation has been how to explain the existence of multiple isolates or strains of prions which have distinct biological properties. Understanding how a protein-only infectious agent could encode such phenotypic information has been of considerable biological interest. However, it is now clear that prion strains can be distinguished by differences in the biochemical properties of PrP^Sc. Prion strain diversity appears to encoded by differences in PrP conformation and pattern of glycosylation.[18] A molecular strain typing approach based on these characteristics has allowed the identification of four main types amongst CJD cases, sporadic and iatrogenic CJD being of PrP^Sc types 1–3, while all vCJD cases are associated with a distinctive type 4 PrP^Sc type.[18,19] A similar PrP^Sc type to that seen in vCJD is seen in BSE and BSE when transmitted to several other species.[18] Such molecular strain typing strongly supported the hypothesis that vCJD was human BSE. This conclusion was strengthened by subsequent transmission studies of vCJD into both transgenic and conventional mice which argued that cattle BSE and vCJD were caused by the same strain.[20,21] Such studies are allowing a molecular classification of human prion diseases; it is likely that additional PrP^Sc types or strains will be identified. This may well open new avenues of epidemiological investigation and offer insights into causes of 'sporadic' CJD. The ability of a protein to encode a disease phenotype has important implications in biology, as it represents a non-Mendelian form of transmission. It would be surprising if this mechanism had not been used more widely during evolution such that prion biology may prove to be of far wider relevance.

Transmission of prion diseases between different mammalian species is limited by a so-called 'species barrier'.[22] Early studies of the molecular basis of the species barrier argued that it principally resided in differences in PrP primary structure between the species from which the inoculum was derived and the inoculated host. Transgenic mice expressing hamster PrP were, unlike wild-type mice, highly susceptible to infection with hamster prions.[23] That most sporadic and acquired CJD occurred in individuals homozygous at *PRNP* polymorphic codon 129 supported the view that prion propagation proceeded most efficiently when the interacting PrP^Sc and PrP^C were of identical primary structure.[13,14] However, it has been long recognized that prion strain type affects ease of transmission to another species. Interestingly, with BSE prions the strain component to the barrier seems to predominate, with BSE not only transmitting efficiently to a range of species, but maintaining its transmission characteristics even when passaged through an intermediate species with a distinct PrP gene.[24,20] The term 'species–strain barrier' or simply 'transmission barrier' may be preferable.[25] Both PrP amino acid sequence and strain type affect the three-dimensional structure of glycosylated PrP which will presumably, in turn, affect the efficiency of the protein–protein interactions thought to determine prion propagation. Contribution of other components to the species barrier are possible and may involve interacting cofactors which mediate the efficiency of prion propagation, although no such factors have yet been identified.

The species barrier between cattle BSE and humans cannot be directly measured but can be modelled in transgenic mice expressing human PrP^C, which produce human PrP^Sc when challenged with human prions.[26] When such mice, expressing both human PrP valine 129 (at high levels) and mouse PrP, are challenged with BSE, three possibilities could be envisaged: these mice could produce human prions, murine prions, or both. In fact, only mouse prion replication could be detected. Although there are caveats with respect to this model, particularly that human prion propagation in mouse cells may be less efficient that that of mouse prions, this result would be consistent with the bovine to human barrier being higher than the bovine to mouse barrier for this *PRNP* genotype. In the second phase of these experiments, mice expressing only human PrP were challenged with BSE. While CJD isolates transmit efficiently to such mice at around 200 days, only infrequent transmissions at over 500 days were seen with BSE, consistent with a substantial species barrier for this human *PRNP* genotype.[27] However, it is important to repeat these studies in mice expressing only human PrP methionine 129 and in heterozygotes. So far, BSE appears to have transmitted only to humans of *PRNP* codon 129 methionine homozygous genotype.

Clinical features and diagnosis

The human prion diseases can be divided aetiologically into inherited, sporadic, and acquired forms with CJD, GSS, and kuru now seen as clinicopathological syndromes within a wider spectrum of disease.

Kindreds with inherited prion disease have been described with phenotypes of classical CJD, GSS, and also with other neurodegenerative syndromes including fatal familial insomnia.[28] Some kindreds show remarkable phenotypic variability which can encompass both CJD- and GSS-like cases as well as other cases which do not conform to either CJD or GSS phenotypes.[29] Cases diagnosed by PrP gene analysis have been reported which are not only clinically atypical but which lack the classical histological features entirely.[30] Significant clinical overlap exists with familial Alzheimer's disease, Pick's disease, frontal lobe degeneration of non-Alzheimer type, and amyotrophic lateral sclerosis with dementia. Although classical GSS is described below it now seems more sensible to designate the familial illnesses as inherited prion diseases and then to subclassify these according to mutation. Acquired prion diseases include iatrogenic CJD, kuru, and now vCJD. Sporadic prion diseases at present consist of CJD and atypical variants of CJD. Cases lacking the characteristic histological features of CJD have been transmitted. As there are at present no equivalent aetiological diagnostic markers for sporadic prion diseases to those for the inherited diseases, it cannot yet be excluded that more diverse phenotypic variants of sporadic prion disease exist. The key clinical features and investigations for the diagnosis of prion disease are given in Table 1.

Sporadic prion disease

Creutzfeldt–Jakob disease

The core clinical syndrome of classic CJD is of a rapidly progressive multifocal dementia usually with myoclonus. The onset is usually in the 45- to 75-year age group with peak onset between 60 and 65. The clinical progression is typically over weeks progressing to akinetic mutism and death often in 2 to 3 months. Around 70 per cent of cases die in under 6 months. Prodromal features, present in around a third of cases, include fatigue, insomnia, depression, weight loss, headaches, general malaise, and ill-defined pain sensations. In addition to mental deterioration and myoclonus, frequent additional neurological features include extrapyramidal signs, cerebellar ataxia, pyramidal signs, and cortical blindness. About 10 per cent of cases present initially with cerebellar ataxia.

Routine haematological and biochemical investigations are normal although occasional cases have been noted to have raised serum transaminases or alkaline phosphatase. There are no immunological markers and acute-phase proteins are not elevated. Examination of the cerebrospinal fluid is normal although raised neuronal specific enolase and S-100 have both been proposed as useful markers, although it is clear that they are not specific for CJD and represent markers of neuronal injury.[31–33] A promising cerebrospinal fluid marker is estimation of 14-3-3 protein, which, while again not a specific disease marker, appears to be a useful adjunct to diagnosis in the appropriate clinical context.[34,35] It is also positive in recent cerebral infarction or haemorrhage and in viral encephalitis, although these conditions do not usually present diagnostic confusion with CJD. Neuroimaging with CT or magnetic resonance imaging (**MRI**) is useful to exclude other causes of subacute neurological illness but there are no diagnostic features; cerebral and cerebellar atrophy may be present. The EEG may, however, show characteristic pseudoperiodic sharp wave activity which is helpful in diagnosis but present only in around 70 per cent of cases. To some extent demonstration of a typical EEG is dependent on the num-

Table 1 Diagnosis of prion disease

Sporadic (classical) CJD

Rapidly progressive dementia with two or more of myoclonus, cortical blindness, pyramidal signs, cerebellar signs, extrapyramidal signs, akinetic mutism

Most cases age 45–75

Serial EEG shows pseudoperiodic complexes in most cases

CSF 14-3-3 protein usually positive

CT and MRI normal, or atrophy, or abnormal signal basal ganglia

PRNP analysis: no pathogenic mutations, most are 129 homozygotes

Brain biopsy in highly selected cases (to exclude treatable alernative diagnoses): PrP immunocytochemistry or Western blot for PrP^{Sc} types 1–3

Iatrogenic CJD

Progressive cerebellar syndrome and behavioural disturbance or classical CJD-like syndrome with history of iatrogenic exposure to human prions (pituitary-derived hormones, tissue grafting, or neurosurgery)

May be young

EEG, CSF, and MRI generally less helpful than in sporadic cases

PRNP analysis: no pathogenic mutations, most are 129 homozygotes

Brian biopsy in highly selected cases (to exclude treatable alternative diagnoses): PrP immunocytochemistry or Western blot for PrP^{Sc} types 1–3

Variant CJD (human BSE)

Early features: depression, anxiety, social withdrawal, peripheral sensory symptoms

Cerebellar ataxia, chorea, or athetosis often precedes dementia; advanced disease as sporadic CJD

Most cases in young adults

EEG non-specific slow waves, CSF 14-3-3 may be elevated

MRI: may be high T$_2$-weighted signal in posterior thalamus bilaterally

PRNP analysis: no mutations, all 129MM to date

Tonsil biopsy: characteristic PrP immunostaining and PrP^{Sc} on Western blot (type 4t)

Inherited prion disease

Varied clinical syndromes between and within kindreds; should consider in all presenile dementias and ataxias irrespective of family history

PRNP analysis: diagnostic, codon 129 genotype may predict age at onset in presymptomatic testing

ber of EEGs performed, and serial EEG is indicated to try and demonstrate this appearance.

Prospective epidemiological studies have demonstrated that cases with a progressive dementia, and two or more of the following: myoclonus, cortical blindness, pyramidal, cerebellar, or extrapyramidal signs, or akinetic mutism, in the setting of a typical EEG, nearly always turn out to be confirmed as histologically definite CJD if neuropathological examination is performed.

Neuropathological confirmation of CJD is by demonstration of spongiform change, neuronal loss, and astrocytosis. PrP amyloid plaques are usually not present in CJD although PrP immunohistochemistry, using appropriate pretreatments,[36] will nearly always be positive. Protease-resistant PrP, seen in all the currently recognized prion diseases, can be demonstrated by immunoblotting of brain homogenates. *PRNP* analysis is important to exclude pathogenic mutations. Genetic susceptibility to CJD has been demonstrated in that most cases of classical CJD are homozygous with respect to the common 129 polymorphism of PrP (see discussion of aetiology above).

Atypical forms of Creutzfeldt–Jakob disease

Atypical forms of CJD are well recognized. Around 10 per cent of cases of CJD have a much more prolonged clinical course with a disease duration of over 2 years.[37] These cases may represent the occasional occurrence of CJD in individuals heterozygous for PrP polymorphisms.[38] Around 10 per cent of CJD cases present with cerebellar ataxia rather than cognitive impairment, so-called ataxic CJD.[39] Heidenhain's variant of CJD refers to cases in which cortical blindness predominates with severe involvement of the occipital lobes. The panencephalopathic type of CJD refers to cases with extensive degeneration of the cerebral white matter in addition to spongiform vacuolation of the grey matter and has been predominantly reported from Japan.[39]

Amyotrophic variants of CJD have been described with prominent early muscle wasting. However, most cases of dementia with amyotrophy are not experimentally transmissible[40] and their relationship with CJD is unclear. Most cases are probably variants of motor neurone disease with associated dementia. Amyotrophic features in CJD are usually seen in late disease when other features are well established.

Acquired prion diseases

While human prion diseases can be transmitted to experimental animals by inoculation, they are not contagious in humans. Documented case-to-case spread has only occurred during ritual cannibalistic practices (kuru) or following accidental inoculation with prions during medical or surgical procedures (iatrogenic CJD).

Kuru

Kuru reached epidemic proportions amongst a defined population living in the Eastern Highlands of Papua New Guinea. The earliest cases are thought to date back to the early part of the century. Kuru affected the people of the Fore linguistic group and their neighbours with whom they intermarried. Kuru predominantly affected women and children (of both sexes), with only 2 per cent of cases in adult males[41] and was the most common cause of death amongst women in affected villages. It was the practice in these communities to engage in consumption of dead relatives as a mark of respect and mourning. Women and children predominantly ate the brain and internal organs, which is thought to explain the differential age and sex incidence. Preparation of the cadaver for consumption was performed by the women and children such that other routes of exposure may also have been relevant. It is thought that the epidemic related to a single sporadic CJD case occurring in the region some decades earlier. Epidemiological studies provided no evidence for vertical transmission, since most of the children born after 1956 (when cannibalism had effectively ceased) and all of those born after 1959 of mothers affected with or incubating kuru were unaffected.[41] From the age of the youngest affected patient, the shortest incubation period is estimated as 4.5 years, although may have been shorter, since time of infection was usually unknown. Currently, two to three cases are occurring annually, all in individuals aged 40 or more, consistent with exposure prior to 1956

and indicating that incubation periods can be 40 years or more (unpublished data).

Kuru affects both sexes and onset of disease has ranged from age 5 to over 60. The mean clinical duration of illness is 12 months with a range of 3 months to 3 years; the course tends to be shorter in children. The central clinical feature is progressive cerebellar ataxia. In sharp contrast to CJD, dementia is usually absent, even in the latter stages, although in the terminal stages many patients have their faculties obtunded.[41] The occasional case in which gross dementia occurs is in marked contrast to the clinical norm. Detailed clinical descriptions have been given by a number of observers and the disease does not appear to have changed in features at different stages of the epidemic. A prodrome and three clinical stages are recognized as follows.

Prodromal stage
Kuru typically begins with prodromal symptoms consisting of headache, aching of limbs, and joint pains which can last for several months.

Ambulatory stage
Kuru was frequently self-diagnosed by patients at the earliest onset of unsteadiness in standing or walking, or of dysarthria or diplopia. At this stage there may be no objective signs of disease. Gait ataxia, however, worsens and patients develop a broad-based gait, truncal instability, and titubation. A coarse postural tremor is usually present and accentuated by movement; patients characteristically hold their hands together in the midline to suppress this. Standing with feet together reveals clawing of toes to maintain posture. This marked clawing response is regarded as pathognomonic of kuru. Patients often become withdrawn at this stage and occasionally develop a severe reactive depression. Prodromal symptoms tend to disappear. Astasia and gait ataxia worsen and the patient requires a stick for walking. Intention tremor, dysmetria, hypotonia, and dysdiadochokinesis develop. Although eye movements are ataxic and jerky, nystagmus is rarely seen. Strabismus, usually convergent, may occur particularly in children. This strabismus does not appear to be concomitant or paralytic and may fluctuate in both extent and type sometimes disappearing later in the clinical course. Photophobia is common and there may be an abnormal cold sensitivity with shivering and piloerection even in a warm environment. Tendon reflexes are reduced or normal and plantar responses are flexor. Dysarthria usually occurs. As ataxia progresses the patient passes from the first (ambulatory) stage to the second (sedentary) stage. The mean clinical duration of the first stage is around 8 months and correlates closely with total duration.[42]

Sedentary stage
At this stage patients are able to sit unsupported but cannot walk. Attempted walking with support leads to a high steppage, wide-based gait with reeling instability, and flinging arm movements in an attempt to maintain posture. Hyper-reflexia is seen although plantar responses usually remain flexor with intact abdominal reflexes. Clonus is characteristically short-lived. Athetoid and choreiform movements and parkinsonian tremors may occur. There is no paralysis, although muscle power is reduced. Obesity is common at this stage but may be present in early disease associated with bulimia. Characteristically, there is emotional lability and bizarre uncontrollable laughter, which has led to the disease being referred to as 'laughing death'. There is no sensory impairment. In sharp contrast to CJD, myoclonic jerking is rarely seen. EEG is usually normal or may show non-specific changes.[43] This

stage lasts around 2 to 3 months. When truncal ataxia reaches the point where the patient is unable to sit unsupported, the third or tertiary stage is reached.

Tertiary stage

Hypotonia and hyporeflexia develop and the terminal state is marked by flaccid muscle weakness. Plantar responses remain flexor and abdominal reflexes intact. Progressive dysphagia occurs, and patients become incontinent of urine and faeces. Inanition and emaciation develop. Transient conjugate eye signs and dementia may occur. Primitive reflexes develop in occasional cases. Brainstem involvement and both bulbar and pseudobulbar signs occur. Respiratory failure and bronchopneumonia eventually lead to death. The tertiary stage lasts 1 to 2 months.

Iatrogenic Creutzfeldt–Jakob disease

Iatrogenic transmission of CJD has occurred by accidental inoculation with human prions as a result of medical procedures. Such iatrogenic routes include the use of inadequately sterilized neurosurgical instruments, dura mater and corneal grafting, and use of human cadaveric pituitary-derived growth hormone or gonadotrophin. It is of considerable interest that cases arising from intracerebral or optic inoculation manifest clinically as classical CJD, with a rapidly progressive dementia, while those resulting from peripheral inoculation, most notably following pituitary-derived growth hormone exposure, typically present with a progressive cerebellar syndrome, and are in that respect somewhat reminiscent of kuru. Unsurprisingly the incubation period in intracerebral cases is short (19–46 months for dura mater grafts) as compared with peripheral cases (typically 15 years or more). There is evidence for genetic susceptibility to iatrogenic CJD with an excess of codon 129 homozygotes[13] (see discussion of aetiology above).

Epidemiological studies have not shown increased risks of particular occupations that may be exposed to human or animal prions, although individual CJD cases in two histopathology technicians, a neuropathologist, and a neurosurgeon have been documented. While there have been concerns that CJD may be transmissible by blood transfusion, extensive epidemiological analysis in the United Kingdom has found that the frequency of blood transfusion and donation was no different in over 200 cases of CJD and a matched control population.[44] Recipients of blood transfusions who developed CJD had clinical presentations similar to those of sporadic CJD patients and not to the more kuru-like iatrogenic cases arising from peripheral exposure to human prions. Furthermore, experimental transmission studies have shown only weak evidence for infectivity in blood,[45] even when inoculated via the most efficient (intracerebral) route. It cannot be assumed that the same picture will hold for vCJD as this is caused by a distinct prion strain[18] from those causing classical CJD and has a distinct pathogenesis.[46] It is also conceivable that many individuals could currently be incubating this disease.

New variant of human prion disease

In late 1995, two cases of sporadic CJD were reported in the United Kingdom in teenagers.[47,48] Only four cases of sporadic CJD had previously been recorded in teenagers, and none of these cases occurred in the United Kingdom. In addition, both cases were unusual in having kuru-type plaques, a finding seen in only around 5 per cent of CJD

cases. Soon afterwards a third very young sporadic CJD case occurred.[49] These cases caused considerable concern and the possibility was raised that they might suggest a link with BSE. It was clearly of some importance to see if any further such extraordinarily rare cases occurred in the United Kingdom. By March 1996, further extremely young onset cases were apparent and review of the histology of these cases showed a remarkably consistent and unique pattern. These cases were named 'new variant' CJD although it was clear that they were also rather atypical in their clinical presentation; in fact most cases did not meet the accepted clinical diagnostic criteria for probable CJD. Extensive studies of archival cases of CJD or other prion diseases failed to show this picture and it seemed that it did represent the arrival of a new form of prion disease in the United Kingdom. The statistical probability of such cases occurring by chance was vanishingly small and ascertainment bias seemed most unlikely as an explanation. It was clear that a new risk factor for CJD had emerged and appeared to be specific to the United Kingdom. The United Kingdom government Spongiform Encephalopathy Advisory Committee concluded that, while there was no direct evidence for a link with BSE, exposure to specified bovine offal prior to the ban on its inclusion in human foodstuffs in 1989, was the most likely explanation. A case of vCJD was soon after reported in France.[50] Direct experimental evidence that vCJD is caused by BSE was provided by molecular analysis of human prion strains and transmission studies in transgenic and wild-type mice (see aetiology). While it is now clear that vCJD is human BSE, it is unclear why this particular age group should be affected and why none of these cases had a pattern of unusual occupational or dietary exposure to BSE. However, very little is known of which foodstuffs contained high-titre bovine offal. It is possible that certain foods containing particularly high titres were eaten predominately by younger people. An alternative is that young people are more susceptible to BSE following dietary exposure or that they have shorter incubation periods. It is important to appreciate that BSE-contaminated feed was fed to sheep, pigs, and poultry and that although there is no evidence of natural transmission to these species, it would be prudent to remain open minded about other dietary exposure to novel animal prions.

The clinical presentation is with behavioural and psychiatric disturbances and in some cases with sensory disturbance.[51] Initial referral is usually to a psychiatrist and the most prominent feature is depression, but anxiety, withdrawal, and behavioural change is also frequent.[52] Suicidal ideation is infrequent and response to antidepressants poor. Delusions, which are complex and unsustained, are common. Other features include emotional lability, aggression, insomnia, and auditory and visual hallucinations. A prominent early feature in some was dysaesthesiae or pain in the limbs or face or pain which was persistent rather than intermittent and unrelated to anxiety levels. A minority of cases have been noted to have forgetfulness or mild gait ataxia from an early stage, but in most cases overt neurological features are not apparent until some months into the clinical course.[53] In most patients a progressive cerebellar syndrome develops with gait and limb ataxia. Dementia usually developed later in the clinical course with progression to akinetic mutism in the majority of cases. Myoclonus was seen in most patients, in some cases preceded by chorea. Cortical blindness develops in a minority of patients in the late stages of disease. Upgaze paresis, an uncommon feature of classical CJD, has been noted in some patients.[53] The age at onset in the initial 14 cases reported ranged from 16 to 48 years (mean 29 years) and the clinical course was unusually prolonged (9–35 months, median 14 months). The EEG is abnormal, most frequently showing generalized slow-wave activity, but without the pseudoperiodic pattern seen in most sporadic CJD cases. Neuroimaging by CT is either normal or shows only mild atrophy. However, a high signal in the posterior thalamus on T_2-weighted MRI is seen in a proportion of cases.[46,53] The sensitivity and specificity of this sign is unclear at present. Cerebrospinal fluid 14-3-3 protein may be elevated. PrP gene analysis showed that all cases available for study were homozygous for methionine at codon 129. No known or novel pathogenic mutations were found in the coding sequence.[54] Recently it has become clear that vCJD can be diagnosed by detection of characteristic PrP immunostaining and PrP^{Sc}.[46,55] It has long been recognized that prion replication, in experimentally infected animals, is first detectable in the lymphoreticular system, considerably earlier than the onset of neurological symptoms. Importantly, PrP^{Sc} is only detectable in vCJD, and not other forms of human prion disease studied. The PrP^{Sc} type detected on Western blot in vCJD tonsil has a characteristic pattern designated type 4t.[46] A positive tonsil biopsy obviates the need for brain biopsy which may otherwise be considered in such a clinical context to exclude alternative, potentially treatable diagnoses.

The neuropathological appearances of vCJD are striking and consistent. While there is widespread spongiform change, gliosis, and neuronal loss, most severe in the basal ganglia and thalamus, the most remarkable feature was the abundant PrP amyloid plaques in cerebral and cerebellar cortex. These consisted of kuru-like, 'florid' (surrounded by spongiform vacuoles), and multicentric plaque types. The 'florid' plaques, seen previously only in scrapie, were a particularly unusual but highly consistent feature. There was also abundant pericellular PrP deposition in the cerebral and cerebellar cortex. A further highly unusual feature was the extensive PrP deposition in the molecular layer of the cerebellum.

Some of the features of vCJD are reminiscent of kuru, in which behavioural changes and progressive ataxia predominate. In addition, peripheral sensory disturbances are well recognized in the kuru prodrome. Kuru plaques are seen in around 70 per cent of cases and are especially abundant in younger kuru cases. The observation that iatrogenic prion disease related to peripheral exposure to human prions has a more kuru-like than CJD-like clinical picture may well be relevant and would be consistent with a peripheral prion exposure.

The relatively stereotyped clinical presentation and neuropathology of vCJD contrasts sharply with sporadic CJD. This may be because vCJD is caused by a single prion strain and may also suggest that a relatively homogeneous genetically susceptible subgroup of the population with short incubation periods to BSE has been selected to date.

Inherited prion diseases

Gerstmann–Sträussler–Scheinker disease

The first case was described by Gerstmann in 1928 and was followed by a more detailed report on seven other affected members of the same family in 1936.[56] The classical presentation of GSS is with a chronic cerebellar ataxia accompanied by pyramidal features, with dementia occurring later in a much more prolonged clinical course than that seen in CJD. The mean duration is around 5 years, with onset usually in either the third or fourth decades. Histologically, the hallmark is the presence of multicentric amyloid plaques. Spongiform change, neuronal loss, astrocytosis, and white-matter loss are also usually present.

Numerous GSS kindreds from several countries (including the original Austrian family described by Gerstmann, Sträussler, and Scheinker in 1936) have now been demonstrated to have mutations in the PrP gene. GSS is an autosomal dominant disorder which can now be classified within the spectrum of inherited prion disease.

Classification and clinical features of inherited prion diseases

The identification of one of the pathogenic PrP gene mutations in a case with neurodegenerative disease allows not only molecular diagnosis of an inherited prion disease but also its subclassification according to mutation. Pathogenic mutations reported to date in the human PrP gene consist of two groups:

(1) point mutations within the coding sequence resulting in amino acid substitutions in PrP or in one case production of a stop codon resulting in expression of a truncated PrP;

(2) insertions encoding additional integral copies of an octapeptide repeat present in a tandem array of five copies in the normal protein.

A suggested notation for these diseases is 'inherited prion disease (PrP mutation)', for instance: inherited prion disease (PrP 144-bp insertion) or inherited prion disease (PrP P102L).

Missense mutations

PrP P102L This mutation was first reported in 1989 in a British and North American family and has now been demonstrated in many other kindreds worldwide. Progressive ataxia is the dominant clinical feature, with dementia and pyramidal features. However, marked variability both at the clinical and neuropathological level is apparent in some families, and has recently been extensively documented in the original Austrian GSS family.[57] A family with marked amyotrophic features has also been reported.[58] Cases with severe dementia in the absence of prominent ataxia are also recognized. Histological examination reveals PrP immunoreactive plaques in the majority of cases. Transmissibility to experimental animals has been demonstrated.

PrP P105L The Pro–Leu change at codon 105 has been found in four patients from three Japanese families.[59] It has not been reported outside Japan so far. The patients presented with a history of spastic paraparesis and dementia. The clinical duration from onset to the development of akinetic mutism was around 5 years. There was no periodic synchronous discharge on EEG, but MRI scans showed atrophy of the motor cortex. On pathological examination there were plaques in the cerebral cortex, and neuronal loss but no spongiosis. Neurofibrillary tangles were variably present amongst cases and no plaques were found in the cerebellum.

PrP A117V This mutation was first described in a French family[60] and subsequently in a North American family of German origin.[61] The clinical features are presenile dementia associated with pyramidal signs, parkinsonism, pseudobulbar features, and cerebellar signs. Neuropathologically, PrP immunoreactive plaques are usually present. This mutation has also been identified in a large family in the United Kingdom.[62]

PrP Y145STOP This mutation was detected in a Japanese patient who had a clinical diagnosis of Alzheimer's disease. She developed memory disturbance and a slowly progressive dementia at age 38. The duration of illness was 21 years. Histological examination revealed typical Alzheimer pathology without spongiform change.[63] Many amyloid plaques were seen in the cortex along with diffuse neuropil threads of paired helical filaments. However, the plaques were immunoreactive with PrP antisera. A4 immunocytochemistry was negative. The clinicopathological findings in this case emphasize the importance of PrP gene analysis in the differential diagnosis of dementias.

PrP D178N This mutation was originally described in two Finnish families with a CJD-like phenotype (although without typical EEG appearances)[64] and has since been demonstrated in additional CJD families in Hungary, The Netherlands, Canada, Finland, France, and the United Kingdom. The Finnish pedigree included 15 affected members in four generations. The mean age of onset was 47 and mean duration was 27.5 months. Brain biopsy and autopsy specimens showed spongiform change without amyloid plaques.

This mutation was also reported in two unrelated families with fatal familial insomnia (FFI).[65,66] The first cases described had a rapidly progressive disease characterized clinically by untreatable insomnia, dysautonomia, and motor signs, and neuropathologically by selective atrophy of the anterior–ventral and mediodorsal thalamic nuclei. There is marked thalamic astrocytosis. Mild spongiform change is seen in some cases and protease-resistant PrP can be demonstrated, albeit weakly, by immunoblotting. Proteinase-K treatment of extracted PrP^Sc from FFI cases has shown a different sized PrP band on Western blots than PrP^Sc from CJD cases[67] suggesting that FFI may be caused by a distinct prion strain type. In a recent study, Goldfarb *et al.*[68] reported that in all the codon 178 families they studied with a CJD-like disease, the codon 178 mutation was encoded on a valine 129 allele while all FFI kindreds encode the same codon 178 mutation on a methionine 129 allele. They suggested that the genotype at codon 129 determines phenotype. However, they have not demonstrated that the families they describe are unrelated and that therefore their comparison may only be based on two extended families. Insomnia is not uncommon in CJD patients, and FFI and CJD may represent extremes of a spectrum of related disease phenotypes. Recently an inherited case with the E200K mutation, which is normally associated with a CJD-like phenotype, has been reported with an FFI phenotype.[69] An Australian family has also been reported with the FFI genotype but in which affected family members have a range of phenotypes encompassing typical CJD, FFI, and an autosomal dominant cerebellar ataxia-like illness.[70] It is of interest that the CJD-like codon 178 cases have frequently transmitted to experimental animals while the FFI type did not transmit to laboratory primates.[71] Recently, transmission of an FFI case to mice has been reported although this case was unusual in that a single octapeptide repeat deletion was present on the same allele.[72] This individual came from an extensive kindred in which other family members, with the same *PRNP* genotype, had a CJD-like phenotype.[73] However, two cases of FFI, one a British case and the second an Italian case, both with the usual FFI genotype of D178N, 129M, transmitted to transgenic mice expressing human prion protein.[74]

PrP V180I This mutation was identified in two Japanese patients with subacute dementia and myoclonus.[59] The period from onset to akinetic mutism was 6 to 10 months. No family history was noted. EEG did not show pseudoperiodic sharp wave activity. Neuropathological examination demonstrated spongiform change, neuronal loss, and astrocytosis. Interestingly, one of the patients with PrP Ile 180 also had PrP Arg 232 (see later). These were on different alleles. This disease has not been transmitted to laboratory animals.

PrP T183A This mutation was reported in a single Brazilian family with a frontotemporal dementia of mean onset 45 years and duration 4 years.[75] Parkinsonian features were also present in some patients. Neuropathological examination revealed severe spongiform change and neuronal loss in deep cortical layers and putamen while there was relatively little gliosis. PrP immunoreactivity was demonstrated in putamen and cerebellum. No transmission studies have been reported to date.

PrP F198S A variant form of GSS was described in a large Indiana kindred which has been traced back to 1792. Unlike other GSS patients with presenile onset of neurological disability, the Indiana kindred had widespread Alzheimer-like neurofibrillary tangles composed of paired helical filaments in the cortex and subcortical nuclei in addition to amyloid plaques. The amyloid plaques were composed of PrP and not βA4. Affected individuals in this kindred have a codon 198 T-C transition resulting in a phenylalanine to serine conversion.[76] There is an apparent codon 129 effect with this mutation, in that individuals who were heterozygous at codon 129 had a later age of onset than homozygotes. Transmission of this disease to laboratory animals has not yet been reported.

PrP E200K This mutation was first described in families with CJD. Affected individuals develop a rapidly progressive dementia with myoclonus and pyramidal, cerebellar, or extrapyramidal signs and a duration of illness usually less than 12 months. The average age of onset for the disease is 55. Histologically these patients are typical of CJD, plaques are absent but PrP^Sc can be demonstrated by immunoblotting. In marked contrast to other variants of inherited prion disease, the EEG usually shows the characteristic pseudoperiodic sharp-wave activity seen in sporadic CJD. Interestingly, this mutation accounts for the three reported ethnogeographic clusters of CJD where the local incidence of CJD is around 100-fold higher than elsewhere (amongst Libyan Jews and in regions of Slovakia and Chile).[77–80] Now that cases can be diagnosed by PrP gene analysis, atypical forms of this condition are being detected with phenotypes other than that of classical CJD. Of interest also are reports that peripheral neuropathy can occur in this disease.[81] Elderly unaffected carriers of the mutation have been reported. Chapman *et al.*[82] have made a detailed analysis on 52 mutation-carrying patients with definite or probable CJD and 34 unaffected mutation carriers. They conclude that the cumulative penetrance reaches 50 per cent at the age of 60, and 80 per cent by the age of 80. However, there was a group of patients, of ages 69 to 82 with possible CJD containing five proven and two obligate carriers of the mutation. That is to say the patients were demented but did not fulfil the clinical criteria for probable CJD. If the analysis was carried out assuming that these possible cases were actually CJD then the penetrance reaches 100 per cent by the age of 80. Individuals homozygous for the mutation have been identified and are phenotypically indistinguishable from heterozygotes, indicating that this condition is a fully dominant disorder.[77] Patients with this condition have now been reported in several other countries outside the well-recognized clusters, including the United Kingdom. At least one of the British cases does not appear to related to the ethnogeographic clusters mentioned above, suggesting a separate United Kingdom focus for this type of inherited prion disease.[83] Goldfarb *et al.* have found this mutation amongst 46 out of 55 CJD affected families studied at the National Institutes of Health in the United States.[84] The codon 129 genotype does not appear to affect age at onset of this disorder. Transmission to experimental animals has been demonstrated.

PrP R208H This was reported in a single patient with CJD and confirmed at autopsy. No details of the family history or phenotypic details have yet been published.[85]

PrP V210I This mutation has been reported only in a single case in France[86] with a rapidly progressive dementia, cerebellar signs, and myoclonus, with age of onset of 63. EEG showed pseudoperiodic sharp-wave activity. The clinical duration was 4 months and neuropathological examination showed spongiform change, neuronal loss, and astrocytosis. No amyloid plaques were seen. Parents had died at ages of 60 and 66 without dementia. A sister with the mutation had died of colon cancer at age 67. It is possible that this mutation produces a very late onset disease or is incompletely penetrant. Transmission to experimental animals has not been reported.

PrP Q217R Reported to date only in a single Swedish family, the presentation is with dementia followed by gait ataxia, dysphagia, and confusion.[16] As with the inherited prion disease with codon 198 serine mutation (Indiana kindred) there are prominent neurofibrillary tangles. Transmissibility to experimental animals has not yet been demonstrated in this condition.

PrP M232R This mutation was first found on the opposite allele to a codon 180 mutation in a Japanese patient with prion disease.[59] It was further demonstrated in two additional Japanese patients with dementia. Both of the latter cases appeared to present as sporadic cases with no family history of neurological disease. Both patients had progressive dementia, myoclonus, and periodic synchronous discharges in the EEG. The mean duration of illness was 3 months. Neuropathology showed spongiform change, neuronal loss, and astrocytosis. PrP immunostaining revealed diffuse grey-matter staining, but no plaques.

Insertional mutations

PrP 24-bp insertion (one extra repeat) A single octapeptide repeat insertion has been reported in a single French individual who presented at age 73 with dizziness. He later developed visual agnosia, cerebellar ataxia, and intellectual impairment, and diffuse periodic activity was noted on EEG. Myoclonus and cortical blindness developed and he progressed to akinetic mutism. Disease duration was 4 months. The patient's father had died at age 70 from an undiagnosed neurological disorder. No neuropathological information is available.

PrP 48-bp insertion (four extra repeats) This mutation has been reported in a single family from the United States.[87] The proband had a CJD-like phenotype both clinically and pathologically with a typical EEG and an age at onset of 58. However, the proband's mother had onset of cognitive decline at age 75 with a slow progression to a severe dementia over 13 years. The maternal grandfather had a similar late onset (at age 80) and slowly progressive cognitive decline over 15 years.

PrP 96-bp insertion (four extra repeats) A 96-bp insertional mutation, encoding four octapeptide elements, was first reported in an individual who died aged 63 of hepatic cirrhosis.[88] There was no history of neurological illness and it is unclear if this finding indicates incomplete penetrance of this mutation. This is the only recorded case of a *PRNP* insertional mutation other than in an affected individual

with a prion disease or an at-risk individual from an affected kindred. Two separate four-octapeptide repeat insertional mutations have been reported in affected individuals, each differing in the DNA sequence from the original four-repeat insertion, although all three of the mutations encode the same PrP. Laplanche *et al.*[89] reported a 96-bp insertion in an 82-year-old French woman who developed progressive depression and behavioural changes. She progressed over 3 months to akinetic mutism with pyramidal signs and myoclonus. EEG showed pseudoperiodic complexes. Duration of illness was 4 months. There was no known family history of neurological illness. Another 96-bp insertional mutation was seen in a patient with classical clinical and pathological features of CJD with the exception of the unusual finding of pronounced PrP immunoreactivity in the molecular layer of the cerebellum.[90]

PrP 120-bp insertion (five extra repeats) A five additional octapeptide repeat mutation was reported in a North American family with an illness characterized by progressive dementia, abnormal behaviour, cerebellar signs, tremor, rigidity, hyper-reflexia, and myoclonus. The age at onset was 31 to 45, with a clinical duration of 5 to 15 years.[88] EEG showed diffuse slowing only. Histological features were of spongiosis, neuronal loss, and gliosis. Transmission has been demonstrated.

PrP 144-bp insertion (six extra repeats) This was the first PrP mutation to be reported and was found in a small British family with familial CJD.[10] The diagnosis in the family had been based on an individual who died in the 1940s with a rapidly progressive illness characteristic of CJD.[91] The reported duration of illness was 6 months. Pathologically there was gross status spongiosis and astrocytosis affecting the entire cerebral cortex, and this case is used to illustrate classic CJD histology in Greenfield's *Neuropathology*. However, other family members had a much longer duration of GSS-like illness. Histological features were also extremely variable. This observation led to screening of various cases of neurodegenerative disease and to the identification of a case classified on clinical grounds as familial Alzheimer's disease.[92] More extensive screening work identified further families with the same mutation which were then demonstrated by genealogical studies to form part of an extremely large kindred.[29,93] Clinical information has been collected on around 50 affected individuals over seven generations. Affected individuals develop in the third to fourth decade onset of a progressive dementia associated with a varying combination of cerebellar ataxia and dysarthria, pyramidal signs, myoclonus, and occasionally extrapyramidal signs, chorea, and seizures. The dementia is often preceded by depression and aggressive behaviour. A number of cases have a long-standing personality disorder, characterized by aggression, irritability, antisocial and criminal activity, and hypersexuality which may be present from early childhood, long before overt neurodegenerative disease develops. The histological features vary from those of classical spongiform encephalopathy (with or without PrP amyloid plaques) to cases lacking any specific features of these conditions.[30] Age at onset in this condition can be predicted according to genotype at polymorphic codon 129. Since this pathogenic insertional mutation occurs on a methionine 129 PrP allele, there are two possible codon 129 genotypes for affected individuals, methionine 129 homozygotes or methionine 129/valine 129 heterozygotes. Heterozygotes have an age at onset which is about a decade later than homozygotes.[93] Limited transmission studies to marmosets were unsuccessful. Transmission to transgenic mice expressing human prion protein has been achieved (unpublished data). Further families with 144-bp insertions, of different nucleotide sequence, have now been reported in the United Kingdom[94] and Japan.[95]

PrP 168-bp insertion (seven extra repeats) This mutation has been reported in a North American family. The clinical features described include mood change, abnormal behaviour, confusion, aphasia, cerebellar signs, involuntary movements, rigidity, dementia, and myoclonus. The age at onset was 23 to 35 years and the clinical duration 10 to over 13 years. EEG showed diffuse slowing in two cases; a third showed slow-wave burst suppression. Neuropathological examination showed spongiform change, neuronal loss, and gliosis to varying degrees.[88] Experimental transmission has been demonstrated.

PrP 192-bp insertion (eight extra repeats) This mutation has been reported in a French family with clinical features which include abnormal behaviour, cerebellar signs, mutism, pyramidal signs, myoclonus, tremor, intellectual slowing, and seizures. The disease duration ranged from 3 months to 13 years. The EEG findings include diffuse slowing, slow-wave burst suppression, and periodic triphasic complexes. Neuropathological examination revealed spongiform change, neuronal loss, gliosis, and multicentric plaques in the cerebellum.[88,96] Experimental transmission has been reported.

PrP 216-bp insertion (nine extra repeats) The finding of a nine-octapeptide insertional mutation was first reported in a single case from the United Kingdom.[97] The clinical onset was around 54 years with falls, axial rigidity, myoclonic jerks, and progressive dementia.[98] Although there was no clear family history of a similar illness, the mother had died at age 53 with a cerebrovascular event. The maternal grandmother died at age 79 with senile dementia. EEG was of low amplitude but did not show pseudoperiodic sharp-wave activity. Neuropathological examination showed no spongiform encephalopathy but marked deposition of plaques, which in the cerebellum and the basal ganglia showed immunoreactivity with PrP antisera.[98] In the hippocampus there were neuritic plaques positive for both β-amyloid protein and tau. Some neurofibrillary tangles were also seen. In some respects therefore the pathology resembled Alzheimer's disease. Experimental transmission studies have not been attempted. A second (German) family with a nine-octapeptide repeat insertion of different sequence has now been reported.[99]

Presymptomatic and antenatal testing

Since a direct gene test has become available it has been possible to provide an unequivocal diagnosis in patients with inherited forms of the disease. This has also led to the possibility of performing presymptomatic testing of unaffected but at-risk family members, as well as antenatal testing.[100] Because of the effect of codon 129 genotype on the age of onset of disease associated with some mutations it is possible to determine within a family whether a carrier of a mutation will have an early or late onset of disease. Most of the mutations appear to be fully penetrant; however, experience with some is extremely limited. In families with the E200K mutation there are examples of elderly unaffected gene carriers who appear to have escaped the disease.

Genetic counselling in prion disease resembles that of Huntington's disease in many respects and those protocols established for Huntington's disease can be adapted for prion disease counselling. PrP gene analysis may have very important consequences for family members other than the individual tested, and it is preferable to have discussed all the issues with the whole family before testing commences. Following the identification of a mutation the family should be referred for genetic counselling. Testing of asymptomatic individuals should only follow adequate counselling of individuals and will require their full informed consent.

Prognosis and treatment

All forms of prion diseases that are currently recognized are invariably fatal and follow a relentlessly progressive course. No currently available treatment alters the clinical course of the disease and all that can be offered at present is general supportive care for the patient and family with hospitalization in the later stages. The duration of illness in sporadic patients is very short with a mean of 3 to 4 months. However, in some of the inherited cases the duration can be 20 years or more.[30] The prion diseases are now perhaps the best understood of the degenerative brain diseases and the development of rational treatments is appearing realistic. In particular, the development of drugs which selectively bind PrP^{Sc} or which bind to PrP^{C} to inhibit its conversion might be able to block prion propagation. Improved early diagnosis will be crucial.

Secondary prophylaxis after accidental exposure

Certain occupational groups are at risk of exposure to human prions, for instance neurosurgeons and other operating theatre staff, pathologists and morticians, histology technicians, and increasing number of laboratory workers. Because of the prolonged incubation periods to prions following administration to sites other than the central nervous system, which is associated with clinically silent prion replication in the lymphoreticular tissue,[101] treatments inhibiting prion replication in lymphoid organs may represent a viable strategy for rational secondary prophylaxis after accidental exposure. A preliminary suggested regimen is a short course of immunosuppression with oral corticosteroids in individuals with significant accidental exposure to human prions.[102] Urgent surgical excision of the inoculum might also be considered in exceptional circumstances. There is hope that progress in the understanding of the peripheral pathogenesis will identify the precise cell types and molecules involved in colonization of the organism by prions. The ultimate goal will be to target the rate-limiting steps in prion spread with much more focused pharmacological approaches, which may eventually prove useful in preventing disease even after iatrogenic and alimentary exposure.[103]

References

1. Gajdusek, D.C., Gibbs, C.J. Jr, and Alpers, M.P. (1966). Experimental transmission of a kuru-like syndrome to chimpanzees. *Nature*, **209**, 794–6.
2. Gibbs, C.J. Jr, Gajdusek, D.C., Asher, D.M., *et al.* (1968). Creutzfeldt–Jakob disease (spongiform encephalopathy): transmission to the chimpanzee. *Science*, **161**, 388–9.

3. McGowan, J.P. (1922). Scrapie in sheep. *Scottish Journal of Agriculture*, **5**, 365–75.

4. Cuillé, J. and Chelle, P.L. (1936). La maladie dite tremblante du mouton est-elle inocuable? *Comptes Rendus de l'Academie des Sciences*, **203**, 1552–4.

5. Hadlow, W.J. (1959). Scrapie and kuru. *Lancet*, **ii**, 289–90.

6. Beck, E. and Daniel, P.M. (1987). Neuropathology of transmissible spongiform encephalopathies. In *Prions: novel infectious pathogens causing scrapie and Creutzfeldt–Jakob disease* (ed. S.B. Prusiner and M.P. McKinley), pp. 331–85. Academic Press, San Diego, CA.

7. Griffith, J.S. (1967). Self replication and scrapie. *Nature*, **215**, 1043–4.

8. Prusiner, S.B. (1982). Novel proteinaceous infectious particles cause scrapie. *Science*, **216**, 136–44.

9. Jackson, G.S., Hosszu, L.L.P., Power, A., *et al.* (1999). Reversible conversion of monomeric human prion protein between native and fibrilogenic conformations. *Science*, **283**, 1935–7.

10. Owen, F., Poulter, M., Lofthouse, R., *et al.* (1989). Insertion in prion protein gene in familial Creutzfeldt–Jakob disease. *Lancet*, **i**, 51–2.

11. Hsiao, K., Baker, H.F., Crow, T.J., *et al.* (1989). Linkage of a prion protein missense variant to Gerstmann–Straussler syndrome. *Nature*, **338**, 342–5.

12. Collinge, J. (1997). Human prion diseases and bovine spongiform encephalopathy (BSE). *Human Molecular Genetics*, **6**, 1699–705.

13. Collinge, J., Palmer, M.S., and Dryden, A.J. (1991). Genetic predisposition to iatrogenic Creutzfeldt–Jakob disease. *Lancet*, **337**, 1441–2.

14. Palmer, M.S., Dryden, A.J., Hughes, J.T., and Collinge, J. (1991). Homozygous prion protein genotype predisposes to sporadic Creutzfeldt–Jakob disease. *Nature*, **352**, 340–2.

15. Baker, H.E., Poulter, M., Crow, T.J., Frith, C.D., Lofthouse, R., and Ridley, R.M. (1991). Aminoacid polymorphism in human prion protein and age at death in inherited prion disease. *Lancet*, **337**, 1286.

16. Hsiao, K., Dlouhy, S.R., Farlow, M.R., *et al.* (1992). Mutant prion proteins in Gerstmann–Sträussler–Sheinker disease with neurofibrillary tangles. *Nature Genetics*, **1**, 68–71.

17. Brown, P., Cathala, F., Raubertas, R.F., Gajdusek, D.C., and Castaigne, P. (1987). The epidemiology of Creutzfeldt–Jakob disease: conclusion of a 15-year investigation in France and review of the world literature. *Neurology*, **37**, 895–904.

18. Collinge, J., Sidle, K.C.L., Meads, J., Ironside, J., and Hill, A.F. (1996). Molecular analysis of prion strain variation and the aetiology of 'new variant' CJD. *Nature*, **383**, 685–90.

19. Wadsworth, J.D.F., Hill, A.F., Joiner, S., Jackson, G.S., Clarke, A.R., and Collinge, J. (1999). Strain-specific prion-protein conformation determined by metal ions. *Nature Cell Biology*, **1**, 55–9.

20. Hill, A.F., Desbruslais, M., Joiner, S., Sidle, K.C.L., Gowland, I., and Collinge, J. (1997). The same prion strain causes vCJD and BSE. *Nature*, **389**, 448–50.

21. Bruce, M.E., Will, R.G., Ironside, J.W., *et al.* (1997). Transmissions to mice indicate that 'new variant' CJD is caused by the BSE agent. *Nature*, **389**, 498–501.

22. Pattison, I.H. (1965). Experiments with scrapie with special reference to the nature of the agent and the pathology of the disease. In *Slow, latent and temperate virus infections* (ed. C.J. Gajdusek, C.J. Gibbs, and M.P. Alpers), pp. 249–57. NINDB Monograph 2. US Government Printing Office, Washington, DC.

23. Prusiner, S.B., Scott, M., Foster, D., *et al.* (1990). Transgenetic studies implicate interactions between homologous PrP isoforms in scrapie prion replication. *Cell*, **63**, 673–86.

24. Bruce, M., Chree, A., McConnell, I., Foster, J., Pearson, G., and Fraser, H. (1994). Transmission of bovine spongiform encephalopathy and scrapie to mice: strain variation and the species barrier. *Philosophical Transactions of the Royal Society of London. Series B: Biological Sciences*, **343**, 405–11.

25. Collinge, J. (1999). Variant Creutzfeldt–Jakob disease. *Lancet*, **354**, 317–23.

26. Collinge, J., Palmer, M.S., Sidle, K.C.L., *et al.* (1995). Unaltered susceptibility to BSE in transgenic mice expressing human prion protein. *Nature*, **378**, 779–83.

27. Hill, A.F., Desbruslais, M., Joiner, S., Sidle, K.C.L., Gowland, I., and Collinge, J. (1997). The same prion strain causes vCJD and BSE. *Nature*, **389**, 448–50.

28. Medori, R., Tritschler, H.J., LeBlanc, A., *et al.* (1992). Fatal familial insomnia, a prion disease with a mutation at codon 178 of the prion protein gene. *New England Journal of Medicine*, **326**, 444–9.

29. Collinge, J., Brown, J., Hardy, J., *et al.* (1992). Inherited prion disease with 144 base pair gene insertion. II: Clinical and pathological features. *Brain*, **115**, 687–710.

30. Collinge, J., Owen, F., Poulter, M., *et al.* (1990). Prion dementia without characteristic pathology. *Lancet*, **336**, 7–9.

31. Jimi, T., Wakayama, Y., Shibuya, S., *et al.* (1992). High levels of nervous system-specific proteins in cerebrospinal fluid in patients with early stage Creutzfeldt–Jakob disease. *Clinica Chimica Acta*, **211**, 37–46.

32. Otto, M., Stein, H., Szudra, A., *et al.* (1997). S-100 protein concentration in the cerebrospinal fluid of patients with Creutzfeldt–Jakob disease. *Journal of Neurology*, **244**, 566–70.

33. Zerr, I., Bodemer, M., Räcker, S., Grosche, S., Poser, S., Kretzschmar, H.A., and Weber, T. (1995). Cerebrospinal fluid concentration of neuron-specific enolase in diagnosis of Creutzfeldt–Jakob disease. *Lancet*, **345**, 1609–10.

34. Hsich, G., Kenney, K., Gibbs, C.J. Jr, Lee, K.H., and Harrington, M.G. (1996). The 14-3-3 brain protein in cerebrospinal fluid as a marker for transmissible spongiform encephalopathies. *New England Journal of Medicine*, **335**, 924–30.

35. Collinge, J. (1996). New diagnostic tests for prion diseases. *New England Journal of Medicine*, **335**, 963–5.

36. Budka, H., Aguzzi, A., Brown, P., *et al.* (1995). Neuropathological diagnostic criteria for Creutzfeldt–Jakob disease (CJD) and other human spongiform encephalopathies (prion diseases). *Brain Pathology*, **5**, 459–66.

37. Brown, P., Rodgers-Johnson, P., Cathala, F., Gibbs, C.J. Jr, and Gajdusek, D.C. (1984). Creutzfeldt–Jakob disease of long duration: clinicopathological characteristics, transmissibility, and differential diagnosis. *Annals of Neurology*, **16**, 295–304.

38. Collinge, J. and Palmer, M.S. (1994). Molecular genetics of human prion diseases. *Philosophical Transactions of the Royal Society of London. Series B: Biological Sciences*, **343**, 371–8.

39. Gomori, A.J., Partnow, M.J., Horoupian, D.S., and Hirano, A. (1973). The ataxic form of Creutzfeldt–Jakob disease. *Archives of Neurology*, **29**, 318–23.

40. Salazar, A.M., Masters, C.L., Gajdusek, D.C., and Gibbs, C.J., Jr. (1983). Syndromes of amyotrophic lateral sclerosis and dementia: relation to transmissible Creutzfeldt–Jakob disease. *Annals of Neurology*, **14**, 17–26.

41. Alpers, M.P. (1987). Epidemiology and clinical aspects of kuru. In *Prions: novel infectious pathogens causing scrapie and Creutzfeldt–Jakob disease* (ed. S.B. Prusiner and M.P. McKinley), pp. 451–65. Academic Press, San Diego, CA.

42. Alpers, M. (1964). Kuru: age and duration studies. Thesis, Department of Medicine, University of Adelaide.

43. Cobb, W.A., Hornabrook, R.W., and Sanders, S. (1973). The EEG of kuru. *Electroencephalography and Clinical Neurophysiology*, **34**, 419–27.

44. Esmonde, T.F.G., Will, R.G., Slattery, J.M., *et al.* (1993). Creutzfeldt–Jakob disease and blood transfusion. *Lancet*, **341**, 205–7.

45. Brown, P. (1995). Can Creutzfeldt–Jakob disease be transmitted by transfusion? *Current Opinion in Hematology*, **2**, 472–7.

46. Hill, A.F., Butterworth, R.J., Joiner, S., *et al.* (1999). Investigation of variant Creutzfeldt Jakob disease and other human prion disease with tonsil biopsy samples. *Lancet*, **353**, 183–9.

47. Bateman, D., Hilton, D., Love, S., Zeidler, M., Beck, J., and Collinge, J. (1995). Sporadic Creutzfeldt–Jakob disease in an 18-year-old in the UK. *Lancet*, **346**, 1155–6.

48. Britton, T.C., Al-Sarraj, S., Shaw, C., Campbell, T., and Collinge, J. (1995). Sporadic Creutzfeldt–Jakob disease in a 16-year-old in the UK. *Lancet*, **346**, 1155.

49. Tabrizi, S.J., Scaravilli, F., Howard, R.S., Collinge, J., and Rossor, M.N. (1996). Grand Round. Creutzfeldt–Jakob disease in a young woman. Report of a Meeting of Physicians and Scientists, St. Thomas' Hospital, London. *Lancet*, **347**, 945–8.

50. Chazot, G., Broussolle, E., Lapras, C.I., Blattler, T., Aguzzi, A., and Kopp, N. (1996). New variant of Creutzfeldt–Jakob disease in a 26-year-old French man. *Lancet*, **347**, 1181.

51. Will, R.G., Ironside, J.W., Zeidler, M., *et al.* (1996). A new variant of Creutzfeldt–Jakob disease in the UK. *Lancet*, **347**, 921–5.

52. Zeidler, M., Johnstone, E.C., Bamber, R.W.K., *et al.* (1997). New variant Creutzfeldt–Jakob disease: psychiatric features. *Lancet*, **350**, 908–10.

53. Zeidler, M., Stewart, G.E., Barraclough, C.R., *et al.* (1997). New variant Creutzfeldt–Jakob disease: neurological features and diagnostic tests. *Lancet*, **350**, 903–7.

54. Collinge, J., Beck, J., Campbell, T., Estibeiro, K., and Will, R.G. (1996). Prion protein gene analysis in new variant cases of Creutzfeldt–Jakob disease. *Lancet*, **348**, 56.

55. Collinge, J., Hill, A.F., Ironside, J., and Zeidler, M. (1997). Diagnosis of new variant Creutzfeldt–Jakob disease by tonsil biopsy—authors' reply to Arya and Evans. *Lancet*, **349**, 1322–3.

56. Gerstmann, J., Sträussler, E., and Scheinker, I. (1936). Über eine eigenartige hereditär-familiäre Erkrankung des Zentralnervensystems. Zugleich ein Beitrag zur Frage des vorzeitigen lakalen Alterns. *Zeitschrift für Neurologie*, **154**, 736–62.

57. Hainfellner, J.A., Brantner-Inthaler, S., Cervenáková, L., *et al.* (1995). The original Gerstmann–Straussler–Scheinker family of Austria: divergent clinicopathological phenotypes but constant PrP genotype. *Brain Pathology*, **5**, 201–11.

58. Kretzschmar, H.A., Kufer, P., Riethmuller, G., DeArmond, S.J., Prusiner, S.B., and Schiffer, D. (1992). Prion protein mutation at codon 102 in an Italian family with Gerstmann–Straussler–Scheinker syndrome. *Neurology*, **42**, 809–10.

59. Kitamoto, T., Ohta, M., Doh-ura, K., Hitoshi, S., Terao, Y., and Tateishi, J. (1993). Novel missense variants of prion protein in Creutzfeldt–Jakob disease or Gerstmann-Straussler syndrome. *Biochemical and Biophysical Research Communications*, **191**, 709–14.

60. Dohura, K., Tateishi, J., Sasaki, H., Kitamoto, T., and Sakaki, Y. (1989). Pro–leu change at position 102 of prion protein is the most common but not the sole mutation related to Gerstmann–Straussler syndrome. *Biochemical and Biophysical Research Communications*, **163**, 974–9.

61. Hsiao, K.K., Cass, C., Schellenberg, G.D., *et al.* (1991). A prion protein variant in a family with the telencephalic form of Gerstmann–Straussler–Scheinker syndrome. *Neurology*, **41**, 681–4.

62. Mallucci, G.R., Campbell, T.A., Dickinson, A., *et al.* (1999). Inherited prion disease with an alanine to valine mutation at codon 117 in the prion protein gene. *Brain*, **122**, 1823–37.

63. Kitamoto, T., Iizuka, R., and Tateishi, J. (1993). An amber mutation of prion protein in Gerstmann–Straussler syndrome with mutant PrP plaques. *Biochemical and Biophysical Research Communications*, **192**, 525–31.

64. Goldfarb, L.G., Haltia, M., Brown, P., *et al.* (1991). New mutation in scrapie amyloid precursor gene (at codon 178) in Finnish Creutzfeldt–Jakob kindred. *Lancet*, **337**, 425.

65. Lugaresi, E., Medori, R., Baruzzi, P.M., *et al.* (1986). Fatal familial insomnia and dysautonomia, with selective degeneration of thalamic nuclei. *New England Journal of Medicine*, **315**, 997–1003.

66. Medori, R., Montagna, P., Tritschler, H.J., *et al.* (1992). Fatal familial insomnia: a second kindred with mutation of prion protein gene at codon 178. *Neurology*, **42**, 669–70.

67. Monari, L., Chen, S.G., Brown, P., *et al.* (1994). Fatal familial insomnia and familial Creutzfeldt–Jakob disease: different prion proteins determined by a DNA polymorphism. *Proceedings of the National Academy of Sciences of the United States of America*, **91**, 2839–42.

68. Goldfarb, L.G., Petersen, R.B., Tabaton, M., *et al.* (1992). Fatal familial insomnia and familial Creutzfeldt–Jakob disease: disease phenotype determined by a DNA polymorphism. *Science*, **258**, 806–8.

69. Chapman, J., Arlazoroff, A., Goldfarb, L.G., *et al.* (1996). Fatal insomnia in a case of familial Creutzfeldt–Jakob disease with the codon 200Lys mutation. *Neurology*, **46**, 758–61.

70. McLean, C.A., Storey, E., Gardner, R.J.M., Tannenberg, A.E.G., Cervenáková, L., and Brown, P. (1997). The D178N (cis-129M) 'fatal familial insomnia' mutation associated with diverse clinicopathologic phenotypes in an Australian kindred. *Neurology*, **49**, 552–8.

71. Brown, P., Gibbs, C.J., Jr, Rodgers Johnson, P., *et al.* (1994). Human spongiform encephalopathy: the National Institutes of Health series of 300 cases of experimentally transmitted disease. *Annals of Neurology*, **35**, 513–29.

72. Tateishi, J., Brown, P., Kitamoto, T., *et al.* (1995). First experimental transmission of fatal familial insomnia. *Nature*, **376**, 434–5.

73. Bosque, P.J., Vnencak-Jones, C.L., Johnson, M.D., Whitlock, J.A., and McLean, M.J. (1992). A PrP gene codon 178 base substitution and a 24-bp interstitial deletion in familial Creutzfeldt–Jakob disease. *Neurology*, **42**, 1864–70.

74. Collinge, J., Palmer, M.S., Sidle, K.C.L., *et al.* (1995). Transmission of fatal familial insomnia to laboratory animals. *Lancet*, **346**, 569–70.

75. Nitrini, R., Rosemberg, S., Passos-Bueno, M.R., *et al.* (1997). Familial spongiform encephalopathy associated with a novel prion protein gene mutation. *Annals of Neurology*, **42**, 138–46.

76. Dlouhy, S.R., Hsiao, K., Farlow, M.R., *et al.* (1992). Linkage of the Indiana kindred of Gerstmann–Sträussler–Scheinker disease to the prion protein gene. *Nature Genetics*, **1**, 64–7.

77. Hsiao, K., Meiner, Z., Kahana, E., *et al.* (1991). Mutation of the prion protein in Libyan Jews with Creutzfeldt–Jakob disease. *New England Journal of Medicine*, **324**, 1091–7.

78. Goldfarb, L.G., Mitrova, E., Brown, P., Toh, B.K., and Gajdusek, D.C. (1990). Mutation in codon 200 of scrapie amyloid protein gene in two clusters of Creutzfeldt–Jakob disease in Slovakia. *Lancet*, **336**, 514–15.

79. Goldfarb, L.G., Korczyn, A.D., Brown, P., Chapman, J., and Gajdusek, D.C. (1990). Mutation in codon 200 of scrapie amyloid precursor gene linked to Creutzfeldt–Jakob disease in Sephardic Jews of Libyan and non-Libyan origin. *Lancet*, **336**, 637–8.

80. Brown, P., Galvez, S., Goldfarb, L.G., *et al.* (1992). Familial Creutzfeldt–Jakob disease in Chile is associated with the codon 200 mutation of the PRNP amyloid precursor gene on chromosome 20. *Journal of Neurological Science*, **112**, 65–7.

81. Neufeld, M.Y., Josiphov, J., and Korczyn, A.D. (1992). Demyelinating peripheral neuropathy in Creutzfeldt–Jakob disease. *Muscle and Nerve*, **15**, 1234–9.

82. Chapman, J., Ben-Israel, J., Goldhammer, Y., and Korczyn, A.D. (1994). The risk of developing Creutzfeldt–Jakob disease in subjects with the PRNP gene codon 200 point mutation. *Neurology*, **44**, 1683–6.

83. Collinge, J., Palmer, M.S., Campbell, T.A., Sidle, K.C.L., Carroll, D., and Harding, A.E. (1993). Inherited prion disease (PrP lysine 200) in Britain: two case reports. *British Medical Journal*, **306**, 301–2.

84. Goldfarb, L.G., Brown, P., Mitrova, E., *et al.* (1991). Creutzfeldt–Jacob disease associated with the PRNP codon 200Lys mutation: an analysis of 45 families. *European Journal of Epidemiology*, **7**, 477–86.

85. Mastrianni, J.A., Iannicola, C., Myers, R., and Prusiner, S.B. (1995). Identification of a new mutation of the prion protein gene at codon 208 in a patient with Creutzfeldt–Jakob disease. *Neurology*, **45** (Supplement 4), A201.

86. Davies, P.T.G., Jahfar, S., Ferguson, I.T., and Windl, O. (1993). Creutzfeldt–Jakob disease in individual occupationally exposed to BSE. *Lancet*, **342**, 680

87. Goldfarb, L.G., Brown, P., Little, B.W., *et al.* (1993). A new (two-repeat) octapeptide coding insert mutation in Creutzfeldt–Jakob disease. *Neurology*, **43**, 2392–4.

88. Goldfarb, L.G., Brown, P., McCombie, W.R., *et al.* (1991). Transmissible familial Creutzfeldt–Jakob disease associated with five, seven, and eight

extra octapeptide coding repeats in the PRNP gene. *Proceedings of the National Academy of Sciences of the United States of America*, **88**, 10 926–30.

89. Laplanche, J.L., Delasnerie Laupretre, N., Brandel, J.P., Dussaucy, M., Chatelain, J., and Launay, J.M. (1995). Two novel insertions in the prion protein gene in patients with late-onset dementia. *Human Molecular Genetics*, **4**, 1109–11.

90. Campbell, T.A., Palmer, M.S., Will, R.G., Gibb, W.R.G., Luthert, P., and Collinge, J. (1996). A prion disease with a novel 96-base pair insertional mutation in the prion protein gene. *Neurology*, **46**, 761–6.

91. Meyer, A., Leigh, D., and Bagg, C.E. (1954). A rare presenile dementia associated with cortical blindness (Heidenhain's syndrome). *Journal of Neurology, Neurosurgery and Psychiatry*, **17**, 129–33.

92. Collinge, J., Harding, A.E., Owen, F., *et al.* (1989). Diagnosis of Gerstmann–Straussler syndrome in familial dementia with prion protein gene analysis. *Lancet*, **ii**, 15–17.

93. Poulter, M., Baker, H.F., Frith, C.D., *et al.* (1992). Inherited prion disease with 144 base pair gene insertion. I: Genealogical and molecular studies. *Brain*, **115**, 675–85.

94. Nicholl, D., Windl, O., De Silva, R., *et al.* (1995). Inherited Creutzfeldt–Jakob disease in a British family associated with a novel 144 base pair insertion of the prion protein gene. *Journal of Neurology, Neurosurgery and Psychiatry*, **58**, 65–9.

95. Oda, T., Kitamoto, T., Tateishi, J., *et al.* (1995). Prion disease with 144 base pair insertion in a Japanese family line. *Acta Neuropathologica (Berlin)*, **90**, 80–6.

96. Guiroy, D.C., Marsh, R.F., Yanagihara, R., and Gajdusek, D.C. (1993). Immunolocalization of scrapie amyloid in non-congophilic, non-birefringent deposits in golden Syrian hamsters with experimental transmissible mink encephalopathy. *Neuroscience Letters*, **155**, 112–15.

97. Owen, F., Poulter, M., Collinge, J., *et al.* (1992). A dementing illness associated with a novel insertion in the prion protein gene. *Molecular Brain Research*, **13**, 155–7.

98. Tagliavini, F., Giaccone, G., Prelli, F., *et al.* (1993). A68 is a component of paired helical filaments of Gerstmann–Straussler–Scheinker disease, Indiana kindred. *Brain Research*, **616**, 325–8.

99. Krasemann, S., Zerr, I., Weber, T., *et al.* (1995). Prion disease associated with a novel nine octapeptide repeat insertion in the PRNP gene. *Molecular Brain Research*, **34**, 173–6.

100. Collinge, J., Poulter, M., Davis, M.B., *et al.* (1991). Presymptomatic detection or exclusion of prion protein gene defects in families with inherited prion diseases. *American Journal of Human Genetics*, **49**, 1351–4.

101. Aguzzi, A. (1997). Neuro-immune connection in spread of prions in the body. *Lancet*, **349**, 742–3.

102. Aguzzi, A. and Collinge, J. (1997). Post-exposure prophylaxis after accidental prion inoculation. *Lancet*, **350**, 1519–20.

103. Collinge, J. and Hawke, S. (1998). B lymphocytes in prion neuroinvasion: central or peripheral players. *Nature Medicine*, **4**, 1369–70.

4.1.6 Lewy body dementia

I. G. McKeith

Introduction

Lewy bodies are spherical neuronal inclusions, first described by the German neuropathologist Friederich Lewy[1] while working in Alzhei-mer's laboratory in Munich in 1912. In 1961, Okazaki published case reports about two elderly men who presented with dementia and died shortly after with severe extrapyramidal rigidity. Autopsy showed Lewy bodies in their cerebral cortex.[2] Over the next 20 years, 34 similar cases were reported, all by Japanese workers. Lewy body disease was thus considered to be a rare cause of dementia, until a series of studies in Europe and North America, in the late 1980s, identified Lewy bodies in the brains of between 15 and 20 per cent of elderly demented cases reaching autopsy.[3,4] Dementia with Lewy bodies (**DLB**) is unlikely to be a newly occurring disorder, since re-examination of autopsy material collected from elderly demented patients in Newcastle during the 1960s, reveals cortical Lewy bodies in 17 per cent of cases. The recent recognition of DLB as the second most common form of degenerative dementia in old age is largely due to the widespread use of improved neuropathological techniques, in particular antiubiquitin immuno-cytochemistry.

The spectrum of Lewy body disease

Lewy bodies probably do not occur in normal ageing. Their presence indicates neurological disease, the clinical presentation varying according to the site of Lewy body formation and associated neuronal loss.[5] Three main clinicopathological syndromes have been described.

- Parkinson's disease, an extrapyramidal movement disorder—associated with degeneration of subcortical neurones, particularly in substantia nigra.

- Dementia with Lewy bodies, a dementing disorder with prominent neuropsychiatric features—associated with degeneration of cortical neurones, particularly in frontal, anterior cingulate, insular, and temporal regions.

- Primary autonomic failure with syncope and orthostatic hypotension—associated with degeneration of sympathetic neurones in spinal cord.

In clinical practice, elderly patients often have heterogenous combinations of parkinsonism, dementia, and autonomic failure, reflecting pathological involvement at multiple locations.

Clinical features

Table 1 summarizes nine studies which report clinical details of 190 autopsy-confirmed DLB cases.[6] Dementia is usually, but not always, the presenting feature; a minority of patients present with parkinsonism alone, some with psychiatric disorder in the absence of dementia, and others with orthostatic hypotension, falls, or transient disturbances of consciousness. Fluctuation in cognitive performance and functional ability, which is based in variations in attention and level of consciousness, is the most characteristic feature of DLB It is usually evident on a day-to-day basis, and often apparent within much shorter periods. The marked amplitude between best and worst performance distinguishes it from the minor day-to-day variations that commonly occur in dementia of any aetiology. Repeated visual hallucinations are present in about two-thirds of patients. They take the form of vivid, colourful, and sometimes fragmented figures of people and animals,

Table 1 Clinical characteristics of 190 DLB and 261 AD autopsy-confirmed cases (1989–1997)

	DLB[a] (n = 190)		AD[b] (n = 261)	
	Symptoms present early in course of illness	Symptoms present ever during course of illness	Symptoms present early in course of illness	Symptoms present ever during course of illness
Dementia	82 (40–100)	100	100	100
Fluctuation	58 (8–85)	75 (45–90)	6 (3–11)	12 (5–19)
Visual hallucinations	33 (11–64)	46 (13–80)	13 (3–19)	20 (11–28)
Auditory hallucinations	19 (13–30)	19 (0–45)	1 (0–3)	4 (0–13)
Depression	29 (7–75)	38 (12–89)	16 (9–38)	16 (12–21)
Parkinsonism	43 (10–78)	77 (50–100)	12 (5–30)	23 (19–30)
Falls	28 (10–38)	37 (22–50)	9 (5–14)	18 (11–24)
Neuroleptic sensitivity	—	61 (0–100)	—	15 (0–29)

Figures are mean percentages with the range reported in different studies indicated in parentheses.

[a] Male-to-female ratio, 1.7 (0.9–3.5); age of onset, 70 years (62–74 years); duration of illness, 75 months (27–114 months).

[b] Male-to-female ratio, 0.53 (0.3–0.9); age of onset, 71 years (68–76 years); duration of illness, 88 months (61–174 months).

Data from nine studies summarized by McKeith.[6]

which are usually described in great detail. Emotional responses vary from intense fear to indifference or even amusement. Although patients may respond to their hallucinations, for example trying to feed an imaginary dog, they later often have good insight into their unreality. Others develop elaborate systematized delusions, usually persecutory or of a phantom boarder. Auditory hallucinations are much less frequent, and only a small minority of patients have olfactory or tactile experiences. Depressive symptoms are common and about 40 per cent of patients will have a major depressive episode, similar to the rate in Parkinson's disease and significantly greater than in Alzheimer's disease (AD). The frequency and severity of spontaneous motor features of parkinsonism varies greatly from one clinical setting to another. Bradykinesia, limb rigidity, and gait disorder are the most common manifestations, rest tremor occurring in only 20 per cent or less. Less than half of DLB cases have parkinsonism at presentation and a quarter continue to have no evidence at any point in their illness. Clinicians, particularly in non-movement disorder specialties, must therefore be prepared to make the diagnosis of DLB in the absence of extrapyramidal motor features—if they do not, their case detection rates will be unacceptably low. Recurrent falls and syncope occur in up to a third of DLB cases, reflecting autonomic nervous system involvement. Transient disturbances of consciousness, in which patients are found mute and unresponsive for periods of several minutes, may represent the extreme of fluctuation in attention and arousal and are often mistaken for transient ischaemic attacks despite a lack of focal neurological signs.

Classification

Pathological

Lewy bodies are composed of intermediate neurofilament proteins, which are abnormally truncated and phosphorylated. Their presence indicates that a neurone is attempting to eliminate damaged proteins from its cytoplasm, a process which is usually followed by cell death.[5] Ubiquitin, α-synuclein, α- and β-crystalin, and associated enzymes are the main chemical constituents. Subcortical Lewy bodies have a dense hyaline core surrounded by a halo of radiating filaments, and are easily seen with conventional histopathological techniques. Cortical Lewy bodies lacking this characteristic core and halo appearance remained difficult to detect until the recent development of specific antiubiquitin immunocytochemical staining methods,[7] allowed their true prevalence to be appreciated.

Recommendations have been made[8] about which brain regions to examine for the presence of Lewy bodies, and a simple semiquantitative scoring system devised. These scores are added to generate three pathological categories.

1. Brainstem-predominant DLB: predilection sites are substantia nigra, locus coeruleus, and dorsal nucleus of vagus.

2. Limbic (or transitional) DLB: predilection sites are anterior cingulate and transtentorhinal cortex.

3. Neocortical DLB: predilection sites are frontal, temporal, and parietal cortex.

Of DLB cases presenting via psychiatric clinics, 69 per cent have extensive neocortical Lewy body pathology,[9] but this is not essential for the development of dementia or other psychiatric symptoms, both of which may occur in the presence of disease limited to limbic structures (24 per cent of cases) or the brainstem (7 per cent).

A distinctive pattern of neuritic degeneration has additionally been identified in Lewy body disease. 'Lewy neurites' are seen in the substantia nigra, hippocampal region CA2/3, dorsal vagal nucleus, basal nucleus of Meynert, and transtentorhinal cortex. Ubiquitin immunocytochemistry and α-synuclein-specific, monoclonal antibody stains are beginning to reveal the extensive nature of these neuritic changes,[10] which are probably more relevant for symptom formation than the relatively sparsely distributed Lewy bodies.

Unresolved issues in classification

Two heated debates have developed around the classification of DLB. The first concerns the interpretation of coexistent Alzheimer-type pathology.[11] High senile plaque counts are found in 80 to 90 per cent of DLB cases, diffuse and neuritic β-amyloid plaques occurring in similar proportions as in pure AD. Significant tau pathology is absent, however, in 80 to 90 per cent of DLB cases, whether measured biochemically or by counting neocortical neurofibrillary tangles. Most DLB cases are therefore classified as 'the Lewy body variant of AD'[3] if AD is defined by increased plaque density. Conversely, if AD is defined by frequent neocortical neurofibrillary tangles, equivalent to Braak stages 5 and 6, then 85 to 90 per cent of DLB cases will not fulfil such criteria.[4,11] (The pathological classification of AD is also discussed in Chapter 4.1.3.) Minor vascular pathology is additionally present in 30 per cent of DLB cases.[9]

The second controversy centres upon the classification of patients who present with motor symptoms of Parkinson's disease and later develop the typical features of DLB, sometimes after many years of severe motor disability. Antiparkinsonian medications are usually held responsible for hallucinations and confusion in Parkinson's disease, but research findings do not support this clinical impression. Factors associated with the development of visual hallucinosis are the later age of onset of Parkinson's disease, total duration of illness, and the presence of cognitive impairment. Patients who do or do not hallucinate are distinguished neither by the severity of their motor disability nor by the dosage of antiparkinsonian medication. Those with early-onset hallucinations are particularly likely to subsequently develop DLB.[12] The DLB consensus statement recommends[8] that if a syndrome meeting diagnostic criteria for DLB develops in a patient who has had motor Parkinson's disease for at least 12 months prior to the onset of neuropsychiatric features, a diagnosis of Parkinson's disease plus DLB, should be made. This 12-month period is purely arbitrary, and a more pragmatic approach may simply be to apply a clinical diagnosis which best describes the patient's current clinical presentation. The neurobiological basis of dementia in Parkinson's disease is discussed in detail in Chapter 4.1.7.

Table 2 Consensus criteria for the clinical diagnosis of *probable* and *possible* dementia with Lewy bodies (DLB)

1. The central feature required for a diagnosis of DLB is progressive cognitive decline of sufficient magnitude to interfere with normal social or occupational function. Prominent or persistent memory impairment may not necessarily occur in the early stages but is usually evident with progression. Deficits on tests of attention and of frontal-subcortical skills and visuospatial ability may be especially prominent.

2. **Two** of the following core features are **essential** for a diagnosis of *probable* DLB, **one** is **essential** for *possible* DLB
    (a) Fluctuating cognition with pronounced variations in attention and alertness
    (b) Recurrent visual hallucinations which are typically well formed and detailed
    (c) Spontaneous motor features of parkinsonism

3. Features **supportive** of the diagnosis are
    (a) Repeated falls
    (b) Syncope
    (c) Transient loss of consciousness
    (d) Neuroleptic sensitivity
    (e) Systematized delusions
    (f) Hallucinations in other modalities

4. A diagnosis of DLB is **less likely** in the presence of
    (a) Stroke disease, evident as focal neurological signs or on brain imaging
    (b) Evidence on physical examination and investigation of any physical illness, or other brain disorder, sufficient to account for the clinical picture

Data from McKeith *et al.*[15]

In summary, there appear to be at least three recognizable anchor points along a spectrum of neurodegenerative disorders. Parkinson's disease is characterized by subcortical Lewy bodies and nigrostriatal degeneration. More extensively distributed Lewy bodies and significant senile plaque formation typify DLB. Lewy bodies are absent in AD, which is best defined by the presence of neocortical neurofibrillary tangles. Cerebrovascular and systemic disease frequently contribute to these pathological and clinical profiles.

Diagnosis and differential diagnosis

Patients with DLB may present to psychiatric services (cognitive impairment, psychosis, or behavioural disturbance), internal medicine (acute confusional states or syncope), or neurology (movement disorder or disturbed consciousness). The details of clinical assessment and differential diagnoses will, to a large extent, be shaped by these symptom and specialty biases.[13] In all cases, a detailed history from the patient and reliable informants should document the time of onset of relevant key symptoms, the nature of their progression, and their effects on social, occupational, and personal function.

The recent consensus criteria for the clinical diagnosis of DLB are shown in Table 2. Particular emphasis needs to be given to recognizing

Table 3 Conditions to be considered in the differential diagnosis of dementia with Lewy bodies

Other causes of dementia
Alzheimer's disease
Vascular dementia
Creutzfeldt–Jakob disease

Other causes of delirium
Infective/pharmacological/metabolic/inflammatory

Other neurological syndromes
Parkinson's disease
Progressive supranuclear palsy (Steele–Richardson–Olszewski syndrome)
Multisystem atrophy
Corticobasal degeneration
Recurrent syncope/unexplained falls
Transient ischaemic attacks
Complex partial seizures

Late-onset functional psychiatric disorders
Delusional disorder (late paraphrenia)
Depressive psychosis
Mania

the characteristic dementia syndrome. Attentional deficits and prominent frontosubcortical and visuospatial dysfunction are the main features—symptoms of persistent or prominent memory impairment are not always present early in the course of illness, although they are likely to develop in most patients with disease progression. Patients with DLB perform better than AD on tests of verbal recall, but relatively worse on tests of copying and drawing.[14] With the progression of dementia, the selective pattern of cognitive deficits may be lost, making differential diagnosis based on clinical examination difficult during the later stages.

Probable DLB can be diagnosed if any two of the three key symptoms (fluctuation, visual hallucinations, spontaneous motor features of parkinsonism) are present. Fluctuation is undoubtedly the most difficult symptom to establish. Some patients identify the variable cognitive state themselves, but generally the most productive approach is to interview a reliable informant. Questions such as 'Are there episodes when his/her thinking seems quite clear and then becomes muddled?' may be useful probes. Substantial changes in mental state and behaviour may be seen within the duration of a single interview or between consecutive examinations. Parkinsonism and visual hallucinations pose fewer problems of identification.

Categories of disorder

There are four main categories of disorder that should be considered in the differential diagnosis of DLB (Table 3).

Other causes of dementia

Of autopsy-confirmed DLB cases, 65 per cent meet the NINCDS–ADRDA clinical criteria for probable or possible AD,[15] and this is the most frequent clinical misdiagnosis of DLB patients presenting with a

primary dementia syndrome. This suggests DLB should routinely be excluded when making the diagnosis of AD. Up to one-third of DLB cases are additionally misclassified as vascular dementia by the Hachinski Ischaemic Index, by virtue of items such as the fluctuating nature and course of illness.[15] Pyramidal and focal neurological signs are, however, usually absent. The development of myoclonus in patients with a rapidly progressive form of DLB may lead the clinician to suspect Creutzfeldt–Jakob disease.[8]

Other causes of delirium

In patients with intermittent delirium, appropriate examination and laboratory tests should be performed during the acute phase to maximize the chances of detecting infective, metabolic, inflammatory, or other aetiological factors. Pharmacological causes are particularly common in elderly patients. Although the presence of any of these features makes a diagnosis of DLB less likely, comorbidity is not unusual in elderly patients and the diagnosis should not be excluded simply on this basis.

Other neurological syndromes

In patients with a prior diagnosis of Parkinson's disease, the onset of visual hallucinations and fluctuating cognitive impairment may be attributed to side-effects of antiparkinsonian medications, and this must be tested by dose reduction or withdrawal. Other atypical parkinsonian syndromes associated with poor levodopa response, cognitive impairment, and postural instability include progressive supranuclear palsy and multisystem atrophy. Syncopal episodes in DLB are often incorrectly attributed to transient ischaemic attacks, despite an absence of focal neurological signs. Recurrent disturbances in consciousness accompanied by complex visual hallucinations may suggest complex partial seizures (temporal lobe epilepsy), and vivid dreaming with violent movements during sleep may meet criteria for REM-sleep behaviour disorder. Both these conditions have been reported as uncommon presenting symptoms of autopsy-confirmed DLB.[16,17]

Late-onset functional psychiatric disorder

DLB should be considered if a patient spontaneously develops parkinsonian features or cognitive decline (or shows excessive sensitivity to neuroleptic medication) in the course of late-onset delusional disorder, depressive psychosis, or mania.[16]

Investigations

Prominent atrophy of the medial temporal lobes on CT or magnetic resonance imaging is indicative of AD rather than DLB.[18] Single-photon emission CT (**SPECT**) HMPAO imaging shows generalized reductions in cortical uptake, similar to AD. [$^{(123)}$I]IBZM and [$^{(123)}$I]FP-CIT are novel SPECT ligands that label postsynaptic D_2 receptors and the presynaptic dopamine transporter site, respectively. Both show marked changes in the caudate-to-putamen ratio in DLB, reflecting nigrostriatal dysfunction, and may prove to be sensitive and specific in the discrimination from AD and other non-Lewy body disorders.[19] Early slowing of dominant electroencephalography rhythms is characteristic of DLB, being associated in 50 per cent of cases with focal delta-wave transient activity in temporal regions.[20]

Diagnostic accuracy

The predictive validity of the consensus criteria for DLB have not yet been fully established. When retrospectively applied to clinical records of autopsy-confirmed cases[21] they had a sensitivity of 0.75 and specificity of 0.79. Inter-rater reliability was acceptable for all key symptoms with the exception of fluctuation ($\kappa = 0.25$–0.36). In the first prospective validation study[9] the consensus criteria show a tendency to clinically underdiagnose DLB (sensitivity 0.83); false-positive diagnoses are uncommon (specificity 0.95). Although it is possible within a specialist centre to diagnose DLB with an accuracy similar to that for AD or Parkinson's disease, further clarification of the criteria would assist in their routine clinical use, particularly for the items relating to fluctuating cognition.

Epidemiology

Several studies in a range of settings have suggested that DLB accounts for just under 20 per cent of all cases of dementia referred for neuropathological autopsy.[3,4,8] The male-to-female ratio in these autopsy series is 1.5:1, but it is unclear to what extent this represents increased male susceptibility or reduced survival. Age at onset ranges from 50 to 83 years and an age at death of between 68 and 92 years.[22] In all, 26 per cent of clinical referrals for dementia to an old age psychiatry service[23] and 24 per cent of demented day-hospital attenders met the clinical criteria for DLB.[24] No estimates of prevalence and incidence in primary-care and community-based samples have been reported. Epidemiological surveys using memory-based screening instruments are likely to miss early DLB cases in whom memory function is relatively intact.

Aetiology

The aetiopathogenesis of Lewy bodies is poorly understood. They presumably form from an interplay between environmental stimuli and the intrinsic responsiveness of neurones.[5] Dementia with Lewy bodies, like Parkinson's disease, does not appear to have a strong heritable component, although the possession of an apolipoprotein *e4* allele appears to confer a risk of developing DLB rather than Parkinson's disease. An inactive allelic variant of cytochrome oxidase (CYP2D6B) is more frequent in Parkinson's disease than controls, but there is disagreement whether the same is true for DLB.

Course and prognosis

Table 1 indicates the typical symptom profiles of DLB at presentation and at any time. Progression is usually more rapid than in AD, typically 1 to 5 years from onset to an endstage of profound dementia and parkinsonism. Men appear to have a worse prognosis than women. Even in the early stages, personal and social function and performance in daily living skills may be markedly impaired by a combination of cognitive, psychiatric, and neurological disability.[25] Psychotic symptoms, particularly visual hallucinations, tend to be very persistent throughout the whole course of illness. There have been three overlapping stages of the illness described.[16]

The first stage is often recognized only in retrospect, and may extend back 1 to 3 years' prepresentation with occasional minor episodes of forgetfulness, sometimes described as lapses of concentration or 'switching off'. A brief period of delirium is sometimes noted for the first time, often associated with genuine physical illness and/or surgical procedures. Disturbed sleep, nightmares, and daytime drowsiness often persist after recovery.

Progression to the second stage frequently prompts psychiatric or medical referral. A more sustained cognitive impairment is established, albeit with marked fluctuations in severity. Recurrent confusional episodes are accompanied by vivid hallucinatory experiences, visual misidentification syndromes, and topographical disorientation. Extensive medical screening is usually negative. Attentional deficits are apparent as apathy, and daytime somnolence and sleep behaviour disorder[17] may be severe. Gait disorder and bradykinesia are often overlooked, particularly in elderly subjects. Frequent falls occur due either to postural instability or syncope.

The third and final stage often begins with a sudden increase in behavioural disturbance, leading to requests for sedation or hospital admission by perplexed and exhausted carers. The natural course from this point is variable and obscured by the high incidence of adverse reactions to neuroleptic medication. For patients not receiving, or not tolerating, neuroleptics a progressive decline into severe dementia with dysphasia and dyspraxia occurs over months or years, with death usually due to cardiac or pulmonary disease. During this terminal phase patients show continuing behavioural disturbance including vocal and motor responses to hallucinatory phenomena. Lucid intervals with some retention of recent memory function and insight may still be apparent. Neurological disability is often profound, with fixed flexion deformities of the neck and trunk and severe gait impairment. Parkinsonian signs and paraplegia in flexion may also occur in advanced AD and other dementias. Parkinsonism occurring for the first time late in the course of a dementia is therefore consistent with a diagnosis of DLB, but not specific for it.

Treatment

Review of evidence

Pharmacological treatment strategies are based upon our knowledge of the neurochemical deficits underlying specific symptoms in DLB.[13] The most clearly established is a correlation between substantia nigra neurone loss and severity of parkinsonism. Levodopa responsiveness is less predictable in DLB than in Parkinson's disease.[22] Activity of the cholinergic enzyme choline acetyltransferase is lower in DLB than AD, particularly in temporal and parietal cortex.[26] Clouding of consciousness, confusion, and visual hallucinations are recognized effects of anticholinergic drug toxicity, and the summative effects of subcortical and cortical cholinergic dysfunction probably play a major role in the spontaneous generation of similar fluctuating symptoms in DLB. Reductions in choline acetyltransferase activity are correlated with the severity of cognitive impairment,[27] and hallucinations may be related to hypocholinergic and (relatively) hypermonoaminergic neocortical neurotransmitter function.[28]

There have been several reports that patients who respond well to cholinesterase inhibitor treatments are more likely to have DLB than AD at autopsy.[25,29,30] This is consistent with the neurochemical profile of DLB and the fact that postsynaptic cortical muscarinic receptors

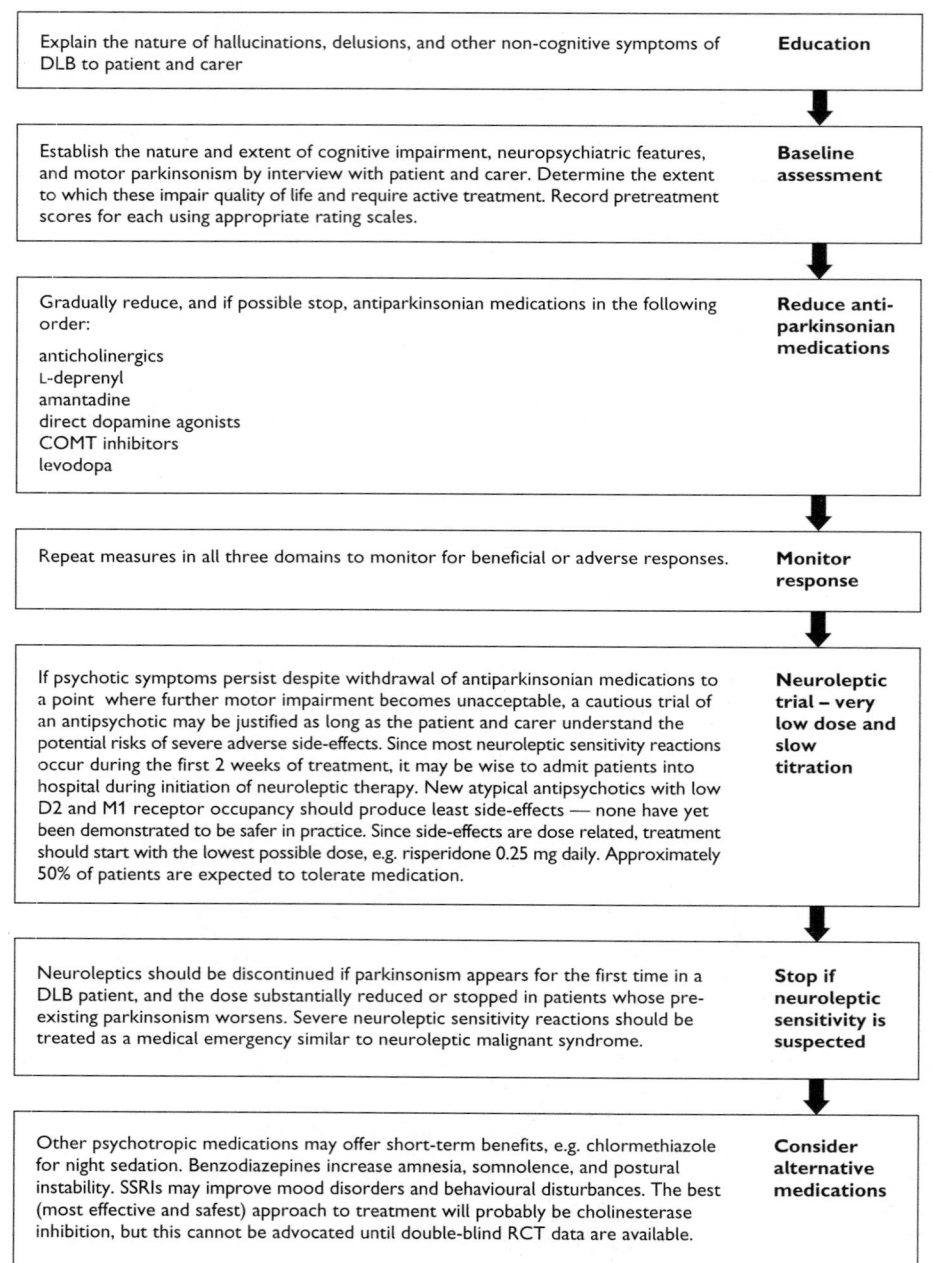

Explain the nature of hallucinations, delusions, and other non-cognitive symptoms of DLB to patient and carer	**Education**
Establish the nature and extent of cognitive impairment, neuropsychiatric features, and motor parkinsonism by interview with patient and carer. Determine the extent to which these impair quality of life and require active treatment. Record pretreatment scores for each using appropriate rating scales.	**Baseline assessment**
Gradually reduce, and if possible stop, antiparkinsonian medications in the following order: anticholinergics L-deprenyl amantadine direct dopamine agonists COMT inhibitors levodopa	**Reduce anti-parkinsonian medications**
Repeat measures in all three domains to monitor for beneficial or adverse responses.	**Monitor response**
If psychotic symptoms persist despite withdrawal of antiparkinsonian medications to a point where further motor impairment becomes unacceptable, a cautious trial of an antipsychotic may be justified as long as the patient and carer understand the potential risks of severe adverse side-effects. Since most neuroleptic sensitivity reactions occur during the first 2 weeks of treatment, it may be wise to admit patients into hospital during initiation of neuroleptic therapy. New atypical antipsychotics with low D2 and M1 receptor occupancy should produce least side-effects — none have yet been demonstrated to be safer in practice. Since side-effects are dose related, treatment should start with the lowest possible dose, e.g. risperidone 0.25 mg daily. Approximately 50% of patients are expected to tolerate medication.	**Neuroleptic trial – very low dose and slow titration**
Neuroleptics should be discontinued if parkinsonism appears for the first time in a DLB patient, and the dose substantially reduced or stopped in patients whose pre-existing parkinsonism worsens. Severe neuroleptic sensitivity reactions should be treated as a medical emergency similar to neuroleptic malignant syndrome.	**Stop if neuroleptic sensitivity is suspected**
Other psychotropic medications may offer short-term benefits, e.g. chlormethiazole for night sedation. Benzodiazepines increase amnesia, somnolence, and postural instability. SSRIs may improve mood disorders and behavioural disturbances. The best (most effective and safest) approach to treatment will probably be cholinesterase inhibition, but this cannot be advocated until double-blind RCT data are available.	**Consider alternative medications**

Fig. 1 Management of the non-cognitive symptoms of DLB.

are functionally intact.[28] Case reports suggest that cholinesterase inhibitors can reduce psychotic symptoms in DLB,[31] and placebo-controlled studies are in progress.

Advice about management

The most important practice point in the management of a patient with DLB is caution in (or preferably avoidance of) the use of neuroleptic medications, which are the mainstay of antipsychotic treatment in other patient groups. Severe neuroleptic sensitivity reactions[16,32] can precipitate irreversible parkinsonism, further impair consciousness level, and induce autonomic disturbances reminiscent of neuro-

leptic malignant syndrome. They occur in 40 to 50 per cent of neuroleptic-treated DLB cases and are associated with a two- to three-fold increased mortality. Acute D2 receptor blockade is thought to mediate these effects; and, despite initial reports, atypical antipsychotics seem to be as likely to cause neuroleptic sensitivity reactions as older drugs. A scheme for the management of the non-cognitive symptoms of DLB is given in Fig. 1.

Until safe and effective medications become available, there is no doubt that the mainstay of clinical management is to educate patients and carers about the nature of their symptoms and to suggest coping strategies. The clinician must ascertain which symptoms are most troublesome for the sufferer and explain the risks and benefits associated with changes in medication.[33] In these circumstances where the clinician is walking a therapeutic tightrope between parkinsonism and psychosis, the best outcome is invariably a compromise between a relatively mobile but psychotic patient and a non-psychotic but immobile individual. The patient and his carers may only be able to decide which is the lesser of these evils after experiencing both states.

Possibilities for prevention

Since the aetiopathogenesis of Lewy body and neurone loss are unknown, specific disease slowing or prevention strategies for DLB are lacking, a situation analogous to Parkinson's disease. The overlap with Alzheimer-type and vascular pathologies suggests that the range of putative neuroprotectives for these disorders, including anti-inflammatories and antioxidants, may confer some advantages in DLB. L-Deprenyl, used for disease slowing in Parkinson's disease, is prone to precipitate hallucinations and is best avoided.

References

1. Lewy, F.H. (1912). Paralysis agitans. I. Pathologische anatomie. In *Handbuch der Neurologie*, Vol. 3 (ed. M. Lewandowsky), pp. 920–33. Springer, Berlin.
2. Okazaki, H., Lipton, L.S., and Aronson, S.M. (1961). Diffuse intracytoplasmic ganglionic inclusions (Lewy type) associated with progressive dementia and quadrapesis in flexion. *Journal of Neurology, Neurosurgery and Psychiatry*, **20**, 237–44.
3. Hansen, L., Salmon, D., Galasko, D., *et al.* (1990). The Lewy body variant of Alzheimer's disease: a clinical and pathologic entity. *Neurology*, **40**, 1–8.
4. Perry, R.H., Irving, D., Blessed, G., Fairbairn, A., and Perry, E.K. (1990). Senile dementia of Lewy body type. A clinically and neuropathologically distinct form of Lewy body dementia in the elderly. *Journal of Neurological Sciences*, **95**, 119–39.
5. Lowe, J.S., Mayer, R.J., and Landon, M. (1996). Pathological significance of Lewy bodies in dementia. In *Dementia with Lewy bodies* (ed. R. Perry, I. McKeith, and E. Perry), pp. 195–203. Cambridge University Press, New York.
6. McKeith, I.G. (1998). Dementia with Lewy bodies: clinical and pathological diagnosis. *Alzheimer's Reports*, **1**, 83–7.
7. Lennox, G., Lowe, J., Landon, M., Byrne, E.J., Mayer, R.J., and Godwin-Austen, R.B. (1989). Diffuse Lewy body disease: correlative neuropathology using anti-ubiquitin immunocytochemistry. *Journal of Neurology, Neurosurgery and Psychiatry*, **52**, 1236–47.
8. McKeith, I.G., Galasko, D., Kosaka, K., *et al.* (1996). Consensus guidelines for the clinical and pathologic diagnosis of dementia with Lewy bodies (DLB): report of the consortium on DLB International Workshop. *Neurology*, **47**, 1113–24.
9. Perry, R.H., Jaros, E., Ince, P.I., *et al.* (1998). Dementia with Lewy bodies: histopathological aspects of differential diagnosis. *Neurobiology of Aging*, **19** (4S), S203.
10. Trojanowski, J. (1998). Dementia with Lewy bodies: diagnostic accuracy using consensus criteria. *Neurobiology of Aging*, **19** (4S), S4.
11. Hansen, L.A. and Samuel, W. (1997). Criteria for Alzheimer's disease and the nosology of dementia with Lewy bodies. *Neurology*, **48**, 126–32.
12. Goetz, C.G., Vogel, C., Tanner, C.M., and Stebbins, G.T. (1998). Early dopaminergic drug-induced hallucinations in parkinsonian patients. *Neurology*, **51**, 811–14.
13. McKeith, I.G., Galasko, D., Wilcock, G.K., and Byrne, E.J. (1995). Lewy body dementia—diagnosis and treatment. *British Journal of Psychiatry*, **167**, 709–17.
14. Gnanalingham, K.K., Byrne, E.J., Thornton, A., Sambrook, M.A., and Bannister, P. (1997). Motor and cognitive function in Lewy body dementia: comparison with Alzheimer's and Parkinson's diseases. *Journal of Neurology, Neurosurgery and Psychiatry*, **62**, 243–52.
15. McKeith, I.G., Fairbairn, A.F., Perry, R.H., and Thompson, P. (1994). The clinical diagnosis and misdiagnosis of senile dementia of Lewy body type (SDLT). *British Journal of Psychiatry*, **165**, 324–32.
16. McKeith, I.G., Perry, R.H., Fairbairn, A.F., Jabeen, S., and Perry, E.K. (1992). Operational criteria for senile dementia of Lewy body type (SDLT). *Psychological Medicine*, **22**, 911–22.
17. Boeve, B.F., Silber, M.H., Ferman, T.J., *et al.* (1998). REM sleep behaviour disorder and degenerative dementia: an association likely reflecting Lewy body disease. *Neurology*, **51**, 363–70.
18. Barber, R., Gholkar, A., Scheltens, P., Ballard, C., McKeith, I.G., and O'Brien, J.T. (1999). Medial temporal lobe atrophy on MRI in dementia with Lewy bodies: a comparison with Alzheimer's disease, vascular dementia and normal ageing. *Neurology*, **52**, 1153–8.
19. Walker, Z., Costa, D.C., Janssen, A.G., Walker, R.W., Livingstone, G., and Katona, C.L. (1997). Dementia with Lewy bodies: a study of post-synaptic dopaminergic receptors with iodine-123 iodobenzamide single-photon emission tomography. *European Journal of Nuclear Medicine*, **24**, 609–14.
20. Briel, R. (1999). EEG findings in dementia with Lewy bodies and Alzheimer's disease. *Journal of Neurology, Neurosurgery and Psychiatry*, **66**, 401–3.
21. Mega, M.S., Masterman, D.L., Benson, F., *et al.* (1996). Dementia with Lewy bodies: reliability and validity of clinical and pathologic criteria. *Neurology*, **47**, 1403–9.
22. Papka, M., Rubio, A., and Schiffer, R.B. (1998). A review of Lewy body disease, an emerging concept of cortical dementia. *Journal of Neuropsychiatry and Clinical Neurosciences*, **10**, 267–79.
23. Shergill, S., Mullan, E., D'ath, P., and Katona, C. (1994). What is the clinical prevalence of Lewy body dementia? *International Journal of Geriatric Psychiatry*, **9**, 907–12.
24. Ballard, C.G., Mohan, R.N.C., Patel, A., and Bannister, C. (1995). Idiopathic clouding of consciousness—do the patients have cortical Lewy body disease? *International Journal of Psychogeriatrics*, **8**, 571–6.
25. Byrne, E.J., Lennox, G., Lowe, J., and Godwin-Austen, R.B. (1989). Diffuse Lewy body disease: clinical features in 15 cases. *Journal of Neurology, Neurosurgery and Psychiatry*, **52**, 709–17.
26. Samuel, W., Alford, M., Hofstetter, C.R., and Hansen, L. (1997). Dementia with Lewy bodies versus pure Alzheimer disease: differences in cognition, neuropathology, cholinergic dysfunction, and synapse density. *Journal of Neuropathology and Experimental Neurology*, **56**, 499–508.
27. Perry, E.K., Haroutunian, V., Davis, K.L., *et al.* (1994). Neocortical cholinergic activities differentiate Lewy body dementia from classical Alzheimer's disease. *NeuroReport*, **5**, 747–9.
28. Perry, E.K. and Perry, R.H. (1996). Altered consciousness and transmitter signalling in Lewy body dementia. In *Dementia with Lewy bodies* (ed. R. Perry, I. McKeith, and E. Perry), pp. 397–413. Cambridge University Press, New York.
29. Levy, R., Eagger, S., Griffiths, M., *et al.* (1994). Lewy bodies and response to tacrine in Alzheimer's disease. *Lancet*, **343**, 176.
30. Wilcock, G.K. and Scott, M.I. (1994). Tacrine for senile dementia of Alzheimer's or Lewy body type. *Lancet*, **344**, 544.
31. Shea, C., Macknight, C., and Rockwood, R. (1988). Donepezil for treatment of dementia with Lewy bodies: a case series of nine patients. *International Psychogeriatrics*, **10**, 229–39.
32. McKeith, I., Fairbairn, A., Perry, R., Thompson, P., and Perry, E. (1992). Neuroleptic sensitivity in patients with senile dementia of Lewy body type. *British Medical Journal*, **305**, 673–8.
33. Harrison, R.H. and McKeith, I.G. (1995). Senile dementia of Lewy body type—a review of clinical and pathological features: implications for treatment. *International Journal of Geriatric Psychiatry*, **10**, 919–26.

4.1.7 Dementia in Parkinson's disease
R. H. S. Mindham

Introduction

The psychiatric complications of Parkinson's disease have attracted attention for two reasons: first, they are of practical importance in the management of patients suffering from this disease and, second, their study provides insight into a range of psychiatric conditions.

The nature of dementia in Parkinson's disease

There have been numerous reports of the impairment of specific cognitive functions in patients with Parkinson's disease. Some of the impairments described are often only identifiable by specially designed methods of assessment, but some are revealed by tests of cognitive function that are in widespread use. Mortimer and his colleagues have reported a very high prevalence of cognitive impairment—93 per cent in a substantial group of patients with Parkinson's disease.[1] Examination of their data showed neither a clear distinction between impaired groups nor the presence of subtypes of Parkinson's disease in which cognitive impairment was a more frequent occurrence. Their findings led them to propose that cognitive impairment in Parkinson's disease lies on a continuum of severity, rather than arising as a feature of particular subgroups. The impairments identified include deficits in memory, language, visuospatial functioning, abstract reasoning, slowness in intellectual tasks, and difficulty in shifting from task to task. Not only are these deficits widespread among patients with Parkinson's disease but they have been shown to occur at a very early stage of the disorder.[2,3]

A proportion of patients with Parkinson's disease show impairment of a range of cognitive functions, which is more akin to the global impairment seen in dementing disorders such as Alzheimer's disease.[4] However, the pattern of this impairment is frequently less severe than that seen in Alzheimer's disease where the pathological changes in the brain are known to be widespread. This observation, together with the occurrence of cognitive impairment in a range of movement disorders where the main neuropathological changes reside in the subcortical region of the brain, has led to the concept of 'subcortical dementia'—a form of intellectual impairment of lesser degree than in Alzheimer's disease, but affecting several cognitive functions and associated with a disorder of movement. In 1974 Albert and his colleagues gave a description of the syndrome in which the main features were listed as emotional or personality changes, impaired memory, defective ability to manipulate acquired knowledge, and a striking slowness in the rate of information processing.[5]

This concept has carried some conviction, as the impairment seen in many subjects with disease in the subcortical region of the brain shows a pattern of cognitive impairment distinctly different from that of Alzheimer's disease. However, many issues have arisen as to the nature of 'subcortical dementia'. Is subcortical dementia a clinical or a pathological concept? Is the difference between this and other forms of dementia simply one of degree? Do the pathological changes occur in the subcortical region of the brain alone? Is the syndrome of cognitive impairment distinctly different from other dementias or does the presence of motor features of the disorder simply give the intellectual impairment a distinct character? Is subcortical dementia a stable condition or a transitional state leading eventually to global dementia? Opinion has ranged from full acceptance of 'subcortical dementia' as a distinct form of cognitive impairment to scepticism.[6–8]

McHugh[9] has gone further than Albert *et al.*,[5] suggesting that the subcortical region subserves functions not only in motor control and cognitive function but also in the control and display of mood. He suggests that some syndromes arising from subcortical disease represent a 'subcortical triad' of symptoms. This combination of symptoms is most convincingly seen in Huntington's disease. A notable difference between this concept and that of Albert and his colleagues is that the pathological disturbance of mood is only intermittently present, whereas the motor and cognitive changes are persistent.

Cummings[10] has suggested a useful development of the concept of 'subcortical dementia'. He believes that the concept is applicable to disorders of movement to varying degrees. He suggests that cognitive impairment in Parkinson's disease takes three forms: a form which is relatively mild and meets the criteria for subcortical dementia, a more severe form showing wider impairment of cognitive function but neuropathologically distinct from senile dementia Alzheimer type (**SDAT**), and a severe form which shows neuropathological changes in both the subcortical region of the brain and in the cortex, the latter of Alzheimer type. This proposal does not resolve some of the questions that have arisen over the nature of subcortical dementia, but it does provide a basis for viewing cognitive changes in Parkinson's disease, albeit provisional.

Many reports have suggested that global dementia occurs in Parkinson's disease. Whether such a severe change in cognitive function can be regarded as an intrinsic feature of this disease, whether it implies an extension of a neuropathological process more widely in the brain, or whether it suggests a different neuropathology from the outset which initially presented with disordered movement is, as yet, uncertain.

The methodology of studies of dementia in Parkinson's disease

Research to establish the status of dementia in Parkinson's disease has confronted a range of methodological issues.[11]

A major problem in research on dementia in Parkinson's disease has been in the diagnosis of Parkinson's disease itself. The original description of paralysis agitans by Parkinson was, in fact, the identification of a syndrome rather than of a disease. The part played by such agents as heavy metals, infection, and vascular disease was recognized more than 50 years ago. More recently, the importance of drug-induced parkinsonism, where patients generally recover following withdrawal of the drug, has been recognized. The term Parkinson's disease had come to be regarded as synonymous with idiopathic Parkinson's disease and paralysis agitans, and to be a degenerative disease of unknown cause. In spite of the use of standardized methods of diagnosis, recent studies have shown that a substantial proportion of patients diagnosed as suffering from Parkinson's disease in life do not show the expected findings in the brain postmortem.[12,13] In the study by Hughes et al.,[12] 80 per cent of cases were shown to have neuropathological changes of Parkinson's disease after death and over 20 per cent were diagnosed as having suffered from progressive supranuclear palsy, multiple system atrophy, or Alzheimer's disease. Furthermore, some dementing illnesses may show movement disorder as a clinical feature, often late in the course of the disease, but further confusing the issue of diagnosis.

Studies of dementia in Parkinson's disease

Cases of dementia in Parkinson's disease have been reported for over a hundred years. Frequently, the relationship between dementia and this disease in reported cases is impossible to discern.

A number of cross-sectional or prevalence studies of dementia in Parkinson's disease have been carried out. The frequency of dementia reported ranges from zero to 81 per cent. In a review of 17 studies Brown and Marsden found that, overall, 35 per cent of subjects were regarded as demented.[14] However, if more stringent criteria for dementia were applied then the proportions demented fell to between 15 and 20 per cent. The authors regarded these figures to be more realistic, and this level has proved to be in keeping with more recent cross-sectional studies.

Follow-up studies have great advantages in studying the frequency of dementia in Parkinson's disease: they allow the diagnosis of Parkinson's disease to be checked; repeated assessment reduces errors in the recognition of dementia; the pattern of evolution of dementia may be followed; the underestimation of dementia by selective loss through death is avoided; and they reveal the incidence rather than the prevalence of the condition. The problems of follow-up studies include the difficulties in the choice of those methods of diagnosis and assessment that will remain appropriate throughout the period of the follow-up.

No prospective controlled study of the incidence of dementia in Parkinson's disease has been entirely satisfactory in its methodology. Probably the most satisfactory is that reported by Biggins et al.,[15] and subsequently after a longer period of follow-up by Hughes et al.[16] Although this study employed satisfactory methods in most respects, its greatest weakness was in the selection of the original samples of both patients and controls. Biggins et al.[15] reported an incidence of dementia of 19 per cent after 4.5 years observation, or 48 per 1000 person-years of observation. A later report on the same cohorts of subjects showed an incidence of dementia of 47.8 per cent after 10 years of observation, or 46.9 cases per 1000 person-years of observation. The study shows a substantial incidence of dementia in Parkinson's disease increasing with the passage of the years. The control group showed cases of cognitive impairment but none amounting to dementia, thereby demonstrating a substantial excess risk in those subjects with Parkinson's disease.

The findings shown in Fig. 1 are broadly in keeping with the few other reported prospective studies.[17,18]

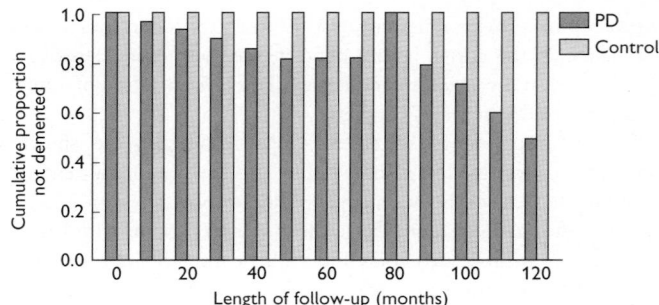

Fig. 1 Comparison of the incidence of dementia in Parkinson's disease with a control group of healthy subjects matched for age and sex. Note that the figure shows the percentage *not* demented. (Data from Biggins et al.[15] and Hughes et al.[16])

Prediction of dementia in Parkinson's disease

There is a consensus from a number of studies as to which of those subjects with Parkinson's disease are most likely to suffer from dementia: older people, patients with Parkinson's disease of longer duration, subjects who have a greater severity of motor symptoms and signs of Parkinson's disease, and those who show greater physical disability.[15,16] Some studies have shown that Parkinson's disease in men or of late onset is more likely to be associated with dementia.[19] In parkinsonism, as distinct from Parkinson's disease, the likelihood of dementia is closely related to the pathological changes that underlie the symptoms of parkinsonism, which include diseases in which dementia is a leading feature, such as Alzheimer's disease. The explanation of an apparent association between the treatment of Parkinson's disease with levodopa and dementia is probably that successful treatment of the motor symptoms of Parkinson's disease prolongs life and thereby increases the risk of dementia.

Neuropathology

The characteristic neuropathological changes of Parkinson's disease were described before the Second World War. The basic lesion is the degeneration of the pigmented neurone cells in the pars compacta of the substantia nigra in the brainstem, the presence of Lewy bodies, and accompanying gliosis. There is also a degeneration of neurones in the striatum and globus pallidus, but these changes may be secondary.[20] Clinical Parkinson's disease does not appear until about 80 per cent of the nigro striatal dopaminergic neurones have died. A correlation between the extent of cell loss in the pars compacta and the severity and duration of Parkinson's disease has been demonstrated. Lewy bodies had come to be regarded as pathognomonic of Parkinson's disease, but are now known to be present in other diseases (see Chapter 4.1.6).

Although the degenerative changes in the substantia nigra are known to be closely linked with decreased dopaminergic neurotransmission in the brain, and that it is this deficiency which leads to the main motor features of the disease, other neurotransmitters are also deficient. Some of these deficiencies are of a type that has been associated with cognitive impairment in other disorders, including a deficiency in acetylcholinesterase in the cortex, a deficiency of nor-adrenaline in the cortex, and a deficiency of serotonin (5-hydroxy-tryptamine) in the striatum and cortex. The concentration of a range of neuropeptides may also be altered.

The neuropathology of cases of Parkinson's disease showing dementia is inconsistent; some show neuropathological changes extending to parts of the brain beyond the subcortical region, whereas in others the changes are similar to those seen in patients with Parkinson's disease without dementia and with neuropathological changes restricted to the subcortical region. In some patients with dementia the neuropathological diagnosis is of Alzheimer's disease or of other recognized degenerated conditions of the brain.[21] An interesting case is that of Lewy body disease, which is dealt with in Chapter 4.1.6.

Just as there are difficulties in isolating Parkinson's disease from other conditions which closely resemble it, there are problems in understand the interrelationships of dementing disorders. At present, the aetiology of Parkinson's disease is unknown. Parkinson's disease shares this situation with a number of 'neurodegenerative' disorders, including Alzheimer's disease. Several distinct neurodegenerative diseases share some aetiological factors, which may represent an inter-action between environmental factors and the ageing process but with differing end results arising from specific factors in the process.[22,23] Problems in the diagnosis of Parkinson's disease, the shrinking cat-egory of idiopathic Parkinson's disease, and the difficulties encoun-tered in explaining the occasional development of dementia in this disease, suggests that the interrelationship between causative agents, the clinical features of disorders of movement, the occurrence of cog-nitive impairment, and the neuropathology of this group of disorders requires substantial further work before it is understood.

The influence of dementia on mortality

Dementia of any origin is associated with an increased risk of pre-mature death. A number of studies have shown an increased mortality in Parkinson's disease to be associated with age, late age of onset of this disease, cognitive impairment, dementia, and, in some studies, male sex. Certain medications have been associated with increased mortal-ity. Many of the studies that have been carried out have been methodo-logically faulty, making comparisons between studies and the identification of the effect of particular factors, including dementia, problematic. A study, meeting most of the requirements for an accur-ate assessment of mortality, showed a hazard ratio for Parkinson's dis-ease compared with controls of 1.64, in general, and of 1.94 for Parkinson's disease with dementia.[24] The occurrence of depression with Parkinson's disease led to increased mortality even more than dementia, with a hazard ratio of 2.66.

Clinical aspects of Parkinson's disease with dementia

The recognition of cognitive impairment in patients with Parkinson's disease has major implications for their management. Although pro-spective studies of patients with Parkinson's disease show that the ill-ness usually follows a course extending over many years, dementia brings with it important changes in the care a patient will require and in their life expectancy. These needs will progressively increase and will place an increasing burden upon the patient's immediate family and carers. The timing of wills and other legal procedures may be affected.

The most important step in the recognition of dementia in Parkin-son's disease is to suspect its presence. There are many features of Par-kinson's disease that tend to obscure the appearance of new clinical features of the disease. The typical blank facial expression seen in Par-kinson's disease may obscure a decline in intellectual activity, slowness in movement may conceal intellectual slowness, and sadness may sug-gest that morbid depression of mood is the reason for a reduction in liveliness. These clinical features may seem to account for increasing disability. The clinical picture can usually be clarified by careful exam-ination of the mental state. Examination of cognitive functions by more extensive standardized psychological tests may be useful in some cases.

The clinical importance of dementia in Parkinson's disease is that there is a marked increase in disability, with problems arising in areas of functioning not previously affected by motor impairment alone. The development of drug treatments for dementia makes its recog-nition in Parkinson's disease especially important. Dementia may be accompanied by an increased liability to confusional episodes from the toxic effects of drugs and other causes.

Management of dementia is similar to that for patients suffering from other dementing disorders, but with attention to the presence of a movement disorder.

References

1. Pirozzolo, F.J., Hansch, E.C., and Mortimer, J.A. (1982). Dementia in Parkinson's disease: a neuropsychological analysis. *Brain and Cognition*, **1**, 71–83.
2. Levin, B.E. and Katzen, H.L. (1995). Early cognitive changes and non-dementing behavioural abnormalities in Parkinson's disease. *Advances in Neurology*, **65**, 85–95.
3. Owen, A.M., James, M., Leigh, P.N., *et al.* (1992). Fronto-striatal cognitive deficits at different stages of Parkinson's disease. *Brain*, **115**, 1727–51.
4. Pollack, M. and Hornabrook, R.W. (1966). The prevalence, natural history and dementia of Parkinson's disease. *Brain*, **89**, 429–48.
5. Albert, M.L., Feldman, R.G., and Willis, A.L. (1974). The 'subcortical dementia' of progressive supra-nuclear palsy. *Journal of Neurology, Neurosurgery and Psychiatry*, **37**, 121–30.
6. Mayeux, R., Stern, Y., Rosen, J., and Benson, D.F. (1983). Is 'subcortical dementia' a recognisable clinical entity? *Annals of Neurology*, **14**, 278–83.
7. Whitehouse, P.J. (1986). The concept of cortical and subcortical dementia: another look. *Annals of Neurology*, **19**, 1–6.
8. Brown, R.G. and Marsden, C.D. (1988). Subcortical dementia: the neuropsychological evidence. *Neuroscience*, **25**, 363–87.
9. McHugh, P.R. (1990). The basal ganglia: the region, the integration of its systems and implications for psychiatry and neurology. In *Function and dysfunction in the basal ganglia* (ed. A.J. Franks, J.W. Ironside, R.H.S. Mindham, R.J. Smith, E.G.S. Spokes, and W. Winlow), pp. 259–69. Manchester University Press.
10. Cummings, J.L. (1988). The dementia of Parkinson's disease: prevalence, characteristics, neurobiology, and comparison with dementia of the Alzheimer type. *European Neurology*, **28**, 15–23.
11. Mindham, R.H.S. The place of dementia in Parkinson's disease: a methodological saga. *Advances in Neurology*, in press.
12. Hughes, A.J., Daniel, S.E., Kilford, L., and Lees, A.J. (1992). Accuracy of diagnosis of idiopathic Parkinson's disease: a clinico-pathological study of 100 cases. *Journal of Neurology, Neurosurgery and Psychiatry*, **55**, 181–4.

13. Anonymous (1992). Parkinson's disease: one illness or many syndromes? (Editorial). *Lancet*, **339**, 1263–4.

14. Brown, R.G. and Marsden, C.D. (1984). How common is dementia in Parkinson's disease? *Lancet*, **ii**, 1262–5.

15. Biggins, C.A., Boyd, J.L., Harrop, F.M., *et al.* (1992). A controlled longitudinal study of dementia in Parkinson's disease. *Journal of Neurology, Neurosurgery and Psychiatry*, **55**, 566–71.

16. Hughes, T.A., Ross, H.F., Musa, S., *et al.* (1998). The incidence and associations of dementia in Parkinson's disease. *Journal of Neurology, Neurosurgery and Psychiatry*, **65**, 422.

17. Rajput, A.H., Offord, K.P., Beard, M., and Kurland, L.T. (1987). A case–control study of smoking habits, dementia, and other illnesses in idiopathic Parkinson's disease. *Neurology*, **37**, 226–32.

18. Mayeux, R., Chen, J., Mirabello, E., *et al.* (1990). An estimate of the incidence of dementia in idiopathic Parkinson's disease. *Neurology*, **40**, 1513–17.

19. Mahieux, F., Fénelon, G., Flahault, A., Manifacier, M-J., Michelet, D., and Boller, F. (1998). Neuropsychological prediction of dementia in Parkinson's disease. *Journal of Neurology, Neurosurgery and Psychiatry*, **64**, 178–83.

20. Harding, A.E. (1993). Movement disorders. In *Brain's diseases of the nervous system* (10th edn) (ed. J. Walton), pp. 393–425. Oxford University Press.

21. Gibb, W.R.G. (1989). Dementia and Parkinson's disease. *British Journal of Psychiatry*, **154**, 596–614.

22. Calne, D.B., McGeer, E., Eisen, A., and Spencer, P. (1986). Alzheimer's disease, Parkinson's disease and motor neurone disease abiotrophic interactions between ageing and environment. *Lancet*, **ii**, 1067–70.

23. Ben-Shlomo, Y., Whitehead, A.S., and Smith, G.D. (1996). Parkinson's, Alzheimer's, and motor neurone disease. Clinical and pathological overlap may suggest common genetic and environmental factors. *Lancet*, **312**, 728.

24. Hughes, T.A. (1998). A controlled study of dementia and mortality in Parkinson's disease. Thesis, University of Leeds.

4.1.8 Dementia due to Huntington's disease

Susan Folstein

Introduction

Huntington's disease was first described in 1872 by an American physician who lived on Long Island, New York. His father and grandfather practised medicine in the same community, and thus he had access to case notes from several generations of families living in the area. This long period of record keeping allowed him to document a hereditary form of chorea, similar to 'common (Sydenham's) chorea', but progressing over many years to death. Its sufferers had a tendency to insanity and suicide. Huntington's brief essay, which also included a clear description of the autosomal dominant inheritance of this disorder, remains one of the classical descriptions of a medical disorder.[1]

Clinical features and course of illness

Huntington's disease is an inherited neuropsychiatric disorder mainly affecting the striatum and its direct connections. It is characterized by a triad of clinical features that are common to most diseases of the striatum and its direct connections: a non-aphasic dementia, depression and other disorders of mood, and a variety of dyskinesias, most typically chorea.[2,3] Chorea, from the Greek word for 'dance', describes involuntary non-stereotyped jerky movements. The illness, insidious in onset, may begin with any of these three features. Patients who present initially to psychiatrists usually have depression, often with suicidal thoughts or attempts, dementia, or loss of temper. The onset may occur at any time from early childhood to old age, most frequently between 35 and 45 years of age. Once the illness begins, sufferers gradually deteriorate over many years in their cognitive and motor functioning and end in a persistent vegetative state with almost complete loss of voluntary motor function. Death occurs after about 16 years (although some patients live much longer) and is usually caused by inanition or aspiration pneumonia. Some patients die earlier from suicide or subdural haematoma caused by a fall.

Pathology and genetics

The earliest visible neuropathology is in the striosomes of the caudate/putamen,[4] followed by a dorsal-to-ventral progressive loss of almost all striatal output neurones. There can also be milder neuronal loss in some brainstem nuclei and the deep layers of cortex.

The disorder, with a point prevalence of about 6/100 000,[5] is caused by the expansion of an unstable triplet repeat sequence (CAG) in the first exon of a gene near the telomere of chromosome 4p.[6] Normally, this triplet sequence contains from about 7 to 30 repeats; when the number rises above 37, Huntington's disease occurs. The abnormal gene is transcribed and appears to function abnormally, causing a 'gain of function' (see Chapter 2.4.2). It is transmitted as an autosomal dominant trait; if one parent is affected, each offspring (regardless of sex) has an independent 50 per cent chance of having inherited the abnormal gene. Those who inherit the gene will almost certainly develop Huntington's disease. The mutation rate is low, so that most patients will have an affected parent. However, it can be difficult to obtain an accurate family history. The pathophysiology may be related to the accumulation of fragments of the abnormal huntington protein (called 'huntingtin') in the nucleus of striatal neurones or the protein's abnormal interaction with other proteins.[7]

Like most disorders caused by the expansion of unstable trimeric repeat sequences, the number does not remain stable at meiosis. In Huntington's disease, the number of CAG repeats is more likely to increase when the gene is transmitted by fathers. As the number of repeats increases, the age at onset is earlier. Thus paternal transmission is often associated with 'anticipation', earlier onset in subsequent generations, and most cases with childhood onset have affected fathers.[8]

Diagnosis

Despite the availability of genetic testing, the diagnosis of Huntington's disease remains dependent on a thorough psychiatric history, including a detailed family history and history of changes in social adjustment, neurological examination, and mental state examination, including a cognitive examination. The clinical presentation changes as the disease progresses.[9]

Diagnosis of patients with early symptoms

Patients with Huntington's disease who initially consult psychiatrists usually present with depression or irritability, and occasionally with bipolar disorder, obsessive–compulsive disorder, schizophrenia, or excessive anxiety. When associated with Huntington's disease, these psychiatric syndromes are clinically indistinguishable from idiopathic psychiatric disorders and may persist as the only manifestation of the illness for several years. It is often during this prodromal phase that patients commit suicide, which may occur even if the patient does not know of his risk for Huntington's disease.[10] Additional presenting symptoms must often be elicited from an informant because the patient minimizes them or is embarrassed about them. These include loss of efficiency at work, which may have precipitated demotion or warnings from superiors stemming from loss of work speed and accuracy; a tendency to become irritated or physically aggressive in response to annoying stimuli that would not have elicited such a response in the past; and a decrease in interest in activities. Most of these symptoms and behaviours are common in psychiatric disorders, but the cognitive inefficiency and irritability may seem to be out of proportion in their severity, relative to the patient's other symptoms. On cognitive examination, the patient may have difficulty recalling dates of important life events and more difficulty than expected with 'serial sevens'. There may be motor restlessness (easily misinterpreted as a manifestation of anxiety), as well as motor signs on neurological examination, but these may be subtle: slightly slow saccadic eye movements,[11] writhing movements of the protruded tongue or of the fingertips when the arms are held at 90°, or mild disdiadochokinesis. Diagnosis can be further complicated by the apparent lack of a family history of Huntington's disease. The family may not have been informed about the affected parent's diagnosis even if it had been made, or may know only that a parent died in a psychiatric institution or committed suicide.

Usually, the cognitive changes are easier to notice after the psychiatric disorder is treated, which can usually be accomplished using standard medications. However, unlike idiopathic disorders, cognitive inefficiency and difficulties at work, apathy (if present), and sometimes irritability remain even after the patient's mood, energy, and sleep patterns have returned to normal. When this happens in the course of treatment of depression, a dementia work-up should be considered and the family history further scrutinized through hospital records and other family informants. If the family history is actually negative (this is quite uncommon for Huntington's disease) or unobtainable (often the case for adopted individuals who frequently present in childhood), the diagnosis may be confirmed by testing the patient's DNA for the expanded trimeric repeat in the Huntington's disease gene.

When Huntington's disease starts in childhood or early adolescence,[12] motor signs are limited to voluntary, parkinsonian-like motor slowness, with lead pipe or cogwheel rigidity and very slow saccades. Occasional children have a coarse tremor, and later myoclonus is seen. Cognitively, there is slowing in the rate of learning in school, deterioration of handwriting, and often loss of interest in school and social activities.[13] Of the patients who present with a schizophrenic syndrome, most are adolescents. Psychosis and loss of cognitive capacity may be the only clinical feature for several years before motor impairment begins. Children with Huntington's disease may have seizures, which are usually grand mal. Sometimes myoclonus is mistaken for seizures.

It is important to make the diagnosis of Huntington's disease as early as possible in persons who are employed. Poor function at work (or in schoolwork or household duties) occurs early in the illness, and patients are at risk of losing their jobs, often on suspicion of drug or alcohol abuse. This can usually be avoided if the diagnosis is made known to the family and employer, allowing the patient to retire on disability grounds. Prompt diagnosis does not mean that the patient needs to be informed of the diagnosis at that same time. Some patients are too depressed to do this safely; others indicate that they do not wish to be told. Treatment can usually proceed despite the patient's reluctance to label the disorder.

Diagnosis of patients with well-established signs and symptoms

After a few years of illness, diagnosis is easier. The signs and symptoms will have worsened, and usually the motor disorder has become obvious. A typical patient who has been ill for about 5 to 7 years is unable to work or manage finances, but lives at home and is able to handle personal needs. Some patients remain active and energetic, continuing to participate as fully in life as their cognitive and motor disabilities allow; others are apathetic most of the time, but irritable when disturbed; still others have severe depression with delusions, obsessions, or compulsions, and most are anxious and easily upset by changes of routine. An uncommon, but very troublesome, feature of Huntington's disease is sexual abnormality. While most patients become impotent or uninterested in sex, a few are hypersexual and may develop paraphilias.[14] While these may begin in the early years of illness, they are usually most troublesome in the middle stages.

Cognitively, patients complain of forgetfulness and becoming easily distracted. Thinking is slow; patients have difficulty following a conversation and cannot complete a multistaged task. On cognitive examination, Mini Mental State Examination scores[15] may still be above the usual 23 cut-off score, but serial sevens will be very poor, and one or two items will be missed on recalling words after a distraction. On neuropsychological testing, IQ will be lower than expected for education, and there will be difficulty learning word lists and on tests that require changing sets.

Most patients will have obvious involuntary choreic movements, as well as difficulty with control of voluntary motor movements, as seen by clumsiness, slowness, dysarthria, and an unsteady gait. The involuntary movements will wax and wane with the level of arousal. Speech will have an irregular staccato, often laboured, quality. Saccadic eye movements will be slow or irregular, and the patient will be obviously clumsy on diadochokinesis and finger–thumb tapping, although finger-to-nose testing is normal. Gait will be wide based and irregular, with difficulty with tandem walking. Reflexes are usually brisk.

Diagnosis of patients with advanced disease

After 10 years of illness, dementia is more severe, with poor performance on all aspects of the cognitive examination except naming. Speech is dysfluent with long lapses between the examiner's question and the patient's reply, rather like Brocca's aphasia. Some patients will be virtually unable to speak, although language is relatively preserved.

Patients (if they are co-operative) can carry out commands and will recognize relatives and nursing staff. Often irritability and depression have improved, but some patients continue to make suicide attempts or be physically aggressive. Physical disabilities are much worse. Patients often need to be fed, toileted, and helped with most daily needs. They have difficulty in walking and are at risk for falls that can cause further disability through broken limbs or subdural haematomas. Chorea often stabilizes and may even subside,[9] but the ability to carry out voluntary movements is more severely impaired. If they survive long enough, patients become unable to initiate speech, swallow with great difficulty, are unable to walk, and have such severely rigid muscle tone that they may be nearly unable to move their bodies. Clonus and positive Babinski signs are present. Patients in this sort of 'persistent vegetative state'[16] are difficult to distinguish from individuals with other movement disorders or dementias; as in early disease, eliciting a positive family history may be the only way to make a confident diagnosis without genetic testing.

Differential diagnosis

The differential diagnosis of Huntington's disease is theoretically quite large,[3] but only a few of the disorders for which it can be mistaken are very common.[2] This includes other dementias, other movement disorders, and other psychiatric disorders. The most frequent subcortical dementia is **Parkinson's disease**, which has a similar motor slowness, but a pill-rolling tremor and festinating gait are rare in Huntington's disease. The dementia associated with **late-life depression** can look very similar to Huntington's disease. **Alzheimer's disease** is easily distinguished by the lack of motor signs during the first several years of illness and more prominent difficulty with memory and language, as opposed to attention and calculation. Perhaps most difficult to distinguish clinically are the **frontal dementias**, which present with prominent behavioural disturbances and a positive family history. The clinical presentation may be insufficient to distinguish these various dementias in patients with advanced disease, since they may all progress to a persistent vegetative state. The family history and the duration of illness (which is longer for Huntington's disease than Alzheimer's disease or frontal dementia) can be helpful.

Several **other diseases classified as movement disorders** include all the features of the subcortical triad. They often have an autosomal dominant inheritance pattern, and some are caused by expansion of unstable trimeric repeat sequences. These include Fahr's syndrome (calcification of the striatum), some forms of spinocerebellar degeneration, chorea acanthocytosis, and dentato–rubral–pallido–lusian atrophy (**DRPLA**). The latter two disorders, while much rarer than Huntington's disease, can look so similar that they can only be diagnosed confidently by genetic testing (in the case of DRPLA) and by a blood smear for acanthocytes (in the case of chorea acanthocytosis). The most common movement disorder that resembles Huntington's disease is **tardive dyskinesia**. Patients with Huntington's disease occasionally have several years of a schizophrenia syndrome before the movement disorder begins. If they have been treated with neuroleptics, the involuntary movements of Huntington's disease are often mistaken for tardive dyskinesia. On the other hand, the choreoathetotic involuntary movements of severe tardive dyskinesia often involve the trunk and extremities as well as the face and look very much like Huntington's disease. Usually, it is possible to distinguish the patients with

tardive dyskinesia by their normal saccadic eye movements, normal tandem gait, and fluid and fluent speech.[17] However, DNA testing for Huntington's disease is sometimes appropriate. Wilson's disease also presents with the subcortical triad and should be considered when neither parent is affected. It is inherited as a recessive, so that the only affected relatives are siblings. Very-late-onset Huntington's disease may be diagnosed as 'senile chorea' because the family history appears to be negative. Family members will also present symptoms only late in life and may have died before their manifestation.

The differential diagnosis of nearly all **psychiatric disorders** includes Huntington's disease. The first clinical manifestation can be bipolar affective disorder, unipolar depression, schizophrenia (particularly in adolescents), obsessive–compulsive disorder, or anxiety disorder. As described above, the differential diagnosis is aided by a family history of Huntington's disease, but some families only know that a parent committed suicide or died in an institution, a history that is equally compatible with Huntington's disease or other psychiatric disorders.

Treatment and management

Currently, no treatment influences the course of illness of Huntington's disease, although advances in research on the function of the Huntington's disease gene may change that. Nevertheless, psychiatric treatments can relieve some of the troublesome symptoms. Clinical experience suggests that the depression, anxiety, and obsessive–compulsive disorder associated with Huntington's disease usually respond to the pharmacological treatments used for the similar idiopathic disorders. Because some patients seem unaware of their depressed mood (just as they can be unaware of their involuntary movements) an informant is needed to elicit the symptoms. It is also important to distinguish depression (from which the patient is miserable and sleepless) and apathy, which does not cause the patient distress. Occasionally, mood and anxiety disorders are chronic and unresponsive to treatment. Severe, unresponsive depression can be treated successfully with electroconvulsive therapy.[18] Bipolar disorder in patients with Huntington's disease does not usually respond to lithium, but may improve with carbamazepine or valproic acid, which is also helpful for severely irritable patients. Lithium is difficult to administer because Huntington's disease patients require high volumes of liquid and easily become lithium toxic if fluid intake is insufficient. In one case report, high doses of sertraline were very effective for intractable aggression.[19] Schizophrenic symptoms can be relatively unresponsive to treatment. Sometimes a combination of clozaril and antidepressants can provide some relief. Small doses of neuroleptics can be helpful in decreasing involuntary movements in the first stages of the illness.[20] Persons with advanced disease are often unresponsive to most medication, probably because few striatal receptors remain.

As with most dementias, psychopathology influences, and is influenced by, the patient's environment. Patients do best in a calm highly predictable environment. Patients whose jobs have become cognitively taxing can be irritable, especially towards their family. Often stopping work will alleviate this almost entirely. Huntington's disease seriously damages family relationships, which in turn affects the patient. The well spouse becomes responsible for supporting the family, caring for children and the patient, and making family and financial decisions. Spouses naturally find this very burdensome and may become irritable and resentful. Some patients are unwilling to give up financial and family decision making, even though they may make very poor decisions that damage family relationships and finances. Some patients neglect their children or treat them badly. If the other parent cannot prevent this, it is wisest to remove the patient from the home. There is no research on the treatment of sexual aggression, but the author has successfully treated a few males using progesterone.

Helping persons at risk for Huntington's disease

People at risk for Huntington's disease vary in their abilities to deal with the burden of uncertainty, depending on their personal attributes and their personal experience with the illness in a relative. A few consult physicians for reassurance, but most avoid doctors until they become ill, and even then many resist medical attention, claiming against all evidence that they are perfectly well. Relatively few persons at risk decide to have genetic testing to see whether they have the Huntington's disease gene, but persons who choose testing usually handle the results well, regardless of the test outcome.[21] They are often people who like to plan for the future; for them uncertainty is worse than bad news. Testing should always be preceded by genetic counselling that includes a discussion of the person's motivations. These usually include childbearing, educational and job decisions, or providing the information to their young adult offspring. Many individuals who come for testing have not seriously considered the possibility that they will have a bad outcome test, so that role playing about various outcome scenarios is important. Occasionally, persons request testing who have recently been told about Huntington's disease in their families or who are depressed or under unusual stress for other reasons. Such persons should be encouraged to delay testing until their situation becomes more settled. Finally, some people who request testing already have symptoms of Huntington's disease, yet do not wish to have a diagnosis. Considerable care is required to decide how best to support individuals in this situation, and family members or other close friends of the person should be consulted.[22]

References

1. Huntington, G. (1872). On chorea. Reprinted in *Advances in Neurology*, **1**, 33–5 (1973).
2. Folstein, S. (1989). *Huntington's disease. A disorder of families*. Johns Hopkins University Press, Baltimore, MD.
3. Harper, P. (ed.) (1991). *Huntington's disease*, Vol. 22. W.B. Saunders, London.
4. Hedreen, J.C. and Folstein, S.E. (1995). Early loss of neostriatal striosome neurons in Huntington's disease. *Journal of Neuropathology and Experimental Neurology*, **54**, 105–20.
5. Folstein, S.E, Chase, G.A., Wahl, W.E., McDonnell, A.M., and Folstein, M.F. (1987). Huntington disease in Maryland: clinical aspects of racial variation. *American Journal of Human Genetics*, **41**, 168–79.
6. Huntington's Disease Collaborative Research Group (1993). A novel gene containing a trinucleotide repeat that is expanded and unstable on Huntington's disease chromosomes. *Cell*, **72**, 971–83.
7. Ross, C.A., Russell, L.M., Becher, M.W., *et al.* (1998). Pathogenesis of neurodegenerative diseases associated with expanded glutamine repeats: new answers, new questions. *Progress in Brain Research*, **117**, 398–419.
8. Ranen, N.G., Stine, O.C., Abbott, M.H., *et al.* (1995). Anticipation and

9. Folstein, S.E., Leigh, R., Parhad, I.M., and Folstein, M.F. (1986). The diagnosis of Huntington's disease. *Neurology*, **36**, 1279–83.
10. Folstein, S.E., Abbott, M.H., Franz, M.L., Huang, S., Chase, G.A., and Folstein, M.F. (1983). The association of affective disorder with Huntington's disease in a case series and in families. *Psychological Medicine*, **13**, 537–42.
11. Leigh, R.J., Newman, S.A., Folstein, S.E., Lasker, A.G., and Jensen, B.A. (1983). Abnormal ocular motor control in Huntington's disease. *Neurology*, **33**, 1268–75.
12. Kosky, R. (1981). Children and Huntington's disease: some clinical observations of children at risk. *Medical Journal of Australia*, **1**, 405–7.
13. Nance, M. (1997). Genetic testing of children at risk for Huntington's disease. *Neurology*, **49**, 1048–53.
14. Federoff, J.O., Peyser, C.E., Franz, M.L., and Folstein, S.E. (1994). Sexual disorders in Huntington's disease. *Journal of Neuropsychiatry and Clinical Neuroscience*, **6**, 147–53.
15. Folstein, M.F., Folstein, S.E., and McHugh, P.R. (1975). 'Mini-Mental State': a practical method for grading the cognitive state of patients for the clinician. *Journal of Psychiatric Research*, **2**, 189–98.
16. Walshe, T.M. and Leonard, C. (1985). Persistent vegetative state: extension of the syndrome to include chronic disorders. *Archives of Neurology*, **42**, 1045–7.
17. David, A.S., Jeste, D.V., Folstein, M.F., and Folstein, S.E. (1987). Voluntary movement dysfunction in Huntington's disease and tardive dyskinesia. *Acta Neurologica Scandinavia*, **75**, 130–9.
18. Ranen, N.G., Peyser, C.E., and Folstein, S.E. (1994). ECT as a treatment for depression in Huntington's disease. *Journal of Neuropsychiatry and Clinical Neurosciences*, **6**, 154–9.
19. Ranen, N.G., Lipsey, J.R., Treisman, G., and Ross, C.A. (1996). Sertraline in the treatment of severe aggressiveness in Huntington's disease. *Journal of Neuropsychiatry and Clinical Neuroscience*, **8**, 338–40.
20. Barr, A.N., Fischer, J.H., Koller, W.C., Spunt, A.L., and Singhal, A. (1988). Serum haloperidol concentration and choreiform movements in Huntington's disease. *Neurology*, **38**, 84–8.
21. Codori, A.M., Slavney, P.R., Young, C., Miglioretti, D.L., and Brandt, J. (1997). Predictors of psychological adjustment in genetic testing for Huntington's disease. *Health Psychology*, **16**, 36–50.
22. Scourfield, J., Soldan, J., Gray, J., Houlihan, G., and Harper, P.S. (1997). Huntington's disease: psychiatric practice in molecular genetic prediction and diagnosis. *British Journal of Psychiatry*, **170**, 146–9.

4.1.9 Vascular dementia

Timo Erkinjuntti

Introduction

Vascular dementia is the second most frequent cause of dementia.[1,2] Because vascular causes of cognitive impairment are common, may be preventable, and the patients could benefit from therapy, early detection and accurate diagnosis of vascular dementia is desirable.[3]

Vascular dementia is not only multi-infarct dementia, but is related to other other vascular mechanisms and pathological changes in the brain, and has other causes and clinical manifestations. Vascular dementia is not a disease, but a syndrome. The origin of of this syndrome reflects complex interactions between vascular aetiologies (cerebrovascular disorders and vascular risk factors), changes in the

instability of (CAG)n repeats in IT-15 in parent–offspring pairs with Huntington's disease. *American Journal of Human Genetics*, **57**, 593–602.

brain (infarcts, white-matter lesions, atrophy), host factors (age, education), and cognition.[4–8]

Conceptual issues related to of vascular dementia include the definition of the cognitive syndrome (type, extent, and combination of impairments in different cognitive domains), and the vascular causes (vascular aetiologies and changes in the brain). Variations in these definitions has led to different estimates of point prevalence, to different groups of patients, and to reports of different types and distribution of brain lesions.[9–11] The cognitive syndrome of vascular dementia is characterized by predominate executive dysfunction rather than deficits in memory and language function.[12] Although the course of cognitive decline may be stepwise, it is often slowly progressive, and may include periods of stability or even some improvement.

The relationship between vascular lesions in the brain and cognitive impairment is important, but which type, extent, side, site, and tempo of vascular lesions in the brain relates to different types of vascular dementia is not established in detail.[4–6,13]

Current criteria for vascular dementia are based on the concept of cerebral infarcts. For example the widely used NINDS-AIREN criteria include dementia, cerebrovascular disease, and a relationship between these two disorders. The main tools for the diagnosis include detailed history, neurological examination, mental state examination, relevant laboratory examinations, and preferably magnetic resonance imaging of the brain.

Vascular dementia research, until recently overshadowed by that into Alzheimer's disease, is now developing rapidly. There is great promise for intervention. Developments in classification, diagnosis, and treatment are likely.

Aetiology and pathophysiology

Aetiology

The main causes of vascular dementia are cerebrovascular disorders and their risk factors. The prevalent cerebrovascular disorders include large artery disease (artery-to-artery embolism, occlusion of an extra- or intracranial artery), cardiac embolic events, small vessel disease (lacunar infarcts, ischaemic white-matter lesions) and haemodynamic mechanisms.[13–15] Less frequent causes include specific arteriopathies, haemorrhage (intracranial haemorrhage, subarachnoidal haemorrhage), haematological factors, venous disease, and hereditary disorders. There may be as yet undiscovered causes.

In most patients diagnosed with vascular dementia, several aetiological factors are involved. However, the roles these factors play have not been identified in detail, and it is not certain which of these mechanisms distinguish vascular dementia from cerebrovascular disease without dementia.[4,5,7,16,17]

Risk factors for vascular dementia can be divided into vascular factors (e.g. arterial hypertension, atrial fibrillation, myocardial infarction, coronary heart disease, diabetes, generalized atherosclerosis, lipid abnormalities, smoking), demographic factors (e.g age, education), genetic factors (e.g. family history, individual genetic features), and stroke-related factors (e.g. type of cerebrovascular disease, site and size of stroke).[18,19] Hypoxic ischaemic events (cardiac arrhythmias, congestive heart failure, myocardial infarction, seizures, pneumonia) may be an important risk factor for incident dementia in patients with stroke.[20]

Changes in the brain

Vascular dementia is related to both ischaemic and non-ischaemic changes in the brain.[4,5,13,14] The ischaemic lesions include arterial territorial infarct, distal field (watershed) infarct, lacunar infarct, ischaemic white-matter lesions, and incomplete ischaemic injury. Incomplete ischaemic injury incorporates laminar necrosis, focal gliosis, granular atrophy, and incomplete white-matter infarction.[21,22] In addition, both focal (around the ischaemic lesion) and remote (disconnection, diaschisis) functional ischaemic changes relate to vascular dementia, and the volume of functionally inactive tissue exceeds that of focal ischaemic lesions in vascular dementia.[23] Limitation in current clinical methods have hampered the detection of both incomplete ischaemic injury and functional ischaemic changes related to vascular dementia. Atrophy is the non-ischaemic factor related to vascular dementia. However, there are no methods to distinguish between ischaemic and degenerative causes of atrophy.

Brain imaging findings

Work on the relationship between brain lesions and cognition in vascular dementia has used varying definitions and measures of cognitive impairment, varying techniques to reveal brain changes, and varying criteria for the selection of patients.[17]

CT and magnetic resonance imaging (**MRI**) studies on vascular dementia have shown that bilateral ischaemic lesions are important.[4,5,7,17] Some studies emphasize deep infarcts in the frontal and limbic areas, while others report cortical lesions especially in the temporal and parietal areas. There is disagreement about the number and volume of the infarcts, as well as the extent and location of atrophy. Diffuse and extensive white-matter lesions have been suggested as an important factor leading to functional disconnection of cortical brain areas. Some general conclusions on brain lesions in vascular dementia may be drawn.

1. There is no single pathological feature, but a combination of infarcts, ischaemic white-matter lesions of varying size and type, and atrophy of varying degree and site.

2. Infarcts associated with vascular dementia tend to be bilateral, multiple (more than two), and located in the dominant hemisphere and in the limbic structures (frontolimbic or prefrontal-subcortical and medial-limbic or medial-hippocampal circuits).

3. White-matter lesions on CT or magnetic resonance imaging (**MRI**) associated with vascular dementia are extensive, extending in periventricular white matter, and confluent to extending in the deep white matter.

4. It is doubtful whether a single small lesion on imaging can be accepted as evidence for vascular dementia.

5. Absence of cerebrovascular lesions on CT or MRI is contrary to a diagnosis of vascular dementia.

Pathophysiology

To what extent pathological changes in the brain cause, compound, or only coexist with the vascular dementia syndrome is still not known precisely. The vascular changes in the brain can be the main cause of cognitive impairment (as assumed in vascular dementia[24,25]), they can contribute to the clinical picture of other dementia syndromes including Alzheimer's disease,[7,26] or they may be coincidental.

It is not certain which are the critical changes in the brain leading to the clinical picture of vascular dementia. the syndrome has been related to the volume of brain infarcts (with a critical threshold), the number of infarcts, the site of infarcts (bilateral, in strategic cortical or subcortical, or affecting white matter), to other ischaemic factors (incomplete ischaemic injury, delayed neuronal death, functional changes), to the atrophic changes (origin, location, extent), and finally to the additive effects of other pathologies (Alzheimer's disease, Lewy body dementia, frontal lobe dementias). But it is uncertain which type, extent, side, site, and tempo of vascular lesions in the brain, and which combinaton with other pathologies, relate to vascular dementia.[4-6,13]

Classification and clinical criteria

Classification

Vascular dementia has been divided into subtypes on the basis of clinical, radiological, and neuropathological features. It is uncertain whether these subtypes are distinct disorders, with separate pathological and clinical features, and responses to therapy.[27] If homogenous subtypes could be identified the comparability of research studies would be greater and multicentre studies easier.[28]

The subtypes of vascular dementia included in most classifications include multi-infarct dementia (cortical lesions), small-vessel dementia (subcortical deep lesions), and strategic infarct dementia.[12,14,27,29-32] Many include also hypoperfusion dementia.[12,14,30,33] Further suggested subtypes include haemorrhagic dementia, hereditary vascular dementia, and combined or mixed dementia (Alzheimer's disease with cerebrovascular disease).

DSM-IV[34] does not specify subtypes. ICD-10[35] includes six subtypes (acute onset, multi-infarct, subcortical, mixed cortical and subcortical, other, and unspecified). The NINDS-AIREN criteria[30] include, without detailed description, cortical vascular dementia, subcortical vascular dementia, Binswanger's disease, and thalamic dementia.

Main subtypes

Multi-infarct dementia or cortical vascular dementia, and small-vessel dementia or subcortical vascular dementia are the two common subtypes, although their frequencies vary in different series.[12,14,31]

Cortical vascular dementia relates to large-vessel disease, cardiac embolic events, and hypoperfusion. Infarcts are predominantly in the cortical and corticosubcortical arterial territories, and their distal fields (watershed). Typical clinical features are lateralized sensimotor changes and the abrupt onset of cognitive impairment and aphasia.[31] A combination of different cortical neuropsychological syndromes has been suggested to occur in cortical vascular dementia.[36]

Subcortical vascular dementia, or small-vessel dementia, incorporates the entities 'lacunar state' and 'Binswanger's disease'. It relates to small-vessel disease and hypoperfusion, with predominately lacunar infarcts, focal and diffuse ischaemic white-matter lesions, and incomplete ischaemic injury.[31,36,37] Clinically, small-vessel dementia is characterized by pure motor hemiparesis, bulbar signs, dysarthria, depression, and emotional lability, and especially deficits in executive functioning.[36-39]

Table 1 The DSM-IV definition of vascular dementia

Focal neurological signs and symptoms (e.g. exaggeration of deep tendon reflexes, extensor plantar response, pseudobulbar palsy, gait abnormalities, weakness of an extremity, etc.)

or

Laboratory evidence of focal neurological damage (e.g. multiple infarctions involving cortex and underlying white matter)

The cognitive deficits cause significant impairment in social or occupational functioning and represent a significant decline from a previously higher level of functioning

The focal neurological signs, symptoms, and laboratory evidence are judged to be aetiologically related to the disturbance

The deficits do not occur exclusively during the course of delirium

Course characterized by sustained periods of clinical stability punctuated by sudden significant cognitive and functional losses

Clinical criteria

Since the 1970s several clinical criteria for vascular dementia have been published.[11,40,41] The most widely used include those in DSM-IV,[34] ICD-10,[35] and NINDS-AIREN.[30]

The two cardinal elements of any clinical criteria for vascular dementia are the definition of the cognitive syndrome[42] and the definition of the cause.[11,41,43] All clinical criteria are consensus criteria, derived neither from prospective community-based studies on vascular factors affecting the cognition, nor on detailed natural histories.[28,30,40,41,44] All these criteria are based on the concept of ischaemic infarcts. They are designed to have high specificity, but have been poorly validated.[40,44] An important consequence of the different definitions of the dementia syndrome,[9,42] and the vascular cause,[10,11] is that the different diagnostic criteria identify different populations.

The DSM-IV definition of vascular dementia (Table 1) requires focal neurological signs and symptoms or laboratory evidence of focal neurological damage clinically judged to be related to the disturbance.[34] The course is specified by sudden cognitive and functional losses. The DSM-IV criteria do not detail brain imaging requirements. The DSM-IV definition of vascular dementia is reasonably broad and lacks detailed clinical and radiological guidelines.

The ICD-10 criteria[35] (Table 2) require unequal distribution of cognitive deficits, focal signs as evidence of focal brain damage, and significant cerebrovascular disease judged to be aetiologically related to the dementia. The criteria do not detail brain imaging requirements. The ICD-10 criteria specify six subtypes of vascular dementia (Table 3). The ICD-10 criteria for vascular dementia have been shown to be highly selective and only some of those fulfilling the general criteria for ICD-10 vascular dementia can be classified into one of the subtypes.[11,43] The shortcoming of these criteria include lack of detailed guidelines (e.g. of unequal cognitive deficits and changes on neuroimaging), lack of aetiological criteria, and heterogeneity.[11,43]

The NINDS-AIREN research criteria for vascular dementia[30] include a dementia syndrome, cerebrovascular disease, and a relationship between these (Table 4). Cerebrovascular disease is defined by the presence of focal neurological lesions and brain imaging evidence of ischaemic changes in the brain. A relationship between dementia and

Table 2 The ICD-10 criteria for vascular dementia

Unequal distribution of deficits in higher cognitive functions with some affected and others relatively spared. Thus, memory may be quite markedly affected while thinking, reasoning, and information processing may show only mild decline

There is evidence for focal brain damage, manifest as at least one of the following: unilateral spastic weakness of the limbs, unilaterally increased tendon reflexes, an extensor plantar response, pseudobulbar palsy

There is evidence from the history, examination, or test of significant cerebrovascular disease, which may reasonably be judged to be aetiologically related to the dementia (history of stroke, evidence of cerebral infarction)

cerebrovascular disorder is inferred from the onset of dementia within 3 months following a recognized stroke, or on abrupt deterioration in cognitive functions, or fluctuating stepwise progression of cognitive deficits. The criteria include a list of features consistent with the diagnosis, as well as a list of features that make the diagnosis uncertain or unlikely. Also, different levels of certainty of the clinical diagnosis (probable, possible, definite) are included. The NINDS-AIREN criteria recognize heterogeneity[45] of the syndrome and variability of the clinical course in vascular dementia, and highlight detection of ischaemic lesions and a relationship between lesion and cognition, as well as stroke and dementia onset.

Table 3 Characteristics of the vascular dementia subtypes in ICD-10

Acute onset (F01.0)

The dementia develops rapidly (i.e. usually within 1 month but within no longer than 3 months) after a succession of strokes, or (rarely) after a single large infarction

Multi-infarct (F01.1)

The onset of the dementia is more gradual (i.e. within 3–6 months) following a number of minor ischaemic episodes. Comments: it is presumed that there is an accumulation of infarcts in the cerebral parenchyma. Between the ischaemic episodes there may be periods of actual clinical improvement

Subcortical (F01.2)

A history of hypertension, and evidence from clinical examination and special investigations of vascular disease located in the deep white matter of the cerebral hemispheres, with preservation of the cerebral cortex.

Mixed cortical and subcortical (F01.3)

Mixed cortical and subcortical components of vascular dementia may be suspected from the clinical features, the results of investigation, or both

Other (F01.8)
Unspecified (F01.9)

In the ICD-10 criteria no specific diagnostic guidelines are given for these two vascular dementia sybtypes

Table 4 The NINDS-AIREN criteria for probable vascular dementia

I. The criteria for the clinical diagnosis of PROBABLE vascular dementia include *all* of the following

1. *Dementia*
2. *Cerebrovascular disease*, defined by the presence of focal signs on neurological examination, such as hemiparesis, lower facial weakness, Babinski sign, sensory deficit, hemianopia, dysarthria, etc. consistent with stroke (with or without history of stroke), and evidence of relevant CVD by brain imaging (CT or MRI) including multiple large-vessel strokes or a single strategically placed infarct (angular gyrus, thalamus, basal forebrain, PCA or ACA territories), as well as multiple basal ganglia and white-matter lacunes or extensive periventricular white-matter lesions, or combinations thereof
3. *A relationship between the above two disorders*, manifested or inferred by the presence of one or more of the following
   (a) Onset of dementia within 3 months following a recognized stroke
   (b) Abrupt deterioration in cognitive functions, or fluctuating stepwise progression of cognitive deficits

II. Clinical features consistent with the diagnosis of PROBABLE vascular dementia include the following
   (a) Early presence of a gait disturbance (small-step gait or *marche à petits-pas*, apraxic–ataxic or parkinsonian gait)
   (b) History of unsteadiness and frequent unprovoked falls
   (c) Early urinary frequency, urgency, and other urinary symptoms not explained by urological disease
   (d) Personality and mood changes, abulia, depression, emotional incontinence, other subcortical deficits including psychomotor retardation and abnormal executive function

III. Features that make the diagnosis of vascular dementia uncertain or unlikely include the following
   (a) Early onset of memory deficit and progressive worsening of memory and other cognitive functions such as language (transcortical sensory aphasia), motor skills (apraxia), and perception (agnosia), in the absence of corresponding focal lesions on brain imaging
   (b) Absence of focal neurological signs, other than cognitive disturbance
   (c) Absence of cerebrovascular lesions on brain CT or MRI

CVD, cerebrovascular disease; PCA, posterior cerebral artery; ACA, anterior cerebral artery.

The NINDS-AIREN criteria are currently most widely used in clinical drug trials on vascular dementia. In a neuropathological series, sensitivity of the NINDS-AIREN criteria was 58 per cent and specificity 80 per cent.[47] The criteria successfully excluded Alzheimer's disease in 91 per cent of cases, and the proportion of combined cases misclassified as probable vascular dementia was 29 per cent.[47] The inter-rater reliability of the NINDS-AIREN criteria is moderate to substantial ($\kappa = 0.46$–0.72).[48]

These three sets of criteria for vascular dementia are not interchangeable; they identify different numbers and clusters of patients. The DSM-IV criteria are less restrictive than the ICD-10 and NINDS-AIREN criteria.[11,46]

Clinical features

Cognitive syndrome

The cognitive syndrome of vascular dementia is characterized by memory deficit, dysexecutive syndrome, slowed information processing, and mood and personality changes. These features are found especially among patients with subcortical lesions. Patients with cortical lesions often have additional cortical neuropsychological syndromes.[36]

The memory deficit in vascular dementia is often less severe than in Alzheimer's disease. It is characterized by impaired recall, relatively intact recognition, and more benefit from cues.[49] The dysexecutive syndrome in vascular dementia includes impairment in goal formulation, initiation, planning, organizing, sequencing, executing, set-sifting and set-maintenance, as well as in abstracting.[12,36,49] The dysexecutive syndrome in vascular dementia relates to lesions affecting the prefrontal subcortical circuit including prefrontal cortex, caudate, pallidum, thalamus, and the thalamocortical circuit (capsular genu, anterior capsule, anterior centrum semiovale, and anterior corona radiata).[50] Typically, personality and insight are relatively preserved in mild and moderate cases of vascular dementia.

Features that make the diagnosis of vascular dementia disease uncertain or unlikely include early and progressive worsening of memory, and other cognitive cortical deficits in the absence of corresponding focal lesions on brain imaging.[30]

Neurological findings

Frequent neurological findings indicating focal brain lesion early in the course of vascular dementia include mild motor or sensory deficits, decreased co-ordination, brisk tendon reflexes, Babinski's sign, visual field loss, bulbar signs including dysarthria and dysphagia, extrapyramidal signs (mainly rigidity and akinesia), disordered gait (hemiplegic, apraxic–ataxic, or small-stepped), unsteadiness, unprovoked falls, and urinary frequency and urgency.[30,31,37–39] Features that make the diagnosis of vascular dementia uncertain or unlikely include absence of focal neurological signs, other than cognitive disturbance.[30]

In cortical vascular dementia, typical clinical features are lateralized sensorimotor changes and abrupt onset of cognitive impairment and aphasia, and in subcortical vascular dementia disease pure motor hemiparesis, bulbar signs, and dysarthria.[31]

Behavioural and psychological symptoms of dementia

Depression, anxiety, emotional lability and incontinence, and other psychiatric symptoms are frequent in vascular dementia. Depression, abulia, emotional incontinence, and psychomotor retardation are especially frequent in subcortical vascular dementia disease.[12,36]

Ischaemic scores

Cardinal features of vascular dementia disease are incorporated in the Hachinski Ischaemia Score[51] (Table 5). In a recent neuropathological series, stepwise deterioration (odds ratio, 6.0), fluctuating course (odds ratio, 7.6), history of hypertension (odds ratio, 4.3), history of stroke (odds ratio, 4.3), and focal neurological symptoms (odds ratio,

Table 5 Hachinski Ischaemia Score

Item	Score value
Abrupt onset	2
Stepwise deterioration	1
Fluctuating course	2
Nocturnal confusion	1
Relative preservation of personality	1
Depression	1
Somatic complaints	1
Emotional incontinence	1
History of hypertension	1
History of strokes	2
Evidence of associated atherosclerosis	1
Focal neurological symptoms	2
Focal neurological signs	2

4.4) differentiated patients with definite vascular dementia from those with definite Alzheimer's disease.[52] Nocturnal confusion and depression did not discriminate. However, the ischaemia score was unable to differentiate the Alzheimer's disease patients with cerebrovascular disease from those with vascular dementia.

Course and prognosis

Traditionally, vascular dementia has been characterized by a relative abrupt onset (days to weeks), a stepwise deterioration (some recovery after worsening), and fluctuating course (e.g. differences between days) of cognitive functions. These features are seen in patients with repeated lesions affecting cortical and corticosubcortical brain structures, i.e. large-vessel multi-infarct vascular dementia, and with watershed infarcts related to haemodynamic problems. However, in patients with small-vessel dementia, i.e. subcortical vascular dementia, the onset is more insidious and course more slowly progressive.[28,30,37,53]

The mean duration of vascular dementia is around 5 years.[2] In most studies survival is less than for the general population or those with Alzheimer's disease.[54,55] Surprisingly little is known about the rate and pattern of cognitive decline, either overall or among different subgroups of vascular dementia.[56] This underlines the lack of studies detailing the natural history of vascular dementia.

Diagnosis and differential diagnosis

The clinical evaluation of patients with memory impairment has two stages, the symptomatic diagnosis, i.e. evaluation of the type and extent of cognitive impairment, and the aetiological diagnosis, i.e. evaluation of vascular cause(s) and related factors. The symptomatic categories other than dementia include delirium, circumscribed neuropsychological syndromes (e.g. aphasia) and functional psychiatric disorders (e.g. depression).[44] Stages of aetiological diagnosis include diagnosis of the specific causes, especially the potentially treatable conditions, evaluation of secondary factors able to affect the cognitive functioning, and more detailed differentiation between specific causes, especially that between vascular dementia disease and Alzheimer's disease.

Clinical evaluation

The cornerstone in the evaluation of a patient with suspected vascular dementia is detailed clinical and neurological history and examination, including interview of a close informant. Assessment of social functions, activities of daily living, as well as psychiatric and behavioural symptoms, is part of the basic evaluation. These patients are challenging and enough time should be allocated time for the consultation, often 40 to 60 min.

Mental status examination

Bedside mental status examination includes the Mini-Mental State Examination.[57] However, this has limitations as it emphasizes language, does not include timed elements and the recognition portion of the memory tests, is insensitive to mild deficits, and is influenced by education and age. Other proposed screening instruments for vascular dementia include a ten-word memory test with delayed recall, cube drawing test for copy, verbal fluency test (number of animals named in 1 min), Luria's alternating hand sequence, or finger rings and letter cancellation test (neglect).[30]

Frequently a more detailed neuropsychological test is needed. It should cover the main cognitive domains including memory functions (short- and long-term memory), abstract thinking, judgement, aphasia, apraxia, agnosia, orientation, attention, executive functions, and speed of information processing.[42,58]

Brain imaging

Brain imaging should be performed at least once during the initial diagnostic workout. MRI is preferred because it has high sensitivity and the ability to demonstrate medial temporal lobe and basal forebrain areas. Depending on the criteria of vascular dementia used, focal brain infarcts have been revealed in 70 to 100 per cent, and more extensive white-matter lesions in 70 to 100 per cent of cases.[13,25,30,59,60]

Single-photon emission CT and positron-emission tomography may reveal patchy reduction of regional blood flow and metabolism, as well as decreased white-matter flow and metabolism.[61]

Other investigations

Chest X-ray, elelectrocardiography, and screening laboratory tests are part of the basic evaluation.[15,62,63] In selected cases extended laboratory investigations, analysis of the cerebrospinal fluid, and EEG are performed, as well as examinations of the extra- and intracranial arteries and detailed cardiological investigations.[15,62,63]

In vascular dementia EEG is more often normal than in Alzheimer's disease, and if abnormal more frequently suggests a focal abnormality. Abnormalities increase with more severe intellectual decline both in vascular dementia disease and Alzheimer's disease.[53]

At present there is no specific laboratory test for vascular dementia. Tests may reveal risk factors and concomitant disorders such as hyperlipidaemia, diabetes, and cardiac abnormality.[53] Apolipoprotein E_4 is a established risk factor for Alzheimer's disease, but its relationship to vascular dementia has not been consistent.[64] Determination of apo-lipoprotein E status is currently not part of clinical evaluation in vascular dementia.

Differential diagnosis of vascular dementia disease

Alzheimer's disease

Typical Alzheimer's disease is characterized by insidious onset and slowly progressive intellectual deterioration, absence of symptoms and signs indicating focal brain damage, and absence of any other specific disease affecting the brain.[65] Alzheimer's disease has typical clinical stages ranging from early changes to profound dementia.[66,67]

When patients with vascular dementia have a clinical history, neurological examination, and brain imaging findings compatible with ischaemic changes of the brain, the differentiation from Alzheimer's disease can be made clinically.[25]

Diagnostic problems arise when Alzheimer's disease is combined with cerebrovascular disease. Difficult clinical problems include stroke unmasking Alzheimer's disease in patients with post-stroke dementia, insidious onset, and/or slow progressive course in vascular dementia patients, and cases where it is difficult to assess the role of white-matter lesions or of infarcts found on neuroimaging. This clinical challenge may be solved when a sensitive and specific ante-mortem marker for Alzheimer's disease is available. The distinction would be less difficult if there were more detailed knowledge of the sites, type, and extent of ischaemic brain changes critical for vascular dementia, and the extent and type of medial temporal lobe atrophy critical for Alzheimer's disease.

Other important conditions to be diffentiated from vascular dementia include normal pressure hydrocephalus,[68] white-matter lesions and dementia,[17,30] frontal lobe tumours and other intracranial masses,[15] Lewy body dementia,[69] frontotemporal dementia,[70] Parkinsons's disease and dementia,[71] progressive supranuclear palsy,[72] and multisystem atrophy.[73]

Epidemiology

Vascular dementia is the second most common cause of dementia accounting for 10 to 50 per cent of cases, depending on the geographic location, patient population, and clinical methods used.[1,2] The prevalence of vascular dementia is from 1.2 to 4.2 per cent of persons aged 65 years and older, and the incidence is 6 to 12 cases per 1000 persons aged over 70 years per year.[2] The prevalence and the incidence of vascular dementia disease increases with increasing age, and men seem to have a higher prevalence of vascular dementia than women. Epidemiology of vascular dementia has been affected by variations in the definition of the disorder, the clinical criteria used, and the clinical methods applied.[18,74,75]

The frequency of vascular dementia disease has been higher than previously reported in recent series comprising older subjects.[10] Stroke and cerebrovascular disorders relate also to a high risk of cognitive impairment and dementia.[24,76] Finally, vascular factors such as stroke and white-matter lesions have a clinical effect on Alzheimer's disease.[26] Thus, vascular factors may even be the leading cause of cognitive impairment worldwide.[77]

Treatment

The objectives of targeted treatment of vascular dementia include symptomatic improvement of core symptoms (e.g. cognitive, behavioural), slowing progression of the disorder, and treatment of secondary factors affecting cognition (e.g. depression, anxiety, agitation).

A number of drugs have been studied in the symptomatic treatment of vascular dementia including cerebro- and vasoactive drugs, nootropics, and some calcium antagonists, but largely these studies have shown negative results.[78] Studies on symptomatic improvement in vascular dementia have mostly had small numbers, short treatment periods, variations in diagnostic criteria and tools, mixed populations, and have had variation in clinical endpoints applied.

Recently nimodipine,[79] memantine,[80] and propentofylline[81] have raised expectations for a symptomatic treatment of vascular dementia. A number of phase 3 double-blind randomized placebo-controlled trials in patients with vascular dementia using these compounds are in progress.[82]

Possibilities for prevention

For primary prevention the target is the brain at risk of cerebrovascular disease and cognitive impairment. The methods relate to the treatment of putative risk factors of vascular dementia, and the promotion of potential protective factors. Risk factors include those related to cerebrovascular disorders and stroke, to vascular dementia, to post-stroke dementia, to white-matter lesions, and to cognitive impairment or dementia, and also those related to Alzheimer's disease.[8] The vascular risk factors include arterial hypertension, atrial fibrillation, myocardial infarction, coronary heart disease, diabetes, generalized atherosclerosis, lipid abnormalities, and smoking. The demographic factors include age and education. One putative protective factor is oestrogen.[83]

Knowledge of effects of primary prevention on these risk factors in populations free of cognitive impairment is still scant.[8,84] In a European study, treatment of mild systolic hypertension decreased the incidence of dementia.[85] Positive effects in primary prevention of stroke support the idea that action on vascular risk factors could reduce the numbers of patients with vascular dementia.

For secondary prevention the target is the brain already affected by cerebrovascular disease and at risk of vascular dementia. Actions include diagnosis and treatment of acute stroke in order to limit the extent of ischaemic brain changes, prevention of recurrence of stroke, and treatment of risk factors. Treatment is guided by the aetiology of cerebrovascular disorder such as large artery disease (e.g. aspirin, dipyridamole, carotid endarterectomy), cardiac embolic events (e.g. anticoagulation, aspirin), small-vessel disease (e.g. antiplatelet therapy), and haemodynamic mechanisms (e.g. control of hypotension and cardiac arrhythmias).[15,29,44] Hypoxic ischaemic events (cardiac arrhythmias, congestive heart failure, myocardial infarction, seizures, pneumonia) are an important risk factor for incident dementia in patients with stroke and should be taken into account in the secondary prevention of vascular dementia.[20]

Detailed knowledge of the effects of secondary prevention of vascular dementia is lacking. In a small series of patients with established vascular dementia, control of high arterial blood pressure,[86] cessation of smoking,[86] and use of aspirin[87] improved or stabilized cognition.

It has been suggested that lowering of plasma viscosity could also have an effect in vascular dementia.[88] The absence of progressive cognitive decline in patients receiving placebo in treatment trials of vascular dementia may also reflect an effect of intensified risk factor control.[81]

References

1. Rocca, W.A., Hofman, A., and Brayne, C., *et al.* (1991). The prevalence of vascular dementia in Europe: facts and fragments from 1980–1990 studies. EURODEM-Prevalence Research Group. *Annals of Neurology*, **30**, 817–24.
2. Hebert, R. and Brayne, C. (1995). Epidemiology of vascular dementia. *Neuroepidemiology*, **14**, 240–57.
3. Bowler, J.V. and Hachinski, V. (1995). Vascular cognitive impairment: a new approach to vascular dementia. *Baillières Clinical Neurology*, **4**, 357–76.
4. Tatemichi, T.K. (1990). How acute brain failure becomes chronic. A view of the mechanisms and syndromes of dementia related to stroke. *Neurology*, **40**, 1652–9.
5. Chui, H.C. (1989). Dementia: a review emphasizing clinicopathologic correlation and brain–behavior relationships. *Archives of Neurology*, **46**, 806–14.
6. Desmond, D.W. (1996). Vascular dementia: a construct in evolution. *Cerebrovascular and Brain Metabolism Reviews*, **8**, 296–325.
7. Pasquier, F. and Leys, D. (1997). Why are stroke patients prone to develop dementia? *Journal of Neurology*, **244**, 135–42.
8. Skoog, I. (1998). Status of risk factors for vascular dementia. *Neuroepidemiology*, **17**, 2–9.
9. Pohjasvaara, T., Erkinjuntti, T., Vataja, R., and Kaste, M. (1997). Dementia three months after stroke. Baseline frequency and effect of different definitions of dementia in the Helsinki Stroke Aging Memory Study (SAM) cohort. *Stroke*, **28**, 785–92.
10. Skoog, I., Nilsson, L., Palmertz, B., Andreasson, L.A., and Svanborg, A. (1993). A population-based study of dementia in 85-year-olds. *New England Journal of Medicine*, **328**, 153–8.
11. Wetterling, T., Kanitz, R.D., and Borgis, K.J. (1996). Comparison of different diagnostic criteria for vascular dementia (ADDTC, DSM-IV, ICD-10, NINDS-AIREN). *Stroke*, **27**, 30–6.
12. Cummings, J.L. (1994). Vascular subcortical dementias: clinical aspects. *Dementia*, **5**, 177–80.
13. Erkinjuntti, T. (1996). Clinicopathological study of vascular dementia. In *Vascular dementia*. *Current concepts* (ed. I. Prohovnik, J. Wade, S. Knezevic, T.K. Tatemichi, and T. Erkinjuntii), pp. 73–112. Wiley, Chichester.
14. Brun, A. (1994). Pathology and pathophysiology of cerebrovascular dementia: pure subgroups of obstructive and hypoperfusive etiology. *Dementia*, **5**, 145–7.
15. Amar, K. and Wilcock, G. (1996). Vascular dementia. *British Medical Journal*, **312**, 227–31.
16. Pantoni, L. and Garcia, J.H. (1995). The significance of cerebral white matter abnormalities 100 years after Binswanger's report. A review. *Stroke*, **26**, 1293–301.
17. Erkinjuntti, T. and Hachinski, V.C. (1993). Rethinking vascular dementia. *Cerebrovascular Disease*, **3**, 3–23.
18. Skoog, I. (1994). Risk factors for vascular dementia: a review. *Dementia*, **5**, 137–44.
19. Gorelick, P.B. (1997). Status of risk factors for dementia associated with stroke. *Stroke*, **28**, 459–63.
20. Moroney, J.T., Bagiella, E., Desmond, D.W., Paik, M.C., Stern, Y., and Tatemichi, T.K. (1996). Risk factors for incident dementia after stroke. Role of hypoxic and ischemic disorders. *Stroke*, **27**, 1283–9.
21. Pantoni, L. and Garcia, J.H. (1997). Pathogenesis of leukoaraiosis: a review. *Stroke*, **28**, 652–9.
22. Englund, E., Brun, A., and Alling, C. (1988). White matter changes in

dementia of Alzheimer's type. Biochemical and neuropathological correlates. *Brain*, 111, 1425–39.

23. Mielke, R., Herholz, K., Grond, M., Kessler, J., and Heiss, W.D. (1992). Severity of vascular dementia is related to volume of metabolically impaired tissue. *Archives of Neurology*, 49, 909–13.

24. Tatemichi, T.K., Paik, M., Bagiella, E. *et al.* (1994). Risk of dementia after stroke in a hospitalized cohort: results of a longitudinal study. *Neurology*, 44, 1885–91.

25. Erkinjuntti, T., Haltia, M., Palo, J., Sulkava, R., and Paetau, A. (1988). Accuracy of the clinical diagnosis of vascular dementia: a prospective clinical and post-mortem neuropathological study. *Journal of Neurology, Neurosurgery and Psychiatry*, 51, 1037–44.

26. Snowdon, D.A., Greiner, L.H., Mortimer, J.A., Riley, K.P., Greiner, P.A., and Markesbery, W.R. (1997). Brain infarction and the clinical expression of Alzheimer disease. The Nun Study. *Journal of the American Medical Association*, 277, 813–17.

27. Wallin, A. and Blennow, K. (1994). The clinical diagnosis of vascular dementia. *Dementia*, 5, 181–4.

28. Chui, H.C., Victoroff, J.I., Margolin, D., Jagust, W., Shankle, R., and Katzman, R. (1992). Criteria for the diagnosis of ischemic vascular dementia proposed by the State of California Alzheimer's Disease Diagnostic and Treatment Centers. *Neurology*, 42, 473–80.

29. Konno, S., Meyer, J.S., Terayama, Y., Margishvili, G.M., and Mortel, K.F. (1997). Classification, diagnosis and treatment of vascular dementia. *Drugs and Aging*, 11, 361–73.

30. Roman, G.C., Tatemichi, T.K., Erkinjuntti, T., *et al.* (1993). Vascular Dementia: Diagnostic Criteria for Research Studies. Report of the NINDS-AIREN International Work Group. *Neurology*, 43, 250–60.

31. Erkinjuntti, T. (1987). Types of multi-infarct dementia. *Acta Neurologica Scandinavica*, 75, 391–9.

32. Loeb, C. and Meyer, J.S. (1996). Vascular dementia: still a debatable entity? *Journal of the Neurological Sciences*, 143, 31–40.

33. Sulkava, R. and Erkinjuntti, T. (1987). Vascular dementia due to cardiac arrhythmias and systemic hypotension. *Acta Neurologica Scandinavica*, 76, 123–8.

34. American Psychiatric Association (1994). *Diagnostic and statistical manual of mental disorders* (4th edn). American Psychiatric Association, Washington, DC.

35. World Health Organization (1993). *ICD-10 classification of mental and behavioural disorders: diagnostic criteria for research*. World Health Organization, Geneva.

36. Mahler, M.E. and Cummings, J.L. (1991). The behavioural neurology of multi-infarct dementia. *Alzheimer's Disease and Associated Disorders*, 5, 122–30.

37. Roman, G.C. (1987). Senile dementia of the Binswanger type. A vascular form of dementia in the elderly. *Journal of the American Medical Association*, 258, 1782–8.

38. Babikian, V. and Ropper, A.H. (1987). Binswanger's disease: a review. *Stroke*, 18, 2–12.

39. Ishii, N., Nishihara, Y., and Imamura, T. (1986). Why do frontal lobe symptoms predominate in vascular dementia with lacunes? *Neurology*, 36, 340–5.

40. Rockwood, K., Parhad, I., Hachinski, V., *et al.* (1994). Diagnosis of vascular dementia: Consortium of Canadian Centres for Clinical Cognitive Research consensus statement. *Canadian Journal of Neurological Sciences*, 21, 358–64.

41. Erkinjuntti, T. (1994). Clinical criteria for vascular dementia: the NINDS-AIREN criteria. *Dementia*, 5, 189–92.

42. Erkinjuntti, T., Ostbye, T., Steenhuis, R., and Hachinski, V. (1997). The effect of different diagnostic criteria on the prevalence of dementia. *New England Journal of Medicine*, 337 (23), 1667–74.

43. Wetterling, T., Kanitz, R.D., and Borgis, K.J. (1994). The ICD-10 criteria for vascular dementia. *Dementia*, 5, 185–8.

44. Erkinjuntti, T. (1997). Vascular dementia: challenge of clinical diagnosis. *International Psychogeriatrics*, 9 (Supplement 1), 51–8.

45. Erkinjuntti, T. (1994). Clinical criteria for vascular dementia: the NINDS-AIREN criteria. *Dementia*, 5, 189–92.

46. Verhey, F.R., Lodder, J., Rozendaal, N., and Jolles, J. (1996). Comparison of seven sets of criteria used for the diagnosis of vascular dementia. *Neuroepidemiology*, 15, 166–72.

47. Gold, G., Giannakopoulos, P., Montes-Paixao, J.C., *et al.* (1997). Sensitivity and specificity of newly proposed clinical criteria for possible vascular dementia. *Neurology*, 49, 690–4.

48. Lopez, O.L., Larumbe, M.R., Becker, J.T., *et al.* (1994). Reliability of NINDS-AIREN clinical criteria for the diagnosis of vascular dementia. *Neurology*, 44, 1240–5.

49. Desmond, D.W., Erkinjuntti, T., Sano, M., *et al.* The cognitive syndrome of vascular dementia: implications for clinical trials. *Alzheimer's Disease and Associated Disorders*, in press.

50. Cummings, J.L. (1993). Fronto-subcortical circuits and human behavior. *Archives of Neurology*, 50, 873–80.

51. Hachinski, V.C., Iliff, L.D., Zilhka, E., *et al.* (1975). Cerebral blood flow in dementia. *Archives of Neurology*, 32, 632–7.

52. Moroney, J.T., Bagiella, E., and Desmond, D.W., *et al.* (1997). Meta-analysis of the Hachinski Ischemic Score in pathologically verified dementias. *Neurology*, 49, 1096–105.

53. Erkinjuntti, T. (1987). Differential diagnosis between Alzheimer's disease and vascular dementia: evaluation of common clinical methods. *Acta Neurologica Scandinavica*, 76, 433–42.

54. Mölsä, P.K., Marttila, R.J., Rinne, U.K. (1995). Long-term survival and predictors of mortality in Alzheimer's disease and multi-infarct dementia. *Acta Neurologica Scandinavica*, 91, 159–64.

55. Skoog, I., Nilsson, L., Palmertz, B., Andreasson, L.-A., and Svanborg, A. (1993). A population-based study on dementia in 85-year-olds. *New England Journal of Medicine*, 328, 153–8.

56. Chui, H.C., and Gonthier, R. (1999). Natural history of vascular dementia. *Alzheimer's Disease and Associated Disorders*, Supplement (December).

57. Folstein, M.F., Folstein, S.E., and McHugh, P.R. (1975). 'Mini-Mental State': a practical method for grading the cognitive state of patients for the clinician. *Journal of Psychiatric Research*, 12, 189–98.

58. Pohjasvaara, T., Erkinjuntti, T., Ylikoski, R., Hietanen, M., Vataja, R., and Kaste, M. (1998). Clinical determinants of poststroke dementia. *Stroke*, 29, 75–81.

59. Erkinjuntti, T., Ketonen, L., Sulkava, R., Sipponen, J., Vuorialho, M., and Iivanainen, M. (1987). Do white matter changes on MRI and CT differentiate vascular dementia from Alzheimer's disease? *Journal of Neurology, Neurosurgery and Psychiatry*, 50, 37–42.

60. Erkinjuntti, T., Ketonen, L., Sulkava, R., Vuorialho, M., and Palo, J. (1987). CT in the differential diagnosis between Alzheimer's disease and vascular dementia. *Acta Neurologica Scandinavica*, 75, 262–70.

61. Launes, J., Sulkava, R., Erkinjuntti, T., *et al.* (1991). 99mTC-HM-PAO SPECT in suspected dementia. *Nuclear Medicine Communications*, 12, 757–65.

62. Orrell, R.W. and Wade, J.P.H. (1996). Clinical diagnosis: how good is it and how should it be done? In *Vascular dementia. Current concepts* (ed. I. Prohovnik, J. Wade, S. Knezevic, T.K. Tatemichi, and T. Erkinjuntii), pp. 143–63. Wiley, Chichester.

63. Erkinjuntti, T. and Sulkava, R. (1991). Diagnosis of multi-infarct dementia. *Alzheimer Disease and Associated Disorders*, 5, 112–21.

64. Slooter, A.J., Tang, M.X., van Duijn, C.M., *et al.* (1997). Apolipoprotein E epsilon4 and the risk of dementia with stroke. A population-based investigation. *Journal of the American Medical Association*, 277, 818–21.

65. McKhann, G., Drachman, D., Folstein, M., Katzman, R., Price, D., and Stadlan, E.M. (1984). Clinical diagnosis of Alzheimer's disease: report of the NINCDS-ADRDA Work Group under the auspices of Department of Health and Human Services Task Force on Alzheimer's Disease. *Neurology*, 34, 939–44.

66. Petersen, R.C. (1995). Normal aging, mild cognitive impairment, and early Alzheimer's disease. *Neurologist*, 1, 326–44.

67. Braak, H. and Braak, E. (1991). Neuropathological staging of Alzheimer-related changes. *Acta Neuropathologica (Berlin)*, **82**, 239–59.

68. Roman, G.C. (1991). White matter lesions and normal-pressure hydrocephalus: Binswanger disease or Hakim syndrome? *American Journal of Neuroradiology*, **12**, 40–1.

69. McKeith, I.G., Galasko, D., Kosaka, K., *et al.* (1996). Consensus guidelines for the clinical and pathologic diagnosis of dementia with Lewy bodies (DLB): report of the Consortium on DLB International Workshop. *Neurology*, **47**, 1113–24.

70. Anonymous (1994). Clinical and neuropathological criteria for frontotemporal dementia. The Lund and Manchester Groups. *Journal of Neurology, Neurosurgery and Psychiatry*, **57**, 416–18.

71. Marder, K., Tang, M.X., Cote, L., Stern, Y., and Mayeux, R. (1995). The frequency and associated risk factors for dementia in patients with Parkinson's disease. *Archives of Neurology*, **52**, 695–701.

72. Tolosa, E., Valldeoriala, F., and Marti, M.J. (1994). Clinical diagnosis and diagnostic criteria of progressive supranuclear palsy (Steel–Richardson–Olsewski syndrome). *Journal of Neurological Transmission*, **52** (Supplement), 15–31.

73. Wenning, G.K., Be-Sholomon, Y., Magalhaes, M., Daniel. S.E., and Quinn, N.P. (1995). Clinicopathological study of 35 cases of multiple system atrophy. *Journal of Neurology, Neurosurgery and Psychiatry*, **58**, 160–6.

74. Jorm, A.F., Korten, A.E., and Henderson, A.S. (1987). The prevalence of dementia: a quantitative integration of the literature. *Acta Psychiatrica Scandinavica*, **76**, 465–79.

75. Rocca, W.A., Hofman, A., Brayne, C., *et al.* (1991). The prevalence of vascular dementia in Europe: facts and fragments from 1980–1990 studies. *Annals of Neurology* **30**, 817–24.

76. Tatemichi, T.K., Desmond, D.W., Mayeux, R., *et al.* (1992). Dementia after stroke: baseline frequency, risks, and clinical features in a hospitalized cohort. *Neurology*, **42**, 1185–93.

77. Hachinski, V. (1992). Preventable senility: a call for action against the vascular dementias. *Journal of the American Geriatrics Society*, **340**, 645–8.

78. Knezevic, S., Labs, K.H., Kittner, B., *et al.* (1996). The treatment of vascular dementia: problems and prospects. In *Vascular dementia. Current concepts* (ed. I. Prohovnik, J. Wade, S. Knezevic, T.K. Tatemichi, and T. Erkinjuntii), pp. 301–12. Wiley, Chichester.

79. Pantoni, L., Carosi, M., Amigoni, S., Mascalchi, M., and Inzitari, D. (1996). A preliminary open trial with nimodipine in patients with cognitive impairment and leukoaraiosis. *Clinical Neuropharmacology*, **19**, 497–506.

80. Görtelmeyer, R. and Erbler, H. (1992). Memantine in treatment of mild to moderate dementia syndrome. *Drug Research*, **42**, 904–12.

81. Rother, M., Erkinjuntti, T., Roessner, M., Kittner, B., Marcusson, J., and Karlsson, I. (1998). Propentofylline in the treatment of Alzheimer's disease and vascular dementia. *Dementia*, **9** (Supplement 1), 36–43.

82. Erkinjuntti, T. (1999). Cerebrovascular dementia: a guide to diagnosis and treatment. *CNS Drugs*, **12**, 35–48.

83. Mortel, K.F. and Meyer, J.S. (1995). Lack of postmenopausal estrogen replacement therapy and the risk of dementia. *Journal of Neuropsychiatry and Clinical Neurosciences*, **7**, 334–7.

84. Skoog, I. (1997). The relationship between blood pressure and dementia: a review. *Biomedicine and Pharmacotherapy*, **51**, 367–75.

85. Forette, F., Seux, M.L., Staessen, J.A., *et al.* (1998). Prevention of dementia in randomised double-blind placebo-controlled Systolic Hypertension in Europe (Syst-Eur) trial. *Journal of the American Geriatrics Society*, **352**, 1347–51.

86. Meyer, J.S., Judd, B.W., Tawaklna, T., Rogers, R.L., and Mortel, K.F. (1986). Improved cognition after control of risk factors for multi-infarct dementia. *Journal of the American Medical Association*, **256**, 2203–9.

87. Meyer, J.S., Rogers, R.L., McClintic, K., Mortel, K.F., and Lotfi, J. (1989). Randomized clinical trial of daily aspirin therapy in multi-infarct dementia. A pilot study. *Journal of the American Geriatrics Society*, **37**, 549–55.

88. Lechner, H. (1998). Status of treatment of vascular dementia. *Neuroepidemiology*, **17**, 10–13.

4.1.10 Dementia due to HIV disease

Mario Maj

Introduction

The first description of a syndrome consisting of cognitive, motor and behavioural disturbances in patients with AIDS was reported in 1986.[1] The syndrome was named 'AIDS dementia complex'. A rating scale for the syndrome, ranging from 0 (normal) to 4 (endstage), was proposed by Price *et al.*[2] in 1988. In 1990, the World Health Organization introduced the term 'HIV-associated dementia',[3] pointing out that subclinical or mild cognitive and/or motor dysfunctions without impairment of performance in daily living activities, corresponding to stages 0.5 and 1 on the scale of Price *et al.*, cannot be subsumed under the term 'dementia'. The expression 'mild cognitive/motor disorder' was proposed for those conditions. The same distinction was made in 1991 by the American Academy of Neurology,[4] which identified an 'HIV-associated dementia complex' and an 'HIV-associated minor cognitive/motor disorder'.

The present chapter is concerned with the dementia syndrome associated with HIV infection. For minor cognitive/motor disorder, the reader is referred to Maj *et al.*[5]

Clinical features

The onset of HIV-associated dementia is usually insidious. Early cognitive symptoms include forgetfulness, loss of concentration, mental slowing, and reduced performance on sequential mental activities of some complexity (the subject misses appointments, or needs lists to recall ordinary duties; loses track of conversations or his or her own train of thought; needs additional time and effort to organize thoughts and to complete daily tasks). Early behavioural symptoms include apathy, reduced spontaneity and emotional responsivity, and social withdrawal (the subject becomes indifferent to his or her personal and professional responsibilities; his or her work production decreases, as well as the frequency of social interactions; the subject complains of early fatiguability, malaise, and loss of sexual drive). Depression, irritability or emotional lability, agitation, and psychotic symptoms may also occur. Early motor symptoms include loss of balance and co-ordination, clumsiness, and leg weakness; the subject is less precise in normal hand activities, such as writing and eating, drops things more frequently than usual, trips and falls more frequently than usual, and perceives the need to exercise more care in walking.[1,6]

Routine mental status tests, in this early stage, may be normal or show only slowing in verbal or motor responses and/or difficulty in recalling a series of objects after 5 min or more. Neurological examination may show tremor (best seen when the patient sustains a posture, such as holding the arms and fingers outstretched), hyperreflexia (particularly of the lower extremities), ataxia (usually seen only on rapid turns or tandem gait), slowing of rapid alternating movements (of the fingers, wrists or feet), frontal release signs (snout reflex, palmar grasp), dysarthria. Tests of ocular motility may show interruption of smooth pursuits, and slowing or inaccuracy of saccades.

In the late stages of the disease, there is usually a global deterioration of cognitive functions and a severe psychomotor retardation. Speech is slow and monotonous, with word-finding difficulties and possible progression to mutism. Patients become unable to walk, due to paraparesis, and usually lie in bed indifferent to their illness and their surroundings. Bladder and bowel incontinence are common. Myoclonus and seizures may occur. Pedal paraesthesias and hypersensitivity may appear, due to concurrent sensory neuropathy. The level of consciousness is usually preserved, except for occasional hypersomnolence.

Classification

The World Health Organization (**WHO**) criteria for HIV-associated dementia[3] are as follows.

1. The research criteria for dementia of the ICD-10[7] are met, with some modifications:

    (a) decline in memory may not be severe enough to impair activities of daily living;

    (b) decline in motor function may be present, and is verified by clinical examination and, when possible, formal neuropsychological testing;

    (c) the minimum requested duration of symptoms is 1 month;

    (d) aphasia, agnosia and apraxia are unusual.

2. Laboratory evidence for systemic HIV infection is present.

3. No evidence of another aetiology from history, physical examination, or laboratory tests should be present (specifically, cerebrospinal fluid analysis and either CT or magnetic resonance imaging (**MRI**) should be done to exclude active central nervous system opportunistic processes).

The American Academy of Neurology criteria[4] require the following.

1. Laboratory evidence for systemic HIV infection.

2. Acquired abnormality in at least two of the following cognitive abilities (present for at least 1 month): attention/concentration, speed of processing of information, abstraction/reasoning, visuospatial skills, memory/learning, and speech/language.

3. At least one of the following:

    (a) acquired abnormality in motor function or performance;

    (b) decline in motivation or emotional control or change in social behaviour.

4. Absence of clouding of consciousness during a period long enough to establish the presence of (2).

5. Absence of evidence of another aetiology.

Both WHO and American Academy of Neurology criteria distinguish three levels of severity of the dementia syndrome (mild, moderate, and severe), on the basis of the degree of the impairment in activities of daily living.

Diagnosis and differential diagnosis

Neuropsychological tests

Neuropsychological examination supports the clinical diagnosis of HIV-associated dementia, by providing evidence of cognitive and motor dysfunction. Moreover, it may be useful in the differential diagnosis with a depressive syndrome.

The most prominent impairment is observed on tests of fine motor control (finger tapping, grooved pegboard), rapid sequential problem solving (trail-making A and B, digit symbol), visuospatial problem solving (block design), spontaneity (verbal fluency), and visual memory (visual reproduction). In contrast, naming and vocabulary skills are largely preserved even in the most advanced cases. This pattern has been regarded as consistent with the clinical picture of a 'subcortical dementia'.

The signs that should alert to the possible presence of a depressive 'pseudodementia' are as follows:[8]

(1) the intratest variability of performance (i.e. missing easy items and then correctly answering more difficult questions);

(2) mood-congruent complaints, which are at odds with objective performance (i.e. the subject complains of having difficulties with a test, whereas his or her performance is near perfect);

(3) responses of 'I don't know' or giving up, which are followed by the correct answer, when the subject is further urged to respond.

It should be considered, however, that dementia and depression may coexist in HIV-seropositive subjects.

Brain imaging

Brain imaging provides additional support to the diagnosis of HIV-associated dementia, especially by excluding central nervous system opportunistic processes, in particular cerebral toxoplasmosis and primary central nervous system lymphoma.

The predominant finding in HIV-associated dementia is cerebral atrophy; both CT and MRI demonstrate widened cortical sulci and, less commonly, enlarged ventricles. Furthermore, MRI frequently shows high-intensity signal abnormalities on the T_2-weighted image (diffuse widespread involvement, patchy localized involvement, focal distinct areas of involvement, or punctuate white-matter hyperdensities). These lesions are without mass effect and are most commonly located in the periventricular white matter and the centrum semiovale (less frequently, in the basal ganglia or in the thalamus).

As to differential diagnosis, both CT and MRI are able to demonstrate the multiple bilateral ring enhancing lesions that are characteristic of cerebral toxoplasmosis, and the contrast-enhancing mass lesions of primary central nervous system lymphoma.

Cerebrospinal fluid analysis

Cerebrospinal fluid analysis can support the clinical diagnosis of HIV-associated dementia, especially by excluding several central nervous system opportunistic infections, in particular cryptococcal meningitis.

The most frequent cerebrospinal fluid findings in HIV-associated dementia are the increase of total proteins and of the IgG fraction and index. A mononuclear pleocytosis may occur. The presence of the HIV core antigen p24 can be detected, although this finding is possible also in neurologically normal subjects. HIV RNA can be demostrated in the cerebrospinal fluid by using the polymerase chain reaction; the levels of HIV RNA in the cerebrospinal fluid correlate with the severity of dementia.[9] Increased cerebrospinal fluid levels of neopterin, β_2-microglobulin and quinolinic acid (non-specific markers of immune activation), as well as of several cytokines (interleukin 1β, interleukin 6, tumour necrosis factor-α), have been reported, but may be detected also during central nervous system opportunistic infections.

As to differential diagnosis, Indian ink staining, cryptococcal antigen titres, and fungal culture can be decisive for the identification of cryptococcal meningitis. Other central nervous system opportunistic infections that can be identified by cerebrospinal fluid analysis include central nervous system tuberculosis, cytomegalovirus encephalitis, and neurosyphilis.

Epidemiology

Estimates of the prevalence and incidence of HIV-associated dementia vary widely, depending on the source from which patients are recruited and the criteria used for the diagnosis.[5]

A recent prospective study, carried out on a cohort of homosexual men in the United States, found that the diagnosis was made concurrently with that of the initial AIDS-defining illness in 3 per cent of cases, and that the incidence of the dementia syndrome during the first 2 years after the diagnosis of AIDS was 7 per cent per year, with 15 per cent of patients developing dementia during the course of the disease.[10]

Several risk factors for the development of HIV-associated dementia have been reported, including older age, decreased body mass, decrements in haematocrit, and a history of intravenous drug abuse. However, avalaible data are not consistent.

Pathogenesis

The pathogenesis of HIV-associated dementia is at present incompletely understood. In the brain, productive infection is almost exclusively restricted to macrophages and microglia. Neuronal injury (most probably apoptosis) is currently believed to be produced by toxic products released directly by HIV-infected macrophages and microglia or by activated astrocytes. Some of these factors have been identified: they include the platelet-activating factor, quinolinic acid, nitric oxide, and some metabolites of arachidonic acid, which are neurotoxic, and tumour necrosis factor-α, which is toxic for oligodendrocytes and can cause demyelination.

The strains of HIV which are isolated from the brain have in common the characteristic of infecting macrophages but not lymphocytes. This macrophage tropism corresponds to what was initially regarded as neurotropism. Macrophage tropism is related to a mutation in a specific region of gp120, the external glycoprotein of the virus. In the late stages of the infection, when active replication of the virus generates more mutants and the compromised immune system permits the escape of these mutants, the development of macrophage-trophic strains is more likely to occur, and this probably represents the limiting step for the occurrence of HIV encephalopathy and dementia.[11]

Course and prognosis

The course of HIV-associated dementia is variable, and no predictor of the pace of progression is currently available. The syndrome often progresses rapidly to severe deterioration and death, especially in patients with advanced systemic disease, but it may also have prolonged stable phases, or may fluctuate, with reversible deterioration occurring in concomitance with opportunistic infections. Death usually occurs as a result of inanition, aspiration pneumonia, or systemic opportunistic infections.

Treatment

Review of evidence

Antiretroviral drugs

Zidovudine is a reverse transcriptase inhibitor which crosses the blood–brain barrier and reaches effective concentrations in the cerebrospinal fluid. It is able to inhibit HIV replication in macrophages and seems to produce an improvement of the symptomatology in patients with HIV-associated dementia, although this effect appears to be transient (i.e. to dissipate after 6–12 months of treatment).

The only double-blind randomized controlled trial[12] comparing zidovudine with placebo in patients with HIV-associated dementia used high doses (either 1000 or 2000 mg/day) of the drug (the standard dosage is 500–600 mg/day). After 16 weeks of treatment, the combined average neuropsychological test z-scores showed a significant improvement in patients receiving zidovudine; the effect was significantly more pronounced in patients taking 2000 mg/day than in the 1000 mg/day group. The improvement was also significant after 32 and 64 weeks of treatment. Adverse side-effects were not documented.

In an open 12-month prospective trial, Tozzi et al.[13] used three different dosages of zidovudine (500, 750, or 1000 mg/day, depending on the haematological state) in 30 patients with HIV-associated dementia. An improvement in the stage of dementia was observed in 15 patients after 1 month and 25 patients after 6 months. Following an initial improvement, eight patients deteriorated in dementia staging after 6 to 12 months of treatment (five of them had received the dosage of 500 mg/day). Two patients dropped out because of adverse side-effects, eight developed haematological toxicity requiring temporary discontinuation of the drug, and five required a reduction of dosage due to bone marrow toxicity.

The decline after initial improvement of cognitive performance in AIDS patients after 6 to 12 months of treatment with zidovudine has been confirmed in other open trials.[14]

Among the other reverse transcriptase inhibitors, didanosine does not seem to have an impact on the progression of HIV-associated dementia, whereas no studies are available on the efficacy of zalcitabine, stavudine, or lamivudine. No trial has tested the efficacy of protease inhibitors; according to currently available evidence, these drugs do not reach effective concentrations in the cerebrospinal fluid.

Drugs under investigation

Drugs whose beneficial effect on cognitive performance in patients with HIV infection has been preliminarily documented in published studies include the monoamine oxidase inhibitor deprenyl (a putative antiapoptotic agent) and peptide T (a neurotrophic peptide). Other investigational drugs include memantine and nitroglycerin (which are N-methyl-D-aspartate receptor antagonists), nimodipine (a calcium-channel blocker) and pentoxifylline (an inhibitor of the production and activity of tumour necrosis factor-α). No published trial in patients with HIV-associated dementia is currently available for any of these drugs.

Drugs for behavioural symptoms

The psychostimulant methylphenidate (at doses ranging from 10 to 90 mg/day) has been repeatedly found to improve cognitive symptoms in patients with AIDS, producing relatively mild side-effects. The available studies, however, have several limitations, including small patient samples, open design, and inclusion of depressed patients. No systematic research has been conducted in patients with HIV-associated dementia.

Patients with AIDS, when treated with typical antipsychotic drugs for the presence of psychotic symptoms or behavioural dyscontrol, are particularly prone to develop extrapyramidal side-effects and neuroleptic malignant syndrome. According to preliminary research evidence, the atypical antipsychotic risperidone is well tolerated even by patients who had to stop standard neuroleptics due to extrapyramidal side-effects.

AIDS patients with depressed mood have been found to respond to tricyclic antidepressants and selective serotonin reuptake inhibitors as well as HIV-seronegative subjects. There is a preliminary evidence that SSRIs (or at least some of them) are better tolerated than tricyclic antidepressants, except in patients with diarrhoea. Current evidence does not support the idea that tricyclic antidepressants may worsen HIV-related cognitive impairment or precipitate delirium, although no specific study is available in patients with HIV-associated dementia.

Advice about management

At the present state of knowledge, patients with HIV-associated dementia should be treated with zidovudine. Although there is uncertainty about the most appropriate dosage, the standard doses of 500 to 600 mg/day should be tried first. If the patient does not respond, the dosage should be increased to 1500 or 2000 mg/day.

Psychosocial interventions should include maintenance of a structured daily schedule, titration of external stimuli, restriction to familiar environments, frequent orienting interactions with significant others, and monitoring of personal and financial affairs.

The care of patients with HIV-associated dementia will make increasing demands on health services, as well as on volunteer and community support systems. It is uncertain, at present, whether such care is best provided in specialized units (e.g. inpatient AIDS units), or within general psychiatric or medical services. Special management problems may arise when the behavioural disturbance (e.g. poor impulse control, sexual acting-out behaviour) is such as to constitute a risk for other patients or staff members. Placement of patients in the terminal stage of the disease may also represent a problem: the lack of appropriate options in the community may obstruct their timely and humane discharge from the hospital.

Possible preventive measures

Several studies suggest that long-term treatment with zidovudine may produce a prophylactic effect in symptomatic patients with HIV infection, reducing the risk for development of HIV-associated dementia. This effect, however, seems to be time limited: in a recent retrospective study carried out on a longitudinal cohort of 1109 patients with AIDS,[15] the use of zidovudine for a period of 6 to 18 months was associated with a reduced risk of dementia, whereas treatment for longer than 18 months was not beneficial.

References

1. Navia, B.A., Jordan, B.D., and Price, R.W. (1986). The AIDS dementia complex: I. Clinical picture. *Annals of Neurology*, **19**, 517–24.
2. Price, R.W., Brew, B., Sidtis, J., Rosenblum, M., Scheck, A.C., and Clearly, P. (1988). The brain in AIDS: central nervous system HIV-1 infection and AIDS dementia complex. *Science*, **239**, 586–92.
3. World Health Organization (1990). *Report of the Second Consultation on the Neuropsychiatric Aspects of HIV-1 Infection, Geneva, 11–13 January 1990.* World Health Organization, Geneva.
4. American Academy of Neurology AIDS Task Force (1991). Nomenclature and research case definitions for the neurological manifestations of human immunodeficiency virus type-1 infection. *Neurology*, **41**, 778–85.
5. Maj, M., Starace, F., and Sartorius, N. (1993). *Mental disorders in HIV-1 infection and AIDS.* Hogrefe and Huber, Bern.
6. Maj, M. (1990). Organic mental disorders in HIV-1 infection. *AIDS*, **4**, 831–40.
7. World Health Organization (1993). *The ICD-10 classification of mental and behavioural disorders: diagnostic criteria for research.* World Health Organization, Geneva.
8. Van Gorp, W.G., Satz, P., Hinkin, C., Evans, G., and Miller, E.N. (1989). The neuropsychological aspects of HIV-1 spectrum disease. *Psychiatric Medicine*, **7**, 59–78.
9. McArthur, J.C., McClernon, D.R., Cronin, M.F., *et al.* (1997). Relationship between human immunodeficiency virus-associated dementia and viral load in cerebrospinal fluid and brain. *Annals of Neurology*, **42**, 689–98.
10. McArthur, J.C., Hoover, D.R., Bacellar, H., *et al.* (1993). Dementia in AIDS patients: incidence and risk factors. *Neurology*, **23** (Supplement), S34–7.
11. Price, R.W. and Perry, S.W. (ed.) (1994). *HIV, AIDS, and the brain.* Raven Press, New York.
12. Sidtis, J.J., Gatsonis, C., Price, R.W., *et al.* (1993). Zidovudine treatment of the AIDS dementia complex: results of a placebo-controlled trial. *Annals of Neurology*, **33**, 343–9.
13. Tozzi, V., Narciso, P., Galgani, S., *et al.* (1993). Effects of zidovudine in 30 patients with mild to end-stage AIDS dementia complex. *AIDS*, **7**, 683–92.
14. Melton, S.T., Kirkwood, C.K., and Ghaemi, S.N. (1997). Pharmacotherapy of HIV dementia. *Annals of Pharmacotherapy*, **31**, 457–72.
15. Baldeweg, T., Catalan, J., and Gazzard, B.G. (1998). Risk of HIV dementia and opportunistic brain disease in AIDS and use of zidovudine. *Journal of Neurology, Neurosurgery and Psychiatry*, **65**, 34–41.

4.1.11 The neuropsychiatry of head injury

Simon Fleminger

Head injury 'imparts at a blow both physical and psychological trauma,'[1] and the consequences are often devastating and enduring.[2] Not infrequently head injury leads to a psychiatric consultation, which will need to take into account the interplay between the brain and its injuries as well as the psychodynamic processes that follow from the injury.

In the immediate aftermath of the head injury the management rests with the acute surgical and medical team.[3] The psychiatrist is usually not involved at this stage. Nevertheless, to understand the later neuropsychiatric effects of head injury it is first necessary to know what happens to the brain when it is injured.

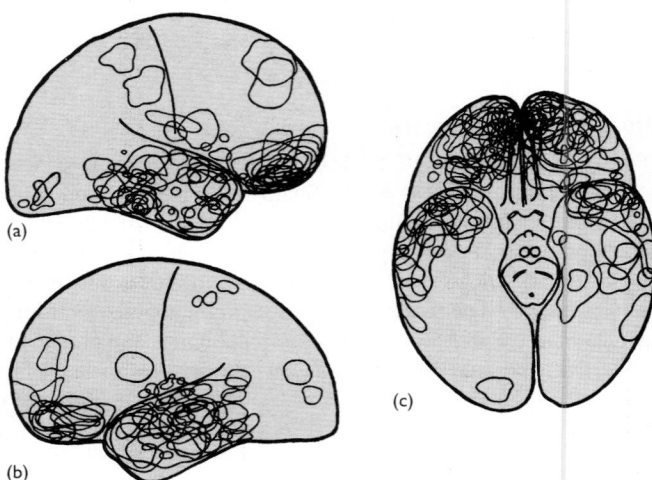

Fig. 1 A composite of the contusions found in 50 cases of people dying from head injury. (Reproduced with permission from C.B. Courville (1937). *Pathology of the central nervous system*, Part IV. Pacific Press, Mountain View, CA.)

Neuropathology

Immediate and early effects

Open head injuries

In open head injuries there is penetration of the skull often with considerable destruction of brain tissue local to the trauma, but relatively less at a distance—particularly for lower-velocity injuries such as stabbing. Open head injuries may therefore be associated with little, if any, loss of consciousness, which is generally a marker of diffuse brain injury.

Closed head injuries

Contusions

In closed head injuries acceleration/deceleration forces and shearing forces damage the brain. The soft brain moves within its hard bony box and is damaged. Contusion of the brain occurs, ranging from slight localized small vessel bleeding into surrounding tissue to almost complete local destruction of the brain.

The medial orbital frontal cortex and the tips and undersurface of the temporal lobes are particularly vulnerable to contusions (Fig. 1). The brain becomes traumatized on adjacent bone of the floor of the skull. Contrecoup localization of contusions is sometimes evident.

Intracerebral haemorrhage

Contusions are often associated with localized haemorrhage into the brain. Scattered intracerebral haemorrhages are also often found at the interface between grey and white matter and are thought to be associated with diffuse axonal injury (see below). A large isolated haematoma suggests that a blood vessel has ruptured.

In very severe injury haemorrhages are also found round the aqueduct in the brainstem, perhaps caused by distortion of the brainstem as a result of cerebral herniation into the posterior fossa due to raised intracranial pressure. They are associated with the vegetative state or death.

Extradural and subdural haemorrhage

Haemorrhage into the extradural or subdural space will act as a space-occupying lesion and contribute to raised intracranial pressure. The extradural haemorrhage, being under high pressure, can rapidly cause coma and death. The patient may 'talk and die', regaining consciousness after the head injury, only to lapse a few hours later into severe coma. Without acute neurosurgical intervention to drain the blood these patients will die.

Subdural haematomas tend to run a subacute course and as such are of more interest to the psychiatrist. They may present with a failure to improve, or fluctuating drowsiness, weeks or months after the head injury. They may regress spontaneously or may require surgical drainage, but they do have a propensity to recur.

Diffuse axonal injury

Diffuse axonal injury occurs in the white matter tracts of the cerebral hemispheres, including the corpus callosum, and the brainstem, particularly the cerebellar peduncles. Axons break up over the course of the first 24 to 48 h following brain trauma with the formation of 'retraction balls'—globular structures at the end of transected axons.[4]

Oedema and ischaemia

Oedema of damaged brain occurs over the first few hours following brain injury. The resulting raised intracranial pressure compromises the cerebral circulation and results in ischaemia, which may further contribute to brain injury. Cerebral oedema tends to resolve over the course of a few days or weeks.

Amyloid

Amyloid precursor protein may be an acute-phase reactant to traumatic brain injury[5] and results in β-amyloid deposition in 30 per cent of fatal brain injuries. Apolipoprotein E (*APOE*) genotype may influence the degree to which amyloid is deposited, being greater in those with the *e4* allele.[6]

Late effects

Hydrocephalus following head injury may be due to cerebral atrophy, which may develop over the weeks and months following injury. Diffuse ventricular enlargement is often associated with atrophy of the corpus callosum, and is usually attributed to diffuse axonal injury. More localized atrophy is observed when contusions resolve to leave a loss of brain tissue.

Of greater importance is hydrocephalus resulting from the residual effects of subarachnoid blood interfering with the normal cerebrospinal fluid flow and preventing it from escaping into the venous system. This may require insertion of a ventriculo-peritoneal shunt to prevent deterioration in cognitive function.

Fractures to the floor of the skull, particularly if they are associated with cerebrospinal fluid leaks, may allow infection into the subarachnoid space, causing meningitis sometimes years after injury. Cerebral abscesses may take months before they become clinically evident.

Loss of consciousness following head injury

The mechanism of loss of consciousness after mild blows to head is poorly understood. Some researchers suggest, based on animal work, that activation of cholinergic nuclei in the pons results in loss of consciousness.[7]

Loss of consciousness lasting for more than a few minutes is likely to be due to damage either to cortical areas necessary for consciousness, or the subcortical arousal systems. Raised intracranial pressure, partly as a result of compromising cerebral circulation, causes coma. Large or multiple haematomas are likely to be associated with a period of coma, particularly if they are associated with cerebral oedema.

Some patients, however, show prolonged coma with little to be found on brain scan apart from some evidence of generalized cerebral oedema. In these patients diffuse axonal injury may be the cause of their coma, possibly by damaging the white matter tracts that carry arousal signals from the brainstem to the cortex.

Remember that the head injury may have been caused by an accident triggered by a loss of consciousness, for example due to hypoglycaemia, alcohol intoxication, or an epileptic fit. Systemic effects (e.g. hypoxaemia or fat emboli) may exacerbate unconsciousness due to head trauma, as may drug intoxication.

Head injury severity

It is surprisingly difficult to predict the degree of brain injury from the size of the blow to the head. Some patients after a severe blow to the head sustain little injury to the brain. Others will suffer severe brain injury associated with prolonged unconsciousness, merely as a result of hitting their head on the ground by falling over from the standing position. There is anecdotal evidence that significant brain injury can result from a head injury with no, or momentary, loss of consciousness (see postconcussion syndrome below). The presence of a skull fracture says little about the severity of the brain injury incurred.

There are several clinical indicators of head injury severity (Box 1). Of these the duration of retrograde amnesia is probably the least valuable: it correlates very poorly with head injury severity. The duration of the retrograde amnesia tends to shrink as the patient recovers.

Box 1

Clinical indicators of head-injury severity

- The duration of retrograde amnesia—the period leading up to the injury for which memories have been lost

- The depth of unconsciousness as assessed by the worst score on the Glasgow Coma Scale—a score of 3 indicates absent responses, 15 is normal consciousness

- The duration of coma—this may be difficult to ascertain because of routine sedation and ventilation following severe head injuries

- Neurological evidence of cerebral injury—abnormality on neuroimaging or EEG

- The duration of post-traumatic amnesia—interval between injury and the return of normal day-to-day memories

The duration of post-traumatic amnesia is the best marker of outcome.[8] This is particularly useful because it can be measured retrospectively quite accurately. Most patients with a post-traumatic amnesia of less than 1 week will be left with little if any disability, while a duration of more than 1 month indicates that there is likely to be enduring and significant disability.

Predictors of a bad outcome after head injury are a previous head injury, older age, *APOE e4* status, and alcohol dependence.

There is no universally accepted classification of head injury severity. However, the most widely used grading system is based on the lowest rating of the Glasgow Coma Scale (**GCS**)[9] following injury.

- Mild: GCS score 13 to 15. Likely to be associated with a loss of consciousness of less than 20 min and a post-traumatic amnesia of less than 24 h. There must be clinical evidence of concussion.

- Moderate: GCS score 9 to 12. Likely to be associated with a loss of consciousness of more than a few minutes but less than 24 h and a post-traumatic amnesia of more than 1 day but less than 1 week.

- Severe: GCS score 3 to 8. Likely to be associated with a loss of consciousness of more than 1 day or a post-traumatic amnesia of more than 1 week.

Epidemiology

On average 200 to 300 per 100 000 population attend hospital with a head injury every year.[10] Socio-economic and cultural factors may have a two- to threefold effect on the rates of head injury, and even larger effects on the individual causes of head injury. About one-sixth of those people attending hospital will be admitted. This reflects the fact that, in most series, about 80 per cent of head injuries are mild, 10 per cent moderate, and 10 per cent severe.

At greatest risk are 15 to 25-year-olds. The sex ratio is about two to three males to one female. Risk factors included alcohol misuse as well as lower socio-economic class. Road traffic accidents are the largest single cause of head injury in most civilian cohorts, followed by assaults and falls. A significant proportion will sustain their head injury as a result of deliberate self-harm.

The prevalence rate for those experiencing considerable disability as a result of head injury is in the order of 100 per 100 000.[11]

Investigations

Neuroimaging

Modern neuroimaging has transformed the investigation of head injury. Skull radiographs are now rarely performed if magnetic resonance imaging (**MRI**) or CT brain scanning is available.

MRI scans cannot be performed if there is any magnetic material present either in the body (e.g. a pacemaker) or attached to the body. Therefore on the trauma unit CT brain scanning is the preferred investigation, with its faster acquisition time and good visualization of subdurals and extradurals.

However, in the postacute setting MRI is the better instrument.[12] Often cerebral contusions are found near the bone–brain interface (see above) where the image quality of CT is poor because of imaging artefacts from the adjacent bone. MRI has no such limitation. MRI is also able to detect, on T_2-weighted images, changes in signal associated with a diffuse axonal injury when the white matter appears normal on CT brain imaging. The better image resolution of MRI is also in its favour.

Despite its greater sensitivity a normal MRI does not rule out significant brain injury. On the other hand, particularly in the elderly, MRI may detect abnormalities unrelated to the head injury.

The MRI scan can be normal and yet functional imaging of cerebral metabolism using single-photon emission computed tomography or positron-emission tomography will detect abnormalities.[13,14] In general, changes on functional imaging correlate better with neuropsychological test performance than do lesions found on structural imaging.[15] However, abnormalities on functional imaging are not necessarily due to brain injury. Hypometabolism may be seen in mental illness without brain injury, for example in depression. There is a recent report of marked hypometabolism on positron-emission tomography imaging in a man with cognitive impairment occurring immediately after a psychological trauma.[16] He had sustained no head injury.

Electroencephalography

If brain imaging is available the role of electroencephalography (**EEG**) is largely confined to the investigation of a deteriorating conscious level and an unexpectedly prolonged unconsciousness, as well as the investigation of unusual behavioural disturbances that may be attributable to epilepsy. However, EEG is not a good predictor of post-traumatic epilepsy.

Non-specific changes are seen on EEG after head injury. An early sign is suppression of the alpha rhythm, while more severe injuries produce diffuse slowing. Haematomas produce localized reduction in amplitude and slowing. Improvements of the EEG correlate with clinical improvement, but the EEG is not a valuable prognostic marker.

Neuropsychological assessment

A neuropsychological assessment is an invaluable accompaniment to the psychiatric history and examination, and good liaison with the neuropsychologist is essential. Areas of impaired performance can be documented and quantified. This is often useful as a baseline for future assessments and to guide rehabilitation.

The National Adult Reading Test, for people whose first language is English, gives a good estimate of preinjury IQ.[17] The present performance can then be compared with this preinjury estimate to see if there has been a drop in performance because of the head injury.

If subtle neuropsychological impairments are found, which are not obvious clinically, this suggests that the patient may have more problems when they return to work than would otherwise have been expected. On the other hand, if there is clinical evidence of underperformance, and standard neuropsychological test results are normal, then tests of executive function should be offered.[18]

Recovery of impairment, disability, and handicap

Psychological symptoms far outstrip neurophysical symptoms (e.g. hemiparesis or dysarthria) as determinants of chronic disability and suffering, both of the patient and their carer, following brain injury.

The ideas encapsulated in the International Classification of Impairments, Disabilities and Handicaps (**ICIDH**)[19] are important for understanding recovery from brain injury.

- Impairments are abnormalities of structure, or physiological or psychological function. Thus poor performance on a test of memory or on a test of co-ordination is an impairment.

- Disability refers to the behaviour of the person and their ability to perform activities. Several impairments may contribute to a single disability.

- Handicap reflects the limitations on fulfilling the person's normal social role and participation in society. External factors (e.g. personal support systems or the availability of appropriate transport) play a large part in determining handicap. Handicap depends partly on the expectations of the individual patient.

The term 'disability' will probably be replaced by 'activity', and 'handicap' by 'participation', in the next version of ICIDH.

Recovery of impairment is usually complete by 1 year, with improvement in neurophysical impairments tending to stop before neuropsychological impairments.

However, the level of disability may continue to fall long after the recovery of the underlying impairment has stopped. This reduction in disability largely reflects improved coping strategies and these will be the focus of inpatient cognitive and behavioural rehabilitation. Once the person is back to living in the community then the rehabilitation team can focus on minimizing handicap, for example by improving access to local shops.

Psychiatric symptoms and quality-of-life measures do not fit easily into the ICIDH model. Psychiatric symptoms, with their multifactorial aetiology, show no simple pattern of recovery.

Psychological sequelae of head injury

To understand the mental symptoms that follow head injury it is necessary to know about the person who was injured, what brain injuries they sustained, and the consequences. However, the interaction between these three antecedents is complex and poorly understood.

Antecedents

Pretraumatic factors

People who take risks or get into fights are more likely to sustain a head injury; therefore these personality traits, present before injury, are over-represented in head injury survivors. Young men are at high risk, as are those who have already had a head injury or have cognitive dysfunction.[20]

The poor social adjustment of many patients before the head injury partly explains why so many run into behavioural problems afterwards. But premorbid characteristics do not strongly predict who will develop emotional and behavioural problems. Nevertheless, traumatic brain injury probably has the potential to turn preinjury personality traits into postinjury personality disorders.

The trauma

The extent of brain injury probably explains less than 10 per cent of the variance in the amount of psychiatric morbidity that follows brain injury.[21] In general, early psychiatric symptoms, within weeks and months of the injury, correlate better with the extent and location of brain injury than do late psychiatric symptoms. Left hemisphere damage seems to be associated with greater psychiatric morbidity. Specific relationships between the location of brain injury and the psychiatric symptoms are discussed below.

But the head injury is also a psychological trauma. Amnesia for the event, as a result of the head injury, protects against post-traumatic stress disorder (see Chapter 5.3.8). However, it is a mistake to believe that amnesia for the event prevents a psychological stress reaction to the event itself.

- The meaning of the event may be distressing to the patient.[22] In the case of assaults, the head injury may act as a marker of the potential for further assaults. An accident may have been life threatening and a shocking reminder to the patient that they are mortal. They may feel aggrieved by an employer's negligent action that caused the accident.

- The patient may be amnesic for the event, lacking explicit memories of what happened, but retain implicit memory of what happened. The consequences of these implicit memories may be akin to those observed in one of Claperède's amnesic patients.[23] The doctor shook the patient's hand, pricking it while doing so with a concealed drawing pin. The next day the patient could not remember having met the doctor, but flinched from shaking his hand when it was offered.

- They may have islets of intact memories that may be extremely frightening.[24]

Post-traumatic factors

Post-traumatic factors deserve special attention because they are most likely to be amenable to intervention. The psychiatrist needs to consider the patient's reaction to any disability, as well as the consequences of the disability on the role of the patient in the family and society. There may be reinforcing cycles of maladaptive behaviour, and compensation claims may complicate the picture.

Cognitive impairment

Cognitive impairment correlates with measures of head injury severity better than any of the other mental sequelae. For example, there is a strong correlation between the duration of post-traumatic amnesia and the severity of cognitive impairment.

Recovery

Recovery of cognitive function, by and large, occurs within the first year.[25] After 2 years most improvement is a result of improved coping strategies, for example memory aids enabling return to work. Continuing improvements in participation in social life and work take place 5 to 10 years after head injury.[26] But sometimes early gains are made, for example as a result of being in a return-to-work rehabilitation programme, which are subsequently lost over the longer term.

Attention and concentration

Non-specific cognitive impairments include slowness and reduced concentration. With severe injury the patients are likely to be stimulus bound, i.e. responding to each and every stimulus they are exposed to in a rather concrete way. At the same time they may show perseveration, with previous responses inappropriately interfering with the answers to subsequent questions, or when the topic of a conversation has been changed.

Dysexecutive syndrome

More specific impairments, generally referred to as the dysexecutive syndrome, result from a disturbance of the executive system responsible for organizing, planning, scheduling, prioritizing, and monitoring cognitive activities.[27] In some patients with isolated medial orbitofrontal lesions the dysexecutive syndrome may stand alone. Disturbance of the executive system also results in difficulties in attending to two things at once, and distractibility.

Patients with the dysexecutive syndrome may be much more impaired in everyday life than is predicted by their performance on standard neuropsychological tests. They can manage with the clear instructions of the well-structured and constrained test situation. But in the real world these are absent; priorities have to be set, a strategy planned, decisions taken, and the unexpected dealt with, all without guidance. In the real world, impairment of the executive system may be catastrophic. Tests of the dysexecutive syndrome have been developed in order to be better predictors of these real-life problems.[18]

Memory impairment

Memory impairment is perhaps the most common cognitive impairment that follows head injury, and can be very disabling.[28] People will have problems remembering where they put things, what to do next, how to get home from shops, what they did yesterday, or what their cousin is called. The term anterograde amnesia is used to refer to these enduring memory problems, and must be distinguished from retrograde and post-traumatic amnesia (see Box 1).

No consistent pattern of brain injury is associated with anterograde amnesia and it seems likely that it is the combined damage to several areas which causes the amnesia. Frontal injury may be particularly implicated and this may be because frontal injury results in failure of the executive processes required for normal memory, for example in memory retrieval. As with most amnesic states the amnesia following brain injury is for explicit memories, namely those which are consciously remembered. Implicit memory, for example remembering and learning a motor skill, generally remains intact.

Anterograde amnesia is often characterized by distortions and inaccurate recall with poor monitoring and insight. Confabulations are often seen.

Communication

Dysphasia is quite common after head injury, and may be rather different from that seen after stroke.[29] The more diffuse and widespread injury of traumatic brain injury results in additional cognitive impairments which colour the picture. Monitoring language errors is often particularly poor and the patient may demonstrate a jargon aphasia in which they are apparently unaware that their speech is completely incomprehensible.

Dysprosody, in which the normal rhythms and intonations of speech are lost, is also seen, more so after right hemisphere damage. This interferes with social communication because the voice sounds flat and fails to convey emotion. Social communication is disrupted for other reasons, for example the patient fails in the turn-taking necessary for normal conversation. Word-finding difficulties are very common.

Visuospatial impairments

Visuospatial impairments are seen and may contribute to spatial disorientation. Visual agnosia is easy to miss in someone with quite widespread cognitive impairments.

Decline in cognitive function

Accelerated cognitive decline, but insufficient to result in dementia, has been found in head-injured soldiers 25 years later.[30] The reduced reserve of the injured brain probably makes it vulnerable to the effects of ageing. Follow-up and case–control studies have shown an association between head injury and subsequent Alzheimer's disease. Individuals with the *APOE e4* allele may be at special risk.[31] However, the evidence for both an accelerated cognitive decline and an increased risk of Alzheimer's disease is inconsistent.

Personality change

Personality change after head injury results in more suffering than any other single sequel.[32,33] In general, the personality change goes hand in hand with cognitive impairment. However, a severe personality change is occasionally found in somebody with almost no impairment of cognitive function. Normal test scores for memory and intellect do not rule out brain injury as a cause of personality change after head injury.

Aetiology

It is not easy to predict who will develop a change in personality after head injury. Sometimes a personality trait present before the injury becomes much more troublesome, but often there is no obvious predisposition. The site of the brain injury may play a role. Convexity lesions, on the lateral surface of the brain, can produce impairments of drive. Orbitofrontal lesions may cause a more troublesome personality change with impairments in social behaviour.

Post-traumatic factors also need to be considered. Some patients seem to learn maladaptive patterns of behaviour; for example the response of the carers may unwittingly reinforce unwanted behaviours. Chronic mental illness may be manifest as personality change, which may be aggravated by chronic psychosocial stressors. Dependence on drugs, particularly alcohol, frequently confounds the picture.

Characteristics of the personality change

Changes in personality[34] include apathy and impairment of motivation and ambition. Patients are often described as childish; this covers a range of traits including impulsivity, poor tolerance of frustration, being demanding and self-centred, and generally lacking the ability to take on the adult role in terms of independent decision-making. Patients may be fatuous and facetious. Antisocial behaviours (see below) and disinhibition are severe handicaps that make integration back into the community very difficult. Sexual disinhibition of any type is particularly worrisome. A spectrum of severity is seen, ranging from being inappropriately flirtatious through to indiscriminate sexual assaults. Head injury is a risk factor for borderline personality disorder.[35]

In acquired antisocial personality disorder[36] the person is often self-centred and relatively oblivious to the needs of others. They are likely to be tactless and, on occasion, offensively rude. Irritability and aggression and impulsive behaviour are seen. They may show a lack of remorse for the violent behaviour. These personality traits often are accompanied by the dysexecutive syndrome. Thus not only does the person show disturbed social decision-making, resulting in antisocial behaviours, but also disruption of the planning and organizational skills needed for cognitive tasks. For example, helpful and supportive friends may be alienated in favour of disreputable acquaintances, at the same time as money is impulsively spent, and lost, on risky projects without any attempt to weigh up the options.

Effects on family and carers

Families find personality change particularly difficult to cope with.[37] Children may be ignored and the partner's needs, particularly emotional needs, forgotten. The healthy balance of the relationship with the partner may be destroyed, with the head-injured person now unable to take an effective part in the household. The partner becomes a carer and the change in roles may have a serious impact on the sexual relationship. Divorce frequently follows. However, parents may find the childish personality of the brain-injured person easier to cope with; they revert to taking on the parental role.

Personality change may deteriorate. Supportive social networks are lost and social isolation and financial problems may contribute to depression or alcohol abuse, which then cause a deterioration in the behavioural problems associated with the personality change. Follow-up studies lend some support to this argument. Some behavioural problems are found to have deteriorated at 5 years after head injury[38], and family burden increases over this period.

Early mental symptoms following brain injury

On recovery of consciousness many patients after a severe head injury go through a period of delirium with clouding of consciousness. This may resolve, leaving a confusional state in clear consciousness with disorientation and thought disorder consisting of muddled thinking, rambling talk, and perseverations. The mental state is dominated by misperceptions and misrecollections as they flit from one false observation to another.[39] Fear is common.

Distortions of memory

Confabulations, brief-lived false memories, emerge at about this time.[24] Confabulations occur particularly in association with memory disturbance associated with frontal injury. The patient almost invariably shows poor insight into their memory problems, and is likely to be disorientated.

Occasionally after a severe head injury there are islets of memory in the dense amnesic period immediately around the time of the injury. These may be recollections of something that was consciously experienced at the time. On the other hand, the memories may have been fabricated from information subsequently given to the patient about what happened, or the memories may have no basis in reality and be properly described as a delusional memory.

Alterations of mood and perception

In the early recovery period oneroid states may be seen. The patient may be perplexed. He or she may feel that the trauma never occurred and that the whole event, including being in hospital, is a fabrication. Derealization/depersonalization may be associated with prominent anxiety, with the patient constantly asking for reassurance. Agitation is often observed in this early recovery period.

Hallucinations, particularly visual, are occasionally observed, whereas illusions of familiarity commonly occur after brain injury. The patient may have a sense of *déja vu*, or that he or she has met clinical staff or patients before. Distortions of the sense of familiarity also seem to be implicated in many of the delusions observed early after brain injury.

Apathetic states

In many patients the recovery period lacks the positive features described above and is dominated by an apathetic withdrawn state.

Psychosis after brain injury

Early psychosis

Delusions involving the misidentification of place, persons, objects, and events may be observed early in the course of recovery. These delusions are often associated with more generalized disturbances of insight, in particular denial of illness (anosognosia), impaired judgement, and disorientation. The best evidence for this comes from a study of delusions after right temporoparietal strokes.[40]

The vast majority of the delusions occurring during the recovery period will themselves remit spontaneously and not relapse. However, in some patients who have recovered from these early delusions amylobarbitone produced a return of symptoms.[41] This suggests that generalized disturbance of brain function plays an important part in the development of early delusions.

Reduplicative paramnesia

Perhaps the delusion that is most pathognomonic of brain injury, and which is also associated with postictal confusional states, is reduplicative paramnesia. The term reduplicative paramnesia covers a range of phenomena, which are often observed concurrently. Pick[42], who introduced the term, used it to describe a patient who believed she had visited a duplicate hospital. Other phenomena covered by the term include the following:

- any delusion involving duplication, for example that events have been duplicated or that the patient has a second left leg

- delusions involving misidentification of place, with or without duplication, including delusional disorientation for place.

Delusional disorientation for place may involve the belief that the current location is a duplicate of the true location or in some way displaced, for example that the hospital is in a different country. The patient may have two incompatible attitudes to orientation; this is sometimes referred to as a double orientation. For example, a patient who lives in Edinburgh acknowledges that he is in a hospital in London, but says that his home is just a few yards down the road.

Capgras syndrome and other delusional misidentifications of person

Whereas isolated delusional misidentifications of place are rare in the absence of manifest organic brain disease, most cases of delusional misidentification of person (e.g. Capgras syndrome) are to be found in schizophrenia. Delusional misidentifications of person may also be observed following brain injury, often alongside a reduplicative paramnesia. (See also Chapter 4.4.)

Organic and psychological factors in delusional misidentification

Delusional misidentification syndromes can best be understood as the result of an interaction between organic brain disease and psychological disorder.[43] Lesions of the right hemisphere, often in combination with frontal injury or more diffuse evidence of brain disease, are particularly associated with delusional misidentification.

Late psychosis

Schizophrenia-like psychosis

A psychotic illness may develop long after the acute confusional state has resolved, which is difficult to distinguish from psychotic illness occurring in the absence of manifest organic brain disease. The patient may develop a typical schizophrenia indistinguishable from idiopathic schizophrenia. Would he or she have developed schizophrenia regardless of having had a head injury?

The best estimate of the increased risk of developing a schizophrenia-like psychosis as a result of a head injury comes from Davison and Bagley's study of 30 years ago.[44] They estimated a two- to threefold increased risk compared with the general population. There were large variations in the different studies they examined, and most were cohorts of war veterans. It is not clear whether the same relative risk will be found in civilian cohorts with mainly closed head injuries. Those who develop schizophrenia after head injury may be at high risk anyway, for example due to a family history of schizophrenia or schizoid personality traits, but the findings are not consistent.

Conversely, case–control studies of patients with schizophrenia show increased rates of childhood head injuries.[45]

The association between head injury and subsequent schizophrenia does not mean that head injury is causing the schizophrenia; they could both be linked to something else, such as behavioural problems. However, specific patterns of brain injury are associated with the development of schizophrenia-like states, and this suggests that brain injury plays a causal role. Late schizophrenic-like psychosis after brain injury is particularly associated with temporal lobe injury and to a lesser extent post-traumatic epilepsy.[44] However, these associations are weak.

Paranoid psychosis

Paranoid psychoses may emerge after brain injury. Not infrequently this occurs relatively early and in a patient with severe cognitive impairment and personality change. Memory impairment will facilitate the development of persecutory ideas; for example, the patient believes that belongings have been stolen. Persecutory ideas or delusions of reference are a fairly common cause of aggression and may be hidden by communication difficulties.

Effects of head injury on schizophrenia

The cognitive and behavioural problems of schizophrenia overlap considerably with those produced by traumatic brain injury. Antisocial behaviours, apathy and lack of spontaneity, and erratic mood swings are common to both. Both will show cognitive problems including disorders of communication, memory, and planning. Will a head injury therefore aggravate these more negative symptoms of schizophrenia? Given that a significant proportion of head trauma is found in people with schizophrenia who have jumped from a height, the question arises from time to time. As yet there are no studies of the outcome.

Mood disorders, including anxiety disorders

Depression

The study of depression after head injury raises two fundamental questions about the nosological status of depression. First, with a severe disability should the belief that life is not worth living be regarded as a symptom of depression or a 'rational' reaction to an intolerable predicament? Second, what is one to make of symptoms of apathy or anhedonia when the brain pathways involved in generating spontaneous behaviour or the experience of pleasure have been damaged? Most of the biological symptoms of depression can be produced by brain injury.

The diagnosis of depression therefore relies heavily on identifying a depressive mood. Symptoms like self-deprecation or guilt are also particularly helpful in diagnosis. Estimates of the prevalence of depression after head injury vary, partly because of the lack of uniformity in defining depression. Perhaps 25 per cent of patients meet DSM-IIIR criteria for major depression 1 month after injury.[46] The majority have recovered from their depression by 6 months, while at 1 year 10 to 20 per cent of those previously not depressed have become depressed.

Aetiological factors include a personal history of depression, which is twice as common in those who become depressed, and lack of social support. Left frontal injury predicts the development of depression within 3 months of a closed head injury, but does not predict those who are depressed at 1 year. Two large follow-up studies have found that after penetrating injuries depression at 1 year is associated with right hemisphere damage, particularly of the frontal lobes.

Depression after head injury interferes with rehabilitation, and is associated with aggression. It may exacerbate cognitive impairment and in some cases produce a pseudodementia.

Emotional lability may occur, particularly after severe head injury, and is frequently associated with the presence of depression.

Mania

Manic illness after head injury is much less common than depression. It needs to be distinguished from the neurobehavioural symptoms of, for example, disinhibition and fatuous behaviour that may follow frontal injury. There is some evidence for a link with right hemisphere lesions and with post-traumatic epilepsy. Mania is particularly associated with aggressive and assaultive behaviour following brain injury.

Anxiety disorder

Anxiety disorders are found in about 30 per cent of patients after head injury, and are at least as common in those who have suffered mild injury.[47]

Early symptoms may be observed in relation to derealization/depersonalization symptoms, or perplexity. Early on, the amnesic period surrounding the injury may cause great distress. In the catastrophic reaction, which is observed in patients with moderate to severe cognitive impairment, sudden distress occurs when they fail to perform a task, or because of their inability to communicate.

Anxiety symptoms, particularly those with a mild head injury, may develop over the weeks and months following a head injury. It is then more likely to be associated with depression, post-concussion syndrome, and with post-traumatic stress disorder. Phobic avoidance is seen, for example travel anxiety following a road traffic accident. Apprehension is a common complaint, perhaps reflecting problems caused by cognitive impairments, and the person may be indecisive. Therefore anxiety symptoms may emerge on return to work. Anxiety symptoms will be inflated in the presence of financial or family stress.

Obsessive–compulsive disorder is a recognized sequela of head injury. This may partly reflect the inflexibility and rigidity of the brain-injured person, or a response to doubt resulting from memory disorder.

Suicide

The risk of suicide is increased following head injury. In a study of Finnish soldiers who suffered brain injuries during the Second World War and were followed up for 25 years, 1.6 per cent had killed themselves, about a threefold greater risk than the general male population.[48] A meta-analysis of six civilian cohorts followed up over 40 years found a threefold risk compared with standard mortality rates.[49] The increased risk attributable to head injury is probably slightly less than these estimates.

Agitation and aggression

The psychiatrist is more likely to be asked to advise about the management of agitation and aggression following head injury than any other psychological symptom.

Agitation in the early recovery period after severe brain injury will generally spontaneously improve over the course of days or weeks.[50] Usually no specific cause is found and it is a marker of a generalized disturbance of brain function. Epilepsy may be contributing, and partial complex seizures may not be immediately obvious clinically. The milder the head injury the more likely it is that psychological factors will be found. The patient's worries and fears need to be explored, and phobic anxiety disorder considered. Drugs may make agitation worse and paradoxical effects of sedative medication occur if the medication increases confusion or disinhibition, or results in akathisia. The patient may be in a withdrawal state having stopped a drug they were taking regularly before the head injury.

Early agitation may be followed by more intractable aggressive behaviour.[51] A major predictor of aggression is antisocial behaviour before the head injury. Other predictors of aggressive behaviour include confusion and disorientation, personality change with disinhibition or impulsivity, and epilepsy and anticonvulsant use.[52]

Otherwise the predictors of aggressive behaviour are by and large no different from those found in the absence of head injury. Symptoms of mental illness, however, may not be immediately obvious because of communication difficulties. It is therefore necessary to search for evidence of persecutory delusions, mania, depression, and anxiety. Drug and alcohol dependence may be especially problematic.

If the aggressive behaviour emerges early, namely during the confusional state or shortly after it resolves, then this suggest that the aetiology is largely organic. A pattern of aggression that is highly stereotyped, or erupts over seconds with no or trivial triggers, or is bizarre, and is against a background of calm behaviour, suggests the possibility of epilepsy.

Alcohol and head injury

Alcohol dependence complicates the management of the head-injured person several-fold. The person may have suffered several previous head injuries, as well as the effects of alcoholic brain damage before the head injury. A blow to the head may result in much greater brain injury for reasons that are poorly understood.[53] Poor physical health is likely to prejudice immediate management after the head injury. Subdural haematomas may be problematic. Alcohol craving may interfere with medical care and rehabilitation.[54] Social networks are often poor, thus complicating discharge from hospital.

Very occasionally a head injury seems to cure the alcohol dependence. Unfortunately alcohol dependence often gets worse, indeed some patients develop alcohol dependence when they find that alcohol relieves their anxiety symptoms.

Postconcussion syndrome

Sometimes called post-traumatic syndrome, the postconcussion syndrome is poorly defined.[55] The term is perhaps most usefully reserved to describe a constellation of symptoms that may result in surprisingly severe disability after mild head injury. These symptoms may be observed after moderate and severe head injuries, in which case they are likely to be in the company of other symptoms more readily understood as resulting from brain injury. There is no consistent relationship between the prevalence of postconcussion symptoms and injury severity.

Phenomenology

Early symptoms tend to have a more neurological flavour and include headache, dizziness, and occasionally diplopia. Mild head injury fairly consistently results, in the immediate aftermath, in impairment of speed of information processing and concentration. Fatigue is also evident from early on, along with symptoms of noise sensitivity. Anxiety, depression, and irritability are common and may appear after a latent period. The symptoms of postconcussion syndrome overlap with those of post-traumatic stress disorder, and chronic fatigue. Other symptoms occasionally reported include tinnitus, unsteadiness, and muscle pain.

In general, symptoms, particularly the more neurological symptoms, will have recovered by 2 to 6 months. But a few patients, often after a latent period, develop persistent symptoms that last for years. This suggests that psychological factors, as well as brain injury, are important.

Aetiology

Brain injury

Several observations support the contribution of brain injury. Microscopic lesions in the brain have been described at postmortem, following mild head injury.[56] Imaging, including functional imaging with single-photon emission CT or positron emission tomography, may show small abnormalities which are attributed to the mild head injury. Delayed brainstem auditory evoked potentials have been found and may predict chronicity of symptoms.[57]

Psychological factors

Psychosocial factors have also been found to play a part in postconcussion syndrome, more so in those with symptoms lasting longer than 1 year. If the accident occurs at work, particularly if the person blames their employer, symptoms are more likely. A meta-analysis of the effects of compensation on symptoms, any symptom, after head injury concluded that, on average, being involved in compensation claims increases symptoms by about 25 per cent.[58]

Model of interaction

Lishman has proposed a model in which early disturbance of brain function after mild head injury results in the early symptoms of postconcussion syndrome.[1] In most patients these gradually resolve and a good recovery is made. However, the postconcussion syndrome may develop if psychological effects interfere with the normal process of recovery. Anxiety is thought to play a large part in impeding recovery; the patient worries about the symptoms and focuses on them. These may be aggravated if the patient is vulnerable to somatization, or there are compensation issues at stake. The symptoms may cause secondary disability provoking yet more anxiety, which will be made worse if there are additional psychosocial stressors.

The role of psychological factors is greatest in those with very mild head injuries and very chronic symptoms. For example, studies looking at the effects of compensation generally show more powerful effects in those with milder injuries.

Post-traumatic epilepsy

Early fits, within the first week, are relatively benign, sensitive to prophylactic anticonvulsants, and are only weak predictors of later epilepsy.

Only about 5 per cent of closed head injuries go on to develop late seizures, compared with 30 per cent after an open head injury. The majority of these late seizures start in the first and second year following injury. By the time 5 years have elapsed without seizures any subsequent seizure development may be unrelated to the head injury.[59]

The likelihood of developing seizures in patients with a closed head injury is increased by the presence of a depressed skull fracture, intracranial haematoma, and early seizure, as well as by the severity of the injury. Mild head injuries result in only a small increased risk of epilepsy above population norms. Children are at increased risk of post-traumatic epilepsy. The EEG is generally not a good predictor of post-traumatic epilepsy (see above).

Post-traumatic epilepsy increases psychiatric morbidity, particularly mood disorders, behavioural problems, and psychotic illness, and may increase the risk of late dementia.

Prophylactic anticonvulsants have no effect on reducing the incidence of late post-traumatic epilepsy.[60] Carbamazepine, rather than phenytoin, is the drug of choice if an anticonvulsant is needed because it has less effect on cognition.[61] Half of all patients with post-traumatic epilepsy from open head injuries are found to be in remission by 5 to 10 years.

Head injury in children

It is possible that the greater potential for plasticity, which may be present in the younger child's brain, will result in a better outcome after head injury. There is some evidence for this for mild and moderate head injuries. However, children with severe head injuries are likely to be left with persistent cognitive deficits and behavioural problems. The quality of parenting has a powerful effect on outcome; those with poor parenting are much more likely to develop behavioural problems.

Children often sustain a bilateral prefrontal injury, which may explain the deficits in concentration, controlling impulsivity, and self-monitoring. The commonest psychiatric disorders that follow childhood head injuries are personality changes, attention-deficit hyperactivity disorder, and obsessive–compulsive disorder.[62] Children who develop attention-deficit hyperactivity disorder after head injury tend to demonstrate less hyperactivity than is seen in the idiopathic form of this disorder. In the long term the head-injured child may be at increased risk of developing schizophrenia. Children are more likely to develop post-traumatic epilepsy than adults.

Boxing

Between 10 and 20 per cent of professional boxers go on to develop a chronic traumatic encephalopathy,[63] the punch-drunk syndrome, with damage to the extrapyramidal system as well as cerebellar and pyramidal pathways. They are slow and ataxic. Cognitive impairment, in particular memory impairment, is a frequent accompaniment and dementia is present in about half of the cases.

Upper brainstem lesions may explain the neurological symptoms, while cerebral atrophy, white matter changes, and damage to diencephalic structures may account for cognitive changes. Perforation of the septum pellucidum, which separates the two lateral ventricles, is a characteristic finding in boxers' encephalopathy. *APOE e4* status increases vulnerability to the punch-drunk syndrome,[64] and this is consistent with the finding that amyloid is present.

Professional footballers may show evidence of subtle impairments of thinking, raising the possibility that repeated blows to the head from heading the ball may be sufficient to cause slight brain injury.

Management

The reader is referred to Chapter 4.1.14 for many of the management principles relevant to patients with a head injury.

Management of early neurobehavioural problems

Behavioural problems, and mental symptoms, arising in the days and weeks following a brain injury should be regarded as a flag to indicate the need to check on the progress of recovery. The history needs to be reviewed, paying attention to the period leading up to injury. The patient will need to be examined physically, paying particular attention to the possibility of fever, and given a reasonably thorough neurological examination. It is essential to document the conscious level and orientation. Routine blood tests should be performed, and blood gases and a chest radiograph considered. The medication needs to be scrutinized. A neurological or neurosurgical opinion may be needed with a view to considering neuroimaging or an EEG. A lumbar puncture, for example looking for meningitis, should probably not be done without specialist advice.

Specific causes of deterioration after head injury are listed in Box 2. Once these have been excluded then the principle of care should be to allow recovery to take place in a safe environment, paying attention to the general principles of the care of the delirious or demented patient as indicated. Explanation to the patient and his or her family of what is happening, is required.

Box 2

Causes of deterioration in cognitive function after brain injury

Specific
- Subdural haematoma
- Hydrocephalus
- Epilepsy, particularly complex partial status
- Late intracranial infection, including cerebral abscess

Non-specific
- Systemic illness, including fat emboli and pain
- Drug intoxication
- Severe mental illness, in particular depression
- The patient 'gives up' as he or she gains insight
- Independent dementing process

Management of late mental sequelae

General management principles

Good medical and surgical care, followed by transfer to appropriate rehabilitation services is required to optimize recovery from head injury. In addition, the individual and their family should have access to support as they try to adjust to the changes forced on them by the head injury. Education, and access to information, is an important part of the strategy.[65] Not infrequently psychological problems arise if any part of this process has not gone smoothly, or is perceived to have failed. The psychiatrist should explore any such concerns.

It is often necessary to find out what services are available in the area that might provide rehabilitation or support. Access to suitable programmes of rehabilitation, or vocational training, or appropriate support, may relieve mental symptoms. A social worker should be asked to undertake a community care assessment, which may identify the need for respite care or modifications to the home.

Specific neuropsychiatric interventions

It is important early on to ascertain the degree of brain injury that has been sustained. If there is any doubt then this may need to include a neuropsychological assessment. The severity of brain injury will suggest whether a particular symptom is mainly due to brain injury or to psychological processes. This will influence management.

Cognitive-behavioural treatment will play a key part in the management of neurobehavioural symptoms. Behavioural strategies are particularly relevant to behavioural problems arising from brain injury.[66] The crucial task is to identify the responses of carers or family that seem to be reinforcing the behaviour.

Pharmacological management

Perhaps the majority of patients who suffer a traumatic brain injury, needing hospital treatment, are given psychotropic drugs,[67] despite the fact that animal studies suggest that some may interfere with recovery from brain injury. Patients should be given psychotropics only if absolutely necessary, using the principles described in Box 3 and avoiding multiple drugs given concurrently.

Box 3

Prescribing psychotropics in brain injury

Small doses—start low, go slow

Only continue treatment if definite evidence of effect

Drug profile—choose drugs with less potential for:

- lowering seizure threshold—avoid chlorpromazine and clozapine
- anticholinergic activity—to minimize potential for increasing confusion
- extrapyramidal side-effects—
    especially akathisia, parkinsonism, and neuroleptic malignant syndrome
- Enzyme induction or other pharmacodynamic interaction with other drugs

Regular medication with long-acting drugs, compared with short-acting drugs as required is less likely to produce:

- withdrawal syndrome
- development of addiction
- reinforcement of unwanted behaviour

Agitation and aggression

Because of the lack of controlled trials, prescribing for agitation and aggression after brain injury is very much trial and error, requiring good monitoring and documentation of the behaviour. If there is no evidence of benefit then the drug should be withdrawn and another drug tried. Be wary of responding to every episode of aggression by increasing the dose or adding a new drug.

Of all the drugs used in the management of agitation and aggression only β-blockers, in very large doses, have been exposed to randomized controlled trials,[68] which showed a slight effect in favour of medication.

Nevertheless, for many psychiatrists carbamazepine is the drug of first choice for aggression after brain injury. It has the advantage of anticonvulsant properties, as well as mood-stabilizing effects. Perhaps a third of patients will respond. Some clinicians recommend sodium valproate.

Antipsychotics should be used in the presence of delusions or persecutory ideas of reference, and possibly when the patient demonstrates undue suspiciousness. Otherwise they should not be the first-line treatment, partly because of the danger that akathisia may perpetuate agitated behaviour which would otherwise have resolved spontaneously. Sulpiride and olanzapine can be recommended as first-line drugs, with risperidone and other new antipsychotic agents held in reserve.

Antidepressants may be helpful, and selective serotonin-reuptake inhibitors should be given in preference to tricyclics. Trazodone, which is sedative, may be particularly useful.

Benzodiazepines and chlormethiazole should be considered for agitation and aggression during the early recovery from severe head injury. But be wary of increasing the confusion, and paradoxical violence due to disinhibition. Because of the potential for addiction, benzodiazepines should not be given to a patient with a chronic aggressive disorder.

Mood disorders and psychosis

Clinically, one has the impression that depression after a head injury is more difficult to treat. This is consistent with the observation that depression, in those who have not suffered a head injury, is more difficult to treat if the patient is found to have evidence of brain damage. However, some studies in head-injured depressed patients have found good response rates. The selection of an antidepressant is no different from that used to treat depression in the absence of brain injury, provided that the principles given in Box 3 are taken into account.

There has been no good trial of antipsychotic drugs in the treatment of psychotic patients after head injury. A case series has shown a good response in the majority of psychotic patients, and this fits with the clinical impression that some delusions and hallucinations do respond. The choice of drug is the same as that for the management of aggression (see above).

Apathy

Bromocriptine and methylphenidate may be useful for treating apathetic states. An initial effect wears away in some patients, but in others a beneficial effect is maintained despite removal of the drug. Methylphenidate, with its risk of addiction and troublesome side-effects, should only be prescribed if bromocriptine has not been successful, under consultant supervision.

Insight, compliance, competence, and detention in hospital

Lack of awareness of deficits is a common problem for the head-injured person[69] and affects compliance with the treatment. As a result, the psychiatrist may be called when the patient demands to leave hospital, even though they would be at risk returning home. If there is evidence of mental disorder then it may be possible to justify detention under the Mental Health Act 1983 (England and Wales), but not if the purpose of doing so is merely to treat a physical condition.

Insight and capacity to consent to treatment should be assessed. Only the very exceptional patient who is demanding to leave hospital following a head injury, and who as a result would be putting his or her health severely at risk, will be found to be competent. In this situation, in England and Wales, it may be possible to detain patients in hospital under common law in their best interests for treatment of a physical condition.

The patient's capacity to give informed consent to any treatment that is being offered may need to be reviewed. They should also be assessed to see whether they are capable of managing their domestic and financial affairs. If they are not, appropriate legal arrangements should be made; in the United Kingdom a receiver may need to be appointed to protect their interests. The prospect of compensation should be considered and, if appropriate, they should be enabled to pursue a personal injury claim.

Service provision for the head-injured

Head-injury services tend to be very heterogeneous and poorly co-ordinated.[70] A head injury co-ordinator or team who identify patients at the outset, i.e. shortly after admission to hospital, is the best solution. They can identify the appropriate services for that individual and ensure continuity of service provision. It helps if there is a named local psychiatrist interested in neuropsychiatry for them to liaise with. The psychiatrist should also be part of the liaison service for the district general hospital, in particular to the trauma unit and neurosurgery. A regional neurobehavioural unit, managing challenging behaviour arising from head injury and other acquired brain injuries, should be available.

Generally brain-injury services are poorly funded. It is often difficult to find services to refer the patient to. In the United Kingdom a recent trial of case management failed to show a beneficial effect, probably because there were insufficient local resources to take on the patients' care.

Further reading

Damasio, A.R. (1994). *Descartes' error: emotion, reason and the human brain.* Grosset/Putnam, New York.

Eames, P. (1997). Traumatic brain injury. *Current Opinion in Psychiatry* **10**, 49–52.

Levin, H.S., Eisenberg, H.M., and Benton, A.L. (1989). *Mild head injury.* Oxford University Press, New York.

Lishman, W.A. (1998). *Organic psychiatry: the psychological consequences of cerebral disorder* (3rd edn). Blackwell Science, Oxford.

Silver, J.M., Yudofsky, S.C., and Hales, R.E. (1994). *Neuropsychiatry of traumatic brain injury.* American Psychiatric Press, Washington, DC.

Wood, R.L. (1990). *Neurobehavioural sequelae of traumatic brain injury.* Taylor and Francis, New York.

References

1. Lishman, W.A. (1988). Physiogenesis and psychogenesis in the 'post-concussional syndrome'. *British Journal of Psychiatry*, **153**, 460–9.
2. Kapur, N. (1997). *Injured brains of medical minds: views from within.* Oxford University Press.
3. Teasdale, G.M. (1995). Head injury. *Journal of Neurology, Neurosurgery and Psychiatry*, **58**, 526–39.
4. Fitzpatrick, M.O., Maxwell, W.L., and Graham, D.I. (1998). The role of the axolemma in the initiation of traumatically induced diffuse axonal injury. *Journal of Neurology, Neurosurgery and Psychiatry*, **64**, 285–7.
5. Sheriff, F.E., Bridges, L.R., and Sivaloganathan, S. (1994). Early detection of axonal injury after human head trauma using immunocytochemistry for B-amyloid precursor protein. *Acta Neuropathologica*, **87**, 55–62.
6. Nicholl, J.A.R., Roberts, G.W., and Graham, D.I. (1995). Apolipoprotein E e4 allele is associated with deposition of amyloid B-protein following head injury. *Nature Medicine*, **1**, 135–7.
7. Hayes, R.L., Lyeth, B.G., and Jenkins, L.W. (1989). Neurochemical mechanisms of mild and moderate head injury; implications for treatment. In *Mild head injury* (ed. H.S. Levin, H.M. Eisenberg, and A.L. Benton), pp. 54–79. Oxford University Press.
8. Bishara, S., Partridge, F., Godfrey, H., *et al.* (1992). Post-traumatic amnesia and Glasgow Coma Scale related to outcome in survivors in a consecutive series of patients with severe closed head injury. *Brain Injury*, **6**, 373–80.
9. Teasdale, G. and Jennett, B. (1974). Assessment of coma and impaired consciousness. A practical scale. *Lancet*, **ii**, 81–4.
10. Jennett, B. (1996). Epidemiology of head injury. *Journal of Neurology, Neurosurgery and Psychiatry*, **60**, 362–9.
11. Bryden, J. (1989). How many head injured? The epidemiology of post head injury disability. *Models of brain injury rehabilitation* (ed. R.L. Wood and P. Eames), pp. 17–27. Chapman & Hall, London.
12. Levin, H.S., Williams, D.H., Eisenberg, H.M., *et al.* (1992). Serial MRI and neurobehavioural findings after mild to moderate closed head injury. *Journal of Neurology, Neurosurgery and Psychiatry*, **55**, 255–62.
13. Ruff, R.M., Buschbaum, M.S., Troster, A.I., *et al.* (1989). Computerised tomography, neuropsychology, and positron emission tomography in the evaluation of head injury. *Neuropsychiatry, Neuropsychology and Behavioural Neurology*, **2**, 103–23.
14. Wilson, J.L.T. and Wyper, D. (1992). Neuroimaging and neuropsychological functioning following closed head injury: CT, MRI, and SPECT. *Journal of Head Trauma Rehabilitation*, **7**, 29–39.
15. Goldenberg, G., Oder, W., Spatt, J., *et al.* (1992). Cerebral correlates of disturbed executive function and memory in survivors of severe closed head injury: a SPECT study. *Journal of Neurology, Neurosurgery and Psychiatry*, **55**, 362–8.
16. Markowitsch, H.J., Kessler, J., Van Der Van, C., Weber-Luxenburger, G., Albers, M., and Heiss, W.D. (1998). Psychic trauma causing grossly reduced brain metabolism and cognitive deterioration. *Neuropsychologia*, **36**, 77–82.
17. Nelson, H.E. and Willison, J.R. (1991). *National adult reading test* (2nd edn). NFER-Nelson, Windsor.
18. Wilson, B.A., Alderman, N., Burgess, P.W., Emslie, H., and Evans, J.J. (1996). *Behavioural assessment of the dysexecutive syndrome.* Thames Valley Test Co., Bury St Edmunds, Suffolk.
19. World Health Organization (1980). *International classification of impairments, disabilities, and handicaps.* World Health Organization, Geneva.
20. Teasdale, T.W. and Engberg, A. (1997). Duration of cognitive dysfunction after concussion, and cognitive dysfunction as a risk factor: a population study of young men. *British Medical Journal*, **315**, 569–72.
21. Lishman, W.A. (1968). Brain damage in relation to psychiatric disability after head injury. *British Journal of Psychiatry*, **114**, 373–410.
22. Pilowsky, I. (1985). Cryptotrauma and 'accident neurosis'. *British Journal of Psychiatry*, **147**, 310–11.
23. Claparède, E. (1911). Récognition et moïté. *Archives of Psychology (Genève)*, **11**, 79–90.
24. Whitty, C.W.M. and Zangwill, O.L. (1966). Traumatic amnesia. In *Amnesia* (ed. C.W.M. Whitty and O.L. Zangwill), pp. 92–108. Butterworths, London.
25. Ruff, R. M., Young, D., Gautille, T., *et al.* (1991). Verbal learning deficits following severe head injury: heterogeneity in recovery over 1 year. *Journal of Neurosurgery*, **75**, S50–S58.
26. Wilson, B. (1992). Recovery and compensation strategies in head injured memory impaired people several years after insult. *Journal of Neurology, Neurosurgery and Psychiatry*, **55**, 177–80.
27. Shallice, T. and Burgess, P.W. (1991). Deficits in strategy application following frontal lobe damage in man. *Brain*, **114**, 727–41.

28. Brooks, D.N. (1975). Long and short term memory in head injured patients. *Cortex*, **11**, 329–40.

29. Adamovich, B.B. and Henderson, J.A. (1990). Traumatic brain injury. In *Aphasia and related neurogenic disorders* (ed. L. La Pointe), pp. 196–209. Thieme Medical, New York.

30. Corkin, S., Rosen, J., Sullivan, E.V., and Clegg, R.A. (1989). Penetrating head injury in young adulthood exacerbates cognitive decline in later years. *Journal of Neuroscience*, **9**, 3876–83.

31. Mayeux, R., Ottoman, R., Maestre, G., *et al.* (1995). Synergistic effects of head injury and apolipoprotein e4 in patients with Alzheimer's disease. *Neurology*, **45**, 555–7.

32. Lezak, M.D. (1978). Living with the characterologically altered brain injured patient. *Journal of Clinical Psychiatry*, **39**, 592–8.

33. Parker, R.S. (1996). The spectrum of emotional distress and personality changes after minor head injury incurred in a motor vehicle accident. *Brain Injury*, **10**, 287–302.

34. Alexander, M.P. (1982). Traumatic brain injury. In *Psychiatric aspects of neurologic disease*, Vol. 2 (ed. D.F. Benson and D. Blumer), pp. 219–49. Grune and Stratton, New York.

35. Streeter, C.C., Van Reekum, R., Shorr, R.I., and Bachman, D.L. (1995). Prior head injury in male veterans with borderline personality disorder. *Journal of Nervous and Mental Disease*, **183**, 577–81.

36. Damasio, A.R. (1996). The somatic marker hypothesis and the possible functions of the prefrontal cortex. *Philosophical Transactions of the Royal Society London B*, **351**, 1413–20.

37. Thomsen, I.V. (1974). The patient with severe head injury and his family: a follow-up study of 50 patients. *Scandinavian Journal of Rehabilitation Medicine*, **6**, 180–3.

38. Olver, J.H., Ponsford, J.L., and Curran, C.A. (1996). Outcome following traumatic brain injury: a comparison between 2 and 5 years after injury. *Brain Injury*, **10**, 841–8.

39. Symonds, C.P. (1937). Mental disorder following head injury. *Proceedings of the Royal Society of Medicine*, **30**, 1081–94.

40. Levine, D.N. and Grek, A. (1984). The anatomic basis of delusions after right cerebral infarction. *Neurology*, **34**, 577–82.

41. Weinstein, E.A. and Kahn, R.L. (1951). Patterns of disorientation in organic brain disease. *Journal of Neuropathology and Clinical Neurology*, **1**, 214.

42. Pick, A. (1903). Clinical studies. III: on reduplicative paramnesia. *Brain*, **26**, 260–7.

43. Fleminger, S. and Burns, A. (1993). The delusional misidentification syndromes in patients with and without evidence of organic cerebral disorder: a structured review of case reports. *Biological Psychiatry*, **33**, 22–32.

44. Davison, K. and Bagley, C.R. (1969). Schizophrenia-like psychoses associated with organic disorders of the central nervous system: a review of the literature. In *Current problems in neuropsychiatry: schizophrenia, epilepsy, the temporal lobe* (ed. R.N. Herrington), *British Journal of Psychiatry* Special Publication No. 4, pp. 113–84. Headley Brothers, Ashford.

45. Wilcox, J.A. and Nasrallah, H.A. (1987). Childhood head trauma and psychosis. *Psychiatry Research*, **21**, 303–6.

46. Jorge, R.E., Robinson, R.G., Arndt, S.V., Starkstein, S.E., Forrester, A.W., and Geisler, F. (1993). Depression following traumatic brain injury: a 1 year longitudinal study. *Journal of Affective Disorder*, **27**, 233–43.

47. Epstein, R.S. and Ursano, R.J. (1994). Anxiety disorders. In *Neuropsychiatry of traumatic brain injury* (ed. J.M. Silver, S.C. Yudofsky, and R.E. Hales), pp. 285–311. American Psychiatric Press, Washington, DC.

48. Achté, K.A., Lönnqvist, J., and Hillbom, E. (1970). Suicides of war brain-injured veterans. *Psychiatrica Fennica*, **1**, 231–9.

49. Harris, E.D. and Barraclough, B. (1997). Suicide as an outcome for mental disorders. A meta-analysis. *British Journal of Psychiatry*, **170**, 205–28.

50. Brooke, M.M., Questad, K.A., Patterson, D.R., *et al.* (1992). Agitation and restlessness after closed head injury: a prospective study of 100 consecutive admissions. *Archives of Physical Medicine and Rehabilitation*, **73**, 320–3.

51. Mysiw, W.J. and Sandel, M.E. (1997). The agitated brain injured patient. Part 2: Pathophysiology and treatment. *Archives of Physical Medicine and Rehabilitation*, **78**, 213–20.

52. Galski, T., Palasz, J., Bruno, R.L., and Walker, J.E. (1994). Predicting physical and verbal aggression on a brain trauma unit. *Archives of Physical Medicine and Rehabilitation*, **75**, 380–3.

53. Rönty, H., Ahonen, A., Tolonen, U., Heikkilä, J., and Niemelä, O. (1993). Cerebral trauma and alcohol abuse. *European Journal of Clinical Investigation*, **23**, 182–7.

54. Sparadeo, F.R. and Gill, D. (1989). Effects of prior alcohol use on head injury recovery. *Journal of Head Trauma Rehabilitation*, **4**, 75–82.

55. Rutherford, W.H. (1989). Postconcussion symptoms: relationship to acute neurological indices, individual differences and circumstances of injury. In *Mild head injury* (ed. H.S. Levin, H.M. Eisenberg, and A.L. Benton), pp. 217–28. Oxford University Press, New York.

56. Povlishock, J.T. and Coburn, T.H. (1989). Morphological change associated with mild head injury. In *Mild head injury* (ed. H.S. Levin, H.M. Eisenberg, and A.L. Benton), pp. 37–53. Oxford University Press, New York.

57. Montgomery, E.A., Fenton, G.W., McClelland, R.J., MacFlynn, G., and Rutherford, W.H. (1991). The psychobiology of minor head injury. *Psychological Medicine*, **21**, 375–84.

58. Binder, L.M. and Rohling, M.L. (1996). Money matters: a meta-analytic review of the effects of financial incentives on recovery after closed-head injury. *American Journal of Psychiatry*, **153**, 7–10.

59. Annegers, J.F., Grabow, J.D., Groover, R.V., Laws, E.R., Elveback, L.R., and Kurland, L.T. (1980). Seizures after head trauma: a population study. *Neurology*, **30**, 683–9.

60. Schierhout, G. and Roberts, I. (1998). Prophylactic antiepileptic agents after head injury: a systematic review. *Journal of Neurology, Neurosurgery and Psychiatry*, **64**, 108–12.

61. Wroblewski, B.A., Glenn, M.B., Whyte, J., and Singer, W.D. (1989). Carbamazepine replacement of phenytoin, phenobarbital and primidone in a rehabilitation setting: effects on seizure control. *Brain Injury*, **3**, 149–56.

62. Max, J.E., Robin, D.A., Lindgren, S.D., *et al.* (1997). Traumatic brain injury in children and adolescents: psychiatric disorders at two years. *Journal of the American Academy of Child and Adolescent Psychiatry*, **36**, 1278–85.

63. Roberts, A.H. (1969). *Brain damage in boxers*. Pitman, London.

64. Jordan, B.D., Relkin, N.R., Ravdin, L.D., *et al.* (1997). Apolipoprotein E e4 associated with chronic traumatic brain injury boxing. *Journal of the American Medical Association*, **278**, 136–40.

65. Wade, D.T., King, N.S., Wenden, F.J., Crawford, S., and Caldwell, F.E. (1998). Routine follow up after head injury: a second randomised controlled trial. *Journal of Neurology Neurosurgery and Psychiatry*, **65**, 177–83.

66. Mateer, C.A. and Ruff, R.M. (1990). Effectiveness of behavior management procedures in the rehabilitation of head-injured patients. In *Neurobehavioural sequelae of traumatic brain injury* (ed. R. L. Wood), pp. 277–302. Taylor and Francis, New York.

67. Goldstein, L.B. (1995). Prescribing of potentially harmful drugs to patients admitted to hospital after head injury. *Journal of Neurology, Neurosurgery and Psychiatry*, **58**, 753–5.

68. Brooke, M.M., Patterson, D.R., Questad, K.A., Cardenas, D., and Farrel-Roberts, L. (1992). The treatment of agitation during initial hospitalization after traumatic brain injury. *Archives of Physical Medicine and Rehabilitation*, **73**, 917–21.

69. Prigatano, G.P. and Schacter, D.L. (1991). *Awareness of deficit after brain injury: clinical and theoretical issues*. Oxford University Press, New York.

70. Greenwood, R.J. and McMillan, T.M. (1993). Models of rehabilitation programmes for the brain injured adult. 1: Current provision, efficacy and good practice. *Clinical Rehabilitation*, **7**, 248–55.

4.1.12 Alcohol-induced dementia (alcohol-induced cognitive impairment)

Jane Marshall

Introduction

Alcoholic brain damage was, until fairly recently, viewed as existing in two major forms: the alcoholic Korsakoff syndrome and alcoholic 'dementia'. Most 'alcoholics' suffering long-term cognitive impairment were thought to fit into the clearly defined Korsakoff category. A smaller proportion, with 'widespread cerebral dysfunction of an uncertain nature' was included in the poorly defined category of alcoholic 'deterioration' or 'dementia'.[1,2]

The alcoholic Korsakoff syndrome, caused by thiamine deficiency, has been the focus of comprehensive research (it should be noted that the chronic Korsakoff syndrome does not respond to thiamine). Research into the aetiology of alcoholic 'dementia' has been less rigorous, but evidence for the direct neurotoxic effect of alcohol has been suggested by neuropathological and neuroimaging studies, and by animal experiments. (The Korsakoff syndrome is considered in Chapter 4.1.13.)

Diagnostic criteria

Diagnostic criteria for 'substance-induced persisting dementia' are included in DSM-IV[3] (Table 1), which also states that there must be evidence from the history, physical examination, or laboratory findings that the deficits are aetiologically related to the persisting effects of substance use (in this case alcohol). The amnesic (Korsakoff) syndrome is listed separately in ICD-10,[4] whereas alcoholic 'dementia' is included under the 'residual and late-onset psychotic disorder' category, where diagnostic guidelines can be found.

Neuropathology

Early neuropathological studies of the alcoholic brain described fairly uniform cerebral atropy, mainly over the dorsolateral frontal regions, widened sulci, a narrowed cortical ribbon, and enlargement particularly of the anterior horns of the lateral ventricles.[1] Air encephalographic studies indicated that between half and three-quarters of subjects showed cortical changes or ventricular enlargement.[5,6] In comparison with controls, brain weights of alcoholics are reduced at autopsy.[7,8] Brain volume, estimated by the volume of the pericerebral space—the cerebrospinal fluid-filled region between the brain and the skull—is also reduced.[9] This indirect measure of cerebral atrophy is, however, mostly described in alcoholics with liver disease or Wernicke's encephalopathy.

The reduction in cerebral volume seen in the alcoholic brain is due mainly to the loss of white matter in the cerebral hemispheres.[10,11] The corpus callosum, in particular, is reduced in thickness.[12] Cortical grey matter appears also to be affected, although the evidence is more equivocal. The selective neuronal loss in the superior frontal cortex reported in one study[13] was not confirmed in another.[11] However, there is evidence that individual neurones are shrunken in regions where neuronal numbers are normal, such as the superior frontal, cingulate, and motor cortices.[13,14]

Animal research suggests that alcohol has a direct neurotoxic effect on the brain. Chronic ingestion of ethanol by well-nourished rats has been shown to be toxic to cholinergic projection neurones[15] and to reduce the complexity of dendritic arborization in hippocampal pyramidal neurones.[16] In the former study, transplantation of cholinergic neurones into the hippocampus and neocortex corrected the cholinergic deficits and memory abnormalities. In the latter, abstinence led to an increase in dendritic arborization.

Structural neuroimaging

Neuroimaging studies (CT and magnetic resonance imaging (**MRI**)) comparing recently detoxified alcoholics without obvious cognitive impairment with age-matched controls confirm that the alcoholics show evidence of reduced cortical brain volume affecting both grey and white matter, and also increased cerebrospinal fluid spaces.[17] These changes in brain structure are evident in young 'social drinkers',[18] but are more prominent in older age groups. Women appear to be particularly vulnerable. However, clinico-radiological comparisons have been equivocal, with measures of radiological change failing to correlate consistently with either duration of drinking or the severity of cognitive impairment. The role of concurrent liver disease is likewise poorly understood. Abstinence leads to reversibility of brain shrinkage;[19] this is most marked in younger individuals and in women.[20] However, many abstinent alcoholics continue to have enlarged ventricles. CT studies have also reported altered absorption densities in the alcoholic brain,[2] the significance of which is not fully understood.

MRI studies have reported volume reductions in localized cortical

Table 1 DSM-IV diagnostic criteria for substance-induced persisting dementia

A. The development of multiple cognitive deficits manifested by both
   (1) memory impairment (impaired ability to learn new information or to recall previously learned information)
   (2) one (or more) of the following cognitive disturbances:
      (a) aphasia (language disturbance)
      (b) apraxia (impaired ability to carry out motor activities despite intact motor function)
      (c) agnosia (failure to recognize or identify objects despite intact sensory function)
      (d) disturbance in executive functioning (i.e. planning, organization, sequencing, abstracting)

B. The cognitive deficits in criteria A1 and A2 each cause significant impairment in social or occupational functioning and represent a significant decline from a previous level of functioning

C. The deficits do not occur exclusively during the course of a delirium and persist beyond the usual duration of substance intoxication or withdrawal

D. There is evidence from the history, physical examination, or laboratory findings that the deficits are aetiologically related to the persisting effects of substance use (e.g. a drug of abuse, a medication)

and subcortical structures, especially the frontal lobes,[21] the mesial temporal lobe structures,[22] the anterior hippocampus,[23] mammillary bodies and cerebellum,[24,25] and corpus callosum,[26] particularly in older age groups. A controlled 5-year follow-up study of alcohol-dependent ($n =16$) and control ($n = 26$) subjects found that both groups showed evidence of age-related reductions in cortical grey matter at follow-up (especially in the prefontal cortex), also enlargement of the lateral and third ventricles.[27] While the alcohol-dependent subjects showed additional loss in the anterior superior temporal cortex, the alcohol-dependent subjects who maintained sobriety over the follow-up period had similar rates of change in ventricular volume as the controls. Continued alcohol abuse in the dependent group resulted in cortical grey-matter volume loss, the degree of which was predicted by the amount of alcohol consumed.

Functional neuroimaging

Functional imaging studies have shown hypometabolism in the frontal and parietal cortices of chronic alcoholics without major neurological impairment when compared with normal controls.[28–30] These abnormalities improve following abstinence,[30,31] mainly during the 16 to 30 days after the last use of alcohol. Metabolic recovery is most marked in the frontal area.[30]

Proton magnetic resonance spectroscopy can be combined with MRI, allowing *in vivo* insight into brain metabolism.[32–34] The metabolic changes observed in the few magnetic resonance spectroscopy studies that have been carried out suggest neuronal loss and compensatory gliosis.

Neuropsychological deficits

Many individuals with a history of chronic excessive alcohol consumption show evidence of moderate impairment in short- and long-term memory, learning, visuoperceptual abstraction, visuospatial organization, the maintenance of cognitive set, and impulse control.[35] This tendency for alcoholics to show proportionally greater visuospatial than language-related impairments suggests that alcohol might have a selective effect on the right hemisphere : the so-called 'right hemisphere hypothesis'.[36] However, right hemisphere functions also decline with ageing and the current view is that the functional lateralities of 'alcoholics' and ageing individuals are similar to normal controls.[36]

Neuropsychological performance improves with abstinence but impairments are still detectable even after 5 years of abstinence.[37] Performance on neuropsychological tests has generally been poorly correlated with structural imaging changes,[19,38] particularly with changes in grey-matter volume. However, one MRI study reported significant correlations between cortical (sulcal) and subcortical (ventricular) fluid volumes and some cognitive measures.[22] Another study using a combination of structural (CT or MRI) and functional imaging (positron emission tomography) together with neuropsychological tests in older alcohol-dependent patients who were abstinent found a significant correlation between degree of atrophy/metabolic functioning in the cingulate gyrus, and performance on the Wisconsin Card Sort Test.[39]

Neuropsychological test scores do not predict outcome in alcohol-dependent patients.[40,41]

Conclusion

Individuals with alcohol-induced brain damage and cognitive impairment are a heterogeneous group. The underlying mechanisms are probably numerous, complex, and interrelated. Alcohol and acetaldehyde neurotoxicity, thiamine depletion, and metabolic factors, such as hypoxia, electrolyte imbalance, and hypoglycaemia, which result from acute or chronic intoxication and withdrawal are all important. Recurrent alcohol withdrawal has been hypothesized to have a kindling effect.[42] During alcohol withdrawal there is increased *N*-methyl-D-aspartate (**NMDA**) function which is postulated to lead to increased neuronal excitability and to glutamate-induced neurotoxicity.[43] The way in which alcohol interferes with glutamatergic neurotransmission, especially through the NMDA receptor, is probably central to an understanding of its long-term effects on the brain.

References

1. Lishman, W.A. (1981). Cerebral disorder in alcoholism. Syndromes of impairment. *Brain*, **104**, 1–20.
2. Lishman, W.A. (1990). Alcohol and the brain. *British Journal of Psychiatry*, **156**, 635–44.
3. American Psychiatric Association (1994). *Diagnostic and statistical manual of mental disorders* (4th edn). American Psychiatric Association, Washington, DC.
4. World Health Organization (1992). *International statistical classification of diseases and related health problems, 10th revision*. WHO, Geneva.
5. Brewer, C. and Perrett, L. (1972). Brain damage due to alcohol consumption: an air-encephalographic, psychometric and electroencephalographic study. *British Journal of Addiction*, **66**, 170–82.
6. Haug, J.O. (1968). Pneumoencephalographic evidence of brain damage in chronic alcoholics. *Acta Psychiatrica Scandinavic, Supplementum*, **203**, 139–43.
7. Harper, C.G. and Blumbergs, P.C. (1982). Brain weights in alcoholics. *Journal of Neurology, Neurosurgery and Psychiatry*, **45**, 838–40.
8. Torvik, A., Lindboe, C.F., and Rogde, S. (1982). Brain lesions in alcoholics: a neuropathological study with clinical correlations. *Journal of Neurological Science*, **56**, 233–48.
9. Harper, C.G. and Kril, J.J. (1985). Brain atrophy in chronic alcoholic patients—a quantitative pathological study. *Journal of Neurological and Neurosurgical Psychiatry*, **48**, 211–17.
10. Harper, C.G., Kril, J.J., and Holloway, R.L. (1985). Brain shrinkage in chronic alcoholics: a pathological study. *British Medical Journal*, **290**, 510–14.
11. Jensen, G.B. and Pakkenburg, B. (1993). Do alcoholics drink their neurones away? *Lancet*, **342**, 1201–4.
12. Harper, C.G. and Kril, J.J. (1988). Corpus callosal thickness in alcoholics. *British Journal of Addiction*, **83**, 577–80.
13. Harper, C.G., Kril, J.J., and Daly, J.M. (1987). The specific gravity of the brains of alcoholic and control patients: a pathological study. *British Journal of Addiction*, **82**, 1349–54.
14. Kril, J.J. and Harper, C.G. (1989). Neuronal counts from four cortical regions in alcoholic brains. *Acta Neuropathologica*, **79**, 200–4.
15. Arendt, T.A., Allen, Y., Sinden, J., *et al.* (1988). Cholinergic-rich brain transplants reverse alcohol-induced memory deficits. *Nature*, **332**, 448–50.
16. McMullan, P.A., Saint-Cyr, J.A., and Carlen, P.L. (1984). Morphological alterations in rat CA1 hippocampal pyramidal cell dendrites resulting from chronic ethanol consumption and withdrawal. *Journal of Comparative Neurology*, **225**, 111–18.
17. Charness, M.E. (1993). Brain lesions in alcoholics. *Alcoholism: Clinical and Experimental Research*, **17**, 2–11.

18. Cala, L.A., Jones, B., Burns, P., *et al.* (1983). Results of computerised tomography, psychometric testing and dietary studies in social drinkers, with emphasis on reversibility after abstinence. *Medical Journal of Australia*, **2**, 264–9.

19. Ron, M.A. (1983). *The alcoholic brain: CT scan and psychological findings*. Psychological Medicine Monograph 3. Cambridge University Press.

20. Carlen, P.L. and Wilkinson, D.A. (1987). Reversibility of alcohol-related brain damage: clinical and experimental observations. *Acta Medica Scandinavica*, **222** (Supplement 717), 19–26.

21. Pfefferbaum, A., Sullivan, E.V., Mathalon, D.H., and Lim, K.O. (1997). Frontal lobe volume loss observed with magnetic resonance imaging in older chronic alcoholics. *Alcoholism: Clinical and Experimental Research*, **21**, 521–9.

22. Jernigan, T.L., Butters, N., and Di Traglia, G. (1991). Reduced cerebral gray matter observed in alcoholics using magnetic resonance imaging. *Alcoholism: Clinical and Experimental Research*, **15**, 418–27.

23. Sullivan, E.V., Marsh, L., Mathalon, D.H., Lim, K.O., and Pfefferbaum, A. (1995). Anterior hippocampal volume deficits in nonamnesic, ageing chronic alcoholics. *Alcoholism: Clinical and Experimental Research*, **19**, 110–22.

24. Davila, M.D., Shear, P.K., Lane, B., Sullivan, E.V., and Pfefferbaum, A. (1994). Mammillary body and cerebellar shrinkage in chronic alcoholics: an MRI and neuropsychological study. *Neuropsychology*, **8**, 433–44.

25. Shear, P.K., Sullivan, E.V., Lane, B.J., and Pfefferbaum, A. (1996). Mammillary body and cerebellar shrinkage in chronic alcoholics with and without amnesia. *Journal of the International Neuropsychological Society*, **2**, 34–5.

26. Pfefferbaum, A., Lim, K.O., Desmond, J.E., and Sullivan, E.V. (1996). Thinning of the corpus callosum in older alcoholic men: a magnetic resonance imaging study. *Alcoholism: Clinical and Experimental Research*, **20**, 752–7.

27. Pfefferbaum, A., Sullivan, E.V., Rosenbloom, M.J., Mathalon, D.H., and Lim, K.O. (1998). A controlled study of cortical grey matter and ventricular changes in alcoholic men over a 5-year interval. *Archives of General Psychiatry*, **55**, 905–12.

28. Sachs, H., Russell, J.A.G., Christman, D.R., and Cook, B. (1987). Alteration of regional cerebral glucose metabolic rate in non-Korsakoff chronic alcoholism. *Archives of Neurology*, **44**, 1242–51.

29. Volkow, N.D., Hitzemann, R., Wang, G.-J., *et al.* (1992). Decreased brain metabolism in neurologically intact healthy alcoholics. *American Journal of Psychiatry*, **149**, 1016–22.

30. Volkow, N.D., Wang, G.-J., Hitzemann, R., *et al.* (1994). Recovery of brain glucose metabolism in detoxified alcoholics. *Americal Journal of Psychiatry*, **151**, 178–83.

31. Nicolas, J.M., Catafau, A.M., Estruch, R., *et al.* (1993). Regional cerebral blood flow—SPECT in chronic alcoholism: relation to neuropsychological testing. *Journal of Nuclear Medicine*, **34**, 1452–9.

32. Fein, G., Meyerhoff, D.J., Di Sclafani, V., *et al.* (1994). ^{1}H magnetic resonance spectroscopic imaging separates neuronal from glial changes in alcohol-related brain atrophy. In *Alcohol and glial cells*, pp. 227–41. Research Monograph 27. National Institutes of Health, Bethesda, MD.

33. Martin, P.R., Gibbs, S.J., Nimmerrichter, A.A., Riddle, W.R., Welch, L.W., and Willcott, M.R. (1995). Brain proton magnetic resonance spectroscopy studies in recently abstinent alcoholics. *Alcoholism: Clinical and Experimental Research*, **4**, 1078–82.

34. Seitz, D., Widmann, U., Seeger, U., *et al.* (1999). Localised proton magnetic resonance spectroscopy of the cerebellum in detoxifying alcoholics. *Alcoholism: Clinical and Experimental Research*, **23**, 158–63.

35. Oscar-Berman, M. (1990). Learning and memory deficits in detoxified alcoholics. *NIDA Research Monographs*, **101**, 136–55.

36. Ellis, R.J. and Oscar-Berman, M. (1989). Alcoholism aging, and functional cerebral asymmetries. *Psychological Bulletin*, **106**, 128–47.

37. Brandt, J., Butters, N., Ryan, C., *et al.* (1983). Cognitive loss and recovery in long term alcohol abusers. *Archives of General Psychiatry*, **40**, 435–42.

38. Carlen, P.L., Wilkinson, D.A., and Wortzman, G., *et al.* (1981). Cerebral atrophy and functional deficits in alcoholics without clinically apparent liver disease. *Neurology*, **31**, 377–85.

39. Adams, K.M., Gilman, S., Koeppe, R.A., *et al.* (1993). Neuropsychological deficits are correlated with frontal hypometabolism in positron emission tomography studies of older alcoholic patients. *Alcoholism: Clinical and Experimental Research*, **17**, 205–10.

40. Alterman, A.I., Kushner, H., and Holahan, J.M. (1990). Cognitive functioning and treatment outcome in alcoholics. *Journal of Nervous and Mental Disorders*, **178**, 494–9.

41. Leenane, K.J. (1988). Patients with alcohol-related brain damage: therapy and outcome. *Australian Drug and Alcohol Review*, **7**, 89–92.

42. Ballenger, J.C. and Post, R.M. (1978). Kindling as a model for alcohol withdrawal syndromes. *British Journal of Psychiatry*, **33**, 1–14.

43. Tsai, G., Gastfriend, D.R., and Coyle, J.T. (1995). The glutamatergic basis of human alcoholism. *American Journal of Psychiatry*, **152**, 332–40.

4.1.13 **Amnesic syndromes**

Michael D. Kopelman

Introduction

Amnesic disorders can be broadly classified across two orthogonal dimensions. Along the first dimension, there can be transient or discrete episodes of amnesia as opposed to persistent memory impairment. On the second dimension, memory loss can result from either neurological damage or psychological causation, although admixtures of these factors are, of course, very common. The notion of confabulation has traditionally been associated with amnesic syndromes, particularly the Korsakoff syndrome, although it may have a separate basis, and false memories are now known to arise in a number of different situations. With the advent of drugs purporting to influence memory, there is increasing interest in the psychopharmacology of memory disorders. In this chapter, these topics will be considered in turn.

Transient amnesias

Transient global amnesia

Transient global amnesia most commonly occurs in the middle-aged or elderly, more frequently in men, and it results in a period of amnesia lasting several hours. It is characterized by repetitive questioning, and there may be some confusion, but patients do not report any loss of personal identity (they know who they are). It is sometimes preceded by headache or nausea, a stressful life event, a medical procedure, or vigorous exercise. Hodges and Ward[1] found that the mean duration of amnesia was 4 h and the maximum was 12 h. In 25 per cent of their sample, there was a past history of migraine, which was considered to have a possible aetiological role. In a further 7 per cent of the sample, the patients subsequently developed unequivocal features of epilepsy (there had been no focal signs or features of epilepsy during the original attack) and the memory loss was therefore attributed, in retrospect, to previously undiagnosed epilepsy. There was no association with either a past history of vascular disease, clinical signs suggestive of vascular pathology, or known risk factors for vascular disease. In particular, there was no association with transient ischaemic attacks. In 60 to 70 per cent of the sample, the underlying aetiology was unclear.

In instances where neuropsychological tests have been administered to patients during their acute episode of transient memory loss,[1,2] the patients showed a profound anterograde amnesia, as expected, on tests of both verbal and non-verbal memory. However, performance on tests of retrograde memory was variable. Follow-up studies showed either complete or almost complete recovery of memories, several weeks to months after the acute attack.

The general consensus is that the amnesic disorder results from transient dysfunction in limbic–hippocampal circuits, crucial to memory formation. For example, Stillhard et al.[3] reported severe bitemporal hypoperfusion during an episode of transient global amnesia using single-photon emission CT (SPECT). Positron emission tomography (PET) in patients with transient global amnesia gives findings consistent with the SPECT results.

Transient epileptic amnesia

This refers to the minority of patients with transient global amnesia in whom epilepsy appears to be the underlying cause of the syndrome.[1] Where epilepsy has not previously been diagnosed, the main predictive factors for an epileptic aetiology are brief episodes of memory loss (an hour or less) with multiple attacks.[1] It is important to note that standard electroencephalography (EEG) and CT findings are often normal. However, an epileptic basis to the disorder may be revealed on sleep EEG recordings.[4]

Patients with transient epileptic amnesia may show residual deficits in between their attacks, associated with their underlying neuropathology. Kopelman et al.[4] found a moderate degree of residual anterograde memory impairment in their patient. Multiple small regions of signal alteration were subsequently found in the medial temporal lobes in this patient, as well as medial temporal hypometabolism on a fluorodeoxyglucose (FDG) PET scan. Kapur et al.[5] described a single case, in whom they found a residual interictal retrograde amnesia, in the presence of only minor anterograde memory impairment. They interpreted this as a case of 'isolated retrograde amnesia'.

Epilepsy may, of course, give rise to automatisms or postictal confusional states. Where there is an automatism, there is always bilateral involvement of the limbic structures involved in memory formation, including the hippocampal and parahippocampal structures bilaterally as well as the mesial diencephalon. Consequently, amnesia for the period of automatic behaviour is always present and is usually complete.

Head injury

In head injury, it is important to distinguish between a brief period of retrograde amnesia, which may last only a few seconds or minutes, a longer period of post-traumatic amnesia, and islands of preserved memory within the amnesic gap.[6,7] Occasionally post-traumatic amnesia may exist without any retrograde amnesia, although this is more common in cases of penetrating lesions. Sometimes there is a particularly vivid memory for images or sounds occurring immediately before the injury, on regaining consciousness, or during a lucid interval between the injury and the onset of post-traumatic amnesia.

Post-traumatic amnesia is generally assumed to reflect the degree of underlying diffuse brain pathology, in particular rotational forces giving rise to axonal tearing and generalized cognitive impairment. The length of post-traumatic amnesia is predictive of eventual cognitive outcome,[8] psychiatric outcome,[7] and social outcome.[8] However, the duration of post-traumatic amnesia is often not well documented in medical records, and these relationships are often weaker than is generally assumed. In addition, contusion to the frontal and anterior temporal lobes is a common consequence of head injury. Various authors have described a disproportionate degree of retrograde memory loss associated with damage to these structures, although an interaction of psychological and neurological factors cannot be excluded in such cases.

Post-traumatic amnesia needs to be distinguished from the persisting anterograde memory impairment, which may be detected on clinical assessment or cognitive testing long after the period of post-traumatic amnesia has ended. Moreover, forgetfulness is a common complaint within the context of a post-traumatic syndrome, which may include anxiety, irritability, poor concentration, and various somatic complaints. Commonly, these complaints persist long after the settlement of any compensation issues.[9]

Alcoholic blackouts

Alcoholic blackouts are discrete episodes of memory loss for significant events, which should not be confused with withdrawal seizures or other ictal phenomena. Alcoholic blackouts are associated with severe intoxication, usually in the context of a history of prolonged alcohol abuse. Goodwin et al.[10] described two types of blackout—the fragmentary and the en bloc. However, alcohol-induced state-dependent experiences can be viewed as related phenomena, and it has been suggested that the three represent gradations of alcohol-induced memory impairment. In state-dependent effects, subjects when sober cannot remember events or facts from an episode of intoxication, which they recall easily when they again become intoxicated. In fragmentary blackouts, the subjects are aware of their memory loss on being told later of an event, there are islands of preserved memory, and the amnesia tends to recover partially through time by shrinkage of the amnesic gap. In en bloc blackouts there is an abrupt beginning and end to the period of memory loss, and the lost memories are very seldom recovered. Blackouts may be more common in binge drinkers, because they are related to a high blood alcohol level. Hypoglycaemia may also be a contributory factor, at least in some cases.

After electroconvulsive therapy

This is an iatrogenic form of transient amnesia. Benzodiazepines[11] and anticholinergic agents[12] can also give rise to transient memory loss in more moderate form.

Subjects tested within a few hours of electroconvulsive therapy (ECT) show a retrograde impairment for information from the preceding 1 to 3 years, a pronounced anterograde memory impairment on both recall and recognition memory tasks, and an accelerated rate of forgetting.[13] When retested approximately 6 to 9 months after completion of a course of ECT, memory returns to normal on objective tests. However, complaints of memory impairment can persist, and they may be evident three or more years after a course of ECT has been completed.[14] It seems that patients with persistent complaints of memory loss tend to be those who have recovered least well from their depression,[13,14] although their complaints tend to focus upon the period for which there was an initial retrograde and anterograde amnesia.

Verbal memory appears to be particularly sensitive to disruption. Unilateral electroconvulsive therapy to the non-dominant hemisphere produces considerably less memory impairment than bilateral ECT, although it is important to identify the non-dominant hemisphere by a valid procedure. Recent studies have attempted to minimize memory disruption by either making changes in premedication or the concomitant administration of other substances, for example glycopyrrolate, physostigmine, thyroxine, dexamethasone, acetylcholine, or other substances. In general, these agents have produced little or no benefit. The most effective methods of avoiding memory deficit consist of either electrode placement over the frontal rather than the temporal lobes or ECT to the non-dominant temporal lobe. In the view of this author, any marginal therapeutic benefits of bilateral ECT are outweighed by the minimization of adverse effects using the non-dominant unilateral technique.

Post-traumatic stress disorder

This clinically important syndrome is described in Chapter 4.6.2. As is well known, it is characterized by intrusive thoughts and memories about the traumatic experience. However, there may be instances of brief memory loss, distortions, or even frank confabulations. For example, a victim of the *Herald of Free Enterprise* disaster at Zeebruge described trying to rescue a close friend still on board the ship, when other witnesses reported that the close friend had, in fact, not been seen by the victim from the moment the ship turned over. These cases are, of course, confounded by other factors, such as head injury or hypothermia. Nevertheless, it is of interest that post-traumatic stress disorder symptoms can occur, even when a subject is completely amnesic for an episode.[15] Post-traumatic stress disorder victims can show deficits in anterograde memory on formal tasks many years after the original trauma, and there is also evidence that they may show loss of hippocampal volume on magnetic resonance imaging (**MRI**) brain scan. The latter has been attributed to effects upon glucocorticoid metabolism, although these findings have to be interpreted with caution in view of the rather crude measurements employed and the wide variability in MRI hippocampal volume estimates even in healthy subjects.

Psychogenic fugue

A fugue state is a syndrome consisting of a sudden loss of all autobiographical memories and knowledge of personal identity, usually associated with a period of wandering, for which there is a subsequent amnesic gap on recovery. Characteristically, fugue states last a few hours or days, although there are descriptions of complaints of autobiographical memory loss lasting much longer. Whenever such complaints persist, the suspicion of simulation must arise. Fugue states differ from transient global amnesia or transient epileptic amnesia in that the subject does not know who he or she is, and repetitive questioning is not a characteristic feature in fugues.

As discussed elsewhere,[16] fugue states are always preceded by a severe precipitating stress. Second, depressed mood is also an extremely common antecedent for a psychogenic fugue state, and may be associated with manifest suicidal ideas just before or following recovery from the fugue. Third, various authors have noted that there

is often a past history of a previous transient neurological amnesia, such as epilepsy or head injury. In brief, it appears the patients who have experienced a previous transient organic amnesia, and who become depressed and/or suicidal, are particularly likely to go into a fugue in the face of a severe, precipitating stress. That stress may consist of marital or emotional discord, bereavement, financial problems, a criminal charge, or stress during wartime. Fugues have been described as a 'flight from suicide'.

Amnesia for offences

This is a phenomenon commonly brought to the attention of psychiatrists, particularly forensic psychiatrists, although the empirical literature on this disorder is scanty. Amnesia is claimed by 25 to 45 per cent of offenders in cases of homicide, approximately 8 per cent of perpetrators of other violent crimes, and a small percentage of non-violent offenders.[16,17] It is necessary to exclude underlying neurological or organic factors such as an epileptic automatism, postictal confusional state, head injury, hypoglycaemia, or sleep walking. Underlying organic pathology can be grounds for a so-called 'insane' automatism in English law (if the result of an internal brain disease) or a 'sane' automatism (if the consequence of an external agent), but otherwise amnesia *per se* does not constitute grounds for alleviation of responsibility for an offence.

Amnesia for an offence is most commonly associated with the following.

1. States of extreme emotional arousal, in which the offence is unpremeditated, and the victim usually a lover, wife, or family member. This is most commonly seen in homicide cases ('crimes of passion').

2. Alcohol intoxication (sometimes in association with other substances), usually involving very high peak levels as well as a long history of alcohol abuse. The victim is not necessarily related to the offender, and the offence may vary from criminal damage, through assault, to homicide.

3. Florid psychotic states or depressed mood. Occasionally offenders describe a delusional account of what has happened, quite at odds with what was seen by other observers, and sometimes resulting in confessions to crimes that the person could not actually have committed (a paramnesia or delusional memory). In many other cases, depressed mood is associated with amnesia for an offence, just as it is a common associate of psychogenic fugue.

It should be noted that many of the factors associated with poor recall in offenders (high emotional arousal, alcohol intoxication, violent crime) are similar to those which have been implicated in poor recall by the victims or eye-witnesses of offences. It should certainly not be assumed that offenders claiming amnesia are malingering.

Persistent memory disorder

The amnesic syndrome can be defined as follows.

> An abnormal mental state in which memory and learning are affected out of all proportion to other cognitive functions in an otherwise alert and responsive patient.[18]

The Korsakoff syndrome can be defined in the same way but with the addition of the following phrase:

> ...resulting from nutritional depletion, notably thiamine deficiency.

In fact, Victor et al.[18] used the first description as a definition of the Korsakoff syndrome, but the present author feels that it is important to distinguish between amnesic syndromes in general (for which the Victor et al. definition suffices) and the particular clinical condition described by Korsakoff,[19] whose cases can all be viewed (with hindsight) as having suffered nutritional depletion, whether of alcoholic or non-alcoholic causation. Various disorders can give rise to an amnesic syndrome.

The Korsakoff syndrome

As mentioned, this is the result of nutritional depletion, namely a thiamine deficiency. Korsakoff[19] described this condition as resulting from alcohol abuse or from a number of other causes, but by far the most common nowadays is alcohol abuse.

Diagnosis

There are frequent misunderstandings about the nature of this disorder. 'Short-term memory', in the sense that psychologists employ it, is intact but learning over more prolonged periods is severely impaired, and there is usually a retrograde memory loss which characteristically extends back many years or decades.[20] Korsakoff himself noted that his patients 'reason about everything perfectly well, draw correct deductions from given premises, make witty remarks, play chess or a game of cards, in a word comport themselves as mentally sound persons'.[19] However, he also noted repetitive questioning, the extensive nature of the retrograde memory loss, and a particular problem in remembering the temporal sequence of events, associated with severe disorientation in time. As will be discussed below, he gave examples of confabulation reflecting the problem with the temporal sequence memory, such that real memories were jumbled up and retrieved inappropriately, out of temporal context.

Many cases of the Korsakoff syndrome are diagnosed following an acute Wernicke encephalopathy, involving confusion, ataxia, nystagmus, and opthalmoplegia. Not all these features are always present, and the opthalmoplegia responds rapidly to treatment with high-dose vitamins. These features are often associated with a peripheral neuropathy. However, the disorder can also have an insidious onset, and such cases are more likely to come to the attention of psychiatrists; in these cases, there may be either no known history of or only a transient history of Wernicke features. There are also reports that the characteristic Wernicke–Korsakoff neuropathology (see below) is found much more commonly at autopsy in alcoholics than the diagnosis is made in life, implying that many cases are being missed.

Pathology

The characteristic neuropathology in what is often known as the Wernicke–Korsakoff syndrome consists of neuronal loss, microhaemorrhages, and gliosis in the paraventricular and periaqueductal grey matter.[18] However, there has been debate as to which particular lesions are critical for the manifestation of chronic memory disorder. Victor et al.[18] pointed out that all 24 of their cases in whom the medial dorsal nucleus of the thalamus was affected had a clinical history of persistent memory impairment (Korsakoff syndrome), whereas five cases in whom this nucleus was unaffected had a history of Wernicke features without any recorded clinical history of subsequent memory disorder. By contrast, the mammillary bodies were implicated in all the Wernicke cases, whether or not there was subsequent memory impairment. However, Mair et al.[21] provided a careful pathological and neuropsychological description of two patients with the Korsakoff syndrome, whose autopsies showed lesions in the mammillary bodies and the midline and anterior portion of the thalamus, but not in the medial dorsal nuclei. Mair et al. suggested that the lesions they described might 'disconnect' a critical circuit running between the temporal lobes and the frontal cortex, and put forward a hypothesis concerning the functional significance of this circuit. Mayes et al.[22] obtained very similar findings in two further patients with the Korsakoff syndrome, who had also been very carefully described both neuropsychologically and at autopsy. Taken together, these findings suggest that the mammillary bodies, the mammillothalamic tract, and the anterior thalamus may be more important to memory dysfunction than the medial dorsal nucleus of the thalamus, but the issue remains controversial.

There is also evidence of general cortical atrophy particularly involving the frontal lobes in patients with the Korsakoff syndrome, and this is associated with neuropsychological evidence of 'frontal' or 'executive' test dysfunction in these patients.[23]

There have been a number of neuroimaging studies of the Korsakoff syndrome. CT scan studies indicated a general degree of cortical atrophy, particularly involving the frontal lobes.[24] MRI studies have indicated more specific atrophy in diencephalic structures. The findings in SPECT and PET studies have been more variable, some showing widespread hypoperfusion and hypometabolism, other studies showing very little change relative to healthy controls, but (usually) some degree of frontal hypometabolism.

Prognosis

Victor et al.[18] reported that 25 per cent of patients with the Korsakoff syndrome 'recover', 50 per cent show improvement through time, and 25 per cent remain unchanged. Whilst it is unlikely that any established patient shows complete recovery, the present author's experience is that substantial improvement does occur over a matter of years; if restated, it is probably correct to say that 75 per cent of these patients show a variable degree of improvement, whilst 25 per cent show no change.

Herpes encephalitis

This can give rise to a particularly severe form of amnesic syndrome.[25] The majority of cases are said to be primary infections, although there may be a history of a preceding 'cold sore' on the lip. Characteristically, there is a fairly abrupt onset of acute fever, headache, and nausea. There may be behavioural changes. Seizures can occur. The fully developed clinical picture with neck rigidity, vomiting, and motor and sensory deficits seldom occurs during the first week.[26] Diagnosis is by finding a raised titre of antibodies to the virus in the cerebrospinal fluid, but often this is missed and a presumptive diagnosis is made on the basis of the clinical picture as well as severe signal alteration, haemorrhaging, and atrophy in the temporal lobes on MRI brain imaging.

Neuropathological and neuroimaging studies show that there is extensive bilateral temporal lobe damage,[27] although, occasionally, the changes are surprisingly unilateral. There are often frontal changes, most commonly in the orbitofrontal regions, and there is a variable degree of general cortical atrophy. The medial temporal lobe structures are particularly severely affected, including the hippocampi, amygdalae, entorhinal and perirhinal cortices, and other parahippocampal structures. Evidence from studies of bilateral temporal lobectomy as well as animal lesion studies has indicated that these structures are particularly critical in memory formation.

The chronic memory disorder in herpes encephalitis is often very severe,[25] but it shows many resemblances to that seen in the Korsakoff syndrome, consistent with the fact that there are many neural connections between the thalami, mammillary bodies, and the hippocampi.[28] Encephalitis, like head injury, can also implicate basal forebrain structures which give cholinergic outputs to the hippocampi; since these are thought to modulate hippocampal function, this may further exacerbate the damage. Contrary to what was postulated in the 1980s, there appears to be no difference between patients with the Korsakoff syndrome and those with herpes encephalitis in terms of rates of forgetting or in the relative effect upon recall versus recognition memory. The patients with herpes appear to have better 'insight' into the nature of their disorder and a 'flatter' temporal gradient to their retrograde memory loss (i.e. less sparing of early memories), and they may have a particularly severe deficit in spatial memory when the right hippocampus is involved.[20] However, the similarities in the episodic memory disorder tend to outweigh the differences.

On the other hand, a more extensive involvement of semantic memory is characteristic in herpes encephalitis, and this results from the widespread involvement of the lateral, inferior, and posterior regions of the temporal lobes. Semantic memory refers to a knowledge of facts, concepts, and language (see Chapter 2.5.2). Left temporal lobe pathology in herpes encephalitis commonly gives rise to an impairment in naming, reading (a so-called 'surface dyslexia'), and other aspects of lexicosemantic memory. Right temporal lobe damage may lead to a particularly severe impairment in face recognition memory or knowledge of people.

Severe hypoxia

Severe hypoxia can give rise to an amnesic syndrome following carbon monoxide poisoning, cardiac and respiratory arrests, or suicide attempts by hanging or poisoning with the exhaust gases from a car. Drug overdoses may precipitate prolonged unconsciousness and cerebral hypoxia, and this quite commonly occurs in heroin abusers. Zola-Morgan et al.[29] described a patient with repeated episodes of hypoxia and/or cardiovascular problems who developed a moderately severe anterograde amnesia. At autopsy 6 years later, this patient was shown to have a severe loss of pyramidal cells in the CA1 region of the hippocampi bilaterally, with the rest of the brain appearing relatively normal. Hippocampal atrophy on MRI has been reported in amnesic patients in whom hypoxia may have been the cause. The author's research group has also produced evidence of medial temporal lobe atrophy in hypoxic patients, but this same group has also found thalamic hypometabolism in hypoxic patients on FDG-PET scanning, and this finding is consistent with other reports. In brief, the memory disorder is likely to result from a combination of hippocampal and thal-

amic changes, related to the many common neural pathways between these two structures.[28]

There have been claims that selective damage to these circuits produces an impairment in recall memory, but not in recognition memory.[28] However, there are many commonalities in the pattern of episodic memory impairment between patients who have experienced severe hypoxic episodes and those whose amnesic disorder results from the more extensive temporal lobe damage found in herpes encephalitis.

Vascular disorders

Two types of vascular disorder can particularly affect memory, as opposed to general cognitive functioning, namely thalamic infarction and subarachnoid haemorrhage.

In an elegant CT scan study, von Cramon et al.[30] showed that damage to the anterior thalamus was critical in producing an amnesic syndrome. When the pathology was confined to the more posterior regions of the thalamus, memory function was relatively unaffected. The anterior region of the thalamus is variably supplied by the polar or paramedian arteries in different individuals: both of which are, ultimately, branches of the posterior cerebral artery, that also supplies the posterior region of the hippocampi. When there is a relatively pure lesion of the anterior thalamus, anterograde amnesia without an extensive retrograde memory loss commonly results. However, cases in whom there is also retrograde memory loss, or even a generalized dementia, have been described following thalamic infarction, and this presumably relates to the extent to which thalamic projections are also implicated in the infarction.

Subarachnoid haemorrhage following rupture of a beri aneurysm can result in memory impairment, whether the anterior cerebral or posterior cerebral circulation from the Circle of Willis is involved. Most commonly described in the neuropsychological literature have been ruptured aneurysms from the anterior communicating arteries, because these affect ventromedial frontal structures and the basal forebrain. Gade[31] has argued that it is whether or not the septal nuclei of the basal forebrain are implicated in the ischaemia which determines whether a persistent amnesic syndrome occurs in such patients. Others have attributed the florid confabulation, which these patients often exhibit, to concomitant ventromedial damage.[32]

Head injury

As discussed above, severe head injury can produce a persistent amnesia which may or may not be associated with generalized cognitive impairment. There may be direct trauma to the frontal and anterior temporal lobes, resulting in contusion and haemorrhaging, contrecoup damage, intracranial haemorrhage, and axonal tearing and gliosis following rotational forces. Memory function is commonly the last cognitive function to improve following an acute trauma, and patients can show the characteristic features of an amnesic syndrome. The phenomenon of 'isolated retrograde amnesia' has been described in other cases of head injury. In many of the latter cases, there appears to have been a differential rate in recovery between an initially severe anterograde memory loss and the retrograde component; in other cases, it is not at all clear that the neurologists and neuropsychologists describing the patients have taken sufficient account of an interaction between psychological and neurological factors. Traumatic head injury is considered in more detail in Chapter 4.1.11.

Other causes of an amnesic syndrome

Deep midline cerebral tumours can give rise to an amnesic syndrome,[7] and this may be exacerbated by surgical or irradiation treatment for pituitary tumours. Other infections, such as tuberculous meningitis or HIV, may, on occasion, give rise to an amnesic syndrome. In the very early stages, Alzheimer dementia may manifest itself as a focal amnesic syndrome.[33] Surgical treatment to the temporal lobes for epilepsy can result in profound amnesia, if there is bilateral involvement. There is increasing evidence that focal lesions in the frontal lobes can also produce severe memory impairment on aspects of anterograde and retrograde memory.[20] This can occur even in the absence of basal forebrain involvement, but it probably results from particular aspects of memory being implicated, including planning and organization, source and context monitoring, and particular aspects of retrieval processes.[34]

Neuropsychological aspects

The terms 'short-term' and 'long-term' memory should be abolished from psychiatric discourse, as they cause confusion across disciplines. It is more useful to consider current or recent memory versus remote or autobiographical memory. In addition, 'prospective memory' refers to remembering to do something.

Concepts of memory are considered in Chapter 2.5.2. As described in that chapter, a distinction is generally drawn between so-called 'working memory', which holds information for brief periods (a matter of several seconds) and allocates resources, and secondary memory, which holds different types of information on a permanent or semipermanent basis. Secondary memory, in turn, can be subdivided into an episodic (or 'explicit') component, semantic memory, and implicit memory. Episodic memory refers to incidents or events from a person's past, and is characteristically severely affected in the amnesic syndrome. As mentioned previously, semantic memory refers to a knowledge of facts, concepts, and language. The learning of new semantic memories may be affected in the amnesic syndrome. Other aspects of semantic memory (naming, reading, well-established general knowledge, mental calculation, comprehension) are affected in disorders where there is concomitant widespread temporal lobe or generalized cortical pathology, such as herpes encephalitis, Alzheimer dementia, and semantic dementia (a form of frontotemporal dementia). Implicit memory refers to procedural perceptuomotor skills, and to the facilitation of responses in the absence of explicit memory, known as 'priming'. Both these aspects are characteristically spared in the amnesic syndrome,[35] although the precise extent of sparing does depend on particular features in the experimental design.[36]

Over the years, there has been extensive debate concerning whether the primary deficit in the amnesic syndrome lies in the initial encoding of information, or some kind of physiological 'consolidation' into secondary memory, or accelerated forgetting of that information, or in retrieval processes.[37] There is still very little agreement about this debate, but, if anything, the consensus is that retrieval problems are secondary to initial encoding and consolidation impairments,[37] at least in anterograde amnesia. Retrieval deficits may be more important where there is an extensive retrograde memory loss,[20] which might account for why there is a poor correlation between scores on anterograde memory measures and retrograde memory measures.

More recently, there has been an emphasis on the specific functions of the hippocampi, prompted by the need in neuroimaging studies to differentiate their role from that of the frontal lobes. One possibility is that the hippocampi particularly contribute to the binding of complex associations;[38] another is that they are involved in the binding together of the distributed features of an episode as a coherent trace, whilst ensuring that there is sufficient pattern separation of similar episodes.[39] The hippocampi may be especially involved in novel or incremental learning,[40] and they may also contribute to retrieval processes.[41] PET and MRI activation studies have emphasized the role of the frontal lobes in learning processes.[42] The frontal lobes are generally thought to contribute to planning and organization in memory, aspects of context and source memory, awareness of memory performance (metamemory), and to particular aspects of retrieval processes.[34]

There are also many controversies concerning the nature of the extensive retrograde memory loss found in many of the above disorders. Modern neuropsychological studies have confirmed that this retrograde memory loss can extend back many years or decades, but that it characteristically shows a 'temporal gradient' with relative sparing of early memories. The gradient is characteristically steeper in the amnesic syndrome than in dementing disorders such as Alzheimer dementia or Huntington's disease. The relative sparing of early memories may result from their greater salience and rehearsal, such that they have become assimilated within semantic memory. However, differing patterns of retrograde memory loss can certainly occur. Left temporal lobe damage seems to characteristically affect memory for facts and for the more linguistic components of remote memory,[20] whereas right temporal lobe damage more commonly affects memory for the incidents in a person's life.[20]

Confabulation disorders

Confabulation can be subdivided into 'spontaneous' confabulation, in which there is a persistent, unprovoked outpouring of erroneous memories, and 'momentary' or 'provoked' confabulation, in which fleeting intrusion errors or distortions are seen in response to a challenge to memory, such as a memory test.[43]

Confabulation is widely believed to be particularly associated with the Korsakoff syndrome, but this is incorrect. Confabulation arises in confusional states and in frontal lobe disease.[44] The link with frontal lobe pathology has been established in many investigations.[32,45] Spontaneous confabulation is often seen in the confusional state of a Wernicke encephalopathy, but it is rare in the more chronic phases of the Korsakoff syndrome.[18,43] On the other hand, fleeting intrusion errors or distortions ('momentary confabulation') do occur in the chronic phase of a Korsakoff syndrome, when memory is challenged. However, such intrusion errors are also seen in healthy subjects when memory is 'weak' for any reason, such as a prolonged delay until recall.[43] They are also seen in Alzheimer dementia and other clinical amnesic syndromes, and they are certainly not specific to the Korsakoff syndrome.

There has been considerable interest of late in the nature of spontaneous confabulations. Moscovitch and Melo[32] argued that it is a product of the following: (i) faulty cue-retrieval, meaning that cues can be ambiguous, resulting in retrieval errors in normal subjects but more particularly in subjects whose memory is impaired; (ii) impaired strategic search, producing misleading cues and thereby inappropriate memories; (iii) defective monitoring, meaning that the resulting errors are not edited out. Similar hypotheses have been put forward by Burgess and Shallice[46] and by Schacter et al.[39] A second approach to this topic emphasizes problems in the temporal ordering of memories. This is a very old theory, put forward by Korsakoff himself, as well as many other authorities (see, for example, Victor et al.[18]). In a particularly elegant study, Schnider et al.[47] found that a group of 'spontaneous confabulators' could be differentiated from other amnesic patients and controls on the basis of their errors on a temporal context memory task, but not on other memory or executive tests. There have been two recent studies that provide some support for this viewpoint, but they also make it clear that temporal and other context memory deficits cannot account for all instances of spontaneous confabulation. In an analysis of a severely confabulating patient's errors,[48] it was evident that many confabulations (particularly in episodic memory) may plausibly have resulted from the conflation and inappropriate retrieval of 'real' memory fragments out of temporal sequence, but that others resulted from perseverations (particularly in semantic memory) or from the patient giving instantaneous, ill-considered, and unchecked responses to immediate environmental and social cues. Likewise, Johnson et al.[49] found that several measures of context memory failed to discriminate between a severely confabulating patient and three other patients with frontal lobe lesions. Johnson et al. concluded that confabulation may reflect an interaction between a vivid imagination, an inability to retrieve autobiographical memories systematically, and source or context monitoring deficits.

The notion of 'confabulation' or 'false memory' has now been extended to a variety of other disorders, including delusional memory, confabulation in schizophrenia, false confessions, apparently false memories for child sexual abuse, pseudologia fantastica, and dissociative identity disorder. Whilst each of these can potentially be accounted for in terms of a general model of memory and executive function, provided that the social context and some notion of 'self' is incorporated, there are likely to be differing mechanisms which give rise to these different types of false memory.[50]

Neurochemistry and neuropharmacology of memory disorders

The Korsakoff syndrome is relatively unusual among memory disorders in that there is a distinct neurochemical pathology with important implications for treatment. Since animal studies in the 1930s and 1940s, and the important observations of De Wardener and Lennox[51] and others in malnourished prisoners of war, it has been known that **thiamine depletion** is the mechanism which gives rise to the acute Wernicke episode, followed by a Korsakoff memory impairment. However, the genetic factor that predisposes some heavy drinkers to develop this syndrome before they develop hepatic or gastrointestinal complications of alcohol abuse remains unclear. In many other alcoholics, the problems are the other way around. There has been much speculation about a transketolase gene, as transketolase is the enzyme which requires thiamine pyrophosphate (**TPP**) as a cofactor. The transketolase gene was identified in 1993, but no particular allelic variation was found that could account for the biochemical properties of the enzyme. Furthermore, it is not clear how thiamine depletion pro-

duces the particular neuropathology found in Wernicke–Korsakoff patients. Thiamine depletion affects six neurotransmitter systems, either by reduction of TPP-dependent enzyme activity or by direct structural damage. Of these neurotransmitters, four (acetylcholine, glutamate, aspartate, and GABA) are directly related to glucose metabolism. Whatever the precise mechanism, treatment as soon as possible with high doses of parenterally administered multivitamins is essential in patients with the Wernicke–Korsakoff syndrome. The Wernicke features respond well to high doses of vitamins, and such treatment almost certainly prevents the occurrence of a chronic Korsakoff state.[7,18] The small risk of anaphylaxis is completely outweighed by the high risk of severe brain damage and the appreciable risk of litigation (not an exaggeration) if such treatment is not administered.

There has been an extensive literature on the effects of **cholinergic antagonists** (such as scopolamine) upon memory. Kopelman and Corn[12] found a pattern of impairment in anterograde memory that closely resembled that seen in the amnesic syndrome. It has been argued that cholinergic blockade produces an effect upon the 'central executive' component of working memory, but Rusted[52] has concluded that this is not sufficient to account for the drug effect upon memory processes. Although some have argued that the predominant effect of scopolamine is on attention, Curran et al.[53] found that co-varying for the sedation or psychomotor effects of the drug did not eliminate the strong drug effects on episodic memory tests, and a similar finding was obtained by Kopelman and Corn.[12] The anticholinesterases physostigmine, tacrine, and donepezil have, of course, been developed and licensed for their effects in Alzheimer dementia, but, in the absence of unequivocal evidence of cholinergic depletion in amnesic syndromes, they have seldom been employed in these disorders.

Despite their very differing pharmacological action, the effects of the **benzodiazepines** upon memory and attention are remarkably similar to those of scopolamine. When recall or recognition is tested after a delay, benzodiazepines produce a marked anterograde impairment in explicit or episodic memory, similar to scopolamine.[53] As with scopolamine, however, once learning has been accomplished, the rate of forgetting is normal, and benzodiazepines do not produce any retrograde deficits. Procedural learning tasks for both benzodiazepines and scopolamine show similar effects, with learning curves on the active drug generally paralleling those for placebo.[12,54] Benzodiazepine effects can be attenuated by coadministration of the benzodiazepine antagonist, flumazenil.

The effects of **catecholamines** upon memory have been studied for many years, but the general consensus is that they act upon 'tonic attentional processes' rather than directly upon the storage or retrieval of memories. In an elegant study, Cahill et al.[55] examined the effects of the β-adrenergic receptor antagonist propranolol on memory for an emotionally arousing story, compared with a carefully matched neutral story. As expected, subjects given a placebo recalled more of the emotional than the neutral story, when tested 1 week later. Subjects given propanolol recalled the neutral story as well as the placebo subjects, but were impaired on the emotional story. Cahill et al.[55] concluded that the enhanced memory for emotional experience is mediated by the β-adrenergic system. However, it is possible that the enhanced memory was mediated by arousal, and that the effect of the drug was on arousal rather than directly upon memory. It has been claimed that clonidine (an adrenergic agonist) produced a small, but statistically significant, benefit in patients with the Korsakoff syndrome on tests of memory and attention, but this finding has not been replicated.

Similarly, some years ago, there was interest in the **serotonergic system** and alcohol-induced memory impairment. Early reports suggested that zimelidine, a serotonin reuptake inhibitor, reversed the memory impairment in healthy volunteers after the administration of ethanol. Later, it was claimed that fluvoxamine improved memory performance in five patients with the Korsakoff syndrome, and that the improvements correlated significantly with reductions in a cerebrospinal fluid breakdown product. The samples were small, the benefits were minor, and the informal use of this drug by the present author has not produced any noticeable benefit. Nevertheless, 3,4-methylenedioxymethamphetamine (ecstasy) has been reported to produce memory impairments either by direct or indirect effects. My colleagues and I have described one case of severe toxicity, in which a profound amnesic syndrome resulted; the memory impairment in this case was attributed to hypometabolism in the thalamus, particularly the anterior thalamus, which is a serotonin-rich brain region.

Conclusions

Systematic clinical descriptions of amnesic disorders and their underlying pathology have become more detailed and rigorous over the years. In particular, recent advances in neuroimaging (structural, metabolic, and activation) have provided the opportunity to relate particular cognitive abnormalities to specific changes in brain function. The use of pharmacological agents, in parallel with such imaging techniques, may promote the development of pharmacological agents more potent than the meagre array that we have at present for the treatment of severe memory disorder.

Further reading

Hodges, J.R. (ed.) (1991). *Transient amnesia: clinical and neuropsychological aspects*. W.B. Saunders, London.

Kopelman, M.D. (1995) The Korsakoff syndrome. *British Journal of Psychiatry*, 166, 154–73.

Kopelman, M.D. (1995) The assessment of psychogenic amnesia. In *Handbook of memory disorders* (ed. A. Baddeley, B. Wilson, and F. Watts), pp. 427–48. Wiley, Chichester.

Kopelman, M.D. (1999). Varieties of false memory. *Cognitive Neuropsychology*, in press.

Parkin, A.J. and Leng, N.R.C. (1993). *Neuropsychology of the amnesic syndrome*. Erlbaum, Hove.

Schacter, D.L., Norman, K.A., and Koutstaal, W. (1998). The cognitive neuroscience of constructive memory. *Annual Review of Psychology* 49, 289–318.

References

1. Hodges, J.R. and Ward, C.D. (1989). Observations during transient global amnesia: a behavioural and neuropsychological study of five cases. *Brain*, 112, 595–620.
2. Kritchevsky, M., Squire, L.R., and Zouzounis, J.A. (1988). Transient global amnesia: characterization of anterograde and retrograde amnesia. *Neurology*, 38, 213–19.
3. Stillhard, G., Landis, T., Schiess Regard, M., and Sialer, G. (1990). Bitemporal hypoperfusion in transient global amnesia: 99m-Tc-HM-PAO SPECT and neuropsychological findings during and after an attack. *Journal of Neurology, Neurosurgery and Psychiatry*, 53, 339–42.
4. Kopelman, M.D., Panayiotopoulos, C.P., and Lewis, P. (1994). Transient epileptic amnesia differentiated from psychogenic 'fugue': neuropsychological, EEG and PET findings. *Journal of Neurology, Neurosurgery and Psychiatry*, 57, 1002–4.
5. Kapur, N., Young, A., Bateman, D., and Kennedy, P. (1989). Focal retrograde amnesia: a long term clinical and neuropsychological follow-up. *Cortex*, 25, 387–402.
6. Russell, W.R. and Nathan, P.W. (1946). Traumatic amnesia. *Brain*, 69, 280–300.
7. Lishman, W.A. (1998). *Organic psychiatry: the psychological consequences of cerebral disorder* (3rd edn). Blackwell Science, Oxford.
8. Brooks, N. (1984). Cognitive deficits after head injury. In *Closed head injury: psychological, social and family consequences* (ed. N. Brooks), pp. 44–73. Oxford University Press.
9. Tarsh, M.J. and Royston, C. (1985). A follow-up study of accident neurosis. *British Journal of Psychiatry*, 146, 178–25.
10. Goodwin, D.W., Crane, J.B., and Guze, S.E. (1969). Phenomenological aspects of the alcoholic 'blackout'. *British Journal of Psychiatry*, 115, 1033–8.
11. Curran, H.V. (1991). Benzodiazepines, memory and mood: a review. *Psychopharmacology*, 104, 1–8.
12. Kopelman, M.D. and Corn, T.H. (1988). Cholinergic 'blockade' as a model for cholinergic depletion: a comparison of the memory deficits with those of Alzheimer-type dementia and the alcoholic Korsakoff syndrome. *Brain*, 111, 1079–110.
13. Frith, C.D., Stevens, M., Johnstone, E.C., Deakin, J.F.W., Lawler, P., and Crow, T.J. (1983). Effects of ECT and depression on various aspects of memory. *British Journal of Psychiatry*, 142, 610–17.
14. Squire, L.R. and Slater, P.C. (1983). ECT and complaints of memory dysfunction: a prospective three-year follow-up study. *British Journal of Psychiatry*, 142, 1–8.
15. McNeil, J.E. and Greenwood, R. (1996). Can PTSD occur with amnesia for the precipitating event? *Cognitive Neuropsychiatry*, 1, 239–46.
16. Kopelman, M.D. (1996). Transient disorders of memory and consciousness. In *Neuropsychiatry: a comprehensive textbook* (ed. B.S. Fogel, R.B. Schiffer, and S.M. Rao), pp. 615–24. Williams and Wilkins, Baltimore, MD.
17. Taylor, P.J. and Kopelman, M.D. (1984). Amnesia for criminal offences. *Psychological Medicine*, 14, 581–8.
18. Victor, M., Adams, R.D., and Collins, G.H. (1971). *The Wernicke–Korsakoff syndrome*. F.A. Davis, Philadelphia, PA.
19. Korsakoff, S.S. (1889). Psychic disorder in conjunction with peripheral neuritis. Translated and republished by M. Victor and P.I. Yakovlev (1955). *Neurology*, 5, 394–406.
20. Kopelman, M.D., Stanhope, N., and Kingsley, D.E.P. (1999). Retrograde amnesia in patients with diencephalic temporal lobe or frontal lesions. *Neuropsychologia*, in press.
21. Mair, W.G.P., Warrington, E.K., and Weiskrantz, L. (1979). Memory disorder in Korsakoff's psychosis; a neuropathological and neuropsychological investigation of two cases. *Brain*, 102, 783.
22. Mayes, A.R., Meudell, P.R., Mann, D., and Pickering, A. (1988). Location of lesions in Korsakoff's syndrome: neuropsychological and neuropathological data on two patients. *Cortex*, 24, 367–88.
23. Jacobson, R.R., Acker, C., and Lishman, W.A. (1990). Patterns of neuropsychological deficit in alcoholic Korsakoff's syndrome. *Psychological Medicine*, 20, 321–34.
24. Jacobson, R.R. and Lishman, W.A. (1990). Cortical and diencephalic lesions in Korsakoff's syndrome: a clinical and CT scan study. *Psychological Medicine*, 20, 63–75.
25. Wilson, B.A. and Wearing, D. (1995). Prisoner of consciousness: a state of just awakening following herpes simplex encephalitis. In *Broken memories* (ed. R. Campbell and M.A. Conway), pp. 14–30. Blackwell Science, Oxford.

26. Juel-Jenson, B.E. (1987). The herpes virus. In *Oxford textbook of medicine* (ed. D.J. Weatherall, J.G.G. Ledingham, and D.A. Warrell), pp. 559–67. Oxford University Press.

27. Hierons, R., Janota, I., and Corsellis, J.A.N. (1978). The late effects of necrotizing encephalitis of the temporal lobes and limbic areas: a clinico-pathological study of 10 cases. *Psychological Medicine*, **8**, 21–42.

28. Aggleton, J.P. and Saunders, R.C. (1997). The relationships between temporal lobe and diencephalic structures implicated in anterograde amnesia. *Memory*, **5**, 49–71.

29. Zola-Morgan, S., Squire, L.R., and Amaral, D.G. (1986). Human amnesia and the medial temporal region: enduring memory impairment following a bilateral lesion limited to field CA1 of the hippocampus. *Journal of Neuroscience*, **6**, 2950–67.

30. von Cramon, D.Y., Hebel, N., and Schuri, U. (1985). A contribution to the anatomical basis of thalamic amnesia. *Brain*, **108**, 997–1008.

31. Gade, A. (1982). Amnesia after operations on aneurysms of the anterior communicating artery. *Surgical Neurology*, **18**, 46–9.

32. Moscovitch, M. and Melo, B. (1997). Strategic retrieval and the frontal lobes: evidence from confabulation and amnesia. *Neuropsychologia*, **35**, 1017–34.

33. Becker, J.T., Bajulaiye, O., and Smith, C. (1992). Longitudinal analysis of a two-component model of the memory deficit in Alzheimer's disease. *Psychological Medicine*, **22**, 437–46.

34. Shimamura, A.P. (1994). Memory and frontal lobe function. In *The cognitive neurosciences* (ed. M.S. Gazzaniga), pp. 803–14. MIT Press, Cambridge, MA.

35. Schacter, D.L. (1987). Implicit memory: history and current status. *Journal of Experimental Psychology: Learning, Memory and Cognition*, **13**, 501–18.

36. Ostergaard, A.L. (1994). Dissociations between word priming effects in normal subjects and patients with memory disorders: multiple memory systems or retrieval? *Quarterly Journal of Experimental Psychology: Section A: Human Experimental Psychology*, **47**, 331–64.

37. Meudell, P. and Mayes, A.R. (1982). Normal and abnormal forgetting: some comments on the human amnesic syndrome. In *Normality and pathology in cognitive functions* (ed. A.W. Ellis), pp. 203–38. Academic Press, London.

38. Mayes, A.R. and Downes, J.J. (1997). What do theories of functional deficit(s) underlying amnesia have to explain? *Memory*, **5**, 3–36.

39. Schacter, D.L., Norman, K.A., and Koutstaal, W. (1998). The cognitive neuroscience of constructive memory. *Annual Review of Psychology*, **49**, 289–318.

40. Kopelman, M.D., Stevens, T.G., Foli, S., and Grasby, P. (1998). PET activation of the medial temporal lobe in learning. *Brain*, **121**, 875–87.

41. Schacter, D.L., Alpert, N.M., Savage, C.R., Rauch, S.L., and Albert, M.S. (1996). Conscious recollection and the human hippocampal formation. *Proceedings of the National Academy of Sciences of the United States of America*, **93**, 321–5.

42. Grasby, P.M., Frith, C.D., Friston, K.J., Bench, C., Frackowiak, R.S., and Dolan, R.J. (1993). Functional mapping of brain areas implicated in auditory-verbal memory function. *Brain*, **116**, 1–20.

43. Kopelman, M.D. (1987). Two types of confabulation. *Journal of Neurology, Neurosurgery and Psychiatry*, **50**, 1482–7.

44. DeLuca, J. and Cicerone, K.D. (1991). Confabulation following aneurysm of the anterior communicating artery. *Cortex*, **27**, 417–23.

45. Baddeley, A.D. and Wilson, B. (1986). Amnesia, autobiographical memory, and confabulation. In *Autobiographical memory* (ed. D.C. Rubin), pp. 225–52. Cambridge University Press, Cambridge.

46. Burgess, P.W. and Shallice, T. (1996). Confabulation and the control of recollection. *Memory*, **4**, 359–411.

47. Schnider, A., von Däniken, C., and Gutbrod, K. (1996). The mechanisms of spontaneous and provoked confabulations. *Brain*, **119**, 1365–75.

48. Kopelman, M.D., Stanhope, N., and Kingsley, D. (1997). Temporal and spatial memory in patients with focal frontal, temporal lobe, and diencephalic lesions. *Neuropsychologia*, **35**, 1533–45.

49. Johnson, M.K., O'Connor, M., and Cantor, J. (1997). Confabulation, memory deficits, and frontal dysfunction. *Brain and Cognition*, **34**, 189–206.

50. Kopelman, M.D. (1999). Varieties of false memory. *Cognitive Neuropsychology*, in press.

51. De Wardener, H.E. and Lennox, B. (1947). Cerebral beriberi (Wernicke's encephalopathy): review of 52 cases in a Singapore PoW hospital. *Lancet*, **i**, 11–17.

52. Rusted, J. (1994). Cholinergic blockade and human information processing: are we asking the right questions? *Journal of Psychopharmacology*, **8**, 54–9.

53. Curran, H.V., Schifano, F., and Lader, M. (1991). Models of memory dysfunction? A comparison of the effects of scopolamine and lorazepam on memory, psychomotor performance and mood. *Psychopharmacology*, **103**, 83–90.

54. Bishop, K.I., Curran, H.V., and Lader, M. (1996). Do scopolamine and lorazepam have dissociable effects upon human memory? A dose–response study with normal subjects. *Experimental and Clinical Psychopharmacology*, **4**, 292–9.

55. Cahill, L., Prins, B., Weber, M., and McGaugh, J.L. (1994). Beta-adrenergic activation and memory for emotional events. *Nature*, **3H**, 702–4.

4.1.14 **The management of dementia**

Simon Fleminger

Introduction

The term dementia is used in two different ways. First there are the **dementias**. These are **diseases** that cause progressive and diffuse cerebral damage, of which Alzheimer's disease is the most common. Second, dementia can be used to refer to a **clinical syndrome**. Thus dementia is 'an acquired global impairment of intellect, memory, and personality, but without impairment of consciousness'.[1] For clinicians this is the preferred usage, and the one adopted in this chapter. It demands that the cause of the dementia is explored, and makes no comment on the likely prognosis.

This chapter will describe the management of people who suffer dementia, whatever the cause. Aspects of management specific to the individual diseases that produce dementia will not be discussed. The discussion will not be limited to older patients, and will, for example, include dementia due to head injury or metabolic disorders. Patients who suffer the dementia before 18 years of age will, by and large, not be included; their needs are often best met by services provided for people with mental retardation.

The first stage of the management of a person with dementia is to try to identify the cause, particularly treatable causes.

Assessment

Assessment serves a twofold purpose: first to establish whether dementia is present, and second, if dementia is present, to determine its cause.

Screening for dementia

History and examination

The history is crucial, and an informant will be needed who should be given the opportunity of being interviewed alone in case there are matters they are reluctant to divulge in front of the patient. The diagnosis hinges on the identification of a change in performance, particularly on cognitive tasks including memory, but also in terms of personality. Functional impairment of occupation or social life, and carer complaints about the patient's memory, are better predictors of dementia than are subjective complaints of poor memory.[2] Subjective memory complaints are more associated with depression.

A patient with a moderately severe dementia may nevertheless be bright-eyed, alert, and have preserved the social banter and etiquette necessary to meet someone and be interviewed. At first sight they can appear normal. The patient should therefore be asked questions that demand informative replies and whose veracity can be determined. Doing this while taking the history allows even quite mild memory problems to be detected, because to give a good account of recent events is quite demanding of memory. It is also a good way to examine patients, often those with depressive pseudodementia who perform poorly when directly confronted with tests of memory and cognition, yet do not do too badly when unaware they are being tested.

Delirium is an important differential diagnosis of dementia, and it is therefore important to look for an impaired or fluctuating level of consciousness.

Screening assessments and investigations

A screening assessment is a useful complement to the standard mental state examination. The Mini-Mental State Examination (**MMSE**)[3] is probably as good as any; when used to detect Alzheimer's disease, sensitivities and specificities of greater than 80 per cent are to be expected using a cut-off of 23 or less (out of 30).[4] It is possible that equivalent specificity and sensitivity is achieved by a brief assessment of orientation to time, serial sevens, and recall of three items.[5]

The results of a screening test need to be interpreted in the light of the history, physical findings, and the prevalence of dementia in the population being tested. For example, in younger patients screening tests will identify proportionately more false positives, who in fact do not suffer from dementia.

Investigations should be targeted at identifying treatable causes. Table 1 suggests the investigations that should routinely be performed in someone with a dementia whose cause has not yet been identified.[6]

The younger patient will demand a more thorough physical examination and investigations, and referral to a neurologist is often appropriate.

A rating of depression may help in the diagnosis of depressive pseudodementia. It is also important to rate depression because it often coexists with dementia and may make the disability worse. The Cornell scale[7] or the Geriatric Depression Rating Scale[8] can be used.

Risk assessment is an important part of the management of patients with dementia and Table 2 suggests various areas of risk that need to be considered. A good history from carers and others involved in the patient's care is essential for a full risk assessment, which is rarely complete without an assessment by an occupational therapist.

It is important to use the outcome of risk assessment to facilitate independence. This is done by introducing appropriate strategies to

Table 1 Investigations for dementia

Routine

Full blood count
Erythrocyte sedimentation rate
Urea and electrolytes
Liver function tests
Calcium and phosphate
Thyroid function
Urinalysis
B_{12} and folate

Worth considering

Syphilis serology
HIV status
Chest radiograph
ECG
CT or MRI brain scan
Electroencephalogram
Neuropsychological assessment

More specialist investigations may be needed, for example cerebrospinal fluid examination, copper studies, genetic studies, investigations for prion diseases, etc.

minimize risk. In addition, a risk–benefit analysis may demonstrate that it is appropriate to run a risk of some adverse event happening if there are clear benefits of doing so. For example, a patient may be at risk of wandering and getting lost from his or her home; however, if the strategy to prevent this involves moving the patient to new accommodation away from family and familiar surroundings, then this may itself be regarded as a sufficiently adverse event to make transfer inappropriate.

Communication and consent

Early suspicions of a dementing disease should generally be discussed with the patient and their family. If the dementia is progressive leaving these discussions until the diagnosis is certain may be too late; the patient's ability to take part in decisions about their future treatment, and their family's future, may by then be jeopardized by cognitive decline. Only early in the course of the illness will they be able to make an enduring power of attorney, settle their will, and discuss with their doctors how they wish to be treated once the disease is well advanced.

The person with dementia will have the best chance of assimilating information if it is given in small chunks, with simple messages. Write down a summary of what has been said. Make it easy for them to express themselves by asking simple questions—if possible, ones that can be answered by yes or no. Make it difficult for them to forget appointments; inform several key people of the time and date. If possible, always have a carer present when discussing important information.

If language is impaired then be aware that the patient is likely to rely more on non-verbal cues. Avoid quick gestures and direct face-to-face confrontation if the patient appears threatened by this. A calm steady voice with the gentle use of touch will help the person understand that they are in safe and caring company.

Table 2 Risk assessment in dementia

Consider the following areas

Antisocial and other behaviour

- Violence/aggression
  Towards others
  Towards self

- Sexual disinhibition/assault

- Other antisocial behaviours that may provoke assaults (e.g. argumentative, spitting, etc.)

- Wandering/agitation

Safety associated with impaired memory and cognition and poor judgement

- Home safety
  Leaving kettles, fires, etc. on
  Leaving doors/windows etc. open
  Cigarettes

- Out and about
  Getting lost
  Road safety (pedestrian, driving)

- Financial
  Not able to handle money, loses money
  Inappropriately spends money, poor judgement

- Work
  Fails to monitor and check for errors
  Unsafe with dangerous machinery

- Supervising others, especially children (and consider aggression/ sexual behaviour)

Vulnerability to

- Abuse by others
  Physical, sexual, emotional, and financial

- Self-neglect
  Including not eating, squalor

Physical health

- Falls

- Managing illness (e.g. diabetes, diet)
  Taking medication (note risk of abruptly stopping anticonvulsants or steroids)
  Drug dependence

- Epilepsy

The normal doctor–patient alliance comes under scrutiny once a diagnosis of dementia becomes likely, and thus the psychiatrist should make an assessment of the patient's capacity to consent. If the patient is unable to give informed consent then it is particularly important to discuss the management on offer with family and carers. Nevertheless, the autonomy of the person with dementia should, as far as possible, be respected.[9]

Cognitive symptoms

Cognitive impairment is a core feature of dementia. Most cognitive rehabilitation is aimed at reducing the disability and handicap resulting from cognitive impairment, rather than improving the impairment itself (see Chapters 1.10.1 and 4.1.11 for a discussion of impairment, disability, and handicap).

Psychological techniques

The management of memory impairment is discussed elsewhere (see Chapter 2.5.2).

Elderly people

Reality orientation attempts to improve the cognitive performance of people with dementia through repeated presentation of orientation information. This can be done using patient groups to discuss the day's events, and/or reality orientation boards displaying information about the day, for example the date, the weather, and the name of the next meal. A systematic review[10] suggests that the method is effective in improving measures of cognition and orientation, but has little impact on behaviour. But the gains are not large and may be lost once the treatment is discontinued, and some have argued that it may adversely affect mood.

Other psychological strategies used in the elderly with dementia include reminiscence therapy[11] and validation therapy.[12] In both these therapies discussions of autobiographical memories are used to improve mood, and foster a sense of well being and worth. There is little good evidence that these therapies produce anything more than short-lived and modest gains in mood, cognition, and behaviour.[13]

Younger people with dementia

Other cognitive techniques have been tried in younger patients with dementia following an acquired single-incident brain injury. These include attention training, for example repeated practice to detect a moving target,[14,15] and computer-mediated cognitive rehabilitation.[16] The evidence that any of them work is inconsistent. Return-to-work programmes should be offered to younger patients with mild and relatively static dementia. Though they have not been evaluated using randomized, controlled trial methodology, a comparison of the employment status of patients before entering such a programme with their status after completing the programme, suggests that return-to-work programmes are effective.[17]

Pharmacotherapy

When drug treatments are described throughout this chapter it is always important to bear in mind the general principles of pharmacotherapy in the person with brain damage, whether caused by injury or disease, which are discussed in Chapter 4.1.11.

Donepezil, an anticholinesterase inhibitor, probably produces an improvement in cognition in a proportion of patients with mild to moderate Alzheimer's disease. It takes a few weeks to take effect,[18] and improvements may be sustained for at least a year on continued treatment. At the time of writing the published evidence only comes from one research group. Donepezil seems to be without serious untoward effects, but it is expensive and its effect should be monitored and reviewed at 12 weeks. Treatment should continue only for those who show benefit.[19] More recently, rivastigmine has been introduced as an alternative to donepezil in dementia.[20] A recent case series suggests that donepezil may also be effective in patients with brain injury.[21]

Systematic reviews, to be found in the 1998 Cochrane Library, find no support for the use of piracetam, nimodipine, or lecithin in dementia. There is some support for the use of selegiline (deprenyl) in Alzheimer's disease, but this is insufficient to recommend its routine clinical use. Vitamin E may slow the rate of functional decline in moderately impaired patients with Alzheimer's disease, and given its limited potential to cause adverse side-effects its use can possibly be justified.[13] It has been suggested that hydergine, a mixture of four derivatives of ergotoxine, is effective, particularly if there is evidence of a vascular dementia, but the evidence is fragile.[22] Many patients take an extract of the leaves of the maidenhair tree (*Ginkgo biloba*), whose mechanism of action is unknown but may be similar to that of hydergine. It probably does no harm, but there is no good evidence that it does any good.[23]

Non-cognitive symptoms

Aggression and agitation

Assessment

Agitation is common in elderly patients with dementia[24] and following brain injury (see Chapter 4.1.11). Agitation and aggression are often associated with confusional states with disorientation, with misidentification, and with delusions.

Medical causes of a deterioration in the cognitive state need to be excluded. Sources of pain and fear should be considered, as well as the possibility of sleep loss or constipation, cold or hunger. A history from the family may indicate phobic disorder, which is now manifest as agitation, or a lifelong tendency to aggression. Alcohol or other drug abuse must be addressed. Enquiry about the behavioural disturbance and examination of the mental state should look for evidence of anxiety, depression, or psychosis and persecutory delusions, as well as the patient's explanation for their aggression.

Psychosocial and behavioural management

Treatment should initially rely on psychological interventions implemented by the carers or nursing team.[25] Agitation may respond to a change in the environment to reduce loneliness or boredom. Avoid overstimulation, which commonly occurs on general medical or surgical wards. A calm predictable environment with no unexpected changes in routine, and with no unnecessary rules and restrictions, is likely to help. The patient may require admission to a psychiatric unit, or a brain-injury unit if the dementia results from brain injury. They may need to be transferred from a medical or surgical ward where they are having to be sedated to stop them interfering with the care of other patients.

For inpatients, it helps to have plenty of staff available if the patient suddenly becomes agitated or aggressive. This will help to maintain the confidence of the nursing team. Nursing should be proactive; reactive nursing, only responding when the patient is demanding, will

reinforce the unwanted behaviours. Confrontation should be avoided; it may be possible to distract the patient or change the subject. Good communication is likely to lessen agitation and aggression; the patient should be told what is happening and messages should be repeated and written down. The family should be encouraged to help if appropriate.

Nursing interventions, in particular for personal care, are often the focus of aggressive behaviour.[26] It may be appropriate to cover such high-risk periods using physical restraint, for instance padded gloves to prevent scratching, for short periods, or brief sedation with medication. These will need to be documented and kept under review, as well as being discussed openly with appropriate parties, including of course the patient and the patient's family. The nursing team needs to be skilled in handling aggressive behaviour and also to be aware of the patient's potential for aggression. Policies for raising the alarm and seeking help, for example using panic buttons, need to be rehearsed. A risk assessment for the management of the agitated/aggressive behaviour needs to be undertaken, both with regard to the patient's safety and the health and safety of staff and others.

Anger management should be offered for more chronic aggressive behaviour. This will include an assessment and, if appropriate, treatment for any anxiety disorder. A behavioural programme may be necessary, but this is usually difficult to implement except in a specialist unit. The programme starts with a situational, or ABC, analysis.

- Antecedents—what was happening before the behaviour started?
- Behaviour—a clear description of the behaviour.
- Consequences—what happened as a result of the behaviour, particularly looking for possible reinforcers of the behaviour?

This analysis may suggest that a specific behavioural strategy is appropriate. The frequency and severity of the behaviour then need to be charted as a baseline before introducing the specific intervention.

Many programmes rely on the differential reinforcement of other behaviour (**DRO**); this involves positive reinforcement of other, appropriate behaviours, with the hope that these will then replace the aggressive behaviour. A useful technique to be used alongside DRO is 'time out on the spot' (**TOOTS**), in which the unwanted behaviour is met with immediate withdrawal of social contact; appropriate behaviours receive warm social contact. The whole nursing/multidisciplinary team must be aware of the principles of reinforcement and extinction of behaviour, because behavioural programmes are unlikely to be effective unless consistently applied across the team. The evidence that such behavioural techniques work is based largely on A–B–A–B design, single-case studies, and case series.[27]

Drug treatment of agitation and aggression

Use drugs only if psychosocial strategies have failed, and only if absolutely necessary. Do not rush in with drug treatment; the behaviour may spontaneously remit. Start low and go slow, titrating to the minimum effective dose. If a drug is not effective then abandon it; do not allow cocktails to build up. Review prescriptions regularly looking for side-effects.

Major tranquillizers are frequently prescribed for patients with dementia, even if the patient has no evidence of psychosis.[28] There is good evidence that antipsychotic drugs are sometimes prescribed too readily in nursing homes. One study found that it was possible to greatly reduce antipsychotic drug use in nursing homes without any adverse effects on the patient.[29]

However, randomized controlled trials have consistently shown that antipsychotics, for example thioridazine and haloperidol, are effective treatments for agitation in dementia, though the size of the effect is modest.[30] There is no empirical evidence to suggest that any one antipsychotic is particularly effective. It is recommended that small doses are used, and as little as 2 to 3 mg of haloperidol a day can produce good response rates.[31] Antipsychotics are a reasonable first-line treatment for the management of agitation in dementia, particularly as a large proportion of agitated patients will have evidence of psychosis. There is some evidence that risperidone is effective in reducing behavioural disturbance;[32] other new atypical antipsychotics, including olanzapine, are also worth considering.

Adverse effects of antipsychotics may be troublesome, particularly in the elderly. The risk of falls may be increased. Confusion may deteriorate, particularly with drugs with anticholinergic effects, and sedation may be problematic. Extrapyramidal side-effects are particularly common in the elderly person with dementia, particularly Lewy body dementia. Clozapine may be worth trying if extrapyramidal side-effects are bad and the use of very low doses may reduce the risk of agranulocytosis, which is otherwise increased in the elderly. New atypical antipsychotics should also be considered. Demented elderly patients are at increased risk of developing tardive dyskinesia.

If antipsychotics do not work then benzodiazepines may be effective, particularly if there is evidence of anxiety. Short-acting benzodiazepines, for example oxazepam or lorazepam, are recommended by some because they are less likely to result in steadily accumulating blood levels. On the other hand, short-acting drugs may produce highly variable blood levels, perhaps increasing the risk of dependence or the reinforcement of untoward behaviour. Behavioural reinforcement can occur, for example if an anxious patient learns that if he becomes aggressive he will immediately be given a dose of benzodiazepine giving dramatic relief of his anxiety. Side-effects of benzodiazepines, for instance an increasing risk of falls, may limit the dose. On the other hand, if there is prominent depression or labile mood disturbance then it is worth considering using carbamazepine or a sedative antidepressant. Buspirone may be worth trying in mild agitation associated with anxiety. High-dose propranolol is worth considering, but blood pressure and the ECG need to be closely monitored.

Wandering

Many people with dementia will wander, and others will abscond or demand to leave. A risk assessment may be needed to determine their safety outside, for example assessing road safety and their ability to find their way back home.

First exclude causes of agitation. Ensure that the patient has plenty of opportunity for physical exercise and is encouraged to take walks. Identify any motivation that may be driving the wandering behaviour, for example the belief that they must get back to work, or that their family is in danger, or a craving for alcohol. At home additional locks or safeguards may be needed, A 'Stop!' sign on the front door may be effective. Some units have number entry locks which the patient with dementia cannot use. Identification bracelets or tagging systems which sound an alarm if the patient leaves the unit are perhaps a last resort. An inpatient or residential unit will need both an absent without leave policy, which will include the protocol for informing family and

police, and a locked door policy which must take into account what happens if there is a fire. Detention under the Mental Health Act 1983, or its equivalent, may need to be considered.

Mood disturbance

Depression

Although depression in people with dementia is quite common, it may be difficult to diagnose because of impaired communication. It is therefore important to consider depression as a cause for almost any change in function or behaviour, and to look for risk factors for depression, for example a recent bereavement, in the history. A screening test to detect depression may be appropriate (see above).

If the patient is depressed then review the general medical state, including any drugs that may produce depression. Make sure that all general psychosocial issues have been addressed, for example appropriate support services, leisure activities, and housing. Specific psychological therapy, for instance cognitive therapy, for depression in people with dementia is generally unavailable. Innovative counselling programmes are now being offered in some centres, but it is not known whether they make any difference.

Therefore antidepressant medication is the main therapeutic strategy. The limited evidence suggests that the antidepressant treatment of depression in patients with dementia is effective.

In antidepressant therapeutic trials, which usually are of a few weeks' duration, about one in two elderly patients with dementia plus depression show an antidepressant response.[33] This rather poor response rate may be little different from that seen in depressed elderly patients without dementia, and may reflect enduring somatic symptoms, for instance poor appetite, which are to be found in the elderly regardless of depression or dementia. On the other hand, the poor response rate may reflect the fact that depressed patients with dementia take longer to respond. It may therefore be worth persisting with antidepressant treatment for longer than a few weeks before concluding that the depression is resistant to treatment with that drug.

The choice of antidepressant drugs depends largely on their side-effect profile. Newer antidepressants, having less anticholinergic activity and less cardiotoxicity, are generally preferred. Of the newer drugs only citalopram and moclobemide have actually been evaluated in dementia, both being found to be effective in relieving symptoms of depression.[33]

Some method to evaluate the effectiveness of the treatment needs to be in place, preferably before treatment is started to get a baseline measure. For example, a measure of activities of daily living may be the target outcome to see whether it improves with antidepressant treatment.

Dementia is not a contraindication for electroconvulsive therapy, though the response is perhaps more varied. However, many patients with dementia develop troublesome confusion, disorientation, and increasing memory impairment, especially if treated with bilateral electroconvulsive therapy.

Apathy

Apathy may be both a symptom of depression and a consequence of organic brain disease affecting those brain systems involved in motivation. It is not yet clear if there is value in distinguishing between these two routes to apathy. If there is any evidence for depressive symptoms alongside the apathy then use an antidepressant. If, however, symptoms of apathy are found in the absence of depression then consider prescribing bromocriptine or methylphenidate. Case series suggest that bromocriptine and methylphenidate are effective, though clinical experience indicates that the effects may be short-lived. Methylphenidate needs to be prescribed under close supervision, given its potential for abuse and the development of mental and motor side-effects.

Mania

Mania is not particularly common in dementia, though there is possibly a specific association with Huntington's chorea. It needs to be distinguished from the irritable, disinhibited, and agitated states that may follow frontal lobe injury. Nevertheless, it is important to consider mania as a cause of aggressive behaviour, particularly after brain injury. There is no evidence to suggest that the treatment of mania in a person with dementia be any different from normal protocols.

Psychotic symptoms

There are few hard data on which to base decisions about antipsychotic drug prescribing for relieving psychotic symptoms in dementia. The choice of antipsychotic is therefore likely to be determined by its profile of side-effects. For example, psychotic patients who are also agitated may need a more sedative drug, while the newer atypical antipsychotics with less extrapyramidal side-effects will be required if these side-effects of the older drugs become troublesome.

Psychosocial measures also need to be considered. For example, delusions of theft, common in people with dementia[34], may be founded on memory impairment, which results in the patient losing things and then attributing the loss to someone having stolen the item. Strategies to help the person keep tags on where they put things etc. may then be helpful.

A risk assessment is an important part of the management plan. Are the psychotic symptoms associated with worrying behaviours, or are they, for example, just one manifestation of general disorientation and confusion? Given the risks of treatment with antipsychotics the risk–benefit analysis for starting antipsychotics needs to be considered and discussed with the patient and his or her family/carers.

Disorders of sexual behaviour

Impotence or reduced libido

Reduced sexual activity and interest is the most common disorder of sexual behaviour associated with dementia, though it is the least likely to come to the attention of the clinician. It probably plays a part in the high rates of divorce seen, for example, in young couples after one partner has sustained a brain injury. Psychological effects, in particular the change in the patient's role in the partnership as a result of dementia, as well as the physiological effects of brain injury on erectile function, contribute to impotence and reduced libido.

The first and most important step is to recognize the problem and talk about it. The couple may wish to be referred to a sexual disorders clinic. If reduced libido is part of a more generalized apathy or depression then it may respond when these features are appropriately treated (see above).

Sexual disinhibition and overactivity

Any display of sexual disinhibition is likely to become a major management issue and needs a thorough, well-documented assessment detailing what behaviour has been observed and when. Occasionally it may be part of a Klüver–Bucy-like syndrome with hyperorality and excessive eating. The Klüver–Bucy syndrome is particularly associated with damage to the temporal lobes and may be seen following herpes encephalitis or head injury, and with Pick's disease. Some symptoms of the syndrome are not uncommon in Alzheimer's disease, particularly in the later stages.[34] Sexual disinhibition and overactivity may very occasionally result from dopamine therapy or epilepsy.[1]

Sexual disinhibition may respond to psychosocial strategies. It may, for example, be necessary to ensure that only men nurse the patient if all the sexual disinhibition is directed towards female staff. A full behavioural programme to try to extinguish the behaviour may be effective, but if the behaviour involves touching and groping then it is essential to discuss and monitor the programme with those involved in the hands-on care of the patient. Staff often find such behaviour particularly upsetting.

Antipsychotics may reduce sexually disinhibited behaviour. The antiandrogens, cyproterone acetate and medroxyprogesterone (Depo-Provera), should be tried if all else fails.

Sleep disturbance

Assessment

Patients with dementia often have a disturbed sleep pattern and this is most troublesome when the sleep–wake cycle is inverted, with the patient asleep during the day but awake at night. The confusion, which frequently accompanies nocturnal waking, makes the problem all the more difficult; the patient may wander or create a disturbance in the middle of the night. This symptom may require urgent intervention if the family is demanding that the patient be admitted into residential accommodation unless they get some peace at night. On the other hand, if the patient is already in a setting that can cope with their nocturnal wakening, does it matter that they are awake at night?

In the assessment it is worth considering restless legs as a cause of sleep disturbance. Does the patient have to get up at night to empty his or her bladder? The normal antidiuresis at night may be lost following damage to the hypothalamus. A late evening dose of desmopressin (1-deamino-8-D-arginine vasopressin) may suppress urine production and result in a good night's sleep for these patients. Are there any other medical reasons why the patient may be waking at night, for example because of pain from a duodenal ulcer? Sleep apnoea, which is more common in the elderly, produces sleep disturbance and is a contraindication for benzodiazepines and other drugs that may suppress respiration. Is sleep disturbance due to depression? Has there been any recent change to the sleeping arrangements; if so any sleep disturbance may be self-limiting.

Sleep hygiene

Because hypnotics are likely to have deleterious effects on cognition it is particularly important that these drugs should only be considered after techniques to improve sleep hygiene have been tried. Minimize daytime sleeping by making sure there is an active programme with plenty to do, both physically and mentally. Make sure that fluids, diuretics, and caffeine are avoided in the evening. Try to introduce calming bedtime rituals, for example having a bath or listening to music. Look at the sleeping arrangements to make sure that they are quiet, warm, and, if possible, familiar or at least away from perceived danger, for example from another threatening resident.

Hypnotics

There is little definite evidence to guide the clinician as to which hypnotic to select in patients with dementia. Comorbid mental symptoms are therefore probably the best guide to which drug to choose. If anxiety or depression is present trazodone is a useful sedative antidepressant for people with dementia. Sedative antipsychotics should be tried in the presence of psychotic symptoms. Benzodiazepines and chloral hydrate should, if possible, not be given indefinitely; particular caution should be taken if the patient already shows disinhibition.

Hypnotics are likely to have a deleterious effect on cognition and this should be monitored, along with an assessment of the impact of treatment on function and activities of daily living.

Incontinence

Dementia in the elderly roughly doubles the risk of urinary incontinence.[35] To minimize incontinence, toilets should be easily identifiable and readily accessible. Clothing may need attention to ensure that it is easy to remove. If urinary incontinence is present then reversible causes, such as urinary tract infection, constipation, and medication (such as diuretics or drugs with anticholinergic side-effects causing urinary retention and overflow) should be excluded.

A diary recording frequency of voiding on the toilet and frequency of incontinence should be kept to see if toileting times can be adjusted to minimize incontinence. Prompted voiding (asking the person hourly if they want to go to the toilet and giving praise for successful toileting) is effective for some individuals.[36] A behavioural programme may be needed for the patient who urinates or defecates in inappropriate places.

If incontinence persists get the advice of a continence advisor before considering drug treatment.

Carers

Support for the family and carers starts with education about the cause of the dementia, the possible prognosis, and the symptoms—both current and those which may develop. They may want to discuss the risks to other members of the family. Family and friends need to understand that cognitive and behavioural symptoms arise from damage to the brain and are part of the illness.

Carers need advice on the principles of care, for example ensuring that communication is simple and direct, avoiding changes to routine, not arguing with the patient, but on the other hand not endorsing false beliefs. They will need guidance on when and how to call on professional advice. Addresses of self-help groups, and the address of information on the Internet, should also be available (e.g. http://www.dementia.ion.ucl.ac.uk). Carers may need help to obtain appropriate citizens advice, help at home (including cleaning, nursing, and meals-on-wheels), as well as legal and financial advice.

If a behavioural programme is being set up then consider what role the carer is going to take; it is difficult to be both a partner and a therapist. Also be aware of potential conflicts of interest. Sometimes it will be inappropriate for the next of kin to have control of the patient's money.

The burden of caring for someone with a dementia may result in depression and other signs of stress. The carer should have the opportunity of talking about any problems they have, if necessary getting their own psychiatric care. Improving the mental health of the carer may reduce the likelihood of institutional care for the patient.

A systematic review of various interventions designed to support carers of people with Alzheimer's disease found little evidence that any of them actually work.[37] Offering spouses help in coping with the disease was found to be effective in one study. Overall the authors of the review concluded that the evidence was inconclusive and did not warrant withdrawal of services providing carer support.

A caregiver's handbook, giving excellent advice to carers, is available on the Internet (http://www.biostat.wustl.edu/lists/alzheimer/Caregivers_Handbook). The handbook ends with a discussion of when it is time to stop and hand over to institutional care; this sensitive issue should be raised with the carer well in advance.

Carers who are under stress are probably more likely to abuse, either physically or emotionally, the person with dementia. Try to ensure that any physical and emotional abuse of the demented person is picked up early. It helps if everybody involved in the person's care knows how to report any concerns they may have about what is happening.

Ensure that professional carers are well supervised and that their employers comply with local standards.

Service provision and liaison

General principles

Health services

Neurologists, geriatricians, old age psychiatrists, medical rehabilitation physicians, as well as general adult psychiatrists, all may be involved in looking after patients with dementia. It is therefore useful if protocols for management are drawn up locally, for example defining who will look after patients with presenile (that is to say an onset before 65 years of age) progressive dementia, or patients with dementia following from brain injury in adult life. Alcoholic dementia is particularly likely to cause debate amongst local professionals. Such debates are best answered by matching the patient's needs to the skills and support that can be offered by the various services. General practitioners may wish to take a central role in dementia care.[38]

Social and other services

Social workers play a major part in dementia care. They will need to advise both the patient and family about financial entitlements and opportunities for support, for example at local day centres or using carers coming into the patient's home. Respite and long-term residential care will need to be considered. They are likely to be partly responsible for ensuring the quality of residential care, for example checking that local registration requirements are met.

Social services may provide a link with self-help organizations, advocacy services and, for the younger patient with dementia, employment services.

Table 3 An effective dementia care system

The following should be put in place[39]

- A system for identifying people with dementia and assessing their needs

- Good continuity of care (seamless)

- A system to ensure that no patient falls between service boundaries

- 24-hour advice and support—medical, psychiatric, and social

- Continuing care arrangements for the life of the patient, with review, monitoring, and planning ahead

- Involvement of voluntary and local community organizations and other agencies to maximize community access and participation

- Advocacy for the patient, maximizing independence and protecting their rights and liberties as well as guarding against abuse

- Carer support

An integrated dementia care system

Local health and social services, and other interested parties including those from the voluntary sector, should work together to define the local strategy for dementia care[39] (Table 3). The strategy for younger adults with dementia (usually arising from a single-incident acquired, brain injury) will be very different from that for older people with dementia who will usually have a progressive disease. Appropriate funding arrangements may be the key to ensuring good liaison between services, for example by defining a joint pool of funding which services only have access to if they are working together.

The individual patient

For the individual patient make sure that all his or her various needs have been assessed by the appropriate specialist. Close liaison with the general practitioner is, of course, essential. Vigilance is important: the doctor must be constantly alert to the possibility that a change in behaviour is due to poor vision or hearing, or pain or infection, or other medical problems. Indeed, a strategy for ensuring regular check-ups of teeth, eyesight, and hearing, as well as general health may be appropriate.

Case conferences, particularly if the patient is living in the community, are necessary to ensure that all agencies know what is being done and to identify unmet needs. These conferences will facilitate liaison with social services who, in the United Kingdom at least, play a large part in case management, and can be expected to undertake a community care assessment.

Further reading

American Psychiatric Association (1997). Practice guidelines for the treatment of patients with Alzheimer's disease and other dementias of late life. *American Journal of Psychiatry*, **154** (Supplement 5), 1–39.

Burns, A. and Levy, R. (1994). *Dementia*. Chapman & Hall, London.

Eccles, M., Clarke, J., Livingstone, M., *et al.* (1998). North of England Evidence Based Guidelines Development Project: guideline for the primary care management of dementia. *British Medical Journal*. **317**, 802–8.

Rossor, M.N. (1994). Management of neurological disorders: dementia. *Journal of Neurology, Neurosurgery and Psychiatry*, **57**, 1451–6.

References

1. Lishman, W.A. (1998). *Organic psychiatry: the psychological consequences of cerebral disorder* (3rd edn). Blackwell Science, Oxford.
2. Tobiansky, R., Blizard, R., Livingston, G., and Mann, A. (1995). The Gospel Oak study stage IV: the clinical relevance of subjective memory impairment in older people. *Psychological Medicine*, **25**, 779–86.
3. Folstein, M.F., Folstein, S.E., and McHugh, P.R. (1975). 'Mini-Mental State': a practical method for grading the mental state of patients for the clinician. *Journal of Psychiatric Research*, **12**, 189–98.
4. Siu, A.L. (1991). Screening for dementia and investigating its causes. *Annals of Internal Medicine*, **115**, 122–32.
5. Klein, L.E., Roca, R.P., McArthur, J., *et al.* (1985). Diagnosing dementia: univariate and multivariate analyses of the mental status examination. *Journal of the American Geriatrics Society*, **33**, 483–8.
6. National Institutes of Health (1987). Differential diagnosis of dementing diseases. *National Institutes of Health Consensus Statement*, **6**, 1–27. [http://text.nim.nih.gov/nih/cdc/www/63txt.htm]
7. Alexopoulos, G.S., Abrams, R.C., Young, R.C., *et al.* (1988). Cornell scale for depression in dementia. *Biological Psychiatry*, **23**, 271–8.
8. Yesavage, J.A., Brink, T.L., Rose, T.L., *et al.* (1983). Development and validation of geriatric depression screening scale: a preliminary report. *Journal of Psychiatric Research*, **17**, 37–49.
9. Norman, A. (1989). Models of care in dementia: defining adequate standards. In *Dementia disorders. Advances and prospects* (ed. C.L.E. Katona), pp. 192–210. Chapman & Hall, London.
10. Spector, A. and Orrell, M. (1998). Reality orientation for dementia: a review of the evidence of effectiveness (Cochrane review). In *The Cochrane Library, Issue 3*. Update Software, Oxford.
11. Burnside, I. and Haight, B. (1994). Reminiscence and life review: therapeutic interventions for older people. *Nurse Practitioner*, **19**, 55–61.
12. Jones, G.M.M. (1997). A review of Feil's validation method for communicating with and caring for dementia sufferers. *Current Opinion in Psychiatry*, **10**, 326–32.
13. American Psychiatric Association (1997). Practice guidelines for the treatment of patient's with Alzheimer's disease and other dementias of late life. *American Journal of Psychiatry*, **154** (Supplement 5), 1–39.
14. Ruff, R., Mahaffey, R., Engel, J., Farrow, C., Cox, D., and Katzmark, P. (1994). Efficacy of THINKable in the attention and memory retraining of traumatically head-injured patients. *Brain Injury*, **8**, 3–14.
15. Wood, R.Ll. and Fussey, I. (1987). Computer-based cognitive retraining: a controlled study. *International Disability Studies*, **9**, 149–53.
16. Chen, S.H., Thomas, J.D., Glueckauf, R.L., and Bracy, O.L. (1997). The effectiveness of computer-assisted cognitive rehabilitation for persons with traumatic brain injury. *Brain Injury*, **22**, 197–209.
17. Wehman, P., Sherron, P., Kregel, J., Kreutzer, J., Tran, S., and Cifu, D. (1993). Return to work for persons following severe traumatic brain injury. Supported employment outcomes after five years. *American Journal of Physical Medicine and Rehabilitation*, **72**, 355–63.
18. Rogers, S.L., Farlow, M.R., Doody, R.S., Mohs, R., and Friedhoff, L.T. (1998). A 24-week, double-blind, placebo-controlled trial of donepezil in patients with Alzheimer's disease. *Neurology*, **50**, 136–45.
19. Standing Medical Advisory Committee (1998). *The use of donepezil for Alzheimer's disease*. Department of Health/Pfizer, London.
20. Rosler, M., Anand, R., Cicin-Sain, A., *et al.* (1999). Efficacy and safety of rivastigmine in patients with Alzheimer's disease: international randomised controlled trial. *British Medical Journal*, **318**, 633–8.

21. Taverni, J.P., Seliger, G., and Lichtman, S.W. (1998). Donepezil medicated memory improvement in traumatic brain injury during post acute rehabilitation. *Brain Injury*, **12**, 77–80.

22. Olin, J., Schneider, L., Novit, A., and Luczak, S. (1998). Efficacy of hydergine for dementia (Cochrane review). In *The Cochrane Library, Issue 3*. Update Software, Oxford.

23. Kleijnen, J. and Knipschild, P. (1992). *Ginkgo biloba* for cerebral insufficiency. *British Journal of Clinical Pharmacology*, **34**, 352–8.

24. Folstein, M., Anthony, J.C., Parhad, L., *et al.* (1985). The meaning of cognitive impairment in the elderly. *Journal of the American Geriatrics Society*, **33**, 228–35.

25. Yeager, B.F., Farnett, L.E., and Ruzicka, S.A. (1995). Management of the behavioural manifestations of dementia. *Archives of Internal Medicine*, **155**, 251–60.

26. Bridges-Parlet, B., Knopman, D., and Thompson, T. (1994). A descriptive study of physically aggressive behaviour in dementia by direct observation. *Journal of the American Geriatrics Society*, **42**, 192–7.

27. Eames, P. and Wood, R.Ll. (1985). Rehabilitation after severe brain injury: a follow-up study of a behaviour modification approach. *Journal of Neurology, Neurosurgery and Psychiatry*, **48**, 613–19.

28. Ancill, R.J., Embury, R.P.N., McEwan, G.W., and Kennedy, J.S. (1988). The use and misuse of psychotropic prescribing for elderly psychiatric patients. *Canadian Journal of Psychiatry*, **33**, 585–8.

29. Ray, W.A., Taylor, J.A., Meador, K.G., *et al.* (1993). Reducing antipsychotic drug use in nursing homes: a controlled trial of provider education. *Archives of Internal Medicine*, **153**, 713–21.

30. Schneider, L.S., Pollock, V.E., and Lyness, S.A. (1990). A metaanalysis of controlled trials of neuroleptic treatment in dementia. *Journal of the American Geriatrics Society*, **38**, 553–63.

31. Devanand, D.P., Marder, K., Michaels, K.S., *et al.* (1998). A randomized placebo-controlled, dose-comparison trial of haloperidol for psychosis and disruptive behaviors in Alzheimer's disease. *American Journal of Psychiatry*, **155**, 1512–20.

32. Ballard, C. and O'Brien, J. (1999). Treating behavioural and psychological signs in Alzheimer's disease. *British Medical Journal*, **319**, 138–9.

33. Roth, M., Mountjoy, C.Q., Amrein, R., and the International Collaborative Study Group (1996). Moclobemide in elderly patients with cognitive decline and depression. An international double-blind, placebo-controlled trial. *British Journal of Psychiatry*, **168**, 149–57.

34. Burns, A., Jacoby, R., and Levy, R. (1990). Psychiatric phenomena in Alzheimer's disease. I: Disorders of thought content. *British Journal of Psychiatry*, **157**, 72–6.

35. Skelly, J. and Flint, A.J. (1995). Urinary incontinence associated with dementia. *Journal of the American Geriatrics Society*, **43**, 286–94.

36. Schnelle, J.F., Traughber, B., Sowell, V.A., Newman, D.R., Petrilli, C.O., and Ory, M. (1989). Prompted voiding treatment of urinary incontinence in nursing home patients. A behavior management approach for nursing home staff. *Journal of the American Geriatrics Society*, **37**, 1051–7.

37. Thomson, C. and Thomson, G. (1998). Support for carers of people with Alzheimer's type dementia (Cochrane review). In *The Cochrane Library, Issue 3*. Update Software, Oxford.

38. Eccles, M., Clarke, J., Livingstone, M., *et al.* (1998). North of England evidence based guidelines development project: guideline for the primary care management of dementia. *British Medical Journal*, **317**, 802–8.

39. Murphy, E. (1997). Dementia care in the UK: looking towards the Millenium. In *Advances in old age psychiatry: chromosomes to community care* (ed. C. Holmes and R. Howard), pp. 128–34. Wrightson Biomedical, Petersfield.

4.2 Substance use disorders

4.2.1 Pharmacological and psychological aspects of drugs of abuse

David J. Nutt and Fergus D. Law

Drug abuse, misuse, and addiction are major issues in society because of their enormous personal, social, and economic costs. They also have important psychiatric components. Many drug treatment programmes are run by psychiatrists, and the evidence strongly supports the notion that a significant proportion of severe drug abusers are psychiatrically ill. Moreover, drug misuse is becoming more frequent in patients with other psychiatric disorders, where it can lead to problems in treatment and a poor outcome. It is therefore essential for all psychiatrists and related health professionals to have a good understanding of the basis of drug misuse.

Why do people take drugs?

A very common misconception is that drug misuse is simply a search for fun. In fact, people take drugs for many reasons other than to get the buzz or high. Indeed, studies have shown that straightforward pleasure seeking is the primary reason for initiation of drug use in fewer than 20 per cent of individuals. While the high or buzz is the most obvious pleasurable effect, many people also describe using drugs to feel comfortably numb, pleasantly drowsy, or full of energy and confidence. Many others will be chasing the high or buzz that they first experienced, always trying to attain the intensity of their initial experiences. Still others will be self-medicating for anxiety, strong emotions such as anger, for pain, boredom, lack of motivation, lack of self-confidence, and many other aversive states including withdrawal.

The main reason to try to ascertain the reasons for drug use is that in many cases identification of the cause can lead to effective interventions. For example, many alcoholics will point to anxiety as their reason for drinking;[1] indeed, social anxiety is one of the most common causes of alcoholism in young men.[2] If this can be treated (e.g. by selective serotonin reuptake inhibitors) then they are frequently able to become abstinent or even drink normally. Social anxiety is also a common reason for the use of stimulants by the young. Another psychiatric disorder associated with drug misuse is depression, which is particularly likely to lead to excess alcohol intake. A vicious cycle then develops because both alcohol and its withdrawal are depressogenic. Alcohol is also one of the most serious risk factors for suicide. There is increasing use of stimulants and cannabis by schizophrenic patients. In part this reflects the behaviour of their peer group but the use of stimulants may be in part due to the fact that they can offset some of the more negative aspects of neuroleptic treatment, especially the loss of drive and motivation. As both types of drug can worsen psychotic illness, dealing with drug misuse in this group is a priority.

Other factors affecting drug use may be less amenable to psychiatric intervention, such as pressure from peers or others. For instance, female opiate addicts often have a male partner who also uses drugs or even deals drugs. Following her withdrawal from drugs, relapse is almost certain to occur if she continues to live with this partner. Another reason for drug use is to reduce pain or boredom, the latter being a common reason given by disadvantaged youth in areas of high unemployment and poor environmental quality such as inner cities or out-of-town housing estates.

Other reasons for drug use, generally of psychedelics, include the search for meaning or for mystical experiences. Whilst not directly relevant to psychiatry, this use can precipitate psychotic episodes in susceptible individuals and may act as the trigger for schizophrenia.

Finally, it is important to remember that the reasons for use are not static. An opiate addict may use the same dose of heroin to get going in the morning, to 'top off' a pleasant experience later in the day, to deal with angry feelings when they occur, and to promote sleep at night. Similarly during a drug-using career different motivations may become dominant. This has been well characterized in opiate users where for many the initial exploration was for pleasure or escape. Over months, as physical dependence becomes increasingly apparent, drug use becomes driven by the need to avoid withdrawal and feel normal at all costs.

Drug use and misuse

It is possible to view the issue of drug abuse from different perspectives, which range from the molecular and genetic through the pharmacological to the psychological and social. Each view has its merits and is important, but there is little doubt that an integrated view is necessary, because for most drugs and for most societies no one perspective can explain all the known features of drug abuse. However,

Table 1 Potential problems with drug use

	Examples/effects
Therapeutic use	
Adverse effects	
Drug interactions	
Withdrawal	Anticonvulsants/epilepsy
	Analgesics/pain
Misuse/problem use	
Illegality	Criminal records; social stigmatization
Intoxication	Physical/social damage
Excessive regular use	Physical/social damage
Dependence	
Tolerance	Dose escalation
Withdrawal	Physical dependence
Urge to use/cannot abstain	Psychological dependence
Craving/drug seeking	Drug dominates life
Drug becomes dominant life goal	Personal/social decline
Reinstatement on relapse	Cycles of dependency

for the purposes of this chapter we have concentrated on the psychological and pharmacological.[3]

Problem use, addiction, dependence, and craving

These are some of the most commonly used terms in discussions of drug misuse but at the same time they are also the most problematic. The use of drugs in any circumstance, therapeutic or otherwise, can be associated with problems, although the nature and scale of these varies (see Table 1). The terms problem use and misuse usually refer to use of drugs (presciption or other) for pleasure but with disregard for the personal or social dangers. For example, alcohol misuse can lead to irresponsible behaviour whilst intoxicated and, if prolonged, to liver, gastric, and nervous system damage without the individual neccessarily being addicted or dependent. Another important current example of potentially problematic excessive regular drug use is ecstasy, which may be neurotoxic at doses that are commonly used.

Addiction is a term that had become so misused in general parlance and had acquired such a pejorative edge, that in the past two decades attempts have been made to remove it from the psychiatric lexicon. Unfortunately, the replacement terminology of dependence, or the dependence syndrome, has been similarly devalued by popular usage to the point where it is also almost meaningless. Journalists and even some 'experts' mention dependence on drugs such as caffeine in the same breath as that on heroin. The reality is that there exists a spectrum of dependence ranging from physiological supplementation (as insulin in diabetes mellitus) through to life-altering dependence on illicit drugs such as heroin (see Table 1). Addiction is still a useful construct if it is reserved for the collection of phenomena that occur at the extreme end of the dependence spectrum, and includes concepts such as the social and personal decline as well as tolerance and withdrawal symptoms (cf. DSM-IV and ICD-10).

Another area of some confusion is the distinction between physical and psychological dependence, with its dualistic overtones. When ori-

ginally conceived, this distinction was helpful in that it emphasized that drug dependence was more than just physical adaptation to drugs as manifest by withdrawal symptoms—psychological processes, especially drug liking, were also important. However, drugs without obvious physical withdrawal syndromes (e.g. stimulants) also result in physiological withdrawal changes which clinically are manifested as psychological withdrawal symptoms. In addition, new neuroimaging techniques such as positron emission tomography (**PET**), single-photon emission CT, and functional magnetic resonance imaging are beginning to reveal the brain circuits underlying the pleasurable effects of drugs, and this has resulted in a blurring of the differentiation between the physical and psychological processes. For example, Plate 13 shows a PET scan of heroin addicts in which the brain regions showing increased blood flow activated by craving for heroin are illuminated using the radiotracer oxygen-15. Similar studies have revealed the brain regions involved in the pleasurable effects of opiates and stimulants.[4] Thus there is a clear convergence in terms of mechanisms, but in terms of treatment regimens the distinction between physical and psychological remains.

Craving is also a term that is widely used yet ill defined. Most commonly it is taken to mean a strong and sometimes irresistible desire to use a drug. The emotional valence of craving is not necessarily pleasurable. Craving can reliably be elicited in situations of negative valence. It is commonly found in withdrawal, when it can lead to relapse. Craving can also be present as an urge or desire to use a drug although the sufferer may be actively denying or resisting its presence. The complex interplay of physical and psychological processes is well exemplified by the physical responses that craving can produce. For example when opiate-dependent subjects are shown drug-related paraphernalia they may experience emotions that range from pleasurable anticipation to early withdrawal (shaking, tearing of the eyes, pupil dilatation, etc.). Each one of these experiences can lead to a desire to use the drug, i.e. craving.

Studies in both animals and humans have demonstrated that conditioning occurs to both the positive and negative aspects of craving.[5,6] Tolerance is to a large extent a conditioned response, particularly related to the environmental context in which a drug has been taken.[7] Thus an environmental context which is drug familiar results in physiological changes in the brain in preparation for the drug effect, and thus less actual drug effect occurs (i.e. tolerance). However, in a novel context, such preparatory changes do not occur so that a standard drug dose will result in a larger drug effect and a potentially fatal outcome.[8] Thus the lethality of a drug is largely dependent on the environment in which it is taken.

Attempts have been made to dissect out the subcomponents of craving using questionnaires. The best known of these are the set designed by Tiffany et al.[9] which independently rate the five main subcomponents of craving—urges and desires to use, intention and planning to use, anticipation of positive outcome, anticipation of relief from withdrawal or negative outcome, and loss of control over use. Ongoing neuroimaging studies are beginning to support this multiprocess view of craving by revealing activation or inhibition of different brain regions to be correlated with individual symptom clusters.

There is also increasing evidence that the particular cognitive sets of patients may be important for treatment, especially during withdrawal. Just as panic disorder patients have high anxiety sensitivity and related catastrophic cognitions, addicted patients may have a high fear of craving and other withdrawal symptoms in association with related catastrophic cognitions. This detoxification fear has been measured in opiate addicts, and shown to predict outcome.[10] Other expectations also play a significant role,[11] and a 15- to 30-min explanation of what the opiate detoxification involves may reduce the measured withdrawal distress by over one-third.[12] Indeed, such is the strength of psychological factors in addiction treatment, there is little doubt that drug treatments should always be combined with the appropriate psychological interventions.

Psychological processes and treatment implications

One of the most influential models in addiction treatment is known as the stages of change model.[13,14] The stage of change that a person can be identified as being at determines the therapeutic approach and type of treatment offered. Thus at the precontemplation stage where there is no recognition of a need for treatment, there is no point in offering intensive treatment interventions. Similarly, at the contemplation stage when treatment is being considered, the appropriate intervention is to help the person clarify their views and build their motivation to change rather than offering active treatment. Indeed, it is only in the decision and action stages that treatment should be actively offered and facilitated.

The brief counselling technique of motivational interviewing[15,16] has been proved to improve outcome effectively, and ties in well with the stages of change model. In the early stages the therapy is focused on encouraging the patient to reduce or resolve their ambivalence which acts as their psychological barrier to treatment. The patient in a client-centred but focused therapy is facilitated to discover the solutions to their own problems themselves. This approach of accepting the client's current level of thinking (rather than offering ready-made solutions, or confronting them, or trying to argue them into the solution) has been shown to be surprisingly effective in the clinical trials.[17] The effectiveness of this technique has resulted in a new understanding of motivation, which is seen as a dynamic state rather than as a fixed state, and one which can be influenced by the therapeutic stance.

Other cognitive therapies also make significant contributions to treatment. Relapse prevention involves the teaching of cognitive and behavioural strategies for dealing with high-risk situations and mental states.[18,19] Other cognitive–behavioural therapies, including extinction of conditioning, contingency management, community reinforcement techniques,[20] and indeed Beck's cognitive therapy,[21] have been effectively applied to substance misuse. The recent very large Project MATCH (matching alcoholism treatments to client heterogenity) study of alcohol treatments compared three types of treatment and found that motivational enhancement, 12-step facilitation, and cognitive–behavioural therapy were equally effective overall, although each therapy excelled in certain subgroups.[22,23] Based on these results it seems likely that specific therapies targeted at specific issues of importance in patients with addiction are roughly equally effective overall, but that we do not yet know enough to confidently match specific patient subtypes to specific therapies.

A number of other therapies have also been shown to be effective, particularly in the alcohol field, including self-control training, self-help groups, marital and family therapy, coping and social skills training, anxiety and stress management, aversion therapies, and brief intervention strategies.[24,25]

Personality variables and the genetics of addiction

The role of personality in addiction is a major issue, with some believing in an 'addictive personality' and others suggesting different personality types might predispose to different aspects or forms of drug misuse.[26,27] In this highly controversial field a few facts are generally agreed. Predisposition to experiment with both licit and illicit drugs is more likely in those with sensation-seeking or impulsive behaviour traits, and in extroverts rather than introverts. However, once drug dependence is established, those with obsessional, dependent, or anxious characteristics find it hardest to stop.[28]

The genetics of drug abuse are beginning to be unravelled and already these studies have thrown up some important insights in relation to personality. The best studied dependence is that on alcohol, where the Scandinavian adoption studies have found the risk of alcoholism in male children of male alcoholics is the same regardless of whether the child is reared with the alcoholic father or by a non-drinking adoptive family. Building on these data, Cloninger[27] has identified two main forms of alcoholism. Type I is the late-onset form that has low inheritance and is associated with anxiety and stress which drinking is used to relieve, often in binges. In contrast, type II alcoholism starts at a younger age with a heavy regular intake and is associated with antisocial personality traits and criminality. This form is male limited, is associated with impulsivity, and may be related to underfunctioning of brain 5-hydroxytryptamine systems, as genetic polymorphisms of 5-hydroxytryptamine receptors and enzymes have been found in these subjects.[29]

How abused substances affect the brain

The brain works by transmitting information between neurones using the primary neurotransmitters. The primary neurotransmitters are glutamate, which is stimulatory (i.e. it turns cells on), and the closely related amino acid γ-aminobutyric acid (GABA) which is inhibitory (i.e. it turns neurones off). The appropriate balance between these neurotransmitters leads to the brain processes underlying action, sensation, learning, and memory. Secondary transmitters are the monoamines and peptides such as dopamine, 5-hydroxytryptamine, noradrenaline (norepinephrine), acetylcholine, and endogenous opiates. These add the tone, valence, and emotion to the primary processes, and some such as noradrenaline are important in memory formation. All 'drugs' (probably even solvents through indirect effects) act by interfering with these neurotransmitters in ways summarized in Table 2.[30,31] However, it is important to realize that the brain has its own 'addictive' neurotransmitters. The best known are the endogenous opioid peptides such as the endorphins and enkephalins, but there are also endogenous cannabinoids (anandamide) and probably others.[32] It is not yet known whether these endogenous substances

Table 2 Drugs and transmitters

Drug class	Endogenous transmitter	Treatment implications
Mimic natural transmitters		
Opiates	Endorphins/encephalins	Antagonists (naltrexone), partial agonists (buprenorphine)
Cannabis	Anandamide/others	Antagonists
Alcohol	GABA	GABA modulators?, acamprosate
Benzodiazepines/barbiturates	GABA	Partial agonist benzodiazepines, antagonists (flumazenil)
Nicotine	Acetylcholine	Antagonists (mecamylamine)
Release transmitters		
Cocaine (buproprion)	Dopamine	Other uptake site blockers D_2-receptor antagonists
Amphetamines	Dopamine	As cocaine
Nicotine	Dopamine	As cocaine
Ecstasy	5-HT, dopamine	5-HT uptake blockers/ antagonists
Alcohol, solvents?	NA/DA	NA/DA uptake blockers
Block transmitters		
Alcohol	Glutamate	Glutamate modulators (acamprosate)
Barbiturates	Glutamate	Glutamate modulators
LSD/other psychedelics	5-HT	Antagonists

DA, dopamine; GABA, γ-aminobutyric acid; 5-HT, 5-hydroxytryptamine; NA, noradrenaline.

are mediators of addiction to cannabis or other drugs, although this would certainly seem possible.

What is certain is that some of the most addictive agents (especially the full agonist opiates such as heroin/morphine) act on the endogenous opioid neurotransmitter pathway, but with a much greater effect than the natural transmitter. The profound ability of opiates such as heroin to produce addiction is because these drugs highjack the natural transmitter system leaving normal levels of stimulation seeming tame by comparison, especially early in withdrawal. Treatment with partial agonist opiates such as buprenorphine offer a compromise in that they are less addicting than heroin yet restore some of the brain's deficiency of opiate tone. They also have the advantage of being much safer than full agonists in overdose and rarely cause death from respiratory depression. Other drugs, in particular alcohol, seem to act in part by indirectly stimulating the endogenous opioid system, which is why opioid antagonists such as naltrexone can be useful treatments.[33]

Other drugs act on the natural stimulant transmitter dopamine. Dopamine deficiency (for instance in Parkinson's disease) has long been known to limit motor behaviour. Stimulant drugs increase energy and stamina by increasing the synaptic levels of dopamine, either by increasing the release or by blocking its reuptake in the basal ganglia. Many drugs of addiction can also increase dopamine availability in other brain regions, the two most important being the nucleus accumbens and the prefrontal cortex.[34] A huge body of evidence points to the nucleus accumbens as being a critical gateway in drug misuse. Almost all abused substances (the only exception being the benzodiazepines) act to increase dopamine release in this area.

How they do this varies; cocaine and nicotine act at the level of the dopamine terminals, while heroin and alcohol activate the cell bodies on the brain stem. The net effect is to increase dopamine transmission out of the nucleus accumbens into the basal ganglia and thalamus, frontal cortex, amygdala, and hypothalamus.[26,30]

This circuit is the one that was shown by Olds in the 1950s to sustain electrical self-stimulation and is the brain's own reward circuit. It is normally activated by positive reinforcers, such as food, water, and sex, that are critical to survival. Because drugs of abuse produce greater effects than the natural reinforcers, the resultant effect is that the brain directs its normal drives away from the natural reinforcers and towards the more pleasurable drugs. In severe addiction, which frequently occurs with the most powerful reinforcers (such as heroin and cocaine), all natural drives may be subsumed to an overwhelming search for and use of the drug. Thus addicts may give up sex, grooming, hygiene, and work, hardly eat or drink, and ignore health problems.

The routes and risks of addiction

In addition to the impact of drug misuse on the social aspects of life, it can lead to significant medical problems. The dangers of drug abuse relate to two main factors; the route of use of the drug and the effects it has in the brain outside of the reinforcement circuit.

For most drugs of abuse the faster the drugs reach their target site in the brain the better they are liked and the more psychologically reinforcing they are. Indeed, the 'pharmaceutical' history of most abused drugs illustrates the progressive refinement of their preparation, in order to accelerate their rate of entry into the brain. A good example is cocaine. The Andean Indians originally used it by chewing coca leaves which produced low levels of cocaine over a period of time. An increase in vigour and a resistance to fatigue is produced, but little pleasure. Over the centuries cocaine has become more refined, first to paste and then to cocaine hydrochloride powder (snow) which when taken nasally produces high levels in the brain within 5 to 10 minutes and a clear 'high.' Further refinement to the free base produces a more lipophilic form (crack) that can be smoked, resulting in entry into the brain in seconds. Intravenous drug use also serves the same purpose of getting the drug to the active site very fast.[35]

A similar process of pharmaceutical refinement to accelerate brain entry has taken place with the opiates. Smoking opium is a method of delivering morphine and related substances reasonably quickly but in low amounts. Refining opium into its active constituents (e.g. morphine) means that higher doses are more easily ingested. However, morphine crosses the blood–brain barrier relatively slowly and has therefore been largely supplanted by opiates such as heroin that cross more rapidly. Heroin is a diacetylated synthetic derivative of morphine that is more lipophilic, meaning that it is able to enter the brain more rapidly and give a better rush. Interestingly, the active form of heroin is morphine; heroin has to be deacetylated before it can act, which proves that pharmacokinetic differences are the critical variable with opiate preference. Similarly, codeine is also inactive until metabolized to morphine, but because this happens very slowly codeine has less abuse potential than morphine.

The benzodiazepines were abused relatively rarely until the advent of gel-filled capsules of temazepam. These provided experienced intravenous opiate users with a convenient source of a concentrated drug which they began to experiment with in the late 1980s. In an attempt to stop this, the drug was reformulated in wax. Unphased by this change, the users started heating up the caplets until they melted and then injecting the hot solution into their veins (hot lining). At body temperature the wax solidified and tended to block the veins and arteries (with missed injections) into which it was administered. Severe ischaemia leading to gangrene and the loss of the limb sometimes resulted. Since there are no therapeutic advantages of temazepam over other benzodiazepines that are much less abusable, this drug has recently been put under a higher degree of control in order to deter its prescription.

As well as affecting the relative reinforcing actions of abused drugs, the rate of brain entry also contributes to risk. A very rapid drug entry makes dose adjustments difficult or impossible and so predisposes to overdose. This is most obvious for intravenous use of opiates where respiratory depression is the main cause of death, but is less common with smoked opiates as intake can more easily be titrated to the desired effect.

The route of use also affects risk, most notably with the risk of infection from intravenous use, especially when needles are not cleaned or are shared. The majority of current intravenous users are hepatitis C positive and we can therefore expect cirrhosis to become a major cause of their death in the next decade or so. This also raises ethical and economic issues; interferon treatment significantly reduces the progression of the disease but is costly and its routine use in addicts would be massively expensive and likely to cause public disquiet. The other main infections are hepatitis B and AIDS. The fright-

Table 3 Addictiveness of various agents

	Pleasure giving	Physical withdrawal problems	Psychological withdrawal problems
Opiates	+++	+++	+++
Amphetamines	++	+	++
Crack/cocaine	+++	++	+++
Cannabinoids	+	+	+
Barbiturates	++	+++	++
Benzodiazepines	+	++	++
Ecstasy	++	+	0
Psychedelics	++	+	0
Cigarettes	+++	+	+++
Alcohol	++	+++	++
Caffeine	+	+	+
Gambling	++	0	++

0, none; +, slight; ++, moderate; +++, strong.

ening rise of AIDS in drug abusers, where it occurred faster than in any other group, was the main impetus to the harm-reduction approach becoming the treatment style of the 1990s. Needle-exchange programmes and increased methadone availability were both proven to reduce the spread of AIDS and have become the cornerstone of treatment in many countries.

Relative risks of abused drugs

This is a critical issue in relation to directing legal as well as medical inputs into drug abuse. There are four main factors which have to be taken into account in determining relative risk:

- risk due to the route of use
- risk of the drug itself
- extent drug controls behaviour (addictiveness)
- ease of stopping.

The risks due to the route have been covered above. The risks of the drugs themselves are determined by standard tests and clinical experience and can be encapsulated in concepts such as the therapeutic index. This is the ratio of toxic dose to therapeutic (or usual) dose. The ratio is very low for heroin and similar opiates, for cocaine especially crack, and for intravenous temazepam and oral ecstasy. It is quite high for psychedelics, cannabis, benzodiazepines, and orally used stimulants such as amphetamines. Another important consideration is the health complications of long-term use which by and large reflects the therapeutic index. An exception to this is the opiates, which, provided sterile administration is used, are thought to have little detrimental effect, even when used chronically and intravenously. Chronic cocaine can lead to cardiac damage, and heavy cannabis smoking causes precancerous change in the same way as tobacco smoking, as well as causing greater levels of chronic bronchitis.

The degree of control over behaviour the drug elicits is a major factor in drug dependence, and is the closest concept to addictiveness. Although the route of administration is another critical variable, we can make some reasonable generalizations. Strong opiates and cocaine are the most addictive, being in the same class as nicotine. The benzodiazepines, ecstasy, and psychedelics are the least addictive, and are significantly less addictive than alcohol.

There are three main factors contributing to drugs gaining control over behaviour, all of which affect the ease with which a drug may be stopped. The first is the pleasure a drug produces—the positive drive for use (pleasure giving and seeking). The others both involve the pain of abstinence—withdrawal in both physical and psychological terms—which leads to drug use to relieve it (discomfort escape). The pattern of drug use during an addiction career generally begins with the quest for pleasure and progressively evolves into the escape from withdrawal pain as neuroadaptive processes develop. In this context it may be thought that withdrawal discomfort is best limited to symptoms with a clear physical symptomatology, i.e. the autonomic symptoms indicative of physical dependence. But in terms of addictiveness, psychological withdrawal may in fact be more important than physical withdrawal. This is illustrated by the finding that those dependent on opiates for medical reasons, although physically dependent, experience little craving and risk of relapse once detoxified, provided the reason for being on the opiate resolves. The ease of stopping the drug thus depends on both the physical and psychological withdrawal symptoms, as well as the ability of the drug to provide positive reinforcement.

It is possible to provide rough guides for these three processes for each drug so that the overall addictiveness potential can be gauged (Table 3). For completeness, the main licit drugs are also shown as well as another highly motivated behaviour which can produce a state of addiction/dependence, i.e. gambling.

References

1. George, D.T., Nutt, D.J., Dwyer, B.A., and Linnoila, M. (1990). Alcoholism and panic disorder: is the comorbidity more than coincidence? *Acta Psychiatrica Scandinavica*, **81**, 97–107.
2. Marshall, J.R. (1994). The diagnosis and treatment of social phobia and alcohol abuse. *Bulletin of the Menninger Clinic*, **58**, 58–66.
3. Medical Research Council (1994). *Field review of the basis of drug dependence*. Medical Research Council, London.
4. Schlaepfer, T.E., Strain, E.C., Greenberg, B.D., *et al.* (1998). Site of opioid action in the human brain: mu and kappa agonists' subjective and cerebral blood flow effects. *American Journal of Psychiatry*, **155**, 470–3.
5. McLellan, A.T., Childress, A.R., Ehrman, R., O'Brien, C.P., and Pashko, S. (1986). Extinguishing conditioned responses during opiate dependence treatment: turning laboratory findings into clinical procedures. *Journal of Substance Abuse Treatment*, **3**, 33–40.
6. O'Brien, C.P., Testa, T., O'Brien, T.J., Brady, J.P., and Wells, B. (1997). Conditioned narcotic withdrawal in humans. *Science*, **195**, 1000–2.
7. Goudie, J.G. and Demellweek, C. (1986). Conditioning factors in drug tolerance. In *Behavioral analysis of drug dependence* (ed. S.R. Goldberg and I.P. Stolerman), pp. 225–85. Academic Press, New York.
8. Siegel, S., Hinson, R.E., Krank, M.D., and McCully, J. (1982). Heroin overdose death: contribution of drug-associated environmental cues. *Science*, **216**, 436–7.
9. Tiffany, S.T., Singleton, E., Haertzen, C.A., and Henningfield, J.E. (1993). The development of a cocaine craving questionnaire. *Drug and Alcohol Dependence*, **34**, 19–28.
10. Schumacher, J.E., Milby, J.B., Fishman, B.E., and Higgins, N. (1992). Relation of detoxification fear to methadone maintenance outcome: 5-year follow-up. *Psychology of Addictive Behaviors*, **6**, 41–6.
11. Phillips, G.T., Gossop, M., and Bradley, B. (1986). The influence of psychological factors on the opiate withdrawal syndrome. *British Journal of Psychiatry*, **149**, 235–8.
12. Green, L. and Gossop, M. (1988). Effects of information on the opiate withdrawal syndrome. *British Journal of Addiction*, **83**, 305–9.
13. Prochaska, J.O. and DiClemente, C. (1983). Stages and processes of self-change of smoking: towards a more integrative model of change. *Journal of Consulting and Clinical Psychology*, **51**, 390–5.
14. Prochaska, J.O. (ed.) (1994). *Changing for good*. Avon Books, New York.
15. Rollnick, S. and Miller, W.R. (1995). What is motivational interviewing? *Behavioural and Cognitive Psychotherapy*, **23**, 325–34.
16. Miller, W.R. and Rollnick, S. (ed.) (1991). *Motivational interviewing: preparing people to change addictive behaviour*. Guilford Press, New York.
17. Noonan, W.C. and Moyers, T.B. (1997). Motivational interviewing. *Journal of Substance Misuse*, **2**, 8–16.
18. Marlatt, G.A. and Gordon, J.R. (ed.) (1985). *Relapse prevention: maintenance strategies in the treatment of addictive behaviors*. Guilford Press, New York.
19. Wanigaratne, S., Wallace, W., Pullin, J., Keaney, F., and Farmer, R. (ed.) (1990). *Relapse prevention for addictive behaviours: a manual for therapists*. Blackwell, London.
20. Stitzer, M.L. and Higgins, S.T. (1995). Behavioral treatment of drug and alcohol abuse. In *Psychopharmacology: the fourth generation of progress* (ed. F.E. Bloom and D.J. Kupfer), pp. 1807–19. Raven Press, New York.
21. Beck, A.T., Wright, F.D., Newman, C.F., and Liese, B.S. (ed.) (1993). *Cognitive therapy of substance abuse*. Guilford Press, New York.
22. Project MATCH Research Group (1997). Matching alcoholism treatments to client heterogenity: Project MATCH postreatment drinking outcomes. *Journal of Studies on Alcohol*, **58**, 7–29.
23. Project MATCH Research Group (1997). Project MATCH secondary *a priori* hypotheses. *Addiction*, **92**, 1671–98.
24. Miller, W.R., Brown, J.M., Simpson, T.L., *et al.* (1995). What works? A methodological analysis of the alcohol treatment outcome literature. In *Handbook of alcoholism treatment approaches: effective alternatives* (2nd edn) (ed. R.K. Hester and W.R. Miller), pp. 12–44. Allyn and Bacon, Boston, MA.
25. Edwards, E. and Dare, C. (ed.). (1996). *Psychotherapy, psychological treatments and the addictions*. Cambridge University Press.
26. Altman, S.J., Everitt, B.J., Glautier. S., *et al.* (1996). The biological, social and clinical bases of drug addiction: commentary and debate. *Psychopharmacology*, **125**, 285–345.
27. Cloninger, C.R. (1987). Neurogenetic adaptive mechanisms in alcoholism. *Science*, **236**, 410–16.
28. Tyrer, P. (1989) Risks of dependence on benzodiazepine drugs: the importance of patient selection. *British Medical Journal*, **298**, 102–5.
29. Nielsen, D.A., Goldman, D., Virkkunen, M., Tokola, R., Rawlings, R. and Linnoila, M. (1994). Suicidality and 5-hydroxyindoleacetic acid concentration associated with a tryptophan hydroxylase polymorphism. *Archives of General Psychiatry*, **51**, 34–8
30. Nutt, D.J. (1997). Neuropharmacological basis for tolerance and dependence. In *Drug addiction and its treatment: nexus of neuroscience and behavior* (ed. B.A. Johnson and J.D. Roache), pp. 171–86. Raven Press, New York.
31. Nutt, D.J. (1999). Alcohol and the brain: pharmacological insights for psychiatrists. *British Journal of Psychiatry*, **174**, 114–19.
32. Nutt, D.J. (1996). Addiction: brain mechanisms and their treatment implications. *Lancet*, **347**, 31–6.
33. Volpicelli, J.R., Alterman, A.I., Hayashida, M. and O'Brien, C.P. (1993). Naltrexone in the treatment of alcohol dependence. *Archives of General Psychiatry*, **49**, 876–80.
34. Di Chiara, G. (1995). The role of dopamine in drug abuse viewed from the perspective of its role in motivation. *Drug and Alcohol Dependence*, **38**, 95–137.
35. Nutt, D.J. (1994). The changing pharmacology of addiction. In *Addictions: process of change* (ed. G. Edwards and M. Lader), pp. 33–49. Oxford University Press.

4.2.2 Alcohol use disorders
4.2.2.1 Aetiology of alcohol problems

Juan C. Negrete

Introduction

Alcohol is one of the most widely used psychoactive substances; approximately eight out of every 10 persons living in Europe and the Americas would report drinking in their lifetime.[1] The norm is for drinking to start in adolescence: close to 50 per cent of American students have had drinking experiences by the age of 13 years and the rate increases to 81.7 per cent at age 17.[2] In Canada, 78 per cent of persons aged 15 years or more are current alcohol users, with 12 per cent of the men and 3 per cent of the women falling within the drinker-at-risk category (i.e. 14 units per week or more). This is the level of use associated with the highest probability of occurrence of untoward consequences. Higher frequencies of drinking (i.e. four or more times per week) are observed in the older age groups, while a heavy intake per single drinking occasion (i.e. five units or more) is more often reported by the population younger than 35 years of age.[3]

The figures displayed in Table 1 are from a random selection of general population surveys of alcohol abuse and alcohol dependence, conducted in four separate countries. The rates elicited indicate that the largest proportion of alcohol users do not develop those clinical disorders. In fact, it has been shown that drinkers who limit their average intake to no more than two standard units per day may even derive some health benefits from alcohol, such as a lower risk of coronary disease.[4] Screening questionnaires such as CAGE, a four-item instrument which rates the probability of alcoholism, identify around 20 per cent of the adult population as probable alcohol misusers. More stringent procedures, which apply full diagnostic criteria, yield point prevalence rates ranging from 5.4 to 7.4 per cent, depending on whether the clinical disorder surveyed is strictly alcohol dependence or any form of harmful drinking (i.e. dependence plus alcohol abuse). These figures are total population percentages; the rates for men are about double those for women.

Alcohol can be used in a relatively harmless manner and there exist public health guidelines on 'safe' drinking practices. The recommendations vary considerably from country to country, but they all assume a greater vulnerability to alcohol effects in the female gender. In the United Kingdom, for instance, hazardous drinking is thought to start at 21 units/week for men and 16 units/week for women;[5] in Canada the upper limit for moderate drinking is estimated at 14 and 12 units/week respectively[6] and in the United States the equivalent guidelines are 14 and 7 drinks per week.[7]

The expression 'alcohol problems' encompasses a wide range of untoward occurrences, from maladaptive, impaired, or harmful social behaviours, to health complications and the condition of alcohol dependence. Alcohol problems are not incurred just by chronic excessive drinkers, but also by persons who drink heavily on isolated occasions (e.g. accidents, violence, poisoning, etc.). Given their high frequency and social costs, these consequences of acute inebriation represent the most significant public health burden of drinking.[8]Figure 1 This section focuses rather on the causes of problems of a clinical nature, the ones presented by individuals who engage in patterns of repeated excessive drinking, i.e. 'alcohol dependence' and 'alcohol abuse' (DSM-IV nomenclature) or 'harmful drinking' (ICD-10 nomenclature).

Alcohol misuse is a bio-psychosocial phenomenon *par excellence*; it results from the contribution of multiple individual and environmental risk factors. Causal mechanisms have been proposed by researchers in fields as diverse as social sciences, behavioural psychology, psychopathology, genetics, pharmacology, toxicology, and neurobiology. But none of them, in isolation, provides a complete explanation for the

Table 1 Prevalence of alcohol misuse

Site/criterion	Year	Sample	Rates (%)		
			Men	**Women**	**Total**
USA/ICD-10 alcohol dependence	1990	General population age 18+	7.8	3.4	5.4
USA/DSM-IV alcohol abuse and dependence	1992	General population age 18+	11.0	4.1	7.4
New Zealand Question: 'Felt the need to cut down but unable to'	1988	General population age 14–65	9.0	6.0	7.5
Austria/CAGE score ≥ 2 score = 4	1995–1996	General population 'adults'	— —	— —	20.0 2.2
England/CAGE score ≥ 2 Question (morning drinking)	1993–1994	Heavier drinking adults (♂ 21+ units; ♀ 14+ units/week)	19.0 15.0	16.0 10.0	—

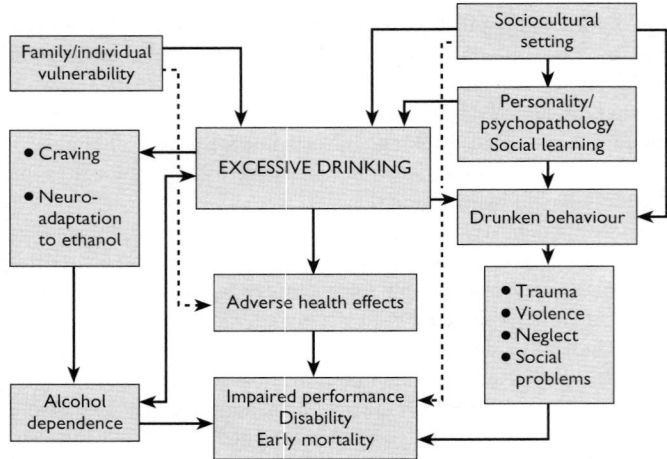

Fig. 1 The causality of alcohol problems.

occurrence of this problem. is a depiction of the interactions assumed to play a role in the genesis of alcoholism. It identifies excessive drinking as the *sine qua non* component in the equation. Heavy drinking is sometimes fostered by sociocultural conditions, but it might result also from individual predispositions of a genetic, neurobiological, or psychopathological nature. It is usually the combined effect of several of these factors that determines the development of an alcohol dependence, or the occurrence of harmful drunken behaviour in a given individual.

Background to the current notions of alcoholism

Two very different schools of thought attract the largest following at the moment—the social learning and the disease models of alcoholism. The former is a relatively recent development, mainly since the 1970s.[9] It contends that alcohol misuse is an acquired behaviour which the individual is capable of correcting with adequate cognitive–behavioural training; even to the point of relearning to drink in a 'controlled' manner.[10] Thus, the learning model tends to play down the importance of predisposing factors, and to ignore the variance in individual biological responses to alcohol, or the brain changes caused by chronic intoxication. Indeed, it assumes that all alcoholics are basically the same and that they are not different from any other drinker in their capacity to exert control over alcohol use.

In marked conceptual contrast, the inability to restrict the quantity or frequency of drinking is a key notion in the disease or 'medical' model of alcoholism.[11] This anomaly is thought to result from heavy alcohol exposure, or else to pre-exist in constitutionally vulnerable individuals. This model further suggests that, once in place, such loss of control over drinking is irreversible.

Learning theorists currently object to the disease concept on scientific grounds, but this modern argument is very much the continuation of old ideological debates on the nature of alcoholism. Pioneer medical authors such as T. Trotter in the early 1800s, Magnus Huss, who coined the term alcoholism in 1849, and the founders of the American and British Societies for the Study of Inebriety towards the end of the nineteenth century had already maintained that the disorder involves the loss of voluntary control over drinking,[12] and this is still the opinion of an important sector of the scientific community today.[13] Moralists of the turn of the century opposed that notion

because it exempts the drinker from personal blame. Of course, they viewed any form of drinking as intrinsically wrong, and alcohol itself as an evil which should be eliminated through prohibition.

The leaders of the 1960s 'antipsychiatry' movement thought this disease entity to be nothing but a self-serving concoction of the medical profession.[11] According to these ideologists, alcoholics are always capable of choosing whether or not to drink, and must assume full responsibility for their behaviour. Thus, by denying the existence of a pathological process, today's supporters of the social learning model find themselves defending the same ideas as the old temperance preachers and the detractors of psychiatry.

This chapter is an eclectic summary of the aetiological theories on alcoholism, most of which view alcohol dependence as ill health.

Sociocultural factors

It is an undisputed fact that the prevalence of alcohol problems varies markedly across different cultural and social settings; that certain environmental conditions appear to facilitate their occurrence while others seem to prevent them.[14] Macrocultural influences such as values, beliefs, and mores; social role functions; local economy; customs and dietary habits; rapid social change; and cultural stress do shape and dictate the way alcohol is used in human societies. But even within a single society, there is variance in the alcohol problems profile of different subgroups. For instance, drinking, heavy drinking, alcohol use disorders, and treatment for alcoholism are more frequently recorded in men than women,[1] the risk of hospital admission for alcoholic psychosis, acute intoxication, and liver cirrhosis is elevated in unskilled and blue collar workers when compared with higher occupational categories,[15] alcoholics are over-represented in occupations with flexible work schedules, in those less supervised, and in the ones which facilitate access to alcohol,[16] and although there are a larger proportion of regular alcohol users among the older, the wealthier, and the better educated, frequency of heavy drinking (i.e. episodes of intoxication, 5+ drinks at a time) is inversely correlated with age, income, and level of education.[3,17]

Cultural beliefs about drinking and related social norms largely determine the manner in which alcohol is used. Disorderly conduct and drunken violence are more likely to occur in societies which, while allowing drinking, do view alcohol as an evil substance.[18] Similar consequences can be expected if drunkenness is culturally considered as a 'time out,' when socially unacceptable behaviours are tolerated or excused.[19] In fact, the social condoning of drunkenness is considered as an epidemiological risk factor.[14]

The very availability of alcohol and the social promotion of frequent or heavy drinking are examples of social risk. But environmental facilitation *per se* does not explain the genesis of an alcohol dependence in specific individuals. This disorder is best understood as the result of social prompting and individual vulnerabilities. However, an individual predisposition is likely to play a lesser role in high availability societies with strong drinking traditions. Conversely, in 'dry' cultures, where drunkenness or even drinking itself are viewed as deviant behaviours, alcohol abusers would tend to be more 'abnormal' individuals capable of disregarding the stronger social barriers against drinking.[12]

Box 1

Sociocultural risk factors

- Male role
- Lower education
- Lower income
- Marital breakdown
- Certain occupations
- Idleness
- Cultural ambivalence towards drinking
- Self-fulfilling prophesy
- Socially condoned drunkenness
- Anomie/marginalization
- Social stress

Individual vulnerability

Genetic influences

The most powerful predictor of alcohol misuse in any individual is the occurrence of alcoholism in first-degree relatives. Men and women belonging to families with alcoholic parents and/or siblings are twice as likely to develop the disorder than those without such family history. The risk is threefold when the disorder is present also in second- or third-degree relatives.[20] More comprehensive analyses demonstrate that family aggregation is true as well for addictive substances other than alcohol.[21] The excess probability observed within single family groups suggests that alcohol misuse could be a genetically transmitted behaviour, and several research approaches have been used to explore this aetiological pathway.

Twin studies

The comparison of concordance rates for alcoholism in monozygotic and dizygotic twins permits to test the genetic basis of the disorder. Since monozygotic pairs have a common genetic stock, while dizygotic ones share on average only 50 per cent of their genes, any condition of genetic origin would be found to co-occur more in them than in fraternal twins. Most studies to date have elicited significantly higher concordance in identical twins, although the rates never reach the perfect 100 per cent level.

Using general population prevalence rates as reference, to have an alcoholic monozygotic sibling markedly increases the chances of developing alcoholism; risk ratio values ranging from 11.8 to 3.9 have been found.[22] Dizygotic co-twins of alcoholics also present elevated risk ratios, but to a lesser degree, in keeping with their lower concordance rates.[22] The earlier studies included male twins only and the applicability of their findings to female siblings was uncertain. However, more recent data from a large sample of female twins indicates an equally strong genetic influence in women's alcoholism.[23]

The significance of those observations notwithstanding, it must be noted that between 40 and 70 per cent of the identical co-twins of alcoholics do not present the disorder, and that such variance can only be due to non-genetic causes.

Adoption studies

The study of adopted-away children of alcoholic parents is a powerful approach to the elucidation of the nature of the family transmission of alcoholism. A genetic vulnerability, of course, should express itself even when such children are brought up by non-alcoholic adoptive parents. All adoption studies consistently report an increased risk in these offspring, regardless of the family environment where they grow up. The probability of occurrence in the probands is much higher than in the control adoptees. This was demonstrated with Danish (risk ratio 3.6), Swedish (risk ratio 1.3), and American (risk ratios 3.5 and 3.6) samples.[22] As in the case of the twin studies, the original research with adoptees was inconclusive with respect to female alcoholism, either because women were excluded from the samples or because their small numbers limited the power of statistics. However, additional work has demonstrated the significant influence of parental alcoholism on women as well, particularly when the affected biological parent is the mother.[23,24]

The offspring of alcoholic parents are unquestionably exposed to an excess risk, but the understanding of the exact pathway of familial transmission is still limited. A more detailed analysis of the adoption data shows that the biological parents of alcoholic adoptees, when compared to the controls, are not only more likely to present alcoholism but also antisocial behaviour.[25] Antisocial personality is also significantly more prevalent in alcohol-abusing adoptees than in controls. The evidence indicates that the alcoholism–antisocial personality tandem is much more 'inheritable' than alcoholism alone. In decreasing order of significance, alcohol abuse in adoptees is predicted by their own antisocial personality, biological parents' alcoholism, biological parents' antisocial history, and, to a much lesser degree, history of alcoholism or psychopathology in the adoptive parents.

Biological predisposition

Alcohol sensitivity

Compared to controls, a significantly larger percentage of men with family history of alcoholism present a lesser physiological response to alcohol; in terms of both subjective sensations and objective measurements (postconsumption plasma cortisol levels and body sway). A lower sensitivity is assumed to lead to heavier drinking and predicts the eventual development of alcoholism. The authors of this prospective follow-up study concluded that the 'innate' low response to alcohol is an independent risk factor, regardless of family history.[26]

Related research findings indicate that men with multigenerational family history of alcoholism tend to derive a greater anxiolytic effect from alcohol. Under experimental conditions, and after drinking an intoxicating dose, their cardiovascular response to acute stress is more attenuated than that of controls.[27] Such increased effects can be expected to reinforce heavy drinking.

Biochemical markers

On average, alcoholics have lower than normal levels of platelet serotonin and of its metabolite 5-hydroxyindole acetic acid in cerebrospinal fluid; especially the problem drinkers who exhibit impulsive and violent behaviour. This serotonin deficiency profile was also found to be abnormally prevalent in young adults with a family history of alcoholism.[28]

The monoamine oxidase enzyme is of interest to alcohol researchers because it participates in the breakdown of neurotransmitters which are involved in the brain action of alcohol. Abnormally low levels of monoamine oxidase platelet activity were found to be linked to a family history of alcoholism, as well as to an earlier age of onset and a higher severity of the disorder.[29]

Both these biochemical deviations seem to be more significant among male than female subjects, and to be strongly associated with antisocial behaviour.

Neurophysiology

Event-related potentials

Alcoholics have been found to present a lower than normal amplitude of the P300 wave, when such brain potential is evoked through complex visuomotor tasks. The P300 potential is thought to measure attentional and memory processes, and its amplitude tends to increase with age and neurological maturity. Subsequent work demonstrated that low P300 amplitude could be observed also in young offspring of alcoholics, both male and female, who had not yet started drinking. It is consequently suggested that such neurophysiological finding might be a biological marker of biological vulnerability to alcoholism.[30] However, P300 anomalies are not specific to alcoholism and are observed also in other psychiatric disorders.

Molecular genetics

As is the case with most health disorders, a very active search is being conducted to identify the genes responsible for the alcohol misuse phenotype. It was originally reported that a variant (Taql-A1 allele) of the human dopamine receptor gene DRD2 was more prevalent in alcoholics than in controls (linkage disequilibrium), and that this allele could be a marker for heightened responsiveness to pharmacological stimulation (i.e. increased baseline positive reinforcement). However, subsequent research has shown that such genetic variance exists across ethnic groups, and that it is not even a consistent finding in all samples of alcoholics.[31]

There is little doubt that alcohol abuse will be found to be a polygenic disorder. The genetically influenced traits assumed to underlie responses to alcohol are quantitative traits. A section of DNA in a chromosome thought to influence a particular quantitative trait is known as a quantitative trait locus. The mapping of quantitative trait loci permits to locate and measure the effects of a single quantitative trait locus on a trait (phenotype). The quantitative trait locus findings available to date pertain mostly to laboratory animals, and markers of genetically transmitted responses such as alcohol-induced hypothermia and alcohol drinking preference have been reliably located in specific chromosomes.[28]

The first genome-wide screens for alcoholism in humans have produced evidence of several chromosomal regions linked to alcohol dependence. A conclusive finding so far is a 'protective' locus near the alcohol dehydrogenase gene cluster in chromosome 4.[32] Ethanol and acetaldehyde metabolizing enzymes, of course, are known to vary across different ethnic populations, and such heterogeneity is assumed to play a role in the cross-ethnic variance of alcoholism prevalence rates.[33] The Collaborative Study on the Genetics of Alcoholism researchers report[34] that the linkage analysis of *severe* alcohol

dependence has identified a locus on chromosome 16, near the marker D16S675.

Box 2

Evidence of a constitutional predisposition to alcohol misuse

- Significantly increased concordance rates in monozygotic twins
- Elevated risk for children of alcoholics, even when raised by adoptive parents
- Greater innate tolerance for the intoxicating effects of alcohol
- Associated biochemical and neurophysiological anomalies (markers)
- Linkage of both resilient and vulnerable phenotypes with chromosomal loci

Psychological factors

Personality

It is now widely accepted that alcoholics do not present a homogeneous premorbid personality profile. However, some distinctive trait clusters have been identified which seem to characterize different types of alcoholics.[35] One such group (type 1) tend to score low in novelty seeking and high in harm avoidance and reward dependence. Another group (type 2) is formed by the natural thrill seekers, who appear to ignore harmful consequences and punitive responses. This latter cluster, which prevails mostly in males with early-onset alcoholism, is also typical of antisocial personalities. Of all personality features, conduct disorder and antisocial behaviour are the strongest predictors of alcohol misuse.[36] However, more than half the alcoholic population do not have such a personality background, presenting rather with a non-specific mixture of the different personality types described in clusters A, B, and C of the DSM-IV classification.[37]

Psychodynamic processes

In keeping with a 'topographic' notion of psychic structure, early psychodynamic writings viewed alcoholism and other addictions as regressive behaviours caused by unconscious conflicts about libidinal pleasures, homosexuality, and aggression. More recent formulations emphasize ego and self-developmental problems, and consider psychoactive substance abuse as a response to psychological suffering; an attempt at re-establishing homeostasis. This is known as the self-medication hypothesis of addictions,[38] according to which, persons with self-regulatory deficiencies in the areas of self-care, self-esteem, self-object relations, and affect tolerance, would drink to palliate their distress.

Learning

An important sector of the scientific community considers alcohol abuse as a behavioural pattern which has been learned through mechanisms of classical (i.e. Pavlovian) and operant conditioning. According to this interpretation, the perpetuation of heavy drinking results from its association with conditioned stimuli (cues), and from the action of positive (pleasant effects) or negative (stress reduction) behavioural reinforcement.[39] Additional components of this equation are the so-called alcohol 'expectancies'. Alcohol abusers tend to overemphasize the pleasant aspects of drinking and to exclude the negative ones; the learning theory of alcoholism assumes that such a cognitive set is also acquired through social exposure.[28]

Psychiatric comorbidity

Community and clinical epidemiology findings point to the presence of other psychiatric disorders as one of the most significant psychological risk factors in alcoholism. The risk is particularly high in persons with schizophrenia, bipolar disorder, major depression, social phobia, panic disorder, post-traumatic stress, attention-deficit hyperactivity disorder, and antisocial and borderline personality disorders.[40]

A major confounder in the interpretation of these findings is the poor specificity of psychiatric symptoms in the alcoholic population. A large proportion of the disorders diagnosed are alcohol induced and tend to dissipate in conditions of abstinence. This evidence led some authors to conclude that most of the excess psychopathology observed in alcoholics is secondary to alcoholism rather than a pre-existing risk factor.[41] It has also been suggested that the coexistence of alcoholism with other psychiatric illnesses (e.g. affective disorders) does not necessarily mean that one is causing the other, but rather that they both result from a common genetic influence.[42]

Brain dysfunction

Altered neuropsychological function can be seen as an additional risk factor in alcoholism: minimal brain damage, attention deficit, learning disabilities, head injuries, fetal alcohol effects, or the actions of other drugs of abuse are examples of brain conditions likely to increase individual vulnerability. Moreover, a transketolase deficiency (possibly genetic), which affects carbohydrate metabolism in the brain, is believed to predispose towards the occurrence of alcoholic organic brain complications.[43]

Conclusions

Several risk factors have been identified which appear to predict the occurrence of the following alcohol-related phenomena: excessive drinking, untoward drunken behaviour, the development of alcohol dependence and its severity, alcohol-induced organ damage, and some neuropsychiatric complications. However, the causal link between such factors and their putative consequences is only partially established, and a sizeable portion of the variance remains largely unexplained.

References

1. Edwards, G., Anderson, P., Babor, T.F., *et al.* (1994). *Alcohol policy and the public good.* Oxford University Press.
2. National Institute on Drug Abuse (1998). Monitoring the future study: trends in drug use among 8th, 10th and 12th graders. *NIDA Notes*, **13**, 15.
3. Health and Welfare Canada (1992). *Alcohol and other drug use by Canadians: a national alcohol and other drug survey (1989) technical report.* Health and Welfare Canada,. Ottawa.
4. Hanna, E.Z., Chou, S.P., and Grant, B.F. (1997). The relationship between drinking and heart disease morbidity in the United States: results from the National Health Interview Survey. *Alcohol: Clinical and Experimental Research*, **21**, 111–18.
5. Royal College of General Practitioners (1986). *Alcohol—a balanced view.* Royal College of General Practitioners, London.
6. Royal College of Physicians and Surgeons of Canada (1990). *Health and public policy committee statement on alcohol and alcohol-related problems.* Royal College of Physicians and Surgeons of Canada, Ottawa.
7. O'Connor, P.G. and Schottenfeld, R.S.(1998). Patients with alcohol problems. *The New England Journal of Medicine*, **338**, 592–602.
8. Single, E., Robson, L., Xie, X., and Rhem, J. (1996). *The costs of substance abuse in Canada.* Canadian Centre on Substance Abuse, Ottawa.
9. Marlatt, G.A. and Donovan, D.M. (1982). Behavioural psychology approaches to alcoholism. In *Encyclopedic handbook of alcoholism* (ed. E.M. Pattison and E. Kaufman), pp. 560–76. Gardner Press, New York.
10. Annis, H.M. and Davis, C.S. (1988). Assessment of expectancies. In *Assessment of addictive behaviors* (ed. D.M. Donovan and G.A. Marlatt), pp. 84–111. Guilford Press, New York.
11. Keller, M. (1976). The disease concept of alcoholism revisited. *Journal of Studies on Alcohol*, **37**, 1694–717.
12. Jellinek, E.M. (1960). *The disease concept of alcoholism.* Hillhouse Press, New Brunswick, NJ.
13. Lyvers, M. (1998). Drug addiction as a physical disease: the role of physical dependence and other chronic drug-induced neurophysiological changes in compulsive drug self-administration. *Experimental and Clinical Psychopharmacology*, **6**, 107–25.
14. Blacker, E. (1966). Sociocultural factors in alcoholism. *International Psychiatry Clinics*, **3** (2), 51–80.
15. Hemmingsson, T., Lundberg, I., Romelsjo, A., *et al.* (1997). Alcoholism in social classes and occupations in Sweden. *International Journal of Epidemiology*, **26**, 584–91.
16. Mandell, W., Eaton, W.W., Anthony, J.C., *et al.* (1992). Alcoholism and occupations: a review of 104 occupations. *Alcohol: Clinical and Experimental Research*, **16**, 734–46.
17. Dawson, D.A., Grant, B.F., Chou, S.P., *et al.* (1995). Subgroup variation in U.S. drinking patterns: results of the 1992 national longitudinal alcohol epidemiological study. *Journal of Substance Abuse*, **7**, 331–44.
18. Merton, R.K. (1972). *Social theory and social structure.* Free Press, New York.
19. Heath, D.B. (1993). Recent developments in alcoholism: anthropology. *Recent Developments in Alcoholism*, **11**, 29–43.
20. Dawson, D.A., Harford, T.C., and Grant B.F. (1992). Family history as predictor of alcohol dependence. *Alcoholism: Clinical and Experimental Research*, **16**, 572–5.
21. Bierut, L.J., Dinwiddie, S.H., Begleiter, H., *et al.* (1998). Familial transmission of substance dependence: a report from the Collaborative Study on the Genetics of Alcoholism. *Archives of General Psychiatry*, **55**, 982–8.
22. Heath, A.C. (1995). Genetic influences in alcoholism; a review of adoption and twin studies. *Alcohol Health and Research World*, **19**, 166–71.
23. Kendler, K.S., Heath, A.C., Neale, M.C., *et al.* (1994). A twin-family study of alcoholism in women. *American Journal of Psychiatry*, **151**, 707–15.
24. Allgulander, C., Nowak, J., and Rice, J.P. (1992). Psychopathology and treatment of 30 344 twins in Sweden. *Acta Psychiatrica Scandinavica*, **86**, 421–2.
25. Cadoret, R.J., Yates, W.R., Troughton, E., *et al.* (1995). Adoption study demonstrating two genetic pathways to drug abuse. *Archives of General Psychiatry*, **52**, 42–52.
26. Schuckit, M.A., Tsuang, J.W., Anthenelli, R.M., *et al.* (1996). Alcohol challenges in young men from alcoholic pedigrees and control families: a report from the COGA project. *Journal of Studies on Alcohol*, **57**, 368–77.
27. Finn, P.R., Earleywine, M., and Pihl, R.O. (1992). Sensation-seeking, stress reactivity and alcohol dampening discriminate the density of a family history of alcoholism. *Alcoholism: Clinical and Experimental Research*, **16**, 585–90.

28. National Institute on Alcohol Abuse and Alcoholism (1997). *Ninth Special Report to the US Congress on Alcohol and Health From the Secretary of Health and Human Services*. US Department of Health and Human Services, Washington, DC.

29. Anthenelli, R.M., Tipp J., Li, T.K., *et al.* (1998). Platelet monoamino oxidase (MAO) activity in subgroups of alcoholics and controls: results from the COGA study. *Alcoholism: Clinical and Experimental Research*, **22**, 598–604.

30. Hill, S.Y., Steinhouser, S.R., Lowers, L., *et al.* (1995). Eight year longitudinal follow-up of P300 and clinical outcome in children from high risk for alcoholism families. *Biological Psychiatry*, **37** (11), 823–7.

31. Gelernter, J., Kranzler, H., and Cubells, J.F. (1998). DRD2 allele frequencies and linkage disequilibria, including the -141C *Ins/Del* promoter polymorphism, in European-American, African-American and Japanese subjects. *Genomics*, **51**, 21–6.

32. Goate, A.M. and Edenberg, H.J. (1998). The genetics of alcoholism. *Current Opinion in Genetics and Development*, **8**, 282–6.

33. Maezawa, Y., Yamauchi, M., Toda, G., *et al.*(1995). Alcohol metabolizing enzyme polymorphisms and alcoholism in Japan. *Alcoholism: Clinical and Experimental Research*, **19**, 951–4.

34. Foroud, T., Bucholz, K.K., Edenberg, H.J., *et al.* (1998). Linkage of an alcoholism-related severity phenotype to chromosome 16. *Alcoholism: Clinical and Experimental Research*, **22**, 2035–42.

35. Cloninger, C.R. (1987). Neurogenetic adaptive mechanisms in alcoholism. *Science*, **236**, 410–16.

36. Harford, T.C. and Parker, D.A. (1994). Antisocial behaviour, family history and alcohol dependence syndrome. *Alcoholism: Clinical and Experimental Research*, **18**, 265–8.

37. Driessen, M., Veltrup, C., Wetterling, T., *et al.* (1998). Axis I and Axis II comorbidity in alcohol dependence and the two types of alcoholism. *Alcoholism: Clinical and Experimental Research*, **22**, 77–86.

38. Khantzian, E.J. (1985). The self-medication hypothesis of addictive disorders. *American Journal of Psychiatry*, **142**, 1259–64.

39. Wilson, G.T. (1988). Alcohol use and abuse: a social learning analysis. In *Theories on alcoholism* (ed. C.D. Chaudron and D.A. Wilkinson), pp. 239–287. Addiction Research Foundation, Toronto.

40. Kessler, R.C., McConagle, K.A., Zhao, S., *et al.* (1994). Lifetime and 12 month prevalence of DSM-III-R psychiatric disorders in the United States. *Archives of General Psychiatry*, **51**, 8–19.

41. Schuckit, M.A. and Hesselbrock, V. (1994). Alcohol dependence and anxiety disorders: what is the relationship? *American Journal of Psychiatry*, **151**, 1723–34.

42. Winokur, G., Coryell, W., Endicott, J., *et al.* (1996). Familial alcoholism in manic-depressive (bipolar) disease. *American Journal of Medical Genetics*, **67**, 197–201.

43. Martin, P.R., Adinoff, B., Weingartner, H., *et al.* (1986). Alcoholic organic brain disease: nosology and pathophysiologic mechanisms. *Progress in Neuro-Psychopharmacology and Biological Psychiatry*, **10**, 147–64.

4.2.2.2 Alcohol dependence and alcohol problems

Jane Marshall

Introduction

The problem of excessive alcohol consumption is a major cause of public health concern in most countries of the world today. Heavy consumption, which involves far more than 'dependence', can cause untold misery to the individual, who is usually affected by other physical, psychological, and social disabilities as well.

As early as 1950, the World Health Organization (**WHO**) viewed the lack of a commonly accepted terminology as a serious obstacle to international action in the alcohol field.[1]

Definitions of 'alcoholism' have been proposed by a range of professional and other bodies, from biomedical scientists, medical doctors and psychiatrists, psychologists, sociologists, patients in treatment, to the general public.[2] Terms such as 'alcoholism', 'addiction', and 'chemical dependence', have passed into everyday speech, becoming 'popularly enriched' and 'technically impoverished'.[2] These terms mean different things to different people and often have pejorative connotations. The lack of a precise definition of 'drinking problems' has hampered interdisciplinary communication.

In this section the evolution of the term 'alcohol dependence' will be traced and put into context as but one aspect of a wider spectrum of alcohol-related problems. The concept of the alcohol dependence syndrome[3] will be discussed. Its influence on the 10th revision of the *International Classification of Diseases*[4] and the most recent versions of the *Diagnostic and Statistical Manual of Diseases* (DSM-IIIR and DSM-IV)[5,6] will be reviewed. The terms 'harmful use' (ICD-10) and 'alcohol abuse' (DSM-IIIR/IV) will be discussed. Finally the issue of 'alcohol problems' will be introduced.

Formulation of definitions of alcohol dependence: 1948–1974

From the time of its inception in 1948, WHO played a major role in formulating public health definitions of 'alcoholism', 'addiction', and 'dependence' through a series of expert committees. Early definitions stressed the sociological rather than the physical aspects of dependence.[7] 'Alcoholics' were defined as:[7]

> those excessive drinkers whose dependence upon alcohol has attained such a degree that it shows a noticeable mental disturbance or an interference with their bodily and mental health, their inter-personal relations, and their smooth social and economic functioning; or who show the prodromal signs of such developments.

This definition had limited utility for biological research and psychiatric classification.[8] Therefore the 1955 Committee of Experts on Alcohol and Alcoholism highlighted the importance of physical criteria describing 'alcoholism' as:[9,10]

> a 'chronic disease characterised by a fundamental disturbance of the nervous system which is manifested on a behavioural level by a state of physical dependence. The major forms of this dependence are either inability to stop drinking before drunkenness is achieved, or inability to abstain from drinking because of the appearance of withdrawal symptoms'.

'Alcoholism' was classified under 'Other non-psychotic mental disorders' in ICD-8.[11] This definition of 'alcoholism' was generic, and included the subcategories of episodic excessive drinking, habitual excessive drinking, and alcohol addiction. Alcohol addiction was defined as:[11]

> a state of physical and emotional dependence on regular or periodic, heavy, and uncontrolled alcohol consumption, during

Table 1 Key elements of the alcohol dependence syndrome

Narrowing of repertoire
Salience of drinking
Increased tolerance to alcohol
Withdrawal symptoms
Relief or avoidance of withdrawal symptoms by
    further drinking
Subjective awareness of compulsion to drink
Reinstatement after abstinence

Reproduced with permission from G. Edwards and M. M. Gross (1976). Alcohol dependence: provisional description of a clinical syndrome. *British Medical Journal*, **i**, 1058–61.

which the person experiences a compulsion to drink. On cessation of alcohol intake there are withdrawal symptoms, which may be severe.

The alcohol dependence syndrome

Clinical description

In 1976, Edwards and Gross proposed the existence of alcohol dependence within a syndrome model.[3] Their description was based on the clinical observation that certain heavy drinkers manifested an interrelated clustering of signs and symptoms. They hypothesized that dependence was not an all-or-nothing phenomenon but existed in degrees of severity. The elements of the syndrome, as originally formulated, are summarized in Table 1. Not all the elements need always be present, nor always present with the same intensity. Edwards and Gross[3] also acknowledged the fact that not everyone who drinks too much is necessarily dependent on alcohol. They hypothesized that alcohol dependence should be conceptually distinguished from alcohol-related problems.

By drawing a clear distinction between the alcohol dependence syndrome and alcohol-related disabilities, Edwards and Gross introduced the concept of a biaxial model. This was described further in the report of a WHO scientific group published in 1977.[12] Alcohol-related disabilities are defined as comprising those physical, psychological, and social problems that are a consequence of excessive drinking and dependence. Consumption may be viewed on a third axis.

The alcohol dependence syndrome was proposed in the first instance as an empirical formulation. It was hoped that future research would allow a more detailed understanding of the 'latent' processes that produced the covariance of signs, symptoms, prognosis, and response to treatment. Unlike previous models of 'alcoholism' that had observational elements but no theoretical input, the alcohol dependence syndrome was influenced by psychological theory and proposed as a synthesis of both general learning theory and specific conditioning models of dependence.[13,14]

Establishment of the validity of the alcohol dependence syndrome

Since 1976, the alcohol dependence syndrome has assumed a position of increasing importance and has stimulated considerable research. Studies have focused on the degree to which the elements of the syndrome co-occur.[15–19] Other areas of research have included construct validity,[20] concurrent validity,[17,21,22] and predictive validity.[23,24] Field trials conducted as background to the preparation of ICD-10, DSM-IIIR, and DSM-IV, have all contributed to the body of research evidence.[6,25–29] Difficulties have been encountered in operationalizing elements such as narrowing of repertoire, subjective change, and reinstatement.[29]

These studies have shown a remarkable similarity in terms of the coherence and dimensionality of the syndrome, and are particularly impressive because of the diversity of methods and populations used.[13]

Individual elements of the alcohol dependence syndrome

Narrowing of the drinking repertoire

Most drinkers vary their alcohol consumption from day to day and week to week. The pattern of their drinking is influenced by a range of internal cues and external circumstances. Heavy drinkers may initially widen their drinking repertoire. As dependence advances, so a diminished variability in drinking behaviour emerges. The dependent person begins to drink in the same manner every day. The daily pattern established ensures that a relatively high blood-alcohol level is maintained and that symptoms of alcohol withdrawal are avoided. As drinking becomes stereotyped with advanced dependence, so dependent drinkers are able to describe their drinking day in minute detail.

Salience of drinking-seeking behaviour

With advancing dependence, individuals give priority to maintaining their alcohol intake. Alcohol consumption is maintained despite painful direct consequences such as physical illness, rejection by family, and lack of money. They will 'beg, borrow, or steal' to obtain money for alcohol.[3]

Increased tolerance to alcohol

Regular drinkers become tolerant to the central nervous system effects of alcohol and can sustain blood alcohol levels that would incapacitate the non-tolerant drinker. In short, they can 'drink others under the table'. Tolerance may decrease in the later stages of dependence, with individuals becoming intoxicated on much less alcohol than would previously have affected them. Cross-tolerance extends to other drugs, notably barbiturates and benzodiazepines.

Withdrawal symptoms

The term 'alcohol withdrawal' describes a broad range of symptoms and signs, from the relatively trivial to the life-threatening. At first the symptoms are intermittent and mild, but as the degree of dependence increases, so do the frequency and intensity of withdrawal symptoms. Symptoms vary from person to person and do not require abstinence to appear; they can occur when blood-alcohol concentrations are falling. When the picture is fully developed, the dependent drinker typically has severe multiple symptoms every morning on waking; these symptoms may wake him in the middle of the night. Those who are severely dependent usually experience mild withdrawal symptoms during the day whenever their alcohol levels fall.

Withdrawal symptoms cannot occur without a high degree of central nervous system tolerance, but tolerance can occur without clinically manifest withdrawal symptoms.[3]

The spectrum of symptoms is wide, but the four key symptoms are tremor, nausea, sweating, and mood disturbance. A range of other symptoms can also occur, including sensitivity to sound (hyperacusis), ringing in the ears (tinnitus), itching, muscle cramps, sleep disturbance, perceptual distortion, hallucinations, generalized (grand mal) seizures, and delirium tremens.

The four key symptoms will be described in further detail.

Tremor

The first experience of alcohol withdrawal tremor may be recalled vividly: 'One afternoon I went to cut the grass at a friend's house. She gave me a cup of tea and my hands kept shaking. I kept rattling the cup on the saucer and couldn't put the cup to my mouth. I had to put them down and pretend that I had finished.' Men often find it difficult to shave first thing in the morning and merely getting the first drink of the day to the mouth may be an ordeal in itself.

Nausea

Dependent drinkers commonly say that their bodies want to vomit first thing in the morning, but that they have nothing to bring up. This may be described as 'dry retching' or 'the dry heaves'. Typically they find it difficult to eat breakfast and to brush their teeth. The first drink of the day is often vomited back.

Sweating

Dependent drinkers commonly describe waking up in the early morning (3 a.m. or 4 a.m.) to find the bed sheets 'drenched'. In the earlier stages of dependence they may report feeling clammy.

Mood disturbance

This is an important feature of the withdrawal syndrome. Mildly dependent individuals may feel 'a bit edgy'. Severely dependent individuals may present with clinically significant symptoms of anxiety and depression.

Relief or avoidance of withdrawal symptoms by further drinking

In the early stages of dependence individuals may find that they need a lunchtime drink to alleviate discomfort. As dependence progresses there emerges the need for an early morning drink to relieve the symptoms of alcohol withdrawal coming on after a night's abstinence. Later, individuals may wake in the middle of the night for a drink, and alcohol is often kept by the bed. If they have to go for 3 or 4 h without a drink during the day, they value the next drink for its relief effect.

Clues to the degree of dependence can be obtained by taking a detailed history of the first drink of the day. The person drinking from a bottle kept by the side of the bed before they get up is more dependent than the person who has breakfast and reads the paper first. The woman who pours whisky into her first cup of tea is more dependent than the librarian who slips out to the lavatory at midday to drink from a quarter bottle of vodka hidden in her handbag.

Subjective awareness of compulsion to drink

This describes an altered subjective experience of an inability to limit drinking to an acceptable level. Although the familiar term 'loss of control' has been used to denote this element, it is more likely that control has been 'impaired' rather than lost.

Another complex experience is that of 'craving', the subjective experience of which is greatly influenced by environment. Individuals can experience craving of very different intensities on different occasions. Cues for craving include the experience of intoxication, the withdrawal syndrome, mood (anger, depression, elation), or situational cues (being in a pub (bar), passing an off-licence (liquor store)).

Here the key experience may best be described as a compulsion to drink. The desire for a further drink is seen as irrational, and is resisted, but despite this a further drink is taken.

Reinstatement after abstinence

Alcohol dependent individuals who begin to drink again after a period of abstinence invariably relapse back into the previous stage of the dependence syndrome. This process occurs over a variable time course, with moderately dependent individuals perhaps taking weeks or months and severely dependent individuals taking a couple of days.

Influence of the alcohol dependence syndrome on later formulations of dependence

ICD-9

The concept of the alcohol dependence syndrome presented a significant challenge to researchers and clinicians, requiring them to re-think many fundamental concepts and definitions. In ICD-9 the term 'alcoholism' was dropped in favour of the 'alcohol dependence syndrome'.[30] It was, however, still classified under the category 'Other non-psychotic mental disorders'. The ICD-9 definition of alcohol dependence may have been somewhat premature, because the theoretical process was still evolving at that time.[2]

DSM-III

At the same time as WHO was formulating public health definitions of 'alcoholism', 'addiction', and 'dependence', a trend towards formal diagnostic criteria was emerging in the United States. This was driven by practical consideration such as the need for better communication between clinicians, researchers, and the general public. Other influential factors included the growing need to categorize persons in an objective fashion for legal, medical, or psychiatric reasons, to collect and communicate accurate public health information, and to standardize practice nationally and internationally. The first two editions of the *Diagnostic and Statistical Manual* classified 'alcoholism' as a subcategory of personality disorder. In DSM-III,[31] it was included under a new and separate category of 'Substance use disorders'. The terms 'alcoholism' and 'addiction' were dropped and the terms 'dependence' and 'alcohol abuse' used instead. Dependence was distinguished from abuse by the presence of tolerance or withdrawal symptoms.

DSM-IIIR

By the mid-1980s DSM-III and ICD-9 were undergoing reviews for the purposes of revision.[32] The diagnostic criteria for dependence were broadened in DSM-IIIR[5] to incorporate the elements of the alcohol dependence syndrome as hypothesized by Edwards and Gross.[3] Here, nine items were included in the diagnostic criteria for dependence, the majority focusing on evidence of loss of control, overuse of the substance, a willingness to give up important events in order to take the substance, and consumption of alcohol despite consequences. Out of the nine items, three related to the presence of tolerance or withdrawal, but these were not required for a diagnosis as they had been in DSM-III. To meet the criteria for dependence, individuals had to fulfil three of the nine items for a period of at least 1 month.

The essential feature of the DSM-IIIR dependence category is defined in the text as a 'cluster of cognitive, behavioural, and physiological symptoms, indicating that the person has impaired control over drinking and continues to drink despite adverse consequences' (Table 2).

DSM-IV[6]

In view of the major changes in criteria that had occurred between 1980 and 1987, the DSM-IV Substance Use Disorders Work Group was reluctant to make any additional major changes. The nine items in DSM-IIIR were reduced to seven (two separate DSM-IIIR items, those referring to withdrawal and the use of drugs to treat withdrawal were combined into one item; another item was moved from the dependence to the abuse section). The repetitive nature of the problem was highlighted in that three or more of the items should have occurred during the same 12-month period and the associated difficulties must have led to clinically significant impairment or distress. DSM-IV also uniquely allows for the subtyping of dependence with and without physiological dependence (Table 3).

ICD-10[4]

ICD-10 includes six items under dependence, most of which are similar to DSM-IV. For a diagnosis of dependence, three or more items should have occurred in the past year. The 'strong desire or sense of compulsion to take the substance' is viewed as a central descriptive

Table 2 DSM-IIIR criteria for substance dependence

A   At least three of the following
   (1) Substance often taken in larger amounts or over a longer period than the person intended

   (2) Persistent desire or one or more unsuccessful efforts to cut down or control substance use

   (3) A great deal of time spent in activities necessary to get the substance, taking the substance, or recovering from its effects

   (4) Frequent intoxication or withdrawal when expected to fulfil major role obligations at work, school, or home, or when substance use is physically hazardous

   (5) Important social, occupational, or recreational activities given up or greatly reduced because of substance use

   (6) Continued substance use despite knowledge of having a persistent or recurrent social, psychological, or physical problem that is caused or exacerbated by the use of the same

   (7) Marked tolerance

   (8) Characteristic withdrawal symptoms

   (9) Substance often taken to relieve or avoid withdrawal symptoms

B   Some symptoms of the disturbance have persisted for at least one month, or have occurred repeatedly over a long period of time

Table 3 DSM-IV criteria for substance dependence

A maladaptive pattern of substance use, leading to clinically significant impairment or distress, as manifested by three (or more) of the following occurring at any time in the same 12-month period

(1) Tolerance
   (a) Need for markedly increased amounts of the substance to achieve intoxication or desired effect
   (b) Markedly diminished effect with continued use of the same amount of the substance

(2) Withdrawal
   (a) Characteristic withdrawal syndrome for the substance
   (b) The same substance taken to relieve or avoid withdrawal symptoms

(3) Substance is often taken in larger amounts or over a longer period than was intended

(4) Any unsuccessful effort or a persistent desire to cut down or control substance use

(5) A great deal of time is spent in activities necessary to obtain the substance, use the substance, or recover from its effects

(6) Important social, occupational, or recreational activities given up or reduced because of substance use

(7) Continued substance use despite knowledge of having had a persistent or recurrent physical or psychological problem that is likely to be caused or exacerbated by the substance

Specify if
With physiological dependence: evidence of tolerance or withdrawal (i.e. either item 1 or item 2 is present)
Without physiological dependence: no evidence of tolerance or withdrawal (i.e. neither item 1 or item 2 is present)

characteristic of dependence in ICD-10. This compulsive-use indicator is not included in the DSM-IIIR or DSM-IV concept of dependence (Table 4).

Although the DSM-IIIR, DSM-IV, and ICD-10 diagnostic approaches have drawn on the original concept of the alcohol dependence syndrome, and are of value in standardizing psychiatric practice nationally and internationally, they picture dependence as an all-or-nothing phenomenon rather than as a dimensional state.[33]

Comparisons of the DSM-IIIR, DSM-IV, and ICD-10 definitions of alcohol dependence[32]

1. ICD-10 collapses four of the DSM-IIIR and DSM-IV dependence criteria into two:

   (a) the two DSM impaired-control criteria are combined in ICD-10;

   (b) the 'important recreational activities' and 'great deal of time spent drinking' from DSM are combined into progressive neglect of alternative pleasures.

2. ICD-10 includes compulsive use, not included in DSM-IIIR or DSM-IV.

3. DSM-IV and ICD-10 combine withdrawal and avoidance of withdrawal criteria, which are separate items in DSM-IIIR.

4. The inability to fulfil role obligations and hazardous-use criteria of DSM-IIIR are moved to the DSM-IV abuse category and dropped from ICD-10.

5. The 'continued use despite problems' category of DSM-IV and ICD-10 includes physical and psychological problems; the DSM-IIIR category is broader, including social problems.

6. The duration of threshold criteria differs across the systems. In DSM-IIIR some symptoms must have persisted for at least 1 month or occurred repeatedly over a longer period. DSM-IV and ICD-10 do not specify a duration criterion. However, several dependence criteria in DSM-IV must occur repeatedly.

7. DSM-IV allows for subtyping of dependence diagnoses with and without physiological dependence.

Research shows that agreement between the three systems on diagnosis of alcohol dependence is good to excellent for 'past year, prior to past year, and life-time diagnoses, for men and women, different ethnic groups and older and younger respondents'.[32] Thus the international effort to integrate the two major classification systems has been successful with respect to the dependence category. The DSM-IIIR classification is the most inclusive, requiring three of nine positive criteria for diagnosis, and the ICD-10 classification the most exclusive, requiring three of six positive criteria. The DSM-IV classification is intermediate, requiring three of seven positive criteria for diagnosis.

Non-addictive alcohol use disorders

Alcohol abuse

The term 'alcohol abuse' appeared infrequently in the American literature before 1970, when the United States National Institute on Alcohol Abuse and Alcoholism was formed. It was adopted as a formal diagnostic category by DSM-III,[31] which defined abuse as a behavioural concept: 'A pattern of pathological use for at least a month that causes impairment in social or occupational functioning'. Although enshrined in DSM-IIIR and DSM-IV, the term 'abuse' has been variously regarded as 'unscientific and pejorative'[34] and 'opprobrious' and 'vindictive'.[35]

DSM-IIIR

The broadening of diagnostic criteria for alcohol dependence in DSM-IIIR relegated 'abuse' to a residual less serious category. The two criteria for DSM-IIIR abuse are also DSM-IIIR dependence criteria; fulfilment of either criterion leads to a positive diagnosis of dependence, rendering the abuse category residual to the dependence category in this system.[32] The abuse diagnosis also required that the symptoms 'persist for at least one month or occur repeatedly over a longer period of time'.

DSM-IV

The DSM-IV Substance Use Disorders Workgroup carried out extensive analysis in an effort to define abuse more precisely. Accordingly, in DSM-IV, four separate items, not included in dependence, are listed for the diagnosis of abuse, focusing on social, physical, legal, and interpersonal problems associated with alcohol use. These problems must have occurred repeatedly over a 12-month period, and caused 'clinically significant impairment or distress' (Table 5).

Harmful use

ICD-10

The ICD-10 criteria for harmful use of alcohol differ significantly from the DSM-IIIR and DSM-IV abuse classifications. An ICD-10 diagnosis of harmful drinking requires a pattern of drinking that has caused actual physical or psychological harm to the user. This definition is overly restrictive and does not overlap with DSM-IIIR and DSM-IV definitions of alcohol abuse.

Alcohol problems

Not everyone experiencing an alcohol problem or alcohol-related disability will be suffering from alcohol dependence. Both dependent and non-dependent drinkers, particularly binge drinkers, are at risk of problems related to heavy alcohol consumption. Indeed, epidemiological evidence supports the view that most alcohol-related harm in the general population occurs in heavy non-dependent drinkers.

Alcohol problems are extremely diverse. They have been defined as 'those problems that may arise in individuals around their use of beverage alcohol, and that may require an appropriate treatment response for their optimum management'.[36] The phrases 'alcohol problems' or 'alcohol-related problem' contain an assumption of causality.[37] This issue is a complex one, involving individual differences and the social context of drinking as well as the pattern, duration, and intensity of alcohol use.

Alcohol problems can be related to the acute or chronic consumption of alcohol. A fractured ankle sustained by falling over while acutely intoxicated is an example of the former category. Cirrhosis of the liver is an example of a chronic problem. An individual who drinks

---

Table 4 ICD-10 criteria for substance dependence

A diagnosis of dependence should usually be made only if three or more of the following have been experienced or exhibited at some time during the previous year

(a) A strong desire or sense of compulsion to take the substance

(b) Difficulties in controlling substance-taking behaviour in terms of its onset, termination, or levels of use

(c) A physiological withdrawal state when substance use has ceased or been reduced, as evidenced by the characteristic withdrawal syndrome for the substance, or use of the same (or a closely related) substance with the intention of relieving or avoiding withdrawal symptoms

(d) Evidence of tolerance such that increased doses of the psychoactive substance are required in order to achieve effects originally produced by lower doses

(e) Progressive neglect of alternative pleasures or interests because of psychoactive substance use, increased amount of time necessary to obtain or take the substance or to recover from its effects

(f) Persisting with substance use despite clear evidence of overtly harmful consequences, such as harm to the liver through excessive drinking, depressive mood states consequent to periods of heavy substance use, or drug-related impairment of cognitive functioning; efforts should be made to determine that the user was actually, or could be expected to be, aware of the nature and extent of the harm

Table 5 Criteria for abuse or harmful use of substances

DSM-IIIR	DSM-IV	ICD-10
A maladaptive pattern of substance use indicated by one of the following	A. A maladaptive pattern of substance use leading to clinically significant impairment or distress as manifested by one (or more) of the following occurring within a 12-month period	Evidence of physical or psychological harm related to substance use
Evidence of use in hazardous situations or		Harmful use should not be diagnosed if dependence syndrome, a psychotic disorder, or another specific form of alcohol-related disorder is present
Continued intake despite problems in social, occupational, psychological, or physical dimensions	(1) Recurrent substance misuse resulting in failure to fulfil major role obligations at work, school, or home	
	(2) Recurrent substance use in situations in which it is physically hazardous	
	(3) Recurrent substance-related legal problems	
	(4) Continued substance use despite having persistent or recurrent social or interpersonal problems caused by or exacerbated by the effects of the substance	
	B. The symptoms have never met the criteria for substance dependence	

in binges will experience different problems compared with someone who drinks the same amount of alcohol spread out over a week or a month or a year. The way in which a person behaves while intoxicated is another important factor determining the nature of alcohol-related problems. The social consequences of drinking such as job loss, imprisonment, marital and family break-up, and drink-driving have profound effects on the well being of the drinker, their family, and society.[37]

Types of alcohol-related problems

Although somewhat artificial, it is helpful to classify alcohol-related problems in individuals into physical, psychological, and social categories. There is often considerable overlap between these three areas. The more severe the dependence, the greater the likelihood of problems of all three kinds.[22]

Alcohol-related physical and psychological problems are discussed in the next section. Some of the social problems can be included here, for example the acute adverse consequences of drinking such as trauma resulting from road traffic accidents, injuries from fights, and death from overdose.[37]

The social problems that can result from drinking are legion. Alcohol is involved in all types of accidents and contributes to 15 per cent of traffic deaths. It is implicated in 26 to 54 per cent of home and leisure injuries[37] and is associated with domestic violence, child abuse, crime, homicide, and suicide. Alcohol is also related to poor work performance, dismissal, unemployment, debt and housing problems, and crimes of violence.

There is a continuity between moderate and excessive drinking and between harmless drinking and drinking that results in harm or in problems. Such problem-clustering may reflect alcohol dependence, certainly amongst a proportion of these drinkers. Given this hetero-

geneity, no one form of treatment is likely to be effective for all individuals with alcohol problems.[36] A range of treatments is required and it should be possible for non-specialists to offer brief interventions (see Chapter 4.2.2.4).

The study of alcohol-related problems remains underdeveloped, compared with the study of alcohol dependence.[38] There may be several reasons for this, not least the difficulties inherent in measuring alcohol-related problems.[39] Another important issue, central to these difficulties, is the extent to which alcohol is causally related to the problem.[38]

Several questionnaires, measuring a variety of alcohol-related problems, have been developed.[38,40] The Alcohol Problems Questionnaire (APQ)[38] is a standardized inventory, which includes 46 items covering eight problem domains: physical, psychological, friends, finances, police, marital, children, and work. All questions apply to the 6-month period prior to the completion of the questionnaire. The shorter version includes the first five domains. This questionnaire can make a useful contribution to the overall assessment, and is of potential value in outcome research.

Conclusions

An understanding of the concepts of alcohol dependence and alcohol problems is central to the therapeutic process with individual patients.

The development of diagnostic criteria has helped to standardize practice nationally and internationally, and aided interdisciplinary communication. The diagnostic criteria for dependence are imperfect because they view the syndrome as an all-or-nothing phenomenon rather than as a dimensional state. The concepts of abuse and harmful use need further classification. The totality of alcohol problems is a vast area with major implications for the general population, not just dependent drinkers.

References

1. World Health Organization (1951). *WHO technical report series*, No 42. WHO, Geneva.

2. Babor, T.F. (1990). Social, scientific and medical issues in the definition of alcohol and drug dependence. In *The nature of drug dependence* (ed. G. Edwards and M. Lader), pp. 19–36. Oxford Medical Publications, Oxford.

3. Edwards, G. and Gross, M.M. (1976). Alcohol dependence: provisional description of a clinical syndrome. *British Medical Journal*, 1, 1058–61.

4. World Health Organization (1992). *International statistical classification of diseases and related health problems, 10th revision*. WHO, Geneva

5. American Psychiatric Association (1987). *Diagnostic and statistical manual of mental disorders* (3rd edn, revised). American Psychiatric Association, Washington, DC.

6. American Psychiatric Association (1994). *Diagnostic and statistical classification of diseases and related health problems* (4th edn). American Psychiatric Association, Washington, DC.

7. World Health Organization (1952). *Expert Committee on Mental Health, Alcoholism Subcommittee, second report*. WHO Technical Report Series, No. 48. WHO, Geneva.

8. Seeley, J. (1959). The WHO definition of alcoholism. *Quarterly Journal of Studies on Alcohol*, 20, 352–6.

9. World Health Organization (1955). *Expert Committee on Mental Health, Alcoholism Subcommitte report*. WHO Technical Report Series, No. 48. WHO, Geneva.

10. World Health Organization (1955). *Expert Committee on Mental Health, Alcoholism Subcommittee report*. WHO Technical Report Series, No. 94. WHO, Geneva.

11. World Health Organization (1974). *Glossary of mental disorders and guide to their classification: for use in conjunction with the International Classification of Diseases* (8th revision). WHO, Geneva.

12. Edwards, G., Gross, M.M., Keller, M., Moser, J., and Room, R. (1977). *Alcohol-related disabilities*. WHO Offset Publication No. 32. WHO, Geneva.

13. Edwards, G. (1986). The alcohol dependence syndrome: a concept as stimulus to enquiry. *British Journal of Addiction*, 81, 171–83.

14. Babor, T.F., Cooney, N.L., and Lauerman, R.J. (1987). The dependence syndrome concept as a psychological theory of relapse behaviour: an empirical evaluation of alcoholic and opiate addicts. *British Journal of Addiction*, 82, 393–405.

15. Stockwell, T., Hodgson, R., Edwards, G., Taylor, C., and Rankin, H. (1979). The development of a questionnaire to measure alcohol dependence. *British Journal of Addiction*, 74, 79–87.

16. Chick, J. (1980). Alcohol dependence: methodological issues in its measurement, reliability of the criteria. *British Journal of Addiction*, 75, 175–86.

17. Stockwell, T., Murphy, D., and Hodgson, R. (1983). The severity of alcohol dependence questionnaire: its use, reliability and validity. *British Journal of Addiction*, 78, 145–55.

18. Meehan, J.P., Webb, M.G.T., and Unwin, A.R. (1985). The severity of alcohol dependence questionnaire (SADQ) in a sample of Irish problem drinkers. *British Journal of Addiction*, 80, 57–63.

19. Feingold, A. and Rounsaville, B. (1995). Construct validity of the dependence syndrome as measured by DSM-IV for different psycho-active substances. *Addiction*, 90, 1661–9.

20. Heather, N., Rollnick, S., and Winston, M. (1983). A comparison of objective and subjective measures of alcohol dependence as predictors of relapse following treatment. *British Journal of Clinical Psychiatry*, 22, 11–17.

21. Kivlahan, D., Sher, K.J., and Donovan, D.M. (1989) The Alcohol Dependence Scale: a validation study among inpatient alcoholics. *Journal of Studies on Alcohol*, 50, 170–5.

22. Caetano, R. (1993). The association between severity of DSM-III-R alcohol dependence and medical and social consequences. *Addiction*, 88, 631–42.

23. Hodgson, R., Rankin, H.J., and Stockwell, T. (1979). Alcohol dependence and the priming effect. *Behaviour Research and Therapy*, 17, 379–87.

24. Rankin, H., Stockwell, T., and Hodgson, R. (1982). Cues for drinking and degrees of alcohol dependence. *British Journal of Addiction*, 77, 287–96.

25. Grant, B.F., Harfold, T.C., Chou, P., and Pickering, R. (1992). DSM-III-R and the proposed DSM-IV alcohol use disorders. United States 1988. A methodological comparison. *Alcoholism, Clinical and Experimental Research*, 16, 215–21.

26. Cottler, L.B. (1993). Comparing DSM-III-R and ICD-10 substance use disorders. *Addiction*, 88, 689–96.

27. Rapaport, M.H., Tipp, J.E., and Schuckit, M.A. (1993). A comparison of ICD-10 and DSM-III-R criteria for substance abuse and dependence. *American Journal of Drug and Alcohol Abuse*, 19, 143–51.

28. Rounsaville, B.J., Bryant, K., Babor, T., Kranzler, H., and Kadden, R. (1993). Cross system agreement for substance use disorders: DSM-III-R, DSM-IV and ICD-10. *Addiction*, 88, 337–48.

29. Cottler, L.B., Phelps, D.L., and Compton, W.M. (1995) Narrowing of the drinking repertoire criterion: should it have been dropped from ICD-10? *Journal of Studies on Alcohol*, 56, 173–6.

30. World Health Organization (1978). *Mental disorders: glossary and guide to their classification in accordance with the Ninth Revision of the International Classification of Diseases*. WHO, Geneva.

31. American Psychiatric Association (1980). *Diagnostic and statistical manual of mental disorders* (3rd edn). American Psychiatric Association, Washington, DC.

32. Grant, B. (1996). DSM-IV, DSM-III-R, ICD-10 alcohol and drug abuse/harmful use and dependence, United States, 1992: a nosological comparison. *Alcoholism, Clinical and Experimental Research*, 8, 1481–8.

33. Edwards, G., Marshall, E.J., and Cook, C.C.H. (1997). *The treatment of drinking problems* (3rd edn). Cambridge University Press.

34. Edwards, G., Arif, A., and Hodgson, R. (1981). Nomenclature and classification of drug- and alcohol-related problems: a WHO memorandum. *Bulletin of the World Health Organization*, 50, 225–42.

35. Keller, M. (1982). On defining alcoholism: with comment on some other relevant words. In *Alcohol, science and society revisited* (ed. E.L. Gomberg, H.R. White, and J.A. Carpenter), pp. 119–33. University of Michigan Press, Ann Arbor, MI.

36. Institute of Medicine (1990). *Broadening the base of treatment for alcohol problems: report of a study by a Committee of the Institute of Medicine, Division of Mental Health and Behavioural Medicine*. National Academy Press, Washington, DC.

37. Edwards, G., Anderson, P., Babor, T.F., Casswell, S., Ferrence, R., and Giesbrecht, N. (1994). *Alcohol policy and the public good*. Oxford University Press.

38. Drummond, D.C. (1990). The relationship between alcohol dependence and alcohol-related problems in a clinical population. *British Journal of Addiction*, 85, 357–66.

39. Room, R. (1977). Measurement and distribution of drinking patterns and problems in general populations. In *Alcohol-related disabilities* (ed. G. Edwards, M.M. Gross, M. Keller, J. Moser, and R. Room), pp. 61–87. WHO, Geneva.

40. Chick, J., Ritson, B., Connaughton, J., Stewart, A., and Chick, J. (1988). Advice versus extended treatment for alcoholism: a controlled study. *British Journal of Addiction*, 83, 159–70.

4.2.2.3 Alcohol and psychiatric and physical disorders

Karl F. Mann

Intoxication

Clinical symptoms of alcohol intoxication depend on the blood alcohol concentration (**BAC**) as well as on the individual's level of tolerance. Whereas in healthy persons without alcohol tolerance it is possible to distinguish mild intoxication (BAC ≤ 100 mg per cent), medium intoxication (BAC 100–200 mg per cent), and severe intoxication (BAC > 200 mg per cent), this schema is too simple for alcoholics. In these people, different levels of tolerance can lead to completely different clinical pictures despite their having similar blood alcohol concentrations. Thus, psychopathology is more important than blood alcohol concentrations for estimating the severity of an acute intoxication state. With increasing BAC we observe elated mood, disinhibition, impaired judgement, belligerence, impaired social and occupational functioning, mood lability, cognitive impairment, reduced attention span, slurred speech, incoordination, unsteady gait, nystagmus, and stupor or coma.

The term 'pathological intoxication' can still be found in the older literature (reviewed by Lishman[1]). It was described as an outburst of aggression and uncontrollable rage, which might have led to serious destructions. As a rule, this behaviour, which was not typical for the individual, ended in terminal sleep and subsequent amnesia. However, since there is not enough empirical evidence for the existence of this syndrome, it was no longer considered in DSM-IV.[2]

Alcoholic-induced amnesias ('blackouts')

This term refers to a transient state of amnesia after a drinking excess. Usually patients' behaviour is no different from their behaviour during other periods of intoxication without blackouts. Nevertheless, the memory gap usually lasts for hours, but may be as long as a day or more. In extreme cases, patients find themselves in strange places with no recollection of how they got there.

Withdrawal

Withdrawal without complications

When alcohol is completely withdrawn or substantially reduced a characteristic withdrawal syndrome can develop. It includes autonomic hyperactivity like hand tremor, insomnia, sweating, tachycardia, hypertension, and anxiety. The symptoms generally occur between 6 and 12 h after the last alcohol consumption. Depending on their severity they may last for up to 4 or 5 days. The neurobiological basis for withdrawal is a gradual upregulation of *N*-methyl-D-aspartate receptors under the influence of chronic alcohol use. As soon as the alcohol, which acts as a central nervous system depressant, is withdrawn, we observe an overwhelming excitatory action on the brain mediated by the glutamatergic system.

Withdrawal with perceptual disturbances

The individual usually experiences more discomfort and anxiety if transient visual, tactile, or auditory hallucinations or illusions are present. In this state, reality testing is still intact: the person still knows that the hallucinations are induced by the substance. If this is no longer true, a substance-induced psychotic disorder or a delirium tremens is likely.

Withdrawal with grand mal seizures (alcoholic convulsions, 'rum fits')

In about 30 per cent of the cases the typical grand mal seizures are followed by a delirium tremens. The electroencephalograph picture is only abnormal at the time of the fits. Before and after it is normal, so that alcohol convulsions have nothing to do with a latent epilepsy.

Alcohol-induced psychosis (delirium tremens)

In delirium tremens the symptoms of alcohol withdrawal described earlier are accompanied by a reduced level of consciousness, disorientation in time and place, impairment of recent memory, insomnia, and perceptual disturbances. The latter include misinterpretation of sensory stimuli and hallucinations; most are visual, but auditory and haptic hallucinations also occur. The hallucinations may be Lilliputian or of normal size, and may be of complex, frightening, and extremely realistic scenes. The patient is restless and fearful, and may become severely agitated. There is marked tremor, and ataxia when standing. Some patients experience vestibular disturbance. Autonomic disturbance includes sweating, tachycardia, raised blood pressure, and dilated pupils. There may be a mild pyrexia. Patients are usually dehydrated, often with abnormal electrolytes, leucocytosis, and impaired liver function. As in other forms of delirium, symptoms are worse at night.

Delirium tremens is the most severe of the states following withdrawal of alcohol, with a reported mortality of up to 5 per cent. In its fully developed form it is uncommon; the more frequent states are acute tremulousness, transient hallucinations with tremor, and uncomplicated fits. Delirium tremens usually begins after 3 to 4 days of abstinence from alcohol, although occasionally it starts while drinking continues. In the latter cases it is assumed that alcohol levels have fallen below some critical level. It is not known by what mechanism alcohol withdrawal leads to the clinical syndrome. Delirium tremens often appears to start suddenly, although close enquiry may reveal a prodromal stage of restlessness, anxiety, and insomnia. It usually lasts for 2 to 3 days, often ending with deep and prolonged sleep from which the patient wakes symptom free and with little memory of the period of delirium. Rarely, the patient is left with an amnesic syndrome, perhaps the consequence of previous undetected Wernicke's encephalopathy.

Treatment is by sedation, usually with a benzodiazepine, together with fluid replacement under close observation. The possibility of accompanying head injury or infection should be investigated. Sedation should be adequate to prevent withdrawal seizures, with frequent monitoring of the response. High-potency vitamins are usually given to prevent Wernicke's encephalopathy. An anticonvulsant is given when there have been withdrawal seizures in the past. Cardiovascular collapse and hyperthermia occur occasionally and require urgent medical treatment.

Hallucinosis

Alcoholic hallucinosis is a rare condition in which auditory hallucinations are present in clear consciousness and without autonomic over-activity, usually in a person who has been drinking excessively for many years. The hallucinations often begin as simple noises, but are gradually replaced by voices which may threaten, abuse, or reproach the person. Usually the voices speak to the person, but sometimes they discuss him or her in the third person. The voices may be occasional or relentlessly persistent. They may command the patient, who may respond with unrestrained or suicidal behaviour. Delusions are secondary interpretations of the hallucinations. Autochthonous hallucinations suggest schizophrenia, as do thought disorder or incongruity of affect. The patient is usually distressed, anxious, and restless.

In both ICD-10 and DSM-IV, the disorder is classified as a substance-induced psychotic disorder and not, as has been suggested in the past, a form of schizophrenia (released by heavy drinking). The differential diagnosis includes transient auditory hallucinations occurring during withdrawal from a period of heavy drinking, and delirium tremens in which auditory hallucinations may accompany the more prominent visual ones. In both these conditions the auditory hallucinations are transient and disorganized, and in the latter consciousness is impaired. In contrast, the auditory hallucinations of an alcoholic hallucinosis are persistent and organized, and occur in clear consciousness. Other differential diagnoses are depressive disorder with psychotic symptoms and schizophrenia, both of which can be accompanied by heavy drinking.

The hallucinations usually respond rapidly to antipsychotic medication. The prognosis is good; usually the condition improves within days or a couple of weeks provided that the person remains abstinent. Symptoms that last for 6 months generally continue for years.[3]

Psychiatric disorders

Alcohol-dependent patients often present with symptoms of anxiety or depression. These states are generally referred to as comorbid disorders or dual diagnosis. Alcoholism can be a consequence of anxiety and mood disorders ('secondary alcoholism'). It can develop independently after anxiety and depression, or it can precede anxiety and depressive symptoms ('primary'). As the former are discussed elsewhere in this textbook, here we concentrate on the latter.

Alcohol-induced mood disorders

Alcohol is a central nervous system depressant. Taken regularly in high doses it may provoke feelings of sadness. Episodes of withdrawal or relative withdrawal can lead to excitability and nervousness, including anxiety. The more a person drinks, the more likely it is that these symptoms will occur. Finally in the stage of alcohol dependence, up to 80 per cent of people report depressive symptoms at some time in their life. About one-third of male patients and up to 50 per cent of female patients have experienced longer periods of severe depression.[4] These high prevalence rates are noteworthy, since more than 20 per cent of alcoholics have attempted suicide once or more and about 15 per cent die in their attempt. Besides depressive features, alcohol-induced mood disorders may also comprise manic symptoms or mixed features. However, the diagnosis should only be used when the symptoms cause clinically significant impairment or distress in social, occupational, or other areas of functioning.

Concerning treatment, it is interesting to note that despite the vast majority of patients who present with depressive symptoms at the beginning of treatment for alcoholism, only very few need specific antidepressent medication or specific psychotherapy. In most other cases depressive symptoms disappear within weeks of controlled abstinence.[5]

Alcohol-induced anxiety disorders

This diagnosis should only be used when anxiety symptoms are thought to be related to the direct physiological effects of alcohol. The symptomatology may involve anxiety, panic attacks, and phobias. Both alcohol-induced anxiety disorders and mood disorders can develop during intoxication, withdrawal, or up to 4 weeks after cessation of alcohol consumption. During intoxication or withdrawal, the diagnosis should only be given when the symptomatology clearly exceeds what would be expected from anxiety or depressive symptoms during a regular intoxication or withdrawal episode.

Anxiety disorders are among the most common groups of psychiatric disorders in the general population, with prevalence rates of up to 25 per cent.[6] In clinical studies between 20 and 70 per cent of patients with alcoholism also suffer from anxiety disorders.[7] On the other hand, between 20 and 45 per cent of patients with anxiety disorders also have histories of alcoholism.[8] However, it has been argued that the comorbidity figures are overestimated, because in some of the studies the focus was on drinking patterns rather than on alcohol dependence or they describe anxiety symptoms rather than disorders according to diagnostic criteria.[9] Family studies analysing the comorbidity of alcoholism and anxiety disorders might be a means of clarifying this controversy. For instance, in the Yale study the presence of anxiety disorders in the probands slightly increased the risk for alcohol dependence in their relatives, whereas alcohol dependence in the proband did not increase their relative's risk for anxiety disorders.[10] Similarly, Maier et al.[11] demonstrated an increased risk of alcoholism in probands with panic disorders, but not the reverse. Kendler et al.,[12] in a study of female twins, found evidence that common genetic factors may underlie both alcoholism and panic disorder.

Effects on the brain

Cerebral cortex

Chronic alcohol consumption leads to structural and functional changes in the brain. Alcoholic dementia is dealt with in Chapter 4.1.12. Most of the tissue loss from the cerebral hemispheres in alcoholics is accounted for by a reduction in the volume of the cerebral white matter, additionally there is a slight reduction in the volume of the cerebral cortex. This has been demonstrated both pathologically[13] and using magnetic resonance imaging with quantitative morphometry.[14]

Harper et al.[15] documented neuronal loss in alcoholics. There was a 22 per cent reduction in the number of neurones in the superior frontal cortex (Brodmann's area 8), while surviving neurones showed shrinkage in the superior frontal, motor, and frontal cingulate cortices.[16] This finding of cortical damage in alcoholics is consistent with neuroradiological studies.[14]

Ferrer *et al.*[17] examined the dendritic tree of cortical neurones in alcoholic subjects using Golgi-apparatus impregnation techniques. They described a significant reduction in the basal dendritic tree of layer III pyramidal neurones in both the superior frontal and motor cortices. These studies suggest that, even though there is no significant reduction in the numbers of cortical neurones in the motor cortex, there are cellular structural abnormalities that could have important functional implications.

Wernicke's encephalopathy

The best-known features of heavy alcohol consumption in adults are Wernicke's encephalopathy and Korsakoff's syndrome. Wernicke's encephalopathy is directly caused by thiamine deficiency, which results from a combination of inadequate dietary intake, reduced gastrointestinal absorption, decreased hepatic storage, and impaired utilization. Only a subset of thiamine-deficient alcoholics develop Wernicke's encephalopathy, perhaps because they have inherited or acquired abnormalities of the thiamine-dependent enzyme transketolase, which reduces its affinity for thiamine. Wernicke's encephalopathy is characterized by degenerative changes, including gliosis and small haemorrhages in structures surrounding the third ventricle and aqueduct: namely, the mammillary bodies, hypothalamus, mediodorsal thalamic nucleus, colliculi, and midbrain tegmentum. Clinical features associated with the Wernicke–Korsakoff syndrome include memory deficits, ocular signs, ataxia, and global confusional states. Most can be related to damaged functional systems in the hypothalamus, midbrain, and cerebellum. In a large Scandinavian neuropathological study, 12.5 per cent of all alcoholics exhibited signs of Wernicke's encephalopathy.[18]

Korsakoff's syndrome

About 80 per cent of alcoholic patients recovering from Wernicke's encephalopathy develop Korsakoff's amnesic syndrome. It is characterized by marked deficits in anterograde and retrograde memory, apathy, an intact sensorium, and relative preservation of other intellectual abilities. Korsakoff's amnesic syndrome may also appear without an antecedent episode of Wernicke's encephalopathy. Acute lesions may be superimposed on chronic lesions, suggesting that subclinical episodes of Wernicke's encephalopathy may culminate in Korsakoff's amnesic syndrome. The memory disorder correlates best with the presence of histopathological lesions in the dorsomedial thalamus. (Amnesic syndrome is considered further in Chapter 4.1.13.)

Cerebellar degeneration

Many alcoholic patients develop a chronic cerebellar syndrome related to the degeneration of Purkinje cells in the cerebellar cortex. Quantitative studies revealed a significant loss of cerebellar Purkinje cells (by 10–35 per cent) and shrinkage of the cerebellar vermal, molecular, and granular cell layers.[19] Evidence for a direct toxic effect caused by ethanol is provided by animal models.[20] In neuroimaging studies, however, cerebellar ataxia in alcoholics does not correlate with the daily, annual, or lifetime consumption of ethanol. As in Wernicke's encephalopathy, thiamine deficiency due to poor nutrition has also been implicated. Cerebellar atrophy has been reported to occur in about 40 per cent of chronic alcoholics.[19] In a clinical study of alcoholic inpatients, 49 per cent had at least discrete clinical signs of cerebellar atrophy.[21]

The diagnosis of alcoholic cerebellar ataxia is based on the clinical history and neurological examination. The ataxia affects the gait most severely. Limb ataxia and dysarthria occur more often than in Wernicke's encephalopathy, whereas nystagmus is rare. Computed tomography or magnetic resonance imaging scans may show cerebellar cortical atrophy, but a considerable number of alcoholic patients with this finding are not ataxic on examination. Whether these represent subclinical cases in which symptoms will develop subsequently is unclear. It is interesting to note that impaired cerebellar function improves significantly when abstinence is maintained.[22]

Hepatocerebral degeneration

Hepatic encephalopathy develops in many alcoholics with liver disease, and is characterized by altered sensorium, frontal release signs, 'metabolic' flapping tremor, hyper-reflexia, extensor plantar responses, and occasional seizures. Whereas some patients progress from stupor to coma and then death, others recover and suffer recurrent episodes. The brains of patients with hepatic encephalopathy show enlargement and proliferation of protoplasmic astrocytes in the basal ganglia, thalamus, red nucleus, pons, and cerebellum, in the absence of neuronal loss or other glial changes.[23]

Patients who do not recover fully after an episode of hepatic encephalopathy go on to develop a progressive syndrome of tremor, choreoathetosis, dysarthria, gait ataxia, and dementia. Hepatocerebral degeneration may progress in a stepwise fashion, with incomplete recovery after each episode of hepatic encephalopathy, or slowly and inexorably, without a discrete episode of encephalopathy.

Rare disorders

The **Marchiafava–Bignami syndrome** is a disorder of demyelination or necrosis of the corpus callosum and adjacent subcortical white matter. The course may be acute, subacute, or chronic, and is marked by dementia, spasticity, dysarthria, and an inability to walk. Patients may lapse into coma and die, survive for many years in a demential condition, or occasionally recover.

Central pontine myelinolysis is a disorder of cerebral white matter that usually affects alcoholics, but it also occurs in non-alcoholics with liver disease including Wilson's disease, malnutrition, anorexia, burns, cancer, Addison's disease, and severe electrolyte disorders such as thiazide-induced hyponatraemia; however, the majority of cases occur in alcoholics, suggesting that alcoholism may contribute to the genesis of central pontine myelinolysis in, as yet, undefined ways.[23] Myelinolytic lesions can be reduced experimentally by rapid correction of chronic hyponatraemia. Symptoms include loss of pain sensation in the limbs, bulbar palsy, quadriplegia, disordered eye movements, vomiting, confusion, and coma.

Reversibility of brain damage

Alcohol-related neuroanatomical brain changes have been shown to be partially reversible. These findings created an ongoing debate on possible mechanisms and clinical correlates.[22]

Fetal alcohol syndrome

The first description of the fetal alcohol syndrome was given by French scientists in 1968.[24] As a research paradigm, it has a major impact on our understanding of alcohol's effects on the brain. Clinically the syndrome is characterized by: growth retardation involving height, weight, and head circumference; deficient intellectual and social performance and muscular co-ordination; minor structural anomalies of the face, together with more variable involvement of the limbs and the heart.

The basis of this pathology is a cascade of effects exerted by alcohol on the developing cell. Under normal conditions growth factors enhance the growth of cells and their differentiation, but alcohol can diminish these effects.[25] A second way of damaging the developing nerve cell is through the production of free radicals that allow calcium to accumulate in the cells.[26] The induction of free-radical formation is induced by alcohol. The result of both pathogenic processes is a decrease in the overall size of the brain and a diminution in the thickness of the outer layers of the cortex, due to decreases in the total numbers of cells. Impaired nerve cell migration might also play a role in the development of the fetal alcohol syndrome.[27]

The effects of alcohol on the developing brain are clinically measured by assessing the head circumference, which a clear dose-dependent effect.

The fetal alcohol syndrome is considered further in Chapter 9.2.7.

Effects on the body

Malnutrition and vitamin deficiency

Malnutrition can be a consequence of deficient food intake. More important in alcoholics seem to be maldigestion and malabsorbtion ('secondary malnutrition'). Apart from the direct toxic effect of alcohol on most body tissues, malnutrition is an important contributor to organ damage in alcoholics.[28] Vitamin metabolism may be profoundly affected by chronic alcohol consumption. As a consequence, many alcoholics have deficiencies in vitamins B_1 (thiamine), A, D, B_6, and E, and folate. This can lead to a variety of physical consequences, including damage to different organs.

Peripheral neuropathy

Besides its effect on the central nervous system, alcohol also damages motor, sensory, and autonomic nerves that control muscles and internal organs. Symptoms are weakness, numbness, pain, and a prickly feeling or burning of the skin, especially the feet. Usually on neurological examination, the tendon reflexes are diminished or have completely disappeared and skin sensibility is reduced, especially in the feet and in the lower limbs. When patients abstain from alcohol, the progression of the symptoms can be stopped and even partial recovery is possible.

Muscle

Alcohol is toxic to skeletal muscles in a dose-dependent way. Alcoholics often suffer from malnutrition, which adds to the chronic changes in muscles. Chronic myopathy can be found in 40 to 60 per cent of alcohol-dependent patients.[29] Pathophysiological mechanisms of muscle damage include alterations in membrane fluidity, ion channels and pumps, as well as protein synthesis and hormonal dysfunction. Patients complain of pain and weakness. Swelling of the muscle can be easily detected. In chronic states, muscle atrophy is evident. There is no acute treatment for alcoholic myopathy other than

abstinence, when acute myopathy can rapidly disappear; chronic myopathy usually only improves, leaving persistent weaknesses.

Liver

The effects of ethanol on the liver are among the first and best-known symptoms of alcoholism. The first manifestation of alcoholic liver diseases is the fatty liver. It is followed by early fibrosis, which can be associated with alcoholic hepatitis. If the process continues, irreversible damage leading to severe fibrosis and to cirrhosis is observed.[30] These effects occur through heavy alcohol consumption even in the absence of dietary deficiences.

Mortality from liver cirrhosis has long been an important correlate of the per capita consumption in a given population. Liver damage is also important because it produces an increase in liver enzymes such as aspartate transaminase, alanine transaminase, and γ-glutamyl transferase, which again are of great practical value as diagnostic markers of severe alcohol consumption. Alcohol accounts for more than 80 per cent of all cirrhosis deaths, a consequence that seems to be even more pronounced in women.[31]

Pancreas

About 5 per cent of alcoholics develop chronic pancreatitis. Ethanol seems to damage the pancreas slowly. In general, it takes between 10 and 15 years of heavy drinking before pancreatitis becomes clinically apparent. In the presomatic phase certain changes such as fibrosis, calcium deposits, and especially loss of functioning in enzyme- and hormone-producing cells can be demonstrated. The acute symptoms are abdominal pain and vomiting. Chronic complications include weight loss, steatorrhoea, and diabetes mellitus.[32]

Skin

Originally it was believed that skin alterations in alcoholics are due to alcoholic liver desease. However, more recent research has revealed that the skin may be affected much earlier by alcohol misuse.[33] Whereas the palmar erythema and spider naevi are well-known consequences of alcoholic liver disease, which also serve as diagnostic markers for alcoholism, psoriasis and facial erythema have less often been linked with high alcohol consumption. Alcohol clearly has to be on the list of agents known to exacerbate psoriasis. One possible mechanism of the action of alcohol on the skin could be a defect in the immune system.

Heart

Cardiac myopathy is one of the oldest known physical consequences of high alcohol consumption. Similar to ethanol's effects on skeletal muscles, the cells of the heart muscle are damaged by ethanol's influence on ion channels and pumps etc. Atrophy leads to a dilatation of the heart as a whole.

Recently, the effect of alcohol on coronary heart disease has been widely discussed. Indeed, it seems that there is a beneficial effect of moderate alcohol consumption, at least in middle-aged men.[34] It seems that an alcohol-induced increase in high-density lipoproteins and a decrease in low density lipoproteins may play a role in this process—an alteration in platelet aggregation could be one possible mechanism of action. Besides cardiomyopathy, cardiac arrythmias are prominent consequences of alcohol consumption. Close to one-third of all cardiomyopathies can be attributed to alcohol consumption.

Hypertension

A dose–reponse relationship between drinking and diastolic and systolic blood pressure has been shown consistently.[31] It is not clear, however, whether this relationship can only be seen above a threshold level of consumption. As a result, haemorrhagic stroke seems to be correlated with ethanol-induced hypertension.

Cancer

There is very clear evidence that alcohol increases the risk of cancer at the upper bronchodigestive tract. This includes cancer of the mouth, pharynx, larynx, and oesophagus. Additionally, alcohol consumption correlates with primary liver cancer. A possible link between alcohol and breast cancer is still a matter of debate: three recent cohort studies with large sample sizes found an excess risk for breast cancer.[35] The same seems to be true for the correlation between beer drinking and cancer of the rectum.

References

1. Lishman, W.A. (1990). *Organic psychiatry. The psychological consequences of cerebral disorder* (2nd edn). Blackwell Science, Oxford.
2. American Psychiatric Association (1994). *Diagnostic and statistical manual of mental disorders* (4th edn). American Psychiatric Association, Washington, DC.
3. Glass, I.B. (1989). Alcohol hallucinosis: a psychiatric enigma—2. Follow-up studies. *British Journal of Addiction*, **84**, 151–64.
4. Brown, S.A. and Schuckit, M.A. (1988). Changes in depression among abstinent alcoholics. *Journal of Studies on Alcohol*, **49**, 412–17.
5. Stetter, F., Rein, W., and Mann, K. (1991). How depressive are male alcoholic inpatients? Psychometric results from the Tübinger Alkoholismusprojekt. *European Psychiatry*, **6**, 243–9.
6. Kessler, R.C., McGonagle, K.A., Zhao, S., *et al.* (1994). Lifetime and 12-month prevalence of DSM-III-R psychiatric disorders in the United States: results from the National Comorbidity Survey. *Archives of General Psychiatry*, **51**, 8–19.
7. Merikangas, K.R. and Angst, J. (1995). Comorbidity and social phobia: evidence from clinical, epidemiologic, and genetic studies. *European Archives of Psychiatry and Clinical Neuroscience*, **244**, 297–303.
8. Kushner, M.G., Sher, K.J., and Beitman, B.D. (1990). The relation between alcohol problems and the anxiety disorders. *American Journal of Psychiatry*, **147**, 685–95.
9. Schuckit, M.A. and Hesselbrock, V. (1994). Alcohol dependence and anxiety disorders: what is the relationship? *American Journal of Psychiatry*, **151**, 1723–34.
10. Merikangas, K.R., Stevens, D., Fenton, B., *et al.* (1996). Comorbidity and co-transmission of anxiety disorders and alcoholism: results of the Yale Family Study. In *Proceedings of the American Psychiatric Association, May 1996*. American Psychiatric Association, Washington, DC.
11. Maier, W., Minges, J., and Lichtermann, D. (1993). Alcoholism and panic disorder: co-occurence and co-transmission in families. *European Archives of Psychiatry and Clinical Neuroscience*, **243**, 205–11.
12. Kendler, K.S., Walters, E.E., Neale, M.C., Kessler, R.C., Heath, A.C., and Eaves, L.J. (1995). The structure of genetic and environmental risk factors for six major psychiatric disorders in women: phobia, generalized anxiety disorder, panic disorder, bulimia, major depression, and alcoholism. *Archives of General Psychiatry*, **52**, 374–83.
13. de la Monte, S.M. (1988). Disproportionate atrophy of cerebral white matter in chronic alcoholics. *Archives of Neurology*, **45**, 990–2.
14. Jernigan, T.L., Butters, N., Di Tragila, G., *et al.* (1991). Reduced cerebral grey matter observed in alcoholics using magnetic resonance imaging. *Alcoholism, Clinical and Experimental Research*, **15**, 418–27.
15. Harper, C., Kril, J., and Daly, J. (1987). Are we drinking our neurons away? *British Medical Journal*, **294**, 534–6.
16. Harper, C.G. and Kril, J.J. (1989). Patterns of neuronal loss in the cerebral cortex in chronic alcoholic patients. *Journal of Neurology Sciences*, **92**, 81–9.
17. Ferrer, I., Fabregues, I., Rairiz, J., and Galofre, E. (1986). Decreased numbers of dendritic spines on cortical pyramidal neurons in human chronic alcoholism. *Neuroscience Letters*, **69**, 115–19.
18. Torvik, A., Lindbö, C.F., and Rodge, S. (1982). Brain lesions in alcoholics. *Journal of Neurological Sciences*, **56**, 233–48.
19. Torvik, A. and Torp, S. (1986). The prevalence of alcoholic cerebellar atrophy. A morphometric and histological study of an autopsy material. *Journal of Neurological Sciences*, **75**, 43–51.
20. Riley, J.N. and Walker, D.W. (1978). Morphological alterations in hippocampus after longterm alcohol consumption in mice. *Science*, **201**, 646–8.
21. Mann, K. (1992). *Alkohol und Gehirn—über strukturelle und funktionelle veränderungen nach erfolgreicher therapie*. Springer, Berlin.
22. Mann, K., Mundle, G., Strayle, M., and Wakat, P. (1995). Neuroimaging in alcoholism: CT and MRI results and clinical correlates. *Journal of Neural Transmission (General Section)*, **99**, 145–55.
23. Charness, M. (1993). Brain lesions in alcoholics. *Alcoholism, Clinical and Experimental Research*, **17**, 2–11.
24. Lemoine, P., Harousseau, H., Borteyru, J.-P., and Menuet, J.-C. (1968). Les enfants de parents alcooliques: anomalies observées à propos de 127 cas. *Ouest Médical*, **25**, 477–82.
25. Dow, K.E. and Riopelle, R.J. (1985). Ethanol neurotoxicity: effects on neurite formation and neurotrophic factor production *in vitro*. *Science*, **228**, 591–3.
26. Kukreya, R.C. and Hess, M.L. (1992). The oxygen free radical system: from equations through membrane–protein interactions to cardiovascular injury and protection. *Cardiovascular Research*, **26**, 641–55.
27. Miller, M.W. (1993). Migration of cortical neurons is altered by gestational exposure to ethanol. *Alcoholism, Clinical and Experimental Research*, **17**, 304–14.
28. Estruch, R. (1996). Alcohol and nutrition. In *Alcohol misuse: a European perspective*. (ed. T.J. Peters), pp. 41–61. Harwood Academic, London.
29. Urbano-Márquez, A. and Fernández-Solà, J. (1996). Musculo-skeletal problems in alcohol abuse. In *Alcohol misuse: a European perspective* (ed. T.J. Peters), pp. 123–44. Harwood Academic, London.
30. Lieber, C.S. (1998). Hepatic and other medical disorders of alcoholism: from pathogenesis to treatment. *Journal of Studies on Alcohol*, **59**, 9–25
31. Anderson, P., Cremona, A., Paton, A., Turner, C., and Wallace, P. (1993). The risk of alcohol. *Addiction*, **88**, 1493–508.
32. Niebergall-Roth, E., Harder, H., and Singer, M.V. (1998). A review: acute and chronic effects of ethanol and alcoholic beverages on the pancreatic exocrine secretion *in vivo* and *in vitro*. *Alcoholism, Clinical and Experimental Research*, **22**, 1570–83.
33. Higgins, E.M. (1996). Alcohol misuse and the skin. In *Alcohol misuse. A European perspective* (ed. T.J. Peters), pp. 77–87. Harwood Academic, London.
34. Edwards, G., Anderson, P., Babor, T., *et al.* (1994). *Alcohol policy and the public good*. Oxford Medical Publications, Oxford.
35. Tuyns, A.J. (1996). Alcohol and malignancies. In *Alcohol misuse: a European perspective* (ed. T.J. Peters), pp. 163–79. Harwood Academic, London.

4.2.2.4 Treatment of alcohol dependence

Jonathan Chick

A chronic relapsing disorder

Some people repeatedly put themselves or others at risk by drinking. One view is that such people could drink sensibly if they were more considerate and used more will power. Another increasingly accepted view is that many such individuals are in a state, existing in degrees of severity, in which the freedom to decide whether to change their drinking, and to adhere to that decision, is reduced compared with other drinkers. This state partly depends on perceived pay-offs for changing, and on acquired dispositions which are less accessible to conscious control. Such persons become aware of a wish, or urge, to drink which overcomes rational thought. They may then make up an explanation, for example 'No wonder I feel like a drink, I've had a hard day'.

Such individuals benefit from help to unlearn those patterns, and to learn different approaches to problems. Discussion, care, and encouragement from others can bolster their will to do so. Assistance to set up controls within or from outside themselves may help. Some people can do this without external help, and others with the help of Alcoholics Anonymous (**AA**) alone.[1]

This approach argues that dependence on alcohol should be managed like other relapsing disorders, such as diabetes and asthma,[2] by using long-term monitoring coupled with intermittent or continuous treatment. However, social and cultural influences are stronger than in relapsing medical conditions and have more effects on outcome.

Starting treatment

The initial interview

Assessment is the first step of intervention; clumsy interviewing alienates an ambivalent patient. The key to success is accepting that the patient is probably in two minds about the interview and about changing his or her drinking habits. Avoid confrontation. The drinking has probably already shown its resistance to deterrence by fear or pain. Gently nudge the matrix of conflicting motivations in the direction of action.

Patients may or may not have been referred for help with alcohol problems. Even if they have, the interview should begin with enquiry into the patient's current concerns. Reflective listening[3] helps the patient to clarify these concerns, conveys empathy, and avoids premature closure. A spirit of collaborative enquiry helps patients to reach their own conclusions about the role of alcohol in their troubles. This will be more convincing than a recitation of medical advice. People are more likely to believe what they hear themselves say than what others tell them. The interview is less likely to slip into confrontation if the doctor conveys recognition that, for the patient, drinking alcohol has been pleasurable. Therefore the assessment should not proceed in a series of closed questions, such as: 'Do you drink more than you intend to?' 'Does alcohol make you depressed?' Instead, ask open-ended questions: 'Tell me about your pattern of drinking. What are the good

aspects...and what are the disadvantages?' 'How does alcohol fit in with these periods of hopelessness you describe?' The patient may want it understood that at times alcohol has dulled pain. Only then will there be a concession that overall it has worsened mood.

A comment such as 'I'm just a heavy social drinker, not an alcoholic' is not a gauntlet to be seized—an argument about definitions will distract from the work of clarifying and planning how to deal with the current problems. Instead, a response such as 'I gather you don't like labels' may reveal pertinent fears and prejudices (e.g. that alcoholics get locked up in hospital or are failures).

Denial permits dismissal of unpleasant or unwanted facts and feelings. It hurts to admit that you have lost your family's respect, or that you will have to give up alchol which you enjoy. Alcohol problems still carry disgrace. In Islamic cultures, where alcohol is forbidden, denial from shame may be deepened by fear of punishment from the authorities.

Explain symptoms

Help the patient to understand withdrawal symptoms and how they can abort attempts to reduce consumption. Patients frequently attribute withdrawal symptoms to other causes; for example, waking at 4 a.m. with sweats and anxiety may be attributed to worry, and trembling hands in the morning to stress.

Informant

If the partner, a close friend, or a relative is present from the start, the salient points usually emerge more rapidly. However, the patient should also be seen alone because matters to do with the police, an employer, the bank, or a lover may still be unknown to the partner. Relatives should hear the exchange between doctor and patient, otherwise the version they hear later from the patient may be diluted—'The doctor says I'm not an alcoholic'. This can leave relatives even angrier than before, convinced that no-one understands their distress and that the drinker has once again deceived the doctor.

Assessments

The use of a breathalyser or saliva test to measure blood alcohol concentration puts alcohol consumption firmly into the objective arena. Use the test before the individual starts to detail recent drinking—there is nothing to be gained from showing that the patient sometimes minimizes the drinking.

Physical signs may be helpful. Heavy drinking may cause excessive capillarization in the conjunctivae or in the skin of the nose and cheeks. The liver may be enlarged. Look for tremor in the outstretched tongue, which is less commonly concealed (or exaggerated) than tremor in the fingers. Tachycardia is another useful sign of withdrawal. In a hyperaroused fearful patient, who has already been without a drink for 24 h, a pulse of over 110 beats/min may presage delirium tremens.

Clinicians vary in how structured an assessment they prefer, but at some point in the first one or two interviews the following should be noted: drinking patterns, history of withdrawal symptoms, previous attempts to stop drinking, use of drugs (prescribed and not prescribed), physical complications including head injuries, police or court involvement (past and current), dwelling arrangements, problems at home, trouble at work, specifying whether the employer has referred to alcohol and/or started disciplinary action, psychiatric illness, family history, previous treatments, and experience of AA.

Medical assistance for withdrawal

Medical assistance to reduce the short-term discomfort of withdrawal can be the beginning of restructuring of thoughts and lifestyle towards long-term abstinence.

If dependence is severe, especially in an unplanned situation where a very heavy drinker is suddenly deprived of alcohol because of an accident, illness, or police arrest, care must be taken to prevent the life-threatening complications of convulsions or delirium. Anticipation is the key.

When dependence is less marked, withdrawal symptoms are mild and the person can stop drinking by gradual reduction, encouraged by the physician or a friend.

When the patient's aim is 'controlled drinking' (see below), this may also entail an initial stage of withdrawal, as the final goal is more likely to be achieved after abstinence for 2 or 3 months.

The setting

Controlled studies have shown that outpatient withdrawal is safe and effective for mild and moderately dependent alcoholics.[4,5] Advice for patients withdrawing at home is given in Box 1. Hayashida et al.[4] randomly allocated 164 mild to moderately affected patients to either inpatient or outpatient detoxification. Completion was successful in 95 per cent of the former and 72 per cent of the latter; inpatient care cost eight times more than outpatient care.

Admission to hospital is indicated when the home social milieu is inimical to abstinence, or when there is a history of withdrawal convulsions or delirium; it is urgent when there are any signs of Wernicke's encephalopathy.

Medication

A benzodiazepine (see systematic review by Mayo-Smith et al.[6]) is prescribed for two reasons: first, to reduce the risk of severe withdrawal symptoms with delirium or convulsions (indicated if recent consumption has been more than 15 units/day for more than 10 days); second, to assist the individual whose wish to abstain or reduce drinking is overcome by longing for alcohol (craving), shaking, anxiety, insomnia, or nausea and vomiting.

A typical outpatient regimen would be chlordiazepoxide 20 to 30 mg four times daily, reducing to zero over 5 days, with the larger doses given at night (Table 1). Medication is issued on the understanding that the patient does not also take alcohol. If there is any doubt that this instruction will be followed, medication is issued daily and a check made (ideally by breath or saliva tests) that drinking has not been resumed. Chlordiazepoxide is preferred to diazepam for outpatient use because it has a lower street value and is therefore less likely to be sold on. When managing severe withdrawal symptoms with marked agitation and tremor, or incipient delirium, diazepam (starting at 10 mg four times daily) is preferred because it has a more rapid action and can be given parenterally. A benzodiazepine with one metabolite only and a shorter half-life (e.g. oxazepam, lorazepam) is preferred if liver

Box 1

Advice to patient on withdrawing from alcohol at home

If you have been chemically dependent on alcohol, stopping drinking causes you to become tense, edgy, perhaps shaky or sweaty, and unable to sleep. There can be vomiting or diarrhoea. This 'rebound' of the nervous system can be severe. Medication controls the symptoms while the body adjusts to being without alcohol. This usually takes 3 to 7 days from the time of your last alcoholic drink. If you did not take medication, the symptoms would be worst in the first 48 h, and then gradually disappear. This is why the dose starts high and then reduces.

You have agreed not to drink alcohol You may become thirsty. Drink fruit juices and water but do not overdo it. You do not have to 'flush' alcohol out of the body. More than 3 litres of fluid could be too much. Do not drink more than three cups of coffee or five cups of tea. These contain caffeine which disturbs sleep and causes nervousness.

Aim to avoid stress The important task is not to give in to the urge to take alcohol. Help yourself relax by going for a walk, listening to music, or taking a bath.

Sleep You may find that even with the capsules, or as they are reduced, your sleep is disturbed. You need not worry about this—lack of sleep does not seriously harm you, but starting to drink again does. Your sleep pattern will return to normal in a month or so. It is better not to take sleeping pills so that your natural sleep rhythm returns. Try going to bed later. Take a bedtime snack or milky drink. The capsules may make you drowsy so you must not drive or operate machinery. If you become drowsy, miss out a dose.

Meals Even when you are not hungry, try to eat something. Your appetite will return.

function is significantly impaired (i.e. there is jaundice, ascites, oedema, low serum albumin, or raised serum bilirubin).

For inpatients, a benzodiazepine such as diazepam 10 mg may be given every hour until symptoms are controlled (symptom-triggered dosing). This procedure leads to lower total prescription of benzodiazepine, less oversedation, and quicker discharge from hospital.[7]

Table 1 Example of a fixed-dose regime for outpatient alcohol withdrawal using capsules of chlordiazepoxide 10 mg

	First thing	12 noon	6 p.m.	Bedtime
Day 1		3	3	3
Day 2	2	2	2	3
Day 3	2	1	1	2
Day 4	1	1		2
Day 5		1		1

If the patient is vomiting, give metoclopropamide 10 mg intramuscularly 30 min before the first benzodiazepine tablet and/or perhaps choose a benzodiazepine that can be administered parenterally; lorazepam 1 mg is absorbed adequately from the intramuscular site, or diazepam 10 mg can be given intravenously (or rectally).

Treating convulsions

With the aim of preventing further convulsions, the patient who has just had a fit or is in a fit is given 10 mg diazepam. Consider giving 15 to 20 mg in a patient who has been taking benzodiazepines regularly prior to this event, or is much above average weight. It is illogical to commence an anticonvulsant which may take 2 to 3 days to reach a therapeutic serum level. Rather, increase the dose of the benzodiazepines. A convulsion may presage delirium.

Preventing convulsions

Deaths have occurred in hospital, prison, and police cells from repeated alcohol withdrawal fits. When withdrawal is planned in patients with a history of fits of any cause the risk can be reduced by commencing phenytoin (300 mg daily) 4 days before the cessation of drinking. In an acute situation, larger than normal doses of long-acting benzodiazepines are given in the first 36 h without waiting until the blood alcohol level has fallen to zero. The benzodiazepine should be started as soon as the blood alcohol level can be presumed to be falling, even though the patient still smells of alcohol or has a positive breath test, provided that he or she is sober enough to understand and co-operate with the procedure.

Treating delirium tremens

Increasing the dose of the benzodiazepine may be sufficient to control the agitation. If not, the slight epileptogenic effect of antipsychotic drugs should not deter their use, especially if delusions and hallucinations have developed, provided that anticonvulsant protection by a benzodiazepine is in place. Parenteral droperidol plus parenteral lorazepam is usually effective. When a patient's behaviour is uncontrolled or dangerous, transfer to a secure unit may be needed. Authoritative calm nursing reduces the risk of aggression. Hospitals should have an emergency team of sufficient personnel to manage disturbed patients.

Preventing delirium tremens

If confusion and hallucinations develop, this usually occurs 48 to 72 h after the last drink. Sufficient benzodiazepine, given early in the withdrawal, reduces the risk, as does sensitive nursing in a quiet evenly lit environment. Explaining symptoms and orientating the patient reduces anxiety, paranoia, and confusion.

Vitamin therapy

It is reasonable to prescribe thiamine 50 mg orally three times a day for 2 to 3 weeks, as thiamine stores may be depleted because of poor diet and alcohol-impaired gut absorption. Wernicke–Korsakoff syndrome is life-threatening and steps must be taken to avoid it developing.[8] The malnourished patient, or the patient who shows any sign of Wernicke's encephalopathy (confusion, ataxia, ophthalmoplegia, nystagmus—do not wait for the 'triad' of symptoms), must be given immediate parenteral B vitamins. Anaphylactic shock was a very rare complication of some older preparations. It is less likely with intramuscular than intravenous injection; infusion saline drip, when practicable, is probably preferable to slow bolus injection.

Interventions to reduce relapse

The evidence

With appropriate help, withdrawing from alcohol is not the dependent drinker's main difficulty. The main difficulty is avoiding later relapse into further problematic drinking or dependence.

Until recently no treatments had been tested in a randomized controlled trial. Therapists explored with patients possible personality or psychological causes of their excessive drinking—trying to find out 'why?'. However, there was no evidence that this reduced relapse. Indeed, it could have had an adverse effect by creating transference problems which triggered drinking and by reinforcing the drinkers' perception of having a need to drink.[9] Similarly, non-directive counselling could act as a confessional, with a sense of absolution allowing further drinking.

Miller *et al.*[10,11] reviewed 302 controlled trials. A score for each therapy was calculated based on the number of positive and of negative reports and their methodological quality. Some of the apparently most effective treatments, such as systematically helping people anticipate and cope with high risk situations ('relapse prevention'[12,13]) and motivational enhancement,[14] had been tested partly in less severe groups of patients. Other effective treatment, such as community reinforcement,[15] social skills training, cognitive therapy, behaviour contracting, and behavioural marital therapy, had been tested in patients showing a wider range of severity.[10] Miller's review[10,11] of disulfiram studies did not separate those where compliance was assured by supervision (where efficacy was demonstrated) from those where supervision was not in place (where the drug was ineffective).[16]

Abstinence or 'controlled drinking'?

Harmful or hazardous use of alcohol without severe dependence can sometimes revert to risk-free drinking. Patients with social supports (family and job) and without impulsive personalities and many social problems are most likely to succeed. For others, including most of those dependent on alcohol, the goal of abstinence is better. In patients attending specialized outpatient clinics, the proportion who can sustain problem-free drinking for at least 1 year is small—5 per cent is a typical finding.[17–19] A randomized trial comparing the goals of controlled drinking and abstinence did not favour controlled drinking.[20] However, for patients without established dependence, reduction programmes (whether or not towards abstinence) using FRAMES (Table 2) proved to be more effective than no intervention.[21–23] Interventions in primary care are discussed in Chapter 4.2.2.5.

If controlled drinking is the agreed goal, the patient and physician collaborate to monitor the amount and pattern of the drinking as follows.

1. Limit number of days of drinking and number of drinks on any occasion.

2. Slow the rate of drinking, and/or reduce alcoholic strength of drinks.

3. Develop assertiveness skills for refusing drinks.

4. Design reward system when goals are achieved.

5. Develop awareness of triggers to overdrinking.

6. Practise other ways of coping with triggers.

7. Record pattern and amount of drinking, for example in a diary.

8. Physician and patient monitor γ-glutamyl transferase blood test results.

Maintaining motivation and compliance

Enhancing motivation has a place not only at onset, but throughout the clinical contact.[24] Treatment aimed only at enhancing motivation was for most measures equal to cognitive-behavioural therapy, and intensive intervention aimed at linking patients with AA.[25] Randomized controlled studies have shown the advantage of motivational interviewing over traditional supportive therapy.[10,26] The style of the opening interview using motivational interviewing techniques has already been discussed. The patient is encouraged not to forget the harm that drinking caused and the benefits of abstinence, but the losses and problems of being sober are not denied. Strategies for maintaining abstinence emerge from collaborative dialogue, and are owned by patients rather than offered as advice from the clinician. If medication is part of the treatment plan, unwanted effects are actively enquired into, and are recognized and not dismissed, and remedies are sought. Any discrepancies that patients reveal between their present view of themselves and how they would like to be, or between what patients say they believe and how they actually behave, are used as a fulcrum for shifting attitudes and testing alternative strategies. These techniques were elaborated by Miller and Rollnick[3] and enshrined as motivational enhancement therapy[27] by Project MATCH (see below).

Helping motivation: the social matrix

It is said that the only successful way to change your drinking is to do it for yourself. Nevertheless, research and experience shows that those

Table 2 FRAMES: ingredients of a brief intervention

Feedback about personal risk or impairment

Responsibility: emphasis on personal responsibility for change

Advice to cut down or, if indicated because of severe dependence or harm, to abstain

Menu of alternative options for changing drinking pattern

Empathic interviewing

Self-efficacy: an interviewing style which enhances this

Reproduced with permission from T. H. Bien *et al.* (1993). Motivational interviewing with alcoholic outpatients. *Behavioural and Cognitive Psychotherapy*, **21**, 347–56.

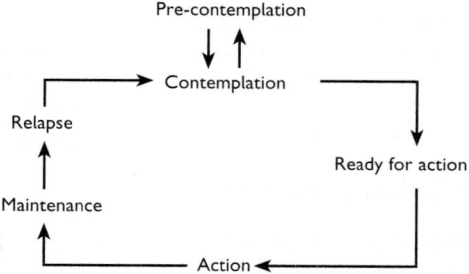

Fig. 1 Wheel of change. (Reproduced with permission from J. Prochaska and C. DiClementi (1984). Stages of change in the modification of problem behaviors. In *Progress in behavior modification*, Vol. 28 (ed. M. Hersen, R. Eisler, and P. Miller), pp. 183–218. Sycamore Publishing, Sycamore, IL.)

dependent on alcohol can start on the road to recovery when their reason is pressure from outside. This may be from the court which is seeking evidence, before deciding on sentence, that offenders have taken steps to alter harmful drinking patterns. The driving licence may have been withdrawn following a drink–drive offence and evidence that drinking is under control is required before its return. Perhaps the partner is ready to take a firm line, even to demand a separation or divorce, or the employer has given a warning.

Friends, partners, colleagues at work, and even employers sometimes adopt an approach that they believe to be motivating but which has the opposite effect and enables the drinker to continue drinking. They may cover up, gloss over, make excuses, or even start blaming themselves for what is going wrong. This cushions drinkers from experiencing the harmful consequences of their drinking or allows them to believe that alcohol is not the chief problem, despite evidence that alcohol is in fact the critical common factor in their downward spiral.

A physician can help the parties improve communication so that important messages are not lost. If the message from the employer or partner, or even the children, is clear and positive, it can have a powerful motivating effect: 'We value our relationship with you. But the way you are drinking is harming that relationship and we will not tolerate it'.

Some physicians are overcautious about confidentiality in this situation. If a doctor is asked by a partner or an employer to comment on the patient's condition, he or she may or may not have permission, or feel it appropriate, to do so. But doctors can usefully help partners or employers clarify for themselves what they want, and then encourage a clear and firm, but positive, message.

Sometimes doctors unwittingly collude in a cover-up. The smokescreen that can be set up by a drinker who is severely dependent and ambivalent about change can be hard to penetrate: 'It's depression, doctor'; 'It's stress at work'; 'If only my wife was more understanding/my sleep was not so disturbed/I didn't get these memory blanks which I think are some kind of stroke'. The doctor may need to wait for that medical moment, perhaps a crisis, to help such an individual. Or, if the doctor has patience, the drip, drip of non-judgemental evidence, and perhaps some social pressure, may bring about the necessary change in the patient's understanding and thus the perceived motivational payoffs. Understanding may lead to action. However, as Fig. 1 shows, that action may not be sustained and the process of helping understanding may need to be repeated many times.[28]

There are few randomized controlled studies allocating patients to different intensities of external motivation. However, the evidence is that alcoholics coerced into treatment do no worse than those attending voluntarily.[29]

Cognitive-behavioural therapies

When incentives are powerful, many newly abstinent patients are able to abstain for short periods. Others lack the skills to cope with the triggers to drinking even when their motivation to abstain has been strong. Cognitive-behavioural therapies seem to improve the coping skills of these patients. If the triggers are in social situations, assertiveness or conversation skills training can help. If the trigger is related to life problems, cognitive therapy may be effective. Other patients are helped by learning to handle frustration and criticism without anger, and to express anger instead of harbouring it. Treatment can be in groups, where the opportunity to discuss these topics with others who have similar problems is appreciated. Groups also enable learning through role playing and by modelling on others.

Relapse prevention therapy

Much of the above is also part of 'relapse prevention therapy'.[12,13] In this therapy patients are shown how to analyse and modify the causes of relapse. They are helped to identify 'seemingly irrelevant decisions', in which a sequence that ended in drinking began with apparently unconnected actions. For example, the person chooses to stop at the supermarket to buy fruit, knowing that there is plenty at home already, and comes out with a bottle of wine. The patient is encouraged to identify seemingly irrelevant decisions, and, by recording thoughts and feelings during the days between therapy sessions, to map out risky emotional or environmental situations and to prepare avoidance and coping tactics. By logging success they can build up their sense of mastery.

Relapse may be preceded by a feeling of deserving a drink or of being deprived. Helping the patient to have more satisfaction in other areas of life helps combat these feelings.

Patients are educated about the abstinence violation effect. The suggestion is that a patient who made a strong commitment to abstain, but has taken one drink, is overcome by a sense of failure and counters this by thinking, for example, 'This shows I'm just a drunk after all!'—which leads to further consumption. The abstinence violation effect predicts that relapse after taking a single drink would be most frequent in those with the strongest resolution to abstain. However, research has found that greater commitment is associated with less risk of relapse after a single lapse.[30] Nevertheless, it seems helpful to prepare patients for a lapse, and to avoid catastrophic thinking.

Cue exposure

The smell or sight of alcoholic drinks can be a powerful stimulus to drinking. Initial studies[31] have shown that 'deconditioning' by exposing inpatients to the sight and smell of their preferred drinks in a laboratory setting, without drinking, was associated in the coming 6 months with a longer period without a relapse. The approach is challenged by those who recognize overconfidence as a precursor of relapse. Although patients should not expect that to be in a bar will inevitably result in heavy drinking, they should not court danger. Bars are places where people go to drink. Cue exposure studies need to be replicated.

Couples should decide together whether to have alcohol in the house. However, patients should not be encouraged to 'test themselves'.

Alcoholics Anonymous

There are many ingredients in the healing process of AA. Newcomers are helped to identify with others as members tell their stories. They see that it is possible to be frank about past errors and the hurt caused to others through the drinking. Telling their own story helps the members not to forget the harm that accrued from drinking. This reduces complacency, which is one of the most common precursors of relapse.

Alcoholism is viewed by AA as a physical, psychological, and spiritual illness, which can be arrested (by avoiding another drink) but cannot be cured. The meetings offer a new social network. Emotional openness is encouraged. Members learn to express warmth, and to accept that they and others have failings. The AA advice on coping with emotions and relationship difficulties has much in common with cognitive-behavioural therapy and relapse prevention therapy. The method has some attractively simple concepts ('Just don't pick up that first drink'; 'HALT'—being alert to four of the most common triggers to relapse, i.e. hunger, anger, loneliness, tiredness). There is a deeper aspect which is to replace preoccupation with self by handing over to the group process, or to a 'Higher Power'.[32]

Accepting that you are 'powerless' to control your drinking is the 'first step' in AA. This entails ceasing the struggle and letting the 'Higher Power' take over. Members vary in their interpretation of the 'Higher Power', and avowed atheists should not be deterred from sampling AA. Residential, outpatient, and day programmes which teach the AA approach are sometimes called 12-step programmes (Box 2). One of their strengths is linking patients to the AA network.

A psychiatrist can introduce patients to AA through a contact member who will tell the patient how AA works, will not ask personal details, and will extend an invitation to a meeting. Doctors are welcome to attend 'open' AA meetings to see how it works. A contact number is given in local telephone directories. AA does not work for everyone, but since it is difficult to predict who will be helped it is good practice to offer contact to all patients with impaired control of their drinking.

A warning, often based on personal experience, may be given at AA meetings about transferring dependence from alcohol to other drugs. This usually refers to use of barbiturates or benzodiazepines, or to the danger of relying on a medication instead of adjusting one's way of living. The use of prescribed medication is not formally disapproved of by AA.

Evidence of efficacy

Naturalistic non-randomized studies have shown that treatment programmes using the AA approach are associated with outcomes in drinking and overall functioning similar to those of programmes using the cognitive-behavioural approach. Patients in 12-step programmes

Box 2

The 12 steps of Alcoholics Anonymous

Step 1 We admitted we were powerless over alcohol—that our lives had become unmanageable.

Step 2 Came to believe that a Power greater than ourselves could restore us to sanity.

Step 3 Made a decision to turn our will and our lives over to the care of God *as we understood Him*.

Step 4 Made a searching and fearless moral inventory of ourselves.

Step 5 Admitted to God, to ourselves, and to another human being the exact nature of our wrongs.

Step 6 Were entirely ready to have God remove all these defects of character.

Step 7 Humbly asked Him to remove our shortcomings.

Step 8 Made a list of all persons we had harmed, and became willing to make amends to them all.

Step 9 Made direct amends to such people wherever possible, except when to do so would injure them or others.

Step 10 Continued to take personal inventory and when we were wrong promptly to admit it.

Step 11 Sought through prayer and meditation to improve our conscious contact with God *as we understood Him*, praying only for knowledge of His will for us and the power to carry that out.

Step 12 Having had a spiritual awakening as a result of these steps, we tried to carry this message to alcoholics and to practise these principles in our affairs.

improve on self-efficacy and coping skills scores much as patients treated by cognitive-behavioural therapy.[33] There are significant associations between AA attendance and positive outcome.[34]

Only two randomized controlled studies of 12-step programmes have been conducted. One compared inpatient treatment (with fewer hours of psychotherapy than many such programmes) with a 12-step inpatient programme (with slightly more hours of therapy). There was a non-significant trend towards a greater total abstinence programme and less relapse in the 12-step programme.[35] In Project MATCH, patients were randomly allocated to cognitive-behavioural therapy, motivational enhancement therapy, or '12-step facilitation', which instructed patients in the tenets of AA, and assisted and encouraged them to attend AA meetings. The three treatments resulted in similar outcomes after 1 and 3 years. However, for those who had been relatively free of psychiatric problems at entry to the study, 12-step facilitation was associated with slightly better outcomes after 1 year. After 3 years the 12-step facilitation led to better outcome for patients who, at entry to the study, had family, social, or work environments bringing them into frequent contact with drinking.[36]

Help for the family

Working with the family

The family of someone with a drinking problem may suffer for years without recognition and can benefit from advice and understanding. They are a vital monitor of the patient's progress. Good family cohesion and low expressed emotion predict better outcome, even after controlling for the predictors of demographic variables and severity of alcohol dependence.

Life in the family becomes increasingly restricted. Finances dwindle. The children fear that the parent may be drunk, and so stop inviting friends to visit. They dread that arguments between mother and father will become violent. The drinker's behaviour becomes slovenly. He or she may wet the bed. Despite these hurts, the drinker may still make the family believe that they are the reason he or she drinks.

The invitation to a family member or partner to attend with the patient may be rejected if the drinker is the messenger, and the message is distorted to: 'The doctor says you're part of the problem'. A direct letter or telephone call from the clinician requesting 'your views on how I can assist' reduces the partner's fear of being burdened with extra guilt or responsibility.

The clinician can help reduce family behaviours, such as hostility or cover-up, that are damaging to the family and counterproductive for the drinker's recovery. Communication between the drinker and the spouse or children has often broken down. In many countries family groups, such as Al-Anon, provide help to families.

Behavioural marital therapy

When the patient is in a relationship, its quality can be motivating or demotivating. Reciprocal contracts are aimed at making the relationship more rewarding for each partner. Although abstinence is a prerequisite, specific agreements should not be contingent on the drinking;[37] otherwise, a relapse means that the partner ceases to work on the relationship. Another prerequisite might be that physical violence is excluded. Contracting could start thus: 'Although you are responsible for not drinking, is there anything that your partner could do more of, or less of, that would help you stick to the plan?' Check that the requests are reasonable and available before the partner is asked to agree. The partner makes reciprocal requests and negotiation follows. Even requests for small changes can start the process.

The partners should give clear messages, owning their statements: 'This is what I would like', 'It makes me feel good if you…'. They will need to be reminded to state the positives and to practise being good listeners, giving non-verbal signals that they are listening, and not butting in with unsolicited good advice.

Violence in the partnership may require specific attention. If the drinker is intoxicated, the partner is advised to back off and avoid argument. Sometimes each partner is asked to sign an agreement that neither will threaten or hit the other. If they do, time-out in another room is agreed in advance to permit slow-breathing to aid calming down, or one of them will leave the house and go to a designated place for 36 to 72 h.

Blaming

The partner 'bringing up the past' can be a major irritant to the drinker. This can be reframed as the partner 'helping the couple not repeat their past'. A partner who feels heard and understood is more ready to look at other ways of achieving these goals.

Efficacy

Behavioural marital therapy produces better outcomes of drinking and marital relations than individual counselling or similar control conditions. The superior effects last for 24 months after treatment. Outcome at 1 year is better if sessions of behavioural marital therapy continue after the end of treatment to reinforce what has been learnt and rehearse relapse prevention plans.[38] This has been reviewed by Miller et al.[10]

Deterrent medication

Disulfiram

If taken in a sufficient dose for at least the preceding 3 to 4 days, disulfiram causes an unpleasant reaction to develop 15 to 20 min after alcohol enters the body. The reaction is due to accumulation of acetaldehyde, the intermediate metabolite of ethanol. The reactions includes flushing, headache, pounding in the chest or head, tightness in breathing, nausea, and sometimes vomiting. Hypotension can occur and is potentially dangerous. (Calcium carbimide has a similar action but is no longer available.) The disulfiram–ethanol reaction varies in intensity. It is recognized practice to increase the dose of disulfiram up to 400 mg daily if the patient has tested the alcohol reaction and it has not been severe enough to act as a deterrent.

Disulfiram is an aid, not a cure. The individual can become used to life without alcohol. This allows time for confidence to recover—personally, in the family, and at work. Patients may object that it is weakness to take a deterrent, and they prefer to show that they can use will power. Explain to the patient that will power is not always there when most needed. With disulfiram a decision to drink or not still has to be made, but only once a day or three times a week.

Unwanted effects which occur even when no alcohol is taken include drowsiness, bad breath, and headache. These make the drug unacceptable to some patients. Concerns that disulfiram can harm the liver are based on a few case reports (the risk is about 1 in 30 000 patient-years). It appears to be a hypersensitivity reaction, and if it is to occur it is likely to be in the first month. Overall, disulfiram is associated with improved liver function tests compared with control groups, presumably owing to reduction of drinking.[39] Peripheral neuropathy (almost always reversible) has been reported following several months at doses of over 250 mg. There are a few reports of psychosis induced by disulfiram, and psychotic illness has been a formal contraindication in the licensing in some countries. The risk is so low and the need to help schizophrenic patients with alcohol problems is sometimes so great that in other countries this contraindication has been changed to a 'caution'. There are many documented cases where improvement has occurred in psychotic patients while taking disulfiram, and in a dose of up to 250 mg daily there are no problems from unwanted actions or interactions with medication for the psychiatric illness.[40]

Efficacy

Disulfiram will only aid recovery if it is taken regularly in a sufficient dose to deter. In randomized controlled studies showing efficacy, a supervisor aided compliance. All reported controlled studies which enhanced compliance in this way showed efficacy.[16] In some of these studies there was a degree of coercion; for example, if the patient ceased taking the disulfiram the partner might withdraw from some agreed item, or disciplinary action at work might be reinstated.

Mode of use

Before prescribing, a physical examination and baseline liver function tests are performed. The patient is encouraged to ask the partner, a nurse or welfare officer at work or at the health centre, or a pharmacist to see that the disulfiram is taken. This can be daily, or three times a week, provided that the total weekly dose is sufficient. The product is in a dispersible form to be taken in water so that it can be seen to be swallowed.

There should be medical follow-up, but there is no consensus as to whether monitoring of liver function tests should be carried out. However, monthly follow-up is appropriate to check for signs of drinking and of liver disease.[39,41]

It is common to prescribe disulfiram for 6 months, but many patients ask to continue for longer and there may be slips when disulfiram is withdrawn, even after long periods of abstinence. Some patients keep a supply to use when they feel an increased risk of drinking, for example on a business trip or at a social event. Occasionally, when abstinence seems stable, a couple agree the opposite, namely that the drinker may have occasional breaks in the disulfiram regimen to permit drinking at a particular event or on a holiday if holidays have not been times of problematic drinking previously. Sometimes this is successful, but at others the wish to drink again regularly can be reawakened.[42] The taking of disulfiram may re-establish an employer's confidence, so that the patient may be reinstated.

Specific neurotransmitter antagonists

Two drugs, sometimes called 'anticraving agents', have been shown in randomized controlled trials to have modest but useful efficacy. However, some methodological problems concerning the conduct and analysis of these studies have been noted.[43–45]

Acamprosate (calcium acetyl homotaurinate)

Acamprosate enhances γ-aminobutyric acid (**GABA**) transmission and antagonizes glutamate transmission, probably by antagonizing N-methyl-D-aspartate receptors (see Chapter 6.2.8). It reduces drinking in alcohol-dependent animals, and reduces the reinstatement of drinking behaviour in animals re-exposed to alcohol after a period of abstinence. Animals do not seek out acamprosate as they do addictive substances, and it does not have mood-altering or drug-abuse potential in humans.[46] It has no deterrent or disulfiram-like effect.

Acamprosate is excreted unchanged in the kidney. It has few unwanted effects; diarrhoea and abdominal discomfort are the only ones reported in more than 10 per cent of patients (up to 20 per cent) and these are mild and transient. It does not exacerbate psychomotor impairment caused by alcohol. There are no known drug interactions.

Efficacy

Acamprosate has a dose-related effect of improving abstinence rates in recently detoxified patients.[47–49] Large randomized controlled studies of acamprosate[50,51] have shown an increase, compared with placebo, in the percentage remaining totally abstinent for 12 months from 10 to 25 per cent to 20 to 50 per cent, a doubling of the time to first relapse, and a halving of total alcohol consumed. There are no studies comparing the advantages of differing lengths of treatment. Systematic follow-up after the end of drug or placebo treatment shows no sudden relapse and no discontinuation symptoms in patients who have received acamprosate for up to 1 year.[51]

Several studies have shown that acamprosate reduces self-reported craving for alcohol; one of these failed to find an effect on drinking.[52] Some newly abstinent patients experience strong craving, but others experience very little.

Acamprosate has only been tested in patients who intend to abstain from alcohol. It has not been shown to assist patients aiming for controlled drinking.

Suggested mode of use

Acamprosate is indicated for patients who have typical severe alcohol dependence requiring medical assistance to withdraw. It is started 2 to 7 days after the last drink. Steady state pharmacokinetics are reached after 5 days. It is given in a dose of 1998 mg daily divided through the day. Patients who relapse while on acamprosate are advised to continue taking the medication and exert effort to limit the lapse. However, acamprosate is not normally continued in patients who relapse more than once despite regularly taking the drug. About 50 per cent or more of patients do not benefit from acamprosate. Those who appear to be benefiting from it should continue the drug for at least 6 months, and up to 1 year if there has been previous relapse in treatment.

Patients taking disulfiram randomly allocated to acamprosate seem to be more successful than patients taking disulfiram and placebo,[53] suggesting that acamprosate's potential to reduce craving in newly abstinent patients may help them to continue taking disulfiram. The reverse procedure, i.e. randomly allocating patients taking acamprosate to disulfiram or control, has not been carried out.

Naltrexone

Naltrexone antagonizes endorphins which are released in one of ethanol's many acute actions on the limbic system. It has been suggested that this action contributes to loss of control.[54] Naltrexone reduces ethanol seeking in dependent animals. It does not exacerbate the psychomotor impairment caused by alcohol.

Efficacy

Two double-blind randomized controlled studies in detoxified outpatients showed that naltrexone 50 mg daily reduces the risk of relapse over a 3-month treatment period.[55,56] A subsequent study failed to find a significant treatment effect in the all-patient intention-to-treat analysis, but found a beneficial effect in a predefined subgroup of compliant patients (who had attended regularly for treatment and received 80 per cent of the prescribed study medication).[57] The effect size of naltrexone treatment in reducing the percentage of days drinking was 0.42 in one study and 0.60 in the other.[58] (For comparison, the mean effect size in meta-analyses of studies of fluoxetine in the treatment of depression is around 0.4.)

Follow-up has not indicated rapid relapse on cessation of these drugs. However, during a 6-month follow-up after 3 months of placebo-controlled treatment, patients relapsed gradually after naltrexone to a final rate similar to that seen in placebo-treated patients.[59]

Mode of action

Some patients who drink while taking naltrexone report that they feel less of the ethanol 'high'. This could lead to less impulse to carry on

drinking.[58,60] However, O'Malley et al.[56] found that more patients reported total abstinence as well as a reduction of drinking overall. It is possible that the reduced craving for alcohol and the reduced likelihood of picking up the first drink occur because the strength of the previous triggers—emotional, cognitive, or environmental—is attenuated.

Reports in the 1970s that naltrexone might cause dysphoria seemed to be supported by statements from heroin addicts given naltrexone to help them abstain from opiates. However, laboratory studies and randomized controlled trials have not found evidence of dysphoria or loss of feelings of pleasure.[61]

Helping women with alcohol problems

It has been said that when a woman has an alcohol problem, there is a man in her life with a similar problem—usually her partner or her father. When the partner also drinks heavily, he should if possible be involved in treatment. Other partners may be overinvolved and have adopted a controlling role, especially if she has been unreliable with the children, money, the car, etc. The woman's resentment at this can fuel the drinking, and it may need months to help her to see how this has come about to help the partner stop checking her behaviour and to restore trust.

Low self-esteem is very common in such women, even in those who were confident before the drinking got out of hand. The partner, while remaining firm about the unacceptability of her drinking, may need help to be more caring and positive, to show interest in what concerns her, and to show appreciation.

Resentments towards family, employer, and partner are common and sometimes lead to depression. Women with alcohol dependence can be helped psychologically to abstain in several ways.

- Help her to stop feeling taken for granted, and to know that she has a right to set limits on what others expect of her.

- Although guilt may be proportional to what she has put her family through by her drinking, it may not help. It may prevent her from asking for the conditions at home or work that would make it easier for her to stop drinking.

- Help her let go of anger.

- Help her find ways of recharging her batteries by, for example, taking up new interests or exercise.

- Talk with the partner, both alone and with her present. He may want to know that she acknowledges the strain on him. While accepting complete responsibility for her drinking, she can let him know what he can do to help her.

- Self-help literature is available in many languages to help women improve self-confidence and self-assertion.[62]

Treatment of coexisting disorders

Affective disorder

Depression is common in patients who are dependent on alcohol. The drinking may have alienated friends, family, or employer, with resulting feelings of hopelessness, guilt, and lack of direction. Alcohol can reduce appetite, energy, and sexual drive. The drinker wakes in the small hours of the night feeling anxious owing to the rebound wakefulness of alcohol withdrawal. Those signs and symptoms suggesting depressive illness commonly clear with abstinence and help in tackling or tolerating personal problems and improving relationships.

Sometimes (more often in women than in men) a depressive episode precedes the alcohol dependence. Alcohol was taken in part as self-medication. Sometimes depressive symptoms continue despite abstinence. In these cases, antidepressants should be offered in the usual way.[63,64] Relapsing alcoholism, secondary to depressive illness, is an indication for long-term antidepressants. Lithium is not a treatment for alcohol dependence itself, but is effective if it is secondary to manic–depressive disorder.

Slightly higher blood levels of antidepressants may result when they are taken concurrently with disulfiram.

Depressed patients who have become dependent on alcohol are susceptible to the nausea and/or agitation which occur with many serotonin-enhancing agents. They may need an antiemetic such as metoclopramide for a few days and a slightly longer time on the reducing benzodiazepine regimen given for alcohol withdrawal. Trials in alcohol-dependent patients of serotonergic drugs with greater $5\text{-}HT_{1A}$ and less $5\text{-}HT_2$ activity, such as mirtazepine, have not yet been reported.

Anxiety and panic disorder

Some patients have had panic attacks for years before discovering that alcohol can end or prevent them. Others have a first panic attack during alcohol withdrawal, but the attacks continue independently even during sustained abstinence. In either case, cognitive-behavioural therapy and/or medication are indicated.

Three studies suggest that the serotonin agonist buspirone can help reduce both drinking and anxiety.[65] Tricyclic antidepressants and selective serotonin-reuptake inhibitors (**SSRIs**) have been shown to be effective in randomized controlled trials of panic disorders, but alcohol dependence has been an exclusion criterion in these trials. Newly abstaining alcohol-dependent patients seem particularly susceptible to the unwanted effects of serotonergic medication (see above).

Some patients with long histories of alcohol dependence and severe panic disorders fail to respond to psychological or antidepressant treatments. For these patients the risk of complications from repeated prescribing of a long-acting benzodiazepine may be less than those from continued excessive drinking. If prescribed (and to do so is controversial), the benzodiazepine should be dispensed in limited amounts. The prescription should be conditional on abstinence from alcohol, which can be aided by disulfiram if necessary. 'As-required' use (e.g. for travelling on public transport) helps to limit the development of tolerance, even though in theory it may perpetuate phobic beliefs. This method probably commits the patient to long-term use and an enduring risk of escalation.

Other comorbidities

Self-harm, sometimes in very severe forms such as self-immolation or disfigurement, may occur when personality disorder accompanies alcohol misuse. Such patients are sometimes helped by antidepressants, lithium, or depot antipsychotic drugs, in conjunction with other relapse prevention measures, and supervised living arrangements.

Attention-deficit hyperactivity disorder in adulthood is associated with alcohol dependence in 25 per cent of cases. There are no trials of methylphenidate in alcohol misuse.

Residential and inpatient treatment

It is debatable whether a period of inpatient treatment can improve the eventual outcome. Some studies have compared outcomes after patients have been randomly allocated to either inpatient or outpatient treatment. Usually no difference has been found. However, the interpretation of these results and their extrapolation to clinical reality has been debated. Finney et al.[66] concluded that the studies often lacked statistical power. Furthermore, the more seriously affected patients had sometimes been excluded before randomization.[66,67] While evidence that it is inpatient treatment rather than intensity of treatment which improves outcome is lacking,[68,69] admission to hospital can provide valuable respite for the drinker and the family when life is severely disorganized because drinking is out of control. Perhaps such respite need not be offered in a relatively expensive medical environment. However, if the patient has become suicidal as difficulties increase or has developed serious medical complications, then hospital admission may be indicated, ideally to specialized facilities if available. Longer stays in hospital are not supported by research. For example, Trent[70] found no evidence of worse outcome when the United States Navy reduced the length of its inpatient alcoholism treatment programme from 6 to 4 weeks. The role of inpatient treatment is considered further in Chapter 4.2.2.5.

Matching patients to treatments

The problem

It is recognized that people with alcohol dependence present a range of problems, come from various backgrounds, and have different personality characteristics. Some have no accompanying emotional disturbance; others have a psychiatric disorder. The poor outcomes of treatment for alcohol dependence have been attributed to their use with unsuitable patient, and better matching of patients to treatments has been sought. A North American study of 1726 outpatients (Project MATCH) set out to test hypotheses about matching treatments to patients. Three treatments were studied, each established in previous randomized controlled trials as more effective than 'supportive therapy': motivational enhancement therapy, cognitive-behavioural therapy, and instruction in the AA approach with encouragement to take part in AA meetings ('12-step facilitation').

Few matching effects reached statistical significance. In patients recruited from outpatient clinics, those who scored high on anger at initial assessment averaged 85 per cent of abstinent days if they had been allocated to motivational enhancement therapy compared with 75 per cent if they had been allocated to 12-step facilitation or cognitive-behavioural therapy.[71] In the first year of follow-up, patients with initially less severe psychiatric symptoms had more abstinent days after the 12-step facilitation than after cognitive-behavioural therapy. Patients with critically high psychiatric severity did no better with cognitive-behavioural therapy.[26]

Another marker of who benefits most from AA emerged in the 3-year Project MATCH data. Patients who came from a social milieu where they mixed a lot with other drinkers owing to family, neighbourhood, or work influences did better if they had received 12-step facilitation than with either cognitive-behavioural therapy or motivational enhancement therapy.[37]

There are several reasons for the absence of evidence of other powerful predictors of treatment outcome in the Project MATCH data. Perhaps the key behaviour—not taking the first drink—can be arrived at in different ways.

Guiding principles

Research into alcoholism spanning 50 years has shown that the attitudes of the agency and the therapist influence patients' outcome, as they may do for many illnesses. Showing respect, enhancing dignity, conveying accurate empathy, adopting objective and not moral criteria, involving the family, and reducing hurdles to seeking help have been shown to improve compliance, and often outcome, for alcohol dependence. The therapeutic alliance is a strong predictor of outcome in the treatment of alcohol dependence.[72] Agencies must set limits on drunken behaviour at the clinic and telephone calls when intoxicated. When relapse is recurrent, resumption of treatment can be made conditional on complying with a new initiative, such as supervision of medication.[73]

Some clinical situations

Morbid jealousy

This is discussed in Chapter 4.4.

The homeless alcohol-dependent person

It is difficult to conduct randomized controlled studies with adequate follow-up to test the efficacy of interventions to reduce drinking and improve social conditions for the homeless, and few answers have been found. A brief hospital admission to 'dry out' and assessment for transfer to residential care may result in transient improvement in physical health and is more humane than prison. However, supporting evidence is lacking. A structured intensive outpatient intervention, called the 'community reinforcement approach' has been shown in a North American study to reduce drinking (corroborated by improvement in serum γ-glutamyl transferase) and increase the number of clients at work and in satisfactory housing.[74] The community reinforcement approach combined an offer of free housing, a place at a 'job club' to assist with finding employment, training in problem-solving skills, communication, goal-setting, refusal of drinks, and independent living. Patients had access to an alcohol-free social club. The housing offer was contingent on sobriety and some evidence of saving money. Continuation in the housing was contingent on sobriety checked by breathalyser. Disulfiram had been shown to improve the effects of the community reinforcement approach.[15,75]

Young people

There is a dearth of evaluation of programmes to help young people with alcohol problems. AA groups may have teenage members. When education or employment are in jeopardy, young people may accept disulfiram, supervised perhaps by the family. However, without the support of a non-drinking peer group (which they would have in AA), most young people will try again and again to resume 'social drinking'. Job or marriage commitments sometimes alter the pay-off matrix sufficiently for recovery to be sustained. Otherwise, it may not be until age 30 that the young person is sufficiently convinced that he or she cannot control drinking and takes serious steps to seek help.

Employment referrals

It is common for individuals to seek help when their drinking has put their job in jeopardy. Having a job helps recovery, and for the person to lose employment while paying only lip-service to treatment is common and disheartening for all. The psychiatrist should find out whether disciplinary procedures are in motion or threatened. It can be helpful if the psychiatrist and the patient are told this directly by the employer. If the consultation is part of an undertaking under a company 'alcohol and drugs policy', the patient may have given permission for the psychiatrist to answer the employer's request to know whether he or she is attending and following advice.

Patients who are on the point of dismissal may offer to take disulfiram supervised in the company's occupational health or welfare department. This can bring about recovery and employment for as long as the threat of dismissal remains, and sometimes afterwards.[76]

The liver transplant candidate

Some transplant centres require a demonstration of months of abstinence, to show commitment, before offering transplant to a patient with alcoholic liver disorder. Other centres have no such restrictions. From 6 to 80 per cent of transplant recipients, varying between centres, have recommenced drinking and exceeded safe limits by the end of the first year. Their eventual outcome in terms of quality of life and psychiatric health is no worse than in other transplant patients, and evidence obtained to date suggests that demanding lengthy preoperative abstinence does not improve outcome.[77]

Physicians as patients

Doctors have a raised rate of alcohol dependence. Their outcome, once in treatment, tends to be better than average, if they can return to their practice. This is probably partly due to the requirement by the licensing body that the 'impaired physician' accept monitoring by an independent specialist to corroborate that he or she is following advice and continuing to progress.[78]

Doctors' reluctance to accept help for their illnesses, and their tendency to treat themselves, is well known and is especially true for substance misuse. Initial denial often means that problems escalate until there are disciplinary or court proceedings, and attempts to treat their own alcohol dependence may result in dependence on other substances.

The alcoholic doctor should be treated in the same way as a lay person. The partner should be invited to be involved. If possible, information should be obtained from the employer or from a colleague about the nature of any problems at work or any disciplinary action, actual or threatened.

In some countries there are support groups for recovering doctors and dentists who meet together and are ready to offer advice and encouragement to individuals and their families.

Follow-up

Systematic follow-up has been shown to improve outcome.[17,79] Early detection of relapse is important, and is aided by regular contact with the family or the workplace, a breathalyser test at interview, and tests for blood markers of drinking (γ-glutamyl transferase or carbohydrate-deficient transferrin).[80] Objective markers are required when a patient requests a report for a court, the driving licence authority, or an employer. Individualized outcome measures can be used, defined by the patient's own goals. This is particularly relevant when the patient's goal is to avoid further health or family problems, to avoid reoffending, or to stay in employment, rather than abstinence *per se*.[81]

References

1. Vaillant, G. (1997). *The natural history of alcoholism revisited*. Harvard University Press, Boston, MA.
2. O'Brien, C.P. and McLellan, A.T. (1996). Myths about the treatment of addiction. *Lancet*, **347**, 237–40.
3. Miller, W.R. and Rollnick, N. (1992). *Motivational interviewing*. Guilford Press, New York.
4. Hayashida, M., Alterman, A.I., McLellan, T., *et al.* (1989). Comparative effectiveness and costs of inpatient and outpatient detoxification with mild-moderate alcohol withdrawal syndrome. *New England Journal of Medicine*, **320**, 358–65.
5. Bennie, C. (1998). A comparison of home detoxification and minimal intervention strategies for problem drinkers. *Alcohol and Alcoholism*, **33**, 157–63.
6. Mayo-Smith, M.F., for the American Society for Addiction Medicine Working Group (1997). Pharmacological management of alcohol withdrawal: a meta-analysis and evidence-based practice guideline. *Journal of American Medical Association*, **278**, 144–61.
7. Foy, A., March, S., and Drinkwater, V. (1988). Use of an objective clinical scale in the assessment and management of alcohol withdrawal in a large general hospital. *Alcoholism: Clinical and Experimental Research*, **12**, 360–4.
8. Cook, C.C. and Thomson, A.D.T. (1997). B-complex vitamins in the prophylaxis and treatment of Wernicke–Korsakoff syndrome *British Journal of Hospital Medicine*, **57**, 461–5.
9. Vaillant, G.E. (1991). An alternative to psychotherapy. In *The international handbook of addiction behaviour* (ed. I.B. Glass), pp. 236–9. Routledge, London.
10. Miller, W.R., Brown, J.M., Simpson, T.L., *et al.* (1995). What works? A methodological analysis of the alcoholism treatment outcome literature. In *Handbook of alcoholism treatment approaches: effective alternatives* (2nd edn) (ed. R.K. Hester and W.R. Miller), pp. 12–44. Allyn and Bacon, Boston, MA.
11. Miller, W.R., Andrews, N.R., Wilbourne, P., and Bennet, M.E. (1998). A wealth of alternatives: effective treatments for alcohol problems. In *Treating addictive behaviours* (2nd edn) (ed. W.R. Miller and N. Heather), pp. 203–16. Plenum Press, New York.
12. Dimeff, L.A. and Marlatt, G.A. (1995). Relapse prevention. In *Handbook of alcoholism treatment approaches: effective alternatives* (2nd edn) (ed. R.K. Hester and W.R. Miller), pp. 176–94. Allyn and Bacon, Boston, MA.
13. Marlatt, G.A. and Gordon, J.R. (1985). *Relapse prevention*. Guilford Press, New York.
14. Miller, W.R., Benfield, R.G., and Tonnegan, J.S. (1993). Enhancing motivation for change in problem drinkers: a comparative outcome study of three controlled drinking therapies. *Journal of Consulting and Clinical Psychology*, **61**, 455–61.
15. Azrin, N.H. (1976). Improvements in the community reinforcement approach to alcoholism. *Behavioural Research and Therapy*, **14**, 339–48.
16. Hughes, J.C. and Cook, C. (1997). The efficacy of disulfiram—a review of outcome studies. *Addiction*, **92**, 381–96.
17. Chick, J., Connaughton, J., Ritson, B., Stewart, A., and Chick, J.A. (1988). Advice versus extended treatment for alcoholism: a controlled study. *British Journal of Addiction*, **83**, 159–70.
18. Helzer, J.E., Robins, L.N., Taylor, J.R., *et al.* (1985). The extent of long-term moderate drinking among alcoholics discharged from medical and psychiatric treatment facilities. *New England Journal of Medicine*, **312**, 1678–82.
19. Vaillant, G.E. (1996). A long-term follow-up of male alcohol abuse. *Archives of General Psychiatry*, **53**, 243–9.
20. Rychtarik, R.G., Foy, D.W., Scott, T., Lokey, L., and Prue, D.M. (1987). Five year follow-up of broad spectrum behavioral treatment for alcoholism: effects of training controlled drinking skills. *Journal of Consulting and Clinical Psychology*, **55**, 106–8.
21. Sanchez-Craig, M., Leigh, G., Spivak, K., and Davila, R. (1989). Superior outcome of females over males after brief intervention for the reduction of heavy drinking. *British Journal of Addiction*, **84**, 395–404.
22. WHO Brief Intervention Group (1996). A cross-national trial of brief intervention with heavy drinkers. *American Journal of Public Health*, **86**, 948–55.
23. Bien, T.H., Miller, W.R., and Tonigan, J.S. (1993). Brief interventions for alcohol problems: a review. *Addiction*, **88**, 315–36.
24. Miller, W.R. (1998). Enhancing motivation for change. In *Treating addictive behaviours* (2nd edn) (ed. W.R. Miller and N. Heather), pp. 121–32. Plenum Press, New York.
25. Project MATCH Research Group (1997). Matching alcoholism treatments to client heterogeneity: Project MATCH posttreatment drinking outcomes. *Journal of Studies on Alcohol*, **58**, 7–29.
26. Bien, T.H., Miller, W.R., and Boroughs, J.M. (1993). Motivational interviewing with alcoholic out-patients. *Behavioural and Cognitive Psychotherapy*, **21**, 347–56.
27. Miller, W.R., Zweben, A., DiClementi, C.C., and Rychtaril, R.G. (1992). *Motivational enhancement therapy manual: a clinical research guide for therapists treating individuals with alcohol abuse and dependence*. NIAAA Project MATCH Monograph Series, Vol. 2. DHHS Publication No. (ADM) 92-1894. US Government Printing Office, Washington, DC.
28. Prochaska, J. and Di Clemente, C. (1992). Stages of change in the modification of problem behaviors. In *Progress in behavior modification*, Vol. 28 (ed. M. Hersen, R. Eisler, and P. Miller), pp. 183–218. Sycamore Publishing, Sycamore, IL.
29. Chick, J. (1998). Treatment of alcoholic violent offenders—ethics and efficacy. *Alcohol and Alcoholism*, **33**, 20–5.
30. Hall, S.M., Havassy, B.E., and Wasserman, D.A. (1990). Commitment to abstinence and acute stress in relapse to alcohol, opiates and nicotine. *Journal of Consulting and Clinical Psychology*, **58**, 175–81.
31. Drummond, C. and Glautier, S. (1994). A controlled trial of cue exposure treatment in alcohol dependence. **62**, 809–17.
32. McCrady, B. (1994). Alcoholics Anonymous and behaviour therapy: can habits be treated as diseases? Can diseases be treated as habits? *Journal of Consulting and Clinical Psychology*, **62**, 1159–66.
33. Oiumette, P.C., Finney, J.W., and Moos, R.H. (1997). Twelve-step and cognitive–behavioural treatment for substance abuse: a comparison of treatment effectiveness. *Journal of Consulting and Clinical Psychology*, **65**, 230–40.
34. Emrick, C. (1987). Alcoholics Anonymous: affiliation processes and effectiveness as treatment. *Alcoholism: Clinical and Experimental Research*, **11**, 416–23.
35. Keso, L. and Salaspuro, M. (1990). In-patient treatment of employed alcoholics: a randomised clinical trial of Hazelden-type and traditional treatment. *Alcoholism: Clinical and Experimental Research*, **14**, 584–9.
36. Longabough, R., Wirtz, P.W., Zweben, A., and Stout, R.L. (1998). Network support for drinking: Alcoholics Anonymous and long-term matching effects. *Addiction*, **93**, 1313–34.

37. O'Farrell, T.J. (1995). Marital and family therapy. In *Handbook of alcoholism treatment approaches* (ed. R.K. Hester and W.R. Miller), pp. 195–220. Allyn and Bacon, Boston, MA.

38. O'Farrell, T.J., Choquette, K.A., and Cutter, H.S.G. (1998). Couples relapse prevention sessions after behavioural marital therapy for male alcoholics: outcomes during the three years after starting treatment *Journal of Studies on Alcohol*, **59**, 357–70.

39. Chick, J. (1998). Safety aspects of disulfiram in the treatment of alcohol dependence. *Drug Safety*, **20**, 427–35.

40. Larson, E.W., Olincy, A., Rummans, T.A., and Morse, R. (1992). Disulfiram treatment of patients with both alcohol dependence and other psychiatric disorders: a review. *Alcoholism: Clinical and Experimental Research*, **16**, 125–30.

41. Wright, C. and Moore, R.D. (1990). Disulfiram treatment of alcoholism. *American Journal of Medicine*, **88**, 647–55.

42. Duckert, F. and Johnsen, J.(1987). Behavioural use of disulfiram in the treatment of problem drinking. *International Journal of the Addictions*, **22**, 445–54.

43. Moncrieff, J. and Drummond, C.D. (1997). New drug treatments for alcohol problems: a critical appraisal. *Addiction*, **92**, 939–48.

44. Moncrieff, J. and Drummond, C.D. (1998). The quality of alcohol treatment research: an examination of influential controlled trials and development of a quality rating system. *Addiction*, **93**, 811–23.

45. *Addiction* (1997). Comments on Moncrieff and Drummond's 'New drug treatments for alcohol problems: a critical appraisal' (seven comments). *Addiction*, **92**, 949–65.

46. Littleton, J. (1995). Acamprosate in alcohol dependence: how does it work? *Addiction*, **90**, 1179–88.

47. Paille, F.M., Guelfi, J.D., Perkins, A.C., Royer, R.J., Steru, L., and Perot, P. (1995). Randomised multicentre trial of acamprosate in a maintenance programme of abstinence after alcohol detoxification. *Alcohol and Alcoholism*, **30**, 239–47.

48. Pelc, I., Verbanck, P., Le Bon, M., Gavrilovic, M., Lion, K., and Lehert, P. (1997). Efficacy and safety of acamprosate in the treatment of detoxified alcohol-dependent patients: a 90-day dose finding study. *British Journal of Psychiatry*, **171**, 73–7.

49. Garbutt, J.C., West, S.L., Carey, T.S., Lohr, K.N., and Crews, F.T. (1999). Pharmacological treatment of alcohol dependence—a review of the evidence. *Journal of the American Medical Association*, **281**, 1318–25.

50. Whitworth, A.B., Fischer, F., Lesch, O., *et al.* (1996). Comparison of acamprosate and placebo in long-term treatment of alcohol dependence. *Lancet*, **347**, 1438–42.

51. Sass, H., Soyka, M., Mann, K., and Zieglgansberger, W. (1996). Relapse prevention by acamprosate: results from a placebo controlled study on alcohol dependence. *Archives of General Psychiatry*, **53**, 673–80.

52. Chick, J., Howlett, H., Morgan, M.Y., and Ritson, B. (2000). United Kingdom Multicentre Acamprosate Study (UKMAS): a 6 month prospective study of acamprosate versus placebo in preventing relapse after withdrawal from alcohol. *Alcohol and Alcoholism*, **35**, in press.

53. Besson, J., Aeby, F., Kasas, A., Lehert, P., and Potgieter, A. (1998). Combined efficacy of acamprosate and disulfiram in the treatment of alcoholism: a controlled study *Alcoholism: Clinical and Experimental Research*, **22**, 573–9.

54. Gianoulakis, C., Krishnan, B., and Thavundayil, J. (1996). Enhanced sensitivity of pituitary β-endorphin to ethanol in subjects at high risk of alcoholism. *Archives of General Psychiatry*, **53**, 250–7.

55. Volpicelli, J.R., Alterman, A.I., Hayashida, M., and O'Brien, C.P. (1992). Naltrexone in the treatment of alcohol dependence. *Archives of General Psychiatry*, **49**, 876–80.

56. O'Malley, S., Jaffe, A.J., Chang, G., Schottenfeld, R.S., Meyer, R.E., and Rounsaville, B. (1992). Naltrexone and coping skills therapy for alcohol dependence. *Archives of General Psychiatry*, **49**, 881–7.

57. Volpicelli, J.R., Rhines, K.C., Rhines, J.S., Volpicelli, L.A., Alterman, A.I., and O'Brien, C.P. (1997). Naltrexone and alcohol dependence: role of subject compliance. *Archives of General Psychiatry*, **54**, 737–42.

58. Volpicelli, J.R., Volpicelli, L.A., and O'Brien, C.P. (1995). Medical management of alcohol dependence: clinical use and limitations of naltrexone treatment. *Alcohol and Alcoholism*, **30**, 789–98.

59. O'Malley, S., Jaffe, A.J., Chang, G., Schottenfeld, R.S., Meyer, R.E., and Rounsaville, B. (1996). Six month follow-up of naltrexone and psychotherapy for alcohol dependence. *Archives of General Psychiatry*, **53**, 217–24.

60. Swift, R.M. (1999). Drug therapy for alcohol dependence. *New England Journal of Medicine*, **340**, 1482–90.

61. Doty, P. and de Wit, H. (1995). Effects of naltrexone pretreatment on the subjective and performance effects of ethanol in social drinkers. *Behavioural Pharmacology*, **6**, 386–94.

62. Jeffers, S. (1987). *Feel the fear and do it anyway*. Century Hutchinson, London.

63. McGrath, P.J., Nunes, E.V., Stewart, J.W., *et al.* (1996). Imipramine treatment of alcoholics with primary depression: a placebo controlled clinical trial. *Archives of General Psychiatry*, **53**, 232–40.

64. Cornelius, J.R., Salloun, I.M., Ehler, J.G., *et al.* (1997). Fluoxetine reduced depressive symptoms and alcohol consumption in patients with comorbid major depression and alcohol dependence. *Archives of General Psychiatry*, **54**, 700–5.

65. Kranzler, H.R., Burleson, J.A., Boca, F.K., *et al.* (1994). Buspirone treatment of anxious alcoholics. *Archives of General Psychiatry*, **51**, 720–31.

66. Finney, J., Hahn, A.C., and Moos, R.H. (1996). The effectiveness of inpatient and outpatient treatment for alcohol abuse: the need to focus on mediators and moderators of setting effect. *Addiction*, **91**, 1773–96.

67. Schuckit, M. (1998). Penny-wise, ton-foolish? The recent movement to abolish inpatient alcohol and drug treatment. *Journal of Studies on Alcohol*, **59**, 5–6.

68. Mattick, R.P. and Jarvis, T. (1994). Inpatient setting and long duration for the treatment of alcohol dependence? Outpatient care is as good. *Drug and Alcohol Review*, **13**, 127–35.

69. Annis, H.M. (1996). Inpatient versus outpatient setting effects in alcoholism treatment: revisiting the evidence. *Addiction*, **91**, 1804–7.

70. Trent, L.K. (1998). Evaluation of a four- versus six-week length of stay in the Navy's alcohol treatment program. *Journal of Studies on Alcohol*, **59**, 270–9.

71. Project MATCH Research Group (1997). Project MATCH secondary a priori hypotheses. *Addiction*, **92**, 1671–98.

72. Connors, G.J., Carroll, K.M., DiClemente, C.C., Longabaugh, R., and Donovan, D.M. (1997). The therapeutic alliance and its relationship to alcoholism treatment participation and outcome. *Journal of Consulting and Clinical Psychology*, **65**, 588–98.

73. Sereny, G., Sharma, V., Holt, S., and Gordis, E. (1986). Mandatory supervised Antabuse therapy in an out-patient alcoholism program: a pilot study. *Alcoholism: Clinical and Experimental Research*, **10**, 290–2.

74. Smith, J.E., Meyers, R.I., and Delaney, H.D. (1998). The Community Reinforcement Approach with homeless alcohol-dependent individuals. *Journal of Consulting and Clinical Psychology*, **66**, 541–8.

75. Azrin, N.H., Sisson, R.W., Meyers, R., and Godley, M. (1982). Alcoholism treatment by disulfiram and community reinforcement therapy. *Journal of Behavior Therapy and Experimental Psychiatry*, **13**, 105–12

76. Robichaud, C., Strickland, D., Bigelow, G., *et al.* (1979). Disulfiram maintenance employee alcoholism treatment: a three phase treatment. *Behaviour Research and Therapy*, **17**, 618–21.

77. Gledhill, J., Burroughs, A., Rolles, K., Davidson, B., Blizard, B., and Lloyd, G. Psychiatric and social outcome following liver transplantation for alcoholic liver disease: a controlled study. *Journal of Psychosomatic Research*, in press

78. Shore, J.H. (1987). The Oregon experience with impaired physicians: an eight year follow-up. *Journal of the American Medical Association*, **257**, 2931–4.

79. Ahles, T.A., Schlundt, D.G., Prue, D.M., and Rychtarik, R.G. (1983). Impact of aftercare arrangements on the maintenance of treatment success in abusive drinkers. *Addictive Behaviours*, **8**, 53–8.

80. Reynauld, M., Hourcade, F., Planche, F., Albuisson, E., Neunier, M.-N., and Planche, R. (1998). Usefulness of carbohydrate-deficient transferrin in alcoholic patients with normal gamma-glutamyl transferase. *Alcoholism: Clinical and Experimental Research*, **22**, 615–18.

81. Patience, D., Buxton, M., Chick, J., Howlett, H., McKenna, M., and Ritson, B. (1997). The SECCAT Survey (II): the alcohol related problems questionnaire as a proxy for resource costs and quality of life in alcoholism treatment. *Alcohol and Alcoholism*, **32**, 79–84.

4.2.2.5 Services for alcohol use disorders

D. Colin Drummond

A spectrum of disorders needing a range of services

The provision of services for alcohol use disorders historically has been driven by the prevailing view of their nature and prevalence. Following the Second World War, the disease concept of alcoholism gained increasing support in both the United States and the United Kingdom.[1] According to this concept, alcoholism is an all-or-nothing phenomenon affecting a relatively small subgroup of the population, and requires intensive specialist treatment. In the United Kingdom this led to the development of specialist alcohol treatment centres with an emphasis on intensive inpatient treatment over several weeks or months, and involving group therapy, often with close affiliation to the Alcoholic Anonymous (**AA**) fellowship. Such programmes tended to be targeted at relatively socially stable, articulate, and affluent males, and universally only catering for the more severely alcohol dependent.[2]

In the 1970s and 1980s, with the development of epidemiological and psychological research, came a recognition that there existed a much wider range of alcohol-related problems in the population than would meet the narrow criteria of alcoholism or alcohol dependence, which might nevertheless benefit from intervention. Further, research began to show that alcohol problems existed on a continuum of severity and thus might not necessarily require intensive specialist treatment with a lifelong goal of complete abstinence from alcohol. Evidence began to emerge that screening and brief intervention with presymptomatic heavy drinkers in the primary care or general hospital medical ward setting could be effective in reducing excessive alcohol consumption and alcohol-related harm.[3,4] This, combined with a degree of pessimism concerning the effectiveness of intensive treatments for more severely dependent drinkers, led to the proposal that greater benefit could be accrued from less intensive approaches aimed at the large number of hazardous drinkers, than more intensive and expensive interventions catering for the minority of very heavy drinkers: the 'preventive paradox'.[5]

In a ground-breaking report, the United States Institute of Medicine advocated 'broadening the base of treatment for alcohol problems'.[6] Recognizing the potential for increased prevention and treatment activity in non-addiction specialist health-care personnel (e.g. general practitioners, physicians, social workers), and the limitations of expanding specialist treatment, particularly in an era of health-care cost containment, the report emphasised the need for an expanded range of locations and methods of intervention, across the spectrum of alcohol use disorders. Importantly however, the report also recognized that alcohol use disorders are heterogeneous, and different types of disorder were likely to require different types or intensities of treatment, i.e. the need to match treatments to the nature of the presenting problem.

In the decade that has followed this report there has been some progress made towards increasing the range and accessibility of treatment. However, in some cases this has been disappointing. This chapter describes the range of treatment approaches and explores the barriers to implementation of a comprehensive system of care for alcohol use disorders. Certain groups in the population may be particularly disadvantaged in terms of access. Finally the cost implications of delivery of treatment services are discussed. The main conclusion of the research evidence is that there remain considerable opportunities to expand and improve treatment services for alcohol use disorders but this will require further training and dissemination initiatives throughout the health system fully to achieve.

Location and intensity of treatment

Specialist treatments

The main treatment response to alcohol use disorders continues to be delivered by specialists. There has been extensive research on the location and intensity of specialist treatment. An early influential study was that of Edwards *et al.*[7] in which 100 alcohol-dependent men referred to the Maudsley Hospital in London were randomized to receive either intensive specialist treatment, including inpatient care in an alcoholism treatment unit, or one session of counselling. At 1-year follow-up there was no difference in outcome between the two treatments. It was concluded that the reliance on intensive treatments up to that time was called into question by the findings. This controversial study gave rise to considerable debate and several studies have subsequently investigated the same issues. Another British study attempted to replicate the Edwards study and found only modest differences between advice only and extended treatment in a randomized controlled trial at 2 years' follow-up.[8] There were, however, no differences between treatments in abstinence rates or alcohol consumption level during follow-up.

In a larger study in the United States, 227 employees identified as abusing alcohol were randomized to one of three options: compulsory inpatient treatment, compulsory AA attendance, or a choice of these two options.[9] At 2-year follow-up there were no differences between the groups in terms of work-related outcome measures. However, on seven drinking-related measures the inpatient group had the best, and the AA group the poorest outcome, with the choice group having an intermediate outcome. The compulsory AA group was more likely than the others to require subsequent inpatient treatment. However, the length of inpatient treatment does not appear to influence outcome significantly.[10,11]

Studies comparing inpatient versus outpatient alcohol detoxification have generally found the two approaches to be equally effective. For example, Hayashida *et al.*[12] randomized 164 male military veterans to inpatient and outpatient detoxification. At 6 months' follow-up no differences in outcome were found between the two groups.

Indeed, outpatient detoxification is generally regarded as the treatment of choice for the majority of patients.[13,14] It should be noted, however, that studies comparing inpatient and outpatient treatment (including detoxification) have tended to exclude patients with particularly poor prognosis (e.g. poor social circumstances, severe psychiatric or physical comorbidity, those at risk of harm to themselves or others). Hence, the clinician needs to interpret the research evidence with caution in the usual clinical setting. However, it is probably safe to assume that in 'uncomplicated' alcohol dependence there is no evidence of an advantage of inpatient over outpatient treatment.

Another important specialist treatment approach used widely in the private or non-statutory treatment sector is residential treatment based upon the Minnesota Model originally developed in the Hazelden Clinic in Minnesota, using an approach closely allied to the AA movement. These approaches, often described as 12-step programmes after the 12 steps of AA, have not generally been subjected to randomized controlled trials.[15,16] One trial in Finland, however, found a higher rate of abstinence at 12 months' follow-up in the Hazelden treatment group compared with traditional residential psychiatric treatment not involving the Minnesota Model approach (26.3 per cent vs. 9.8 per cent).[17] However, the higher abstinence rate was not supported by corresponding reduction in markers of heavy drinking (γ-glutamyl transferase, mean cell volume).

It is also important to note that the self-help movement of AA, which was founded in the United States in 1935, is a major provider of help and support for people with alcohol use disorders, with more than 73 000 groups worldwide.[18] Indeed, a higher proportion of problem drinkers attend AA than formal alcohol treatment programmes.[19] Although this approach is largely unevaluated, because of the difficulty of using conventional randomized controlled trials in this setting, there is evidence that regular AA attendance is associated with better outcomes in those with a high level of alcohol dependence.[20,21] Regular AA attenders are, of course, self-selected.

Overall, the majority of studies that have compared intensive specialist treatment with less intensive treatment have not supported the use of more intensive approaches, with a few important exceptions. However, three points are important to note. Little attention has been paid to the issue of matching effects in these studies: do patients with more severe or complex problems benefit more from intensive treatments, as would seem intuitively reasonable? Second, many of the studies have had important methodological limitations, not least being small sample sizes that increase the risk of type 2 error. Third, as noted above, more complex cases tend to be excluded from research trials, which limits the generalizability of the existing research base. With improved methodology now available and an awareness of the possibility of matching effects, this issue is far from closed.

Community-based specialist treatments

The growth of studies questioning the value of specialist inpatient treatment and a move towards cost containment in health care have led to a shift in resources aimed at treating alcohol use disorders in the community setting. One North American study, for example, found that the proportion of outpatient treatment units more than doubled between 1982 and 1990, consistent with the efforts of managed care organizations to decrease the utilization of inpatient services.[22]

Apart from the potential advantage of lower cost, community-based treatment provides the least social disruption for the individual and offers the opportunity to mobilize existing community resources to support, hopefully, sustained recovery. In the United Kingdom, the past 20 years has seen the widespread development of the community alcohol team model of treatment following the original Maudsley Alcohol Pilot Project.[23] The main principle of the community alcohol team model is that the specialist team (typically consisting of specialist medical, nursing, social work, and psychology staff) work to train and support generic teams, mainly in primary care, to manage alcohol use disorders more effectively. In practice, community alcohol teams have tended to find difficulty in avoiding becoming involved in a more traditional specialist role, often providing direct care for alcohol use disorders in the face of reluctance on the part of primary care personnel to take on this work.[24]

There has been remarkably little research conducted to evaluate the community alcohol team model. One study randomly allocated 40 problem drinkers referred to the specialist alcohol treatment clinic at the Maudsley Hospital to receive either routine specialist treatment or 'shared care'.[25] Following specialist assessment, the shared care group was returned to the care of their general practitioner, who was then supported by the specialist community alcohol team. Shared care within this model included advice and training for the general practitioner, a shared treatment plan, regular phone contact between specialist and general practitioner, and the offer of further specialist care should the patient remain unchanged or deteriorate. At 6 months' follow-up the specialist and shared care groups both showed significant improvements, but there was no difference in outcome between the two groups.

Two other community-based treatment approaches show promise. The 'community reinforcement approach' has been demonstrated to have benefits in the treatment of alcohol dependence.[26] This approach aims to provide reinforcers for abstinence from alcohol including positive family support, help in finding employment, and membership of an alcohol-free social club, including alcohol counselling. The specialist treatment input aims to ensure that these supports are put in place. There is some evidence from small-scale controlled trials[26,27] that this approach is effective in reducing alcohol consumption and improving social adjustment compared to standard treatment, but it has not so far been fully evaluated, and has never been tested in the United Kingdom.

Another variant on the community alcohol team approach has been the evaluation of community psychiatric nurse aftercare following specialist inpatient treatment.[28] One recent study in Northern Ireland evaluated the effectiveness of regular community psychiatric nurse follow-up consisting of weekly 1- to 2-h visits to the patient's home for a period of 6 weeks post-discharge from inpatient care, followed by less frequent visits up to 1 year. The home-based sessions involved advice, support, counselling, partner involvement, and encouragement to attend AA. This was compared to routine 6-weekly hospital appointments. The study, which involved a non-randomized design, found significant improvements in abstinence and engagement in support in the community psychiatric nurse approach compared to the routine aftercare group.

A recent study in Scotland evaluated the efficacy of a home detoxification service compared with minimal intervention in a randomized controlled trial in 95 patients referred by their general practitioner.[29] At 6 months' follow-up the home detoxification group remained abstinent twice as long after treatment than the minimal intervention group.

Overall, the community alcohol team model of alcohol service delivery has been widely implemented in the United Kingdom in advance of clear evidence of its effectiveness. Evidence is now beginning to emerge showing at least the equivalence, and in some cases, the superiority, of outcome from community-based services compared with more traditional hospital-based treatment approaches. However, the community alcohol team approach is implemented in a range of ways in the United Kingdom, and encompasses many different models and specific interventions. More research is needed to evaluate the cost effectiveness of community alcohol team approaches and to identify the specific elements and methods that contribute to treatment effectiveness.

Brief interventions

There has been considerable research interest in the potential of brief interventions in the primary care setting, and to a lesser extent in the general hospital setting.[30] There are several potential advantages in conducting treatment interventions in the primary care setting. Patients with alcohol use disorders consult their general practitioner more frequently than other patients. Alcohol use disorders identified by screening in primary care are largely at an earlier stage in their drinking career and are potentially more likely to benefit from brief early intervention than more severely dependent drinkers. Further, the primary care setting is often seen as less stigmatizing than a specialist clinic.

Several studies have now demonstrated the efficacy of screening and brief intervention in hazardous drinkers in this setting. In a large randomized controlled trial, Wallace et al.[4] found that following screening, brief intervention was more effective than a control treatment in reducing alcohol consumption and γ-glutamyl transferase at 1-year follow-up. Similar findings were obtained in a large World Health Organization multicentre trial[31] and in two recent North American studies.[32,33]

Fewer screening and brief intervention studies have been conducted in the general hospital setting. Two studies, one conducted in the United Kingdom and one in Australia, have found some benefit of brief intervention, although both studies lacked statistical power.[3,34] One study of screening in general hospital and attempted referral to a specialist alcohol service was negative, but again had a small sample size.[35]

Three meta-analyses of brief interventions have all found advantages of brief intervention over control treatments with effect sizes of 10 to 20 per cent on reduced alcohol consumption.[36–38] Effect sizes for men are greater than for women. These reviews have also reached a general conclusion that brief interventions are at least as effective as more intensive specialist treatments. This conclusion has been recently criticized on the basis that studies of opportunistic screening brief intervention are largely not comparable with specialist treatment studies that have included a brief intervention control group, as they involve populations with different characteristics.[39,40] Principally, the former include subjects with less severe alcohol problems, and are not seeking treatment at the point of screening and identification. Further, Drummond[40] has questioned the generalizability of brief intervention research findings in the typical clinical setting, given the large number of exclusions in research studies.

There are barriers to implementation of brief intervention in the non-specialist setting which may limit its effectiveness. In a United Kingdom national survey,[41,42] it was found that general practitioners and primary care practice nurses were reluctant to engage in screening and brief interventions because of a perceived lack of training and support to carry out this work. Effective implementation of large-scale screening and brief intervention programmes will require attention to the training and support needs of non-specialist personnel. Further, screening programmes will identify more severely alcohol-dependent drinkers who may not respond to brief interventions alone. Thus, effective working arrangements between generalists and specialists are needed. An ongoing World Health Organizationcollaborative study aims to identify the most effective ways of engaging primary care personnel in screening and early intervention in alcohol use disorders.

Matching and stepped care

The Institute of Medicine report, while drawing attention to the need for a range of interventions catering for a wider range of alcohol use disorders, also emphasized the need to match the level of intervention to the severity and nature of the presenting problems.[6] There is some empirical evidence of matching effects.[43] Indeed a later follow-up of the Edwards cohort found that more severely dependent drinkers benefited more from intensive treatment.[44] Up until recently, however, matching effects have generally been explored in post hoc analyses in studies that lacked statistical power. The recent large-scale Project MATCH study in the United States aimed to assess a wide range of matching hypotheses in a prospective design, but found no strong matching effects[45] (see Chapter 4.2.2.4). However, it should be noted that most controlled trials, including MATCH, excluded the more severely problematic patients, including those with limited social support and those with severe psychiatric comorbidity. This tends to work against finding matching effects as the study samples lack clinical heterogeneity.[46] Further, many of the patient and treatment programme characteristics likely to mediate treatment matching and treatment effectiveness, remain largely unresearched.

Stepped care[47] is an alternative method of matching treatments to patient needs that has become accepted in the fields of smoking intervention and general medicine. Until now it has received relatively scant attention in the alcohol field. In essence, stepped care involves initially providing relatively low-intensity treatments to all patients, and only offering more intensive treatments to those who fail to respond.[48] This provides a potentially resource-efficient means of delivering treatment, and provides clinicians with clear clinical algorithms in making treatment decisions. However, stepped care in the alcohol field requires evaluation in controlled trials.

Financial considerations

With a general move towards containment of health-care costs in industrialized societies, there has been an increase in the application of health economic research in the alcohol treatment field. The cost of treating alcohol use disorders represents a substantial burden on health-care budgets. It has been estimated that the annual direct treatment costs of alcohol use disorders by specialist treatment agencies amounted to approximately $10.5 billion in the United States and about £400 million in the United Kingdom in 1990.[49,50] Thus there is a need to demonstrate the cost effectiveness of treatments for alcohol use disorders.

Until recently, research on cost effectiveness has been largely speculative and not based on direct estimates of cost benefits. In a landmark study, Holder et al.[51] provided a 'first approximation' of the cost effectiveness of treatment. In their analysis they used a combination of findings of efficacy from clinical trials, typical costs of different treatments, and recommendations from experts and treatment providers about appropriate treatment approaches. While noting the lack of studies directly assessing the cost effectiveness of treatments, they concluded that the treatments with greatest evidence of effectiveness tend to be less costly than those with least evidence of effectiveness. Based on their analysis the cost of care was inversely correlated with evidence of effectiveness. They also noted that those treatments with the highest cost and lowest evidence of effectiveness were amongst the most prevalent in the North American treatment system. While this review has been strongly criticised on methodological grounds, it has stimulated an important debate and has contributed to an increasing number of clinical trials including a health economic component in outcome evaluation.[52,53]

The two recent North American brief intervention primary care studies cited earlier found evidence of reduced postintervention health-care utilization, suggesting the potential of brief intervention in reducing health-care costs. Fleming et al.[32] found that, as well as reducing excessive drinking, there was a reduced length of hospitalization in men during the 12-month follow-up period. In the study by Israel et al.,[33] brief intervention (involving 3 h of counselling by a nurse) led to reduced alcohol-related morbidity and a reduced frequency of physician visits. An earlier study by Kristenson et al.[54] in Sweden found that early intervention and regular follow-up by a physician led to a 'significant reduction' in sickness absences, hospitalizations, and mortality, compared with a control group. All three studies point to the potential cost effectiveness of interventions in the primary care setting, but none of these studies examined cost effectiveness directly.

There has been relatively little research into the cost effectiveness of specialist treatments, and methodologies for examining cost effectiveness is still at an early stage of development in the alcohol field. However, some work has been done. In a 14-year longitudinal study of 'alcoholic' employees within the United States, Holder and Blose[55] found that those who enrolled in treatment incurred 24 per cent less health care costs (including the costs of alcoholism treatment) than those who did not. In fact, there was an increase in health-care costs in treatment non-attenders. This was not a randomized study, however, and the results need to be interpreted with some caution.

The costs of treatment were examined in the trial in which employees were randomized to compulsory AA versus compulsory inpatient treatment, cited earlier.[9] They found that the higher-cost (inpatient) intervention resulted in superior outcomes and was only 10 per cent more expensive than AA referral because many of the AA group subsequently required hospitalization. Another randomized trial by Hayashida et al.[12] examined costs in a comparison of inpatient and outpatient alcohol detoxification in male veterans with mild to moderate alcohol withdrawal and found that the clinical outcome was not significantly different between the two groups. However, inpatient treatment was approximately 10 times the cost of outpatient treatment. The authors concluded that for this group, outpatient detoxification is more cost effective.

A recent analysis based on data from Project MATCH aimed to estimate the relative costs of three psychotherapy approaches.[56] Motivational enhancement therapy, 12-step facilitation, and cognitive-behavioural therapy were assessed on the basis of what they would cost per patient to implement in a typical clinical setting. It was found that although motivational enhancement therapy involved one-third of the number of sessions compared to the other two treatments, it was only approximately 33 per cent less costly to provide. Nevertheless, as all three treatments were found to be equally effective it must be concluded that four sessions of motivational enhancement therapy are more cost effective than 12 sessions of either cognitive-behavioural therapy or 12-step facilitation.

The ideal method of assessing the cost effectiveness of treatment for alcohol use disorders is in the context of a randomized controlled trial. However, the measurement of costs and benefits has so far been restricted mainly to direct treatment costs, and outcomes in terms of drinking-related outcome measures. Also important in establishing cost effectiveness will be estimates of indirect costs including patient out-of-pocket costs, lost productivity, unplanned health-care utilization (e.g. admissions with alcohol-related physical and mental illnesses, primary care utilization), criminal justice costs, accidents, premature deaths, social work involvement, child-care costs, and costs associated with illnesses in relatives and carers.[57,58]

Important in the field of cost effectiveness analysis is the estimation of quality-adjusted life years. This has not so far been adequately studied in the alcohol treatment field. The basic analysis relates the cost of a given intervention to a specific measurable outcome such as quality of life. Quality of life can be measured in a variety of ways (e.g. Euroqol, Short Form 36), but the relationship between quality of life and more typical alcohol-related outcomes, such as alcohol consumption, has not been widely studied.[59,60]

Overall, there is considerable scope for further development of health economic research in the alcohol field. This will prove important in providing health-care purchasers with appropriate information to make rational decisions in the provision of cost-effective evidence-based services for alcohol use disorders. One can expect a considerable expansion of research in this area over the next decade. (For a further account of cost-effectiveness analysis, see Chapter 7.7.)

Access and help-seeking

So far we have concentrated on the effectiveness of interventions at an individual level. However, the overall population impact of treatment interventions is dependent upon the availability and ease of access to treatment programmes, as well as their effectiveness. From a public health perspective the effectiveness of the treatment response to alcohol problems will depend upon the number of people accessing and engaging with interventions. This will be dependent upon two main factors: characteristics of the alcohol-misusing population, and characteristics of the treatment service. There is also likely to be an interplay between these two factors.

Characteristics of the alcohol-misusing population

Specialist alcohol treatment services typically attract younger, male, single patients of lower socio-economic and educational background, with more severe alcohol dependence. Relative to the prevalence of alcohol use disorders in the general population, women, older people, and people from ethnic minorities are typically under-represented, as are the homeless. Further, there are few examples of specific services for young people. This is of particular concern as the prevalence of alcohol use disorders is increasing in these groups in the United Kingdom.

Women

The factors involved in women's help-seeking have recently been the subject of increased research activity. Thom and Green have identified three main factors that may account for the underrepresentation of women in alcohol treatment.[61] Women tend to perceive their problems differently from men, less often identifying themselves as 'alcoholic'. This may in part be related to negative public stereotypes of female drinking and negative attitudes towards female problem drinkers amongst professionals, who, in the medical profession, are still predominantly male. Women have also been found to perceive the 'costs' of entering treatment differently from men. This is particularly in relation to the perceived social stigma as well as other costs, both financial, in relationships, and in terms of losing their children into the care system. Finally, women often find the services offered to be less appropriate in meeting their needs than do men. Often specialist alcohol services do not offer child care or 'women-only' facilities. The latter is particularly relevant in view of the high prevalence of sexual abuse in women seeking alcohol treatment.[62] However, recent evidence suggests that an increasing number of women are seeking help for alcohol use disorders, at least in the United States, on the basis of general population surveys and surveys of treatment populations.[19,22] Nevertheless, more needs to be done to attract women into alcohol treatment by providing services that are sensitive to women's needs. Further, there is a need to develop services catering for pregnant women.[63]

Ethnic minority groups

The evidence concerning help-seeking in ethic minority groups is complex (see Chapter 7.10.3). Harrison et al.[64] have recently provided a review of the evidence. In the United States, Hispanics tend to be under-represented and African-Americans are over-represented in alcohol treatment compared with the general population prevalence. However, interpretation of the evidence is complicated by the fact that household surveys tend to under-represent socially disadvantaged individuals from ethnic minorities. In the United Kingdom, surveys such as the General Household Survey do not examine ethnicity, and estimates of prevalence tend to be based on indirect indicators of alcohol misuse such as cirrhosis mortality. For example, Marmot et al.[65] found that cirrhosis mortality rates were elevated compared to the national average for men from the Asian subcontinent and from Ireland, but lower than average for African-Caribbean men. In women, cirrhosis mortality was lower than average in Asian and African-Caribbean women but higher in Irish women. However, there were few cirrhosis deaths in total in ethnic minorities, which may lead to large errors in extrapolation to the whole population alcohol misuse estimates. Another study found that cirrhosis mortality was higher than expected in Punjabis, Gujuratis, and (perhaps surprisingly) Moslems in the United Kingdom.[66] In terms of alcohol treatment populations, studies have tended to find higher rates of admission (per 100 000 population) in Indian-, Scottish- and Irish-born people than in those born in the Caribbean or Pakistan.[67] Differences in culturally related health beliefs and help-seeking, as well as service factors such as the availability of interpreters or treatment personnel from appropriate ethnic minority groups, may account for some of these differences. There remain few specific services for people from ethnic minorities, although some examples of good practice exist in the United Kingdom.[64]

The homeless

There is a high prevalence of alcohol use disorders (as well as mental and physical health and social problems) amongst the growing homeless population, a group that is not typically well catered for by mainstream alcohol services (see Chapter 7.10.3). The prevalence of alcohol problems in the homeless has been found to be as high as 38 per cent in the United Kingdom[68] and between 2 and 86 per cent in the United States; typically the prevalence is between 20 and 45 per cent in North American studies.[69] This has contributed to the development of specific alcohol services for the homeless and street drinkers, notably 'wet' hostels. In the 'wet' hostel, residents are able to continue drinking but are cared for in an environment that is designed to minimize the harm associated with heavy drinking and to tackle issues associated with homelessness.[70,71] Such facilities tend to be restricted to large urban centres and have restricted places compared to the prevalence of street drinking. Similarly, outreach services and 'crisis centres' have been developed to attract alcohol-misusing homeless people into treatment facilities.[72] Often those entering 'wet' hostels can subsequently be persuaded to undergo alcohol detoxification and progress to 'dry' (or alcohol-free) supported accommodation.

Young people

The prevalence of alcohol use disorders is increasing in young people. The young are over-represented in alcohol-related road traffic accidents, and alcohol is a leading cause of accidental death in this group.[73] Alcohol misuse is also associated with engagement in unprotected sexual activity.[74] Nevertheless, there are few services for young people with alcohol use disorders. Most initiatives have been directed at prevention and health promotion in this group, but the evidence to support this is lacking. This has led to the proposal that individually targeted interventions, for example by the primary health care team, are more likely to be effective.[75]

Relatives and carers

Relatives and carers of people with alcohol use disorders often experience significant social and psychological problems related to the drinking of a 'significant other'. Alcohol use disorders are associated with a high level of domestic violence and child neglect and abuse. Many specialist treatment programmes provide help and support to relatives and carers, and Al-Anon (for adult carers and relatives) and Alateen (for the young), which are affiliates of AA, provide a widely available source of self-help for these groups.

Services for individuals with comorbidity

There is an increasing recognition of the problems associated with alcohol and other drug misuse and mental illness (see Chapter 4.2.2.3). Often alcohol misuse is complicated by multiple substance misuse. For example, in the Epidemiologic Catchment Area Study half of all patients with schizophrenia also had a substance misuse disorder,[76] and a recent British survey of psychotic patients found that 36 per cent misused drugs or alcohol.[77] However, there is currently no consensus on the most appropriate treatment services for patients with comorbidity.[78] Substance misuse can be particularly problematic in the context of mental illness, and is associated with higher rates of violence and poor treatment outcome (see Chapter 11.4.4). Such patients are often non-compliant and disruptive in mental health services, and typically do not engage in alcohol or drug services. Assertive community outreach and integrated service models, covering both mental illness and substance misuse, have been advocated, but evidence for the effectiveness of such services is currently limited.[78,79]

The availability of alcohol treatment services

The availability of alcohol services is likely to affect the overall impact of public health measures to reduce alcohol use disorders. There is some evidence that the availability of alcohol treatment services has an effect on the prevalence of alcohol use disorders at a population level. Mann et al.[80] found that increased treatment services in Ontario, Canada, were associated with decreased hospital discharges for liver cirrhosis. A similar study in North Carolina examining the 20-year period between 1968 and 1987 found an association between increased alcohol treatment admissions and decreased cirrhosis mortality. Further, Mann et al.[81] found a relationship between AA membership and alcohol-related problems including cirrhosis rates in the United States, Canada, and other countries. They estimated that a 1 per cent increase in AA membership was associated with a 0.06 per cent decrease in cirrhosis mortality. These studies of course demonstrate associations rather than causal links between treatment availability and alcohol use disorder prevalence, but do provide support to the hypothesis that access to treatment could lead to potential cost savings in the health care system.[55]

The National Drug and Alcohol Treatment Utilization Survey (**NDATUS**), which is a national census of public and private treatment programmes in the United States, provides a unique data set to study treatment availability. It has been conducted intermittently since 1979 and provides a method to study trends over time. An analysis by the Institute of Medicine found large regional variations in the availability of treatment places.[6] There was no association found between treatment place availability and prevalence of alcohol misuse across States in the United States. This points to the importance of 'needs assessment' in the rational allocation of public resources to fund treatment services. Such an approach usually involves a variety of data sources as indicators of alcohol use disorder prevalence in a particular locality, including general population surveys, mortality statistics (e.g. deaths from hepatic cirrhosis), crime statistics (e.g. public drunkenness and driving whilst intoxicated arrests), and alcohol-related hospital admissions. Such indicators provide indirect measures of relative 'need' in different localities, and can be used to direct resource allocation.[82]

Examining data from repeated NDATUS surveys between 1982 and 1993, Schmidt and Weisner[22] found an overall 190 per cent increase in the number of clients in treatment places. The majority of services (82 per cent) were combined drug and alcohol treatment agencies, however, making it difficult to estimate the number of individuals with alcohol use disorders in treatment. Nevertheless, in a subset of 'alcohol-only' treatment facilities the increase in activity over this period was 147 per cent. In the United States the impact of managed care organizations, which aim to limit access to treatment on the basis of individual need and cost, has yet to be fully established in relation to overall access to alcohol services. Such measures are likely to reduce the availability of inpatient services and to reduce the rate of readmission for those with chronic problems.

In the United Kingdom the introduction of the National Health Service and Community Care Act 1990[83] placed budgets for residential care, including alcohol treatment, under the direct control of the Treasury, with a view to limiting public spending on residential care. The initial impact of this legislation was estimated to be a 23 per cent reduction in residential substance misuse placements, and a 19 per cent reduction in the number of residential 'beds'.[84] As budgets for residential alcohol treatment tend not to be 'ring-fenced', it is likely that further restrictions on public spending will have an impact on the availability of treatment places, which in turn is likely to place more demand upon health-care facilities.

Conclusions

The alcohol treatment field has seen an enormous number of changes over the past 30 years. Some of the changes have been evidence based, and some have been largely politically driven, particularly in the pursuit of containing health-care costs. On the positive side, a shift in policy from a limited number of treatment services catering only for the small minority of severely dependent drinkers, to more community orientated services with a view to early identification and intervention, is to be broadly welcomed. However, in some places a move towards services catering for early-stage 'at-risk' drinkers has been at the expense of losing services for the more severe cases.[40] While the evidence in favour of matching treatments to individual needs is still at a relatively early stage of development, and clear evidence of matching effects is not yet available, clinical practice needs to be guided by pragmatic principles by which more intensive treatments are provided to more complex cases. It must be concluded that, despite a large research effort in evaluating intensive versus less intensive alcohol interventions, there is still a long way to go in developing pragmatic clinical trials that evaluate effectiveness and cost effectiveness of treatment in a way that can best advise practitioners.

Also on the positive side, research has begun to address fundamental health economic issues that are highly relevant to the rational funding of treatment services. Important in this is the development of health economic methods in randomized controlled trials, although this remains at a relatively rudimentary stage. The assessment of the impact of treatment availability on the prevalence of alcohol-related harm also represents a significant advance.

Health services research that does not influence clinical practice fails in its fundamental aim. For example, while there is a now considerable evidence base in support of brief intervention in the primary care setting, there is a resistance within primary care to adopt such approaches, often despite exhortations from governments and professional bodies. Part of the problem may lie in the disparity between the priorities of public health, which is directed towards population level benefits of an intervention, and the priorities of the individual practitioner, whose first duty is to the patient in his or her care.[30] If the individual practitioner remains unconvinced about the value of a particular, usually brief, intervention for the patient, such public health policies are likely to fail even if they are supported by research evidence.

Similarly, as Holder et al.[51] have pointed out, often treatment programmes continue to provide alcohol services that are not supported by an acceptable evidence base. On occasions, but not exclusively, this criticism is levelled at private for-profit agencies, with the implication that their motivation is financial rather than being principally for the benefit of their patients. In many cases, however, the evidence base is lacking because the fundamental research has not yet been conducted. Or, as in the case of self-help organizations such as AA, the methodology necessary adequately to evaluate an intervention would be extremely complex, or perhaps impossible, to conduct to the standard typically expected in evidence-based medicine (i.e. a randomized controlled trial).

Nevertheless, treatment research cannot occur in a vacuum. Research needs to take account of the funding environment in which treatment takes place. Further, treatment research needs to provide answers to the key issues facing purchasers of health care. With the gradual improvement in the quality of treatment research over the past three decades[85] and the development of more advanced health economic methods to evaluate treatment,[57] the treatment research community is in a much better position than ever before to provide evidence to guide the rational development of treatment services for alcohol use disorders.

While many differences between health-care systems exist in different countries, the evidence points to the need for a wide spectrum of services to cater for different needs. The development of low-threshold community-based services should not occur at the expense of more specialized services for more severe alcohol use disorders. Similarly, a treatment system that provides only specialist services for the minority of severe cases misses a significant public health opportunity to reduce the prevalence of alcohol use disorders through early, brief interventions. Further, there is a need for better integration and co-ordination of statutory and non-statutory services to provide a seamless response that best meets the needs of the wide range of presenting alcohol use disorders.

References

1. Jellinek, E.M. (1960). *The disease concept of alcoholism.* Hillhouse, Haven, CT.

2. Edwards, G. (1987). *The treatment of drinking problems: a guide for the helping professions.* Blackwell, London.

3. Chick, J., Lloyd, G., and Crombie, E. (1985). Counselling problem drinkers in medical wards: a controlled study. *British Medical Journal,* **290**, 965–7.

4. Wallace, P., Cutler, S., and Haines, A. (1988). Randomised controlled trial of general practitioner intervention in patients with excessive alcohol consumption. *British Medical Journal,* **297**, 663–8.

5. Kreitman, N. (1986). Alcohol consumption and the preventive paradox. *British Journal of Addiction,* **81**, 353–63.

6. Institute of Medicine (1990). *Broadening the base of treatment for alcohol problems.* National Academy Press, Washington, DC.

7. Edwards, G., Orford, J., Egert, S., *et al.* (1977) Alcoholism: a controlled trial of 'treatment' and 'advice'. *Journal of Studies on Alcohol,* **38**, 1004–31.

8. Chick, J., Ritson, B., Connaughton, J., Stewart, A., and Chick, J. (1988). Advice versus extended treatment for alcoholism: a controlled study. *British Journal of Addiction,* **83**, 159–70.

9. Walsh, D.C., Hingson, R.W., Merrigan, D.M., *et al.* (1991). A randomised trial of treatment options for alcohol-abusing workers. *New England Journal of Medicine,* **325**, 775–82.

10. Trent, L.K. (1998). Evaluation of a four- versus six-week length of stay in the Navy's alcohol treatment program. *Journal of Studies on Alcohol,* **59**, 270–9.

11. Long, C.G., Williams, M., and Hollin, C.R. (1998). Treating alcohol problems: a study of programme effectiveness according to length and delivery of treatment. *Addiction,* **93** (4), 561–71.

12. Hayashida, M., Alterman, A.I., McLellan, A.T., *et al.* (1989). Comparative effectiveness and costs of inpatient and outpatient detoxification of patients with mild-to-moderate alcohol withdrawal syndrome. *New England Journal of Medicine,* **320**, 358–65.

13. Collins, M.N., Burns, T., Van den Berk, P.A.H., and Tubman, G.F. (1990). A structured programme for outpatient alcohol detoxification. *British Journal of Psychiatry,* **156**, 871–4.

14. Stockwell, T., Bolt, L., Milner, I., *et al.* (1991). Home detoxification from alcohol: its safety and efficacy in comparison with inpatient care. *Alcohol and Alcoholism,* **26**, 645–50.

15. Cook, C. (1988). The Minnesota Model in the management of drug and alcohol dependency: a miracle method or myth? Part I. The philosophy and the programme. *British Journal of Addiction,* **83**, 625–34.

16. Cook, C. (1988). The Minnesota Model in the management of drug and alcohol dependency: a miracle method or myth? Part II. Evidence and conclusions. *British Journal of Addiction,* **83**, 735–48.

17. Keso, L. and Salaspuro, M. (1990). Inpatient treatment of employed alcoholics: a randomized controlled clinical trial on Hazelden-type and traditional treatment. *Alcoholism: Clinical and Experimental Research,* **14**, 584–9.

18. Makela, K. (1991). Social and cultural preconditions of Alcoholics Anonymous (AA) and factors associated with the strength of AA. *British Journal of Addiction,* **86**, 1405–13.

19. Weisner, C., Greenfield, T., and Room, R. (1995). Trends in the treatment of alcohol problems in the US general population, 1979 through 1990. *American Journal of Public Health,* **85**, 55–60.

20. Edwards, G., Brown, D., Duckitt, A., *et al.* (1987). Outcome of alcoholism: the structure of patient attributions as to what causes change. *British Journal of Addiction,* **82**, 533–45.

21. Emrick, C. (1987). Alcoholics Anonymous: affiliation processes and effectiveness as treatment. *Alcoholism: Clinical and Experimental Research,* **11**, 416–23.

22. Schmidt, L. and Weisner, C. (1993). Developments in alcoholism treatment. In *Recent Developments in alcoholism,* Vol. 11. *Ten years of progress* (ed. M. Galanter), pp. 369–96. Plenum Press, New York.

23. Shaw, S.J., Cartwright, A.K.J., Spratley, T.A., and Harwin, J. (1978). *Responding to drinking problems.* Croom Helm, London.

24. Clement, S. and Stockwell, T. (ed.) (1987). *Helping the problem drinker: new initiatives in community care.* Croom Helm, London.

25. Drummond, D.C., Thom, B., Brown, C., Edwards, G., and Mullan, M.J. (1990). Specialist versus general practitioner treatment of problem drinkers. *Lancet,* **336**, 915–18.

26. Hunt, G.N. and Azrin, N.H. (1973). A community reinforcement approach to alcoholism. *Behaviour Research and Therapy,* **11**, 91–104.

27. Azrin, N.H., Sisson, R.W., Meyers, R., and Godley, M. (1982). Alcoholism treatment by disulfiram and community reinforcement therapy. *Journal of Behavior Therapy and Experimental Psychiatry,* **13**, 105–12.

28. Patterson, D.G., MacPherson, J., and Brady, N.M. (1997). Community psychiatric nurse aftercare for alcoholics: a five-year follow-up. *Addiction,* **92** (4), 459–68.

29. Bennie, C. (1998). A comparison of home detoxification and minimal intervention strategies for problem drinkers. *Alcohol and Alcoholism,* **33** (2), 157–63.

30. Heather, N. (1998). Brief opportunities for change in medical settings. In *Treating addictive behaviors* (2nd edn) (ed. W.R. Miller and N. Heather), pp. 133–47. Plenum, New York.

31. Babor, T.F. and Grant, B. (ed.) (1992). *Programme on substance abuse: project on identification and management of alcohol related problems. Report on phase II: a randomised clinical trial of brief intervention in primary health care.* World Health Organization, New York.

32. Fleming, M.F., Barry, K.L., Manwell, L.B., *et al.* (1997). Brief physician advice for problem drinkers: a randomized controlled trial in community-based primary care practices. *Journal of the American Medical Association*, **277**, 1039–45.

33. Israel, Y., Hollander, O., Sanchez Craig, M., *et al.* (1996). Screening for problem drinking and counselling by the primary care physician–nurse team. *Alcoholism: Clinical and Experimental Research*, **20**, 1443–50.

34. Heather, N., Rollnick, S., Bell, A., and Richmond, R. (1996). Effects of brief counselling among male heavy drinkers identified on general hospital wards. *Drug and Alcohol Review*, **15**, 29–38.

35. Elvy, G.A., Wells, J.E., and Baird, K.A. (1988). Attempted referral as intervention for problem drinking in the general hospital. *British Journal of Addiction*, **83**, 83–9.

36. Bien, T.H., Miller, W.R., and Tonigan, J.S. (1993). Brief interventions for alcohol problems: a review. *Addiction*, **88**, 315–36.

37. Effective Health Care Team (1993). *Brief interventions and alcohol use.* Effective Health Care Bulletin 7. Department of Health, London.

38. Miller, W.R., Brown, J.M., Simpson, T.L., *et al.* (1995). What works? A methodological analysis of the alcohol treatment outcome literature. In *Handbook of alcoholism treatment approaches: effective alternatives* (2nd edn) (ed. R.K. Hester and W.R. Miller), pp. 12–44. Allyn and Bacon, Boston, MA.

39. Heather, N. (1995). Interpreting the evidence on brief interventions for excessive drinkers: the need for caution. *Alcohol and Alcoholism*, **30**, 287–96.

40. Drummond, D.C. (1997). Alcohol interventions: do the best things come in small packages? *Addiction*, **92**, 375–9.

41. Deehan, A., Templeton, L., Taylor, C., Drummond, D.C., and Strang, J. (1998). Low detection rates, negative attitudes and the failure to meet 'Health of the Nation' targets: findings from a national survey of GPs in England and Wales. *Drug and Alcohol Review*, **17**, 249–58.

42. Deehan, A., Templeton, L., Taylor, C., Drummond, D.C., and Strang, J. (1998). How do general practitioners manage alcohol misusing patients? Results from a national survey of GPs in England and Wales. *Drug and Alcohol Review*, **17**, 259–66.

43. Mattson, M.E., Allen, J.P., Longabaugh, R., *et al.* (1994). A chronological review of empirical studies matching alcoholic clients to treatment. *Journal of Studies on Alcohol*, **12**, 16–29.

44. Orford, J., Oppenheimer, E., and Edwards, G. (1976). Abstinence or control: the outcome for excessive drinkers two years after consultation. *Behaviour Research and Therapy*, **14**, 409–18.

45. Project MATCH Research Group. (1997). Matching alcoholism treatments to client heterogeneity: Project MATCH posttreatment drinking outcomes. *Journal of Studies on Alcohol*, **58**, 7–29.

46. Drummond, D.C. (1999). Treatment research in the wake of Project MATCH. *Addiction*, **94**, 39–42.

47. Orleans, T.C. (1993). Treating nicotine dependence in medical settings: a stepped care approach. In *Nicotine addiction: principles and management* (ed. T.C. Orleans and J. Slade), pp. 145–61. Oxford University Press, New York.

48. Breslin, F.C., Sobell, M.B., Sobell, L.C., Buchan, G., and Cunningham, J.A. (1997). Toward a stepped care approach to treating problem drinkers: the predictive utility of within treatment variables and therapist prognostic ratings. *Addiction*, **92**, 1479–89.

49. Rice, D.P. (1993). The economic costs of alcohol abuse and alcohol dependence: 1990. *Alcohol and Health Research World*, **17**, 10–11.

50. Godfrey, C. and Maynard, A. (1992). *A health strategy for alcohol: setting targets and choosing policies* (YARTIC Occasional Paper 1). Centre for Health Economics and Leeds Addiction Unit, York.

51. Holder, H.D., Longabaugh, R., Miller, W.R., and Rubonis, A.V. (1991). The cost effectiveness of treatment for alcohol problems: a first approximation. *Journal of Studies on Alcohol*, **52**, 517–40.

52. Howard, M.O. (1993). Assessing the cost-effectiveness of alcoholism treatments: a comment on Holder, Longabaugh, Miller and Rubonis. *Journal of Studies on Alcohol*, **54**, 667–74.

53. Finney, J.W. and Monahan, S.C. (1996). The cost effectiveness of treatment for alcoholism: a second approximation. *Journal of Studies on Alcohol*, **57**, 229–43.

54. Kristenson, H., Ohlin, H., Hulton-Nosslin, M.B., Trell, E., and Hood, B. (1983). Identification and intervention of heavy drinking in middle-aged men: results and follow-up of 24–60 months of long term study with randomized controls. *Alcoholism: Clinical and Experimental Research*, **7**, 203–9.

55. Holder, H. and Blose, J. (1992). The reduction of health care costs associated with alcoholism treatment: a 14-year longitudinal study. *Journal of Studies on Alcohol*, **53**, 293–302.

56. Cisler, R., Holder, H.D., Longabaugh, R., *et al.* (1998). Actual and estimated replication costs for alcohol treatment modalities: case study from Project MATCH. *Journal of Studies on Alcohol*, **59**, 503–12.

57. Godfrey, C. (1994). Assessing the cost effectiveness of alcohol services. *Journal of Mental Health*, **3**, 3–21.

58. Healey, A., Knapp, M., Astin, J., *et al.* (1998). Economic burden of drug dependency: social costs incurred by drug users at intake to the National Treatment Outcome Research Study. *British Journal of Psychiatry*, **173**, 160–5.

59. Patience, D., Buxton, M., Chick, J., Howlett, H., McKenna, M., and Ritson, B. (1997). The Seccat survey: II. The alcohol related problems questionnaire as a proxy for resource costs and quality of life in alcoholism treatment. *Alcohol and Alcoholism*, **32**, 79–84.

60. Foster, J.H., Marshall, E.J., and Peters, T.J. (1998). Predictors of relapse to heavy drinking in alcohol dependent subjects following alcohol detoxification: the role of quality of life measures, ethnicity, social class, cigarette and drug use. *Addiction Biology*, **3**, 333–43.

61. Thom, B. and Green, A. (1996). Services for women with alcohol problems: the way forward. In *Alcohol problems in the community* (ed. L. Harrison), pp. 200–22. Routledge, London.

62. Moncrieff, J., Drummond, D.C., Candy, B., Checinski, K., and Farmer, R. (1996). Sexual abuse in people with alcohol problems: a study of the prevalence of sexual abuse and its relationship to drinking behaviour. *British Journal of Psychiatry*, **169**, 355–60.

63. Schorling, J.B. (1993). The prevention of prenatal alcohol use: a critical analysis of intervention studies. *Journal of Studies on Alcohol*, **54**, 261–7.

64. Harrison, L., Harrison, M., and Adebowale, V. (1997). Drinking problems among black communities. In *Alcohol problems in the community* (ed. L. Harrison), pp. 223–40. Routledge, London.

65. Marmot, M., Adelstein, A., and Bulusu, L. (1984). *Immigrant mortality in England and Wales, 1970–78*. HMSO, London.

66. Balarajan, R., Adelstein, A.M., Bulusu, L., and Shukla, V. (1984). Patterns of mortality among migrants to England and Wales from the Indian sub-continent. *British Medical Journal*, **289**, 1185–7.

67. Cochrane, R. and Bal, S. (1989). Mental hospital admission rates of immigrants in England: a comparison of 1971 and 1981. *Social Psychiatry and Psychiatric Epidemiology*, **24**, 2–11.

68. Drake, M., O'Brien, M., and Biebuyck, T. (1981). *Single and homeless*. HMSO, London.

69. Fischer, P.J. (1989). Estimating the prevalence of alcohol, drug and mental health problems in the contemporary homeless population: a review of the literature. *Contemporary Drug Problems*, **16**, 333–89.

70. Harrison, L. and Luck, H. (1997). Drinking and homelessness. In *Alcohol problems in the community* (ed. L. Harrison), pp. 53–75. Routledge, London.

71. Institute of Medicine. (1988). *Homelessness, health, and human needs*. National Academy Press, Washington, DC.

72. Freimanis, L. (1993). Alcohol and single homelessness: an outreach approach. In *Homelessness, health care and welfare provision* (ed. K. Fisher and J. Collins), pp. 44–51. Routledge, London.

73. Royal College of Psychiatrists (1986). *Alcohol: our favourite drug*. Tavistock Publications, London.

74. Fossey, E., Loretto, W., and Plant, M. (1997). Alcohol and youth. In *Alcohol problems in the community* (ed. L. Harrison), pp. 53–75. Routledge, London.

75. May, C. (1993). Young heavy drinkers: is there a problem, is there a solution? *Health and Social Care*, **1**, 203–10.

76. Reiger, D.A., Farmer, M.E., Rae, D.S., *et al.* (1990). Co-morbidity of mental disorder with alcohol and other drug abuse: results from an Epidemiological Catchment Area (ECA) Study. *Journal of the American Medical Association*, **264**, 2511–18.

77. Menzes, P.R., Johnson, S., Thornicroft, G., *et al.* (1996). Drug and alcohol problems among individuals with severe mental illness in South London. *British Journal of Psychiatry*, **168**, 612–19.

78. Weaver, T., Renton, A., Stimson, G., and Tyrer, P. (1999). Severe mental illness and substance misuse. *British Medical Journal*, **318**, 137–8.

79. Lehman, A.F. and Dixon, L.B. (ed.) (1995). *Double jeopardy: chronic mental illness and substance use disorders*. Harwood, Basel.

80. Mann, R.E., Smart, R., Anglin, L., and Rush, B. (1988). Are decreases in liver cirrhosis rates a result of increased treatment for alcoholism? *British Journal of Addiction*, **83**, 683–8.

81. Mann, R.E., Smart, R., Anglin, L., and Adlaf, E. (1991). Reductions in cirrhosis deaths in the United States: associations with per capita consumption and AA membership. *Journal of Studies on Alcohol*, **52**, 361–5.

82. Weisner, C. (1993). Toward an alcohol treatment entry model: a comparison of problem drinkers in the general population and in treatment. *Alcoholism: Clinical and Experimental Research*, **17**, 746–52.

83. Department of Health (1989). *Caring for people: community care in the next decade and beyond*. Cm. 849, HMSO, London.

84. MacGregor, S., O'Gorman, A., Cattell, V., Flory, P., and Savage, R. (1993). *Vulnerable services for vulnerable people*. Alcohol Concern, London.

85. Moncrieff, J. and Drummond, D.C. (1998). The quality of alcohol treatment research: an examination of influential controlled trials and development of a quality rating system. *Addiction*, **93**, 811–23.

4.2.2.6 Prevention of alcohol-related problems

Robin Room

In most developed societies and many developing societies, alcohol consumption is widely distributed in the population, with abstainers in a minority among adults. Those qualifying to be diagnosed with an alcohol use disorder are a minority of drinkers in such societies.

On the other hand, alcohol is causally implicated in a wide variety of health and social problems. The Global Burden of Disease study estimates that alcohol accounts for 10.3 per cent of the total health-related loss of disability-adjusted life-years in developed societies.[1] In terms of where this burden appears in the health system, while psychiatric conditions (including dependence) and chronic physical disease are both important, casualties often play a predominant role. A recent study in Canada calculated that injuries and other acute causes of death accounted for 66 per cent of all potential years of life lost due to alcohol.[2]

The public health importance of acute effects of a particular episode of intoxication underlies what is often described as the 'prevention paradox'. In many societies, a fairly substantial proportion of the population (particularly of males) gets intoxicated at least occasionally, and by that fact is at risk of experiencing and causing social and health harm from drinking.[3] Preventing alcohol problems thus requires looking beyond the considerably smaller segment of the population diagnosable with an alcohol use disorder, or the even smaller segment receiving treatment for such a disorder.

A complication in preventing alcohol problems is that there is also evidence of a health benefit from drinking in terms of reduced cardiovascular disease. This benefit is, however, important mainly for men over 45 and women past menopause, and can be attained with a pattern of very light regular drinking, as little as a drink every second day.[4] There is thus little potential conflict between taking alcohol as a preventive heart medication and any prevention policy short of total prohibition.

Simplifying somewhat, there are seven main strategies to minimize alcohol problems:

(1) educate or persuade people not to use or about ways to use so as to limit harm;

(2) deter drinking-related behaviour with the threat of penalties—a kind of negative persuasion;

(3) operating in the positive direction, provide alternatives to drinking or to drink-connected activities;

(4) somehow insulate the use from harm;

(5) regulate availability of the drug or the conditions of its use—prohibition of supply may be regarded as a special case of such regulation;

(6) work with social or religious movements oriented to reducing alcohol problems;

(7) treat or otherwise help people who are in trouble with their drinking.

We will consider in turn these strategies and the evidence on their effectiveness.

Education and persuasion

In principle, education can be offered to any segment of the population in a variety of venues, but it is usually education of youth in schools which first comes to mind in the prevention of alcohol problems. Community-based prevention programmes, which are often also directed at adults, also may include an educational component.

Education offers new information or ways of thinking about information, and leaves it to the listener to draw conclusions concerning beliefs and behaviour. However, most alcohol education programmes go beyond this. A commonplace of the North American evaluative literature on alcohol education is that 'knowledge-only' approaches do not result in changes in behaviour.[5] School-based alcohol education has thus usually had a persuasional element, aiming to influence students in a particular direction.

Persuasion is directly concerned with changing beliefs or behaviours, and may or may not also offer information. Mass-media campaigns aimed at persuasion have been a very common component of prevention programmes for alcohol-related problems, but persuasion can be pursued also through other media and modalities.

In most societies, public-health-oriented persuasion about alcohol must compete with a variety of other persuasional messages, including those intended to sell alcoholic beverages. The evidence that alcohol advertising influences teenagers and young adults towards increased drinking and problematic drinking is becoming stronger.[6,7] Even where alcohol advertising is not allowed on the mass media, these messages are conveyed to consumers and potential consumers in a variety of other ways.

Evidence on effectiveness

The literature on effectiveness of educational approaches is dominated by studies from the United States on school-based education. This means that the alcohol education has usually been in the context of drug and tobacco education, and that the emphasis has been on abstention,[8] or at least on delaying the start of drinking, in cultural circumstances where the median age of actually starting drinking is about 13, while the minimum legal drinking age is 21. In general, despite the best efforts of a generation of researchers, this literature has had difficulty showing substantial and lasting effects.[9] There is a good argument from general principles for alcohol education in the context of consumer and health education, but there is little evidence from the formal evaluation literature at this point of its effectiveness beyond the short term.

Persuasional media campaigns have also been a favourite modality in many places in recent decades for the prevention of alcohol problems. In general, evaluations of such campaigns have been able to demonstrate impacts on knowledge and awareness about substance use problems, but can show only modest success in affecting attitudes and behaviours. As with school education approaches, there are hints in the literature that success may come more from influencing the community environment around the drinker—in terms of attitudes of significant others, or popular support for alcohol policy measures—than from directly persuading the drinker him- or herself. Thus, media messages can be effective as agenda-setting mechanisms in the community, increasing or sustaining public support for other preventive strategies.[10]

Deterrence

In its broadest sense, deterrence means simply the threat of negative sanctions or incentives for behaviour—a form of negative persuasion. Criminal laws deter in two ways: by general deterrence, which is the effect of the law in preventing a prohibited behaviour in the population as a whole, and specific deterrence, which is the effect of the law in discouraging those who have been caught from doing it again.[11] A law tends to have a greater preventive effect and to be cheaper to administer to the extent it has a strong general deterrence effect.

Prohibitions on driving after drinking more than a specified amount are now in effect in most nations.[12] In many societies there have also been laws against public drunkenness (being in a public place while intoxicated), and against obnoxious behaviour while intoxicated. Other common prohibitions are concerned with producing or selling alcoholic beverages outside state-regulated channels, and with aspects of drinking under a specified minimum age.

Evidence on effectiveness

Drink–driving legislation, such as *per se* laws outlawing driving while at or above a defined blood alcohol level, has been shown to be effective in changing behaviour and reducing rates of alcohol-related problems.[11,13,14] The effect is through both general and specific deterrence. The quickness and certainty of punishment, as well as its severity, are important in the deterrent value (too much severity tends

to undercut its quickness and certainty). Drink–driving is an ideal area for applying general deterrence, since the gains from breaking the law are limited, and drivers typically have something to lose by being caught.

Many English-speaking and Scandinavian countries have had a tradition of criminalizing drinking in public places or public drunkenness as such, but the trend has been to decriminalize public drunkenness. Though there are few specific studies, criminalizing public drunkenness may not be very effective in changing the behaviour of those who have little to lose.

Providing and encouraging alternative activities

Another strategy, in principle involving positive incentives, is to provide and seek to encourage activities which are an alternative to drinking or to activities closely associated with drinking. This includes such initiatives as making soft drinks available as an alternative to alcoholic beverages, providing locations for sociability as an alternative to public houses and bars, and providing and encouraging recreational activities as an alternative to leisure activities involving drinking. Job-creation and skill-development programmes are other examples.

Evidence on effectiveness

'Boredom' and 'because there's nothing else to do' are certainly among the reasons some drinkers give for drinking. There are many good reasons for a general social policy of providing and encouraging alternative activities. However, as has been noted, 'the problem with alternatives to drinking is that drinking combines so well with so many of them'. Soft drinks are indeed an alternative to alcoholic beverages for quenching thirst, but they may also serve as a mixer in an alcoholic drink. Involvement in sports may go along with drinking as well as replace it. The few evaluation studies of providing alternative activities, again from a restricted range of societies, have generally not shown lasting effects on drinking behaviour,[15,16] although they undoubtedly often serve a general social purpose in broadening opportunities for the disadvantaged.[17]

Insulating use from harm

A major social strategy for reducing alcohol-related problems in many societies has been measures to separate the drinking, and particularly heavy drinking, from potential harm. This separation can be physical (in terms of distance or walls), it can be temporal, or it can be cultural (e.g. defining the drinking occasion as 'time out' from normal responsibilities). These 'harm reduction' strategies, as they are called in the context of illicit drugs, are often built into cultural arrangements around drinking, but can also be the object of purposive programmes and policies.[18]

A variety of modifications of the driving environment affect casualties associated with drinking and driving, along with other casualties. These include mandatory use of seat belts, airbags, and improvements in the safety of road vehicles and roads. Many other practical measures to separate intoxication episodes from casualties and other adverse consequences have been put into practice, although usually without formal evaluation.

Evidence on effectiveness

Drink–driving countermeasures are a prime example of an approach in terms of insulating drinking behaviour from harm, since they seek to reduce alcohol-related traffic casualties without necessarily stopping or reducing alcohol use.[19] There is substantial evidence of the success of a range of such countermeasures, including environmental change approaches as well as deterrence.[20,21] Some environmental measures which reduce road casualties in general, for example requiring that seat-belts be worn in cars, providing pavements separated from the road, may prevent casualties associated with intoxication even more than other casualties.

Regulating the availability and conditions of use

In terms of the substantial harms to health and public order they can cause, alcoholic beverages are not ordinary commodities. Governments have thus often actively intervened in the markets for such beverages, far beyond usual levels of state intervention in markets for commodities.

Total prohibition can be viewed as an extreme form of regulation of the market. In this circumstance, where no-one is licensed to sell alcohol, the state has no formal control over the conditions of the sales which nevertheless occur, and there are no legal sales interests, controlled through licensing, to co-operate with the state in the market's regulation.

With a general prohibition, typically the consumption of alcohol does fall in the population, and there are declines also in the rates of the direct consequences of drinking such as cirrhosis or alcohol-related mental disorders.[18,22] But prohibition also brings with it characteristic negative consequences, including the emergence and growth of an illicit market, and the crime associated with this. Partly for this reason, prohibition is not now a live option in any developed society, although it is in some other societies.

The features of alcohol control regimes, regulating the legal market in alcohol, vary greatly. Special taxes on alcohol are very common, imposed often as much for revenue as for public health considerations. Many societies have minimum age limits forbidding sales to underage customers, and regulating forbidding sales to the already intoxicated. Often the regulations include limiting the number of sales outlets, restricting hours and days of sale, and limiting sales to special shops or drinking places. Rationing of alcohol purchases—limiting the amount individuals can buy in a given time period—has also been used as a means of regulating availability. Regulations restricting or forbidding advertising of alcoholic beverages attempt to limit or channel efforts by private interests to increase demand for particular alcoholic beverage products. Such regulations potentially complement education and persuasion efforts. State monopolization of sales of some or all alcoholic beverages at the retail and/or wholesale level has also commonly been used as a mechanism to minimize alcohol-related harm.[23]

The effectiveness of specific types of regulation of availability

The last 25 years have seen the development of a burgeoning literature on the effects of alcohol control measures. Specific types of regulation of the alcohol market, and the evidence on their effectiveness, are discussed below.

Minimum age limits

A minimum age limit is a partial prohibition, applied to one segment of the population. There is a strong evaluation literature showing the effectiveness of establishing and enforcing minimum age limits in reducing alcohol-related problems.[13] However, this literature is North America based, focuses mostly on youthful driving casualties, and mostly evaluates reduction from and increases to age 21 as the limit, a higher minimum age limit than in most societies. The applicability of the literature's findings in other societies and where youth cultures are less car focused has been little tested.

Taxes and other price increases

Generally, consumers show some response to the price of alcoholic beverages, as of all other commodities. If the price goes up, the drinker will drink less; data from developed societies suggests this is at least as true of the heavy drinker as of the occasional drinker.[13] Studies have found that alcohol tax increases reduce the rates of traffic casualties, of cirrhosis mortality, and of incidents of violence.[24,25]

Limiting sales outlets, and hours and conditions of sale

There is a substantial literature showing that levels and patterns of alcohol consumption, and rates of alcohol-related casualties and other problems, are influenced by such sales restrictions, which typically make the purchase of alcoholic beverages slightly inconvenient, or influence the setting of and after drinking.[13] Enforced rules influencing 'house policies' in drinking places on not serving intoxicated customers etc. have also been shown to have some effect.[26]

Monopolizing production or sale

Studies of the effects of privatizing retail alcohol monopolies have often shown some increase in levels of alcohol consumption and problems, in part because the number of outlets and hours of sale typically increase with privatization.[27] From a public health perspective, it is the retail level which is important, while monopolization of the production or wholesale level may facilitate revenue collection and effective control of the market.

Rationing sales

Rationing the amount of alcohol sold to an individual potentially directly impacts on heavy drinkers, and has been shown to reduce levels both of intoxication-related problems such as violence, and of drinking-history-related problems such as cirrhosis mortality.[28,29] But while a form of rationing—the medical prescription system—is well accepted in most societies for psychoactive medications, it has proved politically unacceptable nowadays for alcoholic beverages in developed societies.

Advertising and promotion restrictions

Many societies have regulations on advertising and other promotion of sales of alcoholic beverages.[12] While it is well accepted that advertising can strongly affect consumer choices between products on the market, it has proved difficult to measure the effects of advertising on demand for alcoholic beverages as a whole, in part because the effects are likely to be cumulative and long term, making them difficult to measure. However, the evidence on the effects of advertising and promotion on overall demand has become stronger in the recent literature.[30]

Social and religious movements and community action

Substantial reductions in alcohol-related problems have often been the result of spontaneous social and religious movements which put a major emphasis on quitting intoxication or drinking. In recent decades, there have also been efforts to form partnerships between state organizations and non-governmental groups to work on alcohol problems, often at the level of the local community. There has been an active tradition of community action projects on alcohol problems, often using a range of prevention strategies.[31–34] School-based prevention efforts have also moved increasingly to try to involve the community, in line with general perceptions that such multifaceted strategies will be more effective.[9]

While some of the largest historical reductions in rates of alcohol problems have resulted from spontaneous and autonomous social or religious movements, support or collaboration from a government can easily be perceived as official co-optation or manipulation.[35] Thus, there is considerable question about the extent to which such movements can or should become an instrument of government prevention policies.

Evidence on effectiveness

In the short term, movements of religious or cultural revival can be highly effective in reducing levels of drinking and of alcohol-related problems. Alcohol consumption in the United States fell by about one-half in the first flush of temperance enthusiasm in 1830 to 1845.[18] Rates of serious crime are reported to have fallen for a while to a fraction of their previous level in Ireland in the wake of Father Mathew's temperance crusade.[36] The enthusiasm which sustains such movements tends to decay over time, although they often leave behind new customs and institutions with much longer duration. For instance, although the days when the historic temperance movement in English-speaking societies was strong are long gone, the movement had the long-lasting effect of largely removing drinking from the workplace in these societies.

Treatment and other help

Providing effective treatment or other help for these drinkers who find they cannot control their drinking can be regarded as an obligation of a just and humane society. The help can take several forms: a specific treatment system for alcohol problems, professional help in general health or welfare systems, or non-professional assistance in mutual-help movements. To the extent such help is effective, it is also a means of preventing or reducing future alcohol-related problems.

Treatments for alcohol problems need not be complex or expensive. The evaluation literature suggests that brief outpatient interventions aimed at changing cognitions and behaviour around drinking are as effective in most circumstances as longer and more intensive treatment.[37,38] Positive results from such interventions in a primary

health care settings were shown in a World Health Organization study including a number of countries.[39]

Evidence on effectiveness

In terms of the effects of treatment on those who come for it, there is good evidence of effectiveness of treatment for alcohol problem. Typically, the improvement rate from a single episode of treatment is about 20 per cent higher than the no-treatment condition. Further treatment episodes are often needed. Brief treatment interventions or mutual-help approaches usually result in net savings in social and health costs associated with the heavy drinker (at least where health care is not self-paid), as well as improving the quality of life.[40,41]

The effectiveness of providing treatment as a strategy for reducing rates of alcohol problems in a society is more equivocal. In a North American context, it has been argued that the steep increase in alcohol-related treatment provision and mutual-help group membership in recent decades has contributed to reducing alcohol problems rates.[42] But the strength of the evidence for this contention is disputed.[43,44] A treatment system for alcohol problems is an important part of an integrated national alcohol policy, but as an instrument of prevention—of reducing societal rates of alcohol problems—it is probably not cost-effective.

A note on brief interventions

As noted above, alcohol treatment evaluations have often found that briefer interventions are as effective as longer ones in clinical populations. This finding has fuelled substantial efforts to encourage non-specialists to apply brief interventions to broader populations of problematic drinkers, not only in the context of primary-care medical practice but also in such contexts as college counselling[45] and on-site in public houses and bars.[46] In such contexts, brief interventions may be viewed as a form of targeted persuasion. Results in these expanded frames have been somewhat mixed. Evaluations of brief interventions by medical general practitioners have not always found effects.[47] Persuading general practitioners to use the methods on a sustained basis has not proved easy,[48] and their patients are often unreceptive[49] or recalcitrant.[50] It remains to be seen whether and in what sociocultural circumstances making brief interventions for problematic drinking a routine part of general medical practice is a feasible and effective strategy.

Building an integrated societal alcohol policy

Often the different strategies for preventing alcohol problems appear to be synergistic in their effects.[51] Controls of availability, for instance, are more likely to be adopted, continued, and respected when the public has been successfully persuaded of their effects and effectiveness. But strategies can also work at cross-purposes: a prohibition policy, for instance, makes it difficult to pursue measures which insulate drinking from harm.

In a society where alcohol is a regular item of consumption, in view of the resulting rates of alcohol-related social and health problems, there is a strong justification for adopting a comprehensive policy concerning alcohol, taking into account production, marketing and consumption, and the prevention and treatment of alcohol-related problems.

In terms of strategies we have reviewed for managing and reducing the rates of alcohol problems in society, there is clear evidence for effectiveness and cost-effectiveness of measures regulating the availability and conditions of use, and measures that insulate use from harm. With respect to some aspects of alcohol problems, notably drink–driving, deterrence measures also fall in the same category. Despite their perennial popularity, evidence of the effectiveness of education/persuasion and treatment strategies in reducing societal rates of problems is limited at best. Education and treatment are worthy activities for a society and a government to be doing, but they do not constitute in themselves a public health policy on alcohol. These strategies will nevertheless be pursued in most societies, and they can be best pursued with attention to using cost-effective methods, and to integrating targets and messages with other aspects of alcohol policy.

Physicians and other health workers observe the adverse effects of alcohol in their daily practice, and are well-positioned to argue for public health approaches to reducing the burden of alcohol problems. Reports by colleges of psychiatrists and other physicians have played an important role in such countries as the United Kingdom[52] and Sweden[53] in putting a public health response to alcohol problems on the societal agenda.

References

1. Murray, C.J.L. and Lopez, A.D. (1996). Quantifying the burden of disease and injury attributable to ten major risk factors. In *The global burden of disease: a comprehensive assessment of mortality and disability from diseases, injuries and risk factors in 1990 and projected to 2020.* (ed. C.J.L. Murray and A.D. Lopez), pp. 295–324. Harvard School of Public Health, Cambridge, MA.

2. Single, E., Robson, L., Xie, X., and Rehm, J. (1996). *The costs of substance abuse in Canada.* Canadian Centre on Substance Abuse, Ottawa.

3. Stockwell, T., Hawks, D., Lang, E., and Rydon, P. (1996). Unravelling the preventive paradox. *Drug and Alcohol Review*, **15**, 7–16.

4. Bondy, S., Rehm, J., Ashley, M.J., Walsh, G., Single, E., and Room, R. Low-risk drinking guidelines: the scientific evidence. *Canadian Journal of Public Health*, in press.

5. Botvin, G.J. (1995). Principles of prevention. In *Handbook on drug abuse prevention: a comprehensive strategy to prevent the abuse of alcohol and other drugs* (ed. R.H. Coombs and D. Ziedonis), pp. 19–44. Allyn and Bacon, Boston, MA.

6. Wyllie, A., Zhang, J.F., and Casswell, S. (1998). Positive responses to televised beer advertisements associated with drinking and problems reported by 18- to 29-year-olds, *Addiction*, **93**, 749–60.

7. Wyllie, A., Zhang, J.F., and Casswell, S. (1998). Responses to televised advertisement associated with drinking behaviour of 10–17-year-olds. *Addiction*, **93**, 361–71.

8. Beck, J. (1998). 100 years of 'just say no' versus 'just say know'. *Evaluation Review*, **22**, 15–45.

9. Paglia, A. and Room, R. (1999). Preventing substance use problems among youth: a literature review and recommendations. *Journal of Primary Prevention*, **20**, 3–50.

10. Casswell, S., Gilmore, L., Maguire, V., and Ransom, R. (1989). Changes in public support for alcohol policies following a community-based campaign. *British Journal of Addiction*, **84**, 515–22.

11. Ross, H.L. (1982). *Deterring the drinking driver: legal policy and social control.* Lexington Books, Lexington, MA.

12. Hurst, W., Gregory, E., and Gussman, T. (1997). *International survey: alcoholic beverage taxation and control policies.* Brewers Association of Canada, Ottawa.

13. Edwards, G., Anderson, P., Babor, T.F., *et al.* (1994). *Alcohol policy and the public good.* Oxford University Press.

14. Hingson, R. (1886). Prevention of drinking and driving. *Alcohol Health and Research World*, **20**, 219–26.

15. Moskowitz, J.M., Mailvin, J., Schaeffer, G.A., and Schaps, E. (1983). Evaluation of a junior high school primary prevention program. *Addictive Behaviors*, **8**, 393–401.

16. Norman, E., Turner, S., Zunz, S.J., and Stillson, K. (1997). Prevention programs reviewed: what works? In *Drug-free youth: a compendium for prevention specialists* (ed. E. Norman), pp. 22–45. Garland Publishing, New York.

17. Carmona, M. and Stewart, K. (1996). *Review of alternative activities and alternatives programs in youth-oriented prevention.* Center for Substance Abuse Prevention Technical Report 13. Center for Substance Abuse Prevention, Rockville, MD.

18. Moore, M.H. and Gerstein, D.R. (ed.) (1981). *Alcohol and public policy: beyond the shadow of prohibition.* National Academy Press, Washington, DC.

19. Evans, L. (1991). *Traffic safety and the driver.* Van Nostrand Reinhold, New York.

20. Forsyth, I. (1996). Alcohol and drugs: the role of insurance in promoting effective countermeasures. In *Proceedings of the Road Safety in Europe and Strategic Highway Research Program (SHRP) Conference*, VTI Conference No. 4A, part 3, pp. 45–63. Swedish National Road and Transport Safety Institute, Linkoping, Sweden.

21. Zajac, P.L. (1997). Can technology be used to intervene in behaviour in a human factors engineering approach to drunk driving deterrence? *Dissertation Abstracts International*, **57**, 4126A–7A.

22. Teasley, D.L. (1992). Drug legalization and the 'lessons' of Prohibition. *Contemporary Drug Problems*, **19**, 27–52.

23. Room, R. (1993). The evolution of alcohol monopolies and their relevance for public health, *Contemporary Drug Problems*, **20**, 169–87.

24. Cook, P. (1981). Effect of liquor taxes on drinking, cirrhosis, and auto accidents. In *Alcohol and public policy: beyond the shadow of prohibition* (ed. M.H. Moore and D.R. Gerstein), pp. 255–85. National Academy Press, Washington, DC.

25. Cook, P.J. and Moore, M.H. (1993). Violence reduction through restrictions on alcohol availability. *Alcohol Health and Research World*, **17**, 151–6.

26. Saltz, R.F. (1997). Prevention where alcohol is sold and consumed: server intervention and responsible beverage service. In *Alcohol: minimizing the harm: what works?* (ed. M. Plant, E. Single, and T. Stockwell), pp. 72–84. Free Association Books, New York.

27. Her, M., Giesbrecht, N., Room, R., and Rehm, J. (1999). Privatizing alcohol sales and alcohol consumption: evidence and implications. *Addiction*, **94**, 1125–39.

28. Schechter, E.J. (1986). Alcohol rationing and control systems in Greenland. *Contemporary Drug Problems*, **13**, 587–620.

29. Norström, T. (1987). Abolition of the Swedish alcohol rationing system: effects on consumption distribution and cirrhosis mortality. *British Journal of Addiction*, **82**, 633–41.

30. Casswell, S. (1995). Does alcohol advertising have an impact on public health? *Drug and Alcohol Review*, **14**, 395–404.

31. Giesbrecht, N., Conley, P., Denniston, R., *et al.* (ed.) (1990). *Research, action and the community: experiences in the prevention of alcohol and other drug problems.* DHHS Publication No. (ADM) 89–1651. Office of Substance Abuse Prevention, Rockville, MD.

32. Greenfield, T and Zimmerman, R. (ed.) (1993). *Experiences with community action projects: new research in the prevention of alcohol and other drug problems.* DHHS Publication No. (ADM) 93–1976. Center for Substance Abuse Prevention, Rockville, MD.

33. Holmila, M. (ed.) (1997). *Community prevention of alcohol problems.* Macmillan, Basingstoke.

34. Holder, H.D. (1998). *Alcohol and the community: a systems approach to prevention.* Cambridge University Press.

35. Room, R. (1997). Voluntary organizations and the state in the prevention of alcohol problems. *Drugs and Society*, **11**, 11–23.

36. Room, R. (1983). Alcohol and crime: behavioral aspects. In *Encyclopedia*

of crime and justice, Vol. 1. (ed. S. Kadish), pp. 35–44. Free Press, New York.

37. Finney, J.W. and Monahan, S.C. (1998). Cost-effectiveness of treatment for alcoholism: a second approximation. *Journal of Studies on Alcohol*, **57**, 229–43.

38. Long, C.G., Williams, M., and Hollin, C.R. (1998). Treating alcohol problems: a study of program effectiveness and cost effectiveness according to length and delivery of treatment, *Addiction*, **93**, 561–71.

39. Babor, T.F., Grant, M., Acuda, W., *et al.* (1994). Randomized clinical trial of brief interventions in primary health care: summary of a WHO project (with commentaries and a response). *Addiction*, **89**, 657–78.

40. Holder, H.D., Lennox, R.D.L., and Blose, J.O. (1992). Economic benefits of alcoholism treatment: a summary of twenty years of research. *Journal of Employee Assistance Research*, **1**, 63–82.

41. Holder, H.D. and Cunningham, D.W. (1992). Alcoholism treatment for employees and family members: its effect on health care costs. *Alcohol Health and Research World*, **16**, 149–53.

42. Smart, R.G. and Mann, R.E. (1990). Are increased levels of treatment and Alcoholics Anonymous large enough to create the recent reduction in liver cirrhosis? *British Journal of Addiction*, **85**, 1385–7.

43. Holder, H. (1997). Can individually directed interventions reduce population-level alcohol-involved problems? *Addiction*, **92**, 5–7.

44. Smart, R.G. and Mann, R.E. (1997). Interventions into alcohol problems: what works? *Addiction*, **92**, 9–13.

45. Marlatt, G.A., Baer, J.S., Kivlahan, D.R., *et al.* (1998). Screening and brief intervention for high-risk college student drinkers: results from a 2-year follow-up assessment. *Journal of Consulting and Clinical Psychology*, **66**, 604–15.

46. Reilly, D., Van Beurden, E., Mitchell, E., Dight, R., Scott, C., and Beard, J. (1998). Alcohol education in licensed premises using brief intervention strategies. *Addiction*, **93**, 385–98.

47. Richmond, R., Heather, N., Wodak, A., Kehoe, L., and Webster, I. (1995). Controlled evaluation of a general practice-based brief intervention for excessive drinking, *Addiction*, **90**, 119–32.

48. Richmond, R.L., Novak, K.G., Kehoe, L., Calfas, G., Mendelsohn, C.P., and Wodak, A. (1998). Effect of training on general practitioners' use of a brief intervention for excessive drinkers. *Australian and New Zealand Journal of Public Health*, **22**, 206–9.

49. Conigliaro, J., McNeil, M., Kraemer, K., Conigliaro, R., Joswiak, M., and Maisto, S. (1997). Are patients diagnosed with alcohol abuse in primary care ready to change their behavior? *Journal of General Internal Medicine*, **12** (Supplement 1), 113.

50. Edwards, A.G.K. and Rollnick, S. (1997). Outcome studies of brief alcohol intervention in general practice: the problem of lost subjects. *Addiction*, **92**, 1699–704.

51. DeJong, W. and Hingson, R. (1998). Strategies to reduce driving under the influence of alcohol. *Annual Review of Public Health*, **19**, 359–78.

52. Baggott, R. (1990). *Alcohol, politics and social policy*. Avebury, Aldershot.

53. Sutton, C. (1998). *Swedish alcohol discourse: constructions of a social problem*. Uppsala University Library, Studia Sociologica Upsaliensia 45, Uppsala.

4.2.3 Substance use disorders
4.2.3.1 Introduction to substance use disorders

Philip Robson

Historical review

The yearning to escape reality through intoxication, to enter, albeit briefly, an 'Artificial Paradise',[1] finds expression in the earliest cave drawings, but traces of hallucinogenic black henbane found at sites of mesolithic settlement demonstrate that it predates the ability to record the experience.

The hardy annual which Linnaeus labelled *Cannabis sativa* in 1753 was probably the first non-food crop. A detailed account of its medicinal powers appeared in China almost 5000 years ago, and it subsequently found its way into the pharmacopoeias of each succeeding civilization, including our own. The fibrous stem of the plant was used for rope-making and weaving, and the seeds were a source of oil for food and fuel. 'Indian hemp' reached Europe about 1000 years ago in the pouches of Moorish invaders of Spain and Portugal. It gradually gained a reputation as a rival panacea to opium, but it was not until the eighteenth century that it became a mainstream medicine in Britain and the United States. Recreational use was popular among European artists and intellectuals in the mid-nineteenth century, but in the United States its association in the public mind with the poorest immigrants from Mexico and elswhere demonized its image.

The opium poppy has been the source of humankind's greatest comfort and scourge. From its roots in the pharmacopoeias of the Egyptians, Sumerians, Persians, Greeks, and Romans opium was borne along the arteries of commerce into India, China, and finally Europe in the baggage of returning crusaders at the end of the last millenium. Paracelsus invented a mixture of opium, alcohol, and spices which he called 'laudanum', and this mixture soothed and tormented millions of Europeans over the next 400 years. The conquest of Bengal in 1773 gave Britain a monopoly of Indian opium, which the East India Company aggressively exported to China in exchange for vast quantities of high-quality tea to feed the insatiable British appetite. The Opium Wars which resulted from the Chinese emperor's discontentment at being saddled with 20 million new addicts led to the additional bonus for the British of the ceding of Hong Kong island as a colony 'in perpetuity'. The drug reached North America with the first European settlers, and the first opium-containing patent medicine appeared as early as 1796. American entrepreneurial spirit ensured that by the end of the nineteenth century more than 50 000 such products were available, and the foundations for some collosal modern fortunes were laid in those unregulated times. Concerns about morphine addiction grew, and in 1898 a new treatment was triumphantly introduced—heroin.

The founders of the Babylonian empire were brewing beer 4000 years before the birth of Christ. Wine-making was first described in Egypt, and viticulture had extended throughout Europe by 2500 BC, partially displacing hemp and opium cultivation by Stone Age farmers. The ancient Greeks developed the Symposium as a means of containing heavy drinking within a structure of ritual, and public drunkenness was unusual. But Dionysus evolved into Bacchus; by Nero's time (AD 54) heavy daily drinking was the norm and fuelled the growing atmosphere of savagery and decay. Although the Christian approach to alcohol has always been ambiguous, it was the Christian monasteries which safeguarded the traditions of brewing and viticulture when the Roman Empire collapsed. But around the same time (AD 616) adherents of Islam were forbidden alcohol by the sacred Koran of Mohammed. The process of distillation originated in the Middle East around the twelfth century, but it was not for another 400 years that aqua vitae became easily available alongside wine and beer. Wine-making had become a vast industry in southern Europe, but a new era began in the last quarter of the eighteenth century when Franciscan monks began laying out the Californian vineyards which would form the starting point for the New World wine tradition.

There is no way of knowing when North American Indians might first have incorporated tobacco into social and religious rituals, but the custom was well established by the time Christopher Columbus arrived in 1492. Returning sailors brought back the original duty-free supplies, and tobacco smoking became widespread in mainland Europe. Sir John Hawkins probably imported tobacco to England around 1550, but Sir Walter Raleigh is credited with its popularization throughout society. No country has ever been successful in suppressing tobacco use once the habit has become established, despite dire penalties: hand and foot crushing in Turkey, nostril slitting in Russia, total confiscation of assets in Japan, and a gargle with molten lead in Persia.

Chewing coca leaves has been endemic among South American indians for several thousand years, but it was not until the sixteenth century that coca became known in Europe through the writings of an Italian physician who had observed its use in Peru. Cocaine was isolated in 1859, and soon formed the basis for a plethora of tonics and patent medicines. These rapidly became popular in the United States after 1880 and at about the same time cocaine emerged dramatically as a mainstream medicine. Some practitioners saw it as a veritable wonder-drug, among them Sigmund Freud who wrote a 'song of praise to this magical substance'. According to an advertisement, cocaine could '...supply the place of food, make the coward brave, the silent eloquent, free the victims of alcohol and opium from their bondage...' . Coca-Cola, with a few milligrams in each glassful, was introduced in 1886. Unfortunately, an increasing number people chose to snort or inject cocaine in large amounts, horror stories multiplied, and within a decade or so the public image of the drug had plummetted. Freud moved on to pastures new and caffeine replaced cocaine in Coca-Cola in 1903.

Hallucinogenic substances have been used since prehistory in social and religious rituals. South American shrubs and roots, the skin of certain toads, psilocybin-containing mushrooms, the peyote cactus, mescal beans, thorn apple, sweet flag, deadly nightshade, mandrake root, morning glory seeds, black henbane, jimsonweed—shamans, sorcerers, and witches have never been short of materials able to provide a short-cut to the spirit world. Mystics, including the Delphic Oracle, used naturally ocurring gases or emissions, as well as fumes from perfumes and burning spices, to induce visions and trance states. Peyote extract found its way into some patent medicines, but until Bohemian circles in European cities discovered mescaline soon after its isolation in 1890 purely recreational use was unusual. Albert Hoffman changed all that with the serendipitous discovery of his 'problem child'—lysergic acid diethylamide-25—in 1943.

Legal control of recreational drugs

Until the middle of the nineteenth century there was a free market in drugs in Europe and the United States, with access to everything from alcohol to opium and coca restricted only by the depth of one's pocket. Two developments did much to upset the *status quo*. In 1805, a pharmacist's apprentice separated a chemical from raw opium and named

it morphine after the Greek god of dreams. Isolation of codeine, thebaine, and papaverine soon followed. Then in 1858 a Scottish surgeon invented a device that could deliver a dose of morphine directly to the point of pain, and this became known as a hypodermic syringe. The combination of powerful synthetic drugs and parenteral routes of administration greatly increased the scope for abuse. Combatants on both sides of the American Civil War were issued with morphine and syringes, and for many years afterwards morphine addiction was known as the 'soldiers' disease'.

In Britain, opium dependency was recognized but generally not vilified, although this tolerance extended only to 'opium eaters'; smoking the drug was regarded as a rather vile alien indulgence (as in the United States). Doctors were keen to get into the act, and the medicalization of addiction coincided neatly with the birth of the new specialism of 'psychiatry', which sought to redefine interpersonal and social problems according to moral and medical principles. Concern was growing about the mortality among children sedated with opium when left unattended by women whose efforts fuelled the Industrial Revolution. But the main drive towards the introduction of the Pharmacy Act 1868, which also restricted sales of cocaine, was professional self-interest. Why allow grocers to corner such a profitable market? Controls over patent medicines soon followed, and the Act was made still more restrictive in 1908.

Such controls were slower to arrive in the United States, but in 1906 the Federal Pure Food and Drug Act required ingredients to be specified on the label. Public concern about opiates made the issue a vote winner, and importation of smoking opium became illegal in 1909. America was instrumental in organizing international conferences in Shanghai and The Hague, and in 1912 it was agreed that the 30 participating countries should enact legislation to restrict opiates and cocaine to medical indications on prescription only. The Harrison Act duly entered the United States' statute book in 1914. Then in 1919 the Supreme Court ruled that maintenance prescriptions of morphine or cocaine to addicts did not constitute acceptable medical practice, and a punitive response to addiction was established which lasted until the HIV epidemic in the 1980s forced a change in philosophy. This coercive approach to recreational drugs gathered momentum. A national prohibition of alcohol was enacted in 1919 and was only repealed in 1933 because of a desperate need by the Roosevelt administration for taxation income. Many states banned cannabis, and its use was effectively outlawed nationwide by the Marijuana Tax Act 1937. By the same year, the majority of states had adopted the Uniform Drug Act to standardize their approach to recreational drugs. In a further effort to overcome what was regarded as a fragmented approach to enforcement, the Comprehensive Drug Abuse Prevention and Control Act came into force in 1970.

In Britain, the Establishment was startled out of its *laissez-faire* position during the First World War by the discovery that soldiers were finding life in the trenches more bearable if they had a supply of cocaine to take back after leave in London. The Defence of the Realm Act Regulation 40B (1916) prohibited sale of cocaine or opiates to soldiers. After some fairly sordid newspaper reports of London nightlife in the immediate postwar period, including lurid descriptions of the drug-related death of a well-known actress, this entered civil law as the Dangerous Drugs Act 1920. For a while, the response to drug problems looked set to follow the American penal route, but in 1926 the government-appointed Rolleston Committee recommended that addiction should be regarded as an illness rather than a crime. Long-term maintenance on an opiate prescription for addicts who were unable to abstain was validated, and the 'British system' was born. In deference to the 1925 Geneva Convention, cannabis was outlawed in 1928 but prescription remained possible until final prohibition under the Misuse of Drugs Act 1971.

The United Nations Commission on Narcotic Drugs (**UNCND**) was established in 1946 to take over from the League of Nations the determination of policy for international drug control. The signatory nations to the Single Convention on Narcotic Drugs (1961) and the Convention on Psychotropic Substances (1971) are required to 'limit to medical and scientific purposes the cultivation, production, manufacture, export, import, distribution of, trade in, use and possession of' a long list of drugs which includes opiates, cannabis, stimulants, sedatives, and hallucinogens. UNCND has delegates from each member state of the United Nations and all other signatories of the 1961 Convention.

Most governments are firmly against arguments for legalization or decriminalization, but the Dutch have pioneered a different approach. In 1976, a policy of non-enforcement was initiated whereby possession or trade in small amounts of cannabis (< 30 g) would no longer be prosecuted. The impact of this policy has been assessed by MacCoun and Reuter.[2] Between 1976 and 1983 depenalization resulted in 'little if any effect upon levels of use', but prevalence of cannabis use 'increased sharply' between 1992 and 1996. However, rates increased equally rapidly over this period in countries with rigorous prohibition, and prevalence and street price of cannabis is currently similar in Holland and the United States. But there is some evidence that the Dutch have been succesful in separating 'hard' and 'soft' drugs; only 22 per cent of Dutch cannabis smokers have tried cocaine compared with 33 per cent in the United States. The conclusion is that depenalization did not significantly increase consumption, a finding which has been replicated in several states of the United States, Italy, and Spain. Decriminalization of cannabis in Canberra, Australia, had no impact on prevalence of use among university students.[3] Very few abstaining students would start smoking cannabis if it was legalized.[4] The Dutch surge in prevalence after 1983 is probably explained by increased promotion and commercialization.

Who uses drugs and why?

Recreational drug use is a worldwide phenomenon with considerable national and regional variations. In 1995, 28 per cent of British men and 26 per cent of women admitted to being regular cigarette smokers. The decline in smoking by adults in the developed world has not been mirrored in children, and in particular the rate of initiation among girls under 16 has doubled over the last two decades in the United Kingdom. By the age of 16 years, 94 per cent of young people have tried alcohol, and 78 per cent will have been drunk on at least one occasion.

Sixteen-year-olds from the United States and the United Kingdom topped the league in lifetime experience of any illicit drug in a comparison of 23 countries.[5] Forty-one per cent of British school students admitted using cannabis in comparison with 34 per cent of North American, 19 per cent of Italian, 15 per cent of Spanish, 12 per cent of French, and 2 per cent of Greek students. Overall, around one in four of the British population have tried an illegal drug at some time. Peak use occurs in the late teens and early twenties. Cannabis accounts for 85 per cent of this and most cannabis smokers never use any other illegal drug.

Polydrug use is the norm on the club scene. Among a sample of Scottish clubbers,[6] individuals had consumed a lifetime average of 11 different drugs. Drug use within the past year included alcohol (96 per cent), cannabis (96 per cent), ecstasy (87 per cent), tobacco (86 per cent), LSD (79 per cent), amphetamine (77 per cent), cocaine (59 per cent), 'poppers' (51 per cent), psylocybin mushrooms (47 per cent), temazepam (39 per cent), diazepam (26 per cent), codeine (19 per cent), heroin (11 per cent), ketamine (7 per cent), solvents (6 per cent), and buprenorphine (6 per cent). Other studies confirm that use of LSD, amphetamine, ecstasy, magic mushrooms, and poppers cluster together among young people. A quarter of all 18-year-olds have tried two or more illegal drugs.[7] In a consecutive sample of 100 patients attending an Oxford drug dependency unit, 22 per cent were regularly using three or more street drugs apart from heroin at presentation (unpublished data).

Only 3 per cent of the drug-using population ever injects, but those who do expose themselves to greatly increased risks of accidental overdose, poisoning by adulterants and impurities, and life-threatening infections. Superficial veins progressively thrombose, necessitating recourse to the larger vessels in the neck or groin where damage to an adjacent artery or nerve may threaten life or limb. A sizeable minority persist in exposing themselves to the risk of hepatitis and HIV through the sharing of equipment, and this is particularly prevalent among younger injectors.

Why take drugs? Some have argued that the search for 'altered consciousness' is a basic human appetite,[1, 8] but most young experimenters would simply say that drugs are pleasurable, exciting, or useful for getting into the party spirit. Other reasons include the relief of unpleasant feelings such as shyness or anxiety, fitting in with friends, or revelling in a sense of sophistication, rebellion, or independence.[4] Males are less likely to be total abstainers and tend to consume larger quantities than females. Genetic make-up, psychological factors, family background, and socio-economic circumstances are all influential in shaping the response to an offer of a drug and in determining the cost–benefit equation that will result in cessation, persistance, or abuse.[9]

Risk-taking is an essential part of the process of developing independence and individual identity during the progression through adolescence into adulthood. Because drugs are now part of the environment for most school students, it can no longer be assumed that experimentation is necessarily pathological or abnormal. In a prospective study[10] of 100 American children followed from the age of 3 to 18 years, the subjects broadly fell into three categories with regard to illicit drug use at the end of the investigation: total abstainers, experimenters, or regular users. Those with the healthiest psychological profiles proved to be the experimenters, who had also been in receipt of a significantly higher quality of parenting than either of the other two groups. Psychological traits detectable in the earliest years can predict future drug use, and the triad of alienation, impulsivity, and distress usually precedes abuse. The authors concluded that problem drug use was more likely to be a symptom, rather than a cause, of personal or social maladjustment.

Consequences of drug use for young people

Adverse outcomes can be immediate or deferred. Any form of intoxication carries the risk of accidents and other consequences of impaired judgement or self-concern. The impact of alcohol is terrifying: 1000 British people are killed and more than 20 000 hospitalized by drunk drivers each year; half the reported violent attacks upon strangers and acquaintances, and a third of all domestic violence is perpetrated by people who are drunk at the time.[7] The immediate risks of street drugs are largely related to the low priority to which criminals ascribe to quality control. Variable purity means that accidental overdose is always possible, street drugs often contain toxic by-products, bulking agents, or adulterants, and organic material may be contaminated with pesticides, fungi, or bacteria. The psychological impact of stimulants or hallucinogens can be overwhelming, and young people are at risk from the lifestyle consequences of the street drug scene such as violence or sexual exploitation. In the United States alone more than half a million unborn babies are exposed to illicit drugs each year. Families can be split apart, education disrupted, and careers terminated.

However, most legal and illegal drug users escape such acute disasters, and there is an enormous discrepancy between the large numbers revealed through population surveys to have experimented with various drugs and those who go on to develop problems with them later in life. Prospective studies[11–15] also suggest that modest controlled consumption rarely produces measurable long-term damage. Some people are able to use 'hard' drugs such as heroin, cocaine, and amphetamine in a controlled way, and differ significantly in their personal characteristics and patterns of use from those who surface in clinics or police cells as a result of legal, medical, or social problems.[16]

On the other hand, an early onset of legal or illegal drug use, or regular heavy consumption during the teenage years, is certainly associated with a detrimental impact on mental or physical health later in life, difficult family, social, and sexual relationships, and disrupted education and employment. Such 'problem drug use' is likely to overlap with other undesirable behaviours such as delinquency, teenage pregnancy, and school drop-out, and probably shares many causative factors. Approximately 10 per cent of experimenters with alcohol or drugs will go on to develop problems with them at some time, and vulnerability factors include physiological attributes related to genetics and neurochemical balance, certain personality traits, attitudes, and mood states, parental attitudes and behaviour, peer influences, quality of schooling, socio-economic circumstances, and availability and cost of drugs.[17]

In those who become dependent a chaotic lifestyle will greatly aggravate the damage, particularly if the intravenous route is adopted. Long-term follow-up suggests that opiate dependence is usually a chronic relapsing and remitting condition with a mortality rate of 10 to 15 per cent over 10 years. On the other hand, up to half the subjects will be abstinent from opiates by the end of this period. The relatively benign prognosis in those who survive supports a harm-reduction approach aimed at minimizing day-to-day risks. There is no comparable research that could provide information about outcome for poly-drug users or people dependent upon drugs other than opiates.

Drug and alcohol abuse among the seriously mentally ill is associated with greater consumption of inpatient care and poorer compliance with treatment.[18] The prevalence of violence is higher than in severe mental illness alone.[19] In the United States, specialized services for 'dual-diagnosis' patients have evolved and appear more effective than general psychiatric units.[20]

Do school prevention programmes work?

Outcome research of prevention programmes in the United States has been the subject of a comprehensive review.[21] Programmes should be guided by awareness that the average age of trying alcohol, cigarettes, solvents, or cannabis for the first time is between 11 and 13 years, and that exposure to drugs is now the norm for older teenagers.[22] The two distinct aims are to delay experimentation in younger children and to minimize harm in those over 13, many of whom can be assumed to be dabbling already or to have friends who are doing so. Only those programmes that actively involve students in discussion and debate, and provide relevant skills training such as assertiveness, ways of resisting social pressure, problem solving, stress management, and confidence boosting, have any measurable benefit. Improvement in knowledge without this practical dimension has no effect on behaviour, and scaremongering or moralizing can be actively counterproductive.

Because the large majority of well-integrated children with good familial support are unlikely to sustain long-term damage from transient experimentation, there is a growing awareness of the need to target vulnerable children before serious involvement with drugs or other self-destructive behaviours has been established. A prevention strategy that does not address the social and economic conditions that foster compulsive drug use and ruthless black-marketeering is just tinkering round the margins of the real problem.

What is meant by the harm-reduction approach?

In the early 1980s, a radical departure from the conventional abstinence-oriented approach took place when it was appreciated that 'the spread of HIV is a greater danger to individual and public health than drug misuse'.[23] A harm-reduction philosophy is centred on the belief that it is possible to exert a powerful impact upon morbidity and mortality without necessarily insisting upon abstinence. A hierarchy of aims begins with attempts to make contact with as many problem drug users as possible in order to provide access to clean needles and syringes, advice about safer sex and injecting, basic health care, and help with housing, child care, or legal issues. Then, for some people but not all, a move away from street drugs on to a prescribed oral substitute may be feasible, possibly followed by detoxification and rehabilitation.

Whether through success of this strategy or just good fortune, a serious HIV epidemic among injectors similar to that experienced in the United States and some European countries has not materialized in the United Kingdom. Unfortunately, the same cannot be said about hepatitis C, which is becoming rampant.

References

1. Huxley, A. (1954). *The doors of perception.* Chatto and Windus, London.
2. MacCoun, R. and Reuter, P. (1997). Interpreting Dutch cannabis policy: reasoning by analagy in the legalization debate. *Science*, **278**, 47–51.
3. McGeorge, J. and Aitken, C.K. (1997). Effects of cannabis decriminalisation in the Australian Capital Territory on university students' patterns of use. *Journal of Drug Issues*, **27**, 785–93.
4. Sell, L. and Robson, P. (1998). Perceptions of college life, emotional well-being and patterns of drug and alcohol use among Oxford undergraduates. *Oxford Review of Education*, **24**, 235–43.
5. Hibell, B., Andersson, B., Bjarnasson, T., Kokkevi, A., Morgan, M., and Nanusk, A. (1997). *The 1995 ESPAD report: alcohol and other drug use among students in 26 European countries.* Council of Europe Pompidou Group, Stockholm.
6. Forsyth, A.J.M. (1976). Places and patterns of drug use in the Scottish Dance Scene. *Addiction*, **91**, 511–21.
7. Mirrlees-Black, C., Mayhew, P., and Percy, A. (1996). The 1996 British Crime Survey. *Home Office Statistical Bulletin*, Issue 19/96. Home Office Research and Statistics Directorate, London.
8. Weil, A.T. (1973). *The natural mind.* Jonathan Cape, London.
9. Robson, P. (1999). Why use drugs? In *Forbidden drugs* (2nd edn), pp. 3–18. Oxford University Press.
10. Shedler, J. and Bloch, J. (1990). Adolescent drug use and psychological health. *American Psychologist*, **45**, 612–30.
11. Kandel, D.B., Davies, M., Kams, D., and Yamaguchi, K. (1986). The consequences in young adulthood of adolescent drug involvement. *Archives of General Psychiatry*, **43**, 746–55.
12. Newcomb, M.D. and Bentler, P.M. (1987). The impact of late adolescent substance use on young adult health status and utilization of health services: a structural equation model over four years. *Social Science and Medicine*, **24**, 71–82.
13. Newcomb, M.D. and Bentler, P.M. (1988). Impact of adolescent drug use and social support on problems of young adults: a longitudinal study. *Journal of Abnormal Psychology*, **97**, 64–75.
14. Hawkins, J.D., Catalano, R.F., and Miller, J.Y. (1992). Risk and protective factors for alcohol and other drug problems in adolescence and early adulthood: implications for substance abuse prevention. *Psychological Bulletin*, **112**, 64–105.
15. Newcomb, M.D., Scheier, L.M., and Bentler, P.M. (1993). Effect of adolescent drug use on adult mental health: a prospective study of a community sample. *Experimental and Clinical Psychopharmacology*, **1**, 215–41.
16. Robson, P. and Bruce, M. (1997). A comparison of 'visible' and 'invisible' users of amphetamine, cocaine and heroin: two distinct populations? *Addiction*, **92**, 1729–36.
17. Robson, P. (1999). The nature of addiction. In *Forbidden drugs* (2nd edn), pp. 197–216. Oxford University Press.
18. Bartels, S.J., Teague, G.B., Drake, R.E., *et al.* (1993) Service utilisation and costs associated with substance use disorder among severely mentally ill patients. *Journal of Nervous and Mental Disease*, **181**, 227–32.
19. Smith, J. and Hucker, S. (1994). Schizophrenia and substance abuse. *British Journal of Psychiatry*, **165**, 13–21.
20. Johnson, S. (1997). Dual diagnosis of severe mental illness and substance misuse: a case for specialist services? *British Journal of Psychiatry*, **171**, 205–8.
21. Gerstein, D.R. and Green, L.W. (1993). *Preventing drug abuse: what do we know?* National Academic Press, Washington, DC.
22. Parker, H., Measham, F., and Aldridge, J. (1995). *Drugs futures: changing patterns of drug use amongst English youth.* Research Monograph No. 7. Institute for the Study of Drug Dependence, London.
23. Advisory Council on Misuse of Drugs (1988). *AIDS and drug misuse: Part 1.* HMSO, London.

4.2.3.2 Opiates: heroin, methadone, and buprenorphine

Adam R. Winstock and John Strang

Opium, derived from the ripe seed capsule of the opium poppy (*Papaver somniferum*), has been used for its analgesic and euphoriant effects since antiquity, with Sumerian ideograms of about 4000 BC referring to the poppy as the 'plant of joy'. The extract contains the alkaloid opiate analgesics morphine and codeine. Heroin (diamorphine) is the most commonly abused opiate, usually in the form of black-market powder which is usually injected or smoked ('chasing the dragon'), but is also sometimes snorted. Street purity varies widely (usually 30–60 per cent) and the cost is somewhere between £40 and £90 per gram, depending on purity, type, and geographical location. Daily consumption is commonly in the region of 0.25 to 2 g.

Neurobiology of opiates

Opiate receptors belong to the G family of protein-coupled receptors, and all inhibit adenylate cyclase and calcium channels. Two subtypes, μ and κ, increase potassium conductance. Although the precise mechanisms underlying the development of tolerance to (and dependence on) opiates is not yet clear, there do not appear to be any consistent changes in opiate receptor levels. One contributory mechanism that has been suggested is the downregulation and desensitization of the opiate μ receptor. Acutely, opiates lead to the inhibition of adenylate cyclase with reduced conversion of ATP to cAMP, resulting in reduced firing at noradrenergic neurones located on the locus coeruleus. Following chronic opiate administration, there is compensatory upregulation of cAMP, returning levels towards baseline. On cessation of opiate use (or following opiate receptor antagonism) withdrawal ensues, characterized by a massive surge in unopposed noradrenergic activity (termed the 'noradrenergic storm') from the locus coeruleus. This noradrenergic hyperactivity is thought to underlie many symptoms of opiate withdrawal, and explains the efficacy of the presynaptic α_2 agonists clonidine and lofexidine in the treatment of the symptoms of acute opiate withdrawal.

Although the changes in noradrenergic activity underlie many of the withdrawal symptoms from opiates, it is likely that other neuroadaptive mechanisms and receptor systems are at work in the development of tolerance and dependence, with recent studies indicating roles for both glutamate and γ-aminobutyric acid (**GABA**). For example, positive reinforcement is thought to be mediated via the dopaminergic mesolimbic system. In the ventral tegmental area, GABA inhibits dopaminergic neurones, which in turn are inhibited via μ opiate receptor activation. Consequently, opiate administration leads to increased dopaminergic activity which is thought to mediate the drive to use and its positive reinforcement.[1]

Route of administration

Whilst smoking heroin is probably the most commonly used route of self-administration, many heroin users subsequently climb the ladder of routes which yield increasing bioavailability, intensity, and speed of onset of the effect, moving from snorting intranasally, through smoking and subcutaneous 'skin popping', to intravenous use. Different types of heroin are preferentially used for different routes of administration, which themselves are markedly influenced by cultural bias; for example, chasing is common in Southwest Asia. Brown heroin from the Middle East is poorly water soluble but has a high oil content and 'runs' well on a heated foil, which makes it better for smoking. It may also be cut with caffeine, barbiturate, or methaqualone, which increases the extractability when smoked.[2] In contrast, white heroin from Southeast Asia tends to be more water soluble and better suited for intravenous use, although it may also be snorted or smoked after preparation.

Heroin metabolism

Diamorphine (half-life 2 min) is rapidly metabolized to the psychoactive intermediate 6-mono-acetyl-morphine (the only metabolite that indicates the consumption of heroin specifically as opposed to other opiates) by blood esterases before being converted to morphine (half-life 3 h). Morphine is subsequently metabolized by the cytochrome P-450 system (Cyp2D6) in the liver to codeine which undergoes conjugation before excretion in the urine. In most subjects, about 10 per cent of ingested codeine is converted into morphine, thereby giving a clinically false-positive test result for heroin/morphine.[3]

Patterns of use

Most users who come into contact with services are dependent users who, because of the duration of their use, are often at the greatest risk of opiate-related harm from either the direct pharmacological effects of the drug or the lifestyle changes that accompany drug dependence. Dependent injectors will usually inject three to six times daily to avoid the onset of withdrawal. So-called recreational use of heroin does appear to exist,[4] although this pattern is not the norm.[5]

Epidemiology

The United Kingdom Home Office Addicts Index closed in 1997 (leaving only the informal non-identifiable regional drug misuse databases). At that time there were about 40 000 notified opiate addicts in the United Kingdom. Over the previous decade this figure had increased by approximately 20 per cent annually. Although important as a marker of the prevalence of heroin abuse in the United Kingdom, this centralized resource was of limited value since it only provided information on those who presented to doctors. The current prevalence of heroin use in the United Kingdom is thought to be less than 1 per cent (male-to-female ratio of 2:1), with most new addicts seeking treatment being in their 20s. Other indicators of the level of substance misuse include the number of arrests for possession, Customs' seizures, deaths from opiate abuse, uptake of needle-exchange programmes, and household surveys.

Good epidemiological data regarding opiate misuse among younger people are limited, although recent reports from the North of England highlight new outbreaks of heroin use among this group,[6] often through smoking. Concern over the introduction of heroin into the club scene to help the 'come-down' from stimulant drugs is also a

Table 1 Effects of opiates

Analgesia
Drowsiness and sleep
Mood change (euphoria, intense pleasure)
Respiratory depression
Cough reflex depression
Sensitization of the labyrinth with nausea and vomiting
Decreased sympathetic outflow (bradycardia and hypotension)
Lowering of body temperature
Pupillary constriction
Constipation

potentially worrying new trend. More important perhaps is the relative paucity of treatment services for young people, in terms of both accessibility and the potential consequences of introducing a vulnerable group to adult services where they may meet experienced drug users. The main initiative should be the targeting of individuals who are likely to experience problematic drug use through two main approaches:

(1) a better understanding of the interaction between risk factors and developmental processes may allow the development of early identification and intervention;

(2) a multidisciplinary skill base to address those issues which may be more pertinent in this group (e.g. family and education).

The effects of opiates

The physiological effects of opiate drugs are outlined in Table 1. The acute psychoactive effects vary depending on dose and route, but include euphoria, sedation, emotional numbing, and induction of a dream-like state.

Heroin (and other opiate) withdrawal

Continued use of heroin (or other opiates) tends to lead to dependence and the development of tolerance (with reduced effect from a given dose or, conversely, the need for an increase in dose to achieve the same effect). Once dependence has been established, abrupt cessation or a marked reduction in dose will result in a withdrawal syndrome, much of which can be considered as a rebound from the previous opiate-induced effects. During this time there is an 'undoing' of the neuroadaptation which had occurred during the development of tolerance and dependence. The classic withdrawal syndrome for heroin appears within 4 to 12 h, peaks at 48 to 72 h, and subsides by the end of 7 to 10 days. There is often a period of several hours before frank withdrawal symptoms begin, during which the addict becomes agitated and anxious. Characteristic withdrawal symptoms include aching muscles and joints, dysphoria, insomnia, agitation, diarrhoea, shivering, yawning, and fatigue. More objective measures include tachycardia and hypertension, lacrimation, rhinorrhoea, dilated pupils, and 'goosefleshing' (piloerection) of the skin (hence 'cold turkey' or 'clucking'). Insomnia (with increase in REM sleep) and craving

Table 2 Complications of opiate use

Infections	Cardiorespiratory	Renal	Neurological
Hepatitis and HIV	Pulmonary oedema	Rhabdomyolysis	Peripheral neuropathy
Bacterial endocarditis	Pulmonary emboli	Membranous nephropathy	Transverse myelitis
Septicaemia	Aspiration	Nephrotic syndrome	Brain abscesses
Pneumonia	Pneumothorax		Myopathy
Tuberculosis	Cardiac arrhythmias		Local nerve damage (direct trauma
Skin abscesses	Respiratory depression		and compression)
Cellulitis			
Phlebitis			
Osteomyelitis			

for the drug may persist for weeks. Opiate withdrawal is not usually considered to be life threatening.

Physical complications

The harm from any drug will be a function of both its direct pharmacological effects and the route of administration as well as the effects of any psychoactive adulterants or bulking agents. Problematic contamination with adulterants is rare and particulate matter is more of a problem, although there have been reports of granuloma formation in the lung and liver following injection of preparations containing talc. Approximately 60 per cent of deaths occurring in drug addicts are related to drug use, with the annual mortality for opiate-dependent users being in the region of 1 to 2 per cent, mostly from overdose. Some of the potential complications of opiate use are outlined in Table 2.

The risk of viral transmission (e.g. HIV, hepatitis B and C viruses) is high among injecting drug users, and routine testing with counselling should be available to those at risk. Rates among users show wide geographic variation reflecting differing injecting patterns. Rates of HIV seropositivity amongst injecting drug misusers in the United Kingdom have not increased since the mid-1980s, with recent studies suggesting much lower rates of between 1 and 5 per cent among the injecting population.[7] Much of this reduction in prevalence is believed to be due to the widespread availability of 'needle-exchange' services and provision of services focused towards 'harm minimization'.[8] Rates elsewhere in Europe are considerably higher; those in Italy are between 30 and 80 per cent. Although opiate misusers represent the largest group of injecting drug users, some evidence suggests that rates of HIV infection among those who concurrently inject cocaine/crack or who are intravenous amphetamine users are higher than amongst their peers who use only opiates.[9] Other groups at high risk are prison populations, where injecting is more likely to involve sharing of needles, syringes, and related paraphernalia without the precaution of adequate cleaning of used equipment.[10]

Hepatitis

Recent surveys of intravenous drug users suggest prevalence of levels in the region of 30 to 50 per cent for hepatitis B and 70 to 90 per cent for hepatitis C.[11] Prognosis is worsened by high levels of alcohol consumption, which are common in many methadone maintenance clients.[12] Therefore education and harm-reduction provision must

continue in order to bring about the kind of reduction in prevalence that has been seen with HIV.

Opiate overdose

Most opiate addicts in treatment have experienced an overdose and many have witnessed it in others,[13] with those who inject being far more likely to overdose than those who smoke.[14] Variability in purity, increased central depressant effects following combination drug use (especially alcohol and benzodiazepines), generalized poor health, and high levels of psychiatric comorbidity make this a vulnerable group for both intentional and accidental overdose. There are times in an addict's career which are associated with an increased risk for overdose, for example early on in their dependence or during relapse such as that seen on return to opiate use after a period of abstinence when tolerance has fallen (e.g discharge following treatment or after release from prison). Signs of opiate overdose are listed in Table 3.

The management of opiate overdose should be supportive with standard cardiopulmonary resuscitation and intravenous naloxone (opiate antagonist). However, intravenous access may be problematic in some users, in which case it may be quicker to give naloxone subcutaneously or intramuscularly. Admission to hospital should always be recommended, since the plasma half-life of naloxone is 1 to 2 h with the duration of effect from a single intravenous dose being as short as 45 min compared with 4 to 6 h for the physiological effects of heroin and 24 to 36 h for methadone.

Psychiatric comorbidity

Several studies have found that 70 per cent of addicts meet diagnostic criteria for a current psychiatric disorder, frequently depression, antisocial personality, and alcohol dependency.[15,16] Such diagnoses may be primary or secondary to opiate abuse, and a careful assessment of

Table 3 Signs of opiate overdose

Respiratory arrest with a pulse (almost pathognomic of opiate overdose in adults)

Pinpoint pupils unreactive to light

Snoring giving way to shallow respiration (< 8 breaths/min)

Bradycardia and hypotension

Varying degree of reduced consciousness/coma

mental state and social functioning when opiate free should be performed. Many will have had childhood behavioural problems such as conduct disorder, and studies suggest that attention-deficit hyperactivity disorder, truanting, and juvenile offending are markers for subsequent use.[17] Clearly, comorbid psychiatric disorders should be treated in their own right especially if it is felt that they are important in maintaining opiate use.[18] Opiate dependence is also a strong risk factor for suicide, which accounts for up to a third of all deaths among intravenous drug users.[19]

Social effects

The ramifications among the family and social environment are immense, with high rates of unemployment and divorce. Criminal conviction rates are high (70–80 per cent) with yearly rates of imprisonment being about 2 per cent. Stabilization on methadone or abstinence from opiates is associated with a reduction in associated crime.

Synthetic opiates

Methadone

Methadone is a synthetic orally effective opiate with a longer half-life than heroin (24–36 h), making it suitable for daily administration. It is the mainstay of treatment for heroin dependency in the Western world. A steady state plasma level is reached within 4 to 5 days, and at doses of above 80 mg it is claimed to provide a reasonable level of opiate receptor blockade such that euphoria from illicit opiates 'used on top' is diminished. Deaths have been recorded during the induction phase onto methadone,[20] sometimes when the recipient is not as opiate tolerant as was believed or is using other opiate or central depressant drugs such as alcohol and benzodiazepines. Therefore confirmation of the patient's dependent status is paramount and should be attained by a careful and comprehensive assessment. This should not rely on self-reported drug use, but should also seek objective confirmation by repeated urine drug screens, direct observation of the patient whilst withdrawing, and assessment of the effect of a methadone dose administered on site. Most importantly, addicts starting on methadone should ideally be seen daily during the induction period, especially after three or four consecutive daily doses as a significant increase in steady plasma level is achieved after repeated dosing.

Buprenorphine (Temgesic®, Subutex®)

Buprenorphine is a partial μ-receptor agonist and κ antagonist. It is used medically as an analgesic (usually sublingually), but it does possess abuse potential and may be injected.[21] However, fatal overdose from respiratory depression is believed to be less likely than with full agonist opiates, and buprenorphine is now being developed as a new drug to be in the used in stabilization and detoxification of addicts.[22]

Assessment of the opiate user

A comprehensive assessment of drug use patterns and associated risks forms the basis of any treatment plan. The most important areas are the confirmation of dependence (see below), which is a prerequisite for the commencement of substitute treatment, and an assessment of risk behaviours such as injecting patterns and other substance use. A suggested plan of enquiry that allows both accurate diagnosis and risk assessment is outlined below.

1. **Current consumption** How much heroin (or other opiate) is consumed on a typical day, in terms of either weight or money spent, and for how long has consumption been at this level? Where more than one opiate is being taken, amounts should be quantified, as should the amount of heroin used on a day when no other opiate is taken. The route of use (smoking, intravenous injection), number of administrations per day, and the minimum amount of drug required each day to avoid withdrawal symptoms should also be assessed. The patterns of use (and amounts) of other substances, especially central nervous system depressants such as alcohol, benzodiazepines, and other opiates such as methadone, should be established.

2. **Typical day** By asking users about their typical day one can elicit the appearance of withdrawal symptoms, the use of opiates to relieve these, and very often both the neglect of other interests and the primacy of drug-seeking and drug-using behaviour over other activities. Enquiries should be made about their involvement in risky drug-funding activities, such as theft and prostitution, and about their social network and nutritional intake.

3. **Drug use history** The age of first use and the psychosocial precipitants of use should be established, as should the development of tolerance and craving through increased frequency of use, escalating dose, and where relevant the onset of injecting.

4. **Psycho-sociobiological complications of use** Enquiries should be made about episodes of overdose (intentional or accidental), viral disease, imprisonment, family relationships, employment, etc. Specific attention should be paid to injecting behaviour such as use of needle exchanges, sharing equipment, and use of high-risk injection sites such as the groin and neck. Enquire about comorbid psychiatric conditions, especially depression.

5. **Past treatments and abstinent periods** Have they ever been in contact with treatment services or been maintained on substitute medication? Have they ever been an in- or outpatient at a detoxification unit? What was their longest period of abstinence? What has helped in the past? When and why did relapses occur? What are high-risk situations and other triggers for use?

6. **Motivation for change** Why seek treatment now? What support is needed? Remember that clients with drug problems often present in crisis. The 'five Ls' are often precipitants for seeking treatment and can be used to encourage behavioural change:
   - Livelihood (occupational, financial problems)
   - Life (physical health, overdose)
   - Love life (relationship, family problems)
   - Legal problems (prison, arrest)
   - Losing it (loss of control over use, mental health problems)

Confirmation of dependence

Although a diagnosis of opiate dependence may to some extent be obtainable from a full drug use history, it should be noted that corroborative confirmation of dependence (and tolerance) to opiates should be sought before commencing substitute treatment. This is of paramount importance, as the greatest risk associated with prescribing methadone is the possibility of consumption by a non-tolerant individual. Details should be sought from the general practitioner or other health-care providers. Physical examination may reveal stigmata of injecting drug use such as evidence of recent intravenous injection sites or 'track marks' (linear scarring along veins from repeated intravenous use) on the addict's limbs. Sequential urine testing over a few days may allow the confirmation of regular opiate (although not necessarily heroin) consumption. Physiological changes consequent on opiate use, such as meiosis and sedation, may be observable in the clinic. Objective signs of opiate withdrawal (tachycardia, hypertension, sweating, mydriasis, etc.) following a period of abstinence are also very helpful in confirming dependence, especially if their reversal is observed following a measured dose of opiates administered on site, since this also indicates the level of tolerance.

Management of opiate dependence

There are three major initial considerations in the treatment of the dependent opiate user.

1. How can the client be engaged within the service?
2. What is the aim of the intervention (abstinence or maintenance with harm minimization)?
3. What modalities should be used?

Engagement with statutory services may be through self-referral or from primary care and hospital services. Often 'street' voluntary agencies or outreach workers will be the first point of contact, and such agencies can be important sources of information, needles, and support for the opiate user. Although methadone is often seen as one of the major attractions of engaging with services, the provision of health-care screening as well as legal and social advice can also be useful facilities to offer.

Attainment of either maintenance or abstinence may be achieved using a range of **pharmacological** and **psychosocial** interventions, with the nature of prescribing and counselling determined as much by clients and their current needs as by the agency's treatment philosophy.

Pharmacological interventions for opiate users: maintenance and withdrawal

Methadone may be used as substitute opiate drug, prescribed long term with the aim of achieving stable (non-injecting) opiate dependence (methadone maintenance) or it may be prescribed in the short term to aid withdrawal. In the latter case, a methadone mixture (usually linctus) is prescribed in a reducing dose over 10 to 21 days. Assessing the methadone dose equivalent of reported street heroin use is difficult because of the reliance on self-report and the variable purity of illicit heroin. Broadly speaking, 30 to 40 ml of 1-mg/ml mixture is approximately equivalent to 0.5 g of street heroin. Methadone gives a different urine drug screen test result from heroin with both immunoassay and chromatographic drug screening, thereby allowing non-prescribed opiate use to be identified.

Oral methadone is a cost-effective treatment either as outpatient maintenance or as a means of in- or outpatient detoxification through dose reduction. Studies suggest that a minimum effective dose in excess of 60 mg/day is required to optimize the benefit from maintenance treatment (recommended doses for substitute prescribing are above 50 mg/day), and significantly higher doses will be used in the treatment of many addicts (usual range 40–100 mg/day). However, it must be remembered that these doses are potentially fatal if taken by individuals without tolerance to the effects of opiate drugs.

The benefits of methadone treatment are as follows:

- reduced rates of injecting drugs
- reduced rates of other illicit drug use
- reduced rates of criminal activity
- reduction in suicide/overdose
- allows treatment contact with possibilities of further harm reduction.

Whilst methadone has been shown to be protective against suicide, it is worth noting that there are now proportionately more fatal overdoses involving opiates than 20 years ago. Other substitute opiates such as buprenorphine, dihyrocodeine, and even diamorphine itself have also been used, although problems of diversion of prescribed drugs and risks of continued injecting make the routine prescribing of injectable preparations of diamorphine and other opiates contentious. Clinicians in all specialties should be aware of the misuse potential for all opiate-containing analgesics to develop into iatrogenic dependence. Repeat prescriptions of such analgesics should be carefully reviewed, especially when some preparations may involve the consumption of dangerous amounts of paracetamol.

Substitute prescribing in isolation is of limited efficacy. Like insulin treatment for diabetes in the absence of other lifestyle changes, such as diet and stopping smoking, the effectiveness of methadone in the treatment of opiate dependence will be enhanced by the use of psychosocial support encouraging appropriate behavioural change. Methadone is not a treatment on its own, but encourages engagement with services and forms one part of a multidisciplinary psychosocial pharmacological treatment package.

Management of opiate withdrawal

Although a slow reduction in the dose of a full agonist (or a partial agonist such as buprenorphine) may be used to detoxify dependent users, other methods are now available. The α_2 agonists **clonidine** and **lofexidine** may also be used to alleviate the distress associated with the central noradrenergic hyperactivity that is responsible for many of the symptoms of opiate withdrawal. The dose of lofexidine should be titrated against the symptoms and signs of withdrawal, while being careful to avoid hypotensive episodes. Lofexidine may be used in both outpatient and inpatient settings; it can significantly reduce the discomfort of withdrawal and is as effective in opiate withdrawal as methadone.[23,24] Lofexidine should be considered as the preferred non-opiate method of assisting opiate withdrawal and can safely be used in conjunction with benzodiazepines and simple analgesics. Withdrawal may also be hastened by administering the long-acting opiate antagonist **naltrexone**, which 'kicks' the addict into intense but shorter-lived withdrawal during which symptomatic relief may be given with clonidine and benzodiazepines.[25] In others this precipitant withdrawal is speeded up even further, with the detoxification procedure being completed under general anaesthetic in about 24 h, although this is not without risk.[26] In the future, the use of buprenorphine and the long-acting L-α-acetyl methadol (**LAAM**) as substitute opiates for long-term maintenance may become more widespread.

Prescribing drugs to opiate addicts

In the United Kingdom all doctors may prescribe methadone for the treatment of dependence and other opiates for analgesia or other clinical indications except dependence. Only doctors in possession of a Home Office license are able to prescribe heroin for the treatment of dependence. In recent years there has been growing concern over the diversion of licitly prescribed methadone to the illicit 'grey' market, with such diversion contributing to many of the deaths related to methadone (i.e. in non-tolerant users). Prescriptions for abusable drugs like methadone may contain directives that determine how and when the prescription is dispensed by the pharmacist, and such considerations may limit the diversion of such drugs. For example, the prescription may dictate that the drug is dispensed daily from a named pharmacist or, as is increasingly the case in some areas, methadone is prescribed so that it is taken on site in the pharmacy (supervised administration) or is administered daily from a specialist clinic. Liaison between the pharmacist, the general practitioner, and the specialist is likely to become more important as these shared-care approaches become more commonplace. Supervised daily consumption of methadone and the integration of primary care in treatment delivery to drug users are both recommendations laid out in new United Kingdom government guidelines for the management of drug misuse (the 'Orange Guidelines').[27]

The range of service providers and the impact of treatment

Those who experience problems with opiates may present to wide range of professionals within the health-care, social, and legal systems. The range of treatment options available within statutory and non-statutory agencies will vary, as will the provision of either maintenance or detoxification for opiate dependents depending upon differing treatment philosophies and treatment settings. Partly in response to this diversity of resource provision, an ongoing multicentre prospective outcome study (National Treatment Outcome Research Study) was set up in 1995 to compare the impact of different treatment approaches on subsequent drug use as well as upon psychosocial and physical outcomes. Preliminary results[28] suggested that all four types of intervention (residential rehabilitation, inpatient drug dependency units, methadone maintenance, and reduction) led to reductions in illicit drug use and criminal activity as well as reductions in injecting and sharing behaviours. Least impact was noted on heavy alcohol consumption, which is a particular problem in those with hepatitis C. Recent results from the same group suggest that for every extra £1 spent on treatment, there is a return of more than £3 in cost savings associated with lower levels of victim costs of crime and reduced demands upon the criminal justice system.

Psychological approaches

There are numerous psychological approaches that are currently used in the management of substance misusing individual including cognitive-behavioural therapy, relapse prevention, and psychotherapy (individual, family, and group). The most influential approach in recent years has been the relapse prevention model,[29] which includes identification of cues or triggers for craving (often people, places or paraphernalia, or a certain mood state such as boredom or stress) and learning techniques (distraction , relaxation, imagery) to handle high-risk situations. Recently, motivational interviewing, based on the work of Miller in the United States, has become increasingly popular. It aims to move the client along a 'cycle of change'[30] from pre-contemplator (no interest in changing current using behaviour) to contemplator, and then to determination and action without confrontation.[31] Motivational interviewing is based on five key principles that have utility within the fields of both addiction and eating disorders, but may also be used in any aspect of the doctor–patient relationship where the patient is ambivalent about implementing a change that in the doctors opinion would be beneficial. The five principles are:

- express empathy
- help the client to see discrepancies in their behaviours
- avoid argument
- roll with resistance
- support the patient's sense of self-efficacy.

This is very different from the usual paternalistic and authoritarian approach on which doctors are reared. It is not enough for doctors to expect patients to do something just because the doctor tells them to do it. People only successfully change their behaviours when they perceive that they are able to (perceived competence) and that they will be better for it. Motivational interviewing is a technique that all health-care professionals could utilize to great therapeutic effect, and we strongly recommend anyone interested in improving their ability to assist any of their clients to implement change in a successful manner to read the referenced text.[31] Involvement with Narcotics Anonymous and support groups such as Mainliners should be encouraged.

Physical approaches

Many addicts, especially those who are homeless, do not engage with or have access to primary health care services. High levels of physical and psychiatric morbidity may go undetected or untreated, and increasingly local drug services are finding themselves as stopgap providers of basic medical care ensuring adequate nutrition, contraception, screening, and check-up facilities. Shared care between drug agencies and primary care should be encouraged, with special attention focused on provision of hepatitis testing and vaccination to all users.

Social and educational support

The drug user may stand alone, but all available potential supports should be considered whether family, friends, or support agencies such as Narcotics Anonymous. Educating the drug user about safe practices and harm-reduction techniques is important, as is appropriate liaison with other agencies such as social services or voluntary sector supports. Therapeutic communities and 'concept houses' based on a religious or abstinent theme offer longer-term care.

Special groups

Young people

Young people with opiate problems often have other emotional and/or behavioural problems, and frequently fall between the adult and child psychiatric services as well as the addiction services, compounding difficulties in the delivery of service. In addition to the absence of a dedicated service for young people with substance misuse problems, there is the added problem of engaging this group with services. There is a twofold need to break down the 'us and them' barrier at the patient–doctor and the child–adult level. Service delivery is further compounded by the need to address developmental issues, cognitive and emotional immaturity, education rather than employment problems, and the greater importance of the family and child protection issues. These issues are uncommon in the adult addiction service and this points to the need for the development of a new skill base. Such a service should be comprehensive, competent, child centred, and lawful. Separation of such a service from adult providers would also assist in preventing experienced drug users from influencing more naive users. Ultimately a tiered approach would appear appropriate, since it would allow maximum utility of current services and focused development of new services. Generic services in primary health care could provide accurate screening with initial referral to youth-oriented services within existing departments. Beyond this, referral to specialist and super-specialist regional services could be employed to provide secure environments with the option of residential rehabilitation and therapeutic communities. Full and accurate assessment will be the key issue, with the adage of history, examination, and special investigations being as valid here as elsewhere in medicine. It will only be through early identification and accurate assessment that this vulnerable group will be accessible to service providers. Once engaged they will be able to receive the full range of possible therapies from family work and cognitive-behavioural therapy to pharmacotherapy and self-help groups.

Pregnancy

Maternal opiate use abuse may harm both mother and fetus with damage mediated through the bio-psychosocial consequences of drug use. For the injecting drug user, continued exposure through risk behaviours to pools of infections combined with vertical transmission makes intervention in this group of paramount importance. Increased rates of stillbirth, premature birth, antenatal complications, low birth weight, and neonatal withdrawal are all associated with maternal opiate use, through the pharmacological and lifestyle consequences of drug use. In considering the management of the pregnant drug user, liaison between the primary health care team (especially if also the prescriber) and the drug and pregnancy services is paramount to promote both engagement and compliance with treatment.

General aims of managing the pregnant drug user

- Engage the patient.
- Maintain contact with the patient.
- Promote the health and well being of the mother and fetus.
- Aim to reduce risk-taking behaviours (sharing needles, prostitution).
- Stabilize on non-injectable alternatives such as methadone.
- If considering detoxification, this should be done in the middle trimester.
- Provide good primary health (nutrition) and psychological care.
- Liaise with obstetric, midwifery, and paediatric teams, and with social services where appropriate.

- Social stability and provisions for motherhood.
- Social work/parenting assessment.
- Ensure that other drug and alcohol behaviours are assessed.
- HIV and hepatitis screening (vaccination where appropriate).

Stabilization of the mother on an oral substitute drug should always be the initial aim. Where possible, the mother should be encouraged to become abstinent prior to delivery—indeed this is often what both doctor and mother want. However, such a move may not always be in the best interests of the infant and mother, and it may often be more appropriate to keep the mother in contact with services on low-dose maintenance. The long-term outcome in women who enter methadone treatment programmes during pregnancy is better in terms of their pregnancy, childbirth, and infant development, irrespective of continuing illicit drug use.[27]

Although there is no clear relationship between maternal methadone dose and the intensity of neonatal withdrawal (or likelihood of experiencing it), the pregnant opiate user should be encouraged to try and reduce the dose since lower doses (15 mg) are probably associated with a reduction in severity of neonatal withdrawals. Benzodiazepines and opiates are slowly metabolized by the newborn infant, so that peridelivery administration may result in hypotonia and respiratory depression. Both opiate and benzodiazepine dependence in the mother may be associated with protracted withdrawal syndromes in the infant, with the risk of seizures. There is some evidence to suggest that transferring the pregnant mother onto buprenorphine during the second trimester is associated with lower rates of neonatal withdrawal. Methadone is not a contraindication to breast feeding, although there is wide variation in local recommendations. Issues such as maternal nutritional and viral status also need to be taken into account when deciding whether breast feeding is appropriate.

Prisoners

About one-third of remand prisoners have a substance abuse dependency problem, most commonly alcohol and opiates. Access to illicit substances is not prevented by imprisonment; indeed some users may increase their 'habit' while in prison . Poor levels of identification on screening at entry and as yet inadequate prison treatment services and court diversion schemes for drug-dependent offenders mean that their considerable needs will continue to be unmet. Education and good primary health care are vital. Recent interest in drug treatment and testing orders may allow those dependent users who are convicted of crimes associated with acquisitive offending to receive a treatment order as opposed to a custodial sentence.

Comorbid clients

There are high rates of comorbidity of personality disorders, depression, and anxiety disorders among opiate users, with the severity of premorbid pathology being an important determinate of outcome.[32] Appropriate assessment and treatment of depressive disorders is important in reducing relapse rates and maintaining engagement, remembering that suicide accounts for a high percentage of deaths in opiate users. Again, liaison with adult mental health teams is important.

HIV-positive addicts

Reducing high-risk behaviours by those with HIV is important in limiting the spread of the disease. Stabilization on methadone with abstinence from injecting, needle-sharing, and unprotected sex should be encouraged. Liaison with medical and psychiatric services is important.

Outcome

Outcome in opiate dependence is not unitary. It is a dynamic process with bio-psychosocial facets. Outcome parameters may include the individual's level of alcohol and drug use, his or her personal and social functioning, and the impact upon public health and safety. Figures will depend on the particular population of users that is followed up and on the level of intervention they received. Regarding treatment contact samples, what is clear is that longer treatment contacts are associated with better outcomes.[33] It is thought that methadone treatment has to continue for at least 2 years for significant gains to be made, although earlier health benefits may be seen. Generally, the greater the range of treatment services provided (health care, family therapy, cognitive-behavioural therapy, etc.), the better is the outcome.[34] Abstinence rates following treatment vary widely, but 10 to 40 per cent of treated patients would still be drug free at 6 months.[35] The majority of those who relapse following treatment do so within 3 to 4 months of discharge. The greater the severity of pretreatment psychopathology and dependence the worse is the outcome. Suicide and accidental overdose account for between one-third and half of all deaths of opiate addicts, with risk factors including alcohol use, recent dropout from treatment, and social isolation. A 22-year follow-up of 128 heroin addicts revealed that 43 had died (18 due to drug overdose), with annual mortality running between 1 and 2 per cent, and an excess mortality ratio of about 12.[36] Among the strongest correlates of mortality in this group are level of disability, heavy alcohol use, heavy criminal involvement, and tobacco use.

Long-term follow-up studies suggest that eventual cessation of opiate use is a very slow process and becomes increasingly unlikely if users continue into their late thirties.

References

1. Simonato, M. (1996). The neurochemistry of morphine addiction in the neocortex. *Trends in Pharmacological Science*, **17**, 410–15.
2. Strang, J., Griffiths, P., and Gossop, M. (1997). Heroin in the United Kingdom: different forms, different origins, and the relationship to different routes of administration. *Drug and Alcohol Review*, **16**, 329–37.
3. Wolff, K., Farrell, M., Marsden, J., *et al.* (1999). A review of biological indicators of illicit drug use, practical considerations and clinical usefulness. *Addiction*, **94**, 1279–98.
4. Blackwell, J. (1983). Drifting, controlling and overcoming: opiate users who avoid becoming chronically dependent. *Journal of Drug Issues*, **13**, 219–35.
5. Zinberg, N. (1984). *Drug, set and setting: the basis for controlled intoxicant use.* Yale University Press, New Haven, CT.
6. Parker, H., Burry, C., and Eggington, R. (1998). *New heroin outbreaks amongst young people in England and Wales.* Police Research Group, Home Office, London.
7. Crawford, V. (1997). Injecting drug use. *Current Opinions in Psychiatry*, **10**, 215–19.
8. Stimson, G.V. (1995). AIDS and injecting drug use in the UK, 1987–1993: the policy response and the prevention of the epidemic. *Social Sciences and Medicine*, **41**, 699–716.
9. Hunter, G.M., Donoghue, M.C., and Stimpson, G.V. (1995). Crack use

10. Power, K.G., Markova, I., Rowlands, A., McKee, K.J., Anslow, P.J., and Kilfedder, C. (1992). Intravenous drug use and HIV transmission amongst inmates in Scottish prisons. *British Journal of Addictions*, **87**, 35–45.
11. Fingerhood, M.I., Jasinski, D.R., and Sullivan, J.T. (1993). Prevalence of hepatitis C in a chemically dependent population. *Archives of International Medicine*, **153**, 2025–30.
12. Best, D., Lehmann, P., Marsden, J., Farrell, M., and Strang, J. (1999). Eating too little, smoking and drinking too much; wider lifestyle problems among methadone maintenance patients. *Addiction Research*, **6**, 489–98.
13. Powis, B., Strang, J., Griffiths, P., *et al.* (1999). Self reported overdose among injecting drug users in London: extent and nature of the problem. *Addiction*, **94**, 471–8.
14. Gossop, M., Griffiths, P., Powis, B., Williamson, S., and Strang, J. (1996). Frequency of non-fatal heroin overdose. *British Medical Journal*, **313**, 402.
15. Rounsaville, B.J., Kosten, T.R., Weissman, M.N., and Kleber, H.D. (1986). Prognostic significance of psychopathology in treated opiate addicts: a 2.5 year follow up study. *Archives of General Psychiatry*, **43**, 739–45.
16. Robins, L.N. and Reiger, D.A. (ed.) (1993). *Psychiatric disorders in America: the Epidemiologic Catchment Area Study.* Free Press, New York.
17. Lloyd, C. (1998). Risk factors for problem drug use: identifying vulnerable groups. *Drugs: Education, Prevention and Policy*, **5**, 217–32.
18. Hall, W. and Farrell, M. (1997). Comorbidity of mental illness with substance misuse. *British Journal of Psychiatry*, **171**, 4–5.
19. Frischer, M., Bloor, M., Goldberg, D., Clark, J., Green, S., and McKeganey, N. (1993). Mortality among injecting drug users: a critical reappraisal. *Journal of Epidemiology and Community Health*, **47**, 59–63.
20. Caplehorn, J. and Drummer, O.H. (1999). Mortality associated with New South Wales methadone programs in 1994: lives lost and saved. *Medical Journal of Australia*, **170**, 104–9.
21. Hammersley, R., Lavelle, T., and Forsythe, G.A. (1990). Buprenorphine and temazepam abuse. *British Journal of Addictions*, **85**, 301–33.
22. Ling, W., Charuvastra, C., Collins, J.F., *et al.* (1998). Buprenorphine maintenance treatment of opiate dependence: a multicentre randomised clinical trial. *Addiction*, **93**, 475–86.
23. Bearn, J., Gossop, M., and Strang, J. (1996). Randomised double blind comparison of lofexidine and methadone in the inpatient treatment of opiate withdrawal. *Drug and Alcohol Dependence*, **43**, 87–91.
24. Strang, J., Bearn, J., and Gossop, M. (1999). Lofexidine for opiate detoxification: a review of recent randomised and open controlled trials. *American Journal of Addictions*, **8**, 366–77.
25. Kleber, H.D., Topazian, M., Gaspari, J., *et al.* (1987). Clonidine and naltrexone in the opiate treatment of heroin withdrawal. *American Journal of Drug and Alcohol Abuse*, **13**, 1–17.
26. Bearn, J., Gossop, M., and Strang, J. (1999). Rapid opiate detoxification treatments: a review. *Drug and Alcohol Review*, **18**, 75–81.
27. Department of Health (1999). *Drug misuse and dependence: guidelines on clinical management.* HMSO, London.
28. Gossop, M., Marsden, J., Stewart, D., *et al.* (1997).The NTORS in the UK. Six month follow up outcomes. *Psychology of Addictive Behaviours*, **11**, 324–37.
29. Marlatt, G.A. and Gordon, J.R. (ed.) (1985). *Relapse prevention: maintenance strategies in the treatment of addictive behaviour.* Guilford Press, New York.
30. Prochaska, J.O. and Di Clemente, C.C. (1986). Towards a comprehensive model of change. In *Treating addictive behaviours: process of change* (ed. W.R. Miller and N. Heather). Plenum Press, New York.
31. Miller, W. and Rollnick, S. (1991). *Motivational interviewing.* Guilford Press, New York.
32. Rounsaville, B.J., Wiseman, M.M., Kleber, H., and Wilber, C. (1982).

Heterogeneity of psychiatric diagnosis in treated opiate addicts. *Archives of General Psychiatry*, **39**, 161–6.

33. Simpson, D., Joe, G., and Brown, B. (1997). Treatment retention and follow up outcomes in the Drug Abuse Treatment Outcomes Study (DATOS). *Psychology of Addictive Behaviours*. **11**, 294–307.

34. McLellan, A.T., Arndt, I.O., Metzger, D.S., Wood, G.E., and O'Brien, C.P. (1993). The effects of psychosocial services in substance abuse treatment. *Journal of the American Medical Association*, **269**, 1953–96.

35. McLellan, A.T., Alterman, A.I., Metzger, D., *et al*. (1994). Similarity of outcome predictors across opiate, cocaine and alcohol treatments: role of treatment services. *Journal of Consulting and Clinical Psychology*, **62**, 1141–58.

36. Oppenheimer, E., Tobutt, C., Taylor, C., and Andrew, T. (1994). Death and survival in a cohort of heroin addicts from London clinics: a 22 year follow up study. *Addiction*, **89**, 1229–1308.

4.2.3.3 Disorders relating to the use of amphetamine and cocaine

Nicholas Seivewright

Introduction

Amphetamine and cocaine are classed as stimulant drugs, although the distinction between stimulants and depressants can be criticized on the grounds that the same drug may have both actions in turn.[1] This does indeed occur with amphetamine and cocaine, but the initial desired effects are increased energy and activity, along with elevation in mood. These effects appear to be mainly due to the enhanced central transmission of dopamine and noradrenaline (norepinephrine), with a similar enhancement of serotonin playing a less certain role.

Pharmaceutical preparations of amphetamine were previously widely used for the treatment of depression and obesity, and until the 1970s most misuse of the drug related to such medications. In the period since then of increasing recreational drug use, the powder preparation of 'street' amphetamine (commonly known as 'speed' or 'whizz') has largely displaced the pharmaceutical forms to become one of the most common drugs of misuse in many countries. The powder is typically very impure and constitutes a racemic mixture of D- and L-isomers, with the L-form being relatively inactive. In some countries a more potent street preparation of methylamphetamine is encountered, known as 'ice'. The various forms of the drug may be misused by swallowing (either on its own or in a drink), snorting, or injecting.

The coca shrub is indigenous to several countries in South America, where it is traditional to chew the leaf. Use of the derived cocaine powder has spread to the United States and elsewhere, again most notably since the 1970s. The powder may be injected, sometimes along with heroin, by polydrug users, but probably the best-known usage is by snorting, the image of which became associated with successful executive lifestyles. Cocaine has become more dangerous as usage has gradually transferred in many countries to the 'crack' form, which is made from cocaine hydrochloride powder in a simple chemical process, and is more potent in its effects and withdrawal effects. Very rapid increases in blood levels of the drug can be achieved by smoking crack,

and this is the usual route, although it is injected by committed intravenous drug users.

Of the two drugs, cocaine has generally been much more investigated than amphetamine in terms of epidemiology, effects, and treatment approaches, while there has been a particular interest in the links between amphetamine use and a psychosis resembling schizophrenia.

Clinical features

The effects and withdrawal effects of amphetamine and cocaine can be considered together, as the main features are equivalent. However, amphetamine has a slower onset of action than cocaine and a longer elimination half-life, while crack is the most quickly absorbed of the cocaine preparations. This is reflected not only in the generally more intense effects of cocaine than amphetamine, but in the timescales involved. Thus an amphetamine user may experience desired effects, unwanted mental effects, and withdrawal features over the course of a few days, while a crack user can report the same sequence occurring in a matter of hours or even less. The main effects and withdrawal effects of these two stimulant drugs are shown in Table 1.

The list of effects can be seen as merging from the desired to the undesired. On the whole, these drugs are taken in situations where stimulation is the aim, with sleep not wished for and eating regarded as a hindrance. Mood is elevated, but characteristically this progresses to suspicion, in which true paranoid symptoms may be experienced. This is usually recognized by the individual as indicating that the episode of use should be terminated, but if use persists symptoms may become severe, or a more confused state develop. After stopping the drugs there are typically withdrawal effects of depressed mood, hyperphagia, and hypersomnia; no consensus exists as to whether such features are best viewed as 'rebound' symptoms, a truer withdrawal syndrome, or simply users catching up on sleeping and eating after a period without either.

Such withdrawal features have been delineated most closely in relation to cocaine. A three-stage process has been described:[2] initially agitation, anorexia, and acute craving; second, excessive tiredness, depression, and hyperphagia; finally, a normalization of most features, but a return of craving when triggered by environmental cues. This was the description before the escalation in crack use, and it is widely held that depression, craving, and agitation in particular are much more severe with this form of the drug. While environmental cues are clearly relevant in precipitating the use of any drug, a powerful surge of craving on encountering situations associated with previous use appears particularly characteristic of cocaine and crack.[3] The three-

Table 1 Effects and withdrawal effects of amphetamine and cocaine

Effects	Withdrawal effects
Increased energy	Depression
Hyperactivity	Irritability
Euphoria	Agitation
Reduced appetite	Craving
Insomnia	Hyperphagia
Paranoid symptoms	Hypersomnia
Confusion	

Table 2 Classification of disorders relating to cocaine in ICD-10 and DSM-IV

ICD-10		DSM-IV	
F14.0	Acute intoxication	292.89	Cocaine intoxication
		292.81	Cocaine intoxication delirium
F14.1	Harmful use	305.60	Cocaine abuse
F14.2	Dependence syndrome	304.20	Cocaine dependence
F14.3	Withdrawal state	292.0	Cocaine withdrawal
F14.4	Withdrawal state with delirium		
F14.5	Psychotic disorder	292.11	Cocaine-induced psychotic disorder, with delusions
		292.12	Cocaine-induced psychotic disorder, with hallucinations
		292.84	Cocaine-induced mood disorder
		292.89	Cocaine-induced anxiety disorder
		292.89	Cocaine-induced sexual dysfunction
		292.89	Cocaine-induced sleep disorder
F14.6	Amnesic syndrome		
F14.7	Residual and late-onset psychotic disorder		

stage description of withdrawal features suggests that this phenomenon may occur after months or even years of abstinence.

Are amphetamine and cocaine addictive?

It is commonly observed that amphetamine and cocaine are non-addictive, or cause psychological but not physical dependence. Such observations rest on a distinction in which the condition of addiction, or physical dependence, requires visible bodily withdrawal symptoms, but critics claim that this is of limited meaning now that there is an understanding of the neurobiological basis of drug withdrawal states. The current classification systems do retain some distinctions between physical and psychological dependence, and the issue is largely one of definition and semantics. The credibility of the label 'non-addictive' is certainly tested when individuals are encountered who have injected amphetamine 10 or more times every day for many years, or who spend vast amounts of money using crack in a highly compulsive manner.

Classification

Table 2 shows the classification within ICD-10 and DSM-IV of disorders that may relate to the use of cocaine. In both systems the same diagnoses can be applied to amphetamine, in ICD-10 within a category 'other stimulants'.

Importantly, the list of diagnoses in ICD-10 is a standard one to be used across all psychoactive substances, with the second digit of the code number simply changed according to substance, and so the list itself does not imply that all those conditions can be caused by amphetamine or cocaine. The DSM-IV listing is somewhat more spe-

cific, in that the diagnoses are selected from a wider general list of conditions which can apply to the range of substances. In this way the DSM-IV classification recognizes that cocaine and amphetamine can produce states of dependence and withdrawal, as well as psychosis, affective disorders, and the other conditions included. In both systems there are some more specific subcategories such as intoxication with perceptual disturbances, and categories for 'other' or 'unspecified' substance-related conditions.

Diagnosis

The use of amphetamine or cocaine can be detected by drug screening of a plain urine sample. Laboratory testing is the usual option, while instant testing kits of high specificity and sensitivity are also available. The importance of urine testing as a relatively simple procedure to employ, in any setting, in cases where drug use is suspected must be emphasized, as it is surprisingly often neglected. A limitation of this method, however, is that most drugs of misuse only remain detectable in urine for a few days at maximum, and with cocaine this may be as little as 24 h. In contrast, most drugs stay in the hair for as long as that is present. Although this method of hair analysis has the advantage that drug use may be detected over the period during which hair has grown, it has not been incorporated into routine clinical practice.[4]

Clearly self-reports of drug use are often reliable, especially when it is known that they are to be backed up by testing, but a history may be unavailable in, for example, psychotic states. Testing is therefore indicated, although there may be particular problems of compliance. Where a positive result is obtained in a patient with a psychiatric condition, it is important to realize that drug use may be incidental rather than necessarily causative.[5]

Epidemiology

In most countries, the use of illicit drugs is most common among those of young age, male gender, and lower socio-economic status, in areas with high rates of other social problems. Stimulant use in general reflects this, although of the drugs of misuse, cocaine has been exceptional in the extent of usage by more affluent individuals. With cocaine snorting by that group generally in decline, the transition to the crack form appears to have brought cocaine more into line with other drugs, in terms of the users' general characteristics.

The biggest epidemic of cocaine use outside South America has been in the United States, where it peaked in the mid-1980s.[6,7] Household surveys at that time estimated that approximately one-tenth of the population had used the drug; the same epidemiological method has charted the subsequent general decline in occasional use, but an increase in more dependent use of crack. Cocaine use in other countries does not appear to have spread as widely as was predicted from experience in the United States. In Australia, the population prevalence of cocaine use has remained at around 2 per cent, much of it among inner-city polydrug users,[8] and the United Kingdom picture is similar. Among other factors, it is considered that a rapid rise in cocaine problems is relatively unlikely in countries where there is an established ready availability of amphetamine, as a similar and generally cheaper drug.

Even in areas where it is known that stimulant use is common, such users tend to present relatively rarely to treatment services. This relates to the priority that is generally given to opiate misusers and methadone treatment, and is an important issue for service planners—it also has the effect that treatment statistics will always particularly underestimate stimulant problems. In the United Kingdom, consistently more individuals who are using amphetamine and cocaine as secondary drugs rather than main drugs of preference present to services. Therefore, such statistics in turn overestimate polydrug use, although it is clear from all sources that stimulant users do commonly take other drugs, notably sedatives of various kinds to alleviate withdrawal effects (see the section on course and prognosis below).

Aetiology

Broadly the same familial, social, and psychological factors are relevant in the aetiology of amphetamine and cocaine misuse as in other forms of drug misuse. Overall, approximately two-thirds to three-quarters of drug misusers have an underlying personality disorder,[9] usually of the antisocial type, but the figure has been found to be somewhat lower for stimulant misusers than for those dependent on opiates.[10] This may be partly methodological, to do with the difficulty in distinguishing true personality characteristics from behaviours inherent in the activity of highly dependent drug misuse, but is probably also a reflection of the use of stimulant drugs by a generally broader population.

Course and prognosis

Course

A far greater proportion of amphetamine and cocaine misuse than opiate misuse is recreational in nature, with few significant complications occurring. It is assumed that the vast majority of those who are identified in school and teenage surveys as having used stimulants simply give them up in due course, although little systematic data is available. Complications and involvement with treatment services are more likely where there is dependent usage, and there may be psychiatric contact in episodes of psychosis. A very small proportion of amphetamine injectors progress to high-dose daily usage, while the heavy use of cocaine appears to be less sustainable and is therefore usually periodic in nature.

Other drug use

After being stimulated with amphetamine or cocaine, many individuals will use sedative drugs such as alcohol, benzodiazepines, or cannabis to 'come down' from their drug. Increasingly heroin is being used for this purpose, sometimes to the point of becoming dependent on the opiate, and even requiring methadone treatment. The use of cocaine in particular is commonly encountered as a secondary form of drug misuse in methadone patients,[11] with some individuals appearing to switch their preferred illicit drug from heroin to cocaine when treatment is established.

Prognosis

The drug misuse literature in general would suggest that stimulant use is more likely to progress and become problematic in individuals with associated personal or social difficulties, or psychiatric disorder including personality disorder.[9] There is limited evidence from studies of cocaine misuse treatment that prognosis may be better in women,[12] or when a 'significant other' participates in treatment.[13]

Complications

Many of the complications of amphetamine and cocaine misuse are complications of drug misuse in general, including those related to injecting. The range includes general physical decline, weight loss, dental problems, infective complications ranging from abscesses to hepatitis and infection with the human immunodeficiency virus (HIV), reduced fetal growth in pregnancy, mood disturbances, and various social problems. Complications in the following areas are somewhat more specific to stimulant misuse:

- cardiovascular—hypertension, arrhythmias, myocardial infarction, cerebrovascular accident
- obstetric—premature labour, placental abruption
- psychiatric—anxiety, depression, aggressive behaviours, psychosis.

The cardiovascular problems relate to increased catecholamine secretion produced by stimulants, and were seen at a high rate in the United States cocaine epidemic.[14] With obstetric complications, it is difficult to separate the effects of drugs from other risk factors such as poor diet, smoking, or adverse social conditions, but there appears to be a particular link between stimulants and placental abruption.[15] There are also various psychiatric disorders that are particularly associated with amphetamine and cocaine misuse.

Anxiety is common in relation to the agitation produced by the drugs, while depression is a classic withdrawal effect. An assessment of the true significance of these features therefore requires withdrawal from drugs, while in acute presentations both can be extremely distressing, often requiring pharmacological treatments (see below). Aggressive behaviour may be due to an underlying personality disorder, but it is also characteristic of withdrawal from crack cocaine where severe craving is experienced. Psychosis is such a well-known complication of stimulant misuse that one possible problem is that of overdiagnosis.[5] Psychosis produced by amphetamine usually lasts longer than that due to cocaine, but in either case symptoms can be expected to subside if drug use ceases. A diagnosis of drug-induced psychosis is therefore dubious if definite psychotic symptoms persist when urine drug screens have become negative, although there is no consensus as to the stage at which an alternative diagnosis such as schizophrenia needs to be made.[16]

Treatment

Evidence

There is little evidence in support of any specific clinical treatment in amphetamine and cocaine misuse. The majority of studies are from the United States and concern cocaine, many investigating those medications that may alleviate withdrawal effects.[6,7] Some positive findings have been reported, mainly from uncontrolled studies, relating to the use of the dopaminergic agents bromocriptine and amantadine, and also fluoxetine and other medications. Most studied has been desipramine, with a meta-analysis indicating some benefit in promoting abstinence from cocaine.[17] Inpatient programmes and psychological treatments basically represent modifications of those approaches used across all forms of drug misuse.

Management

Faced with the severe limitations in treatment for these forms of drug misuse that have high morbidity and mortality, drug services have had to consider how best to achieve some benefits in terms of practical management.[18] The factors that appear important in such provision are:

- specific outreach programmes

- harm-reduction approaches

- rapid response where necessary

- targeted use of pharmacological treatments

- admission in severe cases.

To engage stimulant users at all can require specific outreach aimed at the subcultural groups in whom usage is common. Basic harm-reduction measures must be offered, including drug information, education about health risks, advice to reduce damaging injecting practices, and the provision of clean injecting equipment. Counselling of a supportive or more behavioural kind may be provided by various types of agency.

The periodic nature of stimulant problems means that rapid response can be important, for instance in states of acute crack withdrawal or psychiatric disturbance. Use of tranquillizers and antipsychotic medications may be necessary for various presentations, while fluoxetine appears to be increasingly favoured over other antidepressants, due to a possible anticraving effect and good acceptability. Inpatient admission is required relatively frequently in cases where no long-term measure is able to make much impact between acute crises. The possibility of any substitute prescribing in stimulant misuse is highly controversial, with some services seeing a role for oral dexamphetamine in heavily dependent amphetamine users experiencing extreme problems from injecting.[19]

Drug-induced psychosis

The two aspects of management of this complication are the treatment of psychotic symptoms and the withdrawal of the drug which is thought to be causative. The latter can be very problematic other than as an inpatient, and is not guaranteed even then. In practice, ongoing semi-psychotic states in individuals who have not completely stopped drug use are common, and treatment may have to be attempted in such circumstances. The use of antipsychotic medications does not differ significantly from that in psychoses not produced by drugs.

Prevention

The prevention of drug misuse lies largely outside the clinical domain, in the areas of education and enforcement. One experimental clinical

development in cocaine misuse is a vaccine whereby limited exposure produces anticocaine antibodies to subsequently block the drug's effects.[20]

References

1. Nutt, D.J. (1996). Addiction: brain mechanisms and their treatment implications. *Lancet*, **347**, 31–6.
2. Gawin, F.H. and Kleber, H.D. (1986). Abstinence symptomatology and psychiatric diagnoses in cocaine abusers: clinical observations. *Archives of General Psychiatry*, **43**, 107–13.
3. Weddington, W.W., Brown, B.S., Haertzen, C.A., *et al.* (1990). Changes in mood, craving, and sleep during short-term abstinence reported by male cocaine addicts. *Archives of General Psychiatry*, **47**, 861–8.
4. McPhillips, M.A., Strang, J., and Barnes, T.R.E. (1998). Hair analysis. New laboratory ability to test for substance use. *British Journal of Psychiatry*, **173**, 287–90.
5. Poole, R. and Brabbins, C. (1996). Drug induced psychosis. *British Journal of Psychiatry*, **168**, 135–8.
6. Withers, N.W., Pulvirenti, L., Koob, G.F., and Gillin, J.C. (1995). Cocaine abuse and dependence. *Journal of Clinical Psychopharmacology*, **15**, 63–78.
7. Nathan, K.I., Bresnick, W.H., and Batki, S.L. (1998). Cocaine abuse and dependence. Approaches to management. *CNS Drugs*, **10**, 43–59.
8. Hando, J., Flaherty, B., and Rutter, S. (1997). An Australian profile on the use of cocaine. *Addiction*, **92**, 173–82.
9. Seivewright, N. and Daly, C. (1997). Personality disorder and drug use: a review. *Drug and Alcohol Review*, **16**, 235–50.
10. Verheul, R., van den Brink, W., and Hartgers, C. (1995). Prevalence of personality disorders among alcoholics and drug addicts: an overview. *European Addiction Research*, **1**, 166–77.
11. Rawson, R.A., McCann, M.J., Hasson, A.J., and Ling, W. (1994). Cocaine abuse among methadone maintenance patients: are there effective treatment strategies? *Journal of Psychoactive Drugs*, **26**, 129–36.
12. Kosten, T.A., Gawin, F.H., Kosten, T.R., and Rounsaville, B.J. (1993). Gender differences in cocaine use and treatment response. *Journal of Substance Abuse Treatment*, **10**, 63–6.
13. Higgins, St., Budney, A.J., Bickel, W.K., and Badger, M.S. (1994). Participation of significant others in outpatient behavioural treatment predicts greater cocaine abstinence. *American Journal of Drug and Alcohol Abuse*, **20**, 47–56.
14. Galanter, M., Egelko, S., De Leon, G., Rohrs, C., and Franco, H. (1992). Crack cocaine abusers in the general hospital: assessment and initiation of care. *American Journal of Psychiatry*, **149**, 810–15.
15. Hulse, G.K., Milne, G., English, D.R., and Holman, C.D.J. (1997). Assessing the relationship between maternal cocaine use and abruptio placentae. *Addiction*, **92**, 1547–51.
16. Flaum, M. and Schultz, S.K. (1996). When does amphetamine-induced psychosis become schizophrenia? *American Journal of Psychiatry*, **153**, 812–15.
17. Levin, F.R. and Lehman, A.F. (1991). Meta-analysis of desipramine as an adjunct in the treatment of cocaine addiction. *Journal of Clinical Psychopharmacology*, **11**, 371–8.
18. Seivewright, N. (1999). Treatment of non-opiate misuse. In *Community treatment of drug misuse: more than methadone*, Chapter 4. Cambridge University Press.
19. Bradbeer, T.M., Fleming, P.M., Charlton, P., and Crichton, J.S. (1998). Survey of amphetamine prescribing in England and Wales. *Drug and Alcohol Review*, **17**, 299–304.
20. Fox, B.S. (1997). Development of a therapeutic vaccine for the treatment of cocaine addiction. *Drug and Alcohol Dependence*, **48**, 153–8.

4.2.3.4 Disorders relating to the use of phencyclidine and hallucinogens

Henry David Abraham

Phencyclidine

Introduction

Phencyclidine ('angel dust') is one of a class of arylcyclohexylamine dissociative anesthetics, along with ketamine (see Chapter 4.2.3.6). It was first abused in the United States in New York and San Francisco in the 1960s, but abuse declined when a broad range of unpredictable and adverse complications was noted.[1]

Epidemiology

While use of the unadulterated drug occurs, phencyclidine is more frequently mixed with LSD or cannabis. The drug may be ingested or injected, but more commonly it is smoked or snorted. Data suggest greater use in the United States than in Europe.[2] It traffics under a long and colourful list of street names, possibly reflecting the heterogeneity of its psychobiological effects. It has been suggested that any illicit smoked drug with an unrecognized street name (dust, mist, THC, embalming fluid, *inter alia*) should be considered phencyclidine until proven otherwise.

Acute physiological effects

The drug has a delayed onset of activity when taken orally. Unlike the major hallucinogens, phencyclidine requires doses in milligrams to be effective, a factor facilitating toxicological identification. When smoked, the onset of its main effects occurs immediately. The drug operates directly and indirectly at a number of receptor sites. The drug has particular affinity for the sigma opioid receptor, and noncompetitively blocks the *N*-methyl-D-aspartate-type excitatory amino acid receptor. Other effects appear to be mediated indirectly by catecholamine release, cholinergic stimulation, and serotonergic receptors.

DSM-IV lists as criteria for acute phencyclidine intoxication the following: acute onset of agitation, belligerence, impaired judgement, nystagmus, hyperacusis, hypertension, tachycardia, numbness, ataxia, dysarthria, rigidity, salivation, seizures, and coma. It is clear from this daunting inventory that impaired judgement is likely to be present beforehand in any person intentionally choosing to abuse this drug.

Adverse effects

Phencyclidine affects not only adults, but fetuses transplacentally and infants by transmission in breast milk. Undisclosed use by pregnant women is detectable in meconium.[3] Exposure to phencyclidine *in utero* is associated with reduced fetal growth, precipitous labours, and longer hospital stays.[4] Neurological consequences include poor attention, hypertonia, and depressed neonatal reflexes.[5] *In vitro* studies show that phencyclidine causes inhibited axon outgrowth, degeneration, and death in human fetal cerebral cortical neurones.[6]

Pathophysiological effects of phencyclidine toxicity in adults include hypertension, hyperthermia, opisthotonus, cardiac arrhythmia, seizure, and stroke. Phencyclidine is capable of provoking extreme muscular agitation. This condition of heightened muscular activity has been found to cause rhabdomyolysis and secondary renal failure in 2.5 per cent of users.[7] DSM-IV lists psychiatric effects of phencyclidine including intoxication, delirium, phencyclidine-induced psychotic, mood, and anxiety disorders, and phencyclidine abuse and dependence. A criterion for diagnosis is the emergence of the disorder within a month of drug use. While these disorders have been reported in anecdotes, a substantial clinical characterization exists for phencyclidine delirium and psychosis.

Phencyclidine delirium

Unlike acute intoxication with other hallucinogens, phencyclidine delirium is commonly associated with neurological disturbances. A continuum of effects is noted depending on dose.[8] Psychiatric symptoms occur early in drug use, with stupor and coma occurring later. Shortly after drug use, patients appear confused and ataxic. Analgesia in fingers and toes may be described. Phencyclidine can produce complex hallucinations resembling LSD intoxication. Differentiating the two drugs in emergencies is important, since high-potency neuroleptics, which are useful in phencyclidine toxicity, may exacerbate LSD, while the use of benzodiazepines, helpful in acute LSD toxicity, may disinhibit an assaultive phencyclidine patient. Unlike LSD, phencyclidine is readily identified in routine toxicological screening of blood and urine, but such data may not be readily available. One rapid bedside technique to differentiate the two drugs is the palm sign. The examiner asks the patient to describe the names of all the colours seen in the examiner's outstretch palm. A typical LSD patient reports with misplaced awe a vision of multiple colours and images. A phencyclidine patient simply attacks the hand. Dexterity on the part of the examiner is suggested. Unfocused aggression makes phencyclidine delirium a particularly dangerous disorder. The spectrum of violence includes both suicide and homicide.[9] The technique of 'talking down' acutely toxic patients is contraindicated. Environmental stimuli should be minimized, and the patient provided with protective supervision. The use of physical restraints is relatively contraindicated because of the potential for rhabdomyolysis.

Specific treatments involve intravenous naloxone to rule out narcotics overdose, activated charcoal to retard any further gastrointestinal absorption, and acidification of the patient's urine with vitamin C, ammonium chloride, cranberry juice, or all three in combination. Once the urine has been acidified, diuresis can be induced with frusemide (furosemide, Lasix). Antihypertensives may be indicated for uncontrolled blood pressure. For agitation high-potency neuroleptics or barbiturates are indicated. Phencyclidine has mixed agonist and antagonist effects at cholinergic receptors. Anticholinergic drugs may precipitate a synergistic reaction with phencyclidine, worsening delirium. Thus, low-potency neuroleptics, tricyclic antidepressants, and the anticholinergic antiparkinsonian drugs should be avoided.

Phencyclidine-induced psychotic disorder

Phencyclidine delirium may evolve into a chronic phencyclidine psychosis that is differentiated from schizophrenia only with difficulty. Alternatively, a phencyclidine delirium may clear, only to be replaced by the insidious onset of a post-phencyclidine psychotic disorder.

Because phencyclidine-induced psychosis incorporates both positive (e.g. hallucinations and paranoia) and negative (e.g. emotional withdrawal and motor retardation) schizophrenic symptoms, the drug has been considered a molecular model of the latter illness.[10]

Certain features of phencyclidine psychosis, namely neurological abnormalities, dose-related severity of symptoms, and regularity of the length of illness, are not noted with other psychedelic drugs, leading to the suggestion that phencyclidine psychosis is a toxic drug effect rather than a functional illness. Four classes of agents are reported to help phencyclidine psychosis. They are benzodiazepines, neuroleptics, acetylcholinesterase inhibitors, such as physostigmine, and catecholamine depleters, such as reserpine. Otherwise, treatment considerations are those for phencyclidine delirium. The long-term prognosis for this disorder appears to be poor, according to data from a 10-year follow-up of such patients.[11]

Phencyclidine abuse, dependence, and organic mental disorder

Rhesus monkeys will self-administer phencyclidine in a dose-dependent way,[12] suggesting that repeated abuse in humans may be associated with psychophysiological dependence. This in turn is likely to be associated with a decline in social and occupational function characteristic of other forms of addiction. Because of its widespread neuropsychological effects, any intentional, informed use of phencyclidine should be considered maladaptive. For the habituated patient, long-term treatment is indicated. Issues that should be addressed in the process are emotional lability, cognitive defects, depression, and possible phencyclidine withdrawal effects.

Many of the treatments applicable to patients addicted to the opiates, alcohol, and cocaine apply to this population. Several aspects of treating the phencyclidine patient depart from the more conventional addiction treatments. A triad of confusion, decreased cognitive function, and assaultiveness mark an organic mental disorder associated with phencyclidine use. Reduced cognition is a barrier to recovery that must be recognized and addressed in any prospective treatment plan. Neuropsychological assessment is helpful in this regard. Secondly, there is good evidence that phencyclidine is sequestered in fat for extended periods of time.[13] Conditions associated with weight loss are likely to release long-held phencyclidine into the blood and brain.

Hallucinogens

Introduction

Agents that alter perception and mood without disorientation typify hallucinogenic drugs. They have been known and used for millennia for purposes ranging from magical to medical. Anthropologists trace back the earliest use of hallucinogens to palaeolithic Europe, although 80 per cent of extant hallucinogenic plants are to be found in the New World. Galen (AD 130–200) wrote that it was customary to give dinner guests hemp seeds to promote the evening's proceedings. The ergot-bearing fungus *Claviceps purpurea* infected rye in tenth-century France and claimed 40 000 lives. Despite such calamities, ergot continued to be used by midwives in medieval Europe. In search of a benign ergot derivative for use in childbirth, Albert Hofmann synthesized lysergic acid diethylamide (LSD-25) in 1938.

Five years later he accidentally ingested a trace amount of the drug,

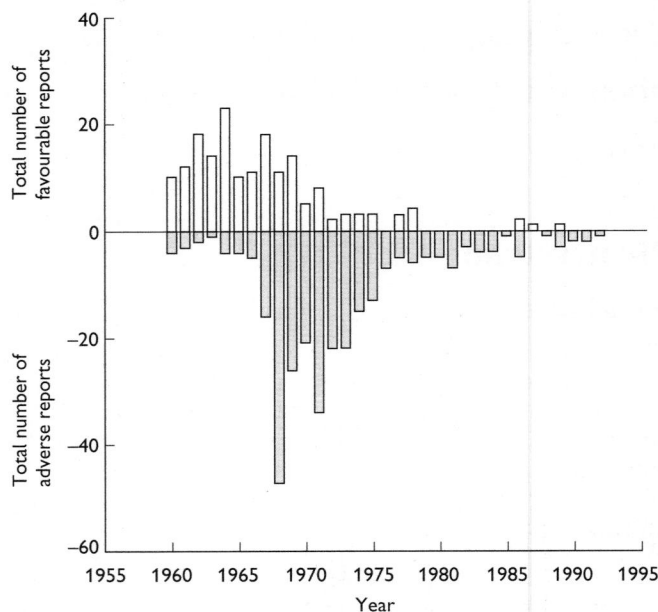

Fig. 1 Scientific problems on LSD in *Index Medicus* between 1960 and 1994. Each human study on LSD was assigned a score of +1 for favourable findings (upward open bars) and –1 for adverse findings (downward shaded bars) when scoring was possible. The curve is measuring not a chemotherapeutic index of the benefits and risks of LSD, but a research trend reflecting a strong cohort-period effect of scientific activity.

and fell into an intoxicated, dream-like reverie in which an uninterrupted stream of imagery flowed before his closed eyes. Three days later he intentionally ingested 250 µg of LSD in an attempt to take notes of his experience. Forty minutes after ingestion he wrote in his laboratory journal, 'Beginning dizziness, feeling of anxiety, visual distortions, symptoms of paralysis, desire to laugh…'. From that point Hofmann's journal is blank. Later he would recall visions and notions that he believed were heralding his insanity.

In 1947 Stoll in Switzerland published the first experimental use of LSD in psychiatry, soon to be followed by Sandison and Elkes in England, Cohen and Eisner in the United States, Leuner in Germany, and Grof in Czechoslovakia. Within a decade the drug moved from scientists to clinicians, clergy, curious professors, and a widening number of students on both sides of the Atlantic. Military investigators in the United States gave the drug surreptitiously to recruits. By the late 1960s LSD and cannabis led the way to a pandemic of drug abuse, particularly among the young. Figure 1 illustrates positive and negative scientific reports regarding LSD from 1960 to 1995. For the majority of the 1960s, LSD earned a positive reputation as a tool for the study and treatment of psychiatric illnesses. From 1968 onward, adverse reports outnumbered positive ones, thus illustrating an axiom that is revisited multiple times throughout history, that new discoveries are often met with inflated enthusiasm, only to be tempered in time by sober reconsideration. The reconsideration of LSD was based on the fact that with the synthesis of high-potency hallucinogenic drugs such as the substituted indole and alkyl amines, a line was crossed separating botanical forms of hallucinogens from those derived solely in the laboratory. The former exist in nature in low concentrations amidst innumerable psychoactive congeners, while laboratory preparations are available in high concentrations and purity. This factor, along with their psychoactive potency in microgram quantities, coupled with the ease with which this class of drugs can be synthesized, transported, and sold, accounts for their enduring role as abusable substances.

Drug preparations

While Hofmann describes 11 classes of hallucinogenic compounds which can be isolated from botanicals, by far the most common hallucinogen of abuse appears to be LSD.[14] Recently the serotonin-2A receptor has been shown to bind strongly to hallucinogenic drugs, and the drugs appear to act as partial agonists.[15] LSD is psychoactive in a single droplet of solvent. The drug is easily dissolved in an aqueous solution. Drops of the drug are placed on sugar cubes or blotting paper stamped with coloured cartoon figures to mark the drug's location. Sheets of the paper are then distributed, and the figures ingested. Injection is not necessary, and seldom used as a means of administration. Dosages commonly range from 25 to 100 µg. A hallucinogenic trip can occur after 75 µg. Other hallucinogens, such as dimethyltryptamine, must be injected. Common botanical hallucinogens include fungi and angiosperms (flower-bearing plants), of which approximately 100 are recognized to possess hallucinogenic properties. Ibogaine is derived from the root of the *Tabernanthe iboga* plant cultivated in Gabon and eaten as a rite of passage. Mescaline (trimethoxyphenylethylamine) is a predominant hallucinogen in the cactus *Lophophora williamsii* of the American Southwest. Strips of cactus are cut from the plant, dried, and eaten. Hallucinogenic mushrooms contain psilocybin and psilocin, which are phosphorylated hydroxylated congeners of dimethyltryptamine. Mushrooms are ingested for their effect, or brewed first and the broth consumed. Not all consumers respond identically. The American psychologist William James reported ingesting several dozen hallucinogenic mushrooms and only experiencing headache. Shulgin has synthesized and tested 179 phenylethylamines for hallucinogenic properties. Their effects on the human brain are complex and largely unknown.

Epidemiology

Recent surveys in the United States and Europe indicate that hallucinogen use is increasing. Johnson *et al.*,[2] for example, reported that the trend for the lifetime prevalence of LSD use among American high school seniors rose from 7.7 to 13.6 per cent from 1988 to 1997. Similarly, a German sample of 3021 adolescents found a twofold increase in LSD and substituted amphetamines from 1990 to 1995.[16] From 1990 to 1992 in East Germany there was a ninefold increase in LSD use, compared to a fivefold increase in all other illegal drugs. In the United Kingdom LSD use increased from 7 per cent in 1989 to 11 per cent in 1993. In Denmark 7.2 per cent of students surveyed reported using hallucinogenic mushrooms in 1993. In surveys of American undergraduates, an 18.4 per cent prevalence of mushroom experimentation was found in the years 1993 to 1994. LSD users tend to start in adolescence, and because this class of drugs lacks the addiction potential of alcohol, cocaine, or opiates, hallucinogen use typically declines in the mid-twenties.

Acute effects

Albert Hofmann, who drew international attention to an accidental ingestion of the drug, classically describes the effects of ingesting LSD.[17] The characteristic LSD trip comprises autonomic arousal, marked mydriasis, and progressive modulations of sensory, more often visual, imagery, which appear to be generated both from external objects and distortions of eidetic imagery. Ordinarily benign objects may take on new emotional meanings. Geometric imagery may rise and fall before one's eyes. A prevalent feeling one experiences is a sense of helplessness to control one's streaming images and emotions, hence the hippie advice of 'going with the flow'. The loss of cognitive, perceptual, and affective control for some users leads to panic, which in turn results in the so-called 'bad trip.' As these effects decline, they may be replaced with a sense of oceanic well being or residual paranoia.

Adverse effects

Adverse reactions to hallucinogens include panic reactions associated with a bad trip, hallucinogen persisting perception disorder, and prolonged psychoses.

Panic reaction

Panic may arise during the acute drug experience. It is characterized by a crescendo of rising anxiety accompanied by autonomic arousal in the context of streaming emotions and imagery. Mydriasis is greater than that seen in non-drug-induced panic. While lay interventionists have encouraged treatment of such panic by 'talking the victim down', the use of an oral benzodiazepine such as diazepam 20 mg is utterly effective in stopping the panic, and bad trip, within an equal number of minutes. The utter efficacy of this class of drugs in aborting a hallucinogenic trip in minutes is strong evidence that the γ-aminobutyric acid-A receptor plays a role in modulating the effects of hallucinogens.

Hallucinogen persisting perception disorder

It became apparent within the first few years of experimentation with LSD that this class of drugs was capable of inducing visual disturbances days to weeks following drug exposure. Subsequent research found that these disturbances, dubbed 'flashbacks' because of their evanescent visual appearance, appeared to be an intermittent form of postdrug visual disorder that in its extreme form was experienced continually. Thus, hallucinogen persisting perception disorder patients are capable of describing a range of visual disturbances that fluctuate in intensity, but are observable from moment to moment. Such imagery includes geometric hallucinations, false perceptions of movement, usually in the peripheral visual field, afterimagery, and the perception of trails of images as an object moves across the visual field. Patients can also visualize myriad clear or coloured pinpoint dots in a bright sky, an experience that they describe as seeing the air ('aeropsia'). These visual disturbances may be intensified by emergence into a dark environment, or by experiencing a variety of psychostimulants such as marijuana, amphetamines, cocaine, anxiety, and the stress of intercurrent illnesses.[18] While recovery may occur over months and years following last drug use, approximately half of the patients so afflicted appear to develop a permanent alteration of the visual apparatus. Neurophysiological studies confirm cerebral disinhibition involving those regions of the cortex processing visual information.[19]

It has been hypothesized that this disorder occurs when a potent hallucinogen such as LSD excitotoxically stimulates and destroys serotonin-2A receptor bearing inhibitory neurones, leading to a chronic disinhibition of visual information processing. That such a response occurs in only a minority of users, while others may apparently use such drugs with impunity, suggests that the disorder may be mediated by a genetic vulnerability to the drug.

Because the disorder is exacerbated by psychological and physiological conditions of arousal, benzodiazepines have been used for management of visual symptoms. The results of these efforts are palliative at best, and complicated by the prospect of treating a drug abuser with an abusable substance. Recent case reports of treatment with sertraline, naltrexone, and clonidine are encouraging.

In addition to pharmacotherapy, hallucinogen persisting perception disorder patients often require supportive psychotherapy to deal with the issues of learning to cope with what may be a permanent alteration in perception. Therapy is also indicated to educate the patient, and prevent the development of common comorbid disorders in hallucinogen persisting perception disorder, namely, major depression, panic disorder, and alcohol dependence.

Psychosis

The suggestion that the use of potent hallucinogens can trigger prolonged psychotic episodes is controversial. Evidence supporting the existence of hallucinogen-induced psychotic disorders is found in a review of longitudinal, cross-sectional, and case studies.[20] Psychiatric patienthood appears to be a risk factor for the development of psychosis following LSD. The clinical picture of post-LSD psychosis resembles schizoaffective disorder more than it does schizophrenia, with the commonly added feature of chronic visual disturbances. Clinically such patients resemble those with good-prognosis schizophrenia, since they possess more affect than those with poor prognosis, have less thought disorder, are more socially related, and appear to have fewer signs of negative schizophrenia. Mystical preoccupations reminiscent of acute drug experiences can predominate. Visual hallucinations often are of the variety that are seen in hallucinogen persisting perception disorder, although in contradistinction to such patients, post-hallucinogen psychotic patients may describe delusions and auditory hallucinations as well.

Atypical pharmacotherapies appear to have an important role in treatment, and in selected cases are preferable to dopamine-blocking neuroleptics. Reports in the literature describe cases responding to electroconvulsive therapy, lithium, anticonvulsants, and the serotonin precursor, l-5-hydroxytryptophan. Long-term supportive psychotherapy is almost always indicated to help the patient and his or her family make painful adjustments to the patient's chronic disappointments in relationships and employment, frequently made all the more poignant by the illness' propensity to preserve the patient's insight as it progresses. This last factor may partially explain the high risk for suicide.[21] No definitive clinical characterization of the disorder exists as yet.

Further reading

Abraham, H.D. (1983). Visual phenomenology of the LSD flashback. *Archives of General Psychiatry*, **40**, 884–9.

Abraham, H.D., Aldridge, A.M., and Gogia, P. (1996). The psychopharmacology of hallucinogens. *Neuropsychopharmacology*, **14**, 285–98.

Hofmann, A. (1980). *LSD: my problem child*. McGraw-Hill, New York.

Johnson, L.D., O'Malley, P.M., and Bachman, J.G. (1998). *National survey results on drug use from the monitoring the future study, 1975–1997*, Vol.

1. Publication No. 98–4345. National Institutes of Health, Rockville, MD.

McCarron, M.M., Schulze, B.W., Thompson, G.A., Conder, M.C., and Goetz, W.A. (1981). Acute phencyclidine intoxication: incidence of clinical findings in 1000 cases. *Annals of Emergency Medicine*, **10**, 237–42.

References

1. McCarron, M.M., Schulze, B.W., Thompson, G.A., Conder, M.C., and Goetz, W.A. (1981). Acute phencyclidine intoxication: incidence of clinical findings in 1000 cases. *Annals of Emergency Medicine*, **10**, 237–42.

2. Johnson, L.D., O'Malley, P.M., and Bachman, J.G. (1998). *National survey results on drug use from the monitoring the future study, 1975–1997*, Vol. 1. Publication No. 98–4345. National Institutes of Health, Rockville, MD.

3. Moore, C., Negrusz, A., and Lewis, D. (1998). Determination of drugs of abuse in meconium. *Journal of Chromatography B: Biomedical and Science Applications*, **713**, 137–46.

4. Tabor, B.L., Smith-Wallace, T., and Yonekura, M.L. (1990). Perinatal outcome associated with PCP versus cocaine use. *American Journal of Drug and Alcohol Abuse*, **16**, 337–48.

5. Golden, N.L., Kuhnert, B.R., Sokol, R.J., Martier, S., and Williams, T. (1987). Neonatal manifestations of maternal phencyclidine exposure. *Journal of Perinatal Medicine*, **15**, 185–91.

6. Mattson, M.P., Rychlik, B., and Cheng, B. (1992). Degenerative and axon outgrowth-altering effects of phencyclidine in human fetal cerebral cortical cells. *Neuropharmacology*, **31**, 279–91.

7. Akmal, M., Valdin, J.R., McCarron, M.M., and Massry, S.G. (1981). Rhabdomyolysis with and without acute renal failure in patients with phencyclidine intoxication. *American Journal of Nephrology*, **1**, 91–6.

8. Milhorn, H.T.J. (1991). Diagnosis and management of phencyclidine intoxication. *American Family Physician*, **43**, 1290–302.

9. Poklis, A., Graham, M., Maginn, D., Branch, C.A., and Gantner, G.E. (1990). Phencyclidine and violent deaths in St. Louis, Missouri: a survey of medical examiners' cases from 1977 through 1986. *American Journal of Drug and Alcohol Abuse*, **16**, 265–74.

10. Javitt, D.C. and Zukin, S.R. (1991). Recent advances in the phencyclidine model of schizophrenia. *American Journal of Psychiatry*, **148**, 1301–8.

11. Wright, H.H., Cole, E.A., Batey, S.R., and Hanna, K. (1988). Phencyclidine-induced psychosis: eight-year follow-up of ten cases. *Southern Medical Journal*, **81**, 565–7.

12. Campbell, U.C., Thompson, S.S., and Carroll, M.E. (1998). Acquisition of oral phencyclidine (PCP) self-administration in rhesus monkeys: effects of dose and an alternative non-drug reinforcer. *Psychopharmacology (Berlin)*, **137**, 132–8.

13. Misra, A.L., Pontani, R.B., and Bartolomeo, J. (1979). Persistence of phencyclidine (PCP) and metabolites in brain and adipose tissue and implications for long-lasting behavioural effects. *Research Communications in Chemistry, Pathology, and Pharmacology*, **24**, 431–45.

14. Schultes, R. and Hofmann, A. (1980). *The botany and chemistry of hallucinogens*. Thomas, Springfield, IL.

15. Glennon, R.A., Titeler, M., and McKenney, J.D. (1984). Evidence for 5-HT2 involvement in the mechanism of action of hallucinogenic agents. *Life Sciences*, **35**, 2505–11.

16. Schuster, P., Lieb, R., Lamertz, C., and Wittchen, H.U. (1998). Is the use of ecstasy and hallucinogens increasing? Results from a community study. *European Addiction Research*, **4**, 75–82.

17. Hofmann, A. (1980). *LSD: my problem child*. McGraw-Hill, New York.

18. Abraham, H.D. (1983). Visual phenomenology of the LSD flashback. *Archives of General Psychiatry*, **40**, 884–9.

19. Abraham, H.D. and Duffy, F.H. (1996). Stable quantitative EEG difference in post-LSD visual disorder by split-half analysis: evidence for disinhibition. *Psychiatry Research and Neuroimaging*, **67**, 173–87.

20. Abraham, H.D., Aldridge, A.M., and Gogia, P. (1996). The psychopharmacology of hallucinogens. *Neuropsychopharmacology*, **14**, 285–98.

21. Bowers, M.B., Jr (1977). Psychoses precipitated by psychotomimetic drugs: a follow up study. *Archives of General Psychiatry*, **34**, 832–5.

4.2.3.5 Misuse of benzodiazepines

Michael Farrell and Sarah Welch

Epidemiology and patterns of use

The rise in benzodiazepine prescribing in the United Kingdom in the 1960s and 1970s was a development that followed the previous period of prescribing of barbiturates and other sedatives. Concerns about the obvious toxicity of barbiturates, and previously other sedatives, in overdose, together with knowledge of their dependence-inducing characteristics, led to their replacement with the safer benzodiazepines as the commonly prescribed anxiolytic and hypnotic drugs. Case reports of patients who escalated their dose of benzodiazepines above the recommended dose, and who experienced convulsions and confusional states on stopping them, began to appear in the 1970s.[1,2] In the mid-1970s and onward, regulatory bodies in the United Kingdom and United States began to recognize the abuse potential of benzodiazepines even in therapeutic doses. Dependence on benzodiazepines was well described in the early literature on the development of these drugs but surprisingly clinical dependence was not reported in the medical literature until the early 1980s.[3,4] Dependence on therapeutic doses of prescribed benzodiazepines is covered in Chapter 6.2.2. In this chapter we are concerned with abuse of and dependence on high doses of benzodiazepines.

The upsurge in the drug epidemic in the 1980s was associated with an increase in misuse of hypnosedatives, and in the late 1980s there was a series of reports on the intravenous use of benzodiazepines, in particular temazepam.[5,6] Because benzodiazepines are the most commonly prescribed anxiolytics and hypnotics it is not surprising to find that they are also reported to be commonly misused. However, patterns of misuse vary, from episodic use of non-prescribed medication with up to 15 per cent of young people reporting some experience with benzodiazepines, to continuous high-dose use. Since the mid-1980s there has been a substantial drop in the prescription of benzodiazepines as anxiolytic agents but use as hypnotics has remained relatively steady with the concentration of long-term use being in the elderly population. Changes in prescribing practices are likely to influence diversion of benzodiazepines to the illicit market.

Reports indicate that supra-therapeutic dose misuse and dependence is strongly associated with polydrug and alcohol abuse and dependence.[7,8] This pattern of benzodiazepine misuse and dependence is probably much less common than iatrogenic benzodiazepine dependence. However, it presents a substantial problem to many clinicians in primary care and specialist settings. In particular, high-dose misuse is likely to be associated with 'doctor shopping' and efforts to extract additional medication on top of that already prescribed. The high doses used present a particular risk because they are often used in combination with other substances such as alcohol, opiates, and stimulants. High doses use may be intermittent in nature (in a 'binge'

pattern), and not associated with dependence (in which case the initiation of a prescription may change a pattern of intermittent binge use to daily dependent use in a manner that entrenches polydrug use; see the section below on guidelines for management). Drug misusers use benzodiazepines in a non-dependent fashion for a variety of reasons. For example, benzodiazepines may be used to enhance the effects of other drugs (such as boosting the euphoria with heroin), or to alleviate unwanted effects from other drugs (to 'cushion' the 'come-down' from cocaine), or to help alleviate withdrawal symptoms when drugs such as heroin are unobtainable, or in attempts at self-detoxification from other drugs. Misuse of benzodiazepines may also arise from injudicious patterns of prescribing for the treatment of alcohol dependence, or from attempts at self-treatment for alcohol dependence. Some drug misusers will also develop a dependent pattern of use of benzodiazepines in their own right. Benzodiazepine dependence may be a factor contributing to poor outcome for patients who are attempting opiate detoxification.

High-dose use is associated with substantial tolerance to the sedating effects of the medication but some of the other effects may not be equivalently protected by tolerance. Thus, some individuals may consume extraordinary high doses, and not appear sedated, but experience profound amnesia for their actions. Such effects of amnesia may also be associated with the reported high rates of risk-taking behaviour, and amnesia may be more pronounced in injecting benzodiazepine users, although there are no good data to confirm this.

The potential of different benzodiazepines for misuse and dependence

In view of the frequency of prescribing of benzodiazepine drugs, it is an important question as to whether some benzodiazepines are more likely to be misused, or to lead to dependence, than others. The similarities between different benzodiazepines are much greater than the differences. Patients may maintain that they need a specific named benzodiazepine, but there is marked cross-tolerance, and patients changed to an equivalent dose of a different benzodiazepine under double-blind conditions show almost complete cross-dependence (i.e. no difference in withdrawal symptoms from those whose medication has been unchanged).[9] However, this cross-dependence was shown for patients who were already benzodiazepine dependent. It is possible that the properties of certain benzodiazepines lead to a stronger motivation for people to desire their effects, to escalate the dose, and to persist with their use.

Factors that have been considered to influence the liability to misuse and development of dependence include the relative potency of the drug, and its elimination half-life.[10] Triazolam, a very short-acting benzodiazepine prescribed for insomnia, was withdrawn from the British market following concerns about the severity of rebound anxiety experienced even after a single dose. Triazolam is a very potent benzodiazepine that binds very readily to benzodiazepine receptors, and experience with its use suggested that it had a more euphoriant effect than other benzodiazepines, resulting in greater potential for misuse and for the development of dependence. Other benzodiazepines that have high potency and have caused concern include flunitrazepam and lorazepam. Flunitrazepam is relatively rarely prescribed in the United Kingdom, but frequently reported as one of the most common benzodiazepines misused in many European countries and in Australia. It is not marketed in the United States. Concerns about its availability on the illicit market continue.[11,12] It has attracted media attention as a drug used to facilitate 'date rape'; it is unclear why this particular benzodiazepine should have this image, although it is a potent drug. Lorazepam, also a potent benzodiazepine, is much more widely prescribed in the United Kingdom, and alprazolam is used in the United States. Some studies suggest that lorazepam and alprazolam may be associated with an earlier and more difficult withdrawal process than diazepam.[9,13] In one European study, triazolam and lorazepam were found to feature more highly among individuals dependent on high doses of benzodiazepine drugs than among those dependent on low or 'therapeutic' doses.[14] In summary, it appears that potency is a contributory factor in the abuse and dependence-inducing potential of benzodiazepine drugs. However, this picture is somewhat complicated by the fact that drugs such as lorazepam tend to have been marketed at higher equivalent doses than some other benzodiazepines. The elimination half-life influences the nature of withdrawal; if it is short, withdrawal symptoms appear more rapidly and may appear more severe, although withdrawal of more insidious onset in longer-acting benzodiazepines may be just as problematic.

As well as properties of the drugs themselves, the abuse potential of different benzodiazepines is also associated with broader prescribing patterns which affect the potential for diversion to illicit market. Diazepam and temazepam have been the most widely prescribed benzodiazepines in the United Kingdom, and are therefore the most likely to be encountered by drug misusers and problem drinkers. Drugs such as clonazepam which tend to be prescribed much less widely, and generally for epilepsy rather than for anxiety or insomnia, seem infrequently to raise concerns about misuse.[10] In other parts of Europe where flunitrazepam is more commonly prescribed, there are reports of its high levels of abuse among the illicit drug-using population.

The potential for misuse by injecting

Drugs such as temazepam and flunitrazepam are more frequently reported to be injected.[7] There are a number of factors that may influence this. These include the availability of the drug, its short-acting nature, and also the formulation of the drug. In the 1980s temazepam was marketed as a liquid-filled capsule, which enabled easy extraction of the contents to put into a syringe for injecting. The later gel formulation was also injected, by heating to liquidize the gel, resulting in very damaging injecting complications. Some medications that come in easily soluble form can also be converted into a form for injecting, such as liquid diazepam.

The injection of benzodiazepine drugs is associated with substantially more harmful drug misuse in a number of respects,[15] with increased rates of reported sharing of injecting equipment,[9,16] increased risks of overdose, and poorer general health.[8]

Benzodiazepine dependence and alcohol dependence: the overlap

There are high reported rates of alcohol dependence among the homeless, and there are substantial reports of benzodiazepine abuse and dependence in this population also. Cross-tolerance between benzodiazepines and alcohol permits individuals who are alcohol dependent to tolerate high doses of benzodiazepines. Patients may be prescribed benzodiazepines to manage alcohol withdrawal, but injudicious prescribing that is not targeted towards the management of alcohol withdrawal symptoms may result in iatrogenic benzodiazepine dependence.

The extensive research on pharmacological interventions for management of alcohol withdrawal in alcohol-dependent patients has been examined in a meta-analysis by Mayo-Smith, who subsequently produced a systematic review with treatment guidelines.[17] This review supports the use of benzodiazepines as the treatment of choice for managing withdrawal symptoms for patients whose symptoms are of sufficient severity to warrant medication. Alternative agents used in withdrawal, such as chlormethiazole and the barbiturate phenobarbital, are less well-supported by controlled trials than benzodiazepines, and carry higher risks of adverse effects.

The potential for misuse of benzodiazepines must be considered in alcohol-dependent patients. However, this is not an adequate reason for avoiding the use of benzodiazepines in the management of withdrawal in view of their superiority in effectiveness, and possibly in potential for harmful misuse, over other treatments. Benzodiazepines with a slower onset of action, such as chlordiazepoxide, appear to have less potential for misuse. The prolonged use of benzodiazepines in withdrawal is rarely necessary or helpful, and evidence for benefits of 'substitute prescribing' of benzodiazepines for alcohol users in the longer term is lacking. Use of benzodiazepines to manage phobic and anxiety disorders associated with alcohol dependence should be strenuously avoided.

Guidelines for management of misuse of non-prescribed benzodiazepines

So far, no clear guidelines have been produced for management of this problem. These are a complex group of patients to manage and in general such patients should be referred for specialist assessment.

Assessment

Assessment should attempt to confirm evidence for benzodiazepine dependence. Assessment over a number of visits should involve obtaining urine specimens to determine objectively the regularity (or intermittent nature) of benzodiazepine consumption. Part of the initial assessment process should identify underlying psychiatric disorders that may have been the trigger for a doctor initiating a prescription or for the patient obtaining drugs for the purpose of self-medication. High levels of psychiatric morbidity have been found among samples of patients with severe benzodiazepine dependence.[18] The commonest conditions are probably anxiety disorders for which anxiolytics have been prescribed injudiciously; however, in some instances major depressive disorders may be treated or self-medicated with benzodiazepines. Thorough assessment should explore for evidence of major depression and if identified, consideration should be given to the use of antidepressant medication combined with cognitive-behavioural therapy.

Treatment

In the presence of polydrug abuse or dependence, caution needs to be exercised about initiating a prescription for benzodiazepines. Where dependence is established, dose titration should aim to ameliorate withdrawal symptoms rather than to match the large doses of medication that the patient reports consuming. Long-acting benzodiazepines such as diazepam are preferred (Chapter 6.2.2), and doses should rarely exceed 40 to 60 mg daily. Where large doses are prescribed these should ideally be dispensed on a daily pick-up basis from the community pharmacist. The prescribing doctor should avoid succumbing to pressure from the patient to increase the dose without a thorough dose assessment and evidence of withdrawal symptoms. Prescriptions issued on a routine 'repeat' basis should be avoided, and the patient should be informed that lost medication will not be replaced. Requests for replacement medication or additional medication should encourage the doctor to review the overall care plan and to consider stopping the benzodiazepine prescription. Virtually all benzodiazepine prescriptions should be time limited and part of a detoxification plan with gradual reduction over a clearly stated and negotiated time period. Alternatively, inpatient detoxification, perhaps with longer admissions, may be the best course of action where reduction regimens fail in the community setting. Reduction regimens with benzodiazepines are very variable and many clinicians opt for a very gradual withdrawal with small dose reduction at wide intervals. There is no evidence to indicate that such a gradual approach is any more effective than 20 to 25 per cent reductions over a shorter more clearly defined time (such as 6 weeks).

Currently there is no evidence base for long maintenance prescribing of benzodiazepines for those who are high-dose injecting polydrug abusers. However, this intervention has not been subject to any structured evaluation and merits further study in the face of the difficulties of managing such patients.

Conclusion

There is a valuable role for benzodiazepines, and a need for vigilance and care in their use, as well as active recognition and management of those who are dependent. However, there is a need for greater awareness of the risks of polydrug dependence with misuse of high doses of benzodiazepines in conjunction with both alcohol dependence and opiate dependence. Caution needs to be used in assessing patients, and benzodiazepine prescribing should be restricted to those where there is clear evidence of dependence.

The risk of synergistic effects with other drugs and consequent overdose should be explained to all patients who are identified as being involved in such behaviour. Community detoxification or inpatient detoxification is the best option based on the evidence of available research and evaluation of current interventions.

References

1. Woody, G.E., O'Brien, C.P., and Greenstein, R. (1975). Misuse and abuse of diazepam: an increasingly common medical problem. *International Journal of Addiction*, **10**, 843–8.
2. Bliding, A. (1978). The abuse potential of benzodiazepines with special reference to oxazepam. *Acta Psychiatrica Scandinavia Supplementum*, **274**, 111–16.
3. Petursson, H. and Lader, M.H. (1981). Benzodiazepine dependence. *British Journal of Addiction*, **76**, 133–45.
4. Hallstrom, C. and Lader, M. (1981). Benzodiazepine withdrawal phenomena. *International Pharmacopsychiatry*, **16**, 235–44.
5. Farrell, M. and Strang, J. (1988). Misuse of temazepam. *British Medical Journal*, **297**, 1402.
6. Ruben, S.M. and Morrison, C.L. (1992). Temazepam misuse in a group of injecting drug users. *British Journal of Addiction*, **87**, 1387–92.
7. Strang, J., Seivewright, N., and Farrell, M. (1992). Intravenous and other novel abuses of benzodiazepines: the opening of Pandora's box? *British Journal of Addiction*, **87**, 1373–5.
8. Ross, J., Darke, S., and Hall, W. (1997). Transitions between routes of benzodiazepine administration among heroin users in Sydney. *Addiction*, **92**, 697–705.
9. Murphy, S.M. and Tyrer, P. (1991). A double-blind comparison of the effects of gradual withdrawal of lorazepam, diazepam and bromazepam in benzodiazepine dependence. *British Journal of Psychiatry*, **158**, 511–16.
10. Tyrer, P. (1993). Pharmacological differences in the dependence potential of benzodiazepines. In *Benzodiazepine dependence* (ed. C. Hallstrom), pp. 77–90. Oxford University Press.
11. Simmons, M.M. and Cupp, M.J. (1998). Use and abuse of flunitrazepam. *Annals of Pharmacotherapy*, **32**, 117–19.
12. Woods, J.H. and Winger, G. (1997). Abuse liability of flunitrazepam. *Journal of Clinical Psychopharmacology*, **17** (Supplement 2), 1S–57S.
13. Rickels, K., Case, W.G., Schweizer, E.E., *et al.* (1986). Low dose dependence in chronic benzodiazepine users; a preliminary report on 119 patients. *Psychopharmacology Bulletin*, **22**, 415–17.
14. Martinez-Cano, H., Vela-Bueno, A., De Iceta, M. *et al.* (1996). Benzodiazepine types in high versus therapeutic dose dependence. *Addiction*, **91**, 1179–86.
15. Darke, S., Hall, W., Ross, M., and Wodak, A. (1992). Benzodiazepine use and HIV risk-taking behaviour among injecting drug users. *Drug and Alcohol Dependence*, **31**, 31–6.
16. Klee, H., Faugier, J., Hayes, C., Boulton, T., and Morris, J. (1990). AIDS-related risk behaviour, polydrug use and temazepam. *British Journal of Addiction*, **85**, 1125–32.
17. Mayo-Smith, M.F. (1997). Pharmacological management of alcohol withdrawal: a meta-analysis and evidence-based practice guideline. *Journal of the American Medical Association*, **278**, 144–50.
18. Busto, U.E., Romach, M.K., and Sellers, E.M. (1996). Multiple drug use and psychiatric comorbidity in patients admitted to the hospital with severe benzodiazepine dependence. *Journal of Clinical Psychopharmacology*, **16**, 51–7.

4.2.3.6 Disorders relating to the use of ecstasy, other 'party drugs', and khat

Adam R. Winstock

Introduction

'Ecstasy' (**MDMA**, 3,4-methylenedioxymethamphetamine) is a ring-substituted amphetamine derivative that has become increasingly popular since it first became associated with the 'rave' music scene during the late 1980s.[1] Incorrectly termed a designer drug, MDMA was first synthesized in 1912 by the Merck Pharmaceuticals as a product of ongoing research, although it never reached the commercial market. It was relatively ignored until the 1950s when United States Army experiments investigated its potential to assist espionage during the Cold War, and it was not until the late 1960s and early 1970s that drug users on the west coast of America began to popularize its recreational use. Although ecstasy is the drug most frequently associated with the term 'party drug' most users of MDMA are polysubstance abusers with experience of cannabis, LSD, amphetamine, amyl nitrate, and cocaine. This chapter is concerned with ecstasy, ketamine, γ-hydroxybutyrate (GHB), khat, and tryptamine derivatives.

Ecstasy (3,4-methylenedioxy-methamphetamine)

Preparation

Unlike most illicit substances of abuse, MDMA is sold in either tablet or capsule form (very occasionally as powder), the composition of which can never be certain. Indeed only half of all tablets sold as ecstasy in the United Kingdom actually contain MDMA, with the rest being either analogues of MDMA, such as methylenedioxyamphetamine (**MDEA**), N-methyl-1-(1,3-benzodioxol-5-yl)-2-butanamine (**MBDB**), and methylenedioxyethylamphetamine (**MDEA**), or combinations of stimulants such as ephedrine or amphetamine and hallucinogens such as LSD or ketamine.[2] The average dose of an ecstasy tablet containing MDMA is about 70 mg (range 50–150 mg).

Mechanism of action

MDMA ingestion leads to an acute increase in central serotonergic effects by causing the calcium-dependent release of serotonin from nerve terminals. To a lesser extent there is also dopamine reuptake blockade. MDMA also results in a rapid inhibition of tryptophan hyrdroxylase, the rate-limiting enzyme in serotonin synthesis, although the mechanism of inactivation in uncertain. This is followed by acute depletion of central serotonin levels which may contribute to the fall in mood that some users notice after use.

Absorption and metabolism

Taken orally the onset of action begins after 30 to 60 min, peaks at between 90 and 120 min with significant effects persisting for a further 3 to 6 h followed by a gradual 'come down' over the subsequent 6 to 12 h. The drug is primarily metabolized by demethylation by the hepatic cytochrome P-450 enzyme, debrisoquine hydroxylase coded for by CYP 2D6.[3] Two phenotypes predominate in the population with 9 per cent being 'poor metabolizers'. The consequence of metabolizer status on patterns of use and toxicity is as yet unknown. The drug may also be taken intranasally (snorted), rectally, and (rarely) intravenously.

Clinical features

Being structurally related to both amphetamine and mescaline,[4] MDMA possesses both stimulant and hallucinogenic properties and is said to 'evoke an easily controlled altered state of consciousness with emotional and sensual overtones'[5] which allows it to be discriminated from other related substances. Some have suggested a new term for this group of drugs 'empathogens' and suggest that the substance's

Table 1 Psychological effects associated with MDMA

Increased empathy and emotional expressiveness
Reduced ability and desire to perform mental tasks
Increased anxiety and restlessness
Increased energy, euphoria with periodic 'rushing' (periodic surges in euphoria)
Reduced defensiveness and decreased aggression
Disinhibition and increased awareness of emotions
Perceptual distortion and hallucinations at higher doses

Adapted from Liester *et al.*[8]

appeal rests in its 'dramatic and consistent ability to induce in the user a profound feeling of attachment and connection'[6] which would be in keeping with its popularity as a social drug within the club scene. It was also these qualities that led to the enthusiasm of a small number of physicians and therapists in the United States who held that it could enhance the therapeutic process.[7] Indeed, it is reported that the Los Angeles dealer who coined the street name 'ecstasy' for MDMA would have preferred the name 'empathy' but he did not feel that his clients would know what it meant.

Psychological effects

As with any psychotropic drug the effects of the drug on a given individual at a particular time are not predictable, depending as it does on the complex interaction of drug dose and type, cognitive set, and environmental setting. As such a wide range of negative psychological effects may also be experienced in addition to the sought-after effects, including anxiety, panic, and paranoia (Table 1).

Physical effects

Physiologically sympathomimetic properties similar to amphetamine predominate including tachycardia, anorexia, increased respiratory rate, blood pressure, increased motor activity, mydriaisis, increased temperature, and sweating. Jaw tightening (bruxism), teeth grinding with molar erosion, and tremor may also be seen.

Patterns of use

The typical pattern of use is a half to two tablets per evening (although the time of use often extends into the next morning) with a usual frequency of between once or twice a week to less than monthly. There has been increasing recognition of a minority of users who take the drug in a binge fashion, consuming up to 30 tablets in a weekend. Although primarily a social drug, MDMA may be used while alone and is not confined to clubs, with use extending to public houses, bars, and football terraces as well as occasional solitary use.

Prevalence

The prevalence of illicit drug use, especially MDMA (ecstasy) and other stimulants, is increasing. For example, recent studies among the younger section of the British population show that 54 per cent of 20- to 22-year-olds had been offered ecstasy at some time and 15 per cent had tried it at least once. Almost twice as many men as women had taken it.[9] In a study of over 3000 second-year university students in the United Kingdom, 13 per cent reported that they had tried MDMA.[10] The number of seizures of MDMA in the United Kingdom rose from 39 000 doses in 1989 to 1 564 000 doses in 1994, and the number of persons found guilty, cautioned or dealt with rose from 286 in 1990 to over 3500 in 1994.[11] Similar findings have been reported from Denmark,[12] Germany,[13] Spain[14] and The Netherlands[15] among others. Australia[16] and America have also seen a rise in use the drug with prevalences of up to 25 per cent having been reported among students in the US.

An association between drug use and musical/subcultural preference has been recognized for many years: cannabis and heroin with jazz and blues, LSD with the 'hippie' movement, and amphetamine sulphate with the punk era.[17] MDMA is associated with the 'dance and club scene'. The particular association between stimulant drugs and the 'dance scene' can be partly explained by the energetic and prolonged dancing that accompanies such music. Stimulants may enhance enjoyment and ability to perform to such music.[18]

Neurotoxicity

Over the last 10 years there has been increasing animal evidence of MDMA's neurotoxicity upon serotonergic neurones with consequent worry over the possible functional implications in humans (for reviews see Steele et al.[4] and Green et al.[19]). After administration of MDMA, animals have reduced levels of 5-hydroxytryptamine (**5-HT**), 5-hydroxyindole acetic acid, and tryptophan hydroxylase. Abnormal 5-HT regrowth has been reported after MDMA-induced damage[20] with a decrease in 5-HT terminal density, suggestive of what has been termed a 'chemical axotomy'. Pathological investigations suggest that 5-HT nerve terminals arising from the dorsal raphe nucleus are specifically involved. The duration and magnitude of these neurotoxic effects are dose dependent and are followed by differential rates of recovery, with 5-HT damage persisting for up to a year in the rat, and dopaminergic damage for up to 3 years in the rhesus monkey.[21] These changes appear to be species specific with primates being more sensitive to the neurotoxic damage than rodents.

Early findings suggesting dose-dependent damage led some to believe that human consumption was at such a level as to make such extrapolations to humans inconsequential. More recent research taking into account species scaling indicates that the average single dose size consumed by humans is indeed near to those levels found to be neurotoxic in animals. Early optimism regarding the risks of use were accompanied by initial expectations of low abuse potential. Subsequent reports suggest that although the majority use low levels of the drug, a significant minority use up to five tablets a night with a lifetime consumption of more than 1000 occasions.[2] With such levels of self-administration and some users reporting a binge pattern, the cumulative doses are certainly reaching the levels found to be neurotoxic in animals and a dependence syndrome similar to that seen with other stimulant drugs remains a possibility. Since the dopaminergic system is influenced by MDMA, the ventral tegmental dopaminergic reward pathway may underlie any reinforcing potential.

Factors other than dose have been implicated in the pathogenesis of neurotoxicity associated with MDMA and some of these have practical relevance for the social context of human use. Core ambient temperature and hydration status have been implicated as key factors in the development of neurotoxicty and malignant hyperthermia respectively. The drug is usually taken during relentless hours of energetic dancing in crowded and poorly ventilated venues. The users sweat excessively and often make inadequate or inappropriate efforts at rehy-

Table 2 Possible markers of 5-HT dysfunction in humans associated with MDMA

Reduced levels of 5-HIAA in CSF
Blunted prolactin and cortisol response to D-fenfluramine challenge
Cardiovascular autonomic dysfunction (impaired Valsalva response)
Decreased brain 5-HT transporter binding on PET scanning
Midweek depression in some users following weekend consumption

5-HIAA, 5-hydroxyindole acetic acid; CSF, cerebrospinal fluid; PET, positron emission tomography.

dration. (Studies on amphetamine aggregation toxicity may be relevant: mice grouped together had enhanced toxic and behavioural effects from amphetamine compared with mice housed alone.) These findings have influenced both public health messages (advising regular isotonic fluid replacement) and the dance club environment with access to 'chill out' rooms and to free water.

The neurochemical mechanism underlying neurotoxicity seems to be dependent upon intact dopaminergic and serotonergic systems since disruption of monoamine transmission in either system protects against MDMA-induced neurotoxicity. Recent studies implicating free radicals in the development of neuronal damage suggest that prior consumption of vitamin C could be protective.

Evidence for 5-HT disruption in humans

Markers for 5-HT damage may be sought either by direct assessment of metabolite levels or indirectly by assessing those functions thought to be dependent on an intact 5-HT system. Subjects with prior exposure to MDMA had lower cerebrospinal fluid 5-hydroxyindole acetic acid than matched controls and lower levels of impulsivity, indirect hostility, and harm avoidance (Table 2). The 5-HT system is implicated in cognition, sex, sleep, and appetite, as well as mood. Uncontrolled human studies have reported cognitive deficits such as impaired immediate and delayed recall in those with a history of MDMA use, and recent work suggests acute mood and cognitive deficit in the days following use.

Further evidence for disruption of the 5-HT system comes from blunted neuroendocrine responses (cortisol and prolactin) to D-fenfluramine in former users of the drug. A study of former users[22] suggested associated personality traits of novelty seeking, depression, and aggressive–impulsive behaviour. The frequency of polysubstance abuse in this population confounds these findings, and the direction of causality in the neuroendocrine, neurochemical, and personality findings is uncertain. Krystal et al.[23] have shown mild to moderate impairment on subtests of the Weschler Memory Scale in nine users, none of whom met clinical criteria for affective disorder. Positron emission tomography studies using novel 5-HT ligands have found results compatible with a decrease in a structural component of brain 5-HT neurones.[24] However, most studies have been of polysubstance users and rely on self-reported histories of drug use, and the control groups were not matched for use of other substances.

Acute psychological problems associated with MDMA use

Increased anxiety[25,26] and panic[27,28] have been described, with the three cases of the latter study complicated by prolonged agorophobia

Table 3 Adverse effects of MDMA use

Cognitive	Motor/physiological	Emotional
Decreased desire to perform mental tasks	Trismus, bruxism, headaches and motor tics	Depressed mood, panic attacks and paranoid ideas
Disorientation and confusion	Nausea/vomiting and anorexia	
Decreased ability to perform mental tasks	Palpitations Delayed or absent orgasm	Increased anxiety and restlessness

which responded to serotonergic antidepressant drugs. Major depressive disorder[29] and prolonged depersonalization with panic and suicide following ingestion[30] have also been described. Numerous cases of MDMA-related psychoses have also been reported[31,32] as well as flashbacks[33,34] and even craving for chocolate.[35] It has been suggested[13,21,22] that such idiosyncratic disturbances are more likely to occur in those already predisposed to psychiatric disorders. It is possible that people predisposed to mood disorders may experience their first episode of psychological disturbance earlier than they would have done had they not taken MDMA. Controlled long-term cohort studies of users, with baseline measures of risk factors, are needed to assess this.

More common adverse effects associated with the use of MDMA are more directly related to the psychostimulant effects of the drug, such as increased restlessness, headaches, and bruxism. Weekend use of MDMA has been shown to be associated with depressed mood mid-week[36] which could reflect depletion of serotonin following the acute elevation that follows ingestion of MDMA. This could be a parallel to the 'crash' reported after abstinence of cocaine use[37] or as a hangover effect. Table 3 lists some of the more common adverse effects that follow MDMA use.

Physical complications from MDMA

Most users of MDMA use other drugs. Concurrent administration of cocaine and amphetamine will potentiate the stimulant effects of MDMA and may increase the likelihood of hyperthermic and cardiac problems. Some users take benzodiazepines and other depressant drugs to treat insomnia and restlessness. Stimulant drugs reduce the individual's awareness of intoxication by alcohol and may lead to higher alcohol consumption and hence increase the risk of accidents.

Other serious physical complications include hepatocellular failure, arterial aneurysms, and cerebral hemorrhages. Of the 70 or so deaths in the United Kingdom reported in association with MDMA use over the last 10 years, most have been from malignant hyperthermia and dehydration, with the remainder secondary to idiosyncratic organ failure involving the heart, liver, and, in several cases, cerebral oedema, possibly linked to the syndrome of inappropriate ADH secretion.[38] The severity of symptoms and potential outcome appear unrelated to dose consumed, suggesting an idiosyncratic response possibly related to genetically determined metabolizer status. The serotonin syndrome and neuroleptic malignant syndrome have also been described. Concurrent consumption of selective serotonin reuptake inhibitors may potentiate the harmful neurochemical and behavioural effects of MDMA. Similar interactions have been noted with monoamine oxidase inhibitors.[39]

Ketamine

Ketamine, a non-barbiturate anaesthetic/analgesic structurally related to phencylidine was developed in the 1960s when it was promoted as an anaesthetic. Unlike inhalational and opiod anaesthetics which work via supresssion of the reticular activating system, ketamine causes functional and electrophysiological dissociation between the thalamocortical and limbic systems. The dissociation results in higher centres being prevented from perceiving auditory, visual, or painful stimuli, i.e. 'a lack of responsive awareness'. The effect has been described as somataesthetic sensory blockade with amnesia and analgesia.

The major clinical use of ketamine is in veterinary surgery and anaesthetic induction, especially in the young and in emergency situations such as at crashes or war zones where its ability to induce a cataleptic state of muscle rigidity (i.e. a patient placed in one position cannot subsequently move until the drug effects have worn off) is desirable. It has also been reported useful in the management of uncontrollable patients and may augment analgesia with opiates.

In the United Kingdom the drug is not controlled under the Misuse of Drugs Act (being a prescription-only medicine under the Medicines Act) and hence possession is not a criminal offence. It appears that most abused ketamine is obtained through diversion from legitimate sources.

The first reports of ketamine as a drug of abuse appeared in the 1970s. In recent years the drug has become associated with the 'rave' music scene. The drug sold as powder or capsules (average dose 70–150 mg) may be marketed as itself 'Special K' or may be a constituent of tablets purportedly sold as ecstasy, in combination with stimulant drugs.

Ketamine is a potent N-methyl-D-aspartate receptor antagonist but also demonstrates stereospecific binding at opiate receptors. The most common routes of administration outside clinical practice are oral and intranasal. After oral administration, effects appear after 20 min, lasting up to 3 h. The onset of action is more rapid and the duration shorter when the drug is snorted. Sought-after effects include a general stimulating effect ('being put into overdrive'), euphoria, depersonalization, out-of-body 'floating' experiences, perceptual distortion, and hallucinations.

As with all psychoactive drugs the adverse effects result from the interaction between the individual's genetic and physiological makeup, the dose and route of administration, other consumed drugs, the cognitive set, and the environmental setting. Adverse effects include the following:

- 'emergence phenomena' (as awakening from anaesthesia) such as vivid dreams, hallucinations, synaesthesia, and delirium
- tachycardia and hypertension
- nausea and vomiting, hypersalivation, and nystagmus
- numbness (with risk of accidental burning or other traumatic injury), ataxia, and slurred speech
- raised intracranial and intraocular pressure.

Flashbacks have also been reported.

Tolerance to ketamine occurs on repeated administration and a small minority may become 'psychologically' dependent on the experience. There are also reports of psychosis following use as well as chronic memory impairment.

γ-Hydroxybutyrate

γ-Hydroxybutyrate is a naturally occurring fatty acid derivative, derived from γ-aminobutyric acid, which may function as an inhibitory chemical transmitter in the central nervous system. It was synthesized for use as an anaesthetic, although trace amounts may be found in certain fruits such as guava. It has been described as an anabolic steroid since it promotes the secretion of growth hormone during slow-wave sleep and has been abused by body builders. Other recently suggested therapeutic uses include the treatment of narcolepsy and the withdrawal from alcohol and opiates. It is colourless and odourless with an insipid taste, and is available as a liquid or occasionally in powder or capsule form. Concentrations of the drug in these preparations are variable and therefore precise dosing is difficult.

Although not controlled in the United Kingdom under the Misuse of Drugs Act, unauthorized manufacture and sale can be an offence under the Medicines Act.

The sought-after effects are sedative and euphoric as opposed to the stimulant effects described with other dance drugs. The effect begins after 10 to 40 min and lasts 8 to 24 h. At low doses euphoria and disinhibition predominate; with increasing dosage, sedative effects become more evident and there may be nausea and vomiting. There have been several reports of acute physical complications following consumption of the drug, with respiratory depression, seizures (usually petit mal type), and coma (usually with full recovery). γ-Hydroxybutyrate is not detected on routine toxicological screens. Complications are likely to be enhanced when the drug is taken with other substances, especially alcohol. A withdrawal syndrome has been described[40] characterized by insomnia, tremor and anxiety.

Khat (qat)

This perennial shrub, indigenous to Yemen, Ethiopia, and surrounding areas, is used in cultures where alcohol is prohibited. Outside its area of propagation, khat is most commonly used among immigrant Somali communities in the United Kingdom, and elsewhere in Europe and the United States. Concern has grown over recent years regarding possible adverse effects that use of this stimulant herb may have upon both individuals and their societies. For a review of the literature and use in the United Kingdom see Griffiths.[41]

The fresh bitter leaves are usually chewed for their stimulant effect with the extracted juices swallowed and the residue kept within the cheek for some time after. This is a relatively slow mode of administration, requiring prolonged chewing to provide a relatively mild stimulant effect. Less often the leaves may be smoked or infusions prepared. Khat is primarily a social drug and its mild stimulant effects appear to promote social interaction. Users report loquacity, disinhibition, and improved concentration. As with other stimulants, use is associated with anorexia and reduced need for sleep. Although originally used more commonly by men, its use is becoming more common among women.

Khat is a central stimulant, considerably less potent that amphetamine, although it has a similar mechanism of action through the release of presynaptically stored catecholamines. The main stimulant psychoactive components, cathine and the more potent cathinone (both phenylpropylamines), are found in combination with other alkaloids and tannins. Because cathinone is very unstable, fresh leaves are used within a day or two of harvesting.

In the countries in which it is used, assessment of the impact on health is confounded by the poor socio-economic status of many users, and the anorexic effects of use. Reported adverse physical effects include oral problems, constipation, and hepatic and cardiac disturbances. Accidents may occur whilst intoxicated. Khat use has been associated with compulsion to use and dependence, but there does not appear to be a physically characterized withdrawal syndrome. There have been several case reports of short-lived amphetamine-like psychoses among users of khat, although there is little to suggest longer-term psychiatric morbidity among users.

Cathine and cathinone are controlled in the United Kingdom under the Misuse of Drugs Act 1971, as well as under international conventions. However, sale of unprepared khat is not prohibited in the United Kingdom and where legislation does exist it has been difficult to enforce.

Because cathinone decomposes rapidly, the effects are modest, and the drug is usually taken by chewing, unprepared khat is unlikely to enter Western drug use. Cheaper more potent synthetic preparations are better suited and more familiar to groups not culturally associated with its use. A refined preparation of cathinone could be used and there has been an isolated outbreak of use associated with localized manufacture of the derivative methylcathinone in the United States.

Tryptamine derivatives

Tryptamine (1H-indole-3-ethanamine) is a naturally occurring metabolite of tryptophan. It forms the parent nucleus of a wide range of hallucinogenic drugs, some entirely synthetic (LSD, N,N-dimethyltryptamine) but many naturally occurring in plants, fungi (psilocybin—the psychoactive component of 'magic mushrooms'), and occasionally animals. It seems unlikely that many tryptamines other than LSD and psilocybin will be used unduly in dance clubs because they possess few stimulant properties, and need to be smoked or injected because most are inactive by mouth unless taken with a monoamine oxidase inhibitor. An example of the latter is the combination of N,N-dimethyltryptamine (the hallucinogen) and harmine (the activator) in the hallucinogenic drink ayahuasca or caapi used in rituals by South American Indians. Drugs such a N,N-dimethyltryptamine may have adverse effects upon both the cardiovascular system and on temperature regulation. They may induce unpleasant hallucinogenic experiences.

References

1. Forsyth, A.J.M. (1996). Places and patterns of drug use in the Scottish dance scene. *Addiction*, **91**, 511–21.
2. Winstock, A.R. and King, L. (1996). Tablets often contain substances in addition to, or instead of ecstasy. *British Medical Journal*, **313**, 423–4.
3. Tucker, G., Lennard, M.S., Ellis, S.W., *et al.* (1995). The demethylation of methylenedioxymethamphetamine (ecstasy) by debrisoquine hydroxylase (CYP2D6). *Biochemical Pharmacology*, **47**, 1151–6.
4. Steele, T.D., McCann, U.D., and Ricaurte, G.A. (1994). Review: 3,4 methylenedioxymethamphetamine (MDMA, 'ecstasy'): pharmacology and toxicology in animals and humans. *Addiction*, **89**, 539–51.

5. Shuglin, A.T. and Nichols, D.E. (1978). Characteristics of 3 new psychomimetics. In *The pharmacology of hallucinogens* (ed. N.C. Stillman and N.E. Willete). Pergamon Press, Oxford.

6. McDowell, D.M. and Kleber, H.D. (1994). MDMA: its history and pharmacology. *Psychiatric Annals*, **24**, 127–30.

7. Woolfson, P.E. (1986). Meetings at the edge with Adam: a man for all seasons? *Journal of Psychoactive Drugs*, **18**, 329–33.

8. Liester, M.B., Grob, C.S., Bravo, M.D., *et al.* (1992). Phenomenology and sequelae of 3,4 MDMA use. *Journal of Nervous and Mental Disease*, **180**, 345–52.

9. National Drugs Campaign Survey (1996). *Drug realities. Summary of key findings.* Health Education Authority, London.

10. Webb, E., Ashton, C.H., Kelly, P., and Kamali, F. (1996). Alcohol and drug misuse in UK university students. *Lancet*, **348**, 922–5.

11. Home Office (1996). *Source statistics of drug seizures and offenders dealt with, UK, 1995.* Home Office Statistical Bulletin. HMSO, London.

12. Frydenlund Nielsen, J.C., Nicholson, K., Pitzner Jorgensen, B.L., and Under, M. (1995). Abuse of ecstasy (3,4 methylene dioxymethamphetamine)—pharmacological, neuropsychiatric and behavioural aspects. *Ugeskrift for Laeger*, **157**, 724–7.

13. Rakete, G. and Flusmeiser, U. (1996). Use and abuse of ecstasy. *Sucht*, **42**, 358–66.

14. Alvarez-Roldan, A., Gamella, J.F., and Sanchez, J. (1997). Ecstasy in Spain: trends and patterns of use. Paper presented at the Sixth Annual Conference on Drug Use and Policy. Amsterdam, 26–28 September 1996.

15. Sandwijk, J.P., Cohen, P.D.A., and Musterd, S. (1995). *Licit and illicit drug use in Amsterdam II. Report of a household survey in 1994 on the prevalence of drug use among the population of 12 years and older.* Institute for Social Geography, University of Amsterdam.

16. Boys, A., Lenton, S., and Norcross, K. (1997). Polydrug use at raves by a Western Australian sample. *Drug and Alcohol Review*, **16**, 227–34.

17. Griffiths, P. and Vingoe, L. (ed.) (1997). *The use of amphetamines, ecstasy and LSD in the European Community: a review of data on consumption patterns and current epidemiological literature. Synthesis and overview.* European Centre for Drugs and Drug Addiction.

18. Forsyth, A.J.M. (1995). Ecstasy and illegal drug design: a new concept in drug use. *International Journal of Drug Policy*, **6**, 193–209.

19. Green, R.A., Cross, A.J., and Goodwin, G. (1995). Review of the pharmacology and clinical pharmacology of 3,4,methylenedioxymethamphetamine (MDMA or 'ecstasy'). *Psychopharmacology*, **119**, 247–60.

20. Fischer, C., Hatzidimitrou, G., Wlos, J., and Ricaurte, G. (1995). Reorganisation of ascending 5HT axon projections in animals previously exposed to the recreational drug (±)3,4 methylenedioxymethamphetamine (MDMA, 'ecstasy'). *Journal of Neuroscience*, **15**, 576–85.

21. Seiden, L.S. and Sabol, K.E. (1996). Methamphetamine and methylenedioxymethamphetamine neurotoxicity: possible mechanisms of cell destruction. *NIDA-Research Monologue*, **163**, 251–76.

22. Gerra, G., Zaimovic, A., Giucastro, G., *et al.* (1998). Serotonergic function after (+/−)3,4-methylene-dioxymethamphetamine ('ecstasy') in humans. *International Clinical Psychopharmacology*, **13**, 1–9.

23. Krystal, J.H., Price, L.H., Opsahal, C., Ricaurte G.A., and Heniger, G.R. (1992). Chronic 3,4 methylene dioxymethamphetamine (MDMA) use: effects on mood and neuropsychiatric function? *American Journal of Drug and Alcohol Abuse*, **18**, 331–41.

24. McCann, U.D., Szabo, Z., Scheffel, U., Dannals, R.F., and Ricaurte, G.A. (1998). Positron emission tomographic evidence of toxic effect of MDMA ('ecstasy') on brain serotonin neurones in human beings. *Lancet*, **352**, 1433–7.

25. Hayner, G.N. and McKinney, H. (1986). MDMA: the dark side of ecstasy. *Journal of Psychoactive Drugs*, **18**, 341–7.

26. Leister, M., Grob, C., Bravo, G., and Walsh, R. (1992). Phenomenology and sequelae of 3,4 MDMA. *Journal of Nervous and Mental Disease*, **180**, 345–52.

27. McCann, U.D. and Ricaurte, G.A. (1992). MDMA ('ecstasy') and panic disorder: induction by a single dose. *Biological Psychiatry*, **32**, 950–3.

28. Pallanti, S. and Mazzi, D. (1992). MDMA (ecstasy) precipitation of panic disorder. *Biological Psychiatry*, **32**, 91–5.

29. McCann, U.C. and Ricaurte, G.A. (1991). Lasting neuropsychiatric sequelae of (±)3,4 methylenedioxymethamphetamine ('ecstasy') in recreational users. *Journal of Clinical Psychopharmacology*, **11**, 302–5.

30. Cohen, R.S. (1996). Adverse symptomatology and suicide associated with the use of methylenedioxymethamphetamine (MDMA; 'ecstasy'). *Biological Psychiatry*, **39**, 819–20.

31. McGuire, P.K., Cope, H., and Fahy, T.A. (1994). Diversity of psychopathology associated with use of 3,4 methylenedioxymethamphetamine ('ecstasy'). *British Journal of Psychiatry*, **165**, 391–5.

32. Keenan, E., Gervin, M., Dorman, A., and O'Connor, J.J. (1993). Psychosis and recreational use of MDMA ('ecstasy'). *Irish Journal of Psychological Medicine*, **10**, 162–3.

33. McGuire, P.K. and Fahy, T. (1992). Flashbacks following MDMA. *British Journal of Psychiatry*, **160**, 276.

34. Creighton, F.J., Black, D.L., and Hyde, C.E. (1991). 'Ecstasy' psychosis and flashbacks. *British Journal of Psychiatry*, **159**, 713–15.

35. Scifano, F. and Magni, G. (1994). MDMA ('ecstasy') abuse: psychopathological features and craving for chocolate: a case series. *Biological Psychiatry*, **36**, 763–7.

36. Curran, V. and Travill, R.A. (1997). Mood and cognitive effects of ±3,4 methylene dioxymethamphetamine (MDMA, 'ecstasy'): weekend high followed by mid week low. *Addiction*, **92** (7), 821–31.

37. Weddington, W.W., Brown, B.S., Haertzen, C.A., *et al.* (1990). Change in mood, craving and sleep during short term abstinence reported by male cocaine users. A controlled, residential study. *Archives of General Psychiatry*, **47**, 861–8.

38. Milroy, C.M., Clark, J.C., and Forrst, A.R. (1996). Pathology of deaths associated with 'ecstasy' and 'eve' misuse. *Journal of Clinical Pathology*, **49**, 149–53.

39. Lane, R. and Baldwin, D. (1997). Selective serotonin reuptake inhibitor-induced serotonin syndrome: review. *Journal of Clinical Psychopharmacology*, **17**, 208–21.

40. Gantt, P., Galloway, S.L., Frederick, S.L., *et al.* (1997). Gamma-hydroxybutyrate: an emerging drug of abuse that causes physical dependence. *Addiction*, **92**, 89–96.

41. Griffiths, P. (1998). *Qat use in London: a study of qat use among a sample of Somalis living in London.* DPI Publication No. 26. Home Office, London.

4.2.3.7 Disorders relating to the use of volatile substances

Richard Ives

Introduction

Volatile substance abuse (**VSA**) is the deliberate inhalation of products, of which there are many (Table 1), to achieve intoxication. It is also known as 'solvent abuse', and in the United States and elsewhere as 'inhalant abuse'. Amyl (pentyl) and isobutyl nitrites ('poppers') have different patterns of misuse, and so are not discussed here; details can be found elsewhere.[1]

VSA has dose-related effects similar to those of other hypnosedatives. Small doses rapidly lead to 'drunken' behaviour similar to the effects of alcohol, and may induce delusions and hallucinations.

Table 1 Some products that can be abused by inhalation

Product	Major volatile components
Adhesives	
Balsa wood cement	Ethyl acetate
Contact adhesives	Butanone, hexane, toluene, and esters
Cycle tyre repair cement	Toluene and xylenes
Woodworking adhesives	Xylenes
Polyvinylchloride (PVC) cement	Acetone, butanone, cyclohexanone, trichloroethylene
Aerosols	
Air freshener	LPG, DME, and/or fluorocarbons
Deodorants, antiperspirants	LPG, DME, and/or fluorocarbons
Fly spray	LPG, DME, and/or fluorocarbons
Hair lacquer	LPG, DME, and/or fluorocarbons
Paint sprayers	LPG, DME, and/or fluorocarbons and esters
Anaesthetics/analgesics	
Inhalational	Nitrous oxide, cyclopropane, diethyl ether, halothane, enflurane, isoflurane
Topical	FC 11, FC 12, monochloroethane
Dust removers ('air brushes')	DME, FC 22
Commercial dry cleaning and degreasing agents	Dichloromethane, FC 113, methanol, 1,1,1-trichloroethane, tetrachloroethylene, toluene, trichloroethylene (now rarely carbon tetrachloride, 1,2-dichloropropane)
Domestic spot removers and dry cleaners	Dichloromethane, 1,1,1-trichloroethane, tetrachloroethylene, trichloroethylene
Fire extinguishers	Bromochlorodifluoromethane, FC 11, FC 12
Fuel gases	
Cigarette lighter refills	LPG
'Butane'	LPG
'Propane'	Propane and butanes
Nail varnish/nail varnish remover	Acetone and esters
Paints/paint thinners	Acetone, butanone, esters, hexane, toluene, trichloroethylene, xylenes
Paint stripper	Dichloromethane, methanol, toluene
'Room odorizer'	Isobutyl nitrite
Typewriter correction fluids/thinners	1,1,1-Trichloroethane
Whipped cream dispensers	Nitrous oxide

Adapted from Flanagan and Ives.[2]

Some users inhale large quantities; a glue sniffer can consume 6 litres of adhesive weekly.

Long-term effects include listlessness, anorexia, and moodiness. The hair, breath, and clothing may smell of the substance(s) used, and empty product containers (e.g. glue cans, cigarette lighter refills, and aerosol spray cans), and bags used to inhale from, may be found.

Being readily available, volatile substances are, along with alcohol and tobacco, the first drugs tried by teenagers. They may therefore introduce youngsters to intoxication and be 'gateways' to illegal drug use. But VSA does not inevitably lead to the use of other psychoactive substances, and those that 'descend the slippery slope' to problematic misuse have other difficulties in their lives.[3]

History

Inhaling substances to achieve intoxication is not new. Inhaling ether and nitrous oxide ('laughing gas'), as well as commercially available volatile products, has a considerable pedigree.

Public concern is more recent. In the United States during the 1950s and 1960s there was much publicity about glue sniffing; this helped to publicize the possibilities of glue as an intoxicant.[4] Only in the 1970s did public concern about volatile substance abuse emerge in the United Kingdom. By 1983 this reached a peak—there were more press cuttings on the subject than on all other drugs.[5] Since then, public interest has waned, despite evidence of continuing high levels of experimental use.

Prevalence of volatile substance use

Volatile substances are used throughout the world. A World Health Organization report gives an overview of the issue,[6] and a National Institute on Drug Abuse (NIDA) report presents prevalence studies worldwide.[7] A Pompidou Group report[8] indicated that VSA was a pan-European problem. In the United Kingdom, up to 20 per cent of young people have tried sniffing volatile substances.[9] In continental Europe, while prevalence is lower, experimental volatile substance use among teenagers comes second only to cannabis, and in Greece and Sweden it is higher than cannabis use.[10]

Although young people from all socio-economic groups experiment with volatile substances, among the poor and the dispossessed VSA is the drug of choice for some. Worldwide, VSA is a particular problem among people living on the street. In the United Kingdom, VSA is more common among young people looked after by local authorities than in the general population.

VSA deaths

Even for first-time users, death from VSA is an ever-present risk. Death may ensue as a result of convulsions and coma, from inhalation of vomit, or from direct cardiac or central nervous system toxicity. VSA-related deaths can easily be overlooked if sudden deaths of young people are not thoroughly investigated. Postmortem examination usually reveals little, except perhaps acute lung congestion and possibly cold-induced burns to the mouth and throat. Toxicological examination of blood and tissue specimens is used to confirm a diagnosis of VSA-related death.[11]

A long-term study in the United Kingdom identified 1596 VSA-related deaths between 1971 and 1996.[12] The death rate peaked in 1990 with 151 deaths, and declined before increasing once more, with 75 deaths being recorded in 1996.

More than two-thirds of those who die are under 20 years old. Most are male, although the overall proportion of female deaths may be rising; in 1996 female deaths made up 20 per cent of the deaths (in contrast, in prevalence surveys there is little difference in the proportions of boys and girls misusing volatile substances). Volatile-substance-related deaths occur in all social classes in the United

Kingdom. However, '…in deaths of those under 16, there was a marked difference in mortality between social classes I and V, with nearly four times as many deaths occurring in social class V…compared with social class I'.[13]

Health issues

Health effects of volatile substances include the following.

- A sensitization of the heart—so that cardiac arrhythmias may occur if VSA is followed by exertion or fright.

- Cooling of the throat tissues—this is caused by spraying substances directly into the mouth, which may causing swelling and suffocation.

- A risk of fire—many of these products are inflammable, especially when combined with smoking.

- Suffocation—this is a particular danger when large plastic bags are used.

- Most products are mixtures of chemicals, and manufacturers do not list constituents. Changing product formulations make the dangers unpredictable.

- Using on one's own in an isolated place presents special hazards.

- When combined with alcohol or other drugs, the effects can be unpredictable.

- Intoxication itself has potential dangers, for example greater recklessness, doing bizarre things in response to hallucinations, becoming unconscious, and choking on vomit.

Apart from the real risk of death, VSA rarely causes long-term damage. However, some products contain poisonous substances, such as lead in some petrols or n-hexane in some glues. Chronic abuse of toluene-containing products and of chlorinated solvents such as 1,1,1-trichloroethane sometimes causes damage to the liver and kidneys. Damage to the lungs, bone marrow, and nervous system is also known, but is uncommon and generally reversible. Some people are more vulnerable (genetically or otherwise) than others to certain harmful effects. However, the long-term effects of sniffing have not been thoroughly studied, and virtually all reports of chronic toxicity are case studies, so the actual morbidity from VSA is not known.

A review article looking at the possibility of cognitive impairments from volatile substance use concluded that: 'the possibility that permanent structural brain damage, with accompanying psychiatric manifestations, results from solvent abuse remains inconclusive'.[14]

Users develop tolerance. Although no dependence syndrome exists, a few young people develop a more compulsive and long-term habit. The United Kingdom Advisory Council on the Misuse of Drugs suggested that: 'There are…pharmacological reasons for suspecting that persistent exposure to volatile substances might be able to induce a dependence of the so-called depressant type'.[15]

Many users of volatile substances are also users of other drugs, both legal and illegal. Using different drugs in combination may potentiate their effects. Polydrug use makes it difficult to assess the risks of individual substances.

VSA during pregnancy is associated with increased maternal and fetal morbidity.[16] Paternal exposure to volatile substances may also have deleterious effects on their offspring.[17] But the complexities of the chemicals involved—and the complexities of people's lives—make the identification of particular causes of fetal damage difficult.

Treatment of VSA-related disorders

Emergency treatment

The immediate treatment of an intoxicated user requires a calm and firm approach. The product being used should be removed, although not if this would lead to conflict; exertion or high emotion may raise adrenaline to dangerous levels for an oversensitized heart. Therefore an intoxicated user should be kept calm and never chased. It is unlikely that it will be possible to have a serious conversation with an intoxicated abuser, but calming and reassuring talk may help. After 5 to 20 min without inhalation the abuser will sober up, unless alcohol or other drugs have also been used. Subsequently, the user may need medical help; a check-up may identify particular health problems.

Cessation

No special regime is necessary when stopping using volatile substances. Although, being lipid-soluble, the chemicals may be detectable in the body tissues for some weeks after cessation of use, they do not have any psychoactive effect. There is no clearly defined withdrawal syndrome, and special detoxification regimes are unnecessary, but rest and sleep, fresh food, and vitamin supplements may aid recovery.

Dealing with experimental misuse

Most teenagers do not try volatile substances; those who do, use them only a few times, and even most regular users do not continue for long. Experimental or the occasional use of volatile substances occurs mainly from curiosity or as part of peer group activity. Appropriate intervention may be a warning of the dangers plus increased supervision. At this stage, specialist treatment is not required, and may be counterproductive, entrenching an otherwise transient activity.

Dealing with dependent misuse

Biology may predispose to dependent use, but chronic VSA is connected with other problems. As the United Kingdom organization Network VSA puts it:[18]

> Persistent misuse of volatile substances is a complex behaviour…frequently associated with low self-esteem, family problems, isolation and psychological difficulties. These are also factors that may also be associated with the problematic use of legal and illegal drugs, and indeed, a large proportion of people who misuse volatile substances also misuse other drugs. Chronic VSA is thus intertwined with social and psychological problems and with the misuse of illegal drugs. Therefore, counselling services for young people should not be narrowly focused on volatile substances, but should be able to deal with VSA in the context of a range of problematic behaviours.

Often, it is these other problems that first need attention, and until these are dealt with the user—even while recognizing the harm—may not give up. Consequently, giving help to users of volatile substances may best be done by generic services, which can deal more effectively with these broader problems, supported where necessary by specialist agencies. Mental health services, as well as drugs' services, have an important role in giving this support, for example they can contribute to making a dual diagnosis and be involved in the treatment of someone thus diagnosed. Specialist services can also help to identify areas for intervention, but how interventions are pursued will depend on the local organization of services. Interventions must take account of the social and cultural patterns of the user's life.

Drug treatment and prevention services are often reluctant to work with young people who form most of this client group not only because of the legal complications of confidentiality and consent, but also because of workers' lack of training and the supposed difficulty of working with this age group. Jumper-Thurman and colleagues point out that the treatment of volatile substance users:[19]

> has presented a particularly difficult challenge…given the general lack of direction for effective treatment strategies. In addition to the physiological, neurological, and emotional challenges abusers face…[they] bring with them a multitude of other problems— academic, legal, social, and family issues.

The Modified Social Stress Model, developed by the WHO Street Children Project, gives a framework for understanding substance use.[20] Potential for change can be assessed using Prochaska and DiClemente's 'revolving door' model of stages of change.[21]

Families who struggle unaided with problematic VSA by a young family member will also need help. The generic practitioner (doctor, teacher, social worker, youth or play worker) receives very little training on the issue, and may encounter the problem too infrequently to develop much expertise. (The Institute for the Study of Drug Dependence has produced a comprehensive publication designed to give professionals the basic information they need and to help them explore treatment options.[22])

Some groups (such as people living on the street, and indigenous peoples) have special problems with substance use that require different, more holistic, attention. Treatment should work 'with the grain' of the culture, rather than imposing inappropriate 'alien' treatment models. Indigenous peoples are beginning to insist that their cultures have useful perspectives and approaches that can be utilized in the treatment of people with drug and volatile substance problems.[23] Female users of volatile substances may not readily present for treatment and can suffer additional stigmatization.

Follow-up

After-care, long-term rehabilitation, social reinsertion, relapse management, and follow-up of discharged patients are important aspects of the treatment process.

Relapse, which is common, should be treated non-judgementally; not as 'failure' but as an opportunity for learning. Support in maintaining improvements may be helpful; for example events for ex-users of volatile substances to help them to maintain abstinence and to utilize the support of the group.

Wider aspects

Chronic VSA is not an individual problem: it arises not only from individual pathology, but also from failures in social structures. Treatment, in the broadest sense, needs to help the healing of the family, the community, and to assist in making changes in society.

Measuring outcomes

Evaluation and monitoring need careful thought and planning. But treatment interventions have multiple aims and varied outcomes. Aims may alter and be adapted as the work develops, so that outcomes will be difficult to assess in relation to the original aims. Evaluation should handle this complexity: identifying 'success' requires measures beyond the simple calculation of reduction in, or abstention from, substance use.

Building evaluation in from the start, and using it to inform the intervention throughout, makes it part of the process of intervention; the reflection that evaluation encourages can increase the effectiveness of the intervention.

Prevention

There are many different sniffable products, many possibilities for substitution of one product for another, many different chemicals involved, and insufficient information about the relative harm of various products and practices. This makes prevention difficult. Additional difficulties are that volatile substance users are generally young, and that VSA-related deaths are sudden and unpredictable.

Tackling the supply of products

This can be approached in several ways.

- Product elimination—some products are particularly dangerous, and have satisfactory substitutes, but not all volatile substances can be eliminated.

- Product modification—there are three possibilities: changing the formulation of the product to remove the intoxicating substance, adding a chemical to make the product unpalatable, and modifying the container to make misuse difficult.

- Warning labels—these may be helpful, although labelling draws attention to the potential for misuse.

- Education for suppliers—retailers need information and advice about a product's potential for misuse. This is difficult, as the many products are sold through many retail outlets.

- Legal controls on the sale and supply of misusable products— these exist in many countries but are difficult to enforce.

Tackling the demand for products

- Legal controls—in Japan, Singapore, and the Republic of Korea VSA is an offence. However, this is not so in most countries because the criminalization of users of volatile substances is considered counterproductive.

- Information and education—this can be provided through public advertising, leaflets, helplines, and schools. Early education about volatile substances is essential; these products are in most people's homes and therefore (unlike illegal drugs) they can be accessed by very young children. Because many parents are unaware of the misuse potential of household products, information should also be targeted at parents.

All these strategies should be considered; as the Advisory Council on the Misuse of Drugs pointed out, '"good practice" will constitute a layered series of alternative or multiple strategies rather than any one master stroke'.[24]

Further reading

Advisory Council on the Misuse of Drugs (1995). *Volatile substance abuse.* HMSO, London.

Flanagan, R.J., Streete, P.J., and Ramsey, J.D. (1997). *Volatile substance abuse: practical guidelines for the analytical investigation of suspected cases and interpretation of results.* United Nations Drug Control Programme, Vienna.

Ives, R. (1995). *Problems with solutions: a manual for work with solvent sniffers and other young drug users* (pack and video). Institute for the Study of Drug Dependence, London.

Ives, R. (1997). *Drug notes 6: solvents.* Institute for the Study of Drug Dependence, London.

Ron, M. (1986). Volatile substance abuse: a review of possible long-term neurological, intellectual and psychiatric sequelae. *British Journal of Psychiatry*, **148**, 235–46.

Taylor, J.C., Norman, C.L., Bland, J.M., Ramsey, J.D., and Anderson, H.R. (1998). *Trends in death associated with abuse of volatile substances 1971–1996 (Report number 11).* Department of Public Health Sciences, St George's Hospital Medical School, London.

Websites

Information about volatile substance abuse: www.vsa.educari.com

Information on United Kingdom VSA-related deaths: www.sghms.ac.uk/phs/vsamenu.htm

United States of America National Inhalants Prevention Coalition: www.inhalants.org

References

1. Haverkos, H. and Dougherty, J. (ed.) (1988). *Health hazards of nitrite inhalants, NIDA Research Monograph 83.* National Institute on Drug Abuse, Rockville, MD.
2. Flanagan, B. and Ives, R. (1994). Volatile substance abuse. *Bulletin on Narcotics*, **46**, 49–78.
3. Davies, B., Thorley, A., and O'Connor, D. (1985). Progression of addiction careers in young adult solvent misusers. *British Medical Journal*, **290**, 6482.
4. Brecher, E. (1972). How to launch a nation-wide drug menace. In *Licit and illicit drugs*, pp. 321–34. Little, Brown, Boston, MA.
5. Ives, R. (1986). The rise and fall of the solvents panic. *Druglink*, **1** (4), 10–12.
6. WHO Programme on Substance Abuse (1999). *Volatile substance abuse: a global overview.* WHO, Geneva.
7. Kozel, N., Sloboda, Z., and De La Rosa, M. (ed.) (1995). *Epidemiology of inhalant abuse: an international perspective (NIDA Research Monograph series No. 148).* NIDA, Washington, DC.
8. Pompidou Group (1994). *Volatile substance abuse.* Council of Europe, Strasbourg.
9. Miller, P. and Plant, M. (1996). Drinking, smoking and illicit drug use among 15 and 16-year-olds in the United Kingdom. *British Medical Journal*, **313**, 294–7.
10. Ives, R. (1998). *Volatile substance abuse among children.* Rädda Barnen (Swedish Save the Children), Stockholm.
11. Flanagan, R.J., Streete, P.J., and Ramsey, J.D. (1997). *Volatile substance abuse: practical guidelines for the analytical investigation of suspected cases and interpretation of results.* United Nations Drug Control Programme, Vienna.
12. Taylor, J., Norman, C., Bland, J., Ramsey, J., and Anderson, H. (1998).
Trends in deaths associated with abuse of volatile substances 1971–1996. St George's Hospital Medical School, London.
13. Esmail, A., Meyer, L., Pottier, A., and Wright, S. (1993). Deaths from volatile substance abuse in those under 18 years: results from a national epidemiological study. *Archives of Disease in Childhood*, **69**, 356–60 (see p. 358).
14. Ron, M. (1986). Volatile substance abuse: a review of possible long-term neurological, intellectual and psychiatric sequelae. *British Journal of Psychiatry*, **148**, 235–46.
15. Advisory Council on the Misuse of Drugs (1995). *Volatile substance abuse*, paragraph 3.11. HMSO, London.
16. Wilkin, H. and Gabow, P. (1991). Toluene abuse during pregnancy: obstetric complications and perinatal outcomes. *Obstetrics and Gynaecology*, **77**, 504–8.
17. Robaire, B. and Hales, B. (1993). Paternal exposure to chemicals before conception (editorial). *British Medical Journal*, **307**, 341–2.
18. Network VSA (1997). *Network VSA statement about volatile substance misuse.* Network VSA, Blackburn, Lancs.
19. Jumper-Thurman, P., Plested, B., and Beauvais, F. (1992). Treatment strategies for volatile substance abusers in the United States. In *Inhalant abuse: a volatile research agenda* (ed. C. Sharpe, F. Beauvais, and R. Spence), NIDA Research Monograph 129. National Institute on Drug Abuse, Rockville, MD.
20. WHO Programme on Substance Abuse (1997). *Street children, substance use and health: training for street educators*, p. 48. WHO, Geneva.
21. Prochaska, J. and DiClemente, C. (1986). Towards a comprehensive model of change. In *Treating addictive behaviours: processes of change* (ed. W. Miller and N. Heather), pp. 3–27. Plenum Press, New York.
22. Ives, R. (1995). *Problems with solutions: a manual for work with solvent sniffers and other young drug users.* Institute for the Study of Drug Dependence, London.
23. Brady, M. (1992). *Heavy metal. The social meaning of petrol sniffing in Australia.* Aboriginal Studies Press, Canberra.
24. Advisory Council on the Misuse of Drugs (1995). *Volatile substance abuse*, paragraph 5.5. HMSO, London.

4.2.3.8 The mental health effects of cannabis use

Wayne Hall

Cannabis the drug

Cannabis is derived from the female plant of *Cannabis sativa*. Its primary psychoactive constituent is delta-9-tetrahydrocannabinol (**THC**).[1] The THC content is highest in the flowering tops of the plant. Marijuana (THC content 0.5–5 per cent) is prepared from the dried flowering tops and leaves of the plant. Hashish (THC content 2–20 per cent) consists of dried cannabis resin and compressed flowers.[1]

Cannabis is usually smoked in a 'joint', like a tobacco cigarette, or in a water pipe, often mixed with tobacco. Although marijuana and hashish may be eaten, cannabis is usually smoked because this is the most efficient way to achieve the desired level of intoxication.[2]

THC acts on a widely distributed specific receptor in those brain regions involved in cognition, memory, reward, pain perception, and motor coordination.[1] These receptors respond to an endogenous ligand, anandamide, which is considerably less potent and has a shorter duration of action than THC.[1]

Patterns of cannabis use

Cannabis has been tried by many young adults in Europe, the United States, and Australia.[3] Most cannabis users in the United States stop in their middle to late twenties, and very few engage in daily cannabis use over a period of years.[3,4] In the United States and Australian surveys, about 10 per cent of those who ever use cannabis become daily users, and another 20 to 30 per cent use weekly.[3] This pattern of use in developed countries differs from that in traditional cannabis-using countries, such as Egypt and India, where recreational cannabis use is uncommon and heavy cannabis use is confined to small and marginalized groups in the population.[3]

Because of uncertainties about THC content, 'heavy' cannabis use is usually defined as daily or near-daily use.[5] This pattern of use over years places users at the greatest risk of experiencing adverse psychological consequences. Daily cannabis users are more likely to use alcohol and tobacco regularly and to use amphetamines, hallucinogens, psychostimulants, sedatives, and opioids.[2,3]

Acute psychological effects of cannabis use

Cannabis produces euphoria and relaxation, perceptual alterations (including time distortion, and impaired short-term memory and attention), and intensification of ordinary sensory experiences, such as eating and listening to music.[2] The most common unpleasant psychological effects are anxiety and panic reactions.[2] These may be reported by naive users and they are a common reason for discontinuing use.[2]

Cannabis produces dose-related impairments in cognitive and behavioural functions that may potentially impair driving an automobile or operating machinery.[6]

Chronic psychological effects of cannabis use

Cannabis dependence

For much of the 1970s cannabis was not regarded as a drug of dependence because of the apparent absence of tolerance and withdrawal symptoms, and a lack of persons seeking help to stop their cannabis use. There is now evidence that animals and humans develop tolerance to the effects of THC,[1] with some heavy users experiencing withdrawal symptoms on the abrupt cessation of cannabis use.[7] During the 1980s and 1990s there was an increase in the number of persons in the United States, Australia, and Europe seeking help to stop their cannabis use.[2]

There is clinical and epidemiological evidence that a cannabis-dependence syndrome occurs in heavy chronic users of cannabis who report problems in controlling their cannabis use, but who continue despite experiencing adverse personal and social consequences.[8]

The lifetime prevalence of cannabis abuse and dependence (as defined in DSM-IIIR) in the United States has been estimated at 4.4 per cent of adults.[9] Similar estimates have been obtained in New Zealand and Australia.[2] The risk of becoming dependent on cannabis seems to have more similarities with that for alcohol than with that for nicotine or the opioids, with around 10 per cent of those who ever use cannabis meeting criteria for dependence at some point in their lives.[2,9]

It is not clear how cannabis dependence is best managed. Stephens and Roffman[10] have reported controlled trials of cognitive-behavioural relapse prevention and social support. They found rates of abstinence at 12 months of around only 30 per cent, but the rates of use had substantially declined among those who continued to use cannabis.

Cannabis psychosis

High doses of THC have been reported to produce visual and auditory hallucinations, delusional ideas, and thought disorder in normal volunteers.[2] In traditional cannabis-using cultures, such as India, a 'cannabis psychosis' has been reported in which the symptoms are preceded by heavy cannabis use and remit after abstinence.[11,12]

The existence of a 'cannabis psychosis' in Western cultures is still a matter for debate. In its favour are case series of 'cannabis psychoses', and a small number of controlled studies that compare the characteristics of 'cannabis psychoses' with those of psychoses in individuals who were not using cannabis at the time of hospital admission.[13] Critics of the hypothesis emphasize the fallibility of clinical judgements about aetiology, the poorly specified criteria used in diagnosing these psychoses, the dearth of controlled studies, and the striking variations in the clinical features of 'cannabis psychoses'.[14]

Cannabis and schizophrenia

There is good clinical and epidemiological evidence of an association between schizophrenia and cannabis use, which suggests that cannabis use can precipitate schizophrenia or exacerbate its symptoms. But this is not the only explanation of the association. Persons with schizophrenia may use cannabis as a form of self-medication, or there may be other variables that explain both; for example, cannabis use is a marker of other psychotogenic drug use, or of vulnerability to schizophrenia.[2]

There is clinical and epidemiological evidence that cannabis use exacerbates the symptoms of schizophrenia in affected individuals. This includes the findings of a number of prospective studies that have controlled for confounding variables.[12] It is also a biologically plausible relationship. Psychotic disorders involve disturbances in the dopamine neurotransmitter systems, since drugs that increase dopamine release produce psychotic symptoms when given in large doses, and neuroleptic drugs that reduce psychotic symptoms also reduce dopamine levels.[12] Cannabinoids, such as THC, increase dopamine release.[1]

There is good prospective evidence from a Swedish conscript study that cannabis use precipitates schizophrenia in persons who are vulnerable because of a personal or family history of this disorder.[15] This hypothesis is consistent with the stress–diathesis model of schizophrenia,[16] in which the likelihood of its developing is the product of stress acting upon a genetic 'diathesis' to develop schizophrenia.

Although plausible, there is very little direct evidence that genetic vulnerability increases the risk that cannabis users will develop psychosis. McGuire et al.[17] reported that persons with a history of heavy cannabis use who developed a psychosis were 10 times more likely to have a family history of schizophrenia than persons with a psychosis who had not used cannabis. It is difficult to identify a genetic diathesis in the majority of cases of schizophrenia since 81 per cent of persons with schizophrenia will not have a first-degree relative with the disorder, and 63 per cent will not have an affected first- or second-degree relative.[16]

The most contentious issue is whether cannabis use can cause schizophrenia that would not otherwise have occurred. This possibility cannot be excluded, but it is unlikely to account for more than a minority of cases. Most of the 274 Swedish conscripts who developed schizophrenia had not used cannabis, and only 7 per cent, at most, of schizophrenia cases could be attributed to cannabis use. Moreover, the treated incidence of schizophrenia, and particularly of early-onset acute cases, declined (or remained stable) during the 1970s and 1980s[12] when cannabis use increased among young adults in Australia and North America.[3] Although there are complications in interpreting such trends, a large reduction in treated incidence has been observed in a number of countries, while cannabis use has increased.[12]

Other disorders

Cognitive impairment

The fact that cannabis use acutely impairs cognitive functioning has raised the reasonable concern that chronic use may produce chronic cognitive impairment. The available evidence, however, suggests that even the long-term heavy use of cannabis does not produce any severe or grossly debilitating impairment of cognitive function.[18] There is no evidence, for example, that it produces anything comparable to the cognitive impairments found in chronic heavy alcohol drinkers; if it did, it should have been detected by research to date.[2]

However, there is some clinical and experimental evidence that the long-term use of cannabis may produce more subtle cognitive impairment in the higher cognitive functions of memory, attention and organization, and the integration of complex information.[18] The evidence suggests that the longer the period of heavy cannabis use, the more pronounced is the cognitive impairment.[18] None the less, the impairments in performance are subtle, and so it remains to be determined how significant they are for everyday functioning. It is also remains to be investigated whether these impairments can be reversed after an extended period of abstinence from cannabis.

A suspicion that chronic heavy cannabis use may cause gross structural brain damage was raised by a single poorly controlled study using an outmoded method of investigation, which reported that cannabis users had enlarged cerebral ventricles.[19] Since then, a number of better controlled studies using more sophisticated methods of investigation have consistently failed to demonstrate evidence of structural change in the brains of heavy long-term cannabis users.[18] These negative results are consistent with the evidence that any cognitive effects of chronic cannabis use are subtle, and are unlikely to be manifest as gross structural changes in the brain.[18]

An amotivational syndrome

Anecdotal reports that chronic heavy cannabis use impairs motivation and social performance have been described in societies with a long history of cannabis use, such as Egypt, the Caribbean, and elsewhere.[2] Among young American adults who were heavy cannabis users in the early 1970s, there were clinical reports[2] of individuals who became apathetic, withdrawn, lethargic, and unmotivated, apparently as a result of chronic heavy cannabis use. This constellation of symptoms was described as an 'amotivational syndrome'. As these reports were uncontrolled it was not possible to disentangle the effects of chronic cannabis use from those of pre-existing personality and other psychiatric disorders.[2]

Field studies of chronic heavy cannabis users in societies with a tradition of such use, for example Costa Rica and Jamaica,[2] have produced evidence that has usually been interpreted as failing to demonstrate the existence of the amotivational syndrome. Critics have argued that these studies are unconvincing because the chronic users studied have come from socially marginal groups, so that the cognitive and motivational demands of their everyday lives were insufficient to detect any impairment caused by chronic cannabis use.[20]

The status of the amotivational syndrome remains contentious. Many clinicians find the cases of 'amotivational syndrome' compelling, while many researchers are more impressed by the largely negative findings of the field and epidemiological studies. However, the possibility has been kept alive by reports that regular cannabis users experience a loss of ambition and impaired school and occupational performance.[2] Some former cannabis users report that impaired occupational performance was a reason for their stopping.[2] Although heavy users who request assistance to give up report impaired motivation as a symptom of cannabis use, a well-defined amotivational syndrome has not been documented. It may be more parsimonious to explain impaired motivation as a symptom of chronic cannabis intoxication.[2]

Flashbacks

There are a small number of case reports of cannabis 'flashbacks', i.e. experiencing symptoms of cannabis intoxication days or weeks after the individual last used cannabis.[21] Because of their rarity and the fact that many affected individuals have also used other drugs, it is difficult to draw any conclusions about the relationship between these symptoms and cannabis use. It is often difficult to decide whether these are rare events that are coincidental with cannabis use, the effects of other drugs that are often taken together with cannabis, rare consequences of cannabis use that only occur at much higher doses than those used recreationally or that require unusual forms of personal vulnerability, or the results of interactions between cannabis and other drugs.

Behavioural effects in adolescence

There has been understandable societal concern about the effects of adolescent cannabis use on school performance, mental health and adjustment, and the use of other more hazardous drugs.

There is a strong cross-sectional association between heavy cannabis use in adolescence and the risk of discontinuing a high-school education and experiencing job instability in young adulthood.[22] However, the strength of this association is reduced in longitudinal studies when adjustments are made for the fact that heavy cannabis users have lower academic aspirations and poorer high-school performance prior to using cannabis than their peers.[22,23]

There is some evidence that heavy cannabis use has adverse effects upon family formation, mental health, and involvement in drug-related crime.[22] In each case, the strong associations in cross-sectional studies are more modest in longitudinal studies after statistically controlling for associations between cannabis use and other pre-existing characteristics which independently predict these adverse outcomes.[23]

A consistent finding in the United States[4,22] has been the regular sequence of initiation into drug use, in which cannabis use has typically preceded involvement with 'harder' illicit drugs such as stimulants and opioids. The interpretation of this sequence of events remains controversial. The least compelling hypothesis is that cannabis use directly increases the use of later drugs in the sequence. There is better support for two other hypotheses: (i) there is a selective recruitment into cannabis use of non-conforming adolescents who have a propensity to use other illicit drugs; (ii) once recruited to cannabis use, it is the social interaction with drug-using peers and greater access to illicit drug markets that increases the likelihood of using other illicit drugs.[2,23]

Summary

The major adverse acute psychological effects of cannabis use are as follows:

- anxiety, dysphoria, panic, and paranoia, especially in naive users

- impairment of attention and memory, psychomotor impairment while intoxicated

- possibly an increased risk of accident if an intoxicated person attempts to drive a motor vehicle.

The major psychological effects of daily heavy cannabis use over many years remain uncertain, but probably include the following:[24]

- a cannabis-dependence syndrome that is characterized by an inability to abstain from or control cannabis use

- subtle forms of cognitive impairment that affect attention and memory and which persist while the user remains chronically intoxicated, and may or may not be reversible after prolonged abstinence from cannabis

- impaired educational achievement in adolescents with a history of poor school performance, whose achievement may be limited by the cognitive impairments produced by chronic intoxication with cannabis

- among those who initiate cannabis use in the early teens, a higher risk of progressing to heavy cannabis and other illicit drug use, and becoming dependent on cannabis.

References

1. Adams, I.B. and Martin, B.R. (1996). Cannabis: pharmacology and toxicology in animals and humans. *Addiction*, **91**, 1585–1614.
2. Hall, W., Solowij, N., and Lemon, J. (1994). *The health and psychological effects of cannabis use*. National Drug Strategy Monograph Series No. 25. Australian Government Publication Service, Canberra, Australia.
3. Hall, W., Johnston, L., and Donnelly, N. (1999). The epidemiology of cannabis use and its consequences. In *The health effects of cannabis* (ed. H. Kalant, W. Corrigal, W. Hall, and R. Smart), pp. 69–125. Addiction Research Foundation, Toronto.
4. Chen, K. and Kandel, D.B. (1995). The natural history of drug use from adolescence to the mid-thirties in a general population sample. *American Journal of Public Health*, **85**, 41–7.
5. Kandel, D.B. and Davies, M. (1992). Progression to regular marijuana involvement: phenomenology and risk factors for near daily use. In *Vulnerability to drug abuse* (ed. M. Glantz and R. Pickens), pp. 211–53. American Psychological Association, Washington, DC.
6. Chait, L.D. and Pierri, J. (1992). Effects of smoked marijuana on human performance: a critical review. In *Marijuana/cannabinoids: neurobiology and neurophysiology* (ed. A. Murphy and J. Bartke), pp. 387–423. CRC, Boca Raton, FL.
7. Weisbeck, G.A., Schuckit, M.A., Kalmijn, J.A., Tipp, J.E., Bucholz, K.K., and Smith, T.L. (1996). An evaluation of the history of marijuana withdrawal syndrome in a large population. *Addiction*, **91**, 1469–78.
8. American Psychiatric Association (1994). *Diagnostic and statistical manual—fourth edition (DSM-IV)*. American Psychiatric Association, Washington, DC.
9. Anthony, J.C., Warner, L.A., and Kessler, R.C. (1994). Comparative epidemiology of dependence on tobacco, alcohol, controlled substances and inhalants: basic findings from the National Comorbidity Study. *Clinical and Experimental Psychopharmacology*, **2**, 244–68.
10. Stephens, R.S. and Roffman, R.A. (1993). Adult marijuana dependence. In *Addictive behaviors across the lifespan: prevention, treatment and policy issues* (ed. J.S. Baer, G.A. Marlatt, and R.J. MacMahon), pp. 202–18. Sage, Newbury Park, CA.
11. Chopra, G.S. and Smith, J.W. (1974). Psychotic reactions following cannabis use in East Indians. *Archives of General Psychiatry*, **30**, 24–7.
12. Hall, W. (1998). Cannabis and psychosis. *Drug and Alcohol Review*, **17**, 433–44.
13. Boutros, N.N. and Bowers, M.B. (1996). Chronic substance-induced psychotic disorders: state of the literature. *Journal of Neuropsychiatry and Clinical Neurosciences*, **8**, 262–9.
14. Poole, R. and Brabbins, C. (1996). Drug induced psychosis. *British Journal of Psychiatry*, **168**, 135–8.
15. Andreasson, S., Allebeck, P., Engstrom, A., and Rydberg, U. (1987). Cannabis and schizophrenia: a longitudinal study of Swedish conscripts. *Lancet*, **ii**, 1483–6.
16. Gottesman, I.I. (1991). *Schizophrenia genesis: the origins of madness*. W.H. Freeman, New York.
17. McGuire, P., Jones, R., Harvey, I., Williams, M., McGuffin, P., and Murray, R. (1995). Morbid risk of schizophrenia for relatives of patients with cannabis associated psychosis. *Schizophrenia Research*, **15**, 277–81.
18. Solowij, N. (1998). *Cannabis and cognitive functioning*. Cambridge University Press.
19. Campbell, A.M.G., Evans, M., Thomson, J.L.G., and Williams, M.J. (1971). Cerebral atrophy in young cannabis smokers. *Lancet*, **ii**, 1219–24.
20. Cohen, S. (1982). Cannabis effects upon adolescent motivation. In *Marijuana and youth: clinical observations on motivation and learning*. National Institute on Drug Abuse, Rockville, MD.
21. Edwards, G. (1983). Psychopathology of a drug experience. *British Journal of Psychiatry*, **143**, 509–12.
22. Newcombe, T. and Bentler, P. (1988). *Consequences of adolescent drug use: impact on the lives of young adults*. Sage, Newbury Park, CA.
23. Fergusson, D. and Horwood, J. (1997). Early onset cannabis use and psychosocial adjustment in young adults. *Addiction*, **92**, 279–96.
24. World Health Organization (1998). *Programme on substance abuse. Cannabis: a health perspective and research agenda*. World Health Organization, Geneva.

4.2.3.9 Patterns of use, epidemiology, adverse effects, and specific issues concerning treatment for nicotine dependence

Martin Jarvis

Introduction

Cigarette smoking is perhaps the most prevalent form of drug dependence in the world, and certainly the most lethal, eventually killing one in every two persisting users. Tobacco is notorious for the tenacious hold it has on smokers, and nicotine is now regarded by many as the purest pharmacological dependence, the very paradigm of drug addiction. Yet for years cigarette smoking was widely regarded as no more than a social habit and there was little awareness that it delivered a psychoactive drug. At usual dose levels, nicotine does not intoxicate or impair motor or cognitive performance or the ability to interact socially in an appropriate way. It does not induce violence. As a result, it is the most mundane, almost invisible, drug dependence. It presents numerous other paradoxes as well. Nicotine is a stimulant drug which users say calms them down and sedates. Smoking is often viewed as a form of self-medication to cope with stress, but there is little evidence that nicotine possesses any anxiolytic or antidepressant properties. Unlike the case of alcohol, cigarette smoking is usually seen as having little bearing on psychopathology, yet in the general population it is far more strongly associated with adverse mood states and with both neurotic and psychotic disorders.[1] The past decade has seen considerable progress in understanding the neurochemical basis of nicotine's effects and in the development of effective behavioural and pharmacological interventions to promote cessation. Despite this, there is little room for optimism. Worldwide both prevalence and deaths from tobacco continue to increase, and are likely to continue to do so for the foreseeable future.

Patterns of smoking prevalence worldwide

While tobacco use has a long history, with forms such as pipe and cigar smoking, chewing tobacco, and nasal snuff predominating in earlier periods, the manufactured cigarette is essentially a phenomenon of the twentieth century. Annual per capita consumption of cigarettes in adults in developed countries rose steadily from 600 in 1920 to a peak of over 3000 in the mid-1970s, but is now declining.[2] Conversely, in developing countries consumption is increasing sharply. On current trends, per adult consumption in developing countries will exceed that of developed countries shortly after the turn of the century.

Recent World Health Organization estimates show that among men, worldwide smoking prevalence, at 47 per cent, approaches one half of all adults, with particularly high levels in China and in the former socialist countries of Eastern Europe.[2] Globally, women's smoking is at much lower levels (12 per cent), with relatively high prevalence being seen in developed countries and low rates in Africa,

India, China, and other parts of Asia where cultural traditions still frown on female smoking. In countries such as the United States and the United Kingdom where awareness of the health risks is widespread and there have been antismoking policies in place for many years, one-quarter to one-third of adults of both sexes still smoke. Overall the size of the world market continues to increase.

Smoking as a cause of death

Deaths from smoking show a time lag of about 30 to 40 years from the onset of regular smoking. As a result, differing patterns of smoking-related deaths are currently seen in men and women and in the developed and developing worlds. In the United Kingdom, male deaths from smoking are now declining, while in women deaths are increasing and will continue to do so for some years, despite prevalence peaking in the early 1970s.[3]

As at 1995, an estimated 2 million people (1.5 million men and 500 000 women) in developed countries were dying each year from tobacco. About 25 per cent of all male deaths, and 9 per cent of female deaths, in developed countries are currently due to smoking. Smoking-related deaths in the developing world, at present about 1 million per year, are certain to increase sharply in the next two decades. Total deaths worldwide from smoking are estimated to increase to 10 million per year by about 2025. Most of these deaths will be in the developing world.[4]

Diseases caused by smoking

Based on the 20-year follow-up of the British doctors' cohort, it was concluded that a young man who persists in smoking will run a 1 in 4 chance of being killed prematurely by tobacco. More recent studies, including the 40-year follow-up of the British doctors[5] and the second large study of the American Cancer Society[6] have forced a re-evaluation of the extent of the risk. It is now apparent that persistent smokers run a 1 in 2 risk of being killed by cigarettes, losing on average 8 years of life.

Smoking causes some 30 per cent of deaths from cancer, the great bulk of deaths from chronic respiratory disease, and is a major contributor to circulatory diseases. Table 1 summarizes data from the American Cancer Society study of over 1 million men and women aged 35 years and over, giving mortality in cigarette smokers and lifelong non-smokers for the main fatal smoking-related diseases.[6] Smoking is recognized to cause 80 per cent or more of all lung cancers. In addition it is responsible for most cancers of the upper respiratory tract (lip, tongue, mouth, pharynx, and larynx) and for a smaller fraction of cancers of the bladder, pancreas, oesophagus, and kidney. Among both men and women, deaths from cardiovascular disease (ischaemic heart disease, aortic aneurysm, and stroke) outnumber those from all other causes, including lung cancer. Over 70 per cent of chronic obstructive lung disease is attributable to smoking. Findings from the British doctors' study[5] additionally indicate a causal effect of smoking on stomach cancer and leukaemia. Associations between smoking and a number of other diseases including cervical cancer, cirrhosis of the liver, suicide, poisoning, and cancer of the liver have been regarded as being due to confounding.[5]

As well as being the single largest cause of preventable premature

Table 1 Fatal diseases associated with smoking: men and women aged over 35 years (standardized mortality per 100 000 per year)

		Lifelong non-smoker	Current cigarette smoker	Relative risk	Absolute excess risk per 100 000 per year	Attributable (%)
Cancer						
Lung	M	24	537	22.4	513	87
	F	18	213	11.9	195	77
Upper respiratory	M	1	27	24.5	26	89
	F	2	10	5.6	8	58
Bladder	M	18	53	2.9	35	36
	F	8	21	2.6	13	32
Pancreas	M	18	38	2.1	20	25
	F	16	37	2.3	21	29
Oesophagus	M	9	68	7.6	59	66
	F	4	41	10.3	37	74
Kidney	M	8	23	3.0	15	37
	F	6	8	1.4	2	11
Ischaemic heart disease	M	500	970	1.9	470	22
	F	386	688	1.8	302	19
Aortic aneurysm	M	24	98	4.1	74	48
	F	11	52	4.6	41	52
Stroke	M	147	328	2.2	181	27
	F	236	434	1.8	198	20
Chronic obstructive	M	39	378	9.7	339	72
lung disease	F	21	216	10.5	195	74
All diseases	M	788	2520	3.2	1732	40
	F	708	1720	2.4	1012	30

Data from American Cancer Society (CPS II).

death, cigarette smoking is a cause of a number of disabling but generally non-fatal conditions.[7] These include peripheral vascular disease, cataracts, Crohn's disease, gastric and duodenal ulcers, hip fracture in elderly people, and periodontitis, the major cause of tooth loss in adults. Breathing other people's smoke also causes a significant burden of disease in non-smokers, especially infants and children.

Smoking in pregnancy

Smoking is an important hazard in pregnancy, leading to an increased risk of spontaneous abortion and doubling the risk of ectopic pregnancy. Babies of smoking mothers weigh on average 150 to 250 g less at birth than babies of non-smoking mothers. Smoking by mothers is recognized as a major cause of sudden infant death syndrome.

Cigarette smoking and nicotine dependence

Drug taking aspects of cigarette smoking were largely ignored until the 1970s, but since then an accumulation of research findings from a variety of disciplines and from both human and animal work has led to a consensus that cigarette smoking is essentially a form of addiction to nicotine.[8] Understanding of nicotine's role is fundamental to an appreciation of smoking uptake, maintenance, and cessation. It does not follow that cigarette smoking is explicable solely in terms of pharmacological factors. Nicotine effects provide a rich substrate for conditioning and social learning mechanisms, and for broad social, economic, and societal influences. In this respect it is no different from other drug dependencies.

The evidence relevant to nicotine's properties as an addictive drug comes from a number of areas.[9,10] Some of the main lines of evidence are briefly summarized here.

Brain neurochemistry

A variety of cholinergic receptors sensitive to nicotine are present in the brain. Both animal and human studies have shown that chronic nicotine administration leads to an increase in the expression of specific nicotine receptors on neurones.[11] Investigations of brain systems thought to be important in reward mechanisms have shown effects of nicotine on dopamine release similar to those of cocaine.[12,13]

Animal self-administration

Under appropriate schedules of reinforcement nicotine functions as a robust primary reinforcer[14,15] in a variety of animal species. 'Knockout' mice lacking the β_2-subunit of the high affinity nicotinic cholinergic receptor do not show dopamine release in response to nicotine administration and are insensitive to nicotine rewards under contingencies where intact animals self-administer readily.[16]

Pharmacokinetics

Nicotine is absorbed through the skin, and through the lining of the mouth and nose, the rate of absorption being enhanced in an alkaline environment and reduced in an acidic environment. Because of the large surface area of the lungs the mildly acidic smoke of cigarettes is absorbed almost immediately and completely on inhalation, giving rise to high concentration arterial nicotine boli which reach the brain in less than 10 s.[17] Nicotine has a distributional half-life of about 15 min and a terminal half-life in blood of about 2 h.[18] This means that blood levels decline overnight to non-smoking levels, and regular cigarettes are required over the course of the day to maintain elevated blood nicotine concentrations. About 70 to 80 per cent of nicotine is metabolized to cotinine, which has a half-life of around 16 h.

Regulation of blood nicotine intake from different tobacco products and from cigarettes with differing deliveries (titration)

Peak blood nicotine levels among cigarette smokers and dependent users of either oral[19] or nasal[20] snuff are remarkably similar, averaging in each case about 35 ng/ml.

Manufactured cigarettes contain 10 to 14 mg of nicotine, an amount that does not vary greatly between brands. But by techniques such as filtration and ventilation, machine-smoked yields of nicotine range from as little as 0.1 mg to over 1 mg, with concomitant tar ranging from 1 to 15 mg or more. The relevance of these machine-smoked yields to human smoking is open to serious question, since smokers extract a similar amount of nicotine (about 1 mg on average) from cigarettes of widely differing yields.[21] Smokers' characteristic tendency to adjust the way they smoke so as to maintain similar nicotine intakes from cigarettes with widely differing deliveries is termed nicotine compensation or titration.[17] A boundary model of nicotine regulation has been proposed, whereby chronic users seek to avoid the adverse effects of either too little (withdrawal) or too much (overdose) nicotine.[22]

Acquisition of nicotine inhalation in novice smokers

Children take up smoking for mainly psychosocial reasons, but studies have shown that pharmacological motives take on importance very early in the smoking career.[23,24] Already by the time they are smoking on a daily basis, children take in as much nicotine from each cigarette as dependent adult smokers.[25]

Compulsive use

Although a few long-term occasional smokers (so-called 'chippers') are found,[26,27] regular daily smoking is the norm. Some 17 per cent of smokers light up their first cigarette within 5 min of waking, and over 50 per cent within 30 min. At least 80 per cent of smokers meet DSM-IV criteria for dependence.[28] Dependent users of alcohol, heroin, and cocaine rate giving up smoking as at least as difficult as their problem drug.[29] Compulsive use is the key feature characterizing nicotine dependence.

Nicotine withdrawal syndrome

Cessation of smoking reliably leads to a variety of signs and symptoms, with an onset within 12 h or less of last tobacco use, and a duration of 3 weeks or longer. The manifestations are predominantly affective in nature, with subjects reporting irritability, difficulty concentrating, anxiety, restlessness, increased hunger, and depressed mood, as well as craving for tobacco. These symptoms are relieved by nicotine replacement but not placebo.[30–34]

The smoking career: patterns of uptake, maintenance, and cessation of smoking

Recruitment of young people to cigarette smoking

Uptake of smoking typically occurs in adolescence, with few people starting to smoke after the age of 20 years.[35,36] In the United Kingdom, about 25 per cent of teenagers smoke by the age of 15 years, with some evidence that at this age (although not among young adults of 16 years of age and above) girls are more likely to smoke than boys. Rates of smoking in young people have shown no decline over the past 15 years in the United Kingdom, and there is evidence that they are currently increasing in the United States.[37,38]

Initiation of smoking is subject to a number of influences: environmental, behavioural, and personal factors all play a part.[24] Environmental influences include parental smoking (approximately doubling the likelihood of a child starting to smoke), and smoking by siblings and friends. Tobacco advertising and promotions effectively target young people with images of smoking as trendy, sporty, and successful.[39–42] Young people from deprived backgrounds where smoking is the norm are more likely to become smokers, an association which becomes accentuated in adulthood, implying that smoking is a marker for social trajectory.

Cigarette smoking is linked with poor school performance, truancy, low aspirations for future success, and early school leaving or drop-out.[24] Smoking in adolescents is frequently associated with other problem behaviours including alcohol and other drug use and other risk taking or rebellious behaviours, as well as with low self-esteem, anxiety, and depression.[43]

School-based interventions to reduce the uptake of smoking by teenagers have shown some initial success, but longer term follow-up has found that these effects dissipate,[44,45] leading researchers to advocate approaches involving the creation of a wider social environment supportive of non-smoking.[46]

Adult smoking: disadvantage and dependence

The most striking feature of the evolution of smoking in developed Western countries over the past 20 years has been the increasing association of cigarettes with markers of disadvantage, whether it be socioeconomic position, or a range of factors indicating stressful living circumstances.[47] High rates of smoking are seen in the unemployed, lone parents, people who are divorced or separated, the homeless (United Kingdom Office of Population Censuses and Surveys), heavy drinkers,[47] drug users (United Kingdom Office of Population Censuses and Surveys), and prisoners.[48] Cigarette smoking is strongly associated with psychiatric illness, whether it be schizophrenia,[49,50] depressive illness,[51] or a variety of other neurotic disorders.[1] The association of cigarettes with lowered levels of psychological well being is not confined to those with a formal psychiatric diagnosis, but extends also into the general population of smokers.[52,53] Between 1973 and 1994 rates of smoking among affluent people halved in the United Kingdom, but among the poorest groups prevalence remained unchanged at close to 70 per cent.[54]

Treatments to promote cessation

The proportion of ever-smokers who have given up varies greatly by factors such as age, socioeconomic status, and dependence,[54] as well as by country. Only about 1 per cent of Chinese smokers have quit,[55] against nearly 50 per cent of American and United Kingdom ever-smokers. In most instances, smokers who quit do so without any formal help, other than the support of family and friends. But the success rate from a single unaided quit attempt is low, with about 1 per cent remaining abstinent 1 year later.[54] Research into treatment methods to enhance rates of cessation has been very actively pursued over the past two decades and is now bearing fruit in the form of well-validated protocols for both intensive clinic-based approaches and interventions in primary care. Evidence-based clinical practice guidelines have been issued in the United States[56] and the United Kingdom[57] emphasizing both the availability of efficacious and cost-effective treatments, and the need for health professionals to incorporate simple interventions into their routine practice of medicine. The recommended approaches have two underlying themes: the value of pharmacological aids to cessation, and the need for a public health model which ensures that cost-effective interventions are delivered to the bulk of the smoking population rather than to the minority who seek specialized help. Table 2 summarizes recommendations on the key elements of effective interventions by non-specialists from the Agency for Health Care Policy and Research Guidelines.[56]

Brief advice from health professionals

Randomized trials have clearly established the value of brief advice from general practitioners, dentists, and others to their smoking patients.[58] Such advice does not require specialist training, can be given in the doctor's own words, and need take no more than a few minutes of face-to-face contact. Its effect is to motivate more cessation attempts rather than to give any specific help in overcoming withdrawal. The Cochrane Collaboration estimates the increment in successful cessation from such interventions to be 2 per cent. While this may seem low, its value from a public health perspective is that it offers the possibility to reach the 70 per cent or more of smokers who consult a health professional each year.

Nicotine replacement therapy

The rationale for nicotine replacement therapy is that many of the difficulties of cessation stem from problems posed by nicotine withdrawal. Numerous experimental and clinical studies have shown that nicotine replacement therapy reliably attenuates the severity of withdrawal, thereby making it easier for would-be ex-smokers to cope with

Table 2 Recommendations for smoking interventions

Action	Strategies for implementation
Ask about smoking status at every visit and document	Include in vital signs, use stickers on patient's notes, or implement computerized reminder system
Advise all smokers to quit, in a clear, strong, and personalized manner	'Quitting smoking is the most important thing you can do to protect your health' Tie smoking to current illness or impact on children and family
Identify smokers willing to make a quit attempt at this time	If willing, provide assistance (see below) If patient prefers more intensive help or if it is indicated, refer to specialist If unwilling, provide motivational intervention

Assist smoker with a quit plan	Set a quit date
	 Help prepare smoker for quitting
	   Inform family and friends
	   Prepare the environment (discard cigarettes)
	   Review previous quit attempts
	   Anticipate challenges

NRT	Encourage use of NRT unless contraindicated
Give key advice	Total abstinence: 'Not a single puff' Avoid alcohol Other smokers in household: consider quitting with others or make specific plans for maintaining abstinence among smokers
Provide supplementary materials	Booklets etc., culturally, educationally, and age appropriate for the smoker
Arrange follow-up in person or by telephone	First follow-up within 1 week of quit date, second within a month; at follow-up, congratulate success, or use lapses for constructive learning, elicit recommitment to total abstinence, identify problems, anticipate challenges, assess use of NRT

NRT, nicotine replacement therapy.
Adapted from the Agency for Health Care Policy and Research smoking cessation guidelines.[56]

abstinence while unlearning the deeply ingrained habit elements of smoking.

Nicotine replacement products are available in a number of forms, including gum, transdermal patch, nasal spray, lozenge, and inhaler. The various forms of nicotine replacement therapy differ in terms of route of administration and speed of absorption, as well as in the extent to which they offer a situational response to craving and a behavioural ritual to replace the rituals of cigarette smoking. None give the high concentration arterial bolus of nicotine characteristic of cigarette smoking, and the overall dose of nicotine they provide is typically only one-third to one-half of that from cigarettes. This, coupled with the absence of toxic tar and gas phase components of cigarette smoke, gives them a reassuring safety profile.

Randomized trials have established that all forms of nicotine replacement therapy are effective aids to cessation, on average close to doubling the chances of a quit attempt succeeding.[59] There is currently no reliable evidence that any one form of nicotine replacement therapy stands out as more effective than the others, which means that choice of product will depend more on features such as ease of compliance with recommended dosing (the skin patch has a particular advantage here) and on availability. There is some evidence for dose response with either combinations of different nicotine replacement therapy products or higher dosages giving better outcomes. The efficacy of nicotine replacement therapy appears to be largely independent of other elements of treatment: although absolute success rates are higher with more intensive behavioural support, the effect of nicotine replacement therapy in doubling the chance of quitting is found in brief interventions and over-the-counter settings as well as in specialized smokers' clinics. This feature gives nicotine replacement therapy an important role in public health approaches aimed at reaching the bulk of the smoking population.

Non-nicotine pharmacological treatments

Many other drugs to aid smoking cessation have been tested, but most have so far failed to yield evidence of efficacy (including most anxiolytics and antidepressants that have been tested), while in others such as clonidine signs of promise have been offset by an unacceptable side-effect profile. Recently, the drug bupropion, an atypical antidepressant with some noradrenergic and dopaminergic activity, became the first non-nicotine medicine licensed for smoking cessation in the United States, Canada, and Mexico. The mechanism of action appears not to be related to the drug's antidepressant effect but rather to pathways common to addiction. Clinical trials, among non-depressed smokers, have shown clear advantage over placebo,[60] and there is evidence that bupropion and the nicotine skin patch have additive effects in enhancing outcomes.[61]

References

1. Meltzer, H., Gill, B., Pettigrew, M., and Hinds, K. (1995). *The prevalence of psychiatric morbidity among adults living in private households.* OPCS Surveys of Psychiatric Morbidity in Great Britain. Her Majesty's Stationery Office, London.
2. Collishaw, N.E. and Lopez, A.D. (1996). *The tobacco epidemic: a public health emergency.* World Health Organization (WHO) Tobacco Alert. WHO, Geneva.
3. Peto, R., Lopez, A.D., Boreham, J., Thun, M., Heath, C., and Doll, R. (1996). Mortality from smoking worldwide. *British Medical Bulletin*, **52**, 12–21.
4. Peto, R., Lopez, A.D., Boreham, J., Thun, M., and Heath, C. (1994). *Mortality from smoking in developed countries 1950–2000: indirect estimates from national vital statistics.* Oxford University Press.
5. Doll, R., Peto, R., Wheatley, K., Gray, R., and Sutherland, I. (1994). Mortality in relation to smoking: 40 years' observations on male British doctors. *British Medical Journal*, **309**, 901–11.
6. Thun, M.J., Day-Lally, C.A., Calle, E.E., Flanders, W.D., and Heath, C.W. (1995). Excess mortality among cigarette smokers: changes in a 20-year interval. *American Journal of Public Health*, **85**, 1223–30.
7. Wald, N.J. and Hacksaw, A.K. (1996). Cigarette smoking: an epidemiological overview. *British Medical Bulletin*, **52**, 3–11.
8. US Department of Health and Human Services (1988). *The health consequences of smoking: nicotine addiction. A report of the Surgeon General.* DHSS Publication No. (CDC) 88-8406. US Government Printing Office, Washington, DC.
9. Stolerman, I.P. and Jarvis, M.J. (1995). The scientific case that nicotine is addictive. *Psychopharmacology*, **117**, 2–10.
10. Henningfield, J.E. and Keenan, R.M. (1993). The anatomy of nicotine addiction. *Health Values*, **17**, 12–19.
11. Benwell, M.E.M., Balfour, D.J.K., and Anderson, J.M. (1988). Evidence that tobacco smoking increases the density of (-)- (3H)nicotine binding sites in human brain. *Journal of Neurochemistry*, **50**, 1243–7.
12. Pontieri, F.E., Tanda, G., and Orzi, F.G.D. (1996). Effects of nicotine on the nucleus accumbens and similarity to those of addictive drugs. *Nature*, **382**, 255–7.
13. Pich, E.M., Pagliusi, S.R., Tessari, M., Talabot-Ayer, D., Hooft van Huisduijnen, R., and Chiamulera, C. (1997). Common neural substrates for the addictive properties of nicotine and cocaine. *Science*, **275**(5296), 83–6.
14. Spealman, R.D. and Goldberg, S.R. (1982). Maintenance of schedule-controlled behavior by intravenous injections of nicotine in squirrel monkeys. *Journal of Pharmacology and Experimental Therapeutics*, **223**, 402–8.
15. Corrigall, W.A. and Coen, K.M. (1989). Nicotine maintains robust self-administration in rats on a limited-access schedule. *Psychopharmacology*, **99**, 473–8.
16. Picciotto, M.R., Zoll, M., Rimondini, R., *et al.* (1998). Acetylcholine receptors containing the B2 subunit are involved in the reinforcing properties of nicotine. *Nature*, **391**, 173–7.
17. Russell, M.A.H. (1980). Nicotine intake and its regulation. *Journal of Psychosomatic Research*, **24**, 253–64.
18. Benowitz, N.L. (1988). Pharmacologic aspects of cigarette smoking and nicotine addiction. *New England Journal of Medicine*, **319**, 1318–30.
19. Holm, H., Jarvis, M.J., Russell, M.A.H., and Feyerabend, C. (1992). Nicotine intake and dependence in Swedish snuff takers. *Psychopharmacology*, **108**, 507–11.
20. Russell, M.A.H., Jarvis, M.J., Devitt, G., and Feyerabend, C. (1981). Nicotine intake by snuff users. *British Medical Journal*, **283**(6295), 814–17.
21. Benowitz, N.L., Hall, S.M., Herning, R.I., Jacob, P., Jones, R.T., and Osman, A.-L. (1983). Smokers of low-yield cigarettes do not consume less nicotine. *New England Journal of Medicine*, **309**, 139–42.
22. Kozlowski, L.T. and Herman, C.P. (1984). The interaction of psychosocial and biological determinants of tobacco use: more on the boundary model. *Journal of Applied Social Psychology*, **14**, 244–56.
23. McNeill, A.D. (1991). The development of dependence on smoking in children. *British Journal of Addiction*, **86**, 589–92.
24. Lynch, B.S. and Bonnie, R.J. (ed.) (1994). *Growing up tobacco free: preventing nicotine addiction in children and youths.* National Academy Press, Washington, DC.
25. McNeill, A.D., Jarvis, M.J., Stapleton, J.A., West, R.J., and Bryant, A. (1989). Nicotine intake in young smokers: longitudinal study of saliva cotinine concentrations. *American Journal of Public Health*, **79**, 172–5.
26. Shiffman, S. (1989). Tobacco 'chippers'. Individual differences in tobacco dependence. *Psychopharmacology*, **97**, 539–47.
27. Evans, N.J., Gilpin, E., Pierce, J.P., *et al.* (1992). Occasional smoking among adults: evidence from the California Tobacco Survey. *Tobacco Control*, **1**, 169–75.
28. Woody, G.E., Cottler, L.B., and Cacciola, J. (1993). Severity of dependence: data from the DSM-IV field trials. *Addiction*, **88**, 1573–9.
29. Kozlowski, L.T., Wilkinson, A., Skinner, W., Kent, C., Franklin, T., and Pope, M. (1989). Comparing tobacco cigarette dependence with other drug dependencies. Greater or equal 'difficulty quitting' and 'urges to use', but less 'pleasure' from cigarettes. *Journal of the American Medical Association*, **261**, 898–901.

30. Jarvis, M.J., Raw, M., Russell, M.A.H., and Feyerabend, C. (1982). Randomised controlled trial of nicotine chewing-gum. *British Medical Journal*, **285**, 537–40.

31. West, R.J., Jarvis, M.J., Russell, M.A.H., *et al.* (1984). Effect of nicotine replacement on the cigarette withdrawal syndrome. *British Journal of Addiction*, **79**, 215–19.

32. Gross, J. and Stitzer, M.L. (1989). Nicotine replacement: 10-week effects on tobacco withdrawal symptoms. *Psychopharmacology*, **98**, 334–41.

33. Sutherland, G., Russell, M.A.H., Stapleton, J., Feyerabend, C., and Ferno, O. (1992). Nasal nicotine spray: a rapid nicotine delivery system. *Psychopharmacology*, **108**, 512–18.

34. Russell, M.A.H., Stapleton, J.A., Feyerabend, C., *et al.* (1993). Targeting heavy smokers in general practice: randomised controlled trial of transdermal nicotine patches. *British Medical Journal*, **306**, 1308–12.

35. Kessler, D.A. (1995). Nicotine addiction in young people. *New England Journal of Medicine*, **333**, 186–9.

36. Kessler, D.A., Barnett, P.S., Witt, A., Zeller, M.R., Mande, J.R., and Schultz, W.B. (1997). The legal and scientific basis for the FDA's assertion of jurisdiction over cigarettes and smokeless tobacco. *Journal of the American Medical Association*, **277**, 405–9.

37. Glynn, T.J., Greenwald, P., Mills, S.M., and Manley, M.W. (1993). Youth tobacco use in the United States—problem, progress, goals, and potential solutions. *Preventive Medicine*, **22**, 568–75.

38. Giovino, G.A., Henningfield, J.E., Tomar, S.L., Escobedo, L.G., and Slade, J. (1995). Epidemiology of tobacco use and dependence. *Epidemiologic Reviews*, **17**, 48–65.

39. Wills, T.A., Pierce, J.P., and Evans, R.I. (1996). Large-scale environmental risk-factors for substance use. *American Behavioral Scientist*, **39**, 808–22.

40. Altman, D.G., Levine, D.W., Coeytaux, R., Slade, J., and Jaffe, R. (1996). Tobacco promotion and susceptibility to tobacco use among adolescents aged 12 through 17 years in a nationally representative sample. *American Journal of Public Health*, **86**, 1590–3.

41. Pollay, R.W., Siddarth, S., Siegel, M., *et al.* (1996). The last straw—cigarette advertising and realized market shares among youths and adults, 1979–1993. *Journal of Marketing*, **60**, 1–16.

42. DiFranza, J.R., Richards, J. Jr, Paulman, P.M., *et al.* (1991). RJR Nabisco's cartoon camel promotes Camel cigarettes to children. *Journal of the American Medical Association*, **266**, 3149–53.

43. Breslau, N., Kilbey, M.M., and Andreski, P. (1993). Nicotine dependence and major depression: new evidence from a prospective investigation. *Archives of General Psychiatry*, **50**, 31–5.

44. Flay, B.R., Koepke, D., Thomson, S.J., Santi, S., Best, J.A., and Brown, K.S. (1989). Six-year follow-up of the first Waterloo school smoking prevention trial. *American Journal of Public Health*, **79**, 1371–6.

45. Nutbeam, D., Macaskill, P., Smith, C., Simpson, J.M., and Catford, J. (1993). Evaluation of two school smoking education programmes under normal classroom conditions. *British Medical Journal*, **306**, 102–7.

46. Flay, B.R. (1985). What we know about the social influences approach to smoking prevention: review and recommendations. *NIDA Research Monograph Series*, **63**, 67–112.

47. Jarvis, M.J. (1994). A profile of tobacco smoking. *Addiction*, **89**, 1371–6.

48. Bridgwood, A. and Malbon, G. (1995). *Survey of the physical health of prisoners*. HMSO, London.

49. Hughes, J.R., Regier, D.A., Farmer, M.E., *et al.* (1991). Comorbidity of mental disorders and nicotine dependence. 2. *Journal of the American Medical Association*, **265**, 1256–7.

50. De Leon, J., Dadvand, M., Canuso, C., White, A.O., Stanilla, J.K., and Simpson, G.M. (1995). Schizophrenia and smoking: an epidemiological survey in a state hospital. *American Journal of Psychiatry*, **152**, 453–5.

51. Glassman, A.H. (1993). Cigarette smoking: implications for psychiatric illness. *American Journal of Psychiatry*, **150**, 546–53.

52. Schoenborn, C.A. and Horm, J. (1993). *Negative moods as correlates of smoking and heavier drinking: implications for health promotion*. Advance Data from Vital and Health Statistics. National Center for Health Statistics, Hyattsville, MD.

53. Anda, R.F., Williamson, D.F., Escobedo, L.G., Mast, E.E., Giovino, G.A., and Remington, P.L. (1990). Depression and the dynamics of smoking: a national perspective. *Journal of the American Medical Association*, **264**, 1541–5.

54. Jarvis, M.J. (1997). Patterns and predictors of unaided smoking cessation in the general population. In *Progress in respiratory research*. Vol. 28, *The tobacco epidemic* (ed. C.T. Bolliger and K.O. Fagerstrom), pp. 151–64. Karger, Basel.

55. Liu, B.Q., Peto, R., Chen, Z.-M., *et al.* (1998). Emerging tobacco hazards in China. 1. Retrospective proportional mortality study of 1 million deaths. *British Medical Journal*, **317**, 1411–22.

56. Fiore, M.C., Bailey, W.C., Cohen, S.J., *et al.* (1996). *Smoking cessation*. Clinical Practice Guideline No. 18. US Department of Health and Human Services, Agency for Health Care Policy and Research, Rockville, MD.

57. Raw, M., McNeill, A., and West, R.J. (1998). *Smoking cessation guidelines for health professionals*. Health Education Authority, London.

58. Silagy, C. and Ketteridge, S. (ed.) (1997). *The effectiveness of physician advice to aid smoking cessation*. Cochrane Database of Systematic Reviews, updated 3 June 1997. Update Software, Oxford.

59. Silagy, C., Mant, D., Fowler, G., and Lancaster, T. (1997). The effect of nicotine replacement therapy on smoking cessation. In *The tobacco addiction module of the Cochrane Database of Systematic Reviews* (ed. T. Lancaster, C. Silagy, and D. Fullerton). Cochrane Collaboration, Oxford.

60. Hurt, R.D., Sachs, D.P.L., Glover, E.D., *et al.* (1997). A comparison of sustained-release bupropion and placebo for smoking cessation. *New England Journal of Medicine*, **337**, 1195–202.

61. Jorenby, D.E., Leischow, S.J., Nides, M.A., *et al.* (1999). A controlled trial of sustained-release bupropion, a nicotine patch, or both for smoking cessation. *New England Journal of Medicine*, **340**, 685–91.

4.2.4 Assessing need and organizing services for drug misusers

John Marsden and John Strang

Introduction

In this chapter a general account is presented of ways of conceptualizing and assessing the extent and nature of drug misuse problems in a population, together with approaches that may be adopted by treatment service organizations seeking to meet the treatment needs of this population. The drug misuse treatment population is heterogeneous and specific treatment issues relevant to certain groups are noted at different points during the discussion. Inter-organizational and operational issues in a locality are the main focus, rather than intra-organizational development and delivery issues. An epidemiological perspective is used to conceptualize and describe population needs for effective treatment services in the context of local health and social care service commissioning arrangements and structures.[1]

Size and nature of the problem

There is considerable concern about illicit drugs and an international commitment to reducing demand for these products.[2,3] This policy is hampered by considerable imprecision about the number of people using illicit drugs and the number of people who experience problems.

Estimates suggest a global annual population prevalence rate for illicit drug use of between 3 and 4 percent, with a modest decline over recent years. In particular, the global population totals for the use of heroin and cocaine are estimated at approximately 8 million and 13.3 million adults respectively.[4]

In the United Kingdom there have been no representative national population surveys focusing exclusively on drug use. However, the latest British Crime Survey of almost 11 000 participants aged 16 to 59 in England and Wales has provided valuable data on the prevalence of illicit drug use.[5] Lifetime prevalence estimates from the British Crime Survey are as follows: cannabis, 22 per cent; amphetamines, 9 per cent; cocaine hydrochloride, 3 per cent; crack cocaine and heroin, 1 per cent. Six per cent of the sample were defined as current users of any drug (having used in the month prior to interview), with the majority reporting cannabis use. Prevalence rates for drug use vary considerably by age grouping and other factors such as unemployment. For example, approximately 50 per cent of young people sampled between the ages of 16 and 24 years have tried an illicit drug on at least one occasion.[5,6] Figures for lifetime cocaine use are 2 per cent for 16- to 19-year-olds and 6 per cent for 20- to 24-year-olds. Data collected in the United States in 1997 suggest that across the total household population over 12 years old, some 13.9 million people are current users of any illicit drug ('current use' is again defined as use in the month prior to interview).[7] The most widely used substance in the United States is cannabis (11.1 million users), and approximately 1.5 million are thought to be current cocaine users. Rates of heroin use are significantly lower, with estimates of approximately 325 000 current users.

Turning to the nature of the treatment population, data from the United States suggested that cocaine problems account for 43 per cent of all admissions, heroin for 22 per cent of admissions, and cannabis for 18 per cent.[3] In contrast, in the United Kingdom heroin is currently the main substance used amongst people seeking treatment. The Home Office's *Addicts Index* (now discontinued) reported some 43 372 individuals in treatment in 1996, a figure nearly double the reported total from 5 years earlier, while the number of drug users reported to the Department of Health in the same year who had attended treatment services was 24 879 for the previous 6 months, a figure some 48 per cent higher than the corresponding figure for 1993.[2]

Course of drug use disorders

Both the causes and diffusion of problematic drug use are uncertain. Susceptibility to drug use is highest amongst young people, with most individuals embarking on their drug using careers before the age of 20. Drug use is also associated with social and economic deprivation and some individuals, particularly those dependent on opiate and stimulant drugs, may become involved in crime to support their dependence. In the United Kingdom, police surveillance estimates suggest that half of all recorded crime is drug related, with associated costs to the criminal justice system estimated to be £1 billion per annum.[2] The putative link between crime and drug use may also be related to lifestyle aspects of criminality which lead individuals to become deviant in other areas[8] and as a cultural fact of life in areas of economic and social deprivation.[9,10]

It is important to recognize that illicit drug use does not inevitably result in problems and people who do experience problems are not a homogenous group.[11] Studies of the natural history of drug use have made an important contribution to our understanding of how illicit

drug use and dependence is initiated, maintained and terminated. Recovery may be apparently spontaneous and many individuals stop using because of a need to change their lifestyles or because of perceived external pressures, responsibilities, and revised outlooks.[12,13] Nevertheless, for a substantial minority of users, drug use may become problematic and continue for many years, and they will require treatment and rehabilitation. Reflecting the chronic relapsing nature of an illicit drug-oriented lifestyle, many individuals develop a treatment 'career' profile alongside their drug use 'career'.

Assessing and diagnosing drug use disorders

A thorough assessment of a drug use disorder spans personal demographic features, health status, health symptoms, and social functioning considerations together with an appraisal of the specific psychological and social functions which drug use serves the individual.[14] Specific drug-related harms range from minor adverse physical or psychological morbidities which are directly induced by an illicit substance, to acute and chronic health disorders (e.g. circulatory problems) or overdose and death. In addition to assessing the harm arising from drug use itself, the potential of contagion and transmission of HIV infection and other blood-borne diseases has made it important to assess specific risk behaviours (e.g. sharing of drug injection equipment; non-condom penetrative sexual intercourse). The assessment of psychiatric comorbidity should also be considered when conducting assessment. The improvement in psychiatric symptoms is an important treatment goal, but their nature, sequelae, and course amongst this population remains under-researched.

Dependence and abuse criteria

Two core concepts relevant to assessment are 'dependence' and 'abuse' (or 'hazardous use'). Based on the original concept of alcohol dependence, illicit drug dependence is incorporated within both the ICD-10 and the DSM-IV.[15,16] The ICD and DSM classifications include diagnostic criteria which view impairment of control over drug use and negative consequences as primary problems. ICD-10 seeks to provide diagnostic guidelines which distinguish a range of disorders that vary on severity of intoxication, hazardous, harmful use, and dependence dimensions. ICD-10 also makes a distinction between harmful use (discernible psychological and/or physical health damage to an individual) and dependence. DSM diagnoses 'abuse' of a particular substance following the endorsement of one or more of the following: use leading to neglect of personal, social, or occupational roles; use in an unsafe or dangerous situation; use leading to repeated problems with the law; and continued use despite relationship, domestic, occupation, or educational problems. Table 1 shows a brief interviewer- or self-administered screening questionnaire which can be used to establish both ICD and DSM diagnoses in addition to an indication of the severity of dependence.

The questionnaire can be separately administered for different classes of illicit substance. There are two possible ways to score the scale. First, one point is given to each item that is experienced by the client during the past 12 months (i.e. a report of 'once or twice' or

Table 1 DSM/ICD-compatible drug-dependence screening questions

In the past 12 months:

(a) How often did you have a strong or persistent desire or compulsion to use [named drug, e.g. heroin]?

(b) Did you have difficulty in cutting down or controlling how often or how much [named drug] you used?

(c) Did you need to use an increased amount of [named drug] to achieve a desired effect?

(d) Did you find that [named drug] had less of an effect when continuing to use the same amount?

(e) How often did you feel sick or unwell when the effects of [named drug] had worn off?

(f) How often did you take more [named drug] or a similar drug to relieve or avoid withdrawal symptoms?

(g) How often did you use [named drug] in larger amounts or for a longer period of time than you intended?

(h) How often did you take large amounts of time either getting or using or recovering from its effects?

(i) Did you find that [named drug] has led you to neglect/have problems at home or work, or socially?

(j) Did you continue to use [named drug] despite having problems with your use?

Responses to items (b), (c), (d), (i), and (j) are assessed as follows: no = 0 or yes = 1. Responses to items (a), (e), (f), (g), and (h) are assessed with the following scale: no = 0; once or twice = 1; 3–5 times = 2; once every 2 months = 3; monthly = 4; 2–3 times a month = 5; once a week = 6; 2–3 times a week = 7; 4–6 times a week = 8; every day or almost every day = 9.

more often). ICD/DSM dependence is then diagnosed if

$$a + b + (c \text{ or } d) + (e \text{ or } f) + g + h + i + j \geq 3.$$

Secondly, scoring some items using the weights zero to 9 (see footnote to Table 1) yields a severity profile for appropriate symptoms for each type of substance assessed. The latter scoring method reflects the conceptualization of dependence as existing in degrees of severity and is a useful measure for research. The precise wording of each question may be altered for each substance (e.g. providing examples of substance-specific withdrawal phenomena, such as sweating, shakes/tremor, anxiety, etc.).

Several standardized screening questionnaires for routine use of certain aspects of drug abuse and dependence are also available including the brief Severity of Dependency Scale,[17] the Drug Abuse Screening Test,[18] and the Drug Use Screening Inventory.[19] Various biological screening procedures for drugs and their metabolites in samples of urine, blood, hair, and saliva may also be used.[20]

Needs groups and the aims of treatment

The development and organization of treatment services to respond to drug use is ideally based on a thorough understanding of the nature of problems which arise to the individual, his or her family and the wider community. Consequently, treatment responses to drug use disorders have three general aims: to reduce the risks and harms that drug use causes both the user and others; to stabilize and reduce illicit drug consumption; and to facilitate abstinence and promote the rehabilitation and reintegration of drug users into society. In planning for an integrated and effective treatment response, a target population's needs in relation to drug use disorders can be defined as that population's ability to benefit from services and treatments shown or considered to be effective.[1]

It is helpful to identify several different types of individual who may be in need of treatment. The following categories may overlap to a considerable extent, but will be considered in turn: the dependent user, the injector, the user in withdrawal, the recovering dependent user, the user with comorbidity, and the intoxicated user. Other factors will interact with these groups, including gender, age, ethnicity, and socio-economic status.

The dependent user

Numerically, individuals who meet the diagnostic criteria for dependence on one or more illicit psychoactive drugs constitute a major treatment group. In the drug misuse field there has been little study of early intervention treatments for non-dependent users, and specialist treatment services remain oriented to the needs of individuals with illicit heroin and other opiate dependence. It is common for this group to have concurrent problems with other illicit drugs and/or alcohol. Management of drug dependence may be discrete and commonly involves several stages with treatments delivered by one or more providers across community and residential settings. For heroin dependence, opioid substitution using oral methadone hydrochloride in either a reducing or a maintenance regimen is the most widely delivered and evaluated community treatment,[21–23] although there are still many countries in which methadone is entirely unavailable or in which such maintenance programmes are not acceptable.

Treatment services must also deal with dependence on other drugs. An increase in cocaine distribution and prevalence in the United Kingdom since the late 1980s has been accompanied by growing concerns to ensure that services can respond to the treatment needs of dependent cocaine users.[24] Internationally, several psychological treatments for cocaine dependence have been developed, with encouraging results from cognitive–behavioural, relapse prevention, cue-exposure therapy, and contingency reinforcement therapies.[25–27] Substantial effort in the United States has also been devoted to the development of anti-cocaine drug medications (e.g. selegeline) and pharmacotherapies to minimize cocaine withdrawal. Tricyclic antidepressants (notably desipramine) and selective serotonin reuptake inhibitors (such as fluoxetine) have been evaluated but equivocal results have been obtained from several clinical trials.[28]

Consumption of another common illicit stimulant, amphetamine, is also rising in the United Kingdom and internationally.[29] In the United Kingdom there is evidence that the prescription of dexamphetamine sulphate is quite widely undertaken by physicians in the treatment of dependent users.[30] However, there is currently only the most limited research evidence base for treatments for dependent amphetamine users. Contemporary treatment approaches combine counselling, health care for physical and psychological symptoms, and substitution prescribing.[31]

The provision of psychosocial treatments (counselling and support) for dependent users (and for users in recovery) is quite widespread but under-researched. Almost all treatment programmes for drug misusers contain some form of counselling and this tends to be aimed at enhancing personal motivation for change and orientated to problem solving and to providing ongoing support to clients. The methods used can vary quite widely both between programmes and across different programme counsellors. Individual psychotherapy has been found to enhance treatment outcomes when integrated with standard addiction counselling, and has a particular impact with clients with higher levels of psychopathology.[32]

The injector

The most prominent influence on the orientation of treatment services since the mid-1980s has been the sustained risk of blood-borne viral infection amongst drug injectors. In the United Kingdom, the *AIDS and Drug Misuse* reports of the Advisory Council on the Misuse of Drugs[33,34] legitimized a pragmatic objective to reach injectors, including those not motivated to alter their current drug-taking behaviour, and to attract them into treatment in order to reduce the risk of acquiring and transmitting HIV. The importance of preventing and stopping injecting was central to this harm-minimization approach and this resulted in the establishment of syringe-exchange programmes to provide sterile injection equipment.[35] These schemes have been shown to lead to reduced levels of equipment sharing as well as increased contact with treatment services.[36]

The importance of provision of information on ways of cleaning used syringes was also embraced by the United Kingdom Department of Health and has been provided as clinical guidance for physicians.[37] Over the last 5 years, over-the-counter sales of needles and syringes across the country have also become increasingly widespread. In 1995, half of all community pharmacists surveyed in England and Wales dispensed controlled drugs.[38] An indicator of the success of these initiatives is that the United Kingdom has not experienced the spread of HIV that has been seen in other nations; this has been attributed to the combined impact of the syringe-exchange initiatives, flexible prescribing, and collaboration between community services.[39,40]

With identification of the risk of hepatitis B and C infection, as well as HIV, efforts to reduce the likelihood of viral infection and transmission include influencing hygiene and, in particular, avoiding sharing of needles, syringes, and associated injecting paraphernalia. The prevention of hepatitis B infection by either vaccinating high-risk individuals or by universal vaccination is also a priority, and responding to hepatitis C viral infection represents a major contemporary global clinical and public health challenge.

The user in withdrawal

If the regular supply of a psychoactive drug (especially sedative drugs such as opiates, barbiturates, benzodiazepines, and alcohol) is interrupted to the dependent user, a classic withdrawal syndrome is likely to develop (e.g. opiate withdrawal syndrome). The nature of the withdrawal syndrome will be determined by the substance group (e.g. opiates, cocaine, benzodiazepines, etc.) whilst the time course of the syndrome will be determined more by the specific drug used (e.g. methadone, heroin). The user in withdrawal from opiates, hypnotics/sedatives, and in some circumstances cocaine may require special short-term detoxification. Detoxification describes a process of supportive medical care and usually pharmacotherapy for neuroadaptation reversal to facilitate a return to abstinence and physiologically normal levels of functioning.[41] Medically supervised detoxification can be delivered in inpatient, residential, or outpatient settings. Detoxification should not be considered *in itself* a treatment for drug dependence and in isolation it is seldom effective in leading to long-term abstinence. Several drugs and detoxification techniques may be used singly or in combination to manage withdrawal symptoms. For

opiate management, the most commonly used method has involved transferring opiate-dependent patients to oral methadone, followed by a gradual reduction in doses. This is by no means the only withdrawal management strategy, and partial agonist medications (e.g. buprenorphine[42]), as well as a variety of rapid detoxification procedures based on administration of antagonist medications, are also available.[43] Sedatives and benzodiazepine medications may also be useful for the short-term treatment of withdrawal symptoms and patient anxiety. For many detoxified individuals, their successful recovery is complicated by the existence of a protracted withdrawal syndrome which, whilst of less intensity, may sap resolve through persistence of poor sleep, agitation, and malaise. As to the research evidence for the effectiveness of specialist inpatient detoxification treatment, a prospective follow-up study of patients in the United Kingdom found that 51 per cent of patients were drug-free at 6-month follow-up.[44] In the United Kingdom, the National Treatment Outcome Research Study (**NTORS**) has subsequently reported positive improvements in opiate use after inpatient treatment at 6-month follow-up.[45]

The recovering dependent drug user

Dependent drug users who attain abstinence may require continuing specialist treatment delivered in a residential setting. Maintaining the commitment to altering a drug-oriented lifestyle is a major and enduring task for many individuals and there are relatively few contemporary services to support this. The treatment philosophy and operation of residential rehabilitation programmes varies quite widely. In the United States, the majority are therapeutic communities and are based on the 12-step or Minnesota Model. The programme length of therapeutic communities varies from short term (e.g. 6 weeks) with aftercare to long-term programmes with a duration of over 1 year. Common to all therapeutic communities is an emphasis on peers and staff as role models for recovery. For some individuals, detoxification can be a gateway into drug-free counselling. Achieving a drug-free state is necessary for entry into many residential rehabilitation programmes or (for opiate users) to receive relapse prevention treatments using the opiate antagonist naloxone. A range of both short- and longer-term residential rehabilitation programmes are available in the United Kingdom (care funding is rarely available for longer-term programmes in excess of 6 months). The evidence base for the impact of residential treatment points to the considerable success of these services for recovering users. Studies from the United States show that, on average, clients receiving therapeutic community treatment have enduring postdischarge reductions in illicit drug use.[46] Amongst residential treatment clients in the United Kingdom, NTORS has described improvements in abstinence from illicit opiates at one year follow-up from 22 per cent to 50 per cent and increases in abstinence from stimulant use from 30 per cent to 68 per cent at follow-up and marked improvements in health and social functioning.[47] Both United States and United Kingdom studies have shown positive psychosocial benefits after treatment.[47–49] Successful outcome in longer-term residential rehabilitation programmes is related to total time spent in treatment, with episodes of at least 3 months associated with positive outcome.[50,51]

The drug user with comorbidity

There is increasing recognition of the importance of managing individuals with comorbidity and special needs. Particular attention should be paid to comorbidities associated with drug use across physical and psychological health domains. At entry to treatment, many individuals with substance use disorders also experience psychiatric symptoms and disorders.[52,53] Across several countries, large-scale surveys have gathered data that suggest high concordance between drug and alcohol use disorders and affective and personality disorders.[54–57] According to one major study from the United States, approximately one in seven individuals with a current mental health disorder also has a substance use disorder.[55] Special attention may need to be given to the health care needs of drug users who are affected by such comorbidities irrespective of their dependent or non-dependent drug use status. Recognition of the importance of understanding the links between substance use behaviours and psychiatric and physical symptoms and disorders and their implications for treatment services is also gaining momentum.[58]

Drug users may also be at risk of physical comorbidity because of their administration of drugs via injection, where they use infected needles/syringes or an unsafe injecting procedure. These risks include septicaemia, inadvertent overdose, and risks of infection with HIV, hepatitis B and C, and other blood-borne viruses (see above). The nature of this comorbidity may be causal, consequent, or coincidental and will include psychiatric as well as physical comorbidities.

The intoxicated user

There is also a need for health care services for the acute management of individuals who are intoxicated to an extent which threatens their continued well being. Management of intoxication is a discrete event and the individual's needs may advance to those associated with dependence, comorbidity, and withdrawal management and support. Most services provided to the intoxicated drug user will be found outside specialist drug or mental health services. Attention should be paid to assessment of the adequacy of care provided in settings such as accident and emergency departments and in police custody, where the health-care needs of the intoxicated drug user may often be overlooked. Uncertainty about the appropriateness of long-term treatment for such individuals can interfere with consideration of their short-term health-care needs (such as the prompt competent management of developing overdose). All services which have contact with opiate users should have prompt access to the injectable opiate antagonist naloxone which may be administered intravenously, intramuscularly, or subcutaneously and can be life-saving in the event of an opiate overdose.

Commissioning of services and needs assessment

The commissioning and organization arrangements of services for drug misusers vary substantially across and sometimes within the treatment systems in many countries. Against this background of diversity there is a growing recognition of the importance of effective co-ordinated action across health, social care, and criminal justice agencies. Additionally, special initiatives are required alongside targeted prevention and treatment interventions aimed at high-risk groups. Effective needs assessment can play an important role when determining the required array of services and their capacity. In all nations with developed treatment systems, specialist drug services are the main providers of care. Complex referral and assessment procedures are used to determine the appropriate setting for treatment and there are resultant case-mix differences with clients of residential treatments generally having longer and more severe drug use histories.[59] The importance of ensuring direct provision or referral access to advice agencies, harm minimization services, and treatment and rehabilitation programmes is paramount. Securing a seamless 'patient pathway' with interagency co-operation over time according to need is a core objective for developed treatment systems.

Co-ordination at local and government levels

The treatment service commissioning process necessitates involvement and partnership of a diverse range of agencies spanning specialist and generalist health care, social services, criminal justice, and non-statutory bodies as well as various community bodies.

Appraisal of the health-care needs of the target populations and commissioning of strategic service responses should be flexible and adaptive to changing circumstances, including the following:

(1) variations and new trends in drugs use and consumption patterns;

(2) the geographical distribution and concentration of local drug use;

(3) variations in demand for services;

(4) the changing relationship between drug use and other conditions, notably HIV infection and blood-borne viral hepatitis;

(5) changing policy in response to drug strategy and to changes in organization of health services;

(6) the evidence for and availability of new treatment responses.

In many communities a continuum of care should be made available, including direct provision or access to harm-minimization services (needle/syringe exchange, vaccination programmes and safer injecting, and drug use advice), community substitution treatment (methadone or other appropriate opiate agonist prescribing services for stabilization, maintenance, and detoxification), and inpatient and residential programmes (detoxification, therapeutic communities and other rehabilitation programmes, and after-care support). Services providing advice, information, assessment, and referral are an important resource and valuable point of contact for individuals, friends, and families. Structured provision of counselling and support are often made available by these services. Additional gateway services (e.g. outreach services seeking to identify problem users not in touch with treatment services and encouraging referral) are also useful elements of an integrated system.

Needs assessment methodologies

A needs assessment approach is equally valuable for the development of new services as it is for the audit and review of an existing treatment system. There is, however, no single best needs assessment methodology in the drug misuse field.[60] With the identification of priority segments of the drug misusing population, organizations involved with the planning of treatment services should identify the following:

(1) the type and probable size of the subpopulations using different drugs who have a treatment need;

(2) the risks and harm conditions which require a specific intervention;

(3) the methods and providers which are available for their delivery;

(4) the probable service capacity that is required for each intervention modality.

General population surveys have been used to estimate the size of the population in need in several nations.[61,62] These produce reliable data but may not be able to sample from all of the priority needs segments in the population and are expensive to implement. A lower cost capture–recapture methodology may be used as an alternative to population surveys in particular regions, but studies of this type have not generally been able to gather sufficient information about individuals in different samples to estimate their treatment need.

In general the six overlapping needs groups outlined earlier may come into contact with various agencies in a locality. In the absence of reliable data, needs assessment can be estimated by identifying a wide range of contexts or settings in which the above groups come into contact, including specialist treatment services, general practitioners, community pharmacists, hospital accident and emergency departments, general hospital wards, community mental health teams, social services departments, children's services, non-specialist voluntary groups, probation services, police, law courts, and prison. There may be additional contact and screening points which can be identified, including schools, employment settings, and genitourinary medicine clinics. A client pathway or continuum of care perspective can then be applied to each contact point to articulate the required service response to the different subgroups of users encountered.

Conclusions

The provision of effective and well-organized treatment services for drug misusers is a priority in many countries worldwide. Drug use disorders are diverse and are characterized and influenced by individual, social, and environmental factors. There are a variety of access points into treatment in the public health and social care systems, and to an increasing extent in the criminal justice system. In response, an array of specialist and generalist providers of treatment in many countries offer a broad range of treatments. There is a growing evidence base for the effectiveness of several types of well-delivered harm-minimization, substitute prescribing, and detoxification and rehabilitation services, and there should be appropriate access or direct provision of these services. Partnership is vital between agencies spanning specialist drug treatment services, general medical, general practice and across health authorities, social services, non-statutory agencies, and criminal justice agencies. For effective service provision at the local level, service commissioners need to assess population needs, estimate the probable level of requirement for treatment, and make an active and sustained commitment to providing efficient and effective services.

References

1. Strang, J., Marsden, J., Lavoie, D., Abdulrahim, D., Hickman, M., and Scott, S. Epidemiologically-based needs assessment—drug abuse. In *Healthcare needs assessment* (ed. A. Stevens). Radcliffe Medical Press, Oxford, in press.
2. Central Drugs Coordination Unit (1998). *Tackling drugs to build a better Britain. The government's 10-year strategy for tackling drug misuse.* HMSO, London.
3. Office of the National Drug Control Policy (1999). *United States Office of National Drug Control Strategy.* Office of the National Drug Control Policy, Washington, DC.
4. United Nations International Drug Control Programme (1997). *World drug report.* Oxford University Press, New York.
5. Ramsay, M. and Spiller, J. (1997). *Drug use declared in 1996: latest results from the British Crime Survey.* Home Office, London.
6. Health Education Authority/BMRB International (1997). *Drug use in England: results of the 1995 National Drugs Campaign Survey.* Health Education Authority, London.
7. Substance Abuse and Mental Health Services Administration (1998). *Preliminary results from the 1997 National Household Survey on Drug Abuse.* US Department of Health and Human Services, Rockville, MD.
8. Hammersley, R., Forsyth, A., Morrison, V., and Davies, J. (1989). The relationship between crime and opioid use. *British Journal of Addiction*, **84**, 1029–43.
9. Nurco, D.N., Shaffer, J.W., and Cisin, I.H. (1984). An ecological analysis of the interrelationships among drug abuse and other indices of social pathology. *International Journal of the Addictions*, **19**, 441–51.
10. Pearson, G. and Gillman, M. (1994). Local and regional variations in drug misuse: the British heroin epidemic of the 1980s. In *Heroin addiction and drug policy: the British system* (ed. J. Strang and M. Gossop), pp. 102–20. Oxford University Press.
11. Zinberg, N. (1984). *Drug, set and setting.* Yale University Press, New Haven, CT.
12. Biernacki, P. (1986). *Pathways from heroin addiction.* Temple University Press, Philadelphia, PA.
13. Joe, G.W., Chastain, R.L., and Simpson, D.D. (1990). Length of careers. In *Opioid addiction and treatment: a 12-year follow-up* (ed. D.D. Simpson and S.B. Sells), pp. 103–19. Keiger, Malabar, FL.
14. Gossop, M. and Marsden, J. (1996). Assessment and treatment of opiate problems. *Baillière's Clinical Psychiatry*, **2**, 1–15.
15. World Health Organization (1992). *International statistical classification of diseases and related health problems, 10th revision.* WHO, Geneva.
16. American Psychiatric Association (1994). *Diagnostic and statistical manual of mental disorders* (4th edn). American Psychiatric Association, Washington, DC.
17. Gossop, M., Darke, S., Griffiths, P., *et al.* (1995). The Severity of Dependence Scale (SDS): psychometric properties of the SDS in English and Australian samples of heroin, cocaine and amphetamine users. *Addiction*, **90**, 607–14.
18. Skinner, H.A. (1982). The Drug Abuse Screening Test. *Addictive Behaviors*, **7**, 363–71.
19. Tarter, R. and Hegedus, A. (1991). The Drug Use Screening Inventory: its applications in the evaluation and treatment of alcohol and drug abuse. *Alcohol, Health and Research World*, **15**, 65–75.
20. Wolff, K., Farrell, M., Marsden, J., Monteiro, M.G., Ali, R., and Strang, J. (1999). A review of biological indicators of illicit drug use, practical considerations and clinical usefulness. *Addiction*, **94**, 1279–98.
21. Farrell, M.J. Ward, R., Mattick, W., *et al.* (1994). Methadone maintenance treatment in opiate dependence: a review. *British Medical Journal*, **309**, 997–1001.
22. Ward, J., Mattick, R.P., and Hall, W. (1992). *Key issues in methadone maintenance treatment.* New South Wales University Press, Sydney.
23. Marsden, J., Gossop, G., Farrell, M., and Strang, J. (1998). Opioid substitution: critical issues and future directions. *Journal of Drug Issues*, **28**, 231–48.
24. Marsden, J., Griffiths, P., Farrell, M., Gossop, M., and Strang, J. (1998). Cocaine in Britain: prevalence, problems and treatment responses. *Journal of Drug Issues*, **28**, 225–42.
25. Carroll, K.M., Rounsaville, B.J., and Keller, D.S. (1991). Relapse prevention strategies for the treatment of cocaine abuse. *American Journal of Drug and Alcohol Abuse*, **173**, 249–65.
26. Rawson, R., Obert, J., McCann, M.J., Castro, F.G., and Ling, W. (1991).

Cocaine abuse treatment: a review of current strategies. *Journal of Substance Abuse*, **3**, 457–91.

27. Higgins, S.T., Budney, A.J., Bickel, W.K., Badger, G.J., Foerg, F.E., and Ogden, D. (1995). Outpatient behavioural treatment for cocaine dependence. *Experimental and Clinical Psychopharmacology*, **3**, 205–12.

28. Levin, F.R. and Lehman, A.F. (1991). Meta-analysis of desipramine as an adjuct in the treatment of cocaine addiction. *Journal of Clinical Psychopharmacology*, **11**, 374–8.

29. Klee, H. (1998). The love of speed: an analysis of the enduring attraction of amphetamine sulphate for British youth. *Journal of Drug Issues*, **28**, 33–56.

30. Strang, J. and Sheridan, J. (1997). Prescribing amphetamines to drug misusers: data from the 1995 national survey of community pharmacists. *Addiction*, **92**, 833–8.

31. Fleming, P.M. and Roberts, D. (1994). Is the prescription of amphetamine justified as a harm reduction measure? *Journal of the Royal Society of Health*, **114**, 127–31.

32. Woody, GE., Luborsky, L., McLellan, A.T., *et al.* (1983). Psychotherapy for opiate addicts. Does it help? *Archives of General Psychiatry*, **40**, 639–45.

33. Advisory Council on the Misuse of Drugs (1988). *AIDS and drug misuse*, Part 1. Department of Health and Social Security, London.

34. Advisory Council on the Misuse of Drugs (1989). *AIDS and drug misuse*, Part 2. Department of Health and Social Security, London.

35. Stimson, G.V., Alldritt, L., Dolan, K., and Donoghoe, M.(1988). Syringe exchange schemes for drug users in England and Scotland. *British Medical Journal*, **296**, 1717–19.

36. Stimson, G., Donoghoe, M., Lart, R., and Dolan, K. (1990). Distributing sterile needles and syringes to people who inject drugs: the syringe exchange experiment. In *AIDS and drugs misuse* (ed. J. Strang and G. Stimson), pp. 221–31. Routledge, London.

37. Department of Health (1999). *Drug misuse and dependence—guidelines on clinical management*. HMSO, London.

38. Sheridan, J., Strang, J., Barber, N., and Glanz, A. (1996). Role of community pharmacists in relation to HIV prevention and drug misuse: findings from the 1995 national survey in England and Wales. *British Medical Journal*, **313**, 270–4.

39. Stimson, G.V. (1995). Aids and injecting drug use in the United Kingdom, 1987–1993: the policy response and the prevention of the epidemic. *Social Science and Medicine*, **41**, 699–716.

40. Strang, J. (1998). AIDS and drug misuse in the UK—10 years on: achievements, failings and new harm reduction opportunities. *Drugs: Education, Prevention and Policy*, **5**, 293–304.

41. Chang, G.A. and Kosten, T.R. (1997). Detoxification. In *Substance abuse: a comprehensive textbook* (3rd edn) (ed. J.H. Lowinson, P. Ruiz, R.B.A. Millman, and J.G. Langrod), pp. 371–81. Williams and Wilkins, Baltimore, MD.

42. Bickel, W.R., Stizer, M.L., Bigelow, G.E., Liebson, I.A., Jasinski, D.E., and Johnson, R.E. (1988). A clinical trial of buprenorphine comparison with methadone in the detoxification of heroin addicts. *Clinical Pharmacology Review*, **43**, 72–8.

43. Bearn, J., Gossop, M., and Strang, J. (1999). Rapid opiate detoxification treatments. *Drug and Alcohol Review*, **18**, 75–81.

44. Gossop, M., Green, L., Phillips, G., and Bradley, B. (1989). Lapse, relapse and survival among opiate addicts after treatment. *British Journal of Psychiatry*, **154**, 348–53.

45. Gossop, M., Marsden, J., Stewart, D., *et al.* (1997). The National Treatment Outcome Research Study in the United Kingdom: six-month follow-up outcomes. *Psychology of Addictive Behaviors*, **11**, 324–37.

46. DeLeon, G., Andrews, M., Wexler, H., Jaffe, J., and Rosenthal, M. (1979). Therapeutic community dropouts: criminal behaviour five years after treatment. *American Journal of Drug and Alcohol Abuse*, **6**, 253–71.

47. Gossop, M., Marsden, J., and Stewart, D. (1998). *NTORS at one year*. Department of Health, London.

48. DeLeon, G. and Jainchill, N. (1982). Male and female drug abusers: social and psychological status two years after treatment in a therapeutic community. *American Journal of Drug and Alcohol Abuse*, **8**, 465–97.

49. Bennett, G. and Rigby, K. (1990). Psychological change during residence in a rehabilitation centre for female drug misusers. Part I. Drug misusers. *Drug and Alcohol Dependence*, **27**, 149–57.

50. Simpson, D.D. (1997). Effectiveness of drug abuse treatment: a review of research from field settings. In *Treating drug abusers effectively* (ed. J. Egertson, D. Fox, and A. Leshner), pp. 41–73. Blackwell Science, Oxford.

51. Gossop, M., Marsden, J., Stewart, D., and Rolfe, A. (1999). Time in residential treatment programmes and outcomes at one year: results from the national treatment outcome research study. *Drug and Alcohol Dependence*, **57**, 89–98.

52. Hall, W. (1996). What have population surveys revealed about substance use disorders and their co-morbidity with other mental disorders. *Drug and Alcohol Review*, **15**, 157–70.

53. Ward, J., Mattick, R.P., and Hall, W. (1998). Psychiatric comorbidity among the opioid dependent. In *Methadone maintenance treatment and other opioid replacement therapies* (ed. J. Ward, R.P. Mattick, and W. Hall), pp. 419–40. Harwood, Amsterdam.

54. Regier, D.A., Farmer, M.E., Rae, D.S., *et al.* (1990). Comorbidity of mental disorders with alcohol and other drug abuse: results from the Epidemiologic Catchment Area (ECA). study. *Journal of the American Medical Association*, **264**, 2511–18.

55. Kessler, R.C., McGonagle, K.A., Zhao, S., *et al.* (1994). Lifetime and 12 month prevalence of DSM-III-R psychiatric disorders in the United States: results from the National Comorbidity Survey. *Archives of General Psychiatry*, **51**, 8–19.

56. Merikangas, K.R., Mehta, R.L., Molnar, B.E., *et al.* (1998). Comorbidity of substance use disoders with mood and anxiety disorders: results of the international consortium in psychiatric epidemiology. *Addictive Behaviors*, **23**, 893–907.

57. Farrell, M., Howes, S., Taylor, C., *et al.* (1998). Substance misuse and psychiatric comorbidity: an overview of the OPCS national psychiatric morbidity survey. *Addictive Behaviors*, **23**, 909–18.

58. Johnson, S. (1997). Dual diagnosis of severe mental illness and substance misuse: a case for specialist services. *British Journal of Psychiatry*, **171**, 205–8.

59. Gossop, M., Marsden, J., Stewart, D., *et al.* (1998). Substance use, health and social problems of clients at 54 drug treatment agencies: intake data from the National Treatment Outcome Research Study (NTORS). *British Journal of Psychiatry*, **173**, 166–71.

60. DeWit, D. and Rush, B. (1996). Assessing need for substance abuse services: a critical review of needs assessment models. *Evaluation and Program Planning*, **19**, 41–6.

61. World Health Organization (1990). *Composite International Diagnostic Interview (CIDI)* (Version 1.0). World Health Organization, Geneva.

62. Cottler, L.B., Robbins, L.N., Grant, B.F., *et al.* (1991). The CID-core substance abuse and dependence questions: cross cultural and nosological issues. *British Journal of Psychiatry*, **159**, 653–8.

4.3 Schizophrenia and acute transient psychotic disorders

4.3.1 Schizophrenia: a conceptual history

German E. Berrios

According to some, the history of schizophrenia consists of a progression of definitions culminating in the present.[1] However, instead of the 'continuity' implicit in this view, historical research indicates that (a) the history of 'schizophrenia' is a series of unconnected and contradicting research programmes, and (b) the current definition of schizophrenia is a patchwork of features.

The 'continuity' version also includes only alienists making modern-sounding points. This would matter little were it not that it denies researchers access to important aspects of the history of schizophrenia.[2] For example, it is a moot point whether the Kraepelinian view would be as popular as it is had it not been for the untimely death of Wernicke, who by 1905 was developing an exciting neuropsychological classification for the psychoses.

Hence, rather than asking who were the alienists who 'foresaw' the wonders of the present, this chapter will ask what historical factors made some views survive, the point being that 'unsuccessful' views have contributed to the history of schizophrenia as much as 'victorious' concepts. Also, clinical criteria are meaningless if taken out of historical context, an approach sometimes called 'polythetic'[3] For example, 'first-rank symptoms' mean little if separated from Schneider's theoretical views on the 'disorders of the self'.

The 'continuity' version

The 'continuity' version states that for centuries 'insanity' and 'madness' referred to a melee of mental diseases which physicians were unable to separate. In the 1850s, Morel coined the term *démence précoce* to refer to states of cognitive deficit in adolescence. During the second half of the nineteenth century, 'catatonia' was described by Kahlbaum and 'hebephrenia' by Hecker. At the end of the century, Kraepelin realized that both disorders, together with 'dementia paranoides' (which he had himself discovered), were manifestations of the same disease process. Kraepelin called this disease dementia praecox and based it on empirical data kept in follow-up cards. In 1911, Bleuler renamed it 'schizophrenia' and, during the 1930s, Schneider listed diagnostic criteria which, owing to their 'empirical' and 'atheoretical' character, deserved to be enshrined in DSM-IV.

It is also part of the continuity story that European psychiatry was influenced by Kraepelin, while American psychiatry followed Adolph Meyer, Bleuler, and the psychoanalysts[4–6] (although Manfred Bleuler, in an interesting paper approved by his father, wrote:[7] 'Since coming to the United States I have had the valuable experience of realizing that the conceptions of schizophrenia are very different here from those held in our clinic at Burghölzli'). This would explain the confused definitions offered in DSM-I and DSM-II[7] and the diagnostic disparities found between the United Kingdom and the United States (of course, this view does not explain the major differences in the conception of schizophrenia between Germany, Italy, France, Russia, Norway, the United Kingdom, etc.). In the event, Kraepelin and Schneider were discovered in the United States, psychoanalysis was eased out, and this paved the way for the advent of biological psychiatry. After some uncertainties (e.g. DSM-III), DSM-IV now offers the *de facto* official definition of schizophrenia.

The problem with this version of events is that it occurs in a historical vacuum. Neither the alternative definitions of schizophrenia nor the factors that explain the successful views are ever mentioned; indeed, the impression is given that there has been an ineluctable progress towards 'the truth'. However, this flattering narrative is hollow for, given that the current definition of schizophrenia is still made on phenomenological grounds, it is necessary to ask how to decide which of the historical definitions were right and which were wrong.

The 'discontinuity' version

Powerful forces shaped the construction of dementia praecox and schizophrenia during the nineteenth century. For example, 'association psychology' provided the basis for the metaphor of 'splitting' and 'faculty psychology' offered a template (the mind as a bundle of intellectual, emotional, and volitional functions) in terms of which the new mental disorders were defined. 'Neo-Kantianism', in turn, supplied a model of thinking which was to become crucial to 'formal thought disorder'—a central 'symptom' of schizophrenia. Lastly, 'evolutionary theory' provided an explanatory framework. For example, according to Kraepelin,[8] the disease process underlying dementia praecox activated a set of 'pre-formed reactions' (responsible for the clinical picture), all of which were biological and evolutionary in origin. Likewise, Bleuler[9] suggested that the *Schnauzkrampf* of schizophrenia was related to the protrusion of lips seen in chimpanzees (to 'express dissatisfaction').

This chapter is based on the view that ideas about mental symptoms and diseases originate in 'convergences'. By this term is meant the coming together of a *term* (newly coined or recycled), a *behaviour* (putatively related to a brain disturbance or to an allegorical human action), and a *concept* (as a carrier of definitions and explanations and rules).[10,11] These components will be considered in relation to schizophrenia, starting with terms and concepts and then considering behaviour.

History of terms and concepts

Dementia praecox

The term 'dementia' had participated in at least three 'convergences' before it was incorporated into dementia praecox. Up to the seventeenth century, dementia referred to states of psychosocial incompetence, whether inborn or acquired, and had a 'legal' connotation—age and irreversibility were not part of its meaning. By the eighteenth century, dementia became linked to states of acquired intellectual deficit at whatever age and of whatever aetiology, i.e. there was a shift towards clinical usage. By the end of the nineteenth century, dementia was redefined in terms of a loss of cognition (mainly 'memory', since called the 'cognitive paradigm').[12] Most importantly, age of onset, reversibility, and evolution became important, so that cognitive deficits in children or acquired states in younger adults (e.g. after head trauma) were no longer called 'dementia'.[13] By the turn of the century, senile and other forms of dementia had been described.[14,15]

Morel[16] coined the term *démence précoce* to refer to the mental state and behaviour of young patients with *stupidité* (stupor) ('surdi-mutité, faiblesse congénitale des facultés, démence précoce', and 'Une espèce de torpeur voisine de l'hébétude remplaça l'activité première, et lorsque je le revis, je jugeai que la transition fatale à l'état de démence précoce était en voie de s'opérer'), i.e. with a disorder of motility and the will secondary to melancholia.[17] By 'dementia' he meant any state of psychosocial incompetence related to a mental disorder and occurring at any age—the criterion of irreversibility did not yet exist. In this sense, the term *démence précoce* has little relationship to the work of Kraepelin or Bleuler. In his brilliant analysis of the development of the concept of schizophrenia, Minkowski[18] stated: 'An abyss separates Morel's *démence précoce* from that of Kraepelin where the streamlet has become a river which, having forgotten its humble origins, threatened to flood everything'. It would seem, however, that the French themselves encouraged the idea that the history of schizophrenia started with Morel.[19]

By the time Kraepelin used the term dementia praecox, the general concept of dementia had acquired a third meaning different from that of the time of Morel. For example, Gross[20] noted that: 'The meaning of the term dementia has changed in current usage. We have grown accustomed to employing it to denote not only an end state but also a developing state, a process…'. Furthermore, Morel's old term had sunk into oblivion; indeed, there is no evidence that in 1896 Kraepelin knew of its existence. Kraepelin first used the term in the fifth edition of his textbook[21] in 1896. Under *Verblödungsprocesse*, Kraepelin lists three independent conditions: 'Dementia praecox' (mild and severe forms, and hebephrenia), 'catatonia', and 'dementia paranoides'. Nowhere in this text is Morel's name mentioned; it only appeared three editions later. By the time that Kraepelin was writing the fifth edition, the term 'dementia' had already changed its meaning; hence he saw the need to qualify 'dementia' by the term 'praecox', by which he meant 'early', 'not

at the expected age', etc. He only 'acknowledged' the Frenchman for the first time in the last edition of his book, where he wrote: 'The name dementia praecox which had already been used by Morel'.[22] There is, however, the distinct possibility that Kraepelin borrowed it from Arnold Pick who used 'dementia praecox' as early as 1891.[23] For an excellent comparison of the editions of Kraepelin's textbook with regard to the construction of 'dementia praecox', see Hoff.[8]

Schizophrenia

Eugen Bleuler

The term 'schizophrenia' first appeared in print in 1908.[24] In 1911, Bleuler[9] wrote: 'Ich nenne die Dementia praecox Schizophrenie, weil, wie ich zu zeigen hoffe, die Spaltung der verschiedensten psychischen Funktionen eine ihren wichtigsten Eigenschaften ist' ('I call dementia praecox schizophrenia because, as I hope to show, the splitting of the different psychic functions is one of its most important features'). And then: 'In jedem Falle besteht eine mehr oder weniger deutliche Spaltung der psychischen Funktionen: ist die Krankheit ausgesprochen, so verliert die Persönlichkeit ihre Einheit… ('In each case there is a more or less clear splitting of the psychological functions: as the disease becomes distinct, the personality loses its unity'). This seems straightforward, but is not. The meanings he gave to *Spaltung* and to *psychischen Funktionen* are ambiguous and need further historical clarification. By 'splitting', Bleuler meant (a) a deep and general 'primary loosening of associational networks' ('primäre Lockerung des Assoziationsgefüges'), leading to irregular breaking ('unregelmäßigen Zerspaltung') of 'concrete concepts', and (b) a more apparent 'systemic splitting of idea-complexes' ('systematischen Spaltung in bestimmte Ideenkomplexe').[9]

Behind these views there is a new model of the mind and hence, despite Bleuler's claims to the contrary,[9] there is a marked difference between Kraepelin's dementia praecox and Bleuler's schizophrenia. Thus the change was not just one of name. Indeed, a disciple of Bleuler wrote: 'the concepts of Bleuler and Swiss psychiatry are looser than those of Kraepelin and German psychiatry'.[25] Gruhle[26] also felt that there was 'no full correspondence' between the views of Kraepelin and Bleuler. This is confirmed by the fact that in France dementia praecox and schizophrenia were treated as different diseases up to the 1920s![27]

Splitting Originating in early nineteenth century Romantic psychology and the work of Herbart,[28] the mechanism of separating, dividing, breaking, dissociating, divorcing, or splitting of mental functions was a common explanation (in popular literature and in psychology) for any unpredictable or strange human behaviour. For example, it is present in Wigan's two-brains model, Stevenson's *Dr Jekyll and Mr Hyde*, Hartmann's model of the unconscious, Jackson's hierarchical model of the brain, Azam's dissociation, Charcot's hysteria, Freud's splitting of the ego, and Wernicke's 'sejunction'.

The mechanism of 'splitting' (*Spaltung*) was popular in German psychiatry at the time when Bleuler coined the term 'schizophrenia'. Indeed, there were a number of rival words more or less based on the same idea: intrapsychic ataxia, dementia dessecans, dementia sejunctiva, dysphrenia, discordance, etc. However, none was adopted.[29] Neither the new term (schizophrenia) nor its associated concept (splitting) were accepted by everyone. Freud expressed some reservation about both, for splitting 'does not belong exclusively to that disease',[30] and Jaspers observed that splitting could not be observed in some schizophrenic patients.[31]

Kurt Schneider

Schneider is listed as the third major alienist in the history of schizophrenia, for example by Hoenig.[32] Study of Schneider's writings shows that there is a discontinuity between his views on schizophrenia and those proposed by Bleuler. For Schneider, the 'first-rank symptoms' were not pathognomonic but suggested a diagnosis of schizophrenia only if there was no evidence of any other organic psychoses. The 11 first-rank symptoms only gain meaning when sought in the context of three diagnostic perspectives: course, symptomatology, and interaction.[33] Because, as Jaspers[34] proposed, the endogenous psychoses result from a process, there is little point in studying the 'course' of schizophrenia.[35] All that was needed was to find out whether there had been some prodromal symptoms of schizophrenia. 'Symptomatic comprehension' included the search for symptoms resulting from a defect in the integration of the self (hence it is not true to claim that Schneider believed that his first-rank symptoms were 'empirical' and 'atheoretical'). 'Comprehension by interaction' referred to the way in which the patient is perceived by the clinician. In this regard, and without naming it, Schneider described the 'praecox feeling' years before Rümke.[25]

Because Schneider had a cross-sectional view of diagnosis, the notion of 'course' (in Kraepelin's sense) was alien to his thinking. Likewise, his conception of schizophrenia included all the paraphrenias, paranoias, marginal psychoses of Kleist, etc. He also believed that, in addition to schizophrenia and cyclothymia (manic–depressive insanity), the 'endogenous psychosis' encompassed a large number of yet undiscovered diseases.[36]

In summary, there is no continuity between Schneider's notion of schizophrenia and earlier views; hence it is nonsense to choose some criteria from Kraepelin (i.e. course and duration), others from Bleuler (formal thought disorder), and yet others from Schneider (first-rank symptoms). It is nonsense because each of these alienists had a different (and non-additive) definition of schizophrenia, and hence the clinical features that each described only make sense in terms of their own conception and not in a decontextualized form. The DSM-IV definition happens to be a composite of the type that we have just described.

History of behaviours

During the 1980s, and encouraged by the assumption that schizophrenia was a recognizable, real, unitary, and stable 'brain disease', questions were asked about the fact that clear descriptions of the disease seem hard to find before 1800.

Did schizophrenia exist before the eighteenth century?

This question remains 'unresolved'.[37] Based on an 'epidemiological' claim, for which there is no historical evidence, supporters of the so-called 'recency hypothesis' suggested that 'some change of a biological kind occurred about 1800 such that a particular type of schizophrenia thereafter became much commoner'.[38] (Gruhle[26] and Cranefield[39] have reviewed 'possible' earlier cases of schizophrenia.) In the wake of this claim, efforts were made to rediagnose earlier 'cases of schizophrenia' as something else.[40] Interestingly, the 'recency hypothesis' seemed also to be supported by those who believed that

the emergence of 'schizophrenia' coincides with the birth of some 'modern episteme' (which Foucault identified with the Kantian revolution).[41] Foucault defined 'episteme' as the set of discursive practices that make possible the emergence of scientific disciplines. Constituted towards the end of the eighteenth century, 'modern episteme' included a view of man as an 'autonomous being' and is responsible for the development of the so-called human sciences.

However, others believed that schizophrenia 'had existed as long as mankind',[42] and cases were rediagnosed in the relevant direction. For example, Macalpine and Hunter[43] suggested that the seventeenth-century painter Christoph Haitzmann (diagnosed by Freud as a 'demoniacal neurosis' in 1923)[44] was suffering from 'schizophrenia'. Likewise, after re-reporting the case of James Tilly Matthews as 'the earliest clear description of schizophrenia', Carpenter[45] explained that the absence of earlier cases resulted from a 'different selection and description of cases for publication'. Jeste et al.[46] ferreted out, although not as successfully as Gruhle,[26] 'a substantial number of clinical descriptions resembling modern conceptions of schizophrenia'.

A pseudo-problem

Looking back, it seems clear that, in terms of the conceptual parameters accepted by the participants, the debate could not have been resolved. Firstly, there were the issues of what counted as evidence, how many cases would falsify 'the recency hypothesis',[47] or what level of diagnostic clarity was required for a case to qualify as evidence? Secondly, both sides were making unprovable claims; for example, 'schizophrenia has always existed' and 'there was a biological change that brought schizophrenia into life during the nineteenth century'.

The issues here are at the same time simpler and harder than anything that the participants in the debate seem to have envisaged. Some issues concern the clinical focus, i.e. what controls the perception and description of mental symptoms and diseases, others the ontology itself of the RRUS, i.e. what claims are being made about the existence of the entities in question, and yet others the rules of the epistemological game, i.e. what counts as evidence etc. In the actual debate these issues appeared in various combinations and permutations. In this chapter, there is only space for one example.

Let us say that, because of their biological basis, the units of analysis (mental symptoms) have always existed. The current definition of schizophrenia is, at best, the result of the belief that some of these mental symptoms occur more frequently together. The way in which research is carried out today makes it very difficult to decide how often such mental symptoms affect individuals who are not considered as suffering from 'schizophrenia'. Let us now take both extremes—that no case or that thousands of cases of schizophrenia can be found before the nineteenth century. Would these lead to the conclusion that schizophrenia did not, or did, exist before the nineteenth century? In fact, neither inference follows; absence of reports can be explained away by using arguments taken from 'clinical focus' or 'rules of the epistemological game' issues (as mentioned above). However, multiple reports create a problem: Why was the disease not recognized and named before if it has such a frequent and stereotyped presentation?

Therefore it can be concluded that it is not possible to write a sensible history of 'behaviours redolent of schizophrenia' for the period before the nineteenth century.[48] This is because both the current concept of mental symptoms and disease and that of schizophrenia are nineteenth-century constructions. Hence clinical reports before this period will always lack epistemological 'distinctness' (from our perspective). However, such reports make a great deal of sense if assessed in terms of categories such as madness, insanity, lunacy, vesania, melancholia, and mania.

Conclusions

The history of schizophrenia can be best described as the history of a set of research programmes running in parallel rather than seriatim and each based on a different concept of disease, mental symptom, and mind. However, only few of these programmes have been discussed in this short chapter.

Historical research shows that there is little conceptual continuity between Morel, Kraepelin, Bleuler, and Schneider. Two consequences follow from this finding. One is that the idea of a linear progression culminating in the present is a myth. The other is that the *current* view of schizophrenia is *not* the result of one definition and one object of inquiry successively studied by various psychiatric teams, but is a patchwork made out of clinical features plucked from different definitions. More research is needed to find out what led to this sorry state of affairs.

The continuity story should be rejected because its main role has been not to illuminate the past but to justify the present. Hopefully, the discontinuity history will offer uncommitted researchers alternative ideas, for example that there is no such a thing as a unitary disease called schizophrenia but only a collection of mental symptoms, some congenital, some relics from evolution, and others acquired.

References

1. American Psychiatric Association (1994). *Diagnostic and statistical manual of mental disorders* (4th edn), p. 187. American Psychiatric Association, Washington, DC.
2. Berrios, G.E. (1995). Conceptual problems in diagnosing schizophrenic disorders. In *Advances in the neurobiology of schizophrenia* (ed. J.A. den Boer, H.G.M. Westenberg, and H.M. van Praag), pp. 7–25. Wiley, Chichester.
3. Andreasen, N.C. and Akiskal, H.S. (1983). The specificity of Bleulerian and Schneiderian symptoms: a critical reevaluation. *Psychiatric Clinics of North America*, **6**, 41–54.
4. Lewis, N.D.C. (1936). *Research in dementia praecox*, p. 29. Northern Masonic Jurisdiction, New York.
5. Raskin, D.E. (1975). Bleuler and schizophrenia. *British Journal of Psychiatry*, **127**, 231–4.
6. Fullinwider, S.P. (1982). *Technicians of the finite. The rise and decline of the schizophrenic in American thought 1840–1960*. Greenwood Press, London.
7. Bleuler, M. (1931). Schizophrenia. *Archives of Neurology and Psychiatry*, **26**, 610–27.
8. Hoff, P. (1994). *Emil Kraepelin und die Psychiatrie als klinische Wissenschaft*. Springer-Verlag, Berlin.
9. Bleuler, E. (1911). *Dementia praecox oder Gruppe der Schizophrenien*. Franz Deuticke, Leipzig.
10. Berrios, G.E. (1996). *The history of mental symptoms. Descriptive psychopathology since the 19th century*. Cambridge University Press.
11. Berrios, G.E. and Porter, R. (ed.) (1995). *The history of clinical psychiatry*. Athlone Press, London.
12. Berrios, G.E. (1989). Non-cognitive symptoms and the diagnosis of dementia. Historical and clinical aspects. *British Journal of Psychiatry*, **154**, 11–16.
13. Berrios, G.E. (1987). Dementia during the 17th and 18th century: a conceptual history. *Psychological Medicine*, **17**, 829–37.
14. Berrios, G.E. (1990). Alzheimer's disease: a conceptual history. *International Journal of Geriatric Psychiatry*, **5**, 355–65.
15. Berrios, G.E. and Freeman, H. (1991). *Alzheimer and the dementias*. Royal Society of Medicine, London.
16. Morel, B.A. (1860). *Traité des maladies mentales*, pp. 516, 566. Masson, Paris.
17. Berrios, G.E. (1981). Stupor: a conceptual history. *Psychological Medicine*, **11**, 677–88.
18. Minkowski, E. (1925). La génése de la notion de schizophrénie et ses caractères essentiels. *Evolution Psychiatrique*, **1**, 193–236.
19. Lanteri-Laura, G. and Gross, M. (1992). *Essai sur la discordance dans la psychiatrie contemporaine*, p. 13. Epel, Paris.
20. Gross, O. (1904). Dementia sejunctiva. *Neurologische Zentralblatt*, **23**, 1144–6.
21. Kraepelin, E. (1896) *Psychiatrie* (5th edn), pp. 425–71. Barth, Leipzig.
22. Kraepelin, E. (1919). *Dementia praecox and paraphrenia* (transl. R.M. Barclay and G.M. Robertson), p. 4. Livingstone, Edinburgh. (Extracted from 8th and last edition, published in 1910.)
23. Pick, A. (1891). Über primäre chronische Demenz (so. Dementia praecox) intramuscular jugendlichen Alter. *Prager Medicinische Wochenschrift*, **16**, 312–15.
24. Bleuler, E. (1908). Die Prognose der Dementia praecox—Schizophreniegruppe. *Allgemeine Zeitschrift für Psychiatrie*, **65**, 436–64.
25. Rümke, H.C. (1990). The nuclear symptom of schizophrenia and the praecox feeling. *History of Psychiatry*, **1**, 331–41 (first published in Dutch in 1941).
26. Gruhle, H.W. (1932). Geschichtliches. In *Bumke's Handbuch der Geisteskrankheiten*. Part 5, *Die Schizophrenie* (ed. K. Wilmanns), pp. 1–30. Springer, Berlin.
27. Rodiet, A. and Heuyer, G. (1931). *La folie au XXe siècle. Étude médico-sociale*, pp. 90–121. Masson, Paris.
28. Scharfetter, C. (1975). The historical development of the concept of schizophrenia. In *Studies of schizophrenia* (ed. M.H. Lader), pp. 5–8. Headley, Ashford.
29. Berrios, G.E. (1987). The fundamental symptoms of dementia praecox and Bleuler. In *The origins of modern psychiatry* (ed. C. Thompson), pp. 200–9. Wiley, New York.
30. Freud, S. (1953). Psychoanalytical notes upon an autobiographical account of a case of paranoia (dementia paranoides). In *Collected papers* (ed. E. Jones), Vol. III, pp. 387–470. Hogarth Press, London.
31. Jaspers, K. (1963). *General psychopathology* (7th edn) (transl. J. Hoenig and M.W. Hamilton). Manchester University Press.
32. Hoenig, J. (1983). The concept of schizophrenia: Kraepelin–Bleuler–Schneider. *British Journal of Psychiatry*, **142**, 547–56.
33. Schneider, K. (1944). *Conferencias psiquiatricas para médicos*, Orfila, Madrid. (Translation of second German edition published in 1936.)
34. Jaspers, K. (1910). Eifersuchtswahn. Ein Beitrag zur Frage: 'Entwicklung einer Personlichkeit' oder 'Prozeß'. *Zeitschrift für die gesamte Neurologie und Psychiatrie*, **1**, 567–637.
35. Häffner, H. (1993). Prozeß und Entwicklung als Grundbegriffe der Psychopathologie. *Fortschritte der Neurologie Psychiatrie*, **31**, 393–437.
36. Huber, G. (1987). Kurt Schneider. The man and his scientific work. *Zentralblatt für Neurologie und Psychiatrie*, **246**, 177–91.
37. Ellard, J. (1987). Did schizophrenia exist before the eighteenth century. *Australian and New Zealand Journal of Psychiatry*, **21**, 306–14.
38. Hare, E. (1988). Schizophrenia as a recent disease. *British Journal of Psychiatry*, **153**, 521–31.
39. Cranefield, P.F. (1961). A seventeenth case of mental deficiency and schizophrenia: Thomas Willis on 'stupidity or foolishness'. *Bulletin of the History of Medicine*, **35**, 291–316.
40. Hare, E. (1988). Schizophrenia before 1800? The case of the Revd. George Trosse. *Psychological Medicine*, **18**, 279–85.
41. Foucault, M. (1970). *The order of things*. Tavistock Publications, London.

42. Strömgren, E. (1982). Development of the concept of schizophrenia. In *Psychoses of uncertain aetiology* (ed. J. Wing and I. Wind), pp. 17–26. Cambridge University Press.

43. Macalpine, I. and Hunter, R. (1956). *Schizophrenia 1677*. Dawson, London.

44. Freud, S. (1925). A neurosis of demoniacal possession in the seventeenth century. In *Collected papers* (ed. E. Jones), Vol. IV, pp. 436–72. Hogarth Press, London.

45. Carpenter, P.K. (1989). Descriptions of schizophrenia in the psychiatry of Georgian Britain: John Haslam and James Tilly Matthews. *Comprehensive Psychiatry*, **30**, 332–8.

46. Jeste, D.V., del Carmen, R., Lohr, J.B., and Whyatt, R.J. (1985). Did schizophrenia exist before the eighteenth century? *Comprehensive Psychiatry*, **26**, 493–503.

47. Turner, T.H. (1992). Schizophrenia as a permanent problem. *History of Psychiatry*, **3**, 413–29.

48. Allen, D.F. (1995). Vers une perspective axiologique de la schizophrénie (éléments pour une histoire critique). Thèse de la Université de Paris 7.

4.3.2 Descriptive clinical features of schizophrenia

Peter F. Liddle

The clinical features of schizophrenia embrace a diverse range of disturbances of perception, thought, emotion, motivation, and motor activity. It is an illness in which episodes of florid disturbance are usually set against a background of sustained disability. The level of chronic disability ranges from a mild decrease in the ability to cope with stress, to a profound difficulty in initiating and organizing activity that can render patients unable to care for themselves.

Disorders of thought and perception

Delusions

Delusions have traditionally been regarded as the hallmark of insanity. Although there are no features that provide an unambiguous distinction between the delusions of schizophrenia and those of other psychotic illnesses, the delusions that are most typical of schizophrenia have an enigmatic character rarely seen in other disorders. In contrast to the delusions of affective psychosis, which have a content consistent with the prevailing emotional state, in schizophrenia delusions often appear to reflect a fragmentation in the experience of reality. This fragmentation is manifest in several ways.

- The content of the delusional belief often contains contradictions. There is a lack of logical consistency between the components of the belief, or between the belief and common understanding of what is possible. For example, a patient was very distressed by the belief that he had no head and also that there was blood all over his face. Another patient believed that his head was split in two by an axe.

- The relationship between the delusional belief and any action that might flow from it is unpredictable. In some instances, the patient believes he has a special role or identity, yet for the most part, lives a life that is scarcely influenced by the belief. In the words of Bleuler:[1] 'Kings, Emperors, Popes, and Redeemers engage for the most part, in quite banal work, provided they still have any energy at all for activity'. In other instances, patients might act in unexpected ways.

- At least in the chronic phase of the illness, patients often acknowledge that a former delusion was not justified, yet in the same interview they reiterate the delusional belief. Bleuler[1] reported: 'sometimes the patients even produce thoughts which are only understandable if it is assumed that the delusions still retain some reality for these patients even though consciously they may reject them. Sometimes the manner in which the delusion is declared to be senseless shows that in a way it is still alive.'

The mental mechanism of schizophrenic delusions remains to be ascertained. It is not a lack of capacity for logical thought; rather it appears that certain ideas acquire an attribute that exempts them from the normal processes of validation. This phenomenon is illustrated by the historic case of Daniel Schreber,[2] a high-ranking judge from Leipzig, who suffered a late-onset schizophrenic illness. His first episode of illness occurred when he was standing for election to the Reichstag at the age of 42. A second, more protracted, episode occurred when he was facing a heavy burden of work after appointment as Presiding Judge of the Appeal Court in Dresden at the age of 51. After obtaining a court order for his discharge from hospital 9 years later, in 1902, he published his memoirs[3] in a volume that includes his own account of his beliefs, and also the report prepared by the asylum director, Dr Weber, opposing his discharge. Schreber eventually suffered a third episode of illness at the age of 55, after his wife suffered a stroke, and he remained in an uncommunicative disorganized state until his death.

Schreber believed that he had a mission to redeem the world and restore humankind to its lost state of bliss. His system of delusions included the belief that he was being transformed into a voluptuous female partner of God. Dr Weber reported that at the onset of his second episode of illness, Schreber's mental life was dominated by delusions and hallucinations. However, prior to discharge from hospital in 1902, he exhibited lively interest in his social environment, a well-informed mind, and sound judgement, while nonetheless maintaining his delusional beliefs in a manner that would accept no contrary argument. Schreber himself agreed that his beliefs were unchangeable. He considered that they belonged to a domain that was exempt from normal logic: 'I could even say with Jesus Christ: My kingdom is not of this world; my so-called delusions are concerned solely with God and the beyond'. Furthermore, he maintained total conviction in his core beliefs despite recognizing that he had previously suffered distorted perceptions of reality. He had believed that his surroundings had been 'miracled up' by rays. He stated:

> Having lived for months among miracles, I was inclined to take more or less everything I saw for a miracle. Accordingly, I did not know whether to take the streets of Leipzig through which I traveled as only theatre props, perhaps in the fashion in which Prince Potemkin is said to have put them up for Empress Catherine II of Russia during her travels through the desolate country, so as to give the impression of a flourishing countryside.

For the purpose of understanding the nature of delusions in schizophrenia, Schreber's account is of special value because, by virtue of his keen intellect, we have access to his own perceptions of his condition in addition to detailed accounts by his physicians. In particular, his case illustrates the frequently observed phenomenon of a delusion engrossing the patient fully during the acute phase, while in the chronic phase it is still held, but coexists with an acknowledgement that it defies normal logic.

The late onset of Schreber's illness and his high level of professional achievement are unusual for an individual with schizophrenia, and raise questions about the diagnosis. However, the fact that he had delusions that were sustained independently of affective disorder, together with persisting difficulty in coping with stress, and eventually suffered a marked deterioration during his third episode of illness strongly supports the diagnosis of schizophrenia. His keen intellect illustrates a paradoxical feature of schizophrenia that can be discerned across the full spectrum of disability—the coexistence of markedly abnormal mental activity with well-integrated mental function. Even patients with symptoms affecting many domains of mental function exhibit this incongruity. Bleuler[1] noted: 'Even the most demented schizophrenic can under proper conditions exhibit productions of a highly integrated type'.

Adherence to delusional beliefs despite the ability to understand the logic of a counter-argument sometimes creates what appears to be playfulness with logic. Bleuler[1] reports the case of a well-educated socially competent patient who complained that he had made her pregnant while she was asleep, and that he had cut the infant out of her arm. When Bleuler attempted to convince her that in reality he could not have been with her in the night, she asked: 'Then why do you come in the dream?'

In many instances, the delusions of schizophrenia appear to arise from an altered experience of self or of external reality. The phenomena identified by the German psychiatrist, Kurt Schneider[4] as first-rank symptoms of schizophrenia (discussed in greater detail below) include several symptoms that entail an aberrant experience of ownership of one's own thought, will, action, emotion, or bodily function, which the patient attributes to alien influence. In some cases, delusions might arise from a delusional mood, i.e. an altered sense of reality in which the current circumstances acquire an indefinable transcendental quality.

Although the delusions most characteristic of schizophrenia have an incongruous quality, it is not uncommon for schizophrenic patients to have coherent delusions that are internally consistent and produce predictable behavioural responses. In particular, coherent persecutory delusions are common, and can lead to defensive actions such as barracading oneself in one's room with blinds drawn. Ideas of reference and delusions of reference are also prevalent. For example, a patient might report that television programmes refer specifically to him or her. In the International Pilot Study of Schizophrenia[5] conducted by the World Health Organization, ideas of reference were reported in 70 per cent of cases, suspiciousness in 66 per cent, and delusions of persecution in 64 per cent.

Hallucinations

Hallucinations in any modality can occur, but auditory hallucinations are the most prevalent in schizophrenia. Hearing voices speaking in the third person is the most specific. This experience is listed among the Schneiderian first-rank symptoms. Sometimes the content is mundane, as in the instance when a patient of Bleuler[1] heard a voice saying 'Now she is combing her hair' while she was grooming in the morning. In other instances there is an implied criticism, as in the case reported by Schneider[4] of a woman who heard a voice saying 'Now she is eating; here she is munching again', whenever she wanted to eat.

Second-person auditory hallucinations are also common. In the International Pilot Study of Schizophrenia,[5] voices speaking to the patient were reported in 65 per cent of cases. Such voices are often derogatory, although it is not uncommon for a patient to hear both derogatory and comforting voices. Voices might issue commands that the patient obeys. In some instances, the patient engages in a dialogue with the voices.

During the acute phase of illness, auditory hallucinations usually have the same sensory quality as voices arising from sources in the external world. The patient might change accommodation in a fruitless attempt to escape from them. In some instances the voice is attributed to a radio-transmitter implanted in the body, especially in the teeth. In the chronic phase, the voices are often recognized as coming from within the person's own mind. Kraepelin[6] reports: 'at other times they do not appear to the patient as sense perceptions at all; they are "voices of conscience"; "voices which do not speak with words"'. These experiences are pseudohallucinations, but nonetheless they are a significant feature in many cases.

In schizophrenia, visual hallucinations are less common than auditory hallucinations, but do occur. Somatic hallucinations are also relatively common, and often are associated with a delusional misinterpretation. For example, a young man reported sensations in his belly that he attributed to a snake, which he believed had crawled up his anus.

Schneiderian first-rank symptoms

Kurt Schneider[4] identified a set of phenomena that he considered were strongly indicative of schizophrenia in the absence of overt brain disease. These symptoms, listed in Table 1, have become known as first-rank symptoms. Schneider did not consider that the diagnosis could be made simply on the presence of one such symptom; on the contrary, he warned[4], 'a psychotic phenomenon is not like a defective stone in an otherwise perfect mosaic'. Schneider did not define the phenomena precisely, and clinicians have interpreted his writings differently. Mellor[7] formulated a precise set of definitions and found that, according to these strict criteria, 72 per cent of patients with schizophrenia exhibited at least one first-rank symptom. Applying the same criteria, O'Grady[8] found that in a series of cases assessed at admission to hospital, 73 per cent of schizophrenic patients exhibited at least one first-rank symptom, while no cases of affective psychosis did. However, applying less strict criteria, O'Grady found more broadly defined first-rank symptoms in 14 per cent of patients with affective psychosis.

Three of the first-rank symptoms (voices commenting, voices discussing, and audible thoughts) involve auditory hallucinations, while the remainder entail delusional attributions to experiences or perceptions. Although Schneider himself avoided speculating on the theoretical implications of these phenomena, it is notable that most of them involve a disorder of the sense of ownership of one's own mental or

Table 1 Schneiderian first-rank symptoms

Voices commenting	A hallucinatory voice commenting on one's actions in the third person
Voices discussing or arguing	Hallucinations of two or more voices discussing or arguing about oneself
Audible thought	Hearing one's own thoughts aloud
Thought insertion	The insertion, by an alien source, of thoughts that are experienced as not being one's own
Thought withdrawal	The withdrawal of thoughts from the mind by an alien agency
Thought broadcast	The experience that one's thoughts are broadcast so as to be accessible to others
Made will	The experience of one's will being controlled by an alien influence
Made acts	The experience that acts executed by one's own body are the actions of an alien agency, rather than oneself
Made affect	The experience of emotion that is not one's own, attributed to an alien influence
Somatic passivity	Bodily function is controlled by an alien influence
Delusional perception	The attribution of a totally unwarranted meaning to a normal perception

physical activity. Thought broadcast, thought withdrawal, and thought insertion reflect the experience of loss of autonomy over thought, while made will, made acts, made affect, and somatic passivity reflect loss of autonomy over action, will, affect, and bodily function.

Mellor[7] emphasizes that there are two aspects to these phenomena: the experience of loss of autonomy and the delusional attribution to alien influence. As an illustration of made acts, Mellor reports a patient who reported that his fingers moved to pick up objects 'but I don't control them ... I sit there watching them move, and they are quite independent, what they do is nothing to do with me. I am just a puppet ... I am just a puppet who is manipulated by cosmic strings'. To illustrate made affect, Mellor quotes a young woman: 'I cry, tears roll down my cheeks and I look unhappy, but inside I have a cold anger because they are using me in this way, and it is not me who is unhappy, but they are projecting unhappiness into my brain.'

Delusional perception, in which an entirely unwarranted conclusion is drawn from a normal perception, illustrates the incongruity between a delusional idea and concurrent mental activity, which is characteristic of schizophrenia. However, the way in which delusional perceptions often crystallize from a delusional mood indicates that it is not merely a matter of illogical inference; the delusional idea is more like a divine revelation. Mellor[7] gives the example of an Irishman who experienced a sense of foreboding while seated at the breakfast table in a lodging house. When another lodger innocently pushed the salt cellar towards him, he suddenly knew this meant that he must return home to greet the Pope who was visiting his family to thank them because Our Lord was to be born again to one of the women.

Disorders of the form and flow of thought

The speech of schizophrenic patients is often difficult to understand because of abnormalities of form of the underlying thought. However, the clinical assessment of thought form disorder remains a major challenge. This is due in part to the fact the essential features of the impediments to verbal communication in schizophrenia have yet to be defined in a fully satisfactory manner. Furthermore, thought disorder is usually manifest during spontaneous speech, making it difficult to create circumstances in which the phenomena can be elicited reliably.

Bleuler[1] coined the term loosening of associations to describe the weakening of the connections between words and ideas that bind thoughts into a coherent whole. While this term is a useful label for one of the major types of disorder of the form of speech and thought, it does not encompass the entire range of such disorders. In addition to disordered connections between words and ideas, there are oddities in the use of language. One of the most comprehensive catalogues is the Thought, Language, and Communication Scale compiled by Andreasen.[9] This scale includes several items that involve different aspects of the loosening of associations:

- derailment—wandering off the point during the free flow of conversation
- tangentiality—answers to questions that are off the point
- incoherence—a breakdown of the relationships between words within a sentence so that the sentence no longer makes sense
- loss of goal—failure to reach a conclusion or achieve a point.

The Thought, Language, and Communication Scale also includes several items that refer to unusual use of language:

- metonyms—unusual uses of words (e.g. hand-shoe instead of glove)
- neologisms—new words invented by the patient.

The various aspects of loosening of associations and peculiarities of language use are commonly regarded as positive thought disorder. The Thought, Language, and Communication Scale also includes negative thought disorders that entail impoverishment of thinking:

- poverty of speech is a disorder of the flow of speech in which the rate of speech production is reduced
- poverty of content is a disorder in which the amount of information conveyed is relatively little in proportion to the number of words uttered.

The Thought, Language, and Communication Scale has proved to be one of the most successful of recent attempts to define and quantify formal thought disorder, but it has several limitations. Most important of these is that the positive thought disorder items defined in the scale do not discriminate well between manic thought disorder and florid schizophrenic thought disorder.[10] Secondly, the scale is not sensitive to the subtle thought form disorders that occur in first-degree relatives of schizophrenic patients.

These limitations are dealt with, at least partially, in the Thought Disorder Index devised by Holzman.[11] This scale employs ratings based on thought and speech elicited by the Rorschach inkblot figures and during an assessment of IQ. Two categories of disorder, disorganization (comprising vagueness, confusion, and incoherence) and idiosyncratic verbalizations, appear to discriminate fairly well between schizophrenic and manic thought.[11] Furthermore, the Thought Disorder Index is sensitive to subtle thought disorder present in first-degree relatives of schizophrenic patients. Unfortunately, this scale is too cumbersome for routine clinical use.

Positive formal thought disorder is usually a transient feature of acute episodes of illness. Nonetheless, after resolution of the acute episode there is often a subtle residual thought disorder that is manifest as vague, wandering speech or minor idiosyncrasies of word usage or ideas.

Negative formal thought disorder has a greater tendency to be persistent. Chronic poverty of speech is associated with impairment in several domains of cognition[12] including abstract reasoning. It leads to impaired social relationships,[13] although it is also influenced by the social milieu. Transient poverty of speech can occur during acute episodes of illness. It is less strongly associated with cognitive impairment and, at least in some cases, appears to reflect an obstruction of the articulation of speech that is catatonic in character. At its most severe, the patient is mute.

Insight

Lack of insight is one of the defining characteristics of psychotic illness. Lack of insight entails a failure to accept that one is ill and to appreciate that symptoms are due to illness. In the International Pilot Study of Schizophrenia[5] lack of insight was the most prevalent symptom reported in schizophrenic patients. It occurred in approximately 90 per cent of cases. Insight is often partial. In particular, even in instances in which a patient acknowledges suffering from an illness, he or she might fail to accept that psychotic symptoms such as delusions or hallucinations are a manifestation of that illness. Lack of insight is one factor that contributes to unwillingness to accept treatment. However, the clinician should be aware that other factors, including lack of appropriate education about the illness and justified fear of side-effects of treatment, can also impede the development of a therapeutic collaboration between physician and patient.

Impaired cognition

In addition to delusions and disorders of thought form, a wide range of cognitive deficits occur in schizophrenia. These are discussed in Chapter 4.3.3.1. This chapter focuses on the relationship between cognitive impairment and other features of the illness.

In the acute phase of the illness, attentional impairment is common and is often associated with psychomotor excitation and/or formal thought disorder. It might also reflect preoccupation with delusions and hallucinations.

During the chronic phase of illness, many schizophrenic patients exhibit persistent cognitive impairments. Longitudinal studies of individuals who subsequently develop schizophrenia reveal that the deficits are discernible during childhood, suggesting that these deficits are an aspect of the predisposition to schizophrenia. The major cognitive impairments are in the realm of executive function, working memory, and long-term memory. Executive dysfunction includes impaired ability to initiate and select self-generated mental activity. Impaired ability to form and initiate plans is associated with chronic poverty of speech, blunted affect, and lack of spontaneous activity, while impaired ability to inhibit inappropriate responses is associated with chronic formal thought disorder.[12]

Disorders of emotion

An extensive range of disorders of emotion occur in schizophrenia. Blunted affect and inappropriate affect are the most characteristic, and also tend to be the most persistent, but transient excitation, irritability, lability, and depression are also common.

Blunted affect

Blunting of affect is manifest as decreased responsiveness to emotional issues, loss of vocal inflection, and diminished facial expression. These objective signs of affective blunting are sometimes accompanied by awareness of loss of emotional tone that, paradoxically, patients find to be distressing. More commonly, there is a lack of concern and even a lack of awareness of the problem. Affective blunting is one of the hallmarks of chronic schizophrenia. Bleuler[1] remarked that when the affects disappear, the illness becomes chronic. While blunted affect is usually chronic, it can also be a feature of acute episodes of the illness that resolves as the acute episode resolves.

Inappropriate affect

Inappropriate or incongruous affect is the expression of affect that is inappropriate in the circumstances. At its most severe it takes the form of hollow laughter that is unrelated to any apparent stimulus. More common is inappropriate giggling that differs from normal nervous giggling in having a more fatuous character.

Excitation and depression

During acute exacerbations of schizophrenia, excitation, manifest as irritability, sleeplessness, agitation, and motor overactivity, is common. Depression is also common around the time of an acute episode of schizophrenia,[14] and is often a feature of the prodromal phase of the illness. It is not uncommon for patients presenting in the first episode of schizophrenia to report having suffered bouts of minor depressive symptoms over a period of several years.

Depression also occurs during the chronic phase of the illness. Although the cross-sectional rate is approximately 10 per cent in the chronic phase,[15] schizophrenic patients have a high probability of suffering depression at some time during their illness. In a longitudinal study, Johnson[16] found that 65 per cent of schizophrenic patients exhibited an episode of depression in a period of 36 months after a florid psychotic episode.

Motor disorders

Subtle disturbance of motor co-ordination is common in schizophrenia. Home videos of children who subsequently develop schizophrenia demonstrate that even in infancy they are noticeably more clumsy than their siblings, suggesting that disturbed motor co-ordination is an aspect of the predisposition to schizophrenia.[17]

More dramatic than subtle motor incoordination are the rare catatonic motor disorders. Catatonia entails disturbance of voluntary motor activity and posture. The level of activity can be either decreased or increased. In extreme cases of hypoactivity the patient is in a stupor, and is unresponsive to stimuli, but usually retains conscious awareness. In hyperactive states the patient often maintains a stereotypic activity for prolonged periods. Even less common are conditions such as waxy flexibility, in which a patient's body can be moulded into an unusual posture, which is then sustained for lengthy periods, and echopraxia, in which the patient mimics the voluntary motor actions of the examiner.

Disorders of volition

Among the most disabling of the clinical phenomena of schizophrenia are disruptions of motivation and will. Voluntary activity can be disjointed or weakened. Disjointed volition is manifest in poorly organized ill-judged activities which appear to be prompted by impulse. For example, an artistic, intelligent young woman felt cold so she lit a fire on the carpet in her bedroom, even though she was able to appreciate that this was a dangerous thing to do. Weakened volition results in prolonged periods of underactivity. The patient might lie in bed or sit in an armchair for hours.

Anxiety and somatoform disorders

Various forms of anxiety and somatic symptoms are common in schizophrenia. Huber[18] described a non-characteristic defect state which is dominated by anxiety and asthenia. Coenesthesia, in which the patient suffers unusual or debilitating bodily experiences that do not have an apparent somatic cause, occurs frequently.

Dimensions of psychopathology in schizophrenia

Schizophrenia is heterogeneous in its clinical presentation, suggesting that several different pathophysiological processes might contribute to the illness.

Positive and negative symptom dimensions

Positive symptoms are those that reflect the presence of an abnormal mental process, and include delusions, hallucinations, and formal thought disorder. Negative symptoms reflect the diminution or absence of a mental function that is normally present. They include poverty of speech and blunted affect. In schizophrenia, positive symptoms tend to be transient, while negative symptoms tend to be chronic. In an influential hypothesis, Crow[19] proposed that positive symptoms arise from dopaminergic overactivity, while negative symptoms reflect structural brain abnormality. While a substantial body of evidence supports this hypothesis, it does not account adequately for the complexity of the heterogeneity of the clinical features in schizophrenia.

Three dimensions of characteristic symptoms

The preponderance of evidence[12,13,20] from factor analysis of schizophrenic symptoms indicates that the characteristic symptoms of schizophrenia segregate into three syndromes, as shown in Table 2. These syndromes do not reflect separate illnesses, but different dimensions of illness, in the sense that a patient might exhibit more than one of the syndromes. In an individual case, the three syndromes vary

Table 2 Three syndromes of symptoms characteristic of schizophrenia

Reality distortion
Delusions
Hallucinations

Disorganization
Thought form disorder
Inappropriate affect
Bizarre behaviour

Psychomotor poverty (core negative symptoms)
Poverty of speech
Blunted affect
Decreased spontaneous movement

independently in severity over time, while the symptoms from within each syndrome tend to vary in parallel.[20]

The three syndromes embrace only the characteristic symptoms that are given weight in making a diagnosis of schizophrenia. In addition, there are two affective syndromes, depression and psychomotor excitation, that are prevalent in schizophrenia,[12] despite being more characteristic of mood disorders. These affective syndromes are usually transient.

An accumulating body of evidence[12] from brain imaging studies indicates that the three characteristic syndromes are associated with three distinguishable patterns of cerebral malfunction involving the areas of association cortex and related subcortical nuclei, which serve higher mental functions. Overall, the evidence indicates that the heterogeneity of symptom profiles in schizophrenia does not reflect the existence of several discrete illnesses, but rather, the existence of several dimensions of psychopathology, each arising from disorder of a specific neuronal system that serves an aspect of higher mental function. In an individual case, several of these neural systems might be involved.

Although many details of the relationships between the diverse clinical features of schizophrenia remain uncertain, a growing understanding of the neural pathways involved is beginning to provide the foundation for understanding the protean manifestations of this disorder.

References

1. Bleuler, E. (1950). *Dementia praecox or the group of schizophrenias* (trans. J. Zinkin). International Universities Press, New York.
2. Spitzer, R.L., Gibbon, M., Skodol, A.E., Williams, J.B.W., and First, M.B. (ed.) (1989). *DSM-IIIR casebook*. American Psychiatric Press, Washington, DC.
3. Schreber, D.P. (1955). *Denkwurdigkeiten eines Nervenkranken (Memoirs of my nervous illness)* (trans. I. Macalpine and R. Hunter). Dawson, London.
4. Schneider, K. (1959).*Clinical psychopathology* (trans. M.W. Hamilton). Grune & Stratton, New York.
5. World Health Organization (1973). *The international pilot study of schizophrenia*. World Health Organization, Geneva.
6. Kraepelin, E. (1919). *Dementia praecox and paraphrenia* (trans. R.M. Barclay). Facsimile edition, 1971. Kreiger, New York.
7. Mellor, C.S. (1970). First rank symptoms of schizophrenia. *British Journal of Psychiatry*, **117**, 15–23.

8. O'Grady, J.C. (1990). The prevalence and diagnostic significance of first-rank symptoms in a random sample of acute schizophrenia in-patients. *British Journal of Psychiatry*, **156**, 496–500.

9. Andreasen, N.C. (1979). Thought language and communication disorders. I Clinical assessment, definition of terms and evaluation of their reliability. *Archives of General Psychiatry*, **36**, 1315–21.

10. Andreasen, N.C. (1979). Thought, language and communication disorders. II Diagnostic significance. *Archives of General Psychiatry*, **36**, 1325–30.

11. Holzman, P.S., Shenton, M.E. and Solovay, M.R. (1986). Quality of thought disorder in differential diagnosis. *Schizophrenia Bulletin*, **12**, 360–71.

12. Liddle, P.F. (1999). The multi-dimensional phenotype of schizophrenia. In *Schizophrenia in a molecular age* (ed. C.A. Taminga), pp. 1–28. American Psychiatric Press, Washington, DC.

13. Liddle, P.F. (1987). The symptoms of chronic schizophrenia: a re-examination of the positive-negative dichotomy. *British Journal of Psychiatry*, **151**, 145–51.

14. Siris, S.G. (1991). Diagnosis of secondary depression in schizophrenia: implications for DSMIV. *Schizophrenia Bulletin*, **17**, 75–98.

15. Barnes, T.R.E., Curson, D.A., Liddle, P.F., and Patel, M. (1989). The nature and prevalence of depression in chronic schizophrenic inpatients. *British Journal of Psychiatry*, **154**, 486–91.

16. Johnson, D.A.W. (1988). The significance of depression in the prediction of relapse in chronic schizophrenia. *British Journal of Psychiatry*, **152**, 320–3.

17. Walker, E. and Lewine, R.J. (1990). Prediction of adult-onset schizophrenia from childhood home videos of the patients. *American Journal of Psychiatry*, **89**, 704–16.

18. Huber, G., Gross, G., and Schuttler, E. (1975). A long term follow-up study of schizophrenia: psychiatric course of illness and prognosis. *Acta Psychiatrica Scandinavica*, **52**, 49–57.

19. Crow, T.J. (1980). The molecular pathology of schizophrenia: more than one disease process. *British Medical Journal*, **280**, 66–8.

20. Arndt, S., Andreasen, N.C., Flaum, M., Miller, D., and Nopoulos, P. (1995). A longitudinal study of symptom dimensions in schizophrenia. *Archives of General Psychiatry*, **52**, 352–60.

4.3.3 Neuropsychological features of schizophrenia
4.3.3.1 The clinical neuropsychology of schizophrenia

Anthony S. David

Introduction

Neuropsychology forms a bridge between the phenomenology and clinical features of schizophrenia, and the underlying pathology. The cognitive sciences have been increasingly adopted as a framework for discussing such features at the expense of a purely descriptive psychopathology. The advantage of this is that cognitive models strive to be mechanistic and explanatory although, like phenomenology, they sometimes succeed only in displacing one lot of arcane jargon for another. The neuro- prefix is a relatively new addition and simply reflects the often tacit acceptance of a biological basis for the changes observed, but in fact earlier discussions of for instance 'disorders of

attention in schizophrenia' which made no reference to the brain, would now be placed under the heading of neuropsychology.[1]

In his description of dementia praecox, Kraepelin emphasized the presence of clear-cut intellectual decline (see Chapter 4.3.1), whereas Bleuler[2] remarked:

> It shows a complete misunderstanding of the peculiarities of schizophrenia if one believes that schizophrenic dementia can be proved or excluded by means of an 'intelligence test'…The actual amount of knowledge remains preserved…but it is not always available or it is employed in the wrong way.

Paradoxically, both positions are correct. There are aspects of the neuropsychology of schizophrenia which are akin to a dementia (i.e. an apparent decline in function across several cognitive domains) in conjunction with other aspects most unlike a straightforward dementia, such as the variability of test performance across and within individuals, and lack of inexorable progression. However, attempts to distinguish schizophrenia from neurological disorders on the basis of neuropsychological tests have failed—the overlap in test scores is surprisingly large and classification rates on this basis, no better than chance.[3]

It was previously common for all-embracing psychological theories of schizophrenia to be advanced. This is less common nowadays, where empirical findings outweigh theoretical speculation. This chapter is not intended to be a comprehensive review of the work in this area but rather a brief overview of clinically relevant findings in the neuropsychology of schizophrenia. The approach taken here will be to divide the neuropsychology of schizophrenia into premorbid, illness-related, and symptom-related deficits, with discussion of whether these deficits are generalized or specific.

Deficits
Premorbid deficits

The majority of patients with schizophrenia have cognitive impairment.[4] This is not entirely due to 'cognitive decline', but to some extent a lower than average IQ detectable premorbidly. Part of the evidence for this comes from two large population-based cohort studies in the United Kingdom[5,6] and a Swedish conscript cohort.[7] In these studies individuals were given intelligence tests during childhood or adolescence, at which time, none was manifesting signs of schizophrenia. After several years, some of the cohort developed schizophrenia and, as a group, when compared to the remainder, they showed a lower than average IQ (by the equivalent of about 5–10 points). Similarly, when school reports of children who later developed schizophrenia are compared with their classmates or siblings, or best of all, identical twins, the results show the same trend.[8] These premorbid differences on IQ tests are, by definition, generalized although language and planning deficits may be slightly more obvious.

Getting an accurate picture of premorbid deficits in routine clinical practice is difficult unless school reports over many years have been retained. However, a rough idea can be gained simply by establishing the level of education achieved (if clearly within the premorbid period) and contrasting this to family expectations and social norms. Deviation from an expected level or in comparison to siblings can provide additional comparisons. Tests of reading ability such as the National Adult Reading Test,[9] have been shown to be relatively

Table 1 Tasks more or less likely to be affected in schizophrenia

More affected	Less affected
Executive	Non-executive
Effortful	Non-effortful
Controlled	Automatic
Serial	Parallel
Conscious	Unconscious

immune from acquired cognitive decline so may serve as a proxy for premorbid ability.

Illness-related deficits

When individuals with a diagnosis of schizophrenia are studied in contrast with 'normal controls', the neuropsychological gulf between them is (again, on average) wide, much wider than that between those destined to develop the disorder but not identified as abnormal at the time of testing; in fact the discrepancy is of the order of 1.5 to 3.0 standard deviations (**SD**) below the normal control mean[10] (1 SD is equal to 15 IQ points). This applies to established cases, as well as first onset and drug-free patients[11] and there is surprisingly little resolution after the episode has abated.[12] Hence cognitive impairment is not an artefact of medication, chronicity, or 'institutionalization'. Although truly longitudinal neuropsychological studies spanning premorbid and post-onset periods are elusive, the obvious assumption is that the onset of the illness brings with it a further substantial cognitive decline. Such studies carried out in the 1950s and 1960s in North America using conscript cohorts, before the days of reliable diagnosis, confirm an illness-related decline.[13]

Again, the question arises, are these deficits generalized or specific? Different studies provide different answers. All show deficits across the board including visual perception, recognition memory, motor skills, language comprehension and expression, episodic memory, and planning. However, some authors point out that some test scores seem to be disproportionately impaired and other relatively spared; this gives rise to the claim for specific neuropsychological deficits in schizophrenia. Visual perception, recognition, naming, and procedural or motor learning are relatively spared while executive functions (including tasks of set shifting, ignoring irrelevance, doing more than one thing simultaneously, forward planning) and learning and semantic memory tend to be the functions more obviously affected.

There have been several attempts to classify those sorts of tasks more or less likely to be affected in schizophrenia, and these are summarized in Table 1. This tends to translate into difficult versus easy, which undermines the theoretical claims made for the distinctions.

The Wisconsin Card Sorting Test is widely regarded as a specific test of set shifting and patients with schizophrenia do poorly on it as do those with frontal lobe lesions. However, the test requires the subject to shift set, to follow rules, and to keep a record of previous responses so that actions are not repeated. It is therefore not surprising that people with global deficits in IQ find the test difficult.[14] Heinrichs and Zakzanis[15] systematically reviewed studies comparing schizophrenic patients and controls on a variety of neuropsychological tests (including the Wisconsin Test). The result of a meta-analysis of some 204 published studies is that there is little evidence for specific deficits and much evidence for large overlap in performance between patients and controls. The greatest difference in performance was found in tests of verbal memory, bilateral motor skill, and performance (non-verbal) IQ although even these showed that around 25 per cent of patients were above the control median.

These studies of cognition have parallels in structural neuroimaging. Quantitative reviews of the studies on schizophrenia with CT[16] and magnetic resonance imaging show much evidence for generalized loss of tissue (large ventricles and smaller cortical thickness),[17] but more localized abnormalities are less consistently observed, with the possible exception of medial temporal lobe structures.[18]

Symptom- and syndrome-related deficits

Despite problems in showing that particular functions are specifically impaired in the disorder, many models have been put forward which have heuristic value. Instead of attempting to explain the whole of schizophrenia with all its diverse manifestation in terms of a single neuropsychological dysfunction, many such models take as their starting point isolated syndromes or symptoms and seek to account for these in cognitive terms.[19]

Executive function

This is a loosely defined set of cognitive abilities which are thought to involve the integration of subsidiary abilities—such as memory and perception. The idea is that as well as requiring the basic ability to retain information, a complex organism in the social world has to be able to organize information, to know when to rely on memory, and to update its store of information. These are executive skills. Other executive functions include selecting appropriate responses and inhibiting inappropriate ones, generating plans, and solving problems. The maintenance of information on line and its manipulation to aid problem solving comes under the heading of 'working memory' seen by most psychologists as an executive function. These functions are loosely allied with the 'frontal lobes' although such brain-behaviour mapping is an oversimplification. With this broad definition it is easy to see how many of the behaviours and features of schizophrenia can be viewed as 'executive function deficits'. The negative symptoms of lack of spontaneity, poor motivation, and socially inappropriate behaviour, in particular fit into this rubric. Difficulties in selecting relevant stimuli for further processing (selective attention or filtering) have been invoked to explain some positive symptoms like perceptual abnormalities (hallucinations) and, perhaps, ideas of reference. The Stroop paradigm, where the subject is asked to name the colour ink in which an incongruent colour word is printed, is a traditional test of 'selective attention'.

Reality monitoring

The understanding of positive symptoms, particularly hallucinations, has benefited from the concepts of reality and source monitoring. These terms describe the everyday challenge of distinguishing between imagined events and memories for real events (reality monitoring) and in the case of actions or speech, between whether, for example, I said something or merely heard someone saying it to me (source monitoring). Building on the assumption that auditory hallucinations are the products of the subject's own mind (and not from aliens from outer space), reality monitoring provides a model whereby normal inner speech is mislabelled as not coming from the self. Why this occurs is another question. One suggestion is that if inner speech or other internal images are particularly vivid, the subject may confuse them for reality, although evidence for this is lacking. Another model advanced by Frith[20] is that our brains continually monitor or check our actions to see whether they tally with our intentions. If an action occurs (my arm reaches an object or I ask a question) but the brain had not registered a prior intention (owing to some failure of feedback), the action may then be regarded as alien. Again this provides a plausible explanation for auditory hallucinations and passivity phenomena. Frith and colleagues suggest that intentions arise from systems connecting the dorsolateral prefrontal cortex, the anterior cingulate, and the supplementary motor area. Others have argued that the hippocampus is a candidate for the 'comparator' function between intentions and actions.[21]

Misattribution

Fundamental to psychosis is the attribution of the agency for one's own thoughts, actions, impulses, and so on to an 'other'. However, social psychologists[22] have shown that this is not merely a defect but rather a bias towards certain types of information. For example, a tendency to attribute or blame others for bad things that happen in one's life, while accepting the credit for good things is an example of such a bias to which most people are prone. Another is paying more attention to events or ideas which seem to confirm one's prejudices. In the extreme these misattributions can amount to delusions. As well as misattributing events, some people are prone to misattribute intentions. Work from child development has proposed that normal children are adept 'mind readers' in the sense of reading the intentions of others. People with autism frequently fail to infer intentions from social behaviour.[23] Frith[24] has proposed that patients with persecutory delusions do infer such intentions in others, but these are prone to error so that the intentions are invariably felt to be dishonourable.

Psychophysiological and conditioning models

Several techniques, such as measurement of skin conductance, startle responses, early cerebral evoked potentials (P50, a positive deflection in scalp-recorded electrical potentials occurring 50 ms after a stimulus), etc., have been applied to the study of schizophrenia. These have generally supported theories which suggest that patients are abnormally 'aroused' by benign stimuli or, as in attentional theories, are unable to filter or 'gate' sensory inputs, thereby leading to sensory 'overload'. Or, within a learning and conditioning framework, experimental results suggest that patients are unable to distinguish between relevant and irrelevant stimuli. These differ from cognitive theories in that they postulate dysfunction early on in the information processing stream, or with 'unconscious' processes (such as conditioning).

Hemisphere dysfunction

Neuropsychological theories of schizophrenia have arisen by analogy from the effects on cognition and behaviour of neurological lesions. For instance, the disturbances in language production observed in some schizophrenia patients (thought disorder) have been likened to aphasia and hence left hemisphere abnormalities while deficits in affect regulation and perception have been likened to right hemisphere lesions. Integration of information across the hemispheres seemed to be an attractive notion to account for the range of schizophrenic disturbances as well as apparent 'splits' between thoughts and actions,

and thoughts and emotions.[25,26] Such theories suffer from the difficulty described above in establishing disproportionate deficits in the task of interest against other less localizable deficits.

The course taken by Liddle[27] combines a syndromic with a neurological approach. He found that symptoms of schizophrenia aggregated into three broad clusters: psychomotor poverty (affecting speech and movement and blunting of affect), reality distortion (essentially positive symptoms, hallucinations, and delusions), and finally disorganization (including thought disorder and inappropriate affect). Using a battery of tests borrowed from the neurology clinic, he showed that psychomotor poverty was associated with poorer performance on abstract reasoning and long-term memory tests, disorganization or impairments of attention and learning, while the reality distortion symptoms correlated with impaired figure ground perception (traditionally temporoparietal tests). One interpretation of these findings is that the poverty and disorganization syndromes reflect different focal disturbances in frontal function (dorsolateral and ventral, respectively). Functional neuroimaging techniques are able to test these hypotheses *in vivo*.

Subsequent research has offered support for this general scheme, namely that 'negative symptoms' tend to correlate with tests of executive (and memory) deficits,[28] while positive symptoms seem less 'anchored' to neuropsychological impairments as commonly described but rather, productive abnormalities of language (thought disorder), biases in information appraisal (paranoia), and reality monitoring errors (auditory hallucinations).

Finally, the concept of insight into illness or unawareness of illness has become a topic for discussion. Again, arguing from the neurological analogy of anosognosia (the lack of awareness of neurological deficit, most commonly left hemiparesis) a right hemisphere dysfunction has been postulated or alternatively a problem with executive function (part of an ability for self-reflection). The evidence to date again points to generalized neuropsychological impairment being related to lack of insight although there is some evidence for executive deficits as well.[29]

Practical implications

Neuropsychological function has been related to various indices of outcome and predictors of rehabilitation success. In a thorough review of the literature, Green[30] concluded that the most consistent finding was that verbal memory was associated with all types of functional outcome so that deficits in this function could limit the level of outcome. Vigilance was related to social problem solving and skill acquisition, while card sorting predicted the quality of more general functioning in the community.

References

1. David, A.S. and Cutting, J.C. (1994). *The neuropsychology of schizophrenia*. Erlbaum, Hove.
2. Bleuler, E. (1911). *Dementia praecox or the group of schizophrenias* (trans. H. Zinkin). International Universities Press, New York, 1950.
3. Heaton, R.K., Baade, L.E., and Johnson, K.L. (1978).

Neuropsychological test results associated with psychiatric disorders in adults. *Psychological Bulletin*, **22**, 141–62.

4. McKenna, P.J. (1994). *Schizophrenia and related syndromes*. Oxford University Press.

5. Jones, P., Rodgers, B., Murray, R., and Marmot, M. (1994). Child developmental risk factors for adult schizophrenia in the British 1946 birth cohort. *Lancet*, **334**, 1393–402.

6. Crow, T.J., Done, D.J., and Sacker, A. (1995). Childhood precursors of psychosis as clues to its evolutionary origins. *European Archives of Psychiatry. Clinical Neuroscience*, **245**, 61–9.

7. David, A.S., Malmberg, A., Brandt, L., Allebeck, P., and Lewis, G. (1997). IQ and risk for schizophrenia: a population-based cohort study. *Psychological Medicine*, **27**, 1311–23.

8. Aylward, E., Walker, E., and Bettes, B. (1984). Intelligence in schizophrenia: meta-analysis of the research. *Schizophrenia Bulletin*, **10**, 430–59.

9. Nelson, H.E. (1982). *The National Adult Reading Test (NART)*. NFER-Nelson, Windsor.

10. Cannon, T.D., Zorrilla, L.E., Shtasel, D., *et al.* (1994). Neuropsychological functioning in siblings discordant for schizophrenia and healthy volunteers. *Archives of General Psychiatry*, **51**, 651–61.

11. Saykin, A.J., Shtasel, D.L., Gur, R.E., *et al.* (1994). Neuropsychological deficits in neuroleptic naive patients with first-episode schizophrenia. *Archives of General Psychiatry*, **51**, 124–31.

12. Censits, D.M., Ragland, D., Gur, R.C., and Gur, R.E. (1997). Neuropsychological evidence supporting a neurodevelopmental model of schizophrenia: a longitudinal study. *Schizophrenia Research*, **24**, 289–98.

13. Rogers, D.G.C. (1996). The cognitive disorder of psychiatric illness: a historical perspective. In *Schizophrenia: a neuropsychological perspective* (ed. C. Pantelis, H.E. Nelson, and T.R.E. Barnes), pp. 19–29. Wiley, Chichester.

14. Laws, K.R. (1999). A meta-analytic review of Wisconsin Card Sort studies in schizophrenia: a generalised deficit in disguise. *Cognitive Neuropsychiatry*, **4**, 1–35.

15. Heinrichs, R.W. and Zakzanis, K.K. (1998). Neurocognitive deficit in schizophrenia: a quantitative review of the evidence. *Neuropsychology*, **12**, 426–45.

16. Van Horn, J.D. and McManus, I.C. (1992). Ventricular enlargement in schizophrenia. A meta-analysis of studies of the ventricle : brain ratio (VBR). *British Journal of Psychiatry*, **160**, 687–97.

17. Elkis, H., Friedman, L., Wise, A., and Meltzer, H.Y. (1996). Meta-analyses of studies of ventricular enlargement and cortical sulcal prominence in mood disorders. Comparisons with controls or patients with schizophrenia. *Archives of General Psychiatry*, **53**, 1165–7.

18. Nelson, M.D., Saykin, A.J., Flashman, L.A., and Riordan, H.J. (1998). Hippocampal volume reduction in schizophrenia as assessed by magnetic resonance imaging: a meta-analytic study. *Archives of General Psychiatry*, **55**, 433–40.

19. David, A.S. (1993). Cognitive neuropsychiatry? *Psychological Medicine*, **23**, 1–5.

20. Frith, C.D. (1992). *The cognitive neuropsychology of schizophrenia*. Erlbaum, Hove.

21. Gray, J.A., Feldon, J., Rawlins, J.N.P., Hemsley, D.R., and Smith, A.D. (1991). The neuropsychology of schizophrenia. *Behavioural and Brain Sciences*, **14**, 1–84.

22. Bentall, R.P. (1996). Brains, biases, deficits and disorders. *British Journal of Psychiatry*, **167**, 149–58.

23. Baron-Cohen, S. (1997). *Mindblindness: an essay on autism and theory of mind*. MIT Press, Cambridge, MA.

24. Frith, C. (1994). Theory of mind in schizophrenia. In *The neuropsychology of schizophrenia* (ed. A.S. David and J.C. Cutting), pp. 147–61. Erlbaum, Hove.

25. Cutting, J.C. (1985). *The psychology of schizophrenia*. Churchill Livingstone, Edinburgh.

26. Cutting, J.C. (1990). *The right cerebral hemisphere and psychiatric disorders*. Oxford University Press.

27. Liddle, P.F. (1987). The symptoms of chronic schizophrenia: a re-examination of the positive–negative dichotomy. *British Journal of Psychiatry*, **151**, 145–51.

28. Tamlyn, D., McKenna, P.J., Mortimer, A.M., Lund, C.E., Hammond, S., and Baddeley, A.D. (1992). Memory impairment in schizophrenia: its extent, affiliations and neuropsychological character. *Psychological Medicine*, **22**, 101–15.

29. Amador, X.F. and David, A.S. (ed.) (1998). *Insight and psychosis*. Oxford University Press.

30. Green, M.F. (1996). What are the functional consequences of neurocognitive deficits in schizophrenia? *American Journal of Psychiatry*, **153**, 321–30.

4.3.3.2 Diagnosis, classification, and differential diagnosis of schizophrenia

Anthony S. David

The diagnosis of schizophrenia

Until the early 1970s, the diagnosis of schizophrenia was one of the most contentious and fraught issues in the whole of psychiatry. Since then a massive international effort has been put in motion out of which explicit diagnostic criteria emerged. Some achieved widespread and even multinational agreement, allowing the painstaking process of calculating diagnostic specificity, sensitivity, reliability, and (perhaps) validity to begin. Although criticism of the diagnosis of schizophrenia continues, mostly from outside psychiatry, the vast majority of psychiatrists look upon the major sets of diagnostic criteria with weary acceptance, seeing them as flawed but useful and possibly 'as good as it gets' given our current state of knowledge/ignorance.

Throughout the 1970s and early 1980s there was an overabundance of criteria including the St Louis criteria[1] and the Research Diagnostic Criteria,[2] followed by the Present State Examination (PSE-CATEGO), the ICD-9, and finally the DSM-III. Perhaps because of the 'cookbook' explicitness of the DSM-III or the pervasive influence of American psychiatric practice, dubbed by some 'neo-colonial', the DSM, now in its fourth revision, is perhaps the mostly widely used, or at least quoted. The ICD-10 is also used throughout the world, but seldom in North America.

Diagnostic criteria

The signs and symptoms of schizophrenia and related disorders are discussed in detail in Chapter 4.3.2. Also, the diagnostic process is described in general in Chapter 1.10.1. As noted, the signs and symptoms, weighted in terms of their typicality or specificity, combined

Table 1 Major diagnostic criteria for schizophrenia

	DSM-IV	ICD-10
Characteristic symptoms		
One or more for 1 month	1. Bizarre delusions 2. Commenting voice or voices conversing	1. Thought echo/insertion/withdrawal/broadcasting 2. Delusions of control 3. Hallucinatory voices 4. Persistent delusions
Or two or more	1. Delusions 2. Hallucinations 3. Disorganized speech 4. Grossly disorganized or catatonic behaviour 5. Negative symptoms	1. Persistent hallucinations 2. Thought block/disorder 3. Catatonia 4. Negative symptoms 5. Significant personality change
Time course	1 month ('significant proportion') for symptoms listed plus 6 months social/occupational disturbance	1 month (most of the time)
Exclusions	Schizoaffective disorder or brief mood disturbance Direct effect of drugs of abuse/medication or general medical condition	Extensive depressive/manic symptoms or diagnosis of schizoaffective disorder Overt brain disease; drug intoxication/withdrawal

with additional clinical factors such as onset, duration, social consequences, etc., are used to make a diagnosis of schizophrenia and subsequently to classify the disorder into subtypes. The DSM and ICD criteria are described below (Tables 1, 2, and 3).

Another group of psychotic disorders which may be distinguished on the basis of formal phenomenological properties are the delusional disorders[3,4] formally known as paranoia (see Chapter 4.4).

Basis of classification

Atheoretical: Schneider's first-rank symptoms

These are still important for the diagnosis using the ICD-10 frame of reference. They are too rare to achieve high levels of sensitivity and their specificity has been challenged. Nevertheless, first-rank symptoms perform creditably on these parameters when compared to negative symptoms.[5,6] On the other hand, the lack of aetiological and prognostic significance of first-rank symptoms has undermined the prominence claimed for them.[7–9] Negative symptoms relate more consistently to outcome/prognosis and show more stability over time.[10] They have poor diagnostic specificity and must be distinguished from depression and parkinsonism, chronic drug dependence, and organic brain damage.

Theoretical

Attempts at a theoretical classification have been made. The first in the modern era was Crow's Type I and Type II distinction,[11] although it echoes older notions of 'process'—chronic and deteriorating versus 'reactive' (relapsing and remitting) typologies. The innovation was to link the distinction with proposed differences in dopamine receptor hyperactivity (Type I), associated with positive symptoms and good response to dopamine antagonist drugs, and on the other hand, to

neurological damage (Type II) as evidenced by ventricular enlargement on CT brain scans, associated with chronicity, poor premorbid functioning and poor response to treatment.

Building on this was the 'aetiological classification' proposed by Murray et al.[12] which contrasted cases with a presumed genetic aetiology and those who had other putative risk factors such as early brain damage (see Chapter 4.3.5.1). Although these attempts have served as useful stimuli for research, they have not been found to aid clinical decision-making. In fact the search for 'biological markers' which might validate diagnostic distinctions has yet to yield conclusive positive results. For example, the presence of ventricular enlargement or cortical thinning, as detected using CT and now magnetic resonance imaging (MRI), is a case in point. Meta-analyses have confirmed that indices of 'cerebral atrophy' are strongly associated with schizophrenia but the effect sizes are small (approximately 10 per cent).[13] Hence, there is substantial overlap between normal controls and schizophrenia cases.

Positive family history remains an important finding in the psychiatric history of an individual patient. Although none of the diagnostic criteria permits the influence of family history, in clinical settings, 'odd' or withdrawn behaviour takes on a very different meaning if seen in the first-degree relative of someone with a firm schizophrenia diagnosis.

Early diagnosis?

The premorbid personality in schizophrenia is typically described as emotionally and socially detached. Such people have few friends, are often cold and aloof, and engage in solitary occupations. Their behaviour may be eccentric and they are indifferent to praise or criticism. Recent studies, including United Kingdom national cohort studies[14] and a Swedish conscript cohort study[15] indicate that children who

Table 2 Criteria for the diagnosis of schizophrenia subtypes

Schizophrenia subtypes	DSM-IV	ICD-10
Paranoid	One or more delusions plus frequent auditory hallucinations; no prominent thought disorder, catatonia, or negative symptoms	Delusions, hallucinatory voices, hallucinations in other modalities; disturbances of affect, volition, and speech 'inconspicuous'
Disorganized DSM Hebephrenic ICD	Prominent disorganized speech behaviour and flat/inappropriate affect; no catatonia	Prominent disturbances of affect, volition, and thought; 2–3 months duration; adolescents/young adults only
Catatonic	Two of motoric immobility, excessive activity, negativism, peculiar voluntary movements, echolalia/praxia	One or more of stupor, excitement, posturing, negativism, rigidity, waxy flexibility, automatic compliance and perserveration
Undifferentiated	Meets criteria for schizophrenia but none of the above subtypes	Meets criteria for schizophrenia but none of the above subtypes plus residual
Residual	Absence of prominent characteristic symptoms (but two or more must be present in attenuated form); continuing evidence of disturbance including negative symptoms	Prominent negative symptoms; clear-cut episode(s) in past; at least 1 year history; no dementia or depression etc.
Simple	Slowly progressive negative symptoms without other psychotic symptoms	(See schizoid personality disorder)

later develop schizophrenia are more likely to have lower IQs and educational achievements than other children. They are also more likely to have interpersonal and behavioural difficulties. Parents recognize 'pre-schizophrenic' children as being different from their other siblings. However, such characteristics are very common in the general population so have virtually no positive predictive value.

Early diagnosis is only successful when based on psychotic symptoms. Here the diagnosis of schizophreniform psychosis (DSM-IV) and the acute schizophrenia-like psychotic disorder of the ICD-10 are relevant. The former must last for more than 1 but less than 6 months (otherwise the diagnosis is brief reactive psychosis). Hence the dis-order is substantial by any common-sense definition, and unsurprisingly many cases (70 per cent) go on to develop full-blown schizophrenia, affective disorder, or schizoaffective disorder.[16] The temporal stability of the diagnosis is poor, with around 30 per cent recovering over follow-up periods averaging 16 months in one study.

Differential diagnosis

Other psychiatric disorders

Other psychoses

It could be argued that distinguishing schizophrenia from schizoaffective disorder, schizophreniform disorder, delusional disorder, etc. is a largely academic exercise. Until recently, treatment in psychiatry was entirely symptom or syndrome based. Thus manic symptoms respond to antimanic agents including lithium, psychotic symptoms respond to neuroleptics, and depressive symptoms respond to antidepressants.[17,18] Other 'mood-stabilizing' agents are also of value especially when combined with neuroleptics. However, it is possible that with increasing clinical experience and research using the new generation of 'atypical' antipsychotic agents such as clozapine, risperidone, and olanzapine, more specific indications will emerge. A recent report of efficacy of olanzapine in schizoaffective disorder in comparison to haloperidol is a case in point.[19] However, a tendency to reduce all psychotic disorders to 'serious mental illness' is unfortunate. It encourages a sloppy approach to history taking and the mental state examination, and a loose attitude to making a diagnosis and, if pursued, would prevent the discovery of specific treatments.

Table 3 Terminology used to describe the course of schizophrenia in the DSM-IV and ICD-10 classifications

DSM-IV	ICD-10
Continuous	Continuous
Episodic with residual symptoms	Episodic with stable deficit
Episodic with no interepisode symptoms	Episodic remittent
Single episode in partial remission	Incomplete remission
Single episode in full remission	Complete remission
Other	Other Episodic with progressive deficit

Course specifiers in both DSM-IV and ICD-10 require 1 year of observation.

The prognostic significance of a diagnosis of schizophrenia (versus schizoaffective and affective disorders) has been discussed in Chapters 4.3.6 and 4.3.8. Although predicting outcome in individual patients is notoriously difficult[20] because of the influence of idiosyncratic factors such as services, relationships within the family, compliance, intelligence, personality, demographics, etc., the more a disorder approaches 'typical' schizophrenia, the poorer the prognosis tends to be.[21]

That said, schizoaffective disorder is the closest disorder, phenomenologically, to schizophrenia but combines schizophrenic symptoms with affective symptoms. The criteria are discussed in Chapter 4.3.8. Schizophreniform (DSM-IV) or acute schizophrenia-like disorders (ICD-10) differ only in terms of duration, as operationally defined (see Chapter 3.3.9). Delusional disorders (Chapter 4.4) differ from schizophrenia in being based around 'non-bizarre' delusions and few or no hallucinations. The onset and course are characteristically later and more benign respectively.

Affective disorders

Typical presentations of either mania or depression usually cause few diagnostic difficulties. Overdiagnosis of schizoaffective disorder is to be resisted although the distinction from schizophrenia proper remains controversial and debatable. The guidelines given in DSM-IV attempt to exclude transient mood disturbances (< 2 weeks) in people with psychosis as a basis for a schizoaffective diagnosis.

In practice reaching a diagnosis of schizophrenia in a person with evidence of one or more core symptoms of psychosis (listed under the DSM-IV and ICD-10) may be complicated for the following reasons.

The presence of mood-incongruent delusions (or hallucinations)

'Congruence' is somewhat in the eye of the beholder, especially where mood may be labile or where disturbed mood is suspected but fails to follow clinical stereotypes. The clinician should try to determine if a 'grandiose' delusion is being enjoyed by the patient, and whether the content (e.g. elevated status, magical powers, material riches) is seen as justified by the patient. Similarly a delusion of depressive content (e.g. physical illness, imminent death) must be seen as undeserved or inexplicable to be deemed 'incongruent'. Auditory hallucinations may be comforting, complimentary, or, more commonly, hostile and critical. It is probably their complexity and personification which makes them 'schizophrenic' rather than their mood-incongruent content.[22]

The duration and acuteness of onset criteria

A good history may simply not be available. Symptoms may wax and wane. Partial or successful treatment may modify or curtail a potentially long episode, and onset may be complicated by the use of psychoactive drugs.

Social and occupational disturbance

This is critical to the diagnosis of schizophrenia, especially the DSM-IV criteria. Here the difficulty is in distinguishing 'premorbid deficits', an illness prodrome and the illness itself. Premorbid personality factors will obscure or set in relief discontinuities in an individual's social trajectory. Objective information and informant testimony is crucial

as in most of the diagnostic process. Other individual differences such as intelligence will also shape the presentation of schizophrenia. At the extreme, people with mental retardation (learning disability) may manifest psychosis in less obvious ways (see Chapters 10.5.1 to 10.5.3). The old diagnosis of 'simple schizophrenia', retained in the ICD-10 describes 'insidious and progressive development of oddities of conduct' and the 'inability to meet the demands of society' that is, social disturbance of long duration. The progressive element distinguishes it from personality disorder although problems adjusting to changing social demands through the lifecycle may give the appearance of progression in a fixed personality disorder.

Organic conditions

Differentiation of a 'primary' psychotic illness from one secondary to an organic condition may arise in essentially two situations:

- a person with a clear-cut diagnosis of a medical or neurological syndrome in which psychosis is a recognized complication (e.g. epilepsy)

- a person with a presumptive diagnosis of schizophrenia in whom significant abnormalities are detected usually following special investigation (e.g. CT brain scanning).

The list of medical conditions that could potentially give rise to psychosis is enormous. These have been the subject of extensive reviews.[23,24] While it appears that almost any disease that causes a cerebral perturbation can give rise to psychosis, abnormalities affecting the temporal lobes and diencephalon are somewhat more likely to do this.

The time course is obviously important in this context. Chronic inflammatory lesions (e.g. sarcoidosis), degenerative disorders (e.g. presenile dementias), chronic infections (e.g. neurosyphilis, AIDS), space-occupying lesions (e.g. tumour or abscesses), metabolic disorders (e.g. hyper- or hypothyroidism and vitamin deficiencies) may mimic schizophrenia by virtue of a gradual deterioration in social functioning and self-care punctuated perhaps by odd or inexplicable behaviour and rarely hallucinations and delusions. The features of the primary disease are usually evident. Rarer conditions may be misdiagnosed, for example, Wilson's disease (hepatolenticular degeneration). This usually presents with a motor disorder with bulbar features and abnormal liver function, but personality changes and psychotic symptoms are also associated. Diagnosis is made on other associated clinical features (e.g. Kayser–Fleischer rings), copper studies, and liver biopsy. Huntington's disease is characterized by chorea and cognitive decline. Affective disorder and occasionally psychotic symptoms may occur. The main differential diagnosis is with patients with chronic psychosis and tardive dyskinesia and is usually clarified by the family history, inexorable progression, and caudate atrophy on CT or MRI. Neurosyphilis is still encountered from time to time and in the 'general paralysis of the insane' form, may present with chronic delusions (often grandiose) plus dementia. Diagnosis is by appropriate serological testing of blood and cerebrospinal fluid. Finally, metachromatic leukodystrophy, a rare inherited progressive demyelinating condition, has recently been identified as a cause of a schizophrenia-like psychosis, when onset is in childhood or early adult life.[25] Arylsulphatase-A is a diagnostic marker detectable in peripheral white blood cells.

Acute disturbances following head trauma, acute infections (viral encephalitis), cerebrovascular accidents, metabolic abnormalities (e.g.

electrolyte disturbances, porphyria), or drug intoxication or withdrawal (including prescribed medication) (see below) may present with a florid psychotic picture, classically dominated by visual distortions or hallucinations and fluctuating levels of alertness, rather than the stereotyped auditory hallucinations in clear consciousness which are characteristic of schizophrenia.[26]

In practice there are few common conditions that ever give rise to real diagnostic uncertainty. The most important is **epilepsy**. It is well established that epilepsy, particularly focal (complex partial or 'temporal lobe epilepsy') can give rise to psychosis and there are inter-ictal and post-ictal patterns (see Chapter 5.3.3). A survey from a large neurology clinic showed that the incidence of schizophrenia is about nine times that of the rest of the population.[27]

Inter-ictal psychoses include the chronic schizophrenia-like psychoses described by Slater et al.,[28] and Trimble.[29] These almost always arise in people with many years of well-established temporal lobe seizures, while the post-ictal variety occurs earlier in the lifecycle but again in a person with previously diagnosed epilepsy. In post-ictal psychosis the temporal relationship to seizures, sometimes occurring in a cluster, is diagnostic, although a lucid interval is often observed. A clear history and independent description of seizures is the foundation of a diagnosis of epilepsy, with EEG confirmation. Resting EEGs show slight and subtle abnormalities in a substantial minority of patients with schizophrenia which may be accentuated by neuroleptic medication. As such, the EEG may be of limited value in differential diagnosis unless pronounced slowing or frank seizure activity is picked up. (See also Chapter 5.3.3.)

Symptoms

Symptoms of schizophrenic psychosis in relative isolation may give rise to diagnostic difficulties.

Auditory hallucinations may occur in alcoholic hallucinosis (see below and Chapter 4.2.2.2). Hallucinations in the context of dissociation (voices representing figures from the patients past or embodiments of aspects of their personality) must also be distinguished from typical schizophrenic hallucinations. These are often multimodal. Pure auditory hallucinations in organic conditions including epilepsy in the absence of other psychotic features are surprisingly rare.

Certain forms of delusion suggest alternative diagnoses. Transient ill-formed but usually paranoid delusions occur in the context of confusion, memory impairment, or dementia (i.e. things going missing, strange people loitering). Delusions of misidentification are particularly associated with organic illness such as dementia or stroke.

Thought disorder may be confused with a fluent aphasia following stroke or cerebral tumours.

Personality deterioration and inappropriate or disinhibited behaviour can occur in many organic conditions in the absence of overt psychotic features. Isolated frontal lesions may cause diagnostic problems since general cognitive impairments may be absent. The widespread availability of CT and MRI in the more developed world has reduced the likelihood of such patients being misdiagnosed.

A small proportion (approximately 5 per cent) of prevalent and incident cases of schizophrenia, if investigated thoroughly, are found to have a variety of 'organic' conditions which may contribute to the illness.[30] These include metabolic abnormalities, cerebral tumours, multisystem autoimmune disease, cerebrovascular disease, etc. Some of these may be incidental; others may have precipitated the psychosis. The range of diseases counts against any specific aetiological mechanism. Similarly, the phenomenology found in such 'organic' patients is usually indistinguishable from their 'functional' counterparts.[31]

Thanks to increased application of non-invasive neuroimaging techniques to psychiatric patients, particularly those with schizophrenia, another class of organic abnormalities have been noted, namely cerebral anomalies which are often congenital. These include agenesis of the corpus callosum, cavum septum pellucidum, aqueduct stenosis, etc. Again, it is difficult to know how often such findings occur in the normal population and are asymptomatic, although the widespread use of MRI for 'minor' complaints such as mild head injury and headache is uncovering such anomalies. The examples above certainly appear to be associated with psychiatric disorders in general more than would be expected by chance. They tend to be associated with below-average IQ and other neurological problems (epilepsy in the cases of callosal agenesis).[32]

Other factors to be taken into account in the differential diagnosis from organic conditions include the presence of a family history of schizophrenia, and abnormal premorbid personality, both of which weight aetiological judgement in favour of the functional diagnosis. This applies to the psychoses of epilepsy and those related to drug abuse especially. 'Secondary' schizophrenias also tend to have less pervasive effects on the person's personality. Treatment is again based on symptoms with the added complication that neuroleptic drugs lower the epileptic seizure threshold, and will tend to worsen extrapyramidal symptoms in patients with primary movement disorders. Treatment of the primary condition (if this has remained undiagnosed for some time) may be disappointing but should always be attempted especially in the case of chronic infections. Reversal of metabolic abnormalities, even long-standing, can lead to dramatic improvements in the mental state.

Drug-induced psychoses

Many drugs of abuse and prescribed drugs can cause psychotic symptoms. The associations are also considered in Chapters 4.2.3.1 to 4.2.3.9. In the context of a differential diagnosis, drugs of abuse—in adolescents and young adults—must be considered. Chronic amphetamine psychosis may be indistinguishable from schizophrenia. The psychosis is florid and may include visual and auditory hallucinations. Phencyclidine (PCP or angel dust) is a drug of abuse in the United States and causes an acute psychosis with prominent affective symptoms as well as perceptual distortions and depersonalization. Other psychotogenic drugs include cocaine, ecstasy, and LSD.

Cannabis is widely used, especially in large metropolitan areas and by certain ethnic groups (e.g. African-Caribbeans); hence an apparent association with schizophrenia may be a chance finding. Cannabis intoxication is more characterized by perceptual distortions and depersonalization than frank psychosis. Clinical experience suggests that cannabis has a propensity to precipitate psychotic relapse in patients with established schizophrenia, although hard data on this issue are lacking.

Delusions and hallucinations may occur rarely during states of alcohol intoxication but are more commonly associated with withdrawal syndromes (Chapter 4.2.2.3). Alcoholic hallucinosis is a chronic hallucinatory state of uncertain nosological status in which the patient with long-standing alcohol dependence often hears 'voices' which may be derogatory and commenting, in clear consciousness, after a lengthy withdrawal period.

Prescribed medication

Again the list of agents that can cause psychotic reactions to be distinguished from schizophrenia is very long, and psychotropic drugs are particularly liable to cause psychotic reactions. Two classes of drug deserve mention because of their widespread use and relatively high incidence of major psychiatric adverse effects:

- steroids can cause a wide range of psychiatric disturbances including psychosis

- dopamine agonists used in the treatment of Parkinson's disease and some pituitary adenomas.

Frank psychosis and affective disorders may be seen. In the treatment of neurological diseases, such as Parkinson's disease, and the use of steroids for diseases of the central nervous system, there is often an interaction between the agent and the underlying condition which increases the likelihood of a drug-induced psychosis.

The diagnostic process

It used to be argued that a diagnosis of schizophrenia in itself caused disability and morbidity due to social 'labelling' and stigmatization. Evidence that this accounts for schizophrenic disability is lacking but the reality of the stigma of mental illness and negative attitudes towards 'schizophrenics' cannot be denied. Hence, making a diagnosis of schizophrenia should not be taken lightly. In the author's experience, very few psychiatrists spontaneously convey the diagnosis to the patient. If a patient asks whether he or she has schizophrenia, the clinician should first try to understand the motivation behind the question and the patient's knowledge and understanding of the term. Ultimately there is seldom justification in withholding the diagnosis if it is established. A schizophrenic diagnosis can be framed in a relatively positive light—this is a condition which we are now beginning to understand and for which there are effective treatments—and may lessen the burden of responsibility and blame that the patient and his or her family may carry for the disorder.

References

1. Feighner, J.P., Robins, E., Guze, S., Woodruff, R.A., Winokur, G., and Munoz, R. (1972). Diagnostic criteria for use in psychiatric research. *Archives of General Psychiatry*, **26**, 57–62.

2. Spitzer, R.L., Endicott, J., and Robins, E. (1977). *Research diagnostic criteria for a selected group of functional disorders* (3rd edn). Biometrics Research Division, New York State Psychiatric Institution, New York.

3. World Health Organization (1992). F20-F29 Schizophrenia, schizotypal and delusional disorders. *The ICD-10 classification of mental and behavioural disorders. Clinical descriptions and diagnostic guidelines*, pp. 97–109. WHO, Geneva.

4. American Psychiatric Association (1994). Schizophrenia and other psychotic disorders. *Diagnostic and statistical manual of mental disorders, DSM-IV* (2nd edn), pp. 284–306. American Psychiatric Association, Washington, DC.

5. David, A.S. and Appleby, L. (1992). Diagnostic criteria in schizophrenia: accentuate the positive. *Schizophrenia Bulletin*, **18**, 551–7.

6. Andreasen, N.C. and Flaum, M. (1991). Schizophrenia: the characteristic symptoms. *Schizophrenia Bulletin*, **17**, 27–39.

7. Wing, J.K., Cooper, J.E., and Sartorius, N. (1974). *Measurement and classification of psychiatric symptoms*. Cambridge University Press.

8. McGuffin, P., Farmer, A., Gottesman, I.I., *et al.* (1984). Twin concordance of operationally defined schizophrenia: confirmation of familiality and heritability. *Archives of General Psychiatry*, **41**, 541–5.

9. Kendell, R.E., Brockington, I.F., and Leff, J.P. (1979). Prognostic implications of six alternative definitions of schizophrenia. *Archives of General Psychiatry*, **30**, 25–34.

10. Andreasen, N.C. and Olsen, S. (1982). Negative v. positive schizophrenia: definition and validation. *Archives of General Psychiatry*, **39**, 789–94.

11. Crow, T.J. (1980). Molecular pathology of schizophrenia: more than one disease process? *British Medical Journal*, **280**, 1–9.

12. Murray, R.M., Lewis, S.W., and Reveley, A.M. (1985). Towards an aetiological classification of schizophrenia. *Lancet*, **i**, 1023–6.

13. Van Horn, J.D. and McManus, I.C. (1992). Ventricular enlargement in schizophrenia. A meta-analysis of studies of the ventricle/brain ratio (VBR). *British Journal of Psychiatry*, **160**, 687–97.

14. Jones, P. (1997). The early origins of schizophrenia. *British Medical Bulletin*, **53**, 135–55.

15. Malmberg, A., Lewis, G., David, A., and Allebeck, P. (1998). Premorbid adjustment and personality in schizophrenia. *British Journal of Psychiatry*, **172**, 308–13.

16. Strakowski, S.M. (1994). Diagnostic validity of schizophreniform disorder. *American Journal of Psychiatry*, **151**, 815–24

17. Johnstone, E.C., Crow, T.J., Frith, C.D., and Owens, D.G.C. (1988). The Northwick Park 'functional' psychoses study: diagnosis and treatment response. *Lancet*, **ii**, 119–26.

18. Siris, S.G., Bermanzohn, M.D., Gonzalez, A., Mason, S.E., White, C.V., and Shuwall, M.A. (1991). The use of antidepressants for negative symptoms in a subset of schizophrenic patients. *Psychopharmacology Bulletin*, **27**, 331–5.

19. Tran, P.V., Tollefson, G.D., Sanger, T.M., Lu, Y., Berg, P.H., and Beasley, C.M. (1999). Olanzapine versus haloperidol in the treatment of schizoaffective disorder. Acute and long-term therapy. *British Journal of Psychiatry*, **174**, 15–22.

20. Cloninger, C.R., Martin, R.L., Guze, S.B., and Clayton, P.J. (1985). Diagnosis and prognosis in schizophrenia. *Archives of General Psychiatry*, **42**, 15–25.

21. David, A.S. (1997). Atypical psychosis. In *Essentials of postgraduate psychiatry* (3rd edn) (ed. R. Murray, P. Hill, and P. McGuffin), pp. 352–61. Cambridge University Press.

22. Nayani, T.H. and David, A.S. (1996). The auditory hallucination: a phenomenological survey. *Psychological Medicine*, **26**, 177–89.

23. Davison, K. and Bagley, C.R. (1969). Schizophrenia-like psychoses associated with organic disorders of the central nervous system. In *Current problems in neuropsychiatry* (ed. R.N. Herrington). British Journal of Psychiatry Special Publication No 4. Headley Brothers, Ashford, Kent.

24. Lishman, W.A. (1997). *Organic psychiatry: the psychological consequences of cerebral disorder* (3rd edn). Blackwell Science, Oxford.

25. Hyde, T.M., Ziegler, J.C., and Weinberger, D.R. (1993). Psychiatric disturbances in metachromatic leukodystrophy. Insights into the neurobiology of psychosis. *Archives of Neurology*, **50**, 131.

26. Cutting, J. (1987). The phenomenology of acute organic psychosis: comparison with acute schizophrenia. *British Journal of Psychiatry*, **151**, 324–32

27. Mendez, M.F., Grau, R., Doss, R.C., *et al.* (1993). Schizophrenia in epilepsy: seizure and psychosis variables. *Neurology*, **43**, 1073–7.

28. Slater, E., Beard, A.W., and Glithero, E. (1963). The schizophrenia-like psychoses of epilepsy. *British Journal of Psychiatry*, **109**, 95–150.

29. Trimble, M.R. (1990). First-rank symptoms of Schneider. A new perspective? *British Journal of Psychiatry*, **156**, 195–200.

30. Johnstone, E.C., Cooling, N., Frith, C.D., Crow, T.J. and Owens, D.G.C. (1988). Phenomenology of organic and functional psychoses and the overlap between them. *British Journal of Psychiatry*, **153**, 770–6.

31. Johnstone, E.C., Macmillan, J.F., and Crow, T.J. (1987). The occurrence of organic disease of possible or probably aetiological significance in a

population of 268 cases of first episode schizophrenia. *Psychological Medicine*, **17**, 371–9.

32. David, A.S., Wacharasindhu, A., and Lishman, W.A. (1993). Severe psychiatric disturbance and abnormalities of the corpus callosum: review and case series. *Journal of Neurology, Neurosurgery and Psychiatry*, **56**, 85–93.

4.3.4 Epidemiology of schizophrenia

Assen Jablensky

Introduction

Epidemiological research into schizophrenia aims to answer four essential questions.

1. What is the 'true' population frequency of the disorder in various populations and how is it distributed across the various groups within populations?

2. Do the incidence, manifestations, and course of schizophrenia vary in relation to factors of the physical and social environment?

3. Who is at risk and what forces determine or influence the risk of developing schizophrenia?

4. Can the answers to the above questions help explain what causes the disorder and how to prevent it?

The hallmark of the epidemiological method (see Chapter 2.7) is the referral of any numerical findings about the occurrence of a disorder or its associated characteristics to a population base or denominator, such as person-years. The epidemiological study of a disorder usually proceeds from a description of its frequency and associations (establishing rates of occurrence) to testing hypotheses about risk and causes, using analysis of ratios between rates.

Schizophrenia has been studied extensively from an epidemiological perspective over the past hundred years.[1] Kraepelin, who introduced the concept of *dementia praecox* in 1896, anticipated the potential of the epidemiological method to 'throw light on the causes of mental disorder' and proposed comparative population studies of the psychoses and factors predisposing to them across different cultures.[2] In the first half of the twentieth century, epidemiological research into schizophrenia took two divergent paths. While European studies tended to have a strong focus on genetic risks, North American researchers investigated the social ecology of the disorder. A variety of techniques and study designs were explored and applied with considerable success by the pioneers of psychiatric epidemiology, and the contours of the epidemiological map of schizophrenia in Europe and North America were effectively laid down between the two World Wars. The early epidemiological studies were carried out by dedicated researchers who typically spent much of their time collecting data 'door to door' in small communities. Intimate knowledge of the respondents, access to multigenerational records from the local parish registers, and the co-operation of the community often resulted in studies that remain landmarks of psychiatric epidemiology (Table 1).

During the last three decades, the scope of epidemiological studies of schizophrenia has expanded to include populations in Asia, Africa, and South America about which little had been known previously. The World Health Organization (**WHO**) International Pilot Study of Schizophrenia and the subsequent WHO 10-country epidemiological study[10,11] were the first systematic investigations of the comparative incidence, clinical manifestations, and course of schizophrenia in both developing and developed countries. The WHO programme provided an impetus for similar studies to be undertaken in India, China, the Caribbean, and Australia. Two major studies of psychiatric morbidity in the United States, the Epidemiological Catchment Area project and the National Comorbidity Survey, generated data on the prevalence of DSM-III/IIIR schizophrenia and related disorders in representative population samples.[12,13] Recent studies, initiated in the 1980s and 1990s, tend to make use of large existing databases such as cumulative case registers or birth cohorts to test hypotheses about risk factors in case–control designs, or include methods of genetic epidemiology within population-based studies. There is a tendency towards integrating epidemiological approaches with other types of aetiological research in schizophrenia.[14] This predicts an important role for epidemiology in the coming era of molecular biology of mental disorders.

Epidemiological methods and instruments used in the study of schizophrenia

The measurement of the prevalence, incidence, and disease expectancy of schizophrenia depends critically on the sensitivity of the case-finding method (i.e. its capacity to identify all affected persons in a given population) and the availability of a diagnostic instrument or procedure that selects 'true' cases (i.e. those corresponding to an established clinical concept).

Case-finding

Case-finding designs fall into three broad groups: case detection in clinical populations (persons in contact with services), door-to-door surveys (including census investigations of entire communities and surveys of population samples), and birth cohort studies. Each method has its advantages and limitations.

While case-finding through the mental health services provides a relatively easy access to a substantial proportion of all persons with schizophrenia, the cases currently in treatment may not be a representative sample of all individuals with the disorder. Different kinds of bias related to gender, marital status, socio-economic factors, culture, or ethnicity are known to affect the probability of being in treatment at any given time in any given setting. Unless such bias is accounted for, generalizations about schizophrenia based on hospital or clinic samples are liable to error. Many of the deficiencies of case-finding through service contacts can be overcome by using cumulative regional or national psychiatric case registers, where such tools exist. Registers cover defined populations and the capacity for linkage to other databases makes them effective research instruments in low-incidence disorders such as schizophrenia.

Surveys essentially involve accounting for every person at risk within a defined community or a population sample in terms of either

Table 1 Landmarks in the history of the epidemiology of psychoses: methods

Reference	Method	Target population	Case-finding	Assessment
Koller (1895)[3]	The first genetic–epidemiological study of psychoses (also the first case–control study)	Probands with psychoses (n = 287) and non-psychiatric control subjects (n = 370)	Records of psychiatric hospitals and clinics	Genealogical inquiry
Luxenburger (1928)[4]	Methodology of twin research; sampling design	Concordant and discordant monozygotic and dizygotic twin pairs	Census of all inpatients; search of birth registers for twin births	Emphasis on reliability of diagnosis: 'definite' and 'probable'
Klemperer (1933)[5]	Birth cohort study	Random sample (n = 1000) from all births in Munich, 1881–1890	Attempted tracing of all cohort members, 44% successfully traced	Personal examination or key informant interview (271 examined)
Brugger (1931)[6]	Census (door-to-door survey)	Area in Thuringia, population 37 561	Records and key informant consulted to detect 'suspected' cases	Personal examination of all 'suspected' cases and of a control sample
Essen-Möller et al. (1956)[7] Hagnell (1966)[8]	Census followed by repeated follow-up surveys	Rural community, initial population 2550 (+1013 new residents in the course of follow-up)	Complete census	Personal examination (and re-examination) of all residents
Ödegaard (1946)[9]	Cumulative national case register	Entire population of Norway	Registration of all first admissions 1926–1935 (n = 14 231)	Statistical analysis of hospital diagnoses and records

being or not being a case. Face-to-face interviewing (and following up) every resident in delimited, usually small, communities has been a feature of intensive high-quality research, especially in the Scandinavian countries. However, since the size of the population that can be surveyed in this way is limited, the number of detected cases of schizophrenia is usually too small to generate stable estimates of epidemiological parameters. Single-community studies are also vulnerable to the so-called 'ecological fallacy' (erroneously inferring that an association observed at the level of the community—say, between the number of pregnant women exposed to influenza epidemics and the number of offspring eventually developing schizophrenia—will also hold at individual level). Therefore surveys of large populations have advantages. There are two basic designs: a single-phase survey of a probability sample drawn from the general population, and a two-phase survey where a screening test is applied to the entire population at risk and only those scoring as screen-positive proceed to a full assessment. In the instance of schizophrenia, mere logistics dictates a choice between assessing large numbers less rigorously and investigating a smaller sample in greater depth. In the absence of a simple and valid screening procedure for schizophrenia, such as a biological or psychological test, the advantages of the two-phase survey may be offset by poor sensitivity or specificity of the screening device which is usually a questionnaire or checklist.

The study of birth cohorts at ages when their members have passed through the greater portion of the period of risk of developing schizophrenia is accomplished either by direct interviewing or by analysing available case register data. If birth cohorts are well characterized, they are the best tools for the study of the incidence of schizophrenia in relation to specific risk factors. This presumes that the population is relatively stable and that an adequate infrastructure is in place for monitoring mortality and morbidity. However, even in settings where such conditions are met, the size of birth cohorts with prospectively collected research data of interest may not be sufficient for conclusive epidemiological inferences.

All this suggests that there is no single gold standard of epidemiological case-finding methods for schizophrenia that could be uniquely applied across all possible settings and situations. Rather, the assets and liabilities of case-finding procedures need to be evaluated in the context of each particular study. This makes the detailed reporting of case-finding methods and procedures a mandatory prerequisite for an 'evidence-based' epidemiology of schizophrenia.

Diagnosis

Variation in diagnostic concepts and practices always explains a certain proportion of the variation in the results of schizophrenia studies, especially if they involve different populations or different periods. Until the late 1960s, the diagnostic rules used in epidemiological research were seldom explicitly stated. The demonstration by the United States–United Kingdom diagnostic study,[15] that American psychiatrists used a broader definition of schizophrenia than their British counterparts, reinforced suspicions that concepts of schizophrenia in different medical cultures could differ to an extent that might invalidate comparisons.

In response to such concerns, the WHO launched the International Pilot Study of Schizophrenia,[10] which examined diagnostic variation across nine countries by comparing the diagnoses made by psychiatrists using a semistructured clinical interview with a standard reference classification by computer algorithm[16] utilizing the same clinical data. The results were reassuring since in the majority of settings psychiatrists were found to use comparable diagnostic concepts corresponding to the definition of schizophrenia in accordance with the Kraepelin–Bleuler tradition. Furthermore, the core of the diagnostic concept of schizophrenia does not seem to have undergone major changes over time. A reanalysis of a sample from Kraepelin's original clinical material demonstrated that descriptions of dementia praecox and manic–depressive psychosis cases of 1908 could be scored and diagnosed using 'modern' syndrome scales with a resulting agreement of 88.6 per cent between the 1908 diagnosis and the ICD-9 diagnosis assigned by computer.[17] The introduction of explicit diagnostic criteria and rules with the consecutive editions of DSM and the WHO's ICD-10 has resolved some, but not all, diagnostic problems with implications for epidemiology. While ICD-10[18] and DSM-IV[19] tend to agree well on the core cases of schizophrenia, they agree less well on the classification of atypical or milder cases. Such differences may be less important in clinical practice than in epidemiological and genetic studies. By providing somewhat restrictive criteria for the diagnosis of schizophrenia, both classifications aim to select homogeneous patient groups and to minimize false-positive diagnoses. However, this is not an unequivocal advantage for epidemiology. Applying such criteria at the case-finding stage of a survey may result in the rejection of potential cases which fail to satisfy the full set of criteria at the time of initial assessment. Therefore it is desirable to develop less restrictive screening versions of the DSM-IV and ICD-10 criteria for epidemiological research.

Diagnostic problems may also arise in studies using 'historical' databases without direct patient contact, such as information from case registers or birth cohort data. The validity of the original diagnoses in such databases is difficult to ascertain, but several studies in which patient samples have been assessed by research interviews suggest that, in the instance of schizophrenia, serious discrepancies between register and research diagnoses are relatively rare.

Instruments

The diagnostic instruments used in surveys involving interviewing of respondents fall into two categories: fully structured interviews such as the Diagnostic Interview Schedule (**DIS**)[12] and the Composite International Diagnostic Interview (**CIDI**),[20] written to match exactly the diagnostic criteria of DSM-IIIR/IV and ICD-10, and semistructured interview schedules such as the Present State Examination (**PSE**)[16] and the Schedules for Clinical Assessment in Neuropsychiatry (**SCAN**),[21] which cover a broad range of psychopathology and elicit data that can be processed by alternative diagnostic algorithms. While the former can be applied by trained lay interviewers, the latter require clinical judgement and are usually administered by clinicians.

The DIS/CIDI type of instrument is reliable and capable of generating standard diagnoses in a single-phase survey design. However, the range of psychopathology covered is restricted to the diagnostic system to which it is linked, and its clinical validity is open to question because symptoms may not be reported accurately or impairment may be underestimated by the respondent. In contrast, the PSE/SCAN type of interview allows a greater amount of psychopathological data to be elicited but its use in epidemiological studies presupposes the availability of clinically skilled and trained interviewers. While SCAN and other similar interviews are suitable as second-stage diagnostic instruments, there is still a need for a relatively simple and effective screening procedure for case-finding of schizophrenia in field surveys.

Persons, place, time: completing the description of schizophrenia

At present, the epidemiological description of schizophrenia draws on extensive evidence regarding its frequency and age and sex distribution in relatively large populations or population groups. However, less than complete information is available on variations in its epidemiological characteristics that may be found in unusual or isolated populations or on the temporal trends in its occurrence.

Prevalence, incidence, and disease expectancy

Prevalence

Prevalence is defined as the number of cases per 1000 persons at risk present in a population at a given time or over a defined period. Point prevalence refers to the 'active' (i.e. symptomatic) cases on a given date, or within a brief census period. Since asymptomatic cases (e.g. persons in remission) will be missed in a point prevalence survey, it is useful to supplement the assessment of the present mental state with an enquiry about past episodes of the disorder to obtain a lifetime prevalence index. In schizophrenia, which tends to a chronic course, estimates of point and lifetime prevalence will be closer to each other than in remitting illnesses.

An overview of selected prevalence studies of schizophrenia spanning a period of 60 years is presented in Table 2. The studies differ in many aspects of methodology but have in common a high intensity of case-finding. Several of them are repeat surveys in which the original population was reinvestigated following an interval of 10 or more years (the resulting consecutive prevalence figures are indicated by arrows).

The majority of studies have produced prevalence estimates in the range 1.4 to 4.6 per 1000 population at risk. However, these are usually crude prevalence figures that are difficult to compare because of the demographic differences between populations with regard to factors such as age-specific mortality and migration. Therefore the modal prevalence of 1.4 to 4.6 per 1000 is unlikely to reflect the extent of variation that exists in the prevalence of schizophrenia in different populations.

There are populations and groups which deviate from the central tendency. Unusually high rates (two to three times the national or regional rate) have been reported for several genetic isolates such as an area in northern Sweden and several areas in Finland, and for an area in Croatia characterized by a high level of out-migration during the nineteenth and early twentieth centuries (see Table 2). At the other extreme, a virtual absence of schizophrenia and a relatively high rate of depression has been claimed for the Hutterites of South Dakota, a

Table 2 Selected prevalence studies of schizophrenia

Reference	Country	Population	Method	Prevalence per 1000 population at risk
Brugger (1931)[6]	Germany	Area in Thuringia (n = 37 561), age 10+	Census	2.4
Strömgren (1938)[22] Bøjholm and Strömgren (1989)[23]	Denmark	Island population (n = 50 000)	Repeat census	3.9 → 3.3
Lemkau et al. (1943)[24]	USA	Household sample	Census	2.9
Sjögren (1948)[25]	Sweden	Island population (n = 25 000)	Census	4.6
Böök (1953)[26] Böök et al. (1978)[27]	Sweden	Genetic isolate (n = 9000), age 15–50	Repeat census	9.5 → 17.0
Essen-Möller et al. (1956)[7] Hagnell (1966)[8]	Sweden	Community in southern Sweden	Repeat census	6.7 → 4.5
Rin and Lin (1962)[28] Lin et al. (1989)[29]	Taiwan	Population sample	Repeat census	2.1 → 1.4
Bash (1967)[30]	Iran	Rural area (n = 11 585)	Census	2.1
Crocetti et al. (1971)[31]	Croatia	Sample of 9201 households	Census	5.9
Dube and Kumar (1972)[32]	India	Four areas in Agra (n = 29 468)	Census	2.6
Rotstein (1977)[33]	Russia	Population sample (n = 35 590)	Census	3.8
Keith et al. (1991)[34]	USA	Aggregated data across five ECA sites	Sample survey	7.0 (point) 15.0 (lifetime)
Jeffreys et al. (1997)[35]	UK	London health district (n = 112 127)	Census, interviews of a sample (n = 172)	5.1
Jablensky et al. (1999)[36]	Australia	Four urban areas (n = 1 084 978)	Census, interviews of a sample (n = 980)	4.7 (point)[a] 4.0 (period, 1 year)[b]

ECA, Epidemiologic Catchment Area.

[a] All psychoses.

[b] Schizophrenia and other non-affective psychoses.

Protestant sect whose members live in close-knit endogamous communities sheltered from the outside world.[37] Negative selection for schizoid individuals who fail to adjust to the lifestyle of the majority and eventually migrate without leaving progeny has been suggested (but not definitively proven) as an explanation.

Low prevalence rates have also been reported for certain Pacific island populations,[38] but uncertainties about the extent of case-finding makes the interpretation of such reports problematic. Two carefully planned surveys in Taiwan (see Table 3) were separated by 15 years during which major social changes had taken place. While the total mental morbidity increased, the prevalence of schizophrenia decreased from 2.1 to 1.4 per 1000. In both surveys, the aboriginal Taiwanese had significantly lower rates than the mainland Chinese who had migrated to the island after the Second World War.

The results of the Epidemiologic Catchment Area study in the United States,[12] which indicate a higher prevalence rate compared with most other studies, should be treated with caution. There are inconsistencies among the study areas that are difficult to interpret (such as a 13-fold difference in the rates for age group 18–24 years across the sites), which suggests that the diagnostic procedure, involving the DIS administered by lay interviewers, may have elicited a number of false-positive diagnoses. In the more recent National Comorbidity Survey, diagnoses of 'non-affective psychosis' by computer algorithm based on a version of the CIDI were found to agree poorly with clinicians' diagnoses based on telephone reinterviews, resulting in discrepant estimates of the lifetime prevalence of both 'narrowly' and 'broadly' defined psychotic illness.[39]

The question of whether major differences exist in the prevalence

Table 3 Selected incidence studies of schizophrenia

Reference	Country	Population	Method	Rate per 1000
Ödegaard (1946)[9]	Norway	Total population	First admissions 1926–1935 (n = 14 231)	0.24
Walsh (1969)[40]	Ireland	City of Dublin (n = 720 000)	First admissions	0.57 (male) 0.46 (female)
Häfner and Reimann (1970)[41]	Germany	City of Mannheim (n = 330 000)	Case register	0.54
Murphy and Raman (1971)[42]	Mauritius	Total population (n = 257 000)	First admissions	0.24 (Africans) 0.14 (Indian Hindus) 0.09 (Indian Moslems)
Lieberman (1974)[43]	Russia	Moscow district (n = 248 000)	Follow-back of prevalent cases	0.20 (male) 0.19 (female)
Helgason (1977)[44]	Iceland	Total population	First admissions 1966–1967 (n = 2388)	0.27
Lin et al. (1989)[29]	Taiwan	Three communities (n = 39 024)	Household survey	0.17
Castle et al. (1991)[45]	UK	London (Camberwell)	Case register	0.25 (ICD) 0.17 (RDC) 0.08 (DSM-III)
Nicole et al. (1992)[46]	Canada	Area in Quebec (n = 338 300)	First admissions	0.31 (ICD) 0.09 (DSM-III)
Rajkumar et al. (1993)[47]	India	Area in Madras (n = 43 097)	Door-to-door survey and key informants	0.41
Hickling (1991)[48]	Jamaica	Total population (n = 2.46 million)	First contacts	0.24 ('broad') 0.21 ('restrictive')
McNaught et al. (1997)[49]	UK	London health district (n = 112 127)	Two censuses, 5 years apart	0.21 (DSM-IIIR)
Brewin et al. (1997)[50]	UK	Nottingham	Two cohorts of first contacts (1978–1980 and 1992–1994)	0.25 → 0.29 (all psychoses) 0.14 → 0.09 (ICD-10 schizophrenia)

of schizophrenia in different populations has no simple answer. In the great majority of studies the prevalence rates are similar. On the other hand, there are a small number of populations that clearly deviate from the average. However, the magnitude of these deviations is modest compared with the 10- to 30-fold differences in prevalence observed in other multifactorial diseases (e.g. ischaemic heart disease, diabetes, multiple sclerosis) across populations.

Incidence

The incidence rate (the annual number of first onset cases in a defined population per 1000 individuals at risk) is of greater interest for the search of risk factors than the prevalence since it is a better estimate of the so-called force of morbidity (the probability of disease occurrence at a point in time) in a given population. Its estimation depends on how reliably the point of onset can be determined. Since it is not possible at present to determine the time of onset of any cerebral dys-

function or biochemical lesion underlying schizophrenia, onset of the disorder is usually defined as the point in time when its clinical manifestations become recognizable and diagnosable according to specified criteria. The first hospital admission, which has been used in many studies, is not a good approximation to the 'true' onset because of the variable time lag between the earliest appearance of symptoms and the first admission. A better approximation is provided by the first contact, i.e. the point at which any psychiatric or general medical service is accessed by symptomatic individuals for the first time.

Table 3 presents the essential features of 13 incidence studies of schizophrenia. The comparison of studies using a 'broad' definition of schizophrenia (e.g. ICD-8 or ICD-9) suggests that the variation in rates based on first admissions or first contacts is about threefold, in the range from 0.17 to 0.54 per 1000 population per year. Studies using restrictive criteria such as the Research Diagnostic Criteria (**RCD**),[51] DSM-III and its successors, and ICD-10 have reported incidence rates that are two to three times lower than those based on 'broad' criteria.

Table 4 Annual incidence rates per 1000 population at risk (age 15–54) for a 'broad' and a 'restrictive' case definition of schizophrenia in the WHO 10-country study[11]

Country	Area	'Broad' definition (ICD-9)			'Restrictive' definition (CATEGO S+)		
		Male	Female	Both sexes	Male	Female	Both sexes
Denmark	Aarhus	0.18	0.13	0.16	0.09	0.05	0.07
India	Chandigarh (rural area)	0.37	0.48	0.42	0.13	0.09	0.11
	Chandigarh (urban area)	0.34	0.35	0.35	0.08	0.11	0.09
Ireland	Dublin	0.23	0.21	0.22	0.10	0.08	0.09
Japan	Nagasaki	0.23	0.18	0.20	0.11	0.09	0.10
Russia	Moscow	0.25	0.31	0.28	0.03	0.03	0.02
UK	Nottingham	0.28	0.15	0.22	0.17	0.12	0.14
USA	Honolulu	0.18	0.14	0.16	0.10	0.08	0.09

To date, the only study that has generated directly comparable incidence data for different populations is the WHO 10-country investigation.[11] Incidence counts in the WHO study were based on first-in-lifetime contacts with any 'helping agency' (including traditional healers in the developing countries) monitored prospectively over a 2-year period. Potential cases and key informants were interviewed by clinicians using standardized instruments, and the timing of onset was ascertained for the majority of the patients. In 86 per cent of the 1022 patients the first appearance of diagnostic symptoms of schizophrenia was within the year preceding the first contact, and therefore the first-contact incidence rate was accepted as a reasonable approximation to the onset rate. Two definitions of 'caseness', differing in the degree of specificity, were used to determine incidence: a 'broad' clinical class comprising ICD-9 schizophrenia and paranoid psychoses, and a restrictive definition including only 'nuclear' schizophrenia manifesting with so-called Schneiderian first-rank symptoms.[52] The rates for eight catchment areas are shown in Table 4.

The differences between the rates for 'broadly' defined schizophrenia (0.16–0.42 per 1000) were significant ($p < 0.001$, two-tailed test); however, those for 'nuclear' schizophrenia were not. Since the mean incidence rates for the 'nuclear' cases were lower than the mean rates for 'broadly' defined schizophrenia, the confidence intervals for the lower rates would be expected to be wider than the confidence intervals for the higher rates. In fact, the opposite was true, which suggests that 'nuclear' schizophrenia comprises a more homogeneous subset of cases than the 'broad' diagnostic class and occurs with a similar frequency in these different populations. However, no differences were found between cases meeting the 'broad' criteria and the 'nuclear' cases with regard to either age or type of onset (acute or insidious), or 2-year course and outcome. Therefore it is unlikely on clinical grounds that 'nuclear' and 'broadly' defined cases represent two different disorders.

In recent years, replications of the design of the WHO 10-country study, including its research instruments and procedures, have been carried out with very similar results by investigators in India, the Caribbean, and the United Kingdom (Table 3).

Disease expectancy (morbid risk)

This is the probability (usually expressed as a percentage) that an individual born into a particular population will develop the disease if he or she survives the period of risk for that disease. In the instance of schizophrenia the period of risk is defined as either 15 to 44 or 15 to 54 years. If the age- and sex-specific incidence rates are known, disease expectancy can be estimated directly by a summation of the age-specific rates within the period of risk. Disease expectancy can be estimated indirectly from prevalence data.

The estimates of risk produced by a number of studies are fairly consistent across populations and over time. Excluding outliers, such as the northern Swedish isolate (Table 2), the risk ratio (ratio of highest to lowest disease expectancy) is about 5.0; for the WHO study[11] it is 2.9 ('broad' diagnostic class) and 2.0 ('nuclear' schizophrenia). The frequently cited 'rule of thumb' estimate of disease expectancy for schizophrenia at around 1 per cent (or slightly less) seems to be consistent with the evidence.

Associations with age and sex

There is adequate evidence that schizophrenia may have its onset at any age—in childhood as well as past middle age—although the vast majority of onsets indisputably fall within the interval 15 to 54 years of age. Onsets in men peak steeply in the age group 20 to 24 years; thereafter the rate of inception remains more or less constant at a lower level. In women, a less prominent peak in the age group 20 to 24 years is followed by another increase in incidence in age groups older than 35. While the age-specific incidence up to the mid-thirties is significantly higher in men, the male-to-female ratio becomes inverted with age, reaching 1 : 1.9 for onsets after age 40 and 1 : 4 or even 1 : 6 for onsets after age 60. There seems to be no real 'point of rarity' between the symptomatology of late-onset schizophrenia and schizophrenia of an early onset.

The sex differences in mean age at onset are unlikely to be an invariant biological characteristic of schizophrenia. For example, within families with two or more affected members, significant differences in age at onset have not been found between male and female siblings with schizophrenia.[53] In some populations (e.g. India) the male–female difference in the frequency of onsets in the younger age groups is attenuated or even inverted.[54]

The question of whether the total lifetime risks for men and women are about the same, or different, has not been answered definitively. In the WHO 10-country study, the cumulated risks for males and females up to age 54 were found to be approximately equal. Some Scandinavian population-based studies which followed up cohorts at risk into a very old age (over 85) reported a higher cumulated lifetime risk in women than in men.[55]

Male–female differences have been described in relation to the premorbid history (better premorbid functioning in women), the occurrence of brain abnormalities (more frequent in men), course (a higher percentage of remitting illness episodes and shorter hospital stay in women), and outcome (higher survival rate in the community, less disability in women). However, there is no unequivocal evidence of consistent sex differences in the symptom profiles of schizophrenia, including the frequency of positive and negative symptoms. Generally, the sex differences described in schizophrenia are more likely to result from the normal sexual dimorphism in brain development, as well as from gender-related social roles, than from sex-specific aetiological factors.

Fertility, mortality, and comorbidity

Fertility

Earlier studies have described a low fertility in both men and women diagnosed as schizophrenic. The average number of children fathered by schizophrenic men in Sweden was 0.9, and the average number of live births over the entire reproductive period of women treated for schizophrenia in Norway between 1936 and 1975 was 1.8, compared with 2.2 for the general female population.[56] Similar results have been reported from Germany.[57] Yet this phenomenon does not seem to be either universal or consistent over time. For example, according to the WHO 10-country study,[11] the fertility of women with schizophrenia in India did not differ from that of women in the general population within the same age groups and geographic areas. An increase in the fertility of schizophrenic women in more recent decades has been noted and is likely to be sustained as a result of the deinstitutionalization of the mentally ill. Although men with schizophrenia continue to be reproductively disadvantaged, at least one study[58] has found a higher than average fertility among married schizophrenic men. Several studies have examined the fertility of biological relatives of probands with schizophrenia. The results are not entirely consistent, but some of these studies have pointed to a higher than average fertility in parents and siblings of schizophrenic patients.[59]

Mortality

Excess mortality among schizophrenic patients has been extensively documented by epidemiological studies on large cohorts. National case register data for Norway indicate that, while the total mortality of psychiatric patients decreased between 1926–1941 and 1950–1974, the relative mortality of patients with schizophrenia remained unchanged at a level more than twice that of the general population.[9] Results from cohort and record linkage studies in other European countries and North America are similar, reporting standardized mortality ratios of 2.6 or higher for patients with schizophrenia, which corresponds to a reduction in life expectancy of about 20 per cent compared with the general population. A meta-analysis of 18 studies[60] resulted in a crude mortality rate of 189 deaths per 10 000 population per year and a 10-year survival rate of 81 per cent. Mortality among males was significantly higher than among females, and the difference was almost entirely due to an excess in accidents and suicides in males. Unnatural causes apart, the leading causes of death among schizophrenic patients are similar to those in the general population, with the possible exception of a lower than expected cancer mortality in males with schizophrenia.[61] The latter phenomenon has been replicated by case register and record linkage studies[62] and does not appear to be an artefact. Its causes remain unknown.

Data on successive Danish national cohorts[63] suggest an alarming trend of increasing mortality in first-admission patients with schizophrenia. The 5-year cumulated standardized mortality ratios increased from 5.30 (males) and 2.27 (females) between 1971 and 1973 to 7.79 (males) and 4.52 (females) between 1980 and 1982. Particularly striking was the standardized mortality ratio of 16.4 for male schizophrenics in the first year after the diagnosis is made. Similar data on high mortality after a first episode of schizophrenia have been reported in several other studies.

The single most common cause of death among schizophrenic patients at present is suicide (aggregated standardized mortality ratios 9.6 for males and 6.8 for females) which accounts, on the average, for 28 per cent of the excess mortality in schizophrenia.[63] The actual mortality due to suicide is likely to be higher, since a proportion of the deaths classified as accidental or of undetermined cause are probably suicides. Thus the suicide rate in schizophrenic patients is at least equal to, or may be higher than, the suicide rate in major depression. Several risk factors have been suggested as relatively specific to schizophrenic suicide: being young and male, experiencing a chronic disabling illness with multiple relapses and remissions, realistic awareness of the deteriorating course of the condition, comorbid substance use, and loss of faith in treatment.[64] Data from Scotland[65] point to a trend of increasing suicide rate in schizophrenic patients, mostly within the first year after discharge. This trend seems to parallel the significant reductions in the number of psychiatric beds. Whether this new wave of increasing suicide mortality can be attributed to the transition from hospital to community management of schizophrenia remains to be established.

Comorbidity

Comorbidity in schizophrenia comprises, above all, relatively common medical problems and diseases that tend to occur among schizophrenic patients more frequently than the expected chance association. Further, certain rare conditions or abnormalities tend to co-occur with schizophrenia.

Substance abuse is by far the most common comorbid problem among schizophrenic patients[66] and may involve alcohol, stimulants, benzodiazepines, hallucinogens, and antiparkinsonian drugs, as well as caffeine and tobacco. In the WHO 10-country study,[11] a history of alcohol use in the year preceding the first contact was elicited in 57 per cent of the male patients, and in three of the study areas drug abuse (mainly cannabis and cocaine) was reported by 24 to 41 per cent of the patients. Cannabis abuse, which exacerbates the symptoms and may precipitate relapse, was a significant predictor of poor 2-year outcome. The prevalence of cigarette smoking among schizophrenia patients is, on the average, two to three times higher than in the general population, taking sex and age group into account. Recent research on the interactions between the nicotinic receptor and the glutamatergic and dopaminergic systems has led to the hypothesis that smoking in schizophrenic patients could be an attempt at self-medication reinforced by the short-term normalizing effect of nicotine on certain neurocognitive deficits such as defective sensory gating.[67]

Physical disease is common but is rarely diagnosed. Between 46 and 80 per cent of inpatients with schizophrenia, and between 20 and 43 per cent of outpatients, have been found in different surveys to have concurrent medical illnesses, including potentially life-threatening conditions in 7 per cent.[68] In addition to increased susceptibility to infection, and especially pulmonary tuberculosis, schizophrenic patients tend to have a higher than expected rate of common diseases, including diabetes, arteriosclerosis disease, and ischaemic heart disease,[69] as well as some rare genetic or idiopathic disorders such as acute intermittent porphyria and coeliac disease. A lower than expected rate of rheumatoid arthritis has repeatedly been found in schizophrenic patients,[70] although one recent record linkage study[71] failed to replicate this. Numerous studies have reported a significantly increased frequency of dysmorphic features and minor physical anomalies, including high-steepled palate, malformed ears, epicanthus, single palmar crease, and finger and toe abnormalities, which may result from deviations in fetal development during the first gestational trimester.[72]

A variety of rare organic brain disorders and anomalies have been described as occurring in association with schizophrenia, including basal ganglia calcification, aqueductus Sylvii stenosis, corpus callosum agenesis, septal cysts, and cerebral hemiatrophy. However, most of these associations have been reported from single case studies; epidemiological evidence of a higher than chance co-occurrence with schizophrenia has so far only been provided for epilepsy[73] and metachromatic leucodystrophy.[74]

Geographical and cultural variation

To date, no population or culture has been identified in which schizophrenic illnesses do not occur. Also, there is no strong evidence that the incidence of schizophrenia varies widely across populations, provided that the populations being compared are large enough to allow a low-incidence disorder such as schizophrenia to 'breed'. The evidence that psychosocial factors or culture play an aetiological role in schizophrenia is also weak. However, there are well-replicated findings of some significant variation in the course and outcome of schizophrenia across populations and cultures which involves, above all, a higher rate of symptomatic recovery and a lower rate of social deterioration in traditional rural communities. Data supporting this conclusion were provided by the WHO studies[10,11] which found a higher proportion of recovering or improving patients in developing countries such as India and Nigeria than in the developed countries. Sampling bias (e.g. a higher percentage of acute-onset schizophreniform illnesses of good prognosis among Third World patients) was not a likely explanation. A better outcome in the developing countries was found in patients with various modes of onset, and the initial symptoms of the disorder did not distinguish good-outcome from poor-outcome cases. What causes such differences in the prognosis of schizophrenia remains largely unknown. The follow-up in the WHO studies demonstrated that outcome of paranoid psychoses and affective disorders was also better in the developing countries. Such a general effect on the outcome of psy-

chiatric disorders may result from psychosocial factors, such as availability of social support networks, non-stigmatizing beliefs about mental illness, and positive expectations during the early stages of psychotic illness, from unknown genetic or ecological (including nutritional) factors influencing brain development, or from an interaction between cultural and biological factors.

The disease and disability burden of schizophrenia

According to World Bank and WHO estimates,[75] no less than 25 per cent of the total 'burden of disease' in the established market economies is at present attributable to neuropsychiatric conditions. Measured as proportion of the disability-adjusted life-years (**DALYs**) lost, schizophrenia, bipolar affective disorder, and major depression together account for 10.8 per cent of the total, i.e. they inflict on most communities losses that are comparable to those due to cancer (15 per cent) and higher than the losses due to ischaemic heart disease (9 per cent).

Secular trends: a decreasing incidence of schizophrenia?

A number of studies have suggested that a decrease of 40 per cent or more may have occurred in the first admission rates for schizophrenia over the last 30 years in some of the developed countries.[76] The data are not entirely consistent; the drop in rates is more marked in females or in late-onset cases according to some reports, is more pronounced in young males according to others, or is of the same magnitude in both sexes and in all age groups. Downward trends have been identified mainly by using national or regional admission and discharge statistics. Attempts to replicate such trends on a local level using case register data have not produced consistent results, while studies in which research diagnoses were made after a case review show no decline in incidence rates. Other concurrent changes, such as a reduction in the number of psychiatric beds and in the total number of first admissions, have also been noted in many of these studies. However, increases have been reported in the mortality of schizophrenic patients, in first admissions with diagnoses of borderline states, paranoid psychosis, and reactive psychosis, and in the proportion of patients with schizophrenia who are managed without hospital admission.

Various hypotheses have been proposed to explain the putative decrease in the incidence of schizophrenia, but no study to date has taken into account all confounding factors that may influence first admission or first contact rates. These include changes in the administrative definition of 'first admission', and changes in diagnostic practices that may have resulted in a greater reluctance among clinicians to diagnose schizophrenia on first admission. Since schizophrenia has a low incidence, its first admission rate would be highly sensitive to such 'diagnostic drift'. If changes in diagnostic habits play a role, a compensatory increase could be expected to have occurred in diagnoses other than schizophrenia. Such increases have actually been reported for borderline states and affective psychosis. All things considered, the case for a true decline in the incidence rate of schizophrenia is suggestive but not proven.

Factors maintaining the incidence of schizophrenia in populations

Since schizophrenic patients have a reduced rate of reproduction, compared with the general population, the maintenance of a relatively stable rate of schizophrenia in the population requires an explanation. A high mutation rate can practically be ruled out since the rate required for a polygenic disorder would exceed by far the theoretically possible mutation rate. Selective advantages of individuals with schizophrenia (balanced polymorphism)[77] that could offset their low fertility have been suggested, such as resistance to physiological stress or certain diseases, and an increased fertility in their biological relatives has been postulated. None of these hypotheses is at present supported by empirical data, although some evidence of normal or increased fertility among relatives of schizophrenic patients has been reported. However, the whole argument that, in the absence of a reproductive compensation for the low fertility of schizophrenic individuals, the disorder will gradually disappear may be fallacious.[78] The concept of balanced polymorphism, developed to explain the population dynamics of single-gene Mendelian diseases may not be applicable to genetically complex disorders such as schizophrenia where both multiple genetic loci and multiple exogenous factors are likely to be involved. If this is the case, there is no phenomenon requiring an explanation.

An epidemiological perspective on antecedents and risk factors

Studies on clinical samples have proposed a number of possible risk factors in schizophrenia. Considering that clinical samples are vulnerable to bias and may not be representative, epidemiological evidence should be sought to evaluate the significance of such findings. Genetic and environmental risk factors are considered further in Chapter 4.3.5.1.

Genetic risk: necessary and sufficient?

Family aggregation of schizophrenia is at present the only epidemiologically well-established risk factor for the disorder, with a relative risk for first-degree relatives of schizophrenics in the range from 9 to 18. Allowing for diagnostic variation, the risk estimates generated by different studies are similar and suggest a general pattern of descending risk as the proportions of shared genes between any two individuals decrease.[79] The weight of the evidence also suggests that genetic vulnerability is necessary but not sufficient to cause schizophrenia and that environmental factors must play a role. However, the evidence for an environmental contribution to the aetiology of schizophrenia remains indirect, stemming primarily from the observation that the concordance for schizophrenia in monozygotic twin pairs is only about 50 per cent. Three general models of the joint effects of the genotype and the environment have been proposed:[80]

(1) the effects of predisposing genes and environmental factors are additive and increase the risk of disease in a linear fashion;

(2) genes control the sensitivity of the brain to environmental insult;

(3) genes influence the likelihood of an individual's exposure to behavioural pathogens, for example by fostering some personality traits.

Current epidemiological research into possible environmental causes of schizophrenia focuses on three main areas: pre- and perinatal damage, factors affecting early brain development, and factors operating at the level of the social and family environment. (See also Chapter 4.3.5.1.)

Environmental insults at the early developmental stages

Obstetric complications

Maternal obstetric complications are widely cited as an established risk factor in schizophrenia.[81] Several explanatory models have been proposed.

1. Severe obstetric complication, such as perinatal hypoxia and resulting hippocampal damage, can prepare the ground for adult schizophrenia even if genetic liability is weak or absent.

2. A genetic predisposition sensitizes the developing brain to lesions resulting from randomly occurring less severe obstetric complications.

3. A genetic predisposition to schizophrenia leads to abnormal fetal development which in turn causes obstetric complications.

4. Maternal constitutional factors, partially influenced by genes, such as small physique or proneness to risk behaviour (drug use, smoking during pregnancy) increases the risk of obstetric complications and fetal brain damage.

None of these models has been directly tested and the association between obstetric complications and adult schizophrenia remains tenuous.[82] The majority of studies have been of a case–control design and small to moderate size. Many studies have relied on maternal recall of complications during a pregnancy that had occurred decades earlier (invoking a possible 'effort after meaning' effect). Two birth cohort studies[83,84] using obstetric data that had been recorded prospectively by midwives reported inconclusive results regarding the association with schizophrenia. However, findings from another birth cohort study suggest that perinatal brain damage might account for as many as 7 per cent of all cases of schizophrenia in the adult population.[85] Such inconsistencies caution against an unqualified acceptance of obstetric complication as a proven risk factor in schizophrenia. Clarification of their role remains an important priority for epidemiological research.

Further information about studies of obstetric complications and hypoxic–ischaemic damage as risk factors for schizophrenia can be found in Chapter 4.3.5.1.

Season of birth

A 5 to 8 per cent winter–spring excess of schizophrenic births was first described in 1929[86] and since then reported by a large number of studies, mainly in the northern hemisphere (southern hemisphere data are inconsistent). On the strength of the number of positive reports, birth seasonality appears to be a robust finding in the epidemiology of schizophrenia.[87] However, seasonality of births has also been reported for various other disorders including bipolar affective illness, major depression, autism, personality disorders, and mental retardation. A large proportion of these studies did not have the sample size needed either to prove or rule out a seasonal effect, or failed to apply the appropriate statistical procedures. As regards the possible explanatory models, few biologically plausible and testable causal hypothesis have been advanced. One of them is the seasonally increased risk of intauterine exposure to viral infection.

Maternal influenza

In utero exposure to influenza has been implicated as a risk factor since a report that an increased proportion of adult schizophrenia in Helsinki was associated with presumed second-trimester *in utero* exposure to the 1957 A2 influenza epidemic.[88] Over 30 studies have subsequently attempted to replicate the putative link between maternal influenza and schizophrenia. While several studies have replicated the original Finnish findings, negative results have more recently been reported from an increasing number of studies based on large epidemiological samples in different parts of the world.[89,90] Two studies[91,92] in which access to data on actually infected pregnant women was available found no increased risk of schizophrenia among their offspring.

The preschizophrenic person

Premorbid social impairment

Individuals who develop schizophrenia as adults are more likely to manifest difficulties in social interaction during childhood and adolescence than individuals who do not develop schizophrenia. Among children at increased genetic risk (having a parent with schizophrenia), poor social competence at age 7 to12, and passivity and social isolation in adolescence, have been found to be common in those who go on to develop the disorder as adults.[93] The association between such 'schizoid' traits and the risk of adult schizophrenia is not restricted to such high-risk populations. Evidence of early developmental peculiarities in children who develop schizophrenia as adults has been provided by prospectively collected data on a national birth cohort in the United Kingdom.[94] Preschizophrenic children had an excess (odds ratios, 2.1–5.8) of speech and educational problems, social anxiety, and preference for solitary play.

A cohort study from Sweden,[95] involving a 15-year follow-up of 50 087 men conscripted into the army at age 18 to 20, found that poor social adjustment during childhood and adolescence was significantly more common among the 195 individuals who subsequently developed schizophrenia than among the rest of the cohort. However, the early behavioural traits that are associated with schizophrenia in adult life are of such low specificity that their presence in a child or adolescent is of negligible predictive value.

Further information about studies of premorbid social impairment can be found in Chapter 4.3.5.1.

Premorbid intelligence (IQ)

In the same Swedish cohort, the subjects who subsequently developed schizophrenia were compared with the rest of the cohort on the performance of IQ-related tests and tasks at the time of conscription into the army. After controlling for confounding effects, the risk of schizophrenia increased linearly with the decrement of IQ. The effect was mainly attributable to poor performance on verbal tasks and tests of reasoning.[96]

Neurocognitive and neurophysiological markers

Several specific deficits in sustained attention,[97] event-related brain potentials,[98] and saccadic eye-movement control[99] have been found in clinical and laboratory research to be common in schizophrenic patients and also in a proportion of their clinically normal biological relatives, but to be rare in control subjects drawn from the general population (see Chapter 4.3.5.2). Their specificity to schizophrenia needs to be investigated in larger population samples. Should such variables be validated by epidemiological studies as biological markers of schizophrenia, the power of risk prediction at the level of the individual may increase substantially.

The social and family environment

Social class

Since the 1930s, numerous studies in North America and Europe have consistently found that the economically disadvantaged social groups contribute disproportionately to the first admission rate for schizophrenia. Two explanatory hypotheses, of social causation ('breeder') and of social selection ('drift'), were originally proposed.[100] According to the social causation theory, the greater socio-economic adversity characteristic of lower-class living conditions could precipitate psychosis in genetically vulnerable individuals who have a constricted capacity to cope with complex or stressful situations. In the 1960s this theory was considered to be refuted by a single study[101] which found that the social class distribution of the fathers of schizophrenic patients did not deviate from that of the general population, and that the excess of low socio-economic status among schizophrenic patients was mainly attributable to individuals who had drifted down the occupational and social scale prior to the onset of psychosis. As a result, aetiological research in schizophrenia in recent decades has tended to ignore such 'macrosocial' variables. However, the possibility remains that social stratification, socio-economic status, and acculturation stress are important factors in the causation of schizophrenia.

Migrants and ethnic minorities

An exceptionally high incidence rate of schizophrenia (about 6.0 per 1000) has been found in the African-Caribbean population in the United Kingdom.[102,103] This excess morbidity is not restricted to recent immigrants and is, in fact, higher in the British-born second generation of migrants. Similar findings of nearly fourfold excess over the general population rate have been reported for the Dutch Antillean and Surinamese immigrants in Holland.[104]

The causes of the phenomenon remain obscure. Incidence studies in the Caribbean do not indicate any excess morbidity in the indigenous populations from which migrants are recruited. Explanations in terms of biological risk factors have found little support.[105,106] A finding in need of replication is the significant increase of schizophrenia among the siblings of second-generation African-Caribbean schizophrenic probands compared with the incidence of schizophrenia in the siblings of white patients.[107] Such a 'horizontal' increase in the morbid risk suggests that an environmental factor may be modifying (increasing) the penetrance of the genetic predisposition to schizophrenia carried by a proportion of the African-Caribbean population. Psychosocial hypotheses involving acculturation stress, demoralization due to racial discrimination, and blocked opportunities for upward social mobility have been suggested but not yet properly tested (see also Chapter 4.3.5.1).

Urbanization

Earlier hypotheses that urban environments increase the risk of psychosis, either by contributing to causation (the 'breeder' effect) or by attracting vulnerable individuals (the 'drift' effect), have been revived in the light of recent epidemiological findings suggesting that urban birth is associated with a moderate but statistically significant increase in the incidence of schizophrenia, affective psychoses, and other psychoses.[108] It remains unclear whether the effect is linked to a factor operating pre- or perinatally, or a factor influencing postnatal development (see also Chapter 4.3.5.1).

Marital status

There is evidence that marital status is significantly associated with first admission rates, the age at onset, and course and outcome of schizophrenia. Single males appear to be over-represented in schizophrenia samples, including epidemiological studies such as the WHO 10-country study[11] and a large German study.[109] Since both overt schizophrenia and preschizophrenic social impairments reduce the chances of marriage, married schizophrenics may represent a selected group with a milder form of the disease. Alternatively, marriage itself (or living with a partner) may have an effect of delaying the onset of schizophrenia or cushioning its impact. Neither of these two hypotheses can be definitively rejected on the basis of available descriptive epidemiological data. However, a statistical analysis of the WHO data, in which confounding factors such as age, premorbid personality traits, and family history were controlled, found that married men experienced a statistically significant delay (1–2 years) in the onset of psychotic symptoms compared with single men.[110]

Early rearing environment

Support for an effect of the early rearing family environment on the risk of developing schizophrenia is provided by a study of a Finnish sample of adopted children of schizophrenic parents (a high-risk group) and a control sample of adoptees at no increased genetic risk.[111] While the rates of adult psychosis or severe personality disorder were significantly higher in the high-risk group compared with the control group, the difference was entirely attributable to the subset of high-risk children who grew up in dysfunctional or otherwise disturbed adoptive families—a result consistent with the model of genetic control of sensitivity to the environment.

Epidemiological issues for the next decade

The rapid growth in basic knowledge about the human genome and the brain suggests that novel approaches to the study of complex disorders such as schizophrenia, integrating molecular genetics, neuroscience, and epidemiology, are likely to arise within the next decade.

Does the categorical disease concept of schizophrenia constrain aetiological research?

It has been suggested that the categorical disease concept of schizophrenia is no longer tenable and may be an obstacle to further progress in aetiological research.[112,113] The reasons advanced include the variation in the clinical phenotype, the likely genetic heterogeneity, and

the absence, following several complete genome scans in large samples of families, of clear evidence for genetic linkage of the diagnostic entity. Reasons for revising the original formulation of the problem of the psychoses were given by Kraepelin himself, who concluded in 1920 that schizophrenia and manic–depressive illness do not represent particular pathological processes but rather indicate which 'areas of our personality' are affected by them.[114]

Whether schizophrenia is a single disease or a syndrome arising as a 'final common pathway' for a variety of pathological processes, the validity of the concept is supported by the epidemiological evidence. This makes it unlikely that the concept will be abandoned unless a clearly superior alternative is proposed. Existing alternatives include dimensional models derived from factor-analytical clinical studies (e.g. specifying a 'psychotic', a 'disorganized', and a 'deficit' dimension),[115] subtyping schizophrenia according to the presence or absence of particular neurophysiological or neurocognitive abnormalities as 'correlated phenotypes',[116] and subdividing the psychoses into multiple, presumably homogeneous, clusters along the lines proposed by Leonhard.[117] While experimenting with such concepts may generate new aetiological hypotheses, the resulting fragmentation of schizophrenia will reduce the statistical power of epidemiological and genetic studies. It is more likely that the diagnostic concept of schizophrenia will be retained, but will be refined by using some of the above models as complementary, rather than alternative, approaches.

Molecular epidemiology of schizophrenia

Notwithstanding the difficulties accompanying the genetic dissection of complex disorders, novel methods of genetic analysis will eventually identify genomic regions and loci predisposing to schizophrenia. The majority are likely to be of small effect, although one cannot exclude the possibility that genes of moderate or even major effects will also be found, especially in relation to the neurophysiological abnormalities associated with schizophrenia. Clarifying the function of such genes will be a complex task. Part of the solution is likely to be found in the domain of epidemiology, since establishing their population frequency and associations with a variety of phenotypic expressions, including personality traits and environmental risk factors, is a prerequisite for understanding their causal role. Thus a molecular epidemiology of schizophrenia is likely to be the next major chapter in the search for causes and cures.

Can schizophrenia be prevented?

The increasing interest in the early diagnosis and treatment of first episodes of schizophrenic and affective psychoses has raised the questions of whether people likely to develop schizophrenia can be reliably recognized prior to the onset of symptoms, and whether early pharmacological, cognitive, or social intervention can prevent the development of the disorder. While early diagnosis and treatment of symptomatic cases are feasible and may have the potential of improving the short- or medium-term outcome, the pre-onset detection of likely cases with a view to preventative intervention is problematic. It has been proposed that screening young age groups in the population by using predictors of high risk (such as a family history of psychosis, obstetric complications, or abnormal eye tracking) could identify potential patients long before onset.[118] However, the poor specificity of such putative risk factors is likely to result in low positive predictive values. Other candidate risk factors have not been evaluated at all epidemiologically. Problems of reliability of measurement apart, using combinations of such variables would decrease further the positive predictive value of the screening procedure and pose the practical and ethical problem of having to treat a large number of individuals who do not have the disorder. From an epidemiological point of view, presymptomatic detection and preventative intervention in schizophrenia do not appear to be feasible at present.

Summary and conclusions

After nearly a century of epidemiological research, many essential questions about the nature and causes of schizophrenia still await answers. Two major conclusions stand out.

First, the clinical syndrome of schizophrenia is robust and can be identified reliably in diverse populations, regardless of wide-ranging demographic, ecological, and cultural differences among them. This suggests that a common pathophysiology is likely to underlie the characteristic symptoms of schizophrenia. On balance, the evidence suggests that no major differences in incidence and disease risk can be found across populations at the level of large population aggregates. However, the study of 'atypical' populations such as genetic isolates or minority groups may be capable of detecting unusual variations in the incidence of schizophrenia that could provide novel clues to the aetiology and pathogenesis of disorder.

The second conclusion is that no single environmental risk factor of major effect on the incidence of schizophrenia has yet been discovered. Further studies using large samples are required to evaluate potential risk factors, antecedents, and predictors for which the present evidence is inconclusive. Assuming that the methodological pitfalls of risk-factor epidemiology (such as the 'ecological fallacy') can be avoided and that a number of variables will eventually be identified as risk factors of small to moderate effect, the results will complement those of genetic research which also implicate multiple genes. All this suggests that the key to understanding schizophrenia is likely to be found in gene–environment interactions.

References

1. Jablensky, A. (1995) Schizophrenia: the epidemiological horizon. In *Schizophrenia* (ed. S.R. Hirsch and D.R. Weinberger), pp. 206–48. Blackwell Science, Oxford.
2. Kraepelin, E. (1904) Vergleichende Psychiatrie. *Zentralblatt für Nervenheilkunde und Psychiatrie*, **27**, 433–7. English translation: Comparative psychiatry. In *Themes and variations in European psychiatry* (ed. S.R. Hirsch and M. Shepherd), pp. 3–6. John Wright, Bristol, 1974.
3. Koller, J. (1895), Beitrag zur Erblichkeitsstatistik der Geisteskranken im Canton Zürich. Vergleichung derselben mit der erblichen Belastung gesunder Menschen durch Geistesstörungen u. dergl. *Archiv für Psychiatrie*, **27**, 269–94.
4. Luxenburger, H. (1928). Vorläufiger Bericht über psychiatrische Serienuntersuchungen an Zwillingen. *Zeitschrift für die gesamte Neurologie und Psychiatrie*, **116**, 297–326.
5. Klemperer, J. (1933). Zur Belastungsstatistik der Durchschnittsbevölkerung. Psychosehäufigkeit unter 1000 stichprobemässig ausgelesenen Probanden. *Zeitschrift für die gesamte Neurologie und Psychiatrie*, **146**, 277–316.
6. Brugger, C. (1931). Versuch einer Geisteskrankenzählung in Thüringen. *Zeitschrift für die gesamte Neurologie und Psychiatrie*, **133**, 252–390.
7. Essen-Möller, E., Larsson, H., Uddenberg, C.E., and White, G. (1956). Individual traits and morbidity in a Swedish rural population. *Acta Psychiatrica et Neurologica Scandinavica*, Supplement 100.
8. Hagnell, O. (1966). *A prospective study of the incidence of mental disorder*. Svenska Bokforlaget, Lund.
9. Ödegaard, Ö. (1946). A statistical investigation of the incidence of mental disorder in Norway. *Psychiatric Quarterly*, **20**, 381–401.
10. World Health Organization. (1979). *Schizophrenia. An international follow-up study*. Wiley, Chichester.
11. Jablensky, A., Sartorius, N., Ernberg, G., *et al.* (1992). *Schizophrenia: manifestations and course in different cultures. A World Health Organization ten-country study*. Psychological Medicine Monograph Supplement 20. Cambridge University Press.
12. Robins, L.N. and Regier, D.A. (ed.) (1991). *Psychiatric disorders in America. The Epidemiologic Catchment Area Study*. Free Press, New York.
13. Kessler, R.C., McGonagle, K.A, Zhao, S., *et al.* (1994). Lifetime and 12-month prevalence of DSM-IIIR psychiatric disorders in the United States. Results from the National Comorbidity Survey. *Archives of General Psychiatry*, **51**, 8–19.
14. Jones, P. and Cannon, M. (1998). The new epidemiology of schizophrenia. *Psychiatric Clinics of North America*, **21**, 1–25.
15. Cooper, J.E., Kendell, R.E., Gurland, B.J., Sharpe, L., Copeland, J.R.M., and Simon, R. (1972). *Psychiatric diagnosis in New York and London*. Oxford University Press, London.
16. Wing, J.K., Cooper, J.E., and Sartorius N. (1974). *The measurement and classification of psychiatric symptoms*. Cambridge University Press.
17. Jablensky, A., Hugler, H., von Cranach, M., and Kalinov, K. (1993). Kraepelin revisited: a reassessment and statistical analysis of dementia praecox and manic–depressive insanity in 1908. *Psychological Medicine*, **23**, 843–58.
18. World Health Organization (1992). *International statistical classification of diseases and related health problems, 10th revision*. WHO, Geneva.
19. American Psychiatric Association (1994). *Diagnostic and statistical manual of mental disorders* (4th edn). American Psychiatric Association, Washington, DC.
20. Robins L.N., Wing, J., Wittchen, H.U., *et al.* (1988). The Composite International Diagnostic Interview: an epidemiologic instrument suitable for use in conjunction with different diagnostic systems and in different cultures. *Archives of General Psychiatry*, **45**, 1069–77.
21. Wing J.K., Babor, T., Brugha, T., *et al.* (1990). SCAN. Schedules for Clinical Assessment in Neuropsychiatry. *Archives of General Psychiatry*, **47**, 589–93.
22. Strömgren, E. (1938). Beiträge zur psychiatrischen Erblehre, auf Grund von Untersuchungen an einer Inselbevölkerung. *Acta Psychiatrica et Neurologica Scandinavica*, Supplement 19.
23. Bøjholm, S. and Strömgren, E. (1989). Prevalence of schizophrenia on the island of Bornholm in 1935 and in 1983. *Acta Psychiatrica Scandinavica*, **79** (Supplement 348), 157–66.
24. Lemkau, P., Tietze, C., and Cooper, M. (1943) A survey of statistical studies on the prevalence and incidence of mental disorder in sample populations. *Public Health Reports*, **58**, 1909–27.
25. Sjögren, T. (1948). Genetic-statistical and psychiatric investigations of a West Swedish population. *Acta Psychiatrica et Neurologica Scandinavica*, Supplement 52.
26. Böök, J.A. (1953). A genetic and neuropsychiatric investigation of a North Swedish population (with special regard to schizophrenia and mental deficiency). *Acta Genetica*, **4**, 1–100.
27. Böök, J.A., Wetterberg, L., and Modrzewska, K. (1978). Schizophrenia in a North Swedish geographical isolate, 1900–1977: epidemiology, genetics and biochemistry. *Clinical Genetics*, **14**, 373–94.
28. Rin, H. and Lin, T.Y. (1962). Mental illness among Formosan aborigines

as compared with the Chinese in Taiwan. *Journal of Mental Science*, **198**, 134–46.

29. Lin, T.Y., Chu, H.M., Rin, H., *et al.* (1989). Effects of social change on mental disorders in Taiwan: observations based on a 15-year follow-up survey of general populations in three communities. *Acta Psychiatrica Scandinavica*, **79** (Supplement 348), 11–34.

30. Bash, K.W. (1967). Untersuchungen über die Epidemiologie neuropsychiatrischer Erkrankungen unter der handesbevölkerung der Provinz Fars, Iran. In *Beiträge zur vergleichenden Psychiatrie* (ed. N. Petrilowitsch), pp. 162–78. Karger, Basel.

31. Crocetti, G.J., Lemkau, P.V., Kulcar, Z., and Kesic, B. (1971). Selected aspects of the epidemiology of psychoses in Croatia, Yugoslavia, II. The cluster sample and the results of the pilot survey. *American Journal of Epidemiology*, **94**, 126–34.

32. Dube, K.C. and Kumar, N. (1972). An epidemiological study of schizophrenia. *Journal of Biosocial Science*, **4**, 187–95.

33. Rotstein, V.G. (1977). Material from a psychiatric survey of sample groups from the adult population in several areas of the USSR. *Zhurnal Nevropatologii i Psikhiatrii*, **77**, 569–74 (in Russian).

34. Keith, S.J., Regier, D.A., and Rae, D.S. (1991). Schizophrenic disorders. In *Psychiatric disorders in America. The Epidemiologic Catchment Area Study* (ed. L.N. Robins and D.A. Regier), pp. 33–52. Free Press, New York.

35. Jeffreys, S.E., Harvey, C.A., McNaught, A.S., *et al.* (1997). The Hampstead Schizophrenia Survey 1991. I: Prevalence and service use comparisons in an inner London health authority, 1986–1991. *British Journal of Psychiatry*, **170**, 301–6.

36. Jablensky, A., McGrath, J. Herrman, H., *et al.* (1999). *People living with psychotic illness*. National Survey of Mental Health and Wellbeing, Report 4. Commonwealth Department of Health and Aged Care, Canberra.

37. Eaton, J.W. and Weil, R.J. (1955). *Culture and mental disorder. A comparative study of the Hutterites and other populations*. Free Press, Glencoe, IL.

38. Torrey, E.F., Torrey, B.B., and Burton-Bradley, B.G. (1974). The epidemiology of schizophrenia in Papua New Guinea. *American Journal of Psychiatry*, **131**, 567–73.

39. Kendler, K.S., Gallagher, T.J., Abelson, J.M., and Kessler, R.C. (1996). Lifetime prevalence, demographic risk factors, and diagnostic validity of nonaffective psychosis as assessed in a US community sample. *Archives of General Psychiatry*, **53**, 1022–31.

40. Walsh, D. (1969). Mental illness in Dublin—first admissions. *British Journal of Psychiatry*, **115**, 449–56.

41. Häfner, H. and Reimann, H. (1970). Spatial distribution of mental disorders in Mannheim, 1965. In *Psychiatric epidemiology* (ed. E.H. Hare and J.K. Wing), pp. 341–54. Oxford University Press, London.

42. Murphy, H.B.M. and Raman, A.C. (1971). The chronicity of schizophrenia in indigenous tropical peoples. Results of a twelve-year follow-up survey in Mauritius. *British Journal of Psychiatry*, **118**, 489–97.

43. Lieberman, Y.I. (1974). The problem of incidence of schizophrenia: material from a clinical and epidemiological study. *Zhurnal Nevropatologii i Psikhiatrii*, **74**, 1224–32 (in Russian).

44. Helgason, L. (1977). Psychiatric services and mental illness in Iceland. *Acta Psychiatrica Scandinavica*, **53** (Supplement 268), 1–140.

45. Castle, D., Wessely, S., Der, G., and Murray, R.M. (1991). The incidence of operationally defined schizophrenia in Camberwell, 1965–84. *British Journal of Psychiatry*, **159**, 790–4.

46. Nicole, L., Lesage, A., and Lalonde, P. (1992). Lower incidence and increased male:female ratio in schizophrenia. *British Journal of Psychiatry*, **161**, 556–7.

47. Rajkumar, S., Padmavati, R., Thara, R., *et al.* (1993). Incidence of schizophrenia in an urban community in Madras. *Indian Journal of Psychiatry*, **35**, 18–21.

48. Hickling, F.W. (1991). Psychiatric hospital admission rates in Jamaica, 1971 and 1988. *British Journal of Psychiatry*, **159**, 817–21.

49. McNaught, A., Jeffreys, S.E., Harvey, C.A., *et al.* (1997). The Hampstead Schizophrenia Survey 1991. II. Incidence and migration in inner London. *British Journal of Psychiatry*, **170**, 307–11.

50. Brewin, J., Cantwell, R., Dalkin, T., *et al.* (1997). Incidence of schizophrenia in Nottingham. *British Journal of Psychiatry*, **171**, 140–4.

51. Spitzer, R.L., Endicott, J., and Robins, E. (1978). Research Diagnostic Criteria. Rationale and reliability. *Archives of General Psychiatry*, **35**, 773–82.

52. Koehler, K. (1979). First rank symptoms of schizophrenia: questions concerning clinical boundaries. *British Journal of Psychiatry*, **134**, 236–48.

53. DeLisi, L.E., Goldin, L.R., Maxwell, M.E., Kazuba, D.M., and Gershon E.S. (1987). Clinical features of illness in siblings with schizophrenia or schizoaffective disorder. *Archives of General Psychiatry*, **44**, 891–6.

54. Murthy, G.V.S., Janakiramaiah, N., Gangadhar, B.N., and Subbakrishna, D.K. (1998). Sex difference in age at onset of schizophrenia: discrepant findings from India. *Acta Psychiatrica Scandinavica*, **97**, 321–5.

55. Helgason, T. and Magnusson, H. (1989). The first 80 years of life. A psychiatric epidemiological study. *Acta Psychiatrica Scandinavica*, **79** (Supplement 348), 85–94.

56. Ödegaard Ö. (1980). Fertility of psychiatric first admissions in Norway, 1936–75. *Acta Psychiatrica Scandinavica*, **62**, 212–20.

57. Hilger, T., Propping, P. and Haverkamp, F. (1983). Is there an increase of reproductive rates in schizophrenics? *Archiv für Psychiatrie und Nervenkrankheiten*, **233**, 177–86.

58. Lane, A., Byrne, M., Mulvany, F., *et al.* (1995). Reproductive behaviour in schizophrenia relative to other mental disorders: evidence for increased fertility in men despite decreased marital rate. *Acta Psychiatrica Scandinavica*, **91**, 222–8.

59. Srinivasan, T.N. and Padmavati, R. (1997). Fertility and schizophrenia: evidence for increased fertility in the relatives of schizophrenic patients. *Acta Psychiatrica Scandinavica*, **96**, 260–4.

60. Brown, S. (1997). Excess mortality of schizophrenia. A meta-analysis. *British Journal of Psychiatry*, **171**, 502–8.

61. Dupont, A., Jensen, O.M., Strömgren, E., and Jablensky A. (1986). Incidence of cancer in patients diagnosed as schizophrenic in Denmark. In *Psychiatric case registers in public health* (ed. S.H. ten Horn, R. Giel, and W. Gulbinat), pp. 229–39. Elsevier, Amsterdam.

62. Mortensen, P.B. (1994). The occurrence of cancer in first admitted schizophrenic patients. *Schizophrenia Research*, **12**, 185–94.

63. Mortensen, P.B. and Juel, K. (1993). Mortality and causes of death in first admitted schizophrenic patients. *British Journal of Psychiatry*, **163**, 183–9.

64. Caldwell, C.B. and Gottesman, I.I. (1990). Schizophrenics kill themselves too: a review of risk factors for suicide. *Schizophrenia Bulletin*, **16**, 571–89

65. Geddes, J.R. and Juszczak, E. (1995). Period trends in rate of suicide in first 28 days after discharge from psychiatric hospital in Scotland, 1968–92. *British Medical Journal*, **311**, 357–60.

66. Rosenthal, R.N. (1998). Is schizophrenia addiction prone? *Current Opinion in Psychiatry*, **11**, 45–8.

67. Dalack, G.W. and Meador-Woodruff, J.H. (1996). Smoking, smoking withdrawal and schizophrenia: case reports and a review of the literature. *Schizophrenia Research*, **22**, 133–41.

68. Jeste, D.V., Gladsjo, J.A., Lindamer, L.A., and Lacro, J.P. (1996). Medical comorbidity in schizophrenia. *Schizophrenia Bulletin*, **22**, 413–30.

69. Herrman, H.E., Baldwin, J.A., and Christie, D. (1983). A record-linkage study of mortality and general hospital discharge in patients diagnosed as schizophrenic. *Psychological Medicine*, **13**, 581–93.

70. Eaton, W.M., Hayward, C., and Ram, R. (1992). Schizophrenia and rheumatoid arthritis: a review. *Schizophrenia Research*, **6**, 181–92.

71. Lauerma, H., Lehtinen, V., Joukamaa, M.R., Helenius, H., and Isohanni, M. (1998). Schizophrenia among patients treated for rheumatoid arthritis and appendicitis. *Schizophenia Research*, **29**, 255–61.

72. Murphy, K.C. and Owen, M.J. (1996). Minor physical anomalies and their relationship to the aetiology of schizophrenia. *British Journal of Psychiatry*, **168**, 139–42.

73. Bredkjær, S.R., Mortensen, P.B., and Parnas, J. (1998). Epilepsy and non-organic non-affective psychosis. National epidemiologic study. *British Journal of Psychiatry*, 172, 235–8.

74. Hyde, T.M., Ziegler, J.C., and Weinberger, D. (1992). Psychiatric disturbances in metachromatic leucodystrophy. *Archives of Neurology*, 49, 401–6.

75. Murray, C.J.L. and Lopez, A.D. (ed.) (1996). *The global burden of disease. A comprehensive assessment of mortality and disability from diseases, injuries, and risk factors in 1990 and projected to 2020.* Harvard School of Public Health, Cambridge, MA.

76. Jablensky, A. (1995). Schizophrenia: recent epidemiologic issues. *Epidemiologic Reviews*, 17, 10–20.

77. Huxley, J., Mayr, E., Osmond, H., and Hoffer, A. (1964). Schizophrenia as a genetic morphism. *Nature*, 204, 220–1.

78. Haverkamp, F., Propping, P., and Hilger, T. (1982). Is there an increase of reproductive rates in schizophrenia? I. Critical review of the literature. *Archiv für Psychiatrie und Nervenkrankheiten*, 232, 439–50.

79. Jablensky, A. and Eaton, W.W. (1995). Schizophrenia. In *Baillière's clinical psychiatry*, Vol. 1, No. 2, *Epidemiological psychiatry* (ed. A. Jablensky), pp. 283–306. Baillière Tindall, London.

80. Kendler, K.S. and Eaves, L.J. (1986). Models for the joint effect of genotype and environment on liability to psychiatric illness. *American Journal of Psychiatry*, 143, 279–89.

81. Cannon, T.D. (1997). On the nature and mechanisms of obstetric influences in schizophrenia: a review and synthesis of epidemiological studies. *International Review of Psychiatry*, 9, 387–97.

82. Geddes, J.R. and Lawrie, S.M. (1995). Obstetric complications and schizophrenia: a meta-analysis. *British Journal of Psychiatry*, 167, 786–93.

83. Done, D.J., Johnstone, E.C., Frith, C.D., *et al.* (1991). Complications of pregnancy and delivery in relation to psychosis in adult life: data from the British perinatal mortality survey sample. *British Medical Journal*, 202, 1576–80.

84. Buka, S.L., Tsuang, M.T., and Lipsitt, L.P. (1993). Pregnancy/delivery complications and psychiatric diagnosis: a prospective study. *Archives of General Psychiatry*, 50, 151–6.

85. Jones, P.B., Rantakallio, P., Hartikainen, A.L., Isohanni, M., and Sipila, P. (1998). Schizophrenia as a long-term outcome of pregnancy, delivery, and perinatal complications: a 28-year follow-up of the 1966 North Finland general population birth cohort. *American Journal of Psychiatry*, 155, 355–64.

86. Tramer, M. (1929). Über die biologische Bedeutung des Geburtsmonates, insbesondere für die Psychoseerkrankung. *Schweizerischer Archiv für Neurologie und Psychiatrie*, 24, 17–24.

87. Torrey, E.F., Miller, J., Rawlings, R., and Yolken, R.H. (1997). Seasonality of births in schizophrenia and bipolar disorder: a review of the literature. *Schizophrenia Research*, 28, 1–38.

88. Mednick, S.A., Machon, R.A., Huttunen, M.O., and Bonett, D. (1988). Adult schizophrenia following prenatal exposure to an influenza epidemic. *Archives of General Psychiatry*, 45, 189–92.

89. Morgan, V., Castle, D., Page, A., *et al.* (1997). Influenza epidemics and incidence of schizophrenia, affective disorders and mental retardation in Western Australia: no evidence of a major effect. *Schizophrenia Research*, 26, 25–39.

90. Grech, A., Takei, N., and Murray, R.M. (1997). Maternal exposure to influenza and paranoid schizophrenia. *Schizophrenia Research*, 26, 121–5.

91. Crow, T.J. and Done, D.J. (1992). Prenatal influenza does not cause schizophrenia. *British Journal of Psychiatry*, 161, 390–3.

92. Cannon, M., Cotter, D., Coffey, V.P., *et al.* (1996). Prenatal exposure to the 1957 influenza epidemics and adult schizophrenia: a follow-up study. *British Journal of Psychiatry*, 168, 368–71.

93. Cannon, T.D., Mednick, S.A., and Parnas, J. (1990). Antecedents of predominantly negative- and predominantly positive-symptom schizophrenia in a high-risk population. *Archives of General Psychiatry*, 47, 622–32.

94. Jones, P., Rodgers, B., Murray, R., and Marmot, M. (1994). Child developmental risk factors for adult schizophrenia in the British 1946 birth cohort. *Lancet*, 344, 1398–402.

95. Malmberg, A., Lewis, G., David, A., and Allebeck, P. (1998). Premorbid adjustment and personality in people with schizophrenia. *British Journal of Psychiatry*, 172, 308–13.

96. David, A.S., Malmberg, A., Brandt, L., Allebeck, P., and Lewis, G. (1997). IQ and risk for schizophrenia: a population-based cohort study. *Psychological Medicine*, 27, 1311–23.

97. Cornblatt, B.A. and Keilp, J. (1994). Impaired attention, genetics, and the pathophysiology of schizophrenia. *Schizophrenia Bulletin*, 20, 31–46.

98. Freedman, R., Adler, L.E., Myles-Worsley, M., *et al.* (1996). Inhibitory gating of an evoked response to repeated auditory stimuli in schizophrenic and normal subjects. *Archives of General Psychiatry*, 53, 1114–21.

99. Clementz, B.A., McDowell, J.E., and Zisook, S. (1994). Saccadic system functioning among schizophrenia patients and their first-degree biological relatives. *Journal of Abnormal Psychology*, 103, 277–87.

100. Mischler, E.G. and Scotch, N.A. (1983). Sociocultural factors in the epidemiology of schizophrenia: a review. *Psychiatry*, 26, 315–51.

101. Goldberg, E.M. and Morrison, S.L. (1963). Schizophrenia and social class. *British Journal of Psychiatry*, 109, 785–802.

102. Bhugra, D., Leff, J., Mallett, R., Der, G., Corridan, B., and Rudge, S. (1997). Incidence and outcome of schizophrenia in Whites, African-Caribbeans and Asians in London. *Psychological Medicine*, 27, 791–8.

103. Harrison, G., Glazebrook, C., Brewin, J., *et al.* (1997). Increased incidence of psychotic disorders in migrants from the Caribbean to the United Kingdom. *Psychological Medicine*, 27, 799–806.

104. Selten, J.P., Slaets, J.P.J., and Kahn, R.S. (1997). Schizophrenia in Surinamese and Dutch Antillean immigrants to The Netherlands: evidence of an increased incidence. *Psychological Medicine*, 27, 807–11.

105. Hutchinson, G., Takei, N., Bhugra, D., *et al.* (1997). Increased rate of psychosis among African-Caribbeans in Britain is not due to an excess of pregnancy and birth complications. *British Journal of Psychiatry*, 171, 145–7.

106. Selten, J.P., Slaets, J., and Kahn, R. (1998). Prenatal exposure to influenza and schizophrenia in Surinamese and Dutch Antillean immigrants to The Netherlands. *Schizophrenia Research*, 30, 101–3.

107. Hutchinson, G., Takei, N., Fahy, T.A., *et al.* (1996). Morbid risk of schizophrenia in first-degree relatives of White and African-Caribbean patients with psychosis. *British Journal of Psychiatry*, 169, 776–80.

108. Marcelis, M., Navarro-Mateu, F., Murray, R., Selten, J.P., and van Os, J. (1998). Urbanization and psychosis: a study of 1942–1978 birth cohorts in The Netherlands. *Psychological Medicine*, 28, 871–9.

109. Häfner, H., Riecher-Rössler, A., van der Heiden, W., *et al.* (1993). Generating and testing a causal explanation of the gender difference in age at first onset of schizophrenia. *Psychological Medicine*, 23, 925–40.

110. Jablensky, A. and Cole, S.W. (1997). Is the earlier age at onset of schizophrenia in males a confounded finding? Results from a cross-cultural investigation. *British Journal of Psychiatry*, 170, 234–40.

111. Wahlberg, K.E., Wynne, L.C., Oja, H., *et al.* (1997). Gene–environment interaction in vulnerability to schizophrenia: findings from the Finnish adoptive family study of schizophrenia. *American Journal of Psychiatry*, 154, 355–62.

112. Kringlen, E. (1994). Is the concept of schizophrenia useful from an aetiological point of view? A selective review of findings and paradoxes. *Acta Psychiatrica Scandinavica*, 90 (Supplement 384), 17–25.

113. van Praag, H.M. (1993). 'Make-believes' in psychiatry or the perils of progress. Brunner–Mazel, New York.

114. Kraepelin, E. (1920). Die Erscheinungsformen des Irreseins. *Zeitschrift für die gesamte Neurologie und Psychiatrie*, 62, 1–29. English translation: Comparative psychiatry. In *Themes and variations in European psychiatry* (ed. S.R. Hirsch and M. Shepherd), pp. 7–30. John Wright, Bristol, 1974.

115. Liddle, P.F. (1987). The symptoms of chronic schizophrenia: a

re-examination of the positive–negative dichotomy. *British Journal of Psychiatry*, **151**, 145–51.

116. Tsuang, M.T. and Faraone, S.V. (1995). The case for heterogeneity in the etiology of schizophrenia. *Schizophrenia Research*, **17**, 161–75.

117. Leonhard, K. (1979). *The classification of endogenous psychoses* (5th edn). Halsted Press, New York.

118. McGlashan, T.H. and Johannessen, J.O. (1996). Early detection and intervention with schizophrenia: rationale. *Schizophrenia Bulletin*, **22**, 201–22.

4.3.5 Aetiology

4.3.5.1 Genetic and environmental risk factors for schizophrenia

R. M. Murray and D. J. Castle

After many years of fruitlessly seeking a single cause for schizophrenia, sometimes sarcastically termed 'the search for the schizococcus', almost all researchers have come to the conclusion that there is no single cause.

Instead, they have concluded that, like other disorders such as ischaemic heart disease and diabetes mellitus, schizophrenia results from the cumulative effects of a number of risk factors. These may be crudely divided into the familial–genetic and the environmental.

Familial–genetic risk

The most powerful risk factor for schizophrenia is having a relative afflicted with the disorder. Numerous studies have shown that the lifetime risk for broadly defined schizophrenia increases from about 1 per cent in the general population to about 10 per cent in first-degree relatives of patients with schizophrenia and to 48 per cent in those with two parents with the disorder.[1] However, familial aggregation does not prove that a condition is genetically transmitted; speaking in French also runs in families!

Adoption studies

Most children inherit their genes and their family culture from the same set of parents. However, since adoptees do not, adoption studies offer the opportunity of separating the effects of the two. In the first study of schizophrenia, Heston and Denney[2] demonstrated that five out of 47 children of schizophrenic mothers who were adopted away within a few days of their birth, later developed schizophrenia compared with none out of 50 adoptees with no family history of schizophrenia. Similar findings were reported from the Danish–American Study of Rosenthal et al.[3] who found that a significantly higher proportion of the adopted-away offspring of schizophrenic parents from Copenhagen were classified as having schizophrenia or 'borderline schizophrenia', than were control adoptees. This study originated the concept of the schizophrenia spectrum disorder, which has come to include not only frank schizophrenia but also schizophreniform disorder, as well as schizotypal and possibly paranoid personality disorder.

In an extension of the Danish–American collaboration, Kety et al.[4] took all schizophrenic adoptees in Denmark as their starting point, and then examined their biological and adoptive relatives; unlike the earlier adoption studies this one also used operational definitions of the schizophrenia spectrum conditions. Fully 23.5 per cent of the biological first-degree relatives of schizophrenic adoptees received a schizophrenia spectrum diagnosis compared with only 4.7 per cent of the biological relatives of normal control adoptees; the adoptive relatives of both groups of adoptees had very low rates of spectrum disorders.

Finally, Wender et al.[5] studied the grown-up children of normal individuals who, by mischance, had been placed with an adoptive parent who later developed schizophrenia. Thankfully, these unfortunate adoptees did not themselves show an increased risk of the disorder. Thus, adoption studies consistently indicate that the familial aggregation of schizophrenia is determined by individuals inheriting genes from someone with the disorder (or a related spectrum condition) rather than any effect of the intrafamilial culture (e.g. being brought up by a parent with schizophrenia).

Twin studies

Twin studies have come to the same conclusion. Gottesman,[1] who reviewed the literature, calculated the average probandwise concordance rate for broadly defined schizophrenia in monozygotic twins to be 46 per cent, compared with 14 per cent in dizygotic twins. This difference has been taken to be a reflection of the fact that while monozygotic twins share all their genes, dizygotic twins share, on average, only 50 per cent. Further evidence of the effect of heredity comes from the evidence that the concordance rate in 12 pairs of monozygotic twins who were reared apart was 58 per cent.[1]

The above twin studies preceded the introduction of operational definitions of schizophrenia. When studies with such definitions were carried out, the rates for both monozygotic and dizygotic twins were both lower but the disparity between the two remained. Thus, in the latest and largest study, which examined 108 consecutive pairs of twins seen at the Maudsley Hospital in London, Cardno et al.[6] reported probandwise concordance rates for DSM-IIIR schizophrenia of 42.6 per cent in monozygotic twins and 0 per cent in dizygotic twins. As can be seen in Table 1, concordance rates for schizophrenia using other operational definitions were not dissimilar.

What is the range of the clinical phenotype transmitted?

The fact that an individual can have the same genes as their schizophrenic co-twin but have a better than evens chance of remaining non-psychotic indicates that it is not schizophrenia *per se* which is inherited

Table 1 Probandwise concordance rates in the Maudsley twins for three operational definitions of schizophrenia

Operational system	Probandwise concordance (%)	
	Monozygotic	Dizygotic
DSM-IIIR	42.6	0.0
ICD-10	42.0	1.7
RDC	40.8	5.3

but rather a susceptibility to it. Further evidence in support of this comes from a study which showed that the offspring of the identical but well co-twins of schizophrenic individuals have a risk of the disorder similar to that of the offspring of the affected.[7] Thus the predisposition is transmitted without being expressed as schizophrenia.

As noted earlier, sometimes the predisposition may be expressed as non-psychotic spectrum disorders. In addition, family studies show that relatives of schizophrenic patients also have an excess of other psychotic conditions such as schizoaffective disorder, atypical and schizophreniform psychoses, and affective psychosis with mood-incongruent delusions. Thus, the clinical phenotype transmitted encompasses a range of psychotic conditions, as well as schizotypal personality disorder.

Within schizophrenia, researchers have asked whether the classical Kraepelinian subtypes are differentially inherited. The results have in general been negative which is not surprising since clinicians know that an individual patient can appear predominantly hebephrenic on one admission and schizoaffective on another. However, there has been a consensus that paranoid schizophrenia is less familial than other types and is associated with a lower monozygotic twin concordance.

Recently, it has been shown that schizophrenic symptoms can be summarized as three main factors: delusions and hallucinations (reality distortion), negative symptoms (psychomotor poverty), and disorganization or positive thought disorder.[8,9] Is schizotypal personality particularly closely related to one of these three core syndromes? Mata et al.[10] showed that schizotypal personality scores in non-psychotic relatives were significantly correlated with the presence of delusions and hallucinations in the probands; indeed, they were also correlated with premorbid schizoptypal traits in the childhood of the probands. Thus, it seems that certain families transmit schizotypal traits which manifest themselves in childhood; some family members remain schizotypal throughout life but in others this deviant personality type is then compounded by other (genetic or environmental) factors so that the individual passes a threshold for the expression of delusions and hallucinations.

Molecular genetics

For almost 15 years researchers have been using molecular techniques to seek the gene or genes that predispose to schizophrenia. The first technique to be used was that of linkage in which large families with several members affected with schizophrenia are studied to try and find a genetic marker that cosegregates with the disease. Unfortunately, to date no single gene or indeed region has been unequivocally implicated in susceptibility to schizophrenia. Rather, linkage studies suggest that no gene can exist which increases the risk of schizophrenia by more than a factor of 3 but that there may be a number of susceptibility genes. Recent findings suggest that some of these may lie within 'hot spots' on chromosomes 22, 6, or 13 (reviewed by Kirov and Murray[11]).

The second approach, that of association studies, takes a gene that is suspected of involvement in the pathogensis of the disorder (e.g. a gene involved in dopamine metabolism) and then compares the frequency of its various alleles in a series of individuals with schizophrenia as opposed to a control group. Some candidate gene studies imply a weak effect of the D_3 dopamine and $5-HT_{2A}$ receptor genes as well as the HLA locus on chromosome 6.[12]

Other studies have noted that patients in successive generations tend to develop frank schizophrenia at ever earlier ages. This process of 'anticipation' occurs in a number of neurological conditions in which an excess number of trinucleotide repeats occurs, and increases with succeeding generations; some claim that the same occurs in schizophrenia but most studies do not (see Kirov and Murray[11]).

Genetic models

Thus, both statistical and molecular studies indicate that schizophrenia cannot be explained by the inheritance of a single major gene. In any case, such simple Mendelian inheritance would be hard to square with the persistence of schizophrenia in the population. Since people with schizophrenia tend to reproduce less frequently than the rest of the population, one would have expected that a single major gene with such damaging consequences would have been selected out of the gene pool.

The evidence is compatible with oligogenic inheritance (a small number of genes involved) but the most popular model is the polygenic model which postulates that a number of genes of small effect are involved. Further support for this model comes from the fact that the risk to an individual increases with the number of affected relatives[1] and also with the finding of Cardno et al.[6] that the monozygotic concordance rate is higher for those twins who had an early rather than late onset of psychosis.

Family studies also show that the relatives of probands with an early onset have a higher morbid risk of psychosis than the relatives of late-onset patients.[13] These findings are compatible with the idea that schizophrenia is in part a developmental disorder and that some of the susceptibility genes may be involved in the control of neurodevelopment.[14]

Biological abnormalities in the relatives of schizophrenics

Relatives have been examined for some of the biological abnormalities which are found in their schizophrenic kin. Thus, in the Maudsley Family Study, Sharma et al.[15,16] carried out magnetic resonance imaging (**MRI**) scans on families with several members affected with schizophrenia. Both the schizophrenic members and those unaffected relatives who appeared to be transmitting the liability to the disorder (so-called obligate carriers) showed larger lateral ventricles than controls as well as loss of the normal cerebral asymmetry. This latter finding gives some support to Crow's[17] hypothesis that an abnormality in the genetic control of the development of normal asymmetry contributes to schizophrenia.

In the same Maudsley Family Study, the non-psychotic relatives exhibited other neurophysiological abnormalities such as an excess of delayed P300 event-related potentials; their prevalence was not as high as in the patients themselves but higher than in normal controls.[18] Those patients who showed an excess of saccadic distractability errors tended to have relatives with the same eye-tracking abnormalities.[19] The schizophrenic patients and their well relatives from these multiply affected families also showed more integrative neurological abnormalities than controls.[20]

These findings suggest that what is being transmitted is not genes for schizophrenia per se but rather genes for a variety of characteristics (e.g. schizotypal personality, enlarged lateral ventricles, loss of cerebral asymmetry, delayed P300, integrative neurological abnormalities, etc.) which increase the risk of schizophrenia. Individuals can inherit these characteristics without being psychotic; perhaps schizophrenia only ensues when an individual inherits a number of such endophenotypic abnormalities and passes a critical threshold of risk.[21]

Environmental factors

It is evident from the above that genes exert a probabilistic rather than a deterministic effect on the development of schizophrenia; environmental risk factors appear to be necessary for the disease to become manifest in many, if not all, cases.[22] But what are these environmental risk factors?

Pre- and perinatal complications

More than 20 studies have shown that patients suffering from schizophrenia are more likely to have a history of pre- or perinatal complications (collectively termed obstetric complications) than are healthy subjects from the general population, patients with other psychiatric disorders, and their own healthy siblings.[23] Some of the studies which reported these findings were based upon interviews with patients' mothers asking them to recall their pregnancies; such interviews are obviously open to distortion by loss of, or faulty, memory. However, similar findings have been reported by studies examining data collected in obstetric records at the time of birth of patients and controls.[24] A further assessment of the epidemiological studies of obstetric complications as risk factors for schizophrenia is given in Chapter 4.3.4.

Of course, it is possible that the excess obstetric complications in schizophrenia may be the consequence of some pre-existing abnormality. Since the fetus plays an active role in the normal progress of pregnancy and labour, fetal impairment induced by earlier abnormality may itself result in some perinatal complications. Also some studies have shown that women with schizophrenia who become pregnant tend to have more obstetric complications, possibly owing to their behaviour during pregnancy, for example smoking and not attending antenatal visits.

The term of 'obstetric complications' covers a broad range of obstetric events. A recent international collaboration therefore gathered data on more than 700 schizophrenics and a similar number of controls to see whether the general association could be explained by one or two specific complications; low birth weight, prematurity, and resuscitation at birth were particularly increased in the schizophrenics;[23] other complications that have been implicated include retarded fetal growth and rhesus incompatability. Thus, a common characteristic of most of the obstetric complications implicated is that they increase the risk of hypoxia.

Could hypoxic–ischaemic damage be the mechanism that increases the risk of later schizophrenia? Children who were subject to cerebral hypoxia at or before birth show an excess of abnormalities on MRI scan, of minor neurological signs, and of cognitive and behavioural problems, characteristics also found in many preschizophrenic children.[25] As one might predict, studies of monozygotic twins discord-

ant for schizophrenia have shown that the affected twins have larger lateral ventricles and smaller hippocampi than their well co-twins;[26,27] furthermore, those twins who have been subjected to the most severe perinatal difficulties have the largest ventricles and smallest hippocampi.[28]

Similarly, Stefanis et al.[29] compared hippocampal volume in schizophrenics with other affected relatives but no history of obstetric complications, schizophrenics with no affected relatives but a history of significant obstetric complications, and normal controls. Hippocampal volume was normal in the first schizophrenic group but reduced in the second group, implying that it is hypoxic–ischaemic damage rather than genetic predisposition alone that determines decreased hippocampal volume in schizophrenia.

Many studies have shown that more schizophrenic persons are born in late winter and spring than expected; since respiratory viral infections such as influenza tend to occur in autumn and winter, maternal infection might provide the explanation. A number of epidemiological studies have, therefore, addressed the question of whether maternal exposure to influenza during the second trimester of pregnancy is a risk factor for schizophrenia; some but not all studies have suggested that it is.[30] Recently, one study has raised the possibility that prenatal exposure to rubella may have a similar risk-increasing effect for schizophrenia while another implicated maternal malnutrition;[31] neither of these reports has yet been replicated. See also Chapter 4.3.4 for a more cautious assessment of the strength of the evidence that maternal exposure to influenza is a risk factor for schizophrenia.

Childhood risk factors

There is now a wealth of evidence attesting to the fact that a proportion of individuals who later manifest schizophrenia show abnormalities in their early development. The evidence for early developmental abnormalities in schizophrenia come from three main sorts of study:

- high-risk studies in which the offspring of parent(s) with schizophrenia are examined
- follow-back studies where cases of schizophrenia are ascertained, and their early developmental trajectory plotted with the help of history from the individual and family, sometimes also including such evidence as school reports, etc.
- cohort studies, where birth cohorts are followed up prospectively, and individuals who later manifest schizophrenia are compared with the rest of the cohort in terms of their early development.

High-risk studies

Studies of the offspring of schizophrenic mothers, the so-called 'high-risk studies', show that around 25 to 50 per cent show some deviation from normal in terms of their early development (reviewed by Davies et al.[32]). In the neonatal period there is a tendency to hypotonia and decreased cuddliness, in infancy milestones are delayed, in early childhood there is poor motor co-ordination, and in later childhood there are deficits in attention and information processing. Fish et al.[33] followed their cohort of 12 high-risk infants into adulthood. One developed schizophrenia and six showed schizotypal or paranoid personality traits; these authors coined the term 'pandysmaturation' to describe the abnormalities which included delayed motor milestones in the first 2 years of life.

Follow-back studies

High-risk studies have been criticised on the basis that they are unrepresentative because only a minority of people who develop schizophrenia have a mother with the same illness. Therefore researchers have carried out studies of reprentative groups of schizophrenic patients which relied on maternal recall to document the early development of adults with schizophrenia; these have shown impairment of cognitive and neuromotor development and interpersonal problems. These findings are more commonly reported in males than females, and tend to be associated with an early onset of illness.[34] The findings are not specific to schizophrenia, being reported also in the early development of some children who later manifest an affective psychosis.[35] Of course, one of the major criticisms of follow-back studies is the likelihood of recall bias. Studies that have avoided this problem include those which have accessed IQ scores assessed prior to illness onset; these have shown that premorbid IQ is, on average, lower in those, particularly males, who later manifest schizophrenia.[36,37]

Another source has been childhood home videos, which have been reviewed by researchers 'blind' to whether the individual later manifested schizophrenia.[38] In comparison with their healthy siblings, the preschizophrenic children showed higher rates of neuromotor abnormalities (predominantly left-sided) and overall poorer motor skills; the group differences were significant only at age 2 years.

Cohort studies

The publication of a number of cohort studies has overcome many of the criticisms of follow-back studies. In an investigation of the 1958 British Perinatal Mortality cohort, comprising 98 per cent of all children ($n = 15\,398$) born in the United Kingdom in a certain week in March 1958, Done et al.[39] compared those who later manifested schizophrenia ($n = 40$), affective psychosis ($n = 35$), and neurotic illness ($n = 79$) with each other as well as with 1914 randomly selected individuals with no history of mental illness. At age 7 years, teacher ratings showed the preschizophrenic children to have exhibited more social maladjustment than controls; the effect was most marked in boys. The preaffective children differed little from normal controls, whilst the preneurotic children (expressly girls) showed some maladjustment (over- and under-reaction) at age 11 years.

In a similar study of the 1946 British Birth Cohort, Jones et al.[40] determined that 30 out of 4746 individuals had, in adulthood, developed schizophrenia. This group were more likely than the rest of the cohort to show delayed milestones and speech problems, to have a lower premorbid IQ and lower education test scores at ages 8, 11, and 15 years, and to prefer solitary play at ages 4 and 6 years.

Together, such studies provide compelling evidence for a tendency of individuals with schizophrenia to show abnormalities in development which antedate the onset of illness. The findings are compatible with the notion that subtle brain abnormalities (which may be genetically or environmentally mediated, or both) underpin schizophrenia. However, it is also possible that some of the childhood risk factors are independent and act in an additive manner to set individuals on an increasingly deviant trajectory towards schizophrenia. Further information about epidemiological studies linking premorbid impairments and schizophrenia is given in Chapter 4.3.4.

Social and geographic risk factors

In 1939 Faris and Dunham[41] reported that an excess of individuals with schizophrenia was found in certain deprived inner-city areas. These authors suggested that social isolation in poor deprived parts of the city could precipitate schizophrenia. However, subsequently their results were interpreted as a consequence of social drift, i.e. the idea that individuals with this illness 'drift' down the social scale.[42] This effect is postulated to result from not only the illness itself but also its prodroma and consequences such as loss of employment and estrangement from family. A related finding is that of lack of upward social mobility in individuals with schizophrenia. For example, Hollingshead and Redlich[43] reported that individuals with schizophrenia to be less likely than expected to attain the socio-economic status of their fathers.

More recently, research has focused on the apparent excess of individuals who later manifest schizophrenia, who actually start life in a setting which appears to increase the subsequent risk of schizophrenia. Kohn[44] stated that '… in all probability, lower class families produce a disproportionate number of schizophrenics' but the evidence concerning such 'social causation' is contradictory. Thus, Turner and Wagenfeld[45] reported fathers of schizophrenia patients to be themselves over-represented in lower socio-economic groups. However, Jones et al.[40] did not find this.

It may be that it is not so much poverty as being born or brought up in a city which increases the risk of the disorder. For example, Lewis et al.[46] found that Swedish conscripts who later manifested schizophrenia were 1.65 times more likely to have been born in urban than rural areas. Similarly, Marcelis et al.[47] reported that birth in an urban area of Holland carried twice the risk of later schizophrenia of birth in a rural area. Similar findings have come from Denmark where those individuals born in Copenhagen appear to have twice the risk of schizophrenia of those born in rural areas.[48] The exact mechanisms underlying this effect remain unclear.

Immigration

Since the classic study of Odegaard in 1932,[49] many studies have reported that migrants are at increased risk of schizophrenia. There have been many competing explanatory hypotheses, including selective migration, migrant stress, and socio-economic deprivation. A notable example has come from a series of studies of African-Caribbeans resident in the United Kingdom, who show a markedly higher rate of schizophrenia than do their white British-born counterparts.[34,50] This is in the absence of any increased risk to Caribbeans who remain in the West Indies (see Harrison[51]). Of particular interest is that this increased risk also pertains to British-born offspring of Caribbean migrants, discounting an explanation in terms of migration stress. Furthermore, there is a marked increased risk in the siblings but not the parents of this second generation;[52] this suggests an environmental effect operating particularly upon this second generation.

Initial studies sought to ascertain any evidence of developmental disadvantage such as poor maternal nutrition, poor obstetric care, and possible maternal susceptibility to novel viruses. However, these studies have shown that, if anything, African-Caribbean schizophrenic patients in England show less evidence of neurodevelopmental insult than their white counterpart patients. Other research focuses on the possibility that a paranoid reaction to social disadvantage and discrimination may be one factor. Further information about these studies and similar ones from The Netherlands is given in Chapter 4.3.4.

Life events

Brown and Birley[53] reported an excess of life events in the 3 weeks preceding schizophrenic relapse. Further studies were conflicting in their findings, possibly due to methodological problems. The recent study of Bebbington et al.[54] avoided many of the methodological pitfalls, assessing life events in 97 psychotic patients (52 with schizophrenia) and general population controls. There was a significant relationship between life events and onset of relapse of schizophrenia, although it was not as strong as for depressive psychosis. One possibility is that certain types of schizophrenic patients are particularly vulnerable to relapse following adverse life events. For example, Bebbington et al.[54] found females to be particularly prone, whilst van Os et al.[9] found life events to be associated with a less severe good-outcome illness.

There is also evidence that families who exhibit high 'expressed emotion' (comprising critical comments, hostility, and/or overinvolvement) can provide an environment which enhances the risk of relapse in a family member with schizophrenia. Again, cause and effect are difficult to tease apart. Thus, it is possible that patients with more severe and intractable illnesses may induce more expressed emotion in their relatives.

Drug abuse

Numerous studies attest to the fact that illicit substance use is more prevalent in patients with schizophrenia than in the general population; estimates of the prevalence of such comorbidity in individuals with schizophrenia range from 20 to 60 per cent, and are consistently higher than in well controls.[55]

Whether illicit substances actually cause schizophrenia is very contentious. Perhaps the methodologically most sound investigation is the study of Andreason et al.,[56] which followed up 45 570 Swedish conscripts and found that a history of cannabis consumption, at 18 years, was positively correlated with a later admission to hospital with schizophrenia. The cohort design and a dose–response effect (heavy users had the highest risk of later schizophrenia) suggest a causal link. However, it might be that those individuals who did manifest schizophrenia in later life were destined to do so in any event, and their premorbid state made them more likely than their peers to use high doses of cannabis.

Similarly, although clinical wisdom suggests that illicit substance use has a negative impact on the longitudinal course of schizophrenia, there are few methodologically sound studies in this area.[57,58] Indeed, even the finding of an excess of use, and the association of such use with a poor longitudinal course, is potentially explicable by confounding factors such as substance abuse by the patients who are more ill.

Why do individuals with schizophrenia use illicit substances? There are two main competing theories: the social affiliation hypothesis, where individuals reportedly use substances in attempt to help them reintegrate socially, and the self-medication hypothesis, where individuals find that use of substances either improves symptoms (e.g. use of amphetamines to counter depression) or alleviates side-effects of neuroleptic medication.

Risk factors, age of onset, and outcome

Individuals who have been exposed to certain of the risk factors for schizophrenia tend have an earlier onset of psychosis than those who have not. Thus, age of onset is earlier in those whose relatives show a high morbid risk of schizophrenia;[13] similarly, those twin pairs in which the schizophrenia has an early onset show the highest monozygotic concordance.[6]

Schizophrenic patients with an early age at onset of psychosis are also more likely than patients with later onset to have had a history of exposure to obstetric complications,[59] while those schizophrenic individuals who showed childhood deficits such as low IQ also tend to have an early onset.[37] Schizophrenic patients who abuse cannabis have also recently been shown to have an earlier onset than those who do not.[58]

If a factor operates to increase the risk of schizophrenia and to bring on its onset, then it is logical to think that if it is still present then it will be associated with a poor outcome. Thus, a family history of schizophrenia, a history of obstetric complication, childhood low IQ, and continued drug abuse are all associated with a poor outcome. On the other hand, those patients who develop psychosis following stressful life-events tend to have a better outcome than those with no such precipitant.[9]

The risk factor model

Gene–environment interaction

Thus, one way of construing the aetiology of schizophrenia is to see individuals on a stress-vulnerability continuum in which genetic and environmental factors act in an additive manner until a threshold of liability for expression of psychosis is passed. An individual might, for instance, inherit a schizotypal personality but not develop frank psychosis unless exposed to some cerebral insult which causes cognitive impairment; the sum of the two factors could produce the psychotic illness.

Assuming such a model in which a number of genes and environmental factors of small effect act additively, then the heritability of schizophrenia can be calculated to be between 66 and 85 per cent (i.e. a high proportion of liability to the disorder is under genetic influence). However, this assumes that the various factors operate additively, and much evidence is against this assumption. Rather, it seems that there is often an interaction between genetic susceptibility and environmental effects. As van Os and Marcelis[22] point out, it seems that certain individuals exposed to an environmental risk factor have a high risk of developing schizophrenia while others with a different genotype are at low risk.

Thus, the quality of upbringing can interact with genetic predisposition. For example, the Finnish Adoption Study has shown that when the offspring of women with schizophrenia are placed in a well-adjusted family, they have a lower risk of developing a schizophrenia spectrum disorder than if they are placed in a dysfunctional family, i.e the genotype renders the individual susceptible to the adverse effect of an adverse family environment.[60] Obstetric complications also appear to interact with, and compound, a genetic liability; the offspring of schizophrenic parents are more likely to develop increased ventricular size following obstetric complications.

Similarly, there is evidence that individuals with a family loading for schizophrenia may be more susceptible to psychosis following abuse of cannabis.[61] The latter situation may be complicated by the possibility that individuals who inherit a schizotypal personality may be more likely to take drugs such as cannabis to try to alter an unhappy internal mood state, i.e. their genotype renders them more liable to expose themselves to a factor to which they are genetically susceptible.

The implications

Having identified various risk factors for schizophrenia, we can proceed to consider the theoretical possibility of reducing the prevalence of certain risk factors and thus reducing the incidence of the disorder. From the point of view of the public health, rare risk factors which have a big effect are much less important than common risk factors of even small effect. Thus, although familial risk has by far the biggest effect, it makes a smaller contribution to the total incidence of the disorder than environmental effects. Therefore, if all cases with an affected first-degree relative could be prevented, we would eliminate only about 10 per cent of the total cases. However, because being born in an urban area is so common, this small effect accounts for a much greater proportion of the population attributable fraction (33 per cent), i.e. if we could bring down the incidence of schizophrenia in cities to that in the countryside, we could theoretically eliminate one-third of all cases of the disorder. Of course, we could only do this if we knew what the critical urban factors were!

The importance of the evidence that early developmental factors are involved in the aetiology of schizophrenia lies in the fact that at least some of these are preventable. For example, advances in antenatal and perinatal care have reduced the frequency, and toxicity, of some obstetric complications. Similarly, vaccination programmes have reduced exposure to some viral infections in pregnancy and childhood. There could be a link between these developments and the decreased incidence of schizophrenia which has been observed in some western countries over recent decades.[62]

Nevertheless, most babies who are exposed to even severe obstetric complications will not later suffer from schizophrenia. Thus, there is at present no sense in attempting to improve antenatal care with the aim of reducing the occurrence of schizophrenia. There is one important exception. It is indisputable that the children of schizophrenic mothers have a higher risk of the disease if they are also exposed to obstetric complications. Therefore those women with schizophrenia who conceive must have the best possible antenatal care during their pregnancy, and steps should be taken to avoid any event (e.g. prolonged labour) which might lead to hypoxic damage to the baby.

The fact that preschizophrenic children show a number of impairments raises the possibility that predisposed individuals could be identified and 'rescued' by some intervention. Unfortunately, the childhood characteristics of preschizophrenics are non-specific, and their predictive value for the later manifestation of the illness is too low to be of value for any preventative intervention, i.e. many children who show such deviation from normal in terms of early development, do not later manifest schizophrenia, whilst other children who later develop schizophrenia have perfectly 'normal' early development. Furthermore, any such abnormalities must be seen in the total context of development, and it should be remembered that many such abnormalities are not static, but may be evident at some stages of development

and not at others. Thus, with a few exceptions, there is as yet little that can be done systematically to reduce the incidence of schizophrenia.

References

1. Gottesman, I.I. (1991). *Schizophrenia genesis: the origins of madness.* W.H. Freeman, New York.
2. Heston, L.L. and Denney, D. (1968). Interactions between early life experience and biological factors in schizophrenia. In *The transmission of schizophrenia* (ed. D. Rosenthal and S. Kety), pp. 363–76. Pergamon Press, Oxford.
3. Rosenthal, D., Wender, P., Kety, S., *et al.* (1971). The adopted-away offspring of schizophrenics. *American Journal of Psychiatry*, **128**, 307–11.
4. Kety, S.S. *et al.* (1994). Mental illness in the biological relatives of schizophrenic adoptees. Replication of the Copenhagen study in the rest of Denmark. *Archives of General Psychiatry*, **51**, 442–55.
5. Wender, P.H., *et al.* (1974). Cross-fostering: a research strategy for clarifying the role of genetic and experimental factors in the etiology of schizophrenia. *Archives of General Psychiatry*, **30**, 121–8.
6. Cardno, A., Marshak, J., Coid, B., *et al.* (1999). Relationships between symptom dimensions and genetic liability to psychotic disorders in the Maudsley Twin Psychosis Series. *Archives of General Psychiatry*, **56**, 162–8.
7. Gottesman, I.I. and Bertelsen, A. (1989). Confirming unexpressed genotypes for schizophrenia: risks in the offspring of Fischer's Danish identical and fraternal discordant twins. *Archives of General Psychiatry*, **46**, 867–72.
8. Liddle, P.F. (1987). Symptoms of chronic schizophrenia. *British Journal of Psychiatry*, **151**, 145–51.
9. van Os, J. *et al.* (1994). The influence of life events on the subsequent course of psychotic illness: a follow-up of the Camberwell Collaborative Psychosis study. *Psychological Medicine*, **24**, 503–13.
10. Mata, I., Sham, P., and Murray, R.M. Schizotypal correlates of the functional psychosis. Submitted for publication.
11. Kirov, G. and Murray, R.M. (1997). The molecular genetics of schizophrenia: progress so far. *Molecular Medicine Today*, March, 124–30.
12. Wright, P., Donaldson, P., Underhill, J., Choudhuri, K., Doherty, D., and Murray, R.M. (1996). Genetic association of the HLA DRB1 gene locus on chromosome 6p21.3 with schizophrenia. *American Journal of Psychiatry*, **153**, 1530–3.
13. Sham, P. *et al.* (1994). Age at onset, sex and familial psychiatric morbidity in schizophrenia. Report from the Camberwell Collaborative Psychosis Study. *British Journal of Psychiatry*, **165**, 466–73.
14. Jones, P. and Murray, R.M. (1991). The genetics of schizophrenia is the genetics of neurodevelopment. *British Journal of Psychiatry*, **158**, 615–23.
15. Sharma, T. *et al.* (1998). Brain changes in schizophrenia: volumetric MRI study of families multiply affected with schizophrenia—the Maudsley Family Study 5. *British Journal of Psychiatry*, **173**, 132–8.
16. Sharma, T., Lancaster, E., Sigmondson, J., *et al.* (1999). Loss of cerebral asymmetry in familial schizophrenics and their relatives detected by magnetic resonance imaging. *Schizophrenia Research*, **40**, 111–20.
17. Crow, T.J. (1990). The nature of the genetic contribution to psychotic illness. *Acta Psychiatrica Scandinavica*, **81**, 1401–8.
18. Frangou, S. *et al.* (1997). The Maudsley Family Study II: endogenous event-related potentials in familial schizophrenia. *Schizophrenia Research*, **23**, 45–53.
19. Crawford, T., Sharma, T., Puri, B.K., *et al.* (1998). Saccadic eye movements in families multiply affected with schizophrenia. *American Journal of Psychiatry*, **155**, 1703–10.
20. Griffiths, T.D., Sigmundsson, T., Takei, N., Rowe, D., and Murray, R.M. (1998). Neurological abnormalities in familial and sporadic schizophrenia. *Brain*, **121**, 191–203.
21. Wickham, H. and Murray, R.M. (1997). Can biological markers identify

endophenotypes predisposing to schizophrenia? *International Review of Psychiatry*, **9**, 355–64.

22. van Os, J. and Marcelis, M. (1998). The ecogenetics of schizophrenia. *Schizophrenia Research*, **32**, 127–35.

23. Geddes, J.R., Verdoux, H., Takei, N., Lawrie, S.M., and Murray, R.M. (1999). Individual patient data meta-analysis of the association between schizophrenia and abnormalities of pregnancy and labour. *Schizophrenia Bulletin*, **25**, 413–23.

24. Hultman, C.M., Sparen, P., Takei, N., Murray, R.M., and Cnattingius, S. (1999). Prenatal and perinatal risk factors for schizophrenia, affective psychosis and reactive psychosis. *British Medical Journal*, **318**, 421–5.

25. Stewart, A.L., Rifkin, L., Amess, P.N., *et al.* (1999). Brain structure, neurocognitive and behavioural function in adolescents who were born very preterm. *Lancet*, **353**, 1653–7.

26. Reveley, A.M., Reveley, M.A., Clifford, C.A., and Murray, R.M. (1982). Cerebral ventricular size in twins discordant for schizophrenia. *Lancet*, **i**, 540–1.

27. Suddath, R.L. *et al.* (1990). Anatomical abnormalities in the brains of monozygotic twins discordant for schizophrenia. *New England Journal of Medicine*, **322**, 789–94.

28. McNeill, T.F., Cantor-Grace, E., and Weinberger, D.R. (1999). Obstetric complications and brain structure size differences in monozygotic twins discordant for schizophrenia. *American Journal of Psychiatry*, in press.

29. Stefanis, N., Frangou, S., Yakeley, J., *et al.* (2000). Hippocampal volume reduction in schizophrenia is secondary to pregnancy and birth complications. *Biological Psychiatry*, **46**, 697–702.

30. McGrath, J. and Murray, R.M. (1995). Risk factors for schizophrenia: from conception to birth. In *Schizophrenia* (ed. S. Hirsch and D. Weinberger), pp. 187–205. Blackwell Science, Oxford.

31. Susser, E.S. and Lin, S.P. (1992). Schizophrenia after prenatal exposure to the Dutch hunger winter. *Archives of General Psychiatry*, **49**, 938–88.

32. Davies, N., Russell, A., Jones, P., and Murray, R. (1998). Which characteristics of schizophrenia predate psychosis? *Journal of Psychiatric Research*, **32**, 121–31.

33. Fish, B., Marcus, J., Hans, S.L., Auerbach, J.G., and Perdue, S. (1992). Infants at risk for schizophrenia. *Archives of General Psychiatry*, **49**, 221–35.

34. Castle, D.J. and Murray, R.M. (1991). The neurodevelopmental basis of sex differences in schizophrenia. *Psychological Medicine*, **21**, 565–75.

35. Foerster, A., Lewis, S.W., Owen, M.J., and Murray, R.M. (1991). Premorbid personality in psychosis: effects of sex and diagnosis. *British Journal of Psychiatry*, **158**, 171–6.

36. Aylward, E., Walker, E., and Bettes, B. (1984). Intelligence in schizophrenia: meta-analysis of the research. *Schizophrenia Bulletin*, **10**, 430–59.

37. Russell, A.J., Munro, J.C., Jones, P.B., Hemsley, D.A., and Murray, R.M. (1997). Schizophrenia and the myth of intellectual decline. *American Journal of Psychiatry*, **154**, 635–9. Letters and reply: *American Journal of Psychiatry*, **155**, 1633–7 (1998).

38. Walker, E.F., Savoie, T., and Davis, D. (1994). Neuromotor precursors of schizophrenia. *Schizophrenia Bulletin*, **20**, 441–51.

39. Done, J.D., Crow, T.J., Johnstone, E.C., and Sacker, A. (1994). Childhood antecedents of schizophrenia and affective illness: social adjustment at ages 7 and 11. *British Medical Journal*, **309**, 699–703.

40. Jones, P.D., Rodgers, B., Murray, R.M., and Marmot, M. (1994). Child developmental risk factors for adult schizophrenia. *Lancet*, **344**, 1398–1402.

41. Faris, R.B.L. and Dunham, H.W. (1939). *Mental disorders in urban areas. an ecological study of schizophrenia and other psychoses.* University of Chicago Press.

42. Goldberg, S.M. and Morrison, S.L. (1963). Schizophrenia and social class. *British Journal of Psychiatry*, **109,** 785–802.

43. Hollingshead, A.B. and Redlich, F.C. (1954). Schizophrenia and social structure. *American Journal of Psychiatry*, **110**, 695–701.

44. Kohn, M.L. (1975). Social class and schizophrenia: a critical review and reformulation. In *Annual review of the schizophrenic syndrome* (ed. R. Cancro). Brunner–Mazel, New York.

45. Turner, R.J. and Wagenfeld, M.O. (1967). Occupational mobility and schizophrenia: an assessment of the social causation and social selection hypothesis. *American Sociological Review*, **32**, 104–13.

46. Lewis, G., David, A., Andreasson, S., and Allebeck, P. (1992). Schizophrenia and city life. *Lancet*, **340**, 137–40.

47. Marcelis, M., Navarro-Mateu, F., Murray, R., Selten, J.-P., and van Os, J. (1998). Urbanization and psychosis: a study of 1942–1978 birth cohorts in The Netherlands. *Psychological Medicine*, **28**, 871–9.

48. Mortensen, P.B., Pedersen, C.B., Westergaard, T., *et al.*(1999). Effects of family history and place and season of birth on risk of schizophrenia. *New England Journal of Medicine*, **340**, 603–8.

49. Odegaard, O. (1932). Emigration and insanity. *Acta Psychiatrica Scandinavica Supplementum*, **4**.

50. van Os, J., Castle, J., Takei, N., Der, G., and Murray, R.M. (1996). Psychotic illness in ethnic minorities: clarification from the 1991 census. *Psychological Medicine*, **26**, 203–8.

51. Harrison, G. (1990). Searching for the causes of schizophrenia. *Schizophrenia Bulletin*, **16**, 663–72.

52. Hutchinson, G. *et al.* (1996). Morbid risk of psychotic illness in first degree relatives of white and African-Caribbean patients with psychosis. *British Journal of Psychiatry*, **169**, 776–80.

53. Brown, G.W. and Birley, J.L.T. (1968). Crises and life changes and the onset of schizophrenia. *Journal of Health and Social Behaviour*, **9**, 203–14.

54. Bebbington, P. *et al.* (1993). Life events and psychosis: initial results from the Camberwell Collaborative Psychosis Study. *British Journal of Psychiatry*, **162**, 72–9.

55. Meuser, K.T. *et al.* (1990). Prevalence of substance use in schizophrenia. *Schizophrenia Bulletin*, **16**, 31–56.

56. Andreason, S., Allebeck, P., Engstrom, A., and Rydberg, U. (1987). Cannabis and schizophrenia: a longitudinal study of Swedish conscripts. *Lancet*, **ii**, 1483–6.

57. Turner, W.M. and Tsuang, M.T. (1990). Impact of substance use on the course and outcome of schizophrenia. *Schizophrenia Bulletin*, **16**, 87–96.

58. Grech, A. (1998). Drug abuse and psychosis in London and Malta. M.Sc. Thesis, University of London.

59. Verdoux, H. *et al.* (1997). Obstetric complications and age at onset in schizophrenia: an international collaborative meta-analysis of individual patient data. *American Journal of Psychiatry*, **154**, 1220–7.

60. Wahlberg, K.E., Wynne, L.C., Oja, H., *et al.* 1997). Gene–environment interaction in vulnerability to schizophrenia. *American Journal of Psychiatry*, **154**, 355–62.

61. McGuire, P., Jones, P., Harvey, I., *et al.* (1994). Cannabis and acute psychosis. *Schizophrenia Research*, **24**, 995–1011.

62. Der, G., Gupta, S., and Murray, R.M. (1990). Is schizophrenia disappearing? Evidence from England and Wales 1952–1986. *Lancet*, **335**, 513–16.

4.3.5.2 **The neurobiology of schizophrenia**

Paul J. Harrison

The neurobiology of schizophrenia may be divided into functional and structural aspects. Significant progress has been made in both areas as

Table 1 Functional brain abnormalities in schizophrenia

	Strength of evidence
Dopamine	
Increased striatal D_2 receptors	++++[a]
Increased cortical D_3 receptors	+
Increased striatal D_4 receptors	+/−
Decreased cortical D_1 receptors	+
Abnormal configuration ('dimerization') of D_2 receptors	+/−
Altered dopamine receptor–G protein coupling	+/−
Increased dopamine content or metabolism	+++[a]
Increased amphetamine-stimulated dopamine transmission	+++
5-HT	
Decreased cortical $5-HT_{2A}$ receptors	+++
Increased cortical $5-HT_{1A}$ receptors	++
CSF 5-HIAA concentrations related to negative symptoms	+
Glutamate	
Decreased expression of hippocampal non-NMDA receptors	++
Increased cortical expression of some NMDA receptor subunits	+
Decreased markers of glutamate reuptake	+
Decreased synaptic glutamate release	+
Altered concentrations of glutamate and metabolites	++
Cerebral metabolism	
Subsyndromes have characteristic regional blood flow patterns	+++
Hypofrontality[b]	+++
Increased activity in medial temporal lobe[b]	++
Neuropsychological profile	
Generalized intellectual impairment	+++
Selective impairment in memory domains	++
Selective impairment in executive functions	+
Attentional deficits	++
Other	
Abnormal evoked potentials	+++

+/−, weak; +, moderate; ++, good; +++, strong; ++++, shown by meta-analysis.
CSF, cerebrospinal fluid; 5-HIAA, 5-hydroxyindoleacetic acid.
[a] Though much of the increase is due to psychotic medication.
[b] See text for details.

a result of the development of imaging modalities and the emergence of molecular techniques to study the underlying cellular processes.

Functional neurobiology of schizophrenia

Functional neurobiology encompasses neurochemistry, which can be measured in postmortem brains or *in vivo*, as well as neurophysiological and neuropsychological approaches. The key findings are summarized in Table 1.

Neurochemistry

A wide range of neurochemical systems and parameters have been investigated in schizophrenia, and a diverse collection of abnormalities reported.[1] Discussion is limited here to three areas of current interest.

Dopamine

The dopamine hypothesis of schizophrenia has been neurochemically pre-eminent since the 1960s. It proposes that the symptoms of schizophrenia result from dopaminergic overactivity, whether due to excess dopamine, or to an elevated sensitivity to it, for example because of increased numbers of dopamine receptors. The hypothesis originated with the discovery that effective antipsychotics were dopamine (D_2) receptor antagonists, and that dopamine-releasing agents such as amphetamine produce a paranoid psychosis. It received support from various findings of increased dopamine content and higher densities of D_2 receptors in schizophrenia.[2] However, despite its longevity there is still no consensus as to precisely what the dopamine hypothesis explains, nor the nature of the supposed abnormality. There are two main difficulties. First, antipsychotics have marked effects on the dopamine system, seriously confounding most studies. Second, molecular biology has revealed an unexpected complexity of the dopamine receptor family, increasing the potential sites of dysfunction and mechanisms by which it might occur.

Striatal D_2 receptor densities are increased in schizophrenia, but it is unclear what proportion, if any, is not attributable to antipsychotic medication.[3] Statistical methods have been used to argue that there is a genuine schizophrenia-associated elevation, but this must be balanced against negative positron emission tomography (**PET**) studies of D_2 receptors in drug-naive first-episode cases. For D_1 and D_3 receptors there are reports of their altered expression in schizophrenia, but these are either unconfirmed or contradicted by other studies. Controversy has surrounded the D_4 receptor following a report that it was upregulated several-fold in schizophrenia, seemingly independent of medication. However, the result appears to have been due to a 'D_4-like site' not the true D_4 receptor, and the status of the latter in schizophrenia is unknown.[4] Overall, the position of dopamine receptors in schizophrenia is still contentious and the case for their involvement unproven. In contrast, there is emerging evidence for a presynaptic abnormality, with three studies of drug-free subjects showing elevated dopamine release in response to amphetamine.[5] This implies a dysregulation and hyper-responsiveness of dopaminergic neurones in schizophrenia, a potentially important finding needing further investigation.

5-Hydroxytryptamine

Suggestions of 5-hydroxytryptamine (**5-HT**, serotonin) involvement in schizophrenia arose because the hallucinogen lysergic acid diethylamide (**LSD**) is a 5-HT agonist. Recently, interest has focused on the $5-HT_{2A}$ receptor.[4] A high affinity for the receptor may explain the therapeutic advantages of atypical antipsychotics, and variants in the gene are a minor risk factor for non-response to clozapine and for schizophrenia. Many studies have found a lowered $5-HT_{2A}$ receptor expression in the frontal cortex in schizophrenia, and there is a blunted neuroendocrine response to $5-HT_2$ agonists. Elevated cortical $5-HT_{1A}$ receptors are also a replicated finding. The $5-HT_{1A}$ and $5-HT_{2A}$ receptor abnormalities are both seen in subjects not on medication at death, but neither has been investigated in drug-naive or first-episode patients.

Hypotheses for the involvement of 5-HT in schizophrenia include the trophic role of the 5-HT system in neurodevelopment, interactions between 5-HT and dopaminergic neurones, and impaired 5-HT$_{2A}$ receptor-mediated activation of the prefrontal cortex.[6]

Glutamate

Phencyclidine and other non-competitive antagonists of the N-methyl-D-aspartate (**NMDA**) subtype of glutamate receptor produce a psychosis closely resembling schizophrenia. This has driven the hypothesis of glutamatergic dysfunction in schizophrenia.[7] In support, there is now considerable evidence for glutamatergic abnormalities in schizophrenia (Table 1). In the medial temporal lobe, for example, glutamatergic markers are decreased and there is reduced expression of non-NMDA glutamate receptors. However, a different pattern is seen in other brain regions and affecting other glutamate receptor subtypes, precluding any simple conclusion regarding the nature of the abnormality in schizophrenia. Mechanisms proposed to explain glutamatergic involvement in schizophrenia centre on its interactions with dopamine, and subtle forms of glutamate-mediated neurotoxicity.

Interpretation of the neurochemical data

In addition to the three neurotransmitters mentioned above, schizophrenia is associated with alterations in many other systems, including γ-aminobutyric acid (**GABA**), neuropeptides, adrenoreceptors, and second messengers.[1] However, there is still no clear picture as to the cardinal neurochemical deficits. One important point, relating to the neuropathology to be discussed below, is that the presence of structural abnormalities, however slight, must be taken into account. That is, a change in the level of a neurotransmitter, receptor, or any other molecule, may be due to dysfunction of the neurones producing it, or a change in the cellular constituents of the tissue, rather than being indicative of a specific abnormality. This applies to *in vivo* functional imaging as well to postmortem neurochemistry. While an obvious point to make, it has not always been appreciated in schizophrenia research, perhaps because of the belief that the brain is structurally normal.

Cerebral activity

Cerebral activity in schizophrenia has been extensively investigated using PET to measure regional cerebral blood flow and glucose utilization (see Chapter 2.3.6). Single-photon emission CT and functional magnetic resonance imaging (**MRI**) have also been applied.

Hypofrontality—decreased activity in the frontal lobes—has been widely studied in schizophrenia since the first report in 1974. The current view is that, whilst hypofrontality does occur in unmedicated subjects,[8] it is not an invariable finding,[9] and its interpretation is still debated.[10] It is seen most clearly when subjects are performing tasks, such as the Wisconsin Card Sorting Test, which require activation of the frontal lobes.

The most comprehensive analysis correlating regional cerebral activity with the clinical features of schizophrenia is that by Liddle and colleagues, showing that the three subsyndromes of chronic schizophrenia identified by factor analysis have their own characteristic patterns of blood flow.[11] For example, subjects with psychomotor poverty are hypofrontal whereas those with prominent positive symptoms have increased activity in the temporal lobe, especially in the hippocampus. Other studies show that the latter region does not activate normally during cognitive tasks.

One conclusion drawn from these studies is that there is no one site of dysfunction in schizophrenia. Rather, its pathophysiology reflects abnormalities in various distributed circuits integrating specific cortical areas and subcortical nuclei.[8,12] The model of schizophrenia as a disorder of disturbed neural connectivity is considered further below.

Neurophysiology

There are two aspects of sensorimotor functioning in schizophrenia relevant to the study of its neurobiology. First, evoked potentials (electrical activity in the brain measured after a brief sensory stimulus) are altered. In particular, the P300 component is reduced and delayed in response to auditory and visual stimuli, indicative of impaired sensory processing and further implicating the temporal lobes in the pathophysiology of the disorder.[13] Second, there is a high rate of eye movement abnormalities in schizophrenia,[14] especially affecting smooth pursuit tracking, suggestive of impairment in the neural pathways subserving oculomotor control.

Neuropsychology

Neuropsychological data provide a further line of support for the involvement of certain brain areas and their connections in the neurobiology of schizophrenia.

Intellectual impairment is a feature of schizophrenia.[15] It is present in first-episode, untreated patients, and worsens in the first few years of illness, warranting the label dementia in severe, chronic cases (see below).[16] Against a background of global decrement[17] there is evidence for greater deficits in semantic memory, executive functioning, and attentional domains.[18] Anatomically, this neuropsychological pattern is in keeping with the preferential involvement of temporal lobe and frontostriatal circuits in schizophrenia identified by functional imaging.

Structural neurobiology of schizophrenia

Alzheimer, a colleague of Kraeplin, began the search for the neuropathology of schizophrenia. However, only recently has progress been made. The major advances have come from structural imaging (CT and MRI) scans, and the findings have, in turn, encouraged a renaissance of histopathological studies.

Macroscopic brain changes

Key findings

Contemporary research into the structural basis of schizophrenia can be traced to a seminal report describing dilatation of the lateral ventricles and cerebral atrophy, as seen on CT scans, in chronic schizophrenia.[19] This finding, which was consistent with earlier pneumoencephalographic data, has been followed by many other CT

Table 2 Structural brain abnormalities in schizophrenia

	Strength of evidence
Macroscopic findings	
Enlarged ventricles	++++
Decreased cortical volume	++++
Above changes present in first-episode patients	+++
Cortical volume loss affects grey rather than white matter	++
Disproportionate volume loss from temporal lobe (including hippocampus)	++
Decreased thalamic volume	++
Histological findings	
Absence of gliosis as an intrinsic feature	+++
Smaller cortical and hippocampal neurones	+++
Reduced synaptic and dendritic markers in hippocampus	++
Fewer neurones in dorsal thalamus	+++
Maldistribution of white matter neurones	+
Entorhinal cortex dysplasia	+/–
Cortical or hippocampal neuronal loss	+/–
Disarray of hippocampal neurones	+/–
Miscellaneous	
Pathology interacts with cerebral asymmetries	++
Alzheimer's disease is not more common than expected	++++

+/–, weak; +, moderate; ++, good; +++, strong; ++++, shown by meta-analysis.

and MRI studies with ever-improving resolution and sophistication of analysis. The key results are described below and in Table 2.

There is enlargement of the cerebral ventricles. Comprehensive reviews of the lateral ventricle-to-brain ratio indicate an increase of 20 to 75 per cent, with an effect size of 0.70, corresponding to a 43 per cent non-overlap between cases and controls.[20,21] Volumetric MRI shows a median 40 per cent increase in ventricular size.[22] The ventricular enlargement is accompanied by a loss of cortical volume averaging 3 per cent.[22,23] Greater reductions occur in temporal lobe (4–12 per cent), especially medial temporal structures (hippocampus, parahippocampal gyrus, and amygdala).[24] Several, though not all, postmortem studies of schizophrenia have confirmed these features, which have recently been shown in childhood-onset cases as well.

Monozygotic twins discordant for schizophrenia have provided valuable information. In virtually all pairs, the affected twin has the larger ventricles and smaller cortical and hippocampal size.[25] The discordant-monozygotic twin study design allows two conclusions to be drawn. First, that structural abnormalities are a consistent finding in schizophrenia, their identification being aided by controlling for random genetic and environmental influences on neuroanatomy. Second, that the alterations are associated with expression of the schizophrenia phenotype rather than merely with the underlying shared genotype. Family studies support this interpretation, in that schizophrenics have bigger ventricles and smaller brains than their unaffected relatives. However, relatives who are obligate carriers (that is to say those unaffected by schizophrenia but who seem to be transmitting the gene(s)) have larger ventricles than other relatives; more-over both groups of relatives have larger ventricles and smaller brain structures than control subjects from families without schizophrenia.[26] These data indicate that a proportion of the structural pathology of schizophrenia may be a marker of genetic liability to the disorder. (A similar conclusion applies to the neuropsychological and neurophysiological indices mentioned above.)

Imaging studies have not established clearly whether there are volume differences in subcortical structures in schizophrenia; one firm conclusion is that the striatal enlargement sometimes reported is, unlike all other volume changes, due to antipsychotic medication. Finally, good evidence for a reduced size of the thalamus has emerged from postmortem studies.

Progression, heterogeneity, and clinicopathological correlations

Ventricle-to-brain ratio in schizophrenia follows a unimodal distribution, indicating that ventricular enlargement is not restricted to a subgroup but is present to a degree in all cases.[20] Conversely, it is important to emphasize that, despite group differences, there is a significant overlap between subjects with schizophrenia and controls for every structural parameter. For this reason, and the fact that the changes are of uncertain diagnostic specificity, schizophrenia remains a clinical rather than a neurobiological diagnosis.

The structural abnormalities are present in first-episode cases, excluding the possibility that they are merely a consequence of chronic illness or its treatment. Furthermore, their magnitude does not correlate with duration of the disease, suggesting that the alterations are largely static after onset. However, some longitudinal studies, spanning 4 to 8 years, find continuing divergence from controls. The issue, which remains controversial, is important as it bears upon the timing, progressive nature, and possible heterogeneity of schizophrenia (see below).

Some studies indicate that male schizophrenics show greater structural changes than do females, but other studies do not. Similarly, there are few established correlations between brain structure and the symptoms or course of schizophrenia. For example, the expectation that enlarged ventricles might be a correlate of poor outcome has not been consistently demonstrated.

Neuropathology

Contemporary histological studies have addressed two main areas. First, to clarify the frequency and nature of neurodegenerative abnormalities in schizophrenia. Second, to investigate the cellular organization (cytoarchitecture) of the cerebral cortex and other components of the limbic system (hippocampus, prefrontal cortex, and thalamus).

Neurodegeneration and schizophrenia

Gliosis

The issue of gliosis (reactive astrocytosis) has been extensively investigated since an influential report[27] that gliosis was common in schizophrenia, especially in the diencephalon around the third ventricle. As gliosis is a sign of past inflammation (see Chapter 2.3.5), this finding supported aetiopathogenic scenarios for schizophrenia involving infective, ischaemic, autoimmune, or neurodegenerative processes. However, many subsequent investigations have not found gliosis, and Bruton and colleagues[28] found that it was only present in cases exhibiting coincidental neuropathological abnormalities, indicating that gliosis is not an intrinsic feature of schizophrenia but merely of superimposed pathological changes which occur by chance in some cases.

The gliosis issue is esoteric but has considerable implications. The gliotic response is said not to begin until the end of the second trimester *in utero*, and hence an absence of gliosis is taken as *prima facie* evidence of a disease process occurring before this time. Unfortunately, both the absence of gliosis, and its interpretation, are less clear than often assumed. First, detecting gliosis is surprisingly difficult, and it can be argued that the data do not wholly rule out its occurrence in (a subtype of) schizophrenia. Second, despite the widely cited time point at which the glial response is said to begin, the matter has not been well investigated; therefore it is prudent not to use this to time the pathology of schizophrenia with spurious accuracy. Furthermore, it is a moot point whether the subtle kinds of morphometric disturbance described in schizophrenia, whenever and however they occurred, would be sufficient to trigger detectable gliosis.

Schizophrenia and Alzheimer's disease

The belief that Alzheimer's disease is commoner in schizophrenia (independent of any cognitive impairment) originated in the 1930s. It received some recent support from three uncontrolled, retrospective studies, and tangentially from data suggesting that antipsychotic drugs promote neurofibrillary tangles. However, a meta-analysis shows that Alzheimer's disease is not more common, and may even be rarer, in schizophrenia.[29] This applies even in elderly schizophrenic patients with prospectively assessed severe dementia, who show no evidence of any other neurodegenerative disorder.[30] Nor is there good evidence that antipsychotic drugs cause Alzheimer-type changes. How, therefore, is the cognitive impairment of schizophrenia explained? One possibility is that it is a more severe manifestation of whatever substrate underlies schizophrenia. Or, it may be that the brain in schizophrenia is more vulnerable to cognitive impairment in response to a normal age-related amount of neurodegeneration.

The cytoarchitecture of schizophrenia

If neurodegenerative abnormalities are uncommon in, and probably epiphenomenal to, schizophrenia, it begs the question as to what **is** the pathology of the disorder and how the macroscopic findings are explained at the microscopic level. The answer has been sought in the cytoarchitecture of the cerebral cortex, with measurements of parameters such as the size, location, distribution, and packing density of neurones and their synaptic connections[31] (Table 2).

Studies of neurones

Various cytoarchitectural alterations have been described in schizophrenia, of which three have generated particular interest: abnormal neuronal organization (dysplasia) in the entorhinal cortex, disarray of hippocampal neurones, and an altered distribution of neurones in the subcortical white matter. These findings are important because they support the hypothesis of an early neurodevelopmental anomaly underlying schizophrenia. However, none have been unequivocally and independently replicated, and for each there is at least one non-replication.[31]

A less well known yet seemingly more robust cytoarchitectural feature of schizophrenia is that many neurones are smaller than expected. This has been shown in three studies of pyramidal neurones in the hippocampus, and has also been reported in dorsolateral prefrontal

cortex and cerebellar Purkinje cells. Some studies find that the neurones are also more closely packed. Outside the cerebral cortex, good cytoarchitectural data are limited to the thalamus, with a replicated finding that the dorsomedial nucleus, which is part of a circuit involving the prefrontal cortex (see Chapter 2.3.1), contains significantly fewer neurones than in normal subjects.

In summary, a range of differences in neuronal structure and organization have been reported to occur in schizophrenia. The abnormalities most often taken to be characteristic of the disorder—disarray, displacement, and paucity of hippocampal and cortical neurones—are features which in fact have not been well demonstrated. This undermines attempts to date the pathology of schizophrenia to the second trimester *in utero* based on their presence (see below). In contrast, decreased neuronal size and loss of thalamic neurones have been shown fairly convincingly. Some of the discrepancies in the literature may reflect regional heterogeneity in the cytoarchitectural pathology of schizophrenia; notably, the cingulate gyrus may have a different pattern of changes.[32]

Studies of synapses and dendrites

Synapses and dendrites represent a potential site for pathology undetectable using standard approaches. Because they are hard to visualize directly, proteins localized to these parts of the neurone are used as markers.

A consistent finding is that markers of presynaptic terminals are reduced in the hippocampus in schizophrenia. The magnitude of the loss varies according to the individual synaptic proteins studied, implying that the synaptic pathology is not uniform. There is some evidence for preferential decrements in excitatory connections, in keeping with the indications of glutamatergic involvement mentioned above. Presynaptic markers are also reduced in the dorsolateral prefrontal cortex. Complementing these changes, alterations in dendrites (the postsynaptic elements upon which most synapses project) have been shown in the hippocampus and neocortex. Although unproven, the simplest interpretation is that these changes reflect a reduction in the density of synaptic contacts being formed and received.[31]

Integrating the neuronal and synaptic findings

There is an encouraging convergence between neuronal and synaptic findings in schizophrenia. In particular, the decreases in presynaptic and dendritic markers are in keeping with the smaller neuronal cell bodies, since the size of the latter is proportional to the dendritic and axonal spread of the neurone. It is also consistent with the findings of increased neuronal density, in that dendrites and synapses are the major component of the neuropil and, if this is reduced, neurones will pack more closely together. Moreover, it also corresponds to the results of proton magnetic resonance spectroscopy studies of schizophrenia, which have shown reductions of the neuronal marker *N*-acetylaspartate, as one would predict if the neurones are on average smaller and have less extensive projections.

Postmortem studies are limited to chronic schizophrenia, so it is impossible to prove that the cytoarchitectural abnormalities are not the result of the illness or its treatment. However, several lines of evidence suggest that this is not the case. First, as the structural brain abnormalities and lower *N*-acetyl-aspartate signals occur in unmedicated and first-episode schizophrenia, it is reasonable to assume that the cytoarchitectural differences which putatively underlie them are also present at this time. Second, no correlations with the duration of

Table 3 Neuropathological evidence for a neurodevelopmental origin of schizophrenia

Ventricular enlargement and decreased cortical volume at first presentation
Absence of gliosis and other neurodegenerative features
Cytoarchitectural abnormalities
Increased prevalence of cavum septum pellucidum

disease or medication exposure have been seen in any of the postmortem studies. Third, although antipsychotic treatment does have morphological consequences, the effect is largely restricted to the basal ganglia.[33]

Interpretation of the neuropathology

Neuropathology and neurodevelopment

The neurodevelopmental model of schizophrenia (see Chapter 4.3.5.1) has become the prevailing pathogenic hypothesis; indeed the principle is now largely unchallenged. The neurobiological data form an important component of the evidence in its favour (Table 3).

A specific version of the theory is that the pathology of schizophrenia originates in the middle stage of intrauterine life.[34] An earlier timing is excluded since overt brain abnormalities would be seen if neurogenesis were affected, whilst the lack of gliosis is taken to mean that the changes must have occurred prior to the third trimester. However, this 'strong' form of the neurodevelopmental model is weak on two grounds. First, because of the limitations of the absence-of-gliosis argument mentioned earlier. Second, the types of cytoarchitectural disturbance adduced in favour (neuronal disarray, malpositioning) are those suggestive of aberrant neuronal migration, a process which occurs at the appropriate gestational period; yet, as mentioned, these cytoarchitectural abnormalities have not been unequivocally shown in schizophrenia. By comparison, the other cytoarchitectural findings, such as alterations in neuronal size, synapses, and dendrites, are modifiable throughout life and hence could originate much later.

Other forms of the neurodevelopmental theory advocate processes such as cell adhesion, apoptosis, myelination, and synaptic pruning. Overall, a parsimonious view is that the neuropathological data are indicative merely of an essentially developmental, as opposed to degenerative, disease process, rather than as pointing to a particular mechanism or timing.

Neuropathology and connectivity

Bleuler's view that the key symptoms of schizophrenia are those of 'psychic splitting' now have their counterparts in the functional imaging studies and neuropsychological models described above, which have implicated aberrant functional connectivity between different brain regions as the putative mechanism of psychosis. It is suggested that the cytoarchitectural features of schizophrenia represent its neuroanatomical basis.[31] However, functional connectivity does not presuppose an anatomical substrate, and the pathological evidence in schizophrenia must be considered on its own merits before attempts are made to integrate structure with function. Certainly, schizophrenia is not a disconnectivity syndrome akin to Alzheimer's disease, in which there is a frank loss of synapses and neurones, but rather a dysconnec-

tivity or misconnectivity syndrome resulting from a disturbance in the precise organization of the neural circuitry (Fig. 1).

Cerebral asymmetry and schizophrenia

Many neuropathological, neurochemical, neuropsychological, and electrophysiological studies of schizophrenia report lateralized abnormalities. Although there are also important negative findings, alterations in normal asymmetries and a left-sided preference of the pathology for the brain do seem to be more common than one would expect by chance. Two explanatory hypotheses exist. Crow's evolutionary theory is that schizophrenia, asymmetry, handedness, and language are causally linked to each other and to the same gene.[35] Alternatively, altered asymmetry in schizophrenia is viewed as an epiphenomenon of its *in utero* origins, a process which interferes with subsequent brain lateralization.[36] The issue remains under active investigation.

Summary

Despite the many uncertainties, there are now established facts about the neurobiology of schizophrenia (see Tables 1 and 2). There is ventricular enlargement and decreased brain volume. Although the cellular correlates remain poorly understood, they involve the size, density, and organization of neurones and their synaptic contacts (see Fig. 1). *In vivo* studies show differences in cerebral metabolism and other parameters of cerebral function, with a pattern indicative of aberrant connectivity between brain areas. Dopaminergic, 5-HT, and glutamatergic systems are all affected, but the specific details of their involve-

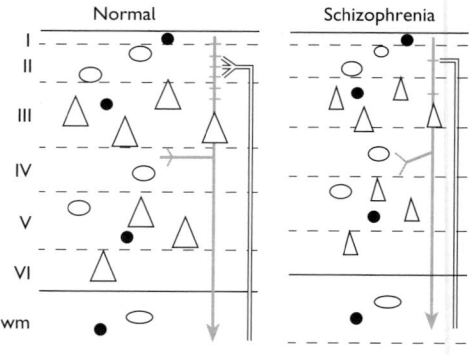

Fig. 1 Diagram of the putative cytoarchitectural features of schizophrenia. The grey matter (labelled I–VI) contains an unchanged number of neurones, but the pyramidal neurones (△) are smaller and more densely packed. The cortex is slightly thinner, especially laminae II and III. Both the reduced neuronal size and increased neuronal density are correlates of a reduced neuropil volume, which in turn reflects abnormalities affecting the axonal (thick vertical lines) and dendritic (thin vertical lines) arborizations of neurones. For example, there may be less extensive, or otherwise aberrant, synaptic connections formed by both incoming corticocortical fibres (hollow lines, shown as having restricted terminations on dendritic spines, which are denoted by thin horizontal lines) and axon collaterals (thick horizontal lines in lamina IV) of efferent pyramidal neurones. Glia (●) are unaffected. Although the figure illustrates the situation in the prefrontal neocortex, a similar diagram could be drawn for the hippocampus. For clarity, possible differences in the distribution and synaptic organization of interneurones (ellipses) and white matter (wm) neurones in schizophrenia are omitted.

ment in schizophrenia, and how they relate to the functional and structural findings, are still frustratingly unclear.

Further reading

David, A.S. and Cutting, J.C. (1994). *The neuropsychology of schizophrenia.* Erlbaum, Hove.

Harrison, P.J. (1999). The neuropathology of schizophrenia: a critical review of the data and their interpretation. *Brain, 122,* 593–624.

Lawrie, S.M. and Abukmeil, S.S. (1998). Brain abnormality in schizophrenia—a systematic and quantitative review of volumetric magnetic resonance imaging studies. *British Journal of Psychiatry, 172,* 110–20.

Owen, F. and Simpson, M.D.C. (1995). The neurochemistry of schizophrenia. In *Schizophrenia* (ed. S.R. Hirsch and D.R. Weinberger), pp. 358–78. Blackwell Science, Oxford.

Weinberger, D.R. and Berman, K.F. (1996). Prefrontal function in schizophrenia: confounds and controversies. *Philosophical Transactions of the Royal Society of London (Biology), 351,* 1495–1503.

References

1. Owen, F. and Simpson, M.D.C. (1995). The neurochemistry of schizophrenia. In *Schizophrenia* (ed. S.R. Hirsch and D.R. Weinberger), pp. 358–78. Blackwell Science, Oxford.

2. Kahn, R.S. and Davis, K.L. (1995). New developments in dopamine and schizophrenia. In *Psychopharmacology: the fourth generation of progress* (ed. F.E. Bloom and D.J. Kupfer), pp. 1193–204. Raven Press, New York.

3. Zakzanis, K.K. and Hansen, K.T. (1998). Dopamine D_2 densities and the schizophrenic brain. *Schizophrenia Research, 32,* 201–6.

4. Harrison, P.J. (1999). Neurochemical alterations in schizophrenia affecting the putative targets of atypical antipsychotics: focus on dopamine (D_1, D_3, D_4) and 5-HT_{2A} receptors. *British Journal of Psychiatry, 174* (Supplement 38), 41–51.

5. Abi-Dargham, A., Gil, R., Krystal, J., *et al.* (1998). Increased striatal dopamine transmission in schizophrenia: confirmation in a second cohort. *American Journal of Psychiatry, 155,* 761–7.

6. Abi-Dargham, A., Laruelle, M., Aghajanian, G.K., Charney, D., and Krystal, J. (1997). The role of serotonin in the pathophysiology and treatment of schizophrenia. *Journal of Neuropsychiatry and Clinical Neuroscience, 9,* 1–17.

7. Tamminga, C.A. (1998). Schizophrenia and glutamatergic transmission. *Critical Reviews in Neurobiology, 12,* 21–36.

8. Andreasen, N.C., O'Leary, D.S., Flaum, M., *et al.* (1997). Hypofrontality in schizophrenia: distributed dysfunctional circuits in neuroleptic-naive patients. *Lancet, 349,* 1730–4.

9. Spence, S.A., Hirsch, S.R., Brooks, D.J., and Grasby, P.M. (1998). Prefrontal cortex activity in people with schizophrenia and control subjects. Evidence from positron emission tomography for remission of 'hypofrontality' with recovery from acute schizophrenia. *British Journal of Psychiatry, 172,* 316–23.

10. Weinberger, D.R. and Berman, K.F. (1996). Prefrontal function in schizophrenia: confounds and controversies. *Philosophical Transactions of the Royal Society of London (Biology), 351,* 1495–503.

11. Liddle, P.F., Friston, K.J., Frith, C.D., Hirsch, S.R., Jones, T., and Frackowiak, R.S.J. (1992). Patterns of cerebral blood flow in schizophrenia. *British Journal of Psychiatry, 160,* 179–86.

12. Buchsbaum, M.S. and Hazlett, E.A. (1998). Positron emission tomography studies of abnormal glucose metabolism in schizophrenia. *Schizophrenia Bulletin, 24,* 343–64.

13. Blackwood, D.H.R., St Clair, D.M., Muir, W.J., and Duffy, J.C. (1991).

14. Hutton, S. and Kennard, C. (1998). Oculomotor abnormalities in schizophrenia. A critical review. *Neurology, 50,* 604–9.

15. Goldberg, T.E., Hyde, T.M., Kleinman, J.E., and Weinberger, D.R. (1993). Course of schizophrenia: neuropsychological evidence for a static encephalopathy. *Schizophrenia Bulletin, 19,* 797–804.

16. Davidson, M., Harvey, P., Welsh, K.A., Powchik, P., Putnam, K.M., and Mohs, R.C. (1996). Cognitive functioning in late-life schizophrenia: a comparison of elderly schizophrenic patients and patients with Alzheimer's disease. *American Journal of Psychiatry, 153,* 1274–9.

17. Blanchard, J.J. and Neale, J.M. (1994). The neuropsychological signature of schizophrenia: generalized or differential deficit? *American Journal of Psychiatry, 151,* 40–8.

18. David, A.S. and Cutting, J.C. (1994). *The neuropsychology of schizophrenia.* Lawrence Erlbaum, Hove.

19. Johnstone, E.C., Crow, T.J., Frith, C.D., Husband, J., and Kreel, L. (1976). Cerebral ventricular size and cognitive impairment in chronic schizophrenia. *Lancet, ii,* 924–6.

20. Daniel, D.G., Goldberg, T.E., Gibbons, R.D., and Weinberger, D.R. (1991). Lack of a bimodal distribution of ventricular size in schizophrenia: a Gaussian mixture analysis of 1056 cases and controls. *Biological Psychiatry, 30,* 887–903.

21. van Horn, J.D. and McManus, I.C. (1992). Ventricular enlargement in schizophrenia. A meta-analysis of studies of the ventricle:brain ratio (VBR). *British Journal of Psychiatry, 160,* 687–97.

22. Lawrie, S.M. and Abukmeil, S.S. (1998). Brain abnormality in schizophrenia—a systematic and quantitative review of volumetric magnetic resonance imaging studies. *British Journal of Psychiatry, 172,* 110–20.

23. Ward, K.E., Friedman, L., Wise, A., and Schulz, S.C. (1996). Meta-analysis of brain and cranial size in schizophrenia. *Schizophrenia Research, 22,* 197–213.

24. Nelson, M.D., Saykin, A.J., Flashman, L.A., and Riordan, H.J. (1998). Hippocampal volume reduction in schizophrenia as assessed by magnetic resonance imaging—a meta-analytic study. *Archives of General Psychiatry, 55,* 433–40.

25. Suddath, R.L., Christison, G.W., Torrey, E.F., Casanova, M.F., and Weinberger, D.R. (1990). Anatomical abnormalities in the brains of monozygotic twins discordant for schizophrenia. *New England Journal of Medicine, 322,* 789–94.

26. Harrison, P.J. (1999). Brains at risk of schizophrenia. *Lancet, 353,* 3–4.

27. Stevens, J.R. (1982). Neuropathology of schizophrenia. *Archives of General Psychiatry, 39,* 1131–9.

28. Bruton, C.J., Crow, T.J., Frith, C.D., Johnstone, E.C., Owens, D.G.C., and Roberts, G.W. (1990). Schizophrenia and the brain: a prospective cliniconeuropathological study. *Psychological Medicine, 20,* 285–304.

29. Baldessarini, R.J., Hegarty, J.D., Bird, E.D., and Benes, F.M. (1997). Meta-analysis of postmortem studies of Alzheimer's disease-like neuropathology in schizophrenia. *American Journal of Psychiatry, 154,* 861–3.

30. Arnold, S.E., Trojanowski, J.Q., Gur, R.E., Blackwell, P., Han, L.Y., and Choi, C. (1998). Absence of neurodegeneration and neural injury in the cerebral cortex in a sample of elderly patients with schizophrenia. *Archives of General Psychiatry, 55,* 225–32.

31. Harrison, P.J. (1999). The neuropathology of schizophrenia: a critical review of the data and their interpretation. *Brain, 122,* 593–624.

32. Benes, F.M. (1995). Is there a neuroanatomic basis for schizophrenia? An old question revisited. *Neuroscientist, 1,* 104–15.

33. Harrison, P.J. (1999). The neuropathological effects of antipsychotic drugs. *Schizophrenia Research,* in press.

34. Bloom, F.E. (1993). Advancing a neurodevelopmental origin for schizophrenia. *Archives of General Psychiatry, 50,* 224–7.

35. Crow, T.J. (1997). Schizophrenia as failure of hemispheric dominance for language. *Trends in Neurosciences, 20,* 339–43.

Auditory P300 and eye tracking dysfunction in schizophrenic pedigrees. *Archives of General Psychiatry, 48,* 899–909.

36. Roberts, G.W. (1991). Schizophrenia: a neuropathological perspective. *British Journal of Psychiatry*, **158**, 8–17.

4.3.6 Course and outcome of schizophrenia and their prediction

Assen Jablensky

Introduction

The course of schizophrenia is as variable as its symptoms. Systematic investigations of the courses of the psychoses were initiated by Kraepelin who believed that, in the absence of demonstrable brain pathology and aetiology, a common outcome into 'psychic weakness' of the clinical syndromes he grouped together as dementia praecox would provide a validity test for the disease entity. Later, Kraepelin revised his claim that the prognosis of dementia praecox was invariably poor and noted that 'permanent cures' had occurred in about 15 per cent of his cases.[1] Subsequent longitudinal studies have confirmed the striking variability of course as one of the salient characteristic of the 'natural history' of schizophrenia.

Methodological issues

The large number of studies on the course and outcome of schizophrenia published since the beginning of the twentieth century might suggest that the longitudinal aspects of the disorder are well established and exhaustively documented. Unfortunately, this is not the case since the methodological difficulties that accompany this type of research are complex and few studies have adequately dealt with all the major sources of error and confounding.[2]

The studies of the course and outcome of schizophrenia comprise statistical reports on admissions and discharges, long-term follow-back studies (in which the initial features of the cases and the course of the disorder are reconstructed retrospectively from admission records), and prospective investigations (in which patients are enlisted at an early stage of the disorder and followed up for a varying length of time). Each design is vulnerable to bias: admission and discharge statistics usually comprise patients at different stages of disease progression, follow-back studies rely on prevalence samples in which chronic cases tend to be over-represented, and prospective studies, though superior to other designs, tend to exclude patients who initially have diagnoses other than schizophrenia and are subsequently rediagnosed as schizophrenic. The methodological issues that need to be considered in interpreting the results from longidutinal research into schizophrenia include the following.

Diagnosis

The use of either 'broad' or 'restrictive' definitions of schizophrenia may result in vastly different samples on which follow-up data are reported. Systems with an inbuilt illness duration criterion, such as DSM-III and DSM-IIIR which require at least 6 months of unremit-

ting symptoms and a decline in functioning, are likely to overselect patients already developing a chronic course. The result would be a greater homogeneity of outcome at the cost of a compromised representativeness of the sample as regards the range of possible outcomes of schizophrenia. Diagnostic systems that emphasize the cross-sectional features of the disorder, such as ICD-10 (which requires 1 month's duration of clinically characteristic symptoms) avoid this limitation, possibly at the expense of including some cases of good prognosis that may be aetiologically or pathogenetically different from poor prognosis schizophrenia. However, until aetiology is elucidated, or a validating pathognomonic lesion is established, the decision as to what constitutes 'true' schizophrenia will remain arbitrary. With regard to prognostic studies, less restrictive systems have the important advantage that a broad spectrum of outcomes would be available at the endpoint of prospective observation, allowing for subgroups to be identified and their characteristics related to the initial manifestations of the disorder and various risk factors.

Definitions and assessment of course and outcome variables

There is no single measure of course and outcome of a complex disorder such as schizophrenia, and blanket terms such as 'recovery', 'improvement', or 'deterioration' tend to conflate substantially different aspects of the evolution of the disorder over time. Most investigators today agree that course (comprising the pathways or trajectories of the disorder) and outcome (the net balance of the clinical and functional descriptors at the endpoint of observation) are multivariate composites. As a minimum, three domains that need not covary over time should be independently assessed: symptom severity, functional impairments including cognitive deficits, and disablement in social and occupational role performance. Each one of these can be further articulated into a number of areas or dimensions. In addition, one must consider extrinsic variables such as measures of environmental and treatment-related influences on course and outcome, as well as subjective experiences commonly described as 'quality of life'. Standardized reliable instruments (interviews, inventories, rating scales) are required for the assessment of most variables. It should not be forgotten, however, that some of the richest sources of information are the perceptive, in-depth case studies based on personal patient contact over many years. Collectively, such single case observations can generate hypotheses for testing in epidemiologically designed studies.

Length of follow-up

The evidence from previous research suggests that very different impressions of the course and outcome of schizophrenia would be gained depending on the duration of prospective observation and the degree of control over the inclusion of patients that are comparable in terms of age and length of previous illness.

Cohort attrition

In any follow-up study, a proportion of cases will be lost to observation because of death, migration, refusal of contact, or other reasons for untraceability. Since such loss of subjects is likely to correlate with particular patterns of course and outcome, it is essential to estimate its possible effect (e.g. by statistical modelling) on the interpretation of the final results, especially if cohort attrition is greater than 15 to 20 per cent of the original sample.

Other aspects of study design

Variation in the sources of recruitment of cases (e.g. any admission to a treatment facility or catchment area sampling), and of information regarding course and outcome variables (e.g. face-to-face interviews or collateral data from case notes or informants), can obviously influence the results of any follow-up study. In addition, subtle variations in study design, such as whether investigators assessing patients' symptoms and functioning at any point in time are 'blind' to data from previous assessments, can influence the final results. Inclusion of a comparison group (e.g. patients with other psychotic disorders) would help evaluate the extent to which any observed patterns of course and outcome are specific to schizophrenia, whereas appropriate controls drawn from the general population can provide reference points for assessing social variables, such as occupational functioning, stressful life events, or habit-related behaviour such as substance use.

Statistical analysis

Longitudinal research poses a number of specific requirements with regard to data analysis. Thus, the problem of multiple comparisons is likely to arise when examining the data for significant associations; time series, survival, or path analysis may be required when observations are made and recorded at successive time points in the evolution of the disorder; and methods of unconfounding are called for at each step of the analysis of longitudinal data. While no single study to date has met all the rigorous methodological requirements, a number of studies have succeeded in controlling at least some of the sources of bias and confounding. The results from previous research are, therefore, not strictly comparable in specific detail, but are informative as regards the general trends and patterns.

The 'natural history' of schizophrenia before the neuroleptic era

Since the great majority of schizophrenic patients are today receiving pharmacological treatment, current and recent studies may not reflect the 'natural' course and outcome of the disorder. Two recent studies in Scotland[3] and India[4] estimated the proportions of never-hospitalized schizophrenic patients at 6.7 per cent and 28.7 per cent respectively. About half of the Scottish patients had been prescribed neuroleptics by their general practitioners while the Indian patients had been virtually untreated. However, in both settings the outcomes of these interesting samples (which presumably approximate the 'natural' history of the disorder) were heterogeneous and, by and large, did not differ from the outcomes in the treated groups. In a historical study of 70 Swedish patients with first admissions in 1925, the lifetime records were retrieved and rediagnosed in accordance with DSM-III.[5] None of these patients had received neuroleptics. The final outcome was rated as good in 33 per cent (but no patient was considered as

completely recovered), as 'profoundly deteriorated' in 43 per cent, and as intermediate in 24 per cent.

Another, long-term perspective on the course of schizophrenia over successive generations is provided by a meta-analysis of 320 outcome studies on schizophrenia or dementia praecox published between 1895 and 1992 and including a total of 51 800 subjects.[6] Overall, about 40 per cent of the patients were reported as improved after an average length of follow-up 5.6 years. There was a significant increase in the rate of improvement during the period 1956 to 1985 compared with 1895 to 1955, clearly related to the introduction of neuroleptic treatment,[7] but a secular trend towards better outcomes with every successive decade had been present for much longer. Coupled with the virtual disappearance of the most malignant or 'catastrophic' forms of schizophrenia resulting in a profound defect state after a first psychotic episode, or death ('lethal catatonia'), these observations suggest that some transition to a less deteriorating course of the disorder had occurred prior to modern pharmacological treatment.[8] Among the factors explaining this shift one should consider improvements in general care, progressive changes in attitudes and hospital regime which occurred in a number of institutions on both sides of the Atlantic in the 1930 and 1940s, as well as heightened expectations that psychosocial measures such as psychotherapy or rehabilitation could result in a cure in some cases.

Long-term prognosis

Results of course and outcome studies published over the last six decades are shown in Table 1. The studies have been selected on the basis of the length of follow-up (>5 years), effective sample size (>50), and intensity of follow-up and assessment.

Three European[12,14,28] and two North American studies,[15,16] in which a total of nearly 1300 patients were followed up for 23 to 37 years, provide a global overview of the long-term course of schizophrenia. Although the studies differ in their design (prospective;[12,14,16] follow-back or retrospective[15,28]), and include patients with onsets in the preneuroleptic era who were later treated with antipsychotic drugs for varying length of time, their results have much in common.

Manfred Bleuler's monograph[12] is the account of an intensive study of 208 patients first admitted in 1942 to 1943 and personally followed up by the author for 22 years or until death. Another 23-year follow-up of 504 patients admitted in 1945 to 1959 has been completed by Huber et al.[14] Ciompi[28] interviewed 289 surviving patients in Switzerland first admitted between 1900 and 1962 (median follow-up length 36.9 years).

Notwithstanding methodological constraints that apply to these studies, their findings are a unique record of what probably represents the closest approximation to the 'natural history' of schizophrenia. In summary, they indicate the following.

- Lasting recovery ('complete cure') occurred in 20 to 26 per cent of the cases—according to Ciompi[28] 43 per cent had either remitted or exhibited mild residual abnormalities which did not interfere with their living in the community.

- Forty-four per cent were still in hospital[28] and severe chronic states had developed in 14 to 24 per cent.

Table 1 Results of selected course and outcome studies in schizophrenia, 1939–1998

Author	Country	Sample size	Length of follow-up (years)	Proportion good outcome[a]
Rennie (1939)[9]	USA	456	1–26	25% recovered
Astrup and Noreik (1966)[10]	Norway	273	5–12	6% recovered; 10% improved
Brown et al. (1966)[11]	UK	273	5	49% functioning well
Bleuler (1972)[12]	Switzerland	208	23	20% complete remission; 33% mild defect
Ciompi and Müller (1976)[13]	Switzerland	289	37	20% recovered; 43% definitely improved
Huber et al. (1980)[14]	Germany	502	22	26% recovered; 31% remission with mild defect
Tsuang et al. (1979)[15]	USA	186	35	46% recovered or improved significantly
Harding et al. (1987)[16]	USA	118	32	62% recovered or improved significantly
Ogawa et al. (1987)[17]	Japan	140	21–27	31% recovered; 46% improved
Shepherd et al. (1989)[18]	UK	107	5	22% recovered, no relapse
Carone et al. (1991)[19]	USA	79	5	17% complete remission
Breier et al. (1991)[20]	USA	58	2–12	20% good outcome
Johnstone et al. (1991)[21]	UK	530	3–13	14% excellent; 18.5% very good social adjustment
Marneros et al. (1992)[22]	Germany	249	25	Full remission in 24% ('broad') or 7% ('pure') schizophrenia
Thara et al. (1994)[23]	India	91	10	12% complete recovery; 62% remission
Mason et al. (1995)[24]	UK	67	13	17% complete recovery; 52% remission
Wieselgren and Lindström (1996)[25]	Sweden	120	5	30% good outcome
Wiersma et al. (1998)[26]	Holland	82	15	27% complete; 50% partial remission
Ganev et al. (1998)[27]	Bulgaria	60	16	32% complete; 5% partial remission

[a] In descriptive categories used by the authors.

- In 50 to 75 per cent of the patients, a clinically stable state set in after the fifth year since onset, with no significant further deterioration.

- Remitting course with multiple episodes and full remissions characterized 22 per cent of the patients;[14] catastrophic course (rapid onset of chronic deterioration) was observed in 1 to 4 per cent.

- The 20-year suicide rate was 14 to 22 per cent.

The two American studies largely concur with these findings. In the Vermont study[16] no less than 62 per cent of the cohort had achieved significant improvement or recovery after an average length of follow-up 32 years; the corresponding proportion in the Iowa 500 study[15] was 46 per cent.

The most striking finding from the long-term follow-up studies is the high proportion of patients who recover, either completely or with mild residual abnormalities, after decades of severe illness. This contrasts with the ingrained image of schizophrenia as an intractable, deteriorating illness that many clinicians tend to adopt on the basis of a limited follow-up horizon and patient samples selected for unfavourable course and treatment response. It is unlikely that the high percentage of recoveries in the long-term studies could be explained by cases of affective illness or brief transient psychoses misdiagnosed as schizophrenia (the retrospective rediagnosis of cases according to Feighner's[29] or DSM-III criteria in the two American studies did not alter significantly the results). Similarly unlikely would be the attribution of all the good outcomes to the antipsychotic treatment many of these patients received in the later stages of their illnesses, since comparable proportions of improvement of recovery had been reported for patients who never received neuroleptics.[5] A tentative conclusion from such follow-up research would be that schizophrenia is not invariably a chronic deteriorating disorder and that the progression of the disease can be arrested, or even reversed, at any stage. The causes of such reversibility remain largely unknown, but research focusing specifically on the recovering cases will undoubtedly provide essential clues for understanding the nature of schizophrenia.

Recent course and outcome studies

Results of longitudinal studies published in the last decade (Table 1) do not add substantially new evidence and tend to corroborate the pattern of outcomes outlined by the earlier studies.

The reported rates of recovery or complete remission vary between 12 per cent[30] and 32 per cent.[27] If the rates of improvement or partial remission are added to those of complete remission, the general improvement rate over 5 to 15 years of follow-up would be no less than 30 per cent and may be as high as 50 per cent. On the other hand, the proportion of patients with an early deteriorating course of illness without clinical remissions is remarkably similar across different studies and is in the order of 20 to 35 per cent. There is a relationship between the length of the follow-up and the proportions of patients who are reported as recovered, remitting, or deteriorating, with a general trend towards higher improvement rates in long-term studies. For example, the proportion of good outcomes increased from 10 per cent at the 2.5-year follow-up to 17 per cent at 5 years in one of the studies;[19] it was 31 per cent in a study with a follow-up of 21 to 25 years[17] and nearly 60 per cent at the end of the 32-year follow-up of the Vermont study.[16]

Patterns and stages of the course of schizophrenia

The great heterogeneity of the course of schizophrenia can be reduced to a limited number of patterns into which cases tend to cluster over time. In the long-term follow-up studies referred to above, eight different categories of course were described by Bleuler[12] and Ciompi,[28] and 12 by Huber et al.[14] These classifications were derived from empirical observation, rather than statistical modelling, and conflated into single categories the mode of onset, longitudinal aspects such as psychotic episodes and remissions, and end states. Treating the various aspects of the longitudinal profile of the illness as independent axes in a multidimensional construct has been recommended.[31,32] However, the complexity of statistical modelling of the course of schizophrenia is such that the development of a classification of course that would be both useful in clinical practice and rigorous in a mathematical sense may not be feasible. Therefore, an heuristic compromise between these two requirements should, as a minimum, define operationally and assess separately the number and duration of discrete episodes of illness, the predominant clinical features of each episode (e.g. psychotic or affective), and the number and length of remissions and their quality (presence/absence of residual negative or deficit symptoms and signs). By combining these variables, several patterns of course have been derived that have found good empirical support in international follow-up studies:[33]

(1) single psychotic episode followed by complete remission;

(2) single psychotic episode followed by incomplete remission;

(3) two or more psychotic episodes, with complete remissions between episodes;

(4) two or more psychotic episodes, with incomplete remissions between episodes;

(5) continuous (unremitting) psychotic illness.

With some modifications, these longitudinal patterns have been incorporated into ICD-10 and DSM-IV as additional descriptors.

Although the components of the course patterns, such as episode, remission, residual symptomatology, etc. almost certainly do not represent 'pure' dimensions, it is desirable to restrict the definition of pattern of course to clinical variables only, in order to be able to examine its correlations with risk factors and predictors, such as premorbid impairments or mode of onset, and with social outcomes. The assessment of social functioning independently of the clinical pattern of course is crucial to the study of illness–environment interactions and the causes of disablement in schizophrenia.

At present it does not seem possible to define with any precision discrete stages in the progression of schizophrenic illnesses using combined clinical and pathological criteria, as in cancer or cardiovascular disease. Nevertheless, a 'softer' form of staging is feasible since there is on the whole a good agreement between the results of different studies on the general pattern of course in schizophrenia. On the basis of long-term follow-up studies, the lifetime course of schizophrenia can be articulated into a premorbid phase (from birth to the onset of psychosis), a phase of acute or positive schizophrenic symptomatology, and

a residual phase.[34] Various substages have been proposed to describe in finer detail the pre-onset period,[35,36] and theorizing about the implications of the so-called neurodevelopmental model of the aetiology of schizophrenia has led to suggestions about backdating the premorbid period to include gestation. However, for most practical and research purposes, a three-stage classification of post-onset course has been proposed:[20]

(1) an early deteriorating phase (the first 5–10 years);

(2) a middle (stabilization) phase;

(3) a gradual improvement phase.

This model agrees well with the empirical evidence and could be useful in the collection and summarizing of data on individual risks and prognosis.

Geographical and cultural variation

Three prospective investigations initiated by the World Health Organization (**WHO**)—the International Pilot Study of Schizophrenia,[33,37] the 10-country study on Determinants of Outcome of Severe Mental Disorders,[38] and the study on Assessment and Reduction of Psychiatric Disability[39]—provide a cross-cultural database for the evaluation of the course and outcome of schizophrenia which comprises extensive initial and follow-up information on a total of 2736 patients in 16 countries, diagnosed as schizophrenic according to strict and comparable criteria. The assessment procedures and instruments used in these studies were identical or similar. Results of the WHO 10-country study (pooled data on 1070 patients in all the research sites) are presented in Table 2. The following general conclusions can be drawn from this research.

1. The striking variability of the course and outcome of schizophrenia has been cross-culturally confirmed. Patients with similar clinical and diagnostic characteristics at the baseline assessment develop a spectrum of outcomes ranging from stable clinical and social recovery after a single psychotic episode to chronic unremitting psychosis and severe impairment. The intensive follow-up and the relatively low cohort attrition lend credibility to the finding of a high proportion (over 30 per cent) of favourable outcomes, a proportion which is in agreement with the results of other longitudinal studies reviewed above.

2. The frequencies of both relapses and remissions tend to increase over time: while at 2-year follow-up of the International Pilot Study of Schizophrenia 11 per cent of the patients had experienced two or more psychotic episodes followed by complete remission and another 18 per cent had two or more episodes followed by residual symptoms and impairments, the corresponding proportions at 5-year follow-up were 15 per cent and 33 per cent.[37]

3. Regardless of the increasing relapse rate, the cumulative proportion of follow-up time during which patients have psychotic symptoms (as a percentage of the total follow-up time), tends to remain stable or decrease. At the end of the 5-year follow-up, 57 per cent of the patients had experienced a total of less than 9 months of active psychosis; only 22 per cent had been psychotic for 45 to 60 months.

Table 2 Two-year course and outcome features of 1070 patients with schizophrenia in the WHO 10-country study

Course and outcome descriptor	Percentage patients in developing countries[a] (*n* = 467)	Percentage patients in developed countries[b] (*n* = 603)
Remitting, complete remissions	62.7	36.8
Continuous or episodic, no complete remission	35.7	60.9
Psychotic <5% of the follow-up	18.4	18.7
Psychotic >75% of the follow-up	15.1	20.2
No complete remission during follow-up	24.1	57.2
Complete remission for >75% of the follow-up	38.3	22.3
On antipsychotic medication >75% of the follow-up	15.9	60.8
No antipsychotic medication during follow-up	5.9	2.5
Hospitalized for >75% of follow-up	0.3	2.3
Never hospitalized during follow-up	55.5	8.1
Impaired social functioning throughout follow-up	15.7	41.6
Unimpaired social functioning >75% of follow-up	42.9	31.6

[a] Colombia, India, Nigeria.
[b] Czech Republic.

4. The levels of social impairment assessed at 2 years changed very little during the subsequent years of follow-up. Overall, most of the observed change in the clinical state and social functioning of patients between the 2-year follow-up and the 5-year follow-up was towards improvement rather than deterioration.

5. While the percentage of patients with continuous, deteriorating illness was similar across the study sites, there were significant differences in the proportions of patients who achieved symptomatic and social recovery. In this respect, outcome was better in the developing countries. This unexpected finding of the follow-up of the International Pilot Study of Schizophrenia patients,[33,37] who had been recruited from consecutive hospital admissions with the attendant possibilities of a selective bias, was subsequently replicated by the 10-country study which had an epidemiological design and recruited only first-contact patients from delimited populations.[38] The better course and outcome in the developing country areas could not be attributed to any particular subtype of the disorder, e.g. cases of acute onset, since it applied equally to the cases of slow, insidious onset. The main outcome difference across the study areas was in the occurrence and average length of symptom-free remissions . Such remissions tended to be more frequent and to last longer in the developing countries. No single factor accounting for this difference could be identified and it is likely that complex interactions between illness and environment are involved that may include, on one hand, population differences in predisposing genes,[40] and on the other hand, cultural differences such as the relative absence of an institutionalized role of the 'schizophrenic' in traditional societies.[41]

Whether the better outcome of schizophrenia in the developing countries is 'transportable' following migration to other settings, remains unclear. Data on immigrants treated for first episodes of schizophrenia in the United Kingdom suggest that while Asian patients have a considerably lower relapse and readmission rate than British-born white people, African-Caribbeans show a higher rate.[42] The marked social and family structure differences between the Asian and the African-Caribbean immigrant communities suggest that the likelihood of a more benign course in the new setting may depend on the degree to which the immigrant group has retained its traditional values and intragroup cohesion.

First-episode psychosis

The recent resurgence of interest in the early detection and treatment of first episodes of psychosis, driven by theoretical considerations and clinical concerns, is supported by empirical evidence suggesting that the course and outcome of the earliest stages of a schizophrenic illness may have a pathoplastic effect on its subsequent course. Specifically, the period between the first onset of psychotic symptoms and the initiation of treatment (duration of untreated psychosis) has been shown to correlate with increased time to remission and poor response to treatment.[43] Plausible clinical considerations have been proposed in support of the view that the first episode of psychosis represents a critical developmental transition that may impact the subsequent course of schizophrenia, possibly by inducing irreversible changes in the connectivity between neural networks and thus preparing the ground for chronic illness.[44] An extension of this mode of thinking is the suggestion that a behavioural or pharmacological intervention prior to the onset of psychotic symptoms could delay or prevent the onset of schizophrenia.[45,46]

None of these hypotheses has been properly tested. However, a number of studies focusing on the earliest manifestations of psychosis have highlighted features such as a presymptomatic drop in cognitive performance and social functioning,[47] early co-occurrence of 'positive' and 'negative' symptoms,[48] as well as a general malleability of such dysfunction in response to appropriate behavioural interventions and low-dose, time-limited pharmacological treatment.[49] This suggests that clinical research bridging the gap between statistical investigations of risk factors or antecedents of disease and individual pathways to psychotic illness may have an important role to play in understanding and, ultimately, influencing the development and course of schizophrenia.

Prognosis of specific clinical symptoms and syndromes

Longitudinal studies suggest that the characteristic symptoms of schizophrenia tend to 'breed true', i.e. only a minority of patients are eventually reclassified into other disease categories because of a significant and lasting change in the predominant symptoms. However, the proportion of cases warranting a rediagnosis seems to increase with the length of follow-up.

Depression in schizophrenia

In the WHO International Pilot Study of Schizophrenia,[33] the proportion of patients with initial schizophrenic symptomatology who developed non-schizophrenic (mostly affective) episodes in the course of time increased from 3 per cent in the first 2 years to 17 per cent at the end of the 5-year follow-up. In contrast, subsequent episodes with schizophrenic features occurred in fewer than 10 per cent of the patients with an initial diagnosis of major depression. Depression is the most common non-schizophrenic syndrome intercurrent with schizophrenia also in those patients who retain the essentially schizophrenic character of their illnesses. The proportion who develop clear-cut episodes of major depression ranges from 15 per cent during a 5-year follow-up[50] to 24 per cent during a 12-year follow-up.[20] This is a much higher period prevalence rate than in the general population, which suggests that depression is part of the clinical spectrum of schizophrenia. Based on such data, a diagnostic rubric of post-schizophrenic depression has been added to the classification of schizophrenia in ICD-10.

Schneiderian first-rank symptoms

Schneider[51] explicitly disclaimed any particular prognostic value for the subjective thought disorder phenomena, passivity experiences, and particular type of auditory hallucinations to which he attributed a 'first-rank' significance in the differential diagnosis between schizophrenic and affective psychoses. However, the first-rank symptoms have a marked tendency to recur in subsequent psychotic episodes. Patients with one or more first-rank symptoms on the initial examination had a threefold increase in the risk of experiencing such symptoms in subsequent episodes compared to patients with no first-rank symptoms on initial examination.[38]

Prognosis of schizophrenia subtypes

The evidence that each of the 'classic' subtypes of schizophrenia is associated with a characteristic patterns of course is generally weak but surprisingly good for some of the subtypes. Thus, consistent differences have been reported between paranoid, hebephrenic, and undifferentiated schizophrenia (diagnosed according to DSM-III) on a long-term follow-up of 19 years.[52] Paranoid schizophrenia tended to have a remittent course, and to be associated with less disability, in contrast to hebephrenia which had an insidious onset and poor long-term prognosis. Undifferentiated schizophrenia occupied an intermediate position. In the WHO International Pilot Study of Schizophrenia,[33] four alternative groupings of the ICD-9 subtypes were tested by a discriminant function for differences with regard to six course and outcome measures. Clear discrimination was achieved between simple and hebephrenic schizophrenia grouped together on the one hand and the schizoaffective subtype on the other. However, the comparison of simple and hebephrenic schizophrenia with paranoid schizophrenia resulted in a considerable degree of overlap.

Better discrimination has been claimed for groups of patients diagnosed according to the criteria of Leonhard.[53] A 5- to 13-year follow-up of 178 patients admitted with a diagnosis of schizophrenia and rediagnosed according to the Leonhardian criteria as systematic schizophrenia, atypical (unsystematic) schizophrenia, cycloid psychosis, or reactive psychosis[54] resulted in marked outcome differences on blind assessment . While only 10 per cent of the cases in the two schizophrenia groups were judged to have 'recovered', the corresponding proportion in the cycloid and reactive psychoses group was 38 per cent. Conversely, the proportions of 'unimproved' cases were 49 per cent and 3 per cent.

The question of whether good-prognosis remitting schizophrenia of an acute onset is a separate subtype that could also be distinguished symptomatologically was addressed in the WHO 10-country study[38] by comparing 274 patients with an initial ICD-9 diagnosis of acute schizophrenic episode and 752 patients with other schizophrenia subtypes. The group of acute cases tended to be younger and had a lower male-to-female ratio, but was no different from the rest of the schizophrenic patients with regard to initial symptomatology. Similar conclusions were reached by Vaillant[55] in a 4- to16-year follow-up of schizophrenic patients who remitted after an acute episode. This argues against acute schizophreniform illness being a discrete syndrome, outside the clinical spectrum of schizophrenia.

The course and outcome data on schizoaffective disorders seem to support their placement within the broad category of schizophrenia. A retrospective and prospective study of 150 schizoaffective patients and 95 bipolar affective patients[56] established general similarities between the two groups but the schizoaffective cases were less likely to achieve a full remission and more likely to develop a residual state (in 57 per cent compared to 24 per cent for the bipolar group). An intermediate outcome between that of schizophrenia and bipolar affective disorder is a common finding.[22]

Predictors of course and outcome

A wide range of variables have been explored as possible predictors of course and outcome in schizophrenia: sociodemographic characteristics; characteristics of the premorbid personality and pre-onset functioning; family history of psychiatric disorder; history of past psychotic episodes and treatments; substance use; characteristics of the onset; features of the initial clinical state and treatment response; variables related to brain morphology and neurocognitive functioning. A synopsis of findings about predictors is presented in Table 3. Table 4 lists the results of statistical analysis of predictors for each of four different measures of 2-year course and outcome in the WHO 10-country study.[38]

Many predictors have been replicated independently by different investigators and there is reasonable agreement on the general direction of their effects. However, the definitions of both the independent (predictor) and the dependent (outcome) variable vary across studies, and the statistical methods employed range from simple descriptive statistics (e.g. *x* per cent of the patients with characteristic *y* developed outcome *z*) to proper statistical models with capacity to quantify the

Table 3 Significant findings about predictors of course and outcome in schizophrenia

Study	Predictor variable	Outcome variable
Harder et al.[57]: 2-year follow-up of 145 patients	Social class Phillips Premorbid Status score (p < 0.001)	Level of functioning; diagnostic severity
Jørgensen et al.[58]: 13-year follow-up of 53 patients	Affective flattening on index admission Diagnosis of schizophrenia on first admission	≥30% of follow-up time as inpatient Readmission risk after first discharge
Vita et al.[59]: 2-year follow-up of 18 patients	Cortical atrophy (but not ventricular enlargement) on index admission	Poor social adjustment
Eaton et al.[60]: combined data from 4 psychiatric case registers in Australia, Denmark, UK, and USA	Age at onset 10–19 Number of prior episodes	Readmission after first hospitalization
Johnstone et al.[61]: 3–13-year follow-up of 342 patients	Fragmentation of family of origin	Duration of hospitalization during follow-up
Harrison et al.[62]: 13-year follow-up of 99 patients	Pattern of course during first 2 years	Global outcome at 13 years
Goldman et al.[63]: 1-year outcome in 59 unmedicated patients	Shorter REM latency on index admission	Poor clinical and social outcome in females
Ho et al.[64]: 2-year follow-up of 50 first-episode patients	Severity of negative symptoms on index admission	Psychosocial functioning, quality of life
Castle et al.[65]: 18-month follow-up of 166 patients	African-Caribbean background	Less illness severity; greater imprisonment risk

independent contribution of individual variables to a specified outcome.

Table 4 Best predictors of 2-year course and outcome in the WHO 10-country study (results of log-linear analysis of 1078 cases)

Predictor	Course and outcome variables			
	Pattern of course	Time in psychosis	Remission/ no remission	Social functioning
Age	NS	NS	NS	*
Sex	*	*	**	**
Marital status	**	***	***	***
Acute versus gradual onset	***	***	***	***
Time since onset (duration of untreated psychosis)	NS	NS	**	***
First-rank symptoms at baseline	NS	NS	NS	NS
Adjustment in childhood	NS	NS	**	***
Adjustment in adolescence	NS	***	***	***
Close friends	*	*	***	***
Street drug use	*	*	***	***
Setting (developing/ developed country)	***	NS	***	***

NS, not significant.
* significant at $p \leq 0.05$.
** significant at $p \leq 0.01$.
*** significant at $p \leq 0.001$.

Limitations of clinical prediction

The explanatory power of any predictor in schizophrenia (in terms of accounting for a proportion of the outcome variance) is likely to vary depending on sample size, setting, homogeneity of patient groups, and measurement error, but generally tends to be limited (rarely exceeding 30 per cent of the outcome variance). This suggests that no single background or premorbid characteristics of the person, and no clinical symptom or sign among the initial manifestations of the disorder, is in a particularly strong association with its prognosis in the longer term. Similarly to the genetic epidemiology of schizophrenia, where non-shared environmental influences account for a greater amount of variance than the shared environment, person-specific emergent life events or changes in the mental state may have a similar or greater impact on outcome than the initial or premorbid predictors. Indeed, variables such as negative symptoms have been shown to gain in predictive power if they are assessed 2 or more years after the onset, or after the patients have received adequate treatment. The predictive capacity of other variables, for example mode of onset[34] or a high index of expressed emotion,[66] tends to become attenuated in the course of time. Thus, there is no fixed set of predictors of the course and outcome of schizophrenia, but rather a number of prognostic indicators which allow a judgement to be made about the probability of one or another type of course over a limited time period (usually not exceeding 5 years).

Medium-range predictors

In first-episode cases, male sex, single marital status, premorbid social withdrawal, and insidious onset have been shown by a number of studies to be relatively robust predictors of a poor outcome in the short to medium term (2–5 years), while female sex, being married, having social contacts outside the home, and acute onset predict a relatively good outcome. No consistent findings have been reported for age at onset as a predictor, and the long-term follow-up studies do not lend support to the view that an early onset is associated with a poor prognosis. Similarly, a history of psychotic illness (including schizophrenia) in a first-degree relative does not predict a worse prognosis. On the contrary, in some studies[61] patients with a high familial load were found on follow-up to have a better outcome than patients with no psychotic illness among their close relatives.

A consistent finding of many studies is that the clinical symptoms in either the early or the advanced stages of schizophrenia have a very limited capacity to predict future course and outcome. An exception is the modest predictive power of any clear-cut negative symptoms appearing early in the course of the disorder, or when assessed under the conditions referred to above.

The sociocultural setting, i.e. a developing country or a developed country, was the best predictor of 2-year and 5-year outcome in the WHO studies.[33,38] Exactly what factors may be underlying these marked cultural differences in the prognosis of schizophrenia remains an unresolved issue.

The predictive status of psychophysiological or neurophysiological variables (such as the electrodermal orienting response or rapid eye movement sleep latency), or neurocognitive measurements (sustained attention, event-related potentials or the pre-pulse inhibition of the startle reflex) has not been sufficiently investigated. At least one study[59] found that brain imaging (computed tomography) evidence of cortical atrophy on first admission was a predictor of poor 2-year clinical and social outcome.

Short-term predictors

There is good agreement between different studies on the factors that help predict a relapse of psychotic symptoms after a period of stabilization or remission. Stressful life events[67] and a high expressed emotion index[66] have attracted considerable interest in this regard but are technically difficult to assess. In addition, the expressed emotion measure is only applicable to patients interacting on a daily basis with family members or other persons in the household. In many settings, such patients would be a minority. By and large, the best predictor of relapse in the short term remains the withdrawal of antipsychotic medication, usually due to non-compliance.[68] Cannabis use on a daily basis has been shown to be associated with an increased risk of relapse in a dose–response relationship.[69] Short-term predictors of a good outcome for the episodes are good initial response to neuroleptics[20] and a positive response to placebo.[70]

Summary and conclusions

Studies conducted over many decades consistently demonstrate that schizophrenia presents a broad spectrum of possible outcomes and course patterns, ranging from complete or nearly complete recovery after acute episodes of psychosis to continuous, unremitting illness leading to progressive deterioration of cognitive performance and social functioning. Between these extremes, a substantial proportion

of patients show an episodic course with relapses of psychotic symptoms and partial remissions during which affective and cognitive change becomes increasingly conspicuous and may progress to gross deficits. Although no less than one-third of all patients with schizophrenia have relatively benign outcomes, in the majority the illness has a profound, lifelong impact on personal growth and development. The initial symptoms of the disorder are not strongly predictive of the pattern of course but the mode of onset (acute or insidious), the duration of illness prior to diagnosis and treatment, the presence or absence of comorbid substance use, as well as background variables such as premorbid adjustment (especially during adolescence), marital status, and availability of a social network allow a reasonable accuracy of prediction in the short to medium term (2–5 years).

One of the most striking aspects of the longitudinal course of schizophrenia is the relatively high proportion of patients who improve substantially, or remit, with ageing. What determines the ultimate outcome is far from clear but the view of schizophrenia as an invariably progressive, deteriorating disorder is certainly too limited and does not accord well with the evidence. Similarly, a model of schizophrenia as a static neurodevelopmental encephalopathy decompensating post-adolescence under the influence of a variety of stressors fits only part of the spectrum of course patterns. In a significant proportion of cases, the disorder exhibits the unmistakable features of a shift-like process with acute exacerbations and remissions which may progress to severe deterioration or come to a standstill at any stage. Whether a single underlying pathophysiology can explain the variety of clinical outcomes, or several different pathological processes are at work, remains obscure. It has been suggested that the longitudinal course of schizophrenia should be seen as an open-ended dynamic life process[71] with multiple, interacting biological and psychosocial determinants. Obviously, such issues cannot be resolved by clinical follow-up studies alone, and require a strong involvement of biological research in prospective investigations of representative samples of cases spanning the entire spectrum of course and outcomes. No such studies have been possible until recently, both because of the technical complexity of such an undertaking and because of the tendency to recruit selectively for biological investigations patients from the severe deteriorating part of the spectrum. Overcoming such limitations will be essential to the uncovering of the mechanisms driving the 'natural history' of schizophrenia.

References

1. Kraepelin, E. (1919). *Dementia praecox and paraphrenia*. Livingstone, Edinburgh.
2. van Os, J., Wright, P., and Murray, R.M. (1997). Follow-up studies of schizophrenia I: natural history and non-psychopathological predictors of outcome. *European Psychiatry* **12** (Supplement 5), 327S-41S.
3. Geddes, J.R. and Kendell, R.E. (1995). Schizophrenic subjects with no history of admission to hospital. *Psychological Medicine*, **25**, 859–68.
4. Padmavathi, R., Rajkumar, S., and Srinivasan, T.N. (1998). Schizophrenic patients who were never treated—a study in an Indian urban community. *Psychological Medicine*, **28**, 1113–17.
5. Jonsson, S.A.T. and Jonsson, H. (1992). Outcome in untreated schizophrenia: a search for symptoms and traits with prognostic meaning in patients admitted to a mental hospital in the preneuroleptic era. *Acta Psychiatrica Scandinavica*, **85**, 313–20.

6. Hegarty, J.D., Baldessarini, R.J., Tohen, M., Waternaux, C. and Oepen, G. (1994). One hundred years of schizophrenia: a meta-analysis of the outcome literature. *American Journal of Psychiatry*, **151**, 1409–16.

7. Wyatt, R.J. (1991). Neuroleptics and the natural course of schizophrenia. *Schizophrenia Bulletin*, **17**, 325–51.

8. Ödegaard, O. (1964). Patterns of discharge from Norwegian psychiatric hospitals before and after the introduction of psychotropic drugs. *American Journal of Psychiatry*, **120**, 772–8.

9. Rennie, T.A.C. (1939). Follow-up study of five hundred patients with schizophrenia admitted to the hospital from 1913–1923. *Archives of Neurology and Psychiatry*, **42**, 877–91.

10. Astrup, C. and Noreik, K. (1966). *Functional psychoses—diagnostic and prognostic models*. Charles C. Thomas, Springfield, IL.

11. Brown, G.W., Bone, M., Dalison, B., and Wing, J.K. (1966). *Schizophrenia and social care*. Oxford University Press, London.

12. Bleuler, M. (1972). *Die schizophrenen Geistesstörungen intramuscular Lichte langjähriger Kranken- und Familiengeschichten*. Thieme, Stuttgart. English translation by S.M. Clemens (1978). *The schizophrenic disorders. Long-term patient and family studies*. Yale University Press, New Haven, CT.

13. Ciompi, L. and Müller, C. (1976). *Lebensweg und Alter der Schizophrenen. Eine katamnestische Langzeitstudie bis ins Senium*. Springer, Berlin.

14. Huber, G., Gross, G., Schüttler, R., and Linz, M. (1980). Longitudinal studies of schizophrenic patients. *Schizophrenia Bulletin*, **6**, 592–605.

15. Tsuang, M., Woolson, R., and Fleming, J. (1979). Long-term outcome of major psychoses: I. Schizophrenia and affective disorders compared with psychiatrically symptom-free surgical conditions. *Archives of General Psychiatry*, **36**, 1295–301.

16. Harding, C., Brooks, G.W., Ashikaga, T., *et al.* (1987). The Vermont longitudinal study of persons with severe mental illness: I. Methodology, study sample, and overall status 32 years later. *American Journal of Psychiatry*, **144**, 718–26.

17. Ogawa, K., Miya, M., Watarai, A., Nakazawa, M., Yuasa, S., and Utena, H. (1987). A long-term follow-up study of schizophrenia in Japan—with special reference to the course of social adjustment. *British Journal of Psychiatry*, **151**, 758–65.

18. Shepherd, M., Watt, D., Falloon, I., *et al.* (1989). The natural history of schizophrenia: a five-year follow-up study of outcome and prediction in a representative sample of schizophrenics. *Psychological Medicine*, Monograph Supplement 15. Cambridge University Press.

19. Carone, B.J., Harrow, M., and Westermeyer, J.F. (1991). Posthospital course and outcome in schizophrenia. *Archives of General Psychiatry*, **48**, 247–53.

20. Breier, A., Schreiber, J.L., Dyer, J., and Pickar, D. (1991). National Institute of Mental Health longitudinal study of chronic schizophrenia. *Archives of General Psychiatry*, **48**, 239–46.

21. Johnstone, E.C. *et al.* (1991). Background, method, and general description of the sample. *British Journal of Psychiatry*, **159** (Supplement 13), pp. 7–20.

22. Marneros, A., Deister, A., and Rohde, A. (1992). Comparison of long-term outcome of schizophrenic, affective and schizoaffective disorders. *British Journal of Psychiatry*, **161** (Supplement 18), 44–51.

23. Thara, R., Henrietta, M., Joseph, A., Rajkumar, S., and Eaton, W.W. (1994). Ten-year course of schizophrenia—the Madras longitudinal study. *Acta Psychiatrica Scandinavica*, **90**, 329–36.

24. Mason, P., Harrison, G., Glazebrook, C., Medley, I., Dalkin, T., and Croudace, T. (1995). Characteristics of outcome in schizophrenia at 13 years. *British Journal of Psychiatry*, **167**, 596–603.

25. Wieselgren, I.M. and Lindström, L.H. (1996). A prospective 1–5 year outcome study in first-admitted and readmitted schizophrenic patients: relationship to heredity, premorbid adjustment, duration of disease and education level at index admission and neuroleptic treatment. *Acta Psychiatrica Scandinavica*, **93**, 9–19.

26. Wiersma, D., Nienhuis, F.J., Sloof, C.J., and Giel, R. (1998). Natural course of schizophrenic disorders: a 15-year follow-up of a Dutch incidence cohort. *Schizophrenia Bulletin*, **24**, 75–85.

27. Ganev, K., Onchev, G., and Ivanov, P. (1998). A 16-year follow-up study of schizophrenia and related disorders in Sofia, Bulgaria. *Acta Psychiatrica Scandinavica*, **98**, 200–7.

28. Ciompi, L. (1980). Catamnestic long-term study on the course of life and aging of schizophrenics. *Schizophrenia Bulletin*, **6**, 606–18.

29. Feighner, J.P., Robins, E., Guze, S.B., Woodruff, R.A., Winokur, G., and Munoz, R. (1972). Diagnostic criteria for use in psychiatric research. *Archives of General Psychiatry*, **26**, 77–83.

30. Thara, R., Henrietta, M., Joseph, A., Rajkumar, S., and Eaton, W.W. (1994). Ten-year course of schizophrenia—the Madras longitudinal study. *Acta Psychiatrica Scandinavica*, **90**, 329–36.

31. Strauss, J.S. and Carpenter, W.T. (1972). The prediction of outcome in schizophrenia. I. Characteristics of outcome. *Archives of General Psychiatry*, **27**, 739–46.

32. Marengo, J. (1994). Classifying the courses of schizophrenia. *Schizophrenia Bulletin*, **20**, 519–36.

33. World Health Organization (1979). *Schizophrenia. An international follow-up study*. Wiley, Chichester.

34. Ciompi, L. (1984). Is there really a schizophrenia? The long-term course of psychotic phenomena. *British Journal of Psychiatry*, **145**, 636–40.

35. McGlashan, T.H. and Johannessen, J.O. (1996). Early detection and intervention with schizophrenia: rationale. *Schizophrenia Bulletin*, **22**, 201–22.

36. Hambrecht, M., Häfner, H., and Löffler, W. (1994). Beginning schizophrenia observed by significant others. *Social Psychiatry and Psychiatric Epidemiology*, **29**, 53–60.

37. Leff, J., Sartorius, N., Jablensky, A., Korten, A., and Ernberg, G. (1992). The International Pilot Study of Schizophrenia: five-year follow-up findings. *Psychological Medicine*, **22**, 131–45.

38. Jablensky, A., Sartorius, N., Ernberg, G., *et al.* (1992). *Schizophrenia: manifestations, incidence and course in different cultures. A World Health Organization ten-country study*. Psychological Medicine Monograph Supplement 20. Cambridge University Press.

39. Jablensky, A., Schwarz, R., and Tomov, T. (1980). WHO collaborative study of impairments and disabilities associated with schizophrenic disorders. *Acta Psychiatrica Scandinavica Supplementum*, **285**, 152–63.

40. Goldman, D., Brown, G.L., Albaugh, B., *et al.* (1994). D$_2$ receptor genotype and linkage disequilibrium and function in Finnish, American Indian, and US Caucasian patients. In *Genetic approaches to mental disorders* (ed. E.S. Gershon and C.R. Cloninger), pp. 327–44. American Psychiatric Press, Washington, DC.

41. Waxler, N.E. (1979). Is the outcome for schizophrenia better in non-industrial societies? The case of Sri Lanka. *Journal of Nervous and Mental Diseases*, **167**, 144–58.

42. Bhugra, D., Leff, J., Mallett, R., Der, G., Corridan, B., and Rudge, S. (1997). Incidence and outcome of schizophrenia in Whites, African-Caribbeans and Asians in London. *Psychological Medicine*, **27**, 791–8.

43. Loebel, A.D., Lieberman, J.A., Alvir, J.M.J., Geisler, S.H., Szymanski, S.R., and Mayerhoff, D.I. (1992). Duration of psychosis and outcome in first-episode schizophrenia. *American Journal of Psychiatry*, **149**, 1183–8.

44. Hoffman, R.E. and McGlashan, T.H. (1993). Parallel distributed processing and the emergence of schizophrenic symptoms. *Schizophrenia Bulletin*, **19**, 119–40.

45. Falloon, I.R.H. (1992). Early intervention for first episodes of schizophrenia: a preliminary exploration. *Psychiatry*, **55**, 4–15.

46. McGorry, P.D., Edwards, J., Mihalopoulos, C., Harrigan, S.M., and Jackson, H.J. (1996). EPPIC: an evolving system of early detection and optimal management. *Schizophrenia Bulletin*, **22**, 305–6.

47. Goldberg, T.E., Hyde, T.M., Kleinman, J.E., and Weinberger, D.R. (1993). Course of schizophrenia: neuropsychological evidence for a static encephalopathy. *Schizophrenia Bulletin*, **19**, 797–804.

48. Gupta, S., Andreasen, N.C., Arndt, S., Flaum, M., Hubbard, W.C., and Ziebell, S. (1997). The Iowa longitudinal study of recent onset psychosis:

one-year follow-up of first episode patients. *Schizophrenia Research*, 23, 1–13.

49. Szymanski, S.R., Cannon, T.D., Gallacher, F., Erwin, R.J., and Gur, R.E. (1996). Course and treatment response in first-episode and chronic schizophrenia. *American Journal of Psychiatry*, 153, 519–25.

50. Sheldrick, C., Jablensky, A., Sartorius, N., and Shepherd, M. (1977). Schizophrenia succeeded by affective illness: catamnestic study and statistical enquiry. *Psychological Medicine*, 7, 619–24.

51. Schneider, K. (1959). *Clinical psychopathology* (transl. M.W. Hamilton). Grune and Stratton, New York.

52. Fenton, W.S. and McGlashan, T.H. (1991). Natural history of schizophrenia subtypes. I. Longitudinal study of paranoid, hebephrenic, and undifferentiated schizophrenia. *Archives of General Psychiatry*, 48, 969–77.

53. Leonhard, K. (1979). *The classification of endogenous psychoses* (5th edn) (transl. R. Berman). Halsted Press, New York.

54. Stephens, J.H. and Astrup, C. (1963). Prognosis in 'process' and 'non-process' schizophrenia. *American Journal of Psychiatry*, 119, 945–53.

55. Vaillant, G.E. (1978). A 10-year follow up of remitting schizophrenics. *Schizophrenia Bulletin*, 4, 78–84.

56. Angst, J., Felder, W., and Lohmeyer, B. (1980). Course of schizoaffective psychoses: results of a follow up study. *Schizophrenia Bulletin*, 6, 579–85.

57. Harder, D.W., Strauss, J.S., Greenwald, D.F., *et al.* (1990). Predictors of outcome among adult psychiatric first-admissions. *Journal of Clinical Psychology*, 46, 120–8.

58. Jørgensen, P.M., Mortensen, P.B., and Machon, R.A. (1991). Hospitalization patterns in schizophrenia. A 13-year follow-up. *Schizophrenia Research*, 4, 1–9.

59. Vita, A. *et al.* (1991). CT scan abnormalities and outcome of chronic schizophrenia. *American Journal of Psychiatry*, 148, 1577–9.

60. Eaton W.W. *et al.* (1992). Long-term course of hospitalization for schizophrenia: Part I. Risk for rehospitalization. *Schizophrenia Bulletin*, 18, 217–27.

61. Johnstone, E.C., Frith, C.D., Lang, F.H., and Owens, D.G.C. (1995). Determinants of the extremes of outcome in schizophrenia. *British Journal of Psychiatry*, 167, 604–9.

62. Harrison, G., Croudace, T., Mason, P., Glazebrook, C., and Medley, I. (1996). Predicting the long-term outcome of schizophrenia. *Psychological Medicine*, 26, 697–705.

63. Goldman, M., Tandon, R., DeQuardo, J.R., *et al.* (1996). Biological predictors of 1-year outcome in schizophrenia in males and females. *Schizophrenia Research*, 21, 65–73.

64. Ho, B.C., Nopoulos, P., Flaum, M., Arndt, S., and Andreasen, N. (1988). Two-year outcome in first-episode schizophrenia: predictive value of symptoms for quality of life. *American Journal of Psychiatry*, 155, 1196–201.

65. Castle, D.J., Wessely, S., van Os, J., and Murray, R.M. (1998). *Psychosis in the inner city: the Camberwell first episode study*. Psychology Press, Hove.

66. Leff, J.P., Wig, N.N., Ghosh, A., *et al.* (1990). Relatives' expressed emotion and the course of schizophrenia in Chandigarh: a two-year follow-up of a first-contact sample. *British Journal of Psychiatry*, 156, 351–6.

67. Brown, G.W. and Birley, J.L.T. (1968). Crises and life changes and the onset of schizophrenia. *Journal of Health and Social Behaviour*, 9, 203–14.

68. Dencker, S.J., Malm, U., and Lepp, M. (1986). Schizophrenic relapse after drug withdrawal is predictable. *Acta Psychiatrica Scandinavica*, 73, 181–5.

69. Linszen, D.H., Dingemans, P.M., and Lenior, M.E. (1994). Cannabis abuse and the course of recent-onset schizophrenic disorders. *Archives of General Psychiatry*, 51, 273–9.

70. Johnstone, E.C., Macmillan, J.F., Frith, C.D., *et al.* (1990). Further investigation of the predictors of outcome following first schizophrenic episodes. *British Journal of Psychiatry*, 157, 182–9.

71. Harding, C.M., Zubin, J., and Strauss, J.S. (1992). Chronicity in schizophrenia revisited. *British Journal of Psychiatry*, 161 (Supplement 18), 27–37.

4.3.7 Treatment and management of schizophrenia

D. G. Cunningham Owens and E. C. Johnstone

Introduction

Historically, therapeutic interventions in patients with psychotic disorders were largely palliative and predicated on essentially psychosocial principles,[1] although the administration of medicines and other physical techniques has been recommended since antiquity[2] and actively employed in Britain for some 300 years.[3]

Over the last 50 to 60 years, a number of physical treatments of schizophrenia have aimed at promoting more specific benefits. Insulin coma, electroconvulsive therapy (**ECT**), and prefrontal leucotomy[4] became widely applied on the basis of enthusiasm rather than scientific study, but since the development of safe and effective medications they have largely fallen into disuse. Since chlorpromazine was introduced in 1952 and shown to have specific antipsychotic properties,[5] numerous antipsychotic agents have come into use, which, along with a range of psychosocial interventions, have been favourably evaluated.

There remains an obvious discrepancy between the generally favourable results of, especially drug, trials in this field and an on-going concern about the difficulties posed by schizophrenia. Some of this can be explained by the difference between responses evident in clinical trials (efficacy) and those that pertain in ordinary circumstances (effectiveness). The unique conditions of the controlled trial provide essential information on which to base rational therapeutic decisions, but not necessarily information that translates to all clinical contexts.

Evidence for efficacy

Drug treatment

Within 15 years of the introduction of chlorpromazine, the efficacy of antipsychotics in schizophrenia became one of the most comprehensively researched areas in psychiatry.[6] In addressing drug efficacy in schizophrenia, however, several different issues need to be considered.[7] These include efficacy in relation to the following:

- 'positive' features
- 'negative' features
- cognitive performance
- non-specific (affective) symptomatology
- behaviour
- maintenance
- treatment resistance.

Table 1 Antipsychotic and placebo response rates in schizophrenia

	Antipsychotic	Placebo
Very much improved	16	1
Much improved	29	11
Improved	16	10
Slightly improved	31	31
Not improved	6	15
Worse	2	33

Data from NIMH Collaborative Study.[9]

'Positive' features

That standard antipsychotic drugs promote resolution of positive symptomatology characterizing acute schizophrenic episodes cannot be doubted. In a review covering the first two decades of antipsychotic use, Davis and Garver[8] found that 86 per cent of controlled studies showed chlorpromazine to be superior to placebo. They also noted that all 26 trials that had used more than 500 mg/day reported chlorpromazine to have definitely greater efficacy than placebo, while in this dose range no trials found only marginal or no benefits.

The question of 'acute' efficacy is now settled to a sufficient degree that further attempts at replication would probably be unethical. Furthermore, this effect, or magnitude of effect, is not shared by other psychotropic agents and can be considered a class effect and a valid basis for classification.

This is not to say that antipsychotics are entirely satisfactory. While these drugs can be dramatically effective in individual cases, overall their efficacy in acute states is only partial. The major first-generation efficacy study,[9] which looked at treatment responses to a phenothiazine of each chemical type (i.e. chlorpromazine, thioridazine, and fluphenazine) in schizophrenic inpatients, showed three things: comparable efficacy for the three active drugs, considerable residual group symptomatology, and a small, but definite, response in the placebo group. Overall, 61 per cent of those who received one of the active drugs were considered 'improved' to 'very much improved'. As a result, it has since been taken that standard antipsychotics produce a satisfactory clinical response in around 60 to 70 per cent of patients with acute schizophrenia, while approximately 6 to 8 per cent do not respond at all.[10] This interpretation is based on exclusion of the placebo response rate (Table 1) which, when taken into account, suggests that significant benefits could be more realistically expected in 40 to 50 per cent of patients. There thus remains substantial room for improvement, even on this primary measure of efficacy.

With one exception, all antipsychotic drugs (standard or new generation) are of equal efficacy on positive schizophrenic symptomatology. The exception is clozapine in treatment-resistant cases, whose advantages may relate only to this specific clinical context.[7]

Despite their limitations, antipsychotics are unquestionably the most satisfactory treatment modality for acute episodes. In a unique study, May[11] compared response rates and outcomes in a large group of schizophrenic patients randomly assigned to one of five treatment regimens: individual psychotherapy alone, antipsychotics alone, individual psychotherapy plus antipsychotics, ECT, and 'milieu' therapy (i.e. a ward environment). Patients who received physical treatments clearly did better in terms of increased rates of discharge, reduced lengths of stay, and decreased need for additional treatments. Two years after discharge, twice as many of those treated with antipsychotics as with psychotherapy were in employment,[12] while in the 3 years post-discharge, the drug-treated patients spent less time back in hospital.[13]

Data from this trial suggested that those not subjected to antipsychotic treatment early on fared less well in terms of long-term outcome than those who had received it in the initial phase of the investigation. This topic has assumed considerable prominence in recent years and the impression is that early intervention is associated with a better outcome than a policy of 'wait and see'.[14] The implication is that antipsychotic drugs achieve their best results when administered as soon after the onset of illness as possible. How long is 'soon' remains unclear, although there is a suggestion that those with first episodes in whom exposure is delayed for longer than 12 months may have a worse long-term outcome than those coming to treatment earlier.[15] This has raised concerns that even brief periods of abstinence, as might be associated with participation in placebo trials, may be detrimental, but available evidence does not support this.[16]

In recent years, a new generation of antipsychotics has been developed, with clozapine the instrument of change. Pharmacologists first applied the term 'atypical' to the benzamides following the widespread launch of sulpiride in the late 1970s, but it was unclear whether the clinical profiles of these drugs were sufficiently different to merit the designation, especially with dose-equivalent usage.[7] Clozapine is unquestionably different and was the first drug that could be legitimately called 'atypical' on clinical grounds. However, a general definition of 'atypicality' remains elusive. Criteria proposed by Lieberman[17] include the following:

(1) enhanced efficacy (i.e. in treatment-resistant cases);

(2) no, or only slight and ill-sustained, elevations of prolactin levels;

(3) most importantly of all, strikingly reduced liability to promote extrapyramidal dysfunction.

The development of new-generation antipsychotics has resulted in a revival of basic and comparative efficacy studies. Results from studies of risperidone,[18] olanzapine,[19] quetiapine,[20] amisulpride,[21] and zotepine[22] (at the time of writing, the compounds that have been commercially launched) have shown each of these drugs to possess antipsychotic efficacy which, on present evidence, appears comparable to each other and a standard comparitor. (Sertindole, an antipsychotic of proven efficacy, was withdrawn in December 1998 amid continuing concerns about its cardiac actions.)

Where the new-generation drugs appear to have advantage is in neurological tolerability,[5] although it is as yet hard to quantify the extent of this. New-generation drugs seem to have a reduced liability to promote acute dystonias, and are associated with lower levels of parkinsonism and akathisia. While it would seem reasonable to conclude that these benefits will translate into reduced rates of tardive motor disorders also, for which some supportive data have been presented,[23,24] firm evidence for this remains to be accrued.

'Negative' features

The issue of whether antipsychotics exert therapeutic efficacy on negative schizophrenic features became of importance largely because of the implications of Crow's type I/type II hypothesis.[25] The inference of this is that drugs exerting beneficial effects on positive features, i.e. antipsychotics, would be unlikely to exert similar therapeutic effects

Table 2 The classification of 'negative' states in schizophrenia

Primary	Authentic schizophrenic state
Secondary	Positive symptomatology
	Depressed mood
	Extrapyramidal disorder
	Early dysphoria
	Bradykinesia
	Psychosocial isolation

After Carpenter et al.[29]

on negative features, owing to the differing pathological substrates proposed for the two states—a structural one for negative states, and a functional (i.e. dopaminergic) disruption for positive symptomatology. Although this hypothesis was originally formulated when only standard drugs were available, the issues it raises have become even more pertinent with the introduction of new-generation compounds.

One of the strongest challenges to Crow's hypothesis came from Goldberg.[26] Reviewing five of the early placebo-controlled American efficacy studies, he clearly demonstrated that what he defined as negative features did respond to antipsychotic treatment. Other investigators, using more modern rating instruments, have also demonstrated similar beneficial effects. However, such findings are not unanimous and, importantly, in some studies, ratings of negative features have been found to covary with positive ratings,[27] raising the question of whether negative features are in fact state dependent.[28]

The key factor is the lack of consensus about what comprises negativity, which makes it difficult to evaluate drug efficacy. Historically, the problem of 'negativity' in schizophrenia was defined longitudinally and primarily in terms of psychosocial functioning. It is the cross-sectional requirements of psychopharmacological research that have raised the conceptual difficulties. Carpenter and colleagues have emphasized the varied clinical states that can present similarly and the need to bear in mind a differential diagnosis[29] (Table 2). If one's concept of negativity encompasses the withdrawal and reserve of those preoccupied with hallucinations or delusions, then negative features are likely to resolve as part of the symptomatic response to antipsychotics—and standardized ratings of each domain will covary. While this is clearly a therapeutic action, it does not address the fundamental issue.

A major confound in assessing trial data in this field is the bradykinesia of drug-related parkinsonism. After nearly half a century, the boundaries of the parkinsonian syndrome associated with antipsychotic drug use remain undefined, particularly in relation to subjective symptomatology.[5] Improvements in negativity on changing from one drug to another may say more about differing liabilities to promote extrapyramidal disorder than about actions on primary negative features.

This issue is of crucial importance in evaluating claims made for new-generation drugs, where improvements in negative features are likely to reflect tolerability rather than efficacy. Sophisticated statistical applications, such as path analysis, which can be used to substantiate a therapeutic action for some new antipsychotics[30,31] do not address the issue, as the problem lies at the clinical, and not the statistical, level. The evidence to date is that even the undoubted benefits of clozapine are restricted to secondary negative symptomatology and reflect that compound's unique neurological tolerability.[32]

Carpenter et al.[33] have also emphasized 'durability' as a defining criterion of the 'deficit' syndrome. By reintroducing longitudinal evaluation, this is much more akin to the historical concept of schizophrenic negativity. It is of interest that this group found the benefits of clozapine on negative features were confined to patients who did not conform to criteria for a 'deficit' state.[34]

Crow's hypothesis has not yet been disproven, and it remains to be shown that antipsychotics exert any therapeutic benefits on primary negative schizophrenic symptomatology. This conclusion applies to new-generation compounds as much as to standard drugs.

Cognitive performance

Recently, attention has focused on the question of whether antipsychotic drugs in general possess, as one of their target actions, therapeutic efficacy on specific aspects of cognition and, increasingly, whether certain compounds exert preferential actions in this regard.[35]

Evaluation of the cognitive effects of antipsychotics faces major methodological problems and the contradictory nature of findings in this field have been highlighted in several reviews.[35–37] Standard antipsychotics have been reported to initially impair aspects of attention and motor behaviour which improve with continued exposure, while working memory and long-term recall do not appear to be fundamentally affected.[35] Beyond this, it is hard to extract a consensus—a conclusion that also applies to studies of new-generation drugs.

In terms of assessment measures, performance tests of executive function that are not timed tend to be insensitive to antipsychotic effects, while paced (i.e. timed) tests are affected.[37] Clearly, certain findings in this field may reflect neurological status.

Non-specific symptomatology

For many schizophrenic patients, affective symptomatology is a prominent part of the clinical picture[38] but the efficacy of antipsychotics on these features has been poorly researched. Their value in the treatment of anxiety experienced during acute episodes has not been systematically addressed and rests largely on clinical wisdom.

There is a long tradition, mainly in Continental Europe, of attributing antidepressant actions to antipsychotic drugs administered in low doses, at which they may exert preferential actions at presynaptic dopaminergic (autoreceptor) sites.[39] Trial evidence has focused on flupenthixol[40] and the L-enantiomer of sulpiride[41] and, more recently, amisulpride. It is unlikely that such an action would be relevant to long-term maintenance in schizophrenia, where the doses used are still considerably above those reportedly associated with antidepressant actions.

A greater concern is whether antipsychotics may contribute to depressive mood change. At one time they were implicated as being 'depressogenic', particularly when administered in depot formulation.[42] This, again, raises the difficulty of distinguishing between similar presentations of pathophysiologically different states. Van Putten and May[43] described a state of dysphoric mood change resembling depression which they referred to as 'akinetic depression'. As this state resolved following administration of an anticholinergic, it is hard to see it as other than a subjective manifestation of bradykinesia.

Depression is a common feature of schizophrenia prior to introduction of medication and it has been shown that depressed mood tends to resolve as positive psychotic symptomatology diminishes.[44]

As with negative states, such findings probably reflect symptom co-variation.

Behaviour

Efficacy studies of antipsychotics seldom consider behaviour as a separate dimension of disorder. It is clear, however, that particular, largely confrontational, behaviours such as hostility, belligerence, and resistiveness do improve with antipsychotic treatment.[6] This is usually taken as secondary to improvements in other domains, especially positive features.

However, behavioural disorganization in schizophrenia may not reflect a single dimension of disorder. In long-stay patients, behavioural disturbance appears to correlate with negative symptomatology and not positive.[45] Antipsychotics are thus unlikely to be efficacious in treating all behavioural disorders with which schizophrenic patients may present.

Maintenance

The long-term use of antipsychotic drugs in the treatment of schizophrenia is most frequently aimed at minimizing the risk of florid exacerbations of a disorder usually characterized by some persisting symptomatology. Hence, the term 'maintenance' is preferable to 'prophylaxis'.

The efficacy of antipsychotics in preventing relapse has also been extensively investigated and is beyond doubt.[46] Despite this, it remains difficult to quantify this effect, as the published literature presents figures that are widely discrepant. Nonetheless, reviewing the randomized, double-blind trials of antipsychotic versus placebo covering variable follow-up intervals, Janicak et al. concluded that on average 55 per cent of those on placebo relapsed compared with 21 per cent on active medication.[46] Statistically, these figures provide overwhelming support for the maintenance action of antipsychotics (1×10^{-7}).

Such comparisons are compelling, but studies addressing the question of long-term maintenance tend to be biased towards patients who have already shown a degree of response. There is reason to question whether the magnitude of the antipsychotic effect, at least over longer than 12 to 24 months, is as great in routine practice as trial-based analyses suggest.[47]

While most studies have concerned patients with established recurrent illness, there is additional evidence that long-term treatment is effective in preventing relapse after first episodes also. In the Northwick Park First Episodes Study,[15] significantly more patients in the placebo group than in the active treatment group relapsed over 2 years (62 per cent versus 46 per cent respectively: $p < 0.002$).

In understanding the benefits and principles of long-term antipsychotic administration, several issues need to be addressed:

- the natural history of relapse
- the history of relapse following successful maintenance/prophylaxis
- practice choices
- the pattern of intervention
- adjunctive measures.

The natural history of relapse

Drawing from three large maintenance studies[48–50] an average constant rate of relapse can be calculated at 11.5 per cent per month. Thus,

in any population of schizophrenic patients around 10 per cent will relapse each month after cessation of antipsychotic treatment.

Davis et al.[51] plotted relapse rates over a 2-year placebo follow-up period and showed that relapses tended to occur along an exponential function. This indicates a progressive and *regular* rate of relapse over time, and suggests that time to relapse may be a fixed aspect of the illness which is characteristic to each individual.

The history of relapse following successful maintenance/prophylaxis

A pertinent clinical question relates to how long medication should be continued in patients in whom stable maintenance has been achieved. Johnson[52] compared patients discontinuing antipsychotics with matched patients remaining on drugs, all of whom had been stable for one of three distinct periods: 1 to 2 years, 2 to 3 years, or 3 to 4 years. Relapse rates at 18 months were similar in all three groups who stopped, regardless of how long they had been stable beforehand (80 per cent, 90 per cent, and 70 per cent, respectively), and substantially higher than those who remained on treatment (35 per cent, 15 per cent, and 19 per cent, respectively). Others have come to the same conclusion using intervals of from 12 months to almost 8 years.[53–55] A similar picture of relapse has also been established in target populations selected on the specific basis of having responded particularly well to long-term medication and hence predicted as being of high likelihood to maintain well being.[56]

The implication seems to be that, no matter the duration or quality of well being on antipsychotic medication, relapse is inevitable following discontinuation in those with an established relapsing–remitting pattern of illness, with a time course that, in general, is consistent for each individual.

Practice choices

There is no evidence that any one drug is better than any other for long-term maintenance if one's 'endpoint' is relapse, although there is persuasive, if largely anecdotal, evidence that in terms of quality-of-life parameters, clozapine offers superior benefits.[57]

There is powerful evidence that the choice of a depot formulation is associated with substantial improvements in relapse prevention. Support for the value of depot over oral administration comes largely form 'mirror-image' studies, which compare a period on depot with a corresponding period prior to starting depot, in terms of, primarily, time spent in hospital. Six such studies were unanimous in showing a substantial reduction of time spent in hospital after the switch to depot (range 55–90 per cent; average 77.8 per cent).[58] There is no evidence that depots are themselves inherently more efficacious in maintenance. Their advantage seems to spring entirely from the enhanced compliance that ensues from their long-term use.

The other treatment practice variable is dosage. There is substantial evidence that long-term, low-dose antipsychotic regimens are associated with an increased risk of relapse. This has been investigated mainly in relation to depots, particularly fluphenazine decanoate. Kane et al.[59] found 1.25 to 5 mg every two weeks to be significantly less effective than 25 mg, a finding supported by other authors and with other preparations.[60–63]

Interpretation of such data is, nonetheless, not clear, and applying a dose–response model, Baldessarini et al.[47] have argued that in long-term treatment the half-maximal effective doses (ED_{50}) may be as low as one-fifth to one-tenth those normally employed. Even the statistical findings of the studies above indicate that *some* individual patients may be successfully maintained on low-dose depot regimens. Kane and colleagues showed that while relapse rates were higher in the low-dose group, neurological adverse effects and psychosocial/quality-of-life parameters were superior.[59] Similarly, the Northwick Park First Episodes Study found that at endpoint, significantly fewer of those treated with active drug achieved some specific advance or attainment in their life than those on placebo.[64] This raises concern that maintenance antipsychotic treatment may have hidden costs.

Pattern of intervention

A further question is whether it is better to support long-term remission via a continuous regimen of administration or whether equal benefits can accrue from interventions targeted on early relapse, identified in prodromal symptomatology. The latter has strong intuitive appeal, especially to patients, but the trial evidence is, alas, not encouraging. None of the controlled studies to investigate the issue found advantage in targeted intervention, and in a meta-analysis of published data, Davis et al.[58] calculated that while relapse rates in those continuously treated were 25 per cent, the corresponding figure for those on targeted intervention was 50 per cent ($p < 1 \times 10^{-20}$). While this approach may have merit in carefully selected individuals, it cannot be recommended as a routine strategy. A further potential caution to the use of intermittent treatment regimens is the increasing concern that this pattern of drug utilization may increase the risk of tardive dyskinesia.[5]

Adjunctive measures

While antipsychotics can clearly protect against relapse, it has also been strongly advocated that additional benefits can be achieved when medication is combined with other forms of management, especially social/family interventions. This principle has considerable support in the literature,[58] although difficulties persist with most studies.

Treatment resistance

Treatment resistance came to prominence following publication of the United States' multicentre clozapine study,[65] one of the most influential studies of recent years. Within an operationally defined concept of treatment resistance, Kane and colleagues found that while 30 per cent of those on clozapine improved, only 4 per cent of those on the comparison regimen of chlorpromazine and benztropine improved ($p < 0.001$). This was the first time that superior efficacy could be attributed to an antipsychotic drug, although the population to which this conclusion applied was circumscribed and the criteria for 'improvement' were modest.

Although enhanced efficacy has been claimed 'by association' for other new-generation antipsychotics (where comparable efficacy has been shown with clozapine as comparitor), specific tests of their advantages in operationally defined treatment resistance have not always shown these drugs to be superior to standard treatments.[66]

Psychosocial interventions

Controlled studies of psychosocial interventions are less extensive than those concerning drug treatments, and assessments in many of the studies have not been blind, but it is possible for the psychosocial therapy of schizophrenia to be evidence based.

The major types of intervention are as follows:

• psychodynamic psychotherapy

• social skills training and illness self-management programmes

• family interventions

• cognitive-behavioural therapy.

A further group, while strictly relating more to administrative measures, may nonetheless be conveniently considered here:

• alternatives to hospitalization.

Psychodynamic psychotherapy

Analytical psychotherapy was widely used in the first half of this century and continues occasionally to be utilized, although usually in combination with antipsychotic medication. The studies of May and colleagues, mentioned above, provide no support for the view that psychotherapy is an appropriate treatment for first-episode schizophrenia.

Gunderson et al.[67] reported a randomized trial comparison of two forms of psychotherapy in schizophrenia: reality adaptive–supportive, which focused on practical problems, and exploratory insight-oriented psychotherapy. The latter was stated to be the more effective in terms of 'ego-functioning' but was clearly less effective than reality adaptive–supportive in terms of measures of rehospitalization and vocational and social adjustment.

Social skills training and illness self-management programmes

Social skills training refers to a structured learning-oriented approach towards the acquisition of skills relevant to the individual and the demands of his or her environment.[68] The studies of Claghorn et al.[69] in which emphasis was put upon tasks of daily living, and of Malm,[70] which stressed communication skills, both demonstrated effectiveness in terms of enhanced insight and socialization. Spencer et al.[71] compared social skills treatment with group discussion in a sample of chronic schizophrenic patients and found that conversational skills were improved in the social skills treatment group but not in the others, with improvements maintained at 2-month follow-up. Hogarty et al.[72] studied family psychoeducation, social skills training, and maintenance chemotherapy in the aftercare of schizophrenic patients, considering the effects after 1 and 2 years. They found an additive beneficial effect of social skills and family therapy after 1 year but this was less after the second year. Dobson et al.[73] randomized 33 schizophrenic patients to social skills training or milieu therapy and found that at 3 months there was a reduction in negative symptoms in the social skills as compared with the milieu therapy group.

Benton and Schroeder[74] conducted a meta-analysis of 27 studies of social skills training and found benefits in terms of assertiveness, general social skills, and speed of discharge. There was a possible reduction in relapse rates and limited evidence for generalization of skills and of their maintenance. Generalization of skills is an important issue for social skills training. Skills are generally taught in a role-play situation, and although some studies have indicated that behaviour learned in this way will generalize to unprompted situations,[75] some reviews have concluded that it is not clear that changes in treatment settings generalize to community settings.[76]

Individuals with substantial cognitive deficits and/or high levels of conceptual disorganization are poor candidates for most social skills training programmes. Illness self-management is an element of a number of these, but this particular area of patients' functioning has been more specifically addressed in separate plans of psychosocial management. Eckman et al.[77] studied the effects of an intensive, twice-weekly group programme directed to illness management which included video modelling, role playing and problem-solving activities. Patients received focused instructions, active coaching, and homework. This package was compared to a similarly intensive, supportive psychotherapy group. The package resulted in improved self-management in medication but little change in symptom levels. Linszen et al.[78] reported that a programme of illness self-management was alone as effective in reducing relapses as it was when combined with a family intervention.

Therefore available trials offer support for various types of social training in relevant skills. In general they have not been assessed on a blind basis. However, it has been shown[66,79] that this can be done successfully using edited video recordings.

Family interventions

Forms of management for schizophrenia focusing upon the patient's family arose from the observation that criticism and hostility on the part of close relatives was an important determinant of relapse.[80] Such criticism and hostility was referred to as high 'expressed emotion', and forms of management designed to reduce this were devised. They combined attempts to improve family interactions with education about the disorder and direct advice about dealing with crises etc. Such packages have been extensively evaluated and their efficacy demonstrated, but which of the diverse elements is necessary for that efficacy is still unclear.[81,82]

Leff and colleagues have published a series of studies comparing education and relatives' groups with family therapy designed to reduce high expressed emotion. They found that relapse rates were reduced in those patients who remained on medication and whose relatives participated in family therapy.[83,84] It was concluded that reduction of expressed emotion and of time in face-to-face contact were important elements in determining the efficacy of this approach, although the authors acknowledge the difficulties of persuading relatives to participate in this type of intervention. Tarrier and colleagues have found essentially similar results.[85,86]

Family education and social skills training were also examined by Hogarty et al.[87] in 103 patients with schizophrenia and schizoaffective psychosis from high expressed emotion households. Relapse rates over 1 year were reduced by about 20 per cent by both treatments. It was concluded that some of the benefit was attributable to high expressed emotion reduction but that on-going antipsychotic medication was essential for schizophrenic patients in high expressed emotion households and that the effect of family therapy was in terms of delaying, rather than preventing, relapse. Glick et al.[88] reported that family education improved symptom ratings over 6 months, while McFarlane et al.,[89] comparing psychoeducation in single family and multiple family treatment styles, showed advantages for the multiple family groups, and suggested that family support may have been the important element.

A meta-analysis of family intervention studies in the Cochrane database found that these reduce relapse rates by about 50 per cent for up to 2 years, and that medication compliance is similarly improved.[90] It was calculated that about six families need to be treated to prevent one relapse. It is therefore clear that family interventions are effective. The extent to which this effectiveness relates to improved compliance with medication, encouragement of realistic expectations, increased family involvement in clinical decision-making, improved family interaction, or indeed reduction of criticism and hostility towards the patient, is unclear.

These issues are underlined by the findings of a large multicentre study in which patients were allocated to one of three antipsychotic drug regimens and either supportive or intensive family treatment strategies.[61] There were clear advantages for standard as opposed to low or intermittent antipsychotic regimens, but no differences could be demonstrated between the two family interventions.

Cognitive-behavioural therapy

In recent years, controlled trials of cognitive-behavioural therapy in schizophrenia have been published. Tarrier et al.[91] randomly allocated 27 patients with residual symptoms on antipsychotic medication to coping strategy enhancement or problem solving, and compared them with 22 patients allocated to a waiting list condition. Both treatments reduced positive symptoms, but not negative symptoms or social functioning. Drury et al.[92] undertook a trial of cognitive-behavioural therapy in drug-treated patients with 'acute non-affective psychosis'. Subjects were randomized to cognitive therapy or equivalent hours of therapeutic input. Of 117 patients, 69 satisfied inclusion criteria and 62 were randomly allocated to the two treatments, but 22 were withdrawn, essentially for non-cooperation. Both groups showed a decline in symptoms, but this was more marked ($p < 0.001$) in the cognitive therapy group. The authors emphasize that the study was not blind and observe that blindness is not possible in studies of psychosocial interventions, though as noted above, this is not now the case.[66,79]

The London–East Anglia randomized controlled trial of cognitive-behavioural therapy for psychosis[93,94] allocated 60 patients with at least one positive schizophrenic symptom resistant to medication to cognitive-behavioural therapy + standard care, or standard care. Fifty per cent of the cognitive-behavioural therapy group, as compared with 31 per cent of the control group, improved over 9 months. A major determinant of improvement with cognitive-behavioural therapy was 'cognitive flexibility concerning delusions'.[94]

Cognitive remediation has recently been applied to the care of schizophrenic patients, where the desired endpoint is not symptom reduction but amelioration of cognitive deficits. Benedict et al.[95] compared 16 patients who received computerized vigilance task training with 17 who did not. The training improved task performance. Vollema et al.[96] found that performance on the Wisconsin Card Sorting Test was improved by training but not financial reward, while Corigan et al.[97] comparing the effects of a 1-h session of vigilance with and without memory training on social cue recognition in 40 patients randomized to these two conditions, found that the combined training had greater benefits. (See also Chapter 6.3.2.4.)

Alternatives to hospitalization

Several randomized controlled trials have demonstrated that alternatives to hospitalization can be successful. Assertive (or intensive) case treatment involves multidisciplinary teams with high staff/patient ratios, working assertively with patients on an 'as-required' basis to avoid hospitalization. Case management involves a designated key worker writing out a care plan for each patient and reviewing progress in meeting their needs via a number of agencies. In randomized controlled studies of mentally ill people not specified as having schizophrenia, Rosenheck et al.[98] and Quinlivan et al.[99] reported that, as compared with standard care, assertive case treatment reduced inpatient service use and reduced overall care costs. Aberg-Wistedt *et al.*[100] studying schizophrenic patients, reported that assertive case treatment (in comparison with standard care) reduced the burden upon relatives and increased the patients' social networks. On the other hand, Telles *et al.*[101] found that case management and a family management programme appeared to be associated with increased symptomatology in schizophrenic patients.

Case management has been the subject of a meta-analysis in the Cochrane database. Marshall *et al.*[102] in a review of nine studies, found that case management does lead to increase in contact with patients but doubles the rates of hospital admission and is not associated with any definite improvements in symptomatology or social functioning.

Principles of treatment and management

Preliminaries

Medically, 'treatment' and 'management' are often used synonymously. In dealing with the complexities of schizophrenia, however, 'treatment', with its narrower, patient-orientated, and medical connotations, is best restricted to primarily psychopharmacological issues targeted on dimensions of efficacy while the latter is more appropriate to broader care issues. The views expressed here are the authors' own and relate to work within the United Kingdom context. They will not be shared by all others, and the strategies we suggest will not always be appropriate in the very different circumstances of some other countries.

The doctor confronted with a patient believed to be acutely psychotic must address three preliminary questions.

(1) Can the clinical situation be dealt with informally or are compulsory powers required?

(2) Does the patient require admission or can they be managed as an outpatient?

(3) Must medication be started immediately or is it legitimate to observe the evolution of the illness over time?

The answer to the first question will depend on a thorough risk assessment. The latter has already been addressed. Research and clinical experience indicate that not all acutely ill patients will require admission, although in certain scenarios admission should be a priority (Table 3).

Admission provides the psychiatrist with a number of advantages, including the following:

• adequate observation to delineate the extent of symptomatology

• comprehensive assessment of risk

• establishing a solid therapeutic alliance

• stabilization of medication in a supervised environment in which rapid changes of plan can be implemented swiftly and safely

• ready opportunities for avoiding or treating psychiatric emergencies.

Table 3 Considerations in relation to admission policies in patients with acute schizophrenia

Supporting admission	Supporting non-admission

Unstable mental state
  Rapidly extending content
  Variable affect
	Mental state disorder stable/slowly evolving

Imperative auditory hallucinations
  To harm self
  To harm others
	Absent/no will to act

Marked affective change
  Suspiciousness, anger
  Depression
	Affective change mild/amenable to reassurance

Behavioural disturbance
  Disorganization
  Dangerousness
  Commission
  Omission
	Minimal behavioural disturbance/risk of harm

Cognitive disturbance
  Lack of insight
  Impaired attention/distractability
  Inability to comprehend advice
  Hopelessness/suicidal ideation
	No barrier to engagement

Inadequate social support
  Living alone
  Vagrancy/neglect
	Good social supports

Any (other) reason for non-compliance	Likelihood of compliance

Medical state
  Intercurrent physical illness
  Substance misuse/dependency
	Physically fit

'Asylum'	Aversion to inpatient care

However, there is an important additional advantage from the patient's, and often the carer's, point of view: inpatient facilities can provide that security and support which define the cardinal elements of 'asylum'.

Identifying goals and defining structure

The key to avoiding confusion and 'decision paralysis' in dealing with the complex clinical situations schizophrenia presents is to delineate the structure within which it is hoped to achieve a series of treatment/management goals.

The acute phase

Goals

The acute phase is characterized by the perception of significant change in well being. The goals of treatment are as follows:

(1) controlling intrusive non-specific symptomatology, such as anxiety, agitation, and, especially, insomnia;

(2) ensuring the safety and well being of the patient and others by containing chaotic and socially damaging behaviour;

(3) engaging the patient in therapeutic recommendations, and gaining consent for treatment plans (mental state permitting);

(4) implementing an appropriate foundation drug regimen;

(5) stabilizing productive symptomatology;

(6) preventing psychiatric emergencies where possible, and treating them appropriately where unavoidable.

Stabilization of 'positive' symptomatology is the ultimate, but not the first, goal of this phase. It is important not to overlook other goals that can be achieved quickly while awaiting specific antipsychotic efficacy.

There is no single first-line drug for the treatment of acute schizophrenic episodes. Choices traditionally reflect individual preferences. Nowadays, one might assume that high-potency compounds are the gold standard, an impression encouraged by the fact that haloperidol has become the first-line choice for comparitor in assessing the efficacy of new agents. Such an assumption would be erroneous. The apparent pre-eminence of high-potency compounds largely springs from the influence of American practice, where these drugs enjoy a prominence less evident elsewhere, although surveys suggest that this represents a relatively recent shift.[47] The multinational phase III efficacy study of risperidone, conducted in 15 countries across the world,[18] suggests that, internationally, low-potency phenothiazines remain the most commonly prescribed.

There are real problems with the use of high-potency drugs in acute-phase treatment. Although relatively safe, the risks of neurological adverse effects are substantially greater than with low-potency compounds, particularly in drug-naive patients. While potency is itself an issue in this, a further factor is that high-potency drugs tend, in relative terms, to be used in higher doses than low-potency compounds.[103] This probably follows from the fact that doses of low-potency drugs are to some extent self-limited by the anti-autonomic and sedative side-effects intrinsic to the group.

There is, however, persistent evidence that, in general, psychiatrists still tend to use higher doses of antipsychotics to treat schizophrenia than are necessary. No studies have been able to demonstrate any therapeutic advantage from high-dose regimens,[46] while neurological side-effects are predictably more prevalent.[5] The complex kinetics of antipsychotics and the variability of both the natural history and response patterns of the illness make it impossible to provide reliable advice on dosage from dose–response data. However, flexible dosing studies suggest that the majority of responses will be achieved in the range of 500 to 600 mg/day of chlorpromazine or its equivalent,[47] with some suggestion that first-episode patients may respond at lower doses.

It has been repeatedly pointed out that there is no evidence to support the view that low-potency drugs are better in the treatment of excited psychotic states. It may be that this is one of those areas in which data from the somewhat idealized circumstances of clinical trials do not travel well to the day-to-day context. In one study of manic patients, which showed no difference at 2 weeks between those treated with chlorpromazine and those on the high-potency thiothixene, subjects were monitored at intervals of 2 h,[104] a level of care which would seem far removed from most routine standards currently.

Controversy persists as to whether antiparkinson medication should, as a matter of routine, be prescribed when standard antipsychotic treatment is started. Coincidental antiparkinson medication does reduce the risk of early extrapyramidal side-effects,[5] although these data relate mainly to high-potency drugs. However, even with these compounds, only a minority will develop significant extrapyramidal disorders, while the most commonly utilized antiparkinson drugs (i.e. anticholinergics) may interfere with antipsychotic actions[105] and have their own profile of unwanted side-effects.[5] Current recommendations are that antiparkinsonian medication should only be prescribed if neurological adverse effects become evident.[5,106]

Perhaps the most taxing question now is the place of new generation drugs. Should they be considered as routine first-line treatments or reserved for specific indications? The core issue is cost and whether the perceived benefits justify the cost implications. With clozapine, the position is clear. This drug is licensed for use in treatment resistance and neurological intolerance only, which removes it from first-line treatment. As for the others currently available, this remains a matter of individual choice and local prescribing policy. However, intolerance to standard antipsychotic regimens relates not only to individual susceptibility, which resides with the patient, but to treatment and management decisions, which reside with the doctor.[5] It is possible to utilize standard antipsychotics with minimal risk of adverse effects in the majority. In the study by Janicak et al.[104] noted above, patients were successfully treated with relatively low doses of medication and none experienced intolerable adverse effects.

In deciding treatment regimens in those with past treatment histories—be advised by the patient! Medications in which they have confidence should always be one's first-line approach in treating acute relapses.

The boundary of the acute phase of treatment is not rigidly defined, nor is it necessarily set by major symptomatic reversals. The important goal is 'stabilization', as evidenced by the psychotic process becoming less 'active'. Should side-effects emerge, it is part of the doctor's on-going efforts at engagement and maintaining consent to explain the issues to the patient, and in the process, educate them about the nature, and possible treatment, of adverse experiences. Psychiatric emergencies are discussed below.

Formulating treatment plans

Initial planning Reasonable, effective treatment plans can be devised around the first-line use of standard antipsychotics and at present, these should be the initial choice in the majority of cases. However, caution is urged with the routine use of high-potency compounds, especially in first-episode patients and those in relapse who have not been receiving medication for some time.

Low-potency regimens

Foundation recommendations With disturbance in both non-specific and behavioural domains, a low-potency drug is a reasonable first choice for the initial treatment plan:

- in the drug-naive or frail, chlorpromazine 50 mg twice daily and 100 mg at night

- in those with prior exposure, chlorpromazine 100 mg three times daily or 100 mg twice daily and 150 mg at night.

Added flexibility 'As-required' prescriptions allow nursing colleagues to intervene at their discretion, in the face of increasing disturbance. These should be carefully prescribed with indications, maximum frequencies, dosages, and modes of administration written up separately and unambiguously. A major advantage of 'as-required' prescriptions is to inform the judgement about how far short initial treatment recommendations fall from practical requirements, and information on the use of this component of the plan should be incorporated into each revision. In order to avoid polypharmacy, choices of drug for 'as-required' prescription should, as far as possible, be limited to additional doses of the initial compound.

Adjunctive medications If the initial plan achieves less than was anticipated, it is important to consider adding adjunctive treatments, in order to avoid over-rapid increments in antipsychotic doses. Benzodiazepines are best in this situation.

High-potency regimens

Foundation recommendations Initial plans with these drugs might comprise the following:

- in the drug naive, haloperidol 1.5 to 2 mg twice daily
- in those previously exposed, haloperidol 2.5 to 3 mg twice daily.

Added flexibility It is important with high-potency regimens to be circumspect about the prescription of 'as-required' doses. Additional doses of one's first-choice drug or single doses of another high-potency compound will inevitably lead to rapid dose escalation and the likelihood of neurological adverse effects. A benzodiazepine should again be considered as an alternative.

Fifty per cent of acute dystonias present within 3 days of the start of treatment or dose increments, and features of akathisia can be evident even after single, especially parenteral, doses of high-potency compounds.[5] Prescribing an 'as-required' anticholinergic does allow experienced nursing staff to intervene immediately should such features emerge, although this should only be implemented after medical confirmation of the diagnosis.

Adjunctive medications Reliance on benzodiazepines to achieve early, acute-phase treatment goals may be greater if one's initial plan incorporates a high-potency antipsychotic, as the low introductory doses recommended here may be inadequate to improve sleep and ease anxiety/agitation as swiftly as is ideal.

Where neither non-specific symptomatology nor behavioural disturbance is prominent, advocacy for any particular drug type is more problematic. While the use of standard compounds as the first-line treatment of acute schizophrenic episodes is advocated, there are two scenarios in which new-generation drugs should be considered:

(1) those first-episode patients in whom it is felt particularly important to minimize the risk of adverse effects, especially sedation and the unpleasant subjective experience of neurological adverse effects;

(2) patients in relapse who have been poorly tolerant, especially of extrapyramidal symptomatology, in the past.

Revision Monitoring response to initial treatment decisions involves bringing together information from nursing colleagues, prescription data, mental state examination, and assessment of non-target effects, including extrapyramidal status. Initial treatment plans should be reviewed frequently—a key element in fostering engagement and compliance as well as in refining treatment recommendations.

The markers of early progress in treatment are stabilization and, over several days, containment of non-specific affective symptomatology, improvement in nocturnal sleep without undue daytime drowsiness, and control of overactive, disorganized, and potentially confrontational behaviour.

There are two temptations to avoid in revising early treatment plans. The first is changing drug prematurely and the second is introducing polypharmacy. While intolerance or patient pressure may force an early change of antipsychotic, it is in general important to give each drug an adequate trial, which may take several weeks, while adding other antipsychotics to the foundation drug will increase the antipsychotic 'load' and the neurological risks. Rather than go down either of these roads, it is better to rely on adjunctive medications to temporarily contain difficult situations.

The post-acute phase

Goals

The post-acute phase is characterized by returning stability. The goals now are as follows:

(1) consolidation of clinical improvements

(2) rationalization of the treatment regimen

(3) resocialization.

All schizophrenic symptomatology does not resolve at the same rate and the first signs of improvement should not be taken as evidence that the tide has conclusively turned. Global improvements evident over the broad range of domains must be shown to deepen into specific improvements in particular symptomatology. Furthermore, improvements evident in the ward environment need to be shown to generalize to the patient's routine situation. Although there is no evidence that rationalizing and simplifying the treatment plan contributes to enhanced compliance,[107] this is intuitively sound. This is also the period when resocialization, and if necessary rehabilitation, should be commenced, and secondly, the issue of longer-term treatment raised.

Formulating treatment/management plans

Initial planning In the post-acute phase, there is often great pressure to reduce medication doses radically, but overzealous reductions at this stage are likely to be followed by symptomatic exacerbation. The main task in the early part of this phase is to persuade the patient of the merits of holding the regimen stable while resocialization is being established. As symptomatology begins to settle, those on low-potency regimens are likely to become less tolerant of sedative actions which may compromise resocialization and compliance. A cautious reduction on this basis is certainly justified. With high-potency drugs the problem is more likely to be the apathy and impaired initiative of bradykinesia, which, if not responsive to antiparkinson medication, would also merit dose reduction.

Revision Once the initial steps in resocialization have been achieved, medication can be rationalized. Where multiple drugs continue to be necessary, they should be prescribed at similar times, with as much of the regimen as possible given at night. In addition, the need for adjunctive medications should be re-evaluated.

There is no consensus as to whether or not stopping antiparkinson medication at this stage will result in recrudescence of neurological signs.[5] As it is likely that some patients will not require these treatments, systematic reductions should be started.

If a depot is agreed, this should also be started. Depots are not ideally suited to acute-phase treatment and because of their unusual pharmacokinetics should be commenced 'in parallel' with existing oral medication, which can be discontinued slowly as the depot approaches steady state (i.e. approximately five times the half-life).

The maintenance phase

Goals

The boundary between post-acute and maintenance phases is the least defined but is reached when improvements in all the major domains of disorder are felt to be maximal.

The major goals of maintenance are as follows:

(1) maximum well being with minimum adverse effects

(2) monitoring efficacy/effectiveness and tolerability

(3) continuation or completion of rehabilitation and social reintegration.

Attempts to reduce medication should still be cautious during maintenance, but over the longer term, more determined. The major medical task in this phase is monitoring, to include effectiveness, as well as the narrower efficacy. Any long-term therapeutic regimen can only be properly evaluated by balancing efficacy/effectiveness against tolerability. Exploration of neurological tolerability should involve both an enquiry into subjective effects as well as an examination to elicit signs, and should be undertaken regularly.

The final, and to some extent most intensive, aim of maintenance comprises those management techniques geared towards helping patients attain the highest possible level of psychosocial functioning and carers the greatest degree of understanding and skills for coping.

Formulating treatment/management plans

For the first few months of maintenance, any social and interpersonal difficulties should be addressed with minimal changes to antipsychotic regimens, unless adverse effects are impeding this process. The more determined period of medication reduction should be reserved for the time when a stable set of routines has been established and the patient is considered to be functioning relatively competently. Any reductions should be followed by a prolonged period of observation before further changes are contemplated; because of their long half-lives, this principle especially applies to depots.

Antiparkinsonism medication should be continually justified by attempting dose reductions throughout the maintenance phase, but these should be delayed following reduction of the antipsychotic. Decreases in the clinical features of extrapyramidal disorder will not occur for some weeks after decreases in antipsychotic doses and premature cessation of the antiparkinson agent may result in a false conclusion that it is required long-term.

Depression during the maintenance phase can have as many causes as depression in other contexts, but despite initial pessimism, there is now good evidence that such mood states do respond to traditional (tricyclic) antidepressants[108] and they should be vigorously treated.

An outline plan for the treatment/management of schizophrenia is shown in Fig. 1, and a decision tree for dealing with negative states is shown in Table 4.

Psychiatric emergencies

Those who deal professionally with acutely ill patients must always bear in mind the 'unpredictability factor' and the potential for violent behaviour during acute symptomatic 'shifts'. Risk assessment of dangerousness is an imprecise science, but an attempt should be incorporated into all routine clinical assessments during acute phase treatment. Caution should be exercised with patients who are profoundly suspicious, verbally aggressive, resistant to engagement, whose pattern of disorder does not allow for a comprehensive mental state examination, or whose clinical condition is complicated by substance abuse, and especially (for those in relapse) who have a past history of assaultive or threatening behaviour.

Principles of wider management are crucial in avoiding emergency situations, bearing on the quality of the environment and the amount and quality of support available. However, even with high levels of vigilance, pre-emptive plans, and good quality management, emergency situations may still occur and must be dealt with swiftly.

An outline plan relating to emergency situations is shown in Fig. 2.

Poor response and treatment resistance

Several intervention strategies have been recommended in those whose response to standard regimens is disappointing.

Antipsychotics

Where a patient has failed to respond satisfactorily to an adequate dose (600–800 mg chlorpromazine or its equivalent per day) of the first-choice antipsychotic, given for an adequate time (at least 6 weeks), they might be considered a 'poor responder' but not yet treatment resistant. Alternative plans have been proposed at this stage and include, in order of implementation:

(1) increasing the first-choice drug to a high-dose schedule (i.e. up to 1000 mg chlorpromazine or its equivalent) for 6 to 8 weeks;

(2) changing to a drug of different class, in standard dose ranges, for 6 to 8 weeks, which nowadays might involve changing to (or from) a new-generation compound;

(3) increasing the second-choice drug to a high-dose schedule, for 6 to 8 weeks.

As far as the research literature is concerned, it is only when at least one, and preferably two, of these steps have been tried without notable improvement that the patient would be considered 'treatment resistant'. For routine practice, however, several other interventions can be recommended.

Should it be that antipsychotic doses have escalated almost 'by default', it is worth reducing to average or low average ranges, as sometimes pervasive extrapyramidal symptomatology may be the source of impaired progress.[5] A further strategy is the addition of a depot with a view to transferring the bulk of treatment to this over time. Failure of the initial oral drug(s) may relate to adverse pharmacokinetic parameters, such as poor absorption or enhanced metabolism, which can be bypassed by depot administration.

First-line adjunctive medications

One should, in addition, look to simplifying any complexities that may have entered into the regimen, such as eradicating polypharmacy, reducing or stopping anticholinergics where possible, and assessing the need for other drugs such as antidepressants.

Second-line adjunctive treatments

Lithium

Lithium salts have been particularly recommended for patients with schizoaffective disorders, although at one time were more widely advocated. Although there is indirect evidence to support this general use,

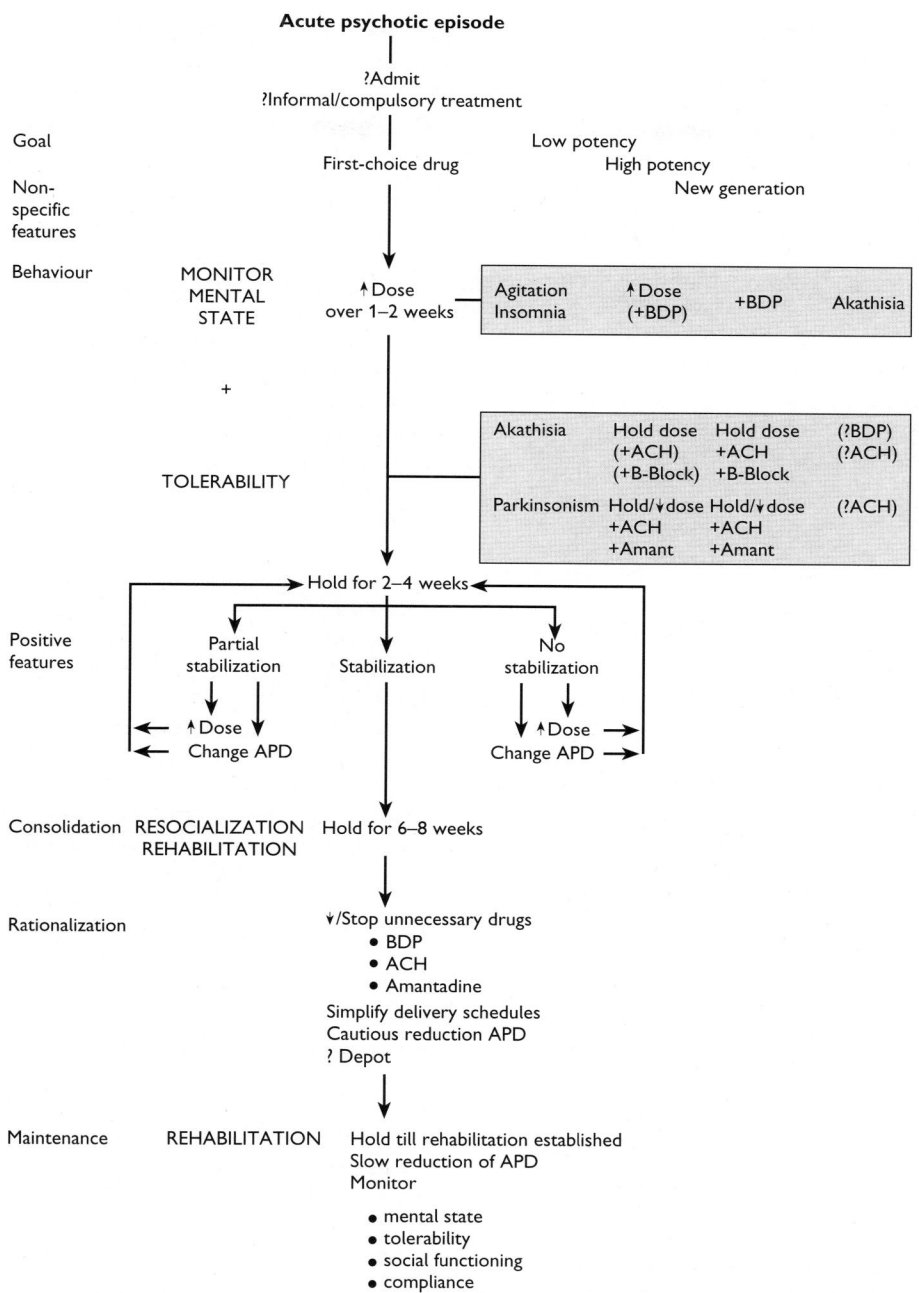

Fig. 1 Outline plan for treatment/management of schizophrenia: APD, antipsychotic drug; BDP, benzodiazepine; ACH, anticholinergic; B-Block, β-blocker; Amant, amantadine.

direct trial evidence is less encouraging[109] and their utilization is best considered as empirical in those with prominent affective symptoms.

Carbamazepine

The use of carbamazepine in schizophrenia has not been systematically researched and rests on anecdotal evidence. It may be considered as an alternative mood stabilizer in those with schizoaffective disorder, although another adjunctive use in schizophrenia may lie with those patients who have intransigent symptomatology, with a perceptual emphasis, reminiscent of temporal lobe disorder, even when the rou-

tine EEG is normal. A further indication may be patients whose EEG abnormalities show a temporal localization without clinical fits. Carbamazepine induces the metabolism of some antipsychotics, which may necessitate raising doses of the latter to prevent a paradoxical deterioration.

High-dose benzodiazepines

High-dose benzodiazepine treatment has been reported as being specifically beneficial in the treatment of acute schizophrenic episodes.[110] It is likely, however, that these benefits, which appear slight

Table 4 Outline management of 'negative' states in schizophrenia

Question	Intervention
1. Is the patient actively psychotic?	Start/increase antipsychotics
	Reduce levels of stimulation
If not:	
2. Is there evidence of extrapyramidal side-effects?	Anticholinergics
	Amantadine
	Reduce antipsychotic doses
	Switch antipsychotic
	New generation
	Low ptency
If not:	
3. Is there evidence of dysphoric mood?	Antidepressants
	Anxiolytics
	Reduce antipsychotics
	Supportive management
	Switch to new-generation antipsychotic
If not:	
4. Has psychosis recently resolved?	Supportive management
If not:	
5. Is the environment impoverished?	Resocialization
	Rehabilitation
If not:	
6. Is the patient receiving long-term medication?	Reduce to reasonable maintenance dose
	Switch to new-generation antipsychotic
	Clozapine
Then:	
7. Is the problem a 'deficit' state?	Adapt expectations to the patient's capabilities

After Carpenter et al.[29]

and inconsistent, result from actions on affective symptomatology or elements of extrapyramidal disturbance, and their adjunctive use in high-dose regimens would not seem justified.

Electroconvulsive therapy

ECT has become less popular as a treatment for schizophrenia, although it can be effective[111] and may still hold a place in the therapeutic armamentarium, but as a third-line treatment.

Comments

While in terms of professional guidelines it would be considered good practice to go through these steps in patients responding poorly or frankly resistant, most are largely empirically derived, and such evidence as there is does not encourage optimism about their overall likelihood of success.

As was noted, the one treatment of established efficacy in resistant schizophrenia is clozapine.[65] While in individual cases impressive benefits may become evident, especially in quality-of-life parameters, improvements attributable to clozapine over standard drugs are far from dramatic. Despite this, clozapine is probably underutilized and should be more readily considered in treatment of resistant cases. (See

Chapter 6.2.5 for further discussion of new-generation antipsychotics.)

Psychosocial interventions in management

While antipsychotic drugs may be considered the cornerstone of the treatment of schizophrenia, the most competent prescribing of these does not provide a comprehensive programme of management. Even if no formal programme is followed, all patients and their relatives will require appropriate information about the nature of the illness and the therapeutic possibilities. They will need support in coming to terms with the limitations that the illness may impose upon the expectations they have had, and guidance about alternative plans. The requirements of individual patients for rehabilitation and resocialization vary greatly, but general rules can be provided in terms of the classification of psychosocial approaches overviewed above.

Antipsychotic drugs can (and indeed overwhelming evidence indicates that they should) be given to all patients in whom the diagnosis of schizophrenia is appropriately made. This is not the case with psychosocial interventions. In general, these require co-operation from patients and/or relatives, and some of them can only be applied to certain types of patient.

There is no evidence for the value of psychodynamic psychotherapy in schizophrenia, but some will nonetheless wish to have it—and may well find it helpful. However, it should only be recommended in combination with treatments of proven effectiveness.

Family interventions have been shown to be of value, although the essential elements of any package remain far from clear. Education and support from trained staff should be offered, although not all families will be willing to accept this in a group format. While social skills training programmes of various kinds have been demonstrated to be efficacious in achieving specific goals in controlled circumstances with selected groups of patients, it is difficult to draw general guidelines about this kind of management. Nonetheless, while the goals may be restricted, enhanced skills in conversation and self-presentation may make a great deal of difference to the success of resocialization. The place of cognitive remediation is less clear and the requirement for it in routine practice cannot yet be said to be established.

Cognitive-behavioural techniques also require the co-operation of the patient and probably a degree of cognitive flexibility in respect of delusions. This again restricts the applicability of such programmes, but the benefits demonstrated by available trials indicate that they should be available for appropriate individuals.

As far as alternatives to hospital care are concerned, assertive case treatment provides benefits in terms of inpatient service utilization costs, and sometimes burden of care, but case management has not been shown to be helpful.

Concluding remarks

Traditionally, psychiatry has not always given to schizophrenia the attention that its complexities and chronicity merit. Views about what really helps in such a disorder are not, at the end of the day, based solely on research evidence, but are informed by personal experience—and, no doubt, personal prejudice. The distinction between theoretical and pragmatic psychiatry is nowhere more evident than in psychiatrists' actions in regard to schizophrenia. As a result, an

IMPENDING EMERGENCY

Non-drug intervention

- Talking down
- Distraction
- Seclusion

Drug intervention

Antipsychotic with sedative properties, orally
e.g. chlorpromazine 50–100 mg liquid/tablet
droperidol 10–20 mg
Low-distribution benzodiazepine
e.g. lorazepam 1–2 mg

Review 30–60 minutes

If no response—repeat
Or
If no response *or* no initial co-operation.

- Talking down
- Distraction
- Seclusion
- Monitor physically

Sedative antipsychotic **IM**
e.g. droperidol 10 mg
chlorpromazine 50–100 mg (with care in
frail, elderly, or drug naive)
Benzodiazepine of low volume of distribution
e.g. lorazepam 1–2 mg

Revise treatment plan—start/increase baseline antipsychotic
Review 30–60 min
If no response—repeat (with higher dose ranges, vital signs permitting)
Revise treatment plan

ESTABLISHED EMERGENCY

Non-drug intervention

- Seclusion
- Talking down
- Monitor vital signs

Drug intervention

Sedative antipsychotic **IM** as above* in adequate doses
±
Low distribution benzodiazepine as above, administered separately
(depending on severity of incident)
High-potency antipsychotic IV
e.g. haloperidol/droperidol 10 mg

Review 30 min
Revise treatment plan
Repeat if necessary (vital signs stable)

*The thioxanthene zuclopenthixol esterified with acetic acid (as the depot
Clopixol Acuphase) has kinetic properties similar to those of an aqueous solution
and is recommended for use in emergency situations. In view of its prolonged effects
(up to 72 h) it should be used with caution, especially in the frail of drug naive.

Fig. 2 Outline plan for treatment/management of psychiatric emergencies.

element of variability in treatment and management recommendations is inevitable. What is often perceived as lacking, however, is less a consistency in practice recommendations than a consistency of personnel. One element sufferers and their families appreciate most is accessible care by experienced professionals, who, by being involved over the long years of illness, know the disorder, the patient, and the families—and are able to attempt some understanding of all three. Combining such an essentially 'primary care' function with rapidly expanding knowledge of pathophysiological mechanisms and a wide, and evolving, array of therapeutic tools, schizophrenia can increasingly be seen as a legitimate and rewarding area for specialist psychiatric practice in which, contrary to widespread belief, the skilled doctor can make a difference.

References

1. Clouston, T. (1884). *Clinical lectures on mental diseases.* Henry Lea, Philadelphia, PA.
2. Adams, F. (1856). *Aretaeus, the Cappadocian: the extant works* (translated and edited by F. Adams). Mulford House, Boston, MA.
3. MacDonald, M. (1981). *Mystical Bedlam: madness, anxiety and healing in seventeenth century England.* Cambridge University Press.
4. Johnstone, E.C. (1998). Psychiatry, its history and boundaries. In *Companion to psychiatric studies* (ed. E.C. Johnstone, C.P.L. Freeman, and A.K. Zealley), pp. 1–10. Churchill Livingstone, Edinburgh.
5. Owens, D.G.C. (1999). *A guide to the extrapyramidal side-effects of antipsychotic drugs.* Cambridge University Press.
6. Klein, D. and Davis, J.M. (1969). *Diagnosis and drug treatment of psychiatric disorders. Baltimore.* Williams and Wilkins, Baltimore, MD.

7. Owens, D.G.C. (1996). Adverse effects of antipsychotic agents: do newer agents offer advantages? *Drugs*, **51**, 895–930.

8. Davis, J.M. and Garver, D.L. (1978). Neuroleptics—clinical use in psychiatry. In *Handbook of psychopharmacology* (ed. L.L. Iversen, S. Iversen, and S. Snyder), pp. 129–64. Plenum Press, New York.

9. Cole, J.O. and the NIMH Psychopharmacology Service Center Collaborative Study Group (1964). Phenothiazine treatment in acute schizophrenia. *Archives of General Psychiatry*, **10**, 246–61.

10. Tuma, A.H. and May, P.R.A. (1979). And if that doesn't work, what next? A study of treatment failures in schizophrenia. *Journal of Nervous and Mental Disease*, **167**, 566–71.

11. May, P.R.A. (1968). *Treatment of schizophrenia: a comparative study of five treatment methods*. Science House, New York.

12. May, P.R.A., Tuma, A.H., Yale, C., Potepam, P., and Dixon, W.J. (1976). Schizophrenia: a follow-up study of results of treatment: II. Hospital stay over two to five years. *Archives of General Psychiatry*, **33**, 481–6.

13. May, P.R.A., Tuma, A.H., Yale, C., and Dixon, W.J. (1981). Schizophrenia: a follow up study of the results of five forms of treatment. *Archives of General Psychiatry*, **38**, 776–84.

14. Wyatt, R.J. (1991). Neuroleptics and the natural course of schizophrenia. *Schizophrenia Bulletin*, **17**, 325–51.

15. Crow, T.J., Macmillan, J.F., Johnson, A.L., and Johnstone, E.C. (1986). The Northwick Park study of first episodes of schizophrenia: II A randomised controlled trial of prophylactic neuroleptic treatment. *British Journal of Psychiatry*, **148**, 120–7.

16. Johnstone, E.C., Crow, T.J., Davis, J.M., and Owens, D.G.C. (1999). Does a four week delay in the introduction of medication alter the course of functional psychosis? *Journal of Psychopharmacology*, **13**, 238–44.

17. Lieberman, J.A. (1993). Understanding the mechanism of action of atypical antipsychotic drugs: a review of compounds in use and development. *British Journal of Psychiatry*, **163** (Supplement 22), 7–18.

18. Peuskins, J., on behalf of the Risperidone Study Group (1995). Risperidone in the treatment of patients with chronic schizophrenia: a multi-national, multi-centre, double-blind, parallel-group study versus haloperidol. *British Journal of Psychiatry*, **166**, 712–26.

19. Tollefson, G.D., Beasley, C.M., Tran, P.V., *et al.* (1997). Olanzapine versus haloperidol in the treatment of schizophrenia and schizoaffective and schizophreniform disorders: results of an international collaborative trial. *American Journal of Psychiatry*, **154**, 457–65.

20. Arvanitis, L.A., Miller, B.G., and the Seroquel Trial 13 Study Group (1997). Multiple fixed doses of 'Seroquel' (quetiapine) in patients with acute exacerbation of schizophrenia: a comparison with haloperidol and placebo. *Biological Psychiatry*, **42**, 233–46.

21. Puech, A., Fleurot, O., Tein, W., and the Amisulpride Study Group (1998). Amisulpride, an atypical antipsychotic, in the treatment of acute episodes of schizophrenia: a dose-ranging study vs. haloperidol. *Acta Psychiatrica Scandinavica*, **98**, 65–72.

22. Pettit, M., Raniwalla, J., Tweed, J., Leutenegger, E., Dollfus, S., and Kelley, F. (1996). A comparison of an atypical and typical antipsychotic: zotepine versus haloperidol in patients with acute exacerbations of schizophrenia: a parallel group, double-blind trial. *Psychopharmacology Bulletin*, **32**, 81–7.

23. Chouinard, G. (1995). Effects of risperidone in tardive dyskinesia: an analysis of the Canadian Multicentre Risperidone Study. *Journal of Clinical Psychopharmacology*, **15** (Supplement 1), 36s–44s.

24. Tollefson, G.D., Beasley, C.M., Tamura, R.N., Tran, P.V., and Potvin, J.H. (1997). Blind, controlled, long-term study of the comparative incidence of treatment-emergent tardive dyskinesia with olanzapine and haloperidol. *American Journal of Psychiatry*, **154**, 1248–54.

25. Crow, T.J. (1980). Molecular pathology of schizophrenia : more than one disease process? *British Medical Journal*, **280**, 66–8.

26. Goldberg, S.C. (1985). Negative and deficit symptoms in schizophrenia do respond to neuroleptics. *Schizophrenia Bulletin*, **11**, 453–6.

27. Tandon, R., Riveiro, S.C.M., DeQuardo, J.R., Goldman, R.S., Goodson, J., and Greden, J.F. (1993). Covariance of positive and negative symptoms during neuroleptic treatment in schizophrenia: a replication. *Biological Psychiatry*, **34**, 495–7.

28. van Kammen, D.P., Hommer, D.W., and Malas, K.L. (1987). Effects of pimozide on positive and negative symptoms in schizophrenic patients: are negative symptoms state dependent? *Neuropsychobiology*, **18**, 113–17.

29. Carpenter, W.T., Heinrichs, D.W., and Alphs, L.D. (1985). Treatment of negative symptoms. *Schizophrenia Bulletin*, **11**, 440–52.

30. Moller, H.-J., Muller, H., Borison, R.L., Schooler, N.R., and Chouinard, G. (1995). A path-analytical approach to differentiate between direct and indirect drug effects on negative symptoms in schizophrenic patients—a re-evaluation of the North American Risperidone Study. *European Archives of Psychiatry and Clinical Neuroscience*, **245**, 45–9.

31. Tollefson, G.D. and Sanger, T.M. (1997). Negative symptoms: a path analytic approach to a double-blind, placebo- and haloperidol-controlled clinical trial with olanzapine. *American Journal of Psychiatry*, **154**, 466–74.

32. Kane, J.M., Safferman, A.Z., Pollack, S., *et al.* (1994). Clozapine, negative symptoms and extrapyramidal side-effects. *Journal of Clinical Psychiatry*, **55** (Supplement B), 74–7.

33. Carpenter, W.T., Heinrichs, D.W., and Wagman, A.M.I. (1988). Deficit and non-deficit forms of schizophrenia: the concept. *American Journal of Psychiatry*, **145**, 578–83.

34. Breier, A., Buchanan, R.W., Kirkpatrick, B., *et al.* (1994). Effects of clozapine on positive and negative symptoms in outpatients with schizophrenia. *American Journal of Psychiatry*, **151**, 20–6.

35. Sharma, T. and Mockler, D. (1998). The cognitive efficacy of atypical antipsychotics in schizophrenia. *Journal of Clinical Psychopharmacology*, **18** (Supplement 1), 12s–19s.

36. King, D.J. (1990). The effect of neuroleptics on cognitive and psychomotor function. *British Journal of Psychiatry*, **157**, 799–811.

37. King, D.J. (1994). Psychomotor impairment and cognitive disturbances induced by neuroleptics. *Acta Psychiatrica Scandinavica*, **89** (Supplement 380), 53–8.

38. Johnstone, E.C., Owens, D.G.C., Frith, C.D., and Leary, J. (1991). Disabilities and circumstances of schizophrenic patients: a follow-up study. III. Clinical findings—abnormalities of the mental state and movement disorder and their correlates. *British Journal of Psychiatry*, **159** (Supplement 13), 21–5.

39. Jenner, P. and Marsden, C.D. (1982). The mode of action of sulpiride as an atypical antidepressant agent. *Advances in Biochemical Psychopharmacology*, **32**, 85–103.

40. Margakis, B.P. (1990). A double-blind comparison of oral amitriptyline and low-dose intramuscular flupenthixol decanoate in depressive illness. *Current Medical Research and Opinion*, **12**, 51–7.

41. Salminen, J.K., Lehtonen, V., Allonen, H., *et al.* (1980). Sulpiride in depression: plasma levels and effects. *Current Therapeutic Research*, **27**, 109–15.

42. de Alarcon, R. and Carney, M.W.P. (1969). Severe depressive mood changes following slow-release intramuscular fluphenazine injection. *British Medical Journal*, **3**, 564–7.

43. Van Putten, T. and May, P.R.A. (1978). 'Akinetic depression' in schizophrenia. *Archives of General Psychiatry*, **35**, 1101–7.

44. Koreen, A.R., Siris, S., Chakos, M., Alvir, J., Mayerhoff, D., and Lieberman, J. (1993). Depression in first-episode schizophrenics. *American Journal of Psychiatry*, **150**, 1643–8.

45. Owens, D.G.C. and Johnstone, E.C. (1980). The disabilities of chronic schizophrenia: their nature and factors contributing to their development. *British Journal of Psychiatry*, **136**, 384–95.

46. Janicak, P.G., Davis, J.M., Preskorn, S., and Ayd, F.J. (1993). *Principles and practice of psychopharmacotherapy*. Williams and Wilkins, Baltimore, MD.

47. Baldessarini, R.J., Cohen, B.M., and Teicher, M.H. (1990). Pharmacological treatment. In *Schizophrenia—treatment of acute episodes* (ed. S.T. Levy and P.T. Ninan), pp. 61–118. American Psychiatric Press, Washington, DC.

48. Caffey, E.M., Diamond, L.S., Frank, T.V., *et al.* (1964). Discontinuation

or reduction of chemotherapy in chronic schizophrenia. *Journal of Chronic Diseases*, **17**, 347–58.

49. Hogarty, G.E., Goldberg, S.C., and Collaborative Study Group (1973). Drug and sociotherapy in the aftercare of schizophrenic patients. *Archives of General Psychiatry*, **28**, 54–64.

50. Prien, R.F., Cole, J.O., and Belkin, N.F. (1969). Relapse in chronic schizophrenics following abrupt withdrawal of tranquilising medication. *British Journal of Psychiatry*, **115**, 679–86.

51. Davis, J.M., Schaffer, C.B., Killan, G.A., Kinard, C., and Chan, C. (1980). Important issues in the drug treatment of schizophrenia. *Schizophrenia Bulletin*, **6**, 70–87.

52. Johnson, D.A.W. (1979). Further observations on the duration of depot neuroleptic maintenance therapy in schizophrenia. *British Journal of Psychiatry*, **135**, 524–30.

53. Hogarty, G.E. and Ulrich, R.F. (1977). Temporal effects of drug and placebo in delaying relapse in schizophrenic outpatients. *Archives of General Psychiatry*, **34**, 297–301.

54. Capstick, N. (1980). Long-term fluphenazine decanoate maintenance dosage requirements of chronic schizophrenic patients. *Acta Psychiatrica Scandinavica*, **61**, 256–62.

55. Cheung, H.K. (1981). Schizophrenics fully remitted on neuroleptics for 3–5 years. *British Journal of Psychiatry*, **138**, 490–4.

56. Morgan, R. and Cheadle, J. (1974). Maintenance treatment of chronic schizophrenia with neuroleptic drugs. *Acta Psychiatrica Scandinavica*, **50**, 78–85.

57. Meltzer, H.Y., Burnett, S., Bastani, B., and Ramirez, L.F. (1990). Effects of six months of clozapine treatment on the quality of life of chronic schizophrenic patients. *Hospital and Community Psychiatry*, **41**, 892–987.

58. Davis, J.M., Metalon, L., Watanabe, M., and Blake, L. (1993). Depot antipsychotic drugs: place in therapy. *Drugs*, **47**, 741–73.

59. Kane, J.M., Rifkin, A., Woerner, M., *et al.* (1983). Low dose neuroleptic treatment of outpatient schizophrenics. *Archives of General Psychiatry*, **40**, 893–6.

60. Marder, S.R., van Putten, T., Mintz, J., Lebell, M., McKenzie, J., and May, P.R.A. (1987). Low- and conventional-dose maintenance therapy with fluphenazine decanoate: two year outcome. *Archives of General Psychiatry*, **44**, 518–21.

61. Schooler, N.R., Keith, S., Severe, J., *et al.* (1997). Relapse and rehospitalization during maintenance treatment of schizophrenia: the effects of dose reduction and family treatment. *Archives of General Psychiatry*, **54**, 453–63.

62. Johnson, D.A.W., Ludlow, J.M., Street, K., and Taylor, R.D.W. (1987). Double blind comparison of half dose and standard-dose flupenthixol decanoate in the maintenance treatment of stabilised outpatients with schizophrenia. *British Journal of Psychiatry*, **151**, 634–8.

63. Davis, J.M., Kane, J.M., Marder, S., *et al.* (1993). Dose response of prophylactic antipsychotics. *Journal of Clinical Psychiatry*, **54** (Supplement 3), 24–30.

64. Johnstone, E.C., Macmillan, F.J., Frith, C.D., Benn, D.K., and Crow, T.J. (1990). Further investigations of the predictors of outcome following first schizophrenic episodes. *British Journal of Psychiatry*, **157**, 182–9.

65. Kane, J.M., Honigfeld, G., Singer, J., Meltzer, H.Y., and the Clozaril Collaborative Study Group (1988). Clozapine for the treatment-resistant schizophrenic: a double-blind comparison with chlorpromazine. *Archives of General Psychiatry*, **45**, 789–96.

66. Mercer, G., Finlayson, A., Johnstone, E.C., Murray, C., and Owens, D.G.C. (1997). A study of enhanced management in patients with treatment resistant schizophrenia. *Journal of Psychopharmacology*, **11**, 349–56.

67. Gunderson, J.G., Frank, A.F., Katz, H.M., Vannicelli, M.L., Frosch, J.P., and Knapp, P.H. (1984). Effects of psychotherapy in schizophrenia. II. Comparative outcome of two forms of treatment. *Archives of General Psychiatry*, **10**, 564–98.

68. Kopelowicz, A., Corrigan, P.W., Schade, M., and Liberman, R.P. (1998). Social skills training. In *Handbook of social functioning in schizophrenia* (ed. K.T. Mueser and N. Tarrier), pp. 307–26. Allyn and Bacon, Needham Heights, MA.

69. Claghorn, J.L., Johnstone, E.E., Cook, T.H., and Itschner, L. (1974). Group therapy and maintenance treatment of schizophrenics. *Archives of General Psychiatry*, **31**, 361–5.

70. Malm, U. (1982). The influence of group therapy on schizophrenia. *Acta Psychiatrica Scandinavica* (Supplement 297), 1–65.

71. Spencer, P.G., Gillespie, C.R., and Ekisa, E.G. (1983). A controlled comparison of the effects of social skills training and remedial drama on the social conversational skills of chronic schizophrenic patients. *British Journal of Psychiatry*, **143**, 165–72.

72. Hogarty, G.E., Anderson, C.M., Reiss, D.J., *et al.* (1991). Family psychoeducation, social skills training and maintenance chemotherapy in the aftercare treatment of schizophrenia. II. Two-year effects of a controlled study on relapse and adjustment. *Archives of General Psychiatry*, **48**, 340–47.

73. Dobson, D.J., McDougall, G., Busheikin, J., and Aldous, J. (1995). Effect of social skills training and social milieu treatment on symptoms of schizophrenia. *Psychiatric Services*, **4**, 376–80.

74. Benton, M.K. and Schroeder, H.E. (1990). Social skills training with schizophrenics: a meta-analytic evaluation. *Journal of Consulting and Clinical Psychology*, **58**, 741–7.

75. Wong, S.E., Martinez-Diaz, J.A., Massel, H.K., *et al.* (1993). Conversational skills training with schizophrenic inpatients: a study of generalisation across settings and conversants. *Behaviour Therapy*, **24**, 285–304.

76. Halford, W.K. and Hayes R. (1991). Psychological rehabilitation of chronic schizophrenic patients: recent findings on social skills and family psycho-education. *Clinical Psychology Review*, **23**, 23–44.

77. Eckman, T.A., Wirshing, W.C., Marder, S.R., *et al.* (1992). Technique for training schizophrenic patients in illness self-management: a controlled trial. *American Journal of Psychiatry*, **149**, 1549–55.

78. Linszen, D., Dingemans, P., Van der Does, J.W., *et al.* (1996). Treatment, expressed emotion and relapse in recent onset schizophrenic disorders. *Psychological Medicine*, **26**, 333–42.

79. Owens, D.G.C., Finlayson, A., Mercer, G., and Johnstone, E.C. (1997). The use of videotaped assessment in relation to a study of enhanced management in treatment resistant schizophrenia. *Journal of Psychopharmacology*, **11**, 357–60.

80. Brown, G.W., Birley, J.L.T., and Wing, J.K. (1972). Influence of family life on the course of schizophrenic disorders. *British Journal of Psychiatry*, **121**, 242–58.

81. Goldstein, M.J., Rodnick, E.H., Evans, J.R., May, P.R., and Steinberg, M.R. (1978). Drug and family therapy in the aftercare of acute schizophrenia. *Archives of General Psychiatry*, **35**, 1169–77.

82. Falloon, I.R.H., Boyd, J.L., McGill, C., Razani, J., Moss, H.B., and Gilderman, A.M. (1982). Family management in the prevention of exacerbations of schizophrenia. *New England Journal of Medicine*, **306**, 1437–40.

83. Leff, J., Kuipers, L., Berkowitz, R., Eberlein-Vries, R., and Sturgeon, D. (1982). A controlled trial of social intervention in the families of schizophrenic patients. *British Journal of Psychiatry*, **141**, 121–34.

84. Leff, J., Berkowitz, R., Shavit, N., Strachan, A., Glass, I., and Vaughn, C. (1990). A trial of family therapy versus a relatives' group for schizophrenia. Two year follow-up. *British Journal of Psychiatry*, **157**, 571–7.

85. Tarrier, N., Barrowclough, C., Vaughn, C., *et al.* (1989). Community management of schizophrenia. A two-year follow-up of a behavioural intervention with families. *British Journal of Psychiatry*, **154**, 625–8.

86. Vaughan, K., Doyle, M., McConaghy, N., Blaszczynski, A., Fox, A., and Tarrier, N. (1992). The Sydney intervention trial: a controlled trial of relatives' counselling to reduce schizophrenic relapse. *Social Psychiatry and Psychiatric Epidemiology*, **27**, 16–21.

87. Hogarty, G.E., Anderson, C.M., Reis, D.J., *et al.* (1986). Family psychoeducation, social skills training, and maintenance chemotherapy in the aftercare treatment of schizophrenia: I. one-year effects of a

controlled study on relapse and expressed emotion. *Archives of General Psychiatry*, **43**, 633–42.

88. Glick, I.D., Clarkin, V., Haas, G.L., and Spencer, J.H., Jr. (1993). Clinical significance of inpatient family intervention: conclusions from a clinical trial. *Hospital and Community Psychiatry*, **44**, 869–73.

89. McFarlane, W.R., Lukens, E., Link, B., *et al.* (1995). Multiple-family groups and psychoeducation in the treatment of schizophrenia. *Archives of General Psychiatry*, **52**, 679–87.

90. Mari, J.J. and Streiner, D. (1996). Family intervention for those with schizophrenia. In *Schizophrenia module of the Cochrane database of systematic reviews* (updated 2 December 1996) (ed. C. Adams, J. De Jesus Mari, and P. White). Available in *The Cochrane Library* (database on disk and CD-ROM). Cochrane Collaboration, Issue 2. Update Software, Oxford. (See also *Psychological Medicine*, **24**, 565–78, 1994; *Evidence-Based Medicine*, **1**, 121, 1996.)

91. Tarrier, N., Beckett, R., Harwood, S., Baker, A., Yusopoff, L., and Ugarteburu, I. (1993). A trial of two cognitive-behavioural methods of treating drug-resistant residual psychotic symptoms in schizophrenic patients. I. Outcome. *British Journal of Psychiatry*, **162**, 524–32.

92. Drury, B., Birchwood, M., Cochrane, R., and Macmillan, J.F. (1996). Cognitive therapy and recovery from acute psychosis: a controlled trial. *British Journal of Psychiatry*, **169**, 593–601.

93. Garety, P., Fowler, D., Kuipers, E., *et al.* (1997). London–East Anglia randomised controlled trial of cognitive-behavioural therapy for psychoses. II. Predictors of outcome. *British Journal of Psychiatry*, **171**, 420–6.

94. Kuipers, E., Fowler, D., Garety, P., *et al.* (1998). London–East Anglia randomised controlled trial of cognitive-behavioural therapy for psychosis. III. Follow-up and economic evaluation at 18 months. *British Journal of Psychiatry*, **173**, 61–8.

95. Benedict, R.H., Harris, A.E., Markow, T., McCormack, J.A., Nuechterlein, K.H., and Asarnow, R.F. (1994). Effects of attention training on information processing in schizophrenia. *Schizophrenia Bulletin*, **20**, 537–46.

96. Vollema, M.G., Geurtsen, G.T., and van Voorst, A.J. (1995). Durable improvements in Wisconsin card sorting performance in schizophrenic patients. *Schizophrenia Research*, **16**, 209–15.

97. Corrigan, P.W., Huschbeck, J.N., and Wilfe, M. (1995). Memory and vigilance training to improve social perception in schizophrenia. *Schizophrenia Research*, **17**, 257–65.

98. Rosenheck, R., Neale, M., Leaf, P., Milstein, R., and Frisman, L. (1995). Multisite experimental cost study of intensive psychiatric community care. *Schizophrenia Bulletin*, **21**, 129–40.

99. Quinlivan, R., Hough, R., Crowell, A., Beach, C., Hofstetter, R., and Kenworthy, K. (1995). Service utilization and costs of care for severely mentally ill clients in an intensive case management program. *Psychiatric Services*, **46**, 365–71.

100. Aberg-Wistedt, A., Cressell, T., Lidberg, Y., Liljenberg, G., and Osby, U. (1995). Two-year outcome of team-based intensive case management for patients with schizophrenia. *Psychiatric Services*, **46**, 1263–6.

101. Telles, C., Karno, M., Mintz, J., *et al.* (1995). Immigrant families coping with schizophrenia. Behavioural family intervention v. case management with a low-income Spanish-speaking population. *British Journal of Psychiatry*, **167**, 473–9.

102. Marshall, M., Gray, A., Lockwood, A., and Green, R. (1997). Family intervention for those with schizophrenia. In *Schizophrenia module of the Cochrane database of systematic reviews* (updated 2 December 1996) (ed. C. Adams, J. De Jesus Mari, and P. White). Available in *The Cochrane Library* (database on disk and CD-ROM). Cochrane Collaboration, Issue 1. Update Software, Oxford. (See also *Evidence-Based Medicine*, **1**, 30, 1995.)

103. Baldessarini, R.J., Katz, B., and Cotton, P. (1984). Dissimilar dosing with high-potency and low-potency neuroleptics. *American Journal of Psychiatry*, **141**, 748–52.

104. Janicak, P.G., Bresnahan, D.B., Sharma, R., Davis, J.M., Comaty, J.E., and Malinick, C. (1988). A comparison of thiothixene with chlorpromazine in the treatment of mania. *Journal of Clinical Psychopharmacology*, **8**, 33–7.

105. Johnstone, E.C., Crow, T.J., Ferrier, I.N., *et al.* (1983). Adverse effects of anticholinergic medication on positive schizophrenic symptoms. *Psychological Medicine*, **13**, 513–27.

106. World Health Organization, Heads of Centres Collaborating in WHO Co-ordinated Studies on Biological Aspects of Mental Illness (1990). Prophylactic use of anticholinergics in patients on long-term neuroleptic treatment: a consensus statement. *British Journal of Psychiatry*, **156**, 412.

107. Fenton, W.S., Blyler, C.R., and Heinssen, R.K. (1997). Determinants of medication compliance in schizophrenia: empirical and clinical findings. *Schizophrenia Bulletin*, **23**, 637–51.

108. Siris, S.H., Morgan, V., Fagerstrom, R., Rifkin, A., and Cooper, T.B. (1987). Adjunctive imipramine in the treatment of post-psychotic depression: a controlled trial. *Archives of General Psychiatry*, **44**, 533–9.

109. Johnstone, E.C., Crow, T.J., Frith, C.D., and Owens, D.G.C. (1988). The Northwick Park 'functional' psychosis study: diagnosis and treatment response. *Lancet*, **ii**, 119–26.

110. Lingjaerde, O. (1991). Benzodiazepines and the treatment of schizophrenia: an updated survey. *Acta Psychiatrica Scandinavica*, **84**, 453–9.

111. Brandon, S., Cowley, P., McDonald, C., Neville, P., Palmer, R.R., and Wellstood-Eason, S. (1985). The Leicester ECT trial: results in schizophrenia. *British Journal of Psychiatry*, **146**, 177–83.

4.3.8 Schizoaffective and schizotypal disorders

Ming T. Tsuang, William S. Stone, and Stephen V. Faraone

Introduction

This chapter focuses on schizoaffective disorder and schizotypal personality disorder, including their clinical features, classification, diagnosis, epidemiology, aetiology, course, prognosis, and possibilities for prevention. Some areas will be emphasized, to reflect controversial issues or new developments. For example, the classification of both these disorders will be stressed to consider the heterogeneity apparent in each of them. The issue is an important one, for at least two reasons. First, it is crucial to develop reliable and valid diagnostic criteria in order to study the aetiology of the disorders and then utilize that knowledge to develop rational and testable treatment strategies. Heterogeneity adds variance to each of these steps that may reduce both the reliability of diagnosis and also the statistical power of experimental designs to detect treatment effects. Second, the development of newer generations of psychopharmacological treatments holds the promise of matching more appropriate and efficacious medications with specific syndromes or types of symptoms. This trend underscores the importance of differential diagnosis in determining what treatment a patient will receive. Heterogeneity within a diagnostic category complicates achievement of this goal. Another area to be emphasized involves the possibility of preventative, as well as palliative, treatments in the near future, for these disorders. In contrast, other areas such as the genetic aetiology of schizoaffective disorder and schizotypal personality disorder, and treatments for schizoaffective disorder, will receive less emphasis here, to avoid redundancies with other chapters in this volume. Each disorder will be considered separately, starting with a review of schizoaffective disorder, the more severe of the two spectrum conditions.

Schizoaffective disorder

Clinical features

Schizoaffective disorder afflicts patients having schizophrenic and affective symptoms. Either they have affective symptoms of sufficient severity and chronicity to exclude an uncomplicated diagnosis of schizophrenia, or they show features of schizophrenia that are sufficient to exclude an uncomplicated diagnosis of an affective disorder. These types of symptoms may or may not occur simultaneously, which underscores the importance of viewing the illness in longitudinal as well as cross-sectional terms. That is, symptom clusters that are primarily affective or primarily schizophrenic may predominate at different times.

Compared with patients with schizophrenia, patients with schizoaffective disorder tend to demonstrate relatively high levels of premorbid function. One of the most common features of the disorder is a precipitating event, such as a life stressor. For example, Tsuang et al.[1] found a higher percentage of such events in schizoaffective disorder (60 per cent) than they did in either schizophrenia (11 per cent), mania (27 per cent), or depression (39 per cent). Marneros et al.[2] also found a higher percentage of precipitating events in schizoaffective disorder (51 per cent) than in schizophrenia (24 per cent), but did not detect a difference between schizoaffective disorder and affective disorder. The nature of the precipitating stressor may vary widely; for instance it may be either physical (e.g. recently giving birth or experiencing a head injury) or interpersonal (e.g. change in an important relationship). The clinical course of the disorder is often characterized by a periodic rapid onset of symptoms that shows a relatively high degree of remission after several weeks or months. As Vaillant pointed out in the 1960s, many of these patients 'recover' completely after an episode, and resume their lives at a premorbid level of function.[3] As will be considered in more detail below, the clinical features of some cases of schizoaffective disorder mainly resemble those of schizophrenia, while the features of other cases are more similar to those of an affective disorder. Regardless of the subtype or variant of the disorder, however, the mortality rate is of special concern. Rates of death, due mainly to suicide or accident, show elevations in this disorder similar to those observed in schizophrenia and in major affective disorders.[4]

In general, the disorder is more common in females than in males.[1,5] The age of onset varies, but tends to be younger than that of unipolar or bipolar disorder. Tsuang et al.[1] found the median age of onset for schizoaffective disorder was 29 years, which was significantly lower than groups with bipolar or unipolar affective disorder, but similar to a group with schizophrenia. Marneros et al.[6] also reported that a median age of onset of 29 years for schizoaffective disorder was lower than the median age for groups with affective disorders (35 years), but also reported that it was higher than a group with schizophrenia (24 years). To an extent, relative differences in the age of onset between schizoaffective and other disorders reflects differences in the diagnostic criteria employed and the heterogeneity of the disorder.

Classification

The classification of schizoaffective disorder has always been controversial. Kraepelin noted in 1919 that patients with both affective and schizophrenic symptoms complicated the differential diagnosis due to the 'mingling of morbid symptoms of both psychoses'. Kasanin first employed the term 'acute schizophrenic psychoses' in 1933 to describe a group of patients who experienced a rapid onset of emotional turmoil and psychotic symptoms, but who recovered after several weeks or months.[5] In other words, the symptoms appeared similar to schizophrenia during periods of exacerbation, but unlike schizophrenia, showed a greater tendency to remit between episodes. These features sparked an ongoing debate by the 1960s about the proper classification of schizoaffective disorder. Much of this discussion involved the possibility that schizoaffective disorder was conceptualized most accurately as follows:

(1) a type of schizophrenia (e.g. 'remitting schizophrenia');

(2) a type of affective disorder;

(3) a unique disorder that was separate from both schizophrenia and bipolar disorder;

(4) an arbitrary categorization of clinical symptoms that masks a continuum of pathology between schizophrenia and affective illness;

(5) a heterogeneous collection of 'interforms' between schizophrenia and affective disorder (i.e. symptoms of both disorders).

The last possibility is not mutually exclusive of the first four; for example, one or more variants of schizoaffective disorder may be related closely to schizophrenia, while another may be related more closely to an affective disorder.

Family and outcome studies provide useful ways of assessing the relative merits of each of the possibilities outlined above. These approaches are informative although interpretations of such studies are complicated at times by the use of different diagnostic criteria across studies.

Family studies

Family studies provide an important tool for assessing the relationship between disorders. In particular, it is a type of genetic study that assumes that related disorders will coaggregate more frequently among biologically related individuals than they would in the general population. Thus, a disorder is concluded to be in the schizophrenia spectrum if it occurs more frequently among the relatives of schizophrenic patients, compared with suitable controls. Similarly, a disorder is considered to be in the affective spectrum if it occurs more frequently among the relatives of patients with affective disorders. Evidence for the inclusion of schizoaffective disorder in the schizophrenia spectrum is discussed in greater detail elsewhere (see Chapter 4.3.5.1). Only representative findings pertinent to the present discussion about the classification of schizoaffective disorder will be summarized here.

Bertelsen and Gottesman[7] summarized a series of seven family studies published between 1979 and 1993, using structured diagnostic criteria. Analyses of risk to the development schizophrenia, schizoaffective disorder, and affective disorder in the first-degree relatives of patients with schizoaffective disorder, were included. In all seven studies, the relatives showed a higher risk of developing an affective disorder than of developing schizoaffective disorder. In five of the seven studies the risks of developing schizophrenia was equal to or greater than the risk of developing schizoaffective disorder. Thus, the relatives of schizoaffective patients showed generally higher risks of developing disorders other than the one with which they were diagnosed. These findings were consistent with a heterogeneous view of schizoaffective disorder, in which individual cases represented subtypes of either schizophrenia or of affective disorder. The findings were also consistent with the possibility that schizoaffective disorder represents a chance collection of 'interforms' between schizophrenia and affective disorder.

These findings were not consistent with the view that schizoaffective disorder represented a continuum between the other two disorders, because in that case, the rate of schizoaffective disorder in first-degree relatives would have been higher, compared with the rates at which these relatives developed schizophrenia or affective disorder. The findings were also inconsistent with the possibility that schizoaffective disorder represented a unique disorder that was independent of either schizophrenia or an affective disorder. In that case, the first-degree relatives of patients with schizoaffective disorder should show relatively high rates of schizoaffective disorder itself, but relatively low rates of the other disorders. Tsuang[8] and others reported similar findings using other definitions of the disorder.[5]

In the series of studies reviewed by Bertelsen and Gottesman,[7] the morbid risk for schizoaffective disorder itself ranged from 1.8 to 6.1 per cent in first-degree relatives of patients with schizoaffective disorder, which was still higher than the rate observed in the general population (see the section on epidemiology below). These results, taken together with the higher risks for both schizophrenia and affective disorder, suggest that schizoaffective disorder is a heterogeneous condition.

The results of family studies allow for a few tentative generalizations concerning the classification of schizoaffective disorder. First, they indicate the likelihood that many cases of the disorder are related to either schizophrenia or affective illness. Results from family studies are less clear about how specific subtypes should be defined.[5] Second, the family studies leave open the possibility that schizoaffective disorder is due to the additive effects of genes for both schizophrenia and affective illness. Third, the rates of schizoaffective disorder are higher among the relatives of schizoaffective patients than would be expected in the general population.

Outcome studies

A majority of outcome studies show that schizoaffective disorder has a better course than schizophrenia, but a poorer course than affective disorder.[9,10] For example, Samson et al.[10] reviewed 10 outcome studies reported between 1963 and 1987 that assessed patients with either schizoaffective disorder or schizophrenia. Global, marital, social, occupational, hospital course, and symptom dimensions of outcome were assessed. In each category, patients with schizophrenia showed poorer outcomes. In contrast, their review of 11 outcome studies comparing schizoaffective disorder with affective disorder showed that affective disorder was associated with equal or better outcomes on almost all dimensions. Thus, despite differences in methodology and diagnostic criteria, schizoaffective disorder was frequently

associated with clinical outcomes that were intermediate between those associated with schizophrenia and those related to affective disorder.

Further evidence for this pattern was provided more recently in an epidemiological family study.[11] Schizoaffective disorder showed levels of impairment that were intermediate between schizophrenia and affective disorder on the Level of Functioning Scale (which includes nine items, such as duration of non-hospital admission, quality of social relations, symptoms, and an overall rating), and on the Scale for the Assessment of Negative Symptoms. These findings, together with family data showing increased rates of both schizophrenia and affective disorder among relatives of schizoaffective patients, were interpreted as additional evidence in favour of the (DSM-IIIR) classification of schizoaffective disorder. They were also interpreted as supportive of the hypothesis that schizoaffective disorder represents an interform of both schizophrenia and affective illness.

Marneros et al.[12] reported on outcomes in the three (modified DSM-IIIR) disorders, as part of the Cologne Longitudinal Study. The outcomes were measured by symptoms in five dimensions (psychotic symptoms, reduction of energetic potential, qualitative and quantitative disturbances of affect, and other disturbances of behaviour) that persisted for at least 3 years. Consistent with the general pattern described thus far, poor outcomes in the schizoaffective group occurred at a rate (49.5 per cent of the sample) that was intermediate between those observed in the schizophrenic (93.2 per cent) and affective groups (35.8 per cent), and differed significantly from both of them.

While these studies show schizoaffective disorder to have intermediate outcomes generally, there are some categories in which it resembles schizophrenia or affective disorder more closely. For example, Samson et al.[10] noted above that outcomes for schizoaffective disorder were equivalent to those for affective disorder in several dimensions. Marneros et al.[13] studied schizophrenic, schizoaffective, and affective subjects who were diagnosed according to narrow, modified DSM-III criteria. On some measures (e.g. psychosocial functioning, as measured by the Global Assessment Scale) the schizoaffective group performed intermediate between the affective group (which was higher) and the schizophrenic group (which was lower). On a measure of social adjustment, however, 70 per cent of the schizoaffective group was rated as good or excellent, which did not differ significantly from the 84 per cent of the affective group who received the same rating. Both groups differed significantly from the schizophrenic group, only 44 per cent of which showed a good or excellent outcome. Moreover, the schizoaffective and affective disorder groups did not differ on a rating scale of psychological impairments (e.g. body language, affect display, conversation skills, and co-operation), although both were rated as significantly less impaired than the schizophrenic group.

Both Kendler et al.[11] and Atre-Vaidya and Taylor[14] reported similarities between some types of psychotic symptoms between schizoaffective disorder and schizophrenia. The former study showed that the two groups did not differ from each other with respect to severity of delusions or positive thought disorder; the latter study showed that the two groups both demonstrated more hallucinations than did an affective disorders group, but did not differ from each other.

These overall differences in outcome further serve to validate the classification of schizoaffective disorder as a separate syndrome. Its heterogeneity, however, raises the issue of whether such intermediate outcomes might reflect the mean of a combination of mainly good and mainly poor outcomes. This in turn leads to the question of whether schizoaffective disorder can be subtyped in a useful and valid manner. If so, are better and worse outcomes associated with different variants of the syndrome?

Vaillant suggested in the 1960s that prognostic indicators, including a good premorbid level of adjustment, the presence of precipitating factors, an acute onset, confusion, the presence of affective symptoms, and a familial history of affective disorder (or the absence of a schizophrenic history), could predict remission in approximately 80 per cent of cases of 'remitting schizophrenia'.[15,16] The inclusion of affective symptoms and a positive family history for affective illness on the list contributed (later) to hypotheses that variants of schizoaffective disorder were related to affective illness and to better outcomes. In contrast, variants associated more with schizophrenic symptoms or family history were likely to be associated with schizophrenia, and with relatively poor outcomes.

There have been a variety of attempts to subtype schizoaffective disorders, based on whether affective or schizophrenic symptoms predominate.[7,16] Tsuang and Fleming[17] also suggested an undifferentiated category. The validity of these attempts has so far remained inconclusive. For example, Bertelsen and Gottesman[7] noted that at best, relatives of individuals with affective type schizoaffective disorder, or schizophrenic type schizoaffective disorder, showed only trends towards higher rates of affective disorder or schizophrenia, respectively. Similarly, Kendler et al.[11] did not detect different rates of schizophrenia or affective illness in first-degree relatives of patients with schizoaffective disorder when the patients were subtyped into bipolar and depressive subgroups. Moreover, the subtypes did not predict differences in outcomes.

Conversely, a latent class analysis of psychotic patients from the Roscommon Study showed that most cases of DSM-IIIR schizoaffective disorder were categorized in either a bipolar schizomania class ($n = 19$), or in a schizodepression class ($n = 13$), rather than in schizophrenia ($n = 1$), major depression ($n = 0$), schizophreniform ($n = 3$), or hebephrenia ($n = 3$) classes.[18] Moreover, Winokur et al.[19] provided indirect evidence for differential outcomes based on subtypes. In that study, subjects were diagnosed with Research Diagnostic Criteria for schizophrenia, affective disorder, or schizoaffective disorder, and evaluated at intake, 1 year later, and 6 years later. Several outcome measures were employed, including 39 Schedule for Affective Disorders and Schizophrenia items. Subjects were then divided into groups that had consistent affective diagnoses (including schizoaffective disorder, affective type) or consistent schizophrenic diagnoses (including schizoaffective disorder, schizophrenic type), at each of the three assessment times. A third group had inconsistent diagnoses. The results showed that recovery from psychosis was more common in the group with consistent diagnoses of affective disorder than it was in the group with consistent diagnoses of schizophrenia. The inconsistent group was intermediate, but was closer to the consistent affective group. Together, these studies show at least some recent support for the subtyping of schizoaffective disorder into mainly affective and mainly schizophrenic variants.

Other factors that may be prognostic of poor outcomes include poor interepisode recoveries,[11] persistent psychotic symptoms in the absence of affective features, poor premorbid social adjustment, chronicity, and a higher number of schizophrenia-like symptoms.[5]

Diagnosis and differential diagnosis

The DSM-IV diagnosis of schizoaffective disorder[20] is listed in the category of 'schizophrenia and other psychotic disorders'. The major feature of the disorder is that, in addition to meeting the clinical criteria for schizophrenia (criterion A), an individual must also experience a major depressive, manic, or mixed episode concurrently. In addition, in the same period of illness, a patient must experience symptoms of psychosis (hallucinations and/or delusions) for a period of at least 2 weeks, in the absence of mood-related symptoms (criterion B). Nevertheless, affective symptoms must comprise a substantial portion of total duration of the illness (criterion C), and symptoms may not be attributable to either substance use or to a major medical condition (criterion D). Two subtypes of the disorder, including bipolar type and depressive type, may be diagnosed.

The criteria for schizoaffective disorder in ICD-10 are similar to those in DSM-IV. The essential requirement is that prominent symptoms of affective disorder and prominent symptoms of schizophrenia are present together for at 2 weeks. Depressive, manic, and mixed subtypes are recognized as in DSM-IV.

The differential diagnosis includes, most prominently, either schizophrenia or affective disorder, which may be differentiated in part by consideration of the longitudinal criteria (criteria B and C), in addition to the cross-sectional criteria (criterion A). The presence of conditions relating to general medication and substance use should also be considered in the differential diagnosis.

Epidemiology

The epidemiological status of schizoaffective disorder is somewhat uncertain compared with schizophrenia, largely because of dilemmas related to the diagnosis and classification of the disorder. To help in the standardization of data from different studies, representative incidence and prevalence estimates will be emphasized from recent investigations that utilized research diagnostic or DSM-IIIR criteria.

Incidence

Earlier studies showed that new cases of 'schizomanic' patients (i.e. manic patients who also demonstrated schizophrenic or paranoid symptoms) numbered approximately 1.7 per 100 000 per year.[5] This was less than the 4 per 100 000 per year shown by 'schizodepressive' patients. The number of schizoaffective cases in this study exceeded the number of manic patients, and made up half of the number of schizophrenic cases. More recently, Tien and Eaton[21] analysed data from the Epidemiologic Catchment Area Study for three non-overlapping groups with psychotic symptoms. One of these groups comprised individuals with 'psychotic affective syndrome', which was similar to schizoaffective disorder except that most members of the group (59 per cent) demonstrated psychotic symptoms only in conjunction with a mood disturbance (essentially DSM-IIIR mood disturbance with psychotic symptoms). The incidence of this disorder was 1.7 per 1000 per year, which was approximately equal to the rate for schizophrenia (2.0 per 1000 per year). Even if the 59 per cent of the group who met the criteria for a mood disorder with psychotic features was excluded, the remaining 41 per cent would still comprise a higher incidence rate than that detected by earlier studies. Differences in sampling procedures (treated versus non-treated samples) may have contributed to the differences observed in the rates. More importantly, however, these studies showed that schizoaffective disorder occurred at 50 to 85 per cent of the rate of schizophrenia, thus confirming that patients with this disorder comprise a clinically significant population.

Prevalence

There are no epidemiological studies of prevalence for schizoaffective disorder, but prevalence estimates are available, based on samples that were treated in clinics. Because a variety of factors influence the decision to enter and remain in treatment, the estimates show substantial variation. For example, Muller-Oerlinghausen et al.[22] showed that the prevalence of schizoaffective disorder assessed in lithium clinics ranged from 7 per cent in Aarhus, to 15 per cent in Berlin, 23 per cent in Vienna, and 32 per cent in Hamilton. Junginger et al.[23] found that 14 per cent of delusional patients met DSM-IIIR criteria for schizoaffective disorder, compared with 60 per cent who met the criteria for schizophrenia and 17 per cent who met the criteria for bipolar disorder. Data from the Cologne Longitudinal Study showed that 28.5 per cent of the sample with psychoses met DSM-IIIR criteria for schizoaffective disorder, which was similar to the rate for affective disorders (30 per cent), but less than the rate for schizophrenia.[24] Prevalence estimates of putative schizoaffective subtypes are subject to the same inconsistencies of diagnosis and selection factors that affect schizoaffective disorder itself. Not surprisingly, there is little consensus about whether manic or schizophrenic subtypes predominate (see also Tsuang et al.[5]).

Review of evidence

Treatments for schizoaffective disorder are the same as those for schizophrenia and affective disorders alone. As the nature and efficacy of those treatments are discussed elsewhere, they will not be considered here. Rather, this section will focus on management issues related to the need to treat symptoms of both disorders simultaneously, or sequentially.

Management

The authors have found it useful to consider its psychopharmacological treatment in terms of its putative subtypes, including affective type schizoaffective disorder and schizophrenic type schizoaffective disorder.

Treatment of affective type schizoaffective disorder will include antipsychotic medication (e.g. clozapine, risperidone or olanzepine), particularly if psychotic symptoms are present. In addition, antidepressants, mood stabilizers (e.g. lithium), or anticonvulsants (e.g. valproate or carbamazepine) may be useful with this group. It will be necessary in such cases to weigh the potential risks of such medications, such as elevated toxicity, against the potential benefits.

In schizophrenic type schizoaffective disorder, combination treatments may also be more effective than a single treatment. We find, however, that antipsychotic treatments alone may be more efficient in many cases. This is particularly true if affective symptoms (i.e. depression) are largely secondary to the experience of having a psychotic condition, and its attendant interpersonal, social, and financial difficulties. In these cases, remediation of the psychotic symptoms may also have the effect of easing the affective problems. For other cases, which include more of a treatment-refractory depression, anti-

psychotic medication may be augmented with lithium[25] or antidepressant medication. Moreover, electroconvulsive therapy may reduce mortality rates in schizoaffective patients.[26]

The authors also note that clinically, it may sometimes be difficult to distinguish the affective subtype from the schizophrenic subtype. In these cases treatment decisions must rest on the presenting symptoms of the patient. Treatment during intermorbid periods is in part dependent on the presence or absence of psychotic symptoms. As noted above, psychotic episodes in this period are associated with relatively poorer outcomes, and are likely to require chronic antipsychotic therapy.

Schizotypal personality disorder

Clinical features

Schizotypal personality disorder is a complex and chronic condition that includes some, but not all, of the features of schizoaffective disorder and schizophrenia. Notably, persistent psychosis is not part of the syndrome, although mild forms of thought disorder may occur (e.g. magical thinking, ideas of reference). Moreover, brief episodes of psychosis may occur in times of stress.

Schizotypal patients show pervasive deficits in social and interpersonal traits. They often demonstrate aloofness, poor eye contact, affective constriction, and suspiciousness. Consequently, close interpersonal relationships are either avoided or cause discomfort and anxiety. Thus, these individuals have few friends. Not surprisingly, schizotypal patients are often deficient in accurately sensing social cues or affective signals from others. Although they can interact with people when necessary, they often prefer not to, and do not become more comfortable in social situations with time.

Schizotypal patients also show magical thinking, ideas of reference, unusual perceptions (e.g. sensing the presence of another person, or that people are talking about them), and/or perceptual illusions (e.g. often perceiving a dimly lit lamp-post as a person). Both their social deficits and these cognitive–perceptual problems contribute to an overall impression of oddness. However, this feature may occur independently of other clinical symptoms,[27] and manifest itself in odd speech or unusual appearance. The oddness or eccentricities evident in these patients are often ego syntonic (i.e. they are not experienced as problems). Moreover, schizotypal patients show deficits in attention, long-term verbal memory, and executive functions. These deficits are qualitatively similar to those seen in schizophrenia, but like many other clinical manifestations of this disorder, they are quantitatively milder.

Like schizophrenia, schizotypal personality disorder is often evident by early adulthood, but schizotypal traits may be evident in late childhood or adolescence.[28] Once it appears, the disorder tends to show a chronic course, but one that includes periodic exacerbations and attenuations of symptoms.

Classification

In contrast to the controversy surrounding the classification of schizoaffective disorder, family, twin, and adoption studies clearly support the view that schizotypal personality disorder is best classified in the schizophrenia spectrum.[29] Nevertheless, it is a complex and chronic disorder that in all likelihood, is also heterogeneous. Kendler[30] pointed out that this heterogeneity was at least partly related to the two primary methods used to study the disorder. One of these involves the 'clinical method', which identifies patients with mild forms of schizophrenic or psychotic-like symptoms. Thaker et al.[31] for example, reported that clinical schizotypal subjects were characterized by relatively high levels of positive psychiatric symptoms (e.g. magical thinking and perceptual distortions).

In contrast, the 'family research method' identifies relatives of patients with schizophrenia who have subtle, schizophrenia-like symptoms. Features associated more with familial than with clinical schizotypal personality disorder include a predominance of negative symptoms (e.g. social withdrawal and impairment, and higher levels of anxiety and poor rapport), cognitive impairments (e.g. impaired language comprehension, eye-tracking, and attentional dysfunctions), and elevated rates of schizophrenia and related disorders in family members.[29] Thaker et al.[31] reported that familial and clinical schizotypal personality disorders were similar on measures of physical or social anhedonia. Also, some neuropsychological deficits are associated with both groups.[32,33]

The concept of familial schizotypal disorder is particularly important because it may share a common genetic basis with schizophrenia. Meehl[34] first proposed the term 'schizotaxia' to describe the genetic vulnerability to schizophrenia, and suggested that individuals with schizotaxia would eventually develop either schizotypal personality disorder or schizophrenia, depending on the protection or liability afforded by environmental circumstances. As the concept evolved, Meehl[35] reformulated it to allow for the possibility that some people with schizotaxia would develop neither schizophrenia nor schizotypal personality disorder. In fact, evidence now shows that the clinical symptoms observed in many non-psychotic, first-degree relatives of people with schizophrenia are similar to those observed in familial schizotypal personality disorder.[29] Psychiatric features in such relatives frequently include an aggregation of negative symptoms that are qualitatively similar to, but milder than, those often cited in schizophrenia.[36] Positive symptoms, however, are usually less evident in these relatives than they are in schizophrenia or in schizotypal personality disorder. Neuropsychological impairments in biological relatives of people with schizophrenia are also qualitatively similar to, but milder than, those seen in people with schizophrenia.[29] In particular, these neuropsychological deficits frequently include problems in working memory/attention, long-term verbal memory, and concept formation/abstraction.

Faraone et al. recently suggested a reformulation of Meehl's concept of schizotaxia that focuses on these features of negative symptoms and neuropsychological deficits.[29] Unlike schizotypal personality disorder, which occurs in less than 10 per cent of the adult relatives of patients diagnosed with schizophrenia, the basic symptoms of schizotaxia occur in 20 to 50 per cent of adult relatives,[37,38] suggesting further that the genetic liability to schizophrenia does not lead inevitably to schizophrenia, schizotypal personality disorder, or schizoid personality disorder.

Diagnosis and differential diagnosis

The DSM-IV criteria for schizotypal personality disorder[20] includes a 'pervasive pattern of social deficits' and 'cognitive or perceptual distortions' and behavioural 'eccentricities' (criterion A). At least five of nine specific symptoms (e.g. ideas of reference, constricted affect, odd behaviour or appearance) must be present to satisfy this criterion. These symptoms must occur by early adulthood. They must not occur exclusively during the course of four other conditions, including schizophrenia, a mood disorder with psychotic features, any other psychotic disorder, or a pervasive developmental disorder (criterion B).

The differential diagnosis includes a variety of other disorders. A key difference between schizotypal personality disorder and schizophrenia, a psychotic mood disorder, or another psychotic condition involves the transient nature of psychotic symptoms in schizotypal personality disorder. It may be distinguished from developmental communication disorders by a lack of compensatory means (e.g. gestures) of communicating, and it may be distinguished from autistic or Asperger's disorders by the relatively greater deficits in social awareness and frequent presence of stereotyped behaviours in those disorders. Schizotypal personality disorder may be confused with several other personality disorders, but it can be distinguished. In particular, it differs from schizoid personality disorder by its pattern of cognitive–perceptual distortions, and by the odd appearance or behaviour shown frequently by schizotypal patients. The pattern of schizotypal symptoms also differs from that manifested in borderline personality disorder, although there are similarities between these conditions. Schizotypal personality disorder differs from borderline personality disorder, however, in that psychotic-like symptoms and social isolation are more likely to persist in the absence of affective turmoil, and schizotypal individuals are less likely to display the impulsive and manipulative traits often associated with borderline personality disorder.

Epidemiology

Incidence

To the authors' knowledge, there are no published incidence studies for schizotypal personality disorder.

Prevalence

Lyons[39] reviewed recent prevalence studies for schizotypal personality disorder. Prevalence rates in non-clinical samples ranged from 0.7 to 5.1 per cent, with a median near 3.0 per cent. Higher rates occurred in clinical samples—2.0 to 64 per cent, with a median of 17.5 per cent. The prevalence of schizotypal personality disorder among the relatives of schizophrenic index cases is as high as 10 per cent.[40]

Treatment

Review of evidence

There is, unfortunately, a dearth of outcome studies involving psychotherapy, psychosocial, or psychopharmacological treatments for schizotypal personality disorder. Published studies often show methodological limitations (e.g. small samples, subjects with mixed diagnoses, inadequate controls, and problems with internal validity), or provide outcome data on only limited aspects of the disorder. Despite these caveats, it is clear that few treatment gains are evident. This is particularly true of studies that utilized psychodynamically oriented therapy, either alone or in combination with other treatments (e.g. group therapy or art therapy) as the primary treatment modality.[41]

For example, McGlashan[42] studied former inpatients approximately 15 years after treatment, who were given retrospective DSM-III diagnoses. The study followed up former patients with a variety of diagnoses, including among others, 'pure' schizotypal personality disorder (*n* = 10). Multiple outcome measures were employed. Because the main purpose of the study was to examine schizotypal personality disorder as a diagnostic entity, there was little emphasis on assessing change in the same measures, which complicates any interpretation. The results showed, however, that most subjects with pure schizotypal personality disorder functioned poorly at follow-up. On one measure of global functioning in which continuously disabled subjects scored zero and normal subjects scored 4 points, the mean score was 1.6.

Several studies investigated the usefulness of medications in treating schizotypal personality disorder, although most investigations employed small numbers of subjects and combined samples of schizotypal and borderline personality disorders.[43,44] For these reasons, conclusions about the effectiveness of treatment must be equivocal. Typical antipsychotic drugs, in particular, have been proposed to reduce positive symptoms or depressed mood in times of acute stress, but the high incidence of adverse side-effects has discouraged their widespread use at other times, including the more chronic stable (i.e. non-crisis) phases of the disorder.[43,45] Other types of medication, including fluoxetine, have shown generally non-specific effects of treatment.[43]

Amoxipine, which has antidepressant and neuroleptic effects, was administered to a small group of personality disordered patients, that included five subjects diagnosed with DSM-III schizotypal personality disorder.[46] After an average treatment duration of 39 days, significant reductions were evident in total scores on the Brief Psychiatric Rating Scale, and on the Hamilton Rating Scale for Depression.

Goldberg et al.[47] administered thiothixine (an antipsychotic medication) to a group of patients that included, among others, DSM-III schizotypal personality disorder (*n* = 6). The Global Assessment Scale and Hopkins Symptom Checklist-90 were among the measures used to assess treatment effects. At the end of 12 weeks of treatment, little therapeutic change was evident within the schizotypal group, but modest improvements were observed in particular areas across groups, such as the psychotic and obsessive–compulsive scales of the Hopkins Symptom Checklist-90.

Hymowitz et al.[48] administered a low dose of haloperidol to 17 outpatients with DSM-III diagnoses of schizotypal personality disorder, for 6 weeks. The initial dose of 2.0 mg was intended to rise to 12.0 mg, but side-effects prevented increases beyond a mean dose of 3.6 mg. Even with lower doses, 50 per cent of the sample withdrew from the study because of side-effects. The 17 subjects who completed 2 weeks of the protocol improved somewhat in ratings of ideas of reference, odd communications, social isolation, and overall functioning.

In summary, the available literature offers few clear indications of effective treatments. The mechanisms of those few treatments that were somewhat effective, remain unclear. Interestingly, improvements in types of symptoms (e.g. psychoticism on the Hopkins Symptom Checklist-90) across diagnoses, rather than within them,[47] suggests that medications may help at least some subgroups of patients. A review of the medications used in these studies also shows the need to find treatments that are well tolerated, and that target negative symptoms and cognitive deficits.

Management

Patients with schizotypal personality disorder often view their worlds as odd and threatening places and may require extended courses of treatment.[45,49] Unfortunately, trust and rapport with the therapist, which are necessary for the success of any therapy, are often difficult to establish in schizotypal personality disorder. The frequent occurrence of paranoia and suspiciousness, together with social aloofness and constricted affect, make exploratory psychotherapeutic approaches less effective than supportive cognitive–behavioural therapies.[45] In fact, these patients may only seek treatment to alleviate circumscribed problems, like anxiety or somatic complaints. Approaches that emphasize concrete, interim goals, and stipulate explicit means of attaining them, thus have the best chances of success. Because individuals with this disorder are vulnerable to decompensation during times of stress and may experience transient episodes of psychosis, they may also benefit from techniques to facilitate stress reduction (e.g. relaxation techniques, exercise, yoga, and meditation). Fortunately, some people with schizotypal features are likely to seek treatment in times of stress.[50] In the short term, brief courses of antipsychotic treatment may be useful if symptoms of psychosis appear.

Cognitive problems are also frequently amenable to concrete goal-oriented approaches to treatment. Patients benefit from an understanding of their cognitive strengths and weaknesses, to help them confront and cope with long-standing difficulties in their lives. For example, problems in attention, verbal memory or organizational skills contribute to failures in educational, occupational, and social endeavours, while reinforcing negative self-images and increasing performance anxiety. Knowledge of circumscribed cognitive problems allows patients to reframe their difficulties in a more positive manner, and facilitate selection of realistic personal, educational, and occupational goals. Moreover, specific cognitive deficits are often subject to partial remediation. For example, standard procedures will attenuate deficits in the acquisition, organization, and retrieval of new information (e.g. writing information down in a 'memory notebook', using appointment books or planners, and rehearsing new information, among others).

Possibilities for prevention

At present, most early intervention programmes involve secondary prevention, which includes the early identification and treatment of clinical (usually psychotic) symptoms.[51] While intervention is necessary to alleviate clinical symptoms at any point during the disorder, it is particularly important early on because it might alter the course of the illness. Patients treated with antipsychotic medication during their first or second hospital admission, for example, show better outcomes than those who are not treated until later in the course of the disorder.[52]

Primary prevention, which involves treatment before the disorder manifests itself clinically, is not yet available for schizoaffective disorder, schizotypal personality disorder, or other disorders in the schizophrenia spectrum. To develop such treatments, it will be necessary to predict who is most likely to develop a disorder. Here, there are some encouraging signs. These include several ongoing 'high-risk' studies, which follow the offspring of schizophrenic parents longitudinally. Such studies help to identify traits early in life that predict which individuals are most likely to experience clinical symptoms in adulthood. In the New York High Risk Project, for instance, problems with attention in childhood predicted social deficits in adolescence and social isolation in adulthood.[53] In another study, Walker and Lewine[54] found that social and neuropsychological impairments characterized children who subsequently developed schizophrenia. This type of study is important because it facilitates formation of homogeneous high-risk groups, which in turn facilitates the development of focused prevention strategies.

With current knowledge, it is difficult to justify preventive treatments—especially medication—for people without symptoms. The authors have argued elsewhere, however, that if people in high-risk groups (like first-degree biological relatives of patients with schizophrenia) show clinically meaningful symptoms, then treatment attempts may be appropriate.[29] The authors recently proposed this course of action for people with 'schizotaxia', and suggested preliminary guidelines for treatment.[55]

Eventually, prevention will be a primary therapeutic approach for the treatment of disorders in the schizophrenia spectrum. While primary prevention has yet to occur, the authors are optimistic that high-risk studies, progress in secondary prevention, and progress in discovering the genetic aetiology of the schizophrenia spectrum, will facilitate primary prevention strategies in the near future.

References

1. Tsuang, M.T., Simpson, S.J.C., and Fleming, J.A. (1986). Diagnostic criteria for subtyping schizoaffective disorder. In *Schizoaffective psychoses* (ed. A. Marneros and M.T. Tsuang), pp. 50–62. Springer-Verlag, Berlin.

2. Marneros, A., Deister, A., and Rohde, A. (1990). Sociodemographic and premorbid features of schizophrenic, schizoaffective and affective psychoses. In *Affective and schizoaffective disorders* (ed. A. Marneros and M.T. Tsuang), pp. 130–45. Springer-Verlag, Berlin.

3. Vaillant, G. (1962). The prediction of recovery in schizophrenia. *Journal of Nervous and Mental Diseases*, **135**, 534–43.

4. Simpson, J. (1988). Mortality studies in schizophrenia. In *Nosology, epidemiology and genetics of schizophrenia* (ed. M.T. Tsuang and J.C. Simpson), pp. 245–73. Elsevier Science, Amsterdam.

5. Tsuang, M.T., Levitt, J.J., and Simpson, J.C. (1995). Schizoaffective disorder. In *Schizophrenia* (ed. S.R. Hirsch and D. Weinberger). Blackwell Scientific, Oxford.

6. Marneros, A., Deister, A., and Rohde, A. (1990). Psychopathological and social status of patients with affective, schizophrenic and schizoaffective disorders after long-term course. *Acta Psychiatrica Scandinavica*, **82**, 352–8.

7. Bertelsen, A. and Gottesman, I.I. (1995). Schizoaffective psychoses: genetical clues to classification. *American Journal of Medical Genetics (Neuropsychiatric Genetics)*, **60**, 7–11.

8. Tsuang, M.T. (1991). Morbidity risks of schizophrenia and affective disorders among first-degree relatives of patients with schizoaffective disorders. *British Journal of Psychiatry*, **158**, 165–70.

9. Angst, J. (1986). The course of schizoaffective disorders. In *Schizoaffective psychoses* (ed. A. Marneros and M.T. Tsuang), pp. 63–93. Springer-Verlag, Berlin.

10. Samson, J.A., Simpson, J.C., and Tsuang, M.T. (1988). Outcome of schizoaffective disorders. *Schizophrenia Bulletin*, **14**, 543–54.

11. Kendler, K.S., McGuire, M., Gurneberg, A.M., and Walsh, D. (1995). Examining the validity of DSM-III-R schizoaffective disorder and its putative subtypes in the Roscommon family study. *American Journal of Psychiatry*, **152**, 755–64.

12. Marneros, A., Rohde, A., and Deister, A. (1998). Frequency and phenomenology of persisting alterations in affective, schizoaffective and schizophrenia disorders: a comparison. *Psychopathology*, **31**, 23–8.

13. Marneros, A., Deister, A., and Rohde, A. (1992). Comparisons of long-term outcome of schizophrenic, affective and schizoaffective disorders. *British Journal of Psychiatry*, **161** (Supplement 18), 44–51.

14. Atre-Vaidya, N. and Taylor, M.A. (1997). Differences in the prevalence of psychosensory features among schizophrenic, schizoaffective, and manic patients. *Comprehensive Psychiatry*, **38**, 88–92.

15. Vaillant, G. (1964). Prospective prediciton of schizophrenic remission. *Archives of General Psychiatry*, **11**, 509–18.

16. Levitt, J.J. and Tsuang, M.T. (1988). The heterogeneity of schizoaffective disorder: implications for treatment. *American Journal of Psychiatry*, **145**, 926–36.

17. Tsuang, M.T. and Fleming, J.A. (1986). Long-term outcome of schizophrenia and other psychoses. In *Search for the causes of schizophrenia*, pp. 88–97.

18. Kendler, K.S., Karkowski, L.M., and Walsh, D. (1998). The structure of psychosis. *Archives of General Psychiatry*, **55**, 492–9.

19. Winokur, G., Monahan, P., Coryell, W., and Zimmerman, M. (1996). Schizophrenia and affective disorder—distinct entities or continuum? An analysis based on a prospective 6-year follow-up. *Comprehensive Psychiatry*, **37**, 77–87.

20. American Psychiatric Association (1994). *Diagnostic and statistical manual of mental disorders* (4th edn). American Psychiatric Association, Washington, DC.

21. Tien, A.Y. and Eaton, W.W. (1992). Psychopathologic precursors and sociodemographic risk factors for the schizophrenia syndrome. *Archives of General Psychiatry*, **49**, 37–46.

22. Muller-Oerlinghausen, B., Ahrens, B., Grof, E., *et al.* (1992). The effect of long-term lithium treatment on the mortality of patients with manic-depressive and schizoaffective illness. *Acta Psychiatrica Scandinavica*, **86**, 218–22.

23. Junginger, J., Barker, S., and Coe, D. (1992). Mood theme and bizarreness of delusions in schizophrenia and mood psychosis. *Journal of Abnormal Psychology*, **101**, 287–92.

24. Marneros, A., Deister, A., and Rohde, A. (1991). Stability of diagnoses in affective, schizoaffective and schizophrenic disorders: cross sectional versus longitudinal data. *European Archives of Psychiatry and Clinical Neurosciences*, **241**, 187–92.

25. de Montigny, C., Cournoyer, G., Morisette, R., Langlois, R., and Caille, G. (1983). Lithium carbonate addition in tricyclic anti-depressant resistant unipolar depression: correlations with neurobiological actions of tricyclic antidepressant drugs and lithium ion on serotonin systems. *Archives of General Psychiatry*, **40**, 1327–34.

26. Tsuang, M.T., Dempsey, G.M., and Fleming, J.A. (1979). Can ECT prevent premature death and suicide in 'schizoaffective patients? *Journal of Affective Disorders*, **1**, 167–71.

27. Battaglia, M., Cavallini, M.C., Macciardi, F., and Bellodi, L. (1997). The structure of DSM-III-R schizotypal personality disorder diagnosed by direct interviews. *Schizophrenia Bulletin*, **23**, 83–92.

28. Olin, S.S., Raine, A., Cannon, T.D., Parnas, J., Schulsinger, F., and Mednick, S.A. (1997). Childhood behavior precursors of schizotypal personality disorder. *Schizophrenia Bulletin*, **23**, 93–103.

29. Faraone, S.V., Green, A.I., Seidman, L.J., and Tsuang, M.T. Clinical implications of schizotaxia: a new direction for research. *Schizophrenia Bulletin*, in press.

30. Kendler, K.S. (1985). Diagnostic approaches to schizotypal personality disorder: a historical perspective. *Schizophrenia Bulletin*, **11**, 538–53.

31. Thaker, G., Moran, M., Adami, H., and Cassady, S. (1993). Psychosis proneness scales in schizophrenia spectrum personality disorders: familial vs. nonfamilial samples. *Psychiatry Research*, **46**, 47–57.

32. Kendler, K.S., Ochs, A.L., Gorman, A.M., Hewitt, J.K., Ross, D.E., and Mirsky, A.F. (1993). The structure of schizotypy: a pilot multitrait twin study. *Psychiatry Research*, **36**, 19–36.

33. Voglmaier, M.M., Seidman, L.J., Salisbury, D., and McCarley, R.W. (1997). Neuropsychological dysfunction in schizotypal personality disorder: a profile analysis. *Biological Psychiatry*, **41**, 530–40.

34. Meehl, P.E. (1962). Schizotaxia, schizotypy, schizophrenia. *American Psychologist*, **17**, 827–38.

35. Meehl, P.E. (1989). Schizotaxia revisited. *Archives of General Psychiatry*, **46**, 935–44.

36. Tsuang, M.T., Gilbertson, M.W., and Faraone, S.V. (1991). Genetic transmission of negative and positive symptoms in the biological relatives of schizophrenics. In *Positive vs. negative schizophrenia* (ed. A. Marneros, M.T. Tsuang, and N. Andreasen), pp. 265–91. Springer-Verlag, New York.

37. Faraone, S.V., Seidman, L.J., Kremen, W.S., Pepple, J.R., Lyons, M.J., and Tsuang, M.T. (1995). Neuropsychological functioning among the nonpsychotic relatives of schizophrenic patients: a diagnostic efficiency analysis. *Journal of Abnormal Psychology*, **104**, 286–304.

38. Faraone, S.V., Kremen, W.S., Lyons, M.J., Pepple, J.R., Seidman, L.J., and Tsuang, M.T. (1995). Diagnostic accuracy and linkage analysis: how useful are schizophrenia spectrum phenotypes? *American Journal of Psychiatry*, **152**, 1286–90.

39. Lyons, M.J. (1995). Epidemiology of personality disorders. In *Textbook in psychiatric epidemiology* (ed. M.T. Tsuang, M. Tohen, and G.E. Zahner), pp. 407–36. Wiley-Liss, New York.

40. Battaglia, M. and Torgersen, S. (1996). Schizotypal disorder: at the crossroads of genetics and nosology. *Acta Psychiatrica Scandinavica*, **94**, 303–10.

41. Tsuang, M.T., Stone, W.S., and Faraone, S.V. Overview of treatments for schizotypal and schizoid personality disorders. *Noos*, in press.

42. McGlashan, T.H. (1986). Schizotypal personality disorder. Chestnut Lodge follow-up study. VI. Long-term follow-up perspectives. *Archives of General Psychiatry*, **43**, 329–34.

43. Coccaro, E.F. (1998). Clinical outcome of psychopharmacologic treatment of borderline and schizotypal personality disordered subjects. *Journal of Clinical Psychiatry*, **59** (Supplement 1), 30–5.

44. Stein, G. (1992). Drug treatment of the personality disorders. *British Journal of Psychiatry*, **161**, 167–84.

45. The Quality Assurance Project (1990). Treatment outlines for paranoid schizotypal and schizoid personality disorders. *Australian and New Zealand Journal of Psychiatry*, **24**, 339–50.

46. Jensen, H.V. and Andersen, J. (1989). An open, noncomparative study of amoxipine in borderline disorders. *Acta Psychiatrica Scandinavica*, **79**, 89–93.

47. Goldberg, S.C., Schulz, C., Schulz, P.M., Resnick, R.J., Hamer, R.M., and Friedel, R.O. (1986). Borderline and schizotypal disorders treated with low-dose thiothixene. *Archives of General Psychiatry*, **43**, 680–6.

48. Hymowitz, P., Frances, A., Jacobsberg, L.B., Sickles, M., and Hoyt, R. (1986). Neuroleptic treatment of schizotypal personality disorders. *Comprehensive Psychiatry*, **27**, 267–71.

49. Stone, M. (1985). Schizotypal personality: psychotherapeutic aspects. *Schizophrenia Bulletin*, **11**, 576–98.

50. Poreh, A. and Whitman, D. (1993). MMPI-2 schizophrenia spectrum profiles among schizotypal college students and college students who seek psychological treatment. *Psychological Reports*, **73**, 987–94.

51. Falloon, I.R.H., Kydd, R.R., Coverdale, J.H., and Laidlaw, T.M. (1996). Early detection and intervention for initial episodes of schizophrenia. *Schizophrenia Bulletin*, **22**, 271–82.

52. Wyatt, R.J. (1995). Early intervention for schizophrenia: can the course of the illness be altered? *Biological Psychiatry*, **38**, 1–3.

53. Dworkin, R.H., Cornblatt, B.A., Friedmann, R., *et al.* (1993). Childhood precursors of affective vs. social deficits in adolescents at risk for schizophrenia. *Schizophrenia Bulletin*, **19**, 563–77.

54. Walker, E. and Lewine, R.J. (1990). Prediction of adult-onset schizophrenia from childhood home movies of the parents. *American Journal of Psychiatry*, **147**, 1052–6.

55. Tsuang, M.T., Stone, W.S., Seidman, L.L., *et al.* Treatment of nonpsychotic relatives of patients with schizophrenia: four case studies. *Biological Psychiatry*, **45**, 1412–18.

4.3.9 Acute and transient psychotic disorders

J. Garrabé and F.-R. Cousin

Historic introduction

Acute and transient psychotic episodes have been described since the end of the nineteenth century. Descriptions have varied from one country to another, so that the exact nosology has not yet been established. The links between acute psychoses (generally defined as having brief obvious psychotic symptomatology) and chronic psychoses (schizophrenic psychoses and psychoses with persistent delusions) are still under discussion.

For instance, sections F20 and F21 in ICD-10[1] are devoted to 'Schizophrenia, schizotypal and delusional disorders'. A specific diagnostic category named 'Acute and transient psychotic disorders' is included, distinct from Schizophrenia (F20), Schizotypal disorder (F21), Persistent delusional disorder (F22), Induced delusional disorder (also called *folie à deux*) (F24), and Schizoaffective disorder (F25).

In this textbook, the acute and transient psychotic disorders (Chapter 4.3.9) appear in the section dedicated to schizophrenia, which also includes schizotypal disorders and schizoaffective disorders (Chapter 4.3.8). However, this section is clearly distinguished from the chapter in which the persistent delusional disorders are discussed (Chapter 4.4). These taxonomic divergences are justified more by the history of acute psychoses than by scientific findings.

In the nineteenth century German psychiatists had already described *akute primäre Verrucktheit*,[2] termed *paranoia acuta* by Karl Westphal. In 1876 (published in 1878), Westphal used this term to describe an acute form of paranoia with an outburst of perceptual hallucinations, consisting mostly of hallucinatory voices and delusions, with clouding of consciousness. In 1890, Meynert repeated the clinical description but named the condition amentia.[3] Sigmund Freud chose this type of acute delusion with hallucinations for his psychoanalytic conception of psychosis.[4]

In the sixth edition of his textbook, published in 1899, Kraepelin[5] included all the paranoias under dementia praecox, and in the eighth edition (1908–1915) he combined manic and melancholic periodic disorders in a single group, leaving acute psychosis with no place between these two diagnostic categories.

In 1911, Bleuler[6] replaced the single disease dementia praecox by the concept of a group of schizophrenias of various clinical forms. He noticed that schizophrenia often began with an acute excitatory episode lasting from a few hours to a few years. He described a wide variation of outcome of acute forms of psychosis, but he separated acute schizophrenias from simple schizophrenia as he believed that acute forms do not necessarily end in deterioration.

In 1916, based on Karl Jaspers' psychopathology, the Danish psychiatrist Wimmer[7] described psychogenic psychosis as a reactive psychosis arising after psychosocial trauma. Mayer-Gross,[8] who proposed an organic aetiology for schizophrenia, described 'oneiroid states' consisting of acute psychotic symptomatology with no other specific organic features.

In 1961, Leonhard[9] used Kleist's concept of marginal psychosis (*Randpsychosen*) to develop his description of 'cycloid psychoses' as endogenous psychoses separate from schizophrenic psychoses and from manic and melancholic psychoses. These cycloid psychoses tend to have a benign and periodic course.

Earlier (1933), Kasanin[10] had described 'acute schizoaffective psychoses', raising questions about the links between schizophrenic and affective diseases.

Langfeldt[11] suggested that observation for 5 years was required to be able to distinguish schizophrenia and what he called schizophreniform psychosis. This long-term observation is a reminder of the Bleulerian concept of acute schizophrenias which could last for several years. Epidemiological studies have led to the presence in modern classifications of a group of acute schizophreniform psychoses under the rubric 'Schizophreniform disorder' (DSM-IV Section 295.40) or 'Acute psychotic disorder schizophrenic-like' (ICD-10 Section F23.2).

In France the concept of *bouffée délirante* led naturally to a specific class of acute psychoses. In 1895, Magnan[12] and his disciple Legrain[13] described *bouffée délirante* or *délire d'emblée* (immediate delusion) within the polymorphic delusions of the chronic insane. This concept is based on Morel's theory of degeneration, commonly accepted in the nineteenth century. The question of whether there is a susceptibility or a predisposition to the occurrence of an acute psychosis remains unanswered.[14]

In 1954, Ey[15,16] described the development of the concept of *bouffées délirantes* and of acute psychoses with hallucinations from the time of Magnan to a symposium devoted to the clinical subdivision of schizophrenic psychoses held at the First World Congress of Psychiatry in 1950, where the various ideas were discussed by Langfeldt, Karl Leonhard, and Aubrey Lewis (Table 1)

Clinical description: psychopathology

The heterogeneous group of acute and transient psychotic disorders are characterized by three typical features, listed below in descending order of priority:

- suddenness of onset (within 2 weeks or less)
- presence of typical syndromes with polymorphic (changing and variable) or schizophrenic symptoms
- presence of associated acute stress (stressful events such as bereavement, job loss, psychological trauma, etc.).

The onset of the disorder is manifested by an obvious change to an abnormal psychotic state. This is considered to be abrupt when it occurs within 48 h or less. Abrupt onset often indicates a better outcome. Full recovery occurs within 3 months and often in a shorter time (a few days or weeks). However, a small number of patients develop persistent and disabling states.

The general (G) criteria for these acute disorders in DCR-10 (Diagnostic Criteria Research of ICD) are as follows.

G1   There is acute onset of delusions, hallucinations, incomprehensible or incoherent speech, or any combination of these. The time

Table 1 Historical development of the terminology of acute and transient psychotic disorders

Historic term	Current terminology
1876 Westphal *Akute primäre Verrucktheit* *Paranoia acuta*	F23.3 Other acute predominantly delusional psychotic disorder
1890 Meynert Amentia	
1895 Magnan and Legrain *Bouffées délirantes*	F23.0 Acute polymorphic psychotic disorder without symptoms of schizophrenia
1899 Kraepelin Dementia praecox	F20.0 Schizophrenia
1909–1913 Kraepelin Paranoia	F22.0 Persistent delusional disorder
1911 Bleuler Acute-onset forms of schizophrenia	F23.1 Acute polymorphic psychotic disorder with symptoms of schizophrenia F23.2 Acute schizophrenia-like psychotic disorder
1916 Wimmer Psychogenic psychosis	F23.3 Other acute predominantly psychotic disorder
1924 Mayer-Gross *Oneroide Erlebnisform*	F23.2 Acute schizophrenia-like psychotic disorder
1933 Kasanin Acute schizoaffective psychoses	F25 Schizoaffective disorders
1939 Langfeldt Schizophreniform states	F23.2 Acute schizophrenia-like psychotic disorder
1954 Ey *Bouffées délirantes et psychoses hallucinatoires aigues*	F23.0 Acute polymorphic psychotic disorder without symptoms of schizophrenia
1961 Leonhard Cycloid psychoses	F23.0 Acute polymorphic psychotic disorder without symptoms of schizophrenia

interval between the first appearance of any psychotic symptoms and the presentation of the fully developed disorder should not exceed 2 weeks.

G2   If transient states of perplexity, misidentification, or impairment of attention and concentration are present, they do not fulfil the criteria for organically caused clouding of consciousness as specified for F05, criterion A.

G3   The disorder does not satisfy the symptomatic criteria for manic episode (F30), depressive episode (F32), or recurrent depressive disorder (F33).

G4   There is insufficient evidence of recent psychoactive substance use to satisfy the criteria for intoxication (F1x.0), harmful use (F1x.1), dependence (F1x.2), or withdrawal states (F1x.3 and F1x.4). The continued moderate and largely unchanged use of alcohol or drugs in the amounts or with the frequency to which the individual is accustomed does not necessarily exclude the use of F23; this must be decided by clinical judgement and the requirements of the research project in question.

G5 There must be no organic mental disorder (F00–F09) or serious metabolic disturbances affecting the central nervous system (this does not include childbirth). (This is the most commonly used exclusion clause.)

A fifth character should be used to specify whether the acute onset of the disorder is associated with acute stress (occurring 2 weeks or less before evidence of first psychotic symptoms):

- F23.x0 without associated acute stress
- F23.x1 with associated acute stress.

For research purposes it is recommended that change of the disorder from a non-psychotic to a clearly psychotic state is further specified as either abrupt (onset within 48 h) or acute (onset in more than 48 h but less than 2 weeks).

Six categories of acute psychoses are presented in ICD-10, and we shall discuss them in order.

F23.0 Acute polymorphic psychotic disorder without symptoms of schizophrenia

The diagnostic criteria are based on the classical symptoms of the true *bouffée délirante* described by Magnan and Legrain.

Suddenness of onset

Bouffée délirante occurs over a period of a few hours or days, usually to young adults and often women in their thirties. The onset of the delirious episode is 'like a thunderbolt in a serene sky'. This aphorism from Legrain has the same meaning as the French classical expression *délire d'emblée* (immediate delusion).

Although premonitory symptoms, such as increasing perplexity and anxiety, may occur, the delusions start suddenly and are always accompanied by a break-up in the individual psychic life. If the onset is preceded by a stressful or traumatic event, such as resettlement or acculturation, this may take place some months previously and the outburst of the delirious episode is delayed. The fifth code character of category F23 is used to specify whether acute stress is associated with the onset of the disorder (e.g. F23.00 has no associated acute stress).

Polymorphic psychotic symptoms

The delusional themes are varied and include grandeur, persecution, influence, possession, body transformation (depersonalization), de-realization, or world alteration; these themes change with time and may combine. Other symptoms are also varied, including hallucinations, illusions, interpretations, and intuitions.

The emotional state

As a consequence of the delusions the patient experiences mood change and emotional turmoil (happiness, ecstasy, anxiety, irritability). However, the criteria for manic episode, depressive episode, schizoaffective disorder, and schizophrenia are not satisfied.

Consciousness fluctuates with the delirious convictions and changes of emotion. There is a specific disorientation with respect to time and place—the passage of time (*temps vécu* according to Eugène Minkowski) and 'temporality' (*Sein und Zeit* according to Ludwig Binswanger) are disturbed. This disorientation, described by Karl

Jaspers as a 'first delirious experience' (*Erlebnisse*), has to be understood as a dreamlike state.

Ey[15,16] differentiated the acute psychoses in terms of the specific alteration in the perception of time rather than their transient course. According to Jacksonian ideas, the acute psychoses are the expression of a destructuring of consciousness to levels related to each acute psychosis.

The duration of the delirious experience

In ICD-10 the criterion of a duration of less than a month distinguishes other categories from schizophrenia (F20) and manic or depressive episodes (F30 and F32).

Short recovery time

In most cases recovery from the acute psychotic disorder occurs within a few weeks or months. However, long-term prognosis is difficult because of the risk of relapse into either a repeated episode or a more chronic disease. If resolution of the symptoms has not occurred after 3 months, the diagnosis should be changed to persistent delusional disorder (F22) or non-organic psychotic disorder (F28).

Suggested criteria

Pull *et al.*[17] have suggested the following empirical criteria for *bouffée délirante*.

- Abrupt or acute onset, with no previous psychiatric disorder except other similar episodes.

- Absence of chronicity: the active stages disappear completely in a few weeks or months. Relapses can occur, but there is no psychiatric disorder between consecutive episodes.

- Specific symptoms: delusions and/or any type of hallucination, depersonalization and/or derealization with or without confusion, and affective disturbance manifesting as depression or euphoria. The symptoms change from day to day and even from hour to hour.

- There is insufficient evidence for organic mental disorder, alcoholism, or drug addiction. The exclusion clauses are less restrictive in ICD-10, since a moderate, continued, and unchanged use of alcohol or drugs in habituated individuals does not excluded the diagnosis.

- The true acute psychotic disorder occurs without any associated psychosocial stress factor. When psychosocial stress factors are found, there is only a temporal link with the so-called 'reactive' acute psychosis.

Long-term evolution

Bleuler[6] described one-third of cases of acute schizophrenic psychoses as single episode, one-third as recurrent episodes with repetition of the same acute and transient psychoses (either manic or depressive), and one-third following a course which developed as schizophrenia.

Between 1976 and 1989, Metzger and Weiber[18] studied 885 cases of acute psychoses. Using the criteria of Pull *et al.*,[17] they found group 303 cases of genuine *bouffée délirante* (two-thirds female, one-third male, average age of 32 years). They followed the course of 191 cases (over an average period of 6.2 years): 34 per cent did not relapse,

24 per cent had recurrent and transient episodes, 34 per cent developed schizophrenia, and over 7 per cent developed a periodic affective disorder (manic and depressive states). The relapse or chronic course rate was higher in the group without triggering factors ($n = 92$) than in the group with triggering factors ($n = 99$). The difference between true *bouffée délirante* (no triggering factors) and other acute and transient psychotic disorders raises questions about their pathogenesis.

In the first 2 years it is essential to distinguish *bouffée délirante* from schizophrenia[19] and other acute psychoses.[20] Follow-up during this period must be very careful.

F23.1 Acute polymorphic disorder with symptoms of schizophrenia (*bouffée délirante* or cycloid psychosis with symptoms of schizophrenia)

This diagnostic category combines the symptoms of acute polymorphic psychotic disorder with some typical symptoms of schizophrenia (F20) present for most of the time. However, the schizophrenic symptoms are not precisely listed. F23.1 can be a provisional diagnosis, which is changed to schizophrenia if the criteria of F20 persist more than a month.

Acute polymorphic disorder with symptoms of schizophrenia satisfies the general criteria for acute and transient psychotic disorders:

- acute onset of less than 2 weeks
- polymorphic delusions and hallucinations or perceptual disturbances leading to incomprehensible or incoherent speech
- clouding of consciousness with impairment of attention or concentration, disorientation, perplexity, etc.
- emotional turmoil and affective symptoms (depressed mood, euphoria, anxiety, irritability) without the symptomatic criteria for manic–depressive or recurrent depressive disorders
- rapid changes of the type and intensity of symptoms
- no evidence of causation by organic or psychoactive substances.

It is also associated with some schizophrenic symptoms which are present most of the time:

- mental automatism (thought echo, insertion, withdrawal, or broadcasting)
- control, influence, passivity referred to body movements, thoughts, actions, or sensations
- hallucinations with commentary
- catatonic behaviour
- negative symptoms.

The ICD-10 clinical criteria give no information about psychotic or schizophrenic symptoms or about the action of antipsychotic drugs on these symptoms.

Leonhard[9] described cycloid psychosis as an episode with clouding of consciousness and a marked alteration of thinking. Many authors have reported follow-up studies of cycloid psychoses,[21–23] which confirm the better prognosis of cycloid psychoses than of schizophrenias and schizoaffective disorders.

F23.2 Acute schizophrenia-like psychotic disorder (schizophreniform psychosis)

This acute psychotic disorder lasts for less than a month and is mostly schizophrenic. The polymorphic psychotic symptoms are stable (no rapid changes, no emotional turmoil or confusion), sometimes with emotional instability.

The duration criterion is the most important. This category is a provisional diagnosis and appears to include such disparate descriptions as oneirophrenia (oneiroid states or *Erlebnisform*[8]), schizophrenic reaction (DSM.IV 298.8, Brief reactive psychoses), and schizophreniform psychosis.[11] In ICD-10, if the first episode lasts for more than a month, it has to be considered as an acute onset of schizophrenia.

The Scandinavian psychiatric school[24] justify the retention of this category because of the very good and rapid recovery, and have tried to determine factors in the personal and family history predicting the onset of schizophrenia.

Schizophreniform disorder remains in DSM-IV (295.40) because the evidence linking it to typical schizophrenia remains unclear, but the duration criterion is less restrictive (up to 6 months). Features suggesting a good prognosis are onset within 4 weeks, confusion at the height of the psychotic episode, previously good social and occupational functioning, and absence of blunted or flat affect.

F23.3 Other acute predominantly delusional psychotic disorders

The main clinical features of this category are delusions and hallucinations. The foreground delusions are mostly persecutory (delusions that the person or close relatives are being malevolently treated or are under external influence, with thought disturbances); auditory hallucinations are present in the background. Despite their stability, these psychotic features do not meet the criteria for schizophrenia (F20).

As for F23.0, the duration of this acute predominantly delusional psychotic episode must be less than 3 months. If the persecutory delusions persist for more than 3 months, the diagnosis changes to persistent delusional disorders (F22). This development from F23.3 to F22 is reminiscent of the classical *paranoia acuta*. Thus both paranoid reaction and psychogenic paranoid psychosis are included in F23.3. Paranoid reaction must be distinguished from induced delusional disorder or *folie à deux* (F24), in which the delusions of the 'dominated' patient disappear when the two people are separated (see Chapter 4.4).

If the background auditory hallucinations persist for more than 3 months, the diagnosis is changed to other non-organic psychotic disorders (F28). This diagnostic category is defined by exclusion: the persistent hallucinatory disorder does not meet the criteria for schizophrenia (F20), persistent delusional disorders (F22), acute and transient psychotic disorders (F23), psychotic types of manic episode (F30.2), or severe depressive episode (F32.3). F28 also corresponds to chronic hallucinatory psychosis, as explicitly noted in ICD-10.

F23.8 Other acute and transient psychotic disorders

This category includes any other acute and transient psychotic disorders with no evidence of organic cause that are not classifiable under previous F23 categories, such as ephemeral delusions or hallucinations and undifferentiated excitement.

F23.9 Acute and transient psychotic disorder unspecified

Brief psychotic disorder (298.8) is defined in DSM-IV as an episode of acute and transient psychotic disorders (delusions and hallucinations with disorganized speech and behaviour) which lasts at least a day but less than a month with eventual full return to previous level of functioning. If the symptoms occur after stressful events in the person's life, brief psychotic disorder with marked stressor(s) has to be specified. If the symptoms occur within 4 weeks postpartum, brief psychotic disorder with postpartum onset has to be specified.

Cultural variants

Other forms of acute psychoses have been observed in both traditional and developing countries, with high prevalence in Asia, Africa, and Latin America. These brief psychotic episodes are culture-bound syndromes, often with immediate precipitating stress or life events.[25] There is disorganized behaviour, delusions, thought disorders, confusion, and mood disorders, usually with full recovery and no relapse in a 1-year follow-up.

The culture-specific disorders[26] and their potentially related syndromes are often acute and transient. The status of these culture-reactive disorders is controversial and needs more clinical and epidemiological research. The mode of assignment to categories in ICD-10 does not suggest category F23.

Appendix I of DSM-IV (Outline for cultural formulation and glossary of culture-bound syndromes) lists 25 syndromes, with a glossary mostly using the local terms (seven in Hispanic languages, five in English, and one in French). *Bouffée délirante*, described only in West Africa and Haiti, is defined as episodes resembling brief psychotic disorder and classified in F23.0. Mezzisch and Lin[25] have suggested that the whole group of culture-bound syndromes should be classified as acute and transient psychotic disorders, although this is justified only for a very few such as *amok* (dissociative episode with persecutory ideas and aggressive behaviour from Malaysia), *shin-byung* (Korean dissociation and possession), and *spell* (trance state in southern United States).

ICD-10 includes the two Malaysian syndromes *koro* and *latah* as well as *dhat* (India) in F48.8, Other specified neurotic disorders.

International follow-up studies have shown that cultural factors can influence the course and prognosis of acute psychotic disorders. In 1979, the World Health Organization compared the course of schizophrenia (295), psychotic depression, mania, and other psychoses in different cultures, using the ICD-9 criteria for the diagnoses. The outcome for the schizophrenic group was better in emerging countries than in the industrialized world. These results probably explain the individualization of category F23 in ICD-10.

Some authors[27] have suggested that short-lived psychotic episodes are expressions of overcharged mechanisms of defence, or of individual psychological fragility. The brief psychosis is an understandable development of the psychic life of the subject and has a cathartic effect.

Culturally related syndromes are discussed further in Chapter 4.16.

Treatment

Short-term treatment

Acute psychotic syndromes require early hospitalization in either an inpatient psychiatric unit or a crisis centre. They are psychiatric emergencies. The decision to admit to hospital is taken in order to make a careful clinical evaluation, to separate the patient from his or her environment, to provide a reassuring setting, and to prevent any suicidal or aggressive tendencies.[28]

Antipsychotic drugs are prescribed.[29] Some clinicians wait for a day or two before starting neuroleptic therapy in order to eliminate an organic cause (a general medical condition or substance abuse disorder can present with acute and transient psychotic symptoms) and prescribe benzodiazepines rather than neuroleptics. More often, however, antipsychotic treatment starts immediately.

The choice of antipsychotic drug depends on the clinician's experience and the clinical features. In cases of major anxiety or agitated behaviour, sedative neuroleptics such as chlorpromazine (100–500 mg/day), loxapine (50–300 mg/day), or levomepromazine (25–300 mg/day) are chosen, or zuclopenthixol acetate (100–300 mg every 3 days by intramuscular injection) is used as a short-acting depot antipsychotic. Parenteral administration (standard intramuscular administration) may be required if the patient refuses oral medication, or if a rapid effect is required because the patient is seriously uncooperative or is too dangerously disturbed.

Predominance of delusions and hallucinations indicates a high-potency antipsychotic agent as haloperidol (5–15 mg/day) or flupenthixol (80–200 mg/day).

Benzodiazepines may be given to potentiate the action of the neuroleptics. Alprazolam (0.5–4 mg/day), clorazepate (50–200 mg/day), and lorazepam (2–5 mg/day) produce rapid sedation in acutely psychotic patients if they are used with a neuroleptic. Some clinicians prefer the combination of two neuroleptics (haloperidol–levomepromazine, haloperidol–cyamemazine). New compounds with fewer adverse effects can be used (amisulpride, 800–1200 mg/day; olanzapine, 5–20 mg/day; quetiapine, 75–500 mg/day; risperidone, 2–10 mg/day).

In culture-bound syndromes the prescription of antidepressants is often recommended as primary treatment. The dosage may be adjusted from low doses and gradually increased, or adjusted to the standard dose after a first loading dose. Frequent monitoring to assess drug response and adverse effects (extrapyramidal side-effects, orthostatic hypotension, anticholinergic effects, and temperature dysregulation) is essential, and corrections and prophylactic prescriptions (e.g. antiparkinsonian medications) may be necessary.

Sociotherapy (occupational or intensive) and psychotherapy (reality–adaptive–supportive) are indicated depending on the state of the patient and his environment, with individual, family or rehabilitation care.

Continuation treatment

The effectiveness of psychopharmacotherapy is usually manifested in the first 6 weeks, with improved sleep, regression of agitation, recovery from anxiety and delusion, and finally disappearance of the psychotic features. When there is no recovery or improvement either another antipsychotic drug should be used or the dosage of the first increased. Worsening of the symptoms, serious side-effects, or a poor response to pharmacotherapy are the main indications for electroconvulsive therapy.

If mood disorders or cyclic episodes occur, treatment with antidepressants, mood stabilizers (lithium or valproate), or an anticonvulsant drug (carbamazepine) may be indicated. Care must be taken to distinguish between a post-neuroleptic depression and the development of a (schizo)affective disorder.

Prevention of recurrence

The possibility that psychotic symptoms may re-emerge has to be borne in mind during the first 2 years of follow-up. Low-dosage pharmacotherapy must be maintained for 1 or 2 years after recovery. During this long-term follow-up, periodic assessment and effective clinical care with social and psychological therapy are essential.

Advice about management

Patients are often hospitalized under constraint because they do not acknowledge the disorder. The initial non-compliance leads to the frequent use of classic intramuscular neuroleptics. After recovery, a switch to a newer antipsychotic drug, which is better tolerated, helps to ensure the acceptance of long-term treatment when the psychotic symptoms have disappeared.

In general, psychotherapy and psychosocial care are more effective in an outpatient setting after recovery has started. A good relationship between patient and psychiatrist together with collaboration with the family practitioner and social workers improve the long-term prognosis. If resources allow, psychotherapy by a trained practionioner, behavioural therapy, or family therapy may be combined with a low-dose pharmacotherapy.

References

1. World Health Organization (1992). *International statistical classification of diseases and related health problems, 10th revision*. WHO, Geneva.
2. Bercherie, P. (1980). L'école d'Illenau. In *Les fondements de la clinique* (ed. Le Seuil), pp. 119–28. Ornicar, Paris.
3. Meynert, T. (1890). *Klinische Vorlesungen über Psychiatrie auf wissenschaftlichen Grundlagen*. Braumüller, Vienna.
4. Freud, S. (1917). Metapsychologie Ergänzung Zurtraumlehre. In *Gesammelte Werke*. Internationales Psychoanalytischer Verlag, Leipzig, 1947.
5. Kraepelin, E. (1899). *Psychiatrie* (6th edn). Barth, Leipzig.
6. Bleuler, E. (1911). Dementia praecox oder Gruppe der Schizophrenien. In *Aschaffenburg Handbuch des Psychiatrie*. Deuticke, Leipzig.
7. Wimmer, A. (1916). Psykogene sindssygdomsformer. In *St. Hans Hospital, Jubilee Publication*. Gad, Copenhagen.
8. Mayer-Gross, W. (1924). *Selbschilderungen der Verwirrtheit (Die oneroïde Erlebnisform)*. Stringler, Berlin.
9. Leonhard, K. (1961). Cycloid psychoses: endogenous psychoses which are either schizophrenic or manic-depressive. *Journal of Nervous and Mental Diseases*, **107**, 633–48.
10. Kasanin, J. (1933). The acute schizo-affective psychoses. *American Journal of Psychiatry*, **13**, 97–126.
11. Langfeldt, G. (1939). *The schizophreniform states*. Oxford University Press, London.
12. Magnan, V. (1893). *Leçons cliniques sur les maladies mentales*. Bataille, Paris.
13. Legrain, M. (1895). *Du délire des dégénérés*. Progrés Medical, Paris.
14. Samuel-Lajeunesse, B. and Heim, A. (1994). Psychoses délirantes aigues. In *Encyclopedie de medecin et de chirurgie*, 37 230, A10. Editions Techniques, Paris.
15. Ey, H. (1954). Bouffées délirantes et psychoses hallucinatoires aigues. In *Etudes psychiatriques*, Vol. III. Desclée de Brower, Paris.
16. Ey, H. (1955). Psychoses délirantes aigues (bouffées délirantes aigues, psychoses hallucinatoires aigues, états oniroïdes), In *Encyclopedie de medecin et de chirurgie*, 37 230, A10, pp. 1–6. Editions Techniques, Paris.
17. Pull, C.B., Pull, M.C., and Pichot, P. (1987). Des critères empiriques français pour les psychoses. II–Consensus des psychiatres français et définitions provisoires. *Encéphale*, **13**, 53–7.
18. Metzger, J.-Y. and Weibel, H. (1991). Les bouffées délirantes. *Congrès de psychiatrie et de neurologie de langue française*. Masson, Paris.
19. World Health Organization (1979). *Schizophrenia: an international follow-up study*. Wiley, Chichester.
20. Guilloux, J. (1987). Psychoses délirantes aigues. Statut nosologique et evolution. *Revue Française de Psychiatrie*, **5**, 9–13.
21. Perris, L. (1974). A study of cycloid psychoses. *Acta Psychiatrica Scandinavica*, Supplement 253, 1–75.
22. Brockington, I.F., Perris, L., Kendell, R.E., Hillier, V.E., and Wainwright, S. (1982). The course and outcome of cycloid psychoses. *Psychiatry in Medicine*, **12**, 97–105.
23. Barcia, D. (1998). *Psicosis cicloides (psicosis marginales, bouffées délirantes)*. Triacastela, Madrid.
24. Strömgren, E. (1963). Schizophreniform psychosis, *Acta Psychiatrica Scandinavica*, **41**, 483–9.
25. Mezzich, J. and Lin, K.M. (1995). Acute and transient psychotic disorders and culture-bound syndromes. In *Comprehensive textbook of psychiatry* (6th edn) (ed. H. Kaplan and B. Sadock), Vol. 1, pp. 1049–57. Williams and Wilkins, Baltimore, MD.
26. World Health Organization (1993). *The ICD-10 classification of mental and behavioural disorders—diagnostic criteria for research*, Annex 2. World Health Organization, Geneva.
27. Cousin, F.R. and Vanelle, J.M. (1987). Défense et illustration du concept de bouffée délirante aiguë. *Information Psychiatrique*, **63**, 315–21.
28. Rochet, T., Daléry, J., and De Villard, R. (1995). Troubles psychotiques aigus et transitoires. In *Thérapeutique psychiatrique* (ed. J.L. Senon, D. Sechter, and D. Richard), pp. 797–803. Hermann, Paris.
29. Janicak, P., Davis, J., Preskorn, S., and Ayd, F. (1997). Management of acute psychosis. In *Principles and practice of psychopharmacotherapy* (2nd edn) (ed. P.G. Janicak, J.M. Davis, S.H. Preskorn, and F.J. Ayd), pp. 110–39. Williams and Wilkins, Baltimore, MD.

4.4 Persistent delusional symptoms and disorders

Alistair Munro

Introduction

Delusional disorder (DSM-IV 297.1 and ICD-10 F22)[1,2] is a psychotic illness with some superficial resemblances to schizophrenia from which, however, it is quite distinct. It presents with a stable and well-defined delusional system which is typically 'encapsulated' from a personality which retains many normal aspects, unlike the situation in schizophrenia where there is widespread personality disorganization in addition to the psychotic features. Nevertheless, although many normal aspects of the personality are preserved, the individual's way of life becomes progressively overwhelmed by the intensity and intrusiveness of the delusional beliefs. Hallucinations may be present but are not usually prominent. This is a chronic disorder, probably lifelong in most instances, which retains an unjustified reputation for being untreatable. Because of the nature of their delusions, many patients are unwilling to accept that they have a mental disorder or that they require psychiatric treatment but, if they can be persuaded to co-operate and accept appropriate medication, the condition can be shown to respond to treatment in a remarkably high proportion of cases.

Delusional disorder is the name now applied to the illness previously known as 'paranoia', and the terms are virtually synonymous. Paranoia and its related disorders were regarded as an important group of psychiatric illnesses until the early part of the twentieth century. Then, because of changing diagnostic and classificatory approaches, especially the tendency in some quarters to overdiagnose schizophrenia, the diagnosis of paranoia and a companion illness, paraphrenia, practically stopped and they all but disappeared from standard classificatory systems. In 1987, paranoia was again officially recognized by DSM-IIIR[3] but was renamed delusional (paranoid) disorder—since simplified to delusional disorder. It is currently the only officially acknowledged member of the old group of paranoid illnesses appearing in DSM-IV and ICD-10.

Although the diagnosis of paranoia almost ceased for many years, the illness and its sufferers did not disappear. When the phenomena of the disorder came to attention, one of two things tended to happen. Either the patient was labelled as schizophrenic or else a specific feature of the delusional symptomatology was seized upon and spurious syndromes were described. Therefore, as will be noted in the brief historical review below, we have a multiplicity of apparently disparate diagnoses such as de Clérambault's syndrome (delusional erotomania), the Othello syndrome (delusional jealousy), querulant paranoia (a form of persecutory delusional disorder), monosymptomatic hypochondriacal psychosis (delusional disorder with somatic preoccu-

pations), and many others. The result has been an extraordinarily scattered literature with cases recorded in a variety of medical and non-medical sources, but very few in psychiatric publications until recently. It is only since the publication of DSM-IIIR that a serious attempt has begun to resolve a profoundly confusing situation and once again to diagnose paranoia/delusional disorder on the basis of its own intrinsic features. Later in this section, some of the problems still bedevilling nomenclature will be discussed.

Jaspers, in discussing paranoia, said: 'Why are the paranoics as defined by Kraepelin so rare, yet when they do occur they are so typical?' This is one of the outstanding paradoxes concerning delusional disorder. There are striking similarities from case to case and the illness has features which clearly distinguish it from other psychoses, yet even now diagnostic practices often lead to its being confused with illnesses such as schizophrenia.

Many psychiatric illnesses are associated with persistent delusions, but DSM-IV and ICD-10 provide criteria to differentiate delusional disorder as an illness in its own right and these are now widely accepted. This section adopts this official approach but with two caveats. The first is that the descriptions are bald and not very helpful to the clinician who has not actually seen cases of the disorder. The second is that the category of delusional disorder (persistent delusional disorders in ICD-10) may well be over-restrictive at present. However, it should be noted that some well-respected authorities[4,5] take a somewhat different approach, regarding 'delusional disorders' as all psychiatric illnesses with delusions and then subcategorizing according to the underlying syndrome, which might be severe mood disorder, schizophrenia, delusional disorder (as in DSM-IV and ICD-10), etc. Therefore the reader must be aware of each author's particular criteria for the diagnosis.

Emil Kraepelin (1856–1926) clearly described paranoia and he included it in a continuum of illnesses with delusional features, which also subsumed paraphrenia and paranoid schizophrenia. This so-called paranoid spectrum will be described later. Paranoid schizophrenia continues to be a widely used diagnosis, but nowadays it officially belongs to the group of schizophrenias rather than with the delusional disorders. Paraphrenia is not officially acknowledged in DSM-IV or ICD-10, but cases fitting its traditional description are not uncommonly seen in practice. A short account of its putative features is provided later in this chapter and an argument advanced for its reacceptance as a discrete disorder within a paranoid spectrum. A somewhat contentious diagnosis—late-onset paraphrenia—has relevance to the contention that paraphrenia does exist, but as a concept it is not widely used outside the United Kingdom; its features will be considered when describing paraphrenia itself.

At present, 'delusional disorder' is both an illness category and essentially the only syndrome contained within that category. In recent years, another diagnosis—delusional misidentification syndrome (**DMIS**)—has come into increasing prominence. This group of disorders was first specifically reported in 1923 by Capgras and Reboul-Lachaux[6] who described the phenomenon of delusional conviction that someone in the patient's environment has been replaced by an almost exact double. For a long time the 'Capgras syndrome' led a rather marginal existence in the literature, sustained mainly by occasional anecdotal descriptions and spurious psychodynamic explanations, but in the past decade there have been considerably more case reports, descriptions have become more objective, and clinical subtypes have been distinguished. Most importantly, sound psychological and neuropathological work has been carried out and there has been an increasing ability to demonstrate scientifically the presence of significant cerebral pathologies in a high proportion of sufferers.

DMIS is not currently recognized by DSM-IV and ICD-10, but it has a number of clinical features similar to those of delusional disorder and there is no doubt that it warrants official acknowledgement and, it is suggested, inclusion in an expanded category of delusional disorders.

Finally, there is an important phenomenon which is found in association with all illnesses with delusions, but is especially prominent in delusional disorder. This is named 'shared psychotic disorder' in DSM-IV and 'induced delusional disorder' in ICD-10, but is often still referred to by its long-established name *folie à deux*. Here, the primary patient has a *bona fide* delusional disorder and a secondary patient comes to accept the abnormal beliefs as true. The secondary patient is usually a highly impressionable individual living in prolonged close contact with the other; he or she is not truly deluded, but retains the beliefs tenaciously as long as the intimate relationship is maintained. A less common variety is when two individuals each have genuine delusional disorders and, through close proximity, come to share identical abnormal beliefs. *Folie à deux* is not uncommon and, as will be explained later, there are very practical reasons why the clinician should be aware of its possible presence and the ways in which it may influence management of the case.

The paranoid spectrum[7]

Since Kraepelin's time, many psychiatrists have believed that paranoia/delusional disorder and paranoid schizophrenia are opposite ends of a continuum of psychotic disorders with delusions as a prominent feature. Therefore a simplified schema of the spectrum is

delusional disorder—paraphrenia—paranoid schizophrenia.

Somewhat anecdotally, the literature suggests that approximately 10 per cent of individuals with delusional disorder or paraphrenia will 'shift to the right' at some stage and deteriorate to schizophrenia. (The proportion may seem higher if the original diagnoses are less than rigorous and if cases of early schizophrenia are included). Otherwise, it seems that the majority of cases of delusional disorder and paraphrenia remain diagnostically stable over a prolonged period.

Several reports have indicated that, as one moves to the left on the spectrum, a family history of schizophrenia becomes progressively less common. The risk for schizophrenia in the close family of a case of delusional disorder appears to be much the same as in the general public.

Although paranoid schizophrenia is invariably grouped with other schizophrenia subtypes, there is still justification for Kraepelin's original concept of its belonging with the delusional disorders. A family history of schizophrenia is approximately half as common in paranoid schizophrenia as in other schizophrenias, and profound disintegration of personality is much less marked. Paraphrenia shares many features with paranoid schizophrenia, but there is even less personality deterioration and the retention of affective warmth and of the capacity for good rapport in paraphrenia make it strikingly different from the emotional coldness and isolativeness of the latter. However, its delusions lack the cohesiveness and encapsulated quality of those in delusional disorder.

When approaching cases in this general area, the clinician may find it helpful to bear in mind the concept of the paranoid spectrum. This, plus a knowledge of the features of its constituent disorders, will make it easier to distinguish delusional disorder from superficially similar conditions. The precise diagnostician will also appreciate its help in recognizing the differences between paraphrenia, paranoid schizophrenia, and other schizophrenias, a process of some importance in pursuing management and deciding on prognosis.

Problems of nomenclature

Although English-speaking psychiatrists (and most members of the general public) customarily use the word 'paranoid' to mean 'persecutory', strictly speaking its meaning is 'delusional'.[8] In many writings on 'paranoia' and 'paranoid' disorders, authors do not make it clear whether delusions are present or not in their cases.

Paranoia used to be an acceptable name for an illness characterized by a well-organized delusional system in a relatively undeteriorated personality, with delusional contents especially of persecution, hypochondriasis, jealousy, erotomania, and grandiosity. Unfortunately, with the passage of time, its usage became so loose that it ceased to have a useful meaning in clinical practice. The term 'paranoia' should now be regarded as historical and be seen as more or less synonymous with delusional disorder.

The term 'paranoid' is still used in the official diagnoses of paranoid schizophrenia and of paranoid personality disorder. The first usage is acceptable enough because the illness is a psychosis and has delusions as a prominent feature, but it is quite illogical in describing a personality disorder which, by definition, does not have delusions. It seems unlikely that the personality disorder will be renamed, and so the reader is warned of the pitfalls in our psychiatric terminology and is again cautioned to read the literature with great care.

A brief historical review of the delusional disorders

Although the form of delusional disorder is remarkably characteristic, the delusional contents and the ways in which cases come to attention are extremely varied. This has led to an extraordinarily complex history. The core description, that of paranoia, gradually crystallized in the second half of the nineteenth century and was definitively delineated by Kraepelin,[9] who recognized subtypes with delusional contents of grandiosity, persecution, erotomania, and jealousy, and also allowed for the possibility of a hypochondriacal content. He clearly differentiated paranoia from *dementia praecox* (later renamed schizophrenia by Bleuler[10]). At first, Kraepelin accepted that auditory hallucinations could occur in paranoia but later (we believe mistakenly) excluded all forms of hallucination from the description. Except that non-prominent hallucinations are now acceptable, Kraepelin's century-old definition of paranoia still largely serves as that of present-day delusional disorder.

Subsequently, Kraepelin[11] introduced the concept of paraphrenia, an illness similar to paranoid schizophrenia but with significantly better preservation of affect and of personality. As already mentioned, he regarded paranoia, paraphrenia, and paranoid schizophrenia as a relatively discrete group of illnesses, later referred to as the paranoid spectrum.

After Bleuler (1857–1939) coined the term 'schizophrenia', he and other authorities gradually widened the definition of this illness, so that first paraphrenia and subsequently most cases of paranoia were absorbed into the overblown category. This process was accentuated by the finding that a proportion of cases of paranoia and paraphrenia (although certainly not all) eventually deteriorated to schizophrenia.[12,13] By the middle of the twentieth century, paraphrenia in the Kraepelinian sense was rarely diagnosed and paranoia had come to be regarded as a curiosity; in fact, many psychiatrists simply denied its existence.

Despite this, various workers continued to contribute to speculation on the nature of delusions and of paranoia. Karl Jaspers (1883–1969) wrote outstandingly on the phenomenology and psychopathology of delusions,[14] and his work continues to influence the views of many psychiatrists. Kretschmer (1888–1964) proposed that paranoid symptoms tended to occur in abnormally sensitive individuals who suffered from lifelong conflict between feelings of inadequacy and of unrequited self-importance and who, after undergoing some 'key experience', were precipitated into a delusional psychosis (*sensitiver Beziehungswahn*).[15] Kretschmer's observations tended to emphasize (perhaps overemphasize) the importance of pre-existing personality disorder in paranoid illness. Sigmund Freud (1856–1939) wrote extensively on paranoia,[16,17] proposing 'latent' homosexuality as the underlying psychopathology, a view no longer widely accepted.

Although these and many other speculations have contributed much to the descriptive phenomenology of delusions, we are left knowing a good deal about delusional contents and little or nothing about the mechanisms underlying delusions and their associated illnesses.[18,19] In particular, we have little idea as to how the unique features of the delusional disorders come about. Most unfortunately, much of the extensive theoretical literature on paranoia appeared at a time when most psychoses, and certainly paranoia, had no effective treatments, and virtually all the authors emphasized the condition's untreatability. This pessimistic view continues over into many modern writings and is quite wrong.

From the 1970s onwards, interest in paranoia began to reappear[20,21] and a more optimistic view of treatment emerged.[22] In 1987, DSM-IIIR returned to a description of the illness which was essentially that of Kraepelin, except that non-prominent hallucinations were allowable, and renamed it delusional (paranoid) disorder, now simplified to delusional disorder in DSM-IV and ICD-10. Paraphrenia has not so far been reaccepted and this diagnosis remains in official limbo.

Despite the vagaries of paranoia during much of the twentieth century, several of its subtypes developed quasi-independent existences. Unfortunately, their recognition depended almost entirely on the content of the abnormal beliefs and the form of the underlying illness was often poorly perceived; this has led to much confusion between cases of paranoia and cases of quite different provenance which happen to share apparently similar beliefs, and the distinction between delusions and overvalued ideas has often been blurred. Nowadays we recognize much more clearly that the 'primary' erotomania of de Clérambault is a subtype of delusional disorder, as are the monodelusional types of pathological jealousy (the Othello syndrome) and hypochondriasis (monosymptomatic hypochondriacal psychosis). In addition, certain cases of persecutory delusional illness and irrational litigiousness (litigious paranoia) prove to be cases of delusional disorder. Since each of these subtypes has developed a literature separate from the others and from the mainstream literature on delusional disorder, tracing the history of the overall concept is a daunting task.

At present the clinical description of delusional disorder is well established, but adequate case series are rare and scientific investigations are in their infancy. The separateness of this illness from schizophrenia is beyond doubt, but its relationship to other disorders within the paranoid spectrum still has to be established. Delusional disorder is no longer regarded as rare, but psychiatrists too often remain ignorant of it and are unaware that many cases are being dealt with by other professionals whose literatures describe typical cases which, however, are often not recognized for what they are.

Delusions: clinical aspects

A delusion may be defined very loosely as a mistaken idea which is held unshakeably by the patient and which cannot be corrected. As will be seen, this is not a satisfactory definition, although it may be a useful starting-point for clinical recognition of a delusional process. This brief exposition is concerned to facilitate clinical recognition rather than to dwell on psychopathological theories which are dealt with in detail elsewhere in this book.

It is a widely held view that delusions are qualitatively different from normal ideas or beliefs and have an all-or-nothing quality. The DSM-IV definition initially seems to accept this viewpoint, stating that a delusion is 'A false belief based on an incorrect inference about external reality that is firmly sustained despite what almost everyone else believes and despite what constitutes incontrovertible and obvious proof or evidence to the contrary. The belief is not one ordinarily accepted by other members of the person's culture or subculture.' But the definition then goes on to say that it is often difficult to distinguish between a delusion and an overvalued idea (in which there is an unreasonable belief or idea but not held with such pathological certitude as in a delusion), and that 'Delusional conviction occurs on a continuum' from normal to abnormal. These two statements markedly lessen the initial description of the absolute nature of the delusional wrongness.

The definition of delusion by Mullen[23] based on the earlier description by Jaspers is widely quoted and its implications are largely accepted by DSM-IV and ICD-10. He characterizes delusions as follows.

1. They are held with absolute conviction.

2. The individual experiences the delusional belief as self-evident and regards it as of great personal significance.

3. The delusion cannot be changed by an appeal to reason or by contrary experience.

4. The content of delusions is unlikely and often fantastic.

5. The false belief is not shared by others from a similar socio-economic group.

Clinicians widely employ the terminology on delusions introduced by Jaspers, for example when they use terms such as 'primary' and 'secondary' delusions, 'delusional mood' (*Wahnstimmung*), and 'delusional memory'. These concepts are of some descriptive and possibly heuristic value, but they do not prove particularly helpful in distinguishing delusions from overvalued ideas in individual cases, nor in deciding whether a particular delusional phenomenon is specific to a given mental disorder.

In a sense, all delusions are secondary in that they are the product of a pathological process in the brain which, in most cases, we can only guess at. It is sometimes useful to differentiate clinically between the 'primary' or 'autochthonous' delusion, which appears fully fledged and relatively suddenly, and the 'secondary' delusion, which is a further development within the delusional system and may sometimes seem to be the individual's way of rationalizing his delusional beliefs although, of course, the rationalization must necessarily be filtered through a mind already thought-disordered and affected by delusions. For example, the initial belief may be that the police are watching him night and day; the secondary delusion 'explains' that this is because he has secret information about aliens which the authorities do not wish divulged. The better organized the delusions, the more convincing are the 'explanations', even to outsiders.

Not all primary delusions arise suddenly and, in fact, it must be presumed that in most cases the suddenness is more apparent than real. Almost certainly, unless the delusion is the result of an acute brain dysfunction such as may follow a head injury or delirium, there is a lead-up process which may be accompanied by the above-mentioned *Wahnstimmung*, a mood state compounded of anxiety, perplexity, and a sense of impending crisis. When the delusion crystallizes, the delusional mood often disappears and is replaced by a sense of revelation and of certainty. It seems likely that this phenomenon occurs in a proportion of delusional disorder patients and it often happens that, at the moment of revelation, some coincidental but irrelevant circumstance is picked upon to explain the appearance of the new belief. For example, a media event, a thunderstorm, a chance telephone call, etc., may thereafter be, in the patient's mind, the 'cause'.

While we regard delusions as one of the most characteristic elements of all the psychotic illnesses and a *sine qua non* in the diagnosis of delusional disorder, clear-cut description and delineation have proved elusive despite many years of study and experiment, especially by clinical psychologists.[24] In fact, Garety and Hemsley[18] point out that, even now, none of the characteristics of delusion which we traditionally accept completely stand up to scientific scrutiny. For example, it turns out that delusions are not necessarily rigidly fixed, but may fluctuate in the intensity with which they are held. They are not totally incorrigible and it has been shown that some at least are modifiable by psychological approaches, and they are certainly not invariably absolute yes–no entities. A delusion need not always be a blind belief and some individuals freely reflect upon the abnormal ideas, even showing some insight at times. In particular, nowadays the so-called bizarreness of a delusion has been shown to have little or no distinguishing value.[25]

Much of the classical work on delusions was done in pretreatment times when the chronic condition was readily available for study in institutions. In the present era our aim is to diagnose psychotic disorders as early as possible, sometimes even before frank delusions are evident, and to begin treatment at once. Neuroleptics rapidly interfere with many psychopathological processes; they certainly suppress delusions, although not necessarily permanently. Of course this makes ongoing experimental observations of delusions, especially acute delusions, all but impossible in clinical circumstances. Psychiatrists find themselves in the paradoxical situation of diagnosing illness because of the presence of delusions whose scientific validity is largely unsubstantiated, and then causing them to disappear before they can be verified properly. Nevertheless, until we have more objective means of making diagnoses it remains essential that, as far as we can, we recognize delusions when they occur and separate them from other abnormal psychopathological appearances.

How can a clinician deal with this? Firstly it seems inescapable that he or she be both experienced and insightful. Given these qualities, it often does seem possible to have an informed sense as to whether a belief is true or false and, if the latter, whether it is being held with delusional intensity. A key element in the decision is a comparison between the patient's current beliefs and those he habitually held, and here a corroborative account from an informed outside source is usually necessary.

The observer's educated suspicion that a delusion is present is the starting point, but it is evident that suspicion has to be aroused by the context of the apparently delusional idea because, no matter how isolated it appears to be, it will usually occur in the setting of a mental disorder whose other features may be typical of a specific psychiatric diagnosis. Illogically, instead of recognizing the delusion and using it to make a specific diagnosis, we often recognize that we are dealing with a probable psychosis and thereafter judge all the patient's utterances in light of that. While he may indeed be experiencing delusions, it is essential that we do not automatically assume that anything the psychotic individual says is of a delusional nature. The following brief case study demonstrates the danger of doing this.

Case Study An elderly man was admitted to hospital, possibly with severe depressive disorder. During history-taking he said that the people upstairs watched him through his ceiling and stole things from him. This was taken as evidence of delusional thinking until a social worker visited his home, which was in a decrepit building. It turned out that there actually was a hole in his ceiling, and that his upstairs neighbours did watch him and did steal from him by reaching down with a walking-stick and lifting belongings from his mantelpiece.

We must accept that we cannot be absolute in our recognition of a delusion. In addition to the illness context we base our estimate on a series of nuances, no one of which is pathognomonic but an accumulation of which becomes increasingly convincing. The abnormalities to be sought are as follows.

1. An idea or belief is expressed with unusual persistence or force.

2. As far as we can tell, the idea is not typical of the individual's previously prevailing thinking and is not shared by his or her social community.

3. The idea appears to exert an undue influence on the person's life and consequently the way of life is altered to an extraordinary degree.

4. Despite the significance to the patient of the belief, he or she often displays secretiveness or resentment when questioned about it.

5. The individual tends to be humourless and oversensitive about the belief.

6. There is a quality of 'centrality'; no matter how strange the belief or its consequences, the patient rarely questions that incredible things are happening to him or her. For example, why should a perfectly ordinary harmless person be singled out for constant surveillance by the security agencies? But this is simply accepted.

7. Attempts to contradict the belief are likely to arouse an inappropriately strong emotional reaction, often with irritability and hostility and with a superciliousness that may be a form of grandiosity.

8. On reflection the belief appears unlikely to the observer, but at the time of history-taking the force of the patient's expression of it may temporarily disguise its improbability.

9. The patient is so emotionally overinvested in the idea that it swamps other elements in the psyche, and many everyday activities are neglected.

10. If the delusion is acted out, uncharacteristic behaviours, sometimes involving violence, will occur which may be partly understood in terms of the abnormal belief.

11. Others who know the patient well will usually observe that his or her thinking and behaviour are alien, unless *folie à deux* is present when, paradoxically, the other person's denials of abnormality may actually tend to confirm the presence of delusion.

12. An odd feature of delusions is that, no matter how strongly they are held, when the patient is given the opportunity to obtain 'proof' he or she persistently evades taking the appropriate action.

13. One must always look for the features which frequently accompany delusions, especially suspiciousness, hauteur, grandiosity, evasiveness, and eccentric or threatening behaviour, as well as evidence of thought disorder, mood change, and hallucinations.

Particular features of delusions in delusional disorder

In addition to any of the above, in delusional disorder we find several other elements which are of importance in leading to the diagnosis.

1. The delusional system is stable and is expressed or defended with intense affect and with highly rehearsed arguments. The form of the logic used by the patient is very consistent but the propositions are based on false premises. Since the individual is so focused on his beliefs he often succeeds in making the enquirer feel inept with his or her self-assurance.

2. The delusional system is markedly 'encapsulated', so that the beliefs therein and their accompanying symptoms are to a considerable extent separate from the rest of the personality which retains a good deal of normal function. However, the compelling force of the delusions often overshadows these normal aspects and this is increasingly so with advancing chronicity of the illness,

when the tendency to express and act out the delusions may well increase.

3. When the individual is preoccupied with the delusional system there is strong emotional and physiological arousal, but when he or she is engaged on neutral topics, the arousal abates and an ordinary conversation can take place. Switching between normal and abnormal 'modes', sometimes very rapidly, is virtually pathognomonic of delusional disorder.

4. Because of the encapsulation of the delusions and the normal–abnormal switch just described, the patient may have phases of relative normality interspersed with psychotic periods. The switch can occur spontaneously or as a result of external provocation; the two are difficult to disentangle since the hypervigilant individual may perceive provocation in almost anything. Since it is a chronic illness the symptoms never remit, but if they are temporarily in the background the patient may converse and function almost normally and may have sufficient quasi-insight to keep the delusions concealed. Total denial of mental abnormality and resistance to psychiatric referral are almost universal in cases of delusional disorder and lead to severe underestimation of the illness's frequency.

4. As a result of the features just described, many delusional disorder patients can continue to exist in society, sometimes with very abnormal but harmless beliefs but in other instances with highly malignant delusions which they may or may not act out.

5. As will be repeatedly emphasized, delusional disorder must be diagnosed on the form of the illness and the content of the delusion is not used to make the primary diagnosis. On the other hand, the particular content is employed to categorize into subgroups, as will shortly be described.

Delusional disorders: clinical features

Official diagnostic criteria

The DSM-IV and ICD-10 criteria are shown in Tables 1 and 2 respectively.

As will be seen, the DSM-IV and ICD-10 descriptions are very similar in overall outline but with a number of rather striking minor differences. The following specific features should be noted.

1. DSM-IV uses the term 'non-bizarre' delusions; this criterion has been shown to have little or no validity.[25]

2. DSM-IV allows the presence of tactile and olfactory hallucinations, while ICD-10 mentions only auditory hallucinations; in practice most modalities may be represented but the important point is that they are relatively non-prominent and usually parallel the content of the delusion(s).

3. DSM-IV says that delusions should have been present for 1 month and ICD-10 insists on 3 months. Both are guesses, but ICD-10 is probably right to err on the side of caution and it provides category F22.8 as a temporary niche until the definitive diagnosis emerges.

4. Both classifications exclude delusional illnesses due to organic brain disorder, medical illnesses, medication effects, or psychoactive substance abuse. In essence this is correct, especially in an

Table 1 DSM-IV delusional disorder (297.1)

Principal features

(a) Non-bizarre delusions of at least 1 month's duration

(b) Criterion A for schizophrenia has never been met, although tactile and olfactory hallucinations may be acceptable if they are related to the delusional theme

(c) Apart from the impact of the delusion(s) or its consequences, functioning is not markedly impaired and behaviour is not obviously odd or bizarre

(d) Concurrent mood episodes, if present, are brief relative to the duration of the delusional disorder

(e) The disturbance is not the direct outcome of a drug or medication or of a medical disorder

Subtypes

Erotomanic
Grandiose
Jealous
Persecutory
Somatic
Mixed (allowing for the presence of more than one of the foregoing)
Unspecified or other

illness of acute onset. However, as will be noted later, an apparently typical delusional disorder may arise as a long-term complication of any of these factors.

Table 2 ICD-10 persistent delusional disorders

Delusional disorder (F22.0)

Principal features

(a) A delusion or set of related delusions, other than those described as typically schizophrenic, must be present; the most common are persecutory, grandiose, hypochondriacal, jealous, or erotic

(b) The delusion(s) must be present for at least 3 months

(c) The general criteria for schizophrenia are not fulfilled

(d) There are no persistent hallucinations, but there may be transitory or occasional auditory hallucinations that are not speaking in the third person or making a running commentary

(e) Depressive symptoms or episodes may be intermittently present, but the delusional symptoms must persist at times when there is no disturbance of mood

(f) There must be no evidence of primary or secondary organic mental disorder or of a psychotic disorder due to psychoactive substance use

Subtypes

Persecutory
Litigious
Self-referential
Grandiose
Hypochondriacal
Jealous
Erotomanic

Other persistent delusional disorders (F22.8)

This is a residual category for persistent disorders with delusions that do not fully meet the criteria for delusional disorder or schizophrenia. Illnesses with prominent delusions accompanied by persistent hallucinatory voices or by psychotic symptoms insufficient to satisfy the criteria for schizophrenia are included here. A delusional disorder of less than 3 months' duration is coded under Acute and Transient Psychotic Disorders (F23) until proven otherwise.

5. DSM-IV and ICD-10 agree emphatically that delusional disorder is not schizophrenia and DSM-IV notes that general functioning is not impaired. Both say that mood disturbance may accompany the delusional illness but is not a cause of it.

6. The list of subtypes according to delusional content is similar in both classifications, although ICD-10 adds self-referential and litigious themes.

7. Neither classification specifies that the essence of delusional disorder is a highly organized delusional system, largely encapsulated from normal aspects of the personality, although DSM-IV hints at this when it comments that functioning is not markedly impaired and behaviour is not obviously odd or bizarre. Neither comments that the patient can demonstrate alternating 'normal' and 'delusional' modes.

8. The ICD-10 category of 'other persistent delusional disorders' is vaguely described and is largely a catch-all heading or, as mentioned above, a temporary holding station. However, it could conceivably be used for the time being to subsume the unofficial delusional disorder diagnoses of paraphrenia and delusional misidentification syndrome which will be described later.

9. Overall, DSM-IV and ICD-10 give rather laconic descriptions of delusional disorder and it will be necessary to flesh them out with relevant clinical details. This will be done immediately after the next section on aetiological considerations.

General aetiological considerations in delusional disorders

It must be stressed that knowledge of aetiology in delusional disorder is scanty and highly speculative, largely because so little modern research has been conducted. What follows is an outline, and certain other factors will be noted when we come to consider the individual subtypes of the illness.

Genetic factors

Changes in definitions of paranoia/delusional disorder over the years and the frequent confusion with schizophrenia make most studies all but impossible to interpret. Conclusions are inferential rather than evidence based. However, it seems well established[26] that delusional disorder and paranoid schizophrenia are less directly inherited than other forms of schizophrenia, and that there is little or no evidence of a genetic link between delusional disorder and schizophrenia.

There may be genetic links with certain severe personality disorders, especially of the paranoid and schizoid varieties, but these are difficult to substantiate. There does seem to be an excess of such disorders in relatives and premorbidly in delusional disorder patients themselves. It is suggested that paranoid and schizoid traits are particularly liable to lead to social isolation and aggravation of delusional tendencies.[27,28]

Organic brain factors

Recent evidence from the study of delusional misidentification syndrome (see later) indicates that delusions of a very specific type may arise in association with certain well-defined brain insults. There are strong hints, but much less supportive evidence, to suggest that organic brain factors may also be important in cases of delusional disorder. For example, head injury may lead to the development of marked paranoid symptoms, and there is a long-established association between chronic alcoholism and pathological jealousy.[29] Old age itself may be linked to the onset of symptoms typical of delusional disorder, and early evidence of brain changes, especially in subcortical areas, is starting to appear in studies of various kinds of senile 'paranoid' illness.[30–32] Amphetamine[33] and cocaine abuse[34] can induce delusional illness, as can therapeutic drugs, including L-dopa and methyldopa, at times. Delusional illness induced by the brain effects of AIDS infection has been documented in recent years.[35]

Gorman and Cummings[36] have proposed that delusional illnesses of organic origin have underlying features in common, particularly temporal lobe or limbic involvement and an excess of dopamine activity in certain areas of the brain.

If organic factors predominate in a particular case, delusions must be seen as a secondary feature of an organic brain disorder. However, if the organic factors are subtle and of long duration, the clinical appearances may be those of a quite typical delusional disorder which, interestingly, may well respond to neuroleptic treatment as effectively as idiopathic cases. (In fact, 'idiopathic' may simply denote organicity at a more subtle level.) It is very possible that organic brain factors are much more common than we suspect in delusional disorder, especially in younger males who have previously abused alcohol or drugs or have suffered a head injury in the past, and in older patients (more commonly female) who suffer from effects of an aging brain.[37]

Interplay with mood factors[38]

We have already seen that DSM-IV and ICD-10 agree that mood symptoms may accompany delusional disorder but not cause it. Delusional and mood disorders are separate illnesses with their own natural histories and responses to treatment, yet there is a complex relationship between them, as is also the case with mood disorder and schizophrenia. For example, it is well documented that some cases of apparently typical mood illness, unipolar or bipolar, can progress to delusional disorder or schizophrenia over time. Conversely, cases which appear to be delusional disorder but with an episodic course may prove to be bipolar illness. There are a number of anecdotal reports of delusional disorder responding to antidepressant treatment, and it is more than likely that these represent a failure to recognize the true nature of a mood disorder associated with delusions.

Both depressive disorder and mania may be complicated by delusions. On the other hand, mood symptoms, especially dysphoria with anxiety, are a common complication of delusional disorder, while individuals with the grandiose subtype may show elation which mimics mania but is far more sustained. In recovering delusional disorder, one may see postpsychotic depression of varying degrees of severity and this is described later. Suicide is not unknown in delusional disorder but its frequency is undetermined.

In many delusional disorder patients the illness is profoundly isolating and sets them at odds with the rest of society, which often generates suspiciousness, dejection, anxiety, and agitation. It seems that a vicious circle results whereby the delusion induces distress and physiological overarousal which, in turn, reinforce the strength of the delusion and progressively diminish reality input.

Psychodynamic theories of causation

The psychodynamic literature continues to discuss aspects of 'paranoia' but often fails to differentiate clearly between trait, symptom, personality disorder, and psychotic illness. Freud postulated that paranoia (by which he probably meant delusional disorder) was the result of regression from the homosexual phase of psychosexual development to a fixation at the primary narcissistic phase. Homosexual feelings unacceptable to the individual are transformed by projection into suspiciousness and rejection—in this theory, an understandable warding-off of supposed homosexual advances. This scenario involving repressed homosexuality is assumed with no convincing proof and there seems to be no established connection between homosexuality and delusional disorder, although cases of delusional disorder in homosexuals are recorded.[39,40]

There are many psychoanalytic references to the central role played by depression in the genesis of paranoia but, as already explained, this does not appear to be true of delusional disorder.[41]

Klein[42] postulated a fixation at the paranoid–schizoid position, said to occur between the sixth and ninth months of life, inducing profound hatred by the infant of the mother, symbolically represented by the maternal breast, and envy of other women, ultimately leading to paranoia. Many other theorists have regarded narcissistic mechanisms as central, with paranoia arising from repeated empathic failures and narcissistic injuries to the developing self.[43] Paranoid delusions have been described as an escape, via projective mechanisms, from shame, guilt, and inadequacy, with persecutory and grandiose beliefs attempting to overcome a prevailing sense of inferiority. A recurring suggestion is of weakness counteracted by paranoid aggressiveness which is projected on to the external object who can then be perceived and blamed as an aggressor.[44]

Much of the psychodynamic literature dwells on the persecutory aspect of paranoia, with only occasional forays into other types of delusional content. Since psychotherapists rarely treat psychotic patients, their experience of delusional phenomena must actually be rare and their knowledge of the features of delusional illness correspondingly scanty.[45] Their theoretical bias is to interpret the origin of paranoia in terms of psychological maldevelopment, ignoring the increasing weight of evidence that faulty brain mechanisms are involved. One must read the psychodynamic literature on this particular topic with an ultracritical approach, since it usually fails to provide adequate illness definitions or clear case reports and generates explanatory theories which are unjustifiably presented as proven facts.

Conclusions regarding aetiology

No systematic research on paranoia took place for more than half a century and modern investigations into delusional disorder are only beginning to appear. Therefore it is premature to propose specific aetiological hypotheses. However, a gathering weight of evidence does suggest a localized and relatively circumscribed brain disorder associated with the possible influence of abnormal neurotransmitter activity, probably involving dopamine overactivity. Whatever the original basis of delusional disorder, it certainly seems that provocative influences such as head injury, alcohol abuse, and ill effects of drugs can evoke the expression of the illness. Hereditary factors and association with inherited personality factors may play a part, but theories of psychological maldevelopment suggest that this is at most a secondary influence. There is an urgent need for the study of extended case series utilizing modern neurophysiological and neuropsychological investigative methods.

Delusional disorder: general features and introduction to the subtypes

We have already outlined the diagnostic criteria for delusional disorder in DSM-IV and ICD-10 and have amplified these with descriptions of many of the clinical phenomena associated with the illness. It has been emphasized that this is a stable and readily recognizable disorder, provided that the clinician is informed of the essential criteria and has dealt with at least several cases to familiarize him- or herself with its very characteristic 'feel'. With this experience it becomes much more possible to delve under the prominent symptoms related to delusional content and to discern the underlying form of the illness. However, it is the predominant delusional content in an individual case, and the symptoms and behaviours related to this, which decide how a patient will present for assessment. Therefore we shall consider the main subtypes in some detail. It cannot be stressed enough that these are not separate types of illness, but variants on a single psychopathological theme.

All cases of delusional disorder occur in clear consciousness and have a stable and persistent delusional system which is relatively encapsulated. Since much of the personality remains remarkably intact, a considerable degree of social functioning is retained in many cases. The patient experiences a heightened sense of self-reference within the delusional context and ordinary events take on extraordinary significance. He or she clings to the delusion with fervid intensity and spurns any suggestion that a mental illness is present. Outside the delusional system the patient shows quite normal thinking, affect, and behaviour, but there is a marked tendency for gradual pushing to one side of these normal aspects. The retention of such a degree of normality makes the illness totally different from schizophrenia.

Earlier it has been indicated that the DSM-IV criterion of 'non-bizarreness' is unhelpful.[25] In all cases of delusional disorder the delusions tend to be well structured, coherent, and consistent, and the logic would often be acceptable if it were not that its basic premises are irrational. Many affected individuals can maintain overtly normal activities, at least in public, but increasing pressure of the delusion tends to cause corresponding responses in behaviour; these may be channelled socially, as in hypochondriacally deluded patients who utilize medical resources, albeit excessively, or antisocially, as in the aggression of the jealously deluded individual. Mood abnormalities are common as a response to the effects of the illness.

Hallucinations do occur in some cases and may affect any modality, but they are often difficult to assess and to differentiate from delusional misinterpretations and illusions. Widespread persistent hallucinations in more than one sensory sphere should make one cautious of the diagnosis of delusional disorder.

The illness appears to affect men and women approximately equally, but it is not clear if this is true of all subtypes. Despite older assertions that the illness is restricted to the middle-aged and elderly, the age of onset can actually be from late adolescence to extreme old age, with male patients appearing on average to experience earlier initiation. Some patients behave in an eccentric or fanatical fashion and, as a group, delusional disorder sufferers are excessively likely to be unmarried, divorced, or widowed, probably reflecting restriction of

affective responses and some asocial tendencies. Despite this, the condition can be compatible with marriage and continued employment. The premorbid personality is usually described as asocial and there may indeed be an excess of long-standing schizoid and paranoid personality disorders. However, when a patient makes a good recovery there may be little evidence of this, and it is possible that in some cases a 'personality disorder' is actually the prolonged and insidious prodrome of the illness.

Onset may be gradual or acute. In the latter the patient often identifies a precipitating stressor which is difficult to confirm (e.g. the person who has a delusion of skin infestation may attribute it to a single insect bite many years previously). While most individuals are secretive about their abnormal beliefs or express them by such means as physical complaints or legal processes, a certain number actually utilize them, perhaps within the context of an extreme religious sect or by becoming an excessively insistent agitator on some social issue. Disinhibited and overtly aggressive behaviour seems usually to be more frequent in males, leading to clashes with authority.

In all cases of delusional disorder, no matter what the nature of the delusional theme, the investigator should look for the relatively unique feature of the illness—the patient's ability to move between normal and delusional modes of thinking. In the former there is relatively calm mood, reasonable rapport, and appropriate emotional reactions, whereas in the latter there is overalerting, suspiciousness, and the sense that the person is being remorselessly driven by the delusional beliefs. This situation is difficult for the inexperienced observer to comprehend, since it is inconceivable to most people that someone who can appear perfectly rational at one moment can almost instantaneously change to a possessed irrational being—and then back again just as quickly. In a sense the same patient is both sane and insane, and when in the latter mode may be ultrapersuasive about the acceptability of his or her beliefs. One may imagine the plight of a lawyer faced with a client who has committed some uncharacteristically outrageous act as a result of a delusion who can then discuss his case with apparent insight and logic, and even remorse, but who nevertheless remains totally self-justifying. As a corollary, the client will usually deny the possibility of mental illness and often refuses to co-operate with psychiatric assessment.

Delusional disorder, when it was known as paranoia, often had a bad reputation because patients were regarded as angry, suspicious, accusatory, and potentially violent. Some undoubtedly are, but as we consider the various subtypes nowadays we realize that many sufferers, perhaps the majority, lead lives of internalized despair in increasingly isolated circumstances. Anger and suspiciousness are often secondary, at least in part, to the perceived neglect of their overwhelming concerns. The illness is chronic and self-reinforcing, and it is likely that only a minority of cases are recognized or helped. Psychiatry does not have an impressive record of recognizing or helping this group of patients.

The subtypes of delusional disorder

As previously noted, DSM-IV recognizes five main subtypes of the illness based on the predominant delusional themes: the erotomanic, grandiose, jealous, persecutory and somatic, and mixed and unspecified types. ICD-10 also recognizes these subtypes, and adds litigious and self-referential. Here, the litigious variety is included under the persecutory group and self-referential cases are not given separate status since self-reference is, in a sense, a feature of the illness as a whole and prominent in all cases.

When delusional disorder was resurrected in DSM-IIIR, single delusional themes were emphasized, but the mixed category in DSM-IV accepts the reality that, for example, a hypochondriacal individual can also feel persecuted and an erotomanic patient can be extremely grandiose. Also, we shall find that there are considerable individual variations within the overall themes, so that in the somatic subtype there are cases involving different body systems. Yet the range of themes does not appear to be all that wide and we have no explanation for this relative restriction in their number. The 'unspecified' category in DSM-IV allows us to accommodate any case whose delusional theme is unusual and to be open to the discovery of other major themes in the future.

In presenting the subtypes, relatively more attention will be given to the somatic form. This should not be taken as an indication that this is the most common variant; rather, it happens to be the one which has been best documented in the recent psychiatric literature. Other types of delusional presentation are much more often described in non-psychiatric and non-medical sources, where the fundamental nature of the illness may be overlooked, and so we are only beginning to correlate such descriptions with modern findings on delusional disorder.

Delusional disorder: persecutory and litigious subtypes

In most people's minds the persecutory type of delusional disorder is the archetype of 'paranoia' and it is usually assumed that it is the most common variety. Therefore it is surprising to find that the literature, while full of speculation, is very lacking in good descriptions of the phenomenology of the illness and, apart from psychoanalytic theory, says relatively little about persecutory delusions themselves.

Clinical features

By definition the illness is a chronic psychotic disorder with a well-systematized delusional system and with relative sparing of the surrounding personality. The persecutory threats may be perceived simply as coming from 'them', but can range from this to descriptions of the most elaborate plots involving a variety of known and unknown adversaries. The beliefs are extremely stable and usually increase in elaboration with the passage of time. There is heightened awareness and misinterpretation of neutral environmental cues and, not unnaturally suspiciousness, extreme anxiety, and irritability are present. Elements of grandiosity are not uncommon, with the individual accepting that he is the centre of focused and malignant attention that would be inexplicable to the normal person. As the illness progresses there is a tendency to involve an increasing number of people in the persecutory system, not uncommonly relatives, physicians, law-enforcement agencies, aspects of government, and others.

As with other subtypes of delusional disorder, many individuals are able to conceal their increasingly insistent delusions at least for some time, but because of fear of harm they are likely to isolate themselves more and more. If they live alone they may come to be regarded as eccentrics, but if they remain in contact with society the suspicion and anger must eventually become evident, so that interactions with family, social agencies, or the authorities become increasingly confronta-

tional.[46] Despite the reputation of 'paranoia' for violence, only a small proportion of these individuals resort to assault, but in those who do the danger may be profound as the individual is without reservation in his beliefs and will act as though genuinely under severe threat. Disinhibition may at times be provoked by alcohol or drug use, which makes such situations even more volatile.

Even in a long-standing illness, islands of normal functioning remain; despite this there is little or no insight and the patient resists any psychological explanation for his beliefs. He usually refuses to see a psychiatrist voluntarily; many patients of this kind are encountered in a forensic setting only after an outburst of unacceptable behaviour and are minimally co-operative.

Case Study Persecutory subtype A single man of 35 was convinced that he had been infected with AIDS by an antagonistic racial minority group. For several years he moved from place to place and from doctor to doctor trying to obtain confirmation of his diagnosis and appropriate treatment. His serology was negative and he appeared physically well, but he refused to accept this and became increasingly frustrated with the medical profession. He sent threatening letters to his family physician, and then one day walked into the latter's office and severely beat him. When charged he said that he was perfectly justified and that this was a deliberate reprimand to physicians in general for their incompetence. He felt sorry for having injured a particular individual, but he had no alternative and would do it again if he was not properly diagnosed. This man was intelligent and well educated, and had no evidence of psychiatric disorder apart from his single, absolutely fixed, delusional system.

Litigious variety of the persecutory subtype (querulous paranoia)[47,48]

In some individuals with delusional disorder there is a profound and persistent sense of having been wronged in some way, and these people endlessly and repetitively seek redress, sometimes personally but often through the legal system. In a proportion of cases there may initially have been a genuine grievance and there may also have been unsatisfactory recompense, but the subsequent pursuit of 'justice' becomes never-ending and also becomes self-reinforcing because no satisfactory resolution is possible.

This group may not be large but it generates considerable media publicity. Reports of cases naturally tend to be in the literature of the legal profession, the law-enforcement agencies, and, to some extent, forensic psychiatry, but rarely from general psychiatry. Because the individual appears relatively high functioning apart from his delusional beliefs, the complaintive behaviour may be regarded as mere eccentricity for a long time. As in many cases of delusional disorder, the immediate complaint and behaviour may seem coherent and not unreasonable but over time their ongoing, never-ending, and extraordinarily demanding quality begin to raise the suspicion of severe underlying psychopathology. Even then, unless the person begins to be perceived as a threat, little may be done and severe harassment of officialdom and the legal system may be accepted for surprisingly long periods. In some national communities (e.g. Germany and the Scandinavian countries) there are legal provisions to stop 'barratry' or unreasonable use of the law by declaring an individual a querulous litigant.

Goldstein[49] has described three typical ways in which 'litigious paranoia' presents. The first is the 'hypercompetent defendant' who knows and uses the letter of the law up to and beyond its limits but pays no heed to its spirit. The second is the 'paranoid party in a divorce proceeding' who is often consumed with jealousy and pursues vendettas against the ex-spouse, the lawyers on both sides, and even the judge. The third is the 'paranoid complaining witness' who endlessly initiates litigation despite repeated adverse judgments. All such individuals pursue their grievances in a driven manner, see conspiracy in every corner, and are often quite unscrupulous in their single-mindedness, blatantly bending facts to fit with their beliefs. Since they hold the delusional belief with total conviction, they can accept no counter-argument or contrary facts. In the past, persistent litigation was virtually a preserve of the rich, but many modern societies provide a variety of avenues for complaintiveness and will even support complaint procedures, and so abnormally litigious behaviour appears to be on the increase.[50]

Case Study Litigious delusional disorder A man in his early forties who is barely literate is well known to local police, the legal system, and the psychiatric profession. He is unmarried and lives alone in squalor. Despite his lack of education, he has developed a remarkable knowledge of the letter of the law. He has insisted for years that neighbours persecute him and he harries them with a noisy radio, by shouting at their house, and occasionally threatening assault. He has repeatedly been cautioned and arrested, but shows a remarkable ability to involve legal aid, the social services, a variety of voluntary agencies, and even the local news media. He is essentially harmless but is a profound public nuisance, and attempts to restrain and incarcerate him always fail in the end. He has never co-operated with any treatment, but several psychiatric examinations have declared him to suffer from delusional disorder of the persecutory/litigious type.

Diagnosis of the persecutory subtype

All the features of a delusional disorder which have been previously described are present. In this subtype, wariness, irritability, suspiciousness, and threatening behaviour are especially prominent, and both impulsive and planned violence may occur. Gaining confidence is extremely difficult, but if this succeeds, the more normal aspects of the individual's personality may become apparent and one may also perceive how chronically afraid and overalerted he or she is.

Differential diagnosis

The illness must be distinguished especially from the following:

- paranoid schizophrenia
- paranoid and antisocial personality disorders
- substance-related disorders
- organic brain disorders, including early dementia and some epileptic disorders
- obsessive–compulsive disorder.

Epidemiology

Virtually nothing is known of the frequency and distribution of persecutory delusional disorder. As with other subtypes it occurs in both sexes, but male cases are probably over-reported because of a readier tendency to violence and antisocial acts. The literature is biased by the reporting of the most overt cases, often in the news media or in legal situations.[51] It is open to speculation how many cases avoid diagnosis; as noted, relatively few come to the detailed attention of psychiatrists other than forensic psychiatrists.

Aetiology

Hypotheses are of the vaguest. There may be an excess of premorbid personality disorder, especially of paranoid and schizoid types. There do not appear to be close genetic links with schizophrenia or major mood disorder. The delusional system can appear suddenly or insidiously and often for no obvious reason, although previous alcohol and other substance abuse and a prior history of head injury may be significant. The psychoanalytic view of 'paranoia' is largely based on the persecutory subtype, but the provenance of cases in that literature is usually vague and speculation far outweighs verifiable fact.

Course and prognosis

Delusional disorder is a very chronic disorder, and it is presumed that cases of the persecutory subtype are as likely as others to be lifelong and to show increasing psychopathology with the passage of time. In a proportion of cases there is always a risk of antisocial behaviour and violence. Since co-operation with treatment is usually minimal, the overall figures for prognosis must be bad, but we have no reliable data to confirm this.

Forensic complications[52,53]

If someone with a generalized psychotic disorder like schizophrenia becomes sufficiently disorganized, functioning in the community becomes impossible. In contrast, many patients with delusional disorder retain a sufficient grasp of reality to continue existing in society, sometimes indefinitely. However, this does not imply that their illness is quiescent. Intellectual ability, capacity for reasoning and the form of thought remain relatively intact, but the delusional process worsens. They retain the ability to brood on their beliefs so that normal thought processes and delusions interweave, as do normal and abnormal behaviours. Anger may express itself explosively, but some individuals may carry out violent actions in a very calculated way, believing that a just vengeance is being exacted. Afterwards there may be real regret and a clear awareness of a wrong against society, but nevertheless the actions are seen as justifiable and necessary.

In 1843 the English legal system devised the McNaghten Rules following the trial of McNaghten, a deluded assassin, and these attempted to define the relationship of delusion to crime. Subsequently they were found to be inadequate, since they dwelt on cognitive misapprehension and largely ignored the rôles of emotion, volition, and the capacity for behavioural control. Nowadays the principal issue in cases of delusionally motivated crime is whether or not the accused appreciated the rightfulness or wrongfulness of his action at the time. In delusional disorder the patient is usually aware that by societal standards his deed is legally and morally wrong, but that awareness resides within the normal non-delusional aspect of his mental functioning. Within the confines of the delusional system, the person unswervingly believes that it was necessary to behave as he did.

In such cases, the judge and jury are placed in a quandary, made worse by the individual's frequent arrogance (which is at least partly grandiosity), self-justification, and ambivalent expression of regret. The ability to acknowledge the wrongness of one's act in general terms and even show remorse for it, while also asserting that it was necessary to carry it out, may well be regarded as indicating wilfulness or hypocrisy. Then, paradoxically, culpability may be determined by the content of the delusion, although this usually has minor relevance to the disinhibition of behaviour. Thus, as Goldstein[51] has pointed out, if the person felt threatened because of a delusional belief and reacted, as he genuinely perceived, in self-defence, his degree of blame may be adjudged to be low. But if he were equally deluded and carefully plotted revenge, this might be seen as highly culpable. Such a distinction cannot be defended logically either in the clinical situation or at law.

Delusional disorder defies any definition of insanity in black or white terms; it is both black and white. Because few psychiatrists, even in the forensic field, are familiar with its detailed characteristics, psychiatry has had limited success in educating the legal profession about the subtleties of the illness or the conundrum that delusions can induce such abnormal behaviour in an individual who superficially appears rational and for significant periods of time is effectively sane even though the illness is always present.

Treatment of the persecutory subtype

Treatment is discussed later in this chapter in the section on overall treatment aspects.

Delusional disorder: somatic subtype (monosymptomatic hypochondriacal psychosis)

Modern society, especially in developed countries, is preoccupied with health concerns. While much of this is positive, there is no doubt that many people worry excessively about health matters and a proportion of these show pathological self-concern. This can shade into hypochondriasis, in which there is a persistent conviction of illness in the absence of objective evidence of its existence, with misinterpretation of bodily sensations as disease and with inability to accept reassurances. In many cases the individual shows some degree of body image disturbance, sometimes of extreme degree.[54,55] Usually we think of hypochondriasis as referring to physical complaints, but nowadays it seems that an increasing number of affected people are also prepared to complain in psychological terms.

Hypochondriasis is common and may be a personality trait, but it can also be an accompaniment to many psychiatric illnesses, both non-delusional and delusional. It is the presenting feature of the somatic subtype of delusional disorder and in different patients we see many varieties of alteration of body image expressed in delusional terms. Certain themes of delusional content tend to predominate and this has meant an unfortunate proliferation of descriptive names scattered across a fragmented literature, leading to many difficulties in conceptualizing the subtype and in separating it from other psychiatric disorders with prominent hypochondriasis. As with all subtypes of delusional disorder, the clinician must bear in mind the advice already given that, for the diagnosis of delusional disorder, it is the characteristic form of the illness that is of prime importance, not the content of the delusional beliefs. The hypochondriasis in delusional disorder may superficially resemble that of somatoform disorder, psychotic depression, or obsessive–compulsive disorder, but careful examination will reveal very different underlying illnesses.

Clinical features

We shall consider the manifestations of the somatic subtype of delusional disorder under four major theme areas:

(1) delusions involving the skin;

(2) delusions of ugliness or misshapenness (dysmorphic delusions);

(3) delusions of body odour or halitosis;

(4) miscellaneous.

Delusions involving the skin[56–58]

In the delusion of skin infestation, the patient insists that he has organisms, usually insects, crawling over the surface of the skin and sometimes burrowing into the skin or under the nails. In most instances he cannot see the creatures, but sometimes there may be graphic descriptions. This may represent a visual hallucination but more usually seems to be a vivid ideational projection.

The delusion of parasites burrowing deeply under the skin is often attributed to worm-like parasites, and internal body sensations or the rippling of small superficial muscles are misinterpreted as evidence of their activities. Sometimes the patient believes that the worms have spread throughout the whole body or intermittently migrate from place to place.

In the delusion of discrete foreign bodies under the skin or nails, these bodies are occasionally described as inanimate, but generally the patient says they are seed-like or believes that they are parasite eggs. In some individuals this is associated with an irresistible desire to pick, and multiple deep excoriations may result. Such people are sometimes labelled as having 'neurotic excoriations' or factitious disorder, but in fact the picking behaviour is delusionally motivated and is an irresistible urge to stem the invasion of the parasites.

Chronic cutaneous dysaesthesia[59] is an unremitting burning sensation of the skin or mucosae, sometimes generalized but at other times largely confined to complaints of glossodynia or vulvodynia. A minority of these patients appear to have a monodelusional complaint.

A subgroup of patients with trichotillomania and onychotillomania[60] have delusional illnesses, and the hair-pulling or nail-picking may be part of the attempt to rid themselves of parasites.

In all the above presentations, the delusion and its associated behaviours typically occur in the setting of many well-retained personality features and the patient can often make very clear-cut and apparently rational complaints, convincing the many physicians they attend, at least for a time, that actual physical disease is present. However, no somatic treatment works and the complaining becomes increasingly frenzied and unreasonable. The sufferer cannot be persuaded that infestation is not present and often becomes very angry at the perceived incompetence of the dermatologists he has visited.

Usually the story of the infestation is presented in great detail, perhaps involving an original event such as an insect bite. 'Proof' is presented by displaying skin lesions, deformed nails, bald patches, etc. The 'matchbox' or 'pill-bottle' sign, in which the patient produces a small container in which 'insect corpses' or 'eggs' are kept, is typical; these nearly always turn out to be dried mucus, skin scrapings, or pieces of lint.[61] Often, there is incessant cleaning of self and surroundings, and repeated demands may be made to local authorities or pest-control agencies for disinfestation of the home. At times bizarre and even dangerous self-treatment is resorted to, such as applying boiling water or corrosive substances to the skin. The more normal part of the psyche is dominated by shame or fear of passing on the infestation, so that progressive social isolation tends to occur, with attendance on doctors as virtually the only outside activity.

Case Study Somatic subtype with a theme of infestation A woman of 67 was referred by a dermatologist because of 'neurotic excoriations'. She had been seen by many physicians over a period of 10 years, complaining of worms which crawled under her skin and laid their eggs, especially around her genital region. She had an irresistible urge to scratch and dig out the 'eggs' and as a result her genital area, buttocks, and thighs were covered with excoriations. She denied any itch and said she dug out the parasites to prevent further spread. No physical treatments had helped. On examination she was alert and showed no evidence of dementia. Her physical health was otherwise good. On most topics she could converse reasonably, but on the 'worms' she was vehement and angrily denied they were 'imagination'. She appeared to have an isolated delusional system of somatic type.

Dysmorphic delusions

'Dysmorphophobia', an old term which implies a morbid fear of being deformed, is still sometimes employed to describe cases in this category but should be abandoned since it has been so loosely used to denote both delusional and non-delusional complaints as well as a variety of very different illnesses.[62] In the present context we are considering only cases typical of delusional disorder which present with a false belief of ugliness or deformity. In some instances there may indeed be some minor deformity, but the complaining is out of all proportion to this and is expressed with unremitting delusional intensity.

A specific feature is often singled out by the individual, such as an overlong nose, prominent ears, over-large or undersized breasts, dissatisfaction with the appearance of the genitalia, a skin blemish, or some other.[63] However, in other cases the total body is perceived as abnormal, and there is evidence that a small subgroup of apparent cases of anorexia nervosa and bulimia nervosa may have an underlying delusional disorder.

Many of the patients with dysmorphic delusions go from surgeon to surgeon demanding cosmetic procedures and usually being refused, but if the surgeon does not perceive the illogicality of the complaint an operation may take place. While some successes have been reported, the general consensus is that most cases need psychiatric rather than surgical intervention and that surgery may seriously worsen the mental disorder in the longer term.

It is sometimes very difficult to distinguish cases of delusional disorder of somatic subtype from severe somatization disorder, and claims have been made that there is a continuum between these illnesses.[64] The evidence for this is minimal and a diagnostic distinction is essential since treatments of the two disorders are very different.

Case Study Somatic subtype with dysmorphic delusion A man aged 35 was seen in psychiatric consultation on a surgical unit. He had been complaining for at least 6 years that an appendicectomy scar was so ugly that it was ruining his life, although he never let anyone other than surgeons see it. He had repeatedly sought cosmetic surgery, but every surgeon who examined him said the scar was normal. The patient gave up work, became reclusive, and ruminated endlessly on his 'deformity'. Finally

he operated on himself, trying to excise the scar, but when he lost a lot of blood he panicked and called for an ambulance. Following operation in hospital he appeared rational on every topic except the scar, was of average intelligence and denied any suicidal feelings. At first he was thought to have a factitious disorder, but his continuing conviction that his life was useless if he could not have reparative surgery proved to be delusional.

Delusion of smell or of halitosis[65–67]

In this category it is often very difficult to distinguish between delusions and hallucinations of smell. The term 'olfactory reference syndrome' is often used to describe olfactory delusions, but in fact it should properly only refer to hallucinatory experiences. Sometimes the deluded patient will say that he or she has not actually experienced the odour, which is usually unpleasant, but 'knows' that it is present because of remarks made by others or their avoidant behaviour. In other cases the stench is described graphically and consistently (like 'burning rubber' or 'faeces') and here a hallucination may be present. There may be no explanation, or else the smell may be attributed to escaping flatus, abnormal sweat secretion, or sinus or dental problems leading to halitosis etc. As is typical, an unending and escalating search for a physical treatment occurs.

Miscellaneous delusional contents

Presumably there is an almost infinite possibility of different themes, but in practice their numbers are somewhat limited. The following have been described.

Dental[68]

Although his dentition is satisfactory, the patient insists that his dental bite is abnormal and obtains repeated corrective treatments from successive dentists, none of which work. This has been termed the 'phantom bite syndrome', and may sometimes be associated with complaints of facial pain for which no physical basis is apparent. There may also be delusional complaints of deformity of the jaw or abnormality of the temporomandibular joint.

Delusion of transmitting non-sexual diseases

Some patients may be convinced that they are causing illnesses in others (e.g. tuberculosis), and they will cite as evidence, for example, that everyone starts coughing when they walk into a room.

Delusion of sexually transmitted disease[69]

Hypochondriasis is, of course, rampant around the topic of sexually transmitted disease. A subgroup of delusional disorder patients develop the conviction that they have venereal disease, often when there is no evidence of risk-taking behaviour having occurred. In the past syphilis was probably the greatest fear, but nowadays it is usually AIDS. Repeated tests showing negative serology have no reassuring effect. Interestingly, a few cases of AIDS have been described in recent years in which a delusional illness with hypochondriasis has emerged, usually due to direct effects of the virus on the brain.

Differential diagnosis of delusional disorder: somatic subtype

First, the presence of a significant physical disorder must be excluded. The illness must be distinguished from the following:

* paranoid schizophrenia

- substance-related disorders (e.g. itching due to alcohol-related liver failure, cocaine abuse, etc.)
- organic brain disorders
- severe depressive disorder with hypochondriacal delusions
- somatoform disorders, especially body dysmorphic disorder
- obsessive–compulsive disorder
- factitious disorder.

Epidemiology

Cases usually present in medical and surgical practices and much less often in a psychiatric context. We have no idea of the frequency because non-psychiatrists make a variety of diagnoses, often untranslatable in psychiatric terms. However, the somatic subtype of delusional disorder is certainly not uncommon, and this is increasingly being revealed as consultation–liaison psychiatry develops.

These cases make a strong impression on physicians and surgeons because of their insistence and unreasonable demands. To date, dermatologists have been most aware of the nature of the delusional complaining and, in some cases, have learned to treat the deluded patients satisfactorily with appropriate medication. Infectious and tropical disease specialists also have an awareness, as do gastroenterologists and some dentists, and they are gradually referring more cases for psychiatric help. Plastic and cosmetic surgeons see a considerable number of cases with dysmorphic delusions, but it is still rather uncommon for them to seek psychiatric consultations. Since the patient with delusional disorder generally refuses to visit a psychiatrist willingly, it is often necessary for us to consult on the other specialists' territory in order to offer practical help and to obtain a better idea of the illness's frequency.

From what we know, the somatic subtype affects both sexes approximately equally and the age of onset may be from late adolescence to extreme old age. The illness is more common in the unmarried, the divorced, and the widowed.

Aetiology

The aetiology is discussed in the section on general aetiological considerations above.

Course and prognosis

Typically the illness is long term with a tendency to worsen with time. Some patients eventually lapse into a rather apathetic state, and some attempt or commit suicide in chronic despair, but the majority continue to demand treatment on their own deluded terms indefinitely.

Treatment of the somatic subtype

Treatment is discussed later in this chapter in the section on overall treatment aspects.

Delusional disorder: jealousy subtype[70,71]

This is sometimes known as the Othello syndrome, but the term is not recommended as it lacks specificity.

The phenomenon of jealousy

Jealousy can arise in various contexts, but here we shall deal with sexual jealousy. This is a virtually universal human emotion, especially when a rival is attempting to lure away someone's sexual partner. Males and females are equally prone to jealousy but may express it differently; Mullen and Martin[72] suggest that men are mainly concerned with losing the partner whereas women worry about the effect of infidelity on the ongoing relationship.

Broadly there are three levels of jealousy. Normal jealousy is understandable in terms of the situation and the individual's perception of it, and its expression can range from pique to severe rage. How it is expressed is largely related to temperament; some people habitually vent anger with slight provocation and others usually bottle up their feelings. On the whole, men tend to act out their jealous anger more physically.

Neurotic jealousy occurs where the mood and its mode of expression are relatively normal but owing to non-psychotic psychiatric illness, including personality disorder, the reaction is impulsive and excessive. Although the individual is reacting to an overvalued idea rather than a delusion, this type of jealousy can be irrational and quite persistent, and may be expressed dangerously.

Psychotic jealousy, such as occurs in delusional disorder, is characterized by a fixed delusional belief which cannot be swayed by reasoned argument or presentation of contrary evidence. This is the most alarming type since there is no dissuasion and there is an inexorability about the way that the individual accuses, controls and even stalks the victim. Since the accusations are usually untrue, the latter is bewildered by them, but occasions do arise when a partner actually has been unfaithful and it is then very difficult for the observer to know at first how much of the jealousy is justified and how much is delusional. Eventually the savageness and unreasonableness of the accusations reveal themselves as undoubtedly abnormal, but meanwhile a frightened partner will have suffered enormous abuse and possibly repeated assault.

When does jealousy become pathological?

Jealousy which appears justifiable is regarded as normal, although perhaps not laudable, and it will usually be accepted by society if its manifestations are not antisocial. Nowadays we increasingly frown on jealous violence, whether provoked or not, but in some communities there is still acknowledgement of the *crime passionel*, the crime committed out of jealous love. However, this is invariably an excuse extended to males, and the jealous woman who commits assault or murder is usually treated more harshly.

Cobb[70] proposed the following as clinical features of pathological jealousy, whether it be neurotic or psychotic.

1. The jealous thinking and behaviour are unreasonable in expression and in intensity.

2. The jealous individual is convinced of the partner's guilt but the evidence is dubious to others.

3. A recognizable psychiatric illness is present which could plausibly be associated with abnormal jealousy.

4. In a proportion of cases, the jealous person has habitual personality characteristics of jealousy, suspiciousness, and overpossessiveness.

5. The jealousy persists unduly and reinforces itself.

6. Pathological jealousy is usually focused on one specific person.

In neurotic jealousy, which in some ways resembles obsessive–compulsive disorder, there is high self-awareness of the emotion and sometimes of its irrationality. In delusional jealousy the person is totally at one with the belief which has come to occupy much of his or her time. Counter-argument or contrary evidence is rejected, yet in delusional disorder the individual may be so high functioning in other areas that he or she is totally convincing to outsiders and may even be able to brainwash the innocent victim into admission of guilt, a form of *folie à deux*.

The impact of pathological jealousy

Delusional jealousy is anguishing to the sufferer and even more so to the sexual partner who is accused of infidelity. The latter is subjected to escalating emotional abuse, and indignation, protest, and proof of innocence are unavailing. Physical violence, especially by males, is common[73] and in a proportion of cases finally ends in homicide, sometimes followed by the suicide of the perpetrator.[74] Subjected to prolonged threat, many victims are too terrified to speak up, and some become housebound in a vain attempt to prevent accusations of philandering. From time to time the situation reveals itself when the desperate partner attempts suicide and talks to a helping professional when recovering.

Clinical features

The person's belief in the other's infidelity is absolute and brooks no contradiction. There is much associated irritability, despondency, and, in some cases, aggressiveness. An ever-increasing proportion of time is spent searching for spurious 'proofs', and 'clues' are pounced upon and misinterpreted; for example, an innocent stain is believed to be semen. The victim is put through endless interrogations and is kept under constant surveillance.

Paradoxically, when the jealous individual is questioned closely about his or her specific charges, details prove vague, there is irritability, and there are self-justifying repetitive statements. Evidence is always about to be produced but rarely materializes. Strangely too, the jealous person often avoids taking the action which might provide definite proof of guilt or innocence, and this passivity in the midst of intensiveness may be evidence of some volitional defect.

As noted, delusional jealousy is more commonly reported in men, but this is probably an artefact due to their greater likelihood of violence. Also, there is a link between chronic alcohol abuse, as well as amphetamine and cocaine abuse, and delusions of jealousy, and it is known that these substance abuses are more common in males.

Epidemiology

The overall prevalence of abnormal jealousy and the specific prevalence of the delusional disorder subtype are unknown and, because of fear on the part of the victim, both are invariably under-reported. Both heterosexual and homosexual cases occur, and family patterns of jealous behaviour have been described, but there is little evidence of direct inheritance.

Aetiology

Psychological, especially psychodynamic, theories of jealousy have failed to distinguish between normal and pathological forms. Freud[16] suggested that delusional jealousy was the result of an unconscious homosexual wish externalized onto the heterosexual partner and the theme of 'latent' homosexuality is again invoked, but with little supportive evidence. Injured narcissism is another recurring speculative theme. Psychological investigations, in general, have raised many questions but provided us with no convincing answers about aetiology.

Inherited temperamental factors may be important[75] but most cases of delusional jealousy do not have a family history of the condition itself. In the jealousy subtype of delusional disorder, it may be fair to postulate a brain abnormality which can express itself over time or when provoked by chronic substance abuse or the effects of brain injury.

Of course, provocative or misunderstood behaviour by the partner may provide a context for the delusion but is never sufficient to account for the illness itself.

Course and prognosis

The condition may appear gradually or suddenly, but even when the onset seems rapid there may have been a previous period of rumination and perplexity of varying duration which probably represents the experiencing of delusional mood or *Wahnstimmung*. When the delusion crystallizes the perplexity vanishes and the patient is then totally sure of his belief.

Delusional jealousy is typical in being chronic and often lifelong. Without treatment the prognosis is poor and the danger to the victim is ever present. Most patients refuse to accept psychiatric treatment and unfortunately may only receive it following incarceration for a violent crime.

Differential diagnosis

The illness must be distinguished from the following:

● actual marital or sexual problems, including spousal infidelity

● mental handicap, where a simple-minded person may develop a 'crush' and be unable to understand that the other person does not reciprocate, or else enters into a sexual relationship and cannot cope with the partner's motives and behaviours

● schizophrenia, especially of the paranoid type

● major mood disorder with delusions, either depressive or manic

● personality disorder, especially of the paranoid, antisocial, borderline, histrionic, and narcissistic types

● obsessive–compulsive disorder

● substance abuse (which may complicate any of the other differential diagnoses)

● organic brain disorders, including dementias and some epileptic disorders

● sexual dysfunction may lead to fears that a normal partner is seeking satisfaction elsewhere.

It should be noted that an important part of the diagnostic process, an accurate collateral history, may be impossible to obtain in cases of delusional jealousy because of the victim's fears.

Forensic complications[51]

In cases of identified physical abuse in a relationship one possibility that must always be considered is delusional disorder of jealous type. Severe assault and even murder are not uncommon, and the physician has a duty to warn and protect the partner if these dangers seem real, perhaps divulging confidential information if necessary. Of course the patient denies that his beliefs are unjustified and may present his case more convincingly than the terrified victim can. If involuntary committal is necessary it may be very difficult to sustain, partly because of the individual's ability to maintain a pseudonormal facade and often because he or she threatens litigation.

Occasionally, cases of stalking, usually of females by deluded males, are jealousy related and the victim is nearly always well aware of the stalker's identity in these instances.

Treatment

This will be discussed when considering the overall treatment approach to delusional disorder. If successful treatment can be achieved, the couple may require considerable psychotherapy and counselling to re-establish a trusting and fear-free relationship.

Case Study Delusional disorder: jealousy subtype A married man aged 47 was arrested by the police after unprovokedly attacking the minister of his church who had been paying a pastoral visit to him and his wife. It emerged that for the past 18 months he had had the growing suspicion that his wife and the minister were having a sexual affair. Lately he had been following her unseen to choir practices and had started to take days off work to observe his own house for secret visits by the minister. Although nothing untoward occurred his conviction grew and his wife reported increasingly alarming jealous outbursts at home. He apparently attacked the minister on the strength of an innocent remark he misinterpreted. On examination in a forensic psychiatric unit he was quiet, mostly rational, and showed some remorse, but still maintained that his wife was committing adultery. He admitted to heavy alcohol use as a young man but not in recent years. Otherwise his history was unremarkable and he was still holding down a steady job. He appeared to have an encapsulated delusional system with jealous content.

Delusional disorder: erotomanic subtype[76–78]

In erotomania the individual has strong erotic feelings towards another person and has the persistent, unfounded belief that this other person is deeply in love with him or her. The belief is usually delusional, though a small number of non-delusional cases have been reported. Occasionally the imagined lover does not actually exist, but more often he or she is a real person who is unaware of the situation. The phenomenon is often referred to as de Clérambault's syndrome, but this usage is obsolete and can be misleading since it is used to describe erotomanic manifestations in a number of different mental illnesses.

De Clérambault[76] distinguished a 'pure' or 'primary' erotomania from other cases which were more symptomatic, and this pure form approximates to the modern description of delusional disorder with erotomanic content. In the older literature it was claimed that eroto-manic delusions were largely confined to women, especially isolated and frustrated elderly spinsters, but more and more cases of male erotomania are being reported nowadays.[79,80] In both sexes the majority of cases described involve heterosexual emotions, but homosexual erotomania is now well documented in both males and females.

Clinical features

The patient yearns for another person and has the unshakeable belief that these feelings are reciprocated. The person is often socially unattainable, may be of higher social status, and can be a celebrity. There has rarely been close contact and the love object will usually be unaware of the situation, but despite this the patient believes that the other initiated the imagined relationship, often with covert signals or utterances. Many patients experience strong erotic feelings, but some insist that the relationship is platonic and that the other person is maintaining a non-sexual attitude of watchful protectiveness.

In many instances the patient makes no attempt to get in touch with the love object, perhaps writing letters or buying gifts but not sending them. When given a chance to make actual contact he or she will frequently avoid doing so and will make spurious excuses such as not wanting to offend the other person's spouse. In those cases where the patient does attempt contact, equally false reasons are presented to explain the almost inevitable rejection that results.

Since this is erotomania in the setting of delusional disorder, the illness will have the typical form of a tightly knit delusional system with preservation of relatively normal personality features and with greater or lesser ability to continue functioning in society. There is often enough insight or inhibition present for the patient to keep the delusional beliefs concealed. However, at times he or she may be profoundly angered by being 'inexplicably' rejected and may act this out, occasionally dangerously. This is more likely to occur in males.

The onset of erotomania can be gradual or apparently sudden. Hallucinations are sometimes present but are not prominent, although the patient may be encouraged by 'hearing' the other person express passionate feelings. Occasionally, the presence of tactile hallucinations leads the patient to believe that a lover has paid a visit during the night (sometimes picturesquely referred to as the 'incubus syndrome')[81]

Diagnosis and differential diagnosis

Many covert examples necessarily go unrecognized and so there is a bias towards diagnosis of cases with some sort of acting-out behaviour. Otherwise the most common situation is one where the patient, after years of silent suffering, becomes unhappy enough to be treated for depression and then, during sympathetic history-taking, lets the delusional belief slip out. There is often much accompanying anguish and perhaps anger, and of course the beliefs are regarded as indisputable. Obviously, if the patient has been very secretive, a confirmatory history may be impossible to obtain. In married patients the spouse may be totally unaware of delusions which have lasted for years.

The following disorders may be associated with secondary erotomanic features.

- Schizophrenia, especially paranoid, in which the erotomania coexists with other delusions, florid hallucinations, and more widespread thought disorder.

- Major mood disorder, in depressive or manic phases.

- Organic brain disorders, including epilepsy, post-head-injury states, following long-term substance abuse, senile dementia, and possibly as a side-effect of steroid treatment.

- Mental handicap, in which misunderstanding occurs regarding another's feelings or intentions. However, we must remember that the mentally handicapped are liable to sexual abuse and we must not unthinkingly dismiss sexually laden remarks that they may make about other individuals. Conversely, we must also remember that mental handicap can coexist with psychotic disorders and delusional expressions.

- Delusional misidentification syndrome has occasionally been described with erotomanic features.

- Non-delusional erotomanic beliefs may emerge in unstable individuals, sometimes complicating transference in the course of psychotherapy. If associated with histrionic traits there may be florid acting out, but the beliefs do not have the qualities of a delusion.

Epidemiology

Nothing is known of the frequency of erotomania in general, or of the erotomanic subtype of delusional disorder. As will be noted below, the more dangerous aspects of the illness are proving to be not uncommon.

Aetiology

Textbooks commonly cite premorbid personality characteristics of oversensitivity, isolativeness, and vulnerability, accompanied by traits of priggishness and prudery, especially in women. They may be correct but the evidence is inferential and slight. Nevertheless a stereotype has been perpetuated of lonely embittered spinsters obtaining vicarious sexual satisfaction with a delusional lover.[15] The truth is that it may be at least as common in younger males whose tendency to aggressiveness can be accentuated by a history of alcohol or drug abuse.

Course and prognosis

Without treatment this is a chronic illness which is likely to worsen gradually over time.

Forensic complications[80,82]

Males who irrationally act out their erotomanic delusions are usually diagnosed as schizophrenic but some prove to have delusional disorder. Often the overt behaviour is in the nature of harassment, but even without violence the individual's persistent intrusiveness and incorrigibility can be thoroughly alarming to the victim, who is bewildered by the situation and by the other's accusations of duplicity.[83]

Severely aggressive behaviour can lead to assault, kidnapping, and even murder, sometimes of the love object or perhaps an acquaintance of the latter who is viewed as a rival. A manifestation which has gained much recent publicity is that of victim stalking, and in a considerable number of cases the victim has no idea who is carrying out the stalking.

While women are generally less prone to aggressive acting out of their delusions, they may sometimes demonstrate their false beliefs in devastating ways. For example, a deluded woman may claim publicly that a physician, counsellor, or teacher has demonstrated strong erotic feelings towards her. This belief may be the result of a delusional memory. If she has an undeteriorated personality, is coherent, totally believes her own story, and presents it with typical vehemence and persistence, it may be virtually impossible to persuade the public and the authorities that the accusations are totally false. Any professional person dealing with deluded patients must be aware of abnormal transference emotions that may arise in the patient during treatment, usually of a heterosexual nature but sometimes homosexual. Great circumspection is then required and the therapist must immediately seek collegial help in dealing with such a situation.

Treatment

Treatment is discussed later in the chapter in the section on the overall treatment of delusional disorder.

Case Study Delusional disorder: erotomanic subtype A woman of 53 was referred for psychiatric opinion by her family doctor because of depressive symptoms. She demanded a female psychiatrist and at first was uncooperative in giving a history. She admitted that she was unhappy and eventually broke down and told the psychiatrist that her unhappiness was due to the fact that she and her gynaecologist were in love but because of his profession he could not declare himself. When she visited his office she knew by his gestures and vocal intonations that he was covertly expressing love and she admitted having orgasmic sensations during pelvic examinations. She had never said anything to him and did not want to break up his or her marriage, but the prolonged stress of unrequited love was causing her depression. No actual depressive illness was present and the symptoms appeared to be those of a delusional disorder, erotomanic subtype. The gynaecologist was discreetly made aware of the situation via the family physician. Fortunately the patient improved with treatment and subsequently agreed to attend a different gynaecologist.

Delusional disorder: grandiose subtype[37]

This is the least well described variant of delusional disorder, not surprisingly in view of its nature. An individual who is habitually elated, even exalted, and who may believe himself or herself rich or powerful is unlikely to seek help, especially psychiatric help. If he or she remains sufficiently high functioning to function in the community, the delusions may be undetected; indeed some people capitalize on their beliefs by belonging to fringe organizations, apocalyptic religious groups, or doomsday sects. Sometimes these groups develop malignant qualities, especially under a deluded but charismatic leader, and one cannot minimize the dangerous qualities of the forceful megalomaniac whose grandiosity is alloyed with persecutory anger. Like-minded and impressionable people are readily drawn in and a kind of mass shared psychotic disorder may result; comparisons with Nazi Germany are not inapt.

Clinical features

This disorder often only emerges over time and with observation. The few cases that we see tend to fall into two categories. The first are those whose state of bliss is so profound that they totally neglect self-care. The rest are usually seen in custody after they have committed an offence under delusional influence. The characteristic underlying features of a delusional disorder have already been well described.

Differential diagnosis

The illness must be distinguished from the following.

- Mania, in which grandiosity is associated with euphoria, overactivity, and, at times, irritability and suspiciousness. As the mood is highly volatile, the grandiose symptoms are unstable.
- Schizophrenia in which there is marked incongruity between ecstatic affect and relative thought poverty.
- Organic brain disorders, especially affecting the prefrontal cerebral lobes, which cause labile mood, disinhibited behaviour, and some degree of cognitive deficit. Cerebral syphilis (general paralysis of the insane) used to be the best-known exemplar.
- Antisocial personality disorder in which the individual feels above the law and may express grandiose ideas and behaviours. In these cases one finds evidence of marked impulsivity, lack of remorsefulness, and a long-standing history of delinquency.

Epidemiology

We have virtually no information. The illness can occur in either sex and apparently at any age from adolescence onwards. It may appear gradually or suddenly.

Aetiology

All that can be said is that the aetiology is probably similar to that of other delusional disorder subtypes and that abnormal brain function is present. Psychoanalysis has suggested that it is due to pathologically inflated narcissism with investment of the self by libido which is usually invested in external objects, as well as a prolongation of the feelings of omnipotence said to occur in the young child. Other theorists have postulated that grandiosity represents a flight from feelings of worthlessness.[84] None of these developmental hypotheses proves helpful in dealing with the clinical case.

Course and prognosis

As far as we know, the grandiose subtype is as chronic and unremitting as the other subtypes of delusional disorder. For many years the presence of grandiosity in any psychiatric disorder has been regarded as a bad prognostic factor. In delusional disorder this may be so, because a grandiose delusional system is particularly likely to be associated with refusal to accept treatment. Even if treatment begins to be effective, the abandoning of highly pleasurable beliefs may not be welcomed by some patients.

There may be forensic complications if grandiose delusions are overtly acted out.

Treatment

Treatment is discussed later in the chapter in the section on the overall treatment of delusional disorder.

Case Study Delusional disorder: grandiose subtype A 78-year-old unmarried woman who had always lived alone was admitted to a geriatric medical unit after being found in unbelievably squalid circumstances. Although unable to care for herself and showing some evidence of malnutrition, she was in reasonable physical health and appeared quite personable in social situations. Her mood was cheerful but not elevated and she was non-demented. It gradually emerged that she believed herself to be a multimillionairess who did not have to care for herself because her affairs were being attended to by multiple servants. Although she appreciated that her home was filthy, she did not see any conflict in this. Her delusions were absolutely fixed but were encapsulated, and she showed marked preservation of personality features. When discussing topics other than herself she was quite reasonable and non-grandiose, and she regularly kept up to date on current affairs via the media.

Delusional disorder: mixed and unspecified subtypes

There is little to be added regarding these categories. When delusional disorder was defined in DSM-IIIR, the emphasis was on single predominant delusional themes such as those that have been described. In DSM-IV it is accepted that more than one theme can exist side by side so that, provided that the form of the illness is that of delusional disorder, it is acceptable that the delusional system may combine themes of, for example, hypochondriasis and persecution, persecution and grandiosity, erotomania and jealousy, etc.

The unspecified type is a residual category and again the illness must have the form of a delusional disorder, but the delusional content is one other than those specifically listed. No systematized data exist on either the mixed or the unspecified subtypes.

Other disorders with persistent delusions

As mentioned previously, ICD-10 has a category for 'other persistent delusional disorders' (F22.8), but this is so loosely worded as to nullify any description as a coherent clinical entity. Under the rubric of 'other disorders with persistent delusions' we shall now discuss two conditions, delusional misidentification syndrome and paraphrenia. Neither of these is officially recognized at present, although paraphrenia could be diagnosed indirectly as a member of category F22.8. It is suggested that both are important diagnoses which belong on the paranoid spectrum and which should be strongly considered for inclusion in it.

Delusional misidentification syndromes (DMIS)[85,86]

The abilities to recognize individual faces and to discriminate between different faces are fundamental human processes and normally we are extraordinarily adept at them. The biological need for face recognition is present from birth and the capacity elaborates throughout earlier life. Changes in a familiar facial appearance can be unsettling and even frightening, not just in children but also in adults. A great deal of sophisticated neurophysiological and neuropsychological investigation has been carried out on normal and abnormal human face-recognition abilities.

A number of clearly defined neurological disorders are associated with very specific abnormalities of face recognition.[87] Since 1923, when Capgras and Reboul-Lachaux[6] first reported the *illusion de sosies* or 'delusion of doubles', there has been growing interest in abnormalities of recognition involving facial and bodily appearance and behavioural characteristics which present as psychiatric, and specifically delusional, disorders. Here we shall emphasize those cases in which a delusion of misidentification is the principal symptom of the disorder and in which the form or structure of the illness is in many ways similar to that of delusional disorder. These are the delusional misidentification syndromes. However, it is important to note that superficially similar presentations may occur as secondary features in cases of schizophrenia, severe mood disorder, or dementia, and in these we refer to a misidentification phenomenon rather than syndrome.

Clinical features[88]

There are four main variants of DMIS:

(1) the Capgras syndrome, in which the patient falsely perceives that someone in his environment, usually a close relative or friend, has been replaced by an almost, but not quite exact, double;

(2) the Frégoli syndrome, where the patient believes that one or more individuals have altered their appearances to resemble familiar people, usually to persecute or defraud him or her;

(3) intermetamorphosis, in which the patient believes that people around have exchanged identities so that A becomes B, B becomes C, and so on;

(4) the syndrome of subjective doubles, where the patient is convinced that exact doubles of him- or herself exist, a kind of *Doppelgänger* phenomenon.

Additional alternative forms have been described and it should be noted that features of more than one variant may occur in an individual case. This is especially true of the subjective doubles phenomenon.

Although the patient is convinced of the deception, typically he is aware that something is wrong and that the replacements are subtly incorrect. Many sufferers are extremely distressed and frightened because they are convinced that the substitution of identity is meant to harm them. In some cases they become enraged and attack the 'impostor' with considerable violence. Their belief is of delusional intensity and they usually cannot be dissuaded by argument or by demonstration of contrary proof.

It is of particular interest that the misidentification is not indiscriminate but involves a limited number of usually familiar people. In some cases, substitution involves not just people but places or objects. An admixture of depersonalization and derealization is not uncommon, especially in the earlier stages.

Classification

Delusional misidentification syndromes have been regarded as something of a curiosity until recently and have not been included in DSM-IV or ICD-10. If a misidentification phenomenon occurs in the setting of another psychotic illness such as schizophrenia, then of course it is regarded as a feature of that illness. However, if it is the principal aspect of a psychosis then it should be regarded as a disorder *sui generis*. In those cases where there is a discrete delusional system occurring in clear consciousness and within a relatively intact personality, it would seem logical to assign the patients to a new status within the Delusional Disorder (DSM-IV) or Persistent Delusional Disorders

(ICD-10) category. In other cases where organic brain disease is more prominent, the proper assignment would be to Mental Disorders due to a General Medical Condition (DSM-IV) or Organic, Including Symptomatic, Mental Disorders (ICD-10).

Diagnosis and differential diagnosis

The diagnosis is based on recognition of the patient's delusional belief, the accompanying agitation, and uncharacteristic behaviours, possibly including violent attacks on people in the environment. A full neurological investigation is mandatory.

Differential diagnosis includes the following:

- schizophrenia
- delusional disorder, persecutory subtype
- major mood disorder with delusions
- organic brain disorder
- substance abuse disorders.

Epidemiology

The frequency of DMIS is unknown. Until the past decade it was regarded as very rare, but an increasing number of cases are being reported. The disorder occurs in both sexes and across a wide age range, but particularly in middle-aged and elderly people.

Aetiology

When DMIS was first recognized, psychological, and especially psychodynamic, explanations were sought for the phenomenon.[89] The fact that the delusion usually involved the patient's nearest and dearest led to the theory that overintense affect towards significant others induced ambivalent feelings, leading to psychological splitting and projection, very much as in theories of paranoia. Such hypothesizing was based entirely on retrospective information, and it has been seriously undermined in recent years by the increasing recognition of significant brain pathology in a high proportion of cases. Also, it has been suggested that the majority of patients tend to be too old at the time of onset for a purely psychological origin to seem feasible. To date, psychodynamic formulation and therapy have not proved useful in practice.

Nowadays we have many reports on brain dysfunction in DMIS[32,90,91] but large case series are lacking. There is some consensus that abnormalities of the right cerebral hemisphere are especially likely to be present, particularly in the right temporoparietal area, but these are not inevitable and lesions in other cerebral locations have been noted. Currently it is acknowledged that at least two-thirds of typical DMIS cases have a demonstrable brain lesion which can be regarded as causal and which may specifically bring about abnormalities of face recognition (a function mediated especially in the right hemisphere). Also, there commonly appears to be dissociation of sensory information from its appropriate affective accompaniment and failure of suppression of inappropriately repetitive behaviours (also a right-sided function). These last two phenomena are very typical of delusional illnesses in general.

We know little of the biological substrate of delusional symptoms, but one proposal is that there may be a dysfunction of the limbic-basal ganglia mechanisms involved in their genesis, with particular emphasis on dopamine overactivity.[92] In DMIS there appears to be a breakdown in integration of information between the right parieto-temporal cortex, the limbic system, and certain basal ganglia, resulting in the specific misidentification quality of the delusion, associated with inappropriate emotion and inability to suppress abnormal thoughts and behaviours. In addition, there is some evidence linking disorders of the limbic lobe with 'paranoid' symptoms in general. Therefore it is possible to postulate a complex brain mechanism which normally integrates sensory and affective impulses and downregulates repetitive behaviour, and whose malfunction results in delusional beliefs, altered judgment, overintense mood, and inability to change or develop insight. The particular delusional content would be determined by the specific site within the mechanism at which the significant abnormality had its predominant affect.

Although the above is simply a paradigm, it is also a model with potential for the study of delusional and concomitant phenomena by modern neurobiological investigative methods. It also allows us to conjecture about the general similarities and specific differences between DMIS and delusional disorder, and perhaps it may help us with the classification of the former.

Course and prognosis

Although DMIS may appear insidiously, it not uncommonly comes on relatively suddenly in a previously normal individual, presumably related to the underlying cerebral pathology. Where brain damage is substantial, the prognosis is that of the brain disease. If the brain dysfunction is more subtle and does not remit, the delusional symptoms may become chronic. Forensic complications may occur if the patient becomes violent,[93] and a small number of murders have been reported in association with DMIS.

Treatment

Acute treatment may involve sedation and antipsychotic medication. Ongoing treatment is by maintenance doses of an antipsychotic with possible addition of an anticonvulsant. Psychological counselling may be beneficial as the patient recovers.

Case Study Delusional misidentification syndrome with Capgras and Frégoli features A man of 63 recovered from a relatively minor stroke with only minimal left-sided weakness. During his convalescence he became very agitated and began accusing his wife of being an impostor. He also thought that visiting relatives were being impersonated by strangers and that this was all part of a plot to deprive him of his money. He frequently threatened to strike others, although he did not actually commit violence. At times he broke down and wept copiously, apologizing to his wife somewhat over-effusively. He was admitted to a psychiatric unit where an electroencephalogram and a CT scan revealed cerebral abnormalities, especially but not exclusively on the right side. His symptoms gradually improved on anticonvulsant treatment. He returned home functioning on a somewhat limited level but apparently free of delusions.

Paraphrenia[11,94]

As noted earlier, paraphrenia is a diagnosis which has fallen out of favour, but its demise has left an uncomfortable gap in the diagnostic repertoire which psychiatrists either ignore by labelling everything as schizophrenia or else ineffectually try to fill with nondescript diagnoses such as 'atypical psychosis' or 'schizoaffective disorder'. The ICD-10 category of 'other persistent delusional disorder' (F22.8) could be used for cases of paraphrenia and would at least denote an illness with links to delusional disorder, but it must be made clear that paraphrenia is not simply a variant of the latter.

Clinical features

Kraepelin's description of paraphrenia[11] was of an illness similar to paranoid schizophrenia, with fantastic delusions and hallucinations but having relatively limited thought disorder and well-preserved affect. Compared with schizophrenia, there was less personality deterioration and volition was less impaired. The patient's ability to communicate with others and to demonstrate rapport and emotional warmth remained good. In contrast with paranoia (now delusional disorder), there was not the encapsulated highly organized quality of the delusional system and the delusions lacked the quasi-logical structure of delusional disorder.

There are few recent descriptions of Kraepelinian paraphrenia[95] and virtually no studies have been carried out on it in the past 60 years. However, a recent investigation by Ravindran et al.[96] appears to confirm that cases of paraphrenia can readily be recognized on predetermined criteria and can be distinguished from schizophrenia. These patients have a disorder which closely fits Kraepelin's original description. In addition, it is noted that agitation and irrational behaviour are prominent in the acute stage, usually an apparent response to vivid delusions and hallucinations. Despite resemblances to paranoid schizophrenia, less than a third had made threats or displayed aggressive behaviour prior to assessment. In fact, nearly half the patients came to notice because of illogical complaints to the authorities, indicating a breakdown in reality testing but some retention of social judgment.

When the immediate psychotic symptoms settle sufficiently to allow better communication, the preservation of emotional warmth and sociability becomes apparent and is in marked contrast to typical schizophrenia, but these individuals still show widespread thought disorder, multiple delusions, and poor insight.

Diagnosis and differential diagnosis

The principal aim is to distinguish paraphrenia from the more deteriorative aspects of schizophrenia on one side and from the encapsulated delusional system characteristic of delusional disorder on the other. Therefore other disorders to be distinguished are:

* paranoid schizophrenia
* delusional disorder
* major mood disorder with delusions
* dementia
* severe schizoid, schizotypal, or paranoid personality disorder
* schizoaffective disorder.

Epidemiology

By inference it appears that cases of paraphrenia are about one-tenth as common as all other cases of schizophrenia in an inpatient psychiatric population, but this tells us nothing about its frequency in a general population. Since personality deterioration is less marked, one might expect cases of paraphrenia to survive better in the community than cases of schizophrenia and to be relatively more common there, but we have no statistics on this.

The illness occurs in both males and females, but the sex ratio is undetermined. Despite their retention of some positive social attributes, many of these patients live alone and experience considerable social isolation. Contrary to the traditional belief that this is an illness of older people, the age of onset can be at any time from early adult life to extreme old age. It is possible that paraphrenia may occur more often in immigrant groups. Schizophrenia is said to be uncommon in the family history, although psychiatric illness in general is frequent in families.

Aetiology

The possible association with immigration has been noted above. Many texts have declared that deafness, and to a lesser extent blindness, are potentially isolative and provocative factors, but evidence for this is uncertain. A family history of psychiatric illness occurs in perhaps half of the cases of paraphrenia and its presence seems to be associated with an earlier onset of the disorder. A prior history of substance abuse and head injury are presumed to have significance in some cases but no statistics are extant.

Course and prognosis

The illness is chronic and is progressive in many cases. Fluctuations in severity occur, but nowadays this may be related to intermittent periods of treatment alternating with non-compliance. Despite their good rapport with staff and fellow patients, paraphrenics often have poor insight and judgement about their illness. As inpatients they co-operate with treatment and usually respond well to neuroleptics, so that superficially they appear remarkably normal at the time of discharge. However, delusional thinking remains covertly active in many cases and a high proportion repeatedly relapse after discharge because they stop their medications. Fortunately many patients remain fairly undeteriorated even after several exacerbations, but in the longer term possibly as many as half will gradually deteriorate towards schizophrenia, particularly of the paranoid type. Consistent compliance with medication is likely to lead to a much more optimistic outcome.

Treatment

In an acute phase the patient usually needs to be admitted for inpatient observation until stabilized on medication. The little evidence that exists suggests that paraphrenics in general respond well to all standard neuroleptics. If relapse occurs, non-compliance is a likely cause. Since the illness is potentially lifelong, the choice of neuroleptic should be influenced by the need to avoid long-term side-effects. Following discharge from hospital it is extremely important to maintain permanent supervision, even when the patient appears appear well, and to remember that these patients can utilize their retained social skills to hide their delusions and their lack of co-operation, at least for a time. The uncooperativeness is often delusionally motivated.

Case Study Paraphrenia A 38-year-old woman was admitted to a psychiatric inpatient unit for the sixth time in 5 years with an initial diagnosis of paranoid schizophrenia. On admission she was restless, disruptive, and grandiose, and she appeared to have severe auditory hallucinations. She had been brought to hospital because she had been virtually camping in the police station demanding action against allegedly persecutory neighbours. This hospital admission was typical of several previous ones. Each time, after some initial resistance, she accepts treatment and rapidly improves. Despite the severity and pervasiveness of her delusions, she

always becomes pleasant and shows remarkable appropriateness and range of mood and a good deal of depth of affect. Rapport with others is good. At discharge she always insists she will comply with treatment, but her insight is poor and she never completely loses her delusional beliefs. Relapse is always the result of stopping her medications. Despite frequent exacerbations and chronicity of the illness, her personality remains remarkably preserved when she takes her treatment, but long-term prognosis is thought to be poor.

Late paraphrenia

This subject is considered in Chapter 8.5.3.

Folie à deux: a phenomenon which may accompany illnesses with delusions[97–99]

This phenomenon is listed as a psychiatric disorder in DSM-IV (Shared Psychotic Disorder, 297.3) and in ICD-10 (Induced Delusional Disorder, F24) but there is a conceptual difficulty in regarding it as a psychotic illness in its own right, as will be discussed shortly.

Folie à deux is a venerable term used to describe a situation in which mental symptoms, usually but not invariably delusions, are communicated from a psychiatrically ill individual (the 'primary patient') to another individual (the 'secondary patient') who accepts them as truth. As noted, DSM-IV and ICD-10 refer to this by different names and there have been several confusing changes of official terminology in recent years. The older name, which is used as an alternative by DSM-IV, is well known to most psychiatrists and is used here by preference. However, *à deux* may sometimes be a misnomer since several people can be involved, and then we read of *folie à trois*, *folie à plusieurs*, *folie à ménage*, etc.

Taking the dyad as the classical situation, the two people are usually closely associated or related, especially husband–wife, siblings, or parent–child, and usually live in social isolation. The content of the shared belief depends on the predominant delusion(s) of the primary patient and can include convictions of persecution, delusional parasitosis, belief in having a child who does not exist, misidentification delusions, and many others. There have been descriptions of shared persecutory and apocalyptic beliefs in quasi-religions and cults apparently originating with a charismatic leader and coming to be shared by gullible followers. In many shared delusional constellations there is a sense of antagonism by 'them' who may be defined or who may be what Cameron[100] referred to as the 'paranoid pseudocommunity', the hovering 'they' who carry out persecution which is evident to the sufferers but not to others.

Once thought rare, *folie à deux* has been increasingly described in the literature. Milder cases may not be recognized and, also, many delusional people strive to avoid psychiatric referral; collusion between primary and secondary patient in this has been noted. The physician should be aware of the phenomenon and not overlook it.

The current official names (above) are open to semantic criticism since 'shared psychotic' and 'induced delusional' disorder imply that both members of the dyad are psychotic. In delusional disorder this is certainly true of the primary patient, but the recipient of the beliefs does not usually have a psychotic illness. Most often, he or she is highly impressionable and perhaps highly dependent and adopts the untrue beliefs because of their prolonged and extraordinarily intense transmission by the primary patient. Social isolation, accentuated by induced mistrust of 'them', prevents adequate reality testing from occurring. Thus one might say that the content of the secondary patient's false belief derives from psychotic thinking, but he or she is not usually psychotic.

Nearly all cases of *folie à deux* are reported in association with schizophrenia, delusional disorder, severe depressive illness with delusions, or early dementia, but it is probable that the condition also sometimes coexists with non-psychotic illnesses such as obsessive–compulsive disorder, somatoform disorder, and histrionic–dissociative personality disorder, in which the beliefs are intensely held and communicated but are not delusional. This makes the DSM-IV and ICD-10 names even less appropriate.

Subtypes

In practice, the great majority of cases are of the type described, often known as *folie imposée* because the belief is impressed on the non-deluded person by the primary patient.

However, one occasionally sees an alternative presentation, the so-called *folie simultanée*, in which two predisposed people develop illnesses with delusions and through long and over-close association come to share identical false beliefs. This is said to be most likely when there is a genetic link (for example two siblings) and the situation may be most common in older people who have lived together in considerable isolation for many years.

Classification

Folie à deux is included with Schizophrenia and Other Psychotic Disorders in DSM-IV and with Schizophrenia, Schizotypal, and Delusional Disorders in ICD-10, and is treated as though it were a separate psychotic illness. It would be better to treat it as an important clinical phenomenon which may be associated with other identifiable mental disorders. However, rather than encourage a pedantic argument, it is best simply to alert the clinician to its existence, its frequency, and, as will be explained, its importance.

Diagnosis

The phenomenon is *sui generis* and is recognized by the identical nature of the two individuals' beliefs, their gross overinvestment of affect in these, and their refusal to accept alternatives even when proof is presented. Careful history taking will usually readily distinguish the primary from the secondary patient, but at times this proves difficult. In the much less common *folie simultanée*, the distinction is largely irrelevant.

Epidemiology

This is unknown except that, by definition, it will occur most often in association with an illness characterized by delusional beliefs or severely overvalued ideas, especially under isolated living conditions, and it is by no means rare. It is extremely important for the clinician to be on the lookout for it. He or she may be convinced that a patient is expressing delusional ideas but be thoroughly perplexed when an apparently rational relative supports the unlikely belief. This can lead to serious mismanagement of the case. Conversely, recognition of *folie à deux* may solve a baffling diagnostic problem and result in appropriate care for both individuals.

Aetiology

Folie à deux appears to arise from a combination of the following:

(1) innate impressionability and marked dependence on the primary patient;

(2) personality traits such as suggestibility, low initiative, poor reality testing, etc. in the secondary patient;

(3) in some cases, low intelligence in the secondary patient;

(4) the intensity of the abnormal beliefs expressed by the primary patient;

(5) the length of time during which the abnormal beliefs are being imposed;

(6) the degree of social isolation.

Course and prognosis

This depends on the outcome of treatment (see below).

Treatment

In *folie imposée* the logical approach is to identify the primary patient and treat his or her mental disorder adequately. It may also be helpful to separate the two individuals for a time, for example by admitting the primary patient to hospital. With both people, every attempt must be made to reduce social isolation and to reintroduce them to reality. If the primary patient's delusions improve with treatment, the secondary patient's beliefs usually also improve. It is rarely appropriate to treat the secondary patient with antipsychotic medication, although this is sometimes mistakenly done.

In *folie simultanée*, both patients require neuroleptic or other active treatment.

Theoretically, treatment is straightforward but in practice it can be problematic. For example, in delusional disorder the primary patient often resists psychiatric help, and subterfuge and resistance by both individuals is common. In group situations, for example a cult, this resistance is likely to be widespread and intense, and will be justified by the participants in terms of religious and social beliefs which they claim are being suppressed and persecuted. The propagators should be separated from the recipients as much as possible, and the treatment team has to expend much time and diplomacy in gaining some confidence and a degree of co-operation. Direct challenge of the beliefs in any shared delusional situation is usually totally counterproductive.

Mass suicide is a reported outcome of shared delusions in some cult situations and any danger of this must be countered with great urgency.[101]

Case Study *Folie à deux* A highly intelligent man in his early fifties had had a brief sexual affair with a woman in his workplace some years before. He felt rather guilty although the liaison ended amicably and his wife did not know about it. About 3 years later he gradually became convinced that the woman involved had generated a plot against him amongst his fellow workers. He became totally preoccupied with this and eventually publicly accused her. She totally denied his charges, but in the next few months he harassed her and fellow employees incessantly, demanding 'proof' and a 'confession'. He was eventually dismissed and it was made clear to him by the company that they found no basis for his suspicion. For the next 2 years he spent all his time at home, endlessly retailing his constantly elaborating beliefs to his wife and neglecting all his normal routines. His equally intelligent wife had become totally convinced by him and was running a campaign with him to force the woman to admit to her alleged provocations. This had resulted in several legal actions against both of them which proved no deterrent. They reluctantly agreed to a psychiatric examination which indicated that he had a delusional disorder of the persecutory subtype and that she suffered from *folie à deux*. Neither accepted the need for treatment.

Treatment of delusional disorder

The treatment approaches to the delusional misidentification syndromes, paraphrenia, and *folie à deux* have been dealt with in their respective sections, but for several reasons the treatment of delusional disorder has been touched on only briefly until now. Firstly, it is necessary for the reader to have a grasp of the disorder's features and to know something of its status within a group of illnesses with delusions. Secondly, there are special aspects to the treatment of delusional disorder which need emphasis, especially since many clinicians are unfamiliar with them.

During the many years when paranoia was all but forgotten many psychiatric illnesses previously regarded as hopeless became readily treatable. When paranoia was again recognized—as delusional disorder—by DSM-IIIR in 1987 it seemed that the therapeutic hopelessness of an earlier era was also revived. Even now most texts state that treatment response is poor and are vague about the specifics of medication approaches. In fact, by far the greatest problem is not treatment responsiveness, but persuading the patient to accept that he needs psychiatric help because his delusions militate against this.

It must be stated categorically that, given careful diagnosis and an approach that encourages the patient to co-operate, delusional disorder is a highly treatable illness.

Unfortunately most of the literature supporting that statement is anecdotal but it shows good consensus on the remediability of the disorder. Virtually all the reports of success refer to psychopharmacological, specifically neuroleptic, treatment.

General aspects of the treatment of delusions[102]

We usually aim to treat the illness of which the delusion is a part, but there is good evidence that delusions themselves, as well as hallucinations, can be considerably modified by a psychological approach. In severe psychotic illnesses the institution of psychological treatment usually has to await the initial controlling of symptoms with medications or, on occasion, electroconvulsive therapy. Thereafter, a cognitive–behavioural approach or, to a much lesser extent, conventional psychotherapy can help the individual to reduce preoccupation with false beliefs, become less isolated from society, and reorientate towards reality.[18,103] However, there is no good evidence that psychological methods by themselves can completely eliminate delusions.

Since many illnesses are associated with delusions we have to tailor the psychopharmacological approach to suit each particular condition. In delusional disorder, the schizophrenias, and schizoaffective disorder, neuroleptics are the mainstay, with antidepressants, mood stabilizers, and electroconvulsive therapy sometimes playing subsidiary roles.

The rate of symptom response to treatment in a psychotic disorder is not uniform.[102] For example, hallucinations often resolve quite quickly, but delusions tend to be much more persistent. Despite vigorous treatment they can last for many months and, in some patients, never fully remit. If the patient continues to be deluded, noncompliance with treatment is likely to be present, especially in delusional disorder where the individual is often expert at concealing his or her lack of co-operation.

Treatment approach[37]

At present it appears that all the subtypes of delusional disorder are potentially responsive to treatment. If treatment fails, consider patient non-compliance first before abandoning the current approach.

The best-attested treatment results refer to the somatic subtype, with smaller literatures on the erotomanic, jealousy, and persecutory subtypes, and virtually nothing on the grandiose form. A wide variety of neuroleptics has been reported upon, but at present pimozide, a diphenylbutylpiperidine neuroleptic, is the drug of first choice.[104] Antidepressants and benzodiazepines are usually ineffective as first-line treatments and monoamine oxidase inhibitor antidepressants are contraindicated as they may worsen the delusions. There is no literature on the use of newer atypical neuroleptics in delusional disorder, but this should certainly be an area of study in the future.

Currently the best estimate of treatment outcomes, admittedly from a very scattered literature, is that, if the diagnosis is correct, the patient compliant, and the treatment adequate, recovery (defined as 'return to full function with total or near-remission of symptoms') occurs in approximately 50 per cent of all patients, no matter which neuroleptic has been used. A further 30 per cent will show substantial but less complete improvement. If pimozide has been the specific neuroleptic the results are a little better and nearly 90 per cent of all patients are reported to be recovered or improved. An unknown proportion of the remainder have failed to improve because they have not taken the medication adequately. Although based on mostly non-blind trials these figures come from a worldwide literature which does show marked consistency in reports of recovery rates.

Practical aspects of treatment

Since so many delusional disorder patients actively resist seeing a psychiatrist, it is best to see them in a non-psychiatric setting where possible, for example in the office of the referring specialist or family physician. The physician who treats cases of delusional disorder needs much patience and tact, and it is common to spend one or more sessions first gaining the individual's confidence and finally persuading him to give a psychotropic medication a trial. Many of them argue vehemently and with well-organized pseudo-logic against the premise that they have a psychiatric illness and use all kinds of sophistry to deny the need for a neuroleptic, but a calm and persistent approach will gain co-operation in a good proportion of cases.

As pimozide does seem to have the best success rate reported so far,[105] its use is recommended, but whatever neuroleptic one prescribes it is essential to begin with the lowest effective dose (e.g. pimozide 1–2 mg daily, haloperidol 1–2 mg daily). This dose is only raised if required and then very gradually to avoid side-effects which are guaranteed to cause cessation of treatment. The patient should be seen at least once a week as an outpatient in the initial stages. Inpatient treatment is not often indicated, although forensic cases will nearly always be seen in an institutional setting.

It is not unusual to observe minor improvements in a few days, such as reduced agitation, a slight increase in well being, improved sleep, and a little less preoccupation with the delusion. On average it is about 2 weeks before the delusional system is significantly ameliorated, but in some patients this may take 6 weeks or longer.

Quite often if this degree of improvement occurs the patient decides that there is no further need for treatment and stops it. Within days or weeks there is an inevitable return of the delusion with its accompanying agitation and preoccupation. It is then that the treating physician must be available to encourage resumption of medication. Although at this stage the patient still believes in his delusions, the experience of improvement followed by relapse makes a deep impression and, given trust in the therapist, often leads to long-term co-operation.

It is striking that good recovery is often relatively rapid and can be surprisingly complete, even when the illness has been present for many years. Some patients return to a considerable degree of intrapsychic, interpersonal, and occupational functioning, with little evidence of the personality disorder that is supposed to be so prevalent in delusional disorder. Also, many patients require surprisingly little counselling or psychotherapy in resuming a reasonable life, although these should always be available if needed. Such results suggest that this profound illness may be due to a relatively circumscribed brain abnormality and also that, in some cases at least, a very insidious onset may cause initial changes which mimic personality disorder.

In most instances, treatment has to be continued for an indefinite period since delusional disorder is potentially a lifelong illness. Naturally the drug dosage should be the lowest which keeps symptoms under control and this maintenance dose is often very low indeed (e.g. 1–2 mg pimozide daily). Perhaps up to one-third of patients can eventually be weaned successfully from medication, but we have no means of predicting who these will be, so that any reduction in treatment must be carried out with extreme caution. Sadly, a proportion of relapses are due to injudicious withdrawal of treatment by a physician and we must assume the need for treatment to be permanent unless proved otherwise. It is interesting that successfully treated patients, whether on maintenance drugs or not, keep a lookout for subsequent recurrences themselves and may report that tension-inducing circumstances provoke some reappearance of symptoms. Such patients may then request to have their medication raised or resumed.

There is no necessary correlation between acquired insight into the desirability of taking one's medication and true insight into the illness itself. Many patients never fully accept the psychotic nature of their experience, but as long as they are benefiting from treatment and are functioning reasonably there is nothing to be gained from challenging them on this. If, despite treatment, the delusions remain intrusive, cognitive–behavioural therapy and counselling should be available, but exploratory psychotherapy is contraindicated.

Throughout treatment, an optimistic and encouraging attitude by the physician is essential. Early on, frequent appointments are necessary and these are scaled down as improvement occurs. In the longer term it is essential that delusional disorder patients have good ongoing supervision; an insightful family physician is excellent for this but a periodic psychiatric review is recommended.

Recognition and treatment of postpsychotic depression[37,106]

Ten per cent or more of delusional disorder patients whose illness responds to neuroleptics experience significant degrees of mood disorder during recovery, sometimes very severe and with suicidal risk.[107] Such postpsychotic depression has also been noted in recovering schizophrenics, or in a few cases, mania.

Various explanations have been proposed such as a medication side-effect or perhaps the achievement of insight which is painful. On the whole the most likely reason is neurochemical, due to rapid changes in neurotransmitter balance.

If the neuroleptic is withdrawn, the depression tends to improve but the delusions return. Therefore the proper approach is to continue with the minimum effective level of neuroleptic and to add an antidepressant drug in a full therapeutic dose. Occasionally, in extremely severe cases, electroconvulsive therapy is indicated. Subsequently the neuroleptic is continued but, in most instances, the antidepressant can be gradually withdrawn.

All cases of delusional disorder should be observed for the possible emergence of mood symptoms during recovery and treatment should be immediately instituted. If suicidal symptoms appear, admission for inpatient observation and treatment is highly recommended.

Conclusions

Paranoia, now delusional disorder, is unique in psychiatry in that it is virtually a newly discovered illness and yet much of the fundamental descriptive work was done a century or more ago. This long hiatus means that most practitioners have scant knowledge or experience of the disorder, and the few who are aware of it usually only see a small part of the fabric. For example, there is the dermatologist who treats a case of delusional parasitosis, the cosmetic surgeon whose difficult patient has a dysmorphic delusion, the lawyer trying to cope with a totally unreasonable litigant, the police officer faced with a jealous murderer or an erotomanic stalker, or the personnel officer who has to deal with an employee who is convinced his fellow workers are persecuting him, and many more. How can we draw all this scattered material together so as to make a whole cloth? The answer at this stage is largely by consciousness raising and education.

Delusional disorder is not rare, but there is good reason to believe that the majority of its sufferers remain in society, still functional to varying degrees, and, even if impaired and suffering, rarely agreeing to be referred to a psychiatrist. Therefore psychiatry's experience of the illness is sketchy and biased, and because of the still-prevailing belief that the illness is untreatable there is little incentive for psychiatrists to seek out cases.

This is a disorder with a considerable impact on society. Somatically deluded patients grossly overuse health services in their demands for inappropriate help. Individuals with persecutory delusions can be very disruptive in their communities, and the law and law-enforcement agencies are involved at various levels with cases which may involve assault and even murder.

To bring order out of the present chaos clinicians must learn to recognize the illness by its characteristic form, using delusional content only afterwards to define the clinical subtypes. Earlier, Jaspers was quoted as saying that delusional disorder is highly recognizable, which is very true, but too many psychiatrists are still seduced by the readily noticeable delusional content and cannot adequately discern the illness underlying it. Not only clinical work on delusional disorder but also research is being held up by lack of clarity in diagnosis.

The delusional disorder which does not yet have official diagnostic status—the delusional misidentification syndrome—has been more clearly defined of late and is being better recognized and more productively researched as a result. It sufficiently resembles paranoia/delusional disorder that one may hope that adaptations of its research methodology could usefully be applied there. This would certainly be facilitated if future DSM and ICD editions included DMIS with delusional disorder in an enlarged category.

The concept of the paranoid spectrum has been discussed earlier in this chapter, and it has been suggested that a significant gap exists in this diagnostic continuum because paraphrenia is currently being ignored. Should paraphrenia be revived in the future it is essential that it not simply be equated with 'late' paraphrenia, a diagnosis that should probably be amalgamated with that of late-onset schizophrenia. Instead, paraphrenia, like delusional disorder, should be recognized as arising in all age groups from early adulthood onwards.

Anyone dealing with the delusional disorders must be aware of two very important associated phenomena, *folie à deux* and postpsychotic depression, and be able to deal competently with the problems that they pose.

Delusional disorder has much to commend it as a focus for research. It is a chronic and stable illness which may well be caused by a focal disturbance of brain function. Many of its sufferers are reluctant to take medication and so their brains are often unaffected by neuroleptics, which is unusual nowadays in a chronic psychotic illness that we wish to investigate. Those patients who do accept treatment often respond quite rapidly, enabling clear-cut studies to be undertaken on pre- and post-treatment states. Those who refuse are still fascinating because the encapsulation of the delusional system allows one to study abnormality and normality at virtually the same time in the same patient.

In this chapter we have attempted to draw together our extremely fragmented knowledge of the delusional disorders and to demonstrate that it is possible to diagnose and classify them with some assurance. Kendler, an authority in this field, has said, 'The paranoid disorders may be the third great group of functional psychoses, along with affective disorder and schizophrenia'.[108] If he is correct, it is clear that this is no trivial task and that the well being of large numbers of patients is dependent on the physician's becoming greatly more skilled and proficient in dealing with the illnesses that have been described.

Further reading

Bhugra, D. and Munro, A. (ed.). (1997). *Troublesome disguises: underdiagnosed psychiatric syndromes.* Blackwell Science, Oxford.

Cash, T.F. and Pruzinsky, T. (ed) (1990). *Body images: development, deviance and change.* Guilford Press, New York.

Garety, P.A. and Hemsley, D.R. (1994). *Delusions: investigations into the psychology of delusional reasoning.* Maudsley Monograph No. 36. Oxford University Press.

Manschrek, T.C. (ed.) (1992). Delusional disorders. *Psychiatric Annals*, **22**, 225–85.

Munro, A. (1999). *Delusional disorder.* Cambridge University Press.

Rix, K.J.B. and Snaith, R.P. (ed.) (1988). The psychopathology of body image. *British Journal of Psychiatry*, **153** (Supplement 2).

Sedler, M.J. (ed.) (1995). Delusional disorders. *Psychiatric Clinics of North America*, **18**, 199–425.

Sharma, V.P. (1991). *Insane jealousy.* Mind Publications, Cleveland, TN.

References

1. American Psychiatric Association (1994). *Diagnostic and statistical manual of mental disorders* (4th edn). American Psychiatric Association, Washington, DC.
2. World Health Organization (1992). *International statistical classification of diseases and related health problems, 10th revision.* WHO, Geneva.
3. American Psychiatric Association (1987). *Diagnostic and statistical manual of mental disorders* (revised 3rd edn). American Psychiatric Association, Washington, DC.
4. Retterstøl, N. (1966). *Paranoid and paranoiac psychoses.* Thomas, Springfield, IL.
5. Berner, P. (1965). *Das Paranoische Syndrom.* Springer, Berlin.
6. Capgras, J. and Reboul-Lachaux, J. (1923). L'illusion des 'sosies' dans un délire systématisé chronique. *Bulletin de la Societé Clinique de Médecine Mentale*, **2**, 6–16.
7. Munro, A. (1997). Paraphrenia. In *Troublesome disguises: underdiagnosed psychiatric syndromes* (ed. D. Bhugra and A. Munro), pp. 91–111. Blackwell Science, Oxford.
8. Fish, F.J. (1974). *Clinical psychopathology.* John Wright, Bristol.
9. Kraepelin, E. (1896). *Lehrbuch der Psychiatrie* (5th edn). Barth, Leipzig.
10. Bleuler, E. (1950). *Dementia praecox or the group of schizophrenias* (trans. J. Ainkia). International Universities Press, New York.
11. Kraepelin, E. (1909–1913). *Lehrbuch der Psychiatrie* (8th edn). Barth, Leipzig.
12. Mayer, W. (1921). Über paraphrene Psychosen. *Zentralblatt für die Gesamte Neurologie und Psychiatrie*, **71**, 187–206.
13. Kolle, K. (1931). *Die Primäre Verrücktheit.* Thieme, Leipzig.
14. Jaspers, K. (1963). *General psychopathology* (7th edn) (trans. J. Hoenig and M. Hamilton). Manchester University Press.
15. Kretschmer, E. (1927). *Der sensitiver Beziehungswahn* (2nd edn). Springer, Berlin.
16. Freud, S. (1958). Extracts from the Fleiss papers. In *Standard edition of the complete psychological works of Sigmund Freud*, Vol. 1 (ed. J. Strachey), pp. 173–280. Hogarth Press, London.
17. Freud, S. (1958). The case of Schreiber. In *Standard edition of the complete psychological works of Sigmund Freud*, Vol. 12 (ed. J. Strachey), pp. 9–82. Hogarth Press, London.
18. Garety, P.A. and Hemsley, D.R. (1994). *Delusions: investigations into the psychology of delusional reasoning.* Maudsley Monograph No. 36. Oxford University Press.
19. Maher, B. (1992). Delusions: contemporary etiological hypotheses. *Psychiatric Annals*, **22**, 260–8.
20. Winokur, G. (1977). Delusional disorder (paranoia). *Comprehensive Psychiatry*, **18**, 511–21.
21. Kendler, K.S. (1980). The nosologic validity of paranoia (simple delusional disorder). *Archives of General Psychiatry*, **37**, 699–706.
22. Munro, A. (1982). Paranoia revisited. *British Journal of Psychiatry*, **141**, 344–9.
23. Mullen, P. (1979). Phenomenology of disordered mental function. In *Essentials of postgraduate psychiatry* (ed. P. Hill, R. Murray, and G. Thorley), pp. 25–54. Academic Press, London.
24. Butler, R.W. and Braff, D.L. (1991). Delusions: a review and integration. *Schizophrenia Bulletin*, **17**, 633–47.
25. Flaum, M., Arndt, S., and Andreasen, N.C. (1991). The reliability of 'bizarre' delusions. *Comprehensive Psychiatry*, **32**, 59–65.
26. Farmer, A.E., McGuffin, P., and Gottesman, I.I. (1987). Searching for the split in schizophrenia: a twin study perspective. *Psychiatric Research*, **13**, 109–18.
27. Kendler, K.S. and Gruenberg, A.M. (1982). Genetic relationship between

paranoid personality disorder and the 'Schizophrenic Spectrum' disorders. *American Journal of Psychiatry*, **139**, 1185–7.

28. Kendler, K.S. (1987). Paranoid disorders in DSM III, a critical review. In *Diagnosis and classification in psychiatry* (ed. G.L. Tischler), pp. 57–83. Cambridge University Press.

29. Michael, A., Mirza, S., Mirza, K.A.H., Babu, V.S., and Vithayathil, E. (1995). Morbid jealousy in alcoholism. *British Journal of Psychiatry*, **167**, 668–72.

30. Feinstein, A. and Ron, M.A. (1990). Psychosis associated with demonstrable brain disease. *Psychological Medicine*, **20**, 793–803.

31. Almeida, O.P., Howard, R., Förstl, H., and Levy, R. (1992). Late paraphrenia: a review. *International Journal of Geriatric Psychiatry*, **7**, 543–8.

32. Flint, A.J., Rifat, S.L. and Eastwood, M.R. (1991). Late-onset paranoia: distinct from paraphrenia? *International Journal of Geriatric Psychiatry*, **6**, 103–9.

33. Connell, P.H. (1958). *Amphetamine psychosis*. Maudsley Monograph No. 5. Chapman & Hall, London.

34. Satel, S.L. and Edell, W.S. (1991). Cocaine-induced paranoia and psychosis-proneness. *American Journal of Psychiatry*, **148**, 1708–11.

35. Reilly, T.M. and Batchelor, D.H. (1991). Monosymptomatic hypochondriacal psychosis and AIDS (letter). *American Journal of Psychiatry*, **148**, 815.

36. Gorman, D.G. and Cummings, J.L. (1990). Organic delusional syndrome. *Seminars in Neurology*, **10**, 229–38.

37. Munro, A. (1998). *Delusional disorder*. Cambridge University Press.

38. Munro, A. (1988) Delusional (paranoid) disorders: etiologic and taxonomic considerations II: a possible relationship between delusional and affective disorders. *Canadian Journal of Psychiatry*, **33**, 175–8.

39. Ovesey, L. (1954). The homosexual conflict: an adaptational analysis. *Psychiatry*, **17**, 243–50.

40. Aronson, T.A. (1989). Paranoia and narcissism in psychoanalytic therapy. *Psychoanalytic Review*, **76**, 329–51.

41. Meissner, W.W. (1978). *The paranoid process*. Jason Aronson, New York.

42. Klein, M. (1957). Envy and gratitude. In *The writings of Melanie Klein*, Vol. 3, pp. 176–235. Hogarth Press, London.

43. Kohut, H. (1977). *The restoration of the self*. International Universities Press, New York.

44. Hesselbach, C.F. (1962). Superego regression in paranoia. *Psychoanalytic Quarterly*, **31**, 341–50.

45. Coen, S.J. (1987). Pathological jealousy. *International Journal of Psycho-Analysis*, **68**, 99–108.

46. Kennedy, H.G., Kemp, L.I., and Dyer, D.E. (1992). Fear and anger in delusional (paranoid) disorder: the association with violence. *British Journal of Psychiatry*, **160**, 488–92.

47. Ungvari, G.S. and Hollokoi, R.I.M. (1993). Successful treatment of litigious paranoia with pimozide. *Canadian Journal of Psychiatry*, **38**, 4–8.

48. Rowlands, M.W.D. (1988). Psychiatric and legal aspects of persistent litigation. *British Journal of Psychiatry*, **153**, 317–23.

49. Goldstein, R.L. (1987). Litigious paranoids and the legal system: the role of the forensic psychiatrist. *Journal of Forensic Sciences California*, **32**, 1009–15.

50. Freckelton, I. (1988). Querulent paranoia and the vexatious complainant. *International Journal of Law and Psychiatry*, **11**, 127–43.

51. Goldstein, R.L. (1995). Paranoids in the legal system: the litigious paranoid and the paranoid criminal. *Psychiatric Clinics of North America*, **18**, 303–15.

52. Reavis, D.J. (1995). *Ashes of Waco: an investigation*. Simon & Schuster, New York.

53. Weightman, J.M. (1984). *Making sense of the Jonestown suicides: a sociological history of the People's Temple*. Edwin Mellen Press, Lewiston, NY.

54. Cumming, W.J.K. (1988). The neurobiology of the body schema. *British Journal of Psychiatry*, **153** (Supplement 2), 7–11.

55. Pruzinsky, T. (1990). Psychopathology of body experience: expanded perspectives. In *Body images: development, deviance and change* (ed. T.F. Cash and T. Pruzinsky), pp. 170–89. Guilford Press, New York.

56. Lyell, A. (1983). Delusions of parasitosis. *Seminars in Dermatology*, **2**, 189–95.

57. Reilly, T.M. and Batchelor, D.H. (1986). The presentation and treatment of delusional parasitosis: a dermatological perspective. *International Clinical Psychopharmacology*, **1**, 340–53.

58. Van Moffaert, M. (1992). Psychodermatology: an overview. *Psychotherapy and Psychosomatics*, **58**, 125–36.

59. Koblenzer, C.S. and Bostrom, P. (1994). Chronic cutaneous dysesthesia syndrome: a psychotic phenomenon or a depressive symptom? *Journal of the American Academy of Dermatology*, **30**, 370–4.

60. Stein, D.J. and Hollander, E. (1992). Low-dose pimozide augmentation of serotonin reuptake blockers in the treatment of trichotillomania. *Journal of Clinical Psychiatry*, **53**, 123–6.

61. Anonymous (1983). The matchbox sign (leading article). *Lancet*, **ii**, 261.

62. Munro, A. and Stewart, M. (1991). Body dysmorphic disorder and the DSM-IV: the demise of dysmorphophobia. *Canadian Journal of Psychiatry*, **36**, 91–6.

63. Cash, T.F. and Pruzinsky, T. (ed.) (1990). *Body images: development, deviance and change*. Guilford Press, New York.

64. McElroy, S.L., Phillips, K.A., Keck, P.E., Hudson, J.I., and Pope, H.G. (1993). Body dysmorphic disorder: does it have a psychotic subtype? *Journal of Clinical Psychiatry*, **54**, 389–95.

65. Pryse-Phillips, W. (1971). An olfactory reference syndrome. *Acta Psychiatrica Scandinavica*, **47**, 484–509.

66. Malasi, T.H., El-Hilu, S.R., Mirza, I.A., and El-Islam, M.F. (1990). Olfactory delusional syndrome with various aetiologies. *British Journal of Psychiatry*, **156**, 256–60.

67. Iwu, C.O. and Akpata, O. (1989). Delusional halitosis: review of the literature and analysis of 32 cases. *British Dental Journal*, **167**, 294–6.

68. Marbach, J.J. (1985). Psychosocial factors for failure to adapt to dental prostheses. *Dental Clinics of North America*, **29**, 215–33.

69. Bhanji, S. and Mahony, J.D.H. (1978). The value of a psychiatric service within the venereal disease clinic. *British Journal of Venereal Disease*, **54**, 266–8.

70. Cobb, J. (1984). Morbid jealousy. In *Contemporary psychiatry* (ed. S. Crown), pp. 68–79. Butterworths, London.

71. Crowe, R.R., Clarkson, C., Tsai, M., and Wilson, R. (1988). Delusional disorder: jealous and nonjealous types. *European Archives of Psychiatric and Neurological Science*, **237**, 179–83.

72. Mullen, P.E. and Martin, J. (1994). Jealousy: a community study. *British Journal of Psychiatry*, **164**, 35–43.

73. Mowat, R.R. (1966). *Morbid jealousy and murder*. Tavistock Publications, London.

74. Fishbain, D.B. (1986). Suicide pacts and homicide. *American Journal of Psychiatry*, **143**, 1319–20.

75. Vauhkonen, K. (1968). On the pathogenesis of morbid jealousy. *Acta Psychiatrica Scandinavica*, **46** (Supplement 202), 1–62.

76. De Clérambault, C.G. (1942). *Les psychoses passionnelles*. Oeuvre Psychiatrique. Presses Universitaires, Paris.

77. Gillett, T., Eminson, S.R., and Hassanyeh, F. (1990). Primary and secondary erotomania: clinical characteristics and follow-up. *Acta Psychiatrica Scandinavica*, **82**, 65–9.

78. Segal, J.H. (1989). Erotomania revisited: from Kraepelin to DSM-IIIR. *American Journal of Psychiatry*, **146**, 1261–6.

79. Taylor, P., Mahendra, B., and Gunn, J. (1983). Erotomania in males. *Psychological Medicine*, **13**, 645–50.

80. Goldstein, R.L. (1987). More forensic romances: de Clérambault's syndrome in men. *Bulletin of the American Academy of Psychiatry and the Law*, **15**, 267–74.

81. Raschka, L.B. (1979). The incubus syndrome, a variant of erotomania. *Canadian Journal of Psychiatry*, **24**, 549–53.

82. Zona, M.A., Sharma, K.K., and Lane, J. (1993). A comparative study of erotomanic and obsessional subjects in a forensic sample. *Journal of Forensic Sciences California*, **38**, 894–903.

83. Pathé, M. and Mullen, P.E. (1997). The impact of stalkers on their victims. *British Journal of Psychiatry*, **170**, 12–17.

84. Swanson, D.W., Bohnert, P.J., and Smith, J.A. (1970). *The paranoid*. Little, Brown, Boston, MA.

85. Ellis, H.D. and Young, A.W. (1990). Accounting for delusional misidentifications. *British Journal of Psychiatry*, **157**, 239–48.

86. Debruille, J.B. and Stip, E. (1996). Syndrome de Capgras: évolution des hypothèses. *Canadian Journal of Psychiatry*, **41**, 181–7.

87. Weinstein, E.A. (1994). The classification of delusional misidentification syndromes. *Psychopathology*, **27**, 130–5.

88. Christodoulou, G.N. (1991). The delusional misidentification syndromes. *British Journal of Psychiatry*, **159** (Supplement 14), 65–9.

89. Berson, R.J. (1983). Capgras' syndrome. *American Journal of Psychiatry*, **140**, 969–78.

90. Cummings, J.L. (1985). Organic delusions: phenomenology, anatomical correlations, and review. *British Journal of Psychiatry*, **142**, 184–97.

91. Förstl, H., Burns, A., Jacoby, R., and Levy, R. (1991). Neuroanatomical correlates of clinical misidentification and misperception in the senile dementia of the Alzheimer type. *Journal of Clinical Psychiatry*, **52**, 268–271.

92. McAllister, T.W. (1992). Neuropsychiatric aspects of delusions. *Psychiatric Annals*, **22**, 269–77.

93. Silva, J.A., Leong, G.B., Weinstock, R., Sharma, K.K., and Klein, R.L. (1994). Delusional misidentification syndromes and dangerousness. *Psychopathology*, **27**, 215–19.

94. Munro, A. (1991). A plea for paraphrenia. *Canadian Journal of Psychiatry*, **36**, 667–72.

95. Naguib, M. (1991). Paraphrenia revisited. *British Journal of Hospital Medicine*, **46**, 371–5.

96. Ravindran, A.V., Yatham, L.N., and Munro, A. (1999). Paraphrenia redefined. *Canadian Journal of Psychiatry*, **44**, 133–7.

97. Gralnick, A. (1942). *Folie à deux*: a psychosis of association. A review of 103 cases and the entire English literature. *Psychiatric Quarterly*, **16**, 230–63.

98. Munro, A. (1986). *Folie à deux* revisited. *Canadian Journal of Psychiatry*, **31**, 233–4.

99. Silveira, J.M. and Seeman, M.V. (1995). Shared psychotic disorder: a critical review of the literature. *Canadian Journal of Psychiatry*, **40**, 389–95.

100. Cameron, N. (1959). The paranoid pseudocommunity revisited. *American Journal of Sociology*, **65**, 57–61.

101. Myers, P.L. (1988). Paranoid pseudocommunity beliefs in a sect milieu. *Social Psychiatry and Psychiatric Epidemiology*, **23**, 252–5.

102. Opler, L.A., Klahr, D.M., and Ramirez, P.M. (1995). Pharmacologic treatment of delusions. *Psychiatric Clinics of North America*, **18**, 379–91.

103. Kingdon, D., Turkington, D., and John, C. (1994). Cognitive behaviour therapy of schizophrenia. *British Journal of Psychiatry*, **164**, 581–7.

104. Munro, A. and Mok, H. (1995). An overview of treatment in paranoia/delusional disorder. *Canadian Journal of Psychiatry*, **40**, 616–22.

105. Opler, L.A. and Feinberg, S.S. (1991). The role of pimozide in clinical psychiatry: a review. *Journal of Clinical Psychiatry*, **52**, 221–33.

106. Mayer-Gross, W. (1920). Über die Stellungsnahme auf abgelanfench akuten Psychosen. *Zeitschrift für die Gesamte Neurologie und Psychiatrie*, **60**, 160–212.

107. Mandel, M.R., Severe, J.B., Schooler, N.R., Gelenberg, A.J., and Mieske, M. (1982). Development and prediction of postpsychotic depression in neuroleptic-treated schizophrenics. *Archives of General Psychiatry*, **39**, 197–203.

108. Kendler, K.S. (1982). Demography of paranoid psychosis (delusional disorder): a review and comparison with schizophrenia and affective illness. *Archives of General Psychiatry*, **39**, 890–902.

4.5 Mood disorders

4.5.1 An introduction to and historical review of mood disorders

Frederick K. Goodwin and S. Nassir Ghaemi

Background

Mood disorders magnify human experiences to larger-than-life proportions. Among their symptoms are exaggerations of normal sadness and fatigue, joy and exuberance, sensuality and sexuality, irritability and rage, energy and creativity. In their diverse forms, mood disorders afflict a large number of people—the exact number depending on how the illnesses are defined and how accurately they are ascertained. First described thousands of years ago, found in widely diverse cultures, manic–depressive illness is the prototypic mood disorder. To those afflicted, it can be so painful that suicide seems the only means of escape; one of every five untreated manic–depressive individuals actually commits suicide.[1]

In this chapter, we draw on and expand our previous descriptions of depression and manic–depressive illness.

Depressive and manic states

What are depression and mania? Ideally, one would first describe 'normal' or average mood. While this can be difficult, an operational definition might be that 'normal' or average mood is the state of not feeling particularly euphoric or sad, except under the right circumstances. For example, if something good happens, one would feel happy for a while, and if something bad were to happen, one would feel sad or down for a while. Most people can relate to this definition. Superficially, depression and hypomania can be viewed as extremes of these normal fluctuations in mood. But clinical depression (or mania) are more than extremes of normal mood. They represent syndromes in which, in addition to mood, there are disturbances in thought, psychomotor state, behaviour, motivation, physiology, and psychosocial function.

Depressive states are sometimes easier to comprehend owing to similarities with non-pathological depression and mourning. Mood is bleak, pessimistic, and despairing. A deep sense of futility is often accompanied, if not preceded, by the belief that the ability to experience pleasures is permanently gone. There is a slowing or decrease in almost all aspects of emotion and behaviour: rate of thought and speech, energy, sexuality, and the ability to experience pleasure. Basic physical 'neurovegetative' activities are affected, such as eating, sleeping, and grooming. Severity varies widely, ranging from mild physical and mental slowing to severe psychosis, with self-denigrating, profoundly negative delusions and hallucinations.

At the outset, manic states often start as hypomania, characterized typically by heightened mood, more and faster speech, quicker thought, brisker physical and mental activity levels, more energy with a corresponding decreased need for sleep, irritability, perceptual acuity, paranoia, heightened sexuality, and impulsivity. As it evolves, it can often progress to frank psychosis with prominent paranoia, grandiose delusions, and even a confused state of delirium, a profoundly disruptive state that generally leads to hospitalization. At the level of hypomania, these changes are generally moderate and tend not to result in serious problems for the person experiencing them. For roughly half of all bipolar patients, the 'high' does not progress beyond hypomania. It is notable that mania can occur without any euphoric mood at all, and simply display an irritable and/or dysphoric quality. In fact, a very common presentation of mania is a 'mixed' episode, where depressive mood predominates. These mixed states can be difficult to distinguish from pure agitated depression. Manic and depressive states underlie the nosology of mood disorders.

History of mood disorders

Graeco-Roman origins: the clinical–empirical tradition

The Hippocratic school performed an essential first service for scientific psychiatry: it argued that these were illnesses of the body, not of supernatural or magical spirits (see Goodwin and Jamison[1] and Alexander and Selesnick[2] for most of the review of ancient and medieval sources discussed below). The Hippocratics described melancholia as a condition 'associated with "aversion to food, despondency, sleeplessness, irritability, restlessness" ',[3] and mania, as a state of high energy and euphoria.

Hippocrates also placed the aetiology of mood disorders in the brain:

> Men ought to know that from the brain and from the brain only arrives our pleasures, joys, laughter and jests, as well as our sorrows, pains, griefs and tears…wherefore, I assert, the brain is the interpreter of consciousness.

This Hippocratic insight was buried for two millennia under the humoral theory, solidified in medicine by Galen (second century AD), which held that melancholia resulted from excessive black bile, and mania from excessive yellow bile. The heart, rather than the brain, also was long thought to be the organ of mood disorders.

In the first century BC, Greek physicians first suggested a connection between melancholia and mania. Regarding treatment, some, like Soranus and Asclepiades, explicitly advocated humane treatment of the mentally ill, while others, like Celsus, 'believed that right treatment would frighten the patient out of mental illness'. Asclepiades famously pledged: 'Curare tuto, celeriter, et jucunde': the cure should be safe, quick, and pleasant. Thus, 'he prescribed bathing, exercise, massages and wine'.[2]

The clinical acumen of that era peaked with Aretaeus of Cappadocia:[4]

> According to Aretaeus, the classical form of mania was the bipolar one: the patient who previously was gay, euphoric, and hyperactive suddenly 'has a tendency to melancholy; he becomes, at the end of the attack, languid, sad, taciturn, he complaints that he is worried about his future, he feels ashamed'. When the depressive phase is over, such patients go back to being gay, they laugh, they joke, they sing, 'they show off in public with crowned heads as if they were returning victorious from the games; sometimes they laugh and dance all day and all night'. In serious forms of mania, called furor, the patient 'sometimes kills and slaughters the servants'; in less severe forms, he often exalts himself: 'without being cultivated he says he is a philosopher…and the incompetent (say they are) good artisans…others yet are suspicious and they feel that they are being persecuted, for which reasons they are irascible.

The Middle Ages

The Greek clinical–empirical tradition survived in the early Middle Ages among Arab Muslims and European Christians, although it later succumbed to religious intolerance. In Europe, monk-physicians, like Cassiodorus (490–585), upheld humane treatment and emphasized the Hippocratic empirical tradition. By the twelfth century, that tradition had given way to a more theological–non-empirical bent. Thus, Roger Bacon, arguing that empirical observation was required for knowledge and that mental illnesses had natural aetiologies, suffered the censure of the church and the condemnation of his colleagues at Oxford University. From the fourteenth century onwards, the Inquisition silenced empiricism as heresy, by intimidating or even killing its advocates.

A similar tension played out in the Middle East. The Hippocratic tradition was exemplified by Rhazes (AD 865–925), a Persian equivalent of Roger Bacon. Adamantly believing that observation was the best guarantor of truth, he ran afoul of the theological status quo, was denounced, and ended his life in penury. Avicenna (AD 980–1037) took a more diplomatic approach and prospered as a moderate synthesizer of Greek, Roman, and religious traditions. His medical synthesis, the Canon of Medicine, engendered near-Galenic respect for centuries, transmitting the view regarding mood disorders that 'undoubtedly the material which is the effective producer of mania is of the same nature as that which produces melancholia'.

The early Islamic tradition, like its Christian counterpart, was humane in its treatment of the mentally ill. The first asylums for the mentally ill, for instance, were built in the eighth century in Fez, Morocco, and in Baghdad. Others were soon added in Cairo and Damascus. As the Baghdad Caliphate became more dogmatic and antirationalistic, the Hippocratic tradition in medicine found refuge in the rival Andalucian Caliphate of Spain, where European and Islamic cultures mixed with fecundity. The first European hospital exclusively organized for the mentally ill was inaugurated in 1409 in the Spanish city of Valencia (for a review of this period, see Alexander and Selesnick[2]).

Beginning in the sixteenth and seventeenth centuries, the Enlightenment gave impetus to medical progress in Europe. The eighteenth century witnessed a flowering of the revival of the clinical–empirical tradition in medicine, with advanced descriptions of mania and melancholia, such as the following by Richard Mead (1751) (quoted by Jackson[3]):

> Medical writers distinguish two kinds of Madness, and describe them both as a constant disorder of the mind without any considerable fever; but with this difference, that the one is attended with audaciousness and fury, the other with sadness and fear: and that they call mania, this melancholy. But these generally differ in degree only. For melancholy very frequently changes, sooner or later, into maniacal madness; and, when the fury is abated, the sadness generally returns heavier than before.

Eighteenth-century medical descriptions were disconnected from one another, however, and many were accompanied by hastily erected classification systems and aetiological speculations.

The nineteenth century turning point: French clinical psychiatry

In 1854, Jean Falret[5] described a circular disorder (la folie circulaire), which for the first time expressly defined an illness in which 'this succession of mania and melancholia manifests itself with continuity and in a manner almost regular'. The same year, Baillarger[6] described essentially the same thing (la folie double forme), emphasizing that the manic and depressive episodes were not different attacks but rather different stages of the same attack. For the first time, manic–depressive illness was conceived as a single disease, clearly anticipating Kraepelin's later synthesis (see Goodwin and Jamison[1]).

Although mild cases of mania had been described by Falret, Esquirol, and other observers, Mendel[7] was the first to define hypomania, a 'form of mania which typically shows itself only in the mild stages, abortively, so to speak.' Around the same time, Kahlbaum[8] described circular disorders (cyclothymia) which were characterized by episodes of both depression and excitement but which did not end in dementia, as chronic mania or melancholia could. Despite these contributions, most clinical investigators continued to regard mania and melancholia as separate entities, chronic in nature, which follow a deteriorating course.

The turn of the twentieth century and the Kraepelinian synthesis

It was left to Emil Kraepelin[9] to segregate psychotic illnesses from each other and clearly draw a perimeter around manic–depressive illness.

As is well known, Kraepelin emphasized those aspects of manic–depressive illness that separated it most clearly from dementia praecox: the periodic or episodic course, the more benign prognosis, and a family history of manic–depressive illness.

Kraepelin's nosology was the first disease model in psychiatry to be backed by extensive and carefully organized observations and descriptions. It did not exclude psychological and social factors, and, in fact, Kraepelin was one of the first to point out that psychological stresses could precipitate individual episodes. By adding 'slight colourings of mood' which 'pass over without sharp boundary into the domain of personal predisposition', Kraepelin also anticipated the later development of spectrum concepts.

While later investigations explored the boundaries between manic–depressive illness and dementia praecox, Kraepelin's revolutionary contribution was unrivalled in the history of affective disorders since Hippocrates. Kraepelin's synthesis is important not because it draws the ultimately 'correct' picture of nature, but rather because it builds a solid and empirically anchored base for future knowledge. This was his major accomplishment.

Unfortunately, Kraepelin and his colleagues did not possess many effective medical treatments for the two conditions they so painstakingly identified. Drug treatments for manic–depressive illness were not available, and the cure of psychosis seemed almost impossible. When Julius von Wagner-Jaurregg, the chief of psychiatry at the University of Vienna, appeared to cure a psychotic patient with malarial blood injections, it was such a feat that he won the Nobel prize. It turned out that Wagner-Jaurregg's patients suffered from neurosyphilis, and his malarial treatment worked by producing intermittent fevers and a decline in the patients' spirochete counts. Penicillin obviously later proved to be a more specific cure. No other psychiatrist has ever won a Nobel prize.[10]

Given these therapeutic difficulties, the Kraepelinian school was criticized for being practically unhelpful. Patients could spontaneously recover from manic–depressive episodes, but there were no treatments available. Dementia praecox, with its deteriorating course was an even greater stimulus to therapeutic nihilism. As Karl Jaspers put it, 'we were therapeutically hopeless but kind'.[11] The psychoanalytic followers of Freud roundly criticized the Kraepelinians on this score. But history returned Kraepelin to favour, at least for now, as the psychopharmacology revolution demonstrated the therapeutic utility of the traditional nosology.

Freud and the psychoanalytic view of mood disorders

For most of the twentieth century, however, the psychoanalytic 'climate of opinion' prevailed. Freud's classic work on mood disorders, 'Mourning and melancholia',[12] set the tone. It argues that melancholia is essentially analogous to the depressive feelings of normal experiences, like bereavement. To Freud, the depressive process in mourning arises from the tension between ambivalent feelings toward the dead parent, like love and aggression. Melancholia was conceived to involve similar ambivalent feelings. Freud's basic insight into the connection between mourning and melancholia was expanded by later psychoanalysts into the general theory that depression is related to feelings of hostility towards another person, often one's parents. These unacceptably hostile feelings turned inwards toward oneself, rather than outwards toward others, leading to depression.

Karl Jaspers' *General Psychopathology*: the phenomenological tradition

Contemporaneously with Kraepelin and Freud, Karl Jaspers wrote *General Psychopathology*,[13] which emphasized the importance of unbiased extensive clinical description of psychopathological states. Jaspers argued that such clinical data needed to be gathered neutrally, free of underlying theories, like Freud's, and free of specific diagnostic paradigms, like Kraepelin's. Jaspers' influence led to more careful description of mood syndromes, as exemplified in the highly influential textbook *Fish's Clinical Psychopathology*,[14] and Max Hamilton's Depression Rating Scale, still in common use today. Jaspers' theoretical work still continues to provide important insights into the conceptual bases of psychiatry.

Mid-twentieth century: Adolf Meyer and the evolution of American psychiatry

During the first half of the twentieth century, the views of Adolf Meyer[15] gradually assumed a dominant position in American psychiatry. Meyer believed that psychopathology emerged from interactions between an individual's biological and psychological characteristics and his or her social environment. While allowing for biological and genetic factors, the Meyerians understood them as part of an individual's vulnerability to specific psychological and social influences. This perspective was symbolized by the rubric 'manic–depressive reaction' in the first official American Psychiatric Association diagnostic manual published in 1952 (DSM-I). Meyer's approach differs from the standard disease model, in which clinical phenomena in a given patient are understood (and, therefore, potentially predictable) in terms of a given disease with a specific natural history and pathophysiology. When the Meyerian focus, considerably influenced by psychoanalysis, turned to manic–depressive illness, the individual and his or her environment became the focus, at the expense of clinical descriptions of symptoms and the longitudinal course of the illness.

Mid-twentieth-century European developments: Bleuler's influence

In Europe, the psychosocial and psychoanalytic traditions continued to develop in relative isolation from the mainstream of psychiatry, which largely retained its medical or disease orientation.

Among the academic psychiatrists, Eugen Bleuler[16] departed from Kraepelin by conceptualizing the relationship between manic–depressive (affective) illness and dementia praecox (schizophrenia) as a continuum without a sharp line of demarcation. Patients were distributed all along this spectrum, and an individual patient could be at different points on the spectrum at different times. Bleuler believed that a patient's location on the spectrum depended on the number of schizophrenic features he or she demonstrated. In that sense, Bleuler considered mood symptoms to be non-specific.

In 1933, Kasanin[17] identified a case series of patients who demonstrated the manic–depressive syndrome, but also displayed psychotic symptoms outside of mood episodes. These conditions seemed to lie outside of Kraepelin's dichotomy, and led to the concept of schizoaffective disorder. Some clinicians continue to see these observations as major challenges to the entire Kraepelinian nosology.[18,19]

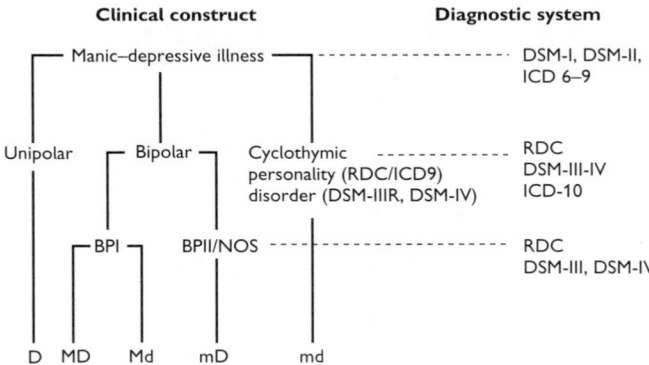

Fig. 1 The evolution of the bipolar–unipolar distinction from manic–depressive illness. D, major depression; d, subthreshold depression; M, mania; m, hypomania. (Adapted from Goodwin and Jamison.[1])

The bipolar–unipolar distinction

In 1957, Karl Leonhard[20] observed that, within the broad category of manic–depressive illness, some patients had histories of both depression and mania, whereas others had depressions only. He then noted that patients with a history of mania (whom he termed bipolar) had a higher incidence of mania in their families when compared with those with depressions only (whom he termed monopolar). In 1966, Jules Angst[21] and Carl Perris[22] independently provided systematic family history data to support Leonhard's distinction, a distinction validated by an independent criterion—family history. Later genetic studies of this distinction proved less consistent with Leonhard's model, suggesting that bipolar and unipolar disorders may lie along a spectrum, with bipolar illness being more severe. Figure 1 displays the evolution of the bipolar–unipolar distinction from Kraepelin's original conceptualization of manic–depressive illness.

The psychopharmacology revolution and the neo-Kraepelinian restoration

After Freud, the object relations theory school made important psychoanalytic contributions to understanding mood disorders. Donald Winnicott,[23] for instance, described the 'depressive position' in infant development, when the infant is helpless and unable to master his or her surroundings. The infant, Winnicott taught, responds to the mother's inability to provide everything for him or her with a necessary phase of depressive mood and activity. Winnicott felt that some adult psychopathology related to a reversion to or inability to conquer that depressive phase of development. Unfortunately, some clinicians translated this hypothesis into the belief that all individuals, pathologically depressed or not, have a tendency to depressive symptoms, and thus depression was conceptualized as a broad spectrum of pathology that existed in everyone.

Unlike the tradition of Kraepelin, where individual psychiatric illnesses were conceived as categorically different based on distinct pathophysiological processes, the Freudian focus was on a psychodynamic theory of instinctual drives and defence mechanisms. This theory, while perhaps useful in certain neuroses, retarded the development of an empirical descriptive basis for psychological categories. Further, when psychodynamic theories were extended to psychoses, the diagnostic distinctions among disorders became even more confused. The

all-encompassing nature of Freudian theory also seemed to lead to impractical conclusions. Everyone, whether ill or not, would seem to benefit from psychoanalysis, and there seemed to be no predetermined limit to how much time and expense was spent in the process. At the other extreme, even the most psychotic patients were felt by some to be treatable by psychoanalysis, and schizophrenia was considered to arise from severe psychosocial childhood trauma. These hypotheses, too long accepted as dogma, have been contradicted by empirical studies.

This ideology, especially when undisciplined, allowed an unbridled optimism: anything, from worried wellness to the most severe schizophrenia, was liable to cure. Freud himself may be exonerated ('*Moi, je ne suis pas Freudiste*', he once said, dissociating himself from some of his more extreme disciples); he directly disavowed the utility of psychoanalysis for schizophrenia and never discussed its use in any systematic manner in manic–depressive illness. But some of his intellectual descendants, like Harry Stack Sullivan,[24] vigorously argued otherwise, perhaps a reflection of American pragmatism and 'can-do' optimism. Unfortunately, this optimism was as uncritically accepted as Kraepelinian nihilism had been.

Contemporary neo-Kraepelinian nosology: DSM-III and DSM-IV

The current nosology, codified in DSM-III in 1980, is neo-Kraepelinian. The empirical evidence for it is based on classical validity studies, deriving from the pioneering work of Robins and Guze,[25] who laid out a groundwork for establishing the validity of a psychiatric diagnosis based on the four criteria of clinical phenomenology, genetics, course, and treatment response. This group of thinkers, centred at the Washington University in St Louis in the 1970s, swam against the tide of psychoanalytic orthodoxy, empirically tested competing nosologies, and developed diagnostic criteria which became the basis for the first empirically based psychiatric nosology. While some studies have failed to find evidence in support of DSM-III's nosology, most of the empirical evidence continues to support the basic structure of the neo-Kraepelinian nosology.[26–28]

Introduction to mood disorders

Given this historical background, we can briefly summarize current views regarding mood disorders.

Diagnostic subtypes of mood disorders in DSM-IV

1. **Major depressive (unipolar) disorder** is characterized by depressive episodes without any hypomanic or manic states: the patient is either depressed or average in mood, but experiences no mania.

2. **Bipolar disorder** is characterized by manic or hypomanic states: the patient is either depressed, euthymic (normal in mood), or hypomanic/manic. Bipolar disorder differs from unipolar disorder by including manic states. No matter how many times a patient is depressed, only one manic/hypomanic episode is required to diagnose bipolar rather than unipolar disorder. Bipolar disorder is further characterized as type I or type II. Type I is diagnosed when at least one manic episode is identified. Usually recurrent depression also occurs, but in 5 to 10 per cent of cases there are no diagnosable major depressive episodes,

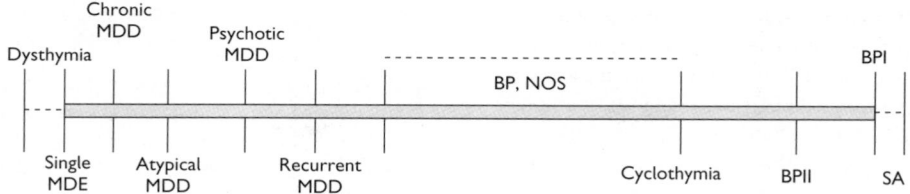

Fig. 2 The affective spectrum: MDD, major depressive disorder; MDE, major depressive episode; BP, NOS, bipolar disorder, not otherwise specified (this could include mania or hypomania only on antidepressants, recurrent MDD with underlying hyperthermia, or recurrent MDD with a first-degree relative with bipolar disorder); SA, schizoaffective disorder, bipolar type, which can be seen as a more severe version of manic–depressive illness.

although almost always there will be minor depressive episodes. Bipolar disorder type II requires the absence of even one manic episode, and instead the occurrence of at least one hypomanic episode and at least one major depressive episode. The critical difference between mania and hypomania, in current DSM-IV nosology, is that mania requires significant social and occupational dysfunction, while in hypomania significant social and occupational dysfunction needs to be excluded. Durational criteria are less strict for hypomania (a minimum of 4 days) than for mania (a minimum of 1 week).

3. **Dysthymia** refers to clinically significant major depressive symptoms that are present for 2 years or more but do not reach the threshold (with respect to severity and/or number of symptoms) for major depression. **Cyclothymia** is a condition in which, like dysthymia, depressive symptoms do not reach the threshold for diagnosis of a major depressive episode, and hypomania is present. Cyclothymia and dysthymia may represent a predisposition to major mood disorders. Lastly, whereas cyclothymia and dysthymia involve some depressive states, 'hyperthymia' is sometimes used to describe chronic mild hypomania (decreased need for sleep, expansive behaviour, marked extroversion, 'the life and soul of the party'). Patients with dysthymia, cyclothymia, or hyperthymia may develop unipolar or bipolar disorder under certain circumstances, such as with antidepressant use (see below).

The affective spectrum

The variations of mood disorders can be conceived along one broad spectrum of affective illness (Fig. 2), with bipolar disorder type I and a single major depressive episode at the extremes. Type II bipolar disorder and cyclothymia display less severe manic symptoms. The area between cyclothymia and recurrent unipolar depression is controversial, corresponding to the DSM-IV diagnosis of 'bipolar disorder, not otherwise specified'. We would suggest that it should include mid-spectrum cases; these might include those who only experience hypomanic or manic episodes with antidepressant medications but not spontaneously, and those with recurrent unipolar major depressive episodes and a first-degree relative with type I bipolar disorder. Some would add those with hyperthymic personality at baseline (i.e. when not depressed) who also experience recurrent unipolar major depressive episodes. Recurrent, psychotic, and atypical unipolar depression may also be closer to the bipolar end of the spectrum, with similarities in underlying pathophysiology and treatment response. At the extreme of the bipolar end of the spectrum, schizoaffective disorder, bipolar

type might be viewed as a more severe psychotic form of bipolar illness (for a review of the data underlying these views, see Goodwin and Jamison[1]).

Moving from 'depression' to diagnosis

A common misperception among some clinicians and patients is to think of 'depression' as being equivalent to unipolar depression, which is then treated with antidepressants. There are a number of reasons for this phenomenon: the first is that patients often lack insight into their manic symptoms; not knowing that they are ill, they deny their manic symptoms to clinicians. Second, depressive symptoms tend to last longer than manic symptoms, sometimes are more frequent, and often are more psychically painful; thus, patients tend to seek assistance when depressed rather than when manic. Third, the many new antidepressants that have become available over the past 10 years have been extensively marketed to physicians at the same time that 'depression awareness' programmes have educated the public about the availability of safe and effective treatments. Simultaneously, few new treatments for bipolar disorder have become available, and there has been scant professional and public education about bipolar illness. For example, the mainstay of bipolar treatment, lithium, is an inexpensive generic drug with minimal funds available for its promotion or for educational efforts.

As with the differential diagnostic process in any medical disease, the diagnosis of mood disorders should start with those disorders that must be ruled out first to those that remain afterwards (Fig. 3). We believe that this process should begin by ruling out depression which is clearly due to another medical or psychiatric disorder, or substance abuse. Such 'secondary depressions' usually involve a single major episode occurring in the absence of prior depressive symptoms or family history, and at a later age of onset than is typical for primary depression. The second rule-out diagnosis is bipolar disorder: first, bipolar I,

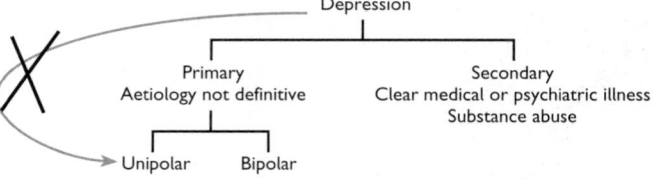

Differential diagnosis of depression

Fig. 3 The differential diagnosis of mood disorders: moving from 'depression' to diagnosis. The order in which diagnoses need to be excluded is as follows: (1) secondary depression; (2) bipolar depression; (3) unipolar depression. Thus, unipolar depression is a diagnosis of exclusion.

then bipolar II, and next bipolar 'not otherwise specified' should be sequentially ruled out before unipolar depression can be diagnosed. Unfortunately, many clinicians and patients jump from the recognition of a major depressive syndrome directly to a diagnosis of unipolar depression without the critical intermediate process of ruling out bipolar conditions. The relevance of this process lies in the underappreciated fact that antidepressants can worsen bipolar illness, either by causing acute mania or by acting as mood destabilizers, counteracting the effects of mood stabilizers, and leading to a long-term rapid-cycling course of illness.[29]

Conclusions

Mood disorders are composed of depressive and manic states that can be conceptualized as unipolar or bipolar conditions and/or along an affective spectrum. Clinical experience with mania and melancholia date to the Hippocratic school, were preserved and connected to humane treatment of the mentally ill in the Middle Ages and Enlightenment, and were systematized in the nineteenth century, culminating in the Kraepelinian nosology. After a de-emphasis of the medical disease model during the psychoanalytic period of influence in the mid-twentieth century, the current nosology has returned to a neo-Kraepelinian structure that is better supported by empirical research. Meanwhile, this nosology has proven useful in targeting new medications produced in the ongoing psychopharmacology revolution.

References

1. Goodwin, F.K. and Jamison, K.R. (1990). *Manic depressive illness.* Oxford University Press, New York.
2. Alexander, F. and Selesnick, S.T. (1966). *The history of psychiatry.* Harper and Row, New York.
3. Jackson, S. (1986). *Melancholia and depression: from Hippocratic times to modern times.* Yale University Press, New Haven, CT.
4. Roccatagliata, G.A (1986). *History of ancient psychiatry.* Greenwood Press, New York.
5. Falret, J. (1854). Memoire sur la folie circulaire. *Bulletin de la Academie Imperiale de Medicin (Paris),* **19**, 382–400.
6. Baillarger, J. (1854). Note sur un genre de folie. *Bulletin de la Academie Imperiale de Medicin (Paris),* **19**, 340–52.
7. Mendel, E. (1881). *Die Manie.* Urban and Schwazenberg, Vienna.
8. Kahlbaum, K. (1882). Uber cyclishes Irresein. *Der Irrenfreund,* **10**, 145–57.
9. Kraepelin, E. (1919). *Manic–depressive insanity and paranoia* (trans. R.M. Barclay). Livingstone, Edinburgh.
10. Valenstein, E.S. (1986). *Great and desperate cures: the rise and decline of psychosurgery and other radical treatments for mental illness.* Basic Books, New York.
11. Jaspers, K. (1986). An autobiographical account. In *Karl Jaspers: basic philosophical writings* (ed. E. Ehrlich, L. Ehrlich, and G. Pepper), pp. 4–8. Humanities Press, Atlantic Highlands, NJ.
12. Freud, S. (1957). Mourning and melancholia. In *Standard edition of the complete psychological works of Sigmund Freud,* Vol. 14 (ed. J. Strachey), pp. 243–58. Hogarth Press, London, 1957.
13. Jaspers, K. (1911). *General psychopathology.* Reprinted by Johns Hopkins University Press, Baltimore, MD, 1998.
14. Hamilton, M. (1974). *Fish's clinical psychopathology.* John Wright, Bristol.
15. Lief, A. (1948). *The commonsense psychiatry of Dr. Adolf Meyer.* McGraw-Hill, New York.
16. Bleuler, E. (1934). *Textbook of psychiatry.* Macmillan, New York.
17. Kasanin, J. (1933). The acute schizoaffective psychoses. *American Journal of Psychiatry,* **116**, 97–126.
18. Crow, T.J. (1986). The continuum of psychosis and its implication for the structure of the gene. *British Journal of Psychiatry,* **149**, 419–29.
19. Kendell, R.E. and Brockington, I.F. (1980). The identification of disease entities and the relationship between schizophrenic and affective psychoses. *British Journal of Psychiatry,* **137**, 324–31.
20. Leonhard, K. and von Trostorff, S. (1964). *Prognostic diagnosis of the endogenous psychoses.* Fischer, Jena.
21. Angst, J. (1966). *Zur Ätiologie und Nosologie endogener depressiver Psychosen.* Springer, Berlin.
22. Perris, C. (1966). A study of bipolar (manic–depressive) and unipolar recurrent depressive psychoses. *Acta Psychiatrica Scandinavica,* **42** (Supplement 194), 15–152.
23. Winnicott, D.W. (1954). *The depressive position in normal emotional development. Through paediatrics to psycho-analysis.* Reprinted by Hogarth Press, London, 1975.
24. Sullivan, H.S. (1954). *The psychiatric interview.* Norton, New York.
25. Robins, E. and Guze, S.B. (1970). Establishment of diagnostic validity in psychiatric illness: its application to schizophrenia. *American Journal of Psychiatry,* **126**, 983–7.
26. Tsuang, M.T., Woolson, R.F., and Fleming, J.A. (1979). Long-term outcome of major psychoses. *Archives of General Psychiatry,* **39**, 1295–301.
27. Kendler, K.S. (1990). Toward a scientific psychiatric nosology. *Archives of General Psychiatry,* **47**, 969–73.
28. Kendler, K.S., Karkowski, L.M., and Walsh, D. (1998). The structure of psychosis. *Archives of General Psychiatry,* **55**, 492–9.
29. Wehr, T.A. and Goodwin, F.K. (1987). Can antidepressants cause mania and worsen the course of affective illness? *American Journal of Psychiatry,* **144**, 1403–11.

4.5.2 Clinical features of mood disorders and mania

Per Bech

Introduction

In both DSM-IV[1] and ICD-10[2] the term 'affective' has been replaced by the term 'mood' to emphasize the duration of the episodes of clinical depression or mania. 'Affective' often refers to emotional states of briefer duration than 'mood' or to milder degrees of symptoms. The duration of depressive mood varies widely from less than 1 month to about 2 years.[3]

Figure 1 shows the spectrum of depression and mania according to both DSM-IV and ICD-10. The diagnosis of the acute forms focuses on the severity of symptoms of the episode itself. However, as indicated in Fig. 1, there are also mixed states of depression and mania. When they recur, these mixed states follow a bipolar pattern.

Non-mixed states of depression and mania are clinical opposites. About 10 per cent of patients will have both depressive and manic recurrence, and the term **bipolar** traditionally refers to recurrent episodes of both depression and mania. (Not all mental disorders showing an episodic course should be classified as mood disorders.) There are also chronic mood disorders. The term chronic major depression is used to describe persistence of the symptoms for more than 2 years which, in accordance with DSM-IV and ICD-10, is the upper limit of a depressive episode. Manic episodes usually last from a week to 6 months. Chronic mania is very rare. However, milder symptoms may persist as depression (dysthymia) and a manic or mixed state (cyclothymia).

It has been argued[4] that the current editions of the DSM and ICD classifications are essentially attempts to standardize the Kraepelinian categories. While this holds true to a large extent, one of the limitations of DSM-IV and ICD-10 is the use of many subcategories resulting in much comorbidity, especially among the depressions. Anxiety is an important symptom of depression and aggression is an important symptom of mania.

Acute depression

Clinical research with symptom rating scales such as the Hamilton Depression Scale (HAM-D) has shown that about ten symptoms are sufficient to characterize the syndrome of most of the acute depressive states.[5] Table 1 shows these ten symptoms of acute depressive disorder as they appear in DSM-IV or ICD-10. The only difference between the two systems is that 'loss of self-esteem' is a separate symptom in ICD-10, whereas in DSM-IV it is included in the symptom of 'feelings of worthlessness and inappropriate guilt'. Thus DSM-IV has nine symptoms and ICD-10 ten symptoms for measuring the severity of depressive states. Mild, moderate (major), and psychotic depressions are considered, on the basis of the number of symptoms, as three different diagnostic categories in DSM-IV and ICD-10.

In the following each of the three diagnostic categories—mild, moderate (major), severe (psychotic)—will be described with reference to Table 1 to illustrate the development of depression from mild to major. A layman's description of these stages is shown in quotations from the American novelist William Styron (Box 1), who at the age of 60 described his own unipolar depressive episode in his memoir *Darkness Visible*.[6] Styron's description shows how anxiety is an important symptom of depression from its onset and continues over several weeks. When the suicidal symptoms became severe, Styron was admitted to the Yale New Hospital.

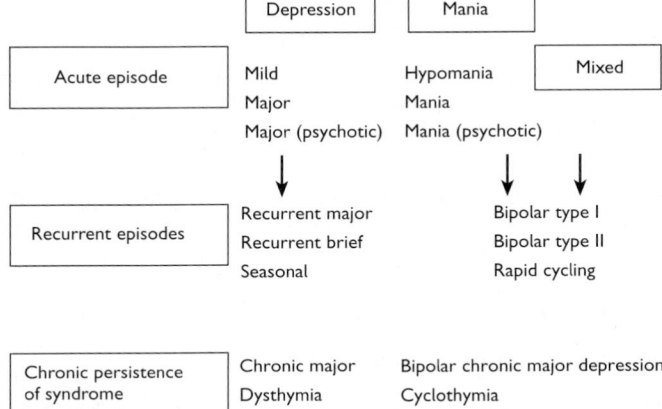

Fig. 1 The manic–depressive spectrum: syndromatic episode, recurrence of episodes, and persistence of syndromes.

Table 1 Acute depression as defined in DSM-IV and ICD-10

	Symptoms of depression	DSM-IV	ICD-10
1	Depressed mood most of the day, nearly every day	+	+
2	Markedly diminished interest or pleasure in all, or almost all, activities most of the day, nearly every day	+	+
3	Loss of energy or fatigue nearly every day	+	+
4	Loss of confidence or self-esteem		+
5	Unreasonable feelings of self-reproach or excessive or inappropriate guilt, nearly every day	+	+
6	Recurrent thoughts of death or suicide, or any suicidal behaviour	+	+
7	Diminished ability to think or concentrate, or indecisiveness, nearly every day	+	+
8	Psychomotor agitation or retardation nearly every day	+	+
9	Insomnia or hypersomnia nearly every day	+	+
10	Change in appetite (decrease or increase with corresponding weight change)	+	+

+ indicates that the symptom is included.

Mild depression

A decrease in positive well being or a lack of interests is often the first symptom of depression: 'walks in the woods, became less zestful' (Box 1). Many patients with mild depression describe themselves as 'distressed' rather than ill. When people describe their feelings in response to life stress, they often speak of anxiety and depression.[7] However, the lowering of mood in the states of distress is much more variable than that in mild depression and lasts for less than a week. The first three symptoms in Table 1 are the core symptoms of mild depression. They are present most of the day, nearly every day, for at least 2 weeks, and a person with a mild depression usually has difficulty in carrying on with his or her normal activities. Diagnosis of mild depression according to ICD-10 requires at least two of the first three symptoms in Table 1, as well as at least two of the remaining seven symptoms. Insomnia and diminished ability to concentrate are common.

Elderly patients with mild depression may experience fatigue, insomnia, and poor concentration associated with ageing rather than with illness. Only about half of patients suffering from depression consult their family doctors, and those who do consult their doctors are more severely depressed.[8] Those patients who are treated for depression have a much better outcome than those who do not consult their doctors.[8]

Major depression with or without melancholia

The cardinal triad of symptoms of depression is as follows: emotional symptoms, psychomotor symptoms, and negative beliefs. Not surprisingly, this triad is more obvious in major depression than in mild depression. Diagnosis of major depression according to DSM-IV

Box 1

The stages from decreased positive well being through mild depression to major depression without psychotic features (from William Styron, *Darkness Visible*[6])

- The shadows of nightfall seemed more sober, my mornings were less buoyant, walks in the woods became less zestful, and there was a moment during my working hours when a kind of panic and anxiety overtook me, just for a few minutes, accompanied by a visceral queasiness . . .

- . . . As the disorder gradually took full possession of my system, I began to conceive that my mind itself was like one of those outmoded small-town telephone exchanges, being gradually inundated by flood-waters . . .

- . . . I particularly remember the lamentable near disappearance of my voice . . . The libido also made an early exit . . . food, like everything else within the scope of sensation, was utterly without savor . . .

- . . . My few hours of sleep were usually terminated at three or four in the morning, when I stared up into yawning darkness . . . I'm fairly certain that it was during one of these insomnia trances that there came over me the knowledge that this condition would cost me my life, if it continued on such a course . . . I had not conceived precisely how my end would come. In short, I was still keeping the idea of suicide at bay . . . What I had begun to discover is that the gray drizzle of horror, induced by depression, takes on the quality of physical pain . . .

requires at least five of the nine symptoms in Table 1, and ICD-10 requires six of the ten symptoms in Table 1. Negative beliefs such as 'loss of self-esteem' or 'inappropriate guilt' are the core symptoms of major depression. Inappropriate guilt is experienced as punishment for past misdeeds (prior to the current episode of depression). The prevailing element of negative beliefs is a sense of loss which is associated with lower self-esteem experienced retrospectively.[9] The symptom which discriminates best between anxiety states and major depressive disorder is guilt.[10]

Psychomotor retardation is more common in younger depressed patients; psychomotor agitation is more common in elderly patients. Psychomotor retardation is manifested not only in decreased motor activity (e.g. fixed facial expression, reduced gestures, and slow movements) but also in decreased verbal activity, concentration difficulties, and emotional withdrawal. Psychomotor agitation can range from hand-wringing and restlessness to almost continuous pacing.

Both in DSM-IV and ICD-10, major depressive states can be further specified as a melancholic or somatic syndrome. In earlier descriptions (including Freud's 'Mourning and melancholia'[11]), endogenous or somatic depression is distinguished from psychogenic or reactive depression by 'early morning awakening' and 'depression regularly worse in the morning'. These two signs are the only features of somatic or melancholic depression not included in the list of symptoms in Table 1. Strictly speaking, diurnal variation in symptoms is not itself a symptom but rather a description of their course. The most 'somatic' symptom in Table 1 is change in body weight (Styron had lost 20 to 25 pounds over a period of 6 weeks, when the illness developed into a major depression).[12]

Styron's depression (Box 1) included the somatic feature of early morning awakening and suicidal thoughts. The latter are not just a consequence of the other symptoms. Styron described how during depression he could still keep '...the idea of suicide at bay...'. At a later stage (not shown in Box 1), just before he was admitted to hospital, Styron tried to write a suicide letter. Suicidal thoughts were often present late at night, when anxiety symptoms had lifted.[12]

Measurements of social behaviour and subjective state have shown that acute major depression is among the most disabling and distressing of medical disorders.[13] The constant mental pain and the suicidal symptoms seriously affect quality of life. The suicidal risk in major depression is especially high when psychomotor retardation is improving under treatment. The treating physician or the relatives typically observe improvement in the depressive symptoms before the patient does, because psychomotor retardation improves before mood state or hopelessness.

The risk is especially high in socially isolated people. Major depression has the highest risk of suicide of all mental disorders, and all patients with major depression should be assessed for the risk of suicide.

Previous editions of DSM and ICD included 'involutional melancholia', which was considered to be a distinct entity, among the late-onset types of depression. However, it is now regarded as a typical major depression.

Major depression with psychotic features

According to DSM-IV or ICD-10, the term 'psychotic depression' is not synonymous with endogenous or melancholic depression. This agrees with Kraepelin[14] and Hamilton[15] who used the term 'psychosis' to refer to the severity of symptoms. As stated by Hamilton:[15] '... a schizophrenic patient, who has delusions is not necessarily worse than one who has not, but a depressive patient who has is much worse ...'. This statement is also valid for mania.

Mood-congruent psychotic features can be considered as a severe degree of symptoms such as guilt and hypochondriasis. Among the case histories selected to illustrate the ICD-10 diagnoses, that of a 35-year-old male patient referred to as the 'Night Walker', illustrates severe depression with mood-congruent psychotic symptoms:[16]

> ...he spoke in a low voice and displayed belief in a fatal illness, from which he was going to die. He said he contaminated others and that he felt guilty about the death of a distant relative...He was evil, worthless, and did not deserve to live... Physical and neurological examinations showed no abnormalities except for the evidence of severe weight loss...

Recurrent depression

Recurrent major depression

After a single episode of major depression around 85 per cent of patients experience recurrent episodes.[17] While the first episode of major depression is often provoked by a negative life event such as loss of job, retirement, marital separation. or divorce, subsequent episodes are often unprecipitated (positive life events can also provoke depression). Depressive episodes typically increase in frequency and duration as they return.[18] This phenomenon has been explained by 'kindling', a process in which repeated stimulation causes an escalating response.[19] Usually, the intervals between episodes of unipolar depression are symptom free, but some patients experience dysthymia between episodes. Such cases have been called 'double depression'.[20]

Recurrent brief depression

The symptoms of recurrent brief depression, which was first described by Angst,[21] are similar to those of major depression (Table 1) with regard to both number and severity. However, they do not meet the requirement that an episode should last for 2 weeks or more. The diagnosis of recurrent brief depression has not been adopted fully in DSM-IV, but it is included in ICD-10. It should be distinguished from recurrent suicidal behaviour, for example in patients with borderline personality disorder.

Reccurrent brief depression occurs in some patients with Parkinson's disease. In contrast, post-stroke depression is similar to major depression.[22]

Seasonal depression

Seasonal depression is seen most frequently in winter, and less frequently in summer. In DSM-IV, seasonal depression has been adopted as a specifier (rather than a diagnostic category) which can be applied not only to recurrent depression but also to bipolar disorder. The seasonal episodes (e.g. winter depression) have to outnumber any non-seasonal depressive episodes in the same patient. In ICD-10 only seasonal depression is briefly mentioned, and that in an annex for disorders under consideration.

According to DSM-IV, the symptoms of seasonal depression are similar to those of major depression. However, Kasper and Rosenthal[23] repeated that the symptoms differ from those of major depression, with hypersomnia, overeating, carbohydrate craving, and weight gain.

In a meta-analysis of 61 studies of seasonal patterns of suicide, Goodwin and Jamison[18] showed that suicide is 10 to 20 times more common in spring (with a peak in May) than in winter or summer. There was also a small peak in October. This pattern is consistent with the peak times of hospital admission for depressive episodes. These findings support the view[23] that seasonal winter depression is an atypical type of major depression.

Chronic depression

In both DSM-IV and ICD-10 'chronic' refers to an episode with a duration of 2 years or more. 'Double depression' is by definition a form of a chronic depression, because dysthymia is defined as lasting for at least 2 years.

Chronic major depression

In DSM-IV, but not in ICD-10, major depression is specified as chronic if the criteria for major depression have been met continuously for at least the past 2 years. Treatment-resistant depression is not

Table 2 Acute mania as defined in DSM-IV and ICD-10

	Symptoms of mania	DSM-IV	ICD-10
1A	Elevated mood	+	+
1B	Irritable mood	+	+
2	Increased self-esteem or grandiosity	+	+
3	Decreased need for sleep	+	+
4	Increased talkativeness	+	+
5	Flight of ideas	+	+
6	Distractibility	+	+
7A	Increased social activities or contacts	+	+
7B	Psychomotor agitation	+	+
8	Risk-taking behaviour	+	+
9	Increased sexual activities		+

+ indicates that the symptom is included.

a diagnosis, but a term that describes many chronic major depressions.

Dysthymia

Both in DSM-IV and ICD-10 dysthymia refers to symptoms of mild depression which have persisted for at least 2 years. The symptoms are similar to those in Table 1, except for 'excessive guilt', 'psychomotor changes', and 'suicidal thoughts'. Symptoms fluctuate more than in major depression, and (in contrast with seasonal depression) they are 'typical' including insomnia, lack of appetite, or poor concentration. In ICD-10, but not in DSM-IV, the symptom of social withdrawal is included as a characteristic symptom of dysthymia. The category 'depressive neurosis' which appeared in earlier editions of the classification included a similar symptom referred to as introversion.[5]

Acute mania

The clinical features of mania form are more distinct than those of depression.[24,25] Symptom rating scales for mania parallel to the Hamilton Scale for Depression have been developed.[26,27]

Table 2 shows the items listed in both DSM-IV and ICD-10. The only difference is that ICD-10 includes 'increased sexual activities' as a separate item, whereas in DSM-IV it is listed under 'risk-taking behaviour'. Hence, ICD-10 has nine items and DSM-IV has only eight items. 'Elevated' and 'irritable' mood are combined in both classifications (item 1, Table 2), as are 'increased social activities' and 'psychomotor agitation' (item 7, Table 2).

Box 2 shows the three stages of mania observed among inpatients before treatment. Whereas most depressive episodes are treated outside hospital, mania is usually treated in hospitals. Therefore most research on mania is still carried out in the hospital setting. The study by Carlson and Goodwin[28] is among the few longitudinal studies in which untreated inpatients have been observed systematically; Box 2 is a modified version of their findings. As in the previous discussion of depression, self-reports will also be referred to.

Box 2

The three stages of the acute manic episode as observed in untreated inpatients

- **Hypomania**
  Increased well being and/or irritable mood, but still with sufficient control over the conditions; more busy; pressured speech; makes more telephone calls; seductive

- **Mania**
  Nearly always pleasant and cheerful. Occasionally losing insight and co-operation, impulsive, angry; very hyperactive, less sleep, more pressure of speech, makes repeated telephone calls; racing thoughts, more expansive, some grandiosity

- **Mania with psychotic features**
  Emotionally labile, can be very angry, very intrusive. Unco-operative, severely agitated, no sleep, very talkative, loud; flight of thoughts, grandiosity, religious delusions 'hearing God', sexually very preoccupied

Modified from Carlson and Goodwin.[28]

Hypomania

Hypomania can be the first stage of a spiralling upswing of mood (Box 2). The main symptom of hypomania is usually intense well being but irritability is also seen. Normal happiness is transient, lasting from minutes to hours. To be diagnosed as hypomania, the elevation of mood must last for at least 4 days. The change of mood is often quite different from any seen when the patient is well.

The cardinal triad of mania comprises emotions, psychomotor symptoms, and expansiveness or increased self-esteem. A slight psychomotor restlessness and some pressured speech are often seen; for example, the person makes more frequent telephone calls. These symptoms are not severe enough to cause marked impairment in social or occupational functioning.

Jamison[29] has described this phase as follows: '…When you're high it's tremendous. The ideas and feelings are fast and frequent …Shyness goes, the right words and gestures are suddenly there, the power to captivate others a felt certainty…Sensuality is pervasive and the desire to seduce and be seduced irresistible'. The shyness or introversion seen in mild depression or dysthymia contrast with the lack of shyness and extraversion seen in the hypomanic patient.

Mania without psychotic features

In mania the elevated spirit seen in hypomania is often mixed with irritability and hostility. Jamison[29] has described the change: 'Humor and absorption on friends' faces are replaced by fear and concern. Everything previously (in the hypomanic state) moving with the grain is now against—you are irritable, angry, frightened, uncontrollable…'.

The psychomotor symptoms of mania are restlessness and less need for sleep. There is pressure of speech; the patient talks more and in a louder voice. There is intrusive behaviour, arguments, and attempts to dominate others. Expansiveness is manifested as increased self-esteem; for example, the patient clearly overestimates his or her own capacities

or hints at unusual abilities. Jamison[29] described how in periods of mania she did not worry about money: 'The money will come from somewhere; I am entitled; God will provide. Credit cards are disastrous, personal cheques even worse … mania is a natural extension of the economy … So I bought precious stones, elegant and unnecessary furniture, three watches within an hour (in the Rolex rather than Timex class)…'.

To be diagnosed as a manic episode, the disorder should last at least a week. The criteria for mania are elevated or clearly irritable mood, and at least three of the symptoms listed in Table 2. These symptoms should be severe enough to cause marked impairment in occupational functioning. Hospital admission is often needed to prevent the patient harming himself or others.

Mania with psychotic features

Psychotic states of mania are characterized by greater pressure of speech, more open hostility, severe agitation, no need for sleep, flight of thoughts, severe distractibility, and grandiose delusions. In younger people psychotic mania is often misdiagnosed as schizophrenia.[30]

In hospital the increased social contact of manic patients is clearly different from the emotional bluntness of schizophrenics. The intrusive behaviour seen in severe mania is of an extremely dominating and manipulative nature, out of context with the setting. Secondary persecutory delusions often develop. The expansive religious delusion 'hearing God' should be differentiated from the schizophrenic patient's religious hallucinations.

Both DSM-IV and ICD-10 differentiate between mood-congruent psychotic symptoms (such as grandiose delusions of religion and voices supporting the patient's superhuman powers) and mood-incongruent psychotic symptoms (which are often the secondary delusions of persecution mentioned above).

Recurrent bipolar episodes

Only about 10 per cent of patients with 'manic–depressive' disorder have mania. Kraepelin, who followed hundreds of patients with manic–depressive illness, observed very few with only recurrent manic episodes.[14] Recurrent manic episodes are more often interspersed with depressive episodes. Mixed states may emerge with the simultaneous presence of depression and manic symptoms (see discussion of acute mixed episodes below). About 85 per cent of patients with an acute episode of mania will run a chronic episodic course.[17]

Bipolar type I disorder

This is the classic manic–depressive illness with episodes of depression fulfilling the criteria of major depression and episodes of mania (with or without psychotic features).

Bipolar type II disorder

This category appears in DSM-IV but not in ICD-10. It is a disorder with episodes of hypomania but not mania, and episodes of major depression. The episodes of hypomania should not be confused with brief states of elevated mood which often follow the remission of a major depression.

Rapid cycling disorder

In DSM-IV rapid cycling disorder is a specifier; in ICD-10 it is mentioned only in an annex for disorders under consideration. In DSM-IV it can be applied to both bipolar type I and bipolar type II disorders. There should have been at least four episodes fulfilling the criteria of major depression, mania, hypomania, or mixed mood disorder in the previous 12 months. The episodes are demarcated by either partial or full remission for at least 2 months or a switch to an episode of opposite kind.

Chronic bipolar disorder

Chronic mania is rarely seen. DSM-IV has a category for chronic bipolar major depression. Both DSM-IV and ICD-10 include cyclothymia.

Chronic bipolar major depression

Chronic major depression can occur in bipolar disorders. However, the diagnosis of chronic bipolar major depression can be applied only if it is the most recent type of mood episode. The criteria of major depression symptoms should have been met continuously for at least the previous 2 years.

Cyclothymia

Previously this was considered to be a personality disorder or the first stage of a bipolar illness. The essential feature of cyclothymic disorder is a persistent fluctuating mood disturbance including numerous periods of depressive symptoms. These are periods, not episodes, of hypomania or depression. Thus it is a disorder of subsyndromal mood swings analogous to dysthymia in unipolar depression. About one-third of patients with cyclothymic disorder will develop bipolar disorder.[18]

Acute mixed episode

Jamison[29] has argued that the term 'bipolar' perpetuates the notion that:

> ...depression exists rather tidily segregated on its own pole, while mania clusters off neatly and discretely on another. This polarisation of two clinical states flies in the face of everything that we know about the fluctuating nature of manic–depressive illness ...and it minimizes the importance of mixed manic–depressive states...

In the acute mixed episode, it is the rapid change from one mood state to the other which is characteristic. The mixture of manic and depressive symptoms is the essential feature of mixed episodes. It is not a bipolar course of symptoms, but the presence of major depression and mania nearly every day. DSM-IV requires that the duration of the mixed episode should be at least 1 week; ICD-10 requires at least 2 weeks.

Kraepelin[31] described transitory mood of depression in acute manic states. Transitory moods of depression have been recorded in manic patients using a rating scale administered by the nursing staff.[32,33] Such short-lived states of 'depression' in patients with acute mania should be referred to as 'microdepressions' and not mixed episodes. Winokur[34] described 'microdepressions' most clearly:

> ...If one allows a manic patient to talk, one will note that he shows fleeting episodes of depression embedded within mania ('microdepressions'). He may be talking in grandiose and extravagant fashion and then suddenly for 30 seconds breaks down to give an account of something he feels guilty about... His eyes will fill with tears but in 15 to 30 seconds he will be back to talking in his expansive fashion.

Conclusion

Frances et al.[35] declared that DSM-IV was moving from reliance on expert consensus to a greater emphasis on empirical evidence. In DSM-III and DSM-IV the diagnostic criteria were based on groups of symptoms which varied together over time. The ICD-10 and DSM-IV criteria for acute and recurrent episodes of mania and depression are in keeping with the accumulating clinical research.[5,18,36] Severity is a key dimension in both depression and mania.[37] The core symptoms of mania and depression shown in Tables 1 and 2 are sufficient to measure the severity of the states and to discriminate between categories.

The former dichotomy between neurotic and endogenous depression has been put aside in favour of the view that, over time, patients can have both 'neurotic' depression (dysthymia) and 'endogenous' (major) depression ('double depression'). Also, only the most severe major depressions are 'psychotic', and not all major depressions are endogenous. Only the dichotomy between unipolar and bipolar disorders remains. This phenomenological approach to the clinical features of affective mood disorders and mania has high interclinician reliability.[5]

Reports from patients themselves have also been included in this chapter. Self-rating scales and questionnaires for depression have shown that depressed patients without psychotic symptoms can give consistent self-reports of their feelings.[5] New questionnaires or scales have been based on the symptoms in Table 1 and 2. For example, the Beck Depression Inventory has recently been modified to cover better the items in Table 1.[38] Another depression questionnaire is based directly on Table 1,[13] as is an interview scale for major depression.[39] A mania scale covering Table 2 has just been released.[40]

All depressed patients should be assessed for the risk of suicidal behaviour. Most answer such questions truthfully. In contrast, the manic patients describe themselves as 'normal'[41] or respond in a so-called 'manic game'.[42] This 'manic game' can develop into potentially dangerous behaviour such as aggressive car driving, foolish business investments, or unusual sexual behaviour. It is a measure of good practice that the psychiatrist has the time and professional skills to convince the manic patient of the need for a short stay in the secure setting of a hospital.

The fluctuating or mixed nature of clinical depression and mania often requires simultaneous use of depression and mania rating scales to measure outcome of treatment (short-term as well as long-term).

References

1. American Psychiatric Association (1994). *Diagnostic and statistical manual of mental disorders* (4th edn). American Psychiatric Association, Washington, DC.

2. World Health Organization (1993). *The ICD-10 classification of mental and behavioural disorders—diagnostic criteria for research.* World Health Organization, Geneva.

3. Angst, J., Baastrup, P., Grof, P., Hippins, H., Pöldinger, W., and Weis, P. (1993). The course of monopolar depression and bipolar psychoses. *Psychiatria, Neurologia, Neurochirurgia,* 76, 489–500.

4. Shepherd, M. (1998). Psychopharmacology: specific and non-specific. In *The psychopharmacologists* (ed. D. Healy), Vol. II, pp. 237–58. Lippincott–Raven, Philadelphia, PA.

5. Bech, P. (1993). *Rating scales for psychopathology, health status and quality of life.* Springer Verlag, Berlin.

6. Styron, W. (1990). *Darkness visible. A memoir of madness.* Random House, New York.

7. Veroff, J., Douran, E., and Kuka, R.A. (1981). *The inner American.* Basic Books, New York.

8. Angst, J. (1998). Treated versus untreated major depressive episodes. *Psychopathology,* 31, 37–44.

9. Beck, A.T. (1967). *Depression: clinical, experimental, and theoretical aspects.* University of Pennsylvania Press, Philadelphia, PA.

10. Breslau, N. and Davis, G.C. (1985). Redefining DSM-III criteria in depression. An assessment of the descriptive validity of criterion symptoms. *Journal of Affective Disorders,* 9, 199–206.

11. Freud, S. (1917). Mourning and melancholia. In *Collected papers,* Vol. 4, pp. 152–70. Basic Books, New York, 1959.

12. West, J.L.W. (1998). *William Styron. A life.* Random House, New York.

13. Bech, P. (1998). *Quality of life in the psychiatric patient.* Mosby–Wolfe, London.

14. Kraepelin, E. (1921). *Manic–depressive insanity and paranoia.* Livingstone, Edinburgh.

15. Hamilton, M. (1960). A rating scale for depression. *Journal of Neurology, Neurosurgery and Psychiatry,* 23, 56–62.

16. Üstün, T.B., Bertelsen, A., Dilling, H., *et al.* (ed.) (1996). *The many faces of mental disorder. Adult case histories according to ICD-10.* American Psychiatric Press, Washington, DC.

17. Angst, J. (1980). Verlauf unipolar depressiver, bipolar manisch-depressiver und schizo-affektiver Erkrankungen und Psychosen. *Fortschift Neurologische Psychiatrie,* 48, 3–30.

18. Goodwin, F.K. and Jamison, K.R. (1990). *Manic–depressive illness.* Oxford University Press, New York.

19. Post, R.M., Uhde, T.W., and Putman, P.W. (1982). Kindling and carbamazepine in affective illness. *Journal of Nervous and Mental Disease,* 170, 717–21.

20. Keller, M.B., Lavori, P.W., and Endicott, J. (1983). 'Double-depression'. Two year follow-up. *American Journal of Psychiatry,* 140, 689–94.

21. Angst, J. (1990). Recurrent brief depression: a new concept of depression. *Pharmacopsychiatry,* 23, 63–6.

22. Wermuth, L., Sørensen, P.S., and Timm, S. (1998). Depression in idiopathic Parkinson's disease treated with citalopram. *Nordic Journal of Psychiatry,* 52, 163–9.

23. Kasper, S. and Rosenthal, N.E. (1989). Anxiety and depression in seasonal affective disorders. In *Anxiety and depression: distinctive and overlapping features* (ed. P.C. Kendall and D. Watson), pp. 341–75. Academic Press, San Diego, CA.

24. Häfner, H., Cesarin, A.C., Cesarion-Krantz, A., *et al.* (1967). Konstanz und Variabilität klinisch psychiatrischer Diagnosen über sechs Jahrzehnte. *Social Psychiatry,* 2, 14–25.

25. Everitt, B.S., Gourlay, A.J., and Kendell, R.E. (1971). An attempt at validation of traditional psychiatric syndromes by cluster analyses. *British Journal of Psychiatry,* 119, 399–412.

26. Bech, P., Rafaelsen, O.J., Kramp, P., and Bolwig, T.G. (1978). The mania rating scale: scale construction and inter-observer agreement. *Neuropharmacology,* 17, 430–1.

27. Young, R.C., Biggs, J.T., Ziegler, V.E., and Meyer, D.A. (1978). A rating scale for mania: reliability, validity and sensitivity. *British Journal of Psychiatry,* 133, 429–35.

28. Carlson, G.A. and Goodwin, F.K. (1973). The stages of mania. A longitudinal analysis of the manic episode. *Archives of General Psychiatry,* 28, 221–8.

29. Jamison, K.R. (1995). *An unquiet mind. A memoir of moods and madness.* Knopf, New York.

30. Mendlewicz, J., Fieve, R.R., Rainer, J., and Fleiss, J.L. (1972). Manic–depressive illness: a comparative study of patients with and without a family history. *British Journal of Psychiatry,* 120, 523–30.

31. Kraepelin, E. (1913). *Psychiatrie* (8th edn), Vol. III. Barth, Leipzig.

32. Biegel, A. and Murphy, D.L. (1971). Assessing clinical characteristics of manic state. *American Journal of Psychiatry,* 128, 688–94.

33. Bech, P., Bolwig, T.G., Dein, E., Jacobsen, O., and Gram, L.F. (1975). Quantitative rating of manic states. *Acta Psychiatrica Scandinavica,* 52, 1–6.

34. Winokur, G. (1981). *Depression: the facts.* Oxford University Press.

35. Frances, A., Pincus, H.A., Widiger, T.A., Davis, W.W. , and First, M.B. (1990). DMS-IV: work in progress. *American Journal of Psychiatry,* 147, 1439–48.

36. Kendell, R.E. (1968). *The classification of depressive illness.* Oxford University Press, London.

37. Goethe, J.W., Fischer, E.H., and Wright, J.S. (1993). Severity as a key concept of depression. *Journal of Nervous and Mental Disease,* 181, 718–24.

38. Beck, A.T., Steer, R.A., Ball, R., and Ranieri, W. (1996). Comparison of Beck Depression Inventories IA and II in psychiatric outpatients. *Journal of Personality Assessment,* 67, 588–97.

39. Bech, P., Stage, K.B., Nair, V.P.V., Larsen, J.K., Kragh-Sørensen, P., and Gjerris, A. (1997). The Major Depression Rating Scale (MDS). Inter-rater reliability and validity across different settings in randomised moclobemide trial. *Journal of Affective Disorders,* 42, 39–48.

40. Bech, P. (1996). *The Bech, Hamilton and Zung scales for mood disorders: screening and listening* (2nd edn). Springer Verlag, Berlin.

41. Platman, S.R., Plutchik, R., Fieve, R.R., and Lawlor, W.G. (1969). Emotion profiles associated with mania and depression. *Archives of General Psychiatry,* 20, 210–14.

42. Janowsky, D.S., Leff, M., and Epstein, R.S. (1970). Playing the manic game. *Archives of General Psychiatry,* 22, 252–61.

4.5.3 Diagnosis, classification, and differential diagnosis of the mood disorders

Gordon Parker

Introduction

Varying expressions and subtypes of depressed and elated mood states make for difficulties in definition, diagnosis, and classification. Some definitional and boundary issues will first be detailed, to assist later consideration of subtyping and differential diagnostic issues.

Definitions

Depression

The term 'depression' can variably define an affect, mood state, a disorder or syndrome, or a specific entity. A depressed 'affect' usually occurs in response to a specific situation and is best defined as a relatively transient state of feeling 'depressed', 'sad', or 'blue'.

A depressed 'mood' is more pervasive, more likely to be experienced as unusual or atypical, associated with negative ideas (e.g. hopelessness, helplessness, pessimism about the future, and feeling like giving up), and may influence behaviour. The quintessential construct defining a depressed mood is lowering of the individual's intrinsic self-esteem and, as a corollary, self-criticism. The extent to which self-esteem is lowered usually defines the severity of the mood disturbance. Depressed mood states are experienced by most people, although in non-clinical subjects they generally last only minutes to days.

A depressive 'condition' (be it a disorder, syndrome, or specific disease entity) is generally distinguished by a longer duration, by more or a greater number of clinical features, and by distinct social impairment. A duration criterion ensures that a transient depressed mood (even if severe) does not alone establish psychiatric 'case' status, with diagnostic criteria sets generally requiring a minimum duration of 2 weeks for conditions other than the so-called 'adjustment disorders'. The addition of several clinical features (detailed shortly) informs us about severity (e.g. 'major' and 'minor' depressive disorders) and subtyping, while the social impairment criterion assists cleavage between 'normal' mood states and psychiatric 'case' status.

At times, depressive conditions are described as 'primary' or 'secondary'. Any such distinction is necessarily imprecise. Thus, we concede 'secondary depression' when depression emerges during the course of a substantive psychiatric condition (e.g. schizophrenia) or medical condition, or following certain aetiologically defined triggers (e.g. organic states; substance abuse, including alcoholism). As depression is commonly associated with certain other psychiatric disorders (e.g. severe anxiety states, personality disorders), it might be logical to also call these 'secondary' depressive disorders. While some authors[1] use the term in this way, formal diagnostic systems operate to the restricted definition.

Mania/hypomania

As described in Chapter 4.5.2, such conditions are the converse of depression and fundamentally represent hedonistic states. Here self-esteem is almost invariably increased, the mood is generally infectious, the individual feels energized or 'wired' (ideas and thoughts race from topic to topic), creativity and religiosity are often enhanced, there is a tendency to spend (or wish to spend) more money, while any psychotic features are generally in synchrony with the mood state.

There is no formal distinction between 'hypomania' and 'mania', and the lack of an agreed definition is regrettable. To some theorists, the presence of psychotic features determines manic (as against hypomanic) status. Goodwin and Jamison[2] suggest that hypomania and mania differ little in mood components, but that cognition, perception, and behaviour differ in severity and manifestation. Both DSM-IV[3] and ICD-10[4] disallow a diagnosis of hypomania if psychotic features are present but, conversely, do not require psychotic features for a diagnosis of mania. ICD-10 views hypomania as 'an intermediate state without delusions, hallucinations, or complete disruption of normal activities'. DSM-IV lists essentially similar clinical criteria for hypomanic and manic episodes, but distinguishes the two by the presence of marked impairment in social functioning, requirement for hospitalization, or the presence of psychotic features in a manic episode.

'Mixed states'

Here the individual with the affective disorder may show depressive features during a manic episode or manic features during a depressive episode. While the term is sometimes used to describe the transition from one polar mood disturbance to another, the more common use is for a genuine coterminous presence of manic and depressive features.

Bipolar/unipolar depression specifics

Turning from cross-sectional to longitudinal definition, the course specifier 'bipolar' has long been applied to describe patients who have had at least one manic or hypomanic episode, whether preceded by any depressive episode or not. Originally, Leonhard[5] introduced the concept of 'monopolar' (or 'unipolar') depression to distinguish those who had had episodes of the melancholic subtype of depression, but no manic episode. Regrettably, the term 'unipolar' depression is now used to define a residual (i.e. non-bipolar) category, so heterogeneous as to be of limited utility for aetiological and treatment studies.

Bipolar categories

In recent years, bipolar disorder has been subcategorized into bipolar I and bipolar II expressions. The DSM-IV definition effectively requires an initial or previous manic episode for the former, while bipolar II disorder requires hypomanic episodes and one or more previous episode of major depression. ICD-10 catalogues a bipolar II disorder (without definition) but does not list or describe a bipolar I disorder.

Depressive disorders: one, two, or three principal types?

The extended debate as to whether the depressive disorders are best conceptualized as comprising one or more distinct disorders warrants overview. The 'unitarian' view posits one depressive disorder, varying essentially by severity. The strict 'binarian' view argues for two separate types.

Debate did not commence this century. Altschule[6] suggested that St Paul distinguished between two types of depression, one 'from God' and the other 'of the world' (Corinthians 7:10), and that several distinguished Christian leaders from the fifth to the eighth century recognized a distinction between 'rational' and 'irrational' depression. Jackson[7] has extensively detailed historic descriptions of melancholic depression from early Roman and Greek views through to the twentieth century, charting the key defining clinical features, with an early emphasis on observable signs—particularly of psychomotor disturbance. Similarly, Berrios[8] informs us that, in classical antiquity 'melancholia was defined in terms of overt behavioural features … [and] that symptoms … were not part of the concept'.

Rich descriptions of melancholia as a depressive condition marked by psychomotor retardation or agitation emerged in the late nineteenth century (e.g. Maudsley[9]), while Kraepelin[10] brought mania and melancholia together as manic–depressive insanity. Kraepelin defined a 'melancholia simplex' condition characterized by a key feature of psychic inhibition, causing paralysis of thought, memory difficulties, and a sense of weariness and enervation, but without psychotic features. He also defined a second melancholic group with delusions and hallucinations in addition to psychomotor retardation or stupor, as well as a third group of 'agitated melancholia' marked by distinct motor agitation. In 1917, Freud[11] published his influential paper on melancholia, and Jackson argued that this changed the descriptive focus of melancholia in the twentieth century, with theorists and analysts then focusing on cognitive and intrapsychic features. Subsequently, and continuing still, clinical description of depression weighted symptoms, and minimized or ignored behavioural signs.

In the 1920s, Mapother[12] argued that it was pointless to distinguish between 'psychotic' and 'neurotic' forms of depression, as both lay along a continuum. This provocative paper, presenting the unitarian position, challenged diagnostic practice. The 'binarians' responded, with Gillespie[13] arguing for two types of depression: first, an 'autonomous' type (previously and subsequently termed 'endogenous depression'), which, once precipitated, tended to run an independent course and be unresponsive to the environment; second, a 'reactive' type, in which the depression was responsive to the environment (although earlier, the concept of 'reactivity' had been tied to onset induced by a psychogenic factor).

The debate was strongly influenced by Lewis's study of 61 patients. Lewis[14] concluded that he could find no clear demarcation between depressive types, examined both cross-sectionally and longitudinally, thus delivering support to the unitarian view. This view prevailed until the introduction of multivariate statistical approaches and computers led to the debate being reactivated in the 1960s, with the so-called Newcastle School arguing strongly that their analyses supported a binary view. In a representative paper, Kiloh and Garside[15] used a factor-analytic strategy to argue for separate 'endogenous' and 'neurotic' depressive conditions. Factor analysis is not ideal for developing a typology, in that it produces dimensions (here symptoms) rather than groupings of patients. Subsequently, more appropriate strategies have been used, such as cluster analysis[16] and latent class analysis,[17] and with those studies providing support for separate classes. Critics suggest, however, that such classes or subgroups could still be determined by severity or, even if subtypes can be identified, question whether subclassification is of any moment.

This latter challenge is fundamental, taking us to the heart of any consideration of the diagnosis and classification of the depressive disorders. To the unitarians (despite evidence of quite varying aetiological factors), depression essentially varies only by degree, allowing treatment decisions (e.g. electroconvulsive therapy (**ECT**), antidepressant drugs, psychotherapy, or cognitive–behavioural therapy) to be decided on the basis of severity or frequency of episode. The opposing argument—for conceding subtypes—has been well put by Kendell,[18] who drew on important historical analogies: distinguishing between cardiac and renal forms of 'dropsy' allowed prediction of those who would respond to digitalis, and it was only when 'the pox' had been identified as comprising smallpox and chickenpox that it was possible to predict who was likely to live or die.

Thus, if there are valid depressive subtypes, the contribution of putative psychosocial and biological risk factors may vary across each, so that the subtypes may have distinctly differing neurobiological determinants and may have differential response to the broad treatment modalities. If this is true, then to force homogeneity by creating dimensionally based categories such as 'major depression' is to ensure muddied results. This is not merely a theoretical objection, when, as noted by Hickie,[19] large numbers of studies of patients with DSM-defined 'major depression' have failed to demonstrate any coherent pattern of neurobiological changes, replicate key biological correlates, and demonstrate any specific pattern of treatment response outside inpatient treatment settings.

How then have the official classificatory systems addressed such a substantive issue? In developing the DSM-III system,[20] the working group was required to make a decision on the competing unitarian or binarian models. While the binarians were at the door, they had, until then, failed to prove their case and the DSM-III committee chose a compromise. Thus, classification was predicated on an initial dimensional component (i.e. major versus minor disorders). If criteria for a major disorder were met, second-order and more categorical decisions about the presence of melancholia or psychotic depression were specified. This model proved unsatisfactory for melancholia. For example, Zimmerman and colleagues[21] noted that the DSM-III melancholia criteria set, unlike the definition provided in the predecessor (DSM-II), 'did not predict treatment response'. Thus, in DSM-IIIR[22] the criteria set for melancholia was revised to include complete recovery after previous episodes, previous good response to somatic treatments, and no significant personality disturbance, to overcome the lack of predictive validity by building into the definition some of the 'givens' held by many clinicians about melancholia. However, the criteria set for melancholia developed for DSM-IV returned essentially to the DSM-III set, with limitations which are considered below. The contrasting system, ICD-10, is essentially based on a dimensional or unitarian view of the depressive disorders.

Thus, there has been an extended debate as to whether a categorical and more 'biological' type of depression exists. There have been many ascriptions to this condition, variably termed 'endogenous', 'endogenomorphic', 'autonomous', and 'melancholic' depression. Definitions over time include a distinctive pattern of symptoms and signs, the greater relevance of genetic and other biological determinants, as contrasted with psychosocial precipitants (so leading to the term 'endogenous depression'), minimal response to placebo, and a selective response to antidepressant medication and ECT. There is evidence to support each of these propositions,[23] although the term 'endogenous' has proved unsatisfactory, as those with melancholia may commonly report antecedent life events. However, only the first issue falls within this chapter's purview, and will be addressed shortly.

Whether psychotic (or delusional) depression is a 'severe' form of melancholia or a separate entity also remains problematic. DSM-III had a category 'major depression with psychotic features' for use when delusions or hallucinations were present or when there was 'depressive stupor (the individual is mute and unresponsive)', thus viewing 'psychotic depression' as a subtype of the generic 'major depression' category rather than a subtype of melancholia. The practical advantage to that definition was in recognizing that psychomotor disturbance can be so severe that some patients will not volunteer or admit to psychotic features—which may only be confirmed by the patient after improvement. While 'depressive stupor' may then be a useful marker or proxy for the condition, this criterion was not retained in DSM-IIIR or DSM-IV, but is included in ICD-10. Two points argue for psychotic depression as a distinct entity: the presence of psychotic features, and its poor response to antidepressant medication alone or neuroleptic medication alone.[24]

A strict interpretation of the 'binary' view would place the non-psychotic and non-melancholic depressive conditions in a pure second class. Variably termed 'neurotic' or 'reactive' depression over time, this class is best regarded as a heterogeneous residue category (i.e. non-melancholic depression), with its heterogeneity expressed widely—across aetiological factors, clinical expression, and natural and treated history.

It is suggested here that there are three relatively separate depressive classes: psychotic, melancholic, and the non-melancholic disorders. Clinical differentiation of each will be described shortly.

Classification of affective mood disorders

Formal classification

For the depressive disorders, both ICD-10 and DSM-IV have multiple conditions and specifiers. The ICD-10 system allows mild and moderate depressive episodes (with or without a 'somatic syndrome' conceptualized as reflecting 'melancholic' features), and severe depressive episode (with or without psychotic symptoms). There are separate codes for a similar set of 'recurrent' disorders, while several 'persistent' mood disorders (including cyclothymia and dysthymia) and residual conditions are listed. DSM-IV has two principal 'stem' disorders (major depressive episode and dysthymia), with the first having a number of optional specifiers including 'with' melancholic, catatonic, psychotic, or atypical features, as well as including disorders showing longitudinal patterns of rapid cycling or a seasonal pattern. Both systems have categories for affective disorders secondary to organic disease, while DSM-IV includes mood disorders due to a general medical condition or substance use, or occurring in the post-partum period. Both classificatory systems include adjustment disorders with depression.

Both ICD-10 and DSM-IV have course specifiers for bipolar disorder containing 10 and four subgroups, respectively. In addition to the number of subgroups, differences include a greater emphasis on distinguishing bipolar I and II in DSM-IV, and cyclothymia being listed as a 'bipolar disorder' in DSM-IV as against being a 'persistent' mood disorder overlapping with a personality style in ICD-10.

For episode disorders, both systems list mania and hypomania, with ICD-10 favouring descriptive diagnostic criteria and DSM-IV specifying duration and required criterion numbers. ICD-10 allows manic subtypes with and without psychotic features, while DSM-IV puts little emphasis on psychotic features in its criterion set, although both favour a duration of at least a week. For hypomania, both DSM-IV and ICD-10 exclude those with psychotic features, and impose a minimum duration (4 days for DSM-IV and 'several days' for ICD-10). DSM-IV requires the presence of at least three specific features, while ICD-10 requires mood and behavioural features to be intermediate between cyclothymia and mania.

Formal classifications are therefore built principally on severity, features of current episode, patterns of disorder expression over time, as well as persistence and recurrence. Few diagnoses are consistent across the ICD-10 and DSM-IV systems and, while each provides definitions that allow a 'shared language' to be used by clinicians and researchers, the extent to which their severity-weighted groupings capture 'meaningful' depressive subtypes remains problematic.

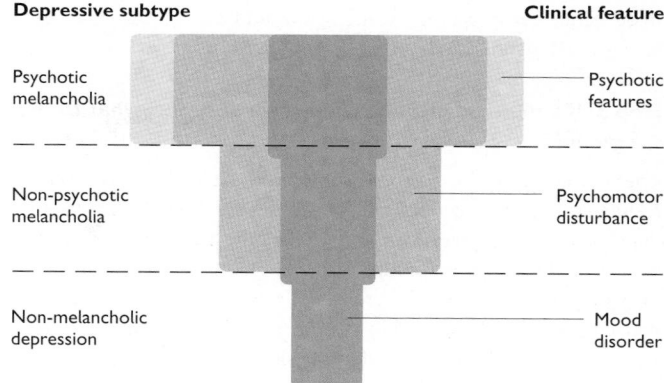

Fig. 1 Hierarchical model for the three principal depressive subtypes comprising an obligatory mood disorder component (albeit varying in severity) and two subtype-specific components of psychomotor disturbance and psychotic features.

Clinical classification—based on a hierarchical or tiered model

This model (see Fig. 1) argues for a shared mood disorder component across three principal subtypes (i.e. from the low-order heterogeneous 'non-melancholic' to the higher order 'melancholic' and 'psychotic' depressive subtypes), and a rationale for the model will be detailed. The first procedural step for the clinician, however, is to determine whether the disorder meets 'caseness' criteria.

Step 1: Is a depressive disorder present?

For all the depressive disorders, the first building block requires evidence of a depressed mood. Useful questions include the following: 'Do you feel depressed?', 'Has there been any change in your self-esteem/the extent to which you generally value yourself?', and 'Are you being more self-critical or harder on yourself than usual?'

The next clinical priority is to determine if the depression is sufficiently severe as to warrant 'case' status, and here the DSM-IV criteria for a major depressive episode have common acceptance. That criteria set lists the following:

- four mood items (depressed mood, loss of interest or pleasure, feelings of worthlessness or inappropriate guilt, recurrent thoughts of death and suicidal ideation)
- weight change
- sleep disturbance
- fatigue
- impaired concentration
- psychomotor disturbance

A positive diagnosis requires five or more of the nine, evidence of functional impairment, and a minimum duration of 2 weeks.

Step 2: If a depressive disorder is present, what subtype?

If 'caseness' criteria are met, the next decision should be to determine the diagnostic subtype. A hierarchical (three-tiered) model is described. As additions to the shared low-order mood construct, evidence of higher-order clinical features (i.e. observable psychomotor disturbance and psychotic features) should be sought to assist definition of melancholic and psychotic depressive subtypes.

Step 3: If a non-melancholic depressive disorder, what clinical subgroup?

There is no generally accepted subtyping system for this essentially residual group (if so defined after excluding psychotic and melancholic depression), and where symptoms reflecting the lower-order mood construct dominate the clinical picture. Historically, terms such as 'neurotic depression' and 'reactive depression' were used, with the former emphasizing a premorbid style of neuroticism and high anxiety, and the latter defining depression developing largely in response to a severe life-event stressor.

Such terminology has not persisted in DSM-IV or ICD-10 where, as described, subtyping proceeds largely on a severity dimension (e.g. 'major' and 'minor') but also on patterns of recurrence and persistence.

A broader clinical approach, albeit proceeding beyond symptoms alone, may have utility here, as various multivariate analytic strategies have identified two non-melancholic subtypes with quite striking consistency. Thus, an early factor-analytic study[25] suggested both a 'hostile' type (evidenced by irritability as well as anxiety) and an 'anxious–tense' type. Blashfield and Morey[26] reviewed 11 cluster analytic studies suggesting separate 'hostile' and 'anxious' depressive subgroups. In an extensive review of the then published studies, Roth and Barnes[27] suggested three principal subgroups, with depression associated with a personality disorder, in addition to 'hostile' and 'anxious' depression.

While such 'hostile' and 'anxious' subgroups have been identified for a lengthy period, clear and consistent descriptions are lacking. Grinker et al.[28] described those with 'hostile' depression as unappreciative, actively angry, provocative, and making excessive demands of and complaints about their therapists. Rosenthal and Gudeman[29] described such group members as having a self-pitying constellation, together with external blame, hypochondriasis, anxiety, demanding and complaining behaviours, irritability, and hostility. They, like Paykel,[16] noted that such patients tended to be younger. The second ('anxiety') subgroup is variably interpreted as defining either those with an anxious personality or temperament, or the presence of significant coterminous anxiety symptoms when primarily depressed.

It is probably most useful to view these two suggested subgroups as 'spectrum disorders', with the term 'spectrum' capturing a continuum between temperament/personality style and symptom states,[30] a model with the temperament component indirectly supported by a recent factor analysis of DSM personality disorders identifying two basic dimensions (i.e. 'hostile' and 'anxious') interpersonal attitudes.[31] The spectrum model allows the possibility that certain biological factors may influence both temperament and personality style, as well as shape surface marker symptoms (here 'hostility' and 'anxiety').

A recent research report[32] suggests that those who develop an 'irritable/hostile' depression tend to be more likely to have a cluster B personality and to report 'acting out' behaviours when stressed (e.g. breaking things, storming around and yelling, being reckless, self-injuring, or otherwise demonstrating a 'short fuse' response to stress). This subgroup was young, so that their 'hostility' may have been a reflection of age. A percentage of the subgroup also had significant anxiety and it may be that, for these, 'irritability' is an externalization of significant anxiety.

By contrast, those with an 'anxious depressive' spectrum disorder appeared more likely[32] to internalize anxiety. They tended to have shown shyness and behavioural inhibition in childhood, to have high rates of lifetime anxiety disorders, score high on trait anxiety, view themselves as 'worriers', 'nervy', or 'tense', and to rate as having a cluster C personality style. They developed their first episode of depression at a young age, had frequent depressive episodes and their depression tended to be highly persistent. They also had a seemingly high rate of becoming dependent on anxiolytic drugs and alcohol, as well as being highly likely to self-injure and attempt suicide. When stressed, they were somewhat more likely to 'act in' by becoming quiet, retiring to their room, crying, and 'stewing'. The clinical picture of their depression was noteworthy for the high frequency of anxiety symptoms. Thus, anxiety was evident both in the temperament pattern and in the prominent symptom profile when depressed.

The suggested profile of these spectrum disorders is not only important for clinical consideration, but in facilitating research into possible neurobiological determinants and to consider any treatment specificity. There have been few studies that have examined the last issue. Blashfield and Morey[33] concluded, from their review, that 'anxious depressives respond well to major and minor tranquillizers but not to tricyclics', while hostile depressives show little improvement with conventional drug therapies', while Fava et al.[34] reported that anxious depressives were more likely to be non-responders to a selective serotonin reuptake inhibitor (**SSRI**) than other depressive subtypes (including 'hostile depressives'). However, as there is currently no formal classification of these suggested groups, research examining for any such treatment specificity or differentiation is rare and limited. Certainly, there is a strong clinical impression that those with an anxious worrying temperament and a non-melancholic depression do well with an SSRI.

'Reactive depression' (or as used in DSM-IV and ICD-10, 'adjustment disorder') is surprisingly difficult to confirm empirically as an 'entity'. This is not to deny that a significant percentage of depressed patients present with a history of having decompensated only as a consequence of a major and stressful life event. Various interpretations have been reviewed,[32] and range from antecedent life events producing, triggering, and maintaining depressive episodes through to life events being epiphenomenal. In an empirical study,[35] the authors were unable to establish clinical, family history, and even life-event stress differences between those with 'situational' and 'non-situational' major depression. In an accompanying editorial, Glass[36] concluded that 'the presence or absence of a precipitant does not seem to be useful for subdividing groups of patients with major depression' and questioned the validity of the intuitively appealing concept of 'situational depression'.

Conflicting evidence of 'reactive depression' may reflect sampling issues. In the community, 'depression' is a common transient response to life-event stress. Thus, most 'normal' people presumably possess mechanisms promoting spontaneous remission of depression within a few days. In clinical samples, where a duration criterion (usually of 2 weeks) is imposed, the utility of the construct is clearly less apparent, and raises the question as to why most patients in clinical samples fail to have a spontaneous remission. A likely explanation is that a significant number have perpetuating factors (e.g. prominent premorbid anxiety) with such factors (here 'worrying' about life-event stressors) tending to maintain the non-melancholic depression. Thus, the life events here act only as provoking factors, seemingly requiring interaction with predispositional or other vulnerability factors.

Thus, while diagnoses of 'reactive depression' and 'adjustment disorder' appear to have clinical validity, they should not be accepted at face value, and should more encourage clinical consideration of predisposing vulnerabilities. The clinician may still seek to assist the patient to resolve or to come to terms with the life-event stressors, but, equally importantly, should seek to identify any predisposing variables that might also benefit from clinical intervention. Common scenarios are the presence of significant anxiety and personality disorder which, if treated or modified, may not only efficiently help resolution of the depression but reduce ongoing vulnerability to further depressive episodes.

Step 4: Distinguishing a melancholic subtype

In DSM-IV, the 'melancholic features specifier' requires, in addition to a base diagnosis of major depression, either one of two A criteria and three (or more) of six B criteria, with most of the latter comprising the so-called 'endogeneity symptoms' (it is therefore another hierarchical model). However, the DSM criteria for melancholia have a number of limitations. Firstly, criterion A (loss of pleasure and/or lack of mood reactivity) is met by most clinically depressed patients, whether 'melancholic' or 'non-melancholic'. Secondly, some of the criterion B features are vague. One, 'distinct quality' is defined as a mood different to that experienced after 'the death of a loved one'. As such, it is a negative definition (akin to defining 'psychiatry' as 'not cardiology'). A second, 'excessive or inappropriate guilt', is a concatenated descriptor, able to subsume the excessive expression of normal guilt, as well as guilt held at an overvalued or delusional level. Several others are non-specific (e.g. early morning wakening, significant anorexia or weight loss), in that they occur commonly in other psychiatric conditions (e.g. anxiety disorders) as well as in other expressions of depression.

Nelson and Charney[37] undertook a review of 33 studies using several multivariate statistical approaches to identify melancholic clinical features or 'endogeneity symptoms'. They found no support for appetite/weight loss and insomnia, little support for early morning wakening and 'distinct quality', but some support for a severely depressed and non-reactive mood, loss of interest in pleasurable activities (or anhedonia), and psychotic features. The most strongly associated feature was psychomotor change (with retardation more consistently associated than agitation). When Rush and Weissenburger[38] examined nine diagnostic systems for diagnosing melancholia or endogenous depression, the only common criterion in all nine was psychomotor retardation (with psychomotor agitation included in six). Our research[39] has established that the specificity of psychomotor disturbance to 'melancholia' is dependent on measuring it as a sign. If assessed as a 'symptom', most depressed patients, independent of depressive type, will admit to feeling 'slowed down' (or, less commonly, agitated), so that its subtyping potential is diffused or lost. If assessed as a sign, its specificity (i.e. presence in melancholic and absence in non-melancholic depression) is impressive.

Thus, and returning to a hierarchical model, differentiation between the non-melancholic and melancholic disorders (on the basis of clinical features) appears assisted principally by the specific feature of behaviourally evident psychomotor disturbance. As measured by the sign-based CORE system,[39] psychomotor disturbance is reflected along three dimensions, essentially assessing motor retardation and

agitation, as well as cognitive processing difficulties, although components are not mutually exclusive. For example, those with significant agitation may have it present for much of the time or, and more commonly, have a base of retardation with intermittent epochs of agitation.

The mood disorder tends to be more severe in melancholic than in non-melancholic depression—either intrinsically or because some of the so-called 'endogeneity symptoms' (e.g. non-reactive mood, anhedonia, diurnal variation in mood and energy) are more severe or more likely to be present in melancholia, but such a difference is dimensional and does not, of itself, allow clear distinction of melancholic and non-melancholic depression.

Step 5: Distinguishing psychotic depression

Proceeding to psychotic (or delusional) depression, here the central mood component generally appears to the clinical observer to be even more severe than in melancholic depression but such patients not uncommonly deny or minimize a depressed mood. A number of 'endogeneity symptoms' are also frequently more severe (particularly non-reactive mood, anhedonia, insomnia, and constipation). One frequent feature in melancholic depression (i.e. diurnal variation of mood) is, however, rarely present at episode nadir in psychotic depression, as the patient is more likely to be consistently depressed across the days. Observable psychomotor disturbance is present and generally markedly more severe than in melancholic depression. In some, the combination of the cognitive processing problems and motor change (retardation in particular) can give the impression of a dementing process, effectively an example of 'pseudodementia'.

The key specific feature, however, that distinguishes psychotic depression from the melancholic and non-melancholic disorders is the presence of psychotic features. Delusions are almost invariably present while hallucinations (auditory most commonly) are present in 10 to 20 per cent according to representative studies. DSM-IV subdivides delusions and hallucinations as 'mood congruent' (where themes of guilt, disease, death, nihilism, and personal inadequacy dominate) and 'mood incongruent' (where psychotic features appear independent of the depressive theme and might include persecutory themes, delusions of control, as well as thought insertion and thought broadcasting) states. It is important to emphasize that mood-incongruent states are common and do not, by themselves, challenge a diagnosis of delusional depression.

A significant percentage (approximately one-third) of patients with psychotic depression develop constipation. In a significant percentage it appears to be a primary feature (not merely a consequence of psychotropic medication), and was so described in historical descriptions[7] of severe depression over the centuries. One term was 'costiveness', with 'costive' being defined as 'slow in action or in expressing ideas, opinions' and derived from the Latin word constipatus. Constipation may serve as a nidus of delusional interpretation (e.g. the depressed patient who believes that their bowels have turned to concrete, or that they have a bowel cancer).

When psychomotor disturbance is extremely severe, it may not be possible for psychotic features to be elicited, particularly if the patient is mute. Many patients are diffident to reveal psychotic material, and here indirect questions can often be useful. In particular, pursuing the presence of 'guilt' can assist, with guilt here defined as a sense of self-blame and not merely self-criticism, together with a sense of remorse for wrong acts or omissions that are independent of any concern about potential evaluation by others. While a high percentage of depressed patients experience guilt, for most it is explainable by circumstances (e.g. the patient concerned by their depression preventing them from optimally looking after their family). In psychotic depression, the guilt is more likely to be held at the level of an overvalued idea or at a formally delusional level. If direct inquiry about guilt does not elicit delusional material, then asking the question 'Do you, in any way, feel any sense that you deserve to be punished?' can often be helpful in eliciting previously unexpressed psychotic material.

Differential diagnosis and ascertainment difficulties

Depression

The three key features of lowered self-esteem, increased self-criticism, and acknowledgment of a depressed mood distinguish depression phenomenologically from states such as grief or bereavement—where there is a distinct sense of 'loss', but no primary 'loss' of self-esteem. They also assist phenomenological differentiation from anxiety, where the individual is more likely to report a sense of insecurity, fear, apprehension, worry, panic, or of 'going mad'. In practice, such features, together with less specific concomitants such as crying, non-reactive mood, and anhedonia, assist in making a diagnosis of depression in the majority of instances.

At the practical level, such a definitional approach may fail in certain groups. The first group comprises some patients with psychotic or melancholic depression, as a percentage appear more emotionally blunted and 'flat' rather than depressed. They may deny depression, self-blame. and worthlessness, and instead note a lack of feeling (or vitality), sluggishness, enervation, or emphasize a physical state, termed 'corporization' by Schneider,[40] with reports of pain or physical sensations in the head, chest, or stomach. As noted earlier, others may have such profound psychomotor disturbance that they do not respond to questioning and appear as if they have a dementia (here a so-called 'pseudodementia'). In such instances, pursuit of proxy items (severe psychomotor disturbance, pathological guilt, overvalued ideas) may assist. If unsuccessful, the diagnosis may require corroborative reports and clinical observation, as well as certain investigations (e.g. CT scans, single-photon emission CT scans, EEG) to exclude a dementia. In a percentage of the elderly, however, a depressive episode and dementia may coexist, and reflect a shared aetiological process.

Secondly, there are some patients and certain cultures where psychological issues are either denied or expressed somatically, although careful and directed questioning about central depressive descriptors will usually clarify the possibility. If unsuccessful, again the diagnosis may require corroborative reports and clinical observation.

Thirdly, it is commonly difficult to define 'clinical depression' in those with a medical illness. Here, general depression criteria sets risk false-positive diagnoses by including certain features which may be secondary to the medical illness (e.g. fatigue, insomnia, anorexia) rather than reflecting depression *per se*. Common corrective strategies include the 'aetiological approach', where only symptoms viewed as independent of the medical condition are counted, the 'exclusive approach', eliminating potentially confounded items such as anorexia, the 'inclusive approach', where all symptoms are counted irrespective of their origin, and the 'substitutive approach', excluding features that could be due to the medical illness and substituting features such as social withdrawal and crying.

In some cases where depression has been established, the salient clinical difficulty is in determining whether depression is or is not the primary disorder in those with concomitant major medical problems, excessive alcohol intake, organic central nervous system disease, and certain psychiatric conditions (e.g. anxiety states, depressive personality disorder). Clinical judgement is generally required with two alternate logical approaches: either weighting the disorders hierarchically or sequentially. The hierarchical approach assumes that the more severe disorder is the primary one, while the sequential approach weights the antecedent condition (e.g. organic disorder, schizophrenia, anxiety). Acceptance of one approach does not logically bind the clinician to any therapeutic consequence (such as necessarily treating only the more severe or primary condition).

Mania/hypomania

The differential diagnoses for manic states essentially include other psychotic conditions (e.g. schizophrenia, drug-induced psychosis) and, rarely, a primary organic state. While cross-sectional dissection of the phenomenology can be helpful, there is wisdom in also weighting the longitudinal course. Thus, those with manic states are more likely to describe complete restoration of function between episodes (of mania and/or depression), while this is less likely for those with schizophrenia. Definitive distinction is not always possible, and a diagnosis of 'schizoaffective' disorder may then be appropriate. In severe mania, an 'organic' picture may be suggested, and require exclusion of a dementia or delirium.

The differential diagnosis of hypomanic states is often quite difficult. Questioned about having 'highs', a number of depressed people will present a remission to a euthymic state as a 'high'. Highly creative people may affirm many hypomanic descriptors when possessed by the muse (e.g. less need for sleep, feeling creative and overconfident, being enthused and energized), as may those with a distinctly extroverted or cyclothymic personality when stimulated. Some patients with a cluster B personality style (especially of the borderline type) may also describe mood states that approximate to hypomania. Regrettably, current criteria sets appear to result in a percentage of patients with a primary personality disorder or even a (healthy) cyclothymic personality style being diagnosed as having a hypomanic (or bipolar II) disorder, risking inappropriate treatment.[41] Clarification is probably best assisted by interview of a corroborative witness to determine if hypomanic behaviours are observable.

Conclusion

Current formal classificatory systems allow a large number of depressive subtypes, with criteria designed to assist diagnostic reliability. Most reflect attempts to create classes on the basis of severity-weighted dimensional models. Terms such as 'major depression' and 'unipolar depression' have achieved acceptance in recent years, for such diagnoses are easily made (and easily reified), but the limitations inherent to their heterogeneity should not be ignored. Until the dissonance between the formal classifications and clinician-derived models has been resolved, practitioners should proceed by recognizing the advantages and limitations to competing approaches.

References

1. Kessler, R.C., Nelson, C.B., McGonagle, K.A., Liu, J., Swartz, M., and Blazer, D.G. (1996). Co-morbidity of DSM-III-R major depressive disorder in the general population: results from the US National Comorbidity Survey. *British Journal of Psychiatry*, **168** (Supplement 30), 17–30.

2. Goodwin, F.K. and Jamison, K.R. (1990). *Manic-depressive illness*. Oxford University Press, New York.

3. American Psychiatric Association (1994). *Diagnostic and statistical manual of mental disorders* (4th edn). American Psychiatric Association, Washington, DC.

4. World Health Organization (1992). *The ICD-10 classification of mental and behavioural disorders—clinical descriptions and diagnostic guidelines*. World Health Organization, Geneva.

5. Leonhard, K. (1957). *The classification of endogenous psychoses* (transl. R. Berman). Irvington, New York.

6. Altschule, M.D. (1967) The two kinds of depression according to St. Paul. *British Journal of Psychiatry*, **113**, 779–80.

7. Jackson, S.W. (1986). *Melancholia and depression: from Hippocratic times to modern times*. Yale University Press, New Haven, CT.

8. Berrios, G.E. (1988). Melancholia and depression during the 19th century. *British Journal of Psychiatry*, **153**, 298–304.

9. Maudsley, H. (1985). *The pathology of the mind: a study of its distempers, deformities and disorders*. Macmillan, London.

10. Kraepelin, E. (1921). *Manic depressive insanity and paranoia*. Livingstone, Edinburgh.

11. Freud, S. (1917). Mourning and melancholia. In *Standard edition of the complete psychological works of Sigmund Freud*, Vol. 14 (ed. J. Strachey), pp. 243–60. Hogarth Press, London, 1957.

12. Mapother, E. (1926). Manic depressive psychosis. *British Medical Journal*, **2**, 872–7.

13. Gillespie, R.D. (1929). The clinical differentiation of types of depression. *Guy's Hospital Report*, **2**, 306–44.

14. Lewis, A. (1934). Melancholia: a clinical survey of depressive states. *Journal of Mental Science*, **80**, 277–378.

15. Kiloh, L.G. and Garside, R.F. (1963). The independence of neurotic depression and endogenous depression. *British Journal of Psychiatry*, **109**, 451–63.

16. Paykel, E.S. (1971). Classification of depressed patients: a cluster analysis derived grouping. *British Journal of Psychiatry*, **118**, 275–88.

17. Parker, G., Hadzi-Pavlovic, P., Mitchell, P., *et al.* (1994). Defining melancholia: properties of a refined sign-based measure. *British Journal of Psychiatry*, **164**, 316–26.

18. Kendell, R.E. (1989). Clinical validity. In *The validity of psychiatric diagnosis* (ed. L.N. Robins and J.E. Barrett), pp. 305–23. Raven Press, New York.

19. Hickie, I. (1996). Issues in classification: III. Utilising behavioural constructs in melancholia research. In *Melancholia: a disorder of movement and mood. A phenomenological and neurobiological review* (ed. G. Parker and D. Hadzi-Pavlovic), pp. 38–56. Cambridge University Press, New York.

20. American Psychiatric Association (1980). *Diagnostic and statistical manual of mental disorders* (3rd edn). American Psychiatric Association, Washington, DC.

21. Zimmerman, M., Black, D.W., and Coryell, W. (1989). Diagnostic criteria for melancholia. The comparative validity of DSM-III and DSM-III-R. *Archives of General Psychiatry*, **46**, 361–8.

22. American Psychiatric Association (1987*). Diagnostic and statistical manual of mental disorders* (3rd edn). American Psychiatric Association, Washington, DC.

23. Rush, A.J. and Weissenburger, J.E. (1995). Melancholic symptom features: a review and options for DSM-IV. In *DSM-IV source book*, Vol. 2. American Psychiatric Press, Washington, DC.

24. Spiker, D.G., Weiss J.C., Dealy, R.S., *et al.* (1985). The pharmacological treatment of delusional depression. *American Journal of Psychiatry*, **142**, 430–5.

25. Overall, J.E., Hollister, C.E., Johnson, M., and Pennington, J. (1966). Nosology of depression and differential response to drugs. *Journal of the American Medical Association*, **195**, 946–8.

26. Blashfield, R.K. and Morey, L.C. (1979). The classification of depression through cluster analysis. *Comprehensive Psychiatry*, **20**, 516–27.

27. Roth, M. and Barnes, T.R.E. (1981). The classification of affective disorders: a synthesis of old and new concepts. *Comprehensive Psychiatry*, **22**, 54–77.

28. Grinker, R.R., Miller, J., Sabshin, M., Nunn, R., and Nunnally, J.C. (1961). *The phenomena of depressions*. Harper and Row, New York.

29. Rosenthal, S.H. and Gudeman, J.E. (1967). The endogenous depressive pattern. An empirical investigation. *Archives of General Psychiatry*, **16**, 241–9.

30. Cassano, G.B., Michelini, S., Shear, M.K., Coli, E., Maser, J.D., and Frank, E. (1997). The panic–agoraphobic spectrum: a descriptive approach to the assessment and treatment of subtle symptoms. *American Journal of Psychiatry*, **154** (Supplement), 27–38.

31. Schotte, C.K.W., de Doncker, D., Vankerckhoven, C., Vertommen, H., and Cosyns, P. (1998). Self-report assessment of the DSM-IV personality disorders. Measurement of trait and distress characteristics: the ADP-IV. *Psychological Medicine*, **28**, 1179–88.

32. Parker, G., Hadzi-Pavlovic, D., Roussos, J., *et al.* (1998). Non-melancholic depression: the contribution of personality, anxiety and life events to subclassification. *Psychological Medicine*, **28**, 1209–19.

33. Blashfield, R.K. and Morey, L.C. (1979). The classification of depression through cluster analysis. *Comprehensive Psychiatry*, **20**, 516–27.

34. Fava, M., Uebelacker, L.A., Alpert, J.E., Nierenberg, A.A., Pava, J.A., and Rosenbaum, J.F. (1997). Major depressive subtypes and treatment response. *Biological Psychiatry*, **42**, 568–76.

35. Hirschfeld, R.M.A., Klerman, G.L., Andreasen, N.C., Clayton, P.J., and Keller, M.B. (1985). Situational major depressive disorder. *Archives of General Psychiatry*, **42**, 1109–14.

36. Glass, R.M. (1985). Situational and neurotic-reactive depression. *Archives of General Psychiatry*, **42**, 1126–7.

37. Nelson, J.C. and Charney, D.S. (1981). The symptoms of major depressive illness. *American Journal of Psychiatry*, **138**, 1–13.

38. Rush, A.J. and Weissenburger, J.E. (1994). Melancholic symptom features and DSM-IV. *American Journal of Psychiatry*, **151**, 489–98.

39. Parker, G. and Hadzi-Pavlovic, D. (1996). *Melancholia: a disorder of movement and mood. A phenomenological and neurobiological review*. Cambridge University Press, New York.

40. Schneider, K. (1920). The stratification of emotional life and the structure of the depressive states. *Zentralblat für Neurologie, Psychiatrie* **59**, 281.

41. Bolton, S. and Gunderson, J.G. (1996). Distinguishing borderline personality disorder from bipolar disorder: differential diagnosis and implications. *American Journal of Psychiatry* **153**, 1202–7.

4.5.4 Epidemiology of mood disorders

Peter R. Joyce

The Global Burden of Disease, which is a comprehensive assessment of mortality and disability from diseases and injuries in 1990 and projected to 2020, highlights the importance of mood disorders for the world. Using the measure of disability-adjusted life years, it was determined that unipolar major depression was the fourth leading cause of disease burden in the world. It was also projected that, in the year

2020, unipolar major depression would be the second leading cause of disease burden in the world. Disability-adjusted life years is based on both mortality and disability. If one looks at disability alone, then unipolar major depression was the leading cause of disability in the world in 1990, and bipolar disorder was the sixth leading cause. Across the world, 10.7 per cent of disability can be attributed to unipolar major depression and, in developed countries, unipolar major depression contributes to nearly 20 per cent of disease burden in women aged from 15 to 44 years.[1]

The mood disorders have received considerable attention in psychiatric epidemiology over the last two decades. These received particular attention in the five-site United States National Institutes of Mental Health Epidemiologic Catchment Area Study (ECA), as well as the epidemiological studies in other countries around the world that used the ECA methodology. Mood disorders also received particular attention in the National Comorbidity Survey (NCS) in the United States and in the National Psychiatric Morbidity Survey of Great Britain. Thus there is substantial data from around the world on the epidemiology of these disorders. In addition, many of the population-based twin registries, such as in Virginia, in the United States, have also paid particular interest to mood disorders and have the additional advantage of being able to consider genetic as well as environmental risk factors.

Bipolar disorders

Diagnostic issues

While classical bipolar disorder with episodes of euphoric mania interspersed with episodes of depression is one of the clearest clinical syndromes in psychiatry, the boundaries of bipolar disorder remain contested. As case definition is central to epidemiology, all the contested boundaries of bipolar disorder could influence prevalence rates and our understanding of risk factors. Some of the major boundary issues for bipolar disorder include the overlap of bipolar disorder with psychotic features, with schizoaffective disorder and schizophrenia, and the overlap of bipolar disorder with unipolar major depression when patients who present primarily with depression have brief or mild episodes of hypomania. There is also the overlap of bipolar disorder with apparent personality disorder, especially Cluster B personality disorders such as borderline and narcissistic, and the issue of when hyperthymic personality merges into bipolar disorder.[2,3]

Another important issue in determining caseness of bipolar disorder for epidemiological surveys is symptom pattern. A number of the diagnostic instruments for assessing bipolarity in population surveys limit the questions on mania to a type of symptom profile characterized by euphoria, grandiosity, increased energy, and decreased sleep. Whether the commonly used epidemiology interviews adequately detect those individuals who have manic episodes characterized by irritability, anger, and activation is very debatable. Furthermore, as insight is sometimes impaired in hypomania and mania, and as these are uncommon disorders, the accuracy of case detection of bipolar disorders in populations remains an issue for further research.[4]

Prevalence

Population studies such as the ECA, and its related cross-national studies, and the NCS reported that the lifetime prevalence of bipolar disorder varies from 0.3 to 1.5 per cent. The NCS data include only bipolar I data, while the ECA includes bipolar I and bipolar II disorder.[4,5] In all studies, the 6-month prevalence is not much lower than the lifetime prevalence of bipolar disorder. These findings reflect the high degree of chronicity and/or recurrence associated with bipolar disorder.

In these population studies, the mean age of onset of bipolar disorder has varied from 17 to 27 years. However, as age of onset is not normally distributed, the mean is a slightly misleading variable; in clinical samples, while the mean age of onset may be in the twenties, the most common age of onset is the late teenage years.[6]

In bipolar disorder, the prevalence in males and females is similar. This is in contrast to the consistent female excess found in major depression.

Comorbidity

In the NCS, all identified bipolar I individuals suffered from at least one, and often up to three or more, comorbid disorders. The most common comorbid disorders included the full range of anxiety disorders, alcohol and drug dependence, and conduct disorder or other antisocial behaviours.

Alcohol and drug abuse and/or dependence are commonly comorbid with bipolar disorder. Old studies found that binge drinking was especially common in bipolar individuals and that this binge pattern of drinking was more associated with manic episodes than with depressive episodes. Clinical studies find that bipolar patients with a comorbid substance dependence are less compliant with prescribed mood stabilizers and have more frequent hospital readmissions.

Individuals with bipolar disorder have the full range of anxiety disorders, including phobias, panic disorder, and obsessive–compulsive disorder. In recent years, the comorbidity of bipolar disorder with panic disorder has received particular attention. In the NCS, for instance, the odds ratio for having panic disorder with major depression was 6.8, but the odds ratio for having panic disorder with bipolar disorder was 13.2. This differential pattern of comorbidity of panic disorder with bipolar disorder and major depression may assist in the search for aetiological or risk factors.

Another area of high comorbidity with bipolar disorder is that of childhood conduct disorder. One of the major issues in understanding this high rate of comorbidity is a diagnostic issue—whether childhood conduct disorder and/or childhood attention-deficit disorder are sometimes the first manifestations or precursors of bipolar disorder. Certainly, if the pattern of conduct-disorder symptoms or attention-deficit symptoms is episodic rather than consistent over time, the issue becomes whether these are not early manifestations of bipolar disorder rather than truly independent comorbid conditions.

Use of health services

In the ECA study, 39 per cent of those with bipolar I or bipolar II disorders received outpatient psychiatric treatment within 1 year and about 10 per cent would receive inpatient treatment within a 6-month period. In the NCS study, 45 per cent of those with bipolar disorder had received psychiatric treatment in the previous 12 months; although 93 per cent reported lifetime treatment for their bipolar disorder. However, both of these studies suggest that more than half the individuals with bipolar disorder are not currently in psychiatric treatment and, given the high morbidity and mortality associated with bipolar disorder, this is of major concern.[4]

Risk factors

In considering the risk factors for the development of bipolar disorder, it is useful to separate risk factors into those that are risk factors for lifetime vulnerability (for example genetic factors) and those that are risk factors for the onset of an episode of depression or mania (for example life events). Thus, in determining risk factors for lifetime vulnerability, genetic factors constitute the largest single risk factor. However, if one is considering who is vulnerable to an episode of mania over the next 6 months, genetic factors will play a relatively smaller part and predictions may best be based on other factors such as past history, childbirth, being treated for depression with antidepressant medication, and the approach of spring or summer. Genetic risk factors are discussed further in Chapter 4.5.5.1.

Organic factors

Although organic factors, such as some type of central nervous system damage, are unusual risk factors in young adults, in late-onset bipolar disorder (age of onset more than 50 years) organic disease of the central nervous system is an increasing factor for the development of mania. In younger adults, AIDS and head injury are two important aetiological factors in a limited number of cases of bipolar disorder.

Other biological factors

A range of other biological factors are particularly relevant risk factors to the onset of episodes of illness, but they may contribute a relatively small part to lifetime vulnerability. Many women have their first episode of depression or mania in the postpartum period. While a limited number of women may have manic episodes limited to the postpartum period, postpartum episodes of mania are more commonly part of a long-term bipolar disorder and these women will have episodes both precipitated by childbirth and at other times in their life. Indeed, in the postpartum period, having a history of bipolar disorder is one of the strongest risk factors for the development of a postpartum psychosis.

There is substantial evidence that seasonal patterns influence the onset of manic and depressive episodes. There are consistent findings of an excess of manic episodes in late spring and early summer. To date, however, the nature of the environmental factors that influence this late spring, early summer peak of manic episodes is less clear.

There is also substantial evidence that disruptions of normal biological rhythms may precipitate the onset of manic or depressive episodes. This has been documented in relation to international travel involving east–west or west–east travel with disruption of circadian rhythms. Disruption of circadian rhythms through shift-work or other factors, which disrupt the normal sleep cycles, may also be important triggers to the onset of episodes of mania. Indeed, this risk factor is now influencing bipolar disorder management plans by including strategies for minimizing disruptions to 24-h biological rhythms.

Life events

Adverse life events have been well documented to be precipitants of manic episodes, as well as depression. It appears that life events are more likely prior to the first or second episode of mania and are less likely later in the course of illness.

Childhood experiences

While there is substantial evidence that adverse childhood experiences contribute to the later development of major depression, there are relatively few data to support the idea that adversity in childhood influences the development of bipolar disorder.

Subthreshold symptoms

While there is a paucity of information from population studies as to how subsyndromal symptoms may be a risk factor for bipolar disorder, family studies have long been suggestive of the fact that individuals may manifest subsyndromal symptoms or syndromes well before the clear onset of bipolar affective disorder. Thus, there are individuals who have 'mini-episodes' of mania or depression who are, presumably, at high risk of the subsequent development of bipolar disorder. Similarly, individuals in their teenage years with a pattern of mood swings and cyclothymia are probably also at increased risk of the development of bipolar disorder. Also, individuals with a hyperthymic personality, particularly if they have had past episodes of depression, are a high-risk group for the subsequent development of bipolar disorder.

Depressive disorders

Diagnostic issues

A key issue for the epidemiology of depressive disorders is defining the boundaries of major depression and dysthymia. Depressive symptoms in the community are common, and defining both the symptom count and the duration at which depressive symptoms count as part of a clinical disorder is arbitrary. Recently, Kendler and Gardner[7] examined the boundaries of major depression as defined by DSM-IV in a population-based twin sample of women. They found that, if a twin had four or fewer depressive symptoms, syndromes composed of symptoms involving no or minimal impairment, and episodes lasting less than 14 days, then the individual's co-twin was still at an increased risk of major depression. Kendler and Gardner concluded that they could find no empirical support for the DSM-IV requirement of duration for 2 weeks, five symptoms, or clinically significant impairment. These authors suggested that major depression, as articulated by DSM-IV, may be a diagnostic convention imposed on a continuum of depressive symptoms of varying severity and duration. Wainwright et al.,[8] using data from the National Psychiatric Morbidity Survey of Great Britain, have also suggested that research should move beyond a binary decision of case versus non-case, and utilize a probablistic measure of psychiatric case status, replacing the arbitrary threshold with a smooth transition. This type of approach allows the benefits of syndrome diagnosis to be retained, while not falling into the dilemma of an arbitrary threshold that may lack validity.

Provided that one accepts the arbitrary definition of major depression, then determining the rates of current depressive disorders is not especially problematic. However, there are major methodological issues involved in determining whether an individual has ever had a lifetime episode of major depression. Lifetime prevalence rates vary from 4.4 per cent in the United States ECA study, to 17.1 per cent in the NCS, and to over 30 per cent in Kendler's Virginia twin sample of women. In part, subjects in the community may forget or fail to report past episodes of major depression, and the manner in which the questions are asked may importantly influence lifetime rates of depression. In the Diagnostic Interview Schedule, which was used in the ECA, respondents were asked about lifetime symptoms, a lifetime diagnosis was made, and then recency of the lifetime diagnosis was determined. More recent diagnostic interview schedules, such as the Composite International Diagnostic Interview, first ask about current depressive symptoms and then, having 'primed' individuals about depressive symptoms, go on to enquire about past depressive episodes. Interviews that follow the schedule of 'priming' before asking about past episodes appear to obtain considerably higher rates of lifetime major depression. Determining lifetime rates of depression with greater precision is an important task, as the vulnerability to depression conferred by risk factors such as genetic factors and childhood experiences may be wrongly estimated if lifetime rates of major depression are imprecise. For instance, when Kendler et al.[9] examined the heritability of major depression and corrected for the moderate reliability of a lifetime diagnosis of major depression, the heritability estimate increased from 40 per cent to over 70 per cent. As concluded by Kendler, major depression is not a disorder of high reliability and moderate heritability, but is a diagnosis of moderate reliability and high heritability.

DSM-IV allows major depression to be further subclassified into subtypes, such as melancholia and atypical and psychotic depression. Most of the traditional epidemiology studies have tended to ignore the issue of subtyping major depression. Recently, however, the issue of the atypical depression subtype has received particular attention in the study of the Virginia twins and in the NCS. In both these studies, latent class analysis suggests that atypical depression is a distinct subtype with several distinctive features, such as higher rates of parental alcohol- and drug-use disorders, higher interpersonal dependency, and higher rates of conduct disorder. If risk factors for atypical depression are, in part, distinct from risk factors for other subtypes of major depression, then for epidemiology to contribute to an understanding of aetiology it will be important to undertake further work on depressive subtypes.[10,11]

Prevalence

In the ECA, the 6-month prevalence of major depression across five sites was 2.2 per 100.[12] In Edmonton, Canada, the 6-month prevalence rate was 3.2 per 100[13] and, in Christchurch, New Zealand, the rate was 5.3 per 100.[14] In the NCS, the 1-month prevalence of a major depressive episode was 6.1 per 100.[15] In the National Psychiatric Morbidity Surveys of Great Britain, the 1-week rate of a depressive episode was 2.1 per 100.[16] Together, these studies would suggest that the current rate of major depression is in the realm of 2 to 5 per cent.

The estimates of the lifetime rate of major depression are much more variable. The lowest rate reported is 4.4 per 100 from the ECA study, while, in the study of Virginia twins, the lifetime rate of major depression is over 30 per cent. It is reasonable to believe that the true lifetime rate of major depression is probably in the realm of 10 to 20 per 100, and so caution should be exercised in expressing lifetime rates of depression with undue precision.

These rates of major depression may also be lower if the rate of bipolar disorder is higher. Isolated clinical studies have found that 1 in 2, not 1 in 10, individuals presenting with depressive disorders have

features of bipolar spectrum disorders. If these figures are correct, then this would presumably lower the rates of major depression, but would correspondingly increase the rates of bipolar disorders.

Over the past decade, one of the controversial findings in the epidemiology of major depression has been whether the rates of depression are increasing, and whether it is occurring at a younger age. The initial suggestions by Klerman and Weissman[17] provoked a variety of studies. Despite methodological concerns about the reliability of lifetime major depression, studies across countries have reasonably consistently documented an increasing rate of major depression with an earlier age of onset.[18] As mood disorders are the single largest risk factor for suicide, it is also of note that, in most Western countries, the rate of suicide, especially in young adults, has increased considerably over the past 20 years.

Risk factors

Genetics

There is now substantial evidence that genetic factors are of major importance as risk factors for vulnerability to major depression. While traditional estimates have put the heritability at about 40 per cent, when Kendler et al.[9] allowed for the moderate reliability of the diagnosis of major depression, the heritability estimate increased to 70 per cent. Of greater interest is that the genes for major depression do not appear to be unique for depression, but overlap with the genes for anxiety and the genes for neuroticism.[19,20] Wilhelm et al.[21] have suggested that the greater prevalence of depression in women is due to the strong association of anxiety and neuroticism with depression, and that the higher rates of anxiety and neuroticism in women lead to higher rates of depression.

Gender

One of the most consistent findings in the epidemiology of major depression is that the ratio of women to men is approximately 2:1. This increased rate of major depression in women arises during puberty, as in childhood there is a slightly higher prevalence of depression in boys than girls. The timing of this transition in rates by gender is related to biological puberty rather than just to age.

Childhood experiences

Early theorizing suggested that the loss of a parent in childhood increased the later risk for major depression; although many studies have examined this issue, they have inconsistently found it to be a risk factor for adult depression.[22] However, studies that examine the nature of child–parent attachment using a measure such as the Parental Bonding Instrument have consistently found that a lack of parental care is associated with increased rates of depression.[23] More recently, childhood sexual abuse has been established as a risk factor for adult major depression.

However, cumulative childhood disadvantage almost certainly poses a greater risk to later depression than any single childhood variable in isolation. Thus, if studies only look at single childhood risk factors, they may miss the full impact of global childhood adversity. The converse of childhood risk factors is childhood resilience, and it is probable that one good relationship with an adult and high intelligence in the child may, in part, protect from other adversities.

Personality

There has been a long history of interest in the likelihood that people with certain personality traits are more vulnerable to depression than others. It is likely that those individuals who are unduly anxious, impulsive, and obsessional may have increased rates of later major depression. The best data exists for neuroticism, which emerges as a clear risk factor for the later development of depressive and anxiety disorders. However, as already mentioned, the same genes seem to contribute to the development of neuroticism and to later anxiety and depressive disorders.

Social environment

There has been considerable interest in the role of marital status as a risk factor for major depression. For men, it appears clear that married men have the lowest rate of depression, while separated or divorced men have the highest rates of major depression. In women, the association is slightly less clear, but in the ECA study the same findings applied for women as for men. Understanding the nature of the association between marital status and rates of depression is more problematic. If personality is a risk factor for depression, then the same traits could interfere with the ability to marry or to stay married. There is little doubt that depression sometimes contributes to marital maladjustment and separation or divorce. Finally, the stresses associated with divorce and separation could increase the likelihood of an episode of depression occurring.

In the classic and influential work of George Brown on working-class women,[24] having three or more children, a lack of paid employment, and the lack of a confidant were risk factors for the development of an episode of depression. Subsequent studies have inconsistently replicated the risk factors of having children or lack of paid employment, but have supported the finding that the lack of a confidant increases the risk of depression.

It is well established that adverse life events, particularly those characterized by loss, increases the risk of an episode of major depression. The increased vulnerability to an episode appears to last for a period of 2 to 3 months following such an event.[25,26]

Early thinking about depression suggested that there would be those depressions that occurred for largely biological reasons and those precipitated by adverse life events; however, it is now clear that such a dichotomous view is incorrect. Kendler et al.[26] showed that there is a significant genotype by environment interaction in the prediction of onset of major depression. They proposed that genetic factors influence the risk of onset of depression, in part, by increasing the sensitivity of individuals to the depression-inducing effects of stressful life events.

Physical illness

Having a chronic or severe physical illness is associated with an increased risk for depression. The mechanisms behind this increased risk may vary depending upon the physical disorder. In disorders such as Parkinson's disease, it is possible that there are shared neurotransmitter abnormalities between Parkinson's disease and depression. In post-stroke depression, there is good evidence that the location of the lesion, at least in part, contributes to the rate of depression, which suggests a neuroanatomical/neurotransmitter connection between the physical illness and the likelihood of depression. For non-central ner-vous system disorders, such as acute myocardial infarction, diabetes, and cancers, the mechanism for this association is less clear. However, at least in the case of patients with cancer, most do not suffer from major depression and, if they do, the key risk factors are family history and a past history of depression. This suggests that the stress associated with a serious or chronic physical illness may act by bringing out an individual's lifetime vulnerability to depression.

An integrated aetiological model

The ultimate purpose of studying risk factors for depressive disorders is to contribute to the development of an integrated aetiological model. The most promising research in this area has been performed by Kendler and colleagues on women from the Virginia Twin Register.[27] In this study, 680 female–female twin pairs of known zygosity were assessed on three occasions at longer than 1-year intervals. Nine predictor variables (genetic factors, parental warmth, childhood parental loss, lifetime traumas, neuroticism, social support, past depressive episodes, recent difficulties, and recent stressful life events) were examined to see how they contributed prospectively to the development of an episode of major depression over the next 12 months. In considering the results from this study, it is important to bear in mind the limitations of this landmark study—including the facts that the sample was limited to women and that variables such as marital status, the presence of young children in the home, and a history of non-affective psychiatric disorders were not included in the analyses. The model was also predicting the onset of an episode over 12 months and not predicting lifetime episode, when a different combination of variables may have been found. However, despite these caveats, Kendler and colleagues developed a model that predicted 50 per cent of the variance in the liability to develop major depression. The four strongest predictors in order of liability to depression were as follows:

- stressful life events
- genetic factors
- previous history of major depression
- neuroticism.

It is of note that some of the risk factors exerted these effects directly, while other effects were largely indirect. Thus, 60 per cent of the effect of genetic factors on liability to depression was direct, but the remaining 40 per cent was indirect and largely mediated by past episodes of depression, stressful life events, and neuroticism. Variables such as perceived parental warmth had no direct effect on liability to develop an episode of major depression, but did impact upon neuroticism, a history of a past depressive episode, recent difficulties, and lifetime traumas.

The most comparable prospective studies looking at risk factors for the development of major depression have been undertaken during the postpartum period, which is a time of increased risk of depression. In this special case, the most consistent risk factors are family history and a past history of depression, and there is lesser support for a lack of social support, neuroticism, and complications during childbirth.

As one of the key tasks of epidemiology is to contribute to an understanding of aetiology, models that integrate risk factors are important strategies for further research. They provide clinicians with predictive power, and can also guide intervention studies to prevent the onset of episodes of depression.

Comorbidity

One of the important contributions of epidemiology to the study of mood disorders over the past 15 years has been the recognition of the extent to which depression and other psychiatric disorders are often comorbid. In both the ECA study and NCS, over two-thirds of all individuals identified as having an episode of major depression also met the criteria for one or more other psychiatric disorders. Not surprisingly, the most common comorbid disorders are anxiety disorders and substance-abuse disorders. In the NCS, the anxiety disorders with the highest odds ratios indicating comorbidity were generalized anxiety disorder, panic disorder, and post-traumatic stress disorder. It is also important to note that for most anxiety disorders, with the exception of panic disorder, the anxiety disorder usually predates the onset of the depressive disorder.[28] This is of considerable importance, as the risk factors for pure major depression differed from the risk factors for comorbid major depression. Furthermore, the cohort effects of increasing rates of major depression were largely attributable to increasing rates of comorbid major depression, rather than to increasing rates of pure major depression. These results raise important issues for prevention, as it may well be that targeting young people with anxiety disorders could be a major step to the prevention of the development of later major depressive disorders.

The second key area of comorbidity with major depression is with alcohol dependence. Data from the Virginia Twin Register suggest that part of this comorbidity is due to shared genetic factors, although there is also a smaller common environmental risk factor to both disorders.

Another area of considerable comorbidity with major depression are the personality disorders. The comorbidity between major depression and these disorders is receiving considerable attention in clinical samples but, to date, there are only limited data in epidemiological samples on the importance of these patterns of comorbidity.

Use of health services

One of the major challenges for psychiatry presented by epidemiological studies of depression has been the consistent finding that the majority of cases of depression in the community are neither recognized, diagnosed, nor treated. In the ECA study, it was found that 65 to 70 per cent of people with depression had visited a health professional in the last 6 months, but only 15 to 20 per cent had had a visit for a mental health reason and only about 10 per cent had seen a mental health specialist. Ormel et al.[29] found that patients with depression who present with largely somatic rather than psychological symptoms are extremely unlikely to be recognized by general practitioners. Similar findings have also been reported in England.[30] Even if major depression is recognized in the primary care setting, it is often not adequately treated. Even when major depression is treated in primary care, there is evidence to suggest that the outcome is worse if treated by the primary physician than when treated by a mental health specialist.[31]

The findings on the non-recognition and low levels of treatment in primary care have prompted national efforts in the United States (Depression Awareness Recognition and Treatment) and the United Kingdom (with a joint project between the College of Psychiatrists and the College of General Practitioners) to improve the recognition and treatment of depression. Given the importance of depression as the leading risk factor for suicide, many countries interested in lowering suicide rates are targeting the recognition and treatment of depression in the community. The Global Burden of Disease study is further evidence of the impact of mood disorders on our populations.

References

1. Murray, C.J.L. and Lopez, A.D. (1996). *The global burden of disease and global health statistics.* Harvard University Press, Boston, MA.
2. Akiskal, H.S. (1996). The prevalent clinical spectrum of bipolar disorders beyond DSM-IV. *Journal of Clinical Psychopharmacology*, **16**, 4s–14s.
3. Blacker, D. and Tsuang, M.T. (1992). Contested boundaries of bipolar disorder and the limits of categorical diagnosis in psychiatry. *American Journal of Psychiatry*, **149**, 1473–83.
4. Kessler, R.C., Rubinow, D.R., Holmes, C., Abelson, J.M., and Zhao, S. (1997). The epidemiology of DSM-III-R bipolar I disorder in a general population survey. *Psychological Medicine*, **27**, 1079–89.
5. Weissman, M.M., Bland, R.C., Canino, G.J., et al. (1996). Cross national epidemiology of major depression and bipolar disorder. *Journal of the American Medical Association*, **276**, 293–9.
6. Joyce, P.R. (1984). Age of onset in bipolar affective disorder and misdiagnosis as schizophrenia. *Psychological Medicine*, **14**, 145–9.
7. Kendler, K.S. and Gardner, C.O. (1998). Boundaries of major depression: an evaluation of DSM-IV criteria. *American Journal of Psychiatry*, **155**, 172–7.
8. Wainwright, N.W.J., Surtees, P.G., and Gilks, W.R. (1997). Diagnostic boundaries, reasoning and depressive disorder, I. Development of a probabilistic morbidity model for public health psychiatry. *Psychological Medicine*, **27**, 835–45.
9. Kendler, K.S., Neale, M.C., Kessler, R.C., Heath, A.C., and Eaves, L.J. (1993). The lifetime history of major depression in women. Reliability of diagnosis and heritability. *Archives of General Psychiatry*, **50**, 863–70.
10. Sullivan, P.F., Kessler, R.C., and Kendler, K.S. (1998). Latent class analysis of lifetime depressive symptoms in the National Comorbidity Survey. *American Journal of Psychiatry*, **155**, 1399–406.
11. Kendler, K.S., Eaves, L.J., Walters, E.E., Neale, M.C., Heath, A.C., and Kessler, R.C. (1996). The identification and validation of distinct depressive syndromes in a population-based sample of female twins. *Archives of General Psychiatry*, **53**, 391–9.
12. Weissman, M.M., Leaf, P.J., Tischler, G.L., et al. (1988). Affective disorders in five United States communities. *Psychological Medicine*, **18**, 141–53.
13. Bland, R.C., Orn, H., and Newman, S.C. (1988). Epidemiology of psychiatric disorders in Edmonton. *Acta Psychiatrica Scandinavica*, Supplement, 1–80.
14. Oakley-Browne, M.A., Joyce, P.R., Wells, J.E., Bushnell, J.A., and Hornblow, A.R. (1989). Christchurch Psychiatric Epidemiology Study, Part 2. Six month and other period prevalences for specific psychiatric disorders. *Australian and New Zealand Journal of Psychiatry*, **23**, 327–40.
15. Blazer, D.G., Kessler, R.C., McGonagle, K.A., and Swartz, M.S. (1994). The prevalence and distribution of major depression in a national community sample: the National Comorbidity Survey. *American Journal of Psychiatry*, **151**, 979–86.
16. Jenkins, R., Lewis, G., Bebbington, P., et al. (1997). The National Psychiatric Morbidity Surveys of Great Britain—initial findings from the household survey. *Psychological Medicine*, **27**, 775–89.
17. Klerman, G.L. and Weissman, M.M. (1989). Increasing rates of depression. *Journal of the American Medical Association*, **261**, 2229–35.
18. Cross National Collaborative Group (1992). The changing rate of major depression. Cross national comparisons. *Journal of the American Medical Association*, **268**, 3098–105.
19. Kendler, K.S., Neale, M.C., Kessler, R.C., Heath, A.C., and Eaves, L.J. (1992). Major depression and generalized anxiety disorder. Same genes (partly) different environment. *Archives of General Psychiatry*, **49**, 716–22.

20. Andrews, G., Stewart, G., Allen, R., and Henderson, A.S. (1990). The genetics of six neurotic disorders: a twin study. *Journal of Affective Disorders*, **19**, 23–9.

21. Wilhelm, K., Parker, G., and Hadzi-Pavlovic, D. (1997). Fifteen years on: evolving ideas in researching sex differences in depression. *Psychological Medicine*, **27**, 875–83.

22. Tennant, C. (1988). Parental loss in childhood. Its effect in adult life. *Archives of General Psychiatry*, **45**, 1045–50.

23. Parker, G. (1983). Parental 'affectionless control' as an antecedent to adult depression. A risk factor delineated. *Archives of General Psychiatry*, **40**, 956–60.

24. Brown, G.W. and Harris, T. (1978). *Social origins of depression: a study of psychiatric disorders in women*. Tavistock Publications, London.

25. Paykel, E.S. (1978). Contribution of life events to causation of psychiatric illness. *Psychological Medicine*, **8**, 245–53.

26. Kendler, K.S., Kessler, R.C., Walters, E.E., *et al.* (1995). Stressful life events, genetic liability and onset of an episode of major depression in women. *American Journal of Psychiatry*, **152**, 833–42.

27. Kendler, K.S., Kessler, R.C., Neale, M.C., Heath, A.C., and Eaves, L.J. (1993). The prediction of major depression in women: toward an integrated etiological model. *American Journal of Psychiatry*, **150**, 1139–48.

28. Kessler, R.C., Nelson, C.B., McGonagle, K.A., Liu, J., Swartz, M., and Blazer, D.G. (1996). Comorbidity of DSM-III-R major depressive disorder in the general population: results from the US National Comorbidity Survey. *British Journal of Psychiatry*, **168**, 17–30.

29. Ormel, J., Koeter, M.W.J., Van den Brink, W., and van de Willige, G. (1991). Recognition, management and course of anxiety and depression in general practice. *Archives of General Psychiatry*, **48**, 700–6.

30. Gater, R. and Goldberg, D. (1991). Pathways to psychiatric care in South Manchester. *British Journal of Psychiatry*, **159**, 90–6.

31. Schulberg, H., Block, H.R., Madonia, M.J., *et al.* (1996). Treating major depression in primary care practice, eight-month clinical outcomes. *Archives of General Psychiatry*, **53**, 913–19.

4.5.5 Aetiology

4.5.5.1 Genetic and social aetiology of mood disorders

D. Souery, S. Blairy, and J. Mendlewicz

Introduction

Advances towards the understanding of the aetiological mechanisms involved in mood disorders provide interesting yet diverse hypotheses and promising models. In this context, molecular genetics has now been widely incorporated into genetic epidemiological research in psychiatry. Affective disorders and, in particular, bipolar affective disorder have been examined in many molecular genetic studies which have covered a large part of the genome; specific hypotheses such as mutations have also been studied. Most recent studies indicate that several chromosomal regions may be involved in the aetiology of bipolar affective disorder. Other studies have reported the presence of anticipation in bipolar affective disorder[1,2] and in unipolar affective disorder.[3] This phenomenon describes the increase in clinical severity and decrease in age of onset observed in successive generations. This mode of transmission correlates with the presence of specific mutations (trinucleotide repeat sequences) and may represent a genetic fac-

tor involved in the transmission of the disorder.[4,5] Large multicentre and multidisciplinary projects are currently under way in Europe and the United States and hopefully will improve our understanding of the genetic factors involved in affective disorders. In parallel to these new developments in molecular genetics, the classical genetic epidemiology, represented by twin, adoption, and family studies, has provided additional evidence in favour of the genetic hypothesis in mood disorders. Moreover, these methods have been improved through models to test the gene–environment interactions.

In addition to genetic approaches, psychiatric research has focused on the role of psychosocial factors in the emergence of mood disorders. In this approach, psychosocial factors refer to the patient's social life context as well as to personality dimensions. Abnormalities in social behaviour such as impairment in social relationships[6–8] and dysfunctional cognitions[9] have been observed during episodes of affective disorders, and implicated in their aetiology. Further, gender and socio-economic status emerged as having a possible impact on the development of affective disorders. Finally, the onset and outcome of affective disorders could also be explained by interactions between the social life context and the individual's temperament and personality. The importance of temperament and personality characteristics in the aetiology of depression has been emphasized in various theories, although disagreement exists with regard to terminology and the aetiology of the characteristics themselves.

While significant advances have been made in these two major fields of research, it appears that integrative models, taking into account the interactions between biological (genetic) factors and social (psychosocial environment) variables, offer the most reliable way to approach the complex mechanisms involved in the aetiology and outcome of mood disorders. This chapter will review some of the most promising genetic and psychosocial hypotheses in mood disorders that can be integrated in interactive models.

Genetic epidemiology of mood disorders

The various strategies available to investigate genetic risk factors in psychiatric disorders belong to the wider discipline of genetic epidemiology. This combines both epidemiological and genetic investigations and has the primary objective of identifying the genetic and non-genetic (environmental) causes of a disease. Genetic epidemiological data in affective disorders has come mostly from family, twin, adoption, and segregation (within families) studies. These classic methods are described in Chapter 2.4.1. Family, twin, and adoption studies are the mainstay in establishing the genetic basis of affective disorders. These methods firstly demonstrated that genetic factors are involved in the aetiology of these disorders.[10] Twin and adoption data may also be used to investigate the relative contributions of genetic and environmental factors to the aetiology of a disease.[11] The exact contribution of these factors is not yet firmly understood for affective disorders but there have been some recent findings.

Adoption studies

The study of adoptees who are separated from their biological parents has consistently favoured the gene–environment hypothesis in the aetiology of diverse psychiatric disorders. One of the recent studies[12] show that major depression in females is predicted by an alcoholic diathesis only when combined with an environmental factor that is characterized by a psychiatrically ill adoptive parent. Other possible environmental factors were identified, such as fetal alcohol exposure, age at the time of adoption, and a family with an adopted sibling who had a psychiatric problem. These findings confirm the importance of the gene–environment interactions in the understanding of aetiological mechanism in mood disorders. The adoption study design is also used to validate clinical entities through the understanding of the gene–environment interactions as aetiological factors. The concept of depression spectrum disease has originally been developed from family studies[13] and further validated in adoption studies. In this model, depressions were divided into pure depressive disease (only depression in the family) and depression spectrum disease (characterized by a family history of alcoholism or antisocial personality). Different adoption studies confirmed this hypothesis, showing that daughters of alcoholics who where not adopted away showed significantly greater depression than control subjects and their female siblings who had been adopted away.[14] An excess of biological mothers with substance abuse was found among adoptees with depression[15] and more alcoholism was observed in the biological relatives of depressed adoptees than in the biological relatives of non-depressed adoptees.[16] These results confirm the significant role of gene–environment interactions in depression spectrum disease and further validate the concept.

Twin studies

The diagnostic validation and the structure of the genetic and environmental risk factors in mood disorders is also approached in twin studies. Using a prospective, epidemiologic, and genetically informative sample of adult female twins, Kendler et al.[17] have been able to identify and validate a typology of depressive syndromes characterized by mild typical depression, atypical depression (increased eating, hypersomnia, frequent, relatively short episodes, and a proclivity to obesity), and severe typical depression (comorbid anxiety and panic, long episodes, impairment, and help seeking). The members of twin pairs concordant for depression had the same depressive syndrome more often than expected by chance and this resemblance was greater in monozygotic than in dizygotic pairs. In order to clarify the interactions between genetic factors and stressful life events in the aetiology of depression, a population-based sample of female–female twin pairs including 2164 individuals where analysed in regard to stressful life events and onset of major depressive episodes in the past year.[18] For severe stressful events, the best-fitting model for the joint effect of stressful events and genetic liability on onset of major depression suggested genetic control of sensitivity to the depression-inducing effects of stressful life events. The authors concluded that genetic factors influence the risk of onset of major depression in part by altering the sensitivity of individuals to the depression-inducing effect of stressful life events.

In a more complex analysis of comorbidity among different psychiatric disorders, a large epidemiological survey of 1030 female–female twin pairs[19] investigated the influence of major genetic and environmental risk factors (separated in different domains: genes, family environment, and individual-specific environment) on comorbidity between different psychiatric disorders (phobia, generalized anxiety disorder, panic disorder, bulimia, major depression, and alcoholism). Each major risk factor domain influenced comorbidity, but in a distinct manner according the disorders investigated and most of the genetic factors that influence vulnerability to alcoholism in women do not alter the risk for development of other common psychiatric disorders.

Family studies

Segregation analysis is used to determine the mode of genetic transmission of a disorder by describing the distribution of phenotypes in affected families. The two principal hypotheses which have emerged from these complex analyses in affective disorders are the single major locus model and the polygenic model involving possible interaction between two or more loci. The exact mode of inheritance is not yet clear.[20] The situation is further complicated by the possible presence of anticipation in families with mood disorder.[1–3] This mode of transmission, which involves dynamic mutations, fits better with the twin and family epidemiological data available in affective disorders and may explain their non-Mendelian pattern of inheritance.

Molecular genetics in affective disorders

The rapid advance in molecular genetic techniques over the last decade has generated a large database of DNA markers across the whole human genome and has enabled chromosomal regions throughout almost the entire genome to be studied in affective disorders. These studies have been performed mainly using linkage and association methodologies. Several markers and chromosomal regions are potentially interesting. Current linkage and association methods investigate heritable factors at a molecular genetic level, and enable genes to be mapped.[21] These approaches are mostly applied to bipolar affective disorder, which is considered to be the 'core' phenotype in affective disorders. Linkage analysis tests the hypothesis that a linkage relationship exists between a known genetic marker and a trait which is known to be genetically determined but has not yet been mapped on a chromosome.[22] Two genetic loci are linked if they are located closely together on a chromosome. In linkage analysis, the distance between a marker locus and the gene under investigation is used for gene mapping. This method was originally designed to explore a major single genetic transmission and to evaluate the extent of co-segregation between genetic markers and the phenotype investigated in pedigrees. The major problems which linkage methodology faces when applied to affective disorders are the complex aetiology and inheritance patterns. More than one locus is probably involved in susceptibility to these disorders, and the exact mode of transmission is not known. Mis-specification of the genetic parameters of the phenotype may lead to errors in linkage studies.[22] Furthermore, the linkage approach fails to detect minor gene effects which contribute to genetic susceptibility to the disorder.[23]

The association method offers an alternative strategy of studying genetic factors involved in complex diseases in which the mode of transmission is not known.[24] The association strategy does not require genetic parameters to be known (non-parametric method). The purpose of association studies is to compare frequencies of genetic marker alleles in patient and control populations in order to detect linkage disequilibrium. Linkage disequilibrium between the disease locus and the marker tested is defined as a level of concordance between the two loci which is higher than would be expected by chance. The major reason for this is their proximity on a chromosome. The major advantage of association studies is that they can detect genes with minor effects other than a single major locus.

The major limitation of this approach is that spurious associations between a genetic marker and a disorder may result from variations in allele frequency between cases and controls observed if the two populations are ethnically different (population stratification). It is important in this case to compare populations which are homogenous in their ethnic background. The haplotype relative risk strategy uses parental data for the control sample and reduces this type of bias. Non-transmitted alleles are selected from parents of the probands for the control population.[25] A further major difficulty in association studies is the interpretation of the precise meaning of the association observed.[26] The result may be interpreted as linkage disequilibrium between the disease locus and the associated marker allele(s). Alternatively, the associated marker may be interpreted as a susceptibility factor which is directly involved in the disease. The candidate gene approach in association studies is a useful method to investigate linkage between markers and diseases. A candidate gene refers to a region of the chromosome which is potentially implicated in the aetiology of the disorder concerned. The possibility of false-positive results must be taken into account, as a very large number of candidate genes now exist. The probability that each of these genes is involved in the aetiology of the disorder is relatively low.

Chromosome 18

Prominent findings with markers in the pericentromeric region of chromosome 18 have been recently published. Berrettini et al.[27] first reported linkage of bipolar affective disorder to chromosome 18 DNA markers in a systematic genome survey including 22 families. These authors' results suggest that a susceptibility gene is present in the pericentromeric region of this chromosome. Results of linkage analysis in individual families indicated possible linkage with some marker loci in this region (18p11). This result is of considerable interest, both because of its significance and also because it is at this location that one finds genes coding for the α unit of a guanosine triphosphate binding protein involved in neurotransmission and the corticotrophin receptor gene. Stine et al.[28] studied 28 nuclear families for markers on chromosome 18 and also found evidence for linkage with bipolar affective disorder. This study also demonstrated evidence of a parent-of-origin effect operating in bipolar affective disorder (an excess of paternally but not maternally transmitted alleles). Gershon et al.,[29] on the other hand, observed linkage with chromosome 18 markers in affected sib-pair analysis only in pedigrees with mixed paternal–maternal transmission. Linkage was not found in pedigrees with exclusively maternal transmission. Chromosome 18 markers have been investigated in two large Belgian pedigrees with bipolar affective disorder.[30] Negative lod scores were found for a marker located in the pericentromeric region. Linkage and segregation analysis in one family suggested that a different region of chromosome 18 (18q21.33–q23) may contain a susceptibility locus for bipolar affective disorder. Freimer et al.[31] used both linkage and association strategies and also reported evidence of linkage with markers in this region (18q23). Despite slight allele sharing with two markers on chromosome 18 (D18S40 on 18p and D18S70 on 18q) in the National Institute of Mental Health genetics initiative bipolar affective disorder pedigrees,[32]

these results were not confirmed in this large genome scan. A negative lod score was found for D18S40 in the study of De Bruyn et al.[30] on 18p markers, indicating exclusion of this region.

Chromosome 11

This region of the genome has been thoroughly investigated in affective disorders because of the presence of genes including those coding for tyrosine hydroxylase (11p15), tyrosinase (11q14–21), dopamine receptor D_2 (11q22–23), dopamine receptor D_4 (11p15.5) and tryptophan hydroxylase (11p15). These proteins play an important role in catecholamine neurotransmission and their genes are considered to be candidate genes in bipolar and unipolar affective disorders. Overall results of linkage studies with tyrosine hydroxylase indicate that the tyrosine hydroxylase gene does not contribute a major gene effect to bipolar affective disorder.[33] Some studies, however, failed to exclude linkage with this gene and suggested that tyrosine hydroxylase should be further investigated using other methods such as allelic association. There are no linkage data for the tyrosine hydroxylase gene in pure unipolar affective disorder families. A possible role for the tyrosine hydroxylase gene was also examined in bipolar affective disorder association studies, all on moderate to small sample sizes.[34] Meta-analysis of the results do not support the tyrosine hydroxylase gene having a major role in the aetiology of bipolar affective disorder, while data suggest that this candidate gene should be examined in larger samples of unipolar affective disorder for which this marker may confer susceptibility to the disease.[34]

Chromosomes 4, 5, 12, and 21

Among the other autosomal DNA markers of interest are findings for chromosome 4, 5, 12, and 21 markers. Blackwood et al.[35] reported linkage between a locus on chromosome 4p (D4S394, 4p16) and bipolar affective disorder in a large family. Dopamine D_5 receptor gene and the α_{2C}-adrenergic receptor gene are located in the same region. Major candidate genes for the affective disorders are located on chromosome 5. Preliminary linkage data including three DNA markers on this chromosome (D5S39, D5S43, and D5S62) suggested linkage with bipolar affective disorder.[36] Two of these markers (D5S62 and D5S43) are located in the distal region of the long arm of chromosome 5 (5q35–q ter) and contain candidate genes contributing to the neurotransmitter receptors for dopamine, noradrenaline (norepinephrine), glutamate, and γ-aminobutyric acid. These two markers, however, had exclusion lod scores in a previous study of 14 families.[37] Dopamine transporter gene (DAT1) is located in a different region of chromosome 5 (5p15). This marker has been investigated in an association study with bipolar affective disorder yet no association was found.[38] Kelsoe et al.[39] recently reported a possible linkage between a locus near the dopamine transporter (DAT) locus on chromosome 5 and bipolar affective disorder.

The Darier's disease region on chromosome 12q23–q24.1 has been investigated in several family studies in bipolar affective disorder, suggesting a possible linkage.[40–43] Two of these studies have been able to report significant lod scores greater than 3.[42,43] To further test the hypothesis that genes containing expanded trinucleotide repeats may contribute to the genetic aetiology of bipolar affective disorder, loci within this region containing CAG/CTG repeat expansions have also been investigated, but no association was found with bipolar affective disorder.[44]

Straub *et al.*[45] detected linkage with the 21q22.3 locus on chromosome 21 in one bipolar family. Overall, however, the 47 families assessed for this genome do not support linkage with this marker.

X chromosome

Mendlewicz *et al.*[46] first reported possible genetic linkage between manic–depressive disorder and coagulation Factor IX (F9) at Xq27 in 11 pedigrees. Linkage with DNA markers on the X chromosome has been excluded, however, in other pedigrees.[33] More recently, Pekkarinen *et al.*[47] evaluated 27 polymorphic markers on the X chromosome (Xq25–28 region) in one large Finnish family. Linkage was found between a marker located on Xq26 (AFM205wd2) and bipolar affective disorder. This marker is located about 7 cM centrimeric to the F9 locus. These results are extremely suggestive of X linkage and confirm the need for further investigation of this region with other markers.

Serotonin markers and affective disorders

Dysfunction of the serotoninergic system has long been suspected in major depression and related disorders. Depression can successfully be treated with selective drugs which target serotonin receptors. The serotonin transporter may also be involved in susceptibility to affective disorders and in the response to treatment with these drugs. Allelic association has been suggested between the serotonin transporter gene (located on chromosome 17q11.1–12) and unipolar affective disorder.[48] The presence of one allele of this gene was significantly associated with a risk of unipolar affective disorder. This study also included a group of bipolar affective disorder patients, although no associations were found with this marker in this patient group compared to normal controls. This preliminary finding may add to our understanding of the possibility of polygenic inheritance in affective disorders. These findings were replicated in two different samples, again showing an association between this marker and unipolar affective disorder (major depression with melancholia)[49] and no association with a group of bipolar affective disorder patients.[50] A linkage study with the functional variant of the serotonin transporter gene in families with bipolar affective disorder could not exclude linkage.[51] More interestingly, a polymorphism within the promoter region of the serotonin transporter gene has been associated to treatment response to fluvoxamine, a typical selective serotonin reuptake inhibitor in major depression with psychotic features.[52] This promising preliminary finding requires to be confirmed. The tryptophan hydroxylase gene, which codes for the rate-limiting enzyme of serotonin metabolism, is also an important candidate gene for affective disorders and suicidal behaviour. Bellivier *et al.*[53] reported a significant association between genotypes at this marker and bipolar affective disorder; no association was found with suicidal behaviour. In a previous study in depressed patients, suicidal behaviour was associated with one variant of this gene.[54]

Anticipation and expanded trinucleotide repeat sequences

Anticipation implies that a disease occurs at a progressively earlier age of onset and with increased severity in successive generations. This may explain the non-Mendelian pattern of inheritance observed in some inherited diseases. This phenomenon has been observed in several neurological diseases including myotonic dystrophy, fragile X syndrome, Huntington's disease, and more recently in spinobulbar muscular atrophy, type 1 spinocerebellar ataxia, and spastic paraplegia.[55] Anticipation has been found to correlate with specific mutations in these syndromes: expanded trinucleotide repeat sequences. An expanded repeat sequence is unstable and may increase in size between family members, leading to increased disease severity of the disorder.

Anticipation has recently been described in bipolar affective disorder[1,2] and in unipolar affective disorder.[3] One recent study highlighted an association between cysteine–adenine–guanine (**CAG**) trinucleotide repeats and bipolar affective disorder in Swedish and Belgian patients.[56] CAG repeats have been detected by the repeat expansion detection method. This study, which was replicated in a different patient population,[57] demonstrated for the first time in a major psychiatric disorder that the mean length of CAG repeats was significantly higher in bipolar affective disorder patients compared to controls. More recently, an association between familial cases (but not sporadic cases) of bipolar affective disorder and CAG length has been observed.[58] This hypothesis has also been tested in a family sample of two-generation pairs with bipolar affective disorder.[59] A significant increase in CAG repeats between parents and offspring generations was observed, however, when the phenotype increased in severity, i.e. changed from major depression, single episode, or unipolar recurrent depression to bipolar affective disorder. A significant increase in CAG repeat length between generations was also found in female offspring with maternal inheritance, but not in male offspring. This is the first evidence of genetic anticipation in bipolar affective disorder families and should be followed by the identification of loci within the genome containing triplet repeats. CTG 18.1 on chromosome 18q21.1 and ERDA 1 on chromosome 17q21.3 are two repeat loci recently identified[60] which can be investigated in such study.

Psychosocial factors in affective disorders

Impairment in social relationships, dysfunctional cognition, gender, economic status, and temperament have been suggested as involved in the emergence of mood disorders. However, empirical studies on psychosocial factors of patients with affective disorders examine psychosocial features assessed after recovery from and/or at the time of episodes of affective disorder. These retrospective studies might not be able to distinguish between premorbid psychosocial patterns and those which result from previous episodes of illness. Further, longitudinal studies focusing on the role of psychosociological factors have involved predictions of recurrence or exacerbation of symptomatology in previously affected people, but not regarding the onset of the diseases. Thus, the demonstration of temporal antecedence to the initial onset of affective disorder is extremely difficult.[61] Thus, the conclusions in terms of aetiological psychosocial factor are limited.

Impairment in social and familial relationships

Difficulties in social functioning are concomitant to depressive disorders.[6,7,62] Previous research found that patients experienced a reduction of **social relationships**, with feeling of social discomfort, loneliness, and boredom.[6] Depressed patients seem lower in social self-confidence, they socialize less, and participate in social interaction less fully than do never-depressed persons.[62] In other words, depressed individuals do not make active effort to develop and sustain reciprocally supportive social relationships. The concept of social support has been widely used to predict general health and more specifically psychiatric symptoms.[63] Previous research revealed that the degree of integration in a social network, or structural support, have a direct positive effect on well being, reducing negative outcomes in both high- and low-stress life events. Among depressed individuals, dysfunctioning in social activities has been found to persist a long time after remission from the depressive episode.[6,64] The social dysfunctioning concerns more specifically marital, parental, and familial relationships.

The relationship between **marital disturbance** and affective disorder has received increased attention over the two past decades. First, descriptive studies have suggested that marital conflict correlates highly with concomitant depression,[65] and marital therapy has been found to be effective in reducing the symptoms of depression, alone[66] as well as in combination with pharmacotherapy.[67] Further, previous research found dysfunctional patterns of communication in couples with a depressed spouse. Specifically, compared with their non-depressed counterparts, depressed couples have been found to exhibit more friction, lack of affection, lower levels of constructive problem solving, mutual self-disclosure, and reciprocal support.[7,68,69] The lack of a confiding and intimate relationships leaves individuals vulnerable to depression.[7,70,71] Finally, marital distress may also exacerbate difficulties experienced in extramarital relationships,[72] thereby increasing introverted behaviour and social isolation. In a similar manner, the absence of a marital partner may hasten the onset of depression among vulnerable individuals.[73]

Parental relationships also seem to have a great impact in the course of affective disorders. A variety of authors have emphasized the importance of the quality of early experiences with parents in the development of adult depression. Beck[74] explicitly attributed the development of negative cognition and negative schemata of self to critical disapproving parents, and later Blatt and collaborators[75] suggested that the vulnerability to depression arises from impairment in relationships with parents. In general, depressive individuals described both mother and father as lacking warmth and a caring attitude, and being overly controlling, which involves intrusiveness, overprotection, and control through guilt.[76,77] For example, Andrews and Brown[78] found that women who became depressed following occurrence of major life events were more likely to report lack of adequate parental care or hostility from their mothers than those who did not become depressed. In summary, perceived lack of parental warmth, acceptance, and affection has consistently been associated with depression, however the evidence for a relationship between parental negative control and affective disorders is less clear. Specifically, some investigators have found that depressed people perceive their mothers to have been overly protective and intrusive, and both parents to have used guilt and anxiety-provoking strategies to exercise control over them; however, contrary findings have also been reported.[79,80]

Studies on parental representation are generally retrospective, i.e. the parental representation of depressed patients is compared to those of non-depressed controls. Consequently, the depressed subjects' negative view of parents may be distortions due to the affective disorder rather than accurate recollections. Gotlib et al.[81] found that the perceptions of maternal caring and overprotectiveness experiences by moderately depressed individuals do not shift with remission of their depressed mood, and may be considered as stable perceptions. Thus,

this study supports the notion that depressed adults had more negative relationships with their parents than have non-depressed persons.

In addition to marital and parental relationships, the quality of the **familial relationships**, in general, has been shown to have a significant impact on mental health.[82,83] When the quality of the family relationships is evaluated, studies have consistently found that when family members are critical, unsupportive, or generally display negative attitudes towards the depressed member, these behaviours lead to less likelihood of recovery or greater likelihood of a relapse of depression for the depressed family member.[84–86]

In summary, the quality of social and familial relationships appear to set the stage of depression. Social maladjustment at recovery may represent a risk factor that predisposes to further recurrent episodes. Individuals who experienced negative parental and familial relationships may be vulnerable to depression, and children exposed to such experiences may become depressed.[87,88] Most of the research to date is correlational, and cannot establish a causal link between negative relationships and the onset of affective disorders. Nevertheless, the associations are robust and well replicated, suggesting that disruption of social relationships may be a critical vulnerability factor for affective disorder.

Dysfunctional cognition

According to the helplessness model of depression,[89] vulnerability to depression derives from a habitual style of explaining the causes of life events, known as attributional style. A large body of research found that individuals suffering from depression think more negatively than healthy individuals. Specifically, depressed patients have a tendency to make internal, stable, and global causal attributions for negative events, and to a lesser extent, the attribution of positive outcomes to external, specific, and unstable causes. In other words, depressed patients have a low self-esteem.[90,91] Thus, when thinking about the self, past, current, and future circumstances, depressed patients emphasize the negative, and this process is likely to contribute to the perpetuation of their depressed mood. However, the role of self-esteem in depression has not yet been well established. A controversy persists as to whether low self-esteem is a consequence of depression or a vulnerability factor of the disease. Lewinsohn et al.[92] assume that low self-esteem neither precedes nor follows depressive episode. Several studies have yielded no evidence of risk of depression associated with pre-depressive cognitions.[93,94] To the contrary, Beck[74] has emphasized the aetiological significance of low self-esteem in depression. According to Beck, the low self-esteem should increase vulnerability to depression by existing in a latent state, to be activated by relatively minor experiences of deprivation or rejection. Brown and collaborators[95–97] have developed a psychosocial model of depression, similar to the Beck's model, in which the importance of the occurrence of both a negative life events and low self-esteem is highlighted. A number of prospective studies using college student samples support the predictive effect of negative attributions on the later development of depression following negative life events.[98] However, Haaga et al.[99] has reviewed five studies, and none of them indicate that negative cognitions added significantly to the prediction of later symptoms. More recently, Staner et al.[100] failed to support the predictive effects of self-esteem on later recurrence of depression in bipolar and unipolar patients. In summary, evidence supports the notion that depressed individuals have lower self-esteem, but less evidence is in favour of a causal role of negative thinking in the development of the disease.

Gender

Evidence for gender differences in responses to depression comes from a large number of studies. Women are consistently reported to have greater prevalence of affective disorders than men.[101–105] The reasons for this gender difference are unclear, and are as likely to be social as biological.

Divergences in the number and quality of **social and occupational roles** have been proposed to explain the greater prevalence of affective disorders among women.[102] In the context of marital relationship, previous research has indicated that, for men, marriage confers a protection against illness, while it appears to be associated with higher rates of depression for women.[106] There has been some evidence that within the marriage the traditional female role is limiting, restricting, and even boring, which may lead to depression.[107,108] For example, the role of child caretaker has consistently been shown to be associated with both high levels of stress and a higher incidence of depression for women.[109] Women are found to have more depressive symptoms when they have young children in the home, and this tends to increase in an almost linear fashion according to the number of children in the household.[110] Further, since women who are employed outside the home also tend to be responsible for household chores,[111] the notion that differentiation in occupational roles partially explains the prevalence of depression for women is supported. Bracke[102] found validity of social role explanations by showing that the gender differences in depression chronicity can partially be explained by differences in employment status, marital status, and educational attainment. However, Weich et al.[105] refute the version of the occupational roles hypothesis, namely that women have a higher prevalence of common mental disorders by virtue of their tendency to be over- or under-occupied compared with men. Specifically, they did not find gender differences in the prevalence of common mental disorders when men and women are adjusted regarding the number or type of roles occupied. In other words, neither the number of social roles, occupancy of traditional 'female' caring and domestic roles, nor socio-economic status explained the gender differences, in their study. In summary, the impact of social and occupational roles as explanation of gender differences in affective disorders is not yet obvious.

Further, to explain why women are more likely than men to manifest depression Nolen-Hoeksema has proposed the **'response style the-ory'.**[104,112] According to this theory, women are more likely than men to have a ruminative response style, which contributes to the perpetuation of their depressed mood.[113–115] Ruminative responses to depression refer to 'behaviours and thoughts that focus one's attention on one's depressive symptoms and on the implications of these symptoms'. Nolen-Hoeksema argued that, when depressed, women are more likely to engage in these ruminative responses, thereby amplifying their depressive symptoms and extending the depressive episode. On the other hand, men are more likely to distract themselves from depressed mood, thereby dampening their symptoms.

Finally, there is some evidence to suggest that the post-partum and the premenstrual periods, with their associated **biological and psychological changes**, represent periods of increased risk of depression among women. However, the extent of the risk imparted by endocrine factors has not yet been determined.[116]

In summary, at similar levels of stress women are probably more vulnerable to affective disorders than men. One explanation of this finding is that women may be more willing than men to admit symptoms and/or men may express their symptoms in different ways through alcohol abuse or 'acting out', for example.

Socio-economic status

Many studies have reported that low socio-economic status is associated with high prevalence of mood disorders.[117] For a long time in social psychiatry, 'social causation' and 'social selection' hypotheses have been accepted explanations of the role of the low socio-economic status in affective disorder. The causation hypothesis suggests that the stress associated with low social position, i.e. exposure to adversity and lack of resource to cope with difficulty, may contribute to the development of the affective disorder,[118,119] while the social selection hypothesis argues that genetically predisposed persons drift down to or fail to rise out of such positions.[120,121] Thus, the social selection hypothesis emphasizes the genetic interpretation of cause, while social causation hypothesis focuses on the aetiological role of the environment. Few longitudinal data sets are available to test the causal hypothesis. Nevertheless, there is evidence that disadvantaged socio-economic status, poverty, or education and occupation can be considered as risk factors for mood disorders.[122,123] Bruce and Hoff[124] found that the effect of poverty is substantially reduced when controlling for degree of isolation from friends and family, suggesting that social isolation mediates some of the relationships between economic status and mood disorders.

In summary, a positive relationship has been found between socio-economic status and vulnerability for affective disorders, with higher rates of vulnerability found among individuals with lower educational and social achievement levels.

Temperament and behaviour

Temperament has been defined in terms of differences in the adaptive systems, i.e. differences in reactivity and self-regulation within the social context.[125–127] According to Derryberry and Rothbart,[126,127] self-regulation refers to the relatively enduring biological make-up of the individual, influenced over time by heredity, maturation, and experience. Reactivity is defined as the functional state of somatic, endocrine, autonomic, and central nervous systems reflecting the response parameters of threshold, latency, intensity, rise time, and recovery time. Self-regulation is a higher-level process functioning to modulate (enhance or inhibit) the reactive state of these systems. Self-regulation was approached in terms of emotion or affective–motivational processes. Indeed, the construct of temperament has traditionally focused upon individual differences in emotionality. When viewed as regulatory, however, affective–motivational processes can be seen to extend beyond the traditional response-oriented domain of emotion, influencing a variety of perceptual and cognitive processes. For example, an emotion such as sadness regulates somatic, autonomic, and endocrine response systems, while at the same time modulating sensory channels converging upon these response system. Thus, the regulatory system of temperament plays a high-level role in co-ordinating attention and response to social context and influences nearly every aspect of experience and behaviour. Many authors[127–129] postulate, to some degree, a stable association between biogenetic dispositions to specific mood and observable temperament traits. Affective disorders are likely to emanate from specific temperament which increases vulnerability to mood disturbances. The relevant literature is vast, and we necessarily limit our coverage to the more influential models.

The model of temperament developed by Eysenck[128] approaches temperament in terms of cortical arousal. Eysenck suggested that individuals differ in their basic arousability and therefore in their optimal level of stimulation. These physiological differences give rise to the primary personality dimension of introversion–extraversion. Introverts are said to possess relatively reactive reticular systems, and thus to attain their optimal level of cortical arousal at relatively low level of stimulation. As a result of their low optimal arousal level, introverts are expected to prefer and seek out mild forms of stimulation and to avoid more intense and novel form of stimulation. In contrast, extraverts are said to possess relatively unreactive reticular systems, to have correspondingly high optimal levels of cortical arousal, and to therefore approach more intense and novel forms of stimulation. While this central form of arousal is seen to influence the affective quality of experience, Eysenck[128] proposed a complementary form of limbic activation influences the intensity of behaviour. Variability in the functioning of the limbic activation system underlies a personality dimension referred to as 'neuroticism–stability'. Individuals with reactive limbic systems (i.e. neurotics) are said to be prone to intense autonomic discharges, while those with less reactive limbic systems (i.e. non-neurotics) are thought to demonstrate autonomic lability. On the basis of their reticular and limbic reactivity, individuals are classified into four basic types: neurotic extravert, stable extravert, neurotic introvert, and stable introvert. In general, neuroticism correlates positively with depressive symptoms while extraversion is inversely related to depression.[129,130] Neuroticism has been shown to be mood dependent,[131] decreasing as depressive symptoms abate. Given the high correlation between neuroticism and anxiety,[132] the decrease in neuroticism may simply reflect the amelioration of anxiety symtoms associated with depressive illness. Although there is some evidence that remitted patients remain abnormally neurotic following recovery from depression, this finding is not consistent across studies, and additional research is required.[133–135] The evidence linking the extraversion–introversion personality dimension with previous dimensions is more consistent. In general it has been found that extraversion scores are not significantly affected by recovery from depression[136] and depressives remain less extraverted than never-depressed people.[137]

The differences between Cloninger's model and other models are that Cloninger assumes relationships between biogenic amine neurotransmitters (noradrenaline, serotonin, and dopamine) and personality dimensions. Specifically, Cloninger defined temperament dimensions in terms of individuals differences in associative learning in response to novelty, danger, or punishment, and reward. Further, he hypothesized a positive correlation between serotoninergic activity and harm avoidance, dopaminergic activity and novelty seeking, and finally between noradrenergic activity and reward dependence. According to this author, these aspects of personality denote traits that are usually considered temperament factors because they are heritable, manifest early in life, and apparently involved in learning. The possible tridimensional combinations of extreme (high or low) variants on these basic stimulus–response characteristics correspond closely to the traditional descriptions of personality disorders. The specific relationship between temperament and mood disorder is not yet understood

satisfactorily. Few studies have been done regarding the Tridimensional Personality Questionnaire scores in relation to mood disorder, the data available suggest that depressed patients have elevated harm avoidance scores.[138–141]

The study of the aetiological role of temperament in mood disorder requires longitudinal research beginning with subjects who have not yet developed the disease. To our knowledge, such issues have not yet been investigated.

The gene–environment hypothesis

Gene–environment interactions

The current relevant data on gene–environment interactions are derived from twin and adoption studies, both providing powerful tools to predict the different ways genetic and environment factors interact. Tree models are commonly used to describe the possible gene–environment relationships.[142] The classical additive models infer that individuals inherit the susceptibility genes for the disease from their parents and that environmental experiences act as an additive effect to cause the disease. In this model, the probability of being exposed to the environmental risk factor is unrelated to the genetic inheritance. In other models, the relationship between genetic factors and environmental factors is more interactive. The 'genetic control of exposure to the environment' refers to possible role of genes conferring a vulnerability to the pathogenic effect of the environment. Genetic factors influence the risk of onset of major depression in part by altering the sensitivity of individuals to the depression-inducing effect of environmental factors. The 'genetic control of exposure to the environment' assumes that genetic factors influence the exposure to the pathogenic environmental factor. Many environmental factors can be considered within these models but very few have been included in twin and adoption studies.

The availability of molecular genetic findings in affective disorders offers new directions in this research field. It is now possible to consider the gene–environment hypotheses using DNA markers as the genetic liability variable. However, it remains difficult to test these hypotheses using classical linkage and association methods.

Molecular genetics and personality traits

Molecular genetics has recently been incorporated into genetic epidemiological research on behavioural traits. Some recent findings in this field may be relevant considering the genetic aspects of psychiatric disorders, particularly affective disorders. The possible role of candidate genes has been investigated in personality traits, in particular dopamine receptor D_4 in novelty-seeking and serotonin transporter in anxiety (see Chapter 4.12.6).

The results of these studies are very interesting since different personality questionnaires and ethnically distinct populations were used. The exact nature of the relationship between behavioural traits and mental disorders has never been investigated using the combined genetic (DNA) determinants. Hence, personality dimensions and their genetic determinants should be considered in future research on genetic aspects of psychiatric disorders in integrative models of gene–environment interactions.

Conclusion

The complexity of affective disorders is a major limitation when their genetic bases are being studied. This could be attributed to their non-Mendelian mode of inheritance. Bipolar affective disorder and unipolar affective disorder are, in fact, phenotypes which do not appear to exhibit classic Mendelian recessive or dominant inheritance involving a single major locus. The presence of both environmental as well as genetic factors and phenotypic heterogeneity also represents important problems when dealing with these disorders. Genetic studies in affective disorder represent a powerful tool for investigating non-genetic factors involved in the aetiology of bipolar affective disorder and unipolar affective disorder. If one or more genes contribute to susceptibility to these common diseases it is reasonable to assume that these will be identified in the near future. Several consistent hypotheses are currently being tested and will, hopefully, lead to major advances. Potential genetic markers have been localized; some of these are directly linked to neurobiological hypotheses of the aetiology of affective disorders. A number of these chromosomal regions actually contain candidate genes for bipolar affective disorder and unipolar affective disorder. Specific mutations and modes of inheritance (trinucleotide repeats and anticipation) have also been implicated in recent studies. Future genetic studies will need to either confirm or refute these findings but should also investigate environmental factors which may be important in affective disorders.

References

1. McInnis, M.G., McMahon, F.J., Chase, G.A., *et al.* (1993). Anticipation in bipolar affective disorder. *American Journal of Human Genetics*, **53**, 385–90.
2. Nylander, P.-O., Engstrom, C., Chotai, J., Wahlström, J., and Adolfsson, R. (1994). Anticipation in Swedish families with bipolar affective disorder. *Journal of Medical Genetics*, **9**, 686–9.
3. Engström, C., Johansson, E.L., Langström, M., *et al.* (1995). Anticipation in unipolar affective disorder. *Journal of Affective Disease*, **35**, 31–40.
4. Lindblad, K., Nylander, P.O., De Bruyn, A., *et al.* (1995). Expansion of trinucleotide CAG repeats detected in bipolar affective disorder by the RED-(rapid expansion detection) method. *Neurobiology of Disease*, **2**, 55–62.
5. O'Donovan, M.C, Guy, C., Craddock, N., *et al.* (1995). Expanded CAG repeats in schizophrenic and bipolar disorder. *Nature Genetics*, **10**, 380–1.
6. Bauwens, F., Tracy, A., Pardoen, D., Vander Elst, M., and Mendlewicz, J. (1991). Social adjustment of remitted bipolar and unipolar out-patients. A comparison with age- and sex-matched controls. *British Journal of Psychiatry*, **159**, 239–44.
7. Bauwens, F., Pardoen, D., Staner, L., Dramaix, M., and Mendlewicz, J. (1998). Social adjustment and the course of affective illness: a one-year controlled longitudinal study involving bipolar and unipolar outpatients. *Depression and Anxiety*, **8**, 50–7.
8. Leader, J.B. and Klein, D.N. (1996). Social adjustment in dysthymia, double depression and episodic major depression. *Journal of Affective Disorder*, **37**, 91–101.
9. Pardoen, D., Bauwens, F., Tracy, A., Martin, F., and Mendlewicz, J. (1993). Self-esteem in recovered bipolar and unipolar out-patients. *British Journal of Psychiatry*, **163**, 755–62.
10. Mendlewicz, J. (1994). The search for a manic depressive gene: from classical to molecular genetics. *Progress in Brain Research*, **100**, 225–59.
11. Vieland, V.J., Susser, E., and Weissman, M.M. (1995). Genetic epidemiology in psychiatric research. In *Genetics of mental disorders*, Part I, *Theoretical aspects* (ed. G.N. Papadimitriou and J. Mendlewicz), pp. 19–46. Baillière Tindall, London.
12. Cadoret, R.J., Winokur, G., Lengbehn, D., *et al.* (1996). Depression spectrum disease, I: the role of gene–environment interaction. *American Journal of Psychiatry*, **153**, 892–9.
13. Winokur, G., Cadoret, R., Dorzab, J., and Baker, M. (1971). Depressive disease: a genetic study. *Archives of General Psychiatry*, **24**, 135–44.
14. Goodwin, D., Schulsinger, F., Knop, J., *et al.* (1977). Alcoholism and depression in adopted-out daughters of alcoholics. *Archives of General Psychiatry*, **34**, 751–5.
15. Van Knorring, A.L., Cloninger, C., Bohman, M., *et al.* (1983). An adoption study of depressive disorders and substance abuse. *Archives of General Psychiatry*, **40**, 943–50.
16. Wender, P., Kttzs, S., and Rosenthal, D. (1986). Psychiatric disorders in the biological and adoptive families of adopted individuals with affective disorders. *Archives of General Psychiatry*, **43**, 923–50.
17. Kendler, K.S., Eaves, L.J., Walters, E.E., *et al.* (1996). The identification and validation of distinct depressive syndromes in a population-based sample of female twins. *Archives of General Psychiatry*, **53**, 391–9.
18. Kendler, K.S., Kessler, R.C., Walters, E.E., *et al.* (1995). Stressful life events, genetic liability, and onset of an episode of major depression in women. *American Journal of Psychiatry*, **152**, 833–42.
19. Kendler, K.S., Walters, E.E., Neale, M.C., *et al.* (1995). The structure of the genetic and environmental risk factors for six major psychiatric disorders in women. Phobia, generalized anxiety disorder, panic disorder, bulimia, major depression, and alcoholism. *Archives of General Psychiatry*, **52**, 374–83.
20. Smeraldi, E. and Macciardi, F. (1995). Association and linkage studies in mental illness. In *Genetics of mental disorders.* Part I: *Theoretical aspects* (ed. G.N. Papadimitriou and J. Mendlewicz), pp. 97–110. Baillière Tindall, London.
21. Weiss, K.M. (1993). *Genetic variation and human disease: principles and evolutionary approaches*, pp. 117–48. Cambridge University Press.
22. Ott, J. (1991). *Analysis of human genetic linkage* (2nd edn). Johns Hopkins University Press, Baltimore, MD.
23. Nothen, M.M., Propping, P., Fimmers, R., *et al.* (1993). Association versus linkage studies in psychosis genetics. *Journal of Medical Genetics*, **30**, 634–7.
24. Hodge, S.E. (1993). Linkage analysis versus association analysis: distinguishing between two models that explain disease-marker associations. *American Journal of Medical Genetics*, **53**, 367–84.
25. Terwilliger, J.D. and Ott, J. (1992). A haplotype-based haplotype relative risk statistic. *Human Heredity*, **42**, 337–46.
26. Hodge, S.E. (1994). What association analysis can and cannot tell us about the genetics of complex disease. *American Journal of Medical Genetics*, **54**, 318–23.
27. Berrettini, W.H., Ferraro, T.N., Goldin, L.R., *et al.* (1994). Chromosome 18 DNA markers and manic-depressive illness: evidence for a susceptibility gene. *Proceedings of the National Academy of Sciences of the United States of America*, **91**, 5918–22.
28. Stine, C., Xu, J., Koskela, R., *et al.* (1996). Evidence for linkage of bipolar disorder to chromosome 18 with parent-of-origin effect. *American Journal of Human Genetics*, **57**, 1384–94.
29. Gershon, E.S., Badner, J.A., Detera-Waldeigh, S.D., *et al.* (1996). Maternal inheritance and chromosome 18 allele sharing in unilineal bipolar illness pedigrees. *American Journal of Medical Genetics (Neuropsychiatric Genetics)*, **67**, 202–7.
30. De Bruyn, A., Souery, D., Mendelbaum, K., *et al.* (1996). Linkage analysis of 2 families with bipolar illness and chromosome 18 markers. *Biological Psychiatry*, **39**, 679–88.
31. Freimer, N., Reus, V., and Escamilla, M. (1996). Genetic mapping using haplotype, association and linkage methods suggests a locus for severe bipolar disorder (BPI) at 18q22-q23. *Nature Genetics*, **12**, 436–41.

32. Detera-Wadleigh, S.D., Badner, J.A., Yoshikawa, T., *et al.* (1997). Initial genome screen for bipolar disorder in the NIMH genetics initiative pedigrees: chromosomes 4, 7, 9, 18, 19, 20 and 21q. *American Journal of Medical Genetics (Neuropsychiatric Genetics)*, **74**, 254–62.

33. Souery, D., Papadimitriou, G., and Mendlewicz, J. (1995). New genetic approaches in affective disorders. In *Genetics of mental disorders. Part I: Theoretical aspects* (ed. G.N. Papadimitriou and J. Mendlewicz), pp. 1–73. Baillière Tindall, London.

34. Furlong, R.A., Rubinsztein, J.S., Ho, L., *et al.* (1999). Analysis and metaanalysis of two polymorphisms within the tyrosine hydroxylase gene in bipolar and unipolar affective disorders. *American Journal of Medical Genetics*, **5**, 88–94.

35. Blackwood, D., He, L., Morris, S., *et al.* (1996). A locus for bipolar affective disorder on chromosome 4p. *Nature Genetics*, **12**, 427–30.

36. Coon, H., Jensen, S., Hoff, M., *et al.* (1993). A genome-wide search for genes predisposing to manic-depression, assuming autosomal dominant inheritance. *American Journal of Human Genetics*, **52**, 1234–49.

37. Detera-Wadleigh, S.D., Berrettini, W.H., *et al.* (1992). A systematic search for a bipolar predisposing locus on chromosome 5. *Neuropsychopharmacology*, **6**, 219–29.

38. Souery, D., Lipp, O., Mahieu, B., *et al.* (1996). Association study of bipolar disorder with candidate genes involved in catecholamine neurotransmission: DRD2, DRD3, DAT1 and TH genes. *American Journal of Medical Genetics (Neuropsychiatric Genetics)*, **67**, 551–5.

39. Kelsoe, J.R., Sadovnick, A.D., Kristbjarnarson, H., *et al.* (1996). Possible locus of bipolar disorder near the dopamine transporter on chromosome 5. *American Journal of Medical Genetics*, **67**, 533–40.

40. Craddock, N., McGuffin, P., and Owen, M. (1994). Darier's disease cosegregating with affective disorder. *British Journal of Psychiatry*, **165**, 272.

41. Dawson, E., Parfitt, E., Roberts, Q., *et al.* (1995). Linkage studies of bipolar disorder in the region of the Darier's disease gene on chromosome 12q23–24.1. *American Journal of Medical Genetics*, **24**, 94–102.

42. Barden, N., Plante, M., Rochette, D., *et al.* (1996). Genome wide microsatellite marker linkage study of bipolar affective disorders in a very large pedigree derived from a homogeneous population in Quebec points to susceptibility locus on chromosome 12. *Psychiatric Genetics*, **6**, 145–6.

43. Ewald, H., Degn, B., Mors, O., and Kruse, T.A. (1998). Significant linkage between bipolar affective disorder and chromosome 12q24. *Psychiatric Genetics*, **8**, 131–40.

44. Franks, E., Guy, C., Jacobsen, N., *et al.* (1999). Eleven trinucleotide repeat loci that map to chromosome 12 excluded from involvement in the pathogenesis of bipolar disorder. *American Journal of Medical Genetics*, **5**, 67–70.

45. Straub, R.E., Lehner, Th., Luo, Y., *et al.* (1994). A possible vulnerability locus for bipolar affective disorder on chromosome 21q22.3. *Nature Genetics*, **8**, 291–6.

46. Mendlewicz, J., Simon, P., Sevy, S., *et al.* (1987). Polymorphic DNA marker on chromosome and manic-depression. *Lancet*, **i**, 1230–2.

47. Pekkarinen, P., Terwilliger, J., Bredbacka, P.-E., Lonnqvist, J., and Peltonen, L. (1995). Evidence of a predisposing locus to bipolar disorder on Xq24–q27.1 in an extended Finnish pedigree. *Genome Research*, **5**, 105–15.

48. Ogilvie, A.D., Battersby, S., Bubb, V.J., *et al.* (1996). Polymorphism in serotonin transporter gene associated with susceptibility to major depression. *Lancet*, **347**, 731–3.

49. Gutierrez, B., Pintor, L., Gasto, C., *et al.* (1998). Variability in the serotonin transporter gene and increased risk for major depression with melancholia. *Human Genetics*, **103**, 319–22.

50. Gutierrez, B., Arranz, M.J., Collier, D.A., *et al.* (1998). Serotonin transporter gene and risk for bipolar affective disorder: an association study in Spanish population. *Biological Psychiatry*, **43**, 843–7.

51. Ewald, H., Flint, T., Degn, B., Mors, O., and Kruse, T.A. (1998). A

52. Smeraldi, E., Zanardi, R., Benedetti, F., *et al.* (1998). Polymorphism within the promoter of the serotonin transporter gene and antidepressant efficacy of fluvoxamine. *Molecular Psychiatry*, **3**, 508–11.

53. Bellivier, F., Leboyer, M., Courtet, P., *et al.* (1998). Association between the tryptophan hydroxylase gene and manic-depressive illness. *Archives of General Psychiatry*, **55**, 33–7.

54. Mann, J.J., Malone, K.M., Nielsen, D.A., *et al.* (1997). Possible association of a polymorphism of the tryptophan hydroxylase gene with suicidal behavior in depressed patients. *American Journal of Psychiatry*, **154**, 1451–3.

55. Miwa, S. (1994). Triplet repeats strike again. *Nature Genetics*, **6**, 3–5.

56. Lindblad, K., Nylander, P.O., De Bruyn, A., *et al.* (1995). Expansion of trinucleotide CAG repeats detected in bipolar affective disorder by the RED-(rapid expansion detection) method. *Neurobiology of Disease*, **2**, 55–62.

57. O'Donovan, M.C, Guy, C., Craddock, N., *et al.* (1995). Expanded CAG repeats in schizophrenia and bipolar disorder. *Nature Genetics*, **10**, 380–1.

58. Oruc, L., Lindblad, K., Verheyen, G., *et al.* (1997). CAG expansions in bipolar and unipolar disorders. *American Journal of Human Genetics*, **60**, 730–2.

59. Mendlewicz, J., Lipp, O., Souery, D., *et al.* (1997). Possible maternal genomic imprinting on expended trinucleotide CAG repeats in bipolar affective disorder. *Biological Psychiatry*, **42**, 1115–22.

60. Lindblad, K., Nylander, P.-O., Zander, C., *et al.* (1998). Two commonly expanded CAG/CTG repeat loci: involvment in affective disorders? *Molecular Psychiatry*, **3**, 405–10.

61. Depue, R.A. and Monroe, S.M. (1986). Conceptualization and measurement of human disorder in life stress research: the problem of chronic disturbance. *Psychological Bulletin*, **99**, 36–51.

62. Hirschfeld, R.M.A, Klerman, G.L., Clayton, P.J., *et al.* (1983). Assessing personality: effects of the depressive state on trait measurement. *American Journal of Psychiatry*, **140**, 695–9.

63. Kendler, K.S. (1997). Social support : a genetic epidemiologic analysis. *American Journal of Psychiatry*, **154**, 1398–404.

64. Shapira, B., Zislin, J., Gelfin, Y., *et al.* (1999). Social adjustment and self-esteem in remitted patients with unipolar and bipolar affective disorder: a case–control study. *Comprehensive Psychiatry*, **40**, 24–30.

65. Crowther, J.H. (1985). The relationship between depression and marital maladjustment: A descriptive study. *Journal of Nervous and Mental Disease*, **173**, 227–31.

66. Beach, S.R.H. and O'Leary, D.K. (1986). The treatment of depression occuring in the context of marital discord. *Behavior Therapy*, **17**, 43–50.

67. Friedman, A.S. (1975). Interaction of drug therapy with marital therapy in depressed patients. *Archives of General Psychiatry*, **32**, 619–38.

68. Kahn, J., Coyne, J.C., and Margolin, C. (1985). Depression and marital disagreement: the social construction of despair. *Journal of Social and Personal Relationships*, **2**, 447–61.

69. Biglan, A., Hops, H., Sherman, L., Friedman, L.S., Arthur, J., and Osteen, V. (1985). Problem-solving interactions of depressed women and their husbands. *Behavior Therapy*, **16**, 431–51.

70. Brown, G.W. and Prudo, R. (1981). Psychiatric disorder in a rural and urban population: 1. Etiology of depression. *Psychological Medicine*, **11**, 581–99.

71. Costello, C.G. (1982). Social factors associated with depression: a retrospective community study. *Psychological Medicine*, **12**, 329–39.

72. Coyne, J.C., and DeLongis, A. (1986). Going beyond social support: the role of social relationships in adaptation. *Journal of Consulting and Clinical Psychology*, **54**, 454–60.

73. Brown, G.W., and Harris T. (1978). *Social origin of depression*. Free Press, London.

74. Beck, A.T. (1967). *Depression: clinical, experimental, and theoretical aspects*. Harper and Row, New York.

75. Blatt, S.J., Wein, S.J., Chevron, E., and Quinlan, D.M. (1979). Parental representations and depression in normal young adults. *Journal of Abnormal Psychology*, **88**, 388–97.

76. Crook, T., Raskin, A., and Eliot, J. (1981). Parent–child relationships and adult depression. *Child Development*, **52**, 950–7.

77. Gerlsma, C., Das, J., and Emmelkamp, P.M. (1993). Depressed patients' parental representations: stability across changes in depressed mood and specificity across diagnoses. *Journal of Affective Disorder*, **27**, 173–81.

78. Andrews, B. and Brown, G.W. (1988). Social support, onset of depression and personality: an exploratory analysis. *Social Psychiatry and Psychiatric Epidemiology*, **23**, 99–108.

79. Crook, T., Raskin, A., and Eliot, J. (1981). Parent–child relationships and adult depression. *Child Development*, **52**, 950–7.

80. Perris, C., Arrindell, W.A., Perris, H., Eisemann, M., Van der Ende, J., and Von Knorring, L. (1986). Perceived depriving parental rearing and depression. *British Journal of Psychiatry*, **148**, 170–5.

81. Gotlib, I.H., Mount, J.H., Cordy, N.I., and Whiffen, V.E. (1988). Depression and perceptions of early parenting: a longitudinal investigation. *British Journal of Psychiatry*, **152**, 24–7.

82. Aneshensel, C. (1986). *Marital and employment role-strain, social support, and depression among adult women*, pp. 99–114. Hemisphere, Washington, DC.

83. Kandel, D.B. and Davies, M. (1982). Epidemiology of depressive mood in adolescents: an empirical study. *Archives of General Psychiatry*, **39**, 1205–12.

84. Hooley, J.M. and Teasdale, J.D. (1989). Predictors of relapse in unipolar depressives: expressed emotion, marital distress, and perceived criticism. *Journal of Abnormal Psychology*, **98**, 229–35.

85. Keitner, G.I., Ryan, C.E., Miller, I.W., Kohn, R., Bishop, D.S., and Epstein, N.B. (1995). Role of the family in recovery and major depression. *American Journal of Psychiatry*, **152**, 1002–8.

86. Swindle, R.W., Cronkite, R.C., and Moos, R.H. (1989). Life stressors, social resources, coping, and the 4-year course of unipolar depression. *Journal of Abnormal Psychology*, **98**, 468–77.

87. Armsden, G.C., McCauley, E., Greenberg, M.T., Burke, P.M., and Mitchell, J.R. (1990). Parent and peer attachment in early adolescent depression. *Journal of Abormal Child Psychology*, **18**, 683–97.

88. Daniels, D. and Moos, R.H. (1990). Assessing life stressors and social resources among adolescents: applications to depressed youth. *Journal of Adolescent Research*, **5**, 268–89.

89. Peterson, C. and Seligman, M.E.P. (1984). Causal explanations as a risk factor for depression: theory and evidence. *Psychological Review*, **91**, 347–74.

90. Tracy, A., Bauwens, F., Martin, F., Pardoen, D., and Mendlewicz, J. (1992). Attributional style and depression: a controlled comparison of remitted unipolar and bipolar patients. *British Journal of Clinical Psychology*, **31**, 83–4.

91. Pardoen, D., Bauwens, F., Tracy, A., Martin, F., and Mendlewicz, J. (1993). Self-esteem in recovered bipolar and unipolar out-patients. *British Journal of Psychiatry*, **163**, 755–62.

92. Lewinsohn, P.M., Steinmetz, J.L., Larson, D.W., and Franklin, J. (1981). Depression-related cognitions: antecedent or consequence? *Journal of Abnormal Psychology*, **90**, 213–19.

93. Hamilton, E.W. and Abramson, L.Y. (1983). Cognitive patterns and major depressive disorder: a longitudinal study in a hospital setting. *Journal of Abnormal Psychology*, **92**, 173–84.

94. Hammen, C., Marks, T., DeMayo, R., and Mayol, A. (1985). Self-schemas and risk for depression: a prospective study. *Journal of Personality and Social Psychology*, **49**, 1147–59.

95. Brown, G.W., Bifulco, A., and Andrews, B. (1990). Self-esteem and depression. IV. Effect on course and recovery. *Social Psychiatry and Psychiatric Epidemiology*, **25**, 244–9.

96. Brown, G.W., Bifulco, A., and Andrews, B. (1990). Self-esteem and depression. III. Aetiological issues. *Social Psychiatry and Psychiatric Epidemiology*, **25**, 235–43.

97. Brown, G.W., Bifulco, A., Veiel, H.O., and Andrews, B. (1990). Self-

98. Metalsky, G.I., Halberstadt, L.J., and Abramson, L.Y. (1987). Vulnerability to depressive mood reactions: toward a more powerful test of the diathesis-stress and causal mediation components of the reformulated theory of depression. *Journal of Personality and Social Psychology*, **52**, 386–93.

99. Haaga, D., Dyck, M., and Ernst, D., (1991). Empirical status of cognitive therapy of depression. *Psychological Bulletin*, **110**, 215–36.

100. Staner, L., Tracy, A., Dramaix, M., *et al.* (1997). Clinical and psychological predictors of recurrence in recovered bipolar and unipolar depressives: a one-year controlled prospective study. *Psychiatry Research*, **69**, 39–51.

101. Bebbington, P.E., Dunn, G., Jenkins, R., *et al.* (1998). The influence of age and sex on the prevalence of depressive conditions: report from the National Survey of Psychiatric Morbidity. *Psychological Medicine*, **28**, 9–19.

102. Bracke, P. (1998). Sex differences in the course of depression: evidence from a longitudinal study of a representative sample of the Belgian population. *Social Psychiatry and Psychiatric Epidemiology*, **33**, 420–9.

103. Kroenke, K. and Spitzer, R.L. (1998). Gender differences in the reporting of physical and somatoform symptoms. *Psychosomatic Medicine*, **60**, 150–5.

104. Nolen-Hoeksema, S.N. (1987). Sex differences in unipolar depression: evidence and theory. *Psychological Bulletin*, **101**, 259–82.

105. Weich, S., Sloggett, A., and Lewis, G. (1998). Social roles and gender difference in the prevalence of common mental disorders. *British Journal of Psychiatry*, **173**, 489–93.

106. Weissman, M.M. (1987). Advances in psychiatric epidemiology: rates and risks for major depression. *American Journal of Public Health*, **77**, 445–51.

107. Gove, W.R. and Tudor, J.F. (1973). Adult sex roles and mental illness. *American Journal of Sociology*, **78**, 1308–14.

108. Ramsey, E.R. (1974). Boredom: the most prevalent American disease. *Harpers*, **249**, 12–22.

109. Thoits, P.A. (1986). Multiple identities: examining gender and marital status differences in distress. *American Sociological Review*, **51**, 259–72.

110. Radloff, L.S. (1975). Sex differences in depression: the effects of occupation and marital status. *Sex Roles*, **1**, 249–65.

111. Rosenfield, S. (1992). The costs of sharing: wives' employment and husbands' mental health. *Journal of Health and Social Behavior*, **33**, 213–25.

112. Nolen-Hoeksema, S.N. (1990). *Sex differences in depression*. Stanford University Press.

113. Nolen-Hoeksema, S.N., Morrow, J., and Fredrickson, B.L. (1993). Response styles and the duration of episodes of depressed mood. *Journal of Abnormal Psychology*, **102**, 20–8.

114. Lyubomirsky, S. and Nolen-Hoeksema, S. (1995). Effects of self-focused rumination on negative thinking and interpersonal problem solving. *Journal of Personality and Social Psychology*, **69**, 176–90.

115. Nolen-Hoeksema, S., Parker, L.E., and Larson, J. (1994). Ruminative coping with depressed mood following loss. *Journal of Personality and Social Psychology*, **67**, 92–104.

116. Abou-Saleh, M.T., Ghubash, R., Karim, L., Krymski, M., and Bhai, I. (1998). Hormonal aspects of postpartum depression. *Psychoneuroendocrinology*, **23**, 465–75.

117. Dohrenwend, B.P., Levav, I., Shrout, P.E., *et al.* (1992). Socioeconomic status and psychiatric disorders: the causation-selection issue. *Science*, **255**, 946–52.

118. Faris, R.E.L. and Dunham, W. (1939). *Mental disorders in urban areas*. University of Chicago Press.

119. Hollingshead, A.B. and Redlich, F.C. (1958). *Social class and mental illness: a community study*. Wiley, New York.

120. Jarvis, E. (1971). *Insanity and idiosy in Massachusetts: report of the commission of Lunacy, 1855*. Harvard University Press, Cambridge, MA.

121. Odegaard, O. (1956). The incidence of psychoses in various occupations. *International Journal of Social Psychiatry*, **2**, 85–104.

122. Bruce, M.L., Takeuchi, D.T., and Leaf, P.J. (1991). Poverty and psychiatric status: longitudinal evidence from the New Haven Epidemiologic Catchment Area Study. *Archives of General Psychiatry*, **48**, 470–4.

123. Gallo, J.J., Royall, D.R., and Anthony, J.C. (1993). Risk factors for the onset of depression in middle age and later life. *Social Psychiatry and Psychiatric Epidemiology*, **28**, 101–8.

124. Bruce, M.L. and Hoff, R.A. (1994). Social and physical health risk factors for first-onset major depressive disorder in a community sample. *Social Psychiatry and Psychiatric Epidemiology*, **29**, 165–71.

125. Cloninger, C.R., Svrakic, D.M., and Przybeck, T.R. (1993). A psychobiological model of temperament and character. *Archives of General Psychiatry*, **50**, 975–90.

126. Derryberry, D. and Rothbart, M.K. (1984). Emotion, attention, and temperament. In *Emotion, cognition, and behavior* (ed. C.E. Izard, J. Kagan, and R.B. Zajonc), pp. 133–66. Cambridge University Press, New York.

127. Derryberry, D. and Rothbart, M.K. (1997). Reactive and effortful processes in the organization of temperament. *Developmental Psychopathology*, **9**, 633–52.

128. Eysenck, H.J. (ed.) (1981). *A model of personality*. Springer-Verlag, New York.

129. Gray, J.A. (1981). A critique of Eysenck's theory of personality. In *A model of personality* (ed. H.J. Eysenck). Springer-Verlag, New York.

130. Lyoo, K., Gunderson, J.G., and Phillips, K.A (1998). Personality dimensions associated with depressive personality disorder. *Journal of Personality Disorder*, **12**, 46–55.

131. Barnett, P.A. and Gotlib, I.H. (1988). Psychosocial functioning and depression: distinguishing among antecedents, concomitants, and consequences. *Psychological Bulletin*, **104**, 97–126.

132. Raikkonen, K., Matthews, K.A., Flory, J.D., Owens, J.F., and Gump, B.B. (1999). Effects of optimism, pessimism, and trait anxiety on ambulatory blood pressure and mood during everyday life. *Journal of Personality and Social Psychology*, **76**, 104–13.

133. Solomon, D.A., Shea, M.T., Leon, A.C., *et al.* (1996). Personality traits in subjects with bipolar I disorder in remission. *Journal of Affective Disorder*, **40**, 41–8.

134. Ulusahin, A. and Ulug, B. (1997). Clinical and personality correlates of outcome in depressive disorders in a Turkish sample. *Journal of Affective Disorder*, **42**, 1–8.

135. Santor, D.A., Bagby, R.M., and Joffe, R.T. (1997). Evaluating stability and change in personality and depression. *Journal of Personality and Social Psychology*, **73**, 1354–62.

136. Hirschfeld, R.M. and Klerman, G.L. (1979). Personality attributes and affective disorders. *American Journal of Psychiatry*, **136**, 67–70.

137. Von Zerssen, D., Asukai, N., Tsuda, H., Ono, Y., Kizaki, Y., and Cho, Y. (1997). Personality traits of Japanese patients in remission from an episode of primary unipolar depression. *Journal of Affective Disorder*, **44**, 145–52.

138. Joffe, R.T., Bagby, R.M., Levitt, A.J., Regan, J.J., and Parker, J.D. (1993). The Tridimensional Personality Questionnaire in major depression. *American Journal Psychiatry*, **150**, 959–60.

139. Kleifield, E.I., Sunday, S., Hurt, S., and Halmi, K.A. (1994). The effects of depression and treatment on the Tridimensional Personality Questionnaire. *Biological Psychiatry*, **36**, 68–70.

140. Nelsen, M.R. and Dunner, D.L. (1995). Clinical and differential diagnostic aspects of treatment-resistant depression. *Journal of Psychiatry Research*, **29**, 43–50.

141. Chien, A.J. and Dunner, D.L. (1996). The Tridimensional Personality Questionnaire in depression: state versus trait issues. *Journal of Psychiatry Research*, **30**, 21–7.

142. Kendler, K.S. (1998). Major depression and the environment: a psychiatric genetic perspective. *Pharmacopsychiatry*, **31**, 5–9.

4.5.5.2 Neurobiological aetiology of mood disorders

Guy Goodwin

Introduction

Neurobiology provides an explanation of behaviour or experience at the level either of systems of neurones or individual cells. There is no particular difficulty now in producing accounts of normal emotion and disorders of emotion, based on the currently available techniques for the investigation of brain function. These accounts remain preliminary, but they are no longer purely speculative. However, there has been a curious divorce between the extensive literature on normal emotion and the predominantly clinical or biochemical accounts of mood disorder. It was probably inevitable that the psychology of normal emotion would take a 'top-down' direction, while clinical approaches would be rather more 'bottom-up', dominated by symptoms and the effects of treatments. However, it now seems certain that one field has the potential to inform the other, and that such unifying activity might well take its origins from contemporary cognitive neuroscience. As well as witnessing conceptual advances, we are at a stage of rapid evolution in the platform technologies of imaging and genetics. These will allow us to improve our accounts of the functional anatomy of the component elements of mood and its disorder, their functional neurochemistry, and, in all probability, give meaning to what a cellular account of depressive illness may eventually mean.

Neurobiology of normal emotion

Any account of function in the human brain must start with its anatomy. Indeed, the most influential modern theory of how emotion is represented within the brain was an essentially anatomical speculation.[1] Building on the observation that decorticate animals could express 'sham rage', Papez argued that areas projecting to the hypothalamus would be essential for the experience of emotion. Movement, thought, and emotion were identified with sensory projections to the striatum, neocortex and limbic system respectively. The limbic cortex had been observed by neuropathologists to be a particular locus for infection with the rabies virus, and the association of early stages of disease expression with psychiatric symptoms was well established. The particular symptoms seen most floridly in rabies are intermittent outbursts of fury or terror.

The term 'limbic cortex or limbic system' is dignified by use, but not by coherent definition. Broca referred to *le grand lobe limbique* as a ring of grey matter bordering the hemispheres lying against the central structures of the brain and arranged in a circular fashion around the interventricular foramen. It is usually taken to include the cingulate gyrus, the hippocampus including dentate gyrus, the subiculum and related areas, the entorhinal cortex, the septum, the olfactory tubercle, and the amygdala. The grouping together of such anatomically different structures of uncertain function has long seemed convenient, but only now are we beginning to accumulate a functional understanding.

The central place of limbic structures in the experience of emotion also emerged from accounts of temporal lobe or psychomotor epilepsy, where a range of phenomena are described that may be relevant to normal emotion and its disorders (see Chapter 5.3.3). The corollary of these observations is the effect induced by stimulation of limbic brain areas in patients with seizures. As well as the simple subjective experiences described in the aura of a seizure, electrical stimulation of cortex exposed prior to surgery produced automatisms of the same type as those involved in spontaneous seizures. This usually required direct activation close to the amygdala for a full range of emotional effects. However, lesions in or stimulation of the inferior frontal and cingulate cortex were also implicated in 'psychomotor' seizures.

These early observations provided the focus for subsequent efforts aimed at understanding the underlying neural mechanisms. Lesions of the amygdala effectively produced the full range of abnormalities described in the Klüver–Bucy syndrome after more extensive temporal lobe excisions, most notably the loss of spontaneous aggression. This and more formal investigation of learning and behaviour after amygdalectomy led to the view that the amygdala was the key structure assigning motivational significance to stimuli. A critical feature of the more recent elaborations of this theory is that some sensory impressions are conveyed to the amygdala independent of the cortex. Such input may deliver unconditioned stimuli (e.g. pain), which allows the amygdala to be critical for conditioning and emotional processing generally. The set of the amygdala is then postulated to be critical in determining the action-repertoire of an individual, from eager readiness for action on the one hand to fearful avoidance or inhibition on the other. Notice how pivotal such a function is and how it may underlie what goes wrong in mood disorder.

In rare clinical cases, bilateral lesions of the amygdala are associated with defective social decision-making and poor recognition of emotional expression.[2] The amygdala appears to be peculiarly adapted to the representation of emotionally significant stimuli. Thus if fearful faces are presented briefly before a neutral face, the conscious perception of the fearful face is prevented–the neutral face masks the fearful face. However, functional magnetic resonance imaging (**MRI**) studies show that the amygdala can still signal the difference between a masked fearful face and a masked happy face.[3] Such subliminal processing could provide the neurological basis for emotional associations that are developed and experienced in particular social circumstances, with specific people, or relating to specific events. The amygdala has extensive projections that can account for effects on autonomic, neuroendocrine, and motor activation.

To study 'emotion' is not necessarily to study mood. Negative and positive mood induction in normal volunteers has been associated with activation or deactivation in a variety of brain areas in different studies. Inferior frontal and temporal cortex, rather than subcortical structures such as the amygdala were the most commonly implicated regions.[4] Differences in experimental design will have contributed to the variability of these findings, which remain difficult to interpret.

Relatively restricted lesions in the inferior frontal cortex have catastrophic consequences for general behaviour without impairing performance on a whole range of knowledge-based tests of higher cognitive function. Damasio[5] has speculatively distinguished 'background feeling' from extremes of emotion in determining this mechanism. Animal experiments suggest that primary reinforcing stimuli, such as taste and smell, are represented in a secondary sensory area directly within the inferior frontal cortex, together with elaborated vis-

ual representations. Efferent projections may regulate autonomic and monoamine projections. Although the objective failures in social or executive activity after such lesions are most obvious, the subjective experience of emotion may also be impaired.[6] Understanding the functions of the amygdala and the inferior prefrontal cortex is likely to prove central to the neurobiology of anxiety, depression, and mania.

As well as a functional anatomy, mood also has a neurochemistry. The original finding that lysergic acid diethylamide (**LSD**) profoundly modified mood and perception formed a critical background to efforts to understand such mechanisms in biochemical terms. The neurotransmitters involved are dopamine and noradrenaline (norepinephrine), together with serotonin (5-hydroxytryptamine, **5-HT**). 3,4-Methylenedioxymethamphetamine (**MDMA**, ecstasy), which more specifically releases 5-HT,[7] has profound effects on mood, activity, and sleep. Ecstasy's particular selectivity for 5-HT neurones may be directly linked to mood modulation; its effects are valued precisely for the sense of contact, happiness, and pleasure that is evoked. Such effects will ultimately be framed in terms of chemical addressing in particular brain regions (see Chapter 4.2.3.6).

The neurobiology of mood disorder

Vulnerability to mood disorder

Genetics

Positional mapping of the genetic loci associated with mood disorder has not yet yielded important clues in searching for fundamental neurobiological causes (see Chapter 4.5.6.1). However, neurobiology informs the genetic search for candidate genes such as the human serotonin transporter (*SERT*) gene.[8,9] Cerebrospinal fluid monoamine levels of the noradrenaline metabolite 3-methoxy-4-hydroxyphenylglycol (**MHPG**) appear to vary in relation to the two *SERT* polymorphisms.[10] This is the sort of finding that, if replicated, will start to illuminate abnormal function in the affected phenotype.

An alternative approach to looking for the heritability of mood disorder itself is to examine the heritability of traits that predispose to its development. Such quantitative trait loci can be sought relatively simply in a normal population (see Chapter 2.4.1). High-trait neuroticism (*N*) accounts for approximately half of the genetic liability to major depression in women.[11] Most importantly, *N* is itself highly heritable and stable in normal populations. Accordingly, individual differences in learning, stress hormone secretion, and a variety of other behaviours lend themselves to genetic studies in animals and ultimately in humans also. The first such successful study showed that 'emotionality' in mice was associated with at least three loci on the mouse genome.[12] These loci may be resolvable to the level of individual genes whose function could represent conserved mechanisms also contributing to human neuroticism. By analogy with other genes linked to common diseases like diabetes, this may lead to the development of novel models of vulnerability to mood disorder which have genuine neurobiological validity.

When animals are selected for differences in emotional behaviour they also show different hypothalamic–pituitary–adrenal (HPA) axis function. Specifically, Roman high- and low-avoidance rats differentially acquire a two-way active avoidance response in a shuttle box. High-avoidance animals show greater prolactin and HPA axis responsivity to stress compared with low-avoidance animals. However, young Roman strain rats show identical HPA axis reactivity, although prolactin responses and behaviour are different.[13] In other words, reactivity to the environment may share a measure of common genetic control across physiological and behavioural domains, but HPA abnormality *per se* develops secondary to emotional experience, or at least is magnified by it. However, the key point is that important differences in stress reactivity may reflect a genetic predisposition and have a biological basis.

Early adverse experience

Adverse childhood experience was identified in genetically uncontrolled studies as a risk factor predisposing women to subsequent depression (Chapter 4.5.6.1) and has been confirmed in genetically informative designs.[11,14] In a clinical context, such developmental or social effects are usually viewed as separable from biology. Indeed, their very existence is usually taken to validate a 'social' approach to psychiatry. From a more unified point of view, however, one would predict measurable neurobiological consequences. In fact, the effects have proved to be more profound than most biologists anticipated.

Variations in maternal care produce individual differences in neuroendocrine responses to stress in rats. The offspring of mothers that exhibited more licking and grooming of pups during the first 10 days after birth showed, in adult life, reduced plasma ACTH and corticosterone responses to acute stress.[15] In addition, there was increased hippocampal glucocorticoid-receptor messenger RNA (**mRNA**) expression, enhanced glucocorticoid feedback sensitivity, and decreased levels of hypothalamic corticotrophin-releasing hormone (**CRH**) mRNA. Greater early maternal attention also substantially reduced subsequent behavioural fearfulness in response to novelty, increased benzodiazepine receptor density in the amygdala and locus coeruleus, increased α_2-adrenoreceptor density in the locus coeruleus, and decreased CRH receptor density in the locus coeruleus. Thus, maternal care serves to programme behavioural responses to stress in the offspring by altering the development of the neural systems that mediate fearfulness.

When BALB/cByJ mice were raised by an attentive C57BL/6ByJ dam, their excessive stress-elicited HPA activity was reduced, as were their behavioural impairments. However, cross-fostering the more resilient C57BL/6ByJ mice to an inattentive BALB/cByJ dam failed to elicit behavioural disturbances. In other words, vulnerable offspring may have their problems exacerbated by maternal behaviour, while early-life manipulations may have less obvious effects in relatively hardy animals.[16] Whether separation or stress paradigms in rodents can be taken as precise models of the mechanisms underlying the risk of mood disorder or other psychiatric problems cannot yet be decided, but their general relevance to the human case seems obvious.

Gene–environment interaction is the likely basis of the neurobiology of mood disorder. In general terms this must be correct. Whether the genetic mechanisms can be brought into sufficient focus to allow specific pathways to be identified remains the major current challenge. There is some reason for caution. The genetic and developmental routes into distal common pathways regulating stress responses may be very numerous. Disorders that are both common and very variable in expression, such as depression, may turn out to have little specificity that is worth talking about. Every illness may be an ensemble of many specific factors, none of which is individually going to lead to a more

focused treatment or a better prediction of treatment response. We shall see.

The neurobiology of life events

Like early adversity, the role of life events in depression has been affirmed in genetically controlled studies.[11,14] Life events are relevant to almost all first episodes of depression, but are less significant in its recurrence. The biology of life events will be subsumed in the biology of stress, at best a clumsy term. In human studies it will always be difficult to isolate the critical ingredients of a particular psychological stress from the individual differences that stressed individuals bring to their experience. There have been several small neurobiological studies of well-defined events such as bereavement. Parents who had experienced the sudden death of a formerly healthy child showed immunological changes (decreased T-suppressor cells, significantly increased T-helper cells) and depression compared with controls, but no difference in cortisol levels.

Disturbances of immune function also occur in depressed patients. The evidence so far is essentially correlational and establishes no direction of effect. Indeed, the functional changes implied by different proportions of active lymphocytes or such similar 'measures' are uncertain. Peripheral and central injections of interleukin 1 and lipopolysaccharide induce the expression of proinflammatory cytokines in animal brain and depress spontaneous and learned behaviours. This may reflect the psychological effects more specifically associated with physical illness, although it is possible that immune mechanisms may sometimes produce psychiatric symptoms, perhaps as part of a more generalized stress response. Drugs that potently modify the immune response should be examined for psychotropic properties. (See also Chapter 2.3.9.)

Biological studies of the depressed state

In the majority of biological studies of affective disorder patients have been studied when ill and compared with normal controls. Over the years, this kind of design has produced a range of positive findings, usually of modest effect. It remains true to say that no biological changes have ever been found that distinguish between depressed patients and controls better than does the clinical assessment of the patients. What is curious, and not a little tantalizing, is the impression that symptoms may, in part, represent biological adaptations directed to put things right. Thus, on the one hand, there may be consistent effects upon hormone secretion or sleep that represent phenomena of illness. On the other, deliberate changes in hormone status or sleep deprivation may modify the state of depression.

The depressed state: functional anatomy

Perfusion or metabolic imaging can indirectly detect changes in neuronal activity (Chapters 2.3.5 and 2.3.8). Signals can be well localized, but they may reflect either reversible changes in function or a permanent loss of neuronal activity. Reductions in function in anterior brain structures have been typical in major depression. Hypoperfusion tends to be greatest in frontal, temporal, and parietal areas and most extensive in older patients; high Hamilton scores tend to be associated with reduced perfusion.[17] Reductions in frontal areas may be more likely in patients with impoverished mental states. Thus, neuropsychological testing in major depression shows evidence of slowing in motor and cognitive domains, with additional prominent effects on mnemonic function that are most marked in the elderly. These effects are correlated with reduced frontal perfusion in the elderly. In younger patients, there may actually be increased perfusion in the frontal and cingulate cortex. Metabolic increases in the cingulate gyrus have been associated with a good treatment response.[18] Highly localizing findings have been unusual, however. The only exceptions have been within-subject changes on recovery in the mesial frontal cortex and perhaps the basal ganglia.[19]

Isotope-based imaging of receptor occupation in depression has so far been limited. Single-photon emission tomography (**SPET**) with the dopamine $D_{2/3}$ ligand [^{123}I]IBZM showed increased binding in the striatum.[20] There were significant correlations between IBZM binding in the left and right striatum and measures of reaction time and verbal fluency, but not of mood as such. Increased $D_{2/3}$ binding in the striatum probably reflects a reduced dopamine function, whether due to a reduced release or secondary upregulation of receptors. Positron emission tomography (**PET**) with the selective radioligand [^{18}F]altanserin maps 5-HT$_2$-receptor distribution; in a small sample of depressed patients, tracer uptake was significantly reduced in the posterolateral orbitofrontal cortex and the anterior insular cortex, and was most marked in the right hemisphere.[21]

In summary, much of the functional imaging work so far completed has been inconclusive. It has served to implicate frontal and limbic rather than posterior brain areas, but this has done little more than broadly confirm anatomical conclusions derived from observing the effects of lesions or brain stimulation.[19] It has failed to illuminate mechanisms underlying the depressed state either at the neuropsychological or neurochemical level. Progress requires that relevant neuropsychological and drug challenges are incorporated into imaging protocols. The likely neuropsychological candidates include the representation of facial emotion; the choice of relevant drug challenges will be guided, as outlined below, by experience in neuroendoncine challenge studies and the pharmacology of effective treatments. Finally, 'functional' abnormalities may importantly predict structural abnormality in depression.

Neuroendocrine challenge tests

Secretion of hormones in the anterior pituitary is under the control, both direct and indirect, of central neuronal cell bodies that may project relatively widely within the brain. The secretion of a given hormone in response to specific precursors or agonists for individual neurotransmitter receptors has been proposed as a way of testing the security of such connections. Hormone secretion provides a bioassay of the system of interest. There is a measure of consensus about the findings in major depression.

Precursor loading of the serotonergic system with intravenous tryptophan produces prolactin and growth hormone secretion. In depressed patients, prolactin and growth hormone responses are blunted but recover with treatment.[22] Responses to intravenous clomipramine, which similarly releases 5-HT by a presynaptic mechanism, are also blunted in depression.[23] The receptors mediating these responses are uncertain, although in any case the requirement for an intact presynaptic system precludes interpretation in terms of receptor subtype.

Appropriately selective agonists with full efficacy are not freely available for testing postsynaptic or presynaptic responses. However, buspirone, gepirone, and ipsapirone are all partial agonists at the 5-HT$_{1A}$ receptor and have been looked at in a preliminary way in depressed patients. There is disagreement about whether postsynaptic (endocrine) responses are or are not blunted, but there is more consensus that presynaptic (hypothermic) responses are blunted.[24]

Noradrenergic and dopaminergic function has been examined using the α_2-adrenoceptor agonist clonidine and the mixed D$_{1/2}$ receptor agonist apomorphine. Growth hormone responses to clonidine are usually reported as being blunted in major depression.[25] Apomorphine-stimulated growth hormone responses are also blunted in depressed patients,[26] while, in symmetry, patients at risk of postpartum psychosis (usually manic in form) have enhanced apomorphine responses.[27]

Cholinergic challenge with an acetylcholinesterase inhibitor such as pyridostigmine or physostigmine produces a secretion of growth hormone; responses in major depression were increased compared with controls.[28]

Neuroendocrine drug challenge suggests attenuated serotonergic function and increased cholinergic function in depression. Reduced responses to adrenergic and dopaminergic challenge also suggest impaired neurotransmission. Interpretation of tests with agonists is always difficult, because blunting may occur in an overactive system that has been downregulated. In addition, if the secretion of the assay hormone itself is actually directly affected by the state of depression, interpretation in terms of specific neurotransmitter abnormalities may be misleading. This is a particular problem for ACTH/cortisol responses (see below). In fact, enthusiasm for neuroendocrine surrogate markers of monoamine transmission within the brain has probably diminished in recent years, but the paradigm of drug challenge nevertheless remains interesting. We must assay brain responses of the monoamine projections more centrally involved in mood regulation.

Hypercortisolaemia

About half of all patients with major depression have a raised cortisol output, which tends to return to normal on recovery. It is most consistently associated with an 'endogenous' pattern of illness (Chapter 4.5.3). While cortisol is always regarded as a 'stress' hormone, and is secreted in response to various types of acute stress, the stresses that commonly result in long-term hypercortisolaemia are poorly understood. The idea that there is a relatively specific link between chronic high cortisol levels and mood disorder is notably persistent. In major depression there is peripheral hypertrophy of the adrenal glands, measurable in MRI body scans, and an enhanced response to corticotrophin. The MRI change, like the hypercortisolaemia itself, reverses on recovery.[29]

Suppression of cortisol secretion occurs normally via glucocorticoid receptor-mediated inhibitory feedback to the hypothalamus; it is readily produced by dexamethasone, which is a potent exogenous glucocorticoid (the dexamethasone suppression test (**DST**)). Nonsuppression of endogenous cortisol after dexamethasone occurs in Cushing's disease for example. It implies either reduced feedback and/or enhanced central drive to release cortisol. It was initially observed that the 1-mg DST showed high specificity (96 per cent) and sensitivity (67 per cent) as a putative diagnostic test for melancholia.[30] At the time this result attracted intense interest, but has since proved difficult to generalize. The high specificity established against normal controls was less against other patient groups. Thus, DST non-suppression has not been accepted as a diagnostic test. This failed effort to give medical respectability to psychiatric diagnosis came to devalue what remains an important observation. Non-suppression usually reflects hypercortisolaemia, which is itself a robust phenomenon of mood disorder that requires explanation like any other core biological symptom. Other symptoms that we identify as part of the depressive syndrome lend themselves less easily to investigation. The DST also has potential clinical uses beyond diagnosis. DST non-suppression predicts a low placebo response rate to drug treatment,[31] and hypercortisolaemia predicts a low rate of clinical response to psychological intervention.[32]

It remains unclear whether cortisol contributes to the clinical state of depression by a direct action on the brain. Exogenous cortisol administration is associated with affective symptoms, and chronic excessive cortisol secretion commonly appears to produce depressive symptoms in Cushing's disease. An HPA axis programmed to hypersecrete cortisol under stress could be a pathogenic mechanism explaining why depression or mania develops. This view has provoked efforts to treat mood disorder by inhibition of cortisol synthesis with metyrapone. Preliminary results suggest this may be effective.

However, when depressed patients are given large doses of cortisol they tend to show acute mood enhancement,[33] and oral dexamethasone has been reported to elevate mood in major depression, especially in hypersecretors.[34] This leads to the converse hypothesis that an HPA axis appropriately adapted to chronic stress early in development might be unable to mount a normal effective response to acute stress later in life. Cortisol may then be seen as a euphoriant (or antidepressant), and hypercortisolaemia as an antidepressant response of the stress-regulating mechanisms of the brain. Based on this view, all cortisol levels seen in depression may be set inappropriately low for the ongoing stress, however high or low they are compared with the normal range.

Whether one supposes cortisol levels to be set too high or too low in depression, it remains inconvenient that either a suppression or an augmentation of steroid effect seems, initially at least, to elevate mood. A way out of this complication may lie in cortisol's action on two receptors in the brain (the glucocorticoid and mineralocorticoid receptors) that may have opposite actions. However, we need better-controlled replicated data on the effects of steroid manipulations.

An increased cortisol production is associated with an increased release of hypothalamic β-endorphin[35] and probably a pulsatile increase in ACTH. The paraventricular nucleus of the hypothalamus represents the highest level of dedicated neurones in the HPA axis. The neurosecretory cells of the paraventricular nucleus release the peptides CRH and AVP into the portal hypophyseal blood. These hormones in turn stimulate the release of ACTH from the anterior pituitary. Major depression is characterized by a blunted ACTH response to CRH,[36] an elevated level of CRH in the cerebrospinal fluid,[37] and increased numbers of neurones expressing CRH mRNA in the paraventricular nucleus of the hypothalamus postmortem.[38] CRH is not confined to the paraventricular nucleus, but is expressed in a variety of other central nuclei whence it can produce anxiogenic behavioural effects. CRH receptors, which exist in two forms, are widely distributed in the hypothalamus and cortex. A related peptide, urocortin, has a similar pharmacology. Knocking out the CRH-1 receptor gene in mice impaired the HPA stress response and reduced anxiety-like behav-

iour.[39] Non-peptide CRH antagonists must be taken seriously as putative anxiolytics or antidepressants and are now in clinical trials. If effective, they will be among the first of a new generation of truly novel treatments based on peptide neurotransmission.

Thyroid abnormalities

In unselected major depression, thyroid hormone levels are usually normal, but there may be abnormalities of the thyrotropin (thyroid-stimulating hormone) response to thyrotropin-releasing hormone. The thyrotropin response is blunted in a significant number of patients, but this effect is poorly understood and has few accepted clinical associations. In contrast, a subgroup of patients may show an enhanced thyrotropin response with normal thyroid hormone levels (referred to as grade II hypothyroidism). These associations and the use of thyroid hormones in treatment suggest that there is more to be learned in this area (see Chapter 4.5.7).

Sleep disturbance

Sleep is often disturbed in depression but in a variety of ways. Early-morning waking is the most typical in endogenous or melancholic depression, with the sleep patterns in such patients being similar to those seen in patients with mania. Trouble getting to sleep, frequent wakings, and unsatisfactorily prolonged sleep are also commonly seen in depression. Like other biological manifestations of the disorder, the extent to which sleep is simply a consequence of the state of depression or a contribution to its biology is uncertain. Patients with severe depression or mania may respond to sleep deprivation with a transient elevation in mood. It implies that the sleep–wake cycle is directly involved with mood regulation and its disorder.

In severe depression (melancholia) the typical effects are a reduction in the total length of slow-wave sleep and a shortened latency in the appearance of rapid eye movement (**REM**) or dreaming sleep.[40] The cholinergic projections from the hindbrain may be REM-ON cells, while serotonergic and noradrenergic cells may be REM-OFF cells. The disturbed sleep of depression could be due to an increased cholinergic and/or a decreased serotonergic/noradrenergic drive; simplistic though it sounds, the experimental evidence is supportive. Depressed patients challenged with a cholinergic agonist in the second non-REM period enter REM significantly faster than psychiatric and normal control subjects.[41] The reduced sensitivity of the noradrenergic system is suggested because clonidine fails to suppress REM in depressed patients compared with controls.[42] Tryptophan depletion (to attenuate 5-HT function) partially mimics the changes seen in depression in recovered patients.[43]

Sleep tends to recover on recovery from depression, and the tricyclic antidepressants in particular suppress REM sleep. However, sleep disturbance may be an early predictor of relapse, and disturbed sleep parameters predict a poor response to cognitive–behaviour therapy.[44] Indeed, depressed patients may have inherently weak slow-wave sleep processes because unaffected subjects with a family history of depression show reduced slow-wave sleep and increased REM density in the first sleep cycle.[45] (See also Chapter 4.14.5.)

Monoamine metabolite turnover

The earliest studies to investigate the actions of tricyclic antidepressants highlighted their actions on the turnover of the monoamine

Table 1 Baseline means of monoamine metabolites in cerebrospinal fluid by sex

	Mean ± SD (pmol/ml (*N*))		
	Depressed	Manic	Control
MHPG			
M	46.2 ± 11.2 (53)	57.8 ± 20.9 (9)	42.5 ± 8.9 (30)
F	49.3 ± 11.5 (46)	63.8 ± 18.8 (5)	44.1 ± 7.9 (31)
Combined	47.6 ± 11.4	59.9 ± 19.6	43.3 ± 8.4
HVA			
M	178.0 ± 59.7 (49)	240.0 ± 88.5 (9)	220.0 ± 68.2 (30)
F	209.0 ± 77.3 (43)[a]	324.0 ± 128.0 (5)	240.0 ± 81.8 (32)
5-HIAA			
M	105.0 ± 29.7 (49)	118.0 ± 43.6 (9)	108.0 ± 22.5 (29)
F	130.0 ± 33.6 (43)[b]	161.0 ± 41.2 (5)	114.0 ± 37.1 (29)

HVA, homovanillic acid; 5-HIAA, 5-hydroxyindoleacetic acid; M, males; F, females.

[a] $F = 4.65$, $p < 0.04$ compared with depressed male subjects.

[b] $F = 14.6$, $p < 0.001$ compared with depressed male subjects.

Reproduced with permission from S.H. Koslow *et al.* (1983). *Archives of General Psychiatry*, **40**, 999–1010.

metabolites in animal brain. The 'monoamine theory of depression' proposed the reduced functioning of monoamine transmission in depression. Therefore it was natural to seek relevant measures of monoamine chemistry in the cerebrospinal fluid of patients and controls. The study of what became irreverently known as 'neural urine' and indeed of urine itself, since peripheral measures of monoamine turnover are also potentially relevant, virtually defined a decade of biological psychiatry in the 1970s and 1980s. Drugs had similar effects on neurotransmitter turnover as seen in animal studies, demonstrating that the human techniques were sufficiently sensitive. Indeed the monoamine theory is, at its best, a theory about drug action because the monoamine and metabolite changes produced by illness in patients have proved remarkably unconvincing.[46] Typical results are summarized in Table 1 from the largest published samples. The findings for the noradrenaline metabolite MHPG and the 5-HT metabolite 5-hydroxyindoleacetic acid were negative. The dopamine metabolite homovanillic acid did show the predicted decrease, but only significantly in women. There were trends to modest increases in all the major metabolites in mania. Although disappointing, cerebrospinal fluid studies could never reflect the activities of smaller groups of neurones localized in areas critical for the modulation of mood. Such a focus is only possible in isotope imaging (PET or SPET) or better post-mortem studies of the brain.

Tryptophan depletion

The most convincing evidence that 5-HT is intimately involved in mood disorder has come from depletion of tryptophan, the amino acid precursor of 5-HT. The level of tryptophan in both peripheral blood and the brain can be driven to very low levels by a short-term low-protein diet and subsequent loading with large neutral amino acids. These compete with tryptophan for access to the brain amino acid transporter and also increase its peripheral metabolism, which results in the reduced synthesis and release of 5-HT. Initial observa-

tions appeared to bear primarily on the mechanism of drug action. Thus, patients who had recovered from major depression while taking a serotonin-selective reuptake inhibitor, experienced a clear-cut return of severe symptoms lasting for several hours after tryptophan depletion. This finding has now been critically extended to patients with a history of recurrent major depression who were euthymic but not taking any medication.[47] Prominent objective symptoms of retardation and cognitive distortion returned in a stereotyped and severe way, reflecting previous symptoms (see Fig. 1). The effects on mood in patients who have had a previous episode of depression are qualitatively different from the more minor changes seen in normal female controls or even subjects with a strong family history. This may imply the formation of a form of neurobiological template, which increases the vulnerability to subsequent relapse or recurrence. The immediacy of the link between neurotransmitter function and symptoms may be the reason why patients with recurrent major depression need long-term treatment with antidepressant drugs to remain well.

Does mood disorder have a functional neuropathology?

Severe mood disorder is virtually defined by its frequent recurrence or its chronicity. The first episodes of severe depression occur more frequently with increasing age and tend to be more refractory to treatment. Severe mood disorder is associated with ventricular enlargement and sulcal prominence[48] and persistent cognitive impairment, again most strikingly in older patients.[49] Therefore something may be permanently wrong in the brains of patients with particularly intractable mood disorder and it may be linked to poor outcome.[50] Indeed, there is an increased rate of white matter lesions, perhaps related to vascular disease, in older patients.[51] However, the key hypothesis must be that it is the particular pattern of functional

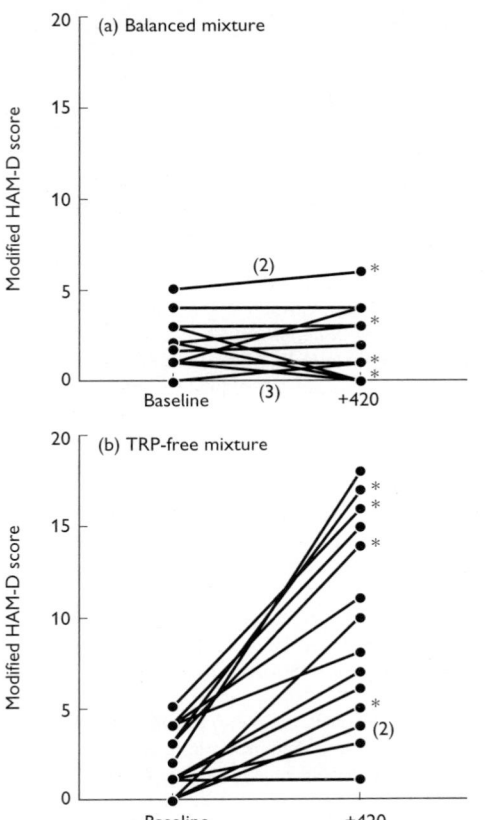

Fig. 1 Changes in modified Hamilton depression (HAM-D) ratings on (a) control and (b) tryptophan (TRP) depletion days over time. (Reproduced with permission from K.A. Smith *et al.* (1997). Relapse of depression after rapid depletion of trytophan. *Lancet*, **349**, 915–19.)

disruption resulting from any cellular pathology that increases the risk of depression. It may be reasonable to describe such a change as a functional neuropathology.

In younger patients with unusual refractoriness and chronicity, MRI scanning again suggested reduced grey matter parameters, most significantly in the left hippocampus but also more diffusely in the left parietal and frontal association cortices (Plate 14). Left hippocampal grey matter density was correlated with measures of verbal memory, supporting the functional significance of the imaging changes. In contrast, patients with severe illnesses fully responsive to treatment showed no differences from controls. Any finding in the chronic group could predate the onset of depression, or be the result of the illness process or its treatment. It is fashionable to attribute structural changes in depression to hypercortisolaemia, but in this study that was not the explanation.[20]

It has been claimed recently that a lobule of inferior frontal cortex, thought to be a critical node for the integration of mood, is atrophic in major depressive illness. Preliminary histopathological assessments of postmortem tissue have suggested that the decrement in grey matter volume is associated with a reduction in glia without an equivalent loss of neurones.[52] This is an unusual finding and requires replication. However, it highlights the fact that postmortem studies of the brain in mood disorder have been rare and seldom focused on 'candidate regions' such as the inferior frontal or cingulate cortex, amygdala, or

hippocampus. Such studies in elderly depression have greater potential validity than the much more numerous investigations of schizophrenia; a definitive study is awaited. (See also Chapter 2.3.5.)

Postmortem studies can also address the neurochemistry, perhaps more directly and completely than other methods. Normal ageing is accompanied by a decline in a variety of indices of monoamine function including presynaptic markers of 5-HT innervation. There is some evidence for a more reduced binding at these sites postmortem in depression,[53] suicide,[54] and cases of Alzheimer's disease with depression.[55] Whether a reduced serotonergic innovation is the critical change that increases the vulnerability to mood disorder of patients with advancing years is not yet established. If so, the potential for MDMA to have long-term effects in heavy users is real and worrying.[56]

In suicide, postmortem findings have broadly paralleled those in depression, with an important emphasis on 5-HT metabolism and neurotransmission (see Chapter 4.15.3). Whether 5-HT neurotransmission, perhaps like that involving the other monoamines, represents a functional domain implicated independently in a variety of psychiatric syndromes and behaviours remains to be well established.

The neurobiology of treatments

It seems quite likely that our understanding of the mechanism of action of drugs or treatments such as electroconvulsive shock, which are antidepressant, antimanic, or mood stabilizing (effective against both poles of bipolar illness), will continue to stimulate ideas about the neurobiology of the illnesses they treat. This approach results from a rather simple linking of the drugs' actions to the possible pathophysiology that they may be correcting. For the first time we are now seeing drugs that have been developed from plausible extrapolations of the neurobiology. The potential of CRH antagonists has already been noticed; neurokinin receptor antagonists that will prevent the action of substance P, another peptide transmitter with a stress profile, also appear to be putative antidepressant drugs.[57]

Conclusions

Mood disorder has an important neurobiological basis. This stretches from a vulnerability, which seems to be attributable to polymorphism in genes critical to stress regulation, through the impact that early experience has on the subsequent programming of the brain for stress responses, to the final responsiveness when encountering particular personal adversity in later life. Biological studies have highlighted the role of key brain areas within the limbic system such as the cingulate cortex and amygdala. We are still a long way from understanding, with any precision, the critical connections and cellular mechanisms, but the function of monoamine neurones generally, and serotonergic projections in particular, is closely associated with mood regulation. Peptide neurotransmitters have long seemed likely to play a central role in stress regulation, and their potential as targets for antidepressant drug action may yet be fulfilled. Finally, observations in the most chronic illnesses and in the elderly with depression have highlighted the possibility of a functional neuropathology underlying severe mood disorder that remains poorly understood.

The approaches of clinicians to the phenomenon of depression still polarize around the biological and the psychosocial. The main purpose is sometimes little more than an assertion of professional territory. This is both regrettable and unnecessary. Any account of depression that claims to be purely social or even psychological misses the point that we are also, in our natures, biological. It is possible to embrace the biology of depressive illness as a fact, while simultaneously acknowledging that it is expressed, and in particular experienced, by patients in psychological terms. Dualism has done psychiatry no favours by teaching us to create a dichotomy between a world of brainless minds and another of mindless brains. The fact that there is an underlying biology which can be unified with a brain-based psychology is, in itself, evidence neither for nor against the likely effect of biological versus psychological treatment. Only with an integrated understanding of the biology and the psychology of mood disorder will we understand the potential and limitations for treatments based on drugs or talking.

References

1. Papez, J.W. (1937). A proposed mechanism of emotion. *Archives of Neurology and Psychiatry*, **38**, 725–43.
2. Adolphs, R., Tranel, D., Damasio, H., and Damasio, A.R. (1995). Fear and the human amygdala. *Journal of Neuroscience*, **15**, 5879–91.
3. Whalen, P.J., Rauch, S.L., Etcoff, N.L., McInerney, S.C., Lee, M.B., and Jenike, M.A. (1998). Masked presentations of emotional facial expressions modulate amygdala activity without explicit knowledge. *Journal of Neuroscience*, **18**, 411–18.
4. George, M.S., Ketter, T.A., Parekh, P.I., Herscovitch, P., and Post, R.M. (1996). Gender differences in regional cerebral blood flow during transient self-induced sadness or happiness. *Biological Psychiatry*, **40**, 859–71.
5. Damasio, A.R. (1995). *Descartes' error. Emotion, reason and the human brain*. Picador, London.
6. Hornak, J., Rolls, E.T., and Wade, D. (1996). Face and voice expression identification in patients with emotional and behavioural changes following ventral frontal lobe damage. *Neuropsychologia*, **34**, 247–61.
7. Green, A.R., Cross, A.J., and Goodwin, G.M. (1995). Review of the pharmacology and clinical pharmacology of 3,4-methylenedioxymethamphetamine (MDMA or 'ecstasy'). *Psychopharmacology*, **119**, 247–60.
8. Battersby, S., Ogilvie, A.D., Smith, C.A.D., *et al.* (1996). Structure of a variable number tandem repeat of the serotonin transporter gene and association with affective disorder. *Psychiatric Genetics*, **6**, 177–81.
9. Heils, A., Teufel, A., Petri, S., *et al.* (1996). Allelic variation of human serotonin transporter gene expression. *Journal of Neurochemistry*, **66**, 2621–4.
10. Jonsson, E.G., Nothen, M.M., Gustavsson, J.P., *et al.* (1998). Polymorphisms in the dopamine, serotonin, and norepinephrine transporter genes and their relationships to monoamine metabolite concentrations in CSF of healthy volunteers. *Psychiatry Research*, **79**, 1–9.
11. Kendler, K.S., Kessler, R.C., Neale, M.C., Heath, A.C., and Eaves, L.J. (1993). The prediction of major depression in women: toward an integrated etiologic model. *American Journal of Psychiatry*, **150**, 1139–48.
12. Flint, J., Corley, R., DeFries, J.C., *et al.* (1995). A simple genetic basis for a complex psychological trait in laboratory mice. *Science*, **269**, 1432–5.
13. Castanon, N., Dulluc, J., Le Moal, M., and Mormede, P. (1994). Maturation of the behavioural and neuroendocrine differences between the Roman rat lines. *Physiology and Behavior*, **55**, 775–82.
14. Kendler, K.S. and Karkowski-Shuman, L. (1997). Stressful life events and genetic liability to major depression: genetic control of exposure to the environment? *Psychological Medicine*, **27**, 539–47.
15. Liu, D., Diorio, J., Tannenbaum, B., *et al.* (1997). Maternal care, hippocampal glucocorticoid receptors, and hypothalamic–pituitary–adrenal responses to stress. *Science*, **277**, 1659–62.
16. Caldji, C., Tannenbaum, B., Sharma, S., Francis, D., Plotsky, P.M., and Meaney, M.J. (1998). Maternal care during infancy regulates the development of neural systems mediating the expression of fearfulness in the rat. *Proceedings of the National Academy of Sciences of the United States of America*, **95**, 5335–40.
17. Goodwin, G.M. (1996). Functional imaging, affective disorder and dementia. *British Medical Bulletin*, **52**, 495–512.
18. Mayberg, H.S., Brannan, S.K., Mahurin, R.K., *et al.* (1997). Cingulate function in depression: a potential predictor of treatment response. *Neuroreport*, **8**, 1057–61.
19. Goodwin, G.M. (1997). Neuropsychological and neuroimaging evidence for the involvement of the frontal lobes in depression. *Journal of Psychopharmacology*, **11**, 115–22.
20. Shah, P.J., Ebmeier, K.P., Glabus, M.F., and Goodwin, G.M. (1998). Cortical grey matter reductions associated with treatment-resistant chronic unipolar depression: controlled magnetic resonance imaging study. *British Journal of Psychiatry*, **72**, 527–32.
21. Biver, F., Wikler, D., Lotstra, F., Damhaut, P., Goldman, S., and Mendlewicz, J. (1997). Serotonin 5-HT-2 receptor imaging in major depression: focal changes in orbito-insular cortex. *British Journal of Psychiatry*, **171**, 444–8.
22. Upadhyaya, A.K., Pennell, I., Cowen, P.J., and Deakin, J.F.W. (1991). Blunted growth hormone and prolactin responses to L-tryptophan in depression; a state-dependent abnormality. *Journal of Affective Disorders*, **21**, 213–18.
23. Anderson, I.M., Ware, C.J., Da Roza, J.M., and Cowen, P.J. (1992). Decreased 5-HT-mediated prolactin release in major depression. *British Journal of Psychiatry*, **160**, 372–8.
24. Cowen, P.J., Power, A.C., Ware, C.J., and Anderson, I.M. (1994). 5-HT (1A) receptor sensitivity in major depression. A neuroendocrine study with buspirone. *British Journal of Psychiatry*, **164**, 372–9.
25. Schittecatte, M., Charles, G., Machowski, R., *et al.* (1994). Effects of gender and diagnosis on growth hormone response to clonidine for major depression: a large-scale multicenter study. *American Journal of Psychiatry*, **151**, 216–20.
26. Pitchot, W., Hansenne, M., Moreno, A.G., and Ansseau, M. (1995). Effect of previous antidepressant therapy on the growth hormone response to apomorphine. *Neuropsychobiology*, **32**, 19–22.
27. Wieck, A., Kumar, R., Hirst, A.D., Marks, M.N., Campbell, I.C., and Checkley, S.A. (1991). Increased sensitivity of dopamine receptors and recurrence of affective psychosis after childbirth. *British Medical Journal*, **303**, 613–16.
28. O'Keane, V., O'Flynn, K., Lucey, J., and Dinan, T.G. (1992). Pyridostigmine-induced growth hormone responses in healthy and depressed subjects: evidence for cholinergic supersensitivity in depression. *Psychological Medicine*, **22**, 55–60.
29. Rubin, R.T., Phillips, J.J., Sadow, T.F., and McCracken, J.T. (1995). Adrenal gland volume in major depression: increase during the depressive episode and decrease with successful treatment. *Archives of General Psychiatry*, **52**, 213–18.
30. Carroll, B.J., Feinberg, M., Greden, J.F., *et al.* (1981). A specific laboratory test for the diagnosis of melancholia. Standardization, validation, and clinical utility. *Archives of General Psychiatry*, **38**, 15–22.
31. Ribeiro, S.C.M., Tandon, R., Grunhaus, L., and Greden, J.F. (1993). The DST as a predictor of outcome in depression: a meta-analysis. *American Journal of Psychiatry*, **150**, 1618–29.
32. Thase, M.E., Dube, S., Bowler, K., *et al.* (1996). Hypothalamic–pituitary–adrenocortical activity and response to cognitive behavior therapy in unmedicated, hospitalized depressed patients. *American Journal of Psychiatry*, **153** (Supplement), 886–91.

33. Goodwin, G.M., Muir, W.J., Seckl, J.R., *et al.* (1992). The effects of cortisol infusion upon hormone secretion from the anterior pituitary and subjective mood in depressive illness and in controls. *Journal of Affective Disorders*, **26**, 73–83.

34. Dinan, T.G., Lavelle, E., Cooney, J., *et al.* (1997). Dexamethasone augmentation in treatment-resistant depression. *Acta Psychiatrica Scandinavica*, **95**, 58–61.

35. Goodwin, G.M., Austin, M.P., Curran, S.M., *et al.* (1993). The elevation of plasma beta-endorphin levels in major depression. *Journal of Affective Disorders*, **29**, 281–9.

36. Heuser, I., Yassouridis, A., and Holsboer, F. (1994). The combined dexamethasone/CRH test: a refined laboratory test for psychiatric disorders. *Journal of Psychiatric Research*, **28**, 341–56.

37. Mitchell, A.J. (1998). The role of corticotropin releasing factor in depressive illness: a critical review. *Neuroscience and Biobehavioral Reviews*, **22**, 635–51.

38. Raadsheer, F.C., Van Heerikhuize, J.J., Lucassen, P.J., Hoogendijk, W.J.G., Tilders, F.J.H., and Swaab, D.F. (1995). Corticotropin-releasing hormone mRNA levels in the paraventricular nucleus of patients with Alzheimer's disease and depression. *American Journal of Psychiatry*, **152**, 1372–6.

39. Timpl, P., Spanagel, R., Sillaber, I., *et al.* (1998). Impaired stress response and reduced anxiety in mice lacking a functional corticotropin-releasing hormone receptor 1. *Nature Genetics*, **19**, 162–6.

40. Berger, M. and Riemann, D. (1993). REM sleep in depression—an overview. *Journal of Sleep Research*, **2**, 211–23.

41. Gillin, J.C., Sutton, L., Ruiz, C., *et al.* (1991). The cholinergic rapid eye movement induction test with arecoline in depression. *Archives of General Psychiatry*, **48**, 264–70.

42. Schittecatte, M., Garcia Valentin, J., Charles, G., *et al.* (1995). Efficacy of the 'clonidine REM suppression test (CREST)' to separate patients with major depression from controls; a comparison with three currently proposed biological markers of depression. *Journal of Affective Disorders*, **33**, 151–7.

43. Moore, P., Gillin, J.C., Bhatti, T., *et al.* (1998). Rapid tryptophan depletion, sleep electroencephalogram, and mood in men with remitted depression on serotonin reuptake inhibitors. *Archives of General Psychiatry*, **55**, 534–9.

44. Thase, M.E., Simons, A.D., and Reynolds, C.F., III. (1993). Psychobiological correlates of poor response to cognitive behavior therapy. Potential indications for antidepressant pharmacotherapy. *Psychopharmacology Bulletin*, **29**, 293–301.

45. Lauer, C.J., Schreiber, W., Holsboer, F., and Krieg, J.C. (1995). In quest of identifying vulnerability markers for psychiatric disorders by all-night polysomnography. *Archives of General Psychiatry*, **52**, 145–53.

46. Schatzberg, A.F., Samson, J.A., Bloomingdale, K.L., *et al.* (1989). Toward a biochemical classification of depressive disorders. X. Urinary catecholamines, their metabolites, and D-type scores in subgroups of depressive disorders. *Archives of General Psychiatry*, **46**, 260–8.

47. Smith, K.A., Fairburn, C.G., and Cowen, P.J. (1997). Relapse of depression after rapid depletion of tryptophan. *Lancet*, **349**, 915–19.

48. Elkis, H., Friedman, L., Wise, A., and Meltzer, H.Y. (1995). Meta-analyses of studies of ventricular enlargement and cortical sulcal prominence in mood disorders: comparisons with controls or patients with schizophrenia. *Archives of General Psychiatry*, **52**, 735–46.

49. Abas, M.A., Sahakian, B.J., and Levy, R. (1990). Neuropsychological deficits and CT scan changes in elderly depressives. *Psychological Medicine*, **20**, 507–20.

50. Simpson, S., Baldwin, R.C., Jackson, A., and Burns, A.S. (1998). Is subcortical disease associated with a poor response to antidepressants? Neurological, neuropsychological and neuroradiological findings in late-life depression. *Psychological Medicine*, **28**, 1015–26.

51. Coffey, C.E., Figiel, G.S., Djang, W.T., Cress, M., Saunders, W.B., and Weiner, R.D. (1988). Leukoencephalopathy in elderly depressed patients referred for ECT. *Biological Psychiatry*, **24**, 143–61.

52. Drevets, W.C., Ongur, D., and Price, J.L. (1998). Neuroimaging abnormalities in the subgenual prefrontal cortex: implications for the pathophysiology of familial mood disorders. *Molecular Psychiatry*, **3**, 220–6.

53. Lawrence, K.M., Kanagasundaram, M., Lowther, S., Katona, C.L.E., Crompton, M.R., and Horton, R.W. (1998). [³H] imipramine binding in brain samples from depressed suicides and controls: 5-HT uptake sites compared with sites defined by desmethylimipramine. *Journal of Affective Disorders*, **47**, 1–3.

54. Mann, J.J. (1998). The neurobiology of suicide. *Nature Medicine*, **4**, 25–30.

55. Chen, C.H., Alder, J.T., Bowen, D.M., *et al.* (1996). Presynaptic serotonergic markers in community-acquired cases of Alzheimer's disease: correlations with depression and neuroleptic medication. *Journal of Neurochemistry*, **66**, 1592–8.

56. Green, A.R. and Goodwin, G.M. (1996). Ecstasy and neurodegeneration. *British Medical Journal*, **312**, 1493–4.

57. Kramer, M.S., Cutler, N., Feighner, J., *et al.* (1998). Distinct mechanism for antidepressant activity by blockade of central substance P receptors. *Science*, **281**, 1640–5.

4.5.6 Course and prognosis of mood disorders

Jules Angst

The importance of course and the limits of our knowledge

An understanding of the course of a disorder is fundamental for doctor and patient when deciding whether to start long-term prophylactic medication and, at a later stage, whether to stop a successful long-term treatment. Course is a crucial factor in estimating the social consequences, suicide risk, and mortality associated with mood disorders.

A distinction should be made between the natural history of a disorder, describing its spontaneous untreated course, and course as observed under treatment, whether of episodes or long term (both episodes and the intervals between them). Most mood disorders have a phasic course, characterized by multiple recurrences; a minority manifest as a single episode or have a chronic course.

The description of course includes the age of onset, episode length, recurrence of episodes, and residual symptoms between episodes and outcome (remission, chronicity, death). All these aspects are discussed in this chapter.

Our understanding of the course of affective disorders is limited for several reasons. The course of bipolar disorder and unipolar depression are markedly different; however, Kraepelin's[1] unification of bipolar disorder[2] with all affective disorders to form the single diagnosis 'manic depressive insanity' resulted in there being very little investigation of the natural history of the two subgroups (bipolar and depressive disorders) before the introduction of modern pharmacotherapy. Moreover, modern studies are carried out on treated patients, and the effect of drug-induced changes on the natural history of disorders is difficult to estimate. Another methodological limitation of modern studies of course is the selection of samples. Traditionally, samples have comprised hospitalized psychiatric patients, with a minority including psychiatric outpatients; studies following patients in primary care or in the community have been rare. Yet another methodological problem is that of memory artefacts. Although a retest study on the age of onset over a time span of 6 months showed good reliability, over the longer term patients significantly forget or misreport the previous history of their disorders, especially the precise age of onset and the number of earlier episodes, and there are no lifelong prospective studies of course in representative samples selected from the community or general practice to compensate for such distortions.

For all these reasons our understanding of the natural history and the course of mood disorders remains limited, especially in milder cases.

Stability of the diagnoses of mood disorders

Ever since Kahlbaum[3] and Kraepelin[1] the course and outcome of mental disorders have played important roles as criteria and validators of psychiatric classification. Mood disorders can be roughly subclassified into bipolar disorder and depressive disorders. The two groups of disorders differ significantly as regards family history and course.[4–6]

Distinguishing between bipolar disorder and unipolar depressive disorder is hampered by the fact that the diagnosis of unipolar depression is always uncertain. A long-term follow-up study over 27 years showed an annual rate of diagnostic change from depression to hypomania of about 1 per cent. The risk of such change seems not to fade but rather to be renewed with each fresh episode during a recurrent course. Therefore most studies conducted on unipolar depressive subjects include an unknown proportion of bipolar cases. For the same reason the exact ratio of bipolar to unipolar depressive subjects is unknown. Modern estimates range from 1:5 to 1:1. Thus many depressives may be hidden bipolar patients; these would include depressives with a positive family history of mania, those who have at some time manifested minor mood swings of hypomania (1–3 days), those who have shown so-called 'drug induced' hypomania, and depressive subjects with a hyperthymic or cyclothymic temperament or a cyclothymic mood disorder.

Today, bipolar disorder is conceptualized as a wide spectrum embracing all the milder forms of the disorder, ranging from cyclothymia and mild and brief hypomania, through hypomania, bipolar II disorder, and bipolar I disorder, to 'pure' mania. Bipolar II disorder shows good diagnostic stability over a 5-year period.[7] Nevertheless, over a patient's lifetime there may be frequent shifts across the diagnostic spectra of bipolar disorder and depressive disorders respectively. In the longer term the diagnosis of major depressive disorder remains stable in only 40 to 50 per cent of cases; in the remainder, diagnostic changes to dysthymia, recurrent brief depression, minor depression, and subthreshold depression are frequently observed, as well as recovery.

Onset of bipolar disorder and depression

In patients admitted to hospital between 1913 and 1940 and not treated by electroconvulsive therapy or modern psychotropic drugs, bipolar disorder clearly manifested earlier than unipolar depression;[8]

this finding is confirmed by modern community studies. Bipolar disorder generally begins during adolescence but may manifest even earlier.

Epidemiological studies identify the age of onset of bipolar disorder as between 15 and 19 years (means), whereas studies of hospitalized patients date its onset in the early twenties or in the thirties. The age-of-onset curve is skewed, and therefore mean values are not representative. In a large Canadian general population study,[9] 95 per cent of manic cases manifested before the age of 26 (males) and 25 (females), and 95 per cent of major depressive episodes before the age of 55 (males) and 43 (females). There was a considerable time lag between the age at onset of the first impairing symptoms (15 years), diagnosis (19 years), first treatment (22 years) and hospitalization (26 years).

Bipolar I illness manifests earlier than bipolar II and psychotic bipolar disorder. Late-onset bipolar disorder is rare but does occur and may be associated with specific neuropathology.

Unlike bipolar disorder, depression may start at any time of life. There is no dichotomy but a continuum from early-onset to late-onset depression, with a systematic decrease in genetic vulnerability and an increase in precipitation by environmental factors. Late-onset depression is more often milder and chronic.

A two-peak distribution of the age of onset has sometimes been described for both bipolar disorder and depression, but there is no second peak linked with the menopause in women.

Prodromal hypomanic and depressive symptoms and subclinical syndromes frequently precede mania and major depression over many years; this is especially true for depression in old age (75 years and more). The first manic and depressive manifestations are commonly mild, brief, or uncharacteristic, and are only diagnosed in retrospect.

Length of episodes

Most bipolar and depressive episodes are short, but a minority become chronic (lasting more than 2 years); the distribution of episode length is log normal, and therefore percentiles and not averages should be used as parameters. Using the data collected a century ago by Mendel[10] and Ziehen[11] on the natural length of episodes of mania and bipolar disorder, mainly among hospitalized patients, it is possible to compute a median length of 4 to 6 months for mania and 5 to 6 months for bipolar disorder. Wertham[12] also reports a median length of 4 to 6 months based on analysis of 2000 manic attacks. These figures do not differ from those obtained today despite a wide range of antimanic and antidepressant treatments. Among hospitalized patients episode length (median) was 4.2 months for bipolars and 5.4 months for major depressives;[13] 25 per cent of bipolar episodes lasted more than 7.3 months and 25 per cent of depressive episodes lasted more than 11 months. By contrast, in the community, where many untreated cases of depression occur, episode duration was considerably shorter; the 25th, 50th, and 75th percentiles were 4 weeks, 12 weeks, and 30 weeks respectively for 71 incident episode duration, and were 4 weeks, 8 weeks, and 16 weeks respectively for 28 recurrent episodes.[14] These subsamples were small and the data on recurrent episodes were not corrected for total number of episodes.

In 10 to 20 per cent of subjects, mood disorders take a chronic course (length over 24 months) without remission.[15] Electroconvulsive therapy can curtail depressive episodes, whereas antimanic and antidepressant drugs only alleviate the symptoms; this is why termination of treatment during an ongoing episode induces a rapid relapse.

It is important to note that the lengths of episodes of bipolar disorder and of depression have probably remained constant for over a century.

Recurrence

Recurrence is typical of mood disorders. It can be characterized by the number of episodes, the length of intervals (measured from remission to the onset of a new episode), and the length of cycles (measured from the beginning of one episode to the beginning of the next). Statistically, a normal distribution of cycle length can be obtained by log n transformation. In prospective studies, the length of the interval is frequently used as a parameter for survival analyses of recurrence.

In both bipolar disorder and unipolar depression the time from the first to the second episode is on average much longer than that from the second to the third. This progressive shortening of cycles and free intervals then levels off and fluctuates around a certain (but still variable) individual limit. Most published data on interval length or cycle length are methodologically flawed because they have not been corrected for the number of episodes/cycles observed, an improvement suggested by Slater[16] as early as 1938. Nonetheless, multiple episodes obviously follow each other in more rapid succession than a few episodes distributed over a lifetime. Even after taking episode numbers into account, there is a clear intraindividual trend to a progressive shortening of cycle length,[17,18] dimming the prognosis for both bipolar disorder and unipolar depression. Cycle length tends to be shorter in late-onset than in early-onset mood disorders, increasing the risk of recurrence in the elderly.

Precipitating events play an important role in the onset of the first few affective episodes; thereafter recurrrence seems to become more autonomous with stressful events contributing little or nothing to the process.[19] Stressors may not only precipitate episodes but also increase a pre-existent vunerability, sensitizing the individual and thereby making him or her more vulnerable to further episodes (kindling effect[20]). In bipolar illness there is no difference in the quality or quantity of stressors precipitating depressive and manic episodes; a legacy or the loss of a relative can induce depression or hypomania.

Counts of single-episode cases of mood disorders depend strongly on whether or not mild and brief hypomania and depression are included and on the length of observation. Single-episode bipolar disorders probably do not occur, and single-episode unipolar depression is observed in only 10 to 15 per cent of cases.

The course of the mood disorders of the overwhelming majority of patients, whether psychiatric inpatients, outpatients, or general practitioner patients, is recurrent; even milder depressive episodes tend to be recurrent.[21]

The pattern of recurrence is irregular. Compared with normal subjects, the daily mood ratings of bipolar subjects were characterized as a low-dimensional chaotic process and true cyclicity was not apparent in the power spectra of either group (normal subjects or bipolars).[22]

Over a lifetime bipolar patients experience twice as many episodes as unipolar depressives, a difference which is not explained by the manifestation of manic episodes in addition to depression. The total number of episodes observed depends on the length of observation. In a 22- to 26-year follow-up study, bipolar patients experienced a median of 10 episodes, whereas depressive patients experienced four episodes.[13] On average, 0.44 episodes per year were observed in bipolar patients and 0.30 in depressive patients.

A follow-up study of manic subjects applying survival analysis demonstrated relapse and recurrence rates of 20 per cent by 6 months, 48 per cent by 1 year, and 81 per cent by 5 years; patients with mixed/cycling features had a 10 per cent higher recurrence rate than pure manics. In a recent large representative Danish record study ($N = 20 350$ first admissions) unipolar depressives had strikingly lower recurrence rates (hospitalizations) than bipolars, both correlating with the number of previous episodes.[18] The authors concluded: 'The course of severe unipolar and bipolar disorder seems to be progressive in nature despite the effect of treatment and irrespective of gender, age and type of disorder'.

Outcome

Incomplete remission

Remission after affective episodes is frequently incomplete. Residual symptoms are common in psychiatric and general practitioner patients and in cases identified in community studies. Comparatively little is currently known about the residual symptoms of mania, although they do exist. Residual symptoms of major depression, defined by a score of 8 or more on the 17-item Hamilton Depression Scale, were found in 32 per cent of 60 patients 12 to 15 months after remission.[23] Residual symptoms represent a strong risk factor for further recurrence; a survival analysis by Paykel et al.[23] found a threefold higher risk of recurrence (76 per cent) in patients with residual symptoms than in those without (25 per cent). Chronic residual symptoms are those typical of depression: mood, anxiety, genital symptoms,[24] insomnia, headaches, neurasthenic complaints, reduced libido, and gastrointestinal symptoms. They are frequently treated by long-term antidepressant medication, which should not be withdrawn until the patient has had 4 months completely free of symptoms.

Long-term outcome

The long-term outcome of mood disorders is usually unfavourable. Five comparable long-term follow-up studies (10 years or more) are listed in Table 1. All re-examined depressive patients, most if not all of whom had originally been admitted to psychiatric hospitals. After 10 years, roughly one-third had been readmitted, and this figure rose to about two-thirds after 20 years. A poor outcome, as operationally defined by Lee and Murray,[25] was observed in 11 to 25 per cent of patients. The outcome was in no way more favourable in the two studies that included psychiatric outpatients.

Bipolar disorder has a poorer outcome than depression. After a follow-up of 22 to 26 years, definitive recovery (at least 5 years with good social adaptation) was found in 25 per cent of 186 depressive subjects, whereas the figure was 16 per cent of the 220 bipolar patients; a chronic course lasting at least 2 years without remission was present in 11.8 per cent of the depressive subjects compared with 14.1 per cent of the bipolars.[29]

Modern treatment may have changed the outcome of mood disorders by reducing chronicity and rehospitalization. A recent 10-year prospective study of 131 hospitalized bipolar patients[30] found that

Table 1 Long-term follow-up studies of depression

Reference	N	Follow-up (years)	Readmitted (%)	Poor outcome (%)	Suicide (%)
Lee and Murray (1988)[25]	89	18	62	25	9[a]
Kiloh et al. (1988)[26]	133	15	56	11	7
Thornicroft and Sartorius (1993)[27]	439[b]	10	35	18	9
Surtees and Barkley (1994)[28]	80[c]	12	60	27	0
Angst and Preisig (1995)[29]	186	22–27	66	13	13

[a] Including probable suicide/suspect unnatural deaths.
[b] 62.8% inpatients.
[c] 87.5% inpatients.

only 4 per cent had developed chronicity, although most patients still had recurrences. The frequency of episodes did not increase with time, so no further kindling effect was observed. Comorbidity with alcoholism, a factor known to correlate with poorer outcome, was found in 30 per cent of the patients. Coryell et al.[7] found that, over 5 years, bipolar II disorder had a better outcome than bipolar I disorder in terms of rehospitalizations; furthermore, the two groups tended to remain diagnostically stable. Episode frequency was comparable in the two groups.

Mortality

Mortality expressed by the standardized mortality ratio (**SMR**) is elevated in subjects suffering from mood disorders, irrespective of the sample selection (community or psychiatric inpatients). An SMR of between 1.37 and 2.49 has been found among mood disorder subjects; in the normal population it is 1.0. Suicide is the main, but not the sole, cause of this elevated mortality. Other over-represented causes of death among patients with mood disorders are accidents, cardiovascular disorders, cerebrovascular disorders, respiratory infections, thyroid disorders, and secondary substance abuse/dependence.[31]

A meta-analysis[32] of 58 studies covering 2257 cases of suicide gave the following SMRs for suicide mortality compared with suicides in the general population (SMR = 1.0): bipolar disorder, 15.05, major depressive disorder/major depressive episode, 20.35; dysthymia, 12.12; depression not otherwise specified, 16.10. Taking all diagnostic categories together, suicide among mood-disorder patients was 13.65 times more frequent than in the general population.

The long-term follow-up studies of severely depressed patients (Table 1) gave suicide rates between zero and 13 per cent. The frequently quoted rate of 12 to 19 per cent[33] may only be valid for hospitalized patient samples, which by definition include many suicidal patients. In community and outpatient samples, suicide accounted for only a small percentage of deaths. Many suicides can probably be prevented by administering long-term antidepressant medication[34] and lithium.[35,36]

Prediction

Predicting course remains an uncertain art. In general, studies of predictors should be prospective and the results replicated, prerequisites which are rarely fulfilled. Most of the reported predictors tend to be hypothetical in value.

The previous course of mood disorders predicts future course, recurrence (number of previous episodes) predicts further recurrence, and the length of episodes and residual symptoms predict recurrence. Acute onset and few attacks predict a better outcome, whereas poor functioning over years predicts a worse outcome.

Age does not seem to have a great effect on outcome, but depression in the elderly, although milder, is often more chronic.

Neuroticism as a measure of emotional and vegetative lability tends to remain stable in depressives, if the effect of ageing is taken into account. High-baseline neuroticism scores predict a poorer outcome in patients, primiparae with postnatal depression, and subjects in the community.

Neuroticism is a risk factor for recurrence perhaps because it includes many items measuring depressive symptoms (and subclinical depression is known to predict incidence and recurrence of depression). The Symptom Check List 90R[37] is also a predictor for recurrence; it correlates closely with neuroticism and includes both emotional and vegetative lability.

Low self-esteem was not found to be a predictor of the first onset of depression but rather a symptom that waxes and wanes with depression itself.[38] Lack of self-confidence predicted the recurrence of depression in a prospective study.[39]

Neurotic depression has a poorer prognosis than endogenous depression and a much poorer prognosis than retarded depression. However, on the whole the subtyping of depression (melancholic, endogenous, simple, delusional) has little predictive value.

Comorbidity of alcoholism and personality disorders with bipolar disorder and depression make for a poorer prognosis and outcome of both.

Course of other subtypes of mood disorders

Minor depression

In the community, measures of the recurrence of minor depression are similar to those for major depression, a fact confirmed by survival analyses.[40]

A diagnostic change from minor to major depression, or the reverse, is frequent during the course of mood disorders. Primary minor depression, like depressive symptoms in general, is a significant risk factor for major depression. It may represent a residual state of major depression and a risk factor for recurrence. Among the elderly, in which age group only about one-third of cases of major depression fully recover, minor depression is common as a residual state of major depression.

Both minor and major depression should be seriously considered as a target for preventive intervention and treatment.[40]

Seasonal affective disorder

Many patients experience affective episodes mainly in the spring or in autumn to winter; others suffer from both types of seasonal recurrence. Seasonal affective disorder (**SAD**) remained seasonal in 70 per cent of 43 cases followed up over 2 to 5 years, but the rate of diagnostic stability of SAD was limited to 26 per cent because 44 per cent of the subjects later developed seasonal subthreshold (subsyndromal) depression and another 20 per cent recovered.[41] In three other studies SAD had a higher diagnostic stability (between 38 per cent and 57 per cent).

Thus the diagnostic stability of SAD is clearly weaker than the seasonality of depressive symptoms and syndromes.

Rapid cycling mood disorder

Rapid cycling is found almost exclusively in bipolar disorder. It is defined by the presence of four or more affective episodes in 12 months, and is more frequent in females and in the bipolar II subtype. Rapid cycling does not appear to represent a chronic endstage form of bipolar disorder; it is often a transient non-familial manifestation of bipolar disorder.[42] A prospective follow-up study conducted over approximately 3 years showed diagnostic stability in about half the cases and the other half had fewer than four further episodes per year; in a control group 10 per cent of the non-rapid-cycling patients converted to rapid cycling.[43]

Rapid cycling does occur in unipolar depression, but is usually a transient and unstable phenomenon. Bipolar rapid cycling takes a very autonomous course and is very hard to treat.

Consequences for treatment

After the initial split into bipolar disorder and unipolar depression, the last 30 years have seen the progressive subdivision of mood disorders into further subgroups: bipolar I, bipolar II, rapid cycling bipolar disorder, minor depression, dysthymia, SAD, and so on. In the process the characteristics of the course of a disorder have been incorporated into the classification, which means that course and prognosis are no longer independent of the diagnostic definition.

The distinction between bipolar disorder and unipolar depression is fundamental. These disorders differ markedly in their course and outcome, with bipolar disorder having an earlier onset, higher episode frequency, slightly shorter episode length, and poorer outcome (fewer full recoveries, slightly more chronicity), but, unexpectedly, probably fewer suicides. All bipolar disorders and most unipolar depressive disorders are recurrent, with a minority having a really good prognosis without residual symptoms and further recurrences. Bipolar II disorders probably have a slightly better prognosis than bipolar I disorders.

Therapeutic decisions on the length of acute treatment will depend on the length of the individual's previous episodes and on the average episode length observed in follow-up studies. The length of affective episodes has probably not changed in 100 years. Antidepressants cannot shorten the episodes but can minimize the symptoms. Treatment should be maintained for the duration of episodes, which are frequently masked; otherwise relapses must be expected.

The choice of a long-term prophylactic medication also has to take into consideration the previous individual course of the disorder plus the general scientific knowledge about course and prognosis, and to keep in mind the increased mortality, especially the high suicide mortality associated with mood disorders.[44] Recurrence is also a feature in mild cases, but in contrast with severe cases the suicide mortality is probably low. Decisions about long-term medication also have to take into account whether there are residual symptoms during the intervals; such symptoms are a strong risk factor for further recurrence. Over the lifetime, each new recurrence is associated with a new risk of suicide. Any cessation of treatment has to take these risks into account. So far there are no positive recommendations for the cessation of prophylactic treatment.

References

1. Kraepelin, E. (1899). *Psychiatrie. Ein Lehrbuch für Studierende und Ärzte* (6th edn). Barth, Leipzig.
2. Falret, J.P. (1851). De la folie circulaire ou forme de maladie mentale caractérisée par l'alternative régulière de la manie et de la mélancholie. *Bulletin de l'Académie de Médecine (Paris)*, **6**, 382–400.
3. Kahlbaum, K. (1863). *Die Gruppirung der psychischen Krankheiten und die Eintheilung der Seelenstörungen*. A.W. Kafemann, Danzig.
4. Angst, J. (1966). *Zur Ätiologie und Nosologie endogener depressiver Psychosen. Monographien aus dem Gesamtgebiete der Neurologie und Psychiatrie*. Springer-Verlag, Berlin.
5. Perris, C. (1966). A study of bipolar (manic–depressive) and unipolar recurrent depressive psychoses. *Acta Psychiatrica Sandinavica*, **194** (Supplement), 1–189.
6. Winokur, G. and Clayton, P.J. (1967). Family history studies. I. Two types of affective disorders separated according to genetic and clinical factors. In *Recent advances in biological psychiatry*, Vol. 9 (ed. J. Wortis), pp. 35–50. Plenum Press, New York.
7. Coryell, W., Keller, M.B., Endicott, J., Andreasen, N.C., Clayton, P.J., and Hirschfeld, R.M.A. (1989) Bipolar II illness: course and outcome over a five-year period. *Psychological Medicine*, **19**, 129–41.
8. Stephens, J.J. and McHugh, P.R. (1991). Characteristics and long-term follow-up of patients hospitalized for mood disorders in the Phipps Clinic. *Journal of Nervous and Mental Diseases*, **179**, 64–73.
9. Bland, R.C., Newman, S.C., and Orn, H. (1988). Age of onset of psychiatric disorders. *Acta Psychiatrica Scandinavica*, **338** (Supplement), 43–9.
10. Mendel, E. (1881). *Die Manie*. Urban and Schwarzenberg, Vienna.
11. Ziehen, T. (1896). *Die Erkennung und Behandlung der Melancholie in der Praxis*. Karl Marhold, Halle.
12. Wertham, F.I. (1929). A group of benign chronic psychoses: prolonged manic excitements. With a statistical study of age, duration and frequency in 2000 manic attacks. *American Journal of Psychiatry*, **9**, 17–28.
13. Angst, J. and Preisig, M. (1995) Course of a clinical cohort of unipolar, bipolar and schizoaffective patients. Results of a prospective study from 1959 to 1985. *Schweizer Archiv für Psychiatrie und Neurologie*, **146**, 5–16.
14. Eaton, W.W., Anthony, J.C., Gallo, J., *et al.* (1997) Natural history of Diagnostic Interview Schedule DSM-IV major depression. The Baltimore Epidemiologic Catchment Area follow-up. *Archives of General Psychiatry*, **54**, 993–9.

15. Angst, J. (1988). Clinical course of affective disorders. In *Depressive illness: prediction of course and outcome* (ed. T. Helgason and R.J. Daly), pp. 1–48. Springer-Verlag, Berlin.

16. Slater, E. (1938) Zur Periodik des manisch-depressiven Irreseins. *Zeitschrift für die Gesamte Neurologie und Psychiatrie*, **162**, 784–801.

17. Angst, J. (1981). Course of affective disorders. In *Handbook of biological psychiatry*. Part IV: *Brain mechanisms and abnormal behavior-chemistry* (ed. H.M. van Praag), pp. 225–42. Marcel Dekker, New York.

18. Kessing, L.V., Andersen, P.K., Mortensen, P.B., and Bolwig, T.G. (1998) Recurrence in affective disorder. I. Case register study. *British Journal of Psychiatry*, **172**, 23–8.

19. Goodwin, F.K. and Jamison, K.R. (1990). *Manic–depressive illness*. Oxford University Press.

20. Post, R.M., Rubinow, D.R., and Ballenger, J.C. (1984). Conditioning, sensitization, and kindling: implications for the course of affective illness. In *Neurobiology of mood disorders* (ed. R.M. Post and J.C. Ballenger), pp. 432–66. Williams and Wilkins, Baltimore, MD.

21. Angst, J. (1990). Depression and anxiety: a review of studies in the community and primary health care. In *Psychological disorders in general medical settings* (ed. J. Costa e Silva, Y. Lecrubier, and U. Wittchen), pp. 60–8. Hogrefe and Huber, Toronto.

22. Gottschalk, A., Bauer, M.S., and Whybrow, P.C. (1995). Evidence of chaotic mood variation in bipolar disorder. *Archives of General Psychiatry*, **52**, 947–59.

23. Paykel, E.S., Ramana, R., Cooper, Z., Hayhurst, H., Kerr, J., and Barocka, A. (1995). Residual symptoms after partial remission: an important outcome in depression. *Psychological Medicine*, **25**, 1171–80.

24. Paykel, E.S. (1998). Remission and residual symptomatology in major depression. *Psychopathology*, **31**, 5–14.

25. Lee, A.S. and Murray, R.M. (1988). The long-term outcome of Maudsley depressives. *British Journal of Psychiatry*, **153**, 741–51.

26. Kiloh, L.G., Andrews, G., and Neilson, M. (1988). The long-term outcome of depressive illness. *British Journal of Psychiatry*, **153**, 752–7.

27. Thornicroft, G. and Sartorius, N. (1993). The course and outcome of depression in different cultures: 10-year follow-up of the WHO Collaborative Study on the Assessment of Depressive Disorders. *Psychological Medicine*, **23**, 1023–32.

28. Surtees, P.G. and Barkley, C. (1994). Future imperfect: the long-term outcome of depression. *British Journal of Psychiatry*, **164**, 327–41.

29. Angst, J. and Preisig, M. (1995). Outcome of a clinical cohort of unipolar, bipolar and schizoaffective patients. Results of a prospective study from 1959 to 1985. *Schweizer Archiv für Psychiatrie und Neurologie*, **146**, 17–23.

30. Tohen, M., Waternaux, C. and Tsuang, M.T. (1990). Outcome in mania. A 4-year prospective follow-up of 75 patients utilizing survival analysis. *Archives of General Psychiatry*, **47**, 1106–11.

31. Angst, F., Sellaro, R., Stassen, H.H., and Angst, J. Mortality of patients with mood disorders: follow-up over 34 to 38 years. In preparation.

32. Harris, E.C. and Barraclough, B. (1997). Suicide as an outcome for mental disorders. A meta-analysis. *British Journal of Psychiatry*, **170**, 205–28.

33. Guze, S.B. and Robins, E. (1970). Suicide and primary affective disorder. *British Journal of Psychiatry*, **117**, 437–8.

34. Angst, F., Sellaro, R., and Angst, J. (1998) The natural history of bipolar disorder. Presented at the Summer Meeting of the British Association for Psychopharmacology, July 1998, Cambridge. *Journal of Psychopharmacology*, **12** (Supplement A to No. 3), A1.

35. Coppen, A., Standish-Barry, H., Bailey, J., Houston, G., Silcocks, P., and Hermon, C. (1991). Does lithium reduce the mortality of recurrent mood disorders? *Journal of Affective Disorders*, **23**, 1–7.

36. Müller-Oerlinghausen, B., Ahrens, B., Grof, E., *et al.* (1992). The effect of long-term lithium treatment on the mortality of patients with manic–depressive and schizoaffective illness. *Acta Psychiatrica Scandinavica*, **86**, 218–22.

37. Derogatis, L.R. (1977). *SCL-90. Administration, scoring and procedures manual I for the R (revised) version and other instruments of the psychopathology rating scales series.* Johns Hopkins School of Medicine, Baltimore, MD.

38. Ernst, C., Schmid, G.B., and Angst, J. (1992). The Zurich Study: XVI. Early antecedents of depression. A longitudinal prospective study on incidence in young adults. *European Archives of Psychiatry and Clinical Neuroscience*, **242**, 142–51.

39. Surtees, P.G. and Wainwright, N.W.J. (1996). Fragile states of the mind: neuroticism, vulnerability and the long-term outcome of depression. *British Journal of Psychiatry*, **169**, 338–47.

40. Kessler, R.C., Zhao, S., Blazer, D.G., and Swartz, M. (1997). Prevalence, correlates, and course of minor depression and major depression in the National Comorbidity Survey. *Journal of Affective Disorders*, **45**, 19–30.

41. Graw, P., Gisin, B., and Wirz-Justice, A. (1997). Follow-up study of seasonal affective disorder in Switzerland. *Psychopathology*, **30**, 208–14.

42. Coryell, W., Endicott, J., and Keller, M. (1992) Rapidly cycling affective disorder: demographics, family history, and course. *Archives of General Psychiatry*, **49**, 126–31.

43. Bauer, M.S., Calabrese, J., Dunner, D.L., *et al.* (1994) Multisite data reanalysis of the validity of rapid cycling as a course modifier for bipolar disorder in DSM-IV. *American Journal of Psychiatry*, **151**, 506–15.

44. Schou, M. (1998). The effect of prophylactic lithium treatment on mortality and suicidal behavior: a review for clinicians. *Journal of Affective Disorders*, **50**, 253–9.

4.5.7 Treatment of mood disorders

E. S. Paykel and J. Scott

This chapter will review evidence on efficacy of treatment and deal with practical management of affective disorders, both unipolar and bipolar.

Evidence

Medication and physical treatments

Acute treatments for depression

Antidepressants: general issues

The first modern antidepressants, tricyclics and monoamine oxidase inhibitors, became available in the late 1950s, coinciding with the introduction of randomized controlled trials in psychiatry, which were therefore widely used for these drugs. A progressive tightening of requirements by drug licensing authorities since has ensured that efficacy evidence is good for most antidepressants in use. Overall efficacy of most antidepressants appears to be similar as does speed of response at effective dose, although newer drugs with lower side-effects may permit more rapid build-up of dose.

The evidence also indicates limitations in the magnitude of efficacy. Differences in proportions of subjects responding well on antidepressant and on placebo are of the order of 30 per cent. Few reviews have used the concept of effect size, but they suggest effect sizes of 0.4 to 0.8.[1] This is partly due to the good response often seen in placebo groups in controlled trials. This group controls for all effects except that of the active medication, including those of spontaneous improvement, and non-specific treatment effects such as those of seeing a helping figure, supportive and specific psychotherapies, and, for inpatients, admission to hospital. For milder depressives, spontaneous remission is common and non-specific effects may be powerful. There is little to suggest that the effects of the inert pill itself contributes a large amount to remission. One meta-analysis of trials of tricyclics against active placebo, predominantly atropine,[1] pointed to smaller effects in these and suggested partial unblinding with inert placebos. This is a possibility in most trials, but the studies reviewed tended to be of only 3 to 4 weeks' duration, too short for full therapeutic effects. Outcome in placebo groups may also vary; it tends to be worse among severely ill inpatients, but here also antidepressants may be less effective, compared with electroconvulsive therapy (**ECT**). Placebo-controlled trials are still mandated by regulatory authorities for new antidepressants, since comparisons between active drugs have a high risk of type 2 error.

Table 1 lists antidepressants and recommended doses. Drugs available vary from one country to another, as may recommended doses, depending on licensing authorities. Readers are advised to check the situation in their own countries.

Tricyclic antidepressants

There have been many reviews of tricyclics, and further studies have accumulated as tricyclics have been used as active comparators in placebo-controlled trials of new antidepressants. An early comprehensive review[2] of the limited selection of tricyclics then available in the United States found 93 placebo-controlled trials, of which 61 found the drug to be better than placebo. The negative studies may partly be due to poor trial methodology, but also reflect the limited therapeutic benefit overall.

Regarding predictor studies of who responds best,[3,4] earlier views that tricyclics were more effective in endogenous and psychotic depressives have not been well supported. There is evidence of effects across a broad spectrum of depressives, including some dysthymics (see Chapter 4.5.8) and extending more widely into anxiety disorders, panic disorder, and obsessive–compulsive disorder. A severity threshold exists at which superiority over placebo develops a little below major depression but excluding mild illness.[5,6]

Selective serotonin reuptake inhibitors

Meta-analyses of selective serotonin reuptake inhibitors (**SSRIs**)[7–10] show efficacy comparable with that of tricyclics. Conclusions differ as to rates at which patients discontinue the drugs because of side-effects. These are probably lower than for older tricyclics, but comparable with other newer antidepressants.[10]

There do not appear to be any major differences in responsive patients within depression, although there is debate, with conflicting evidence, as to whether SSRIs may be less effective than tricyclics and other combined noradrenaline (norepinephrine) and serotonin reuptake inhibitors in severe depression. There is good evidence that SSRIs and clomipramine, the most serotoninergic tricyclic, are more effective than noradrenergic tricyclics in obsessive–compulsive disorder.[11,12]

Monoamine oxidase inhibitors

There are few monoamine oxidase inhibitors available, reflecting their use mainly as second-line treatments by psychiatrists. Following recognition of the cheese reaction, they were withdrawn in some countries, but generally use remained at a lower level.

Controlled trials of the older monoamine oxidase inhibitors[13,14] show superiority to placebo in depression, and in anxiety disorders. Absence of efficacy in some large early studies appears in retrospect to

Table 1 Antidepressant medications[a]

Drug	Usual dose range (mg/day)[b]
Combined serotonin and noradrenaline reuptake inhibitors	
Tricyclics	
Amitriptyline	75–300
Clomipramine	75–300
Desipramine	75–300
Dothiepin	75–300
Doxepin	75–300
Imipramine	75–300
Lofepramine	70–210
Maprotiline	75–225
Nortriptyline	75–150
Protriptyline	15–60
Trimipramine	75–200
Serotonin and noradrenaline reuptake inhibitor	
Venlafaxine	75–375
Selective serotonin reuptake inhibitors	
Fluoxetine	20–80
Fluvoxamine	75–300
Paroxetine	10–50
Sertraline	50–200
Citalopram	20–60
Selective noradrenaline reuptake inhibitor	
Reboxetine	4–10
Monoamine oxidase inhibitors	
Isocarboxazid	30–50
Phenelzine	45–90
Tranylcypromine	20–30
Reversible monoamine oxidase inhibitor	
Moclobemide	300–750
Dopamine and noradrenaline uptake inhibitor	
Bupropion	200–450
Others	
Amineptine	100–500
Amoxapine	100–400
Mianserin	30–90
Mirtazapine	15–45
Nefazodone	100–600
Tianeptine	25–50
Trazodone	150–600
Viloxazine	100–400

[a] This list is not fully comprehensive because of new developments and national differences.
[b] Official dose recommendations vary between different countries and should always be checked.

be due to too low doses or short treatment periods; high doses are necessary. The reversible monoamine oxidase-A selective drug moclobemide has been reviewed more recently.[15] Again, dosage is the key. Doses below 450 mg daily are not superior to placebo, and evidence is best for 600 mg. The older hydrazine monoamine oxidase inhibitors, phenelzine and isocarboxazid, are acetylated in metabolism, and slow acetylators show better clinical response.[16]

From the late 1950s, following the views of Sargant, there have been suggestions that monoamine oxidase inhibitors are preferentially effective in atypical depression, variously regarded as non-endogenous depression, anxiety disorder with depression, or a pattern of reversed vegetative symptoms with increased appetite, increased sleep, evening worsening, reactivity, and other features.[17] The last of these meanings is currently predominant in the United States.

The evidence for selective efficacy is not very strong, but comparative trials of phenelzine and tricyclics point to better effects than tricyclics with anxiety disorders and reversed vegetative symptoms.[14] The latter has emerged in studies from the New York group.[18] On the other hand monoamine oxidase inhibitorss have been used commonly as second-line drugs where other antidepressants have failed, irrespective of clinical picture, and a meta-analysis of trials of moclobemide against tricyclics and other antidepressants showed no selective differential response.[19]

Other antidepressants

Space does not permit full review of efficacy of many other antidepressants of smaller classes. Readers are referred to other textbooks[20,21] and review articles.[22] Modes of action are discussed in Chapter 6.2.3.

Among older drugs, mianserin and trazodone are sedative in side-effects. Mianserin carries a definite although low risk of agranulocytosis which has had limited use since its recognition. Trazodone carries a risk of priapism in males. Bupropion is relatively stimulant and is used primarily in the United States. It has epileptogenic potential.

Among newer drugs, nefazodone[23] is claimed to be relatively free of sexual side-effects. Venlafaxine[24] inhibits reuptake both of serotonin and noradrenaline and is an effective and useful drug in severe depression. Mirtazepine shares some actions of mianserin with additional effects on serotonin receptors; clinically it is sedative. Reboxetine is a specific noradrenaline reuptake inhibitor, similar to desipramine and maprotiline but without tricyclic effects on other receptors. Only limited evidence is available on amineptine, which has effects predominantly on dopamine reuptake,[25] and tianeptine, an atypical drug which enhances serotonin reuptake.[26]

Electroconvulsive therapy

ECT, the earliest of modern treatments, is still the most effective in severe depression. The best efficacy evidence comes from six double-blind trials against simulated ECT carried out in the United Kingdom in the late 1970s and early 1980s (reviewed by Paykel[27]). All were carried out in severely ill inpatients. Earlier, in the 1960s there were a number of non-blind randomized controlled trials of ECT against antidepressants, mainly in hospitalized samples, which overall showed ECT superior to tricyclic antidepressants and markedly superior to monoamine oxidase inhibitors.[27,28]

Early predictor literature on ECT suggesting best effects in psychotic depression has been confirmed. Two of the trials against simulated ECT found best effects in depressives with psychomotor retardation and delusions.[29] There is also some evidence, which is not conclusive, that ECT may benefit mania.[30]

More recent studies of ECT have focused on qualities of the convulsive stimulus. Bilateral ECT is more effective overall than unilateral although it produces more memory disturbance.[31–33] Low-dose electrical stimulus produces weaker response.

A recent experimental approach is transcranial magnetic stimulation—the application of repeated short-lived magnetic stimulation. Preliminary studies suggest some benefit,[34] but samples have been small.

Acute treatments for mania

The treatment of acute mania may include neuroleptics, atypical antipsychotics, and ECT as well as mood stabilizers. A review of 18 uncontrolled and three controlled studies of the use of lithium in acute mania suggested that 60 to 70 per cent of patients respond within 7 to 10 days, compared to 40 per cent of patients receiving placebo.[35] McElroy et al.[36] reviewed trials of valproate in acute mania. Overall, valproate was at least moderately effective in 60 per cent of patients, many of whom had previously failed to respond to lithium. West et al.[37] reviewed five placebo-controlled and two lithium-controlled studies of the treatment of acute mania and found valproate significantly more effective than placebo and as effective as lithium. However, few of the studies met stringent criteria. In a multicentre double-blind randomized controlled study of 179 manic patients, Bowden et al.[38] reported a response rate of 49 per cent on lithium, 48 per cent on valproate but only 25 per cent on placebo.

Controlled studies of carbamazepine in acute mania have been reviewed by Ketter et al.[39] Although many of the studies have methodological weaknesses, the evidence suggests that about two-thirds of acutely manic patients respond to carbamazepine within 7 to 10 days.

Longer-term treatment

Continuation treatment

In recent years, it has become apparent from follow-up studies that the long-term outcome of depression is still often problematic. It is customary to distinguish between relapse, or early symptom return, assumed to be a return of the original episode, and later recurrence of a new episode.[40] In parallel, drug treatment after the acute episode has been divided into earlier continuation treatment, to prevent relapse, and longer-term maintenance treatment to prevent recurrence.

There have been many controlled trials of continuation treatment, in which responders to acute treatment are randomized either to withdraw double blind on to placebo or to continue on active drug for 6 to 8 months. All studies show substantial benefit from continuation.[41] A recent controlled trial of fluoxetine with staged withdrawal showed benefit of continuation for 24 and 38 weeks, but not 62 weeks.[42]

Maintenance treatment

Longer-term maintenance studies of antidepressants including tricyclics, monoamine oxidase inhibitors and SSRIs have mostly employed withdrawal designs but a small number have commenced the maintenance drug after other acute treatment. The withdrawal design may exaggerate therapeutic benefit if withdrawal is abrupt with rebound symptom return, and also because it selects responders to the particular acute treatment, often from samples chosen as highly recurrent beforehand.

The trials show clear benefit from antidepressants in maintenance treatment of unipolar depression.[41] However, benefits are weaker than in continuation treatment and recurrence rates in drug-treated patients have often remained moderately high.

There may be withdrawal reactions if antidepressants are stopped abruptly. There has long been recognition of a transient withdrawal syndrome after abrupt stopping of tricyclics, often in high dose for long periods, with malaise, coryza-like symptoms, vomiting, and diarrhoea. It has been attributed to withdrawal of atropinic effects, but somewhat similar symptoms have been reported recently on withdrawal of SSRIs and other antidepressants.[43]

A number of trials of lithium in maintenance treatment of severe recurrent unipolar depressives also show benefit over placebo.[44] The relative benefits of lithium and antidepressants are not clear, with direct comparisons somewhat evenly balanced. In practice, response to an antidepressant followed by its maintenance is a much more common clinical practice.

Maintenance treatment of bipolar disorder

Maintenance treatment of bipolar disorder has been reviewed extensively.[45–47] Controlled trials of lithium against placebo have been criticized because of the possibility of withdrawal effects,[48] but there is little doubt of therapeutic effects.[49] Lithium is also superior to tricyclic antidepressant alone, particularly because of high rates of mania with the latter.[44] Lithium has not been well evaluated as an active antidepressant, but effects appear to be weak.[50]

It has become clear that there are high rates of early recurrence, particularly of mania, when lithium is discontinued after long-term use.[51,52] This rebound, which may have exaggerated therapeutic benefit in trials, mandates slow withdrawal in practice. One study[53] has indicated greater benefit on residual symptoms for doses producing blood levels 0.8 to 1.0 mmol/l than for 0.4 to 0.6 mmol/l.

There have been fewer long-term studies of anticonvulsants.[50,54] Valproate is approved in the United States for treatment of mania. Controlled trial evidence of efficacy in prophylaxis is sparse although it is commonly used in this circumstance. Carbamazepine has been used for longer. There is good evidence of efficacy in mania[45,54] and there have been longer-term controlled studies which suggest benefit. Other anticonvulsants have also been tried in bipolar patients; lamotrigine is currently the most advanced in evaluation.

Psychological treatments

Acute treatment of depression

Psychological treatments: general issues

There is high public demand for psychotherapies for unipolar depression. Recently, the use of these interventions in bipolar disorder has also been advocated.[55] Guidelines for the use of psychotherapy in depression are less well developed than for pharmacotherapy and are based on less robust empirical data. Early research into the benefits of psychotherapy in depression comprised single case studies, small case series, and open or non-randomized treatment trials. The increase in randomized, controlled trials of psychotherapy for depression can be attributed both to the introduction of 'manualized' (or 'protocol-driven') therapies, enabling consistency of application[56] and valid and reliable evaluations, and to the emphasis on evidence-based medicine and cost-effectiveness.[57]

Almost all the controlled trials of psychotherapy for depression undertaken have employed manualized therapies. The interventions share the common characteristics of being time limited (less than 20 sessions), with primary targets symptom reduction and problem resolution. Cognitive therapy, interpersonal therapy, behavioural therapy, and some models of brief dynamic psychotherapy fall into this category. The largest volume of efficacy research has focused on cognitive therapy (about 50 studies), with fewer studies (about 30 in total) of interpersonal therapy, behavioural therapy, and other dynamic therapies. Sample sizes are often smaller than desirable and many studies have methodological weaknesses including the failure to include pill-placebo control groups.

Meta-analyses

Early meta-analyses were hampered by use in most most outcome studies of 'completer' samples rather than 'intent-to-treat' analyses. A meta-analysis of 81 studies of the treatment of neurotic disorders (mainly depression) (effect size 0.97) showed that specific psychological therapies, particularly cognitive therapy, were more effective than other verbal therapies (effect size 0.74) or waiting-list controls.[58] Other meta-analyses, restricted to acute depressive episodes, found similar trends for superiority of cognitive or behavioural approaches over other therapies.[59,60] Dobson[61] reviewed studies of cognitive therapy using the Beck Depression Inventory as the primary outcome measure. Cognitive therapy gave effect sizes of 2.15 compared to waiting-list controls, 0.46 compared to behavioural therapy, and 0.53 compared to pharmacotherapy. Robinson et al.[62] identified 58 outpatient depression treatment studies. Overall behavioural therapy and cognitive therapy showed moderate effect sizes, with cognitive therapy showing marginal superiority over behavioural therapy. Psychological therapies also showed a small but significant advantage when compared with pharmacotherapy (mean effect size 0.12). However, Robinson et al.[62] found that the results of their meta-analysis became less stable if the allegiance of the researcher to a particular therapeutic model was taken into account. Using regression analysis to partial out the effect of allegiance virtually extinguished differences in treatment outcome.

The most recent meta-analysis of 29 carefully selected controlled trials, employing intent-to-treat design, explored group and individual therapies for major depression, included the National Institute of Mental Health (**NIMH**) study,[63] and also incorporated interpersonal therapy studies for the first time. The study used categorical outcomes (recovered versus not recovered). The efficacies of individual cognitive therapy (response rate, 50 per cent), behavioural therapy (55 per cent), and interpersonal therapy (52 per cent) in the treatment of the acute episode were not significantly different and compared favourably with pharmacotherapy (58 per cent). Brief dynamic psychotherapies, mainly group therapies, were less effective (35 per cent) and only marginally superior to waiting-list controls (30 per cent). Cognitive therapy was less effective in a group format (39 per cent), behavioural therapy was equally effective, and interpersonal therapy was more beneficial when a significant other took part in therapy, rather than one individual alone.

Almost all trials of psychological therapies have been in outpatient depressives, not above moderate severity. Comparisons with pharmacotherapy must be interpreted in this light and do not represent severe or inpatient disorder.

Cognitive therapy

Earlier studies of individual cognitive therapy suggested that it was at least as effective and acceptable as antidepressant drugs (or 'treatment as usual') in the treatment of non-psychotic outpatient unipolar depressives in primary care and hospital outpatient settings (for reviews see Hollon et al.[64] and Scott[56]). Furthermore, severity and endogenicity did not appear to be a contraindication to cognitive therapy. However, most of these studies had significant methodological flaws. The three-centre NIMH study[63] sought to overcome these. A total of 239 patients with major depression were randomly allocated to one of four treatments, imipramine with clinical management, pill placebo with clinical management, cognitive therapy, or interpersonal therapy. Treatments were undertaken by trained and supervised therapists. The primary analysis showed few differences between the active treatments. A secondary analysis which controlled for severity of depression, found that cognitive therapy was not as effective as pharmacotherapy in the more severe disorders within the outpatient range studied. The findings have been subject to debate, particularly over variations between sites and adequacy of therapist supervision.[64] Hollon et al.[65] undertook a well-designed controlled trial of cognitive therapy and pharmacotherapy in 107 patients. The primary and secondary analyses, again controlling for severity, did not demonstrate any significant between-group differences in treatment outcome.

Other psychotherapies

Fewer outcome studies are available regarding the efficacy of interpersonal therapy, behavioural therapy, or brief dynamic psychotherapy. Most data are available for interpersonal therapy. The first randomized study in depressed women[66] found that only antidepressant prevented relapse, whilst interpersonal therapy, started 6 weeks after acute amitriptyline had a significant effect on social functioning. In a later study[67] interpersonal therapy was as effective as amitriptyline in acute treatment of outpatient depression. The NIMH study[63] is the only one that has compared interpersonal therapy with a pill-placebo control. Interpersonal therapy was nearest to the effectiveness of imipramine but a little weaker.

Few acute controlled trials of other therapies have been published. Two large-scale studies of individual behavioural therapy are available. In a comparison of behavioural therapy with insight-orientated therapy, antidepressant drugs, and relaxation, the behavioural approach was more effective than insight-orientated therapy (which tended to fair worst overall), but differences between treatments had largely disappeared at 3 months' follow-up.[68] Hersen et al.[69] randomly allocated 125 depressed females to antidepressant drug treatment, social skills training plus antidepressants, social skills training plus placebo or dynamic therapy plus placebo, and found similar outcome in all groups.

Few high-quality studies exist on marital and family models of psychotherapy. It is clear that cognitive therapy, interpersonal therapy, and brief dynamic psychotherapy can be applied to families, groups or couples, but the only published randomized controlled trials on marital therapy mainly draw on behavioural approaches. For example, O'Leary and Beach[70] demonstrated that behavioural marital therapy or cognitive therapy were both more effective than waiting-list controls in treating women with depression or dysthymia. Furthermore, Jacobson et al.[71] demonstrated an advantage for behavioural marital therapy over cognitive therapy in depressed individuals with marital discord.

Combined psychotherapy and pharmacotherapy

Data on whether the use of a combination of psychotherapy and pharmacotherapy bestows additional benefit over either treatment alone are not conclusive. Overall the studies suggest a small advantage at the level of severity usually studied. Conte et al.[72] in a meta-analysis suggested an advantage for combined treatments, but this review has been criticized.[57] Hollon et al.[64] found a non-significant trend for a higher response rate with a combination of pharmacotherapy and cognitive therapy as opposed to either treatment alone. A similar trend is reported in studies of interpersonal therapy plus medication as compared to either treatment alone.[66,67] However, when these data were included in a single meta-analysis of eight outcome studies, neither cognitive therapy, behavioural therapy, or interpersonal therapy added to antidepressants were any more effective than pharmacotherapy alone.[73]

These analyses have primarily used symptom outcomes. An equally important target of interpersonal therapy and dynamic psychotherapies may be improvement in interpersonal relationships and social adjustment. There is some evidence for interpersonal therapy of preferential benefit on such measures.[74] This may result in benefit from the combination, by effects on different measures.

Longer-term treatment

Follow-up studies

There are few adequately designed studies examining the role of psychotherapy in the prevention of relapse or recurrence of depression. None is available on brief dynamic psychotherapy. Short-term follow-up studies of behavioural therapy[68,69] and interpersonal therapy[75] do not demonstrate any significant differences in outcome between these interventions and the other psychological or pharmacological treatments with which the approaches were compared.

Most cognitive therapy studies comprise naturalistic follow-ups of treatment responders in previously published acute depression studies, sometimes without adequate drug continuation. Better drug continuation was used in the study by Evans et al.[76] which prospectively followed up a cohort of patients treated in a randomized controlled trial of cognitive therapy and pharmacotherapy.[65] In this study the relapse rate in the cognitive therapy group (20 per cent) was no different from that in the drug continuation treatment group (27 per cent) and less than half that of the patients who had drug treatment withdrawn at the time the depression remitted (50 per cent). These findings support trends in the NIMH follow-up[77] and other naturalistic follow-up studies that cognitive therapy reduces relapse rates.

Continuation and maintenance trials

The use of continuation and maintenance psychotherapy is a new concept in psychological treatment studies. In a follow-up study Blackburn et al.[78] offered about five sessions of cognitive therapy over the following 6 months to subjects from an acute treatment study. At 2-year follow-up, the relapse rate in patients who had received acute pharmacotherapy was significantly higher than that in patients who had received cognitive–behavioural therapy either alone or in combination with medication. Blackburn and Moore[79] allocated subjects with recurrent major depression to 16 weeks of acute treatment and 2 years of maintenance treatment which comprised either antidepressants alone, cognitive therapy alone, or antidepressants followed by maintenance cognitive therapy. All groups improved in the acute phase and there were no differences in relapse rates in the maintenance phases, suggesting that cognitive therapy may be a viable alternative to maintenance medication.

Recently there have been two controlled trials designed to test reduction of relapse and recurrence rates by cognitive therapy given after the acute episode in patients with residual depressive symptoms after major depression.[80,81] Both studies compared cognitive therapy with clinical management in patients with residual depression following antidepressant treatment. Both studies found significant worthwhile reduction in relapse and recurrence rates.

There is evidence from a well-designed 3-year study of maintenance interpersonal therapy, undertaken at monthly intervals, that interpersonal therapy may reduce the risk of relapse.[82] However, benefit was much greater from imipramine than from interpersonal therapy. Effects of interpersonal therapy were more substantial where it was rated as of high quality.

Bipolar disorder

Psychotherapy for bipolar disorders has not been systematically studied. No studies are available on psychological interventions in acute mania. Reviews by Scott[55] and by Roth and Fonagy[57] highlight that psychosocial interventions undertaken during other phases of bipolar disorder all resulted in greater symptomatic improvement and social adjustment than treatment with medication alone. However, the studies were poorly designed and the data are weak. The only controlled trial published[83] randomly assigned a small sample of 28 subjects to either six sessions of compliance-oriented cognitive therapy or standard clinic care. In the next 6 months lithium compliance appeared to be enhanced in the cognitive–behavioural therapy group, who also showed fewer hospitalizations. The most promising approaches to bipolar disorders appear to be cognitive therapy, interpersonal therapy–social rhythms therapy, and family therapy, and large-scale controlled trials of these therapies are now underway in the United Kingdom and the United States.

Management

General aspects

The goals of treatment of affective disorders are to alleviate acute symptoms, to restore psychosocial functioning, and to prevent relapse and recurrence. Crucial decisions in clinical management are the appropriate selection of an intervention and treatment setting. Research on which depressed patients will respond to a particular treatment offered in a particular setting does not give a good practical guide.[84] Pragmatic decisions regarding management usually focus on four key issues: the severity of the disorder (including risk of harm to self or others), the availablity of effective treatments (either specific antidepressants or trained therapists), patient preference, and the nature of any associated difficulties.

Severe cases of depression with significant suicidal risk are often best managed in inpatient facilities to allow regular observation and careful monitoring of the patient's mental state. If risk of suicide is lower and the patient has appropriate social support it may be possible to manage severe cases with intensive community support, such as partial hospitalization, day care, or a combination of outpatient and home-based care. Moderate or mild cases of depression can usually be managed in outpatient settings, unless treatment is complicated by comorbidity of severe physical or other mental disorders (including

drug or alcohol misuse) or non-response requires more detailed assessment.

Although severe cases of depression may respond to psychotherapy alone, the rate of recovery is slower than with drugs or ECT.[56] Psychotherapy may be used in addition to drugs or ECT, but should not be used alone. In mild or moderate depressions, treatment choice may be more balanced and depends partly on patient preference and, for psychotherapies, on availability, although when major depression criteria are reached antidepressants should not generally be withheld.

Most patients with affective disorders are treated in primary care or general medical settings. Cases seen by specialist mental health services are usually referred because the disorder is more severe, chronic, treatment resistant, or because other difficulties, such as alcohol misuse or marital difficulties, complicate the clinical picture. In these situations it may be necessary to use combinations of drugs and psychosocial approaches. The rest of this section gives an overview of physical and psychological treatments. Although these approaches are described separately, the treatment of affective disorders rarely involves simply prescribing medication. Education and support of a depressed patient and his or her family are important aspects of any clinical management package.

Medication and physical treatments

Acute treatment of unipolar disorder

The most important indications for use of medication are probably severity and persistence. Two studies[5,6] have shown a threshold a little below major depression at which tricyclic antidepressants start to show superiority over placebo in acute episodes of depression. There is not yet equivalent evidence for SSRIs. Tricyclics are also superior to placebo in dysthymia,[85] but most studies do not separate those dysthymics without added major depression. For mild acute depressive episodes highly reactive to major stress, and for acute grief, prognosis for spontaneous resolution is often good, and medication may be delayed, provided that improvement is occurring. Impairment of function and suicidal feelings in the context of the depressive syndrome are other indications to treat. Recent guidelines[73,86] recommend use in major depression, equivalent to ICD-10 depressive episode. For depressions reaching these criteria, antidepressants should be used irrespective of life stress or symptom pattern: counselling and psychotherapy may be combined with antidepressants where indicated.

Choice of antidepressant

Because the evidence of selective response is weak, and overall efficacy appears equivalent, choice of initial antidepressant legitimately varies considerably among clinicians and countries. Where cost is an important consideration, some older tricyclics are very inexpensive. Where cost minimization is less crucial, SSRIs and newer antidepressants often have advantages in side-effects and tolerability. Irrespective of first choice, troublesome side-effects indicate a change to an antidepressant with a different side-effect profile. Monoamine oxidase inhibitors are little used as first choices. Where there is a previous history of antidepressant response, the best first choice is the antidepressant to which the patient previously responded.

With a few exceptions clinical symptom pattern is not in practice a good guide to treatment. Effects of the tricyclics extend widely across the spectrum of depression and in to anxiety disorders. The place of

SSRIs in very severe depression is still debated. On the other hand their lower incidence of side-effects and absence of sedation can render them easier to use in milder depression. Monoamine oxidase inhibitors are a reasonable first choice in atypical depression. A reversible inhibitor of monoamine oxidase A (moclobemide) is safer.

Comorbidity with anxiety is common in depression. Here the evidence is still too weak to determine treatment choice. For concomitant obsessive–compulsive disorder clomipramine, or the SSRIs, are preferable to noradrenergic antidepressants. Phototherapy for seasonal affective disorder is dealt with in Chapter 6.2.9.2.

Special situations

Some special situations require specific treatment choices. Major suicidal risk, particularly by overdose, points away from tricyclics, most of which carry considerable risk of death by cardiac arrhythmia. SSRIs and most newer antidepressants are comparatively safe in overdose.

Cardiac problems also indicate use of a non-tricyclic antidepressant. Although tricyclics can often be used without major problems, there is risk of arrhythmia, particularly partial or complete heart block, and orthostatic hypotension is common. Monoamine oxidase inhibitors lower blood pressure as a dose-related effect and are also better avoided.

Concomitant epilepsy can often easily be controlled by adjustment of anticonvulsant dose. Tricyclics are epileptogenic and should be avoided. Epileptic potential is usually less with newer antidepressants but is often not clear, and the only antidepressants clearly established to be free of epileptic potential are older monoamine oxidase inhibitors.

The elderly are particularly liable to anticholinergic side-effects, including confusion, and orthostatic hypotension may precipitate falls and fractures. SSRIs and newer antidepressants are preferable to tricyclics.

Antidepressant treatment of patients with medical disorders is often difficult, because of toxicity due to the medical disorder, high blood levels due to impaired metabolism, side-effects, and drug interactions. All antidepressants interact with some other medications, including SSRIs, which affect other medications metabolized by the cytochrome P-450 system. Choice of antidepressant depends on the specific situation.

Pregnancy

The tricyclics have been used in pregnancy and do not carry risk of fetal malformation. For SSRIs and newer antidepressants the situation is less clear as sufficient experience is lacking: they usually carry warnings against use in pregnancy. Accumulating experience suggests that fluoxetine is safe.[87] Mood stabilizers are contraindicated; lithium, carbamazepine, and valproate all have some risk of fetal malformation. Where antidepressants are used at the time of delivery there may be complications of anaesthesia and fetal sedation, and these should be anticipated. Most antidepressants and mood stabilizers appear in breast milk, but in small quantities. Breast feeding should be discussed with the patient.

Clinical use of antidepressants

There is a delay in clinical antidepressant effects of 1 to 3 weeks or longer, although some improvement may be seen earlier. Medication needs to be continued for a minimum duration of 6 weeks at adequate or high dose before treatment can be deemed ineffective.

For most antidepressants, side-effects are most apparent in the early weeks and some tolerance develops so that build-up of dose over 2 to 3 weeks is advisable. Newer drugs, better tolerated, allow more rapid dose escalation. For fluoxetine, the exceptionally long half-life of the active metabolite means that blood levels build up for some weeks, even on a standard dose.

Dose division during the day can be based on pharmacology. Half-lives of most antidepressants are such that, combined with delay in therapeutic effects, one dose per day is adequate, but for most, two doses per day is better; three doses are useful where daytime sedation is an advantage. For fluoxetine only a single dose is appropriate. Moclobemide, as a competitive monoamine oxidase inhibitor which is easily displaced and metabolized, should be given in three doses daily. For sedative antidepressants, administration of two-thirds of the dose at night is beneficial and enables avoidance of hypnotics, although it may leave a little morning 'hangover' sedation. Doses at bedtime of the more stimulant antidepressants, including monoamine oxidase inhibitors and SSRIs, should be avoided.

Common side-effects of tricyclics clinically are sedation and anticholinergic side-effects of dry mouth, blurred near vision, urinary retention, orthostatic hypotension, and confusion in the elderly. Common side-effects of SSRIs are nausea, and other gastrointestinal disturbances, insomnia, and sometimes tension and restlessness. Dose-limiting side-effects of monoamine oxidase inhibitors are hypotension, insomnia, and ankle oedema.

A common problem in use of antidepressants is low dosage. If response does not occur and side-effects are not severe, doses should be progressively increased until either response occurs, severity of side-effects precludes further increase, or dose becomes very high. In the United States, doses of older tricyclics used may be up to 300 mg daily, although in Europe 200 to 250 mg are more common maxima. Monitoring plasma levels of mood stabilizers is an essential part of good clinical practice, but the use of plasma drug levels for other drugs has equivocal support.[88] A single plasma level measurement is less likely to help in management decisions than a short series of two to three measurements, but monitoring may help in the following circumstances:[73] non-response or partial response to therapeutic doses of a particular drug; symptom breakthrough following full response; symptoms of toxicity at low or therapeutic doses; situations of altered metabolism (elderly people, pregnant women, patients with medical illness, psychiatric comorbidity, or receiving other drugs that affect antidepressant metabolism); potential non-compliance.

Electroconvulsive therapy

Extent of clinical use of ECT varies cross-nationally. Many psychiatrists, including ourselves, use it as a first choice treatment in severe depression with psychomotor retardation or mood-congruent depressive delusions. Alternatively an antidepressant may be tried, with a change to ECT if there is poor response or worsening. ECT is also appropriate for moderately severe depressions which have not responded to one or two courses of antidepressant.

An alternative to ECT for the treatment of psychotic (delusional) depression with mood-congruent delusions is combination of neuroleptic and antidepressant. Spiker et al.[89] report that only 35 per cent of psychotic depressions responded to tricyclics alone, but 80 per cent responded to tricyclics plus antipsychotic medications. Neuroleptic–antidepressant combinations are also indicated where there are non-mood-congruent delusions or schizoaffective symptoms.

In the United Kingdom, the Royal College of Psychiatrists[90] has made detailed recommendations on administration of ECT, including equipment, anaesthesia, and the use of stimulus dose titration to achieve a moderately suprathreshold dose.

Non-response and resistant depression

If the first choice of antidepressant medication fails, a change should be made to an antidepressant of a different class, or to ECT. There is little to support change to an alternative antidepressant of the same class. If the second choice fails, a third-class, ECT, or lithium augmentation (see below) are appropriate choices, depending on the circumstances.

If there is still limited response, a more systematic approach to resistant depression should be adopted.

1. Reassess the situation thoroughly, with full history, assessment, and laboratory investigation of thyroid function to ask the following questions.

    (a) Is the diagnosis correct? Wrong diagnosis is in practice unusual.

    (b) Are there perpetuating factors in personality, family environment, or the social setting? It is common where depression has been long term that secondary role loss (including work) and family adaptations to a non-functioning member mean there are no roles or relationships for the patient to return to and remission cannot occur, or is transient, unless psychotherapy, family therapy, and rehabilitation are employed to change the situation.

    (c) Is hypothyroidism impairing response? This may develop as a result of earlier use of lithium.

2. Consider previous treatment. Failure to use high-dose antidepressant is a common reason for apparently resistant depression, or at least was so in the past.[91]

3. Consider drug and other physical treatments.

4. As remission occurs, introduce psychotherapeutic, cognitive, and rehabilitative interventions.

The actual choices depend on what has been used before. A common sequence is to start with the most promising antidepressant suggested by the history and to push it to a very high dose. Clomipramine has in the past been used by many psychiatrists for this purpose. Our clinical experience suggests that venlafaxine, with similar actions but lower side-effects, is an appropriate substitute, with monitoring of blood pressure for elevation as high doses are reached. Whatever the antidepressant, doses in excess of officially recommended levels may be required.

The next intervention is to use an augmentation strategy. Lithium augmentation is the easiest and probably most effective. There is good evidence of efficacy.[92,93] Blood levels required for augmentation are not established, but are probably similar to those for maintenance. Tremor may be a troublesome side-effect with tricyclics, particularly clomipramine. If response occurs, it is our practice to continue the lithium for some months, but not as long as antidepressant, although controlled trial evidence is lacking. Care should be taken to monitor for a serotonin syndrome (excitability, restlessness, temperature elevation), particularly with SSRIs.

There is some evidence that L-tryptophan may potentiate monoamine oxidase inhibitors and the more serotoninergic uptake inhibitors.[94] This amino acid was withdrawn from the market because of eosinophilic myalgia, but is now available again in some countries. Its effect is weak, but may be combined with lithium potentiation.

Thyroid hormone, particularly tri-iodothyronine,[95] may also potentiate antidepressants. It is used less frequently in clinical practice; care must be exercised if there are cardiac problems.

There is accumulating evidence that pindolol, which has effects in blocking 5-HT$_{1A}$ autoreceptors, can accelerate speed of antidepressant response.[96] Augmentation of amount of response is less clear, but it may have a place in this circumstance.

At one time combinations between tricyclics and monoamine oxidase inhibitors were often used in resistant depression. Although two controlled trials suggested that the combination was not superior to single antidepressant,[97,98] subjects were not resistant cases. It occasionally still has a place, combined with lithium. Serotoninergic uptake inhibitors are contraindicated because of the risk of serotonin syndrome. Tricyclics other than clomipramine may be combined with older monoamine oxidase inhibitors or moclobemide, with gradual dose increase of both. In ordinary clinical practice 1 to 2 weeks should intervene between stopping an older monoamine oxidase inhibitor and starting a reuptake inhibitor, because of the risk of interaction until new monoamine oxidase is synthesized.

When vigorous medication regimens have still not produced a response, it is often helpful to add bilateral ECT to maximal drug therapy, even when ECT alone has not helped in the past. When all else fails in intractable severe chronic depression, psychosurgery still has an occasional place. In spite of the absence of controlled trials, it does appear sometimes to be helpful, when followed by active rehabilitation.

Longer-term treatment

Continuation therapy

In view of the strong evidence from controlled trials, continuation for approximately 6 months is recommended as routine practice following response to acute treatment of major depression.[73,86] There is one trial in dysthymia showing similar benefit.[99] Although clear evidence is lacking, it should also probably be routine in milder acute episodes treated with antidepressants, unless there is strongly suggestive evidence that the response is non-pharmacological, for example occurring on very low dose, developing very early after treatment commencement, or closely related in timing and context to reversal of a major stress.

Continuation is particularly important where there has been partial remission with residual symptoms, or a history of previous relapse or recurrence. There is good evidence of high rates of relapse where residual symptoms are present.[100] One study showed particular superiority of drug over placebo in this situation;[101] in another study relapse after stopping antidepressant only occurred where 4 months completely free of symptoms had not supervened. Sometimes continuation antidepressant or lithium may be required after ECT, where relapse has occurred.

The dose used for continuation should initially be the same as the acute treatment dose. After 2 to 3 months this may be reduced if side-effects are a problem, but only by a small amount, to avoid symptom return.

The usual length of antidepressant continuation should be about 6 months after response. The patient should also be completely free of residual symptoms for 4 months. Withdrawal should then be carried out slowly, over 2 to 3 months, to minimize the risk of relapse, and of withdrawal symptoms.

In some patients, complete withdrawal, or achievement of a low dose, will be followed by return of depressive symptoms. This phenomenon usually reflects a genuine relapse, and in one study relapse rates on placebo withdrawal and open withdrawal to no drug were the same.[67] If symptoms persist, full dose should be resumed, followed by continuation for a further period of 9 months to a year. Some of these patients relapse again on later drug withdrawal, and long-term maintenance should then be considered.

Maintenance treatment

Longer-term maintenance is indicated where there have been several recurrences. Various recommendations for initiating maintenance have been formulated, such as two episodes in the last 2 years, or three episodes in 5 years.[46,73] This also depends on the severity of episodes, their potential impact on personal life, family life, and career, and the patient's preference and willingness to commit to prolonged drug treatment. Discussion is required with the patient, and where appropriate the family, to reach a joint decision.

For most unipolar depressives the maintenance treatment choice will be whichever antidepressant has been effective and well tolerated. Where antidepressants have not been fully effective, lithium or combination are required. Antidepressant doses should be of the same order as those needed for acute treatment in the particular patient. The length of maintenance is harder to specify, and it depends on the previous history, but it should be at least 3 to 5 years, particularly where there has been a good acute response to antidepressant, persisting through continuation.[102] Drug withdrawal should be attempted at some point thereafter, unless there is clear evidence from previous history that further recurrence has followed previous withdrawal. Withdrawal of antidepressants, lithium, or other drugs after long-term maintenance should always be gradual. Where withdrawal is followed soon after by a recurrence, longer-term maintenance is indicated, and where this sequence has been repeated, lifelong treatment.

Bipolar disorder

Bipolar depression

The treatment of bipolar depression is in principle similar to that of unipolar depression. Lithium may produce some benefit alone, but usually an antidepressant is required in addition. Antidepressants may precipitate mania, and rapid cycling, so that combination with a mood stabilizer is usually desirable. It is a clinical impression that rapid cycling may occur more readily with uptake inhibitors than with monoamine oxidase inhibiting agents including moclobemide. Bipolar depression is often characterized by increased sleep, one feature of an atypical depression. ECT may be indicated, in similar circumstances to those in unipolar depression, and does not appear to lead to rapid cycling.

Acute treatment of mania

A number of mood stabilizers are reported to have an acute antimanic effect, but the Expert Consensus Guideline on the Treatment of Bipolar Disorder[103] advocated either lithium or valproate as the drugs of first choice. Valproate is often preferred for patients with mixed states or rapid cycling disorder. Response to lithium or valproate is usually delayed by 7 to 14 days, so most clinicians also use other drugs such as neuroleptics or atypical antipsychotics. These are effective within a matter of days in controlling the acute symptoms of mania, particularly delusions, hallucinations, thought disorder, or severe agitation. The main problem with the classic combination of haloperidol and lithium is the need for close monitoring, as manic patients are at greater risk of neuroleptic malignant syndrome and a combined lithium–neuroleptic neurotoxicity syndrome has also been reported. Benzodiazepines such as lorazepam and clonazepam are frequently used to treat hyperactivity, insomnia, and agitation.[103]

The loss of insight, impaired judgement, and disinhibited behaviour of manic patients or the level of agitation and hyperactivity often mean that hospitalization is required to ensure the patient's safety and commence an appropriate treatment regimen. For severe cases of mania, ECT may occasionally be used as a first-line treatment.

Continuation and maintenance treatment

Continuation treatment is indicated for at least 6 months after acute bipolar episodes, using the single medication or combination of mood stabilizers, antidepressants, and neuroleptics that has been used in acute treatment. Since neuroleptics have the least specific effects and carry occasional risk of tardive dyskinesia even after short-term treatment, they should be terminated first.

Bipolar disorder is more recurrent than unipolar disorder, and the disinhibition of mania can have catastrophic long-term effects on personal life. The threshold for maintenance treatment is therefore lower than for unipolar disorder. There is a case for 1 to 2 years' maintenance following a first episode of mania.

Choice of mood stabilizer includes an increasingly wide range. Probably lithium is still the drug of first choice, in the absence of major side-effects or patient reluctance. It is usual to recommend doses to achieve blood levels 12 h after the last dose of 0.4 to 0.8 mmol/l. Sometimes higher levels may be necessary to prevent recurrences, and to reduce residual symptoms.[103] After some months of use blood levels are often very stable and only require very occasional monitoring. Advice needs to be given on circumstances which may disturb blood levels (e.g. dehydration, gastrointestinal upset, travel, hot climates). Thyroid function should be monitored every 6 to 12 months, in view of possible insidious onset of hypothyroidism.

Poor or partial responses are not uncommon, and carbamazepine or valproate should be added. They are alternatives as single drugs where the patient prefers. Valproate is increasingly a drug of first choice in the United States. Blood levels for bipolar disorder are not well established but it is usual to target blood levels in the anticonvulsant range. In treatment-resistant cases, there is an increasing trend toward the use of combinations of mood stabilizers (particularly lithium and valproate). The indications and precautions necessary when using such combinations are reviewed by Freeman and Stoll.[104]

Antidepressants can often be slowly withdrawn in bipolars after mood stabilizers are well established, but may be necessary to prevent depression; mood stabilizers, particularly lithium, appear to have better effects in preventing mania. Antidepressants should not usually be used alone for maintenance in bipolars in view of the risk of mania. Neuroleptics, although better avoided in the long term, are sometimes necessary in multiple drug combinations in highly recurrent bipolar disorder. Very occasionally depot neuroleptics are helpful in non-compliant subjects.

Length of maintenance treatment necessarily varies, from a few years, to lifelong where several recurrences have followed withdrawal. There have been fears that withdrawal of lithium might be followed by treatment resistance in recurrences, but a recent study suggested that this is not the case.[105] Withdrawal of lithium should always be slow, over 3 to 6 months, in view of the evidence for rebound mania. In the absence of evidence to the contrary for the anticonvulsants it is best to follow a similar practice.

Psychological treatments

Acute treatment of unipolar disorder

The psychological management of acute depression ranges from basic clinical management, supportive psychotherapy, psychoeducation sessions for the individual with their partner or family present, through to formal psychotherapy. Clinical management and family psycho-education sessions will involve education about the nature of the disorder (including polarity, course, and prognosis), treatment options (including the advantages and disadvantages of psychotherapy, or in the use of drugs, the delay in benefits, and probable side-effects) and an early discussion about the planned length of treatment. These basic sessions can help build a strong alliance between the clinician and the patient, overcome misconceptions about the diagnosis and treatment (such as fears of addiction to antidepressants), reduce tension in inter-personal relationships and significantly reduce barriers to medication compliance.

For some individuals the reduction in symptoms that occurs after the introduction of medication restores them to their previous level of functioning and they are once again able to use their own coping skills to resolve personal problems. However, for others, the disorder is only partially resolved or the nature of problems is such that additional input is required over a longer period of time. Such cases may benefit from longer-term supportive psychotherapy. This may be provided in an outpatient clinic, but might also be provided through day services or visits by a community psychiatric nurse.

Formal psychotherapy may be offered as the only treatment to individuals with milder depressions or in combination with medication in those with moderate and severe disorders. More than 20 per cent of couples report marital discord in association with depressive disorders and so marital or family approaches should always be considered as an alternative to individual therapy. Individual treatments, such as cognitive therapy, may particularly benefit milder depressions. There are a number of features that identify potentially effective psychological approaches to depression.[56] The therapy should be highly structured and based on a coherent model. It should provide the patient with a clear rationale for the interventions made and the therapy should promote independent use of the skills learned. Change should be attributed to the individual's rather than the therapist's skill-fulness and the therapy should enhance the individual's sense of self-efficacy. Clearly cognitive therapy, behavioural therapy, and interpersonal therapy conform to this description. The choice of which of these models to use is less dependent on the patient's presentation than on the availability of a trained and experienced therapist. Adherence to the therapy model, therapists' level of expertise and skill and the provision of regular and adequate supervision to the practitioner are important determinants of outcome and may account for some 30 per cent of the variance in patient's improvement.[57] Furthermore, the more severe or complex the case, the more important therapist factors become.[56,57] It is also likely that more severe or chronic disorders will require a more prolonged course of therapy. Scott and DeRubeis[106] reviewed studies using cognitive therapy plus drugs in patients with non-responsive depression and found that the average response rate (about 44 per cent) was about the same as that achieved with lithium augmentation, but tended to increase with expertise of the therapist and overall duration of treatment.

Acute treatment of mania

Psychotherapy has not been tested in manic patients, but it is important to use clinical management, supportive therapy, and psychoeducational sessions as described previously. Clarkin et al.[107] have demonstrated that the use of inpatient family interventions (about six sessions) with patients who have been stabilized in hospital can have beneficial effects extending beyond discharge.

Longer-term treatment

In day-to-day practice, supportive therapy or other forms of psychological input may extend over considerable periods of time. In addition, people with affective disorders form about 15 to 20 per cent of the long-stay patient populations of mental hospitals in the United Kingdom and the United States. Rehabilitation techniques as applied to schizophrenia and other severe mental disorders are important for instilling hope and developing day-to-day living skills in people with chronic or recurrent affective disorders. Lastly, all individuals with chronic health problems are at high risk (about 50 per cent) of non-compliance with medication.[108] Jamison et al.[109] have identified the potentially critical role of psychotherapy in enhancing medication compliance in bipolar disorder and outlined an intervention programme.[47]

References

1. Moncrieff, J., Wessely, S., and Hardy, R. (1998). Meta-analysis of trials comparing antidepressants with 'active placebos'. *British Journal of Psychiatry*, **172**, 227–31.
2. Morris, J.B. and Beck, A.T. (1974). The efficacy of antidepressant drugs: a review of research. *Archives of General Psychiatry*, **30**, 667–74.
3. Bielski, R.J. and Friedel, R.O. (1976). Prediction of tricyclic antidepressant response: a critical review. *Archives of General Psychiatry*, **33**, 1479–89.
4. Joyce, P.R. and Paykel, E.S. (1989). Predictors of drug response in depression. *Archives of General Psychiatry*, **46**, 89–99.
5. Paykel, E.S., Hollyman, J.A., Freeling, P., and Sedgwick, P.J. (1988). Predictors of therapeutic benefit from amitriptyline in mild depression: a general practice placebo-controlled trial. *Journal of Affective Disorders*, **14**, 83–95.
6. Stewart, J.W., Quitkin, F.M., Liebowitz, M.R., McGrath, P.J., Harrison, W.M., and Klein, D.F. (1983). Efficacy of desipramine in depressed outpatients: response according to Research Diagnostic Criteria and severity of illness. *Archives of General Psychiatry*, **40**, 202–7.
7. Song, F., Freemantle, N., Sheldon, T.A., et al. (1993). Selective serotonin reuptake inhibitors: meta-analysis of efficacy and acceptability. *British Medical Journal*, **306**, 683–7.
8. Montgomery, S.A., Henry, J., McDonald, G., et al. (1994). Selective serotonin reuptake inhibitors: meta-analysis of discontinuation rates. *International Clinical Psychopharmacology*, **9**, 47–53.
9. Anderson, I.M. and Tomenson, B.M. (1995). Treatment discontinuation with selective serotonin reuptake inhibitors compared to tricyclic antidepressants: a meta-analysis. *British Medical Journal*, **310**, 1433–8.

10. Hotopf, M., Hardy, R., and Lewis, G. (1997). Discontinuation rates of SSRIs and tricyclic antidepressants: a meta-analysis and investigation of heterogeneity. *British Journal of Psychiatry*, **170**, 120–7.

11. Goodman, W.K., Price, L.H., Delgado, P.L., *et al.* (1990). Specificity of serotonin reuptake inhibitors in the treatment of obsessive–compulsive disorder: comparison of flovoxamine and desipramine. *Archives of General Psychiatry*, **47**, 577–85.

12. Griest, J.H., Jeffferson, J.W., Kobak, K.A., Katzelnick, D.J., and Serlin, R.C. (1995). Efficacy and tolerability of serotonin transport inhibitors in obsessive–compulsive disorder: a meta-analysis. *Archives of General Psychiatry*, **52**, 53–60.

13. Tyrer, P. (1976). Towards rational therapy with monoamine oxidase inhibitors. *British Journal of Psychiatry*, **128**, 354–60.

14. Paykel, E.S. (1990). Monoamine oxidase inhibitors: when should they be used. In *Dilemmas and difficulties in the management of psychiatric patients* (ed. K. Hawton and P. Cowen), pp. 17–30. Oxford University Press.

15. Paykel, E.S. (1995). Clinical efficacy of reversible and selective inhibitors of monoamine oxidase A in major depression. *Acta Psychiatrica Scandinavica*, **91** (Supplement 386), 22–7.

16. Paykel, E.S., West, P.S., Rowan, P.R., and Parker, R.R (1982). Influence of acetylator phenotype on antidepressant effects of phenelzine. *British Journal of Psychiatry*, **141**, 243–8.

17. Paykel, E.S., Parker, R.R., Rowan, P.R., Rao, B.M., and Taylor, C.N. (1983). Nosology of atypical depression. *Psychological Medicine*, **13**, 131–9.

18. Quitkin, F.M., McGrath, P.J., Steward, J.W., *et al.* (1990). Atypical depression, panic attacks, and response to amipramine and phenelzine: a replication. *Archives of General Psychiatry*, **47**, 935–41.

19. Angst J. and Stabl M. (1992). Efficacy of moclobemide in different patient groups: a meta-analysis of studies. *Psychopharmacology*, **106**, S109–13.

20. Paykel, E.S. (ed.) (1992). *The handbook of affective disorders* (2nd edn). Churchill Livingstone, Edinburgh.

21. Bloom, F.E. and Kupfer, D.J. (ed.) (1995). *Psychopharmacology: the fourth generation of progress*. Raven Press, New York.

22. Frazer, A. (1997). Antidepressants. *Journal of Clinical Psychiatry*, **58** (Supplement 6), 9–25.

23. Davis, R., Whittington, R., and Bryson, H.M. (1997). Nefazodone: a review of its pharmacology and clinical efficacy in the management of major depression. *Drugs*, **53**, 608–36.

24. Holliday, S.M. and Benfield, P. (1995). Venlafaxine: a review of its pharmacology and therapeutic potential in depression. *Drugs*, **49**, 280–94.

25. Garattini, S. (1997). Pharmacology of amineptine, an antidepressant agent acting on the dopaminergic system: a review. *International Clinical Psychopharmacology*, **12**, S15–19.

26. Ginestet, D. (1997). Efficacy of tianeptine in major depressive disorders with or without melancholia. *European Neuropsychopharmacology*, **7**, S341–5.

27. Paykel, E.S. (1989). Treatment of depression: the relevance of research for clinical practice. *British Journal of Psychiatry*, **155**, 754–63.

28. Janicak, P.G., Davis, J.M., Gibbons, R.D., Ericksen, S., Chang, S., and Gallagher, P. (1985). Efficacy of ECT: a meta-analysis. *American Journal of Psychiatry*, **142**, 297–302.

29. Buchan, H., Johnstone, E., McPherson, K., Palmer, R.L., Crow, T.J., and Brandon, S. (1992). Who benefits from electroconvulsive therapy? Combined results of the Leicester and Northwick Park trials. *British Journal of Psychiatry*, **160**, 355–9.

30. Mukherjee, S., Sackeim, H.A., and Schnur, D.B. (1994). Electroconvulsive therapy of acute manic episodes: a review of 50 years' experience. *American Journal of Psychiatry*, **151**, 169–76.

31. DiFelia, G. and Raotma, H. (1975). Is unilateral ECT less effective than bilateral ECT? *British Journal of Psychiatry*, **126**, 83–9.

32. Abrams, R., Taylor, M.A., Faber, R., Ts'o, T.O., Williams, R.A., and Almy,

G. (1983). Bilateral versus unilateral electroconvulsive therapy: efficacy in melancholia. *American Journal of Psychiatry*, **140**, 463–5.

33. Sackheim, H.A., Prudic, J., Devanand, D.P., *et al.* (1993). Effects of stimulus intensity and electrode placement on the efficacy and cognitive effects of electroconvulsive therapy. *New England Journal of Medicine*, **328**, 839–46.

34. George, M.S., Wassermann, E.M., Kimbrell, T.A., *et al.* (1997). Mood improvement following daily left prefrontal repetitive transcranial magnetic stimulation in patients with depression: a placebo-controlled crossover trial. *American Journal of Psychiatry*, **154**, 1752–6.

35. El-Mallakh, R. (1996). *Lithium: actions and mechanisms*, pp. 3–10. American Psychiatric Press, Washington, DC.

36. McElroy, S., Keck, P., and Pope, H. (1992). Valproate in the treatment of bipolar disorder: literature review and clinical guidelines. *Journal of Clinical Psychopharmacology*, **12**, 42–52.

37. West, S., Keck, P., and McElroy, S. (1998). Valproate. In *Mania: clinical and research perspectives* (ed. P. Goodnick), pp. 301–18. American Psychiatric Press, Washington, DC.

38. Bowden, C., Brugger, A., Swann, A., *et al.* (1994). Efficacy of divalproex vs lithium and placebo in the treatment of mania. *Journal of the American Medical Association*, **271**, 918–24.

39. Ketter, T., Post, R., Denicoff, K., *et al.* (1998). Carbamazepine. In *Mania: clinical and research perspectives* (ed. P. Goodnick), pp. 263–300. American Psychiatric Press, Washington, DC.

40. Frank, E., Prien, R.F., Jarrett, R.B., *et al.* (1991). Conceptualisation and rationale for consensus definitions of terms in major depressive disorder. Remission, recovery, relapse and recurrence. *Archives of General Psychiatry*, **48**, 851–5.

41. Paykel, E.S. (1996). Tertiary prevention: longer-term drug treatment in depression. In *The prevention of mental illness in primary care* (ed. T. Kendrick, A. Tylee, and P. Freeling), pp. 281–93. Cambridge University Press.

42. Reimherr, F.W., Amsterdam, J.D., Quitkin, F.M., *et al.* (1998). Optimal length of continuation therapy in depression: a prospective assessment during long-term fluoxetine treatment. *American Journal of Psychiatry*, **155**, 1247–53.

43. Haddad, P., Lejoyex, M., and Young, A. (1998). Antidepressant discontinuation reactions are preventable and simple to treat. *British Medical Journal*, **316**, 1105–6.

44. Paykel, E.S. (1994). The place of antidepressants in long-term treatment. In *Psychopharmacology of depression. British Association for Psychopharmacology Monograph 13* (ed. S.A. Montgomery and T.H. Corn), pp. 218–39. Oxford University Press, New York.

45. McElroy, S.L. and Weller, E. (1997). Psychopharmacological treatment of bipolar disorder across the lifespan. In *Review of psychiatry*, Vol. 16 (ed. L.J. Dickstein, M.B. Riba, and J.M. Oldham), pp. 124–78. American Psychiatric Press, Washington, DC.

46. Prien, R.F. (1992). Maintenance treatment. In *Handbook of affective disorders* (ed. E.S. Paykel), pp. 419–36. Churchill Livingstone, Edinburgh.

47. Goodwin, F.K. and Jamison, K.R. (1990). *Manic depressive illness*. Oxford University Press, New York.

48. Moncrieff, J. (1995). Lithium revisited: a re-examination of the placebo-controlled trials of lithium prophylaxis in manic-depressive disorder. *British Journal of Psychiatry*, **167**, 569–73.

49. Goodwin, G. (1995). Lithium revisited: a reply. *British Journal of Psychiatry*, **167**, 573–4.

50. Calabrese, J.R., Bowden, C. and Woyshville, M.J. (1995). Lithium and the anticonvulsants in the treatment of bipolar disorder. In *Psychopharmacology: the fourth generation of progress* (ed. F.E. Bloom and D.J. Kupfer), pp. 1099–111. Raven Press, New York.

51. Suppes, T., Baldessarini, R.J., Faedda, G.L., and Tohen, M. (1991). Risk of recurrence following discontinuation of lithium treatment in bipolar disorder. *Archives of General Psychiatry*, **48**, 1082–8.

52. Baldessarini, R.J., Tondo, L., Floris, G. and Rudas, N. (1997). Reduced morbidity after gradual discontinuation of lithium treatment for bipolar

I and II disorders: a replication study. *American Journal of Psychiatry*, **154**, 551–3.

53. Keller, M.B., Lavori, P.W., Kane, J.M., *et al.* (1992). Subsyndromal symptoms in bipolar disorder: a comparison of standard and low serum levels of lithium. *Archives of General Psychiatry*, **49**, 371–6.

54. Post, R.M. (1992). Anticonvulsants and novel drugs. In *Handbook of affective disorders* (ed. E.S. Paykel), pp. 387–418. Churchill Livingstone, Edinburgh.

55. Scott, J. (1995). Psychotherapy for bipolar disorders. *British Journal of Psychiatry*, **167**, 581–8.

56. Scott, J. (1995). Editorial: psychological treatments for depression: an update. *British Journal of Psychiatry*, **167**, 28–92.

57. Roth, T. and Fonagy, P. (1996). *What works for whom?*, pp. 57–103. Guilford Press, London.

58. Andrews, G. and Harvey, R. (1981). Does psychotherapy benefit neurotic patients. A re-analysis of the Smith, Glass and Miller data. *Archives of General Psychiatry*, **38**, 1203–8.

59. Steinbrueck, S., Maxwell, S., and Howard, G. (1983). A meta-analysis of psychotherapy and drug therapy in the treatment of unipolar depression with adults. *Journal of Consulting and Clinical Psychology*, **51**, 856–63.

60. Neitzel, M., Russell, R., Hemmings, K., and Gretter, M. (1987). Clinical significance of psychotherapy for unipolar depression: a meta-analytic approach to social comparison. *Journal of Consulting and Clinical Psychology*, **55**, 156–61.

61. Dobson, K. (1988). A meta-analysis of the efficacy of cognitive therapy for depression. *Journal of Consulting and Clinical Psychology*, **57**, 414–19.

62. Robinson, L., Berman, J., and Neimeyer, R. (1990). Psychotherapy for the treatment of depression: a comprehensive review of controlled outcome research. *Psychological Bulletin*, **108**, 30–49.

63. Elkin, I., Shea, M., Watkins, J., *et al.* (1992). National Institute of Mental Health treatment of depression collaborative treatment programme. *Archives of General Psychiatry*, **46**, 971–82.

64. Hollon, S., Shelton, R., and Davis, D. (1993). Cognitive therapy for depression: conceptual issues and clinical efficacy. *Journal of Consulting and Clinical Psychology*, **2**, 270–5.

65. Hollon, S., DeRubeis, R., Evans, M., *et al.* (1992). Cognitive therapy and pharmacotherapy for depression: singly and in combination. *Archives of General Psychiatry*, **49**, 774–81.

66. Klerman, G.L., DiMascio, A., Weissman, M.M., Prusoff, B.A., and Paykel, E.S. (1974). Treatment of depression by drugs and psychotherapy. *American Journal of Psychiatry*, **131**, 186–91.

67. DiMascio, A., Weissman, M., Prusoff, B., Neu, C., Zwilling, M., and Klerman, G. (1979). Differential symptom reduction by drugs and psychotherapy in acute depression. *Archives of General Psychiatry*, **36**, 1451–6.

68. McLean, P. and Hakstian, A. (1990). Relative endurance of unipolar depression treatment effects: longitudinal follow-up. *Journal of Consulting and Clinical Psychology*, **58**, 482–8.

69. Hersen, M., Bellack, A., Himmelhoch, J., and Thase, M. (1984). Effects of social skills training, amitryptiline and psychotherapy on unipolar depressed women. *Behaviour Therapy*, **15**, 21–40.

70. O'Leary, K. and Beach, S. (1990). Marital therapy: a viable treatment for depression and marital discord. *American Journal of Psychiatry*, **147**, 183–6.

71. Jacobson, N., Dobson, K., Furzzetti, A., and Schmaling, K. (1991). Marital therapy as a treatment for depression. *Journal of Consulting Clinical Psychology*, **59**, 547–57.

72. Conte, H., Plutchik, R., Wild, K., and Karasu, T. (1986). Combined psychotherapy and pharmacotherapy for depression. *Archives of General Psychiatry*, **43**, 471–9.

73. Depression Guideline Panel (1993). *Clinical practice guideline no 5: depression in primary care*, Vol. 2. *Treatment of major depression*, pp. 71–123. US Department of Health and Human Services, AHCPR Publications, Rockville, MD.

74. Paykel, E.S. (1995). Psychotherapy, medication combinations and compliance. *Journal of Clinical Psychiatry*, **56** (Supplement 1), 24–30.

75. Weissman, M., Klerman, G., Prusoff, B., Sholomskas, D., and Padian, N. (1981). Depressed outpatients: results one year after treatment with drugs and/or interpersonal psychotherapy. *Archives of General Psychiatry*, **38**, 51–5.

76. Evans, M., Hollon, S., DeRubeis, R., *et al.* (1992). Differential relapse following cognitive therapy and pharmacotherapy for depression. *Archives of General Psychiatry*, **49**, 802–8.

77. Shea, M.T., Elkin, I., Linber, S., *et al.* (1992). Course of depressive symptoms over follow-up. *Archives of General Psychiatry*, **49**, 782–7.

78. Blackburn, I., Euson, K., and Bishop, S. (1986). A two year naturalistic follow-up of depressed patients treated with cognitive therapy, pharmacotherapy or both. *Journal of Affective Disorders*, **109**, 67–75.

79. Blackburn, I. and Moore, R. (1997). Controlled acute and follow-up trial of cognitive therapy and pharmacotherapy in outpatients with recurrent depression. *British Journal of Psychiatry*, **171**, 328–34.

80. Fava, G.A., Grandi, S., Zielezny, M., Rafanelli, C., and Canestrari, R. (1996). Four-year outcome for cognitive behavioural treatment of residual symptoms in major depression. *American Journal of Psychiatry*, **153**, 945–7.

81. Paykel, E.S., Scott, J., Teasdale, J., *et al.* (1999). Prevention of relapse in residual depression by cognitive therapy: a controlled trial. *Archives of General Psychiatry*, **56**, 829–35.

82. Frank, E., Kupfer, D., Perel, J., *et al.* (1990). Three year outcomes for maintenance therapies in recurrent depressions. *Archives of General Psychiatry*, **47**, 1093–9.

83. Cochran, S. (1984). Preventing medical non-compliance in the outpatient treatment of bipolar affective disorders. *Journal of Consulting and Clinical Psychology*, **52**, 873–8.

84. Sotsky, S., Glass, D., Shea, M., *et al.* (1991). Patient predictors of response to psychotherapy: findings in the NIMH treatment of depression collaborative research programme. *American Journal of Psychiatry*, **148**, 997–1008.

85. De Lima, M.S., Hotoph, M., and Wessely, S. (1999). The efficacy of drug treatments for dysthymia: a systematic review and meta-analysis. *Psychological Medicine*, **29**, 1273–89.

86. Paykel, E.S. and Priest, R.G. (1992). Recognition and management of depression in general practice: consensus statement. *British Medical Journal*, **305**, 1198–202.

87. Altschuler, L., Cohen, L., Szuba, M.P., Burt, V.K., Gitlin M., and Mintz, J. (1996). Pharmacologic management of psychiatric illness during pregnancy: dilemmas and guidelines. *American Journal of Psychiatry*, **153**, 592–606.

88. Scott, J. (1995). Review: managing treatment resistant depression. *Primary Care Psychiatry*, **1**, 141–52.

89. Spiker, D., Weiss, J., Dealy, R., *et al.* (1985). The pharmacological treatment of delusional depression. *American Journal of Psychiatry*, **142**, 430–6.

90. Freeman, C.P. (ed.) (1995). *Council report CR39: the ECT handbook. The second report of the Royal College of Psychiatrist' Special Committee on ECT*. Royal College of Psychiatrists, London.

91. Scott, J. (1988). Chronic depression. *British Journal of Psychiatry*, **153**, 287–97.

92. Austin, M.-P., Souza, F.G.M., and Goodwin, G.M. (1991). Lithium augmentation in antidepressant-resistant patients: a quantitative analysis. *British Journal of Psychiatry*, **159**, 510–14.

93. Katona, C.L.E., Abou-Saleh, M.T., Harrison, D.A., *et al.* (1995). Placebo-controlled trial of lithium augmentation of fluoxetine and lofepramine. *British Journal of Psychiatry*, **166**, 80–6.

94. Cowen, P. (1990). L-Tryptophan and the eosinophilia–myalgia syndrome. *Psychiatric Bulletin*, **14**, 738–9.

95. Aronson, R., Offman, H.J., Joffe, R.T., and Naylor, D. (1996). Triiodothyronine augmentation in the treatment of refractory depression: a meta-analysis. *Archives of General Psychiatry*, **53**, 842–8.

96. McAskill, R., Mir, S., and Taylor, D. (1998). Pindolol augmentation of antidepressant therapy. *British Journal of Psychiatry*, **173**, 203–8.

97. Young, J.P.R., Lader, M.H., and Hughes, W.C. (1979). Controlled trial of trimipramine, monoamine oxidase inhibitors and combined treatment in depressed outpatients. *British Medical Journal*, **279**, 1315–17.

98. Razani, J., White, J., Simpson, G., Sloane, R.B., Rebal, R., and Palmer, R. (1983). The safety and efficacy of combined amitriptyline and tranylcypramine antidepressant treatment. *Archives of General Psychiatry*, **40**, 657–61.

99. Kocsis, J.H., Friedman, R.A., Markowitz, J.C., *et al.* (1996). Maintenance therapy for chronic depression: a controlled clinical trial of desipramine. *Archives of General Psychiatry*, **53**, 769–74.

100. Paykel, E.S., Ramana, R., Cooper, Z., Hayhurst, H., Kerr, J., and Barocka, A. (1995). Residual symptoms after partial remission: an important outcome in depression. *Psychological Medicine*, **25**, 1171–80.

101. Mindham, R.H., Howland, C., and Shepherd, M. (1973). An evaluation of discontinuation therapy with tricyclic antidepressants in depressive illness. *Psychological Medicine*, **3**, 5–17.

102. Kupfer, D.J., Frank, E., Perel, J.M., *et al.*(1992). Five-year outcome for maintenance therapies in recurrent depression. *Archives of General Psychiatry*, **49**, 769–73.

103. Kahn, D., Ross, R., and Rush, A. (1996). Expert consensus treatment guidelines for bipolar disorder. *Journal of Clinical Psychiatry*, **57**, 1–8.

104. Freeman, M. and Stoll, A. (1998). Mood stabilizer combinations: a review of safety and efficacy. *American Journal of Psychiatry*, **155**, 12–21.

105. Coryell, W., Solomon, D., Leon, A.C., *et al.* (1998). Lithium discontinuation and subsequent effectiveness. *American Journal of Psychiatry*, **155**, 8895–8.

106. Scott, J. and DeRubeis, R. (2000). The role of cognitive therapy and psychosocial interventions in chronic and refractory mood disorders. In *Textbook on refractory mood disorders*. Cambridge University Press.

107. Clarkin, J., Glick, I., Haas, G., *et al.* (1990). A randomized clinical trial of inpatient family intervention: results for affective disorder. *Journal of Affective Disorder*, **18**, 17–28.

108. Sackett, D. and Snow, J. (1979). The magnitude of compliance and non-compliance. In *Compliance in health care* (ed. R. Haynes, D. Taylor, and D. Sacket), pp. 11–22. Johns Hopkins University Press, Baltimore, MD.

109. Jamison, K., Gerner, R., and Goodwin, F. (1979). Patient and physician attitudes toward lithium: relationship to compliance. *Archives of General Psychiatry*, **45**, 217–24.

4.5.8 Dysthymia, cyclothymia, and related chronic subthreshold mood disorders

Hagop S. Akiskal

Subthreshold affective conditions

Long before psychiatry moved to the outpatient arena in the latter part of the twentieth century, psychiatrists had observed milder mood disturbances among the kin of patients hospitalized for endogenous or psychotic depressions or mania. Some were described as sullen, morose, or otherwise moody, but without discrete episodes; others reported self-limited episodes, but often went untreated. With the advent of modern treatments, practitioners are being increasingly consulted by patients presenting with attenuated affective disturbances. Although the relationship of these ambulatory mood disorders and more classical severe affective states has not been resolved, there is emerging sleep electroencephalography (**EEG**) and familial-genetic evidence[1–4] that a continuum exists between them. Along the same lines, studies conducted in the United States and Germany[5,6] into what were once described as 'neurotic' depressions have revealed a progression to more endogenous, psychotic, or otherwise severe, mood states—even bipolar switching in 18 per cent of patients. For these and related reasons, current official classification systems such as the ICD-10 and DSM-IV, have dropped the neurotic–endogenous dichotomy. Sceptics would perhaps argue that the new categorization of depressive disorders into dysthymic and major subtypes is not much of an improvement. None the less, the new terminology has drawn attention to a large universe of human suffering that had been neglected in the past, and the conceptualization of dysthymia as a variant of mood disorder has had a far-reaching impact on diagnostic and therapeutic habits of clinicians worldwide.[7] The emerging concept of the bipolar spectrum,[8] which does include manic, cyclic depressive (bipolar II), cyclothymic, and related conditions, is beginning to have a similar impact on practice.[9]

The subthreshold mood disorders are not only in continuum with more pathological mood states, but they also provide a bridge with normal affective conditions. In this context, temperament, as a construct encompassing affective personalities, is currently enjoying a renaissance as one of the possible substrates for the origin of mood disorders.[10] Temperament classically refers to an adaptive mixture of traits which, in the extreme, can lead to illness or modify the expression of superimposed affective states. The subthreshold conditions covered in this chapter represent the extreme expressions of these temperaments.

In the current literature, various items such as 'minor affective states', 'intermittent depression', 'hysteroid dysphoria', and 'atypical depression' are often used for subthreshold disorders.[11] These terms are avoided here, because in contemporary practice these conditions are at least as 'typical' as major mood disorders: their impact on the sufferer is not time-limited, nor minor, and involves more than a state of demoralization and moral foible. The following passage from Sir Aubrey Lewis[12] is *à propos*:

> …Severe emotional upsets ordinarily tend to subside, but mild emotional states…tend to persist, as it were, autonomously. Hence the paradox that a gross blatant psychosis may do less damage in the long run than some meagre neurotic incubus: a dramatic attack of mania or melancholia, with delusions, wasting, hallucinations, wild excitement may have far less effect on the course of man's life than some deceptively mild affective illness which goes on so long that it becomes inveterate. The former comes as a catastrophe and when it has passed the patient takes up his life again…while with the latter he may never get rid of his burden.

It is a curious fact that most subthreshold affective conditions, while symptomatologically attenuated, tend to pursue a chronic course. This raises the question, partially addressed in this chapter, that these conditions in their trait expressions might serve some useful function, even as they burden the individual with cares and instability which could predispose to full-blown affective disease. By their very chronicity, these subaffective conditions pose difficult conceptual and clinical questions about their differentiation from personality disorders.[13] Sceptics might argue that subthreshold affective conditions are nothing more than expressions of 'neuroticism'. Actually, a close examination of the Eysenck personality inventory, which ranges over a large terrain of depressiveness, anxiousness, emotionality, and mood lability among others,[14] reveals low-grade intermittent affective symptomatology.[15] And at least one genetic investigation has reported that neuroticism and major depression in women share substantial genetic underpinnings.[16] None the less, clinicians have always preferred categorical constructs, because neuroticism and related personality constructs do not do justice to the rich clinical phenomenology of disorders within the subaffective realm.[17]

The dysthymic spectrum

History

The term 'dysthymia' (meaning 'bad mood') originated in classical Greek and is still in current use in that country with the same connotation.[18] In the Hippocratic school, it was considered as part of the broader concept of melancholia (meaning 'black bile'). A temperament predisposed to melancholia was also delineated, and referred to individuals who were lethargic, brooding, and insecure. It was not until the early nineteenth century that dysthymia was reintroduced into medicine by the German physicians Stark and Fleming to describe depressions in inpatients that pursued a chronic course. Eventually, dysthymia came to subsume all mood disorders. The major residue of dysthymia in the latter sense in Europe today is the French rubric of *les dysthymies*, as a synonym for *troubles de l'humeur*; the DSM-IV or ICD-10 'dysthymic disorder' in that country is translated as *le trouble dysthymique*.

The more direct lineage of our current usage of the term dysthymia is to be found in the latter part of the nineteenth century in the work of Kraepelin, who delineated the depressive disposition as one of the constitutional foundations of affective episodes.[19] The condition often began early in life, such that by adolescence many showed an increased sensitivity to life's sorrows and disappointments: they were tormented by guilt, had little confidence in their abilities, and suffered from low energy. As they grew into adulthood, they experienced 'life with its activity [as] a burden which they habitually [bore] with dutiful self-denial without being compensated by the pleasures of existence'. In some, these temperamental peculiarities were so marked that they could be considered 'morbid without the appearance of more severe, delimited attacks…' (clearly foreshadowing the modern concept of trait dysthymia). In other cases, recurrent melancholia arose from this substrate without definite boundaries (again anticipating the concept of 'double-depression').

Subsequently, Kurt Schneider in his opus *Psychopathic Personalities*[20] devoted considerable space to a depressive type whose entire existence was entrenched in suffering. Building on this rich phenomenological tradition, our research in Memphis[21] helped in operationalizing the core characteristics of such patients encountered in contemporary practice: gloomy, sombre, and incapable of having fun; brooding, self-critical, and guilt-prone; lack of confidence, low self-esteem, preoccupation with failure; pessimistic, easily discouraged; easy to tire, sluggish, and bound to routine; non-assertive, self-denying, and devoted; shy and sensitive. These traits have excellent internal consistency and discriminatory ability.[22,23] Similar concepts have also appeared in the Japanese literature,[24] with particular emphasis on self-critical attitudes, persistence in work habits, and devotion to others. Finally, the French construct of *la depression constitutionelle*[25] has emphasized the lethargic aspects with a sense of inadequacy.

The classical tenet in psychiatry has been that affectively ill patients recover from their acute episodes with relatively little symptomatic residua and dysfunction. Community psychiatry, which has given renewed visibility to the temperamentally expressed low-grade fluctuating depressive disorders, has challenged this classic view. With the advent of DSM-III, such patients are now officially designated as 'dysthymic.' In the ICD-10 classification, the low-grade depressive baseline is considered the main pathology; only an occasional superimposed depressive episode is permitted, provided that it is mild. In the latest American Psychiatric Association revision (DSM-IV), at least two patterns have been described: pure dysthymia uncomplicated by major depression, and a more prevalent pattern of dysthymia complicated by major depressive episodes that could be even moderate or severe in intensity (and which has been dubbed 'double depression').

The mystery of this incapacitating depressive subtype[26]—long recognized, but only recently sanctioned in official diagnostic manuals—is that, in their habitual condition, sufferers lack the classical 'objective' or 'major' signs of acute clinical depression, such as profound changes in psychomotor and vegetative functions. Instead, patients consult their doctors for more fluctuating complaints consisting of gloominess, lethargy, self-doubt, and lack of *joie de vivre*; they typically work hard, but do not enjoy their work; if married, they are deadlocked in bitter and unhappy marriages which lead neither to reconciliation nor separation; for them, their entire existence is a burden: they are satisfied with nothing, complain of everything, and brood about the uselessness of existence. As a result, in the past those who could afford it were condemned to the couch for what often proved to be interminable analysis. The legitimization of dysthymia as a clinically significant variant of affective disorder in both the United States and WHO classifications has helped the cause of more cost-effective treatments.

To sum up, for nearly 2500 years physicians have described individuals with a low-grade chronic depressive profile marked by gloominess, pessimism, low enjoyment of life, relatively low drive, yet endowed with self-critical attitudes and suffering for others. This constellation is as much a virtue as it is a disposition to melancholy, and many dysthymic patients presenting clinically have various admixtures of major depression. This is compatible with a spectrum-concept of depressive illness, which defines various degrees of severity.

Clinical picture and diagnostic considerations

Diagnostic criteria for dysthymia in both DSM-IV and ICD-10 stipulate a 2-year duration of low-grade depressive symptoms, exclusive of such indicators of severity as suicidality and psychomotor disturbances. Dysthymia is distinguished from chronic major depressive disorder by the fact that it is not a sequel to well-defined major depressive episodes. Instead, patients often complain that they have always been depressed.[27] Most are of early onset (less than 20 years). A late-onset subtype[28] first manifesting after the age of 50 is much less prevalent and has not been well characterized clinically, but it has been identified largely through studies in the community.

At their best, dysthymic individuals invest whatever energy they have in work, leaving none for leisure or social activities. According to Tellenbach,[29] such dedication to work represents an overcompensation against depressive disorganization. Kretschmer[30] had earlier suggested that such persons were the backbone of society, devoting their lives to jobs that require dependability and great attention to detail. These features represent the obsessoid facet of dysthymia. Such individuals may seek outpatient counselling and psychotherapy for what some clinicians might consider 'existential depression': individuals who complain that their life lacks lustre, joy, and meaning. Others present clinically because of an intensification of their gloom to the level of clinical depression; history of lifelong low-grade depressive symptoms would distinguish them from episodic major depressive patients.

The proverbial dysthymic patient will often complain of having been 'depressed since birth'.[21] In the eloquent words of Kurt Schneider,[20] 'they view themselves as belonging to an "aristocracy of suffering"'. These hyperbolic descriptions of suffering in the absence of more objective signs of depression earn such patients the label of 'characterological depression'.[27] The description is further reinforced by the fluctuating depressive picture that merges imperceptibly with the patient's habitual self, leading to the customary clinical uncertainty as to whether dysthymic disorder belongs to the affective or personality disorder domains.

At their worst, patients with low-grade depression having an intermittent course can present such instability in their life, including suicidal crises, that some clinicians would entertain the diagnosis of borderline personality disorder. This is not consistent with the classic picture of dysthymia arising from a temperamental type with more mature ego structure[31] described above. Depressives with unstable (that is to say, 'borderline') personality structure more often belong to the irritable cyclothymic–bipolar II spectrum.

The greatest overlap of dysthymia is with major depressive disorder, but differs from it in that symptoms tend to outnumber signs (more subjective than objective depression). Thus, marked disturbances in appetite and libido are uncharacteristic, and psychomotor agitation or retardation is not observed. Nonetheless, subtle 'endogenous' features are not uncommonly reported: inertia, lethargy, and anhedonia that are characteristically worse in the morning.[27] Because many patients with dysthymia presenting clinically fluctuate in and out of a major depression, the core DSM-IV criteria for dysthymia tend to emphasize vegetative dysfunction, whereas the alternative criterion B for dysthymia in a DSM-IV appendix lists cognitive symptoms; although the latter appear more characteristic of trait dysthymia, the DSM-IV field trial[32] could not demonstrate their specificity for dysthymia.

A recent Italian investigation[33] of a large sample from community and primary-care medical settings revealed that negative mood (by definition), along with low energy, poor concentration, low self-esteem, sleep and appetite disturbance, and hopelessness (in descending order) were the most common symptoms of dysthymia. These data suggest that the cognitive and somatic symptoms are not easily separable in practice. None the less, this study did raise the possibility that factors could be discerned along two different axes: 'negative affectivity' and 'lassitude with poor concentration'. In our experience, patients loading on the latter factor often complain of hypersomnia and may exhibit subtle bipolar signs; alternatively, they might have some link to the poorly defined constructs of neurasthenia, chronic

Table 1 The core characteristics of dysthymia

Long-standing subthreshold depression of a fluctuating or persistent nature
Gloomy and joyless disposition
Brooding about the past and guilt prone
Low drive and lethargy
Low self-esteem and preoccupation with failure
Identifies suffering as part of the habitual self

Summarized from Akiskal.[26]

fatigue syndrome, and fibromyalgia. In terms of differential diagnosis, patients with chronic fatigue syndrome present with disabling fatigue and, typically, deny depressive symptoms; patients with fibromyalgia complain of pain; by contrast, the typical patient with dysthymia cannot stop relating to the physician his or her litany of depressive symptoms. Polysomnography, though not yet definitive, may shed some light on differentiating fibromyalgia from dysthymia proper.[34]

Although dysthymic disorder represents a more restricted concept than does its parent, neurotic depression, it is still quite heterogeneous. Anxiety is not a necessary part of its clinical picture, yet dysthymia is sometimes diagnosed in patients with anxiety and neurotic disorders. That clinical situation is perhaps to be regarded as a secondary or 'anxious dysthymia' or, as some British authors seem to prefer, as part of a 'general neurotic syndrome'[35] (an implicit partial return to the now defunct concept of neurotic depression).

The clinical picture of dysthymic disorder that emerges from the foregoing descriptions is quite varied, with many who fluctuate in and out of major depression,[36] whereas in others the pathology is woven into the habitual self.[27] These considerations suggest that a clinically satisfactory operationalization of dysthymia must include both symptoms and trait characteristics (Table 1). The following vignette illustrates this more prototypical form of dysthymic suffering.

Case Study This 37-year-old never-married male teacher presented with the complaint that he was 'tired of living' and was considering 'ending it all'. He said that much of his life had been 'wasted', he had never known any joy, that all human existence for him was a 'tragic mistake of God'. He was known to be a dedicated and talented teacher, but he felt all his efforts had been 'useless and in vain'. He said he probably was 'born depressed', because he had not known any happiness and that the only utility he could have for mankind was 'to serve as a specimen to be researched—to shed light on human misery'. Although he conceded that some women found him interesting, even intellectually stimulating, he said he could not enjoy physical intimacy, that even orgasm lacked passion; nonetheless, he masturbated frequently, fantasizing about married female teachers—only to feel guilty. We could not document any major affective episodes. He stated that he had always functioned at a 'mediocre level' (which was at variance with the good feedback students had given him year after year); but did admit he 'appreciated work, because there was nothing else to do'. He denied alcohol and drug habits. There had never been any periods of hypomania, but one of his maternal aunts had been treated for a 'cyclical depression' and was apparently doing well on lithium. The patient's mother was a sombre serious work-oriented woman who had raised three children and had done voluntary work for the church, but had no depressive complaints. His father had died from a coronary attack, but his side of the family was otherwise unremarkable.

Although both DSM-IV and ICD-10 omit suicidal preoccupations

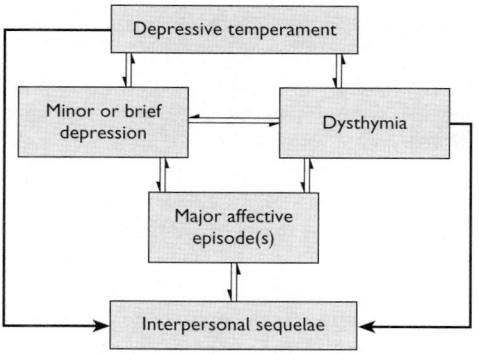

Fig. 1 Diagram to show putative relationships within a broad depressive spectrum.

in their diagnostic criteria for dysthymia, as testified by the above case, this is what often brings patients to clinical attention.

Course

An insidious onset of depression dating back to late childhood or the teens, preceding any superimposed major depressive episodes by years, even decades, is the most typical developmental background of dysthymic disorder. A return to the low-grade depressive pattern is the rule following recovery from superimposed major depressive episodes, if any—hence the designation 'double depression'.[36]

A long-term prospective study of prepubertal children[37] has revealed an episodic course of dysthymia with remissions and exacerbations, and eventual complication by major depressive episodes, as well as hypomanic, manic, or mixed episodes postpubertally. Persons with dysthymic disorder presenting clinically as adults tend to pursue a chronic 'unipolar' course, which may or may not be complicated by major depression: they rarely develop spontaneous hypomania or mania. However, when treated with antidepressants, some adult patients with dysthymia may experience brief hypomanic switches[38] that typically disappear when the antidepressant dose is decreased. Although ICD-10 and DSM-IV would not 'allow' the occurrence of such switches in dysthymia, systematic clinical observation[39,40] have verified their occurrence in between 10 and 30 per cent of dysthymic patients. In that special dysthymic subgroup, the family histories are typically positive for bipolar disorder.[38] Such patients, often conforming to the double depressive pattern, represent a clinical bridge between major depressive disorder and bipolar II.[8]

A recent 12-year prospective study[41] has shown that patients with major depressive disorder spent 44 per cent of their course in low-grade depression (versus 15 per cent of time in major depressive episodes). This suggests that major depression, dysthymia, or otherwise subsyndromal depression constitute somewhat artificial conventions on the threshold and duration of depressive illness, representing alternative manifestations of the same diathesis. In this context, residual intermorbid depressive symptoms have been confirmed as being strongly predictive of a rapid relapse into a new major depressive episode. Various 'major' and 'minor' depressive conditions described in DSM-IV and its appendix must not be viewed as distinct depressive subtypes, but part of a symptomatic continuum.[42] Figure 1 shows a diagram of these putative relationships within a broad depressive spectrum.

Epidemiology

From 1966 to 1980, *Index Medicus* listed no more than 10 articles on chronic depressions. Since 1980, when dysthymia was first introduced in DSM-III, at least 200 articles have appeared on chronic depression, mostly on dysthymia. This phenomenal growth in research interest parallels the increasing public health significance of this disorder. It is estimated that 3 per cent of the North American population is suffering from this condition;[43] the figures in other parts of the world are comparable, at least on average.[44] Like major depressive disorder, dysthymia is twice as common in women as in men. Because of its chronicity, dysthymia is among the most common clinical presentations of a psychiatric condition. Dysthymia is more disabling, as far as quality of life in social and personal areas, work, and leisure, than depression in the setting of a severe anxiety disorder like agoraphobia.[45] Celibacy is also common in early-onset dysthymia,[46] but not for long; modern successful treatments often lead to a change in marital status!

Other research in primary care[47] has focused on depressive symptoms falling short of the major depressive threshold, as far as symptom intensity is concerned, as well as falling short of the 2-year duration criterion for dysthymia. Despite its chronicity, 50 per cent of people remain unrecognized by general practitioners. Despite the low-grade nature of their depressive complaints, these patients report high degrees of morbidity and impairment in a variety of health domains and quality of life, including 'bed days' (namely the number of days per year they stayed ill in bed). Actually, these impairments are generally more pronounced than those of patients with a variety of medical conditions, such as hypertension, diabetes, arthritis, and chronic lung disease; only coronary artery disease exceeded the disability of low-grade depression in several domains.

In light of the foregoing developments, both the World Psychiatric Association[48] and the World Health Organization[49] have developed programmes to address the challenges of educating general practitioners in the proper recognition and treatment of dysthymia.

Aetiological considerations

Some sensitivity to suffering, a cardinal feature of the depressive temperament, represents an important attribute in a species like ours, where caring for young and sick individuals is necessary for survival. This temperament, historically the *Anlage* of dysthymia, in the extreme often leads to clinical depression. The constitutional viewpoint, while dominant in the early part of the twentieth century,[19] gradually disappeared from psychiatric thinking. One reason was that Kurt Schneider[20] preferred to conceptualize this form of pathology as 'psychopathy', by which he meant abnormal personality development. Independently, Freud's disciples took this one step further and, eventually, in outpatients, all milder depressions with a tendency to chronicity came to be considered as the expressions of a character neurosis.[50] In support for this position, these authors could point to the long-standing nature of the interpersonal difficulties in the lives of these individuals. When, and if, antidepressants were prescribed, they were given in homeopathic doses; worse, many patients received stimulants or benzodiazepines rather than genuine antidepressants. Failure to respond to these incorrectly chosen pharmaceutical agents seemed to further reinforce the notion of a 'character' defect.

Table 2 Evidence for considering dysthymia as a variant of major depressive disorder

Familial affective loading
Phase advance of rapid eye-movement sleep
Diurnality of inertia, gloominess, and anhedonia
Thyroid-releasing hormone–thyroid-stimulating hormone challenge test abnormalities
Prospective course complicated by recurrent major depressive episodes
Positive response to selected thymoleptics
Treatment-emergent hypomania

Updated from Akiskal.[26]

Several lines of observation have challenged the concept of 'character neurosis' as an explanation for low-grade depression, and thereby forced a return to the more classical European concept of temperament with its biological underpinnings. First, in a 1980 study of rapid eye movement (**REM**) latency (normally 90 min, measured from sleep onset to the first REM period) conducted in 'depressive characters' who were not in a state of major depression, we reported that REM latency was less than 60 min, and sleep was redistributed to the early part of the night[27] (which was the reverse of what we observed in chronic anxious patients[51]). Moreover, a family history for major affective illness (including bipolar) was significantly high in short-REM latency patients.[38] (The reverse was true for those with familial alcoholism and sociopathy.) The sleep findings were so reminiscent of those seen in major affective illness that we were compelled to give our patients systematic open trials with desipramine and nortriptyline (the best-tolerated secondary amine tricyclics in those days) or lithium carbonate if antidepressants failed (based on the observation of familial bipolar disorder in some).[27] Nearly 40 per cent remitted, of whom one out of three developed brief hypomania. The sleep findings have been replicated in other laboratories,[52] and Rihmer[39] has shown that patients with dysthymia experience transient lifting of their mood with sleep deprivation. Klein et al.[53] have shown high rates of affective illness in a systematic familial investigation of dysthymic probands. There also exist dysthymic patients whose lifelong suffering and discontent appear, in retrospect,[38] a legacy of an unsatisfactory childhood marked by deprivation or abuse at the hands of alcoholic and/or sociopathic parents or step-parents. Although it is clinically attractive to invoke the notion of 'learned helplessness' secondary to such inescapable childhood traumata, an alternative hypothesis[54] is that the helplessness of these individuals might develop secondary to an inherited diathesis which biases these children's early experiences in a dysphoric direction.

As for neuroendocrine markers,[52] thyroid-releasing hormone–thyroid-stimulating hormone challenge and electrodermal activity similar to those with major depressive disorders are the main findings; by contrast, dexamethasone suppression and catecholamine metabolism are essentially unaltered in dysthymia. These observations, along with the REM latency findings, suggest that dysthymia represents trait depression. Coupled with the family history data, this traitness can be postulated to be of constitutional origin. Certainly, the occurrence of major affective episodes in the long-term course of dysthymia, in both community and clinical samples,[50,51] is in line with this position. It is, therefore, of great theoretical and practical significance that shortened REM latency has been reported in the offspring of the affectively ill.[55,56] Table 2 summarizes the foregoing links between dysthymia

and major depressive disorder, and which support its inclusion within the family of mood disorders.

There are also medical and neurological factors that may contribute to dysthymic symptom formation.[52] Actually, joint medical–neurological and non-affective psychiatric disease is often contributory to extreme refractoriness among the chronic depressive states of these patients. Such patients are at risk for suicide, especially those with epilepsy or progressive degenerative neurological disease. Interestingly, living with a medically disabled spouse or family member, too, can be associated with some chronicity of depression.

The emergence of pathogenetic understanding, as outlined above, is all the more impressive, given the controversies on the very nature of dysthymia and its legitimacy as a nosological entity.[57]

Treatment

The trait nature of dysthymia can be further observed in the fact that dysthymia often pursues an unrelenting course towards chronicity.[11] Thus, spontaneous recovery has been shown to occur in no more than 13 per cent of subjects in the community over 1 year.[58] In outpatient clinics, the outcome is somewhat better, but this is probably due to the treatment received and a longer follow-up.[11]

Evidence

Most classes of antidepressants[59–66] have been shown to be effective in dysthymia in double-blind studies (Table 3). The rationale for using classic antidepressants such as tricyclic compounds was the observation of shortened REM latency in dysthymic subjects in our sleep laboratory.[27] Irreversible monoamine oxidase inhibitors such as phenalzine were used because of the belief that non-classical depressions respond preferentially to this class of drugs;[61] the same can be said for the reversible inhibitors of type A monoamine oxidase.[66] Ritanserin[62] (now withdrawn because of cardiotoxicity) and amisulpride[65] were tried, because both compounds reverse 'negative' symptoms in schizophrenia and, by analogy, it was hypothesized that the low motivation and lethargy seen in some patients with dysthymia reflected a shared underlying dimensional transnosological pathology. The selective serotonin re-uptake inhibitors (**SSRIs**) were used empirically,[63,64] because of good tolerance compared with the tricyclic antidepressants, and later it was suggested that improvement in dysthymia correlates with normalization of serotonergic indices.[67] The foregoing trials, conducted in different countries during the past 12 years represent the most eloquent evidence for the increasing worldwide acceptance of the concept of dysthymia as a clinically significant variant of affective disorder.

Table 3 Major controlled pharmacological trials in dysthymia worldwide

Reference	Country	Medication
Vallejo et al. (1987)[59]	Spain	Phenelzine versus imipramine
Kocsis et al. (1988)[60]	USA	Imipramine versus placebo
Stewart et al. (1989)[61]	USA	Phenelzine versus placebo
Bakish et al. (1993)[62]	Canada	Ritanserin versus placebo
Thase et al. (1996)[63]	USA	Sertraline versus imipramine
Vanelle et al. (1997)[64]	France	Fluoxetine versus placebo
Lecrubier et al. (1996)[65]	France	Amisulpride versus placebo
Versiani et al. (1997)[66]	Brazil	Moclobemide versus imipramine

Clinical management

The treatment of dysthymia should continue in most cases for 2 years or more. Tricyclic antidepressants have too many side-effects in clinically effective doses (desipramine equivalent of 150 mg or more per day). Given dietary and medication prohibitions, monoamine oxidase inhibitors are also not practical as first-line drugs. Overall good tolerance in long-term use, despite sexual side-effects, has made the SSRIs the first-line intervention treatment for dysthymia; given that many people with dysthymia are young individuals who should be eager to form families, their acceptance of long-term SSRI use is an indication that the alleviation of the depressive suffering of dysthymia is genuine and far outweighs the sexual dysfunction. However, 75 to 150 mg bupropion-SR (an antidepressant available in the United States) can be taken in the morning on the desired day of sexual union, but preferably no more than once a week. If severe, sexual dysfunction can be reversed by switching to nafazodone with sex-sparing 5-HT$_2$ action (which might work on clinical grounds, though its antidysthymic action is still under investigation). Moclobemide also spares sexual function, but seems more effective in anxious and milder cases of dysthymia. Amisulpride, which rarely causes amenorrhoea and/or galactorrhoea, is otherwise well tolerated in dysthymia in the more lethargic forms of the illness seen in general medical practice.

The dosage of nearly all antidepressants in dysthymia is in the full range for that recommended for major depression (20–40 mg for fluoxetine). In the case of amisulpride, the dosage is low (25–50 mg), because at this dosage the drug is a dopamine agonist, believed to be the necessary ingredient for its mechanism of action in dysthymia. Both dysthymia and double depression respond equally well, and the duration of underlying dysthymia does not seem to matter. The main difference in treatment for these two course patterns is that dysthymia need not be treated for a lifetime, but double depression should probably be treated indefinitely. Women seem to have a preferentially better response to SSRIs,[46] which have the added benefit of treating the premenstrual accentuation of dysthymic symptoms. Borderline thyroid function (e.g. a high baseline thyroid-stimulating hormone level) preferentially occurs in women with dysthymia, so that these women would benefit from thyroid augmentation (levothyroxine 175 mg/day) of the antidepressant. In those patients who oversleep in the morning, terminal sleep deprivation and/or morning phototherapy represent useful adjuncts to antidepressants. Although there are no controlled studies in children, our clinical experience indicates that SSRIs often prove effective in this population, with the appropriate dosage reduction for body-weight. In adults, concurrent personality disturbances (for instance, obsessoid, avoidant, dependent, and hostile features) do not compromise therapeutic responses.[46] Indeed, more often than not, such personality disturbances recede with the successful alleviation of dysthymic suffering; social function improves in tandem.[68] (However, extremely hostile patients, who may meet symptomatological criteria for 'dysthymia' but whose irritable dysphoria more appropriately belongs to the cyclothymic domain, are best managed with mood-stabilizing anticonvulsants, for example divalproex 600 to 1200 mg/day.)

Together with Haykal, we have shown that, with the judicious use of the foregoing modalities in private practice,[46] three out of four patients with dysthymia engulfed in gloom for much of their lives had sustained remissions for five or more years. Depressive episodes and suicidal preoccupation and/or crises were prevented, in tandem with

Table 4 Psychotherapeutic principles in dysthymia

Provide a deliverable (and believable) dose of optimism
Optimize compliance to pharmacotherapy
Limit destructive expression of negative feelings
Address accumulated conflicts
Combat postdepressive resignation and inertia
Provide support for patient and significant others
Be aware of countertransference feelings
Consult experts with extensive experience in treating chronic depression
Gradually, mobilize patient's skills and resources

Updated from Akiskal.[76]

the alleviation of the dysthymia. Approximately 15 per cent experienced 'overcorrection' of their dysthymia in the direction of mild hypomania; this is particularly likely in the presence of inhibited-social phobic traits as part of dysthymia, and when the family history is bipolar. The hypomania is typically short-lived, and tends to disappear when the antidepressant dose is reduced; in some cases, it is necessary to provide lithium (600–900 mg/day) or valproate augmentation (500–750 mg/day). The question has been raised whether selective serotonin-reuptake inhibitors, in particular fluoxetine, change the personality in a hyperthymic direction. In our experience, most observed changes are compatible with adaptive behaviour that emerge as a result of alleviation of depressive suffering; the more distinctly protracted hypomanic changes nearly always require familial bipolar diathesis.[46] It is, nonetheless, true that with SSRIs we have entered an era of 'dimensional psychopharmacology', whereby the clinician could dose the patient to a desired end from a functional standpoint.[69] Many become care-less rather than careless.[70] The present author has also encountered some patients treated with SSRIs who view a life without cares as negative; in such cases, one should opt for very low doses and a more gradual lifting of the dysthymia, and help the patient adjust to a new self-image of normalcy.

As for psychotherapy, there is little credible evidence for its efficacy as a monotherapy in the treatment of dysthymia.[71] Actually, a panel of female experts[72] has argued that exploration of one's mental inadequacies, in the 'passive' psychoanalytical situation, is particularly negative for women; the more 'active' cognitive–behavioural approaches, which encourage thinking, and behaviours reinforcing for the individual, are preferable. Many clinicians profitably use the latter strategy along with pharmacotherapy—to boost the self-esteem of the patient. In a more practical vein, there are clinical management strategies[73] that are specifically useful for both the patients and their clinicians (Table 4). It is particularly important for the clinician not to be submerged by the negative thinking of the patient, and it is even more crucial for the therapist to recognize that a relative lack of progress can generate feelings of 'impotence' and countertransference; periodic consultation with more experienced clinicians in the treatment of chronic depression would be desirable.

Interpersonal psychotherapy has been used in medication failures by Markowitz.[71] This is best viewed as a more practical abbreviation of psychodynamic psychotherapy, with a strong emphasis on support and encouragement for patients with dysthymia who seek help at a time of loss or role transition in their lives. Knowledge of the interpersonal context of depression is obviously important in formulating how the clinician would stage the psychological recovery process from dysthymia. None the less, there are some suggestions that SSRIs often lead to improved coping behaviour, even without formal psychotherapy. Indeed, it has been shown by Ravindran and colleagues[74] that a successful response to SSRIs is often associated with decreased emotion-focused coping and decreased perception of daily hassles, as well as alleviation of the sense of loneliness one experiences in chronic depression.

No matter what the active ingredients in antidysthymic treatments, there is little doubt that for the first time we have potent practical treatments to alleviate a major source of chronic human suffering, including what were once deemed depressive characterological attributes inseparable from the habitual self. Helping patients attain a new homeostasis of the self is an art unparalleled in the history of medical science. It does not constitute 'cosmetic psychopharmacology'.[75]

Prevention opportunities

Community subjects with pure dysthymia have been found in two prospective studies[76,77] to be at risk for major depressive episodes. Because dysthymia often makes its first appearance in juvenile years, identifying the disorder at this early stage represents a special opportunity for prevention in child psychiatry and paediatrics.

In still another group of patients, low-grade chronic depressive developments occur in the setting of disabling systematic medical and neurological disorders, and are best categorized as 'secondary dysthymias'.[78] For instance, poliomyelitis may not only lead to deformities in musculoskeletal structures in children, but could permanently scar the sufferer's sense of enjoyment, fulfilment, and outlook of life. Likewise, low-grade chronic depressive development often complicates neurodegenerative cerebrovascular disease later in life. In both situations, psychological factors might be operative, yet the contribution of specific cerebral lesions to the subthreshold mood disturbance may be substantial. This group as a whole is not well captured by the conventional depressive categories in ICD-10 and DSM-IV. In these subacute dysthymic-like conditions, the affective state is often disabling, yet symptomatologically less severe than major depression; it is low grade, yet not as chronic as dysthymia. 'Minor depression' would not capture the clinical significance of their condition. Indeed, there is emerging data that treating these subacute dysthymias may improve the prognosis of the underlying neurological disorder.[49]

Cyclothymic disorder and labile–irritable variants

History

Kraepelin[19] included the cyclothymic disposition as one of the temperamental foundations from which manic–depressive illness arose. Kretschmer[30] went one step further and proposed that this constitution represented the core characteristic of the illness: some patients were more likely to oscillate in a sad direction, while others would more readily resonate with cheerful situations; these were merely viewed as variations in the cyclothymic oscillation between these two extremes. Kurt Schneider,[20] who did not endorse the concept of 'temperament', instead referred to 'labile psychopaths' whose moods constantly changed in a dysphoric direction, and who bore no relationship to patients with manic depression. To confuse matters further, Schneider used the term 'cyclothymia' as a synonym for all manic depressive illness, from the mildest to the most severe psychotic forms. Today,

Table 5 Discriminatory biphasic characteristics of cyclothymic disorder

Lethargy alternating with eutonia
Shaky self-esteem alternating between low self-confidence and overconfidence
Decreased verbal output alternating with talkativeness
Mental confusion alternating with sharpened thinking
Unexplained tearfulness alternating with excessive punning and jocularity
Introverted self-absorption alternating with uninhibited people-seeking

Summarized from Akiskal et al.[23,80]

'cyclothymia' is still sometimes used in this broader sense in Germanophone psychiatry. But in much of the rest of the world, cyclothymia (short for 'cyclothymic disorder') is reserved for a form of extreme temperament related to bipolar disorder.

Cyclothymia, which in ICD-9 and DSM-II was subsumed under the affective personalities, was first introduced into DSM-III and DSM-IV and subsequently into ICD-10 as a form of attenuated chronic mood disorder. The diagnosis is not commonly made in clinical practice, because it is almost always seen when a patient presents with major depressive episodes, warranting the designation of 'bipolar II'.[8,18] None the less, the construct is of great theoretical and practical significance as one of the possible substrates for major mood disorders. Moreover, it could shed light on social and occupational maladjustment and/or addictive behaviours that could otherwise be misattributed to personality disorder.

Clinical features and diagnostic considerations

By definition, individuals with cyclothymia report short cycles of depression and hypomania that fail to meet the sustained duration criterion for major affective syndromes. At various times, they exhibit the entire range of manifestations required for the diagnosis of depression and hypomania, but only from a few days at a time up to 1 week, rarely longer.[79] These cycles follow each other in an irregular fashion, often changing abruptly from one mood to another, with only rare interposition of 'even' periods. The unpredictability of mood swings is a major source of distress for cyclothymes, as they do not know from moment to moment, how they will feel.[80] As one patient put it, 'my moods swing like a pendulum, from one extreme to another'. The rapid mood shifts, which undermine the patients' sense of self, may lead to the misleading diagnostic label of borderline personality. But unlike a personality disorder, the mood changes in cyclothymes have a circadian component. One patient described it as follows: 'I would go to bed in a cheerful mood and wake up down in the dumps'. This observation is in line with psychophysiological data on mood-switching occurring out of the rapid eye movement sleep phase, as reported in more typical cases of manic depression.[81]

The mood swings of cyclothymes are biphasic: eutonia versus anergic periods; people-seeking versus self-absorption; sharpened thinking versus mental paralysis. Table 5 provides an empirically tested set of criteria. In addition, the following presentations characterize their roller-coaster biography.

Irritable periods

At one time or another, labile angry or irritable moods are observed in virtually all these patients.[80] Cyclothymes, unlike patients with epilepsy, are aware of their 'fits of anger', which lead to considerable personal and social embarrassment after they subside. The patients often feel 'on edge, restless, and aimlessly driven'; family and friends report that during these periods patients seem inconsiderate and hostile toward people around them. The contribution of alcohol and sedative-hypnotic drugs to these moods cannot be denied, but the moods often occur in the absence of drugs. Electroencephalography typically reveals no seizure or subseizure activity. The interpersonal costs of such unpredictable interpersonal explosiveness can be quite damaging. One of our patients reported frequent periods where he would start unprovoked fights with very close friends, only to shift into periods of prolonged 'soul-searching, guilt, shame, and embarrassment'. In other patients, outbursts of anger are 'reactive' to minor interpersonal disputes[82]—but once in full force, they are like emotional avalanches with the distinct potential to destroy relationships. Should they dominate the clinical picture, especially among young women who hurt themselves in response to interpersonal contexts, the problematic diagnosis of borderline personality disorder is often invoked (more so in North America than elsewhere). Although controversial, contemporary research suggests that many 'borderline' patients represent a severe labile–irritable variant of cyclothymia on the border of manic–depressive psychosis.[17,83,84] On the other hand, bizarre episodes of self-harm, recurrent illusions, and dissociative symptoms of the post-traumatic stress disorder type are uncharacteristic of cyclothymia, and suggest other diagnoses.

Romantic–conjugal failure

It is easy to understand how individuals with mercurial moods would charm others when in an expansive people-seeking mode, and rapidly alienate them when dysphoric. In effect, the life of many of these patients is a tempestuous chain of intense but brief romantic liaisons,[80] often with a series of unsuitable partners. Some rationalize their behaviour on the grounds that their spouse or partner is 'too conservative in sex, too unimaginative, too unaware of the intensity' needed to stimulate them. As expected, frequent marital separations, divorces, and remarriage to the same person occur.

Uneven school and work record

Repeated and unpredictable shifts in work and study habits occur in most people with cyclothymia, giving rise to a dilettante biography.[79,80] Although some do better during their 'high' periods—for example, one car salesman would sell cars only 'when up'—for others, the occasional 'even' periods were more conducive to meaningful work. It is sometimes unappreciated by clinicians inexperienced with bipolarity that the hypomanic period can be one of disorganized and unpatterned busyness that could easily lead to a serious drop in net productivity. For instance, one insurance salesman related that he was less successful when 'high', because he tended to enter into unproductive arguments with his clients. When 'down', productivity obviously abates, although two creative individuals in our case series[80]—one inclined poetically, the other towards painting—produced their better work when coming out of mini-depressions.

Alcohol and drug abuse

An alternating pattern of the use of 'uppers' and 'downers' occurs in at least 50 per cent of patients.[79] We have clinically evaluated at least five cyclothymes who 'sold dope' to maintain their habit: two went to prison. These and other observations[85–87] suggest that a proportion of substance-abusing, especially stimulant-abusing, patients might be suffering from subtle or cryptic forms of bipolar disorder. The bipolar nature of mood swings in alcohol- or substance-abusing individuals can be documented by demonstrating mood swings well past the period of detoxification; in some cases, escalating mood instability makes its first appearance following abrupt drug or alcohol withdrawal. The DSM-IV criteria for drug-induced or drug withdrawal-induced mood disorder are, in our opinion, biased against the diagnosis of otherwise treatable bipolar spectrum disorders.[8]

Financial extravagance

One patient in our case series reported going to bars and buying people drinks because he wanted everybody to feel like him. Another patient intermittently showered his lovers with expensive jewellery. In general, however, the extravagance of the cyclothymic group reflects gregariousness and tends to occur on a smaller scale compared to the psychotic manner in which manic patients bring financial ruin to themselves and their families.

The social warmth observed among most people with cyclothymia distinguishes them from adult attention-deficit hyperactivity disorder (**ADHD**). Also, elation and inflated self-confidence, which occur periodically in cyclothymia, are uncharacteristic of ADHD; the moodiness in the latter is largely depressive in nature. Finally, antidepressants and stimulants typically worsen the moods in cyclothymia; they treat ADHD. In rare cases, however, cyclothymia and ADHD coexist.[80]

Course patterns

In cyclothymia, hypomania and mini-depression alternate with each other from adolescence. For instance, the optimistic, overconfident, people-seeking phase can give way to self-absorption, self-doubt, pessimism, and a sense of futility, emptiness, and suicidal ideation. More commonly, depressive periods dominate the clinical picture, interspersed by 'even', 'irritable', and occasional hypomanic periods. Indeed, most people with cyclothymia who present clinically do so because of depression.[80] These depressions are typically short-lived, yet unrelenting in their cyclic course, creating much interpersonal havoc for the patient. The following vignette illustrates the cardinal clinical features of cyclothymia that has not yet progressed to major depression.

Case Study This 24-year-old songwriter presented with the chief complaint of 'depression so bad that I become totally dysfunctional—I cannot even get out of bed'. Since her mid-teens she had experienced periods lasting from a few days up to a week, during which she would withdraw into herself, losing confidence and interest, feeling drained of energy, and crying when approached by anybody. These periods were particularly prevalent during the autumn and winter months, but they did not coincide with the premenstrual phase. All she needed sometimes was restful sleep to 'feel alive again'; at other times she would have little sleep, and would wake up 'wired', 'ready to go', 'open to experience all the joy waiting for me out there'; she would exude confidence, 'sensuality and sexual aroma'. These occurred less frequently than the 'down' periods and usually lasted for 1 to 3 days, but were not associated with creative spurts. The latter came as she was descending from 'highs' into a more 'mellow depression'. Her success in music had been sporadic, paralleling the sporadic nature of her 'muses' that visited her on the descending limb of 'hypomania merging with tears'. However, the major toll of her mood swings had been in her personal life, the intensity of her moods had driven away most men she

Table 6 Prospective 1- to 2-year course of cyclothymic subjects

Clinical affective episode	Cyclothymic subjects (%) (N = 50)	Non-affective controls (%) (N = 50)	p
Drug-free course			
Major depression	26	4	
Protracted hypomania	16	0	
Mania	6	0	
Total	36	4	0.001
Course on TCAs[a]			
Protracted hypomania	44	0	0.001

[a] Tricyclic antidepressants (TCAs) were prescribed, when clinically warranted, to 25 of 50 cyclothymic patients—11 (44%) developed hypomania. This was very similar to the rate of 35% (not shown) in bipolar controls and both were found to be highly significantly different from the non-affective personalities by chi-square test. Summarized from Akiskal.[80]

had loved, of whom she had lost count. She described periods of such intense sexual arousal, that sometimes she would go to bed with anybody, including 'women of all ages, shapes, and description'. But, she added: 'I am not a lesbian—oral love is just one way of relating to these women— why not?' She had also experimented with drugs, such as stimulants, which had made her moodiness worse. More recently, she had been prescribed at least two SSRIs, which after a period of 'success' for a few months, had made her depressive swings more frequent and lower in amplitude, leading to the present consultation in our clinic.

As documented in this case, sexual excesses with both sexes are often readily admitted by patients. Winter accentuation or clustering of depressive periods, as exemplified here, is not uncommon in cyclothymia. We also would like to point out the special relationship of the moods to artistic productivity which occur in up to 8 per cent of cyclothymic depressions.[88] The 4-day threshold for hypomania in the official diagnostic manuals is too conservative; as shown in this case, most patients with cyclothymia (and bipolar II disorder) report a threshold of 1 to 3 days (though on occasion, one would observe a hypomanic duration of 1 week or longer).[79,89] It is also noteworthy that the episodes are short-lived and do not reach the duration threshold for rapid cycling. Sometimes, the term 'ultra rapid cycling' is used for these patients, but we prefer to reserve this for extremely severe cases who require hospitalization. The short cycle length in cyclothymia is, in part, a selection artefact: the universe of patients with bipolar disorder is composed of an extreme variety of overlapping patterns.[8]

The relationship of a cyclothymic temperament to the bipolar spectrum is more complex than that of dysthymia to major depressive disorder. Although cyclothymia can be observed in some patients with full-blown manic–depressive illness (bipolar I with severe or hospitalized mania), it is more commonly associated with the bipolar II pattern (of recurrent major depression with self-limited hypomanias). In a recent French national study of patients with major depression,[9] 88 per cent of those with a cyclothymic disposition belonged to the bipolar II subtype. (Mania, by contrast, has been reported to more likely represent either an extension of hyperthymic traits, or a reversal from a depressive temperamental baseline.[90])

One-third of patients with cyclothymia studied by us on a prospective basis, progressed to spontaneous affective episodes with more protracted hypomanias and clinical (major) depression (Table 6).

Thus, 6 per cent of the original cyclothymic cohort could be reclassified as bipolar I, and 30 per cent as bipolar II. The tendency to switch to hypomania was further augmented by the administration of antidepressants. A larger and more recent National Institute of Mental Health study[91] of patients with major depression who switched to bipolar II during a prospective observation period of up to 11 years, found that a temperamental mix of 'mood-labile', 'energetic-active', and 'daydreaming' traits (reminiscent of Kretschmer's concept of the cyclothymic temperament[30]) were the most specific predictors of such outcome. Limited data[92] also exist on the importance of these temperamental factors in predicting which of the offspring of bipolar probands will progress to clinical episodes.

The foregoing clinical and course characteristics suggest that a cyclothymic temperament leading to major depressive recurrences represents a distinct longitudinal pattern of 'cyclothymic depression', and which appears to capture the core features of bipolar II disorder in contemporary clinical practice.[8,91] Because hypomanic episodes cannot be easily ascertained by history, assessing cyclothymia in clinically depressed patients represents a more sensitive and specific approach to the diagnosis of bipolar II.

Epidemiology

An excess of interpersonal difficulties and psychiatric consultations distinguish people with cyclothymia in the community from controls; excessive use patterns of stimulants, caffeine, nicotine, and alcohol, have also been well documented.[93,94] Explosive traits, probably representing the irritable component of cyclothymia, have been reported to be prevalent in the community in a British study.[95] More recently, we found that 6.3 per cent of a national cohort of 1010 Italian students between the ages of 14 and 26 years of age[22] scored above two standard deviations for cyclothymia; this was more prevalent in females, with a ratio of 3:2. Overall, the foregoing data testify to the fact that a cyclothymic and/or labile disposition can be accurately measured, is prevalent, and represents a population at risk for affective disorders. Table 7 summarizes the rates in different populations.[22,79,93–96]

Aetiological aspects

The flamboyant behaviour and the restless pursuit of romantic opportunities in cyclothymia suggest the hypothesis that its constituent traits may have evolved as a mechanism in sexual selection. Even their creative bent—in poetry, music, painting, or fashion design—may have evolved to subserve such a mechanism. Cyclothymic traits appear to lie

Table 7 Prevalence of cyclothymic and related mood-labile temperaments

Reference	Population (country)	Rate (%)
Akisal et al. (1977)[79]	Mental health centre (USA)	10
Weissman and Myers (1978)[96]	Community (USA)	4
Depue et al. (1981)[93]	College students (USA)	6
Casey and Tyrer (1986)[95]	Community (UK)	6
Wicki and Angst (1991)[94]	Community (Zurich)	4
Placidi et al. (1988)[22]	14–26-year-old students (Italy)	6

on a polygenic continuum between excessive temperament and manic depression. Indeed, clinically identified cyclothymes have patterns of familial affective illness, as one would expect for a *forme fruste* disorder.[79]

Cyclothymia has also been observed in the offspring of manic–depressive probands, with onset in the postpubertal period.[92] Finally, family studies of patients with a bipolar disorder have revealed an excess of cyclothymia.[97] Hypothetically, this temperament might represent one of, if not the most important, inherited trait diathesis for bipolar disorder. For instance, moody-temperamental individuals are over-represented in the 'discordant' monozygotic co-twins of manic–depressives.[98] Alternatively, and in a more theoretical vein, manic–depressive illness might be the genetic reservoir for the desirable cyclothymic traits in the population at large.

Clinical management

The proper pharmacological treatment for cyclothymic excesses is low doses of lithium (600–900 mg/day) or valproate (500–750 mg/day). These are based on open systematic studies.[80,99,100] There is some data from a controlled trial with lithium about the prevention of depression in cyclothymic individuals.[101] Similarly controlled data exist for a related construct—'labile personality'.[102] Generally speaking, patients with cyclothymia object to the 'overcontrol' that may come from mood stabilizers, and this is particularly the case with lithium.

Patients should be taught how to live with the extremes of their temperamental inclinations, and to seek professions where they determine the hours that they work.[103] Marriage to a rich older spouse might sustain them for a while, but eventually interpersonal friction and sexual jealousy terminate such marriages. The artistically inclined among them should be encouraged to live in those parts of a city inhabited by artists and other intellectuals, where temperamental excesses are better tolerated. Ultimately, the decision to use mood stabilizers in such individuals should balance any benefits from decreased mood instability against the social and creative spurts that the cyclothymic disposition can bring to them. Their clinical management represents a challenging task for the psychiatrist who is willing to learn about the lifestyle of these individuals, not prejudging them by the more mundane norms of society. But the psychiatrist should also be there to help them during the multiple crises of their lives. Low-dose sedating neuroleptics, both classical (e.g. thioridazine 50 mg at bedtime) and atypical (e.g. olanzapine 2.5 mg at bedtime) may temporarily help to diffuse such crises. It is only when a clinician has earned therapeutic alliance with a patient that the latter will permit limit-setting on his or her extravagant or outrageous behaviour. Parents might also benefit from some counselling, because the dilettante life of their children is often a source of great sorrow for them. Rarely, parents or spouses are rewarded by great artistic or intellectual achievement, which does not necessarily reduce the pain that the volatile cyclothymes bring to their loved ones.

Kurt Schneider[20] admonished the kin of labile individuals (who might approximate the contemporary concept of borderline personality disorder) 'on their bad days…to keep out of their way as far as possible'. Cyclothymes with some insight into their own temperament would give the same advice to their loved ones. A cautious trial of anticonvulsants will often prove effective in those distressed enough by their behaviour to comply with such treatment.

Prevention

The offspring of patients with bipolar disorder who exhibit a cyclothymic level of temperamental dysregulation represent a logical population for prevention studies.[92] This is a challenge for the twenty-first century. Presumably molecular genetic testing will one day identify those moody individuals who carry the genes for bipolar disorder. At present, it would be useful to conservatively follow-up the cyclothymic offspring of people with bipolar disorders and provide them with psychoeducation about the necessity of avoiding stimulants and sleep deprivation. It may not be entirely possible to prohibit the use of moderate alcohol consumption, but benzodiazepines should not be used. It is also imperative, should they get depressed, to protect them from the indiscriminate prescription of antidepressants.

Mood-labile female prisoners, commonly given the diagnosis of antisocial or borderline personality disorder,[104] may represent affective variants with irritable cyclothymic features. Formal studies are needed in prison populations, to assess more precisely the rates of preventable cryptic bipolarity among female and male offenders.

Complications of the hyperthymic temperament

History

Although well described by classical German psychiatrists (e.g. Schneider[20]), the hyperthymic type appears neither in DSM-IV nor in ICD-10. A lifelong disposition, hyperthymia must be distinguished from short-lived hypomanic episodes. Alternatively, this disposition can be characterized as trait hypomania. It derives from the ancient Graeco-Roman sanguine temperament, believed to represent the optimal mixture of behavioural traits. They are full of zest, fun-loving, and prone to lechery: their habitual disposition is one of buoyant action-orientation, extraverted people-seeking, overconfidence, and swift thinking. Typically short sleepers, they possess boundless energy to invest in sundry causes and projects, which often earn them leadership positions in the various professions and politics, yet their carefree attitudes and propensity for risk-taking can bring them to the brink of ruin; this is particularly true for their finances and sexual life, which can be marred by scandal.[105] A hyperthymic lifestyle is so reinforcing that some resort to 'augmenting' it with stimulants such as amphetamines or cocaine. In brief, while a hyperthymic temperament *per se* does not constitute affective pathology—indeed, it represents a constellation of adaptive traits—in excess it could lead to undesirable complications. The latter will be our main focus here.

Epidemiology

The foregoing considerations partly explain why such a temperament has received scant research attention in the community. Extrapolating from studies on intermittent hypomania in the community,[94,106] if strictly limited to hypomania with early onset and persistent course, the prevalence of hyperthymic temperament can be estimated to be slightly under 1 per cent. On the other hand, the traits that constitute the hyperthymic profile are so desirable that normal individuals tend to endorse them; in a recent Pisa–San Diego collaboration[22] involving 1010 students aged between 14 and 26, of whom 8.2 per cent met the full criteria for hyperthymic temperament, all participants scored between the first and second positive standard deviation. Thus, more work needs to be done on the psychometric standardization of this temperamental construct; on the other hand, all studies are consistent in showing marked male predominance.

Diagnostic aspects

On the positive side, hyperthymic individuals are enterprising, ambitious, and driven, often achieving considerable social and vocational prominence.[105] Abuse of stimulants is not so much an attempt to ward off depression and fatigue as an effort to enhance their already high-level drive and, sometimes, to further curtail their already reduced need for sleep. Hyperthymic individuals typically marry three or more times. Others, without entering into legally sanctioned matrimony, form three or more families in different cities; these men are capable of maintaining such relationships for long periods, testifying to their financial and personal resourcefulness, as well as their generosity towards their lovers and the offspring from such unions. Unlike the antisocial psychopath who is predatory on others and neglects or abuses his women and children, these men care for their loved ones. But obviously the 'arrangement' involving women of different generations is complex, and a fertile soil for jealousy, drama, scandal, and tragedy. Nonetheless, it is not uncommon to see more than three or four women crying profusely and expressing their common grief at the funerals of these men!

Although individuals with hyperthymia optimally enjoy the advantage of their reduced need for sleep (giving more time and energy to invest in work and pleasure), some present clinically because of insomnia. Thus, in a predominantly male sample of executives presenting to a sleep centre,[105] habitual sleep need was 4 to 5 h; however, they had been intermittently bothered by 'nervous energy' and difficulty falling asleep. Now, in late middle age, alcohol was no longer an effective hypnotic. Although they vigorously denied depressive and other mental symptoms—indeed, they had extremely low scores on self-rated depression—spouses or lovers provided collateral information about brief irritable–depressive dips, especially in the morning and, in some cases, more protracted 'fatigue states' of days to weeks during which the subject would vegetate. Despite these depressive dips, these patients were distinguished from the constantly shifting moods of cyclothymic patients by the fact that the depressions arose from a baseline of trait hypomania of a more or less stable course. Our most current diagnostic guidelines for a hyperthymic temperament consist of the following traits on a habitual basis since at least early adulthood: cheerful, overoptimistic, or exuberant; extraverted and people-seeking, often to the point of being overinvolved or meddlesome; overtalkative, eloquent, and jocular; uninhibited, stimulus-seeking, and sexually-driven; vigorous, full of plans, improvident; overconfident, self-assured, and boastful attitudes that may reach grandiose proportions.

A systematic retrospective review of the case records of people with manic depression, whose course was dominated by manic episodes, was recently undertaken in Munich,[107] yielding attributes overlapping with our proposed list: active, vivid, extraverted, verbally aggressive, self-assured, strong willed, engaged in self-employed professions, risk-taking, sensation-seeking, breaking social norms, spendthrift, and generous. The fact that at least 10 per cent of patients with major depression in an Italian study[108] could be characterized as premorbidly hyperthymic, suggests that this temperament has relevance

to both major affective poles. This is an important diagnostic consideration, because rather than being considered narcissistic depressions, these should be recognized as a soft bipolar variant.[8]

Aetiological aspects

It is of interest that Gardner's ethological analysis[109] of what constitutes 'leadership' led to a description that overlaps with a hyperthymic profile: cheerfulness, joking, irrepressible infectious quality, unusual warmth, expansive, strong sense of confidence in one's abilities, scheming, robust, tireless, pushy, and meddlesome. Hypothetically, this temperament evolved in primates whose social life required leadership to better face challenges to the group from within and without.

In the only sleep electroencephalography study conducted to date,[105] REM latency was found to be shortened; similar findings have been reported on the sleep of manic patients,[110] thereby supporting the notion of a trait–state continuum at the neurophysiological level. (Although counterintuitive, this neurophysiological marker appears to be shared between the depressive and hyperthymic poles.) Finally, family history for frank bipolar disorder characterizes many such individuals. The foregoing data, albeit limited, suggest that hyperthymic traits share several key biological underpinnings of affective disorder.

Course and treatment

Little is known about the natural course of the hyperthymic temperament, except what can be reconstructed retrospectively from biographical and clinical studies. Given their overoptimistic and self-assured style of thinking, these individuals feel perfectly fit in all areas of functioning and thus have no need to consult a psychiatrist. They do so only when forced by loved ones. There are no systematic treatment studies on hyperthymia. Anecdotally,[111] low doses of anticonvulsants such as valproate (e.g 500–750 mg/day) can be useful in reducing drivenness, deemed to be damaging to the cardiovascular system, or the enormous sexual appetite that places them at risk for social scandals and, in some cases, exposure to HIV infection.[112] Drug-abusing subjects with hyperthymia can be detoxified with valproate, carbamazepine, or gabapentin. Clinically depressed subjects with a hyperthymic temperament often respond poorly to antidepressants. In our opinion, the efficacy of lithium augmentation in resistant depression is partly based on the high prevalence of hyperthymia in resistant populations;[113] it would be wise to keep the dose of lithium in augmentation in such individuals to a lower to middle range (i.e. 600–900 mg/day).

People with hyperthymia are action-oriented, and are not inclined to any type of self-examination. Furthermore, their hypertrophied sense of denial[114] makes them poor candidates for psychotherapy. The physician must, none the less, attempt psychoeducation about the harm that can come to them and their loved ones because of their temperamental excesses. Alcohol consumption, which is common in these individuals, should not be abruptly interrupted because of the risk of the switch to a suicidal depression. If detoxification is necessary for health reasons, admission to a suitable inpatient facility should be arranged. The occasion might be profitably used for whatever counselling is deemed appropriate for life and health situations confronting them at the time.

References

1. Akiskal, H.S., Judd, L.L., Gillin, J.C., and Lemmi, H. (1997). Subthreshold depressions: clinical and polysomnographic validation of dysthymic, residual and masked forms. *Journal of Affective Disorders*, **45**, 53–63.

2. Meier, W., Lichterman, D., Minges, J., Heun, R., and Mallmayer, J. (1992). The risk of minor depression in families of probands with major depression: sex differences and familiality. *European Archives of Psychiatry and Clinical Neuroscience*, **242**, 89–92.

3. Kendler, K.S., Neale, M.C., and Kessler, R.C. (1992). A population-based twin study of major depression in women: the impact of varying definitions of illness. *Archives of General Psychiatry*, **49**, 257–66.

4. Remick, R.A., Sadovnick, A.D., Lam, R.W., Zis, A.P., and Yee, I.M. (1996). Major depression, minor depression, and double depression: are they distinct clinical entities? *American Journal of Medical Genetics*, **67**, 347–53.

5. Akiskal, H.S., Bitar, A.H., Puzantian, V.R., Rosenthal, T.L., and Walker, P.W. (1978). The nosological status of neurotic depression: a prospective three-to-four year examination in light of the primary–secondary and unipolar–bipolar dichotomies. *Archives of General Psychiatry*, **35**, 756–66.

6. Bronisch, T., Wittchen, H.-U., Krieg, C., Rupp, H.-U., and von Zerssen, D. (1985). Depressive neurosis: a long-term prospective and retrospective follow-up study of former inpatients. *Acta Psychiatrica Scandinavica*, **71**, 237–48.

7. Akiskal, H.S. and Cassano, G.B. (ed.) (1997). *Dysthymia and the spectrum of chronic depressions*. Guilford Press, New York.

8. Akiskal, H.S. (1996). The prevalent clinical spectrum of bipolar disorders: beyond DSM-IV. *Journal of Clinical Psychopharmacology*, **16** (Supplement), 4s–14s.

9. Hantouche, E.G., Akiskal, H.S., Lancrenon, S., *et al.* (1998). Systematic clinical methodology for validating bipolar-II disorder: data in mid-stream from a French national multisite study (EPIDEP). *Journal of Affective Disorders*, **50**, 163–73.

10. Akiskal, H.S. and Akiskal, K. (1996). The temperamental foundations of mood disorders. In *Interpersonal factors in the origin and course of affective disorders* (ed. C.H. Mundt), pp. 3–30. Gaskell, London.

11. Akiskal, H.S. and Weise, R.E. (1992). The clinical spectrum of so-called 'minor' depressions. *American Journal of Psychotherapy*, **46**, 9–22.

12. Lewis, A. (1936). Melancholia: a prognostic study. *Journal of Mental Science*, **82**, 488–558.

13. Herpertz, S., Steinmeyer, E.M., and Sa, H. (1998). On the conceptualisation of subaffective personality disorders. *European Psychiatry*, **13**, 9–17.

14. Eysenck, H.F. (1987). The definition of personality disorders and the criteria appropriate for their description. *Journal of Personality Disorder*, **1**, 211–19.

15. Snaith, R.P. (1991). Measurement in psychiatry. *British Journal of Psychiatry*, **159**, 78–82.

16. Kendler, K.S., Neale, M.C., Kessler, R.C., Heath, A.C., and Eaves, L.J. (1993). A longitudinal twin study of personality and major depression in women. *Archives of General Psychiatry*, **50**, 853–62.

17. Akiskal, H.S. (1981). Subaffective disorders: dysthymic, cyclothymic and bipolar II disorders in the 'borderline' realm. *Psychiatric Clinics of North America*, **4**, 25–46.

18. Brieger, P. and Marneros, A. (1997). Dysthymia and cyclothymia: historical origins and contemporary development. *Journal of Affective Disorders*, **45**, 117–26.

19. Kraepelin, E. (1921). *Manic–depressive insanity and paranoia*. Livingstone, Edinburgh.

20. Schneider, K. (1958). *Psychopathic personalities*. Charles C. Thomas, Springfield, IL.

21. Akiskal, H.S. (1983). Dysthymic disorder: psychopathology of proposed chronic depressive subtypes. *American Journal of Psychiatry*, **140**, 11–20.

22. Placidi, G.F., Signoretta, S., Liguori, A., Gervasi, R., Maremmani, I., and

23. Akiskal, H.S. (1998). The Semi-Structured Affective Temperament Interview (TEMPS-I): reliability and psychometric properties in 1010 14–26 year students. *Journal of Affective Disorders*, **47**, 1–10.

23. Akiskal, H.S., Placidi, G.F., Signoretta, S., *et al.* (1998). TEMPS-I. Delineating the most discriminant traits of cyclothymic, depressive, irritable and hyperthymic temperaments in a nonpatient population. *Journal of Affective Disorders*, **51**, 7–19.

24. Kasahara, Y. (1991). The practical diagnosis of depression in Japan. In *The diagnosis of depression* (ed. J.P. Feighner and W.F. Boyer), pp. 163–75. Wiley, Chichester.

25. Montassut, M. (1938). *La dépression constitutionnelle: l'ancienne neurasthénie dans ses rapports avec la médecine générale; clinique biologie, thérapeutique*. Masson, Paris.

26. Akiskal, H.S. (1996). Dysthymia as a temperamental variant of affective disorder. *European Psychiatry*, **11** (Supplement), 117s–22s.

27. Akiskal, H.S., Rosenthal, T.L., Haykal, R.F., Lemmi, H., Rosenthal, R.H., and Scott-Strauss, A. (1980). Characterological depressions: clinical and sleep EEG findings separating 'subaffective dysthymias' from 'character-spectrum' disorders. *Archives of General Psychiatry*, **37**, 777–83.

28. Devinand, D.P., Nobler, M.S., Singer, T., *et al.* (1994). Is dysthymia a different disorder in the elderly? *American Journal of Psychiatry*, **151**, 1592–9.

29. Tellenbach, H. (1980). *Melancholia*. Duquesne University Press, Pittsburgh, PA.

30. Kretschmer, E. (1936). *Physique and character*. Kegan Paul, Trench, Trubner, London.

31. Kernberg, O.F. (1970). A psychoanalytic classification of character pathology. *Journal of the American Psychoanalytic Association*, **18**, 800–22.

32. Keller, M.B., Klein, D.N., Hirschfeld, R.M.A., *et al.* (1995). Results of the DSM-IV mood disorders field trial. *American Journal of Psychiatry*, **152**, 843–9.

33. Seretti, A., Jori, M.C., Cassadei, J., Ravizza, L., Smeraldi, E., and Akiskal, H.S. Delineating psychopathologic clusters within dysthymia: a study of 512 patients without major depression. *Journal of Affective Disorders*, in press.

34. Madhulika, A., Gupta, M.D., and Moldofsky, H. (1986). Dysthymic disorder and rheumatic pain modulation disorder (fibrositis syndrome): a comparison of symptoms and sleep physiology. *Canadian Journal of Psychiatry*, **31**, 608–16.

35. Tyrer, P., Seivewright, N., Ferguson, B., and Tyrer, J. (1992). The general neurotic syndrome: a coaxial diagnosis of anxiety, depression and personality disorder. *Acta Psychiatrica Scandinavica*, **85**, 201–6.

36. Keller, M.B., Lavori, P.W., Endicott, J., Coryell, W., and Lerman, G.L. (1983). Double depression: two-year follow-up. *American Journal of Psychiatry*, **140**, 689–94.

37. Kovacs, M., Akiskal, H.S., Gatsonis, C., and Parrone, P.L. (1994). Childhood-onset dysthymic disorder: clinical features and prospective naturalistic outcome. *Archives of General Psychiatry*, **51**, 365–74.

38. Rosenthal, T.L., Akiskal, H.S., Scott-Strauss, A., Rosenthal, R.H., and David, M. (1981). Familial and developmental factors in characterological depressions. *Journal of Affective Disorders*, **3**, 183–92.

39. Rihmer, Z. (1993). Dysthymia: a clinician's perspective. In *Dysthymic disorder* (ed. S. Burton and H.S. Akiskal), pp. 112–25. Royal College of Psychiatrists, London.

40. Klein, D.N., Taylor, E., Harding, K., *et al.* (1988). Double depression and episodic major depression: demographic, clinical, familial, personality, and socioenvironmental characteristics and short-term outcome. *American Journal of Psychiatry*, **145**, 1226–31.

41. Judd, L.L., Akiskal, H.S., Maser, J.D., *et al.* (1998). A prospective 12-year study of sub-syndromal and syndromal depressive symptomatology in patients with unipolar major depressive disorder. *Archives of General Psychiatry*, **55**, 694–700.

42. Akiskal, H.S. (1994). Dysthymia: clinical and external validity. *Acta Psychiatrica Scandinavica*, **89** (Supplement), 19–23.

43. Weissman, M.M., Leaf, P.J., Bruce, M.L., and Florio, L. (1988). The epidemiology of dysthymia in five communities: rates, risks, comorbidity, and treatment. *American Journal of Psychiatry*, **145**, 815–19.

44. Waintraub, L. and Guelfi, J.D. (1998). Nosological validity of dysthymia. Part I, historical, epidemiological and clinical data. *European Psychiatry*, **13**, 173–80.

45. Perugi, G., Akiskal, H.S., Musetti, L., Simonini, E., and Cassano, G.B. (1994). Social adjustment in panic-agoraphobic patients reconsidered. *British Journal of Psychiatry*, **164**, 88–93.

46. Haykal, R. and Akiskal, H.S. (1999). The long-term outcome of dysthymia in private practice. Clinical features, temperament, and the art of management. *Journal of Clinical Psychiatry*, **60**, 508–18.

47. Wells, K.B., Stewart, A., Hays, R., *et al.* (1989). The functioning and wellbeing of depressed patients: results from the medical outcomes study. *Journal of the American Association*, **262**, 914–19.

48. The WPA Dysthymia Working Group (1995). Dysthymia in clinical practice. *British Journal of Psychiatry*, **166**, 174–83.

49. Licinio, J., Prilpko, I., and Bolis, C.L. (ed.) (1997). Dysthymia in neurological disorders. In *Proceedings of the WHO Meeting*. World Health Organization, Geneva.

50. Arieti, S. and Bemporad, J. (1978). *Severe and mild depression*. Basic Books, New York.

51. Akiskal, H.S., Lemmi, H., Dickson, H., King, D., Yerevanian, B.I., and VanValkenburg, C. (1984). Chronic depressions: Part 2. Sleep EEG differentiation of primary dysthymic disorders from anxious depressions. *Journal of Affective Disorders*, **6**, 287–95.

52. Howland, R.H. and Thase, M.E. (1991). Biological studies of dysthymia. *Biological Psychiatry*, **30**, 283–304.

53. Klein, D.N., Riso, L.P., Donaldson, S.K., *et al.* (1995). Family study of early-onset dysthymia. Mood and personality disorders in relatives of outpatients with dysthymia and episodic major depression and normal controls. *Archives of General Psychiatry*, **52**, 487–96.

54. Hamburg, S.R. (1998). Inherited hypohedonia leads to learned helplessness: a conjecture updated. *Reviews of General Psychology*, **2**, 384–403.

55. Giles, D.E., Kupfer, D.J., and Roffwarg, H.P. (1988). Polysomnographic parameters in first-degree relatives of unipolar probands. *Psychiatry Research*, **27**, 127–36.

56. Kreig, J.C., Lauer, C.J., and Hermle, L. (1993). Psychometric, polysomnographic, and neuroendocrine measures in subjects at high risk for psychiatric disorders: preliminary results. *Neuropsychobiology*, **23**, 57–67.

57. Burton, S.W. and Akiskal, H.S. (ed.) (1993). *Dysthymic disorder*. Gaskell and Royal College of Psychiatrists, London.

58. McCullough, J.P., McCune, K.J., Kaye, A.L., *et al.* (1994). One-year prospective replication study of an untreated sample of community dysthymia subjects. *Journal of Nervous and Mental Disease*, **182**, 396–401.

59. Vallejo, J., Gasto, C., Catalan, R., and Salamero, M. (1987). Double-blind study of imipramine versus phenelzine in melancholias. *British Journal of Psychiatry*, **151**, 639–42.

60. Kocsis, J.H., Zisook, S., Davidson, J., *et al.* (1997). Double-blind comparison of sertraline, imipramine, and placebo in the treatment of dysthymia: psychosocial outcomes. *American Journal of Psychiatry*, **154**, 390–5.

61. Stewart, J., Quitkin, F.M., McGrath, P.J., *et al.* (1989). Social functioning in chronic depression: effect of 6 weeks of antidepressants treatment. *Psychiatry Research*, **25**, 213–22.

62. Bakish, D., Lapierre, Y.D., Weinstein, R., *et al.* (1993). Ritanserin, imipramine, and placebo in the treatment of dysthymic disorder. *Journal of Clinical Psychopharmacology*, **13**, 409–14.

63. Thase, M.E., Fava, M., Halbreich, U., *et al.* (1996). A placebo-controlled, randomized clinical trial comparing sertraline and imipramine for the treatment of dysthymia. *Archives of General Psychiatry*, **53**, 777–84.

64. Vanelle, J.M., Attar-Levy, D., Poirier, M.F., Bouhassira, M., Blin, P., and

Olié, J.P. (1997). Controlled efficacy study of fluoxetine in dysthymia. *British Journal of Psychiatry*, **170**, 345–50.

65. Lecrubier, Y., Boyer, P., Turjanski, S., and Rein, W. (1997). Amisulpride versus imipramine and placebo in dysthymia and major depression. *Journal of Affective Disorders*, **43**, 95–103.

66. Versiani, M., Amrein, R., and Stabl, M. (1997). Moclobemide and imipramine in chronic depression (dysthymia): an international double-blind, placebo-controlled trial. *Clinical Psychopharmacology*, **12**, 183–93.

67. Ravindran, A.V., Bialik, R.J., and Lapierre, Y.D. (1994). Therapeutic efficacy of specific serotonin re-uptake inhibitors (SSRIs) in dysthymia. *Canadian Journal of Psychiatry*, **39**, 21–6.

68. Kocsis, J.H., Zisook, S., Davidson, J., *et al.* (1997). Double-blind comparison of sertraline, imipramine and placebo in the treatment of dysthymia: psychosocial outcomes. *American Journal of Psychiatry*, **154**, 390–5.

69. Knutson, B., Wolkowitz, W., Cole, S.W., *et al.* (1998). VI. Selective alteration of personality and social behavior by serotonergic intervention. *American Journal of Psychiatry*, **155**, 373–9.

70. Andrews, W., Parker, G., and Barrett, E. (1998). The SSRI antidepressants: exploring their 'other' possible properties. *Journal of Affective Disorders*, **49**, 141–4.

71. Markowitz, J.C. (1994). Psychotherapy of dysthymia. *American Journal of Psychiatry*, **151**, 1114–21.

72. McGrath, E., Keita, G.P., Strickland, B.R., and Russo, N.P. (ed.) (1993). *Women and depression: risk factors and treatment issues*. American Psychological Association, Washington, DC.

73. Akiskal, H.S. (1992). Psychopharmacological and psychotherapeutic strategies in intermittent and chronic affective conditions. In *Long-term treatment of depression* (ed. S.A. Montgomery and F. Rouillon), pp. 245–63. Wiley, Chichester.

74. Ravindran, A.V., Griffiths, J., Waddell, C., and Anisman, H. (1995). Stressful life events and coping styles in relation to dysthymia and major depressive disorder: variations associated with alleviation of symptoms following pharmacotherapy. *Progress in Neuro-Psychopharmacology and Biological Psychiatry*, **19**, 634–53.

75. Kraemer, P.D. (1993). *Listening to Prozac*. Viking Press, New York.

76. Broadhead, W.E., Blazer, D.G., George, L.K., and Tse, C.K. (1993). Depression, disability, and days lost from work in a prospective epidemiological survey. *Journal of the American Medical Association*, **264**, 2524–8.

77. Horwath, E., Johnson, J., Klerman, G.I., and Weissman, M.M. (1992). Depressive symptoms as relative and attributable risk factors for first-onset major depression. *Archives of General Psychiatry*, **49**, 817–23.

78. Akiskal, H.S., King, D., Rosenthal, T.L., Robinson, D., and Scott-Strauss, A. (1981). Chronic depressions: Part 1. Clinical and familial characteristics in 137 probands. *Journal of Affective Disorders*, **3**, 297–315.

79. Akiskal, H.S., Djenderedjian, A.H., Rosenthal, R.H., and Khani, M.K. (1977). Cyclothymic disorder: validating criteria for inclusion in the bipolar affective group. *American Journal of Psychiatry*, **134**, 1227–33.

80. Akiskal, H.S., Khani, M.K., and Scott-Strauss, A. (1979). Cyclothymic temperamental disorders. *Psychiatric Clinics of North America*, **2**, 527–54.

81. Gillin, J.C., Mazure, C., Post, R.M., Jimerson, D., and Bunney, W.E., Jr (1977). An EEG sleep study of a bipolar (manic–depressive) patient with a nocturnal switch process. *Biological Psychiatry*, **12**, 711–18.

82. Akiskal, H.S. (1992). Delineating irritable-choleric and hyperthymic temperaments as variants of cyclothymia. *Journal of Personality Disorders*, **6**, 326–42.

83. Stone, M.H. (1980). *The borderline syndrome: constitution, personality and adaptation*. McGraw-Hill, New York.

84. Levitt, A.J., Joffe, R.T., Ennis, J., MacDonald, C., and Kutcher, S.P. (1993). The prevalence of cyclothymia in borderline personality disorder. *Journal of Clinical Psychiatry*, **51**, 335–9.

85. Gawin, F.H. and Ellinwood, E.H., Jr (1988). Cocaine and other

stimulants. Actions, abuse, and treatment. *New England Journal of Medicine*, **318**, 1173.

86. Mirin, S.M., Weiss, R.D., Griffin, M.L., and Michael, J.L. (1991). Psychopathology in drug abusers and their families. *Comprehensive Psychiatry*, **32**, 36–51.

87. Brady, K.T. and Sonne, S.C. (1995). The relationship between substance abuse and disorder. *Journal of Clinical Psychiatry*, **56** (Supplement), 19–24.

88. Akiskal, H.S. and Akiskal, K. (1988). Re-assessing the prevalence of bipolar disorders: clinical significance and artistic creativity. *Psychiatrie et Psychobiologie*, **3**, 29s–36s.

89. Angst, J. (1998). The emerging epidemiology of hypomania and bipolar II disorder. *Journal of Affective Disorders*, **50**, 143–51.

90. Akiskal, H.S., Hantouche, E., Bourgeois, M., *et al.* (1998). Gender, temperament and the clinical picture in dysphoric mixed mania: findings from a French national study (EPIMAN). *Journal of Affective Disorders*, **50**, 175–86.

91. Akiskal, H.S., Maser, J.D., Zeller, P., *et al.* (1995). Switching from 'unipolar' to bipolar II: an 11-year prospective study of clinical and temperamental predictors in 559 patients. *Archives of General Psychiatry*, **52**, 114–23.

92. Akiskal, H.S., Downs, J., Jordan, P., Watson, S., Daugherty, D., and Pruitt, D.B. (1985). Affective disorders in the referred children and younger siblings of manic–depressives: mode of onset and prospective course. *Archives of General Psychiatry*, **42**, 996–1003.

93. Depue, R.A., Slater, J.F., Wolfstetter-Kausch, H., *et al.* (1981). A behavioral paradigm for identifying persons at risk for bipolar depressive disorder: a conceptual framework and five validation studies. *Journal of Abnormal Psychology*, **90**, 381–437.

94. Wicki, W. and Angst, J. (1991). The Zurich study. X. Hypomania in a 28–30-year-old cohort. *European Archives of Psychiatry and Clinical Neuroscience*, **240**, 339–48.

95. Casey, P.R. and Tyrer, P.J. (1986). Personality, functioning and symptomatology. *Journal of Psychiatry Research*, **20**, 363–74.

96. Weissman, M.M. and Myers, J.K. (1978). Affective disorders in a US urban community, the use of research diagnostic criteria in an epidemiological survey. *Archives of General Psychiatry*, **35**, 1304–11.

97. Gershon, F.S., Hamovit, J., Guroff, J.J., *et al.* (1982). A family study of schizoaffective, bipolar I, bipolar II, unipolar, and normal control probands. *Archives of General Psychiatry*, **39**, 1157–67.

98. Bertelsen, A., Harvald, B., and Hauge, M. (1977). A Danish twin study of manic–depressive disorders. *British Journal of Psychiatry*, **130**, 330–51.

99. Jacobsen, F.M. (1993). Low-dose valproate: a new treatment for cyclothymia, mild rapid cycling disorders, and premenstrual syndrome. *Journal of Clinical Psychiatry*, **54**, 229–34.

100. Deltito, J. (1993). The effect of valproate on bipolar spectrum temperamental disorder. *Journal of Clinical Psychiatry*, **54**, 300–4.

101. Peselow, E.D., Dunner, D.L., Fieve, R.R., and Lautin, A. (1982). Lithium prophylaxis of depression in unipolar, bipolar II, and cyclothymic patients. *American Journal of Psychiatry*, **139**, 747–52.

102. Rifkin, A., Quitkin, F., Carrillo, C., *et al.* (1972). Lithium carbonate in emotionally unstable character disorder. *Archives of General Psychiatry*, **27**, 519–23.

103. Akiskal, H.S. (1994). Dysthymic and cyclothymic depressions: therapeutic considerations. *Journal of Clinical Psychiatry*, **55**, 46–52.

104. Coid, J.W. (1993). An affective syndrome in psychopaths with borderline personality disorder? *British Journal of Psychiatry*, **162**, 641–50.

105. Akiskal, H. (1984). Characterologic manifestations of affective disorders: toward a new conceptualization. *Integrative Psychiatry*, **2**, 83–8.

106. Eckblad, M. and Chapman, L.J. (1986). Development and validation of a scale for hypomanic personality. *Journal of Abnormal Psychology*, **95**, 214–22.

107. Pössi, J. and von Zerssen, D. (1993). A case history analysis of the 'manic type' and the 'melancholic type' of premorbid personality in affectively ill patients. *European Archives of Psychiatry and Neurological Science*, **239**, 347–55.

108. Cassano, G.B., Akiskal, H.S., Savino, M., Musetti, L., Perugi, G., and Soriani, A. (1992). Proposed subtypes of bipolar II and related disorders: with hypomanic episodes (or cyclothymia) and with hyperthymic temperament. *Journal of Affective Disorders*, **26**, 127–40.

109. Gardner, R. Jr (1982). Mechanisms in manic–depressive disorder: an evolutionary model. *Archives of General Psychiatry*, **39**, 1436–41.

110. Hudson, J.I., Lipinski, J.F., Franjenburg, F.R., Grochocinski, V.J., and Kupfer, D.J. (1988). Electroencephalographic sleep in mania. *Archives of General Psychiatry*, **45**, 267–73.

111. Akiskal, H.S. (1997). Chronic disturbances of temperament. *Bibliotheca Psychiatrica (Basel)*, **167**, 29–32.

112. Perretta, P., Akiskal, H.S., Nisita, C., *et al.* (1998). The high prevalence of bipolar II and associated cyclothymic and hyperthymic temperaments in HIV patients. *Journal of Affective Disorders*, **50**, 215–24.

113. Akiskal, H.S. and Mallya, G. (1987). Criteria for the 'soft' bipolar spectrum: treatment implications. *Psychopharmacology Bulletin*, **23**, 68–73.

114. Akhtar, S. (1988). Hypomanic personality disorder. *Integrative Psychiatry*, **6**, 37–52.

4.6 Stress-related and adjustment disorders

4.6.1 Acute stress reactions

Anke Ehlers and Allison G. Harvey

Introduction

Exceptionally stressful life events can cause severe psychological symptoms, including anxiety, feelings of derealization and depersonalization, and hyperarousal. In one of the first studies to comprehensively document acute reactions to extreme stress, Lindemann[1] observed that the symptoms reported by survivors of the Coconut Grove Fire included avoidance, re-experiencing scenes from the fire, reports of derealization, and the experience of anxiety when exposed to reminders of the event. Similarly, acute responses reported by soldiers who fought in the First and Second World Wars included re-experiencing symptoms and dissociative responses such as numbing, amnesia, and depersonalization.[2]

The *International Classification of Diseases* has recognized acute stress reactions since 1948 (ICD-6).[3] In the most recent edition (ICD-10),[4] early reactions to exceptionally stressful life events are diagnosed as acute stress reaction, one of the diagnoses in the section headed 'Reactions to severe stress, and adjustment disorders'.

In contrast, the *Diagnostic and Statistical Manual of Mental Disorders* did not formally recognize that exceptionally stressful life events are a sufficient cause of psychological symptoms until 1980 when its third edition (DSM-III)[5] introduced the diagnosis of post-traumatic stress disorder (**PTSD**). DSM-III did not stipulate a duration for the symptoms, but the revised third version (DSM-III-R)[6] required that the symptoms of PTSD must be present for more than 1 month after the traumatic event. This stipulation precluded the inclusion of acutely traumatized individuals who instead were diagnosed with adjustment disorder.[7] In 1994 the fourth edition of DSM (DSM-IV)[8] formally recognized acute trauma reactions by introducing the new diagnosis of acute stress disorder into the anxiety disorders section.

The diagnoses of acute stress reactions in ICD-10 and of acute stress disorder in DSM-IV have similarities in that they are caused by extreme stress and have some overlap in symptom patterns. They can be considered as two separate points on a continuum from transient to more enduring symptoms. However, there are also differences in the underlying concepts, as we will discuss in this chapter.

Clinical features

Acute stress reactions, as defined in ICD-10, are transient reactions to exceptional physical and/or mental stress. There is an initial stage of a 'daze', including narrowing of attention, inability to comprehend stimuli, and disorientation. This is followed by a rapidly changing picture of symptoms that may include withdrawal from the surrounding situation, flight reactions, panic anxiety and autonomic hyperarousal, depression, anger, or despair. Symptoms usually begin to diminish after 24 to 48 h and should be minimal after about 3 days.

In contrast, acute stress disorder, as defined in DSM-IV, is only diagnosed if the psychological symptoms persist for more than 2 days. Dissociative symptoms dominate the symptom pattern. Dissociation refers to a disruption of the usually integrated feelings of consciousness, memory, identity, or perception of the environment. Symptoms include a subjective sense of numbing or detachment, reduced awareness of surroundings, derealization, depersonalization, or dissociative amnesia. In addition, patients with acute stress disorder experience symptoms that are typical of PTSD, namely re-experiencing aspects of the event, avoidance of reminders of the event, and hyperarousal symptoms. Acute stress disorder is seen in DSM-IV as a precursor of PTSD. If the re-experiencing, avoidance, and hyperarousal symptoms persist for more than 4 weeks, PTSD is diagnosed.

Classification

ICD-10 classifies acute stress reactions (F43.0) among the reactions to severe stress and adjustment disorders (F43) that are primarily caused by stressful events. DSM-IV classifies acute stress disorder (308.3) among the anxiety disorders, like PTSD (see also Chapter 4.6.2).

Diagnosis and differential diagnosis

The main diagnostic criteria for acute stress reactions (ICD-10) and acute stress disorder (DSM-IV) are compared in Table 1.

Stressor criterion

Both ICD-10 and DSM-IV require that acute stress responses must occur in the immediate aftermath of an exceptionally stressful event. ICD-10 uses a broad concept of what qualifies as an 'exceptional mental or physical stressor'. This includes stressors that would be regarded as traumatic (e.g. rape, criminal assault, natural catastrophe) as well as

Table 1 Comparison of criteria for acute stress reaction (ICD-10) and acute stress disorder (DSM-IV)

	Acute stress reaction (ICD-10 research diagnostic criteria)	Acute stress disorder (DSM-IV)
Stressor	Exposure to exceptional mental or physical stress	(1) Exposure to event involving actual or threatened death or serious injury to self or others (2) Experience of fear, helplessness, or horror
Symptoms	*Criterion C: Symptoms of generalized anxiety disorder (at least 4 symptoms)* Palpitations, sweating, trembling, dry mouth, difficulty breathing, choking, chest pain, nausea, dizziness, derealization or depersonalization, fear of losing control, fear of dying, hot flushes, numbness or tingling, muscle tension, restlessness, keyed up, difficulty swallowing, exaggerated startle response, difficulty concentrating, irritability, difficulty getting to sleep *Criterion C: Additional symptoms to determine severity* Social withdrawal, narrowed attention, disorientation, aggression, hopelessness, overactivity, excessive grief	*Criterion B: Dissociation (at least 3 symptoms)* Numbing, reduced awareness, derealization, depersonalization, dissociative amnesia *Criterion C: Re-experiencing (at least one symptom)* Recurrent images, thoughts, dreams, illusions, flashbacks, reliving, distress on exposure *Criterion D: Marked avoidance* Avoidance of thoughts, feelings, conversations, activities, places, people associated with the trauma *Criterion E: Marked anxiety or increased arousal* Difficulty sleeping, irritability, poor concentration, hypervigilance, exaggerated startle response, motor restlessness *Criterion F: Clinically significant distress or impairment in functioning*
Time from trauma	Onset within 1 h	Onset within 4 weeks; lasts for at least 2 days
Time course	Transient; symptoms begin to diminish within 48 h	May result in post-traumatic stress disorder
Relationship to post-traumatic stress disorder	Alternative diagnosis	Precursor
Diagnostic group	Reactions to severe stress	Anxiety disorder
Exclusion criteria	No other concurrent (within last 3 months) mental or behavioural disorder, except for generalized anxiety disorder or personality disorder	(1) Not due to effects of a substance or general medical condition (2) Not better accounted for by brief psychotic disorder (3) Not merely exacerbation of pre-existing Axis I or Axis II disorder

unusually sudden changes in the social position and/or network of the individual (e.g. domestic fire or multiple bereavement). In contrast, DSM-IV uses a narrow definition of stressors that lead to acute stress disorder, which is identical to the stressor criterion of PTSD. It requires (1) that the traumatic event must have involved actual or threatened death or serious injury, or a threat to the physical integrity of self or others, and (2) that the person's response to the traumatic event must have involved intense fear, helplessness, or horror (or disorganized or agitated behaviour in children) (see Chapter 4.6.2 for the rationale underlying this definition).

Symptom patterns

As shown in Table 1, the diagnostic criteria for acute stress reactions (ICD-10) and acute stress disorder (DSM-IV) overlap, in that they include symptoms of dissociation, anxiety, and hyperarousal. DSM-IV puts a much greater emphasis on dissociation, requiring a minimum of three of the dissociative symptoms specified in Table 1 (Criterion B). According to ICD-10, any combination of a minimum of four symptoms of generalized anxiety disorder (specified in Criterion C, Table 1) would be sufficient to establish the diagnosis of acute stress reaction. In addition, DSM-IV, but not ICD-10, requires the individual to have at least one re-experiencing symptom, to show marked avoidance of reminders of the trauma, and to experience significant distress or impairment of functioning.

In contrast to DSM-IV, ICD-10 distinguishes between mild, moderate, and severe forms of acute stress reactions on the basis of additional symptoms (Criterion C, additional symptoms, Table 1) such as social withdrawal, hopelessness, or excessive grief. A mild severity is stipulated when none of these symptoms are present, moderate when two are reported, and severe when four are reported or when there is dissociative stupor.

Time course of symptoms

The two diagnoses cover distinct periods on a continuum from transient to more persistent symptoms. Specifically, to meet the criteria for acute stress reaction (ICD-10), symptoms must be manifest within 1 h of the stressor (Criterion B) and begin to diminish after no more than 8 h for a transient stressor and after no more than 48 h for an enduring stressor (Criterion D).

The diagnostic criteria for acute stress disorder (DSM-IV) require that the disturbance must last for a minimum of 2 days and a maximum of 4 weeks post-trauma, after which a diagnosis of PTSD can be considered.

Assessment instruments

There are three clinician-administered and one self-report measure of acute stress disorder (DSM-IV) available. As yet, there are no established standardized assessment instruments for transient acute stress reactions (ICD-10).

Acute stress disorder interview

This structured clinical interview establishes the presence or absence of 19 symptoms of acute stress disorder.[9] The sum of the symptoms scored as being present indicates acute stress disorder severity. This measure has very good internal consistency ($r = 0.90$), and, with clinician-based diagnoses as the criterion, very good sensitivity (91 per cent) and specificity (93 per cent). Test–retest reliability is strong ($r = 0.88$).

Structured clinical interview for DSM-IV dissociative disorders

This instrument has also been offered as a structured interview for acute stress disorder.[10] It provides a comprehensive assessment of five core dissociative symptoms: amnesia, depersonalization, derealization, identity confusion, and identity alteration. However, it does not fully assess the re-experiencing, avoidance, and arousal symptoms that also constitute the acute stress disorder diagnosis.

Structured clinical interview for DSM-IV (SCID[11])

The SCID interview indexes the presence, absence, or subthreshold presence of each acute stress disorder symptom specified in DSM-IV. An advantage of employing this interview is that it provides a comprehensive assessment of the differential diagnoses and comorbid disorders that can be present in trauma populations.

Stanford acute stress reaction questionnaire

This self-report inventory asks patients to rate the frequency of a range of dissociative, intrusive, somatic anxiety, hyperarousal, attention disturbance, and sleep disturbance symptoms.[12] The questionnaire has very good internal consistency (Cronbach's alpha = 0.90 and 0.91 for dissociative and anxiety symptoms, respectively) and concurrent validity with scores on the Impact of Event Scale ($r = 0.52$ to 0.69).[13,14]. It can be employed as a measure of the severity of symptoms, but does not allow the diagnosis of acute stress disorder to be established as it has not yet been validated against clinician diagnoses.

Differential diagnoses

Both ICD-10 and DSM-IV require that the symptoms are not merely an exacerbation of a pre-existing disorder. In addition, a number of alternative diagnoses need to be considered.

Post-traumatic stress disorder

In ICD-10, PTSD is conceptualized as an alternative diagnosis of acute stress reactions. The definitions of acute stress reaction and PTSD differ in terms of the stressor criterion (exceptionally stressful life event vs. exceptionally threatening or catastrophic event), the time course (symptoms start to diminish within 48 h versus no time limit), and symptom pattern (PTSD, but not acute stress reaction, includes involuntary re-experiencing the traumatic event).

In DSM-IV, acute stress disorder can be distinguished from PTSD by the time-frame covered by the diagnoses. Acute stress disorder refers to the period from 2 days to 1 month post-trauma, after which a diagnosis of PTSD can be considered. The primary difference between the symptom criteria for acute stress disorder and PTSD in DSM-IV is the former's emphasis on dissociative reactions.

Adjustment disorder

This diagnosis covers a wide range of emotional or behavioural symptoms indicative of distress, which are judged to be out of proportion to the stressor experienced. This broad coverage can be contrasted with (1) the specific set of symptoms described by the acute stress disorder and acute stress reaction criteria, and (2) the stipulation that the stressor involves both a threat to life and a subjective response of fear for the acute stress disorder and an exceptional stressor in the case of acute stress reaction.

Brain injury

A number of acute stress disorder symptoms overlap with symptoms of brain injury including reduced awareness, depersonalization, derealization, irritability, and concentration difficulties.[15] While results from neuropsychological and neurological investigations may assist in the differential diagnosis, there appear to be a group of individuals with a mild head injury for whom there are no known tools to differentiate whether the disturbance is due to brain injury or acute stress disorder, or whether both are present.

Brief psychotic disorder

When there is one or more psychotic symptoms present after experiencing an extreme stressor, the brief psychotic disorder diagnosis should be considered.

Dissociative disorders

Given the emphasis on dissociative symptoms in acute stress disorder, it needs to be distinguished from dissociative amnesia and depersonalization disorder. The criteria for these diagnoses stipulate that if the amnesia or depersonalization can be accounted for by acute stress disorder then a dissociative disorder cannot be diagnosed (see Chapter 5.2.4).

Epidemiology

Incidence

There is little research into what proportion of people develop acute stress reactions to severe stress. In a study of accident survivors, 14 per cent experienced a response pattern characterized by derealization, and a further 17 per cent exhibited strong anxiety or dysphoria.[16]

The incidence of acute stress disorder is 13 to 14 per cent in motor vehicle accident survivors,[15,17] 19 per cent in assault victims,[18] and 33 per cent in witnesses of a mass shooting.[19] Given the variable procedures and assessment tools employed across studies, it is difficult to determine whether the different rates of acute stress disorder detected are attributable to differences in method or in the type of trauma.

Comorbidity

Data on comorbidity are sparse. Given the similarities between acute stress disorder and PTSD it is likely that the conditions found to be comorbid with PTSD, in particular depression and substance abuse, will be applicable to acute stress disorder (see Chapter 4.6.2).

Aetiology

Both psychological and biological theories have attempted to explain the symptoms of acute stress disorder. They overlap largely with theories of PTSD (see Chapter 4.6.2). Given that acute stress reaction describes a transient disturbance, there are no specific theories of acute stress reactions as defined in ICD-10.

Psychological theories

Psychological explanations of re-experiencing symptoms

Psychological theories have offered two major explanations for the re-experiencing symptoms following traumatic stress, characteristics of the trauma memory, and the effect of trauma on basic beliefs about the self and the world. Foa and colleagues[20,21] suggested that PTSD is characterized by a pathological network in memory that is particularly large and easily triggered. It contains many stimulus propositions erroneously linked to danger, causing fear responses to harmless stimuli associated with the traumatic event in memory. Ehlers and Clark[22] suggest that re-experiencing occurs because the trauma memory is inadequately linked to its context in time, place, and other autobiographical memories. Stimuli resembling those present during the traumatic event can thus trigger vivid memories and strong emotional responses that are experienced as if the event was happening right now. Brewin *et al.*[23] postulated that dual representations of the trauma are formed in memory. The first, termed verbally accessible memory, contains the conscious recollection of the trauma. The second memory representation, termed situationally accessible memory, which cannot be deliberately accessed, comprises sensory, physiological, and motor aspects of the trauma in the form of codes that enable the re-experiencing of the original experience.

Horowitz[24] explained re-experiencing symptoms as the result of a slow process that helps the traumatized person to adjust their inner models (schemas) of the self and the world to the traumatic experience. Until this process is completed, the information related to the traumatic event is thought to be held in active memory and thus intrudes into consciousness. Similarly, Janoff-Bulman[25] proposed that traumatic events 'shatter' previously held beliefs (for instance, 'The world is a safe place'), and that post-trauma adjustment requires rebuilding basic beliefs about the self and the world. Traumatic events can not only shatter basic beliefs, but also confirm pre-existing negative beliefs.[20,26]

Dissociation and other processes that impede recovery

Psychological models of post-trauma reactions concur that recovery is thought to require 'working through' the trauma memory—in other words, going through the experience again in one's own mind, understanding the meaning of the event, distinguishing which of the stimuli that were present at the time the trauma are dangerous and which are innocuous, and readjusting basic beliefs about the self and the world.

Horowitz[24] suggested that the normal process of recovery involves working through the traumatic experience in a graduated manner, i.e. the individual uses protective cognitive mechanisms such as denial to prevent becoming overwhelmed by the experience. Psychological models concur in that the excessive use of such avoidant strategies (e.g. trying not to think about the trauma, efforts to push intrusive memories out of one's mind, ruminating about how the trauma could have been avoided) prevents recovery.[20,22,24] There is preliminary empirical evidence supporting this hypothesis.[27–29]

The cognitive mechanism that has received the most attention in relation to acute stress disorder is dissociation, as reflected in the DSM-IV criteria. It has been argued that dissociation minimizes the adverse emotional consequences of trauma by restricting awareness of the experience to avoid overwhelming fear and loss of control.[14] Dissociation is thought to prevent recovery because it prevents the integration of the traumatic experience into existing schemas[30] and it prevents the full activation of the trauma memory which is thought to be necessary for its modification.[31] In line with these hypotheses, dissociation during or immediately after a traumatic event predicts PTSD.[13,28,32]

Biological theories

Biological theories propose that extreme stress affects neuronal functions, and that the resulting changes are responsible for the symptoms of acute stress disorder and PTSD. Specifically, there is considerable theoretical speculation concerning the neurotransmitters involved in the responses to traumatic stressors (see also Chapter 4.6.2). Catecholamines, glucocorticoids, serotonin, and endogenous opioids have been studied as potential mediators of post-traumatic stress responses. In one of the few studies of biological correlates of acute stress, Resnick *et al.*[33] found that lower cortisol levels in the acute phase after rape predicted the presence of PTSD 3 months later. These findings are in line with other research showing abnormally low levels of cortisol in PTSD, suggesting that the hypothalamic–pituitary–adrenal axis is set to produce large responses to further stressors in PTSD (see Chapter 4.6.2).

Although some theorists, such as Kolb,[34] have proposed that excessive stimulation of the central nervous system at the time of the traumatic experience can result in permanent neuronal changes, most theories implicate prolonged stress, or the repeated stress of intrusive re-experiencing symptoms, as the major reason for neurophysiological changes.[35]

The degree of acute arousal during the traumatic stressor may be one of the factors that determine longer term trauma reactions. Acute arousal may have direct biological effects, or may reflect levels of distress that mediate persistent intrusive and avoidance patterns.[36]

Course and prognosis

Time course of symptoms

Whereas the ICD-10 criteria define acute stress reactions as a disorder that remits within a few days, DSM-IV conceptualizes acute stress disorder as a marker of those vulnerable to the development of PTSD.[30] Evidence relating to these different assumptions was sparse at the time the diagnoses were established.

Recent evidence supports the assumption that acute stress disorder is a precursor to PTSD.[17–19,37,38] In general, people who have more severe symptoms of PTSD in the weeks following trauma have a poorer prognosis than those with less severe symptoms.[39,40] Nevertheless, there is a substantial rate of spontaneous remission of about 50 per cent in the first year after a traumatic event.[39,40] Whether or not initial dissociative symptoms predict PTSD over and above what can be predicted from the initial PTSD symptoms remains unclear, and a recent prospective study reported negative findings.[18]

Predictors of acute stress disorder

Little is known about predictors of acute stress reactions. A history of psychiatric disorder, depressive and dissociative symptoms prior to the traumatic event, and previous trauma predict acute stress disorder.[38,41,42]

Treatment

Psychological treatments

Debriefing

Critical incident stress debriefing is a widely practised intervention that has the goal of promoting adaptation to traumatic events. Debriefing is generally conducted in a group within 24 to 72 h of the trauma. However, these parameters have been modified to permit more flexible interventions. Mitchell[43] proposes that debriefing comprises seven phases:

(1) an initial outline of the purpose and benefits of debriefing;

(2) the fact phase, in which participants relate what happened to them;

(3) a thought phase, in which participants relate their initial thoughts after the critical incident;

(4) a feeling phase, which requires participants to focus on the worst aspects of the incident and engage in their emotional reactions to the incident;

(5) an assessment phase, in which participants are trained to note their physical, cognitive, emotional, and behavioural symptoms;

(6) an education phase, which provides information about stress responses and ways to manage them;

(7) the re-entry phase, in which the information given is summarized and referral information offered.

These phases may take 1 to 5 h, and are usually co-ordinated by a trained mental health professional.

Anecdotal evidence and clinical reports attest to the efficacy of debriefing. However, despite its widespread use, very few controlled trials have been conducted. A Cochrane review of randomized controlled studies of individual debriefing[44] found that although participants usually found the intervention useful, debriefing had no overall positive effect on psychological symptoms. Out of six studies included in the review, two actually found that the debriefing group had a worse outcome than the control group.[45–47] A recent randomized controlled study confirmed the conclusion that individual debriefing has no beneficial effect on post-trauma symptoms.[48]

In line with these results on individual debriefing, the first two non-randomized controlled studies of the efficacy of group debriefing found that the intervention had no beneficial effects on post-trauma symptoms.[49,50] One of the studies found negative effects of the intervention after 18 months.[50]

Cognitive–behaviour therapy

Cognitive–behavioural interventions are effective in treating PTSD (see Chapter 4.6.2). The results of two randomized controlled studies of rape victims and road traffic accident survivors suggest that a brief four-session version of this treatment is effective in acute stress disorder and prevents the development of chronic post-trauma reactions.[51,52] Treatment involved the following:

(1) education about trauma reactions;

(2) progressive muscle relaxation;

(3) prolonged exposure;

(4) cognitive restructuring of fear-related beliefs;

(5) graded *in vivo* exposure.

However, the results remain preliminary as other studies have shown a significant rate of spontaneous recovery within the first year after trauma.[39,40]

Psychopharmacological treatment

Case studies report on the utility of tricyclic antidepressants,[53] benzodiazepine anxiolytics,[54] and benzodiazepine hypnotics[55] in acutely traumatized individuals. However, no randomized controlled trials have been completed. Research on PTSD suggests that selective serotonin-reuptake inhibitors are, to date, the best pharmacological treatment for persistent reactions to traumatic stress (see Chapter 4.6.2).

Advice about management

Given the transient nature of acute stress reactions (ICD-10) and the doubtful effectiveness of early psychological debriefing, no psychological intervention that focuses on working through the traumatic experience appears to be indicated for this condition. However, clinicians who see acutely traumatized individuals are faced with the pressure to do something to help. Research on the predictors of PTSD suggests that normalization of symptoms and information about their time course, practical help in resuming one's life, and, if possible, facilitation of social support may be helpful (see Chapter 4.6.2). Furthermore, patients may benefit from practical advice about issues such as hospital procedures, police questioning, insurance claims, legal procedures, and media pressure to tell one's story.

If patients with acute stress reactions appear unable to tolerate the anxiety and arousal symptoms, single doses (or a few days) of benzodiazepine treatment may be considered.[54] Hypnotic medication may be considered if the patient is unable to sleep.[55] However, it remains unclear whether these medications have positive or negative effects on long-term recovery. Benzodiazepines are ineffective in treating persistent post-traumatic symptoms.

For more persistent reactions to extreme stress, treatment may be indicated. However, patients with acute stress disorder who have low symptom severity have a good chance of recovering without intervention. For those with more severe acute stress disorder symptoms, a course of cognitive–behavioural treatment may be considered. If the patient is offered cognitive–behavioural treatment, therapists need to be aware that avoidance is a hallmark symptom of acute stress disorder and may reduce the likelihood that an individual will attend treatment sessions regularly. Flexible treatment procedures (e.g. initial contacts by telephone, scheduling sessions around the patient's preferences) and discussions about the ambivalence towards treatment may be helpful. Therapists need to be knowledgeable about the conditions surrounding the traumatic event and be sensitive to the particular sociocultural background of the patient, which will affect the personal meaning of the event. If anger is a major problem, the use of specialized cognitive–behavioural techniques is recommended.[56] This treatment involves the following:

(1) devising an anger-provocation hierarchy based on a period of self-monitoring;

(2) relaxation, breathing, and guided-imagery training to reduce physiological arousal;

(3) restructuring of anger-related cognitions;

(4) training in communication, problem-solving, and assertiveness training.

The lack of randomized controlled trials suggests that pharmacological treatment cannot be considered a front-line treatment for acute stress disorder, but research on PTSD suggests that selective serotonin reuptake inhibitors may be helpful.

Possibilities for prevention

Identifying highly symptomatic individuals with acute stress disorder and providing a cognitive–behavioural intervention from approximately 2 weeks post-trauma may reduce the risk of later PTSD. Additional preventive methods have been explored that prepare individuals 'at risk' (e.g. emergency services and military personnel) for experiencing trauma so as to enhance their coping strategies and reduce the risk of them developing longer term symptomatology. For those individuals at high risk of experiencing a trauma, providing them with training to remain calm, evaluate the situation objectively,[57] to not identify with victims, to utilize social supports, and to express emotional reactions[58] have all been found to be associated with better coping after the trauma. However, evidence remains preliminary.

References

1. Lindemann, E. (1944). Symptomatology and management of acute grief. *American Journal of Psychiatry*, **101**, 141–8.
2. Sargent, W. and Slater, E. (1941). Amnesic syndromes in war. *Proceedings of the Royal Society for Social Medicine*, **34**, 757–74.
3. World Health Organization (1948). *International statistical classification of diseases, injuries, and causes of death* (6th revision). World Health Organization, Geneva.
4. World Health Organization (1992). *The ICD-10 classification of mental and behavioural disorder: diagnostic criteria for research* (10th revision). World Health Organization, Geneva.
5. American Psychiatric Association (1980). *Diagnostic and statistical manual of mental disorders* (3rd edn). American Psychiatric Association, Washington, DC.
6. American Psychiatric Association (1989). *Diagnostic and statistical manual of mental disorders* (3rd edn, revised). American Psychiatric Association, Washington, DC.
7. Pincus, H.A., Frances, A., Davis, W.W., First, M.B., and Widiger, T.A. (1992). DSM-IV and new diagnostic categories: holding the line on proliferation. *American Journal of Psychiatry*, **149**, 112–17.
8. American Psychiatric Association (1994). *Diagnostic and statistical manual of mental disorders* (4th edn). American Psychiatric Association, Washington, DC.
9. Bryant, R.A., Harvey, A.G., Dang, S., and Sackville, T. (1998). Assessing acute stress disorder: psychometric properties of a structured clinical interview. *Psychological Assessment*, **10**, 215–20.
10. Steinberg, M. (1993). *Structured clinical interview for DSM-IV dissociative disorders (SCID-D)*. American Psychiatric Press, Washington, DC.
11. First, M.B., Spitzer, R.L., Gibbon, M., and Williams, J.B.W. (1995). *Structured clinical interview for DSM-IV Axis I disorders—patient version (SCID-I/P, Version 2.0)*. Biometrics Research Department of the New York State Psychiatric Institute, New York.
12. Cardeña, E., Classen, C., and Spiegel, D. (1991). *Stanford acute stress reaction questionnaire*. Stanford University Medical School, Stanford, CA.
13. Koopman, C., Classen, C., and Spiegel, D. (1994). Predictors of post-traumatic stress symptoms among survivors of the Oakland/Berkeley, Calif. firestorm. *American Journal of Psychiatry*, **151**, 888–94.
14. Spiegel, D. (1991). Dissociation and trauma. In *American psychiatric*

press review of psychiatry, Vol. 10 (ed. A. Tasman and S.M. Goldfinger), pp. 261–75. American Psychiatric Press, Washington, DC.

15. Harvey, A.G. and Bryant, R.A. (1998). Acute stress disorder following mild traumatic brain injury. *Journal of Nervous and Mental Disease*, **186**, 333–7.

16. Schnyder, U. and Malt, U.F. (1998). Acute stress response patterns to accidental injuries. *Journal of Psychosomatic Research*, **45**, 419–24.

17. Harvey, A.G. and Bryant, R.A. (1998). The relationship between acute stress disorder and post-traumatic stress disorder: a prospective evaluation of motor vehicle accident survivors. *Journal of Consulting and Clinical Psychology*, **66**, 507–12.

18. Brewin, C.R., Andrews, B., Rose, S., and Kirk, M. (1999). Acute stress disorder and post-traumatic stress disorder in victims of violent crime. *American Journal of Psychiatry*, **156**, 360–6.

19. Classen, C., Koopman, C., Hales, R., and Spiegel, D. (1998). Acute stress disorder as a predictor of post-traumatic stress symptoms. *American Journal of Psychiatry*, **155**, 620–4.

20. Foa, E.B. and Riggs, D.S. (1993). Post-traumatic stress disorder in rape victims. In *Annual review of psychiatry*, Vol. 12 (ed. J. Oldham, M.B. Riba, and A. Tasman), pp. 273–303. American Psychiatric Association, Washington, DC.

21. Foa, E.B., Steketee, G., and Rothbaum, B.O. (1989). Behavioral/cognitive conceptualizations of post-traumatic stress disorder. *Behavior Therapy*, **20**, 155–76.

22. Ehlers, A. and Clark, D.M. A cognitive model of persistent post-traumatic stress disorder. *Behaviour Research and Therapy*, in press.

23. Brewin, C.R., Dalgleish, T., and Joseph, S. (1996). A dual representation theory of post-traumatic stress disorder. *Psychological Review*, **103**, 670–86.

24. Horowitz, M.J. (1997). *Stress response syndromes. PTSD, grief and adjustment disorders*. Jason Aronson, Northvale, NJ.

25. Janoff-Bulman, R. (1992). *Shattered assumptions: toward a new psychology of trauma*. Free Press, New York.

26. Resick, P.A. and Schnicke, M.K. (1993). *Cognitive processing therapy for rape victims*. Sage, Newbury Park, CA.

27. Ehlers, A. and Steil, R. (1995). Maintenance of intrusive memories in post-traumatic stress disorder: a cognitive approach. *Behavioural and Cognitive Psychotherapy*, **23**, 217–49.

28. Ehlers, A., Mayou, R.A., and Bryant, B. (1998). Psychological predictors of chronic post-traumatic stress disorder after motor vehicle accidents. *Journal of Abnormal Psychology*, **107**, 508–19.

29. Harvey, A.G. and Bryant, R.A. (1998). The effect of attempted thought suppression in acute stress disorder. *Behaviour Research and Therapy*, **36**, 583–90.

30. Koopman, C., Classen, C., Cardena, E., and Spiegel, D. (1995). When disaster strikes, acute stress disorder may follow. *Journal of Traumatic Stress*, **8**, 29–46.

31. Foa, E.B. and Hearst-Ikeda, D. (1996). Emotional dissociation in response to trauma: an information-processing approach. In *Handbook of dissociation: theoretical and clinical perspectives* (ed. L.K. Michelson and W.J. Ray), pp. 207–22. Plenum Press, New York.

32. Shalev, A.Y., Peri, T., Canetti, L., and Schreiber, S. (1996). Predictors of PTSD in injured trauma survivors: a prospective study. *American Journal of Psychiatry*, **153**, 219–25.

33. Resnick, H., Yehuda, R., Pitman, R.K., and Foy, D.W. (1995). Effect of previous trauma on acute plasma cortisol level following rape. *American Journal of Psychiatry*, **152**, 1675–7.

34. Kolb, L.C. (1987). Neurophysiological hypothesis explaining post-traumatic stress disorder. *American Journal of Psychiatry*, **144**, 989–95.

35. van der Kolk, B.A. (1996). The psychobiology of PTSD. In *Traumatic stress: the effects of overwhelming experience on mind, body, and society* (ed. B.A. van der Kolk, A.C. McFarlane, and L. Weisaeth), pp. 214–41. Guilford Press, New York.

36. Shalev, A.Y. (1992). Post-traumatic stress disorder among injured survivors of a terrorist attack. *Journal of Nervous and Mental Disease*, **180**, 505–9.

37. Bryant, R.A. and Harvey, A.G. (1998). The relationship between acute stress disorder and post-traumatic stress disorder following mild traumatic brain injury. *American Journal of Psychiatry*, **155**, 625–9.

38. Murray, J., Ehlers, A., and Mayou, R.A. Predictors of acute stress disorder and post-traumatic stress disorder after motor vehicle accidents. Results from two prospective studies, in preparation.

39. Blanchard, E.B., Hickling, E.J., Barton, K.A., Taylor, A.E., Loos, W.R., and Jones-Alexander, J. (1996). One-year prospective follow-up of motor vehicle accident victims. *Behaviour Research and Therapy*, **34**, 775–86.

40. Rothbaum, B.O., Foa, E.B., Riggs, D.S., Murdock, T., and Walsh, W. (1992). A prospective examination of post-traumatic stress disorder in rape victims. *Journal of Traumatic Stress*, **5**, 455–75.

41. Barton, K.A., Blanchard, E.B., and Hickling, E.J. (1996). Antecedents and consequences of acute stress disorder among motor vehicle accident victims. *Behaviour Research and Therapy*, **34**, 805–13.

42. Harvey, A.G. and Bryant, R.A. (1999). Predictors of acute stress following motor vehicle accidents. *Journal of Traumatic Stress*, **12**, 519–26.

43. Mitchell, J. (1983). When disaster strikes. The critical incident stress debriefing process. *Journal of Emergency Medical Services*, **8**, 36–9.

44. Rose, S. and Bisson, J. (1998). Brief early psychological interventions following trauma: a systematic review of the literature. *Journal of Traumatic Stress*, **11**, 697–710.

45. Bisson, J.I., Jenkins, P.L., Alexander, J., and Bannister, C. (1997). Randomised controlled trial of psychological debriefing for victims of acute burn trauma. *British Journal of Psychiatry*, **171**, 78–81.

46. Hobbs, M., Mayou, R., Harrison, B., and Worlock, P. (1996). A randomised controlled trial of psychological debriefing for victims of road traffic accidents. *British Medical Journal*, **7**, 1438–9.

47. Mayou, R.A., Ehlers, A., and Hobbs, M. A three year follow-up of a randomised controlled trial of psychological debriefing for road traffic accident victims. Submitted for publication.

48. Rose, S., Brewin, C., Andrews, B., and Kirk, M. A randomised trial of psychological debriefing for victims of violent crime. Submitted for publication.

49. Kenardy, J.A., Webster, R.A., Lewin, T.J., Carr, V. J., Hazell, P.L., and Carter, G.L. (1996). Stress debriefing and patterns of recovery following a natural disaster. *Journal of Traumatic Stress*, **9**, 37–49.

50. Carlier, I.V.E., Lamberts, R.D., van Uchelen, A.J., and Gersons, B.P.R. (1998). Disaster-related post-traumatic stress in police officers: a field study of the impact of debriefing. *Stress Medicine*, **14**, 143–8.

51. Foa, E.B., Hearst-Ikeda, D., and Perry, K.J. (1995). Evaluation of a brief cognitive–behavioural program for the prevention of chronic PTSD in recent assault victims. *Journal of Consulting and Clinical Psychology*, **63**, 948–55.

52. Bryant, R.A., Harvey, A.G., Dang, S.T., Sackville, T., and Basten, C. (1998). Treatment of acute stress disorder: a comparison of cognitive behaviour therapy and supportive counselling. *Journal of Consulting and Clinical Psychology*, **66**, 862–6.

53. Blake, D.J. (1986). Treatment of acute postraumatic stress disorder with tricyclic antidepressants. *Southern Medical Journal*, **79**, 201–4.

54. Ashton, H. (1994). Guidelines for the rational use of benzodiazepines. *Drugs*, **48**, 25–40.

55. Mellman, T.A., Byers, P.M., and Augenstein, J.S. (1998). Pilot evaluation of hypnotic medication during acute traumatic stress response. *Journal of Traumatic Stress*, **11**, 563–9.

56. Chemtob, C.M., Novaco, R.W., Hamada, R.S., and Gross, D.M. (1997). Anger regulation deficits in combat-related posttraumatic stress disorder. *Journal of Traumatic Stress*, **10**, 17–36.

57. Hytten, K. (1989). Helicopter crash in water: effects of simulator escape training. *Acta Psychiatrica Scandinavica*, **80** (Supplement), 73–8.

58. Fullerton, C.S., McCarroll, J.E., Ursano, R.J., and Wright, K.M. (1992). Psychological responses of rescue workers: fire fighters and trauma. *American Journal of Orthopsychiatry*, **62**, 371–8.

4.6.2 Post-traumatic stress disorder

Anke Ehlers

Introduction

Clinicians have long noted that traumatic events can lead to severe psychological disturbance. At the end of the nineteenth and the beginning of the twentieth centuries, railway disasters, the World Wars, and the Holocaust prompted systematic descriptions of the symptoms associated with traumatic stress reactions. These include the spontaneous re-experiencing of aspects of the traumatic events, startle responses, irritability, impairment in concentration and memory, disturbed sleep, distressing dreams, depression, phobias, guilt, psychic numbing, and multiple somatic symptoms. A variety of labels were used to describe these reactions including 'fright neurosis', 'combat/war neurosis', 'shell-shock', 'survivor syndrome', and 'nuclearism'.[1–3]

Whether the traumatic event can be considered a major cause of these psychological symptoms, has been the subject of considerable debate. Charcot, Janet, Freud, and Breuer suggested that hysterical symptoms were caused by psychological trauma, but their views were not widely accepted. The dominant view was that a traumatic event in itself was not a sufficient cause of post-trauma symptoms, and experts searched for other causes. Many suspected an organic cause. For example, damage to the spinal cord was suggested as the cause of the 'railway spine syndrome', microsections of exploded bombs entering the brain as the cause of 'shell shock', and starvation and brain damage as causes of the chronic psychological difficulties of concentration camp survivors. Others doubted the validity of the symptom reports and suggested that malingering and compensation-seeking ('compensation neurosis') was the major cause in most cases. Finally, the psychological symptoms were attributed to pre-existing psychological dysfunction. The predominant view was that reactions to traumatic events are transient, and that therefore only people with unstable personalities, pre-existing neurotic conflicts, or mental illness would develop chronic symptoms.[1–3]

It was the recognition of the long-standing psychological problems of many war veterans, especially Vietnam veterans, that changed this view and convinced clinicians and researchers that even people with sound personalities can develop clinically significant psychological symptoms if they are exposed to horrific stressors. This prompted the introduction of post-traumatic stress disorder (**PTSD**) as a diagnostic category in DSM-III.[4] It was thus recognized that traumatic events such as combat, rape, man-made or natural disasters give rise to a characteristic pattern of psychological symptoms. The diagnostic criteria specified the experience of a traumatic event as a necessary condition for the diagnosis. ICD-10[5] emphasized the causal role of traumatic stressors in producing psychological dysfunction even more clearly, in that a specific group of disorders, 'reaction to severe stress, and adjustment disorders', was created. These disorders are 'thought to arise always as a direct consequence of the acute severe stress or continued trauma. The stressful event…is the primary and overriding causal factor, and the disorder would not have occurred without its impact.'

What makes a stressor traumatic?

In everyday language, many upsetting situations are described as 'traumatic', for example divorce, loss of job, or failing an examination. However, a field study designed to establish what kinds of stressors lead to the characteristic symptoms of PTSD, showed that only 0.4 per cent of a community sample developed the characteristic symptoms of PTSD in response to such 'low magnitude' stressors.[6] Thus, in diagnosing PTSD, it appeared necessary to employ a strict definition of what constitutes a traumatic stressor.

Few people would contest that horrific events such as rape or bombings are traumatic. In an attempt to capture the essence of these stressors, the authors of DSM-IIIR required a traumatic stressor to be 'outside the range of usual human experience' and that it 'would be markedly distressing to almost anyone'.[7] However, epidemiological studies showed that stressors that can lead to PTSD are actually quite common, for example road traffic accidents[8] or sexual assault.[9] Thus, the DSM-IIIR definition appeared too restrictive.

ICD-10 uses a broader definition and characterizes traumatic stressors by their exceptional severity and the distress they would cause for the average person 'a stressful event or situation…of an exceptionally threatening of catastrophic nature, which is likely to cause pervasive distress in almost anyone'.[5] Thus, the ICD-10 diagnosis refers to a common-sense understanding of which situations are likely to be extremely distressing.

In contrast, the authors of DSM-IV[10] attempted a specific definition. On the basis of research findings that threat to life or physical integrity during the event is one of the most consistent predictors of PTSD,[11] DSM-IV requires that the person 'experienced, witnessed, or was confronted with an event or events that involved actual or threatened death or serious injury, or a threat to the physical integrity of self or others'. The authors of DSM-IV made a further important step, in that they moved away from a purely situational definition and included the person's subjective response to the situation as an additional criterion, requiring that the 'person's response involved intense fear, helplessness, or horror' (or disorganized or agitated behaviour in the case of children).[10] The latter criterion takes into account that there is a large interindividual variability in the psychological response to the same situation.

The stressor criterion of DSM-IV is still under debate. Recent research suggests that both components of the definition may require extension. First, it may be necessary to include further possible emotional responses to traumatic stressors. There is accumulating evidence that emotional numbing during traumatic events is predictive of PTSD.[12] Furthermore, it has been established that perpetrators of violent crime sometimes develop PTSD. Witnessing or participating in war-related crimes such as torturing or killing prisoners of war and civilians and mutilation of corpses is more closely linked to PTSD in Vietnam veterans than the threat of death associated with combat.[13] The psychological state of the perpetrators during the events that later lead to PTSD has not been studied in detail, but it is doubtful that they would meet the current DSM-IV definition. More likely, feelings of shame or guilt that were experienced at the time or subsequently, may be predictive of PTSD in this group.

Second, the emphasis on threat to life or physical integrity may omit important dimensions of subgroups of traumatic events. The threat to the perception of oneself as an autonomous human being may be a relevant dimension of traumatic events that involve intentional harm by other people.[14] Mental defeat, the perceived loss of all autonomy, was related to PTSD in political prisoners and assault victims,[14,15] independent of other indicators of trauma severity including threat to life and perceived helplessness.

Clinical features

The most characteristic symptoms of PTSD are the re-experiencing symptoms. Patients involuntarily re-experience aspects of the traumatic event in a very vivid and distressing way. This includes: flashbacks in which the person acts or feels as if the event were recurring; nightmares; and intrusive images or other sensory impressions from the event. For example, a women who was assaulted kept seeing the eyes of the perpetrator looking through the letterbox before he broke into her house, and a man involved in a severe car crash at night kept hearing the sound of the impact. Despite these vivid memory fragments, intentional recall of the event is often poor and disorganized, and some patients have amnesia for parts of the event (see also Chapter 4.6.3).

Reminders of the trauma arouse intense distress and/or physiological reactions and are consequently avoided, including conversations about the event. Patients try to push memories of the event out of their mind and avoid thinking about the event in detail, particularly about its worst moments. On the other hand, many ruminate excessively about questions that prevent them from coming to terms with the event, for example about why the event happened to them, about how it could have been prevented, or about how they could take revenge.

The patients emotional state ranges from intense fear, anger, sadness, guilt, or shame to emotional numbness. They often describe feeling detached from other people and give up previously significant activities. Various symptoms of hyperarousal include hypervigilance, exaggerated startle responses, irritability, difficulty concentrating, and sleep problems.

Classification

ICD-10[5] classifies PTSD (F43.1) among the reactions to severe stress and adjustment disorders (F43) that are primarily caused by stressful events. DSM-IV[10] classifies PTSD (309.81) among the anxiety disorders because symptom patterns, psychophysiological responses, family studies, and the efficacy of exposure treatment and serotonergic drugs suggested a relationship with other anxiety disorders. However, some of the symptoms would also suggest a relationship with dissociative disorders (e.g. amnesia) or depression (e.g. loss of interest).[16,17]

Diagnosis and differential diagnosis

Diagnostic criteria in ICD-10 and DSM-IV

Table 1 compares the diagnostic criteria of ICD-10 and DSM-IV.[10] ICD-10 research diagnostic criteria,[18] as well as diagnostic guidelines,[5] are included. The diagnostic systems agree on the core symptoms of PTSD—re-experiencing, avoidance, emotional numbing, and hyperarousal—but differ in the weight assigned to them.

- DSM-IV puts a stronger emphasis on the avoidance/numbing cluster of symptoms by requiring a minimum of three of these symptoms. Although emotional numbing is listed prominently in the ICD-10 diagnostic guidelines, it was not included in the ICD-10 research diagnostic criteria. As a consequence, patients that meet ICD-10 criteria may not fulfil the criteria for a DSM-IV PTSD diagnosis if they have too few of the numbing symptoms. They would be diagnosed as having an adjustment disorder according to DSM-IV.

- The ICD-10 research diagnostic criteria require the patient to either suffer from psychogenic amnesia or hyperarousal symptoms. Thus, in contrast to DSM-IV, a patient could be diagnosed as having PTSD in the absence of hyperarousal symptoms if amnesia is present.

- DSM-IV states two additional criteria that are not included in ICD-10. First, it requires a minimum symptom duration of 1 month because acute stress disorder would be diagnosed before 4 weeks have elapsed. Second, it requires that the symptoms cause significant distress or impaired functioning.

- Thus, although the diagnostic systems largely agree on the type of symptoms that characterize PTSD, DSM-IV criteria are stricter. A recent large-scale study[19] found a prevalence of ICD-10 PTSD of 6.9 per cent, and a prevalence of DSM-IV PTSD of 3 per cent. The concordance between the diagnostic systems was only 35 per cent. The concordance could have been increased to 56 per cent if ICD-10 included a criterion of emotional numbing and if the DSM-IV disability criterion was dropped.

Differential diagnoses

Differential diagnoses are summarized in Table 1. Distinguishing features include the following:

- the type of stressor (adjustment disorders, enduring personality change)

- the symptom pattern (adjustment disorders, enduring personality change)

- the duration of the symptoms (acute stress disorder, acute stress reaction)

- the question of whether the avoidance, numbing, and hyperarousal symptoms were present before the traumatic event occurred (other anxiety or depressive disorders)

- the nature of the intrusive cognitions and perceptual disturbances (obsessive–compulsive disorder, psychotic symptoms, substance-induced symptoms).

Prolonged repeated trauma, such as captivity or repeated childhood sexual abuse, may lead to a more complex pattern of symptoms, 'complex PTSD', that is characterized by somatization, dissociation, affect dysregulation, poor impulse control, self-destructive behaviour, and pathological patterns of relationships.[20] It was debated whether to include a category 'disorders of extreme stress not otherwise specified' (**DESNOS**) into DSM-IV to accommodate these cases, but the decision was not to include it.[16] In ICD-10, the diagnosis 'Enduring personality changes after catastrophic experience' covers such long-standing consequences of enduring trauma.

Table 1 Diagnostic criteria for PTSD in ICD-10 and DSM-IV

ICD-10 diagnostic guidelines	ICD-10 research diagnostic criteria	DSM-IV criteria

Stressor criterion
1. Event or situation of exceptionally threatening or catastrophic nature
 	
2. Likely to cause pervasive distress in almost anyone
	A. 1. Event or situation of exceptionally threatening or catastrophic nature
	
	   2. Likely to cause pervasive distress in almost anyone
		A. 1. The person experienced, witnessed, or was confronted with an event or events that involved actual or threatened death or serious injury, or a threat to the physical integrity of self or others
		  2. The person's response involved intense fear, helplessness, or horror (or disorganized or agitated behaviour in children)

Symptom criteria
Necessary symptom
1. Repetitive intrusive recollection or re-enactment of the event in memories, daytime imagery, or dreams
 	
Other typical symptoms
2. Sense of 'numbness' and emotional blunting, detachment from others, unresponsiveness to surroundings, anhedonia
 	
3. Avoidance of activities and situations reminiscent of trauma
 	
Common symptoms
4. Autonomic hyperarousal with hypervigilance, enhanced startle reaction, insomnia
 	
5. Anxiety and depression
 	
Rare symptoms
6. Dramatic acute bursts of fear, panic, or aggression triggered by reminders
	Necessary symptoms
	B. Persistent remembering or 'reliving' of the stressor in intrusive 'flashbacks', vivid memories, or recurring dreams, and in experiencing distress when exposed to circumstances resembling or associated with the stressor
	
	C. Actual or preferred avoidance of circumstances resembling or associated with the stressor which was not present before exposure to the stressor
	
	D. 1. Inability to recall, either partially or completely, some important aspects or the period of exposure to the stressor
	
	or
	
	  2. Persistent symptoms of increased psychological sensitivity and arousal (not present before exposure to stressor), shown by any two of the following
	    (a) Difficulty in falling or staying asleep
	    (b) Irritability or outbursts of anger
	    (c) Difficulty in concentrating
	    (d) Hypervigilance
	    (e) Exaggerated startle response
		Necessary symptoms
		B. The traumatic event is persistently re-experienced in one (or more) of the following ways
		1. Recurrent and intrusive distressing recollections of the event, including images, thoughts, or perceptions (or repetitive play in which the themes or aspects of the trauma are expressed in children)
		2. Recurrent distressing dreams of the event (or frightening dreams without recognizable content in children)
		3. Acting or feeling as if the traumatic event were recurring (or trauma-specific re-enactment in children)
		4. Intense psychological distress at exposure to internal or external cues that symbolize or resemble an aspect of the traumatic event
		5. Physiological reactivity at exposure to internal or external cues that symbolize or resemble an aspect of the traumatic event
		
		C. Persistent avoidance of stimuli associated with the trauma and numbing of general responsiveness (not present before trauma), as indicated by three (or more) of the following
		1. Efforts to avoid thoughts, feelings, or conversations associated with the trauma
		2. Efforts to avoid activities, places, or people that arouse recollections of the trauma
		3. Inability to recall an important aspect of the trauma
		4. Markedly diminished interest or participation in significant activities
		5. Feeling of detachment or estrangement from others
		6. Restricted range of affect
		7. Sense of foreshortened future

(continued)

ICD-10 diagnostic guidelines	ICD-10 research diagnostic criteria	DSM-IV criteria
		D. Persistent symptoms of increased arousal (not present before the trauma), as indicated by two (or more) of the following 1. Difficulty falling or staying asleep 2. Irritability or outbursts of anger 3. Difficulty concentrating 4. Hypervigilance 5. Exaggerated startle response
Time frame Symptoms should usually arise within 6 months of the traumatic event	Symptoms should usually arise within 6 months of the traumatic event	Symptoms present for at least 1 month
Disability criterion N/A	N/A	The disturbance causes clinically significant distress or impairment in social, occupational, or other important areas of functioning
Differential diagnoses 1. Acute stress reaction F43.0 (immediate reaction in the first 3 days after event) 2. Enduring personality change after a catastrophic experience F62.0 (present for at least 2 years, only after extreme and prolonged stress) 3. Adjustment disorder (less severe stressor or different symptom pattern) 4. Other anxiety or depressive disorders (absence of traumatic stressor or symptoms precedes stressor)	Same as ICD-10 diagnostic guidelines	1. Acute stress disorder (duration of up to 4 weeks) 2. Adjustment disorder (less severe stressor or different symptom pattern) 3. Mood disorder or other anxiety disorder (symptoms of avoidance, numbing, or hyperarousal present before exposure to the stressor) 4. Other disorders with intrusive thoughts or perceptual disturbances (e.g. obsessive–compulsive disorder, schizophrenia, other psychotic disorders, substance-induced disorders)

Furthermore, it is currently being debated whether an additional diagnostic category 'traumatic grief' should be included into the psychiatric classification system.[21,22]

Ongoing research on symptom criteria

Recent research has questioned the symptom clusters of DSM-IV. In particular, it emerges that it may be preferable to assess the emotional numbing symptoms separately from the avoidance symptoms, because these symptoms do not load on the same factor in factor analyses and may have different underlying mechanisms. Furthermore, it may be preferable to include severity criteria for the symptoms rather than relying on counting the presence of symptoms.[23]

Assessment instruments

Several semistructured interviews assess the DSM-IV criteria for PTSD. The Structured Clinical Interview for DSM-IV (**SCID**)[24] allows one to establish the diagnosis of PTSD. The Clinician Administered PTSD Scale (**CAPS**)[25] and the Anxiety Disorders Interview Schedule for DSM-IV (**ADIS-IV**)[26] provide measures of symptom severity as well as establishing the diagnosis of PTSD.

The most widely used self-report measure of PTSD symptoms used to be the Impact of Event Scale.[27] The original scale contained two scales, an intrusion and an avoidance scale. It has recently been expanded to include an additional hyperarousal scale (**IES-R**).[28] The IES-R does not cover all the symptoms of PTSD specified in DSM-IV. This is why new measures that are modelled on the DSM-IV criteria are now commonly used in research studies, for example the Post-traumatic Stress Diagnostic Scale (**PDS**).[29]

Epidemiology

The available epidemiological data so far stem mainly from studies conducted in the United States. It remains to be investigated whether these data replicate in other countries. The prevalence of PTSD may be low in some societies such as Iceland or Hong Kong. One has to bear in mind that the society and natural environment set conditions for exposure to traumatic events. For example, in the last decades, people in developing countries have had a much greater exposure to war and natural disasters than people in industrialized Western societies.[30]

How common are traumatic events in the population?

In a large representative United States' sample, Kessler et al.[31] found that 60.7 per cent of the men and 51.2 per cent of the women had experienced at least one traumatic event meeting DSM-IIIR criteria in their lifetime. The most common types of trauma were witnessing someone being killed or severely injured, accidents, and being involved in a fire, flood, or natural disaster. Using DSM-IV criteria, Stein *et al.*[32] found a lifetime exposure to serious traumatic events of 81.3 per cent for men, and 74.2 per cent for women. Sudden death of a loved person was one of the most frequent traumatic stressors (DSM-IV criteria).[33]

What types of trauma are associated with high PTSD rates?

PTSD rates depend on the type of traumatic event. Rape was associated with the highest PTSD rates in several studies. For example, 65 per cent of the men and 46 per cent of the women who had been raped met PTSD criteria in the Kessler *et al.*[31] study. Other traumatic events associated with high PTSD rates included combat exposure, childhood neglect and physical abuse, sexual molestation; and for women only, physical attack and being threatened with a weapon, kidnapped, or held hostage. Accidents, witnessing death or injury, and fire or natural disasters were associated with relatively low lifetime PTSD rates of less than 10 per cent.[31] Other research has shown high PTSD rates for torture victims,[34] survivors of the Holocaust,[35] and prisoners of war.[36]

The emphasis in DSM-IV on threat to life or physical integrity has led to increasing awareness that medical illness and treatment can lead to PTSD.[37] Waking up during anaesthesia, especially if the patient experienced pain, is an example for such a traumatic event. Epidemiological data for this subgroup of PTSD patients are largely lacking.

What proportion of people develop PTSD in response to a traumatic stressor?

Kessler *et al.*[31] found that the risk of developing PTSD after a traumatic event is 8.1 per cent for men, and 20.4 per cent for women. For young urban populations, higher risks have been reported; Breslau *et al.* found an overall risk of 23.6 per cent,[38] a risk of 13 per cent for men and 30.2 per cent for women.[39]

The figures reported in these studies may be influenced by two types of biases that have opposite effects on probability estimates. First, Breslau *et al.*[33] have pointed out that previous studies overestimated the PTSD-risk imposed by traumatic events because participants reported on the worst trauma that they had experienced. When the symptoms induced by a traumatic event that was randomly selected from the ones that a person had experienced were assessed, the conditional risk of PTSD following exposure to trauma was found to be 9.2 per cent, using DSM-IV criteria.

Second, the retrospective methodology used in the epidemiological studies may have led to underestimation of PTSD rates due to selective recall. For example, the prevalence of PTSD 3 months after road traffic accidents was found to be around 20 per cent in prospective longitudinal studies,[40,41] whereas the retrospective studies found prevalences below 10 per cent.

How prevalent is PTSD in the population?

Kessler *et al.*[31] estimated that the lifetime prevalence of PTSD is 7.8 per cent, using DSM-IIIR criteria. Women had a higher prevalence than men (10.4 versus 5.0 per cent). This was due to both a greater exposure to high-impact trauma (rape, sexual molestation, childhood neglect, and childhood physical abuse) and a greater likelihood of developing PTSD when exposed to a traumatic event. Other studies using DSM-IIIR criteria have yielded similarly high prevalence rates.[9,39] A recent study used DSM-IV criteria and found a past-month PTSD prevalence of 2.7 per cent for women and 1.2 per cent for men.[32]

Earlier studies using DSM-III criteria had reported lower lifetime prevalences of about 1 per cent.[42,43] Besides differences in procedures and sampling methods, the low PTSD prevalence in these earlier studies may be due to the use of an interview schedule with low sensitivity in detecting PTSD.[44] In particular, the interview asked global questions about the occurrence of traumatic events and lacked the repeated probing for specific events or event categories that seems to be necessary in eliciting relevant experiences.

Partial PTSD

Several studies have found substantial levels of distress and disability for traumatized people who met some, but not all, of the PTSD criteria specified in DSM-IV.[32] These people may be at greater risk of developing the full PTSD syndrome than people with fewer symptoms.[40,41]

Comorbidity of PTSD with other disorders and symptoms

PTSD shows a substantial comorbidity with affective disorders, other anxiety disorders, substance-use disorders, and somatization. In the study by Kessler *et al.*,[31] 88.3 per cent of the men and 78.1 per cent of the women with PTSD had comorbid psychiatric diagnoses. Studies of veterans with PTSD have also indicated an enhanced level of problems in family and marital adjustment and violent behaviour,[45] and heavy smoking.[46] Furthermore, reports of poor health and increased rates of various diseases, in particular infectious and nervous system diseases, are associated with PTSD.[47]

Is PTSD primary or secondary to the comorbid diagnoses? There is, as yet, little research into this question. The retrospective accounts obtained by Kessler *et al.*[31] suggested that PTSD was primary to comorbid affective or substance-use disorders in the majority of cases, and PTSD was primary to comorbid anxiety disorders in about half of the cases. Similarly, Breslau *et al.*[39] found that PTSD increased the risks for first-onset major depression and alcohol-use disorder. Conversely, pre-existing major depression also increased vulnerability to the PTSD-inducing effects of traumatic events and risk for exposure to traumatic events. A prospective study confirmed that PTSD increased the risk of subsequent pain, conversion symptoms, and somatization symptoms.[48]

Most of the comorbidity research has concentrated on the nature of the relationship between PTSD and alcohol or drug abuse. A recent longitudinal study[49] of 1007 adults showed that PTSD led to an increased risk of drug abuse or dependence, whereas exposure to traumatic events in the absence of PTSD did not increase the risk. Consistent with the interpretation that drug-use disorders are usually secondary to PTSD, there was no evidence that pre-existing drug abuse or dependence influenced the risk of PTSD after traumatic exposure. Similarly, the majority of studies have found that PTSD precedes the development of alcohol-abuse problems. There are probably several mechanisms for this relationship. In the short term, alcohol is used to self-medicate the symptoms of PTSD, but paradoxically intoxication and withdrawal symptoms may intensify the symptoms in the long term.[50]

Longitudinal studies have produced conflicting findings on whether drug use increases the risk of exposure to traumatic events.[49] However, other studies have suggested that alcohol abuse may increase the likelihood of traumatization because of its association with violence and accidents.[51]

Summary of main findings from epidemiological studies

- The majority of people will experience at least one traumatic event in their lifetime.

- In assessing PTSD history, interviewers should probe for specific events.

- Assault, in particular sexual assault, and combat have a higher impact than accidents and disasters.[31,32]

- If the frequency and impact of traumatic events are considered together, sudden unexpected death of a loved one[33] and road traffic accidents[8] can be considered important causes of PTSD in Western industrialized societies.

- Men tend to experience more traumatic events than women, but women experience higher impact events.[31,32]

- Women are at least twice as likely to develop PTSD in response to a traumatic event than men. This enhanced risk is not explained by differences in the type of traumatic event. The estimated lifetime prevalence for women is approximately 10 to 12 per cent, and for men 5 to 6 per cent.[9,31,38,39]

- Comorbid depression and substance-use disorders appear to be secondary to PTSD in the majority of cases.

Aetiology

There is no single accepted theory of PTSD. Theoretical explanations have focused on psychological and biological mechanisms that are not mutually exclusive.

Psychological processes

Fear conditioning

Mowrer's two-factor conditioning theory of phobias has been applied to PTSD.[52–54] It is suggested that through classical (Pavlovian) conditioning, stimuli that were present at the time of the trauma (unconditioned stimulus) become associated with fear and arousal responses. Subsequently, the conditioned stimuli trigger similar (conditioned) responses when presented on their own. Through stimulus generalization and higher-order conditioning, a wide variety of stimuli become triggers of distress in the aftermath of trauma. Quite naturally, the person will try to avoid the conditioned stimuli and the associated distress. The avoidance behaviour is negatively reinforced (operant or instrumental conditioning) because it leads to a reduction in psychological and physical discomfort. In the long term, however, avoidance

prevents extinction of the conditioned fear responses to reminders of the traumatic event, and thus maintains the problem.

Appraisals of the traumatic event and its sequelae

A traumatic event threatens the person's view of the world, the self, and the future. Several theorists propose that this threat to basic inner models is at the core of PTSD, or of responses to trauma in general. Horowitz[21] explained re-experiencing symptoms as the result of a slow process that helps the traumatized person to adjust their inner models (schemas) of the self and the world to the traumatic experience. Until this process is completed, the information related to the traumatic event is thought to be held in active memory and thus intrudes into consciousness. Similarly, Janoff-Bulman[55] proposed that traumatic events 'shatter' previously held beliefs (e.g. 'The world is a safe place'), and that post-trauma adjustment requires rebuilding basic beliefs about the self and the world. However, PTSD is quite often associated with a confirmation of previously held negative beliefs rather than a shattering of positive beliefs (e.g. 'Bad things always happen to me')[50,56,57] so that recovery requires the modification of these beliefs.

The persistence of PTSD symptoms has been explained by individual differences in the appraisal of the traumatic event: that is to say, in what personal meaning it has for them.[56,58,59] Some people are able to see the trauma as a time-limited terrible experience that does not necessarily have negative implications for the future, and may also be able to find some element of personal growth in it. These people are likely to recover quickly. Individuals with persistent PTSD are characterized by excessively negative appraisals of the event. The nature of predominant emotional responses in PTSD depends on the particular appraisals; for example, appraisals concerning danger lead to fear ('Nowhere is safe'), appraisals concerning others violating personal rules lead to anger ('Others have not treated me fairly'), appraisals concerning responsibility for the traumatic event lead to guilt or shame ('It was my fault', 'I did something despicable'), and appraisals concerning loss lead to sadness ('My life will never be the same again').[58] Such appraisals distinguished between traumatized individuals with and without PTSD.[60]

Negative appraisals involved in maintaining PTSD do not only concern the traumatic event itself, but also its sequelae such as the initial PTSD symptoms or responses of other people in the aftermath of the traumatic event.[58,61,62] In line with this hypothesis, negative interpretations of intrusive recollections (e.g. 'I am going mad') after road traffic accidents were one of the most important predictors of PTSD at 1 year after the event.[41] Perceived negative responses from other people in the aftermath of trauma predicted PTSD in studies of assault and torture victims.[14,15]

Nature of trauma memories

PTSD patients have relatively poor intentional recall of the traumatic event. Their narratives of the event tend to be fragmented and disorganized.[63] With successful treatment, the narratives become elaborated and organized.[64] These observations have led to the hypothesis that insufficient elaboration of the event and its meaning leads to the re-experiencing symptoms of PTSD.[58] Autobiographical memories are normally organized in a way that prevents triggering of very vivid and emotional re-experiencing of an event. Recall is driven by themes and personal time periods, and it is relatively abstract.[65] Ehlers and Clark[58] suggested that re-experiencing in PTSD occurs because the trauma memory is inadequately linked to its context in time, place, and other autobiographical memories. Stimuli that resemble those present during the traumatic event can thus trigger vivid memories and strong emotional responses that are experienced as if the event was happening right now.

Foa and colleagues[56,62] suggested that PTSD is characterized by a pathological network in memory that is particularly large and easily triggered. It contains many stimulus propositions that are erroneously linked to danger, causing fear responses to harmless stimuli associated with the traumatic event in memory. In addition, the person's reactions during the trauma are linked to the belief that the self is incompetent. Activation of components of the trauma memory (for instance, by confrontation to a reminder, by similar bodily sensations, or by thinking about the event) will activate the whole network, including the emotional responses that the person had during the traumatic event.

Brewin and colleagues[66] have proposed that the symptoms of PTSD can only be explained if one assumes several levels of representation of the traumatic event, for example verbally accessible memory and memory that is triggered by situation-specific cues. PTSD is thought to be characterized by easily accessible situationally specific memories.

Patients with PTSD may not only have deficits in their autobiographical memories of the traumatic event, but the organization of the autobiographical memory base in general may be affected.[58] Patients with PTSD have difficulty retrieving specific autobiographical memories and exhibit overgeneral memories, similar to depressed patients.[6] These memory deficits may be linked to poor problem-solving and enhanced stress responses to everyday stressors, a sense of foreshortened future (because the overgeneral memory of the past makes it difficult to envisage a future), and more frequent stimulus-driven retrieval of memories of the traumatic event leading to re-experiencing symptoms.

Behaviours that maintain PTSD symptoms

Whereas many people will recover from initial PTSD symptoms, some do not get better. This has led researchers to specify possible maintaining behaviours. These include avoidance of reminders, suppression of thoughts and memories connected to the event, rumination, safety behaviours, dissociation, and the use of alcohol or drugs. Ehlers and Clark[58] suggested that these behaviours and cognitive strategies maintain PTSD in three ways. First, some behaviours directly lead to increases in symptoms; for example, thought suppression leads to paradoxical increases in intrusion frequency. Second, other behaviours prevent changes in the problematic appraisals; for example, constantly checking one's rear mirror (a safety behaviour) after a car accident prevents change in the appraisal that another accident will happen if one does not check the mirror. Third, other behaviours prevent elaboration of the trauma memory and its link to other experiences. For example, avoiding thinking about the event prevents people from incorporating the fact that they did not die into the trauma memory, and they thus continue to re-experience the fear of dying they originally experienced during the event. Several studies have found that avoidance, safety behaviours, thought suppression, and rumination predict maintenance of PTSD.[15,41]

Some of the cognitive processes that maintain PTSD symptoms are not intentional. Patients with PTSD have an unintentional attentional bias to stimuli that are reminiscent of the traumatic event.[6] Involun-tary selective attention to reminders may be one of the reasons why these patients have frequent re-experiencing symptoms. Rumination is often described by the patient as unintentional. In particular, patients have problems stopping ruminating once they have started. Rumination may represent a cognitive habit that started as an intentional strategy employed to solve problems and that became more automatic with time.

Biological processes

A number of biological factors have been linked to PTSD symptoms. They have the effect that they make people with PTSD hyper-responsive to stressful stimuli, especially stimuli that are reminiscent of the trauma.[67]

Chronic stress reaction

Patients with PTSD show several abnormalities that are consistent with a chronic stress reaction or an enhanced reactivity to minor stressors. There is evidence for a chronically enhanced secretion of adrenaline (epinephrine) and noradrenaline (norepinephrine). In psychophysiological studies, patients with PTSD showed enhanced startle responses and higher baseline heart rates and blood pressure than traumatized controls without PTSD. However, these responses may, in part, reflect anticipatory anxiety related to the expectation of trauma cues. Patients with PTSD exhibit greater physiological reactivity to trauma cues (e.g. sounds, pictures, or guided imagery) than control subjects without PTSD.[6]

Hypothalamic–pituitary–adrenal axis abnormalities

Patients with current PTSD show abnormally low levels of cortisol compared to normal controls and traumatized individuals without current PTSD. In addition, PTSD patients have an increased number of lymphocyte glucocorticoid receptors. When given a low dose of dexamethasone, PTSD patients exhibit hypersuppression of cortisol. Thus, patients with PTSD show a very different pattern of hypothalamic–pituitary–adrenal response than patients with major depression. The pattern of findings suggests that the hypothalamic–pituitary–adrenal axis in PTSD is characterized by enhanced negative feedback.[68] There may also be a downregulation of corticotrophin-releasing factor receptors at the anterior pituitary due to chronic increases in this factor.[69] Overall, the pattern of findings suggests that, in PTSD, the hypothalamic–pituitary–adrenal axis is set to produce large responses to further stressors.

Neuroendocrinological abnormalities

Several neurotransmitter systems seem to be dysregulated in PTSD.[53] Research suggests a sensitization of the noradrenergic system, in particular, a downregulation of α_2-adrenergic receptors, in a subgroup of PTSD patients.[70] The downregulation of the α_2-adrenergic receptors is thought to lead to enhanced locus coeruleus activity and increased levels of noradrenaline. This could cause the symptoms of autonomic hyperarousal and re-experiencing (through the effects on β-adrenergic receptors in the amygdalae and cortical structures). Yohimbine (which blocks the α_2-receptors) provokes flashbacks and panic attacks in a substantial subgroup of PTSD patients.

Another subgroup of PTSD seems to be characterized by a sensitized serotonergic system. They respond to meta-chlorophenylpiper-azine with panic attacks and PTSD symptoms such as flashbacks.[70] In animals, serotonin depletion has been linked to hyperirritability and inability to modulate arousal. These effects parallel the hyperarousal symptoms in PTSD. Serotonin controls the function of the septohip-pocampal behavioural inhibition system. Sensitization of this system will lead to a impaired distinction between reward, punishment, novelty and frustrative non-reward with the consequence that the behavioural inhibition system can be activated by mild everyday stressors.[67]

Endogenous opiates have been suspected to mediate the symptoms of emotional numbing and amnesia. In the animal model, uncontrollable stress leads to the secretion of endogenous opiates that induce analgesia. Patients with PTSD show conditioned secretion of endorphins and analgesia when confronted with reminders of the traumatic event.[67]

Veterans with PTSD show enhanced levels of corticotrophin-releasing factor (**CRF**) in their cerebrospinal fluid compared to normal controls.[69] Intraventricular administration of CRF has been shown to lead to enhanced plasma adrenaline and noradrenaline concentrations and anxiety and fear-related behaviours in animals, and it is thus thought that the enhanced CRF levels could cause these symptoms in PTSD patients.

The dopaminergic, γ-aminobutyric acid, and *N*-methyl-D-aspartate systems have also been implicated in PTSD, but the evidence for these hypotheses is sparse at this stage.

Thyroid function

Some studies have found an increased levels of thyroid hormones in patients with PTSD. These correlated with the severity of hyperarousal symptoms.[67]

Neuroimaging

Magnetic resonance imaging studies have shown a reduced hippocampal volume in veterans and women with a history of childhood sexual abuse. This line of research was prompted by animal studies showing that high levels of cortisol seen during stress are associated with damage to the hippocampus.[71] Disturbances of hippocampal function may lead to enhanced reactivity to stimulation, and may be involved in the deficits in autobiographical memory observed in PTSD patients.[6] It remains unclear whether the decreased hippocampal volume is a risk factor for the development of PTSD or a consequence of chronic PTSD.

It has been suggested that PTSD is characterized by dysfunctions in the amygdalae or the areas that project to them (the hippocampus, septum, and prefrontal cortex), leading to problems in the extinction of fear responses to reminders of the traumatic event.[53] Animal studies established that conditioned fear responses could only be extinguished if the cortex was intact.[72] Consistent with possible deficits in cortical control, positron emission tomography studies have shown a relative decrease in middle temporal blood flow (and several adjacent medial prefrontal areas) in patients with PTSD relative to controls when they imagined the traumatic event or were presented with reminders of it. The middle temporal cortex plays a role in the extinction of fear through inhibition of amygdala function. At the same time, PTSD patients showed increased blood flow in the limbic regions (parahippocampus and cingulate).[71]

Animal models of PTSD

There are biological and psychological parallels between the animal model of inescapable shock and exposure to a traumatic event. The uncontrollability of an aversive event seems to make it particularly traumatic.[73] Inescapable shock leads to changes in the noradrenergic system, the HPA axis, and endogenous opiates that parallel findings in PTSD patients.[53]

However, these effects are usually only observed after repeated exposure to inescapable shock, whereas one traumatic event can be sufficient in inducing PTSD. This is why some authors have suggested that the animal model of kindling or behavioural sensitization is more appropriate in explaining PTSD. Kindling refers to a process whereby intermittent subconvulsive electrical stimulation of the limbic system eventually has the effect that the animal will respond with a seizure to a stimulus that previously was subthreshold. Post *et al.*[74] have suggested that the repeated re-experiencing of the traumatic event may constitute a kindling process, to the effect that PTSD symptoms become more easily triggered with time. Similarly, previous exposure to stressors may sensitize people to respond with PTSD symptoms to a traumatic event.

Animal models suggest that the massive secretion of neurohormones at the time of the trauma, in particular noradrenaline and vasopressin, leads to overconsolidation (long-term potentiation) of the trauma memory. This would have the effect that the conditioned fear responses are particularly difficult to extinguish and that stimuli that resemble those present during trauma are particularly likely to trigger intrusive memories, distress, and/or the corresponding physiological responses.[67]

Genetic factors

Twin studies have found a higher concordance of PTSD among monozygotic than dizygotic twins. There is also an increased prevalence of psychiatric disorders, especially anxiety disorders, affective disorders, sociopathy, and/or substance abuse, among family members of people with PTSD.[75]

Course and prognosis

Time course of symptoms

For the vast majority of PTSD cases, symptoms begin immediately after the traumatic event. Delayed onset is found in a minority (11 per cent or less) of the cases.[6]

A series of prospective longitudinal studies suggest that a large proportion of people who initially develop PTSD recover within the first year after a traumatic event. For example, a study of rape victims found that 94 per cent met PTSD criteria (with the exception of the symptom duration criterion) in the 2 weeks after the trauma, and 65 per cent, 47 per cent, and 42 per cent at 1, 3, and 6 months, respectively.[76] Across different studies, it can be estimated that about 50 per cent of those with initial PTSD symptoms will recover during the first year. Long-term outcome depends on initial symptom severity. People with high initial PTSD severity were more likely to remain symptomatic at follow-up than those with low initial symptom severity.[41]

The substantial rate of initial recovery does not imply, however, that PTSD in general has a good prognosis. A substantial proportion of traumatized individuals will suffer long-standing morbidity after a traumatic event. Retrospective studies suggest that about one-third of people who develop PTSD after a traumatic event will not recover for many years.[31]

Factors that influence the risk of developing PTSD

Demographic variables and pretrauma personality

Women are at greater risk of developing PTSD than men, and black and Hispanic people are at greater risk than Caucasians.[8,31,39,77] As yet, the mechanisms of these relationships remain unclear.

A personal or family history of psychiatric disorders, especially mood and anxiety disorders, increases the risk of PTSD.[38,39,75,78] Previous traumatic experiences, in particular childhood sexual or physical abuse,[38,79,80] childhood separation from parents,[39] and family instability[80] are also associated with a higher risk of PTSD.

Among the personality variables predicting PTSD are low intelligence,[81] neuroticism,[38,78] low self-esteem,[82] external locus of control,[83] and pre-existing negative beliefs about the self and the world.[15] Political activism appears to be protective in torture survivors.[84]

Stressor variables

PTSD risk depends on the severity of the stressor. Prolonged and repeated trauma, exposure to the grotesque aftermath of violence, events that involve intentional harm by another person and abusive violence, and events that involve harm to children are particularly likely to lead to PTSD.[11,59,85,86]

Injury severity is only a weak predictor of PTSD. Long-term health problems and loss of function may play a greater role in maintaining PTSD.[41,85] There are some reports that unconsciousness during a traumatic event may decrease the risk of PTSD,[87] but other studies have found small associations in the opposite direction.[41]

Psychological responses during trauma

PTSD risk depends on the degree of psychological distress the traumatic event caused. The psychological impact of the trauma depends on the perceived threat to life,[11] the perceived loss of control (helplessness),[88] causal attributions[89] and the perceived threat to one's autonomy (mental defeat).[14] Among the psychological responses predicting PTSD are feelings of anger, guilt, or shame[90,91] and dissociation and numbing.[92,93]

Factors affecting recovery from trauma

Recovery environment

Recovery is facilitated by social support and the absence of negative responses from others after the event.[15,83,94,95] Further stressful or traumatic life events impede recovery from PTSD.[95–97] This includes the stress caused by long-lasting negative effects of the event on health and personal appearance, financial difficulties, disruptions in everyday life, and ongoing litigation.[41,87,96]

Psychological processes

Excessively negative appraisals of the traumatic event impede recovery (e.g. 'Nowhere is safe', 'I cannot trust anyone', 'I am inadequate').[15,57,60] If individuals interpret their initial PTSD symptoms as signs that they are going mad or losing control, or as signs of a permanent change for the worse, they are less likely to recover.[15,41]

If individuals engage in behaviours or cognitive coping styles that prevent them from 'working through' and accepting the trauma, they are less likely to recover. Such maladaptive behaviours include avoidance, not talking about the experience, safety behaviours, denial, thought suppression, and rumination.[15,41,83,94,98]

Treatment of PTSD

Several psychological and pharmacological treatments are effective in PTSD. The effect sizes (Cohen's d statistic) given below are taken from a recent meta-analysis of 61 treatment-outcome trials.[99] The difference between the pre- and post-treatment scores is divided by the pooled standard deviation of the pre- and post-treatment scores. An effect size $d = 1$ means that the treatment led to improvement by one standard deviation. In interpreting the effect sizes, one has to bear in mind that PTSD patients in pill-placebo or waiting-list conditions also showed some improvement. Mean effect sizes for these conditions were $d = 0.77$ and $d = 0.75$ for observer-rated PTSD symptoms, and $d = 0.51$ and $d = 0.44$ for self-rated PTSD symptoms.

Psychological treatments

Cognitive-behavioural therapy

Cognitive-behavioural treatments are effective in the treatment of PTSD. The meta-analysis[99] reported mean effect sizes of $d = 1.89$ for observer-rated and $d = 1.27$ for self-rated PTSD symptoms. This analysis included several versions of cognitive-behavioural therapy that are described below.

Education

All versions of cognitive-behavioural therapy include some form of education about the symptoms of PTSD and treatment rationales. Common reactions to trauma are explained to normalize the patient's PTSD symptoms. The therapists explains the necessity of confronting the memory of the traumatic event and of giving up behaviours that maintain the problem such as avoidance and safety behaviours.

Self-monitoring of symptoms

Most cognitive-behavioural therapy treatments include some form of self-monitoring that may in itself be therapeutic. Tarrier *et al.*[100] found that 4 weeks of systematic self-monitoring of intrusive symptoms led to considerable and stable improvement in about 10 per cent of the cases studied.

Exposure

Exposure treatment comprises two components.[62] In imaginal exposure, patients are asked to relive the traumatic event in their imagination, including their thoughts and feelings at the time. This is repeated until the reliving no longer evokes high levels of distress. *In vivo* exposure involves confronting (safe) situations that patients avoid because they remind them of the trauma (e.g. going to the site of the traumatic event, driving again after a road traffic accident). Exposure is repeated until the patient no longer responds with high levels of distress. There are probably several mechanisms for the efficacy of exposure treatment.[58,62] First, patients realize that exposure does not lead to a feared outcome (for example, going to the site of an accident will not mean that another accident will happen; thinking about the trauma will not make them go mad) and thus helps in correcting dysfunctional beliefs about danger of the world and the meaning of PTSD symptoms. Second, the repeated reliving of the event helps them to create an organized memory and facilitates the distinction that intrusive thoughts and images are memories rather than something happening right now.

Exposure treatment is superior to supportive psychotherapy and relaxation treatment.[101,102] Whereas exposure treatment is effective in the majority of cases, a minority of patients become worse.[100] In particular, exposure treatment does not appear suitable for patients whose traumatic memories are about being perpetrators rather than victims.[101] It may also have limits in treating survivors of complex and prolonged traumatic events such as torture, war, or captivity.[103]

Cognitive therapy/restructuring

Cognitive therapy identifies and modifies excessively negative appraisals of the traumatic event and/or its sequelae.[57,104] Methods include discussion of the evidence for and against the appraisals, identification of thinking errors, challenging of appraisals with behavioural tests, and imagery modification. Recent studies have shown that cognitive therapy is effective on its own, without additional exposure treatment.[100,102] When verbal challenging of dysfunctional beliefs was used as an additional treatment after a session of imaginal exposure, it did not lead to additional treatment gains.[102]

Anxiety management (stress inoculation)

The goal of this treatment is to teach the patient a set of skills that will help them cope with stress. Examples include relaxation training, training in slow abdominal breathing, thought stopping of unwanted thoughts, assertiveness training, and training in positive thinking.[59] Anxiety management is more effective than supportive psychotherapy. In the long term it appears to be somewhat less effective than exposure treatment.[101] Relaxation treatment alone is less effective than exposure and cognitive therapy in the short and long term.[102]

Anger management

An anger management programme for PTSD patients with severe anger reactions is more effective in reducing anger than routine clinical care.[105]

Eye-movement desensitization reprocessing

This is a relatively new and controversial treatment.[106] The patient is instructed to focus on a trauma-related image and its accompanying feelings, sensations, and thoughts, while visually tracking the therapist's fingers as they move back and forth in front of the patient's eyes. After a set of approximately 24 eye movements, cognitive and emotional reactions are discussed with the therapist. Coping statements are also introduced while the scene is being imagined. A series of studies have established that eye-movement desensitization reprocessing is effective, at least for self-rated PTSD symptoms. Mean effect sizes were $d = 0.69$ for observer-rated and $d = 1.24$ for self-rated PTSD symptoms. For self-rated symptoms, eye-movement desensitization reprocessing effect sizes were larger than those of control conditions. The mechanism of treatment is not yet understood. Recent studies have shown that the eye movements are not a necessary component of the treatment.[99]

Psychodynamic therapy

The treatment focuses on understanding the meaning of the traumatic event in the context of the patient's previous experiences, personality, and attitudes. The goal of the treatment is to work through and resolve an unconscious conflict which the traumatic event is thought to have provoked. One controlled study of psychodynamic therapy showed an effect size of $d = 0.90$ for self-rated PTSD symptoms.[99] Psychodynamic therapy was more effective than the waiting-list condition in that study. Further uncontrolled reports indicated that psychodynamic therapy may be effective.[101,103] More studies are needed to evaluate whether this holds up in controlled studies.

Hypnotherapy

The patient is given instructions to induce a state of highly focused attention, a reduced awareness of peripheral stimuli, and a heightened suggestibility. The goal of this treatment is to enhance control over trauma-related emotional distress and hyperarousal symptoms and to facilitate the recollection of details of the traumatic event. One controlled study of hypnotherapy showed an effect size of $d = 0.94$ for self-rated PTSD symptoms.[99] Hypnotherapy was more effective than the waiting-list condition in that study. Shalev et al.[103] raise concerns about the use of hypnotherapy in the treatment of PTSD as it may induce dissociative states.

Pharmacological treatments

Selective serotonin-reuptake inhibitors (SSRIs)

SSRIs (sertraline, fluvoxamine, fluoxetine) are effective in the treatment of PTSD symptoms.[107] They affect all the PTSD symptoms, including the avoidance, numbing, and hyperarousal symptoms.[108] The meta-analysis showed mean effect sizes of $d = 1.43$ for observer-rated and $d = 1.38$ for self-rated PTSD symptoms.[99] Across studies, the SSRIs were more effective than all other drug therapies. SSRIs are an attractive choice because they reduce alcohol consumption; a relevant finding given the high comorbidity of PTSD with substance abuse or dependency.[108] Despite the overall impressive effects, SSRIs may not be effective in all populations of PTSD patients. One study showed that fluoxetine was significantly superior to placebo in civilians in a trauma clinic, but not in combat veterans in a Veterans Administration Hospital.[107]

Monoamine oxidase inhibitors (MAOIs)

Phenelzine has shown good effects on re-experiencing symptoms and insomnia, but weak effects on avoidance, numbing, and hyperarousal symptoms.[108] However, the meta-analysis did not find the MAOIs to be significantly more effective than control conditions such as a pill placebo or a waiting list.[99] Effect sizes were $d = 0.92$ for observer-rated and $d = 0.61$ for self-rated PTSD symptoms. Some studies may have underestimated the MAOI effects because of an inadequate length of treatment.[108] Thus, MAOIs such as phenelzine may be useful in the treatment of PTSD, but cannot be considered among the first-choice treatments because of the risks of hypertensive crisis and the necessary dietary restrictions.[107] The development and evaluation of reversible inhibitors of monoamine oxidase type A such as moclobemide for the treatment of PTSD appears promising.[107,108]

Tricyclic antidepressants

Evidence for the efficacy of tricyclic antidepressants is mixed. If at all, they seem to be effective in less severe cases of PTSD.[107] These agents seem to mainly affect the re-experiencing rather than the avoidance, numbing, and hyperarousal symptoms of PTSD.[108] The mean effect sizes across studies were not significantly greater than for pill-placebo or waiting-list controls,[99] $d = 0.86$ for observer-rated and $d = 0.54$ for self-rated PTSD symptoms. Some of the studies may have failed to find a drug effect because the treatment length was insufficient.[107] Two trials of combat veterans administered amitriptyline or imipramine for 8 weeks found that 35 per cent more patients improved with the tricyclic antidepressant than with placebo. However, treatment was less effective the more severe the symptoms were and the greater the combat exposure had been.

Anticonvulsants

Anticonvulsants (carbamazepine, valproate) have shown promising effects in preliminary studies, but have not yet been widely investigated.[108] Effect sizes in a study of carbamazepine were $d = 1.45$ for observer-rated and $d = 0.93$ for self-rated PTSD symptoms.[99] It has been estimated that about 65 per cent of PTSD patients respond to anticonvulsant therapy.[107]

Benzodiazepines

Benzodiazepines do not appear to be effective in the treatment of PTSD. They do not affect the re-experiencing, avoidance, and numbing symptoms, although they may show some effects on insomnia, irritability, and general anxiety and arousal symptoms.[108] The effect sizes in one study were $d = 0.54$ for observer-rated and $d = 0.49$ for self-rated PTSD symptoms,[99] and these were not different from pill-placebo or waiting-list controls. In addition to the poor efficacy, caution is warranted with short-acting benzodiazepines such as alprazolam. They may pose a particular problem with PTSD patients because they may cause a rebound syndrome upon discontinuation including anxiety, sleep disturbance, nightmares, and rage reactions.[107]

Antiadrenergic agents

Although adrenergic dysregulation is associated with chronic PTSD, antiadrenergic agents have received little attention as a treatment option. Several case reports and open trials found positive effects of propanolol or clonidine on PTSD symptoms.[108] It remains to be investigated whether these results hold up in controlled trials.

Advice on management

Diagnosing PTSD

In diagnosing PTSD, clinicians need to ascertain that patients experienced a traumatic event and that they involuntarily re-experience the event. In addition, patients will show symptoms of hyperarousal, avoidance, and emotional numbing. Self-report instruments such as the Post-traumatic Stress Diagnostic Scale[29] or semistructured interviews such as the Clinician Administered PTSD Scale[25] are useful in assessing the symptom pattern. The DSM-IV criterion of a minimum of three avoidance or numbing symptoms appears too strict for clinical purposes. It does not appear justified to withhold treatment if the patient is distressed by the PTSD symptoms but fails to meet this criterion.

Choice of treatment

The best treatment options of PTSD to date are cognitive-behavioural treatments and SSRIs. Effect sizes of these treatments are comparable. Psychological treatments have the advantage of lower drop-out rates. The meta-analysis found that, across studies, 14 per cent of the patients dropped out of psychological treatments, compared with 36 per cent for the SSRIs.[99] An additional advantage of cognitive-behavioural treatments is their established long-term effectiveness. Treatment gains are maintained during follow-up.[99,109] In contrast, long-term follow-up studies are lacking for pharmacological treatments, so that it is not known whether treatment-effects are maintained when medications are withdrawn or when they are continued for long periods. The advantage of SSRIs compared to cognitive-behavioural treatment is that they are more readily available.

Recent expert consensus guidelines concluded that cognitive-behavioural treatments are the treatment of choice for PTSD. For very severe or special cases (e.g. geriatric patients) the combination of these psychological treatments with pharmacotherapy is recommended as an alternative to psychological treatment alone.[110]

Special considerations may apply to subgroups of PTSD patients. The efficacy of psychological treatments in patients with comorbid substance dependence remains to be established. It has been suggested that SSRIs are particularly useful for these patients,[108] but controlled trials are lacking.

Special problems in the management of PTSD patients

Avoidance is one of the main symptoms of PTSD, and it can thus take years for the patient to seek help for this condition. It is important for clinicians to bear in mind that even those who seek help may find it hard to talk about the traumatic experience, and may show signs of avoidance such as irregular attendance or failure to disclose the worst moments of the trauma initially. Therapeutic techniques to deal with this problem include empathy, gradual encouragement, and giving the patient control over the timing and mode of working through the experience (e.g. writing, talking into a tape recorder, reliving with the support of the therapist).

One of the requirements for change is that the patient feels safe. Therapists therefore have to make sure that they establish a good relationship with the patient, and that the therapeutic setting or their behaviour does not remind the patient of the traumatic event. Sometimes support in changing living circumstances may be necessary if they prevent the patient from being safe (e.g. moving house if assaulted by a neighbour).

Patients with PTSD often suffer from poor sleep and concentration, and find it painful to face reminders of the trauma. For these reasons, they have difficulty in dealing with the aftermath of traumatic events such as legal procedures and continuing treatment for physical injuries, including the long delays that this usually involves. Such ongoing stressors impede recovery, and patients may therefore benefit from problem-solving and practical advice.

References

1. Gersons, B.P.R. and Carlier, I.V.E. (1992). Post-traumatic stress disorder: the history of a recent concept. *British Journal of Psychiatry*, **161**, 742–8.

2. Kinzie, J.D. and Goetz, R.R. (1996). A century of controversy surrounding post-traumatic stress-spectrum syndromes: the impact of DSM-III and DSM-IV. *Journal of Traumatic Stress*, **9**, 159–79.

3. Van der Kolk, B.A., Weisaeth, L., and Van der Hart, O. (1996). History of trauma in psychiatry. In *Traumatic stress* (ed. B.A. van der Kolk, A.C. McFarlane, and L. Weisaeth), pp. 47–74. Guilford Press, New York.

4. American Psychiatric Association (1980). *Diagnostic and statistical manual of mental disorders* (3rd edn). American Psychiatric Association, Washington, DC.

5. World Health Organization (1992). *International statistical classification of diseases and related health problems, 10th revision*. WHO, Geneva

6. McNally, R.J. (2000). Post-traumatic stress disorder. In *Oxford textbook of psychopathology* (ed. T. Millon, P.H. Blaney, and R.D. Davis). Oxford University Press.

7. American Psychiatric Association (1987). *Diagnostic and statistical manual of mental disorders* (3rd edn revised). American Psychiatric Association, Washington, DC.

8. Norris, F.H. (1992). Epidemiology of trauma: frequency and impact of different potentially traumatic events on different demographic groups. *Journal of Consulting and Clinical Psychology*, **60**, 409–18.

9. Resnick, H.S., Kilpatrick, D.G., Dansky, B.S., Saunders, B.E., and Best, C.L. (1993). Prevalence of civilian trauma and post-traumatic stress disorder in a representative national sample of women. *Journal of Consulting and Clinical Psychology*, **61**, 984–91.

10. American Psychiatric Association (1994). *Diagnostic and statistical manual of mental disorders* (4th edn). American Psychiatric Association, Washington, DC.

11. March, J.S. (1993). What constitutes a stressor? The 'Criterion A' issue. In *Post-traumatic stress disorder: DSM-IV and beyond* (ed. J.R.T. Davidson and E.B. Foa), pp. 37–56. American Psychiatric Press, Washington, DC.

12. Roemer, L., Orsillo, S.M., Borkovec, T.D., and Litz, B.T. (1998). Emotional response at the time of a potentially traumatizing event and PTSD symptomatology: a preliminary retrospective analysis of the DSM-IV criterion A-2. *Journal of Behavioural Therapy and Experimental Psychiatry*, **29**, 123–30.

13. Yehuda, R., Southwick, S.M., and Giller, E.L. (1992). Exposure to atrocities and severity of chronic post-traumatic stress disorder in Vietnam combat veterans. *American Journal of Psychiatry*, **149**, 333–6.

14. Ehlers, A., Maercker, A., and Boos, A. PTSD following political imprisonment: the role of mental defeat, alienation, and perceived permanent change. *Journal of Abnormal Psychology*, in press.

15. Dunmore, E., Clark, D.M., and Ehlers, A. (1999). Cognitive factors involved in the onset and maintenance of post-traumatic stress disorder (PTSD) after physical or sexual assault. *Behaviour Research and Therapy*, **37**, 809–30.

16. Brett, E.A. (1996). The classification of post-traumatic stress disorder. In *Traumatic stress* (ed. B.A. van der Kolk, A.C. McFarlane, and L. Weisaeth), pp. 117–28. Guilford Press, New York.

17. Davidson, J.R.T. and Foa, E.B. (1991). Diagnostic issues in post-traumatic stress disorder: consideration for the DSM-IV and beyond. *Journal of Abnormal Psychology*, **100**, 346–55.

18. World Health Organization (1993). *The ICD-10 classification of mental and behavioural disorders. Diagnostic criteria for research*. World Health Organization, Geneva.

19. Andrews, G., Slade, T., and Peters, L. (1999). Classification in psychiatry: ICD-10 versus DSM-IV. *British Journal of Psychiatry*, **174**, 3–5.

20. Herman, J.L. (1992). Complex PTSD: a syndrome in survivors of prolonged and repeated trauma. *Journal of Traumatic Stress*, **5**, 377–91.

21. Horowitz, M.J. (1997). *Stress response syndromes. PTSD, grief, and adjustment disorders*. Jason Aronson, Northvale, NJ.

22. Prigerson, H.G., Shear, M.K., Jacobs, S.C., *et al.* (1999). Consensus criteria for traumatic grief. A preliminary empirical test. *British Journal of Psychiatry*, **174**, 67–73.

23. Foa, E.B, Riggs, D.S., and Gershuny, B.S. (1995). Arousal, numbing, and intrusion: symptom structure of PTSD following assault. *American Journal of Psychiatry*, **152**, 116–20.

24. First, M.B., Spitzer, R.L., Gibbon, M., and Williams, J.B.W. (1995). *Structured clinical interview for DSM-IV Axis I disorders—patient version (SCID-I/P, Version 2.0)*. Biometrics Research Department of the New York State Psychiatric Institute, New York.

25. Blake, D.D., Weathers, F.W., Nagy, L.M., *et al.* (1995). The development of a clinician-administered PTSD scale. *Journal of Traumatic Stress*, **8**, 75–90.

26. Brown, T.A., DiNardo, P.A., and Barlow. D.H. (1994). *Anxiety disorders interview schedule for DSM-IV*. Graywind, Albany, NY.

27. Horowitz, M.J., Wilner, N., and Alvarez, W. (1979). Impact of Event Scale: a measure of subjective stress. *Psychosomatic Medicine*, **41**, 209–18.

28. Weiss, D.S. and Marmar, C. R. (1997). The Impact of Event Scale—Revised. In *Assessing psychological trauma and PTSD* (ed. J.P Wilson, and T.M. Keane), pp. 399–411. Guilford Press, New York.

29. Foa, E.B., Cashman, L., Jaycox, L., and Perry, K. (1997). The validation of a self-report measure of post-traumatic stress disorder: the post-traumatic diagnostic scale. *Psychological Assessment*, **9**, 445–51.

30. McFarlane, A.C. and de Girolamo, G. (1996). The nature of traumatic stressors and the epidemiology of post-traumatic reactions. In *Traumatic stress* (ed. B.A. van der Kolk, A.C. McFarlane, and L. Weisaeth), pp. 129–54. Guilford Press, New York.

31. Kessler, R.C., Sonnega, A., Bromet. E., Hughes, M., and Nelson, C.B. (1995). Post-traumatic stress disorder in the National Comorbidity Survey. *Archives of General Psychiatry*, **52**, 1048–60.

32. Stein, M.B., Walker, J.R., Hazen, A.L., and Forde, D.R. (1997). Full and partial post-traumatic stress disorder: findings from a community survey. *American Journal of Psychiatry*, **154**, 1114–19.

33. Breslau, N., Kessler, R.C., Chilcoat, H.D., Schultz, L.R., Davis, G.C., and Andreski, P. (1998). Trauma and post-traumatic stress disorder in the community. *Archives of General Psychiatry*, **55**, 626.

34. Maercker, A. and Schützwohl, M. (1997). Longterm effects of political imprisonment: a group comparison study. *Social Psychiatry and Psychiatric Epidemiology*, **32**, 435–42.

35. Kuch, K. and Cox, B.J. (1992). Symptoms of PTSD in 124 survivors of the Holocaust. *American Journal of Psychiatry*, **149**, 337–40.

36. Engdahl, B.E., Dikel, T.N., Eberly, R., and Blank, A. (1997). Post-traumatic stress disorder in a community group of former prisoners of war: a normative response to severe trauma. *American Journal of Psychiatry*, **154**, 1576–81.

37. Mayou, R.A. and Smith, K.A. (1997). Post traumatic symptoms following medical illness and treatment. *Journal of Psychosomatic Research*, **43**, 121–3.

38. Breslau, N., Davis, G.C., Andreski, P., and Peterson, E. (1991). Traumatic events and post-traumatic stress disorder in an urban population of young adults. *Archives of General Psychiatry*, **48**, 216–22.

39. Breslau, N., Davis, G.C., Andreski, P., Peterson, E.L., and Schultz, L.R. (1997). Sex differences in post-traumatic stress disorder. *Archives of General Psychiatry*, **54**, 1044–8.

40. Blanchard, E.B. and Hickling, E.J. (1997). *After the crash. Assessment and treatment of motor vehicle survivors*. American Psychological Association, Washington, DC.

41. Ehlers, A., Mayou, R.A., and Bryant, B. (1998). Psychological predictors of chronic post-traumatic stress disorder after motor vehicle accidents. *Journal of Abnormal Psychology*, **107**, 508–19.

42. Davidson, J.R.T., Hughes, D., Blazer, D., and George, L.K. (1991). Post-traumatic stress disorder in the community: an epidemiological study. *Psychological Medicine*, **21**, 1–19.

43. Helzer, J.E., Robins, L.N., and McEnvoy, L. (1987). Post-traumatic stress disorder in the general population. *New England Journal of Medicine*, **317**, 1630–4.

44. Solomon, S.D. and Davidson, J.R.T. (1997). Trauma: prevalence, impairment, service use, and cost. *Journal of Clinical Psychiatry*, **58**, 5–11.

45. Jordan, B.K., Marmar, C.R., Fairbank, J.A., *et al.*. (1992). Problems in families of male Vietnam veterans with post-traumatic stress disorder. *Journal of Consulting and Clinical Psychology*, **60**, 916–26.

46. Beckham, J.C., Kirby, A.C., Feldman, M.E., *et al.* (1997). Prevalence and correlates of heavy smoking in Vietnam veterans with chronic post-traumatic stress disorder. *Addictive Behaviors*, **22**, 637–47.

47. Boscarino, J.A. (1997). Diseases among men 20 years after exposure to severe stress: implications for clinical research and medical care. *Psychosomatic Medicine*, **59**, 605–14.

48. Andreski, P., Chilcoat, H., and Breslau, N. (1998). Post-traumatic stress disorder and somatization symptoms: a prospective study. *Psychiatry Research*, **79**, 131–8.

49. Chilcoat, H.D. and Breslau, N. (1998). Post-traumatic stress disorder and drug disorders. *Archives of General Psychiatry*, **55**, 913–17.

50. Stewart, S.H. (1996). Alcohol abuse in individuals exposed to trauma: a critical review. *Psychological Bulletin*, **120**, 83–112.

51. McFarlane, A.C. (1998). Epidemiological evidence about the relationship between PTSD and alcohol abuse: the nature of the association. *Addictive Behaviors*, **23**, 813–25.

52. Mowrer, O.H. (1939). A stimulus-response analysis of anxiety and its role as a reinforcing agent. *Psychological Review*, **46**, 553–65.

53. Charney, D., Deutch, A.Y., Krystal, J.H., Southwick, S.M., and Davis, M. (1993). Psychobiological mechanisms of post-traumatic stress disorder. *Archives of General Psychiatry*, **50**, 294–305.

54. Keane, T.M., Zimering, R.T., and Caddell, J.M. (1985). A behavioral formulation of post-traumatic stress disorder. *Behavior Therapist*, **8**, 9–12.

55. Janoff-Bulman, R. (1992). *Shattered assumptions: toward a new psychology of trauma*. Free Press, New York.

56. Foa, E.B. and Riggs, D.S. (1993). Post-traumatic stress disorder in rape victims. In *Annual review of psychiatry*, Vol. 12 (ed. J. Oldham, M.B. Riba, and A. Tasman), pp. 273–303. American Psychiatric Association, Washington, DC.

57. Resick, P.A. and Schnicke, M.K. (1993). *Cognitive processing therapy for rape victims*. Sage, Newbury Park, CA.

58. Ehlers, A. and Clark, D.M. A cognitive model of persistent PTSD. *Behaviour Research and Therapy*, in press.

59. Meichenbaum, D. (1994). *Treating post-traumatic stress disorder. A handbook and practice manual for therapy*. Wiley, Chichester.

60. Foa, E.B., Ehlers, A., Clark, D.M., Tolin, D.F., and Orsillo, S.M. (1999). The post-traumatic cognitions inventory (PTCI): development and validation. *Psychological Assessment*, **11**, 303–14.

61. Ehlers, A. and Steil, R. (1995). Maintenance of intrusive memories in post-traumatic stress disorder: a cognitive approach. *Behavioural and Cognitive Psychotherapy*, **23**, 217–49.

62. Foa, E.B. and Rothbaum, B.O. (1998). *Treating the trauma of rape. Cognitive–behavior therapy for PTSD*. Guilford Press, New York.

63. Van der Kolk, B.A. and Fisler, R. (1995). Dissociation and the fragmentary nature of traumatic memories: overview and exploratory study. *Journal of Traumatic Stress*, **8**, 505–25.

64. Foa, E.B., Molnar, C., and Cashman, L. (1995). Change in rape narratives during exposure therapy for post-traumatic stress disorder. *Journal of Traumatic Stress*, **8**, 675–90.

65. Conway, M.A. (1997). Introduction: what are memories? In *Recovered memories and false memories* (ed. M.A. Conway), pp. 1–22. Oxford University Press.

66. Brewin, C.R., Dalgleish, T., and Joseph, S. (1996). A dual representation theory of post-traumatic stress disorder. *Psychological Review*, **103**, 670–86.

67. Van der Kolk, B.A. (1996). The body keeps the score. Approaches to the psychobiology of post-traumatic stress disorder. In *Traumatic stress* (ed. B.A. van der Kolk, A.C. McFarlane, and L. Weisaeth), pp. 214–41. Guilford Press, New York.

68. Yehuda, R., Giller, E.L., Levengood, R.A., Southwick, S.M., and Siever, L.J. (1995). Hypothalamic–pituitary–adrenal functioning in post-traumatic stress disorder: expanding the concept of the stress response spectrum. In *Neurobiological and clinical consequences of stress: from normal adaptation to post-traumatic stress disorder* (ed. M.J. Friedman, D.S. Charney, and A.Y. Deutch), pp. 351–65. Lippincott–Raven, Philadelphia, PA.

69. Bremner, J.D., Licinio, J., Darnell, A., *et al.* (1997). Elevated CSF corticotropin-releasing factor concentrations in post-traumatic stress disorder. *American Journal of Psychiatry*, **154**, 624–9.

70. Southwick, S.M., Krystal, J.H., Bremner, J.D., *et al.* (1997). Noradrenergic and serotonergic function in post-traumatic stress disorder. *Archives of General Psychiatry*, **54**, 749–58.

71. Bremner, J.D. (1998). Neuroimaging of post-traumatic stress disorder. *Psychiatric Annals*, **28**, 445–50.

72. LeDoux, J.E. (1992). Emotion as memory: anatomical systems underlying indelible memory traces. In *Handbook of emotion and memory* (ed. S.A. Christianson), pp. 269–88. Erlbaum, Hillsdale, NJ.

73. Foa, E.B., Zinbarg, R., and Rothbaum, B.O. (1992). Uncontrollability and unpredictability in post-traumatic stress disorder: an animal model. *Psychological Bulletin*, **112**, 218–38.

74. Post, R.M., Weiss, S.R.B., and Smith, M.A. (1995). Sensitization and kindling: implications for the evolving neural substrates of post-traumatic stress disorder. In *Neurobiological and clinical consequences of stress: from normal adaptation to post-traumatic stress disorder* (ed. M.J. Friedman, D.S. Charney, and A.Y. Deutch), pp. 203–24. Lippincott–Raven, Philadelphia, PA.

75. Connor, K.M. and Davidson, J.R.T. (1997). Familial risk factors in post-traumatic stress disorder. *Annals of the New York Academy of Sciences*, **821**, 35–51.

76. Rothbaum, B.O., Foa, E.B., Riggs, D.S., Murdock, T.B., and Walsh, W. (1992). A prospective examination of post-traumatic stress disorder in rape victims. *Journal of Traumatic Stress*, **5**, 455–75.

77. Frueh, B.C., Brady, K.L., and Dearellano, M.A. (1998). Racial differences in combat-related PTSD: empirical findings and conceptual issues. *Clinical Psychology Review*, **18**, 287–305.

78. McFarlane, A.C. (1989). The aetiology of post-traumatic morbidity: predisposing, precipitating and perpetuating factors. *British Journal of Psychiatry*, **154**, 221–8.

79. Boney-McCoy, S. and Finkelhor, D. (1996). Is youth victimization related to trauma symptoms and depression after controlling for prior symptoms and family relationships? A longitudinal, prospective study. *Journal of Consulting and Clinical Psychology*, **64**, 1406–16.

80. King, D.W., King, L.A., Foy, D.W., and Gudanowski, D.M. (1996). Prewar factors in combat-related post-traumatic stress disorder: structural equation modeling with a national sample of female and male Vietnam veterans. *Journal of Consulting and Clinical Psychology*, **64**, 520–31.

81. McNally, R.J. and Shin, L.M. (1995). Association of intelligence with severity of post-traumatic stress disorder symptoms in Vietnam combat veterans. *American Journal of Psychiatry*, **152**, 936–8.

82. Darves-Bornoz, J.M., Lépine, J.P., Choquet, M., Berger, C., Degiovanni, A., and Gaillard, P. (1998). Predictive factors of chronic post-traumatic stress disorder in rape victims. *European Psychiatry*, **13**, 281–7.

83. Solomon, Z., Mikulincer, M., and Avitzur, E. (1988). Coping, locus of control, social support, and combat-related post-traumatic stress disorder. *Journal of Personality and Social Psychology*, **55**, 279–85.

84. Basoglu, M., Mineka, S., Paker, M., Aker, T., Livanou, M., and Gök, S. (1997). Psychological preparedness as a protective factor in survivors of torture. *Psychological Medicine*, **27**, 1421–33.

85. Green, B.L. (1994). Psychosocial research in traumatic stress: an update. *Journal of Traumatic Stress*, **7**, 341–62.

86. Clohessy, S. and Ehlers, A. (1999). PTSD symptoms, response to intrusive memories, and coping in ambulance service workers. *British Journal of Clinical Psychology*, **38**, 251–66.

87. Mayou, R.A., Bryant, B., and Duthie, R. (1993). Psychiatric consequences of road traffic accidents. *British Medical Journal*, **307**, 647–51.

88. Baum, A., Cohen, L., and Hall, M. (1993). Control and intrusive

memories as possible determinants of chronic stress. *Psychosomatic Medicine*, **55**, 274–86.

89. Joseph, S., Yule, W., and Williams, R. (1993). Post-traumatic stress: attributional aspects. *Journal of Traumatic Stress*, **6**, 501–13.

90. Andrews, B., Brewin, C.R., Rose, S., and Kirk, M. Predicting PTSD in victims of violent crime. Submitted for publication.

91. Riggs, D.S., Dancu, C.V., Gershuny, B.S., Greenberg, D., and Foa, E.B. (1992). Anger and post-traumatic stress disorder in female crime victims. *Journal of Traumatic Stress*, **5**, 613–25.

92. Koopman, C., Classen, C., and Spiegel, D. (1994). Predictors of post-traumatic stress symptoms among survivors of the Oakland/Berkeley, Calif. firestorm. *American Journal of Psychiatry*, **151**, 888–94.

93. Shalev, A.Y., Peri, T., Canetti, L., and Schreiber, S. (1996). Predictors of PTSD in injured trauma survivors: a prospective study. *American Journal of Psychiatry*, **153**, 219–25.

94. Carr, J.V., Lewin, T.J., Webster, R.A., Hazell, P.L., Kenardy, J.A., and Carter, G.L. (1995). Psychosocial sequelae of the 1989 Newcastle earthquake: I. Community disaster experiences and psychological morbidity 6 months post-disaster. *Psychological Medicine*, **25**, 539–55.

95. King, L.A., King, D.W., Fairbank, J.A., Keane, T.M., and Adams, G.A. (1998). Resilience-recovery factors in post-traumatic stress disorder among female and male Vietnam veterans: hardiness, postwar social support and additional stressful life events. *Journal of Personality and Social Psychology*, **74**, 420–34.

96. Carr, J.V., Lewin, T.J., Webster, R.A., Kenardy, J.A., Hazell, P.L., and Carter, G.L. (1997). Psychosocial sequelae of the 1989 Newcastle earthquake: II. Exposure and morbidity profiles during the first 2 years post-disaster. *Psychological Medicine*, **27**, 167–78.

97. Norris, F.N. and Kaniasty, K. (1994). Psychological distress following criminal victimization in the general population: cross-sectional, longitudinal and prospective analyses. *Journal of Consulting and Clinical Psychology*, **62**, 111–23.

98. Joseph, S., Dalgleish, T., Williams, R., Yule, W., Thrasher, S., and Hodgkinson, P. (1997). Attitudes towards emotional expression and post-traumatic stress in survivors of the Herald of Free Enterprise disaster. *British Journal of Clinical Psychology*, **36**, 133–8.

99. Van Etten, M.L. and Taylor, S. (1998). Comparative efficacy of treatments for post-traumatic stress disorder: a meta-analysis. *Clinical Psychology and Psychotherapy*, **5**, 126–44.

100. Tarrier, N., Pilgrim, H., Sommerfield, C., Faragher, B., Reynolds, M., Graham, E., and Barrowclough, C. (1999). A randomised trial of cognitive therapy and imaginal exposure in the treatment of chronic post traumatic stress disorder. *Journal of Consulting and Clinical Psychology*, **67**, 13–19.

101. Foa, E.B. and Meadows, E.A. (1997). Psychosocial treatments for post-traumatic stress disorder: a critical review. *Annual Review of Psychology*, **48**, 449–80.

102. Marks, I.M., Lovell, K., Norshirvani, H., Livanou, M., and Trasher, S. (1998). Treatment of post-traumatic stress disorder by exposure and/or cognitive restructuring. *Archives of General Psychiatry*, **55**, 317–25.

103. Shalev, A.Y., Bonne, O., and Eth, S. (1996). Treatment of post-traumatic stress disorder: a review. *Psychosomatic Medicine*, **58**, 165–82.

104. Beck, A.T. (1976). *Cognitive therapy and the emotional disorders.* International Universities Press, New York.

105. Chemtob, C.M., Novaco, R.W., Hamada, R.S., and Gross, D.M. (1997). Cognitive–behavioral treatment for severe anger in post-traumatic stress disorder. *Journal of Consulting and Clinical Psychology*, **65**, 184–9.

106. Shapiro, F. (1995). *Eye movement desensitization and reprocessing: basic principles, protocols, and procedures.* Guilford Press, New York.

107. Davidson, J.R.T. (1997). Biological therapies for post-traumatic stress disorder: an overview. *Journal of Clinical Psychiatry*, **58**, 29–32.

108. Friedman, M.J. (1998). Current and future drug treatment for post-traumatic stress disorder. *Psychiatric Annals*, **28**, 461–8.

109. Sherman, J.J. (1998). Effects of psychotherapeutic treatments for PTSD: a meta-analysis of controlled clinical trials. *Journal of Traumatic Stress*, **11**, 413–35.

110. Foa, E.B., Davidson, J.R.T., and Frances, A. (1999). The Expert Consensus Guideline Series. Treatment of post traumatic stress disorder. *Journal of Clinical Psychiatry*, **60** (Supplement 16).

4.6.3 **Recovered memories and false memories**

Chris R. Brewin

Clinicians working with survivors of traumatic experiences have frequently noted the existence of memory loss with no obvious physical cause and the recovery of additional memories during clinical sessions, although little systematic research has been conducted until recently. Indeed, amnesia is described in diagnostic manuals as a feature of post-traumatic stress disorder, although its presence is not necessary for this diagnosis. In the majority of these cases, people forget details of the traumatic event or events, or forget how they reacted at the time, although they remember that the event happened. They typically report that they have endeavoured not to think about the event, but have never forgotten that it occurred. In the critical cases currently being debated, memories of traumatic events appear to be recovered after a long period of time in which there was complete forgetting that they had ever happened. Although some of Britain's leading psychologists and psychiatrists described this kind of memory loss when treating soldiers in the last two world wars, the controversy has largely erupted in the context of recovered memories of child sexual abuse. It has been suggested that many, if not all, of these apparent recovered memories are the product of inappropriate therapeutic suggestion. This argument has been promulgated in particular by the False Memory Syndrome Foundation in the United States, by its counterpart, the British False Memory Society, and by their scientific advisors.

The 'false memory' position

Loftus[1] suggested that at least some of the memories of child sexual abuse recovered in therapy after apparent total amnesia may not be veridical, but may be false memories encouraged or 'implanted' by therapists who have prematurely decided that the patient is an abuse victim and who use inappropriate therapeutic techniques to persuade him or her to recover corresponding 'memories'. The false memory societies have claimed that there are many cases known to them in which previously happy families have been disrupted by accusations of abuse that were only triggered when an adult child entered therapy. Particular scepticism has been levelled at reports of repeated abuse, all of which has apparently been forgotten, and it has been claimed that such reports are contradicted by what is known scientifically about memory. Reports of 'repressed' memories of childhood abuse are generally regarded as clinical speculations and the psychoanalytical concept of repression as one that has no credible scientific support. Several reviewers claim that there is no empirical support for repression or dissociative amnesia in trauma victims.[2–4]

Loftus[1] and Lindsay and Read[5,6] have marshalled evidence to suggest that the creation of false memories within therapy is a possibility that must be taken seriously. For example, they review experimental studies conducted with non-clinical subjects concerning the fallibility and malleability of memory, and note the potential for inaccurate recall involved in techniques such as hypnosis. Experiments have demonstrated that people are sometimes confused about whether a recent event in the laboratory actually happened, or whether they only imagined it happening. Other experiments have repeatedly succeeded in implanting apparent childhood memories of single non-abusive events in approximately 25 to 30 per cent of subjects, particularly in those who score highly on measures of hypnotizability or suggestibility. These studies have tended to use repeated suggestion, sometimes backed up by 'corroboration' from a family member—one kind of event used in these studies involved being lost in a shopping mall as a child.

Critics have argued that these experiments are a long way from being evidence that therapists could implant false memories of child abuse, and even the experimental studies have shown that successful suggestion depends on the plausibility of the event subjects are asked to believe in. Nevertheless, although no one has performed experiments in an attempt to implant the notion that abuse occurred, it is reasonable to argue that some patients may be highly suggestible and inclined to go along with the beliefs of therapists who may be their only source of support. If their therapist was convinced that abuse had occurred, put overt or covert pressure on their patient to 'remember' this abuse, and was insufficiently alert to the unreliability of memory, there would be a greatly increased risk of false memories occurring.

In conclusion, the recently developed 'false memory' position goes beyond previous concerns of a general nature about errors in memory, and specifically identifies a process whereby errors arise after a person has been subjected to repeated suggestive influences that the explanation for their symptoms lies in forgotten child sexual abuse. These influences are usually thought to occur in therapy, although it has been proposed that exposure to certain books or broadcast media may have the same effect. This position relies partly on information from the false memory societies about their members, and partly on experimental evidence from non-traumatic procedures in the laboratory. There has been little independent scrutiny of the data from members of false memory societies, and many of their claims, for example that parents have been falsely accused, that accusations only follow entry into therapy, or that there is a 'false memory syndrome', are anecdotal and have not been empirically verified.[7]

Evidence for genuine 'recovered memories'

Over 20 longitudinal and retrospective studies have now found that a substantial proportion of people reporting child sexual abuse (somewhere between 20 and 60 per cent) report periods in their lives (often lasting for several years) when they could not remember that the abuse had taken place.[8,9] Although the rates vary between studies, broadly similar findings have been obtained by clinical psychologists, psychiatrists, and cognitive psychologists in both clinical and community samples. As has been pointed out by critics of these studies, this evidence supports the forgetting of trauma, but does not yet have much to say about the mechanism (for example 'repression') by which it

occurs. Thus it would be true to say that while there is evidence for forgetting, there is little evidence for 'repression' as such.

Three main factors support the argument that these apparently forgotten memories are not necessarily false.

1. Surveys have also found recovered memories of other traumatic experiences such as witnessing accidents, experiencing medical procedures, physical abuse in childhood, and combat or war exposure including events connected to the Holocaust.[10] It is unclear how these could have been brought about by suggestion.

2. A number of studies have found that apparent recovered memories occur prior to any therapy, and in the absence of any obvious prolonged suggestive influence.[11,12] Again, it is unclear how these could have been brought about by suggestion.

3. Surveys of psychologists,[12] therapists,[10] and patients reporting childhood trauma[13] found that approximately 40 per cent of those with apparent recovered memories reported corroborative evidence for the content of the memories, such as abusers' confessions, testimony from other victims, and court records. Although the quality of this corroboration has been criticized, it seems unlikely that all these cases can be summarily dismissed. There are also substantial numbers of case studies reporting more detailed corroborative evidence for apparent recovered memories, some of this evidence of reasonably high quality.[14–16]

The quality of the research evidence supporting genuine recovered memories is mixed, and almost all the studies can be argued to have some flaws, but taken together the evidence for genuine memories of major traumatic events is far more extensive than the evidence for false memories of such events. Moreover, these observations need not, as has sometimes been claimed, contradict what we know about memory. Cognitive psychology recognizes that ordinary memory relies as much for its efficiency on the ability to inhibit unwanted material as on the ability to gain rapid access to relevant material. Experimental studies clearly demonstrate the inhibition of memory retrieval and the existence of a subgroup of individuals with poor memories for negative experiences.[17]

But even if forgetting of single traumas occurs, it is far from clear how repeated traumas could be completely forgotten. A hypothesis put forward by trauma researchers is that children learn to 'dissociate' during the abuse, that is to say they are in an altered mental state in which they are less aware of the abuse and of any associated fear and pain. In this state they may, for example, report feeling numb, feeling as though they are observing events from outside their own body, or feeling that they have escaped into an alternative private world. This altered state may make the abuse easier to forget.

This hypothesis has received indirect support from the accounts of adults and children with known traumatic experiences, and from neurobiological research on the effects of extreme stress on memory. Whereas high levels of arousal often make events more difficult to forget, it has been argued by several well-known neuroscientists that extraordinarily high levels of catecholamines or other neuropeptides at the time of the trauma, perhaps in combination with a failure to release sufficient cortisol, may produce amnesia.[18,19] Several studies have demonstrated that the hippocampus, an area of the brain involved in memory, is smaller in traumatized subjects.[20] Changes in hippocampal volume have also been found in stressed animals, and these potentially reversible anatomical effects may have important implications for memory functioning under stress. Again, much of the evidence is indirect and not yet compelling. The intimate neuro-anatomical connections between brain circuits involved in emotion and those involved in memory do, however, provide a good reason for believing that memory may not behave in the same way under conditions of extreme real-world stress as it does in ordinary laboratory experiments.

Why the debate?

From a purely scientific point of view, it should be evident that the quality of the available evidence is insufficient to justify any extreme position at present. However, scientific considerations have been secondary to the passionate advocacy practised by parents who claim to be falsely accused, and by accusers who claim that their memories of abuse are being ignored. Psychiatrists and psychologists have become caught up in the debate and in some cases have abandoned any pretence at neutrality. In the face of these overwhelming and desperately painful personal concerns, the quality of much of the argument has become debased. Thus, supposedly scientific contributions on both sides of this debate have questioned the motives and integrity of people with whom they disagree and have attempted to disparage opponents' professional abilities. Some of these same authors have made exclusive claims for the scientific legitimacy of their own perspective, subjecting opposing data to fierce scrutiny while being relatively uncritical of studies that support their point of view. Much of the literature is obfuscatory and confusing. Logical errors abound, seen for example in the conclusion that because a memory has been recovered in therapy, the practitioner must have been using 'recovered memory therapy'.

A good example of the debate in action is the article by Pope *et al.*[4] on the evidence for dissociative amnesia in trauma victims and the commentary that follows it.[21] These articles demonstrate how widely differing conclusions can be drawn from the same set of studies, depending on the way terms are defined, on assumptions about what evidence should be given the most weight, and on the rigour with which alternative explanations are evaluated.

An emerging scientific and professional consensus

What should be clear by now is that extreme views, claiming that either false memories or genuine recovered memories are rare or impossible, cannot be supported by the available data. Nevertheless, the dispute continues about whether traumatic events, and particularly repeated traumas, can be forgotten and then remembered with essential accuracy. In my view it is safe to conclude from the evidence reviewed that the hypothesized implantation of false memories by practitioners cannot account for more than a subset of recovered memories (and at present it is entirely unclear how large or small this subset might be). False memories may certainly arise in other circumstances, but as yet there is little pertinent evidence. On the other hand, there is a great deal of plausible evidence supporting the existence of genuine recovered memories.

Although members of the advisory boards of false memory societies mostly remain sceptical, on the basis of the kind of evidence reviewed above many commentators now appear to accept that traumatic events can be forgotten and then remembered. For example, cognitive psychologists Lindsay and Read[6] concluded: 'In our reading, scientific evidence has clear implications…memories recovered via suggestive memory work by people who initially denied any such history should be viewed with scepticism, but there are few grounds to doubt spontaneously recovered memories of common forms of child sexual abuse or recovered memories of details of never-forgotten abuse. Between these extremes lies a grey area within which the implications of existing scientific evidence are less clear and experts are likely to disagree'. Similarly, the consensus view among independent commentators, repeated in the 1995 report of the British Psychological Society's Working Party on Recovered Memories and the 1995 interim statement of the American Psychological Association's Working Group on Investigation of Memories of Childhood Abuse, is that memories may be recovered from total amnesia and they may sometimes be essentially accurate. Equally, such 'memories' may sometimes be inaccurate in whole or in part.

In practical terms, the debate has had two major effects. First, proponents of 'recovered memory therapy' are now almost impossible to find within the ranks of leading psychiatrists and psychologists. Despite the small amount of empirical support, there is widespread agreement that situations in which there is sustained suggestive influence, such as therapy, do have the potential to induce false memories. Active attempts to recover suspected forgotten memories may sometimes be appropriate in unusual or extreme cases, but both the client and the therapist must be aware of the risk of false memories. Techniques such as hypnosis and guided imagery should not be used without safeguards against potential suggestive influence. Second, good practice now requires both the therapist and the client to adopt a critical attitude towards any apparent memory that is recovered after a period of amnesia, whether or not this is within a therapeutic context, and not to assume that it necessarily corresponds to a true event. Even highly vivid traumatic memories (sometimes known as 'flashbacks') may be misleading or inaccurate in some cases. Clinical guidelines are now available to help the practitioner avoid the twin perils of uncritically accepting false memories as true or summarily dismissing genuine recovered memories.[9,22]

References

1. Loftus, E.F. (1993). The reality of repressed memories. *American Psychologist*, **48**, 518–37.
2. Brandon, S., Boakes, J., Glaser, D., and Green, R. (1998). Recovered memories of childhood sexual abuse. *British Journal of Psychiatry*, **172**, 296–307.
3. Pope, H.G. and Hudson, J.I. (1995). Can memories of childhood abuse be repressed? *Psychological Medicine*, **25**, 121–6.
4. Pope, H.G., Hudson, J.I., Bodkin, J.A., and Oliva, P. (1997). Can trauma victims develop 'dissociative amnesia'? The evidence of prospective studies. *British Journal of Psychiatry*, **172**, 210–15.
5. Lindsay, D.S. and Read, J.D. (1994). Psychotherapy and memories of childhood sexual abuse. *Applied Cognitive Psychology*, **8**, 281–338.
6. Lindsay, D.S. and Read, J.D. (1995). 'Memory work' and recovered memories of childhood sexual abuse: scientific evidence and public, professional and personal issues. *Psychology, Public Policy and the Law*, **1**, 846–908.
7. Pope, K.S. (1996). Memory, abuse and science: questioning claims about the False Memory Syndrome epidemic. *American Psychologist*, **51**, 957–74.

8. Freyd, J.J. (1996). *Betrayal trauma: the logic of forgetting childhood abuse.* Harvard University Press, Cambridge, MA.

9. Mollon, P. (1998). *Remembering trauma: a psychotherapist's guide to memory and illusion.* Wiley, Chichester.

10. Andrews, B., Brewin, C.R., Ochera, J., *et al.* The characteristics, context, and consequences of memory recovery among adults in therapy. *British Journal of Psychiatry,* in press.

11. Andrews, B., Morton, J., Bekerian, D., Brewin, C.R., Davies, G.M., and Mollon, P. (1995). The recovery of memories in clinical practice. *Psychologist,* **8**, 209–14.

12. Feldman-Summers, S. and Pope, K.S. (1994). The experience of 'forgetting' childhood abuse: a national survey of psychologists. *Journal of Consulting and Clinical Psychology,* **62**, 636–9.

13. Herman, J.L. and Harvey, M.R. (1997). Adult memories of childhood trauma: a naturalistic clinical study. *Journal of Traumatic Stress,* **10**, 557–71.

14. Cheit, R. (1998). *The recovered memory project.* Internet posting http://www.brown.edu/Departments/Taubman_Center/Recovmem/Archive.html.

15. Schooler, J.W. (1994). Seeking the core: the issues and evidence surrounding recovered accounts of sexual trauma. *Consciousness and Cognition,* **3**, 452–69.

16. Schooler, J.W., Bendiksen, M., and Ambadar, Z. (1997). Taking the middle line: can we accommodate both fabricated and recovered memories of sexual abuse? In *Recovered memories and false memories* (ed. M.A. Conway), pp. 251–92. Oxford University Press.

17. Brewin, C.R. and Andrews, B. (1998). Recovered memories of trauma: phenomenology and cognitive mechanisms. *Clinical Psychology Review,* **18**, 949–70.

18. Bremner, J.D., Krystal, J.H., Charney, D.S., and Southwick, S.M. (1996). Neural mechanisms in dissociative amnesia for childhood abuse: relevance to the current controversy surrounding the 'false memory syndrome'. *American Journal of Psychiatry,* **153** (Supplement), 71–82.

19. Yehuda, R. and Harvey, P. (1997). Relevance of neuroendocrine alterations in PTSD to memory-related impairments of trauma survivors. In *Recollections of trauma: scientific evidence and clinical practice* (ed. J.D. Read and D.S. Lindsay), pp. 221–42. Plenum Press, New York.

20. Stein, M.B., Koverola, C., Hanna, C., Torchia, M.G., and McClarty, B. (1997). Hippocampal volume in women victimized by childhood sexual abuse. *Psychological Medicine,* **27**, 951–9.

21. Brewin, C.R. (1998). Commentary: questionable validity of 'dissociative amnesia' in trauma victims. *British Journal of Psychiatry,* **172**, 216–17.

22. Pope, K.S. and Brown, L.S. (1996). *Recovered memories of abuse: assessment, therapy, forensics.* American Psychological Association, Washington, DC.

4.6.4 Adjustment disorders

James J. Strain, Jeffrey Newcorn, and Angela Cartagena-Rochas

Introduction

The psychiatric diagnoses that arise between normal behaviour and the major psychiatric morbidities constitute the problematic subthreshold disorders. These subthreshold entities are also juxtaposed between problem-level diagnoses and more clearly defined disorders. They present major taxonomical and diagnostic dilemmas in that they are often poorly defined, overlap with other diagnostic groupings, and have indefinite symptomatology. It is therefore not surprising that issues of reliability and validity prevail. One of the most commonly employed subthreshold diagnosis that has undergone a major evolution since 1952 is adjustment disorder (**AD**) (Table 1). The advantage of the indefiniteness of these subthreshold disorders is that they permit the classification of early or prodromal states when the clinical picture is vague and indistinct, and yet the morbid state is in excess of that expected in a normal reaction and this morbidity needs to be identified. Therefore AD has an essential place in the psychiatric taxonomy:

(1) normal state

(2) problem-level diagnoses (V Codes)

(3) adjustment disorders

(4) disorders not otherwise specified (**NOS**)

(5) major psychiatric disorders.

Adjustment disorder would 'trump' problem-level disorders, but would be 'trumped' by a specific diagnosis even if it were in the NOS category. The aetiological and dynamic attributes of the diagnosis of AD make it an important diagnostic category that bridges normality and pathology.

Many questions prevail with regard to the concept of the adjustment disorder diagnosis: the role of stressors and the place of specific stressors; the importance of age; the role of concurrent medical morbidity, for example comorbidity of Axis I and Axis III morbidity; the specificity of the diagnostic criteria; the unavailability of a list of symptoms; uncertainty as to optimal treatment protocols; undocumented

Table 1 DSM-IV criteria for adjustment disorders

A. The development of emotional or behavioural symptoms in response to an identifiable psychosocial stressor(s), which occurs within 3 months of the onset of the stressor(s)

B. These symptoms or behaviours are clinically significant as evidenced by either of the following

  (1) Marked distress that is in excess of what would be expected from exposure to the stressor

  (2) Significant impairment in social or occupational (academic) functioning

C. The stress-related disturbance does not meet the criteria for any specific Axis I disorder and is not merely an exacerbation of a pre-existing Axis I or Axis II disorder

D. The symptoms do not represent bereavement

E. Once the stressor (or its consequences) has terminated, the symptoms do not persist for more than an additional 6 months

Specify if:

Acute: if the disturbance lasts less than 6 months.

Persistent/chronic: if the disturbance lasts for 6 months or longer

Table 2 ICD-10 definition of adjustment disorder

A. Onset of symptoms must occur within 1 month of exposure to an identifiable psychosocial stressor, not of an unusual or catastrophic type

B. The individual manifests symptoms or behavioural disturbances of the types found in any of the affective disorders (except for delusions and hallucinations), any disorders in F40–F48 (neurotic, stress-related, and somatoform disorders) and conduct disorders, but the criteria for an individual disorder are not fulfilled. Symptoms may be variable in both form and severity

The predominant feature of the symptoms may be further specified by use of a fifth character:

Brief depressive reaction
Prolonged depressive reaction
Mixed anxiety and depressive reaction
With predominant disturbance of other emotions
With predominant disturbance of conduct
With mixed disturbance of emotions and conduct
With other specified predominant symptoms

C. Except in prolonged depressive reaction, the symptoms do not persist for more than 6 months after the cessation of the stress or its consequences. However, this should not prevent a provisional diagnosis being made if this criterion is not yet fulfilled

---

outcomes or prognosis. Research data regarding these questions will be examined.

AD is a stress-related phenomenon in which the stressor precipitates maladaptation and symptoms that are time limited until the stressor is attenuated or a new state of adaptation occurs (Table 2). At the same time that AD was evolving, other stress-related disorders, for example post-traumatic stress disorder and acute stress disorder, have been described. (Acute stress disorders were formulated by Spiegel during the development of the DSM-IV.[1,2]) Acute stress reactions could result from involvement in a natural disaster such as a flood, or an avalanche, or a cataclysmic personal event, for example loss of a body part. The stress-related disorders are unique in that they are psychiatric diagnoses with a known aetiology—the stressor—and this aetiology is central to the diagnosis. (Three other diagnostic categories also invoke aetiology in their diagnostic criteria: organic mental disorders (aetiology—physical abnormality); substance abuse disorders (aetiology—ingestion of substances); post-traumatic and acute stress disorders (aetiology—an identifiable stressor).) The DSM was conceptually designed with an atheoretical framework to encourage psychiatric diagnoses to be derived on phenomenological grounds with an avowed dismissal of pathogenesis or aetiology as diagnostic imperatives. In frank contradiction of this atheoretical algorithm, the stress-induced disorders require the inclusion of an aetiological significance to a life event—a stressor—and the need to relate the stressor's effect on the patient in clinical terms.

The diagnosis of AD also requires a careful titration of the timing of the stressor in relation to the adverse psychological sequelae that ensued. Maladaptation and disturbance of mood should obtain within 3 months of the patient experiencing the stressor. Until the DSM-IV criteria, the ADs were regarded as transitory diagnoses that should not

exceed 6 months in duration. Thereafter, that appellation could not be employed and the diagnosis had to be changed to a major psychiatric disorder or dropped.

In summary, AD is a diagnosis that has been insufficiently researched but is, however, commonly employed in clinical practice. The utilization of the AD diagnosis is attributable to several issues:

(1) in a diagnostic system that is principally atheoretical, AD remains one of the few conditions which is linked to an aetiologic event;

(2) the concept that adjustment problems stem from stressful events has been a precept of psychodynamic thinking, and often underlies the approach of psychotherapeutic treatment;

(3) because the development of transient psychiatric symptoms in the context of stress is virtually a universal experience, AD is considered by many to be a non-stigmatizing diagnosis to assign when making a patient's psychiatric status public.

Definition and history

Wise,[3] who described the history of AD since 1945, states that the AD diagnostic concept initially included the idea of a transient situational disturbance, classified by developmental epochs (Table 3). It then evolved to embody a disorder of adjustment characterized by maladaptation, for example work (or academic) inhibition, accompanied by a mood state, for example depressed, anxious, mixed (DSM-III).[4] In 1987 with the advent of DSM-IIIR, another category of adjustment disorders was included, i.e. physical complaints.[5]

With the opportunity in 1994 to develop another evolutionary step of the DSM, i.e. DSM-IV,[4] the authors were asked to re-examine the subthreshold diagnostic category of AD with the goal of improving its acknowledged 'shortcomings.' The research included review of the literature, reanalysis of existing studies of AD and their data sets, and examination of field studies (e.g. minor depression, minor anxiety) to observe if there was sufficient differentiation among these minor disorders from the ADs (e.g. how often was a stressor identified in those patients assigned the diagnosis minor depression or minor anxiety?). From these three sources and consultations, modifications for DSM-IV and their rationale were formulated based on the best evidence extant.

Changes in the criteria for adjustment disorder in DSM-IV

The review of the literature and the reanalysis of the Western Psychiatric Institute and Clinic data supported the following changes in the DSM-IV.

1. Enhance the understanding of the language.

2. Describe the time of the reaction to reflect duration: acute (less than 6 months) or chronic (6 months or greater).

3. Allow for the continuation of the stressor for an indefinite period; psychological reactions to chronic stress states (e.g. chronic arthritis, HIV, abuse by an alcoholic spouse) do not necessarily terminate at 6 months, nor do they necessarily lead to a major psychiatric disorder.

4. Eliminate the subtypes of mixed emotional features, work (or academic) inhibition, withdrawal, and physical complaints (as they were rarely employed by diagnosticians).

Table 3 Development of the classification of adjustment disorder

DSM-I (1952): Transient situational personality disorder
Gross stress reaction
Adult situational reaction
Adjustment reaction of infancy
Adjustment reaction of childhood
Adjustment reaction of adolescence
Adjustment reaction of late life
Other transient situational personality disturbance

DSM-II (1968): Transient situational disturbance
Adjustment reaction of infancy
Adjustment reaction of childhood
Adjustment reaction of adolescence
Adjustment reaction of adult life
Adjustment reaction of late life

DSM-III (1980): Adjustment disorder
Adjustment disorder with depressed mood
Adjustment disorder with anxious mood
Adjustment disorder with mixed emotional features
Adjustment disorder with disturbance of conduct
Adjustment disorder with mixed disturbance of emotions and conduct
Adjustment disorder with work (or academic) inhibition
Adjustment disorder with withdrawal
Adjustment disorder with atypical features

DSM-IIIR (1987): Adjustment disorder
Adjustment disorder with depressed mood
Adjustment disorder with anxious mood
Adjustment disorder with mixed emotional features
Adjustment disorder with disturbance of conduct
Adjustment disorder with mixed disturbance of emotions and conduct
Adjustment disorder with work (or academic) inhibition
Adjustment disorder with withdrawal
Adjustment disorder with physical complaints
Adjustment disorder not otherwise specified (NOS)

DSM-IV (1994): Adjustment disorder
These follow the criteria contained in Table 1 and the subtypes listed in Table 4

Although it might be argued that ADs could be placed in a new category of 'stress response syndromes', the literature and research reports did not support this taxonomical organization. AD could be eliminated altogether, with the advantage of maintaining the atheoretical approach of DSM, and substitute in its place the appropriate minor or NOS categories. However, this solution does not seem beneficial in view of the recent findings that demonstrate AD to be a valid frequently employed diagnosis.[6] AD was diagnosed in over 60 per cent of burned inpatients,[7] over 20 per cent of patients in early stages of multiple sclerosis,[8] and over 40 per cent of poststroke patients.[9] Furthermore, evaluations of patients in a psychiatric walk-in clinic showed a significant difference in the symptom profile of those assigned AD and the others, including minor diagnoses.[10] (The McArthur field trials on the prospective assessment of minor depressive and anxiety disorders and which collected data on the occurrence of stressors immediately preceding the outbreak of symptoms are important databases that need further study to establish whether stress *per se* is a distinguishing characteristic between AD and the other minor mood disorders.)

Problems with the adjustment disorder diagnosis

The symptom profile

Two issues remain as fundamental confounds in the diagnosis of AD. First, because of the lack of any quantitative behavioural or operational criteria, the problem of reliability and validity are paramount. Criterion reference was evaluated by Aoki *et al.*[11] who reported that three psychological tests, Zung's Self-Rating Anxiety Scale,[12] Zung's Self-Rating Depression Scale,[13] and the Profile of Mood States,[14] were useful tools for the diagnosis of AD in physical rehabilitation patients. While these measures succeeded in reliably differentiating AD patients from normal patients, they were not able to distinguish them from patients with major depression or post-traumatic stress disorder. The second confounding factor is that the classification of syndromes that do not fulfill the criteria for a major mental illness but present with serious (or incipient) symptomatology that requires intervention and/or treatment may be viewed, by default, as 'subthreshold' and hence attract a subthreshold interest by health-care workers and third-party payers. Thus the construct of AD is designed as a means for classifying psychiatric conditions having a symptom profile that is (as yet) insufficient to meet the more specifically operationalized criteria for the major syndromes but that is:

(1) clinically significant and deemed to be in excess of a normal reaction to the stressor in question;

(2) associated with impaired vocational or interpersonal functioning;

(3) not solely the result of a psychosocial problem (V Code) requiring medical attention (e.g. non-compliance, phase of life problem, etc.).

Attention to minor mental symptomatology (and psychiatric morbidity) may forestall the evolution to more serious disorders and allow remediation before relationships, work, and functioning have been so impaired that they are disrupted or permanently impaired. Yet in the 'grey area' where early diagnosis may take place and has enormous value with modest therapeutic investment, guidelines are the most tenuous. It is the professionals at the 'front door'—those involved in primary care, triage, and emergency room treatment—who must be assisted to make this most difficult call: is there sufficient psychiatric morbidity to warrant mental health assessment and/or intervention? A number of studies state that because of the subthreshold nature of the AD diagnosis and the absence of a symptom checklist, non-psychiatric physicians and nurses have more difficulty making the AD diagnosis than that for a major psychiatric disorder.[7,15–17] However, the concurrence of medical illness, which is a frequent comorbidity of AD, does not have the same impact on evaluating a symptom profile as occurs in the major disorders with checklists. For example, in major affective disorders, if seminal symptoms which are key to the diagnosis (e.g. those of appetite, sleep, energy, libido) are attributable to a medical diagnosis, they cannot be used to support a psychiatric diagnosis. At times the attribution of the symptoms (physical or psychological) cannot be determined and therefore the quantitative assessment of prescribed symptoms supporting one diagnosis or another is problematic. However, field studies are being performed[18] to assess whether a reliable checklist from an elaborate list of symptoms associated with AD can be constructed (Table 4). (The V Codes—a problem level of diagnoses—are understandably devoid of a symptom-based diagnostic schema.)

Table 4 DSM-IV subtypes of adjustment disorder

Adjustment disorder with depressed mood
Adjustment disorder with anxious mood
Adjustment disorder with mixed anxiety and depressed mood
Adjustment disorder with disturbance of conduct
Adjustment disorder with mixed disturbance of emotions and
    conduct
Adjustment disorder unspecified

The meaning of 'maladaptive'

The imprecision of the diagnostic criteria for AD is immediately apparent in the DSM-IV description of this disorder as a maladaptive reaction to an identifiable psychosocial stressor, or stressors, that occurs within 3 months after onset of the stressor. It is assumed that the disturbance will remit soon after the stressor ceases or, if the stressor persists, when a new level of adaptation is achieved.[1] In addition to the problem of no symptom checklist, difficulties are inherent within each of these diagnostic elements.

First, with regard to the 'maladaptive reaction', it is unclear how this concept can or should be operationalized. The social, vocational, and relationship dysfunctions that are qualitatively or quantitatively unspecified lend themselves neither to reliability, nor to validity, nor even to clinical agreement when maladaptation is present. The concept of a maladaptive reaction is confounded by physical status, perception, and especially by culture, i.e. the reactions expected to occur within a specific cultural environment, gender responses, developmental level differences, and the 'meaning' of events to an individual. The concepts of 'average expectable environment' and 'the patient's explanatory belief model' are examples of assessing cultural and subjective differences that can effect an individual's mental state and reaction.[19] The variable of culture was not included in the decision-making algorithm of DSM-IV. Is the assessment of maladaptation subjective or objective? Who makes the decision—a third party, a mental health professional, the patients themselves, or an admixture of these? Is this decision 'culture bound?' Succinctly when does an individual cross the threshold into 'patienthood,' and who will make the decision?

The patient's functional status evaluation (Axis V) is not linked via an algorithm to the AD construct in DSM-IV. Fabrega et al.[20] contend that both subjective symptoms and decrement in social function can be considered 'maladaptive,' and that the severity of either of these is subject to great individual variation. Utilizing data from Axis V and their newly constructed 'Axis VI'—an additional and more specific functional status axis on their Initial Evaluation Form[10]—these authors could not conclude that the level of psychopathology correlates with impaired functioning.(The functional status measure, involving seven levels of impairment, is used to assess 'current functioning' of patients in three dimensions: 'at work or at school, with family, and with other person or groups'.[20]) However, Bodlund et al.[21] found that the use, according to Axis V, of the Global Assessment of Functioning Scale self-report was a poor predictor for an AD with depressive symptoms as these patients, more than others, tended to score themselves lower.

The stressor

Obviously, the stressor and its effect are central to the AD diagnosis. The second major confound emanates from the fact that the DSM-IV presents no criteria or 'guidelines' to quantify stressors or to assess their effect or meaning for a particular individual at a given time. Furthermore, the assessment of stress is not linked by an algorithm to Axis IV—a statement of stress during the previous year—and so internal consistency or reinforcement within the diagnostic lexicon is not mandated (D. Schafer, personal communication, 1990). Many of the confounds expressed regarding the assessment of maladaptation above apply to the evaluation of stressors as well.[22–24] Mezzich et al.[10] attempted to classify and quantify the psychosocial stressors in 13 specific domains: health, bereavement, love and marriage, parental, family stressors for children and adolescents, other familial relationships, other relationships outside the family, work, school, financial, legal, housing, and miscellaneous. Such specificity has not been defined in DSM-IV and the construct is vague and generic with minimal opportunity to achieve quantification. Despland et al.[25] observed that the type of stressor may indeed be of help in diagnosing AD. His study demonstrated that AD with depressed mood and mixed mood was associated with more marital problems than major depressive disorders. AD with anxiety could be distinguished from the major anxiety disorders by the quantity of family and marital problems.

The time course

The time course and chronicity of both stressors and their consequent symptoms were left vague in DSM-IIIR and were not consistent with the clinical situation. The modifications introduced in DSM-IV, which differentiate between acute and chronic forms of AD, solved the problem of the 6-month limitation of the AD diagnosis in DSM-IIIR and was more in keeping with what is observed in the clinical situation. This change was validated by Despland et al.[25] who observed that 16 per cent of patients with AD required treatment longer than 1 year—the mean exceeded the prior limitation of 6 months.

Other problems of definition

With all the limitations presented—the diagnosis of AD is not scientifically rigorous—it is just this imprecision that paradoxically makes the diagnosis so empirically useful to psychiatry. The identification of an emerging illness in its early stages, where the diagnosis of AD can serve as a 'temporary' diagnosis modifiable with evolving information from longitudinal evaluation and treatment, allows the 'marking' of an individual for possible difficulty, before the psychiatric morbidity becomes more apparent and at times destructive.

Even serious symptomatology (e.g. suicidal behaviour) that is not regarded as part of a major mental disorder needs treatment and a 'diagnosis' under which it can be placed, for example a V Code, 'Phase of Life Problem,' AD, acute stress response, etc. De Leo et al.[26,27] reported on AD and suicidality. Recent life events, which would constitute an acute stress, were commonly found to correlate with suicidal behaviour in a patient cohort which included those with AD.[28] Spalletta et al.[29] observed the assessment of suicidal behaviour to be an important tool in the differentiation among major depression, dysthymia, and AD. AD patients were found to be among the most common recipients of a deliberate self-harm diagnosis, with the majority involving self-poisoning.[30] Thus deliberate self-harm is more common in AD patients,[30] while the percentage of suicidal behaviour was found to be higher in AD patients with depressed mood.[29]

The AD DSM-IV Work Group suggested that suicide and deliberate self-harm could be subtypes of AD. However, there were concerns that patients with other diagnoses, for example major affective disorder, borderline personality disorder, etc. and suicide behaviour, would be assigned the AD diagnosis since there was a specific placement for suicidal ideation and behaviour and that would be a predominant reason to use AD. The final decision was to place the problem of suicidal symptomatology without a psychiatric diagnosis in the DSM-IV F Code section for other problems 'that may be a focus of clinical attention.' A subthreshold diagnosis, AD, does not necessarily imply the presence of subthreshold symptomatology!

Boundaries with other disorders

Finally, the issue of boundaries among depression NOS, anxiety NOS, and AD remains problematic. How often are the major syndromes associated with a stressor and maladaptation? How different are the symptom profiles of depression and anxiety NOS from those of AD? How often does AD have a vegetative symptom (e.g. decreased appetite, libido, fatigue) or an ideational symptom (e.g. guilt, suicidality, hopelessness)? Much uncertainty about diagnostic boundary definition remains. The diagnosis of AD was consistently associated with shorter length of stay compared with major psychiatric diagnoses.[25,31] But, while Despland et al.[25] found a significantly greater number of Axis II comorbidities in AD patients compared with patients with other psychiatric diagnosis, Spalletta et al.[29] observed the prevalence of Axis II personality disorder to be lower in patients with AD with depressed mood than in those diagnosed as having major depression or dysthymia.

'Splitting' and 'lumping' continues; the subthreshold diagnosis of mixed anxiety–depressive disorder is a new category included in the DSM-IV. This disorder is very similar to AD with mixed mood; a boundary between the two is difficult to demarcate. The main difference between the two diagnoses was the chronicity of the mixed anxiety–depressive disorder (as was noted in the mixed anxiety–depression field trial).[32] The change in criterion C for AD—allowing a chronic or recurrent disturbance—confounds the differentiating of these two subthreshold diagnoses. This uncertainty is further complicated by the question of treatment. Is this an anxiety accompanied by depression which should be treated with anxiolitics, such as benzodiazapines, or is this a depression accompanied by anxiety, which should be treated with an antidepressant, such as a selective serotonin reuptake inhibitor? Furthermore, it is commonly viewed that the majority of patients with AD should be treated with psychotherapy or counselling as the initial approach.

Another potential mood disorder, subsyndromal symptomatic depression (**SSD**), has been suggested.[33] It joins AD in the grey area of subthreshold diagnoses. However, there are two critical differences between SSD and AD: SSD employs a symptom checklist, and it is not associated with a stressor. As was stated, AD trumps a problem-level diagnosis, but will be trumped by a specific psychiatric diagnosis, even if it is in the NOS category. By definition, 'SSD is the simultaneous presence of any two or more symptoms of depression, persistent for most or all of the time for a duration of at least two weeks, associated with social dysfunction, and occurring in patients who do not meet the criteria for minor depression, major depression, and/or dysthymia'.[33] In some cases, the SSD diagnosis is the same as the DSM-IV diagnosis for minor depression, termed by the authors 'SSD with mood disturbance', and has to be documented as such. In other cases, the disorder is SSD 'without mood disturbance'. By definition SSD with mood disturbance, i.e. minor depression, would trump AD. But should SSD without mood disturbance trump AD? Research is neces-

sary to demarcate the boundaries between the problem level, subthreshold, minor, and major disorders, and, in particular, with regard to the role of stressors as aetiological precipitants, concomitants, or essentially unrelated variables.

Age and medical comorbidity

In contrast with DSM-IIIR, DSM-IV has tried to accommodate the presence of comorbid medical illness. DSM-IIIR was regarded as 'medical illness and age unfair' (i.e. inadequate consideration of age and/or medical illness) (L. George, personal communication, 1981).[34] To enhance reliability and validity, there will need to be a psychiatric taxonomy that takes into account medical illness and symptomatology and developmental epochs (e.g. children and adolescents, adults, 'young' elderly, and 'old' elderly). It is clear from the Western Psychiatric Institute studies that the symptom profile for children and adolescents is very different from that for adults with regard to the entire spectrum of diagnoses. It is also apparent that symptoms secondary to a medical illness are not to be 'counted' in the algorithm for psychiatric diagnoses (e.g. anorexia, decreased energy) but they are extremely difficult to differentiate from the same symptoms which may be psychiatrically induced. As a possible solution Endicott[35] recommends replacing vegetative with ideational symptoms when evaluating depressed patients with medical illness. Rapp and Vrana[36] confirmed Endicott's proposed changes in the diagnostic criteria for depression in medically ill elderly persons and observed a maintenance of specificity and sensitivity respectively when substituting ideational for vegetative symptoms. With regard to age, recent studies report AD patients to be significantly younger compared with those with major psychiatric diagnosis.[25,37] Zarb's study[38] suggests that in cognitively impaired elderly, using individual items of the Geriatric Depression Scale, AD could be differentiated from major depression. In addition, Despland et al.[25] showed that patients labelled AD with depressive or mixed symptoms included more women: a sex ratio resembling that seen in major depression or dysthymia. The future evolution of the DSM needs to consider the effect of developmental epochs, gender, and medical comorbidity on symptom profiles in the various diagnostic categories.

Epidemiology

The Epidemiologic Catchment Area Study did not include AD in its historic survey of patients in the population of five major settings in the United States. Most studies are of smaller or more discrete samples and have the problem of generalization. Andreasen and Wasek[39] reported that 5 per cent of an inpatient and outpatient sample at the university hospital and clinics in Iowa were labelled as having AD. Fabrega et al.[20] reported that 2.3 per cent of a sample of patients presenting to a walk-in clinic (diagnostic and evaluation centre) met criteria for AD, with no other diagnoses on Axis I or Axis II; when patients with other Axis I diagnoses (i.e. Axis I and II comorbidities) were included, 20 per cent had the diagnosis of AD. In general hospital inpatient psychiatric consultation populations, AD was diagnosed as 21.5 per cent, 18.5 per cent and 11.5 per cent respectively.[40–42] D. Schafer (personal communication, 1990) noted that up to 70 per cent of children in the psychiatric setting may be given the diagnosis of AD in a variety of mental health care environments. Faulstich et al.[43]

reported the prevalence of DSM-III conduct and AD for adolescent psychiatric inpatients. Andreasen and Wasek,[39] utilizing a chart review, reported that more adolescents than adults experienced acting out and behavioural symptoms, but adults had significantly more depressive symptomatology (87.2 per cent versus 63.8 per cent). Anxiety symptoms were frequent at all ages.

Mezzich and coworkers[10,20] evaluated 64 symptoms currently present in three cohorts: subjects with specific diagnoses, those with AD, and those who were not ill. Vegetative, substance use, and characterological symptoms were greatest in the specific-diagnosis group, intermediate in the AD group, and least in the group with no illness. The symptoms of mood and affect, general appearance, behaviour, disturbance in speech and thought pattern, and cognitive functioning had a similar distribution. The AD group was significantly different from the no-illness group with regard to more 'depressed mood' and 'low self-esteem' ($p \leq 0.0001$). The AD and no-illness groups had minimal pathology of thought content and perception. A positive response on the suicide indicators was obtained in 29 per cent of AD compared with 9 per cent of the no-illness group. The three cohorts did not differ on the frequency of Axis III disorders.

Associated features of adjustment disorder

Andreasen and Wasek[39] observed that in their AD cohorts 21.6 per cent of the adolescents' fathers and 11.8 per cent of the adults' fathers had problems with alcohol. Greenberg et al.[31] report more substance abuse in adults with diagnosed AD compared with all those with other diagnoses. Breslow et al.,[44] comparing patients with AD and other psychiatric diagnoses, observed that alcohol or substance use/abuse did not help to differentiate between diagnostic groups. Thus, higher rate of substance use at this time does not serve as an incontrovertible prediction factor for the diagnosis of an AD diagnosis.

Aetiology—the role of stress

Nature of the stressor

Hirschfeld[45] and Winokur[46] discussed both sides of the controversy regarding 'neurotic' depression (i.e. related to a stressor) and 'endogenous' depression (i.e. not related to a stressor). From the examination of several studies, it has been difficult to demonstrate a significant temporal link between the onset of an identified stressor and the occurrence of depressive illness.[45–51]

Andreasen and Wasek[39] described the differences between the chronicity of stressors found in adolescents compared with those in adults: present for a year or more, 59 per cent and 35 per cent; present for 3 months or less, 9 per cent and 39 per cent. Fabrega et al.[20] reported that their AD group had greater registration of stressors compared with other diagnoses and the non-illness cohorts. Compared with other diagnoses and the non-illness patients, AD was overrepresented in the 'higher stress category'. In their consultation cohort, Popkin et al.[40] found that in 68.6 per cent of the cases the medical illness itself was judged to be the primary psychosocial stressor. Snyder and Strain[42] observed that stressors as assessed on Axis IV were significantly higher ($p = 0.0001$) for consultation patients with AD than for patients with other diagnostic disorders.

Modifiers of stress

Stress has been described as the aetiological agent for AD. Vulnerability to stress is another risk factor. Diverse variables and modifiers are involved regarding who will experience AD following a stress. Cohen[22] argues as follows:

(1) acute stresses are different from chronic stresses in both psychological and physiological terms;

(2) the meaning of the stress is affected by 'modifiers' (e.g. ego strengths, support systems, prior mastery);

(3) manifest and latent meanings of the stressor(s) may be associated with differential impact (e.g. loss of job may be a relief or a catastrophe).

AD with maladaptive denial of pregnancy, for example, can be a consequence of a stressor such as separation from a partner.[52] An objectively overwhelming stress may have little impact on one individual, whereas a minor stress could be regarded as cataclysmic by another. A recent minor stress superimposed on a previous underlying (major) stress that has no observable effect on its own may have a significant additive impact (i.e. concatenation of events) (B. Hamburg, personal communication, 1990).

The chronological relationship of the stressor and symptoms has been examined less extensively. Depue and Monroe[53] and Skodol et al.[54] identified significant methodological problems in evaluating the quality, quantity, and timing of both stressors and symptoms. Depue and Monroe[53] and Rahe[55] state that the model of a single stressor impinging on an undisturbed individual to cause symptoms at a single point in time is insufficient to account for the many presentations of stress and illness in the clinical situation.

Confounds: assessing stress

Limitations of the current construct of stress for research have been described.[22] Holmes and Rahe[56] assigned relative values to specific stressors, but there has been much concern about their methodology and the results obtained.[22] Other life-event scales[51,57,58] have also been shown to be inconsistent in their ability to link stress and illness. As discussed above, many authors have cautioned that the vulnerability of the individual (e.g. ego strengths, support system, underlying personality disorders, the timing and concatenation of the stress(es), the issue of control over the stressor, and the desirability of the event, etc.) need to be evaluated to ascertain the impact of the stressor on the individual. Axis IV of DSM-III was included to allow the clinician to assess the presence of stress in the multiaxial diagnoses of psychiatric disorders, but it has been confounded by low reliability.[59–61] Despland et al.[25] reported that stressors were present on Axis IV in 100 per cent of those assigned AD with depressed mood, while it was present in 83 per cent of those with major depression, 80 per cent of those with dysthymia, and 67 per cent of those with non-specific depression, which emphasizes the importance of stressors in the AD diagnosis.

Clinical features

Nine different types of AD are listed in DSM-IV.[1] As in DSM-III, AD is classified in DSM-IIIR according to the predominant symptom picture. In DSM-IV, AD has been reduced to six types that, again, are classified according to their clinical features:

(1) AD with depressed mood;

(2) AD with anxious mood;

(3) AD with mixed anxiety and depressed mood;

(4) AD with disturbance of conduct;

(5) AD with mixed disturbance of emotions and conduct;

(6) AD not otherwise specified.

In their study, Despland et al.[25] suggested reducing the subtypes even further, demonstrating identical profiles for AD with depressed mood and AD with mixed mood, and proposing assimilation of mixed mood into the depressed mood category. Fifty-seven per cent of their sample were represented by these two groups; the remainder were accounted for by AD with 'anxiety' and 'other' categories.

Treatment

Psychotherapy and counselling

Treatment of AD initially focuses on psychotherapeutic and counselling interventions to reduce the stressor, enhance the capacity to cope with a stressor that cannot be reduced or removed, and establish a system of support to maximize adaptation. The patient needs to be made aware of the significant dysfunction that the stressor has caused and consider strategies to manage the disability. Some stressors, for example taking on more responsibility than can be managed by the individual, or putting oneself at risk (e.g. unprotected sex with an unknown partner), can be avoided or minimized. Other stressors may elicit an over-reaction on the part of the patient (e.g. abandonment by a lover). The patient may attempt suicide or become reclusive, damaging his or her source of income. In this situation, the therapist would assist the patient to verbalize his or her disappointed feelings and rage rather than behaving destructively. The role of verbalization in minimizing the discomfort of the stressor and enhancing coping cannot be overestimated. It is necessary to clarify and interpret the meaning/reality of the stressor for the patient. For example, if a mastectomy has devastated a patient's feelings about her body and herself, it is mandatory to articulate that the patient is still a woman, capable of having a fulfilling relationship, including a sexual one, and that recurrence of the cancer may not occur. Without the correction of distortions, the patient's pernicious fantasies—'all is lost'—may occur as sequelae to the stressor (i.e. the mastectomy) and intensify incapacitation at work and/or sex, as well as a profound disturbance of mood.

Counselling, psychotherapy, crisis intervention, family therapy, and group treatment are utilized to encourage the verbalization of fears, anxiety, rage, helplessness, and hopelessness to the stressors imposed upon a patient. As mentioned above, the goal of treatment is to expose the concerns and conflicts that the patient is experiencing, identify means to reduce the stressor(s), enhance the patient's coping skills, and clarify the patient's perspective on the adversity, and enable the establishment of supporting relationships. The primary treatment for AD is talking.

Psychopharmacotherapy

Small doses of antidepressants and anxiolytics may sometimes be appropriate for AD patients when dysphoria remains profound despite several sessions of psychological treatment.

No randomized controlled trials of pharmacological treatment of AD are available. Although formal psychotherapy is presently the treatment of choice,[62] psychotherapy combined with benzodiazapines is utilized, especially for patients with severe life stress(es) and an unrelenting anxious component.[62] Tricyclic antidepressants or buspirone were recommended in place of benzodiazepines for AD patients with current or past excessive alcohol use because of their greater risk of dependence.[62] The use of antidepressants may assist some patients if their maladaptation is debilitating and the accompanying mood is pervasive.

Course and prognosis

Adults and adolescents

Andreasen and Hoenk[63] report that the long-term outcome of AD has a good prognosis for adults, but that a majority of adolescents eventually have major psychiatric disorders. Follow-up at 5 years after original diagnosis of AD revealed that 71 per cent of adults were completely well, 8 per cent had an intervening problem, and 21 per cent had developed a major depressive disorder or alcoholism. However, in adolescents at 5-year follow-up, only 44 per cent were without a psychiatric diagnosis, 13 per cent had an intervening psychiatric illness, and 43 per cent went on to develop major psychiatric morbidity (e.g. schizophrenia, schizoaffective disorders, major depression, bipolar disorder, substance abuse, and personality disorders). In contrast with the adults, the chronicity of the illness and the presence of behavioural symptoms in the adolescents were the strongest predictors for major psychopathology 5 years after the initial AD diagnosis. The number and type of symptoms were less useful than the length of treatment and chronicity of symptoms as predictors of future outcome.

As Chess and Thomas[64] have reported, it is important to note that AD with disturbance of conduct, regardless of age, has a more guarded outcome. In agreement with the findings of Andreasen and Wasek.[39] Chess and Thomas[64] emphasize that:

> a significant number [of AD adolescents] did not improve or even grew worse in adolescence and early adult life. It was not possible to predict the developmental course of the disorder in the early period after its first identification. Hence, we would suggest active appropriate therapeutic intervention in all cases but especially adolescents [and adequate follow-up].

Spalletta et al.[29] report that suicidal behaviour and deliberate self-harm are important predictors in the diagnosis of AD. As mentioned before, these are obviously not subthreshold symptoms; they can lead to the most dire consequence—death. This outcome, when reached, can be neither corrected nor resolved. These behaviours mandate immediate and protective interventions. The diagnosis of AD may suggest that the patient has minor symptomatology. Such assessment may be life-threatening. There needs to be a definite split from viewing a diagnosis as subthreshold, and therefore the attendant symptoms as subthreshold. It is similar to labelling a patient with hypochondriasis, which in some settings can influence a more casual physical assessment, when such a patient could have serious physical morbidity concomitant with their hypochondriacal Axis I pathology.

As mentioned earlier, the diagnosis of an AD may be in the early phase of an evolving disorder that has not yet developed to the extent that full-blown symptoms are evident to reach threshold for a major psychiatric disorder. If a patient continues to worsen, becomes more symptomatic, and does not respond to treatment, it is critical to review the diagnosis for the presence of a major disorder.

Conclusions

The domains of diagnostic rigour and clinical utility seem at odds for AD. Studies that employ reliable and valid instruments (e.g. depression or anxiety rating scales, stress assessments, length of disability, treatment outcome, family patterns, etc.) would enhance more exact specification of the parameters of the AD diagnosis. Identification of the time course, remission or evolution to another diagnosis, and the evaluation of stressors (characteristics, duration, and the nature of adaptation to stress) would enhance the understanding of the aetiology, mechanisms, and mediators of a stress-response illness.

Studies with adequate symptom checklists rated independently from the establishment of the diagnosis would clarify the threshold between major and minor depression and anxiety, as well as guide an entry threshold to employ the AD diagnosis. Although the upper threshold is established by the specified criteria for the major syndromes, the entry threshold between an AD and problem-level diagnoses and normality is undesignated with operational criteria. The careful examination of associated demographic and treatment outcome variables would also enable clinicians to describe more specifically the boundaries among subthreshold diagnoses, problem-level diagnosis, and normal behaviour. Associated features such as family history, biological correlates, treatment response, long-term course, and so forth, are all critical to establishing the authenticity of a diagnosis. The theory and practice of medicine have demonstrated the need for a comprehensive multidimensional formulation of all these physiological and functional variables to describe an illness and develop the most appropriate working diagnosis.

Subthreshold syndromes can encompass significant psychopathology that must not only be identified but treated (e.g. suicidal ideation/behaviour). Cross-sectionally, AD may appear to be the incipient phase of an emerging major syndrome. Consequently, AD, despite its questionable reliability and validity, serves an important diagnostic function in the practice of psychiatry. Problem- and subthreshold-level diagnoses are critical to the function of any medical discipline. Because this may be the initial phase, or a mild form, of a dysfunction that is not yet fully developed, there is a need to describe the relationship of this incipient state to other potential diagnoses. This lack of specificity and questionable reliability and validity are the hallmark of interface disorders and subthreshold phenomena, whether they be in diabetes mellitus, hypertension, or depression.

Should drugs be used in the treatment of AD? The pharmacological studies are not conclusive. The diagnostic dilemmas of the AD present sufficient difficulty in and of themselves.[65–67] It would be preferred that cautious psychotropic drug administration be employed, to avoid subjecting the patient to the risk of unfavourable drug–psychotrophic drug interaction. Psychotrophic drug treatment will not be necessary if the condition resolves. If it evolves into a major psychiatric illness then drug treatment needs to be considered.

As mentioned earlier, the characteristics of a mental disorder vary over the lifecycle, and this is clearly illustrated by AD. Certain developmental epochs may be associated with a particular symptom profile, as seen with acute myocardial infarction or appendicitis. The effect of the stressor may vary, and the assessment of functioning must be 'measured' according to the demands of the developmental stage (e.g. school (adolescents), work (adults), self-care and maintenance (elderly)). The symptom characteristics and functional assessment of other diagnoses may also vary along the developmental schema from birth to senescence; illnesses such as major depressive disorders, organic mental disorders, sexual dysfunctions, and eating disorders need to be 'recast' in another hierarchy to incorporate the stage of the lifecycle extant at the time of the assessment, and symptom profiles adjusted accordingly. The normal variations across developmental epochs would make AD and the other psychiatric disorders more reliable and valid across the lifecycle. Similarly there needs to be a consideration of a possible concomitant state of medical illness. The result would be a taxonomy tempered by the vicissitudes of development and medical illness.

A taxonomy which considers the development epoch and the presence of medical illness would be more useful to child psychiatrists, paediatricians, geriatricians, geriatric psychiatrists, and primary care specialists, who often are convinced that a patient does not conform with today's psychiatry's lexicon. A significant number of their patients remain at the problem level of diagnoses with their somatic complaints as well. It is not uncommon for a fever of unknown origin to not be diagnosed, or for a chest pain to remain unspecified. It is the art of medicine that makes it a profession, and a most difficult one, at the interface of medicine and psychiatry, or at the interface of normality and pathology. Anna Freud[68] has emphasized the difficulty of understanding normality and pathology in her assessments of childhood. This important advice would obtain across the lifecycle and be an important challenge to the developers of the subthreshold diagnoses (e.g. AD) and the future evolution of the DSM.

References

1. American Psychiatric Association (1994). *Diagnostic and statistical manual of mental disorders* (4th edn). American Psychiatric Association, Washington, DC.
2. Spiegel, D. (1994). *DSM-IV options book*. American Psychiatric Association, Washington, DC.
3. Wise, M.G. (1988). Adjustment disorders and impulse disorders not otherwise classified. In *American Psychiatric Press textbook of psychiatry* (ed. J.A. Talbot, R.E. Hales, and S.C. Yudofsky), pp. 605–20. American Psychiatric Press, Washington, DC.
4. American Psychiatric Association (1980). *Diagnostic and statistical manual of mental disorders* (3rd edn). American Psychiatric Association, Washington, DC.
5. American Psychiatric Association (1987). *Diagnostic and statistical manual of mental disorders* (3rd edn, revised). American Psychiatric Association, Washington, DC.
6. Kovacs, M., Ho, V., and Pollock, M.H. (1995). Criterion and predictive validity of the diagnosis of adjustment disorder: a prospective study of youths with new-onset insulin-dependent diabetes mellitus. *American Journal of Psychiatry*, **152**, 523–8.
7. Perez-Jimenez, J.P., Gomez-Bajo, G.J., Lopez-Catillo, J.J., *et al.* (1994). Psychiatric consultation and post-traumatic stress disorder in burned patients. *Burns*, **20**, 532–6.
8. Sullivan, M.J., Winshenker, B., and Mikail, S. (1995). Screening for major depression in the early stages of multiple sclerosis. *Canadian Journal of Neurological Science*, **22**, 228–31.
9. Shima, S., Kitagawa, Y., Kitamura, T., *et al.* (1994). Poststroke depression. *General Hospital Psychiatry*, **16**, 286–9.

10. Mezzich, J.E., Dow, J.T., Rich, C.L., et al. (1981). Developing an efficient clinical information system for a comprehensive psychiatric institute, II: Initial Evaluation Form. Behavioral Research Methods and Instrumentation, 13, 464–78.

11. Aoki, T., Hosaka, T., and Ishida, A. (1995). Psychiatric evaluation of physical rehabilitation patients. General Hospital Psychiatry, 17, 440–3.

12. Zung, W. (1971). A rating intrument for anxiety disorders. Psychosomatics, 12, 371–9.

13. Zung, W. (1965). A self-rating depression scale. Archives of General Psychiatry, 12, 63–70.

14. McNair, D.M., Lorr, M., and Doppelman, L.F. (ed.) (1971). Manual for the Profile of Mood States. Educational and Industrial Testing Service, San Diego, CA.

15. Margolis, R.L. (1994). Nonpsychiatrist house staff frequently misdiagnose psychiatric disorders in general hospital inpatients. Psychosomatics, 35, 485–91.

16. Fincannon, J.L. (1995). Analysis of psychiatric referrals and interventions in an oncology population. Oncology Nursing Forum, 22, 87–92.

17. Silverstone, P.H. (1996). Prevalence of psychiatric disorders in medical inpatients. Journal of Nervous and Mental Disease, 184, 43–51.

18. Strain, J.J., Newcorn, J., Mezzich, J., et al. (1998). Adjustment disorder: the McArthur reanalysis. In DSM-IV source book, Vol. 4, pp. 404–24. American Psychiatric Association, Washington, DC.

19. Kleinman, A. (1980). Patients and healers in the context of culture: an exploration of the borderland between anthropology, medicine, and psychiatry. University of California Press, Berkeley, CA.

20. Fabrega, H. Jr, Mezzich, J.E., and Mezzich, A.C. (1987). Adjustment disorder as a marginal or transitional illness category in DSM-III. Archives of General Psychiatry, 44, 567–72.

21. Bodlund, O., Kullgren, G., Ekselius, L., et al. (1994). Axis V—Global Assessment of Functional Scale. Evaluation of a self-report version. Acta Psychiatrica Scandinavica, 90, 342–7.

22. Cohen, F. (1981). Stress and bodily illness. Psychiatric Clinics of North America, 4, 269–86.

23. Perris, H., von Knorring, L., Oreland, L., et al. (1984). Life events and biological vulnerability: a study of life events and platelet MAO activity in depressed patients. Psychiatry Research, 12, 111–20.

24. Zilberg, N.J., Weiss, D.S., and Horowitz, M.J. (1982). Impact of Event Scale: a cross-validation study and some empirical evidence supporting a conceptual model of stress response syndromes. Journal of Consulting and Clinical Psychology, 50, 407–14.

25. Despland, J.N., Monod, L., and Ferrero, F. (1995). Clinical relevance of adjustment disorder in DSM-III-R and DSM-IV. Comprehensive Psychiatry, 36, 456–60.

26. De Leo, D., Pellegrini, C., and Serraiotto, L. (1986). Adjustment disorders and suicidality. Psychology Reports, 59, 355–8.

27. De Leo, D., Pellegrini, C., Serraiotto, L., et al. (1986). Assessment of severity of suicide attempts: a trial with the dexamethasone suppression test and two rating scales. Psychopathology, 19, 186–91.

28. Isometsa, E., Heikkinen, M., Henriksson, M., et al. (1996). Suicide in non-major depressions. Journal of Affective Disorders, 36, 117–27.

29. Spalletta, G., Troisi, A., Saracco, H., et al. (1996). Symptom profile: Axis II comorbidity and suicidal behaviour in young males with DSM-III-R depressive illnesses. Journal of Affective Disorders, 39, 141–8.

30. Vlachos, I.O., Bouras, N., Watson, J.P., et al. (1994). Deliberate self-harm referrals. European Journal of Psychiatry, 8, 25–8.

31. Greenberg, W.M., Rosenfeld, D.N., and Ortega, E.A. (1995). Adjustment disorder as an admission diagnosis. American Journal of Psychiatry, 152, 459–61.

32. Zinbarg, R.E., Barlow, D.H., Liebowitz, M., et al. (1994). The DSM-IV field trial for mixed anxiety–depression. American Journal of Psychiatry, 151, 1153–62.

33. Judd, L.L., Rapaport, M.H., Paulus, M.P., et al. (1994). Subsyndromal symptomatic depression: a new mood disorder? Journal of Clinical Psychiatry, 55 (Supplement), 18–28.

34. Strain, J.J. (1981). Diagnostic considerations in the medical setting. Psychiatric Clinics of North America, 4, 287–300.

35. Endicott, J. (1984). Measurement of depression in patients with cancer. Cancer, 53, 2243–9.

36. Rapp, S.R. and Vrana, S. (1989). Substituting nonsomatic for somatic symptoms in the diagnosis of depression in elderly male medical patients. American Journal of Psychiatry, 146, 1197–200.

37. Mok, H. and Walter, C. (1995). Brief psychiatric hospitalization: preliminary experience with an urban sort-stay unit. Canadian Journal of Psychiatry, 40, 415–17.

38. Zarb, J. (1996). Correlates of depression in cognitively impaired hospitalized elderly referred for neuropsychological assessment. Journal of Clinical and Experimental Neuropsychology, 18, 713–23.

39. Andreasen, N.C. and Wasek, P. (1980). Adjustment disorders in adolescents and adults. Archives of General Psychiatry, 37, 1166–70.

40. Popkin, M.K., Callies, A.L., Colón, E.A., et al. (1990). Adjustment disorders in medically ill patients referred for consultation in a university hospital. Psychosomatics, 31, 410–14.

41. Foster, P. and Oxman, T. (1994). A descriptive study of adjustment disorder diagnoses in general hospital patients. Irish Journal of Psychological Medicine, 11, 153–7.

42. Snyder, S. and Strain, J.J. (1989). Differentiation of major depression and adjustment disorder with depressed mood in the medical setting. General Hospital Psychiatry, 12, 159–65.

43. Faulstich, M.E., Moore, J.R., Carey, M.P., et al. (1986). Prevalence of DSM-III conduct and adjustment disorders for adolescent psychiatric inpatients. Adolescence, 21, 333–7.

44. Breslow, R.E., Klinger, B.I., and Erickson, B.J. (1996). Acute intoxication and substance abuse among patients presenting to a psychiatric emergency service. General Hospital Psychiatry, 18, 183–91.

45. Hirschfeld, R.M.A. (1981). Situational depression: validity of the concept. British Journal of Psychiatry, 139, 297–305.

46. Winokur, G. (1985). The validity of neurotic-reactive depression: new data and reappraisal. Archives of General Psychiatry, 42, 1116–22.

47. Akiskal, H.S., Bitar, A.H., Puzantian, V.R., et al. (1978). The nosological status of neurotic depression: a prospective three- to four-year follow-up examination in light of the primary-secondary and unipolar–bipolar dichotomies. Archives of General Psychiatry, 35, 756–66.

48. Andreasen, N.C. and Winokur, G. (1979). Secondary depression: familial, clinical, and research perspectives. American Journal of Psychiatry, 136, 62–6.

49. Benjaminsen, S. (1981). Stressful life events preceding the onset of neurotic depression. Psychological Medicine, 11, 369–78.

50. Garvey, M.J., Tollefson, G.D., Mungas, D., et al. (1984). Is the distinction between situational and nonsituational primary depression valid? Comprehensive Psychiatry, 25, 372–5.

51. Paykel, E.S., Prusoff, B.A., and Uhlenhuth, E.H. (1971). Scaling of life events. Archives of General Psychiatry, 25, 340–7.

52. Brezinka, C., Huter, O., Biebl, W., et al. (1994). Denial of pregnancy: obstetrical aspects. Journal of Psychosomatic Obstetrics and Gynecology, 15, 1–8.

53. Depue, R.A. and Monroe, S.M. (1986). Conceptualization and measurement of human disorder in life stress research: the problem of chronic disturbance. Psychological Bulletin, 99, 36–51.

54. Skodol, A.E., Dohrenwend, B.P., Line, B.G., et al. (1990). The nature of stress: problems of measurement. In Stressors and the adjustment disorders (ed. J.D. Noshpitz and R.D. Coddington), pp. 3–22. Wiley, New York.

55. Rahe, R.H. (1990). Psychosocial stressors and adjustment disorder: Van Gogh's life chart illustrates stress and disease. Journal of Clinical Psychiatry, 51 (Supplement), 13–19.

56. Holmes, T.H. and Rahe, R.H. (1967). The Social Readjustment Rating Scale. Journal of Psychosomatic Research, 11, 213–18.

57. Dohrenwend, B.S., Krasnoff, L., Askenasy, A.R., et al. (1978). Exemplification of a method for scaling life events: the PERI Life Event Scale. Journal of Health and Social Behaviour, 19, 205–29.

58. Tennant, C. (1983). Life events and psychological morbidity: the evidence from prospective studies (editorial). *Psychological Medicine*, **13**, 483–6.

59. Rey, J.M., Stewart, G.W., Plapp, J.M., *et al.* (1988). DSM-III Axis IV revisited. *American Journal of Psychiatry*, **145**, 286–92.

60. Spitzer, R.L. and Forman, J.B.W. (1979). DSM-III field trials, II: initial experience with the multiaxial system. *American Journal of Psychiatry*, **136**, 818–20.

61. Zimmerman, M., Pfohl, B., Coryell, W. *et al.* (1987). The prognostic validity of DSM-III Axis IV in depressed inpatients. *American Journal of Psychiatry*, **144**, 102–6.

62. Uhlenhuth, E.H., Balter, M.B., Ban, T.A., *et al.* (1995). International study of expert judgment on therapeutic use of benzodiazepines and other psychotherapeutic medications: III. Clinical features affecting experts' therapeutic recommendations in anxiety disorders. *Psychopharmacology Bulletin*, **31**, 289–96.

63. Andreasen, N.C. and Hoenk, P.R. (1982). The predictive value of adjustment disorders: a follow-up study. *American Journal of Psychiatry*, **139**, 584–90.

64. Chess, S. and Thomas, A. (1984). *Origins and evolution of behavior disorders: from infancy to early adult life.* Brunner–Mazel, New York.

65. Hosaka, T., Aoki, T., and Ichikawa, Y. (1994). Emotional states of patients with hematological malignancies: preliminary study. *Japanese Journal of Clinical Oncology*, **24**, 186–90.

66. Oxman, T.E., Barrett, J.E., Freeman, D.H., *et al.* (1994). Frequency and correlates of adjustment disorder relates to cardiac surgery in older patients. *Psychosomatics*, **35**, 557–68.

67. Hugo, F.J., Halland, A.M., Spangenberg, J.J., *et al.* (1996). DSM-III-R classification of psychiatric symptoms in systemic lupus erythematosus. *Psychosomatics*, **37**, 262–9.

68. Freud, A. (1968). *Normality and pathology: assessment of childhood.* International Universities Press, New York.

4.7 Anxiety disorders

4.7.1 Generalized anxiety disorders

David A. Spiegel and David H. Barlow

Anxious apprehension and over-concern are common to many anxiety and mood disorders. Prior to 1980 in the American DSM diagnostic system, and 1992 in the international ICD system, individuals who experienced those symptoms in the absence of a realistic focus of concern were classified as having an 'anxiety neurosis' (DSM-II) or 'anxiety state' (ICD-9). In DSM-III, panic disorder was split off from that classification, and the residual category was renamed generalized anxiety disorder (**GAD**). A similar nomenclature was adopted in ICD-10.

Since its inception, GAD as a nosological entity has been troubled by problems of poor reliability and high comorbidity. Those concerns have prompted several revisions of the DSM criteria and also have raised more basic questions regarding the validity of GAD as a disorder distinct from other anxiety and mood states. The question of what is GAD is still being debated. Unfortunately, most of the information we have about it, including the majority of the published treatment studies, is based on criteria that are now outdated.

Clinical features

Individuals with GAD experience persistent anxiety and worry that is out of proportion to actual events or circumstances. Typically, the anxiety and worry involve minor or everyday matters, such as work, finances, relationships, the health or safety of loved ones, and routine tasks. Often, the focus of worry shifts from one concern to another. Although people with GAD do not always consider their worries to be unrealistic or excessive, they do find them difficult to control. Consequently, the worries often interfere with concentration and performance.

Associated with the anxiety and worry, individuals with GAD have a variety of cognitive and somatic symptoms, including trembling, feeling shaky, aching in the back and shoulders, tension headaches, chest tightness, restlessness, exaggerated startle, irritability, insomnia, fatigue, dry mouth, sweating, urinary frequency, trouble swallowing, nausea, and diarrhoea. In addition, GAD may be accompanied by other conditions typically associated with stress, such as irritable bowel syndrome or atypical chest pain.

Classification

Diagnosis

DSM criteria

In DSM-III, GAD was essentially a residual category for individuals with somatic symptoms of anxiety who did not meet diagnostic criteria for another, more specific, anxiety disorder. Diagnosis required the presence, for at least a month, of symptoms from three of four symptom clusters: motor tension, autonomic hyperactivity, apprehensive expectation, and vigilance and scanning. Unfortunately, clinicians had difficulty applying those criteria. Even in studies that used structured diagnostic interviews, kappa coefficients reflecting rates of agreement between independent evaluators were low (0.47 to 0.57).[1,2] In addition, because GAD was not diagnosed if another anxiety disorder was present, its diagnosis also depended on the application of the criteria for other diagnoses.

In DSM-IIIR, apprehensive expectation was removed from the diagnostic symptom clusters, was redefined as unrealistic or excessive anxiety and worry about two or more life circumstances, and was made the essential feature of GAD. In addition, the duration criterion was changed from 1 to 6 months, and the hierarchical exclusion rule was dropped, allowing GAD to be diagnosed in addition to other disorders.

Despite those changes, the diagnostic reliability of GAD remained essentially unchanged.[3] Investigations revealed that the new worry criterion was problematic. Interviewers commonly disagreed as to whether two distinct spheres of worry were present, whether the worry was unrealistic or excessive, or whether the focus of the worry could be construed to be part of the symptomatology of another disorder. Moreover, studies indicated that patients with GAD did not differ substantially from control subjects in the content of their worries.[4,5] The main difference between patients and controls was that the former experienced their worrying to be uncontrollable while the latter did not.

Based on those and other findings, the GAD criteria were revised again in DSM-IV. The 'unrealistic' descriptor and the requirement for anxiety or worry to involve at least two spheres of life circumstances were deleted, and a new criterion was added that the worry must be experienced as difficult to control. In addition, the associated symptom criterion was modified to require only three of six symptoms from the previous motor tension and vigilance and scanning clusters (Table 1). For additional information about the evolution of the DSM criteria for GAD, see Barlow and Wincze[6] or Brown et al.[7]

Table 1 DSM-IV inclusion criteria for GAD

A. Excessive anxiety and worry, occurring more days than not for at least 6 months, about a number of events or activities

B. The person finds it difficult to control the worry

C. The anxiety and worry are accompanied by at least three of the following six symptoms (one in children): restlessness or feeling keyed up or on edge; being easily fatigued; difficulty concentrating or mind going blank; irritability; muscle tension; sleep disturbance

D. The anxiety, worry, or physical symptoms cause significant distress or functional impairment

ICD-10 criteria

Like DSM-IIIR and DSM-IV, ICD-10 requires a period of 6 months of generalized anxiety and worry accompanied by certain somatic symptoms (Table 2). The specified symptoms include 16 of the 18 DSM-IIIR GAD symptoms plus six additional symptoms that are listed under panic attacks in the American classification system (feeling of choking, chest pain or discomfort, derealization or depersonalization, fear of losing control or going crazy, and fear of dying). Most of the symptoms ICD-10 shared with DSM-IIIR were in the autonomic hyperactivity cluster, which was deleted during the 1994 DSM revision. Thus, of the 22 symptoms listed in ICD-10, 16, including the four that comprise the essential autonomic arousal cluster, do not appear in DSM-IV. One DSM-IV symptom (being easily fatigued) does not appear in ICD-10, nor does ICD-10 require that the person find it difficult to control the worry, which is an essential criterion in DSM-IV.

Differential diagnosis

Everyone experiences anxiety and worry sometimes, and some people describe themselves as born worriers. GAD differs from these non-pathological anxiety experiences in that it is both persistent and severe enough to cause significant distress or interference. Typically also, the

Table 2 ICD-10 inclusion criteria for GAD

A. At least 6 months of prominent tension, worry, and feelings of apprehension about everyday events and problems

C. At least four of the following 22 symptoms must be present, at least one of which must be from the autonomic arousal cluster

Autonomic arousal symptoms: palpitations or pounding heart or accelerated heart rate; sweating; trembling or shaking; dry mouth (not due to medication or dehydration)

Symptoms involving the chest and abdomen: difficulty in breathing; feeling of choking; chest pain or discomfort; nausea or abdominal distress

Symptoms involving mental state: feeling dizzy, unsteady, faint, or lightheaded; derealization or depersonalization; fear of losing control, 'going crazy', or passing out; fear of dying

General symptoms: hot flushes or cold chills; numbness or tingling sensations

Symptoms of tension: muscle tension or aches and pains; restlessness and inability to relax; feeling keyed up, on edge, or mentally tense; a sensation of a lump in the throat, or difficulty in swallowing

Other non-specific symptoms: exaggerated response to minor surprises or being startled; difficulty in concentrating, or mind 'going blank' because of worrying or anxiety; persistent irritability; difficulty getting to sleep because of worrying

Table 3 General medical conditions that can cause symptoms resembling anxiety

Cardiac conditions: arrhythmias, coronary insufficiency, mitral valve prolapse, heart failure

Endocrine conditions: hyperthyroidism, hypoparathyroidism, hypoglycaemia

Neurological conditions: temporal lobe epilepsy, vestibular nerve disease

Respiratory conditions: asthma, hypoxia, hyperventilation, obstructive lung disease, pulmonary embolism

Other conditions: porphyria, carcinoid tumour, systemic lupus erythematosus, pellagra

worries are more pervasive and difficult to control than normal worries and are associated with physical symptoms of anxiety and tension.

A number of **general medical conditions** can present with signs and symptoms resembling GAD (Table 3). In addition, **substances** such as caffeine, alcohol, other drugs of abuse, toxins, and some medications (Table 4) can cause anxiety-like symptoms either as a direct effect or as part of a withdrawal syndrome. These causes may be established on the basis of a medical and substance use history, physical examination, or laboratory tests.

GAD is distinguished from other psychiatric disorders, in part, by the focus of the anxiety and worry, which is not limited to a feature of another disorder. For example, the worry is not only about the possible occurrence or implications of panic attacks (as in **panic disorder**), or about negative evaluations by others (**social phobia**), gaining weight (**anorexia nervosa**), or having a serious illness (**hypochondriasis**). In **obsessive–compulsive disorder**, the anxiety and worry are associated with intrusive thoughts, images, or impulses that are distressing.

Generalized anxiety commonly occurs in **depression**, and GAD and depression also share associated symptoms such as sleep disturbance, fatigue, restlessness, and poor concentration. When the associated symptoms could fit with either disorder, the distinction is made on the basis of the presence and time course of depressed mood relative to anxiety. In DSM-IV, GAD is not diagnosed if its features occur exclusively during a mood disorder.

Epidemiology

Prevalence estimates of GAD vary considerably with the diagnostic criteria used. For example, in one study, the prevalence of GAD among women was 11.5 per cent using DSM-III criteria but only 2.4 per cent

Table 4 Medications that can cause symptoms resembling anxiety

Psychotropics: antidepressants, neuroleptics (akathisia), sedative-hypnotics (withdrawal syndrome), disulfiram

Respiratory drugs: β-adrenergic stimulants, bronchodilators

Cardiovascular drugs: antiarrhythmics, antihypertensives

Neurological disorder medications: anticonvulsants, anticholinergic agents, L-dopa

Anaesthetic drugs: pre-anaesthetics, general anaesthetics (post-anaesthetic syndrome)

Other drugs: thyroid hormone, antibiotics, non-steroidal anti-inflammatory drugs, anticancer drugs

Table 5 Prevalence of comorbid disorders in 109 patients with GAD

Any additional lifetime disorder	74%
Two disorders	20%
Three or more disorders	17%
Current anxiety or mood disorder[a]	
Social phobia	23%
Simple phobia	21%
Panic disorder	11%
Dysthymia	8%
Past major depression	42%
Past substance abuse	24%

[a] Patients with current major depression were excluded.
Data from Brawman-Mintzer et al.[15]

when the duration requirement was increased to 6 months.[8] Other studies have found two- to fourfold higher prevalence rates using ICD-10 criteria than using DSM-IIIR criteria.[9,10]

In the American-based Epidemiologic Catchment Area Study, which used DSM-III criteria, the 12-month prevalence of GAD in a community sample was 3.8 per cent.[11] A surprisingly similar rate (3.1 per cent) was found in the National Comorbidity Survey, using DSM-IIIR criteria.[12] The lifetime prevalence in the National Comorbidity Survey was 5.1 per cent using DSM-IIIR criteria and 8.9 per cent using ICD-10 criteria.[10] In both studies, GAD was more common among women than men. Estimates of GAD among patients presenting to primary care clinics are about three times higher than the general population figures, probably reflecting increased utilization of health care services by individuals with GAD.[13,14]

Comorbidity

GAD usually coexists with other anxiety and mood disorders. In the major epidemiological surveys, nearly two-thirds of individuals with GAD had additional DSM Axis I diagnoses.[10,12] Most common among these were simple (21–59 per cent) and social (16–59 per cent) phobias, followed by panic disorder (3–27 per cent) and depression (8–39 per cent). In the largest clinical sample to date,[15] which excluded patients with current major depression, 74 per cent of patients with a primary DSM-IIIR diagnosis of GAD had one or more additional lifetime diagnoses (Table 5). There is less information about the prevalence of personality disorders among patients with GAD. One study found a prevalence of 49 per cent.[16]

Is GAD a valid disorder?

The findings of only fair diagnostic reliability and high comorbidity for GAD have been interpreted as indicating poor discriminant validity of the disorder, suggesting that differentiating GAD from other anxiety and mood disorders may be artifactual. In considering those arguments, it is important to distinguish the diagnostic criteria sets specified in the DSM and ICD classification systems from the clinical syndromes they are intended to identify. Low discriminant validity for a disorder may be due to problems with the former rather than the latter. To establish the construct validity of a syndrome, one must demonstrate that it has a consistent set of features, the pattern of

which separates it from other related syndromes. One approach to doing that is to compare the profiles of patients with different diagnoses across various illness dimensions.

In one such study, data from patients who took part in the DSM-IV mixed anxiety–depression field trial were examined.[14] Using factor analyses of patients' scores on 73 items from the Hamilton anxiety and depression rating scales, four clusters were identified that corresponded to the dimensions of anxiety, depression, physiological arousal, and general negative affect (containing items that loaded on both the anxiety and depression factors). Patients with a principal diagnosis of GAD had a unique profile (high on negative affect and anxiety, low on physiological arousal and depression) that distinguished them from individuals with panic disorder, major depression, anxiety or depressive disorder not otherwise specified, or no mental disorder.

A subsequent study, using an anxiety clinic sample and an expanded array of measures, yielded similar results.[17] In this case, five primary factors (corresponding to panic, agoraphobia, social anxiety, obsessions/compulsions, and general anxiety) and a higher-order factor (negative affect) were identified. Again, patients with GAD had a unique factor profile.

Recently, the findings of the preceding studies were replicated and extended in an independent sample of patients.[18] As in the earlier studies, GAD was found to be distinct from other anxiety syndromes and depression, although it had the highest degree of overlap with other syndromes, especially depression. In addition, GAD was strongly associated with the non-specific dimension of negative affect, which is common to anxiety and depression. The authors suggest that GAD may represent a 'basic emotional disorder,' because it consists of features that are present to varying degrees in all anxiety and mood disorders.

Finally, all three of the preceding studies (and a variety of others, e.g. Barlow et al.[19]) support the differentiation of symptoms of autonomic arousal, which are characteristic of panic attacks, from somatic symptoms related to central nervous system tension, which form the DSM-IV-associated symptom cluster of GAD.

Aetiology

Genetic factors

In a family study that used DSM-III criteria, GAD (but not other anxiety disorders) was five times more prevalent (19.5 per cent versus 3.5 per cent) among first-degree relatives of patients with GAD than among relatives of controls.[20] However, two twin studies using the same criteria found concordance rates for GAD were no higher among monozygotic than dizygotic twins.[21,22] Two subsequent studies that used DSM-IIIR criteria found a shared heritability for GAD and mood disorders.[23–25] At present, it appears that genetic factors play a modest role in the aetiology of GAD, and one that is more closely related to vulnerability for depression than for other anxiety disorders.

Neurobiological mechanisms

A variety of neuroanatomical, neurochemical, neuroendocrine, and neurophysiological systems have been implicated in the pathogenesis of anxiety states. Much of this information has come from animal models and research on the effects of stress. Studies of neurobiological functioning in humans with GAD are limited. Some of the physical systems that may be involved in the emotion of anxiety are summarized below. Additional information may be found in reviews by Brawman-Mintzer and Lydiard,[26] Connor and Davidson,[27] and Gray and McNaughton.[28]

The noradrenergic nervous system

Noradrenergic pathways (the **locus coeruleus–noradrenaline–sympathetic nervous system**) have long been associated with fear and arousal and play an important role in the body's response to threat. However, their role in persistent anxiety states is not clear. Resting catecholamine levels in patients with GAD appear to be normal. On the other hand, GAD patients exhibit subnormal responses to both stimulation[29] and blockade[30] of α_2-adrenergic receptors and a reduced density of α_2-receptors in platelets.[31] Those findings could reflect downregulation of the α_2-receptors due to initially high levels of noradrenaline (norepinephrine).

Consistent with those neurochemical findings, somatic measures of autonomic nervous system function (e.g. skin conductance, respiratory rate, heart-rate variability, blood pressure) in patients with GAD tend to show normal resting values with blunted and sometimes prolonged responses to stressful stimuli.[31,32] Those findings may indicate diminished autonomic nervous system responsiveness in individuals with GAD.

The hypothalamic–pituitary–adrenal axis

The **hypothalamic–pituitary–adrenal axis** and its end-product, cortisol, also are involved in reactions to stress. Activity in the hypothalamic–pituitary–adrenal axis is subject to a variety of influences. Primary control is by means of hypothalamic secretion of corticotrophin-releasing factor, which stimulates pituitary secretion of ACTH, which in turn stimulates adrenal secretion of cortisol. Circulating cortisol, and analogues such as dexamethasone, exert inhibitory feedback at the level of the pituitary gland and apparently also by means of receptors on the hippocampus.

In rats, chronic exposure to stress or exogenous steroids results in a reduction of corticosteroid receptors in the hippocampus and a consequent decrease in feedback inhibition by cortisol.[33] These animals exhibit reduced dexamethasone suppression of cortisol secretion and greater or more prolonged adrenocortical responses to stress. Reduced dexamethasone suppression also has been observed in approximately one-third of patients with DSM-III-diagnosed GAD.[34] This reduction in the normal regulatory control of cortisol secretion may be one mechanism through which chronic or repeated stress can lead to persistent anxiety.

The amygdala and the bed nucleus of the stria terminalis

LeDoux[35,36] and others have demonstrated the central role played by the **amygdala** in the mediation of fear reactions. The amygdala is thought to be responsible for the detection of potential threats to the organism and the mobilization of a range of defensive responses (Fig. 1). Through connections with the hypothalamus, it can activate the sympathetic nervous system and hypothalamic–pituitary–adrenal axis. Through efferent fibres to the central grey area of the midbrain, it can mediate behavioural defence responses such as the fight-or-flight response and behavioural 'freezing.' Through connections to the nucleus reticularis pontis caudalis, it can enhance the defensive startle reflex.

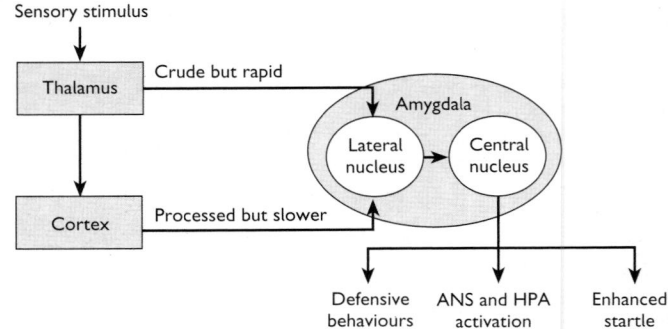

Fig. 1 Fear pathways (based on descriptions by LeDoux[36] and Davis[37]): ANS, autonomic nervous system; HPA, hypothalamic–pituitary–adrenal axis.

The extent to which these pathways are involved in the neurobiology of anxiety (as opposed to fear) is unclear. However, a structure closely related to the amgdala, the **bed nucleus of the stria terminalis**, may be involved in this emotion. The bed nucleus resembles the amygdala in its neurotransmitter content, cell morphology, and hypothalamic and brainstem connections and, like the amygdala, it exerts a modulating effect on the startle reflex.[37] Studies of this latter effect implicate it in the experience of anxiety.

Administration of corticotrophin-releasing factor into the cerebral ventricles of rats produces a state of generalized arousal resembling anxiety. Under those conditions, the startle reflex also is enhanced. Exposing rats to bright light for 5 to 20 min has similar effects. These effects are not blocked by damage to amygdala but are by lesions to the bed nucleus of the stria terminalis and by treatment with benzodiazepines or buspirone. Conversely, infusion of corticotrophin-releasing factor directly into the bed nucleus of the stria terminalis, but not the amygdala, produces a rapid increase in startle. Based on these observations, Davis[37] has suggested that the stria terminalis may play a role in anxiety analogous to that of the amygdala in fear reactions and, further, that prolonged or repeated stimulation of the stria terminalis by corticotrophin-releasing factor during periods of stress might lead to sustained activation and thus to persistent anxiety.

The septohippocampal system (behavioural inhibition system)

The bed nucleus of the stria terminalis is part of the larger septohippocampal system.[38] In 1982, based on data from several lines of research, Gray hypothesized that the septohippocampal system, together with the Papez circuit (a neural loop connecting the subicular area in the hippocampal formation to the mammillary bodies, anterior thalamus, cingulate cortex, and back to the subiculum), is responsible for mediating the emotion of anxiety as well as the major effects of anxiolytic drugs.[38] Gray called this network the **behavioural inhibition system**, because he believed that, when activated, it interrupts ongoing behavior and redirects the organism's attention to signs of possible danger.

According to Gray's model,[28,38] the behavioural inhibition system receives information about the environment from the sensory cortex via the temporal lobe and hippocampal formation. The system checks the information for consistency with predictions, which are updated continuously by the Papez circuit based on preceding information and stored patterns, as well as for consistency with the immediate goals of the organism. When a mismatch is found, or if a predicted event is aversive, the outputs of the behavioral inhibition system are activated, resulting in a constellation of emotional and behavioural effects consistent with anxiety (Fig. 2).

The activation of the behavioural inhibition system appears to be moderated by ascending noradrenergic and serotonergic projections to the septohippocampal complex, providing a possible mechanism for the anxiolytic actions of some drugs. The amygdala also provides inputs to the behavioural inhibition system and may relay its outputs to the hypothalamus and autonomic nervous system, thereby mediating anxious arousal. Sustained activation of the behavioural inhibition system might therefore account for many of the features of GAD.

The benzodiazepine–γ-aminobutyric acid system

The powerful anxiolytic and sedative effects of benzodiazepines are believed to be mediated by benzodiazepine recognition sites located on γ-aminobutyric acid (**GABA**) type A receptor complexes in the central nervous system. When bound to those complexes, benzodiazepines allosterically modulate the GABA receptors to enhance the normal inhibitory effects of GABA on neurotransmission. Activation of **central benzodiazepine–GABA receptor complexes** also suppresses hypothalamic–pituitary–adrenal axis axis activity and, consequently, cortisol levels.

In addition to these central receptor complexes, benzodiazepine recognition sites of a different type are present widely in cells outside the central nervous system. These so-called **peripheral benzodiazepine receptors** are believed to be instrumental in controlling the synthesis of regulatory steroids. Their role in the anxiolytic actions of benzodiazepines is unknown; although they bind some drugs (e.g. diazepam), they have low affinity for others (e.g. clonazepam). Interestingly, peripheral benzodiazepine receptors are decreased in blood cells of individuals with untreated GAD but return to normal levels after successful treatment with benzodiazepines. Their numbers also vary in response to stress, being elevated following acute stressors and reduced during chronic stress.

A possible explanation for those changes has been suggested by Rocca *et al.*[39] The investigators note that peripheral benzodiazepine

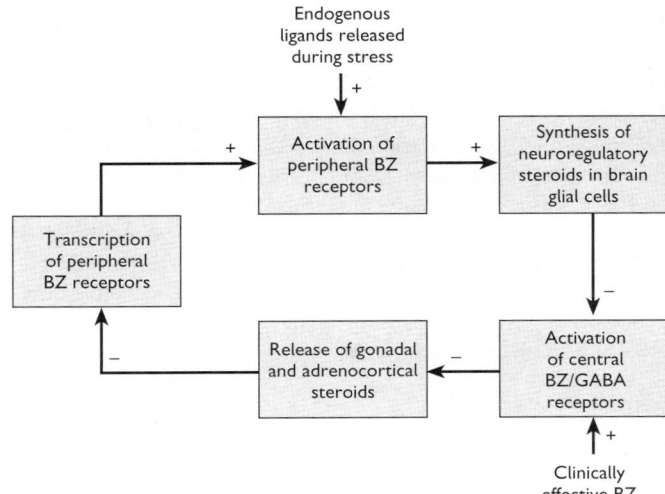

Fig. 3 Possible involvement of peripheral benzodiazepine receptors in acute and chronic stress reactions (based on descriptions by Rocca *et al.*[39]): BZ, benzodiazepine.

receptors in brain glial cells control the production of neurosteroids that act as modulators of GABA$_A$ receptor sensitivity. Their effect on GABA functioning appears to be opposite to that of clinically effective benzodiazepines, that is, they *decrease* rather than increase the inhibitory effects of GABA. It is hypothesized that an endogenous ligand of these glial cell receptors (possibly diazepam binding inhibitor) is released during stress, initiating the cycle of events depicted in Fig. 3.

The immediate effect of these events would be to enhance the stress-induced release of cortisol. However, prolonged cortisol excess is hypothesized to downregulate peripheral benzodiazepine receptors, resulting in the reduced receptor densities found in GAD. Administration of a clinically effective benzodiazepine drug would interrupt the proposed pathway at the point of the central GABA receptor, lowering cortisol levels and restoring synthesis of peripheral benzodiazepine receptors.

Other neurotransmitter systems

Individuals with GAD have been reported to have reduced serotonin levels in the cerebral spinal fluid[40] and decreased platelet binding of paroxetine, a selective serotonin reuptake inhibitor.[41] In addition, drugs that affect serotonergic transmission (e.g. buspirone and venlafaxine) are effective in the treatment of GAD. These findings suggest that serotonin regulation may be abnormal in GAD.

Cholecystokinin neuropeptides (CCK-4 and CCK-8S) have been implicated in the genesis of arousal and fear responses.[42] It is unclear how those effects are mediated; however cholecystokinin interacts with several neurotransmitters and systems believed to be involved in anxiety responses, including the noradrenergic nervous system, the hypothalamic–pituitary–adrenal axis, the benzodiazepine–GABA system, and serotonin.

Psychosocial mechanisms

Data from twin studies suggest that at least 70 per cent of the variance in liability to GAD comes from environmental factors.[23] Several such factors have been implicated.

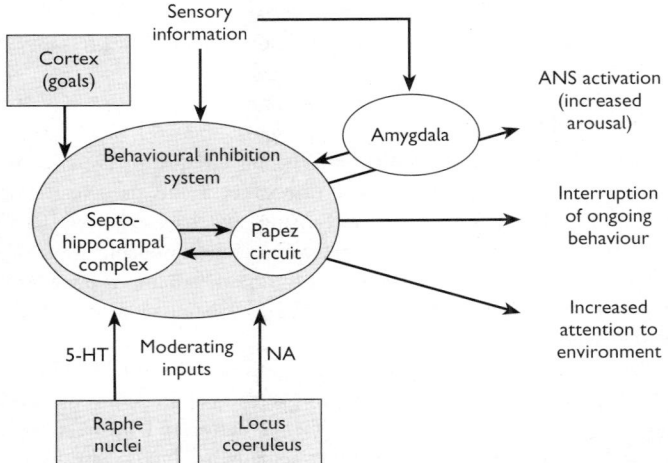

Fig. 2 Behavioural inhibition system (based on descriptions by Gray and McNaughton[28]): ANS, autonomic nervous system; 5-HT, serotonin; NA, noradrenaline.

Stressful life events

Several studies have found an association between stressful or traumatic life events and GAD. In a subset of participants in the Epidemiologic Catchment Area Study, men who reported experiencing four or more stressful life events during the preceding year were more than eight times as likely to meet DSM-III criteria for GAD than those reporting three or fewer stressful life events.[43] The experience of even one very important unexpected negative event was associated with a threefold increase in GAD in both men and women. A variety of stressors have been associated with increased risk of GAD, including early parental death,[44] rape or combat,[45] and chronically dysfunctional marital and family relationships.[46]

Parenting

There is an extensive literature on the influences of early environmental factors on the development of anxiety and other negative emotions in children (for an integrative review, see Chorpita and Barlow[47]). Attachment theory holds that parents or other consistent caregivers serve an important function in a child's development by providing a protective and secure base from which the child can operate. Disruption of this base is hypothesized to lead initially to anxious apprehension and dependency and, if the disruption is severe, subsequently to withdrawal and depression.

An important aspect of a healthy parent–child relationship is its ability to foster in the child a sense of control over events. According to Chorpita and Barlow,[47] an individual who lacks sufficient early experiences of control may develop a general perception of personal inefficacy which may predispose him or her to chronic negative emotional states such as GAD. Two aspects of parenting appear to be important in providing a child with opportunities to experience control: responsiveness to the child's efforts at engagement and encouragement of the child to explore and manipulate the environment. A parenting style characterized by excessive control of the child's environment (overprotection) coupled with a lack of warmth and responsiveness toward the child would deprive the child of such opportunities and thus, theoretically, could contribute to the development of anxiety.

Consistent with this theory, mothers of anxious preschool children were found to be more critical and intrusive and less responsive to their children than mothers of non-anxious children.[48] In addition, adults who rated their parenting as more protective and less caring had higher trait anxiety scores than other individuals surveyed.[49] A similar pattern was found to distinguish patients meeting DSM-IIIR criteria for GAD or panic disorder from controls.[50] One hypothesis is that the relationship of these early parenting experiences to the subsequent development of anxiety (or depression) is mediated by the early formation of cognitive vulnerability best described as a sense of uncontrollability regarding future events in one's life (Fig. 4).[47]

Course and prognosis

GAD is a chronic and disabling condition. The Harvard/Brown Anxiety Research Program study provides information on the course and impact of GAD among patients treated naturalistically over a 3-year period.[51,52] The mean age at onset of GAD was 21 years (range 2–61 years), and the average duration of illness at initial evaluation was 20 years. Excluding patients with comorbid panic disorder, one-

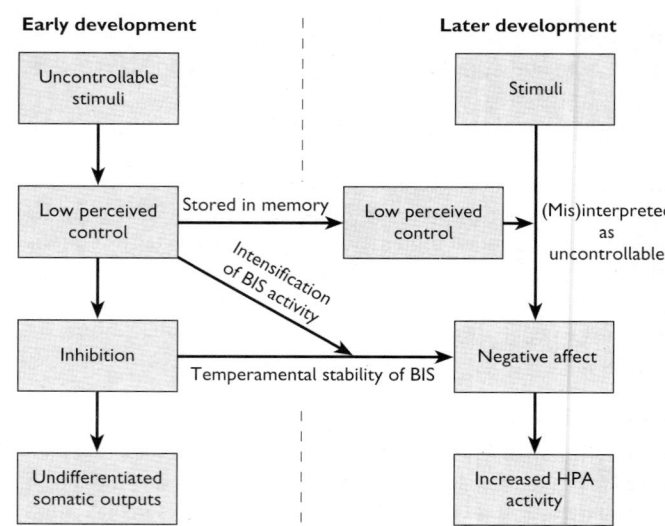

Fig. 4 Model of the development of vulnerability for anxiety and depression. BIS, behavioural inhibition system[28]; HPA, hypothalamic–pituitary–adrenal axis. (Reproduced with permission from B.F. Chorpita and D.H. Barlow (1998). The development of anxiety: the role of control in the early environment. *Psychological Bulletin*, **124**, 3–21.)

third of subjects had never married and another 17 per cent were separated, widowed, or divorced. Unemployment was higher than average, and 37 per cent of subjects had received public financial assistance. Despite the fact that more than 80 per cent of patients received treatment during the study period, remission from GAD was uncommon (15 per cent at 1 year, 27 per cent by 3 years). Among patients with comorbid psychiatric disorders, the proportions achieving remission from GAD and coexisting anxiety disorders were only 8 per cent and 17 per cent at 1 and 3 years, respectively.

Treatment

Pharmacotherapy

Several pharmacological agents have been shown to be effective for the treatment of GAD (for a review, see Connor and Davidson[27]). Chief among these are the benzodiazepines, azapirones, and antidepressants. (See also Chapter 6.2.2.)

Benzodiazepines

Benzodiazepines have for decades been the most frequently prescribed medications for anxiety. Compared with other agents used to treat anxiety disorders, they are safe, fast-acting, and have relatively few side-effects. All currently available benzodiazepines probably are efficacious for GAD. Approximately two-thirds of patients experience moderate to marked improvement, with effects being evident within the first 1 or 2 weeks of treatment.[53]

Benzodiazepines appear to be more effective for the somatic symptoms of GAD than for psychic symptoms such as apprehensive worry and irritability, possibly because of their sedative and myorelaxant properties. In some studies, irritability actually has increased during treatment with benzodiazepines.[54] Consequently, these drugs may be better for patients whose complaints are more somatic than psychic, whereas other agents may be better when the reverse is true.

Azapirones

In recent years, azapirone drugs have become a popular alternative to benzodiazepines for the treatment of GAD. These drugs lack the sedative and muscle relaxant properties of the benzodiazepines as well as their ability to potentiate the effects of alcohol. However, improvement is somewhat slower (2–4 weeks) than with benzodiazepines. The most widely-used of these agents is buspirone, whose efficacy and safety have been demonstrated in several well-controlled trials (see Rickels[55] for a review). It is as effective as benzodiazepines for general anxiety and may reduce some of the associated features of GAD as well, including depression and agitation. Ipsapirone, an azapirone with somewhat greater affinity and selectivity for the 5-hydroxytryptamine-1A receptor and fewer side-effects than buspirone also appears to be effective.[56] Other drugs in this class include gepirone, tandospirone, and flesinoxan.

Antidepressants

Both imipramine and trazodone have been superior to placebo for the treatment of GAD in controlled trials. In one trial, the two drugs were comparable to each other and to diazepam in reducing anxiety after the first 2 weeks of treatment.[53] In another study, imipramine was as effective as chlordiazepoxide overall and produced greater reductions in associated depression.[57] Nefazadone, an agent related to trazodone but less sedating, was effective for GAD in a small open trial.[58]

One of the most promising new antidepressant drugs for GAD is venlafaxine, a serotonin and noradrenaline reuptake inhibitor. Preliminary reports of two large multicentre trials indicate that venlafaxine is as effective as buspirone, with declines in anxiety being evident in some cases by the end of the first week of treatment. The efficacy of selective serotonin reuptake inhibitors for GAD has yet to be determined, although clinical experience and a small open trial of paroxetine suggest that they may be helpful if excessive stimulation can be avoided.

Psychosocial treatment

Early psychological treatments for GAD consisted mostly of non-specific interventions such as supportive psychotherapy, relaxation training, and biofeedback. In general, those treatments were not very effective. More recently, treatments have been developed that specifically target cognitive (e.g. worry) and behavioural (e.g. avoidance) features of GAD. These treatments are typically administered in a dozen or so sessions, and can be conducted in group or individual formats. In controlled trials, these newer cognitive and cognitive-behavioural treatments have been more effective than no treatment or a psychological or drug placebo treatment and at least as effective as benzodiazepines (for a review, see Barlow et al.[59]). Attrition is low (10–15 per cent), and reductions in anxiety average about 50 per cent, with gains being maintained at follow-up. Currently, the most successful treatments combine relaxation training with cognitive interventions focused on making the worry process more controllable.

Consistent with the findings of individual studies, meta-analyses have found moderate to large treatment effects (effect sizes of 0.73 to 1.54) favouring cognitive and cognitive-behavioural treatments over waiting-list or placebo controls.[60] Treatments that combined both cognitive and behavioural interventions had a larger average effect size than those using cognitive or behavioural interventions alone. As in individual trials, meta-analytic comparisons of effective drug and psychosocial treatments for GAD show the two modalities to be equally effective. Cognitive therapy for anxiety disorders is considered further in Chapter 6.3.2.1.

Combined pharmacotherapy and psychotherapy

Although common in clinical practice, little is known about the effects of combining pharmacotherapy and psychotherapy for GAD. In the only published study to date, Power et al.[61] compared cognitive-behavioural therapy, diazepam, a pill placebo, cognitive-behavioural therapy plus diazepam, and cognitive-behavioural therapy plus a pill placebo in a sample of DSM-III-diagnosed GAD patients. At post-treatment and follow-up, patients in all three cognitive-behavioural therapy conditions were more improved than those who received diazepam or placebo alone. Although the cognitive-behavioural therapy groups did not differ significantly from each other on any measure, the cognitive-behavioural therapy plus diazepam group improved earliest and had the largest percentage of patients achieving a criterion of clinically significant change on all measures. Unfortunately, the use of DSM-III criteria in this study makes its relevance to GAD as it is currently defined uncertain. In addition, the cognitive-behavioural therapy used was briefer (seven sessions) and less specific than the currently recommended forms.

Effect of comorbidity on treatment outcome and vice versa

Owing to the residual nature of GAD in DSM-III, until recently most treatment trials excluded patients with comorbid Axis I disorders. A review of 48 GAD studies published between 1980 and 1991 found that only eight reported including patients with other psychiatric disorders.[62] When comorbid disorders have been permitted, their effect on treatment outcome generally has not been evaluated. In the Harvard–Brown Anxiety Research Program study, the presence of a comorbid psychiatric disorder reduced response rates at 1 and 3 years by nearly 50 per cent. In addition, two studies found that concurrent personality disorders impair outcome of treatment for GAD.[63,64] In one of these studies,[64] improvement was comparable among treatment completers with or without Axis II disorders, but attrition was greater in the former (44 per cent) than the latter (19 per cent) group.

On the other hand, successful treatment of GAD in patients with comorbid disorders often reduces the severity of the other disorders as well. Borkovec et al.[65] examined the effect of various psychosocial treatments for GAD on coexisting anxiety and mood disorders (except panic disorder or severe depression, which were excluded from the study). Across treatments, patients whose GAD improved exhibited reductions as well in other anxiety disorders (mostly social and simple phobia) and dysthymia. Only four of 13 successfully treated patients who had additional disorders at pretreatment continued to have them at post-treatment.

Clinical management

Many anxious patients do not meet diagnostic criteria for GAD. These patients often respond to conservative measures. If the symptoms are minor or are related to a situational stressor, brief psychotherapy and support is the treatment of first choice. In one study, patients who initially reported physical or minor emotional complaints responded better to counselling than to diazepam, even when counselling was limited to only 3 h.[66] Often, an explanation of the relationship of physical symptoms to stress is reassuring to patients and can interrupt a spiral of symptoms leading to anxiety and worry about health, leading to increased symptoms, and so on. Simple behavioural interventions such as relaxation training for patients with prominent muscle tension or breathing exercises for those with dyspnoea or hyperventilation may be helpful as well.

For patients with marked adrenergic symptoms or insomnia, the temporary (a few days to a few weeks) use of a benzodiazepine may be helpful as an adjunct to psychotherapy. In some cases, a hypnotic drug alone is sufficient. In general, as-needed use of benzodiazepines should be discouraged, because it is more likely than scheduled use to foster reliance on drugs as the principal means of coping with anxiety. For the same reason, the drug dose should be kept as low as possible and should be tapered as therapy proceeds.

For patients meeting diagnostic criteria for GAD, treatment with an empirically validated form of psychosocial therapy for GAD is strongly recommended. Such treatments are available in manualized form with accompanying patient workbooks.[67,68]

When medication treatment is preferred, a trial of buspirone is a good initial choice. Exceptions are patients with comorbid panic disorder or marked adrenergic symptoms, for whom benzodiazepines may be better if they are not contraindicated (see below). The typical starting dose of buspirone is 15 mg/day in divided doses (5 mg thrice daily or 7.5 mg twice a day), which is increased by 5 mg/day every few days to a target dose of 30 mg/day. If the response is insufficient after 2 to 4 weeks at that amount, or if the patient is experiencing significant depressive symptoms, the dose may be advanced gradually to a maximum of 60 mg/day. Improvement may continue for up to 3 months.

It is important to inform patients of the typical side-effects and response time of buspirone (see Chapter 6.2.2). Patients who have taken benzodiazepines previously may expect prompt relief and sedative side-effects from the medication and may become discouraged when these are absent. When switching from a benzodiazepine to buspirone, it may be helpful to continue the benzodiazepine during the first month of buspirone therapy before initiating a gradual taper. Remember that buspirone will not prevent benzodiazepine withdrawal symptoms.

Failing a course of buspirone, or in patients with comorbid major depression, trials of antidepressant medications (e.g. imipramine, venlafaxine, trazodone) would be a reasonable second choice. Venlafaxine may be effective at doses as low as 75 mg/day (the usual starting dose). Because of its short metabolic half-life, the extended-release form is preferred, which allows once-per-day dosing and thus may improve compliance. The dose typically is advanced by 75 mg/day every 2 weeks to a maximum of 225 mg/day. Dosing for other antidepressants is the same as for the treatment of depression.

Because of the risk of dependence and (uncommonly) abuse, long-term use of benzodiazepines generally is reserved for patients who do not respond sufficiently to other options. Relative contraindications include a need to be alert (e.g. drivers and machinery operators), a personal or family history of alcoholism or drug abuse, and prominent aggressiveness or irritability. Generally, longer half-life benzodiazepines (e.g. diazepam, clonazepam), which can be taken once or twice daily, are preferred. A typical starting dose is 5 to 10 mg/day of diaze-

pam or equivalent, which is advanced every few days to a maximum of 40 mg/day.

In instances where pharmacotherapy is the primary treatment, responders should be continued on medication for at least 6 months before a gradual drug taper is attempted. Even so, a substantial proportion will relapse after drug discontinuance and will require further treatment. Discontinuing pharmacotherapy in the context of effective psychosocial treatment may improve success rates.

Conclusions

Based on current knowledge, GAD seems to be the exaggerated expression of the human potential to apprehensively anticipate future misfortune. As such, it may represent a 'basic' disorder, a better understanding of which may shed light on other anxiety and mood disorders.[7] Unfortunately, the development of treatments for GAD, as well as more basic psychopathological and pathopysiological research, has lagged behind that of other disorders such as panic disorder and depression. This is despite the fact that GAD, and the closely related subsyndromal condition, mixed anxiety–depressive disorder, affect substantially more individuals than other anxiety disorders, particularly in primary care settings.[14] For these reasons, facilitating more accurate clinical recognition and devoting more resources to treatment development and associated research deserve higher priorities than heretofore accorded.

References

1. DiNardo, P.A., O'Brien, G.T., Barlow, D.H., Waddell, M.T., and Blanchard, E.B. (1983). Reliability of DSM-III anxiety disorder categories using a new structured interview. *Archives of General Psychiatry*, **40**, 1070–4.
2. Barlow, D.H. (1987). The classification of anxiety disorders. In *Diagnoses and classification in psychiatry: a critical appraisal of DSM-III* (ed. G.L. Tischler), pp. 223–42. Cambridge University Press.
3. DiNardo, P.A., Moras, K., Barlow, D.H., Rapee, R.M., and Brown, T.A. (1993). Reliability of DSM-III-R anxiety disorder categories: using the Anxiety Disorders Interview Schedule—Revised (ADIS-R). *Archives of General Psychiatry*, **50**, 251–6.
4. Abel, J.W. and Borkovec, T.D. (1995). Generalizability of DSM-III-R GAD to proposed DSM-IV criteria and cross validation of proposed changes. *Journal of Anxiety Disorders*, **9**, 303–15.
5. Craske, M.G., Rapee, R.M., Jackel, L., and Barlow, D.H. (1989). Qualitative dimensions of worry in DSM-III-R generalized anxiety disorder subjects and nonanxious controls. *Behavior Research and Therapy*, **27**, 189–98.
6. Barlow, D.H. and Wincze, J. (1998). DSM-IV and beyond: what is generalized anxiety disorder? *Acta Psychiatrica Scandinavica*, **98** (Suppl. 393), 23–9.
7. Brown, T.A., Barlow, D.H., and Liebowitz, M.R. (1994). The empirical basis of generalized anxiety disorder. *American Journal of Psychiatry*, **151**, 1272–80.
8. Breslau, N. and Davis, G.C. (1985). DSM-III generalized anxiety disorder: an empirical investigation of more stringent criteria. *Psychiatric Research*, **14**, 231–38.
9. Wacker, H.R., Mullejans, R., Klein, K.H., *et al.* (1992). Identification of cases of anxiety disorders and affective disorders in the community according to ICD-10 and DSM-III-R using the Composite International Diagnostic Interview (CIDI). *International Journal of Methods in Psychiatric Research*, **2**, 91–100.

10. Wittchen, H.-U., Zhao, S., Kessler, R.C., and Eaton, W.W. (1994). DSM-III-R generalized anxiety disorder in the National Comorbidity Survey. *Archives of General Psychiatry*, **51**, 355–64.

11. Blazer, D.G., Hughes, D., George, L.K., Swartz, M., and Boyer, R. (1991). Generalized anxiety disorder. In *Psychiatric disorders in America: the Epidemiologic Catchment Area Study* (ed. L.N. Robins and D.A. Regier), pp. 180–203. Free Press, New York.

12. Kessler, R.C., McGonagle, K.A., Zhao, S., *et al.* (1994). Lifetime and 12-month prevalence of DSM-III-R psychiatric disorders in the United States: results from the National Comorbidity Survey. *Archives of General Psychiatry*, **51**, 8–19.

13. Shear, M.K., and Schulberg, H.C. (1995). Anxiety disorders in primary care. *Bulletin of the Menninger Clinic*, **59**, A73–85.

14. Zinbarg, R.E., Barlow, D.H., Liebowitz, M., *et al.* (1994). The DSM-IV field trial for mixed anxiety–depression. *American Journal of Psychiatry*, **151**, 1153–62.

15. Brawman-Mintzer, O., Lydiard, R. B., Emmanuel, N., *et al.* (1993). Psychiatric comorbidity in patients with generalized anxiety disorder. *American Journal of Psychiatry*, **150**, 1216–18.

16. Sanderson, W.C., Wetzler, S., Beck, A.T., and Betz, F. (1994). Prevalence of personality disorders in patients with anxiety disorders. *Psychiatry Research*, **51**, 167–74.

17. Zinbarg, R. and Barlow, D.H. (1996). Structure of anxiety and the anxiety disorders: a hierarchial model. *Journal of Abnormal Psychology*, **105**, 181–93.

18. Brown, T.A., Chorpita, B.F., and Barlow, D.H. (1998). Structural relationships among dimensions of the DSM-IV anxiety and mood disorders and dimensions of negative affect, positive affect, and autonomic arousal. *Journal of Abnormal Psychology*, **107**, 179–92.

19. Barlow, D.H., Chorpita, B.F., and Turovsky, J. (1996). Fear, panic, anxiety, and disorders of emotion. In *Nebraska Symposium on Motivation*. Vol. 43, *Perspectives on anxiety, panic, and fear* (ed. D.A. Hope), pp. 251–328. University of Nebraska Press, Lincoln, NE.

20. Noyes, R., Clarkson, C., Crowe, R.R., *et al.* (1987). A family study of generalized anxiety. *American Journal of Psychiatry*, **144**, 1019–24.

21. Andrews, G., Stewart, S., Allen, R., *et al.* (1990). The genetics of six neurotic disorders: a twin study. *Journal of Affective Disorders*, **19**, 23–9.

22. Torgersen, S. (1983). Genetic factors in anxiety disorder. *Archives of General Psychiatry*, **40**, 1085–9.

23. Kendler, K.S., Neale, M.C., Kessler, R.C., Heath, A.C., and Eaves, L.J. (1992). Generalized anxiety disorder in women: a population-based twin study. *Archives of General Psychiatry*, **49**, 267–72.

24. Kendler, K.S., Neale, M.C., Kessler, R.C., Heath, A.C., and Eaves, L.J. (1992). Major depression and generalized anxiety disorder: same genes, (partly) different environments? *Archives of General Psychiatry*, **49**, 716–22.

25. Skre, I., Onstad, S., Torgersen, S., Lygren, S., and Kringlen, E. (1993). A twin study of DSM-III-R anxiety disorders. *Acta Psychiatrica Scandanavica*, **88**, 85–92.

26. Brawman-Mintzer, O. and Lydiard, R.B. (1997). Biological basis of generalized anxiety disorder. *Journal of Clinical Psychiatry*, **58** (Supplement 3), 16–25.

27. Connor, K.M. and Davidson, J.R.T. (1998). Generalized anxiety disorder: neurobiological and pharmacotherapeutic perspectives. *Biological Psychiatry*, **44**, 1286–94.

28. Gray, J.A. and McNaughton, N. (1996). The neuropsychology of anxiety: a reprise. In *Nebraska Symposium on Motivation*. Vol. 43, *Perspectives on anxiety, panic, and fear* (ed. D.A. Hope), pp. 61–134. University of Nebraska Press, Lincoln, NE.

29. Charney, D.S., Woods, S.W., Heninger, G.R., *et al.* (1989). Noradrenergic function in generalized anxiety disorder: effects of yohimbine in healthy subjects and patients with generalized anxiety disorder. *Psychiatry Research*, **27**, 173–82.

30. Abelson, J.L., Glitz, D., Cameron, O.G., Lee, M.A., Bronzo, M., and Curtis, G.C. (1991). Blunted growth hormone response to clonidine in patients with generalized anxiety disorder. *Archives of General Psychiatry*, **48**, 157–62.

31. Cameron, O.G., Smith, C.B., Lee, M.A., *et al.* (1990). Adrenergic status in anxiety disorders: platelet alpha two-adrenergic receptor binding, blood pressure, pulse, and plasma catecholamines in panic and generalized anxiety disorder patients and in normal subjects. *Biological Psychiatry*, **28**, 3–20.

32. Thayer, J.F., Friedman, B.H., and Borkovec, T. (1996). Autonomic characteristics of generalized anxiety disorder and worry. *Biological Psychiatry*, **39**, 255–66.

33. Jacobson, L. and Sapolsky, R. (1991). The role of the hippocampus in feedback regulation of the hypothalamic–pituitary–adrenocortical axis. *Endocrine Reviews*, **12**, 118–34.

34. Tiller, J.W.G., Biddle, N., Maguire, K.P., *et al.* (1988). The dexamethasone suppression test and plasma dexamethasone in generalized anxiety disorder. *Biological Psychiatry*, **23**, 261–70.

35. LeDoux, J. (1996). *The emotional brain: the mysterious underpinnings of emotional life*. Simon and Schuster, New York.

36. LeDoux, J. (1998). Fear and the brain: where have we been, and where are we going? *Biological Psychiatry*, **44**, 1229–38.

37. Davis, M. (1998). Are different parts of the extended amygdala involved in fear versus anxiety? *Biological Psychiatry*, **44**, 1239–47.

38. Gray, J.A. (1982). *The neuropsychology of anxiety*. Oxford University Press, New York.

39. Rocca, P., Beoni, A.M., Eva, C., Ferrero, P., Zanalda, E., and Ravizza, L. (1998). Peripheral benzodiazepine receptor messenger RNA is decreased in lymphocytes of generalized anxiety disorder patients. *Biological Psychiatry*, **43**, 767–73.

40. Brewerton, T.D., Lydiard, R.B., Johnson, M.R., *et al.* (1995). CSF serotonin: diagnostic and seasonal differences. In *New research abstracts of the 148th meeting of the American Psychiatric Association*, Abstract NR385:151. American Psychiatric Press, Washington, DC.

41. Iny, L.J., Pecknold, J., Suranyi-Cadotte, B.E., *et al.* (1994). Studies of neurochemical link between depression, anxiety, and stress from [3H]imipramine and [3H]paroxetine binding on human platelets. *Biological Psychiatry*, **36**, 281–91.

42. Bradwejn, J., Koszycki, D., Couetoux du Tertre, A., *et al.* (1992). The cholecystokinin hypothesis of panic and anxiety disorders: a review. *Journal of Psychopharmacology*, **6**, 345–51.

43. Blazer, D., Hughes, D., and George, L.K. (1987). Stressful life events and the onset of a generalized anxiety syndrome. *American Journal of Psychiatry*, **144**, 1178–83.

44. Torgersen, S. (1986). Childhood and family characteristics in panic and generalized anxiety disorders. *American Journal of Psychiatry*, **143**, 630–2.

45. Steketee, G. and Foa, E.B. (1987). Rape victims: post traumatic stress responses and their treatment: a review of the literature. *Journal of Anxiety Disorders*, **1**, 69–86.

46. Ben-Noun, L. (1998). Generalized anxiety disorder in dysfunctional families. *Journal of Behavior Therapy and Experimental Psychiatry*, **29**, 115–22.

47. Chorpita, B.F. and Barlow, D.H. (1998). The development of anxiety: the role of control in the early environment. *Psychological Bulletin*, **124**, 3–21.

48. Dumas, J.E., LaFreniere, P.J., and Serketich, W.J. (1995). 'Balance of power': a transactional analysis of control in mother–child dyads involving socially competent, aggressive, and anxious children. *Journal of Abnormal Psychology*, **104**, 104–13.

49. Parker, G. (1979). Reported parental characteristics in relation to trait depression and anxiety levels in a non-clinical group. *Australian and New Zealand Journal of Psychiatry*, **13**, 260–4.

50. Silove, D., Parker, G., Hadzi-Pavlovic, D., Manicavasagar, V., and Blaszczynski, A. (1991). Parental representations of patients with panic disorder and generalised anxiety disorder. *British Journal of Psychiatry*, **159**, 835–41.

51. Massion, A., Warshaw, M., and Keller, M. (1993) Quality of life and psychiatric morbidity in panic disorder versus generalized anxiety disorder. *American Journal of Psychiatry*, **150**, 600–7.

52. Yonkers, K.A., Warshaw, M.G., Massion, A.O., and Keller, M.B. (1996). Phenomenology and course of generalised anxiety disorder. *British Journal of Psychiatry*, **168**, 308–13.

53. Rickels, K., Downing, R., Schweizer, E., and Hassman, H. (1993). Antidepressants for the treatment of generalized anxiety disorder: a placebo-controlled comparison of imipramine, trazodone, and diazepam. *Archives of General Psychiatry*, **50**, 884–95.

54. Rosenbaum, J.E., Woods, S.W., Groves, J.E., *et al.* (1984). Emergence of hostility during alprazolam treatment. *American Journal of Psychiatry*, **141**, 792–3.

55. Rickels, K. (1990). Buspirone in clinical practice. *Journal of Clinical Psychiatry*, **51** (Supplement 9), 51–4.

56. Cutler, N.R., Sramek, J.J., Keppel-Hesselink, J.M., *et al.* (1993). A double-blind, placebo-controlled study comparing the efficacy and safety of ipsapirone versus lorazepam in patients with generalized anxiety disorder: a prospective multicenter trial. *Journal of Clinical Psychopharmacology*, **13**, 429–37.

57. Kahn, R.J., McNair, D.M., Lipman, R.S., *et al.* (1986). Imipramine and chlordiazepoxide in depressive and anxiety disorders; II: efficacy in anxious outpatients. *Archives of General Psychiatry*, **43**, 79–85.

58. Hedges, D.W., Reimherr, F.W., Strong, R.E., Halls, C.H., and Rust, C. (1996). An open trial of nefazodone in adult patients with generalized anxiety disorder. *Psychopharmacology Bulletin*, **32**, 671–6.

59. Barlow, D.H., Esler, J.L., and Vitali, B.A. (1997). Psychosocial treatments for panic disorders, phobias, and generalized anxiety disorder. In *A guide to treatments that work* (ed. P.E. Nathan and J.M. Gorman), pp. 288–318. Oxford University Press, New York.

60. Gould, R.A., Otto, M.W., Pollack, M.H., and Yap, L. (1997). Cognitive-behavioral and pharmacological treatment of generalized anxiety disorder: a preliminary meta-analysis. *Behavior Therapy*, **28**, 285–305.

61. Power, K.G., Simpson, R.J., Swanson, V., Wallace, L.A., Feistner, A.T.C., and Sharp, D. (1990). A controlled comparison of cognitive-behaviour therapy, diazepam, and placebo, alone and in combination, for the treatment of generalized anxiety disorder. *Journal of Anxiety Disorders*, **4**, 267–92.

62. Swinson, R.P., Cox, B.J., and Fergus, K.D. (1993). Diagnostic criteria in generalized anxiety disorder treatment studies. *Journal of Clinical Psychopharmacology*, **13**, 455.

63. Rickels, K. and Schweizer, E. (1997). The clinical presentation of generalized anxiety in primary-care settings: practical concepts of classification and management. *Journal of Clinical Psychiatry*, **58** (Supplement 11), 4–10.

64. Sanderson, W.C., Beck, A.T., and McGinn, L.K. (1994). Cognitive therapy for generalized anxiety disorder: significance of comorbid personality disorders. *Journal of Cognitive Psychotherapy*, **8**, 13–18.

65. Borkovec, T.D., Abel, J.L., and Newman, H. (1995). Effects of psychotherapy on comorbid conditions in generalized anxiety disorder. *Journal of Consulting and Clinical Psychology*, **63**, 479–83.

66. Boulenger, J., Fournier, M., Rosales, D., and Lavallée, Y. (1997). Mixed anxiety and depression: from theory to practice. *Journal of Clinical Psychiatry*, **58** (Supplement 8), 27–34.

67. Craske, M.G., Barlow, D.H., and O'Leary, T.A. (1992). *Mastery of your anxiety and worry: client workbook*. Graywind Publications/The Psychological Corporation, San Antonio, TX.

68. Zinbarg, R.E., Craske, M.G., and Barlow, D.H. (1993). *Mastery of your anxiety and worry: therapist guide*. Graywind Publications/The Psychological Corporation, San Antonio, TX.

4.7.2 Social and specific phobias

David M. Fresco, Brigette A. Erwin, Richard G. Heimberg, and Cynthia L. Turk

Introduction

Great strides have been made in our knowledge of phobic disorders. As our classification systems have been refined, we have come to view social phobia and specific phobia as distinct disorders, with divergent patterns of prevalence, aetiology, and course. Moreover, treatments for these disorders have become increasingly sophisticated. This chapter presents an overview of the current state of the field with regard to social and specific phobias.

Social phobia

Social phobia only recently became an official diagnostic category. In the first and second editions of the *Diagnostic and Statistical Manual of Mental Disorders* (**DSM**),[1,2] all phobias were grouped together. However, in 1966, Marks and Gelder[3] observed that various phobias had different ages of onset and surmised that they might be distinct disorders, providing the initial impetus for the inclusion of social phobia in DSM-III.[4] Nevertheless, research into the nature and treatment of social phobia lagged behind that for other anxiety disorders, leading to its description as the neglected anxiety disorder.[5] Over the past decade, however, attention to the conceptualization, definition, and classification of social phobia has increased dramatically.

Clinical presentation

Almost everyone experiences anxiety in situations involving potential evaluation by others (e.g. job interviews, public-speaking engagements, first dates). However, for individuals with social phobia, these situations are typically associated with incapacitating levels of anxiety and a desire for escape or avoidance. Many individuals with social phobia are self-critical and perfectionistic—attempting to conduct themselves according to extreme and exacting standards to avoid the negative evaluation of others that they may perceive as epidemic. Commonly, persons with social phobia experience somatic symptoms such as blushing, trembling, dry mouth, or perspiring, which they believe will be noticed by others and provide further evidence of their incompetence. By leaving anxiety-provoking situations (escape) or by foregoing them entirely (avoidance), individuals with social phobia may reduce or prevent the immediate experience of anxiety, but this relief may also reinforce their belief in their inadequacies. This cycle may serve to maintain the person's social anxiety in the absence of objective threat.[6,7]

Functional impairment

Individuals with social phobia experience significant impairment in social, educational, and vocational functioning.[5,8] They may find it difficult to initiate or maintain social or romantic relationships, avoid classes that require public presentations, discontinue their education prematurely, or take jobs below their ability to avoid social or performance demands. They are more likely to be single, less well educated, and to receive financial assistance than persons without the disorder.[9] They are also more likely to contemplate suicide.[9]

Despite the profound impairment associated with social phobia, it rarely leads someone to seek treatment. For example, Stein (unpublished observations) found that 7 per cent of 511 primary-care patients met criteria for social phobia. While these individuals reported more days lost from work and more days of decreased productivity in the past month due to 'nerves or emotional problems' than those without a psychiatric disorder, only one in six had received appropriate treatment for their anxiety.

Classification

DSM and ICD

While DSM is widely used in North America, the *International Classification of Mental and Behavioural Disorders* (**ICD**) is commonly used in other parts of the world. Social phobia first appeared in ICD-10[10] 12 years after its appearance in DSM-III. The ICD-10 criteria for social phobia are less detailed and more circumscribed than those in DSM-IV.[11] Specifically, DSM-IV requires an excessive fear of humiliation or embarrassment in social or performance situations, anxiety provoked by exposure to feared situations, recognition that the fear is excessive, avoidance of situations or endurance with distress, and significant distress or impairment. Furthermore, the fear and avoidance cannot be better accounted for by another psychiatric disorder, a general medical condition, or the effects of a substance. In contrast, ICD-10 requires only that the symptoms be representative of anxiety and not another psychiatric disorder, that the anxiety occurs in relation to social situations, and that avoidance of anxiety-provoking situations be present. Because most published research on social phobia relies on DSM rather than ICD criteria, this chapter will also do so.

Diagnostic issues

DSM-III originally described social phobia as a fear of embarrassment, humiliation, and scrutiny by others in one or two specific performance situations. It also stated that social phobia rarely led to substantial impairment. However, research and clinical experience suggest that individuals whose fears are limited in this way represent a minority of persons with social phobia who present for treatment. More commonly, those presenting for treatment endorse multiple fears and significant impairment.[5] In recognition of the heterogeneity of persons with social phobia, DSM-IIIR[12] and DSM-IV include subtypes of social phobia. The generalized type is specified when 'most social situations' are feared. Persons whose fears do not extend to most social situations are grouped together into the non-generalized subtype of social phobia. While these criteria are ambiguous, persons with generalized and non-generalized social phobia differ on several dimensions, including symptom severity, functional impairment,[13] and physiological symptoms when exposed to feared situations.[13,14] However, conclusive differences between subtypes in the course and response to treatment remain to be demonstrated.[15,16]

Like social phobia, avoidant personality disorder (**APD**) first appeared in DSM-III and has undergone significant revision. While DSM-III regarded social phobia as an irrational fear of a limited number of performance situations, it regarded APD as an instance of severe interpersonal anxiety. Furthermore, the presence of APD pre-empted a diagnosis of social phobia. Later, DSM-IIIR allowed an individual to receive concurrent diagnoses of social phobia and APD, and the criteria for APD became more similar to those of social phobia. The core disturbance of APD was changed to an extreme fear of negative evaluation rather than discomfort in interpersonal relationships.[17] Changes to the criteria for APD, as well as the evolution of the social phobia criteria, have led researchers to question whether the two categories represent distinct disorders or whether they differ only in degree. Indeed, research supports the position that social phobia and APD belong on a continuum that is artificially divided at the boundary between Axes I and II.[17] Individuals with APD almost always have social phobia, while many individuals with social phobia do not meet the criteria for APD. Individuals with generalized social phobia (median = 58 per cent) are more likely than individuals with non-generalized social phobia (median = 18 per cent) to meet the criteria for APD.[17] Many investigators have concluded that the co-occurrence of generalized social phobia and APD describes those persons with the most severe social phobia and the poorest global functioning.[18]

The *DSM-IV* task force considered other refinements to the criteria of social phobia. The parenthetical name 'social anxiety disorder' was added to acknowledge the significant impairment associated with social phobia and its differentiation from specific phobia. The criteria were also modified to include features specific to children.[11] There must be evidence that children are capable of forming social relationships, and anxiety must be evident in peer relationships. It is also acknowledged that children may manifest their anxiety differently than adults: they may cry, throw tantrums, freeze, or shrink from interactions with strangers, and they may not acknowledge that their fears are irrational. Also, social anxiety may develop as a result of some medical conditions. For example, persons may become excessively anxious or avoid social situations because of obesity, acne, benign essential tremor, stuttering, or Parkinson's disease. These conditions are not considered exemplars of social phobia in DSM-IV because anxiety developed secondary to the medical condition. Instead, they are assigned to the category 'anxiety disorder not otherwise specified'. However, persons who experience secondary social anxiety are often responsive to pharmacological or cognitive-behavioural treatments that demonstrate efficacy for social phobia.[19] While there was substantial discussion about this issue in the DSM-IV workgroup, this loophole in the diagnostic criteria was not closed.

Comorbidity and differential diagnosis

Social phobia may increase the risk for other psychiatric disorders.[9,20,21] In the National Comorbidity Survey (**NCS**), 81 per cent of persons with primary social phobia met the criteria for at least one other lifetime psychiatric disorder.[22] Odds ratios for other DSM-IIIR disorders given social phobia were 7.75 for simple phobia, 7.06 for agoraphobia, 4.83 for panic disorder, 3.77 for generalized anxiety disorder, 2.69 for post-traumatic stress disorder, 3.69 for major depression, 3.15 for dysthymia, and 2.01 for substance abuse.[22] In persons with comorbid diagnoses in the Epidemiological Catchment Area Study (**ECA**), social phobia preceded the comorbid disorder in 76.8 per cent and onset in the same year in 7.2 per cent of cases.[9]

Differential diagnosis is complicated by the fact that certain Axis I disorders both resemble and co-occur with social phobia. However, the distinction among disorders is clinically important because pharmacological and psychological treatments may be differentially efficacious.

Panic disorder with agoraphobia (**PDA**) can be differentiated from social phobia in several ways. While many individuals with social phobia experience panic attacks, their anxiety occurs in anticipation of being evaluated negatively by others; for persons with panic disorder, panic attacks are often unexpected, may not be associated with specific cognitions, and can be nocturnal.[5] The age of onset for social phobia tends to be earlier than that for PDA.[23] Persons with social phobia presenting for treatment either show an equal gender distribution or are slightly more likely to be male;[24,25] those with PDA presenting for treatment are substantially more likely to be female.[5,26] Persons with social phobia are more likely to experience blushing and muscle twitches, while individuals with PDA are more likely to experience symptoms such as blurred vision, headaches, chest pain, and ringing in the ears and to fear that they will die or go crazy.[5,26] Finally, persons with social phobia report feeling more comfortable when alone, while persons with PDA may feel more comfortable in the presence of others.[23]

Individuals with generalized anxiety disorder endorse higher levels of social anxiety than individuals with anxiety disorders other than social phobia.[24] Although individuals with either social phobia or generalized anxiety disorder may devote excessive amounts of time to worrying and ruminating, the focus of the worries in social phobia is specific to social or performance situations, while the hallmark feature of worry in generalized anxiety disorder is a heightened focus on possible catastrophic consequences across several domains of life. Patterns of anxiety symptoms also differentiate the two. Sweating, flushes, and breathing problems are more common in social phobia, while headaches, insomnia, and fear of dying are more common in generalized anxiety disorder.[27,28]

Social phobia and depression may share the characteristic of withdrawal from social situations.[26] In differentiating between social phobia and depression, one must consider the reason for the withdrawal. Persons with depression do so because they fail to experience pleasure in or lack the energy for social engagement. Persons with social phobia fear the negative evaluation they believe is associated with such situations. Persons with depression may be indifferent about engaging in social situations, while persons with social phobia often have a strong desire to affiliate with others which is hampered by anxiety.

Schizophrenia spectrum disorders are also characterized by symptoms that may resemble those of social phobia. For example, persons with schizophrenia, schizotypal personality, and schizoid personality are socially avoidant. However, they do not typically desire social relationships.[26] Similarly, persons with paranoid personality disorder may avoid others because they are suspicious of and fear harm from other persons.

Epidemiology

Prevalence

Lifetime rates of social phobia vary from 2.4 per cent in ECA[9] to 13.3 per cent in the NCS.[20] The NCS rates make social phobia the third most common psychiatric disorder behind major depression and alcohol abuse. However, rates for all disorders differ depending on how one defines caseness.[29] For example, ECA utilized the more restrictive DSM-III criteria, while the NCS utilized DSM-IIIR criteria. Furthermore, the NCS probed six potentially fear-evoking situations,

while ECA probed only three. Given the greater similarity between DSM-IIIR and the current DSM-IV, lifetime rates of DSM-IV social phobia are probably closer to those estimated in the NCS. The 12-month prevalence rate estimates the number of individuals in a given year who experience social phobia. The NCS reported a 7.9 per cent 12-month prevalence rate of social phobia.

Age at onset/age of treatment seeking

Social phobia often begins early in life. Findings from ECA suggest that its onset is bimodal, with peaks before the age of 5 years and between 11 and 15.[9] Despite the early onset, persons with social phobia often do not present for treatment until 30 years of age or later, after enduring the symptoms of social phobia for many years.[30]

Gender differences

Although men and women with social phobia who seek treatment do so in relatively equal numbers,[24,25] epidemiological studies suggest that women are more likely than men to have social phobia.[9,20] Furthermore, in a clinical sample, women reported fear of more social situations and scored higher on several social phobia assessment measures.[31] Thus, it appears that, although women are more likely to experience social anxiety, men are more likely to seek treatment and may do so when troubled with less severe symptoms. While little research has directly addressed this issue, it may be that social phobia impairs the expected role-functioning of men to a greater extent than it does for women.

Aetiology of social phobia

Both genetic and environmental factors contribute to the emergence of social phobia. Studies of first-degree relatives of probands with social phobia have clearly established that it runs in families. One of the first proband studies interviewed 83 first-degree relatives of individuals with social phobia and 231 first-degree relatives of individuals with no psychiatric history to assess their lifetime history of DSM-IIIR disorders.[32] Of relatives of individuals with social phobia, 16 per cent met the criteria for social phobia compared with only 5 per cent of relatives of individuals with no psychiatric history. Rates for all other anxiety disorders were similar among relatives of the two proband groups. Similarly, first-degree relatives of probands with DSM-IIIR simple phobia, social phobia, and panic disorder with agoraphobia most frequently met the criteria for the proband's anxiety disorder, but were not more likely to meet the criteria for the other disorders.[33] Further, in a study of psychopathology in the children of individuals with social phobia, 27 out of 47 children met the criteria for at least one anxiety disorder, with overanxious disorder (30 per cent) and social phobia (23 per cent) the most common.[34] Finally, two studies found rates of social phobia in first-degree relatives of probands with generalized social phobia higher than in relatives of probands with non-generalized social phobia or with no psychiatric history.[35,36]

Much less work has considered the relative contributions of genetic and familial factors to social phobia. However, the Virginia Twin Study examined concordance rates of several DSM-III disorders in 2163 female twins.[37] The concordance rate for social phobia among monozygotic twins (24.4 per cent) was greater than that for dizygotic twins (15.3 per cent). Nevertheless, genetic factors accounted for less than one-third of the variance in the transmission of social phobia. Taken together, twin and proband studies suggest that a general predisposition towards interpreting situations as dangerous may be conferred genetically, while environmental factors influence the specific processing and interpretation of social cues.[6]

Course of social phobia

Scant information is available on the course of social phobia. In the only prospective study to date, social phobia persisted throughout adulthood.[38] Furthermore, course was unrelated to gender, age of onset, duration of illness, level of functioning at intake, lifetime history of anxiety disorders, or current comorbidity of anxiety or depressive disorders.[38,39] To date, no studies have followed individuals across their entire lifespan. Most other information on course is derived from retrospective accounts of individuals with social phobia. In an epidemiological sample, individuals with social phobia had, on average, met the criteria for the disorder for 19.4 years.[21] In ECA, 15.5 per cent of participants reported that they had experienced symptoms of social phobia throughout their whole lives.[9]

In childhood, two related conditions emerge and are relatively stable into adulthood. Individuals who had been shy as children exhibited overall lower levels of functioning when assessed 30 years later.[40] Similarly, behavioural inhibition, or the tendency to withdraw from novel people, settings, or objects, was more prevalent in the children of individuals with anxiety disorders; this remained relatively stable for over 7 years in children initially assessed between the ages of 21 and 31 months.[41] These findings suggest that behavioural inhibition may be an early expression of social phobia.[41]

In sum, social phobia is a chronic disorder that is unlikely to remit without treatment. However, individuals can gain relief from social phobia with both somatic and psychological treatments. The next section describes and summarizes treatments that have demonstrated efficacy.

Empirically evaluated treatments

The randomized double-blind design and the utilization of blind assessors represents the 'high-water mark' in the evaluation of pharmacotherapies. Although it is difficult to keep the patient and therapist uninformed about the psychotherapy being administered, independent and multimodal assessments are increasingly common in research on psychosocial treatments as well. Open trials and uncontrolled case series provide little empirical information compared with these more sophisticated approaches. Therefore, in the following sections, we focus on those studies that evaluate treatments in comparison with placebo and other control conditions.

Pharmacotherapy

The efficacy of traditional monoamine oxidase inhibitors, reversible inhibitors of monoamine oxidase, selective serotonin reuptake inhibitors, benzodiazepines, β-blockers, and buspirone have all been evaluated in placebo-controlled studies.

Monoamine oxidase inhibitors

Phenelzine sulphate has been studied extensively, and its efficacy has been repeatedly demonstrated. However, this therapy requires patients to adhere to strict dietary restrictions. Briefly, phenelzine produces long-lasting, irreversible inhibition of monoamine oxidase, which in turn potentiates a number of substrates including tyramine, dopamine, tryptophan, and other amines.[42] Ingesting foods rich in tyramine (e.g. most aged cheeses, red wine, beer, and broad beans) can increase the risk of rapidly escalating blood pressure (often referred to as a 'hypertensive crisis'). Persuading a patient with social phobia to take phenelzine can be challenging,[43] but the costs of monoamine oxidase therapy seem justified, especially if other treatments with more benign side-effect profiles prove ineffective. To date, four controlled trials support the efficacy of phenelzine.

Liebowitz et al.[44] compared phenelzine, atenolol (a cardioselective β-blocker), and a pill placebo. After 8 weeks, independent assessors classified 64 per cent (16/25) of patients receiving phenelzine as treatment responders compared with 23 per cent (6/26) of patients given placebo. After maintenance treatment for an additional 8 weeks, the overall response rate among patients treated with phenelzine remained superior to that of patients given a placebo.

Versiani et al.[45] compared phenelzine, moclobemide (a reversible inhibitor of monoamine oxidase), and placebo. After 8 weeks, patients who received phenelzine endorsed significantly greater reductions in self-reported social anxiety and were rated as less impaired by clinicians than patients given a placebo. Many phenelzine effects were evident after only 4 weeks. In the first 8 weeks, patients prescribed phenelzine reported more side-effects than patients who received placebo. In order of frequency, among the phenelzine patients (versus patients given placebo) these reported side-effects were sleepiness (50.0 per cent versus 11.5 per cent), orthostatic hypotension (42.3 per cent versus 3.8 per cent), dry mouth (38.5 per cent versus 8 per cent), constipation (38.5 per cent versus 8 per cent), reduced libido (26.9 per cent versus 0 per cent), impaired ejaculation (19.2 per cent versus 0 per cent), insomnia (15.4 per cent versus 0 per cent), vertigo (11.5 per cent versus 4 per cent), and headaches (10.2 per cent versus 3.8 per cent). Most side-effects persisted for the duration of treatment.

In one study, 65 patients were randomly assigned to phenelzine, alprazolam, cognitive-behavioural group therapy, or pill placebo.[46] All groups exhibited significant improvement between pre- and post-treatment, with few differences between conditions. Patients receiving phenelzine reported lower trait anxiety after treatment than other patients. They also achieved significantly greater reductions in work and social disability as rated by clinicians (administered only to patients given medication or placebo). After treatment had been discontinued for two months, clinicians continued to rate patients taking phenelzine as less impaired than patients given placebo.

Heimberg et al.[47] compared the efficacy of phenelzine with that of cognitive-behavioural group therapy, pill placebo, and a credible placebo psychotherapy. A more detailed review of this study is presented below. However, phenelzine again appeared to be an efficacious treatment for social phobia. Independent assessors classified 77 per cent (20/26) of patients receiving phenelzine who completed 12 weeks of treatment, compared with 41 per cent (11/27) of patients given placebo, as responders. In an intent-to-treat analysis, these rates were 65 per cent and 33 per cent, respectively.

Reversible inhibitors of monoamine oxidase

These newer agents do not require dietary restrictions. Moclobemide and brofaramine have been evaluated in social phobia. In the study by Versiani et al.,[45] phenelzine was superior to moclobemide on several measures after 4 weeks, but the two treatments were equally effective after 8 weeks. Furthermore, moclobemide was better tolerated than phenelzine. Patients given moclobemide reported the following side-effects: insomnia (19.2 per cent), sleepiness (15.4 per cent), dry mouth (15.4 per cent), vertigo (11.5 per cent), headache (11.5 per cent), constipation (7.7 per cent), orthostatic hypotension (3.8 per cent), and loss of libido (3.6 per cent). Only sleepiness (11.8 per cent) persisted after week 8.

Two other placebo-controlled studies have evaluated moclobemide. In an industry-supported trial,[48] 578 patients were randomly assigned to receive either 300 or 600 mg/day of moclobemide or placebo. All groups demonstrated an improvement after 12 weeks. Almost half (47 per cent) the patients treated with 600 mg were classified as much or very much improved compared with 41 per cent of patients treated with 300 mg and 34 per cent of patients given placebo. However, only the 600-mg group was statistically superior to placebo. Finally, Schneier et al.[49] reported considerably more modest results in a placebo-controlled trial. Only 7 out of 40 (17.5 per cent) patients in the moclobemide group, compared with 5 out of 37 (13.5 per cent) patients given placebo, were classified as responders after 8 weeks. Brofaramine showed promise in controlled trials,[50,51] but is no longer being manufactured. Thus, while reversible inhibitors of monoamine oxidase result in fewer adverse effects than traditional monoamine oxidase inhibitors, they have not secured a place in the social-phobia formulary.

Selective serotonin reuptake inhibitors

The selective serotonin reuptake inhibitors fluvoxamine,[52] paroxetine,[53,54] and sertraline[55] have demonstrated efficacy in placebo-controlled trials. A controlled trial still underway suggests that fluoxetine has a similar efficacy.[56]

A total of 30 patients were randomly assigned to 12 weeks of either fluvoxamine or placebo treatment.[52] Independent assessors classified 46 per cent (7/15) of fluvoxamine completers as significantly improved compared with 7 per cent (1/13) of placebo completers.

In an industry-supported trial,[53] 183 patients with generalized social phobia received either paroxetine or placebo. In an intent-to-treat analysis, 55 per cent (50/91) of patients receiving paroxetine, compared with only 23.9 per cent (22/92) of patients given placebo, were much or very much improved after 11 weeks. Patients tolerated paroxetine well, as indicated by relatively modest levels of attrition (15 per cent; 14/91). In an earlier study,[54] patients with generalized social phobia were treated for 11 weeks with paroxetine. Of these, 16 responders were then randomly assigned to 12 additional weeks of paroxetine or pill placebo following a step-down discontinuation: five patients given placebo, but only one paroxetine patient, relapsed following discontinuation.

Favourable results were reported for a small cross-over trial of sertraline and placebo (n = 12).[55] Patients receiving sertraline first endorsed reductions in both clinician- and self-rated measures of social anxiety that were maintained after being switched to placebo. Patients receiving placebo first showed no changes on these measures until they received sertraline.

Finally, preliminary findings from an ongoing trial comparing fluoxetine, placebo, cognitive-behavioural therapy, cognitive-behavioural therapy plus fluoxetine, and cognitive-behavioural therapy plus placebo in the treatment of generalized social phobia indicate that all treatments exceed the efficacy of placebo.[56]

Benzodiazepines

As described above, Gelernter et al.[46] randomly assigned 65 patients to alprazolam, phenelzine, cognitive-behavioural treatment, or placebo. Of the patients assigned to the alprazolam group, 38 per cent made significant improvements on self-ratings of social fear. However, 2 months after medication was discontinued, most patients experienced a re-emergence of symptoms.

In another trial, 75 patients were randomly assigned to receive clonazepam or placebo.[57] Patients given clonazepam endorsed improvements on clinician-rated and self-report measures of social anxiety after 6 weeks. After 10 weeks, 78 per cent of clonazepam patients, compared with 20 per cent of patients given placebo, were classified as responders. Clonazepam-treated patients endorsed significantly more side-effects than patients given placebo: anorgasmia (44 per cent versus 6 per cent), forgetfulness (44 per cent versus 21 per cent), unsteadiness (62 per cent versus 21 per cent), and impaired concentration (35 per cent versus 15 per cent).

β-Blockers

Phenelzine was superior to both atenolol and placebo after 8 weeks.[44] After 8 additional weeks of maintenance treatment, the atenolol group was improved, but it still failed to surpass placebo. Turner et al.[58] randomly assigned 72 patients to 12 weeks of behaviour therapy (imaginal and in vivo exposure), atenolol, or placebo. Atenolol was inferior to behaviour therapy and again failed to surpass placebo.

Buspirone

In one study, 34 performance-anxious musicians were randomly assigned to 6 weeks of buspirone, placebo, cognitive-behavioural therapy, or buspirone plus cognitive-behavioural therapy, and it was found that buspirone was no better than placebo.[59] Another study randomly assigned 30 patients to 12 weeks of buspirone or placebo;[60] only one patient from each condition qualified as a responder.

Psychological interventions

Cognitive-behavioural treatments have been subjected to the most thorough empirical evaluation. Treatments that utilize exposure and exposure combined with cognitive restructuring are the focus of our review.

Exposure

Exposure requires individuals to imagine (imaginal exposure) or directly confront (in vivo exposure) feared stimuli. Relatively little research has examined the effectiveness of imaginal exposure for social phobia, although in vivo exposure has repeatedly demonstrated efficacy. In preparation for in vivo exposures, patients rank-order problematic social situations from least to most feared. Then, on their own or with therapist assistance, they enter these situations, typically beginning with a situation rated as eliciting moderate fear. When, after repeated and prolonged exposure, the situation no longer elicits a distressing level of fear, the individual turns to the next most feared situation. This process is repeated until the anxiety associated with all problematic situations is reduced.

Individuals with social phobia treated with exposure alone have been shown to make greater improvements than individuals receiving relaxation training,[61,62] pill placebo,[58] or delayed treatment.[63] However, exposure alone may not produce optimal outcomes in terms of cognitive change or treatment durability.[64] Several theorists[18,65] suggest that exposure alone may not be sufficient to treat social phobia, because the core feature of the disorder is essentially a cognitive construct (for example, fear of negative evaluation). Specifically, exposure alone may not provide patients with exposure to the disapproval they fear or, more importantly, to the information that other people are seldom as critical as they expect.[65] Contemporary cognitive-behavioural models of social phobia propose that anxiety is largely maintained by dysfunctional beliefs and information processing biases, and that successful treatment will be associated with modification of these difficulties.[6,7]

Exposure combined with cognitive restructuring

Cognitive restructuring is an intervention originating from Beck's cognitive therapy[66] and Ellis's rational emotive therapy.[67] In cognitive restructuring, individuals are taught the following:

(1) to identify negative thoughts that occur during stressful or anxiety-provoking situations;

(2) to evaluate the accuracy of those thoughts as compared with objective information derived via repeated questioning or as a result of planned 'behavioural experiments';

(3) to derive rational alternative thoughts based on the acquired information.

By engaging in this process and utilizing the alternative thoughts on exposure to feared situations, patients can 'undo' habitual ways of viewing these situations, and, in turn, lessen the anxiety they experience.

Several studies have demonstrated equivalent outcomes for exposure alone and exposure plus cognitive restructuring.[68,69] Other studies have found combined treatments to be superior on several post-treatment measures, to result in greater protection against relapse, or to provide additional gains during the follow-up period.[70,71] In two recent meta-analyses, cognitive restructuring plus exposure and exposure alone resulted in similar attrition rates and yielded similar effect sizes at post-treatment and follow-up.[72,73] However, a third meta-analysis comparing six conditions (waiting-list control, placebo, exposure alone, cognitive restructuring without exposure, cognitive restructuring with exposure, social skills training) painted a somewhat different picture. While all active therapies and placebo produced greater effect sizes than the waiting-list control, only cognitive restructuring combined with exposure had a significantly larger effect size than placebo.[69]

Various explanations have been proposed to account for the mixed findings regarding whether or not cognitive techniques enhance treatment gains beyond those attained with exposure alone. One possibility is that they do not, and that positive findings have been due to chance.[74] Alternatively, cognitive techniques may lead to better outcomes, but the effect size is moderate and inconsistently detected in a literature characterized by inadequate statistical power.[75] Another possibility is that some patients benefit adequately from exposure alone but that other patients require cognitive restructuring to achieve optimal outcomes, and we do not know how to differentiate these two types of patients.[76]

Whether cognitive techniques are ultimately shown to be necessary to maximize treatment gains, cognitive change, however achieved, may be central to good clinical outcomes. Changing maladaptive beliefs may be necessary to reduce fear and avoidance of social situations over the long term. Exposure alone may provide sufficient disconfirmatory information to alter maladaptive beliefs for some patients, and it is not unusual to find evidence of cognitive change in exposure-only treatments.[63,68,77]

Cognitive-behavioural group therapy

In this section, we describe cognitive-behavioural group therapy (**CBGT**)[78] (our treatment protocol, which integrates cognitive techniques and exposure in the treatment of social phobia) and briefly review the literature supporting its efficacy.

Most commonly, this form of therapy is conducted in weekly sessions of approximately 2.5 h for 12 weeks. The optimal number of patients is six. Effort is taken to balance the group in terms of age, gender, and social phobia subtype. Ideally, male and female co-therapists lead the groups to allow for maximum flexibility in constructing within-session exposure exercises. In the first two sessions, patients receive the rationale and instructions for exposure, cognitive restructuring, and homework assignments as well as opportunities to practise cognitive restructuring skills. Thereafter, therapists lead patients through individualized exposures that are preceded and followed by therapist-directed cognitive restructuring exercises. Patients are also coached in rational thinking during the exposure itself. At the end of each session, therapists work with each patient to develop homework assignments for completion during the coming week. Homework typically consists of exposures to real-life situations and patient-directed pre- and postexposure cognitive restructuring.

Several controlled studies have evaluated the efficacy of CBGT. In one study, 49 patients were randomly assigned to CBGT or educational-supportive group therapy—a credible placebo treatment consisting of lectures, discussions, and social support.[79] Following treatment, 75 per cent of patients who received CBGT were classified as having made a significant improvement by clinical assessors, compared with 40 per cent of patients given educational-supportive group therapy. The CBGT patients also reported less anxiety before and during an individualized behaviour test than did the educational-support patients. Both groups showed similar improvement over baseline on self-report measures. At a 6-month follow-up visit, a greater number of patients in the cognitive-behavioural group demonstrated durable treatment gains on self-report and assessor ratings. Of the patients treated in this study, 19 were reassessed 4.5 to 6.25 years later.[80] Independent assessors classified 89 per cent of these patients as no longer exhibiting significant impairment compared with 44 per cent of the education-support group. Furthermore, the patients who received CBGT reported less social anxiety and were rated by independent judges as less anxious and more socially skilled during an individualized behaviour test.

In another study, 133 patients were randomly assigned to CBGT, phenelzine, pill placebo, or education support, and 107 patients completed 12 weeks of treatment.[47] At post-test, independent assessors classified 21/28 CBGT completers (75 per cent) and 20/26 phenelzine completers (77 per cent) as having made clinically significant response (intent-to-treat analysis, CBGT 58 per cent, phenelzine 65 per cent). In general, CBGT and phenelzine produced response rates higher than the pill placebo and education support, but not different from each other. Many patients receiving phenelzine classified as responders after 12 weeks of treatment had achieved gains by the midtreatment assessment, while this was less common among patients assigned to the CBGT group. Patients receiving phenelzine were also more improved than the CBGT group of patients on a subset of measures after 12 weeks.

In the second phase of this study, patients who responded to CBGT or phenelzine received a further 6 months of maintenance treatment and a 6-month follow-up period (Liebowtiz and Heimberg, unpublished observations). Thereafter, 50 per cent of previously responding patients taking phenelzine had relapsed, compared with only 17 per cent of the CBGT group of patients. The difference in relapse between treatments was especially pronounced for patients with generalized social phobia. The overall pattern of results suggests that phenelzine might have slightly greater immediate efficacy, but that cognitive-behavioural treatment may confer greater protection against relapse.

Social skills training

Social skills training is based on the assumption that individuals with social phobia lack the basic skills for social interaction. This deficit provokes negative reactions from others, and social interactions become unpleasant and anxiety-provoking for the patient.[81] Research examining whether socially anxious individuals exhibit deficits in social performance is mixed, with some studies suggesting that their performance is poorer than non-anxious controls[82,83] and other studies finding no differences.[84–86] Even if an individual with social phobia does perform poorly, this may be the result of inhibition caused by anxiety or maladaptive beliefs rather than poor social skills (i.e. a lack of knowledge or ability to carry out the appropriate behaviours). Nevertheless, the effectiveness of social skills training in the treatment of social phobia has been examined both alone[87] and as part of multicomponent treatment packages.[88] Social skills training commonly includes therapist modelling, behavioural rehearsal, corrective feedback, social reinforcement, and homework assignments. In the only controlled study of social skills training alone, patients receiving 15 weeks of treatment did not exhibit improvements in social anxiety, social skills, or overall adjustment beyond patients in a delayed treatment group.[87] However, Turner et al.[88] have developed a multicomponent treatment package, 'social effectiveness training', that combines exposure with social skills training and education delivered both in group and individual sessions. A pilot study of 17 patients with generalized social phobia revealed significant improvements in self-reported and clinician-rated social anxiety, as well as anxiety experienced during behavioural tests for the 13 treatment completers. Of these 13 patients, eight participated in a 2-year follow-up.[89] Self-report and clinician ratings indicated maintenance of treatment gains or additional improvement during follow-up, although three of the eight patients had received additional treatment in the interim.

Relaxation strategies

Relaxation strategies are based on the notion that individuals with social phobia experience extreme physiological arousal that interferes with performance. Applied relaxation involves training in three skills. First, the patients learn to attend to the physiological sensations of anxiety. Second, the patients learn to relax quickly while engaging in everyday activities. Finally, the patients learn to apply relaxation skills in anxiety-provoking situations.[90] Applied relaxation thus combines relaxation and exposure to help individuals cope with anxiety-provoking situations. Treatment studies suggest that applied relaxation is superior to delayed treatment[91] and as effective as social skills training.[92] However, applied relaxation was less effective than cognitive treatment in one study.[91] Research has demonstrated minimal improvement in social phobia symptoms when relaxation techniques are not combined with exposure.[61,62]

Management of social phobia

Several statements can be made regarding the management of social phobia. First, several classes of medication (monoamine oxidase inhibitors, selective serotonin reuptake inhibitors, clonazepam) and cognitive-behavioural therapies that include an exposure component may effectively provide symptom relief. These treatments generally work equally well for individuals with non-generalized and generalized social phobia, although individuals with generalized social phobia may require a longer course of treatment to reach an optimal endstate. Second, pharmacologically treated individuals tend to get relief from social anxiety symptoms quickly—perhaps as quickly as a few weeks after initiation of treatment. Third, patients treated with cognitive-behavioural therapy may not respond as quickly as individuals treated with these medications, but they may be less likely to relapse than medication responders.

Comorbid psychiatric conditions may complicate phenelzine therapy if the patient's ability to adhere to dietary restrictions is compromised. In addition to the risk of hypertensive crisis, there may also be a risk of behavioural disinhibition during treatment. In some instances, patients treated with phenelzine experience decreases in fear and avoidance of situations to such a degree that they exhibit signs of expansiveness, grandiosity, and other features of mania.[93] While disinhibition may occur in individuals without a history of bipolar spectrum depression, individuals with a documented history may be more prone to disinhibition. Consequently, careful monitoring may be required during treatment with phenelzine.[93]

Benzodiazepine treatment may be contraindicated among patients with a history of alcohol or substance abuse or dependence. It may also be difficult for patients whose jobs require a state of high alertness. Given these concerns and their more benign side-effect profile, the selective serotonin-reuptake inhibitors are increasingly regarded as the first-line medication, with the benzodiazepines and monoamine oxidase inhibitors held in reserve for non-responding patients. We know little at this point of the appropriate duration of medication treatments in social phobia, and more research is needed. In our own research, 9 months of phenelzine treatment was associated with relapse among 50 per cent of patients.

To date, few studies on the combination of medication and cognitive-behavioural treatments have been conducted, and it is unclear whether combined treatment will emerge as superior. However, combined treatments are common in clinical practice. Therefore, it is important to consider whether treatments should be administered simultaneously or sequentially. For instance, sequential treatments might capitalize on a rapid medication response for quick relief and phased-in cognitive-behavioural treatment for superior relapse prevention. Cognitive-behavioural treatments may also be utilized to help patients discontinue medical regimens after an initial drug response.

Finally, comorbid anxiety and mood disorders do not appear to degrade a patient's response to cognitive-behavioural treatment (Erwin, Heimberg, Juster, and Mindlin, unpublished observations). However, the effects of other comorbid conditions have not been examined, and there is no evidence that comorbid conditions improve during cognitive-behavioural or pharmacological treatment for social phobia. In some cases, the most sensible clinical decision will be to treat the comorbid condition before the social phobia. This may be the decision if substance dependence prevents the patient from engaging in exposure or other therapeutic activities. In other cases, a comorbid condition might become the focus after social phobia treatment. Patients who abuse substances in order to 'treat' their social anxieties are often reticent to give up their substances before other 'coping strategies' are made available. In summary, the management of comorbid conditions in individuals with social phobia depends on the analysis of the relationships between the disorders, and varies from case to case.

Prevention of social phobia

Few studies to date have specifically examined ways of preventing social phobia. However, the evidence for familial aggregation and for a large degree of environmental influence is strong. Furthermore, recent evidence suggests that parents may reinforce anxious children for making avoidant choices,[94] and these data suggest that anxious children may benefit from the inclusion of their parents in treatment, family-oriented treatment interventions, or successful treatment of their parents' anxiety.

Since social phobia has an early age of onset, the treatment of children and adolescents should help to prevent social phobia from becoming a chronic condition. In a more purely prevention-oriented mould, the Queensland Early Intervention and Prevention of Anxiety Project, administered by Dadds, Barrett, and colleagues is a model for the future. These investigators implemented a 10-week school-based child- and parent-focused psychosocial intervention for child anxiety and compared it to a monitoring-only intervention.[95] A 2-year follow-up documents that the programme was successful in reducing the rate of existing anxiety disorder and preventing the onset of new disorder compared with the monitoring-only programme.[96]

Specific phobia

Clinical features and functional impairment

The hallmark feature of specific phobia, which prior to DSM-IV was called simple phobia, is a 'marked and persistent fear that is excessive or unreasonable, cued by the presence or anticipation of a specific object or situation'. Commonly feared/avoided objects include animals, aspects of nature, or blood. Most individuals may endorse a degree of fear of these stimuli. However, in specific phobia, fear and avoidance cause significant interference with an individual's normal routine, career, academic pursuits, or social/interpersonal activities. Nevertheless, some individuals with specific phobias maintain a relatively normal routine by pursuing a lifestyle that minimizes exposure to the phobic stimulus. Consequently, they may present for treatment only when life changes occur that force them to face the previously avoided situation or object. More frequently, specific phobias accompany a more impairing primary disorder, which is the stimulus for seeking treatment.[97]

Classification

DSM and ICD

There is greater similarity between DSM-IV and ICD-10 criteria for specific phobia than for social phobia. Both diagnostic systems view the fear as associated with exposure to a specific object or situation,

which leads to acute autonomic and psychological symptoms of anxiety. However, DSM-IV also stipulates that anxiety may be cued by the anticipation of the feared object or situation, while there is no mention of anticipatory anxiety in ICD-10. As for social phobia, our review of specific phobia follows DSM conventions. Mention of simple phobia refers to DSM-III or DSM-IIIR criteria, while specific phobia refers to DSM-IV criteria.

Specific phobia subtypes

DSM-IV classifies specific phobias into five subtypes:

- animals
- aspects of the natural environment
- blood, injection, injury
- situational
- other (e.g. dental/medical procedures, choking, etc.).

With the exception of blood–injection–injury phobias, exposure to the phobic stimulus evokes intense anxiety that may meet the criteria for a situationally bound panic attack. Additionally, there is extreme apprehension and desire to escape or avoid the phobic stimulus.[98] By contrast, individuals with blood–injection–injury phobias exhibit a biphasic anxiety reaction (vasovagal syncope), characterized by initial short-lived sympathetic arousal followed by parasympathetic arousal that may result in fainting.[99] Furthermore, the subjective experiences of these individuals tend to be characterized by disgust and repulsion rather than pure apprehension.[98]

Comorbidity

The vast majority (83.4 per cent) of individuals with a specific phobia experience at least one other lifetime psychiatric disorder.[22] In the NCS, individuals with simple phobia were five times more likely to have at least one additional disorder than individuals who had never met the criteria for a phobic disorder. Odds ratios for simple phobia ranged from 2.08 (alcohol abuse) to 10.05 (mania). The odds ratios for anxiety disorders ranged from 7.25 (panic disorder) to 7.87 (social phobia). Odds ratios for unipolar mood disorders were 4.55 (major depression) and 3.42 (dysthymia). Alcohol abuse without dependence and drug abuse without dependence were the only disorders assessed in the NCS with non-significant odds ratios. In most cases, simple phobia preceded the onset of the other disorder.

Epidemiology

Prevalence

The NCS reported a lifetime prevalence rate of 11.3 per cent and a 12-month prevalence rate of 8.8 per cent for simple phobia.[20] A recent study of over 700 adults[100] found situational/environmental phobias to be the most common (13.2 per cent), followed by animal phobias (7.9 per cent), and blood–injection–injury phobias (3.0 per cent).

Age at onset/age of treatment-seeking

Specific phobia tends to begin earlier than other anxiety disorders,[22,101] with a median age of 15 years in the NCS. However, age at onset varies as a function of phobia subtype. For example, animal phobias onset earliest (age 7), followed by blood phobias (age 9), dental phobia (age 12), and claustrophobia (age 20).[102] Despite a relatively early age of onset, individuals with phobic disorders rarely seek help for the condition.[103] A recent secondary analysis of NCS data revealed that only 10 per cent of individuals with a phobic disorder (simple, social, or agoraphobia) approached a service provider about their condition in their onset year (compared with approximately half of NCS participants with panic disorder). Similarly, cumulative probabilities of telling a service provider increased significantly less rapidly for phobic disorders (1.4 per cent per year) than for generalized anxiety disorder (5.9 per cent per year).[103] Because this study did not report these rates separately for simple, social, or agoraphobia, these data cannot be directly applied to simple phobia. However, they highlight the tendency of persons with certain irrational fears to delay professional consultation.

Gender distribution

Women receive diagnoses of specific phobia more often than men. Lifetime rates for simple phobia in the NCS were 15.7 per cent for women but only 6.7 per cent for men.[20] In one study, women reported higher rates of animal and situational/environmental phobias, but rates of blood–injection–injury phobia did not differ.[100] In ECA, there were no gender differences with regard to age of onset or willingness to report symptoms, although women were more likely than men to endorse certain fears (for example, fear of 'being near any harmless or dangerous animal that couldn't get to you').[104]

Aetiology of specific phobia

There is considerable evidence for a familial/genetic transmission of specific phobia.[33,37] Specifically, 31 per cent of first-degree relatives of persons with simple phobia also met the criteria for simple phobia.[33] Further, rates of simple phobia were higher among first-degree relatives of persons with simple phobia and no other anxiety disorder than among first-degree relatives of persons who were never mentally ill.[105]

Few twin studies have examined concordance for specific phobia. In the Virginia Twin Study,[37] concordance rates for animal phobia were 25.9 per cent and 11.0 per cent among monozygotic and dizygotic twins respectively. However, concordance rates for situational phobia were quite similar in monozygotic and dizygotic twins (22.2 per cent and 23.7 per cent respectively).

Psychosocial approaches to the aetiology of specific phobia come from a broad range of theoretical orientations. Freud's case of Little Hans[106] is the model for the psychoanalytical understanding of phobias. Freud conceptualized Little Hans's fear of horses as resulting from unconscious Oedipal fears. Little Hans denied these fears and projected them onto horses. Accordingly, symptoms of phobia are thought to be related to unresolved unconscious conflicts. The anxiety of the conflict is experienced, but the source of the anxiety is shifted onto an unrelated and harmless object, and the real source of anxiety is kept from consciousness. The implication that the symptoms of the phobia will not subside unless the real source of the anxiety is addressed lacks empirical support.

Classical conditioning theory[107] holds that phobias are learned through the association of negative experience with an object or situation. Accordingly, Wolpe and Rachman[108] maintained that Little

Hans was not afraid of his father, but rather of horses. Two-factor learning theory[109] introduced avoidance as a critical component of the maintenance of anxiety. Responses of avoidance or escape are learned and serve to decrease the discomfort arising from conditioned stimuli. Repeated negative reinforcement of avoidance behaviour maintains the fear and makes it resistant to extinction.

Some conditioning theorists assert that feared stimuli are not randomly determined. Rather, through natural selection, humans have inherited a predisposition to fear specific stimuli.[37] Marks' 'preparedness' theory[110] maintains that commonly feared objects are those that historically threatened the survival of the individual or the species. In this model, phobias are viewed as instances of 'prepared learning', which is selective, easily acquired, difficult to extinguish, and non-cognitive.[111] However, a large number of studies also suggest that phobias may be acquired via observational learning.

Course of specific phobia

Individuals with specific phobias acquire their fear(s) early in life, and the disorder persists for many years.[112] For many individuals, specific phobias are not sufficiently impairing for them to seek treatment. Often individuals with specific phobias adapt their lifestyle to avoid contact with the feared stimulus, such that only persons with the most severe specific phobias seek treatment. Events that commonly precipitate treatment-seeking include a change in lifestyle such that the feared stimulus becomes intolerable (for instance, accepting a job that requires frequent air travel), and the experience of a panic attack in anticipation or in the presence of the feared stimulus. Improvement in specific phobia is unlikely unless the person seeks effective treatment.

Empirically evaluated treatments

Pharmacotherapy

Drug treatments for specific phobia have consistently been shown to be less effective than behavioural treatments. β-Blockers reduce some symptoms of sympathetic arousal during exposure to feared stimuli. However, they fail to decrease subjective fear.[113] While benzodiazepines may facilitate approach to the feared stimuli, they may also reduce the efficacy of behaviour therapies by inhibiting the experience of anxiety during exposure.[114] Because of the marginal to moderate effects of drug treatments relative to behaviour therapy, little attention has been devoted to the study of drug treatments for specific phobia.

Cognitive-behavioural interventions

Systematic desensitization

Systematic desensitization[115] has been used successfully in the treatment of specific phobias since the mid-1960s. Combining progressive relaxation and graduated imaginal exposure to the feared stimulus, systematic desensitization has been demonstrated to be superior to psychotherapy in some cases[116–118] but not others.[119] Wolpe[115] contended that systematic desensitization works by the principle of reciprocal inhibition, which asserts that the sympathetic response associated with anxiety is incompatible with, and thus inhibited by, the parasympathetic response that occurs during deep muscle relaxation. Therefore, pairing parasympathetic activation with the feared stimulus leads to the conditioning of relaxation to the phobic stimulus. More recently, theorists have taken the position that the exposure component is responsible for the efficacy of systematic desensitization, while the decrease in autonomic arousal achieved by relaxation enhances habituation to the feared stimulus.

Applied relaxation

Two studies have investigated the efficacy of applied relaxation.[120,121] Both studies found that applied relaxation was an effective treatment, especially among patients who demonstrate higher levels of physiological reactivity than behavioural avoidance.

Applied tension

Blood–injection–injury phobia differs from other specific phobias because it is associated with parasympathetic arousal. Applied tension, designed specifically for blood–injection–injury phobia, requires the patient to tense different muscle groups instead of relaxing them, thereby countering parasympathetic arousal. The first trial of applied tension[122] demonstrated that persons with phobias for blood, wounds, and injuries responded equally well to applied tension, applied relaxation, or their combination. A later study demonstrated that a higher percentage of persons treated with applied tension were clinically improved post-treatment and at 1-year follow-up than were patients treated with *in vivo* exposure alone.[123] Similar positive effects were reported for those treated with one versus five sessions of applied tension.[124]

Exposure

Prolonged and repeated *in vivo* exposure to feared stimuli is by far the most studied and effective form of treatment for specific phobia.[125,126] Several studies have attempted to identify those elements of exposure that lead to the fastest and most complete elimination of the phobia.

While *in vivo* exposure is generally believed to be more effective than imaginal exposure for specific phobia, some studies have found these techniques to be similarly effective.[127] Modelling in the form of observing another patient receive treatment has been shown to enhance the effects of exposure and to increase the speed at which positive outcomes are attained.[128] Multiple exposure sessions are considered more effective than one exposure session, although some studies report quite positive outcomes for one-session treatments.[129] One-session group *in vivo* exposure treatment has produced gains similar to those of one-session individual *in vivo* exposure treatment.[129] However, self-directed treatments are less effective than therapist-directed treatments.[130,131] Effects of therapist-directed *in vivo* exposure have been shown to endure for up to 1 year.[132]

In vivo exposure situations can sometimes be difficult to arrange; imaginal exposure may not achieve the reality or intensity that is needed to elicit an anxiety response. For these reasons, virtual reality treatment may greatly enhance the efficacy of exposure sessions. Immersive computer-generated virtual reality treatment involves the three-dimensional simulation of feared situations. Occasionally, the salience of virtual environments can be augmented by instructing patients to touch real objects (e.g. toy spiders), which correspond with the virtual environment. Recent case studies have reported on the efficacy of virtual reality exposure either alone[133,134] or in combination with anxiety management training[135] in the treatment of specific phobia. Virtual reality exposure techniques are beginning to be supported by controlled studies.[136]

Cognitive restructuring

Phobia-specific irrational thoughts may contribute to the development of the phobia, maintain avoidance behaviour, and contribute to physiological symptoms.[137] Cognitive restructuring treatments help patients to monitor irrational thoughts and change underlying beliefs, so that they are better able to enter feared situations. When combined with exposure to feared stimuli, cognitive restructuring has been demonstrated as effective.[138] However, there are relatively few studies of cognitively oriented treatments for specific phobia.

Management of specific phobia

Several investigations suggest that tailoring treatment to individual response patterns will improve outcome. For example, patients with a profile of heightened physiological reactivity may respond preferentially to applied relaxation, while patients with a profile characterized by avoidance may respond better to *in vivo* exposure.[121] Patients who experience their anxiety primarily in the form of anxious thoughts may respond better to cognitive techniques than patients whose symptoms are characterized more by somatic arousal.[139]

Prevention of specific phobia

Children with specific phobia were included in the Queensland Early Intervention and Prevention of Anxiety Project, but no other preventive efforts have been mounted. It is tempting to speculate that children could be 'inoculated' against a variety of the more common specific phobias by systematic exposure to potentially feared objects or situations.

References

1. American Psychiatric Association (1952). *Diagnostic and statistical manual of mental disorders*. American Psychiatric Association, Washington, DC.
2. American Psychiatric Association (1968). *Diagnostic and statistical manual of mental disorders* (2nd edn). American Psychiatric Association, Washington, DC.
3. Marks, I.M. and Gelder, M.G. (1966). Different ages of onset in varieties of social phobia. *American Journal of Psychiatry*, **123**, 218–21.
4. American Psychiatric Association (1980). *Diagnostic and statistical manual of mental disorders* (3rd edn). American Psychiatric Association, Washington, DC.
5. Liebowitz, M.R., Gorman, J.M., Fyer, A.J., and Klein, D.F. (1985). Social phobia, review of a neglected anxiety disorder. *Archives of General Psychiatry*, **42**, 729–36.
6. Rapee, R.M. and Heimberg, R.G. (1997). A cognitive–behavioural model of anxiety in social phobia. *Behaviour Research and Therapy*, **35**, 741–56.
7. Clark, D.M. and Wells, A. (1995). A cognitive model of social phobia. In *Social phobia, diagnosis, assessment, and treatment* (ed. R.G. Heimberg, M.R. Liebowitz, D.A. Hope, and F.R. Schneier), pp. 69–93. Guilford Press, New York.
8. Schneier, F.R., Heckelman, L.R., Garfinkel, R., *et al.* (1994). Functional impairment in social phobia. *Journal of Clinical Psychiatry*, **55**, 322–31.
9. Schneier, F.R., Johnson, J., Hornig, C.D., Liebowitz, M.R., and Weissman, M.M. (1992). Social phobia: comorbidity and morbidity in an epidemiological sample. *Archives of General Psychiatry*, **49**, 282–8.

10. World Health Organization (1992). *The ICD-10 classification of mental and behavioural disorders: clinical description and diagnostic guidelines.* World Health Organization, Geneva.

11. American Psychiatric Association (1994). *Diagnostic and statistical manual of mental disorders* (4th edn). American Psychiatric Association, Washington, DC.

12. American Psychiatric Association (1987). *Diagnostic and statistical manual of mental disorders* (3rd edn revised). American Psychiatric Association, Washington, DC.

13. Heimberg, R.G., Hope, D.A., Dodge, C.S., and Becker, R.E. (1990). DSM-III-R subtypes of social phobia: comparison of generalized social phobics and public speaking phobics. *Journal of Nervous and Mental Disease*, **173**, 172–9.

14. Levin, A.P., Saoud, J.B., Strauman, T., *et al.* (1993). Responses of 'generalized' and 'discrete' social phobics during public speaking. *Journal of Anxiety Disorders*, **7**, 207–21.

15. Heimberg, R.G., Holt, C.S., Schneier, F.R., Spitzer, R.L., and Liebowitz, M.R. (1993). The issue of subtypes in the diagnosis of social phobia. *Journal of Anxiety Disorders*, **7**, 249–69.

16. Kessler, R.C., Stein, M.B., and Berglund, P. (1998). Social phobia subtypes in the National Comorbidity Survey. *American Journal of Psychiatry*, **155**, 613–19.

17. Heimberg, R.G. (1996). Social phobia, avoidant personality disorder and the multiaxial conceptualization of interpersonal anxiety. In *Trends in cognitive and behavioural therapies*, Vol. 1 (ed. P.M. Salkovskis), pp. 43–61. Wiley, Chichester

18. Turk, C.L., Fresco, D.M., and Heimberg, R.G. (1999). Social phobia: cognitive behavior therapy. In *Handbook of comparative treatments of adult disorders* (2nd edn) (ed. M. Hersen and A.S. Bellack), pp. 285–316. Wiley, New York.

19. Schneier, F.R., Liebowitz, M.R., Beidel, D.C., *et al.* (1998). MacArthur data reanalysis for DSM-IV: social phobia. In *DSM-IV sourcebook* (ed. T.A. Widiger, A.J. Frances, H.A. Pincus, *et al.*), pp. 307–28. American Psychiatric Press, Washington, DC.

20. Kessler, R.C., McGonagle, K.A., Zhao, S., *et al.* (1994). Lifetime and 12-month prevalence of DSM-III-R psychiatric disorders in the United States: results from the National Comorbidity Survey. *Archives of General Psychiatry*, **51**, 8–19.

21. Davidson, J.R., Hughes, D.L., George, L.K., and Blazer, D.G. (1993). The epidemiology of social phobia: findings from the Duke Epidemiological Catchment Area Study. *Psychological Medicine*, **23**, 709–18.

22. Magee, W.J., Eaton, W.W., Wittchen, H.U., McGonagle, K.A., and Kessler, R.C. (1996). Agoraphobia, simple phobia, and social phobia in the National Comorbidity Survey. *Archives of General Psychiatry*, **53**, 159–68.

23. Mannuzza, S., Fyer, A.J., Liebowitz, M.R., and Klein, D.F. (1990). Delineating the boundary of social phobia: its relationship to panic disorder and agoraphobia. *Journal of Anxiety Disorders*, **4**, 41–59.

24. Rapee, R.M., Sanderson, W.C., and Barlow, D.H. (1988). Social phobia features across the DSM-III-R anxiety disorders. *Journal of Psychopathology and Behavioral Assessment*, **10**, 287–99.

25. Solyom, L., Ledwidge, B., and Solyom, C. (1986). Delineating social phobia. *British Journal of Psychiatry*, **149**, 464–70.

26. Heckelman, L.R. and Schneier, F.R. (1995). Diagnostic issues. In *Social phobia: diagnosis assessment, and treatment* (ed. R.G. Heimberg, M.R. Liebowitz, D.A. Hope, and F.R. Schneier), pp. 3–20. Guilford Press, New York.

27. Cameron, O.G., Thyer, B.A., Nesse, R.M., and Curtis, G.C. (1986). Symptom profiles of patients with DSM-III anxiety disorders. *American Journal of Psychiatry*, **143**, 1132–7.

28. Reich, J., Noyes, R., and Yates, W. (1988). Anxiety symptoms distinguishing social phobia from panic and generalized anxiety disorders. *Journal of Nervous and Mental Disease*, **176**, 510–13.

29. Stein, M.B., Walker, J.R., and Forde, D.R. (1994). Setting diagnostic thresholds for social phobia: considerations from a community survey of social anxiety. *American Journal of Psychiatry*, **151**, 408–12.

30. Rapee, R.M. (1995). Descriptive psychopathology of social phobia. In *Social phobia: diagnosis, assessment, and treatment* (ed. R.G. Heimberg, M.R. Liebowitz, D.A. Hope, and F.R. Schneier), pp. 41–66. Guilford Press, New York.

31. Turk, C.L., Heimberg, R.G., Orsillo, S.M., *et al.* (1998). An investigation of gender differences in social phobia. *Journal of Anxiety Disorders*, **12**, 209–23.

32. Fyer, A.J., Mannuzza, S., Chapman, T.F., Liebowitz, M.R., and Klein, D.F. (1993). A direct interview family study of social phobia. *Archives of General Psychiatry*, **50**, 286–93.

33. Fyer, A.J., Mannuzza, S., Chapman, T.F., Martin, L.Y., and Klein, D.F. (1995). Specificity in familial aggregation of phobic disorders. *Archives of General Psychiatry*, **52**, 564–73.

34. Mancini, C., van Ameringen, M., Szatmari, P., Fugere, C., and Boyle, M. (1996). A high-risk pilot study of the children of adults with social phobia. *Journal of the American Academy of Child and Adolescent Psychiatry*, **35**, 1511–17.

35. Mannuzza, S., Schneier, F.R., Chapman, T.F., Liebowitz, M.R., Klein, D.F., and Fyer, A.J. (1995). Generalized social phobia: reliability and validity. *Archives of General Psychiatry*, **52**, 230–7.

36. Stein, M.B., Chartier, M.J., Hazen, A.L., *et al.* (1998). A direct-interview family study of generalized social phobia. *American Journal of Psychiatry*, **155**, 90–7.

37. Kendler, K.S., Neale, M.C., Kessler, R.C., Heath, A.C., and Eaves, L.J. (1992). The genetic epidemiology of phobias in women: the interrelationship of agoraphobia, social phobia, situational phobia, and simple phobia. *Archives of General Psychiatry*, **49**, 273–81.

38. Reich, J., Goldenberg, I., Vasile, R., Goisman, R., and Keller, M. (1994). A prospective follow-along study of the course of social phobia. *Psychiatry Research*, **54**, 249–58.

39. Reich, J., Goldenberg, I., Goisman, R., and Vasile, R. (1994). A prospective, follow-along study of the course of social phobia. II: Testing for basic predictors of course. *Journal of Nervous and Mental Disease*, **182**, 297–301.

40. Caspi, A., Edler, G.H., Jr., and Bem, D.J. (1988). Moving away from the world: life-course patterns of shy children. *Developmental Psychology*, **24**, 824–31.

41. Rosenbaum, J.F., Biederman, J., Hirshfeld, D.R., Bolduc, E.A., and Chaloff, J. (1991). Behavioral inhibition in childhood: a possible precursor to panic disorder or social phobia. *Journal of Clinical Psychiatry*, **52** (Supplement), 5–9.

42. Potts, N.L.S. and Davidson, J.R.T. (1995). Pharmacological treatments: literature review. In *Social phobia: diagnosis, assessment, and treatment* (ed. R.G. Heimberg, M.R. Liebowitz, D.A. Hope, and F.R. Schneier), pp. 334–65. Guilford Press, New York.

43. Schneier, F.R., Marshall, R.D., Street, L., Heimberg, R.G., and Juster, H.R. (1995). Social phobia and specific phobia. In *Treatments of psychiatric disorders* (ed. G.O. Gabbard), pp. 1453–75. American Psychiatric Press, Washington, DC.

44. Liebowitz, M.R., Schneier, F.R., Campeas, R., *et al.* (1992). Phenelzine vs atenolol in social phobia: a placebo-controlled comparison. *Archives of General Psychiatry*, **49**, 290–300.

45. Versiani, M., Nardi, A.E., Mundim, F.D., Alves, A.B., Liebowitz, M.R., and Amrein, R. (1992). Pharmacotherapy of social phobia: a controlled study with moclobemide and phenelzine. *British Journal of Psychiatry*, **161**, 353–60.

46. Gelernter, C.S., Uhde, T.W., Cimbolic, P., *et al.* (1991). Cognitive–behavioral and pharmacological treatments of social phobia: a controlled study. *Archives of General Psychiatry*, **48**, 938–45.

47. Heimberg, R.G., Liebowitz, M.R., Hope, D.A., *et al.* (1998). Cognitive–behavioral group therapy versus phenelzine in social phobia: 12-week outcome. *Archives of General Psychiatry*, **55**, 1133–41.

48. The International Multicenter Clinical Trial Group on Moclobemide in Social Phobia (1997). Moclobemide in social phobia: a double-blind, placebo-controlled clinical study. *European Archives of Psychiatry and Clinical Neuroscience*, **247**, 71–80.

49. Schneier, F.R., Goetz, D., Campeas, R., Fallon, B., Marshall, R., and Liebowitz, M.R. (1998). Placebo-controlled trial of moclobemide in social phobia. *British Journal of Psychiatry*, **172**, 70–7.

50. van Vliet, I.M., den Boer, J.A., and Westenberg, H.G. (1992). Psychopharmacological treatment of social phobia: clinical and biochemical effects of brofaromine, a selective MAO-A inhibitor. *European Neuropsychopharmacology*, **2**, 21–9.

51. Fahlen, T., Nilsson, H.L., Borg, K., Humble, M., and Pauli, U. (1995). Social phobia: the clinical efficacy and tolerability of the monoamine oxidase-A and serotonin uptake inhibitor brofaromine: a double-blind placebo-controlled study. *Acta Psychiatrica Scandinavica*, **92**, 351–8.

52. van Vliet, I.M., den Boer, J.A., and Westenberg, H.G.M. (1994). Psychopharmacological treatment of social phobia: a double blind placebo controlled study with fluvoxamine. *Psychopharmacology*, **115**, 128–34.

53. Stein, M.B., Liebowitz, M.R., Lydiard, R.B., Pitts, C.D., Bushnell, W., and Gergel, I. (1998). Paroxetine treatment of generalized social phobia (social anxiety disorder). A randomized controlled trial. *Journal of the American Medical Association*, **280**, 708–13.

54. Stein, M.B., Chartier, M.J., Hazen, A.L., *et al.* (1996). Paroxetine in the treatment of generalized social phobia: open-label treatment and double-blind placebo-controlled discontinuation. *Journal of Clinical Psychopharmacology*, **16**, 218–22.

55. Katzelnick, D.J., Kobak, K.A., Greist, J.H., Jefferson, J.W., Mantle, J.M., and Serlin, R.C. (1995). Sertraline for social phobia: a double-blind, placebo-controlled crossover study. *American Journal of Psychiatry*, **152**, 1368–71.

56. Kozak, M., Foa, E., Amir, N., *et al.* (1988). *Efficacy of comprehensive cognitive–behavioral therapy versus fluoxetine in generalized social phobia: preliminary findings of a multi-center trial.* Association for the Advancement of Behavior Therapy, Washington, DC.

57. Davidson, J.R., Potts, N., Richichi, E., *et al.* (1993). Treatment of social phobia with clonazepam and placebo. *Journal of Clinical Psychopharmacology*, **13**, 423–8.

58. Turner, S.M., Beidel, D.C., and Jacob, R.G. (1994). Social phobia: a comparison of behavior therapy and atenolol. *Journal of Consulting and Clinical Psychology*, **62**, 350–8.

59. Clark, D.B. and Agras, W. S. (1991). The assessment and treatment of performance anxiety in musicians. *American Journal of Psychiatry*, **148**, 598–605.

60. van Vliet, I.M., den Boer, J.A., Westenberg, H.G., and Pian, K.L. (1997). Clinical effects of buspirone in social phobia: a double-blind placebo-controlled study. *Journal of Clinical Psychiatry*, **58**, 164–8.

61. Al-Kubaisy, T., Marks, I.M., Logsdail, S., and Marks, M.P. (1992). Role of exposure homework in phobia reduction: a controlled study. *Behavior Therapy*, **23**, 599–621.

62. Alström, J.E., Nordlund, C.L., Persson, G., Hårding, M., and Ljungqvist, C. (1984). Effects of four treatment methods on social phobic patients not suitable for insight-oriented psychotherapy. *Acta Psychiatrica Scandinavica*, **70**, 97–110.

63. Newman, M.G., Hofmann, S.G., Trabert, W., Roth, W.T., and Taylor, S. (1994). Does behavioral treatment of social phobia lead to cognitive changes? *Behavior Therapy*, **25**, 503–17.

64. Juster, H.R. and Heimberg, R.G. (1995). Social phobia: longitudinal course and long-term outcome of cognitive–behavioral treatment. *Psychiatric Clinics of North America*, **18**, 821–42.

65. Butler, G. (1985). Exposure as a treatment for social phobia: some instructive difficulties. *Behaviour Research and Therapy*, **23**, 651–7.

66. Beck, A.T. (1976). *Cognitive therapy and the emotional disorders.* International Universities Press, New York.

67. Ellis, A. (1962). *Reason and emotion in psychotherapy.* Lyle Stuart, New York.

68. Hope, D.A., Heimberg, R.G., and Bruch, M.A. (1995). Dismantling cognitive–behavioural group therapy for social phobia. *Behaviour Research and Therapy*, **33**, 637–50.

69. Taylor, S. (1996). Meta-analysis of cognitive–behavioral treatment for social phobia. *Journal of Behavior Therapy and Experimental Psychiatry*, **27**, 1–9.

70. Mattick, R.P., Peters, L., and Clarke, J.C. (1989). Exposure and cognitive restructuring for social phobia: a controlled study. *Behavior Therapy*, **20**, 3–23.

71. Butler, G., Cullington, A., Munby, M., Amies, P., and Gelder, M. (1984). Exposure and anxiety management in the treatment of social phobia. *Journal of Consulting and Clinical Psychology*, **52**, 642–50.

72. Feske, U. and Chambless, D.L. (1995). Cognitive behavioral versus exposure only treatment for social phobia: a meta-analysis. *Behavior Therapy*, **26**, 695–720.

73. Gould, R.A., Buckminster, S., Pollack, M.H., Otto, M.W., and Yap, L. (1997). Cognitive–behavioral and pharmacological treatment for social phobia: a meta-analysis. *Clinical Psychology: Science and Practice*, **4**, 291–306.

74. Scholing, A. and Emmelkamp, P.M. (1993). Exposure with and without cognitive therapy for generalized social phobia: effects of individual and group treatment. *Behaviour Research and Therapy*, **31**, 667–81.

75. Taylor, S., Woody, S., Koch, W.J., McLean, P., Paterson, R.J., and Anderson, K.W. (1997). Cognitive restructuring in the treatment of social phobia: efficacy and mode of action. *Behavior Modification*, **21**, 487–511.

76. Scholing, A. and Emmelkamp, P.M. (1996). Treatment of generalized social phobia: results at long-term follow-up. *Behaviour Research and Therapy*, **34**, 447–52.

77. Mattick, R.P. and Peters, L. (1988). Treatment of severe social phobia: effects of guided exposure with and without cognitive restructuring. *Journal of Consulting and Clinical Psychology*, **56**, 251–60.

78. Heimberg, R.G. and Becker, R.E. *Treatment of social fears and phobias.* Guilford Press, New York, in press.

79. Heimberg, R.G., Dodge, C.S., Hope, D.A., Kennedy, C.R., Zollo, L.J., and Becker, R.E. (1990). Cognitive behavioral group treatment for social phobia: comparison with a credible placebo control. *Cognitive Therapy and Research*, **14**, 1–23.

80. Heimberg, R.G., Salzman, D.G., Holt, C.S., and Blendell, K.A. (1993). Cognitive–behavioral group treatment for social phobia: effectiveness at five-year followup. *Cognitive Therapy and Research*, **17**, 325–39.

81. Lucock, M.P. and Salkovskis, P.M. (1988). Cognitive factors in social anxiety and its treatment. *Behaviour Research and Therapy*, **26**, 297–302.

82. Halford, K. and Foddy, M. (1982). Cognitive and social skills correlates of social anxiety. *British Journal of Clinical Psychology*, **21**, 17–28.

83. Stopa, L. and Clark, D.M. (1993). Cognitive processes in social phobia. *Behaviour Research and Therapy*, **31**, 255–67.

84. Clark, J.V. and Arkowitz, H. (1975). Social anxiety and self-evaluation of interpersonal performance. *Psychological Reports*, **36**, 211–21.

85. Glasgow, R.E. and Arkowitz, H. (1975). The behavioral assessment of male and female social competence in dyadic heterosexual interactions. *Behavior Therapy*, **6**, 488–98.

86. Rapee, R.M. and Lim, L. (1992). Discrepancy between self- and observer ratings of performance in social phobics. *Journal of Abnormal Psychology*, **101**, 728–31.

87. Marzillier, J.S., Lambert, C., and Kellet, J. (1976). A controlled evaluation of systematic desensitization and social skills training for socially inadequate psychiatric patients. *Behaviour Research and Therapy*, **14**, 225–38.

88. Turner, S.M., Beidel, D.C., Cooley, M.R., Woody, S.R., and Messer, S.C. (1994). A multicomponent behavioural treatment for social phobia: social effectiveness therapy. *Behaviour Research and Therapy*, **32**, 381–90.

89. Turner, S.M., Beidel, D.C., and Cooley-Quille, M.R. (1995). Two-year follow-up of social phobics treated with social effectiveness therapy. *Behaviour Research and Therapy*, **33**, 553–5.

90. Öst, L.G. (1987). Applied relaxation: description of a coping technique and review of controlled studies. *Behaviour Research and Therapy*, **25**, 397–409.

91. Jerremalm, A., Jansson, L., and Öst, L.G. (1986). Cognitive and physiological reactivity and the effects of different behavioural methods in the treatment of social phobia. *Behaviour Research and Therapy*, **24**, 171–80.

92. Öst, L.G., Jerremalm, A., and Johansson, J. (1981). Individual response patterns and the effects of different behavioural methods in the treatment of social phobia. *Behaviour Research and Therapy*, **19**, 1–16.

93. Liebowitz, M.R. and Marshall, R.D. (1995). Pharmacological treatments: clinical applications. In *Social phobia: diagnosis, assessment, and treatment* (ed. R.G. Heimberg, M.R. Liebowitz, D.A.Hope, and F.R. Schneier), pp. 366–83. Guilford Press, New York.

94. Barrett, P.M., Rapee, R.M., Dadds, M.R., and Ryan, S.M. Family enhancement of cognitive style in anxious and aggressive children: threat bias and the FEAR effect. *Journal of Abnormal Child Psychology*, in press.

95. Dadds, M.R., Spence, S.H., Holland, D.E., Barrett, P.M., and Laurens, K.R. (1997). Prevention and early intervention for anxiety disorders: a controlled trial. *Journal of Consulting and Clinical Psychology*, **65**, 627–35.

96. Dadds, M.R., Holland, D.E., Laurens, K.R., Mullins, M., and Barrett, P.M. (1999). Early intervention and prevention of anxiety disorders in children: results at 2-year follow-up. *Journal of Consulting and Clinical Psychology*, **67**, 145–50.

97. Barlow, D.H., DiNardo, P.A., Vermilyea, B.B., Vermilyea, J., and Blanchard, E.B. (1986). Co-morbidity and depression among the anxiety disorders: issues in diagnosis and classification. *Journal of Nervous and Mental Disease*, **174**, 63–72.

98. Merckelbach, H., de Jong, P.J., Muris, P., and van den Hout, M.A. (1996). The etiology of specific phobias: a review. *Clinical Psychology Review*, **16**, 337–61.

99. Thyer, B.A., Himle, J., and Curtis, G.C. (1985). Blood–injury–illness phobia: a review. *Journal of Clinical Psychology*, **41**, 451–9.

100. Fredrikson, M., Annas, P., Fischer, H., and Wik, G. (1996). Gender and age differences in the prevalence of specific fears and phobias. *Behaviour Research and Therapy*, **34**, 33–9.

101. Scheibe, G. and Albus, M. (1992). Age at onset, precipitating events, sex distribution, and co-occurrence of anxiety disorders. *Psychopathology*, **25**, 11–18.

102. Öst, L.G. (1987). Age of onset in different phobias. *Journal of Abnormal Psychology*, **96**, 223–9.

103. Kessler, R.C., Olfson, M., and Berglund, P.A. (1998). Patterns and predictors of treatment contact after first onset of psychiatric disorders. *American Journal of Psychiatry*, **155**, 62–9.

104. Bourdon, K.H., Boyd, J.H., Rae, D.S., Burns, B.J., Thompson, J.W., and Locke, B.Z. (1988). Gender differences in phobias: results of the ECA community survey. *Journal of Anxiety Disorders*, **2**, 227–41.

105. Fyer, A.J., Mannuzza, S., Gallops, M.S., *et al.* (1990). Familial transmission of simple phobias and fears: a preliminary report. *Archives of General Psychiatry*, **47**, 252–6.

106. Freud, S. (1909). Analysis of a phobia in a five-year-old boy. In *Standard edition of the complete psychological works of Sigmund Freud*, Vol. 10 (ed. J. Strachey), pp. 5–149. Hogarth Press, London.

107. Pavlov, I.P. (1927). *Conditioned reflexes*. Oxford University Press, London.

108. Wolpe, J. and Rachman, S. (1960). Psychoanalytic evidence: a critique of Freud's case of Little Hans. *Journal of Nervous and Mental Disease*, **130**, 198–220.

109. Mowrer, O.H. (1939). Stimulus response theory of anxiety. *Psychological Review*, **46**, 553–65.

110. Marks, I.M. (1969). *Fears and phobias*. Academic Press, New York.

111. Seligman, M.E. (1971). Phobias and preparedness. *Behavior Therapy*, **2**, 307–20.

112. Boyd, J.H., Rae, D.S., Thompson, J.W., *et al.* (1990). Phobia: prevalence and risk factors. *Social Psychiatry and Psychiatric Epidemiology*, **25**, 314–23.

113. Campos, P.E., Solyom, L., and Koelink, A. (1984). The effects of timolol maleate on subjective and physiological components of air travel phobia. *Canadian Journal of Psychiatry*, **29**, 570–4.

114. Sartory, G. (1983). Benzodiazepines and behavioural treatment of phobic anxiety. *Behavioural Psychotherapy*, **11**, 204–17.

115. Wolpe, J. (1973). *The practice of behavior therapy* (2nd edn). Pergamon, New York.

116. Gelder, M.G. and Marks, I.M. (1966). Severe agoraphobia: a controlled prospective trial of behaviour therapy. *British Journal of Psychiatry*, **112**, 309–20.

117. Gelder, M.G., Marks, I.M., and Wolff, H.H. (1967). Desensitization and psychotherapy in the treatment of phobic states: a controlled inquiry. *British Journal of Psychiatry*, **113**, 53–73.

118. Gelder, M.G. and Marks, I.M. (1968). Desensitization and phobias: a cross-over study. *British Journal of Psychiatry*, **114**, 323–8.

119. Klein, D.F., Zitrin, C.M., Woerner, M.G., and Ross, D.C. (1983). Treatment of phobias: II. Behavior therapy and supportive psychotherapy: are there any specific ingredients? *Archives of General Psychiatry*, **40**, 139–45.

120. Jerremalm, A., Jansson, L., and Öst, L.G. (1986). Individual response patterns and the effects of different behavioural methods in the treatment of dental phobia. *Behaviour Research and Therapy*, **24**, 587–96.

121. Öst, L.G., Johansson, J., and Jerremalm, A. (1982). Individual response patterns and the effects of different behavioural methods in the treatment of claustrophobia. *Behaviour Research and Therapy*, **20**, 445–60.

122. Öst, L.G., Sterner, U., and Fellenius, J. (1989). Applied tension, applied relaxation, and the combination in the treatment of blood phobia. *Behaviour Research and Therapy*, **27**, 109–21.

123. Öst, L.G., Fellenius, J., and Sterner, U. (1991). Applied tension, exposure *in vivo*, and tension-only in the treatment of blood phobia. *Behaviour Research and Therapy*, **29**, 561–74.

124. Öst, L.G., Hellstrom, K., and Kaver, A. (1992). One versus five sessions of exposure in the treatment of injection phobia. *Behavior Therapy*, **23**, 263–82.

125. Chambless, D.L. (1990). Spacing of exposure sessions in treatment of agoraphobia and simple phobia. *Behavior Therapy*, **21**, 217–29.

126. Marks, I.M. (1987). *Fears, phobias, and rituals: panic, anxiety, and their disorders*. Oxford University Press.

127. Hecker, J.E. (1990). Emotional processing in the treatment of simple phobia: a comparison of imaginal and *in vivo* exposure. *Behavioural Psychotherapy*, **18**, 21–34.

128. Gotestam, K.G. and Berntzen, D. (1997). Use of the modeling effect in one-session exposure. *Scandinavian Journal of Behaviour Therapy*, **26**, 97–101.

129. Öst, L.G. (1996). One-session group treatment of spider phobia. *Behaviour Research and Therapy*, **34**, 707–15.

130. Hellstrom, K. and Öst, L.-G. (1995). One-session therapist directed exposure vs two forms of manual directed self-exposure in the treatment of spider phobia. *Behaviour Research and Therapy*, **33**, 959–65.

131. Öst, L.G., Salkovskis, P.M., and Hellstrom, K. (1991). One-session therapist-directed exposure versus self-exposure in the treatment of spider phobia. *Behavior Therapy*, **22**, 407–22.

132. Doctor, R.M., McVarish, C., and Boone, R.P. (1990). Long-term behavioral treatment effects for the fear of flying. *Phobia Practice and Research Journal*, **3**, 33–42.

133. Carlin, A.S., Hoffman, H.G., and Weghorst, S. (1997). Virtual reality and tactile augmentation in the treatment of spider phobia: a case report. *Behaviour Research and Therapy*, **35**, 153–8.

134. North, M.M., North, S.M., and Coble, J.R. (1997). Virtual reality therapy for fear of flying. *American Journal of Psychiatry*, **154**, 130.

135. Rothbaum, B.O., Hodges, L., Watson, B.A., Kessler, G.D., and Opdyke, D. (1996). Virtual reality exposure therapy in the treatment of fear of flying: a case report. *Behaviour Research and Therapy*, **34**, 477–81.

136. Rothbaum, B.O., Hodges, L.F., Kooper, R., Opdyke, D., Williford, J., and North, M.M. (1995). Effectiveness of computer-generated (virtual

reality) graded exposure in the treatment of acrophobia. *American Journal of Psychiatry*, **152**, 626–8.

137. Thorpe, S.J. and Salkovskis, P.M. (1995). Phobia beliefs: do cognitive factors play a role in specific phobias? *Behavior Research and Therapy*, **33**, 805–16.

138. Greco, T.S. (1989). A cognitive–behavioral approach to fear of flying: a practitioner's guide. *Phobia Practice and Research Journal*, **2**, 3–15.

139. Norton, G.R. and Johnson, W.E. (1983). A comparison of two relaxation procedures for reducing cognitive and somatic anxiety. *Journal of Behavior Therapy and Experimental Psychiatry*, **14**, 209–14.

4.7.3 Panic disorder and agoraphobia

James C. Ballenger

Introduction

Panic disorder draws its name from the Greek god Pan, god of flocks. Pan was known for suddenly frightening animals and humans 'out of the blue'. The spontaneous 'out of the blue' character of panic attacks is the principal identifying characteristic of panic disorder and central to its recognition and diagnosis.

We know the syndrome that we currently call panic disorder with and without agoraphobia has probably existed since the beginning of recorded history. Hippocrates presented cases of obvious phobic avoidance around 400 BC.[1] One of the first modern descriptions was by Benedikt around 1870, describing individuals who developed sudden anxiety and dizziness in public places. Panic disorder is thought to occur in almost all cultures, and one of the earliest and clearest descriptions comes from a syndrome experienced by Eskimo hunters. When preparing to hunt polar bears, these hunters would occasionally have sudden spontaneous episodes of extreme fright and tachycardia which we now know as panic attacks. They described this as 'kayak angst' in the early 1900s.[2]

Certainly, our current modern ideas of panic disorder evolved essentially simultaneously in the United States and Europe in the early to mid-1960s. Donald Klein in the United States described in 1964 the panic syndrome and reported that it was responsive to imipramine.[3] Isaac Marks in the United Kingdom also described panic attacks and agoraphobic avoidance, and treating the syndrome effectively with behaviour therapy.[4]

Until the last couple of decades, panic disorder and agoraphobia were actually thought to be rare syndromes. It is now clear that individuals with these difficulties are anything but rare. In fact, panic disorder is one of the most common presenting problems in individuals seeking mental health treatment. It is also the fifth most common problem seen in primary care settings.[5] It was thought to be a mild problem, but we now know that it is associated with significant dysfunction. The disability in social, occupational, and family life is in fact comparable to major depression.[6]

Although there are differences in the understandings of panic disorder and its treatments across the world, this chapter will review the current, almost universal, understanding about panic disorder, its characteristics, diagnosis, aetiology, and treatments.

Clinical features

One of the earliest and most accurate descriptions of panic attacks was provided by Charles Darwin in 1872 as he described his own episodes:

> The heart beats quickly and violently so that it palpitates and knocks against the ribs…the skin instantly becomes pale as during incipient faintness…under a sense of great fear…in connection with the disturbed action of the heart, the breathing is hurried…one of the best marked symptoms is the trembling of all the muscles of the body.[7]

The most characteristic type of panic attack is the spontaneous 'out of the blue' episode of extreme anxiety. Other 'situational panic attacks' occur immediately upon exposure, or in anticipation of exposure to particular situations, usually where panic attacks have occurred previously. Some individuals have panic attacks in certain situations some of the time, but not always, and these are labelled 'situationally predisposed panic attacks'.

Panic attacks also occur in other anxiety syndromes and are more or less the same in whatever syndrome when they do occur. However, spontaneous panic attacks tend to have more dizziness, paraesthesia, shaking, chest pain, and fears of going mad. Shortness of breath is more common in panic attacks in agoraphobia. Certainly blushing is particularly characteristic of panic attacks in social phobia.

The symptoms of panic attacks in order of their frequency are palpitations, pounding heart, tachycardia, sweating, trembling or shaking, shortness of breath or smothering, feeling of choking, chest pain or discomfort, nausea or abdominal distress, feeling dizzy, unsteady, lightheaded or faint, derealization or depersonalization, fear of losing control or going mad, fear of dying, paraesthesia, and chills or hot flushes.

Panic attacks by definition generally involve four or more of the above symptoms to meet diagnostic criteria for panic disorder in the DSM-IV. The anxiety is crescendo in nature, building to a peak in 10 min in most cases. Panic attacks usually last for several minutes, but in some patients they can last for hours. The frequency and severity of panic attacks varies greatly between individuals and, at times, in individuals. Some have only one to three panic attacks per year, whereas others may have multiple panic attacks each day. Some individuals have bursts of panic attacks and then an absence of all attacks for a period of time. Across a large panic disorder clinical trial, the typical patient described one to two panic attacks per week.[8]

Panic attacks with fewer than four symptoms have been labelled 'limited-symptom attacks' or 'little panic attacks', and most individuals with panic disorder have these, as well as panic attacks with four or more symptoms. The threshold of four symptoms was chosen for DSM-IV because individuals with panic attacks with four symptoms or more had more disability than patients with one- to three-symptom attacks. This threshold is clearly arbitrary, and patients having panic attacks with fewer symptoms do have significant morbidity.

Panic attacks are extremely frightening and patients develop an essentially logical fear of having more panic attacks. Patients develop worry and anxiety about the possibility of panic attacks recurring. This anxiety between attacks has been called 'anticipatory anxiety' and can be almost constant, and characteristically increases prior to exposure to situations previously associated with panic attacks (e.g. having to shop in the supermarket where a panic attack has occurred).

A significant number of people with panic attacks go on to develop fear and avoidance of situations associated with previous panic attacks. They fear these situations where escape would be difficult or embarrassing, or where help might not be available. Most patients mistakenly believe they become incapacitated and incapable of taking care of themselves during a panic attack and therefore feel unsafe in multiple situations. Many go on to develop pervasive avoidance of a variety of situations. Factor analytical studies demonstrate that there is a cluster of situations associated with avoidance. These typically include public transportation (e.g. buses, trains, planes), riding in or driving a car, especially on heavily travelled roads, crowds (e.g. the cinema, a football match, large shopping centres), shopping (especially in supermarkets), particularly where one must stand in queues, and bridges, tunnels, elevators, and other enclosed spaces.[9] People often have an overwhelming need to escape or return to a place of safety such as home. Therefore they fear situations where escape is difficult or impossible, e.g. airplanes, traffic jams on a bridge, dental appointments, etc. On closer examination, it is clear that patients do not actually fear the situation itself but rather reason 'what if' the panic feelings occur while in that situation. This has led to the syndrome being called the 'what if' syndrome, emphasizing that there is actually a 'fear of the fear'.[10]

Patients tend to avoid such situations or force themselves to endure them in distress or take a companion along 'to help'. Others limit their travel to short distances from home or take longer routes where they perceive help would be available (e.g. police, doctors' offices, fire stations, etc.).

Some patients develop agoraphobic avoidance following their first attack, some only after frequent and severe attacks, and some never develop agoraphobic avoidance. In community samples, one-third to one-half of patients who meet criteria for panic disorder also have significant agoraphobic avoidance. The rate is higher (75 per cent) in most clinical samples. A minority (5 per cent) ultimately become unable to leave their homes and are housebound.

It appears that certain cognitive factors may differentiate those who develop agoraphobic avoidance. If patients believe the occurrence of a panic attack is evidence of a catastrophic medical problem such as a heart attack, they are much more likely to develop agoraphobia.[11]

Some patients have panic attacks that awaken them from sleep (**nocturnal panic attacks**). These are in fact quite common and the majority of panic disorder patients experience them. These occur during slow wave sleep early in sleep. These panic attacks are essentially identical to traditional panic attacks that occur during the day, except for occurring during sleep.

There is a group of patients who have what are called **non-fearful panic attacks**. These involve the sudden onset of physiological symptoms without the cognitive components of fear or anxiety. These primarily are medical patients, usually cardiac, who might have episodes of sudden tachycardia and palpitations but no fear.[12]

Symptoms of panic attacks do differ across cultural groups. Although heart pounding is the most common symptom across all groups studied, other symptoms differ in frequency across ethnic lines.[13]

Classification

The earliest modern accounts of what is almost certainly the panic disorder syndrome began appearing in the mid-1900s. There were accounts beginning in 1866 of paroxysmal anxiety episodes that did not use the term 'panic attack'. During the American Civil War, patients were diagnosed with 'irritable heart syndrome' or 'Da Costa syndrome' (1871) with clear descriptions of what we now know as panic disorder. Westphal in Germany in 1872 clearly described patients having panic attacks and agoraphobic avoidance of wide open spaces.[14] Again, in the First World War (1918) the syndrome 'neurocirculatory asthenia' was described which had most of the features of panic disorder.

It was, in fact, Freud in *Case IV of Katharina*, published in 1895, who set the background for the modern classification of panic disorder.[15] However, it was the Feighner criteria published in the United States in 1972 that give the first formal diagnostic recognition to the syndrome.[16] The Research Diagnostic Criteria (**RDC**) which followed in 1978 first split panic disorder away from what we now call generalized anxiety disorder (**GAD**). In the RDC, panic disorder had panic attacks while GAD did not. These diagnoses were made part of the DSM-III diagnostic scheme in 1980.

It was the conceptualization of panic disorder by Donald Klein in 1964 in the United States that led to the predominant view of the syndrome, certainly in the United States.[17] Klein argued that panic attacks were the core of the syndrome, and the remaining clinical phenomena were consequences of the panic attacks. Therefore, he conceptualized that anticipatory anxiety was the fear of the possible recurrence of panic attacks, and similarly that agoraphobia was the subsequent fear and avoidance of situations where panic attacks had occurred. The bringing together of these three phenomena into one concept was accepted in the DSM-IIIR, and more recently in the DSM-IV in the United States.[18]

The biological findings that typical panic attacks could be elicited in panic disorder patients with infusions of lactate (oral or intravenous), doses of caffeine, or breathing 35 per cent CO_2 supported this conceptualization of the syndrome as primarily centred around panic attacks. This idea of a core syndrome centred around recurrent panic attacks was further supported by epidemiological findings of essentially the same illness around the world.[19]

However, this idea remains controversial across the different sides of the Atlantic. The American DSM-IIIR and DSM-IV diagnostic schema continues to utilize the idea that panic attacks are pre-eminent and created two diagnoses: panic disorder and panic disorder with agoraphobia. In Europe and in the ICD-10, agoraphobia is conceptualized as dominant over panic attacks. Therefore, when agoraphobia and panic attacks are both present, the diagnosis is conceptualized as a phobia and that condition is diagnosed as agoraphobia with panic attacks. At the heart of this theoretical debate is whether the treatment should be aimed first at panic attacks (in the United States concept) or at agoraphobic avoidance, for example with exposure therapy (in the European schema). Of further practical importance, in some countries that still utilize the ICD-9 and the diagnosis of anxiety neurosis, all patients with GAD and panic disorder are lumped together under that diagnosis.

Diagnosis

The most recently revised diagnostic schema for this syndrome is the DSM-IV. Changes from the DSM-IIIR and DSM-IV were made following two principles:

(1) any new empirical data that required changes be made;

(2) an attempt to make the DSM-IV and ICD-10 more compatible.

For the diagnoses of panic disorder and agoraphobia, an attempt was also made to more nearly describe the prototypic patient and to move away from the pseudoquantification of using number of panic attacks per week.[18]

The DSM-IV clarified that panic attacks occurred in multiple syndromes including social phobia, obsessive–compulsive disorder, depression, and others. However, DSM-IV utilized the distinction that only in panic disorder were there recurrent spontaneous panic attacks not bound to any particular situations. The diagnosis of panic disorder has several requirements including the following.

- Recurrent, unexpected panic attacks (situational panic attacks could also occur but there would need to be at least two unexpected panic attacks by history).

- Panic attacks needed to be followed by at least 1 month of persistent anxiety about potential recurrence of further panic attacks, implications of these attacks (e.g. going mad, something wrong medically), or a significant behavioural change because of these attacks. This was necessary because some patients had panic attacks and completely changed their lives but denied that they were worried about experiencing more panic attacks or the implications of the panic attacks.[18]

The agoraphobia criteria remained largely unchanged, but it was made more clear that the diagnosis was based on persistent fear and avoidance of certain clusters of situations and listed the most common. Again, patients could have panic disorder alone, or it could be complicated by agoraphobia.

The controversial diagnosis of agoraphobia without a history of panic disorder was retained until further clarification is obtained through research. Our current understanding is that these patients generally have never fully met criteria for panic disorder because their panic-like symptoms have not met the diagnostic criterion requiring four full symptoms for a panic attack. Available research suggests that these patients are otherwise very much like typical patients with panic disorder and agoraphobia, except that their anxiety attacks involve fewer symptoms. Some patients actually have only one or two symptoms (e.g. fear of loss of bladder or bowel control or only tachycardia).

Perhaps the most difficult diagnostic issue is the frequent comorbidity. The Epidemiologic Catchment Area study documented that approximately 50 per cent of panic disorder patients over their lifetime have another anxiety disorder.[20] Certainly one of the most common is panic disorder associated with agoraphobia, which across multiple cultures averages 15 to 20 per cent; however, in multiple studies it has been shown to be as high as 50 to 60 per cent.[21]

In actuality, depression is more commonly comorbid with panic disorder than even agoraphobia and suggests a close relationship

Table 1 Influence of comorbidity on suicide attempts in panic disorder

	Prevalence of suicide attempts (%)
No psychiatric disorder	1
Panic disorder	7–17.1
Panic disorder plus	
Depression (lifetime) or	23.6–50.0
Alcoholism and/or substance abuse or	46.2
Major depression plus alcoholism and/or substance abuse	72.2

Data from Weissman et al.,[26] Johnson et al.,[27] and Lépine et al.[28]

between these syndromes. Comorbid depression ranged from 22.5 to 68.2 per cent in various samples. Lifetime rates vary from 35 to 91 per cent.[21] Major depression ranged from 3.8 to 20.1 per cent. Although approximately half the patients developed panic disorder and depression at essentially the same time, one-quarter develop depression before panic disorder and one-quarter panic disorder before depression.[22] Surprisingly, bipolar illness has been reported to be as high as 20.8 per cent.[23]

Easily one-third of panic disorder patients abuse alcohol.[24] The percentage in clinical samples is much higher with 13 to 43 per cent of panic disorder patients also meeting criteria for alcoholism.[25]

Differential diagnosis

It is particularly important to determine whether agoraphobic avoidance is present, because its treatment usually requires some sort of exposure therapy. Patients will often not volunteer that they are avoiding certain situations out of embarrassment. As mentioned earlier, depression and panic disorder often occur together and again patients often do not describe the other syndrome, but rather describe the syndrome which is most painful to them at that time. However, proper recognition of comorbid depression is especially important because of the marked increase (fourfold) in suicide attempts in patients with panic disorder and depression (Table 1).

The difference between panic disorder and GAD depends on whether patients have panic attacks and whether they have multiple, unrealistic, and excessive worries about most aspects of life, not just panic attacks. These worries in GAD often concern money, health, children, work problems, etc. The differential with social phobia centres not around the occurrence of panic attacks, but whether they are confined entirely to social situations where the individual fears embarrassment and humiliation. Specific phobias involve panic attacks, but they occur in very specific situations (high places) or in the presence of specific objects (e.g. animals, snakes). The post-traumatic stress disorder patient may have many panic-like symptoms, but their illness begins quite specifically after a traumatic experience 'outside the range of usual human experience' where they feel threatened with death or serious injury. Finally, obsessive–compulsive disorder can involve panic attacks but only in the specific context of obsessional concerns (e.g. contamination etc.). In these patients, panic attacks are also dwarfed in importance by typical obsessions and compulsions/ rituals concerning contamination, symmetry, bad events, etc.

Table 2 Medical conditions that produce panic-like symptoms

Endocrine	Respiratory
Hyperthyroidism	Chronic obstructive
Hypoparathyroidism	pulmonary disease
Hypoglycaemia	Asthma
Phaeochromocytoma	
Carcinoid syndrome	**Substance-induced**
Cushing's disease	Caffeine
	Cocaine
Cardiovascular	Theophylline
Arrhythmias	Amphetamines
Atypical chest pain	Steroids
Mitral valve prolapse	Alcohol/sedative
	withdrawal
Neurological	
Seizures	**Haematological**
Vestibular disease	Anaemia

Medical conditions

Panic-like symptoms do occur in various medical conditions (hyperthyroidism, phaeochromocytoma, seizures, cardiac arrhythmias, chronic obstructive pulmonary disease) (Table 2). Also, the typical panic disorder patient does report a large number of physical symptoms and usually to a non-psychiatric physician. This leads to very frequent misdiagnosis, generally because of how frequently these patients present in general medicine where there is a general lack of awareness of this syndrome.

As mentioned, there are medical conditions that can mimic panic disorder (Table 1). There is also evidence that there are slightly increased rates of certain illnesses, for example hyperthyroidism (11–13 per cent)[29] and perhaps mitral valve prolapse.[30] However, these are uncommon in panic disorder patients. Most experts recommend a relatively conservative approach medically. Generally, the most valuable part of a medical examination is a careful history with follow-up of any strongly suggested possibilities, supplemented by a few laboratory tests (complete blood count, thyroid function tests, metabolic screen, and ECG, especially if the patient is over 40 years of age).

Panic disorder in the general medical setting

Conservative estimates of panic disorder in primary care have ranged from 3 to 8 per cent with at least 50 per cent going unrecognized.[31] The average panic disorder patient in general medicine takes 10 years for a correct diagnosis to be made with an escalation of the use of health care services over this period.[32] In general, the presence of panic disorder leads to a threefold increase in utilization of general medical services.

The percentage of panic disorder patients is also markedly higher in certain medical groups. These include the very prevalent but most difficult to diagnose patients with vague symptoms such as fatigue, back pain, headache, dizziness, chest pain, etc.[33] or multiple symptoms (more than five).[34]

In a classic study of unrecognized panic disorder patients who were referred for a psychiatric consultation from primary care, 39 per cent had cardiovascular symptoms, 33 per cent gastrointestinal symptoms, and 44 per cent neurological.[35] It is now clear that 16 to 25 per cent of patients presenting to the emergency room with chest pain have panic disorder. Fully 25 per cent of cardiology practice involves panic disorder, usually unrecognized with 80 per cent of patients with chest pain and normal angiograms ultimately diagnosed with panic disorder. We could also increase our yield of recognizing panic disorder patients in certain procedure-oriented situations. For instance, 28 per cent of patients referred for Holter monitoring for palpitations have panic disorder, as do 66 per cent of patients undergoing a work-up to rule out phaeochromocytoma.[36] Also, 44 per cent of irritable bowel syndrome and 15 per cent of patients with headache symptoms seeing a physician have panic disorder, and these are both very prevalent disorders.

Comment

A recent large study sponsored by the World Health Organization (**WHO**) studied primary care patients in 14 different countries.[31] Of patients in that study who had a single panic attack in the previous month, 99 per cent had an anxiety disorder or depression, or a subthreshold anxiety disorder or depressive disorder.[37,38] The occurrence of a single panic attack also predicted the onset of panic disorder in two-thirds of the patients studied in the next year, a fourfold increase in depression (51 per cent) in the next year, and marked increases in alcoholism, social phobia, and obsessive–compulsive disorder. If replicated, it would appear that the occurrence of even a single panic attack may well represent the 'tip of the iceberg' and should serve as a signal for increased scrutiny for anxiety and depressive syndromes.

Epidemiology

Surveys largely utilizing DSM diagnoses have found wide agreement and generally equal prevalences of panic disorder across many countries (Table 3).[21,28] The recent United States Epidemiologic Catchment Area study[39] and National Comorbidity Study[40] have been the most carefully performed and therefore the most informative. Utilizing specific criteria for panic attacks, prevalence for panic attacks has generally averaged 7 to 9 per cent of the population (range 1.8–15.6 per cent). However, if criteria for panic attacks are liberalized somewhat ('fearful spells') in terms of the number of times and severity, the prevalence doubles.

There is a striking uniformity worldwide for the observed prevalence of panic disorder. In 10 community studies involving over 40 000 subjects, the majority of studies found lifetime prevalence rates for panic disorder averaging 1.5 to 2.5 per cent, with a yearly prevalence of around 1 per cent. In clinical samples there is greater variability. In the previously mentioned WHO survey of 14 countries, the prevalence for panic disorder ranged from a low of 1.4 per cent to a high of 16.5 per

Table 3 Prevalence of panic symptoms and panic attacks

	Prevalence (%)
Intense fearful spells (past year)	11.3
Previous month	5.8
DSM-IIIR panic attacks (lifetime)	7–9
Previous month	2.2
Recurrent panic attacks	4.2

Data from National Cohort Study[40] and Epidemiologic Catchment Area Study.[39]

cent for panic attacks and 0 to 3.5 per cent for panic disorder itself.[31] The average was 1.1 per cent (currently) and 3.5 per cent (lifetime), which is surprisingly similar to the community samples. As mentioned, rates are much higher in specialized medical clinics and range from 15 per cent in dizziness clinics, to 16 to 65 per cent in cardiology practices, to 35 per cent in hyperventilation clinics, etc.

Risk factors

Panic disorder has been uniformly observed to be at least two times more prevalent in females than males. The Epidemiologic Catchment Area study demonstrated a prevalence of 3:2.[41] In clinical samples it is generally 3:1. The onset of panic disorder appears to fall into two peaks. The first occurs in the early to mid-twenties (15–24 years old) with a second peak at 45–54 years of age. The onset of panic disorder after the age of 65 is rare (0.1 per cent).

The highest rates of panic disorder and agoraphobia occur in widowed, divorced, or separated individuals living in cities. Limited education, early parental loss, and physical or sexual abuse are also risk factors.[42] Agoraphobia is clearly more prevalent in females, and females make up three-quarters of the sample with extensive avoidance. Males tend to have longer duration of illness but less agoraphobia and depression, and less frequent help seeking. Perhaps the greater necessity to perform in the workplace ameliorates avoidance in males.

Aetiology

Genetic predisposition

Certainly the preponderance of evidence suggests there is a genetic contribution to the predisposition to develop panic attacks and agoraphobia. There are increased rates of panic disorder in first-degree relatives with 7.9 to 41 per cent versus 8 per cent or less in control populations. The overall increased risk in first-degree relatives ranges from two- to 20-fold with the median seven- to eightfold. Overall, studies suggest that another affected relative can be found 25 to 50 per cent of the time, two times as commonly in female relatives. The increased familial aggregation is specific for panic disorder.[43] These findings are certainly consistent with a modest genetic transmission with relatively high specificity.

Although twin studies are limited, Torgersen[44] did find increased concordance in monozygotic twins (31 per cent versus zero). Skre et al.[45] found a twofold increase of panic disorder in monozygotic twins, while Andrews et al.[46] failed to find an increased incidence. In the largest sample of interviewed female twins, a several-fold increase was again found (23.9 per cent versus 10.9 per cent).[47]

Overall, evidence from family and twin studies suggests that panic disorder involves modest inheritability of around 30 to 40 per cent. The best model suggests 50 per cent genetic and 50 per cent environmental influences.[48] Recent linkage studies to confirm these hypotheses have been contradictory but do suggest that single-gene transmission is unlikely. This leaves the possibilities of either heterogeneity across families and/or a polygenic inheritance.

Several converging lines do link childhood anxiety with adult anxiety, consistent with a genetic predisposition.[49] This is particularly true for separation anxiety in children.[50] Kagan et al.[51] have prescribed that 10 per cent of Caucasian children are born with height-

ened anxiety which they call behavioural inhibition. Behavioural inhibition is higher in children of anxiety-disordered parents,[52] and there are high rates of anxiety disorders in children of adults with panic disorder.[53] As behaviourally inhibited children have aged, they have been found to show higher rates of anxiety and phobic disorders. Currently, this is probably the best model of an inherited anxiety predisposition. A variant of this type model proposes that there is an ethological factor involving an evolutionarily determined vulnerability to unfamiliar territory.[54] This might explain why the seemingly inherited anxiety is to specific situations. This is also consistent with the high rate of precipitating events prior to the onset of clinical difficulties. In this model an evolutionarily/genetically determined vulnerability, would be clinically 'activated' by critical stressors in genetically vulnerable individuals.

Precipitating events have been reported in 60 to 96 per cent of cases. These have often centred on separation or loss, relationship difficulties, taking on new responsibility, and physiological stressors (e.g. childbirth, surgery, hyperthyroidism).[55] This is certainly consistent with a diathesis/vulnerability model with the illness being precipitated in a predisposed individual in adulthood.

There are also many studies suggesting that traumatic early events may figure in the vulnerability leading to panic disorder. The majority of children in some studies have experienced early parental separation.[42] A traumatic event in childhood has been retrospectively reported in at least two-thirds of children, a threefold increase.[56] Early sexual abuse before the age of 5 may even be specific for the subsequent development of panic disorder.[57] The most common adult disorder following sexual abuse before the age of 5 is in fact a 44 per cent incidence of agoraphobia.[58]

There is some evidence in a prospective study involving over 3000 individuals that dependent personality traits were later associated with the development of anxiety disorders.[59] There are also retrospective data that adult panic disorder patients describe their parents as being overly protective and less caring.[60] It is difficult to separate the effects on individuals of the anxiety disorders themselves which create dependent behaviour, or overprotectiveness in the parents producing dependent personality traits.

Biological models

Noradrenaline

There is considerable evidence implicating the brain noradrenaline (norepinephrine) brain systems and panic disorder.[61] The noradrenergic agents yohimbine and isoproterenol stimulate panic attacks in panic disorder patients, suggesting a possible subsensitivity of presynaptic α_2 inhibitory adrenoreceptors. Both these drugs increase the firing rate of the locus ceruleus, thought by some to be the brain alarm system. It is also true that most effective medications in the treatment of panic disorder in fact decrease locus ceruleus firing rate and most panicogenic stimuli increase the locus ceruleus firing rate.

Serotonin

Findings with serotonin brain systems in panic disorder are quite contradictory, probably because of the different 5-hydroxytryptamine circuits in different areas of the brain. Most investigators believe, however, that an increase in 5-hydroxytryptamine transmission decreases panic disorder. The principal evidence for this is that the selective serotonin reuptake inhibitors are effective and that they increase 5-hydroxytryptamine release after long-term use. Whether this increased release in fact leads to downregulation of a supersensitive postsynaptic receptor is one logical possibility, but is as yet unproven.

γ-Aminobutyric acid

The γ-aminobutyric acid (GABA) system is almost certainly involved in panic disorder with perhaps the strongest evidence being that benzodiazepine agonists such as alprazolam and clonazepam are clearly effective treatments for panic disorder.[62] Also GABA antagonists such as flumezanil have increased panicogenic effects in panic disorder patients, and reverse benzodiazepine agonists such as β-carbolines can cause panic attacks. Also, positron emission tomography data have demonstrated decreased benzodiazepine binding in the inferior brain areas, including the inferior parietotemporo-occipital areas.[63]

Cholecystokinin–pentagastrin

Cholecystokinin is clearly involved in anxiety in animals. Also, panic disorder patients develop panic attacks in a dose-dependent fashion with administration of pentagastrin. However, cholecystokinin antagonists have not yet been shown to be effective in humans.[64]

A biological deficit in panic disorder is supported by a series of studies: abnormalities in the mesotemporal region on magnetic resonance imaging have been observed,[65] decreased benzodiazepine sensitivity is present in panic disorder patients,[66] and the benzodiazepine antagonist flumezanil causes panic attacks in panic disorder patients, but not in normal subjects, suggesting a change in the set point for the benzodiazepine receptors.[61]

Psychological factors

Many critics disagree with the importance of biological findings in panic disorder, principally, various European workers and the cognitive theorists. They argue that panic attacks are not 'biological' and that a phobic attitude is required, and/or certain temperamental factors. Others attempt an integrated model utilizing both findings of biological differences and psychological factors of temperament and child-rearing practices.

Course and prognosis

There is limited evidence with appropriate population-based samples to clearly delineate the course of panic disorder. Available evidence suggests that panic disorder is a stable but chronic condition once criteria for the disorder are met. Most patients seeking treatment have experienced chronic, frequently chronically worsening, illness generally for 10 to 15 years prior to diagnosis.[67,68] However, other evidence does suggest that there is heterogeneity in terms of course.

As previously mentioned, the Klein model suggests that spontaneous panic attacks are the first manifestation of the illness, followed by anticipatory anxiety, and agoraphobia in some individuals. However, for most panic disorder patients examined closely, a panic attack is rarely the first symptom. In some studies, over 90 per cent of patients have had mild phobic or hypochondriacal, milder symptoms prior to the onset of their first panic attack.

The first panic attack is usually in a 'phobogenic' situation such as a public place, street, store, public transportation, crowd, elevator, tun-

nel, bridge, or open space. As mentioned, these are often preceded by stressful life events.[69]

The earliest studies indicated low recovery rates with chronic waxing and waning in most patients. Some individuals have outbreaks of symptomatology with less difficulty in between, but the majority of patients seem to have a more or less continuous symptom picture which ranges from mild to severe.

Recovery rates vary from 25 to 75 per cent for 1 to 2 years' follow-up.[70] Over a 5-year follow-up, only 10 to 12 per cent had fully recovered in one study and 30 per cent in another. The most common picture is about 50 per cent of patients are neither well nor very sick with mild symptoms most of the time or on and off.[71] After diagnosis and some sort of treatment, functional recovery occurs in the majority of patients.

In acute pharmacological trials, 50 to 70 per cent of patients have excellent acute responses with another 20 per cent having a moderate response. With effective behavioural therapy, again the majority of patients recover[72] and in some trials over 75 per cent of patients are much improved 1 to 9 years following therapy, with an average decrease in symptoms of 50 per cent.[73]

Poor responses were most consistently associated with initial high symptom severity and high agoraphobic avoidance at baseline. Poor response is also associated with low socio-economic status, less education, longer duration, limited social networks, death of a parent, divorce or unmarried status, and personality disorders.

Treatment

Introduction

Multiple effective treatments have been developed since the early 1960s and include both psychological and pharmacological treatments. Both exposure-based treatments and imipramine were shown to be effective in treating panic disorder and agoraphobia in the early 1960s.[3,74] Psychological-based treatments have moved increasingly toward cognitive-behavioural therapy with efficacy roughly comparable to pharmacological treatments.

Imipramine and monoamine oxidase inhibitors (**MAOIs**) were the first medications shown to effectively treat panic disorder in the 1960s. The high-potency benzodiazepines (alprazolam and clonazepam) were also shown to be effective in the 1980s. Most now agree that the selective serotonin reuptake inhibitors (**SSRIs**) are the treatment of choice.[75,76]

Medication treatments

Selective serotonin reuptake inhibitors

The most extensively studied SSRIs are clomipramine, fluvoxamine, and most recently paroxetine. However, sertraline, citalopram, and fluoxetine have also been shown to be effective.[77]

Clomipramine

Although clomipramine is an SSRI, its actions are not as specific to the serotonin system as the other SSRIs. Based on extensive experience in Europe, many have considered it to be the so-called 'gold standard' in Europe, although it has not been extensively utilized in the United States for the treatment of panic disorder. From the earliest studies, approximately 75 per cent of patients had a good response which often began by week 2 at surprisingly low doses (40–50 mg/day).[78] The first methodologically rigorous trial consisted of a double-blind placebo-controlled trial involving 108 patients, all of whom had panic disorder. In this trial, as well as those to follow, clomipramine reduced panic attacks, anxiety, agoraphobic avoidance, and depression. In fact, two trials suggested that clomipramine was the best treatment because it appeared to be better than imipramine. In these trials clomipramine was better on some efficacy measures.[79,80] Also, this response was observed earlier, appearing at week 4, while imipramine's effects began at week 8, typical of previous trials. Doses in these studies and others suggest an average dose of 100 to 150 mg/day.

In one modern comparison of clomipramine to a true SSRI (fluvoxamine), both medications led to resolution of panic symptomatology in approximately 60 per cent of the patients.

Fluvoxamine

There are several double-blind placebo-controlled 8-week trials in large samples demonstrating fluvoxamine's superiority to placebo. Effective doses ranged from 200 to 250 mg/day, with good response in approximately two-thirds of the patients by week 3.

Paroxetine

Paroxetine has been extensively the most studied, leading to its being the first SSRI to be licensed for the treatment of panic disorder in 1995. The first trial was in seven Danish centres involving a 12-week comparison with placebo, with all patients receiving standard cognitive-behavioural therapy. Eighty-two per cent of the paroxetine group versus 50 per cent of placebo demonstrated a 50 per cent reduction of panic attacks. In the paroxetine group, 36 per cent had no panic attacks (placebo 16 per cent) at the end of the trial, with average numbers of panic attacks per week falling from 21.2 to 5.2 in the paroxetine group, versus 26.6 to 16.4 on placebo.

The most definitive trial in the field involved 39 centres in 13 countries, mostly in Europe. A sample of 367 were randomly assigned to paroxetine, clomipramine, and placebo. Beginning at a dose of 10 mg with ultimate dosing of 20 to 60 mg/day of paroxetine and 50 to 100 mg/day of clomipramine, paroxetine was significantly superior to placebo at weeks 6, 9, and 12 for percentage of patients having no panic attacks (50.9 per cent paroxetine, 36.7 per cent clomipramine, 31.6 per cent placebo at week 12). Paroxetine's effect was significantly greater on several measures than clomipramine at weeks 6 and 9. Measures of other symptomatic domains (anxiety, agoraphobia, functional disability) all improved on paroxetine and clomipramine greater than on placebo. There were significantly greater side-effects from clomipramine than paroxetine, especially gastrointestinal and central nervous system side-effects.

Interestingly, in contrast to early experience with SSRIs, in all these studies with paroxetine (and the other SSRIs to follow) initial hyperstimulation reactions were not observed. This was probably because patients were started on low doses (e.g. 10 mg/day paroxetine) initially.

In the only trial establishing a target dose for an SSRI, paroxetine at 10 mg, 20 mg, and 40 mg/day were compared with placebo. Only the 40-mg group was significantly greater than placebo on most outcome measures. At the end of the trial, the highest percentage free of panic attacks was on 40 mg/day (86 per cent) versus 20 mg (65.2 per cent), 10 mg (67.4 per cent), and placebo (50 per cent). Global measures, as well as ratings for anxiety and depression, were more improved in the 40-mg group.

Sertraline

Sertraline has been studied in two double-blind, placebo-controlled, flexible dose trials with a combined sample of 342. These were 10-week trials conducted in United States and Canada with doses of sertraline between 50 and 200 mg/day. when a new measure called Panic Attack Burden (panic attack frequency × severity) was utilized, there were significant differences from placebo by week 1 and panic attack frequency by week 2. There were significantly greater decreases in global measures (avoidance and anxiety) and quality-of-life measures on sertraline. Sertraline patients had greater improvement in work, household, family, social, hobbies, and overall satisfaction with the medicine and life. It was well tolerated with the usual SSRI side-effects (nausea, dry mouth, diarrhoea, sexual difficulties, etc.).

Initial hyperstimulation was not observed with 25 mg but a higher early drop-out rate was observed, (10.5 per cent) versus placebo (0 per cent), suggesting that even lower initial doses might be helpful.

Another large multicentre fixed-dose trial compared 50, 100, and 200 mg/day but failed to find significant differences between the groups. The 100-mg cell did have the largest drop in number of panic attacks. Although there is no clear evidence of a target dose or dose–response relationship, suggested dosage is between 100 and 150 mg/day.

Fluoxetine

Controlled trials are currently in progress but not yet published; however, there is considerable clinical evidence from small trials that fluoxetine is an effective treatment of panic disorder. The biggest issue has been a high incidence of initial hyperstimulation reactions because most patients were initially begun at 20 mg, or even when at 10 mg. To avoid this effect, most clinicians begin fluoxetine in panic disorder patients at 2.5 to 5.0 mg/day. There is no clear dose–response relationship, but most patients are treated with 10 to 30 mg/day.

Comparison of the SSRIs

There is little well-controlled evidence comparing SSRIs. In the trials mentioned comparing paroxetine and clomipramine, paroxetine was certainly better tolerated and had a somewhat faster onset and somewhat greater reduction of symptoms and disability in the 1-year maintenance trial. Certainly, the greatest issue is the comparison between the tricyclic antidepressants and SSRIs. SSRIs are much better tolerated (less weight gain, sedation, anticholinergic symptoms) except for the increased sexual dysfunction noted with SSRIs.

Benzodiazepines

Alprazolam

Currently the best-studied benzodiazepine for panic disorder is alprazolam, with over two dozen controlled trials which led to its approval in the United States and some European countries.[81] Almost all trials show greater efficacy of alprazolam over placebo and decreased panic attacks, higher percentage of patients free of panic attacks, reduced agoraphobic avoidance, anxiety, depression, and associated disability. Its effects are demonstrated to be equivalent to imipramine and other benzodiazepines such as clonazepam, lorazepam, and diazepam.

Effective doses in the acute treatment of panic disorder have ranged from 0.5 to 10 mg/day with 4 to 6 mg/day being the average. Doses

Table 4 Advantages and disadvantages of various antipanic agents

	Advantages	Disadvantages
SSRIs	Well-tolerated antidepressant Safe in overdose Little weight gain Once-daily dosing	Initial activation Nausea, headache, asthenia, insomnia Sexual side-effects
Benzodiazepines	Rapid efficacy Reduces anticipatory anxiety Well tolerated No initial activation Safe in overdose	Sedation Memory problems Withdrawal Abuse potential Sexual dysfunction
Tricyclic antidepressants	Single daily dose Less expensive Long experience Antidepressant	Initial activation Anticholinergic side-effects Weight gain Orthostatic hypotension Dangerous in overdose Sexual dysfunction
MAOIs	More effective (against comorbid depression)? Antidepressant	Dietary restrictions Hypertensive crises Initial activation Onset delayed Orthostatic hypotension Dangerous in overdose Sexual dysfunction

have generally been reduced into the 1 to 3 mg/day range after 6 months of treatment.

The greatest difference is certainly the rapid response, with some patients responding within the first few days.[82] The principal side-effects with alprazolam have included sedation and fatigue, which usually improve over the first few weeks. There are rare difficulties with intoxication, aggressive behaviour, mania, and depression.

Clonazepam

Because of the longer half-life of clonazepam compared with alprazolam, it can be given once per day with less inner-dose anxiety breakthrough.[83] Doses are generally one-third to one-half those of alprazolam with most patients being treated with 1 to 3 mg/day. The principal drawback with clonazepam has been some reports of depression.

Diazepam

Controlled trials with diazepam have now demonstrated that diazepam's effectiveness is comparable to alprazolam with sufficiently high doses. In the three best controlled trials, the mean effective dose of diazepam was 43, 44, and 56 mg/day. In an 8-week trial with 241 patients, the percentage free of panic attacks were 62.8 per cent with diazepam, 71.4 per cent with alprazolam, and 37.5 per cent with placebo, a highly significant difference from placebo.

Other benzodiazepines

Several other benzodiazepines appear to be effective as well, including clobazam (50 ± 17 mg/day) and lorazepam 3.8 ± 1.3 mg/day.

Conclusion

The benzodiazepines remain the most frequently utilized treatment for panic disorder worldwide, probably because of their quick onset of action, increased efficacy against anticipatory anxiety, low cost, and because they are well tolerated (Table 4). Interestingly, they are not associated with the frightening initial hyperstimulation reactions, an important difference. The principal drawback to benzodiazepines is the general concern with their abuse potential, particularly in alcoholics and opiate or pill addicts. Although there does appear to be increased risk in drug abusers, the risk for abuse in patients with uncomplicated panic disorder actually appears to be small. The more realistic issue is the high rate of withdrawal symptoms and relapse following discontinuation of benzodiazepines. Even with a 30-day taper in the large Cross-National Panic Trial, 35 per cent had significant withdrawal symptoms after only 8 weeks of treatment.[84] After 8 months of treatment, 47 of 88 patients were unable to complete a taper on time, while 20 per cent had severe withdrawal symptoms. In another trial of 50 patients treated for 8 months and tapered slowly, there was a 70 to 80 per cent relapse with alprazolam.[85] However, in a subsequent trial with a very slow taper over 2 to 4 months, withdrawal symptoms were almost eliminated. Overall, it appears that the critical issues concerning withdrawal are the rate of taper and physician and patient attitudes towards discontinuation and withdrawal symptoms.[86]

Tricyclic antidepressants

It was probably the early demonstration of imipramine's effectiveness in panic disorder that established the field of panic disorder and certainly its treatment with medication. There are now over a dozen well-controlled placebo trials, all but one of which have demonstrated significantly greater effects than placebo.[87]

It was with imipramine that the initial hyperstimulation effect was first observed. As with other medications that cause this initial frightening increase in anxiety symptoms, with lower initial doses (e.g.

10 mg/day imipramine), this frightening reaction can generally be managed or avoided.

The beneficial effects of imipramine (and all effective medications) are against all aspects of the panic disorder syndrome; however, with imipramine significant effects are rarely observed before 4 weeks and often require 8 to 12 weeks.

Some of the most important advantages of imipramine is how well studied it is, that it can be given once per day, and its lower cost (Table 4). Its principal difficulties are the hyperstimulation reactions and significant weight gain with long-term use and danger in the case of overdose. Dosing should begin at 10 mg/day and be increased gradually until the patient responds or a maximum of 300 mg/day is reached. In the large, Multinational Phase II Cross-National Panic Study with a flexible dose design, 70 per cent (endpoint) of patients were panic free (78 per cent of completers) at a mean dose of 155 mg/day.[19]

Monoamine oxidase inhibitors

The greatest experience with the MAOIs has been with phenelzine (Nardil®), although tranylcypromine has also been demonstrated to be effective.[88] The most definitive trial was an early comparison of phenelzine and imipramine in the mid-1970s. Both medications were approximately equally effective, although phenelzine was more effective in several of the global symptom measures. This was the first trial to suggest that the MAOIs might be the most effective medication class, perhaps especially if the panic disorder patient is depressed.

Effective doses of Nardil have ranged from 45 to 90 mg/day, usually beginning at 15 mg/day and increased in twice a day dosage to 45 or 60 mg/day. Approximately 70 to 80 per cent of patients have responded in acute trials.

Certainly the major issue is the need for a patient to be on a restricted diet and the danger of hypertensive crisis if the diet is not followed (Table 4). There are also dangers if certain other medications are used, especially certain analgesics and other antidepressants.

Most United States clinicians are reluctant to use MAOIs, although this reluctance is less prominent in other countries. In general, MAOIs are reserved for patients who have failed to respond to other treatments. The principal side-effects are insomnia, weight gain, postural hypotension, anticholinergic side-effects, and sexual dysfunction.

The reversible MAOIs, brofaramine and meclobemide, have stimulated recent interest because they require no restrictive diet. However, recent trials with meclobemide were unable to distinguish medication from placebo and despite promising early results with brofaramine, its development has been discontinued.

Other medications

Although acute trials with tricyclic antidepressants, MAOIs, benzodiazepines, and SSRIs have approximately 75 per cent positive responses in acute treatment,[89] complete resolution of symptoms and functional difficulties as well as side-effects and comorbid problems occur in somewhat fewer than 50 per cent of patients.[90] This has led to attempts to find better medications that have been generally unsuccessful to date.

Certainly several small trials have demonstrated that valproic acid is effective in panic disorder with an effect similar to traditional agents.[91] Although buspirone has been demonstrated to be ineffective, small trials have suggested that the azapirone gepirone and the imidazopyridines may be effective.

Psychological treatments

Psychodynamic psychotherapy

Although psychodynamic psychotherapy remains a popular treatment for all psychiatric disorders including panic disorder, there has been very little research demonstrating its efficacy in panic disorder. There is one large case-report study of patients with panic disorder reporting that most patients did respond well. One trial compares clomipramine with clomipramine plus 15 weekly sessions of brief dynamic psychotherapy. Patients in both groups responded well with 75 per cent of the patients in the clomipramine group being panic free and all of the patients in the combination group. Also, only 20 per cent of the combination group relapsed following discontinuation of the clomipramine, whereas 75 per cent of the clomipramine-alone group relapsed.

In an extension of this work, an emotion-focused treatment for panic disorder has been developed which explores typical fears of being abandoned or trapped as stimuli for panic attacks. This often involves a 12-session acute treatment with six sessions of monthly maintenance in which patients are encouraged to identify, reflect upon, and attempt to change problematic feelings and their responses. Although there are no rigorously controlled trials, emotion-focused treatment has been compared with cognitive-behavioural therapy. Both treatments were found to be equally effective. This has led to a specific form of dynamic psychotherapy entitled 'panic-focused psychodynamic psychotherapy' which is generally applied in 3-month increments, in some cases longer.[92] Although not empirically tested, this is a promising use of traditional psychodynamic principles in treatment of panic disorder.

Behavioural treatments

Exposure treatments

Behavioural treatments which utilize *in vivo* exposure to phobic situations have been the mainstay of the behavioural treatments of panic disorder. They are based on the theory and evidence that patients who enter a feared situation experience habituation of their anxiety whether they are exposed slowly or suddenly and extensively (flooding). The critical nature of exposure for improvement was made clear in one study in which patients being treated with imipramine received no improvement from imipramine when given anti-exposure instruments. However, they significantly improved if it were simply suggested that they re-expose themselves to their previously phobic situations when ready.

A large number of studies have documented the effectiveness of exposure-based treatments with 58 to 83 per cent of patients improving, with the treatment gains continuing or improving for several years (2 to 9).[89]

Studies which have compared use of exposure to cognitive-behavioural therapy, the other empirically documented treatment, and have found them to be essentially equal in efficacy.[89,93] There appears to be little benefit from the combination although the drop-out rate was lower (zero versus 14 per cent for cognitive-behavioural therapy and 20 per cent for exposure). However, others have documented positive combination effects with a higher percentage of patients doing very well and in fact more rapidly.[94]

One consistently observed effect of exposure-based treatments is its long-lasting effects. In one trial with 110 individuals treated with 12 weeks of exposure-based treatment, fully 74 per cent achieved panic-free status and this improvement was maintained in almost all patients throughout a 7-year follow-up.

Evidence supporting the importance of exposure-based treatments is very clear but it too is not the ideal treatment. Many patients remain symptomatic and because it is a significantly anxiety-provoking treatment, many studies report between 10 per cent and 25 per cent of patients drop out.

Cognitive-behavioural therapy

Cognitive-behavioural therapy is based on the theory that patients with panic disorder interpret physical symptoms in a catastrophic way and these cognitive distortions need to be challenged and changed. Treatment generally involves an initial education component which is followed by identification of these critical misinterpretations of panic symptoms. Patients are then taught ways in which they can challenge and correct these misinterpretations. This includes evaluating how likely (or unlikely) the imagined consequences are and how in fact catastrophic it would be, even if their worst fears did occur. Most cognitive-behavioural therapy is also combined with interoceptive exposure to the physical symptoms that frighten them. For instance, a patient fearful of dizziness might be spun in a chair. Someone fearful of an increased heart rate might be asked to exercise and then challenge their fears about the resultant tachycardia. Cognitive-behavioural therapy of panic disorder evolved from early work of Aaron Beck, but has been applied to panic disorder primarily by Barlow and colleagues working in the United States[95] and by Clark in the United Kingdom (see Chapter 6.3.2.1).

In a recent direct comparison of cognitive-behavioural therapy, imipramine, applied relaxation, and 3-month waiting-list controls were compared. At 3 months, cognitive-behavioural therapy patients were doing better than either of the other two active conditions, although cognitive-behavioural therapy and imipramine were approximately equal at 6 months. However, again at follow-up, more imipramine patients had relapsed than cognitive-behavioural therapy patients.

Although applied relaxation has been shown to be somewhat effective in panic disorder, other studies have demonstrated that cognitive-behavioural therapy, especially combined with interoceptive exposure, is more effective. There is some suggestion that this be called panic-control therapy, and it has now been shown to be effective in other sites beyond the Barlow group responsible for its initial development. In an 8-week comparison with waiting-list controls, 85 per cent of the panic-control therapy group were panic free compared with less than one-third of the waiting-list group. These improvements were maintained at 6 months' follow-up. Studies are now underway to see if the panic-control therapy can be shortened to 10 h or as little as 4 h, and these have been promising.

There is the suggestion from several studies that the panic-control therapy or cognitive-behavioural therapy may in fact be more effective than medication, although this remains controversial.

The most carefully performed trial was a multicentre 11-week acute trial with a 6-month follow-up for responders and a 6-month follow-up after discontinuation of treatment.[96] This trial compared imipramine with cognitive-behavioural therapy, their combination, and placebo. All the active treatment cells were approximately equal at the end of the acute trial and significantly greater than placebo on most measures. This was also true at the 6-month follow-up. Interestingly, responders to imipramine had a more robust response than responders to cognitive-behavioural therapy alone. The combination of imipramine plus cognitive-behavioural therapy was not significantly better than either treatment alone, although there was a trend suggesting greater improvement. Significantly, at follow-up 6 months after ending treatment, significantly more imipramine patients had experienced relapse. This study is consistent with the general findings in the field that imipramine's effects tend to wear off in a small group of responders (probably 20–30 per cent). This trial provided evidence that cognitive-behavioural therapy applied early in treatment did not offer protective effects against imipramine relapse. However, some data suggest that it is protective if given during the discontinuation period.

Continuation/maintenance treatments

There are now a series of studies utilizing antidepressants or benzodiazepines as maintenance treatment for 6 and 12 months for panic disorder and agoraphobia. In each trial to date, treatment gains from acute treatment are almost always maintained, and generally are extended while the medication is continued. After treatment with clomipramine for 6 months, 93 per cent of patients became panic free, compared with 60 per cent on placebo. In a 12-month trial comparing clomipramine and placebo, the clomipramine group continued to improve and tolerated the medication well. On various outcome measures, there was 82 to 100 per cent improvement. Placebo patients who were switched to active medication matched the good responses of the clomipramine group.

In one of the earliest trials, clonazepam was continued for a year in 20 patients and 18 had a positive response at a mean dose of 2.3 ± 1.6 mg/day. In a 6-month continuation study of alprazolam patients following an 8-week initial trial, the group maintained their efficacy with a dose at the end of the 8-week trial of 5.1 ± 2.3 mg/day. This decreased to 4.7 ± 2.1 mg/day at week 32 and subsequent follow-up 1 to 2 years later found most patients' doses had drifted down to 1 to 2 mg/day.

In the large follow-up to the Phase II Cross-National Panic Trial, there was a 32-week double blind comparison of alprazolam, imipramine, and placebo in 181 patients. Again, efficacy was maintained in both medications with no escalation of dose. Patients on both active treatments generally extended their improvement, although the placebo patients tended to lose some efficacy and certainly had a higher drop-out rate. The most recent long-term extension continued paroxetine, clomipramine, and placebo in 176 patients following an acute trial.[77] During the 1-year extension, both the paroxetine and clomipramine patients continued to improve and, similar to the previous trial mentioned, placebo patients tended to lose some of their initial response.

As evidence has accumulated of the high relapse rate with discontinuation of effective medication treatments for panic disorder, longer-term treatment, generally 6 to 18 months, has become routine.[68,97] Although not well documented, perhaps one of the more important issues is that it appears that patients not only continue to improve for the first 6 months but that improvement continues to be extended the longer patients are on treatment, perhaps even throughout the first 2 years of treatment.[68]

Prevention of recurrence

Available evidence remains inconclusive about the percentage of patients who will relapse if effective pharmacotherapy of panic disorder is discontinued. However, early estimates suggested that most patients relapse. It remained the prevailing opinion that 35 to 85 per cent of patients relapse after antidepressants or benzodiazepines were discontinued. However, one trial reported almost no relapse after discontinuation of clomipramine patients, perhaps because they used a gradual taper. There is certainly a strong suggestion that rapid taper of benzodiazepines produces significant withdrawal symptoms which probably stimulates relapse.

The early trial by Zitrin et al. reported only 26 per cent relapse.[98] In a modern trial comparing imipramine and cognitive-behavioural therapy, the imipramine relapse rate was 40 per cent.[99] One of the most carefully performed relapse prevention trials followed the fixed-dose study of paroxetine described above. After acute treatment, patients were re-randomized in double-blind fashion to receive either paroxetine at their prior dose, or to placebo for an additional 3 months of treatment. Interestingly, only 30 per cent of the patients randomized to placebo relapsed, compared with 5 per cent relapse if paroxetine was continued.[77] The relapse in the placebo patients occurred over each of the initial 4 weeks after discontinuation. In the large multicentre trial recently completed, patients were also carefully discontinued and followed up. Again of interest, the relapse rate appeared comparable to that of the paroxetine study. Although these studies certainly need replication, it suggests that the relapse rate may be lower than previously estimated if patients are slowly tapered and carefully followed.

There is one small study that suggests that the relapse rate is lower if treatment is longer. Mavissikalian followed a small group of patients who responded to imipramine, discontinuing some after 6 months of treatment and the other group after 18 months of treatment.[100] In these patients, there was an 80 per cent relapse rate in the 6-month treatment group, but only 20 per cent in the 18-month treatment group. This suggestive finding is consistent with clinical experience but certainly needs replication; however, it is certainly supportive of the general recommendation of continued treatment for 12 to 18 months if effective.

Management

The suggestions for management in this section are based on evidence of the empirically based treatments in panic disorder and agoraphobia, much of which has been reviewed above. However, as in treatment of all patients, there are suggestions that also involve the 'art' of treating these patients which have evolved, but have not been empirically studied or confirmed.

Management of the uncomplicated patient

As reviewed above, it appears clear that the average patient with panic disorder can be treated with multiple medications or exposure-based and/or cognitive-behavioural treatments designed for panic disorder with approximately equal efficacy. Patients also present for treatment often with clear ideas how they wish to be treated or believe they will be better treated. There are some people who have strong feelings or prejudices for or against both medication and cognitive-behavioural

treatments. Given that situation, as well as the lack of any clear reason to choose one treatment over the other, ethical practice would dictate offering patients a choice of treatment. There is also some evidence that patients will respond better to the treatment they 'believe in'. Unfortunately, the two types of treatments are not equally available in all settings or all countries. Psychiatrists tend to use medication treatment with education, exposure, and cognitive-based work of a less systematic nature than psychologists and other non-physician caregivers. Although many behaviourally and cognitively oriented psychologists do affiliate with psychiatrists and other physicians to provide medications, for many this ease of combination treatment is not readily available.

As mentioned, most psychiatrists utilize one of the medications mentioned above, supplemented by clear educational efforts with the patient and pertinent family members. This generally includes use of some written material which the patient and spouse read and discuss with the psychiatrist. Education is also a critical part of the initial treatment of patients in exposure-based treatments and cognitive-behavioural therapy. These educational efforts are almost always very helpful and in the more mildly symptomatic patients may suffice for treatment.

For the patient who will be prescribed medication, it is most reasonable to offer a discussion of which medications might be appropriate, and the pros and cons of each. As outlined in Table 4, each medication is different, and depending upon the individual patient's needs and previous experience any of the four classes of medications might be appropriate. As mentioned, current opinion would suggest that the medication of first choice at this point in time, if possible, would be an SSRI. We have the most experience with paroxetine, fluvoxamine, citalopram, and sertraline, although fluoxetine appears to be effective as well. In a recent meta-analysis of all the effective medications utilized in the treatment of panic disorder, the SSRIs were shown to be more effective than the other classes.[101] Coupled with their greater tolerability, lack of weight gain, and safety in overdose, they would appear to be the logical first choice if available.

For clinical and other practical issues, all patients should be told initially that whatever medication is the initial treatment, there are multiple other effective medications. It is important to emphasize that there is little way of knowing which specific medication is most appropriate for which patients and that the initial choice may not be effective, but subsequent choices could very well be effective.

There are few data to direct the choice of the medications beyond those favouring the SSRIs mentioned above. There is only one trial documenting a difference in patient type leading to a choice of medication. In the large cross-national comparison of imipramine, alprazolam, and placebo, patients with predominantly respiratory symptoms responded better to imipramine.[102] Similarly, patients with a predominantly cardiovascular symptom picture responded better to alprazolam than imipramine. Otherwise, there are no data suggesting a particular medication for a specific patient beyond the various advantages and disadvantages listed in Table 4.

Once medication is chosen, it is prudent to begin at the lowest dose possible. This would include utilizing paroxetine 10 mg/day, imipramine 10 mg/day, sertraline 25 mg/day, fluoxetine 2.5 to 5 mg/day, etc. This beginning low dose also extends to the benzodiazepines but is less critical since they are not associated with an initial hyperstimulation reaction. This is one of the reasons why benzodiazepines are easier to utilize and often more popular with patients who somehow realize that from previous experience or feedback from other patients that they are not associated with the initial worsening of symptoms.

At a practical level, management of the worries about the initial hyperstimulation reaction is one of the most important issues in the psychopharmacological management of panic disorder patients. If handled incorrectly, this issue can lead to a drop-out rate that reaches 25 to 50 per cent. With proper reassurance and close follow-up of patients, this drop-out rate can be reduced to almost zero. Patients need to be told that hyperstimulation can occur in up one-third of patients but is transient and not dangerous. Because of the inherent anxiety and even phobia about taking medications, this reassurance is not usually sufficient and patients need to be invited to contact the treating physician with any anxiety or questions they might have about taking medications with a quick response to their concerns.

After initial tolerance of medication is established, the dose can be slowly raised over several weeks to a target level. Obviously, if a patient does not show a response at lower doses, the medication should be raised to maximum doses.

It is important for the patient and physician alike to keep in mind that effectiveness of medications often requires a significant amount of time. The antidepressants as a class routinely take 2 to 6 weeks and with certain medications and patients as much as 6 to 12 weeks before significant effectiveness is established. This is less an issue with benzodiazepines, where initial effectiveness is generally seen in the first week or two, but there too the appropriate doses must be obtained, which often takes several weeks. Higher doses of all medicines are needed to reduce agoraphobic avoidance.

As mentioned, if agoraphobic patients do not gradually re-expose themselves to situations they fear, their avoidance fears will not be decreased. This exposure to their actual phobic situations can be accomplished in many ways. Some patients are capable of gradually re-exposing themselves after they understand the principles of exposure and the need to remain in the situation until their fears diminish. They may need help in establishing a hierarchy of their fears, and although it is not necessary that they in fact do work up the hierarchy in a gradually increasing fashion from 'least feared' to 'most feared', it is often easier for most patients to conceptualize and accomplish it in this fashion.

Many therapists develop a hierarchical list and then monitor the patient's progress on a regular basis. There is evidence that the exposure must be regular, and extensive, often on a daily basis. Also, encouragement from the therapist and partner have both been shown to be important. Some patients can re-enter their phobic situations better if supported by their partner, or other phobics from a support group. If they are particularly afraid, an *in vivo* therapist (often recovered phobics) can be very helpful. The critical issues appear to be approaching their fears in a consistent systematic basis in the real phobic situations accompanied by encouragement and support.

In a similar fashion, many psychiatrists combine principles of cognitive-behavioural therapy without embarking on a formal cognitive-behavioural therapy programme. As mentioned, cognitive-behavioural therapy routinely initially involves education about the illness and its treatments. Other elements of identification and challenge of catastrophic thinking are widely applied by psychiatrists, but in a less systematic fashion than in formal cognitive-behavioural therapy protocols.

It is important that from the beginning that most patients be told that if treatment is effective, the expectation is to continue the medi-cation it for 12 to 18 months. An important issue to negotiate with the patient is how, when, and if effective pharmacotherapy should be tapered and discontinued.[103] Most evidence and experience suggests that patients be continued long enough to receive maximum benefit from medication treatment. In that context, patients should have experienced symptomatic and functional recovery to a maximum extent possible before discontinuation is considered. Patients should have regained a sense of confidence and control of their symptoms and lives. This might be conceptualized as a 'period of normal living' after attainment of symptomatic control before consideration is given to discontinuing an effective treatment. Because the principal danger of discontinuation is relapse, the time should be carefully chosen. This should be a time when potential disruption from discontinuation symptoms and/or relapse would be least problematic.

There are strong suggestions in the literature, some of which is reviewed above, that all medications, and certainly the benzodiazepines, should be tapered very slowly, probably over 2 to 6 months if possible. This is both to minimize frightening withdrawal symptoms and to observe for relapse symptoms as medications are slowly tapered.

The strongest reasons for discontinuing effective pharmacotherapy are the problematic side-effects and expense. Because this is a syndrome frequently seen in young women, the most important reason is the wish to conceive a child or onset of pregnancy. Certainly, routine practice is to try to taper and discontinue all medications during pregnancy, but sometimes this is not possible. There are now a series of women who have delivered normal children after having tried unsuccessfully to discontinue medication during pregnancy.

Many patients want to manage their own symptoms without the use of medications, and this is also a reasonable reason to taper and discontinue medications, if strongly felt by the patient. The therapist should explore, however, unreasonable prejudices against the use of medications stimulated by reading, television shows, relatives, or even well-meaning physicians. Most in the field now believe that panic disorder and agoraphobia are conditions similar to hypertension and diabetes in the sense that patients do not like the thought that they are ill and resist compliance with medication treatment. However, treatment is beneficial and not harmful, and patients often need encouragement and education in order to agree to a programme where they continue medications rather than press to discontinue them.

If medications are discontinued, the patient should be followed closely, at least by telephone, for difficulties that could include withdrawal symptoms, especially with benzodiazepines, or incipient relapse. If relapse does occur, evidence suggests that patients will respond to reinstitution of the same medication treatment regimen. If symptoms and/or functional disability associated with relapse are problematic, patients should be offered retreatment with the same medication or offered other effective non-medication treatments.

Psychological treatments

Management of patients with predominantly psychological treatments also begins with the use of educational materials, as is frequently the case with medication treatment of panic disorder. Almost all psychological treatments involve some sort of exposure-based treatment. In some, this is the predominant modality with considerable variation on how exposure to feared situations is accomplished. Although some initial exposure therapy in particularly frightened patients may be accomplished in imagination prior to *in vivo* exposure, most exposure treatments are usually attempted *in vivo* from the outset. Most treatments have been shown to be effective if they involve *in vivo* exposure according to therapist's inclinations, available resources, and patient preferences. Gradual exposure is the norm, although some programmes use very rapid exposures often called 'flooding', which involves exposure to multiple phobic situations rapidly over several days. Most programmes involve therapist-assisted exposure, sometimes utilizing professional *in vivo* therapists or volunteers who accompany phobics into their feared situations. Partners of patients are often enlisted as assistants and there is some evidence that this more effective than non-partner exposure aides.

Most exposure-based treatments involve frequent, often daily practices involving several hours. Often the critical issue is adequate support of the patient to accomplish this much exposure 'homework', as well as encouragement and praise.

Almost anything that can help the patient accomplish the actual exposure appears to be useful and helpful. For instance, manuals and computer programs, as well as telephone-based supervision and encouragement have been shown to be effective. Although many therapists utilize relaxation techniques, applied relaxation has been the most widely utilized and effective. Many therapists employ breathing retraining, encouraging people who hyperventilate to slow their breathing by utilizing their diaphragm. Although both have been shown to be effective and are widely utilized, other studies suggest they may not be essential components of treatment, and their use does vary.

Cognitive-based treatments involving education, breathing retraining, and applied relaxation primarily involve a systematic programme of cognitive restructuring and interoceptive exposure.[95] Cognitive restructuring involves the patient and therapist identifying the so-called 'automatic thoughts' they have with and after each panic attack. These are the misinterpretations that patients make about what these symptoms mean. For instance, the patient and therapist together identify that these symptoms often trigger thoughts that they are very ill, having a heart attack, or perhaps even dying. Over several sessions, these are identified and it is made clear to the patient the power these thoughts have to frighten them. At that point a number of strategies can be tried to try to correct these cognitions. Some studies involve attempts to compute the actual probability of the catastrophic consequences that patients fear. Others involve 'decatastrophizing' in which the ultimate consequences that patients fear are exposed, and generally can then be disavowed by the patient as extremely unrealistic. Patients can be taught to correct these thoughts or substitute more positive statements in their place. These skills are then worked on as 'homework', including actual exposure in which negative thoughts are identified and challenged *in vivo*.

The other usual aspect of cognitive-behavioural therapy for panic disorder is interoceptive exposure, in which physical symptoms that frighten patients are identified and then they are taught to habituate to those symptoms and challenge the negative cognitions that arise with them. For instance, if the patients are afraid of dizzy feelings, they can be spun in a chair and learn to handle those feelings. If they have fears of fast heart beat, they can undergo normal exercise and then habituate to the tachycardia, challenging the negative cognitions that arise.

Both exposure-based treatments and cognitive-behavioural therapy often are delivered in an 8- to 16-week treatment format, with varying frequencies of follow-up. Many attempts are underway to shorten these treatments and make them more efficient, most of which have been effective. It may be that effective treatment can be delivered with 3 to 4 h of therapy involvement with various self-help supplements to that treatment.

Treatment of comorbid patients

Treatment of the panic disorder patient comorbid with substance abuse is probably the most difficult challenge. In general, the substance abuse problem tends to be predominant even if it were temporally secondary to panic disorder symptoms. Therefore, treatment of substance abuse generally has to be initiated and completed first, although as soon as possible treatment of panic disorder needs be initiated.

Treatment of comorbid social phobia, obsessive–compulsive disorder, or GAD has recently been made somewhat simpler with the demonstration that the SSRIs are effective in these other conditions as well. Although not yet empirically demonstrated, it is reasonable to expect that an SSRI would effectively treat the panic disorder as well as the other comorbid anxiety disorders. This is an important area for future research. Behavioural treatments specific to obsessive–compulsive disorder and to social phobia may well be needed in addition to medication treatment.

The most common comorbidity is with depression and again one of the advantages of antidepressants is probable dual treatment of panic disorder and depression. Perhaps the most important management issue is recognition that comorbid depression carries with it a marked increase in suicide risk which needs to be a part of the psychiatric management of comorbid depressed patients. As mentioned, there is some evidence that depressed panic disorder patients respond better to an MAOIs, and this should be considered.

Resistance to treatment

There are relatively few systematic data about treatment options for patients resistant to initial medication or to exposure- or cognitive-behavioural-based treatments. Generally, however, most patients can be tried on another medication, often with success. If they are on medicine and have not tried exposure or cognitive-behavioural therapy, that should definitely be added. The converse is also true. Non-response can often be traced to inadequate doses or blood levels of the medication or an inaccurate length of trial. Comorbid psychiatric and particularly comorbid medical conditions need to be ruled out. Apparent resistance is often related to concomitant personality disorders or failure of agoraphobics to actually attempt exposure treatments. True resistance to one medication is sometimes overcome by a switch to another medication or to two medications at a time. If the combination of an antidepressant and benzodiazepine has not been tried, that is often the first attempted combination. In highly resistant patients, sometimes a combination of tricyclic and SSRI antidepressants are indicated.

Ethical issues

The principal ethical issues concern the availability of treatment. Because the two types of effective treatments (medications and exposure or cognitive-behavioural therapy) are not widely or equally distributed in all practices or locations, sometimes caregivers face a difficult ethical choice of having only one type of treatment available.

In these instances, patients should be informed of the limitations and participate in the choices made.

Most of the treatment experience and certainly the empirical evidence has been in Caucasian patients. We do know that symptoms are different across ethnic groups and that response is often less positive in non-Caucasian groups. Treatments need to be tested and developed for all ethnic and national groups as part of the ethical development of the field.

Possibilities for prevention

The best evidence now suggests that panic disorder is often preceded by an anxiety pattern in childhood. In Kagan's model of behaviourally inhibited children, there is certainly a tendency for the pattern to persist throughout life, but some children appear to lose this trait along their development. This may well be related to parental child-rearing practices in which children are encouraged to face issues they fear rather than be withdrawn and fearful. Research is needed to explore whether different parental rearing practices or educational efforts with these children can reduce later development of anxiety disorders. If so, these efforts at the public health and school level need to developed.

The other major aetiological consideration for panic disorder and agoraphobia has been the evidence of negative traumatic events occurring in the childhood of adults with panic disorder. Preventative efforts need to be aimed at these issues through public education and education of caregivers of children. Also, one of the intervention goals in helping a traumatized child should be to prevent future development of anxiety disorders and other problems.

References

1. Hippocrates (1870). *On epidemics V.* Section 82 (translated by S. Farrar). Cadel, London.
2. Benedikt, M. (1870). Uber Platzschwindel. *Allgemeine Wiener Medizinische Zeitung,* **15,** 488.
3. Klein, D.F. (1964). Delineation of two drug responsive anxiety syndromes. *Psychopharmacology,* **5,** 397–408.
4. Marks, I.M. (1969). *Fears and phobias.* Heinemann, London.
5. Klerman, G.L., Weissman, M., Ovellete, R., Johnson, J., and Greenwald, S. (1991). Panic attacks in the community: social morbidity and health care utilization. *Journal of the American Medical Association,* **265,** 742–6.
6. Markowitz, J., Weissman, M.M., Ovellette, R., and Liek, J. (1989). Quality of life in panic disorder. *Archives of General Psychiatry,* **46,** 984–92.
7. Noyes, R., Jr. and Barloon, T.J. (1997). Charles Darwin and panic disorder. *Journal of the American Medical Association,* **277,** 138–41.
8. Ballenger, J.C., Burrows, G.D., Dupont, R.L., *et al.* (1988). Aprazolam in panic disorder and agoraphobia: results from a multicenter trial. I. Efficacy in short-term treatment. *Archives of General Psychiatry,* **455,** 413–22.
9. Burns, L.E. and Thorpe, G.L. (1977). The epidemiology of fears and phobias with particular reference to the national survey of agoraphobics. *Journal of International Medical Research,* **5,** 1–7.
10. Goldstein, A.J. and Chambless, D.L. (1978). A reanalysis of agoraphobia. *Behavioral Therapy,* **9,** 47–59.
11. Thorpe, G.L. and Burns, L.E. (1983). *The agoraphobic syndrome.* Wiley, New York.
12. Beitman, B.D., Kushner, M.G., Lamerti, J.W., and Mukerji, V. (1990). Panic disorder without fear in patients with angiographically normal coronary arteries. *Journal of Nervous and Mental Disease,* **178,** 307–12.
13. Eaton, W.W. and Garrison, R. (1992). Mental health in Mariel Cubans and Haitian boat people. *International Migration Review,* **26,** 1395–1415.
14. Westphal, C. (1872). Agoraphobie, eine neuropahtische Erscheinung. *Archiv für Psychiatrie und Nervenkrankheiten,* **3,** 138–61.
15. Breuer, J. and Freud, S. (1895). *Studien uber Hysterie.* Franz Deuticke, Leipzig. English translation (1961) in *The standard edition of the complete works of Sigmund Freud,* Vol. 2 (ed. J. Strachey), p. 125. Hogarth Press, London.
16. Feighner, J.P., Robins, E., Guze, S.B., Woodruff, R.A., Winokur, G., and Munroz, R. (1972). Diagnostic criteria for use in psychiatric research. *Archives of General Psychiatry,* **38,** 57–63.
17. Klein, D.F. (1964). Delineation of two drug responsive anxiety syndromes. *Psychopharmacology,* **5,** 397–408.
18. Ballenger, J.C. and Fyer, A.J. (1993). Examining criteria for panic disorder. *Hospital and Community Psychiatry,* **44,** 226–8.
19. Cross-National Collaborative Panic Study Second Phase Investigators (1992). Drug treatment of panic disorder. Comparative efficacy of alprazolam, imipramine and placebo. *British Journal of Psychiatry,* **160,** 191–202.
20. Weissman, M.M. (1990). Epidemiology of panic disorder and agoraphobia. In *Frontiers of clinical neuroscience.* Vol. 9, *Clinical aspects of panic disorder* (ed. J.C. Ballenger *et al.*), pp. 57–65. Wiley–Liss, New York.
21. Weissman, M.M., Bland, R.C., Canino, G.J., *et al.* (1997). The cross-national epidemiology of panic disorder. *Archives of General Psychiatry,* **54,** 305–9.
22. Lépine, J.P., Wittchen, H.U., Essau, C.A., and participants of the WHO-ADAMHA CIDI Field Trials (1993). Lifetime and current comorbidity of anxiety and affective disorders: results from the International WHO-ADAMHA CIDI Field Trials. *International Journal of Methods in Psychiatric Research,* **3,** 67–77.
23. Chen, Y.W. and Dilsaver, S.C. (1995). Comorbidity of panic disorder in bipolar illness: evidence from the epidemiologic catchment area survey. *American Journal of Psychiatry,* **152,** 280–2.
24. Regier, D.A., Boyd, J.H., Burke, J.D., *et al.* (1988). One-month prevalence of panic disorders in the United States: based on five Epidemiological Catchment Area sites. *Archives of General Psychiatry,* **45,** 977–86.
25. Lydiard, R.B. and Brady, K. (1993). Association of anxiety and alcoholism. *Psychiatric Quarterly,* **64** (2), 135–49.
26. Weissman, M.M., Klerman, G.L., Markowitz, J.S., *et al.* (1989). Suicidal ideation and suicide attempts in panic disorder and attacks. *New England Journal of Medicine,* **321,** 1209–14.
27. Johnson, J., Weissman, M.M., and Klerman, G.L. (1990). Panic disorder, comorbidity, and suicide attempts. *Archives of General Psychiatry,* **47,** 805–8.
28. Lépine, J.P., Chignon, J.M., and Teherani, M. (1991). Suicidal behavior and onset of panic disorder. *Archives of General Psychiatry,* **48,** 668–9.
29. Lesser, I.M., Rubin, R.T., Pecknold, J.C., *et al.* (1988). Secondary depression in panic disorder and agoraphobia. *Archives of General Psychiatry,* **45,** 437–43.
30. Gorman, J.M., Fyer, M.R., Goetz, R., *et al.* (1988). Ventilatory physiology of patients with panic disorder. *Archives of General Psychiatry,* **45,** 31–9.
31. Sartorius, N., Uestuen, B., Costa e Silva, J.A., *et al.* (1993). An international study of psychological problems in primary care: preliminary report from the World Health Organization Collaborative Project on Psychological Problems in General Health Care. *Archives of General Psychiatry,* **50,** 819–24.
32. Ballenger, J.C. (1998). Treatment of panic disorder in the general medical setting (editorial). *Journal of Psychosomatic Research,* **44,** 5–15.
33. Kroenke, K. and Mangelsdorff, A.D. (1989). Common symptoms in ambulatory care: incidence, evaluation, therapy and outcome. *American Journal of Medicine,* **86,** 262–6.
34. Simon, G.E. and Von Korff, M. (1991). Somatization and psychiatric

disorder in the Epidemiologic Catchment Area study. *American Journal of Psychiatry*, **148**, 1494–500.

35. Katon, W. (1984). Panic disorder and somatization. Review of 55 cases. *American Journal of Medicine*, **77**, 101–8.

36. Ballenger, J.C. (1998). Panic disorder in primary care and general medicine. In *Panic disorder and its treatment* (ed. J. Rosenbaum and M. Pollack), pp. 1–36. Dekker, New York.

37. Lécrubier, Y. and Usten, T.B. (1998). Panic and depression: a worldwide primary care perspective. *International Journal of Clinical Psychopharmacology*, **13** (Supplement 4), S7–11.

38. Ballenger, J.C. (1998). Comorbidity of panic and depression: implications for clinical management. *International Journal of Clinical Psychopharmacology*, **13** (Supplement 4), S13–17.

39. Eaton, W.W., Drymon, A., and Weissman, M.M. (1991). Panic and phobias. In *Psychiatric disorders in America: the Epidemiologic Catchment Area Study* (ed. L.N. Robins and D.A. Regier), pp. 155–79. Free Press, New York.

40. Eaton, W.W., Kessler, R.C., Wittchen, H.U., and Magee, W.J. (1994). Panic and panic disorder in the United States. *American Journal of Psychiatry*, **151**, 413–20.

41. Von Korff, M.R., Eaton, W.W., and Keyel, P.M. (1985). The epidemiology of panic attacks and panic disorder. *American Journal of Epidemiology*, **122**, 970–81.

42. Faravelli, C., Webb, T., Ambonetti, A., Fonnescu, F., and Sessarego, A. (1985). Prevalence of traumatic early life events in 31 agoraphobic patients with panic attacks. *American Journal of Psychiatry*, **142**, 1493–4.

43. Harris, E.L., Noyes, R., Jr., Crowe, R.R., and Chaudhry, D.R. (1983). Family study of agoraphobia: report of a pilot study. *Archives of General Psychiatry*, **40**, 1061–4.

44. Torgersen, S. (1983). Genetic factors in anxiety disorders. *Archives of General Psychiatry*, **40**, 1085–90.

45. Skre, I., Onstad, S., Torgersen, S., *et al.* (1993). A twin study of DSM-III-R anxiety disorders. *Acta Psychiatrica Scandinavica*, **88**, 85–92.

46. Andrews, G., Stewart, G., Allen, R., and Henderson, A.S. (1990). The genetics of six neurotic disorders: a twin study. *Journal of Affective Disorders*, **19**, 23–9.

47. Kendler, K.S., Neale, M.C., Kessler, R.C., *et al.* (1993). Panic disorder in women: a population-based twin study. *Psychological Medicine*, **40**, 397–406.

48. Crowe, R.R., Wang, Z., Noyes, R., Jr, *et al.* (1997). Candidate gene study of eight GABAa receptor subunits in panic disorder. *American Journal of Psychiatry*, **154**, 1096–100.

49. Pollack, M.H., Otto, M.W., Rosenbaum, J.F., *et al.* (1990). Longitudinal course of panic disorder: findings from the Massachussetts General Hospital Naturalistic Study. *Journal of Clinical Psychiatry*, **51**, 12–16.

50. Klein, R.G. (1995). Is panic disorder associated with childhood separation anxiety disorder? *Journal of Clinical Neuropharmacology*, **18** (Supplement), 7–14.

51. Kagan, J., Reznick, J.S., Clarke, C., and Snidman, N. (1984). Behavioral inhibition to the unfamiliar. *Child Development*, **55**, 2212–25.

52. Rosenbaum, J.F., Biederman, J., Gersten, M., *et al.* (1988). Behavioral inhibition in children of parents with panic disorder and agoraphobia: a controlled study. *Archives of General Psychiatry*, **45**, 463–70.

53. Turner, S.M., Beidel, D.C., and Costello, A. (1987). Psychopathology in the offspring of anxiety disorders patients. *Journal of Consulting and Clinical Psychology*, **55**, 229–35.

54. Lelliott, P., Marks, I., McNamee, G., and Tobeña, A. (1989). Onset of panic disorder with agoraphobia. Toward an integrated model. *Archives of General Psychiatry*, **46**, 1000–4.

55. Liebowitz, M.R. and Klein, D.F. (1991). Clinical psychiatric conferences: assessment and treatment of phobic anxiety. *Journal of Clinical Psychology*, **40**, 486–92.

56. Faravelli, C., Pallanti, S., Frassine, R., *et al.* (1988). Panic attacks with and without agoraphobia: a comparison. *Psychopathology*, **21**, 51–6.

57. Laraia, M.T., Stuart, G.W., Frye, L., Lydiard, R.B., and Ballenger, J.C. (1994). Childhood environment of women with panic disorder and agoraphobia. *Journal of Anxiety Disorders*, **8**, 1–17.

58. Saunders, B.E., Villeponteaux, L.A., Lipovsky, J.A., *et al.* (1992). Child sexual assault as a risk factor for mental disorders among women: a community survey. *Interpersonal Violence*, **7**, 189–204.

59. Nystrom, S. and Lyndegard, B. (1975). Predisposition for mental syndromes: a study comparing predisposition for depression, neurasthenia, and anxiety state. *Acta Psychiatrica Scandinavica*, **51**, 69–76.

60. Parker, G. (1981). Parental representations of patients with anxiety neurosis. *Acta Psychiatrica Scandinavica*, **63**, 33–6.

61. Nutt, D.J., Ballenger, J.C., and Lepine, J.P. (1999). Overview and future prospects. In *Panic disorder: clinical diagnosis, management and mechanisms* (ed. D.J. Nutt, J.C. Ballenger, and J.P. Lépine,), pp. 221–8. Dunitz, London.

62. Ballenger, J.C. (1990). Efficacy of benzodiazepines in panic disorder and agoraphobia. *Journal of Psychiatric Research*, **24**, 15–25.

63. Malizia, A.L., Cunningham, V.J., and Nutt, D.J. (1997). Flumazenil delivery changes in panic disorder at rest. *Neuroimage*, **5**, S302.

64. Kramer, M.S., Cutler, N.R., Ballenger, J.C., *et al.* (1995). A placebo-controlled trial of L365,260, a CCKB antagnoist, in panic disorder. *Journal of Biological Psychiatry*, **37**, 118–21.

65. Fontaine, R., Breton, G., Dery, R., *et al.* (1990). Temporal lobe abnormalities in panic disorder: an MRI study. *Journal of Biological Psychiatry*, **27**, 304–10.

66. Roy-Byrne, P.P., Cowley, D.S., Greenblatt, D.J., *et al.* (1990). Reduced benzodiazepine sensitivity in panic disorder. *Archives of General Psychiatry*, **47**, 259–72.

67. Roy-Byrne, P.P. and Cowley, D.S. (1995). Course and outcome in panic disorder. A review of recent follow-up studies. *Anxiety*, **1**, 151–60.

68. Mavissakalian, M.R. and Prien, R.F. (ed.) (1996). *Long-term treatments of anxiety disorders*. American Psychiatric Press, Washington, DC.

69. Faravelli, C. and Pallanti, S. (1986). Recent life events and panic disorder. *American Journal of Psychiatry*, **146**, 622–6.

70. Faravelli, C., Paterniti, S., and Scarpato, M.A. (1995). 5-year prospective, naturalistic follow-up study of panic disorder. *Journal of Comprehensive Psychiatry*, **36**, 271–7.

71. Katschnig, H., Amering, M.A., Stolk, J.M., *et al.* (1991). Long-term follow-up after a drug trial for panic disorder. *British Journal of Psychiatry*, **176**, 487–94.

72. Barlow, D.H., Craske, M.G., Cerny, J.A., and Klosko, J.S. (1989). Behavioral treatment of panic disorder. *Behavior Therapy*, **20**, 261–82.

73. O'Sullivan, G., Noshirvani, H., Marks, I., Monteiro, W., and Lelliott, P. (1991). Six-year follow-up after exposure and clomipramine therapy for obsessive compulsive disorder. *Journal of Clinical Psychiatry*, **52**, 150–5.

74. Marks, I.M. (1987). *Fears, phobias, and rituals*. Oxford University Press, New York.

75. Jobson, K.O. and Poter, W.Z. (1995). International Psychopharmacology Algorithim Project report. *Psychopharmacology Bulletin*, **31**, 457–507.

76. Ballenger, J.C., Davidson, J.R., Lécrubier, Y., *et al.* (1998). Consensus Statement on Panic Disorder from the International Consensus Group on Depression and Anxiety. *Journal of Clinical Psychiatry*, **59**, 47–54.

77. Ballenger, J. (1999). Selective serotonin reuptake inhibitors (SSRIs) in panic disorder. In *Panic disorder: clinical diagnosis, management and mechanisms* (ed. D. Nutt, J. Ballenger, and J.P. Lépine), pp. 159–78. Dunitz, London.

78. Gloger, S., Grunhaus, L., Gladic, D., *et al.* (1989). Panic attacks and agoraphobia: low dose clomipramine treatment. *Journal of Clinical Psychopharmacology*, **9**, 28–32.

79. Cassano, G.B., Petracci, A., Perugi, G., *et al.* (1998). Clomipramine for panic disorder: I. The first 10 weeks of a long-term comparison with imipramine. *Journal of Affective Disorders*, **14**, 123–7.

80. Modigh, L., Westberg, P., and Eriksson, E. (1992). Superiority of clomipramine over imipramine in the treatment of panic disorder: a placebo-controlled trial. *Journal of Clinical Psychopharmacology*, **51**, 53–8.

81. Burrows, G.D. and Norman, T.R. (1999). The treatment of panic disorder with benzodiazepines. In *Panic disorder: clinical diagnosis, management and mechanisms* (ed. D. Nutt, J. Ballenger, and J.P. Lépine), pp. 145–58. Dunitz, London.

82. Ballenger, J.C., Burrows, G., Dupont, R., *et al.* (1988). A multicenter comparison of alprazolam and placebo in short-term treatment of panic disorder and agoraphobia. *Acta Luso-Espanoles de Neurologia, Psiquiatria y Ciencias Afines*, **16**, 55–67.

83. Herman, J.B., Rosenbaum, J.F., and Brotman, A.W. (1987). The alprazolam to clonazepam switch for the treatment of panic disorder. *Journal of Clinical Psychopharmacology*, **7**, 175–8.

84. Cross-National Collaborative Panic Study (1993). Drug treatment of panic disorder: comparative efficacy of alprazolam, imipramine, and placebo. *British Journal of Psychiatry*, **160**, 191–202.

85. Noyes, R., Garvey, M.J., Cook, B., and Suelzer, M. (1991). Controlled discontinuation of benzodiazepine treatment for patients with panic disorder. *American Journal of Psychiatry*, **148**, 517–23.

86. Dupont, R.L., Swinson, R.P., Ballenger, J.C., *et al.* (1992). Discontinuation of alprazolam after long-term treatment of panic-related disorders. *Journal of Clinical Psychopharmacology*, **12**, 352–4.

87. Lydiard, R.B. and Ballenger, J.C. (1987). Antidepressants in panic disorder and agoraphobia. *Journal of Affective Disorders*, **13**, 153–68.

88. Rosenberg, R. (1999). Treatment of panic disorder with tricyclics and MAOIs. In *Panic disorder: clinical diagnosis, management and mechanisms* (ed. D. Nutt, J. Ballenger, and J.P. Lépine), pp. 125–44. Dunitz, London.

89. Ballenger, J.C., Lydiard, R.B., and Turner, S.M. (1997). Panic disorder and agoraphobia. In *Treatments of psychiatric disorders* (2nd edn) (ed. G.O. Gabbard), Vol. 2, pp. 1421–52. American Psychiatric Press, Washington, DC.

90. Roy-Byrne, P.F. and Cowley, D.S. (1995). Course and outcome in panic disorder: a review of recent follow-up studies. *Anxiety*, **1**, 151–60.

91. Keck, P.E., Taylor, V.E., Tugrul, K.C., *et al.* (1993). Valproate treatment of panic disorder and lactate-induced panic attacks. *Biological Psychiatry*, **33**, 542–6.

92. Milrod, B., Busch, F., Cooper, A., and Shapiro, T. (1997). *Manual of panic-focused psychodynamic psychotherapy.* American Psychiatric Press, Washington, DC.

93. Margraf, G., Barlow, D.H., Clark, D.M., and Telch, M.J. (1993). Psychological treatment of panic: work in progress in outcome, active ingredients, and follow-up. *Behaviour Research and Therapy*, **31**, 1–8.

94. Michelson, L.K., Marchione, K.E., Greenwald, M., *et al.* (1996). A comparative outcome and follow-up investigation of panic disorder with agoraphobia: the relative and combined efficacy of cognitive therapy, relaxation training, and therapist-assisted exposure. *Journal of Anxiety Disorders*, **10**, 297–330.

95. Barlow, D.H. and Craske, M.G. (1988). *Mastery of your anxiety and panic.* Center for Stress and Anxiety Disorders, State University of New York at Albany.

96. Barlow, D., Shear, K., Woods, S., and Gorman, J. (1998). A multicenter trial comparing cognitive behavior therapy, imipramine, their combination and placebo. Presented at the Annual Convention of the Anxiety Disorders Association of America, Boston, MA.

97. Ballenger, J.C. (1998). Benzodiazepines. In *Textbook of psychopharmacology* (2nd edn) (ed. A.F. Schatzberg and C.B. Nemeroff), pp. 271–86. American Psychiatric Press, Washington, DC.

98. Zitrin, C.M., Klein, D.F., Woerner, M.G., and Ross, D.C. (1983). Treatment of phobias. 1: Comparison of imipramine hydrochloride and placebo. *Archives of General Psychiatry*, **40**, 125–38.

99. Clark, D.M., Salkovskis, P.M., Hackmann, A., *et al.* (1994). A comparison of cognitive therapy, applied relaxation and imipramine in the treatment of panic disorder. *British Journal of Psychiatry*, **164**, 759–69.

100. Mavissakalian, M. (1990). Sequential combination of imipramine and behavioral instructions in the treatment of panic disorder with agoraphobia. *Archives of General Psychiatry*, **46**, 127–31.

101. Boyer, W. (1995). Serotonin uptake inhibitors are superior to imipramine and alprazolam in alleviating panic attacks: a meta-analysis. *International Clinical Psychopharmacology*, **10**, 45–9.

102. Briggs, A.C., Stretch, D.D., and Brandon, S. (1993). Subtyping of panic disorder by symptom profile. *British Journal of Psychiatry*, **163**, 201–9.

103. Ballenger, J.C. (1992). Medication discontinuation in panic disorder. *Journal of Clinical Psychiatry*, **53**, 26–31.

4.8 Obsessive–compulsive disorder

Iulian Iancu, Pinhas N. Dannon, and Joseph Zohar

Introduction

Obsessive–compulsive disorder (**OCD**) is a common, chronic, and disabling disorder marked by obsessions and/or compulsions that are egodystonic and cause significant distress to the patients and their families. During the last two decades, there has been a resurgence of studies into various aspects of OCD, including epidemiological, pathophysiological, and pharmacological investigations. Moreover, algorithms for the management of these patients have been proposed. The progress in our understanding of OCD is an example of the investment in studies on selective treatments, advanced methodologies of imaging studies (both before and after treatment), and the neurological aspects of OCD and OCD-related conditions, all of which reflect the development of psychiatry in recent years.

Up to the early 1980s, OCD was considered a treatment-refractory chronic condition of psychological origin. Dynamic psychotherapy was of little benefit and several pharmacological treatments were attempted without much success.[1] Since then, several researchers have reported that the prevalence of OCD is around 2 per cent in the general population.[2,3] In addition, numerous studies have reported on the efficacy of various serotonin reuptake inhibitors, and consequently an understanding of the biological basis of OCD has begun to unfold.

The observation that clomipramine, a tricyclic antidepressant with a serotonergic profile, is effective in treating symptoms of OCD[4,5] has increased interest in the relationship between serotonin and OCD. Substantial evidence currently suggests that OCD is almost unique among psychiatric disorders, as only serotonergic medications appear to be effective in this disorder.[6] For example, non-serotonergic drugs, such as desipramine, a potent antidepressant and antipanic agent, are entirely ineffective in OCD.[7–9] This specific response to serotonergic drugs has paved the way for further research on the role of serotonin in the pathogenesis of OCD in particular, and in OCD-related disorders in general.

Epidemiology

The lifetime prevalence of OCD in the general population is between 2 and 3 per cent, and therefore it is more prevalent than schizophrenia.[2,10] This rate has been confirmed across different cultures.[3] The prevalence of OCD among children and adolescents appears to be as high as among adults.[11] However, Nelson and Rice[12] and Stein *et al.*[13] have suggested that the diagnosis of OCD by the Diagnostic Interview Schedule administered by lay people leads to overdiagnosis, and so have proposed lower prevalence rates of 1 to 2 per cent.

Men and women are equally likely to be affected, although some reports have suggested a slight female predominance.[3] During adolescence, boys are more commonly affected than girls. The mean age of onset is about 20 years of age. Single people are more commonly affected, probably representing the difficulty for people with OCD to maintain a relationship.

Patients with OCD are commonly afflicted by other mental disorders; for instance, the lifetime prevalence for a major depressive episode in these patients is around 67 per cent.[3,14] Other common comorbid psychiatric diagnoses include alcohol-use disorders, social phobia, specific phobia, panic disorder, and eating disorders. The comorbidity with schizophrenia and with tic disorders raises interesting pathophysiological and therapeutic implications. The rate of tic disorders approaches 40 per cent in juvenile OCD, and there is an increase in the prevalence of Tourette's syndrome among the relatives of OCD patients.[15]

The relationship between OCD and obsessive–compulsive personality disorder (**OCPD**) has been a focus of debate. Although prospective research is lacking, it appears that OCPD is not a prominent risk factor for developing OCD, as the prevalence of OCPD among patients with OCD is not far from its prevalence in other psychiatric disorders.

Clinical features and diagnosis

The diagnosis of OCD according to DSM-IV criteria is based on the presence of either obsessions or compulsions, which cause marked distress, are time consuming (more than an hour per day), or significantly interfere with the person's normal routine and social and occupational activities. It stipulates that, at some point during the course of the disorder, but not necessarily during the current episode, the person has recognized that the obsessions or compulsions are excessive or unreasonable. However, if the patient does not recognize for most of the time during the current episode that the obsessions and compulsions are excessive or unreasonable, the diagnosis is OCD with poor insight.

If another Axis I disorder is present, it is mandatory that the content of the obsessions or compulsions is not restricted to it (e.g. a preoccupation with food or weight in eating disorders, or guilt feelings in the presence of a major depressive episode). The disturbance should not be due to the direct effects of a substance (e.g. a drug of abuse or a medication) or a general medical condition.

The obsessions are recurrent, intrusive, and distressing thoughts, images, or impulses, whereas the compulsions are repetitive, seemingly purposeful, behaviours that a person feels driven to perform. Obsessions are usually unpleasant and increase a person's anxiety, whereas carrying out compulsions reduces anxiety. Resistance to carrying out a compulsion results in increased anxiety. The patient usually realizes that the obsessions are irrational and experiences both the obsession and the compulsion as egodystonic.

Patients with both obsessions and compulsions constitute at least 75 per cent of the affected patients, with most patients presenting with multiple obsessions and compulsions. The symptoms may shift, so that a patient who had washing rituals during childhood may present with checking rituals as an adult.

OCD can express itself in many different symptoms, but the classical presentations include washing and checking. Recent dimensional approaches have been used to analyse these characteristic subtypes, and present the different symptoms in an innovative way.

The most common pattern is an obsession with dirt or germs, followed by washing or avoiding presumably contaminated objects (doorknobs, electrical switches, newspapers, people's hands, telephones). The feared object is hard to avoid (e.g. faeces, urine, dust, or germs). Patients wash their hands excessively and sometimes avoid leaving home because of their fear of germs. A second common pattern is an obsession of doubt, followed by a compulsion of checking. The person checks whether the oven is turned off or the front and back doors are closed—the checking may involve many trips back home to check the oven. Instead of resolving uncertainty, the checking often contributes to even greater doubt, which leads to further checking. The patients exhibit obsessional self-doubt, and feel guilty for having forgotten or committed some action (for instance, a fear of hurting someone while driving, leading to driving back over the same spot again and again).

Another pattern involves intrusive obsessional thoughts without a compulsion. Such obsessions are usually repetitious thoughts of some sexual or aggressive act that is reprehensible to the patient. Still another pattern is the need for symmetry or precision, which leads to a compulsion of slowness. Patients can take hours to eat a meal or shave, in an attempt to do things 'just right'. Unlike other patients with OCD, these patients do not resist their symptoms. Other patterns include hoarding and religious obsessions.

The gap between the knowledge that the symptoms are irrational and the overwhelming urge to perform them (even after resisting and failing) contributes to the immense suffering associated with OCD.

OCD and schizophrenia

About 25 per cent of patients with chronic schizophrenia may also present with OCD symptoms (range 5 to 45 per cent);[16] 15 per cent of patients with schizophrenia may qualify for the diagnosis of OCD. As in OCD, the OCD symptoms in these patients will not necessarily surface unless specific questions are asked. Many patients with schizophrenia can distinguish the egodystonic, obsessive–compulsive symptoms, perceived as coming from within, from the egosyntonic delusions perceived as introduced from the outside. Follow-up studies demonstrate a diagnostic stability over the years, and it seems that the presence of OCD in schizophrenia predicts a poor prognosis.[16] Sev-

eral studies among patients with schizophrenia and OCD reported an improvement in OCD symptomatology after the addition of a specific anti-obsessive medication.[16]

The poor prognosis of patients with schizophrenia and OCD, preliminary data regarding their response to the unique combination of antipsychotic and anti-obsessive medications, along with the high prevalence of this presentation has led several researchers to suggest that a 'schizo-obsessive' category may be of value.

Differential diagnosis

Personal distress and functional impairment, which are required for the diagnosis, differentiate OCD from ordinary or mildly excessive worries, thoughts, and habits. The medical differential diagnosis includes tic disorders (especially Tourette's syndrome), temporal lobe epilepsy, trauma, and postencephalitic complications.

Psychiatric diagnoses that should be ruled out include schizophrenia, OCPD, phobias, and depressive disorders. OCD can usually be differentiated from schizophrenia by the absence of other schizophrenic symptoms, by the less bizarre nature of symptoms, and by the patients' insight into their disorder. Moreover, patients with OCD usually attempt to resist the obsessions. OCPD does not have the degree of functional impairment characteristic of OCD and it is egosyntonic.

Phobias are distinguished by the absence of a relationship between the obsessive thoughts and the compulsions. The fears in OCD usually involve harm to others rather than harm to oneself. In addition, in OCD, when patients are 'phobic' they are usually afraid of an unavoidable stimulus (for instance, viruses, germs, or dirt) as opposed to the classic phobic objects like tunnels, bridges, or crowds.

Major depressive disorder can sometimes be associated with obsessive ideas, but patients with OCD usually fail to meet all the criteria of the former. Other psychiatric diagnoses closely related to OCD are hypochondriasis, body dysmorphic disorder, and trichotillomania. These patients have repetitive worries or behaviours, but they are focal and dissimilar from the multiple obsessions/compulsions that patients with OCD usually manifest.

Course and prognosis

Many patients with OCD have a sudden onset of symptoms, usually after a stressful event such as pregnancy, a loss, or a sexual problem. Owing to the secretive nature of the disorder, there is often a delay of 5 to 10 years delay before patients come to psychiatric attention, although the delay may shorten due to increased public awareness to the disorder through articles, books, and movies. The course is usually long, but variable; some patients experience a fluctuating course, while others experience a chronic course.[17]

About 20 to 30 per cent of the patients show a significant improvement in their symptoms, and 40 to 50 per cent a moderate improvement. The remaining 20 to 40 per cent become chronic or their symptoms worsen.

Patients are prone to depression and sometimes even to suicide. A poor prognosis is indicated by yielding (rather than resisting) to compulsions, a childhood onset, bizarre compulsions, the need for hospitalization, a coexisting major depressive disorder, delusional beliefs, the presence of overvalued ideas (that is, some acceptance of the obsessions and compulsions), and the presence of personality disorder (especially schizotypal personality disorder). A good prognosis is indicated by good social and occupational adjustment, the presence of a precipitating event, and symptoms of an episodic nature.[17] The obsessional content does not seem to be related to the prognosis.

Aetiology

Neurotransmitters

Many clinical trials of various serotonergic drugs lend support to the hypothesis that a dysregulation of serotonin is involved in OCD. However, this does not necessarily reflect on pathogenesis. Abnormality of the serotonergic system, and particularly the hypersensitivity of postsynaptic 5-HT receptors, constitutes the leading hypothesis for the underlying pathophysiology of OCD.[7,18–31]

Clinical studies have assayed cerebrospinal levels of serotonin metabolites (e.g. 5-hydroxyindoleacetic acid (**5-HIAA**) a 5-HT metabolite that serves as an index of 5-HT turnover)[18,19] and affinities of imipramine binding sites on platelets (labelling with [³H]imipramine shows that it binds to serotonin reuptake sites),[20–23] although results have been inconsistent in patients with OCD. A study supporting the relationship between a decreased function of the serotonergic system and a positive response to selective serotonin reuptake inhibitors (**SSRIs**), demonstrated normalization of the number of platelet 5-HT transporters following treatment with different SSRIs.[24] In an earlier study, patients who responded to clomipramine had higher pretreatment levels of 5-HIAA than the non-responders.[18] Moreover, the clinical improvement was positively correlated with a decrease in the concentration of 5-HIAA in cerebrospinal fluid.[18]

Another approach is to examine peripheral measures of serotonergic and noradrenergic function in patients with OCD. In one study, clinical improvement during clomipramine therapy closely correlated with pretreatment platelet serotonin concentration and monoamine oxidase activity, as well as with the decrease in both measures during clomipramine administration.[25] Moreover, only the plasma levels of clomipramine (a potent 5-HT reuptake inhibitor), but not the plasma levels of its primary metabolite, desmethyl clomipramine (which has noradrenergic properties), correlated significantly with an improvement in OCD symptoms. These findings suggest that the effects of anti-obsessive medications, clomipramine in this study, on serotonin function are pertinent to the anti-obsessional action observed.

Additional support for the importance of serotonin in the therapeutic response to serotonin reuptake inhibitors (**SRIs**) in OCD came from a study by Benkelfat et al.,[31] in which the investigators administered the serotonin receptor antagonist metergoline and placebo to 10 patients with OCD in a double-blind crossover study. Patients receiving clomipramine on a long-term basis responded with greater anxiety to a 4-day administration of metergoline when compared with the placebo phase of the study.

Additional evidence for disturbances of the serotonergic system in OCD was provided by challenge studies. Challenges with L-tryptophan,[26] m-chlorophenylpiperazine (mCPP),[7,27] sumatriptan (a 5-HT$_{1D}$ agonist[6]), ipsapirone (a 5-HT$_{1A}$ receptor ligand[28]), and MK-212 (a 5-HT$_{1A}$ and 5-HT$_{2C}$ agonist[29]), among others, were used to evaluate whether they worsen obsessive–compulsive symptoms or whether they elicit different physiological responses (thermal or neuroendocrine) in patients with OCD compared with controls. Only two compounds (m-chlorophenylpiperazine and sumatriptan) have

shown behavioural hypersensitivity and neuroendocrine hyposensitivity to be characteristic of the OCD challenge response. These studies may have the potential to pinpoint the receptor subtype involved in OCD, raising the possibility that 5-HT$_{1D}$ and 5-HT$_{2C}$ receptors, but not 5-HT$_{1A}$, could be involved in OCD.[30]

Dopamine

The most compelling evidence for dopaminergic involvement in OCD comes from the abundance of OCD symptoms in basal ganglia disorders, such as Tourette's syndrome, Sydenham's chorea, and postencephalitic parkinsonism. The therapeutic benefits obtained with the coadministration of dopamine blockers and SRIs in a subset of patients with OCD and tic disorders[32] has also suggested a role for dopamine dysfunction. A study evaluating levels of platelet sulphotransferase, an enzyme involved in the catabolism of catecholamines (providing a marker of presynaptic dopamine function), reported a decreased level of platelet [³H]imipramine binding and a parallel increase in the level of sulphotransferase activity in OCD compared with controls. This provides further support for the hypothesis of reduced 5-HT activity and increased dopamine transmission in OCD.[21]

Immune factors

Study of autoimmune factors has been prompted by the association of OCD and the autoimmune disease of the basal ganglia, Sydenham's chorea. This complication of rheumatic fever is accompanied by obsessive–compulsive symptoms in over 70 per cent of cases:[33] 10 out of 11 children had antibodies directed against the caudate.[33] These children had a history of obsessive–compulsive symptoms, which started prior to the onset of the chorea, reached a peak in line with the motor symptoms, and declined with their resolution. This is consistent with the hypothesis of basal ganglia dysfunction in OCD.

Antibodies against two peptides of the basal ganglia have also been found.[34] A strong connection was reported between OCD/Tourette's syndrome and the B-cell antibody D8/17, another antibrain antibody.[35] The specificity of these antibodies to OCD is as yet unclear. Cell-mediated immune-function alterations have been reported in OCD, but replication studies are still needed.

Brain imaging studies

The use of positron emission tomography has demonstrated the presence of increased activity (i.e. metabolism and blood flow) in the frontal lobes, the basal ganglia (especially the caudate nucleus), and the cingulum of patients with OCD.[36] Pharmacological and behavioural treatments reportedly reverse those abnormalities.[37] The data from functional imaging studies are consistent with the data from structural brain imaging studies. Both CT and magnetic resonance imaging studies have found decreased sizes of caudates bilaterally. Both functional and structural imaging procedures are also consistent with the observation that neurological procedures involving the cingulum are sometimes effective in the treatment of patients with OCD.

Overall, the brain imaging research suggests a role for the prefrontal cortex–basal ganglia thalamic circuitry. Dysfunction of these circuits can be explored by neuropsychological testing and recording evoked potentials. A recent study of patients with OCD showed that they are slower in performing tasks involving frontocortical systems, suggesting alterations at this level.[38] An evoked potential study showed enhanced processing negativity in the frontal cortex consistent with the prefrontal hyperactivity shown in brain imaging studies.[39]

Genetics

A significantly higher concordance rate was found for monozygotic twins than for dizygotic twins.[40] Of the first-degree relatives of patients with childhood-onset OCD, 35 per cent are also afflicted with the disorder.[41] Although this high rate is possibly related to the early-onset subtype, it nevertheless suggests a genetic component in OCD. Genetic research has yet to find abnormalities at the 5-HT transporter gene level. A recent study exploring the polymorphism of the promoter region of the gene for the 5-HT transporter failed to identify any differences between patients with OCD and controls.[42]

Other biological data

Sleep electroencephalography and neuroendocrine studies have found abnormalities similar to those seen in depression, such as decreased rapid eye movement latency, non-suppression on the dexamethasone suppression test, and decreased growth hormone secretion with clonidine infusions.[43,44]

Behavioural factors

According to the learning theory, obsessions are conditioned stimuli. When a relatively neutral stimulus is coupled with an anxiety-provoking stimulus, through conditioning it will produce anxiety even when presented alone. The compulsions reduce anxiety and the patient repeats them and learns them in order to avoid anxiety. Avoidance strategies are learned and become fixed.

Psychological factors

The dynamic aspects of OCD were first described by Sigmund Freud, who coined the term 'obsessional neurosis'. The disorder was thought to result from a regression from the Oedipal phase to the anal phase, with its characteristic ambivalence. The coexistence of hatred and love towards the same person leaves the patient paralysed with doubt and indecision. Freud originally suggested that obsessive symptoms result from unconscious impulses of an aggressive or sexual nature. These impulses cause extreme anxiety, which is avoided by the defence mechanisms. One of the striking features of patients with OCD is the degree to which they are preoccupied with aggression or cleanliness (anal phase), either overtly in the content of their symptoms or in the underlying associations.

Freud described three major psychological defence mechanisms that are important in OCD: isolation, undoing, and reaction formation. According to the psychoanalytical formulation, OCD develops when these defences fail to contain the anxiety. Isolation is the separation of the idea and the affect that it arouses, when the patient is only aware of the affectless idea. Undoing is a secondary defence to combat the impulse and quiet the anxiety that its imminent eruption into consciousness arouses. Undoing is a compulsive act, performed to prevent or undo the results that the patient irrationally anticipates from a frightening obsessional thought or impulse. Reaction formation is related to the production of character traits rather than symptom formation (characteristic of the above defences). The trait seems highly

exaggerated and inappropriate (i.e. the switch of anger and hate into exaggerated love and dedication).

Summary

The efficacy of the SRIs, together with the lack of efficacy of adrenergic antidepressants in OCD, have suggested that serotonin is involved in the pathophysiology of OCD. This relationship was validated by research on serotonergic markers in OCD and by the challenge paradigm.[6] Which type of serotonergic receptor is involved in the pathogenesis and/or the mechanism of action of anti-obsessional drugs, is still unclear. Further studies are crucial for elucidating the role of serotonin in the pathophysiology and management of OCD.

The pharmacological treatment of OCD

Since the early 1980s, several potent SRIs have been studied extensively in OCD. Aggregate statistics for all SRIs suggest that 70 per cent of treatment-naive patients will improve at least moderately.[45]

Efficacy of serotonergic versus adrenergic antidepressants

Whilst anecdotal reports have suggested that clinical benefit can be obtained with a range of antidepressant medications, consistent effectiveness has only been demonstrated for the SRIs. Several studies have directly compared clomipramine with other antidepressants and a consistent pattern emerges: antidepressant drugs that are less potent SRIs than clomipramine are generally ineffective in OCD.[7–9,18]

In the late 1960s, clomipramine was the first reported effective medication for OCD.[4,5] Since then, numerous placebo-controlled studies have clearly shown clomipramine's effectiveness, and this has been confirmed in a United States multicentre controlled trial ($n = 520$).[46] In this study, after 10 weeks of treatment, 58 per cent of patients treated with clomipramine rated themselves much or very much improved versus 3 per cent of placebo-treated patients.

Besides the SRI clomipramine, the newer non-tricyclic SSRIs, such as fluoxetine, fluvoxamine, paroxetine, sertraline, and citalopram are gaining acceptance as effective alternatives for the treatment of OCD in controlled studies.

Onset of treatment response

It has been suggested that a relatively long period, up to 8 or even 12 weeks, is needed before one can consider clomipramine (or other antiobsessive medication) to be ineffective. Several months' treatment is often needed to achieve a maximum response.

Long-term treatment

Most patients relapse after prematurely discontinuing treatment, but, as stated above, it may take many months for a maximum response to be seen. Pato et al.[47] reported that 16 out of 18 patients with OCD relapsed within 7 weeks after stopping clomipramine, although some had been treated for more than a year (mean, 10.7 months). All patients regained the therapeutic effects when clomipramine was reintroduced. Leonard et al.[9] examined the effect of clomipramine substitution during a long-term clomipramine treatment in 26 children and adolescents with OCD (mean duration of treatment was 17 months). Half the patients were blindly assigned to 2 months of desipramine treatment, and then clomipramine was reintroduced. Almost 90 per cent relapsed during the 2 months' substitution period compared with only 18 per cent of those kept on clomipramine throughout the study. Therefore, it seems advisable that patients with OCD should be maintained on anti-obsessive medications for more than a year before a very gradual attempt is made to discontinue the treatment.

The maintenance dose needed in OCD is also unclear. In a study that examined this issue, Mundo et al.[48] investigated the effect of dose reduction in 30 patients previously treated successfully with clomipramine or fluoxetine. Patients were randomized to receive the same drug dosage, to receive a reduced dose, or a very reduced dose. There was no difference between the groups during the 102 days of the study.

Drug dosage

Higher doses of SSRIs have been used in the treatment of OCD than in the treatment of depression, but empirical data supporting this practice are scant. However, two fixed-dose studies using fluoxetine and one pan-European study with paroxetine have found some advantage with using higher doses, while one fixed-dose study with sertraline has not.[6,30] Therefore it seems reasonable to use higher doses in non-responders or when only partial relief is attained.

Comparative studies of clomipramine versus SSRIs

The introduction of SSRIs has raised the question regarding the comparative efficacy of clomipramine versus that of the SSRIs. SSRIs are important alternatives to clomipramine, since their range of side-effects is clearly different (absence of anticholinergic side-effects, sedation, safety with overdose, etc.). Although SSRIs may provoke nausea, headaches, and sleep disturbances, these side-effects are usually less troublesome to most patients.

Fluoxetine was compared with clomipramine in 11 patients with OCD in a 10-week crossover study.[49] Although no significant differences were noted regarding clinical efficacy, the proportion of fluoxetine non-responders who later responded to clomipramine tended to be higher compared with the clomipramine non-responders who were switched to fluoxetine. However, patients reported significantly fewer side-effects while on fluoxetine. Freeman et al.[50] compared the efficacy of fluvoxamine and clomipramine in a multicentre randomized double-blind parallel-group comparison in 66 patients. Both drugs were equally effective and well tolerated, but fluvoxamine produced fewer anticholinergic side-effects and caused less sexual dysfunction than clomipramine, but more reports of headache and insomnia.

Paroxetine was of comparable efficacy to clomipramine and both were significantly more effective than placebo in a multinational double-blind placebo-controlled parallel-group study of 399 patients with OCD.[51] Bisserbe et al.[52] reported that sertraline (50–200 mg/day) was significantly more effective than clomipramine (50–200 mg/day) in a double-blind study ($n = 160$).

Other pharmacological approaches and neurosurgery

Considered as one of the anxiety disorders according to DSM-IV (but not according to the ICD-10), it is not surprising that anxiolytics have been suggested for the treatment of patients with OCD. Thus alprazo-

lam and clonazepam have been reported as efficient in several uncontrolled studies and case series, and even in a small double-blind randomized multiple crossover study. However, since OCD is a chronic disorder, the long-term use of anxiolytics raises questions of dependency.

Despite reports in open studies regarding the efficacy of trazodone, buspirone, and lithium, results from double-blind studies proved negative. Adding drugs that affect dopamine function, especially the atypical antipsychotics (risperidone), to SRI therapy in patients with treatment-resistant OCD, may result in improvement in patients with a personal or family history of tics.[53]

Neurosurgery has been reported to be effective in some patients with OCD, which involve procedures that disconnect the outflow pathways originating from the orbitofrontal cortex. Cingulotomy can help some intractable patients, but although the immediate results may be striking, the long-term prognosis is more reserved.[54]

Summary of drug treatment for OCD

The first-line treatment consists of either an SSRI or clomipramine. Any one of the five SSRIs in current use constitutes an effective and safe choice, but choosing which SSRI depends on the drug's pharmacokinetic profile, as well as the physician's familiarity with the drug. The dose should be higher than that used for treating depression (e.g. 40–60 mg of fluoxetine) and the trial should last at least 12 weeks. If clomipramine is chosen, cardiovascular problems and closed-angle glaucoma should first be ruled out. Doses of 200 to 300 mg of clomipramine are needed, but titration should last for 1 to 3 weeks and this dose should be continued for at least 12 weeks before determining a response.

If the patient cannot tolerate the first drug (an SSRI) or did not respond, a trial of a drug from the other group is advised (clomipramine and vice versa).

The third stage in non-responders, and in cases of only a partial response, includes small doses of antipsychotics (especially in Tourette's syndrome), a combination of SRIs and clomipramine, or the addition of lithium or trazodone, buspirone or tryptophan. The fourth stage consists of atypical neuroleptics, thyroid supplementation, clonidine, a monoamine oxidase inhibitor, intravenous clomipramine, or clonazepam. In resistant cases, electroconvulsive therapy or neurosurgery should be tried.

Psychological approaches

The effect of a psychodynamic approach in OCD is limited, whereas modern interventions like cognitive and behavioural therapy show promising results.[55] Behavioural therapy is as effective as pharmacotherapy in OCD,[55,56] and some data indicate that the beneficial effects of behavioural therapy are longer lasting.[57] About two-thirds of patients with moderately severe rituals can be expected to improve substantially, but not completely. A combination of behavioural therapy and pharmacotherapy may constitute the optimal treatment for OCD. Recently, two neuroimaging studies found that patients with OCD who are successfully treated with behavioural therapy show changes in cerebral metabolism similar to those produced by successful treatment with SRIs.[38,58]

Behavioural therapy can be conducted in inpatient and outpatient settings. The principal behavioural approaches in OCD are exposure for obsessions and response prevention for rituals (see Chapter 6.3.2.1). Desensitization, thought stopping, flooding, implosion therapy, and aversion conditioning have also been used in patients with OCD. In behavioural therapy the patient must collaborate and perform assignments. In a study of 18 patients with OCD, those receiving exposure and response prevention therapy showed significant improvement, whereas patients on a general anxiety management intervention (control) showed no improvement from baseline.[59] Direct comparisons of behavioural therapy and pharmacotherapy are few and are limited by methodological issues. Cox et al.[60] reported equal efficacy in a meta-analysis.

In thought stopping, the patient (or initially the therapist) shouts 'stop' or applies an aversive stimulus to counteract the obsessional preoccupation. The patient may also imagine a stop sign with a police officer nearby or another image that evokes inhibition at the same time that he or she recognizes the presence of the obsession. Another technique is to 'postpone' the thought until a specified time (e.g. an hour later) and not to think about it until then.

Despite the fact that biological interventions are more efficacious in patients with OCD, psychodynamic factors might be of considerable benefit in understanding what precipitates exacerbations of the disorder and in treating various forms of resistances to treatment, such as non-compliance to medications or to homework assignments. It is important to remember that the symptoms may have important psychological meanings that make patients reluctant to give them up. A psychodynamic assessment of the patient's resistance to treatment may result in improved compliance.

In the absence of controlled studies of insight-oriented psychotherapy for OCD, the anecdotal reports reporting lasting change do not allow generalizations to be made regarding efficacy. Also, the efficacy of medications in producing quick improvement has rendered slow and long-term psychotherapy out of favour.

Supportive psychotherapy has a place in managing patients with OCD, and may help patients improve their functioning and adjustment. The management plan should also include attention to the family members through the provision of emotional support, reassurance, explanation, and advice on how to manage and respond to the patient. Family therapy may reduce marital discord and build a treatment alliance, as well as helping in the resistance to compulsions. Group therapy is useful as a support system for some patients.

Summary

The treatment of OCD was characterized by pessimism until 20 years ago when effective treatments using behavioural therapy and the serotonin reuptake inhibitors were developed. Although introduced for OCD in 1967, it was only in the 1980s that double-blind studies confirmed the efficacy of clomipramine, an SRI. This was followed by the introduction of the selective serotonin reuptake inhibitors, which also proved effective for OCD. The anti-obsessive activity of these drugs was found to be independent from the drugs' antidepressant effect, as established by their efficacy both in depressed and non-depressed patients. Overall, serotonergic therapies have provided a better outlook for these patients and have increased our understanding of the pathophysiology of OCD.[6,7] Previously thought to be a rare and untreatable disorder, OCD is now recognized as common, and there is

good reason to expect that patients with OCD will benefit substantially from behaviour therapy and potent SRIs.

Many patients with OCD do not seek treatment and the disease tends to be chronic. There is a 10-year lag between the onset of symptoms and the seeking of professional help due to feelings of embarrassment. Further delay ensues until the diagnosis and correct treatment are given.[61] Census data suggest that over $8 billion are spent in the United States each year on the management of OCD, one-fifth of that spent on cardiac disease.[62] Because patients with OCD often attempt to conceal their symptoms, it is incumbent on clinicians to screen for OCD in every mental status examination, since appropriate treatment can result in improved quality of life, reduced OCD chronicity, and reduced costs to the individual and society.

References

1. Salzman, L. and Thaler, F.H. (1981). Obsessive compulsive disorder: a review of the literature. *American Journal of Psychiatry*, **138**, 286–96.
2. Robins, L.N., Helzer, J.E., Weissman, M.M., *et al.* (1984). Lifetime prevalence of specific psychiatric disorders in three sites. *Archives of General Psychiatry*, **41**, 949–58.
3. Weissman, M.M., Bland, R.C., Canino, G.J., *et al.* (1994). The cross national epidemiology of obsessive compulsive disorder. *Journal of Clinical Psychiatry*, **55**, (Supplement 3), 5–10.
4. Renynghe de Voxrie, G.V. (1968). Anafranil (G34586) in obsessive compulsive neurosis. *Archives Belges de Neurologie*, **68**, 787–92.
5. Fernandez-Cordoba, E. and Lopez-Ibor, A.J. (1967). La monoclorimipramina en enfermos psiquiatricos resistenses a otros tratamientos. *Actas Lusoespañolas de Neurologia, Psiquiatria y Ciencias Afines*, **26**, 119–47.
6. Dolberg, O.T., Iancu, I., Sasson, Y., *et al.* (1996). The pathogenesis and treatment of obsessive–compulsive disorder. *Clinical Neuropharmacology*, **19**, 129–47.
7. Zohar, J. and Insel, T. (1987). Obsessive–compulsive disorder: psychobiological approaches to diagnosis, treatment, and pathophysiology. *Biological Psychiatry*, **22**, 667–87.
8. Goodman, W.K., Price, L.H., Delgado, P.L., *et al.* (1990). Specificity of serotonin reuptake inhibitors in the treatment of obsessive compulsive disorder: comparison of fluvoxamine and desipramine. *Archives of General Psychiatry*, **47**, 577–85.
9. Leonard, H., Swedo, S.E., Lenane, M.C., *et al.* (1991). A double-blind desipramine substitution during long-term clomipramine treatment in children and adolescents with obsessive–compulsive disorder. *Archives of General Psychiatry*, **48**, 922–7.
10. Karno, M., Golding, J.M., Sorenson, S.B., *et al.* (1988). The epidemiology of obsessive–compulsive disorder in five US communities. *Archives of General Psychiatry*, **45**, 1094–9.
11. Flament, M.F., Whitaker, A., Rapoport, J.L., *et al.* (1988). Obsessive compulsive disorder in adolescence: an epidemiological study. *Journal of the American Academy of Child and Adolescent Psychiatry*, **27**, 764–71.
12. Nelson, E. and Rice, J. (1997). Stability of diagnosis of obsessive compulsive disorder in the epidemiologic catchment area study. *American Journal of Psychiatry*, **154**, 826–31.
13. Stein, M.B., Forde, D.R., Anderson, G., and Walker, J.R. (1997). Obsessive compulsive disorder in the community: an epidemiologic survey with clinical reappraisal. *American Journal of Psychiatry*, **154**, 1120–6.
14. Rasmussen, S.A. and Eisen, J.L. (1992). Epidemiology and clinical features of obsessive–compulsive disorder. In *Obsessive compulsive disorders. Theory and management* (ed. M.A. Jenike, L. Baer, and W.E. Minichiello), pp. 10–27. Year Book, Chicago, IL.
15. Pauls, D. (1992). The genetics of OCD and Gilles de la Tourette's syndrome. *Psychiatric Clinics of North America*, **15**, 759–66.

16. Berman, I., Sapers, B.L., Chang, H.H.J., Losonczy, M.F., Schmilder, Z., and Green, A.I. (1995). Treatment of obsessive–compulsive symptoms in schizophrenic patients with clomipramine. *Journal of Clinical Psychopharmacology*, **15**, 206–10.

17. Ravizza, L., Maina, G., and Bogetto, F. (1997). Episodic and chronic OCD. *Depression and Anxiety*, **6**, 154–8.

18. Thoren, P., Asberg, M., Gronholm, B., *et al.* (1980). Clomipramine treatment of obsessive compulsive disorder. II. Biochemical aspects. *Archives of General Psychiatry*, **27**, 1289–94.

19. Insel, T.R., Mueller, E.A., Alterman, I., *et al.* (1985). Obsessive compulsive disorder and serotonin: is there a connection? *Biological Psychiatry*, **20**, 1174–88.

20. Weizman, A., Carmi, M., Hermesh, H., *et al.* (1986). High affinity imipramine binding and serotonin uptake in platelets of eight adolescent and ten adult obsessive–compulsive patients. *American Journal of Psychiatry*, **143**, 335–9.

21. Marazziti, D., Hollander, E., Lensi, P., *et al.* (1992). Peripheral markers of serotonin and dopamine function in obsessive–compulsive disorder. *Psychiatry Research*, **42**, 41–51.

22. Vitiello, B., Shimon, H., Behar, D., *et al.* (1991). Platelet imipramine binding and serotonin uptake in obsessive–compulsive patients. *Acta Psychiatrica Scandinavica*, **84**, 29–32.

23. Kim, S.W., Dysken, M.W., Pandey, G.N., *et al.* (1991). Platelet 3H-imipramine binding sites in obsessive compulsive behavior. *Biological Psychiatry*, **30**, 467–74.

24. Marazziti, D., Pfanner, C., Palego, L., *et al.* (1997). Changes in platelet markers of obsessive compulsive patients during a double-blind trial of fluvoxamine versus clomipramine. *Pharmacopsychiatry*, **30**, 245–9.

25. Flament, M.F., Rapoport, J.L., Murphy, D.L., *et al.* (1987). Biochemical changes during clomipramine treatment of childhood obsessive–compulsive disorder. *Archives of General Psychiatry*, **44**, 219–25.

26. Charney, D.S., Goodman, W.K., Price, L.H., *et al.* (1988). Serotonin function in obsessive–compulsive disorder: a comparison of the effects of tryptophan and *m*-chlorophenylpiperazine in patients and healthy subjects. *Archives of General Psychiatry*, **45**, 177–85.

27. Hollander, E., DeCaria, C.M., Nitescu, A., *et al.* (1992). Serotonergic function in obsessive–compulsive disorder: behavioral and neuroendocrine responses to oral *m*-chlorophenylpiperazine and fenfluramine in patients and healthy volunteers. *Archives of General Psychiatry*, **49**, 21–8.

28. Lesch, K.P., Hoh, A., Disselkamp-Tietze, J., *et al.* (1991). 5-Hydroxytryptamine 1A receptor responsivity in obsessive compulsive disorder. Comparison of patients and controls. *Archives of General Psychiatry*, **48**, 540–7.

29. Bastani, B., Nash, J.F., and Meltzer, H.Y. (1990). Prolactin and cortisol responses to MK-212, a serotonin agonist, in obsessive–compulsive disorder. *Archives of General Psychiatry*, **47**, 833–9.

30. Sasson, Y. and Zohar, J. (1996). New developments in obsessive–compulsive disorder research: implications for clinical management. *International Clinical Psychopharmacology*, **11** (Supplement), 3–12.

31. Benkelfat, C., Murphy, D.L., Zohar, J., *et al.* (1989). Clomipramine in obsessive compulsive disorder: further evidence for a serotonergic mechanism of action. *Archives of General Psychiatry*, **46**, 23–8.

32. McDougle, J., Goodman, W.K., Price, L.H., *et al.* (1990). Neuroleptic addition in fluvoxamine-refractory obsessive–compulsive disorder. *American Journal of Psychiatry*, **147**, 652–4.

33. Swedo, S.E., Leonard, H.L., and Kiessling, L.S. (1994). Speculations on antineuronal antibody-mediated neuropsychiatric disorders of childhood. *Pediatrics*, **93**, 323–6.

34. Roy, B.F., Benkelphat, C., Hill, J.L., *et al.* (1994). Serum antibody for somatostatin, 14 and prodynorphin 209–240 in patients with obsessive–compulsive disorder, schizophrenia, Alzheimer's disease, multiple sclerosis and advanced HIV infection. *Biological Psychiatry*, **35**, 335–44.

35. Swedo, S.E., Leonard, H.L., Mittelman, B.B., *et al.* (1997). Identification of children with pediatric autoimmune neuropsychiatric disorders associated with streptococcal infections by a marker associated with rheumatic fever. *American Journal of Psychiatry*, **154**, 110–12.

36. Rauch, S.L. (1998). Neuroimaging in OCD: clinical implications. *CNS Spectrum*, **3**, (Supplement), 26–9.

37. Baxter, L.R. Jr, Schwartz, J.M., Bergman, K.S., *et al.* (1992). Caudate glucose metabolic rate changes with both drug and behaviour therapy for OCD. *Archives of General Psychiatry*, **49**, 681–9.

38. Galderisi, S., Mucci, A., and Catapano, F. (1995). Neuropsychological slowness in obsessive–compulsive patients: is it confined to tests involving the fronto-subcortical systems? *British Journal of Psychiatry*, **167**, 394–8.

39. Towey, J.P., Tenke, C.E., Bruder, G.E., *et al.* (1994). Brain event-related potential correlates of over focused attention in obsessive–compulsive disorder. *Psychophysiology*, **31**, 535–43.

40. Rasmussen, S.A. and Tsuang, M.T. (1986). Clinical characteristics and family history in DSM-III obsessive–compulsive disorder. *American Journal of Psychiatry*, **143**, 317–22.

41. Lenane, M.C., Swedo, S.E., Leonard, H., *et al.* (1990). Psychiatric disorders in first degree relatives of children and adolescents with obsessive–compulsive disorder. *Journal of the American Academy of Child and Adolescent Psychiatry*, **29**, 407–12.

42. Billet, E.A., Richter, M.A., King, N., *et al.* (1997). Obsessive compulsive disorder, response to serotonin reuptake inhibitors and the serotonin transporter gene. *Molecular Psychiatry*, **2**, 403–6.

43. Insel, T.R., Gillin, J.C., Moore, A., Mendelson, W.B., Lowenstein, R.J., and Murphy, D.L. (1982). The sleep of patients with OCD. *Archives of General Psychiatry*, **39**, 1372–7.

44. Insel, T.R., Kalin, N.H., Guttmacher, L.B., Cohen, R.M., and Murphy, D.L. (1982). The dexamethasone suppression test in patients with primary OCD. *Psychiatry Research*, **6**, 153–8.

45. Rasmussen, S.A., Eisen, J.L., and Pato, M.T. (1993). Current issues in the pharmacological management of obsessive–compulsive disorder. *Journal of Clinical Psychiatry*, **54**, 4s–9s.

46. Clomipramine Collaborative Study Group (1991). Clomipramine in the treatment of patients with obsessive–compulsive disorder. *Archives of General Psychiatry*, **48**, 730–8.

47. Pato, M.T., Zohar-Kadouch, R., Zohar, J., *et al.* (1988). Return of symptoms after discontinuation of clomipramine in patients with obsessive compulsive disorder. *American Journal of Psychiatry*, **145**, 1521–5.

48. Mundo, E., Barregi, S.R., Pirola, R., *et al.* (1997). Long-term pharmacotherapy of obsessive–compulsive disorder: a double-blind controlled study. *Journal of Clinical Psychopharmacology*, **17**, 4–10.

49. Pigott, T.A., Pato, M.T., Bernstein, S.E., *et al.* (1990). Controlled comparisons of clomipramine and fluoxetine in the treatment of obsessive–compulsive disorder: behavioral and biological results. *Archives of General Psychiatry*, **47**, 926–32.

50. Freeman, C.P.L., Trimble, M.R., Deakin, J.F.W., *et al.* (1994). Fluvoxamine versus clomipramine in the treatment of obsessive compulsive disorder: a multi-center, randomized, double-blind, parallel group comparison. *Journal of Clinical Psychiatry*, **55**, 301–5.

51. Zohar, J. and Judge, R. (1996). Paroxetine versus clomipramine in the treatment of obsessive–compulsive disorder. *British Journal of Psychiatry*, **169**, 468–74.

52. Bisserbe, J.C., Lane, R.M., Flament, M.F., *et al.* (1997). A double-blind comparison of sertraline and clomipramine in outpatients with obsessive–compulsive disorder. *European Psychiatry*, **153**, 1450–4.

53. McDougle, J.C., Goodman, W.K., and Price, L.H. (1997). Dopamine antagonists in tic-related and psychotic spectrum obsessive–compulsive disorder. *Journal of Clinical Psychiatry*, **55** (Supplement), 24–31.

54. Jenike, M.A., Baer, L., Ballantine, T., *et al.* (1991). Cingulotomy for refractory obsessive–compulsive disorder. *Archives of General Psychiatry*, **48**, 548–55.

55. Van Balkom, A.J.L.M., De Haan, E., Van Oppen, P., Spinhoven, P., Hoogduin, K.A.L., and Van Dyck, R. (1998). Cognitive and behavioral therapies alone versus in combination with fluvoxamine in the treatment of obsessive compulsive disorder. *Journal of Nervous and Mental Disease*, **186**, 492–9.

56. Marks, I.M., Hodgson, R., Rachman, S., *et al.* (1975). Treatment of chronic obsessive–compulsive neurosis *in vivo* exposure: a 2-year follow-up and issues in treatment. *British Journal of Psychiatry*, **127**, 349–64.

57. Greist, J.H. (1996). New developments in behaviour therapy for obsessive–compulsive disorder. *International Clinical Psychopharmacology*, **11** (Supplement), 63–73.

58. Schwartz, J.M., Stoessel, P.W., Baxter, L.R., Jr, *et al.* (1996). Systematic changes in cerebral glucose metabolic rate after successful behavior modification treatment of OCD. *Archives of General Psychiatry*, **53**, 109–13.

59. Lindsay, M., Craig, R., and Andrews, G. (1997). Controlled trial of exposure and response prevention in obsessive–compulsive disorder. *British Journal of Psychiatry*, **171**, 135–9.

60. Cox, B.J., Swinson, R.P., Morrison, B., *et al.* (1993). Clomipramine, fluoxetine, and behaviour therapy in the treatment of OCD: a meta-analysis. *Journal of Behavior Therapy and Experimental Psychiatry*, **24**, 149–53.

61. Hollander, E. (1997). Obsessive compulsive disorder: the hidden epidemic. *Journal of Clinical Psychiatry*, **12** (Supplement), 3–6.

62. DuPont, R.L., Rice, D.P., Shiraki, S., *et al.* (1995). Economic costs of obsessive compulsive disorder. *Medical Interface*, April, 102–9.

4.9 Depersonalization disorder

K. W. de Pauw

Depersonalization disorder is an uncommon disorder, characterized by persistent or recurrent episodes of a distressing subjective feeling of unreality or detachment from various aspects of the self. The condition is experienced by sufferers as a sense of disconnection or estrangement from their own body, thoughts, feelings, or behaviour, or from the outside world. In DSM-IV depersonalization disorder is classified as a dissociative disorder (300.6) while ICD-10 places it in the category of neurotic, stress-related, and somatoform disorders under the rubric of depersonalization–derealization syndrome (F48.1).

Clinical features

Patients with depersonalization disorder often report that they feel like a robot or an outside observer, as if watching themselves from a distance, in a film, or on a stage. There may be a sense of the physical body acting while the mind observes and of not being in full control of one's voice, movements, or behaviour. An emotional numbness or inability to experience feelings and a sensation of being in a dream, fog, or trance are often present as well. Some individuals have even described that they were unable to recognize themselves in a mirror. Accompanying derealization may be experienced as alterations in the quality, colour, shape, distance, or size of objects while other people seem unfamiliar, lifeless, or mechanical. Although unpleasant and distressing, patients are usually aware of the unreality of the changes and retain an intact sensorium and capacity for emotional expression.[1]

Primary depersonalization is considered a rare condition, reflected in the scarcity of systematic investigation into its prevalence, sex ratio, course, treatment response, and aetiology.[2] Because of the widespread occurrence of depersonalization, some authors consider it as a non-specific symptom of various psychiatric disorders rather than a separate nosological entity.[3,4] As early as 1935 the variety of identified precipitants caused Mayer Gross to reject psychological theories as being of 'limited value' in explaining the syndrome, suggesting instead that it be regarded as 'an unspecific preformed functional response of the brain'.[5]

Nevertheless, clinical experience, supported by a modest number of individual reports and case series, suggest to some investigators that depersonalization can occur as a primary disorder in its own right.[6,7] In these patients, comorbid symptoms appear to be secondary in intensity and severity without fulfilling syndromal criteria for another Axis I disorder. If a separate disorder is diagnosed, a clear history may indicate that depersonalization either predated it or occurred persistently and extensively beyond its manifestations. It is on this rather doubtful basis that depersonalization disorder is conceptualized as a discrete syndrome with its own onset, phenomenology, clinical characteristic, course, and treatment response.[2]

Differential diagnosis

The diagnosis of depersonalization disorder as a primary condition must be distinguished from symptoms that arise secondary to other psychiatric or general medical disorders.

Symptomatic depersonalization often occurs during the course of a variety of clinical conditions, including schizophrenia and related psychotic states, mood and anxiety disorders, acute intoxication with or withdrawal from alcohol, illicit substances, or medication, and as a physiological consequence of migraine, hypoglycaemia, hyperventilation, epileptic seizures, or structural central nervous system pathology.[4,8,9]

In otherwise normal individuals, brief episodes of depersonalization may be experienced under diverse conditions, such as sleep or sensory deprivation, being in unfamiliar surroundings or when confronted by potentially life-threatening situations. This suggests that the phenomenon occurs on a continuum in the general population, ranging from mild and transient episodes, without clinical significance, to recurrent or persistent episodes associated with considerable morbidity.[1,4,10]

Epidemiology and course

The lifetime prevalence of depersonalization disorder in the community is unknown. However, up to 50 per cent of adults will, at some point in their lives, experience at least one episode of depersonalization symptoms, often, although not invariably, as a response to a distressing event.[4,11] In a large series of psychiatric inpatients it was elicited in 80 per cent of the cases while 12 per cent described disabling and persistent experiences of depersonalization.[3] A recent comprehensive review of a cohort of 30 consecutively recruited individuals found a female to male a ratio of about 2 to 1 and a similar predominance of women was reported by earlier investigators.[2] Whether the higher incidence reflects a selection bias, due to women being more likely to seek treatment, remains uncertain.

According to DSM-IV depersonalization disorder may arise undetected in childhood but it usually has its onset during adolescence or early adulthood. It is rare to occur for the first time in middle or late life. Patients frequently give a vivid account of their first episode. The onset is usually abrupt and often without any clear-cut precipitant. Alternatively, some individuals recall a close association with a specific event, such as the abuse of illicit substances or a distressful, possibly life-threatening, experience.[1,2]

The duration of episodes of depersonalization varies considerably between individual patients. Some are brief and transient while others last hours, weeks, or months, usually resolving gradually in contrast to their sudden onset. The course is usually chronic and marked by remissions and exacerbations. Recurrent episodes may occur in response to real or perceived stressful events, while others pursue an unremitting course with continuous depersonalization lasting for years.

Aetiology

Even if the validity of depersonalization disorder is accepted, the degree of psychiatric comorbidity is considerable. The most prevalent conditions are the various anxiety disorders and unipolar mood disorders. A wide variety of personality disorders are also manifested.[2]

In normal individuals, depersonalization may serve as an adaptive response to overwhelming stress, permitting continuous function by protecting against potentially overwhelming anxiety. Conversely, a lowering of conscious awareness could play an important aetiological role when depersonalization occurs during states of fatigue, sensory isolation, or sleep deprivation.[4] More than 30 per cent of survivors of near fatal accidents report transient experiences,[12] and Roth[13] found severe stress in later life, such as an external threat or a bereavement, to be associated with what he termed the phobic–anxiety depersonalization syndrome.

In DSM-IV, symptoms of depersonalization and derealization are listed among the criteria for panic attacks and are experienced by about 30 per cent of patients with panic disorder. In turn, most patients with depersonalization disorder also manifest symptoms of phobia, anxiety, and panic. Depersonalization in depression is usually restricted to a change in emotional responsiveness but can extend to volition and behaviour as well as to the external world.[1]

Although psychotic states have also been linked with depersonalization, the nature of the association is uncertain and the loss of insight in schizophrenia possibly indicates that this is a qualitatively different experience. Careful mental state examination will often reveal perplexity, affective incongruity, and a tendency to make delusional misinterpretations of subjective experiences and events in the environment.[10] The frequent observation of depersonalization and derealization in patients with Capgras or Frégoli delusions suggests that these phenomena play an important aetiological role in the development of delusional misidentification. Interestingly, the depersonalization symptoms are usually most prominent before or at the onset of the psychosis and disappear or diminish in intensity as the delusion becomes fully manifest.[14]

Several authors have drawn attention to the phenomenological similarities, such as age of onset and chronic course, between obsessive–compulsive and depersonalization disorders. Both are ego-dystonic with a fixed focus and are aggravated by bouts of intense rumination and repeated self-scrutiny.[15] In the adolescent onset of chronic depersonalization appears to be particularly likely to develop, often abruptly, in individuals with conspicuously introspective obses-

sional personalities. Some patients with disorders of impulse control may repeatedly resort to acts of deliberate self-harm in an effort to obtain relief from recurrent or continuous episodes of depersonalization.[1,10]

The occurrence of depersonalization in a variety of structural and metabolic disturbances of central nervous system function provides non-specific evidence for an underlying biological basis. In these cases there may be a disruption of the final integrative mechanisms, located in the parietotemporal cortex and adjacent limbic areas, which are normally responsible for the experience.[16] More specifically, findings such as the association with migraine and the abuse of LSD or cannabis, and neuropsychiatric impairments similar to those reported in obsessive–compulsive disorder, implicate a dysfunction of serotonergic mechanisms in the pathophysiology of depersonalization. Positive responses to serotonin reuptake inhibitors also offer some support to this hypothesis, particularly in view of the frequent refractoriness to treatment of the symptoms to a large variety of pharmacological agents.[2,15]

Psychodynamically, depersonalization has been interpreted as a response of the ego to defend against painful and conflicting memories, impulses, or affects, particularly in patients reporting traumatic experiences during their childhood.[4] However, attributing adult psychopathology primarily to early life events is problematic and studies demonstrating such an association are fraught with methodological difficulties. Despite their ubiquity, assumptions about the aetiological significance of traumatic events in childhood have not received consistent support from empirical research.[17,18]

Treatment

The treatment response of depersonalization disorder is often disappointing and many patients remain quite disabled. Although a variety of therapeutic approaches have been reported in the literature, efficacy remains to be demonstrated convincingly for any particular modality.[2]

Relief of transient episodes of depersonalization was reported in the early literature, using intravenous amphetamines and barbiturates, either separately or in combination. The response to treatment with neuroleptics is unpredictable; some patients obtain benefit while others experience an exacerbation of their symptoms. In view of its frequent association with anxiety and depression, various anxiolytic and antidepressive drugs have been widely used in an attempt to treat depersonalization. However, even when conditions such as major depression and panic disorder are comorbid with depersonalization, the latter may not respond during treatment of the former, which would support its independent diagnostic status. Selective serotonin reuptake inhibitors may prove to be an exception, in at least a proportion of patients.[19]

Positive outcomes have been claimed in individual cases for behavioural treatments, employing techniques such as *in vivo* exposure to exacerbating situations, *in vitro* flooding, paradoxical suggestion to induce an episode and thus gain a sense of control, negative reinforcement by performing a task after each episode, and reward contingency. However, it is unclear whether behaviour therapy is so effective in treating patients with continuous as opposed to episodic depersonalization. Successful psychodynamically orientated therapy has tended to focus on limited practical approaches and goals, that is acceptance and understanding of symptoms, identifying any putative defensive functions, the treatment of any underlying psychopathology, and integrating traumatic experiences and memories.

In patients where symptoms of depersonalization clearly arise against a background history of head injury, seizures, or other central nervous system pathology, appropriate investigations, including brain imaging and an EEG, possibly with nasopharyngeal leads, should be pursued. Treatment is directed towards the underlying condition and may result in symptomatic relief.

References

1. Slater, E. and Roth, M. (1969). *Clinical psychiatry* (3rd edn). Baillière Tindall and Cassell, London.

2. Simeon, D., Gross, S., Guralnik, O., Stein, D., Schmeidler, J., and Hollander, E. (1997). Feeling unreal: 30 cases of DSM-III-R depersonalization disorder. *American Journal of Psychiatry*, **154**, 1107–13.

3. Brauer, R., Harrow, M., and Tucker, G.J. (1970). Depersonalization phenomena in psychiatric patients. *British Journal of Psychiatry*, **117**, 509–15.

4. Sedman, G. (1970). Theories of depersonalisation: a re-appraisal. *British Journal of Psychiatry*, **117**, 1–14.

5. Mayer Gross, W. (1935). On depersonalisation. *British Journal of Medical Psychology*, **15**, 103–22.

6. Davison, K. (1964). Episodic depersonalization: observations on seven patients. *British Journal of Psychiatry*, **110**, 505–13.

7. Shorvon, H.J. (1946). The depersonalization syndrome. *Proceedings of the Royal Society of Medicine*, **39**, 779–92.

8. Cummings, J.L. (1985). *Clinical neuropsychiatry*. Grune and Stratton, Orlando, FL.

9. Kenna, J.C. and Sedman, G. (1965). Depersonalisation in temporal lobe epilepsy and the organic psychoses. *British Journal of Psychiatry*, **111**, 293–9.

10. Hamilton, M. (1974). *Fish's clinical psychopathology: signs and symptoms in psychiatry*. John Wright, Bristol.

11. Dixon, J.C. (1963). Depersonalisation phenomena in a sample population of college students. *British Journal of Psychiatry*, **109**, 371–5.

12. Noyes, R. and Kletti, R. (1977). Depersonalization in response to life-threatening danger. *Comprehensive Psychiatry*, **18**, 375–84.

13. Roth, M. (1959). The phobic-anxiety depersonalization syndrome. *Proceedings of the Royal Academy of Medicine*, **52**, 587–95.

14. Christodoulou, G.N. (1986). Role of depersonalization–derealization phenomena in the delusional misidentification syndromes. *Bibliotheca Psychiatrica*, **164**, 99–104.

15. Cohen, L.J., Simeon, D., Hollander, E., and Stein, D.J. (1997). Obsessive–compulsive spectrum disorders. In *Obsessive–compulsive disorders: diagnosis, etiology, treatment* (ed. E. Hollander and D.J. Stein), pp. 47–73. Dekker, New York.

16. Hill, D. (1989). On states of consciousness. In *The bridge between neurology and psychiatry* (ed. E.H. Reynolds and M.R. Trimble), pp. 56–71. Churchill Livingstone, Edinburgh.

17. Paris, J. (1997). Childhood trauma as an etiological factor in the personality disorders. *Journal of Personality Disorders*, **11**, 34–49.

18. Pope, H.G. (1997). *Psychology astray: fallacies in studies of 'repressed memory' and childhood trauma*. Upton, Boca Raton, FL.

19. Hollander, E., Liebowitz, M.R., DeCaria, C., Fairbanks, J., Fallon, B., and Klein, D.F. (1990). Treatment of depersonalization with serotonin reuptake blockers. *Journal of Clinical Psychopharmacology*, **32**, 468–9.

4.10 Disorders of eating

4.10.1 Anorexia nervosa

Gerald Russell

Introduction: history of ideas

Two different approaches may be discerned in the conceptualization of anorexia nervosa.

1. The medicoclinical approach defines the illness in terms of its clinical manifestations; the main landmarks were the descriptions by William Gull in 1874[1] and Charles Lasègue in 1873.[2]

2. The sociocultural approach is unlike the more empirical clinical approach and takes causation into account by viewing the illness as a response to prevailing social and cultural systems. This was best argued by the social historian Joan Jacobs Brumberg who considers anorexia nervosa simply as a control of appetite in women responding to widely differing forces which may change during historical times.[3] This approach allows flexibility in identifying anorexia nervosa in different historical and cultural settings, but it carries the risk of excessive diagnostic latitude.

There is a strong argument for accepting the original descriptions by Gull (1874) and Lasègue (1873) as containing the essence of anorexia nervosa. They both recognized a disorder associated with severe emaciation and loss of menstrual periods, inexplicable in terms of recognized physical causes of wasting. They were both extremely cautious about the nature of the mental disorder. Gull spoke of a morbid mental state or 'mental perversity', and adopted the more general term anorexia 'nervosa' which has persisted until today. Lasègue also referred to 'mental perversity' but was bold enough to call the condition 'anorexie hystérique, faute de mieux'.

It is probably best to seek a balance between the diagnostic rectitude of the medicoclinical approach and the malleability of anorexia nervosa in response to changing historical and sociocultural settings. Looking back in historical times, it may well be that the self-starvation and asceticism of St Catherine of Siena corresponded to modern anorexia nervosa.[4,5] In more recent times the preoccupations of the patients have altered so that their disturbed experience with their own body[6] or their 'morbid fear of fatness'[7] has earned the distinction of becoming one of the diagnostic criteria. Yet this concern with body size was not remarked upon by Gull or Lasègue. This is an argument for concluding that at least the psychological content, and perhaps also the form, of anorexia nervosa are changeable in response to historical times and sociocultural influences.

Epidemiology

Screening instruments

The most commonly used screening test in the detection of anorexia nervosa is the Eating Attitudes Test (**EAT**).[8] Doubt has, however, been expressed about the predictive value of the EAT in the very populations where its use was introduced, as only a small percentage of the EAT-screened positive scores will have an actual eating disorder.[9] Thus, the EAT has limited usefulness in surveys for detecting anorexia nervosa unless it is supplemented by detailed clinical assessments. A survey depending on initial screening by questionnaire also runs the risk of failing to detect cases of anorexia nervosa as it was found that patients currently receiving active treatment were among the non-respondents, presumably because they wished to conceal their disorder.[10]

Populations surveyed

General population surveys

These are often impracticable when the aim is to detect anorexia nervosa, a relatively uncommon disorder.

Surveys of primary care populations

A useful compromise is that of surveying populations of patients who consult their general practitioners. A Netherlands study was successful because a large population was surveyed (over 150 000) and the general practitioners themselves, after suitable training, were responsible for making the diagnoses.[11]

Populations thought to be more at risk

Surveys of ballet and modelling students were conducted because it was thought likely that there would be a high prevalence of anorexia nervosa among them as a result of pressures exerted to sustain a slim figure in keeping with their professional image.[12,13]

Populations of adolescent schoolgirls have also been surveyed as their susceptibility might be raised by virtue of their age, sex, and the frequency of dieting among the school population.[14,15] The most thorough survey of 15-year-old school-children was that conducted in Göteborg, Sweden.[16]

Surveys based on case registers and hospital records

Data have been obtained on patients referred to inpatient and outpatient psychiatric services,[17,18] or with the addition of patients who had consulted paediatricians, general medical services, or gynaecologists.[19,20]

Results of epidemiological surveys

Incidence of anorexia nervosa

The studies which counted only hospitalized patients tended to yield low estimates of the annual incidence of anorexia nervosa expressed per 100 000 population (e.g. 0.45 in Sweden[17]). Estimates based on case registers of psychiatric patients similarly yielded fairly low incidence rates (e.g. 0.64 in Monroe County, New York[18]). The incidence found in community-based studies was by far the highest (6.3 in The Netherlands[11] and 8.2 in Rochester, Minnesota[21]), presumably because they included the less severe cases.

Prevalence of anorexia nervosa in vulnerable populations

A high prevalence rate was found among Canadian ballet students (6.5 per cent) and modelling students (7 per cent).[12] A similar survey in an English ballet school also showed a high prevalence of 'possible' cases of anorexia nervosa (7.0 per cent).[13]

Surveys among schoolgirls have shown a fairly wide variation in prevalence rates, ranging from zero to 1.1 per cent. In the English studies a consistent difference in prevalence rate was found between private schools (1 per cent) and state schools (0–0.2 per cent).[14,15] This social class distinction was not so definite in the Swedish study where the overall prevalence of 0.84 per cent of schoolgirls, up to and including 15 years of age, represents a high rate for anorexia nervosa.[16]

Age and sex

Epidemiological surveys have confirmed clinical opinion that anorexia nervosa commences most frequently in the young, especially within a few years of puberty. The peak age of onset is 18 years.[14] The illness is less common before puberty, but in a series of patients admitted to a children's hospital the age of onset ranged from 7.75 to 14.33 years.[22]

The marked predominance of females over males was also confirmed, for example 92 per cent in northeast Scotland[19] and 90 per cent among the children in Göteborg.[16]

Social class and socio-economic status

The view has been widely held that anorexia nervosa occurs predominantly in patients with middle-class backgrounds, since Fenwick's classical observation that anorexia nervosa 'is much more common in wealthier classes of society than amongst those who have to procure their bread by daily labour'.[23]

Epidemiological surveys aimed at wider populations leave the question of social class distribution somewhat equivocal. Whereas a high percentage of combined social classes 1 and 2 (Registrar General's categories) were found in clinical studies,[24] a high social class predominance was not found in studies utilizing case registers.[19] On the other hand, the schoolgirl studies mentioned above tended to confirm a high social class predominance.

Has the incidence of anorexia nervosa increased since the 1950s?

Hilde Bruch had no doubt about the answer to this question: 'one might speak of an epidemic illness, only there is no contagious agent; the spread must be attributed to psycho-social factors'. This is an exaggeration as the increase in anorexia nervosa does not merit the term 'epidemic'.[25] Indeed, such a notion was dismissed in an article 'The epidemic of anorexia nervosa: another medical myth?'.[26] It was concluded that there had been an increase in first admissions of patients over 10 years (1972–1981) but that this was due to an increase in the number of young women in the population. This rejection of a true increase in the incidence of anorexia nervosa has in its turn been criticized.[27]

The most reliable evidence for changes in the incidence of anorexia nervosa comes from repeated surveys of the same population. This has been achieved with the surveys conducted in southern Sweden,[17] northeast Scotland,[19] Switzerland,[20] Monroe County, New York,[18] and Rochester, Minnesota.[21] The researchers applied the same methodology to a similar population after an interval of several years, thus controlling for many of the variables that make it impossible to compare surveys conducted in different centres. There was a clear trend for an increase in incidence over time. The most thorough study was in Rochester, Minnesota.[21] The researchers separated female patients aged 15 to 24 years (61 per cent) from the remainder and established an increase in these younger patients, but only in them. They concluded that this increased incidence over time reflected a greater vulnerability of younger female subjects to adverse social factors.

There remains at least one sceptic who has argued that there is no evidence of an increase in anorexia nervosa.[28] He has found statistical imperfections in all epidemiological studies so far, and even questioned the possible significance of changes in diagnostic criteria from DSM-III to DSM-IIIR. He agreed that the Rochester survey had produced robust data, but thought that it still contained unresolved analytic problems.

This issue remains an important one because of its significance in the search for sociocultural factors causing anorexia nervosa. But it is better to pose a different question which renders this controversy unnecessary. We should ask instead whether there has been an increase in the incidence of eating disorders including anorexia nervosa. This is especially relevant in view of the fact that bulimia nervosa is a variant of anorexia nervosa, and in many patients follows an earlier episode of anorexia nervosa.[29] There is strong evidence that bulimia nervosa is a new disorder and has not simply appeared because of improved medical recognition.[30] Moreover, the incidence of bulimia nervosa has risen sharply during the past 20 years, so that it is now about double that of anorexia nervosa (see also Chapter 4.10.2). In conclusion, it is clear that since the 1960s there has been a significant increase in eating disorders, of which the two clearest syndromes are anorexia nervosa and bulimia nervosa.

Aetiology

Aetiological concepts

According to one robust opinion, it is essential to pursue the search for a specific and necessary cause of anorexia nervosa because the currently popular 'multifactorial' approach has little explanatory

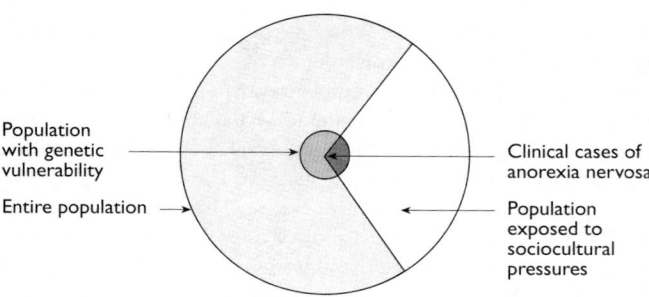

Fig. 1 Diagrammatic illustration of the way that genetic predisposition interacts with sociocultural pressures to cause anorexia nervosa. There is no intention of drawing the different parts of the circle to scale as the relative sizes of the populations are not known.

power.[31] Accordingly the failure to identify a necessary causal element is regrettable. Many of the factors within a wide range of psychological, social, and physical causes so far studied may therefore only be relevant in predisposing to anorexia nervosa. The patients 'become terribly afflicted victims of an often-incurable illness whose causes still elude clarification'.[31]

The multidimensional approach to anorexia nervosa

It is precisely because we do not know the fundamental (necessary) cause of anorexia nervosa that recourse has to be had to a multidimensional approach, *faute de mieux*. Although it has its limitations, a multidimensional approach permits one to consider a range of possible causal factors which not only act in an additive manner but may combine in a specific manner to bring about the illness: 'It is the interaction and timing of these phenomena in a given individual which are necessary for the person to become ill'.[32]

It is useful to provide a simple model of the way that two broad sets of factors may interact and augment each other (Fig. 1). The outer circle represents the entire population in a developed 'Westernized' country. Within the circle there is a large sector representing females within an age range of 10 to 50 years who experience prevailing social pressures to acquire a slender body shape through dieting. Evidently only a small proportion of these women develop the illness. It is likely that for anorexia nervosa to develop it is also necessary to possess a genetic predisposition, represented by the small inner circle. The intersection of the inner circle and the large sector produces a small sector of females who have the genetic predisposition and also experience sociocultural pressures to lose weight, interacting to cause clinical anorexia nervosa.

Causal factors may not only interact as explained above, but they can also influence the content of the illness, its 'colouring', and its form. This modelling function is described by the term 'pathoplastic' which was introduced by Birnbaum.[33] Pathoplastic features are to be distinguished from the more fundamental causes of psychiatric illness, but they do exert a predisposing tendency as well as a modelling role.

Sociocultural causes

The cult of thinness

The pathoplastic sociocultural causes of eating disorders have been subsumed under the term 'the modern cult of thinness' prevalent in

Westernized societies.[30] Vulnerable patients are likely to respond to this pressure by experimenting with weight-reducing diets which carry a degree of risk, and anorexia nervosa is arguably but an extension of determined dieting.[34]

It is proposed that the cult of thinness is responsible for the increase in the incidence of eating disorders since the 1950s. The social pressures which lead to dietary restraint include the publication of books and magazines advising weight-reducing diets, the fashion industry which caters mainly for the slimmer figure, television attaching sexual allure and professional success to the possession of a svelte figure, and the emphasis on physical fitness and athleticism.[3]

Changes in the psychopathology of anorexia nervosa

At the beginning of this chapter it was pointed out that the psychological content and the form of anorexia nervosa have changed over historical time and in response to sociocultural influences. Whereas Gull and Lasègue spoke only of 'anorexia nervosa' and 'anorexie hystérique' respectively, more recent descriptions of the psychopathology of anorexia nervosa have stressed a disturbed experience of one's own body,[6] a weight 'phobia',[35] or a morbid dread of fatness.[7] It is precisely the modern anorectic's dread of fatness that is most in keeping with today's cult of thinness. It is arguable therefore that modern societal pressures have determined the patients' preoccupations and contributed to their food avoidance. The beliefs are held obstinately and amount to overvalued ideas.

Anorexia nervosa as a culture-bound syndrome

The proposition that anorexia nervosa is a culture-bound syndrome has much support.[36–38] An intense fear of becoming obese is as culture bound as the disorder koro (a fear of shrinkage of the genitals) in Malaysia and South China.[36]

> A culture-bound syndrome may be defined as a collection of signs and symptoms which is not to be found universally in human populations, but is restricted to a particular culture or group of cultures. Implicit is the view that culture factors play an important role in the genesis of the symptom cluster ...[37]

Anorexia nervosa meets these criteria, first because it is limited to Westernized or industrialized nations, and secondly because it is clear that the psychosocial pressures on women to become thin constitute a powerful cultural force leading to anorexia nervosa.

In order to allow for exceptions to the rule, when anorexia nervosa occurs in non-Westernized countries, the illness may be understood as arising from cultures undergoing rapid cultural change.[38] Anorexia nervosa is thus a 'culture-change syndrome', explaining its increased incidence in Japan and Israel. Anorexia nervosa remains rare in Asia (particularly India), the Middle East (with the exception of Israel), and generally in poorly developed countries.

Young female immigrants who move to a new culture may suffer from an increased prevalence of eating disorders. For example, children with anorexia nervosa were found among Asian families living in Britain. This was linked with an exposure to a conflicting set of sociocultural norms in comparison with their parents and grandparents.[39]

Adverse life events

Anorexia nervosa may be precipitated by adverse life events. Early clinical studies depended solely on the patient's reports of an adverse life event preceding the onset of the illness. These varied widely in severity and included the death of grandparents, a father's remarriage, a severe physical illness, stress or failure of school examinations, or being teased about being overweight.[24]

Recent studies have relied on more objective measurements of adverse life events and comparisons with control groups. In one such study,[40] life events were rated according to the Bedford College Life Events and Difficulties Schedule and included the death of a close relative, a poor relationship with parents, or an unhappy marriage. Fairly severe life events and lasting difficulties were found in the majority of patients with a late onset (after 25 years), whereas they were only found in a minority of patients with an early onset (before 25 years) or in patients with a 'chronic' course.

Anorexia nervosa can also be precipitated by sexual experiences and conflicts. In a series of 31 adolescent and young women it was observed that in 14 first sexual intercourse had occurred before the illness.[41] Sexual problems were seen by 13 patients as major precipitants of their illness; 10 of them had experienced intercourse. The authors concluded that a specific aetiological role of sexual factors seemed unlikely, but there might be a direct relationship between the onset of eating difficulties and concurrent sexual problems.

In a series of 15 patients, anorexia nervosa developed during pregnancy or, more often, during the postnatal period when it was accompanied by depression.[42] Risk factors included ambivalence about motherhood, a large weight gain during the pregnancy, physical complications during pregnancy, postnatal depression, and past psychiatric illness.

Childhood sexual abuse

Since it was reported that a high proportion of patients in a treatment programme for anorexia nervosa gave histories of sexual abuse in childhood, it has been supposed that this trauma would be a contributory causal factor.[43] It would be better if this history could be corroborated, but for obvious reasons it is often difficult to do so. Investigators often stress that their patients' accounts are convincing and that they should be believed. Hence this subject raises unusual difficulties in judging the reliability of the data. Child sexual abuse is also discussed in the chapter on bulimia nervosa (Chapter 4.10.2).

In a careful study of childhood sexual experiences reported by women with anorexia nervosa, the authors classified the events according to the seriousness of the sexual act in childhood and concentrated on sexual experiences with someone at least 5 years older.[44] They found surprisingly high rates (about one-third) of adverse sexual experiences in women with eating disorders, and, unlike other investigators, they did not find that the frequency of these reports was less in anorexia nervosa than bulimia nervosa. They concluded that it was plausible that childhood sexual contact with an adult may in some cases contribute to a later eating disorder.

The complexity of this subject has been increased by a study on the relationship between sexual abuse, disordered personality, and eating disorders.[45] The authors found that 30 per cent of patients referred to an eating disorders clinic (a majority with anorexia nervosa) gave a history of childhood sexual abuse. In addition, they found that 52 per cent of their patients had a personality disorder. A significantly higher proportion of women with a personality disorder had a history of childhood sexual abuse, compared with those without a personality disorder. Surprisingly they still concluded that in patients with eating disorders it was not possible to show a clear causal link between child sexual abuse and personality disorder.

In a review of the subject a number of hypotheses were examined on the relationship between childhood sexual abuse and eating disorders.[46] One hypothesis is that child sexual abuse is more common in bulimia nervosa than in anorexia nervosa. The authors had to concede that the findings remain inconclusive. They also examined the question of whether child sexual abuse is a specific risk factor for eating disorders. They concluded that this was not the case, as the rates of child sexual abuse in eating disorder patients were similar to or less than those in various other psychiatric comparison groups. Finally, they found strong evidence that patients with eating disorders reporting child sexual abuse were more likely to show general psychiatric symptoms including depression, alcohol problems, or suicidal gestures, in addition to the association with personality disorders already mentioned.

Family factors

Two influential groups of family therapists (Minuchin at the Philadelphia Child Guidance Clinic and Selvini Palazzoli in Milan) have devised family models to explain the genesis of anorexia nervosa.

Minuchin *et al.* identified faulty patterns of interaction between members of the anorexic patient's family; they in turn were thought to lead to the child's attempt to solve the family problems by starving herself:[47] 'The sick child plays an important role in the family's pattern of conflict avoidance, and this role is an important source of reinforcement for his symptoms'. Five main characteristics of family interaction were identified as detrimental to the function of the family: enmeshment (a tight web of family relationships with the members appearing to read each other's minds), overprotectiveness, rigidity, involvement of the sick child in parental conflicts, lack of resolution of conflicts.

Selvini Palazzoli[48] also identified abnormal patterns of communication within these families and in addition described abnormal relationships between the family members. She assumed that anorexia nervosa amounted to a logical adjustment to an illogical interpersonal system. But it remains uncertain whether these abnormal interactions are to blame for the illness or develop as a response by parents faced with a starving child. Careful therapists take pains to reassure parents at the commencement of family therapy: '...we always find it useful to spend some time discussing the nature of the illness, stressing in particular that we do not see the family as the origin of the problem'.[49]

Bruch[25] described girls who developed anorexia nervosa as 'good girls', who previously had a profound desire to please their families to the point of becoming unaware of their own needs. The frequency of broken families in anorexia nervosa is thought to be fairly low. Anorexic families have been found to be closer. They spent most of their spare time together and tended to mix less with people outside the family circle; the patients more often perceived themselves as having happy relationships within the family.[50]

Personality disorders

A sizeable proportion of patients (30 per cent[17] and 32 per cent[24]) were said to have had a 'normal' personality during childhood before their illness. Nevertheless there is general agreement of a close relationship between obsessional personalities and the later development of anorexia nervosa. In fact Janet, who carefully described obsessions and psychasthenia, was dubious about the validity of the diagnostic concept of anorexia nervosa (*anorexie hystérique*). He thought that the patient's fear of fatness was an elaborate obsessional idea.[51]

In a study of patients admitted for treatment they were classified into anorexia nervosa, bulimia nervosa, or a combination of the two disorders.[52] Personality disorders were identified through the Structured Clinical Interview for DSM-IIIR personality disorders (SCID-II). Seventy-two per cent of the patients met the criteria for at least one personality disorder. Anorectics were found to have a high rate of obsessive–compulsive personality disorder. On the other hand, bulimic patients with a history of anorexia nervosa showed high rates of borderline (40 per cent) and histrionic (40 per cent) personality disorder.[52]

There have been attempts to disentangle the features of premorbid personality and illness in order to clarify the personality characteristics predisposing to anorexia nervosa. Women who had recovered from restricting anorexia nervosa were tested at an 8- to 10-year follow-up, using a number of self-report instruments.[53] They were compared with two control groups: normal women and the sisters of the recovered anorexic patients. The women who had recovered from anorexia nervosa rated higher on risk avoidance and conforming to authority. In comparison with their sisters, the recovered women showed a greater degree of self-control and impulse control, and less enterprise and spontaneity.

In a study examining the close relationships between anorexia nervosa and obsessive–compulsive personality traits and disorder, 12 patients who had recovered from anorexia nervosa were examined and compared with normal controls.[54] They continued to exhibit obsessional traits in the weight-restored state and attained significantly higher scores on the Maudsley Obsessive–Compulsive Inventory and the Tridimensional Personality Questionnaire (harm avoidance and reward dependence).

Biomedical factors and pathogenesis

Historical notes

Since the early part of the twentieth century a recurring theme has been the possibility that anorexia nervosa is primarily caused by an endocrine or cerebral disturbance. From 1916 there was much preoccupation with the concept of Simmonds' cachexia,[55] the assumed result of latent disease of the pituitary gland. There was diagnostic confusion between anorexia nervosa and hypopituitarism which was only clarified much later when it became known that in true hypopituitarism weight loss and emaciation are uncommon. Hormonal deficits indicative of impaired pituitary function are indeed common in anorexia nervosa, but are merely a secondary manifestation of prolonged malnutrition.

Interest in the neuroendocrinology of anorexia nervosa led to the formulation of the hypothalamic model.[7,56] From the beginning the model was aimed at explaining pathogenesis rather than aetiology; it was not considered an alternative to the psychological origin for anorexia nervosa, but a means of explaining a constellation of disturbed neural mechanisms, as follows:

(1) a disordered regulation of food intake;

(2) a neuroendocrine disorder affecting mainly the hypothalamic–anterior pituitary–gonadal axis;

(3) a disturbance in the regulation of body temperature.

It was known that these functions all reside within the complex of hypothalamic physiology. A 'feeding centre' had been described in the lateral hypothalamus because bilateral lesions there induced self-starvation and death in rats.[57] A 'satiety centre' in the ventromedial hypothalamus whose destruction caused obesity had previously been described.[58] Over the years it has become clearer that many of the disturbances could be attributed to the patients' malnutrition, as demonstrated by experimental studies in healthy young women who were asked to follow a weight reducing diet. It was found that ovarian function is extremely sensitive to even small restrictions of caloric intake which often lead to impaired menstrual function.[59]

Cerebral lesions and disturbances

Interest in the hypothalamic model was fuelled early on by clinical reports of patients diagnosed as suffering from anorexia nervosa who were later found to have cerebral lesions, especially tumours of the hypothalamus.[60] More recently, occult intracranial tumours have been detected, masquerading as anorexia nervosa in young children.[61]

Neuroimaging studies in anorexia nervosa have led to findings suggestive of an atrophy of the brain. CT has disclosed a widening of the cerebral sulci and less frequently an enlargement of the ventricles.[62] The outer cerebrospinal fluid spaces were enlarged markedly in 36 per cent of the patients. When the CT examination was repeated after weight gain 3 months later, the widening of the sulci had disappeared in 42 per cent of the patients who had previously shown this finding. In other patients, however, the widening remained unaltered for 1 year after body weight had returned to normal.

Functional neuroimaging techniques have also been applied to research in anorexia nervosa. Fifteen children with anorexia nervosa were investigated by means of single-photon emission CT which provides a measure of regional cerebral blood flow.[63] In the majority of the children there was an above-critical difference in the regional cerebral blood flow between the temporal lobes. Hypoperfusion was found on the left side in eight children and on the right side in five. Follow-up scans were undertaken in three children after they had returned to normal weight; the reduced regional cerebral blood flow in the temporal lobe persisted on the same side as the initial scan. The authors concluded that there was an underlying primary neurological abnormality—an imbalance of the limbic system which in turn led to a hypothalamic–pituitary abnormality. Caution is advisable when interpreting functional neuroimaging studies as it is extremely difficult to have a control group with children.

Genetic causes

The strongest argument in favour of a biomedical causation of anorexia nervosa is the evidence that genetic factors have a role to play. The evidence is mainly derived through the classical method of comparing the concordance rates for the illness in monozygotic and dizygotic twins. The first sizeable series of twins studied came from the Maudsley Hospital and St George's Hospital in London, and revealed a higher concordance rate for monozygotic than for dizygotic twins.[64] Among the 30 twin pairs the concordance rates were 56 per cent among monozygotic twins compared with 7 per cent among dizygotic twins. The authors concluded that there is a genetic predisposition to anorexia nervosa.

Tentative calculations of the 'heritability' of anorexia nervosa suggested that it accounts for as much as 80 per cent of the variance.[65] It remains uncertain how the genetic vulnerability to anorexia nervosa expresses itself in terms of the pathogenesis of this disorder. An interesting proposal is that this vulnerability confers a weakness of the homeostatic mechanisms which normally ensure weight restoration after a period of weight loss. This hypothesis would explain why in Western society, where dieting behaviour is common, those who are genetically vulnerable would be likely to develop anorexia nervosa.[65]

There is also evidence for a familial aggregation of anorexia nervosa. This does not necessarily mean that the origin of the disorder is genetic because environmental factors in common must also be considered. In a series of 387 first-degree relatives of 97 probands with anorexia nervosa it was found that the illness occurred in 4.1 per cent of the first-degree relatives of the anorexic probands, whereas no case was found among relatives of the controls who were probands with a primary major affective disorder or with various non-affective conditions.[66] The authors concluded that anorexia nervosa was familial with intergenerational transmission. It was roughly eight times more common in female first-degree relatives of anorexic probands than in the general population, and absent in the relatives of probands with major affective disorder, thus indicating a specificity in the risk of transmission of anorexia nervosa and an absence of shared familial liability with affective disorders.

Neurotransmitters

Since the early 1970s, the hypothalamic model of anorexia nervosa has been transformed from a consideration of anatomical 'centres' to 'systems' involving neurotransmitters. Much evidence has been presented to show that a wide range of neurotransmitters modulate feeding behaviour, and it was only a small conceptual step to suggest that some were involved in the pathophysiology of eating disorders. At first the neurotransmitters considered were mainly the monoamine systems— noradrenaline (norepinephrine), dopamine, and serotonin. In addition, opioids, the peptide cholecystokinin, and the hormones corticotrophin-releasing factor and vasopressin have also been thought to play a part in the pathogenesis of eating disorders. During recent years the main interest has been focused on the role of serotonin (5-hydroxytryptamine, 5-HT) in the control of natural appetite, especially those aspects concerning the phenomenon of satiety, mediated through a range of processes called the 'satiety cascade'.[67] There is now strong evidence that pharmacological activation of serotonin leads to an inhibition of food consumption. It was also postulated that a defect in serotonin metabolism confers a vulnerability to the development of an eating disorder.[67]

A boost to the concept of altered serotonin activity in anorexia nervosa has come from research showing that these patients while still underweight had significant reductions in cerebrospinal fluid 5-hydroxyindoleacetic acid (**5-HIAA**). The levels became normal when the patients were retested 2 months after they reached their target weight.[68] In order to test whether these findings were secondary to malnutrition, the researchers resorted to the ingenious step of studying patients after 'recovery' when they had reached normal weight. They found elevated levels of cerebrospinal fluid 5-HIAA, possibly indicating increased serotonin activity contributing to the abnormal eating behaviour which often persists in patients who have otherwise recovered.[69] The arguments against this simple model of enhanced serotonin activity as a vulnerability trait in anorexia nervosa should be briefly represented. In two recent studies serotonin function

was again assessed in long-term weight-restored anorectics. The investigators used a dynamic neuroendocrine challenge with D-fenfluramine as a specific probe of serotonin function which mediates the release of prolactin. If there were any persistent abnormality in serotonin function, the response to this challenge test should differ from that in normal controls. In fact, the rise in prolactin levels was very similar in former patients and normal controls. Accordingly, these studies failed to support the notion of increased central serotonin function as a vulnerability trait in anorexia nervosa.[70,71]

Clinical features

Classical anorexia nervosa (postpubertal)

The illness usually occurs in girls within a few years of the menarche so that the most common age of onset is between 14 and 18. Sometimes the onset is later in a woman who has married and had children.

By the time the patient has been referred for psychiatric treatment she is likely to have reduced her food intake and lost weight over the course of several months, and her menstrual periods will have ceased. A regular feature of the illness is its concealment and the avoidance of treatment. Most clinicians are reluctant to express themselves frankly on this subject in case their observations sound derogatory. It is to the credit of one French author, that he has said explicitly:[72] 'Denial of the illness, lies, cheating, manipulation, are characteristic of the behaviour of anorectics'. Even after having lost 5 to 10 kg in weight and missed several periods, the patient's opening remark is often 'there is nothing wrong with me, my parents are unduly worried'. It is only when the clinician asks direct questions that she will admit to insomnia, irritability, sensitivity to cold, and a withdrawal from contacts with her friends, including her boyfriend if she has one.

Because of this denial, it is important to enquire from a close relative, as well as the patient, about the most relevant behavioural changes.

1. A **food intake history** is obtained by asking the patient to recall what she has eaten on the previous day, commencing with breakfast which is often missed. An avoidance of carbohydrate and fat-containing foods is the rule. It is likely that pastry, puddings, biscuits, and confectionery are entirely omitted, as are fried foods, butter, and full-cream milk. When asked to explain her restricted choice of food, the patient is likely to defend it on the grounds that she wishes to follow a 'healthy' diet. What remains is an often stereotyped selection of vegetables and fruit. 'Diet' drinks and unsweetened fruit juice are preferred, although some patients are partial to black coffee. It is the mother who will indicate that her daughter finds ways of avoiding meals, preferring to prepare her own food and withdrawing into her bedroom to eat it.

2. The patient is usually willing to provide a **weight history** and has a clear memory of her weight at successive stages of the illness. She may try to conceal her optimum weight before her decision to 'diet', but she is likely to be objective about her current weight, if only to express pride in the degree of 'self-control' she has exerted. The clinician then has an opportunity to enquire into her 'desired' weight by simply asking what weight she would be willing to return to. Her answer will betray a determination to maintain a suboptimal weight.

3. A **history of exercising** should be taken. Again, the patient is likely to conceal the fact that she walks long distances to school or to work rather than use public transport. She may also cycle vigorously or attend aerobic classes. A parent may report that his or her daughter is running on the spot or performing press-ups in the privacy of her bedroom, judging from the noise that can be heard. The amount of exercising may be grossly excessive, with the patient indulging in brisk walks or jogging even in the presence of painful knees or ankles due to soft tissue injuries.

4. **Additional harmful behaviours** which should be enquired into include self-induced vomiting, purgative abuse, and self-injury. Vomiting and purgative abuse are similar to the behaviours that occur in bulimia nervosa (see Chapter 4.10.2). In anorexia nervosa they may occur without the prelude of overeating and the patient's motive is simply to accelerate weight loss. Even so, vomiting is most likely to occur after the patient's frugal meals, and the laxative abuse is often at the end of the day. The favourite laxatives in the United Kingdom are Nylax, Senokot, and Dulcolax, and the patient is likely to take them in increasing quantities to achieve the wanted effect as tolerance develops. Self-injury should also be enquired into, and the skin of the wrists and forearms inspected for scratches or cuts with sharp instruments.

5. **Menstrual history**: the patient may not volunteer the information that her periods ceased, which often occurs soon after commencing the weight-reducing diet. On the other hand she may admit that she is relieved that her periods have stopped as she found them to be a nuisance or unpleasant.

The patient's mental state

Specific psychopathology

Several near-synonyms have been used to describe the specific attitude detectable in the patient who systematically avoids fatness: a 'disturbance of body image',[6] a 'weight phobia',[35] or a 'fear of fatness'.[7] *Magersucht*, or seeking after thinness, was a term applied in the older German literature. The patient will express a sensitivity about certain parts of her body, especially her stomach, thighs, and hips. Not only is she likely to assert that fatness makes her unattractive, but she may add that it is a shameful condition betraying greed and social failure. These distorted attitudes generally amount to overvalued ideas rather than delusions. Occasionally, however, a patient may be frankly deluded, such as one young woman who believed that her low weight was due to thin bones and that fatness was still evident on the surface of her body.

Studies have demonstrated that wasted patients, when asked to estimate their body size, see themselves as wider and fatter than they actually are.[73] Since these early observations, numerous perceptual studies have been undertaken using a variety of methods which have been reviewed and the conclusion drawn that anorexic patients overestimate their body width more often than normal controls. These distorted attitudes are often associated with a negative affect, so that the disturbance might be viewed as one of 'body disparagement'.[74]

The patient's dread of fatness is so common that it is pathognomonic of anorexia nervosa. There are, however, exceptions. Sometimes a patient may simply deny these faulty attitudes. Another exception is the occurrence of anorexia nervosa in Eastern countries where thinness is not generally admired (e.g. Hong Kong and India). The imposition of fear of fatness as a diagnostic criterion on patients from a different culture, where slimness is not valued, may amount to a contextual fallacy, i.e. a failure to understand the illness in the context of its culture.[75]

Depression

Depression of varying severity, including major depressive disorders, is common. The patients express guilt after eating, adding that they do not deserve to have food. A high rate of depression (42 per cent) was found at presentation in one study[24] and the lifetime history of depression in follow-up studies may be as high as 68 per cent.

Obsessive–compulsive features

The patients frequently eat in a ritualistic way, for example restricting their food intake to a narrow range of foods which experience tells them are 'safe' because they will not lead to weight gain. There is often a compulsive need to count the daily caloric intake. One patient rejected prescribed vitamin tablets in case they contained 'calories'. The frequency of obsessive–compulsive disorder in anorexia nervosa was found to be 22 per cent in a clinical series.[24] In studies using structured clinical interviews the frequency ranges from 25 to 70 per cent.

Neuropsychological deficits

These deficits are seldom detected clinically, and an emaciated patient may pursue studies and obtain surprisingly good examination marks. On the other hand, neuropsychological testing has revealed deficits in attention, and impairment of memory and visuospatial function.[76]

The endocrine disorder

The impairment of hypothalamic–pituitary–gonadal function

Amenorrhoea is an early symptom of anorexia nervosa and in a minority of patients may even precede the onset of weight loss. Amenorrhoea is an almost necessary criterion for the diagnosis of anorexia nervosa. An exception is when a patient takes a contraceptive pill which in fact replaces some of the hormonal deficit and may lead her to say she still has her periods.

Generally, when the patient is undernourished, levels of gonadotrophins and oestrogens in the blood are found to be low or undetectable.[77] Not only do malnourished patients show low blood levels of luteinizing hormone and follicle-stimulating hormone, but the secretion patterns of these pituitary hormones regress to patterns of earlier development. For example, severely wasted patients display an infantile luteinizing hormone secretory pattern with a lack of major fluctuations over the course of 24 h. With some degree of weight gain a pubertal secretory pattern appears, consisting first of a sleep-dependent increase of luteinizing hormone at night, and later displaying more frequent fluctuations.[78] When a patient is still malnourished the ultrasound pelvic examination will reveal that ovarian volume is much smaller than in normal women.[79] Three stages can be discerned in the appearance of the ovaries as the patient gains weight:

(1) small amorphous ovaries;

(2) multifollicular ovaries (with cysts 3–9 mm in diameter);

(3) dominant follicle (10 mm or more in diameter).

At the same time there is a corresponding return of hormonal secretion; follicle-stimulating hormone appears first, followed by luteinizing hormone and finally oestradiol which leads to enlargement of the uterus.[80]

These abnormalities signify that the patient is infertile and remains so until endocrine function recovers. Pregnancy occasionally occurs as the patient is still underweight and improving but before the appearance of the first menstrual period.[81] The pregnancy carries a risk of poor fetal growth during the first trimester, albeit with some 'catch-up' growth during the neonatal period.[82] Occasionally an underweight anorexic patient may seek treatment at an infertility clinic. Treatment with gonadotrophin-releasing hormone may restore fertility, but this practice has been severely criticized.[83]

Hypothalamic–pituitary–adrenal and hypothalamic–pituitary–thyroid axes

The emaciated anorexic patient shows an increased 24-h plasma cortisol level which returns to normal with a minimal increase in weight, as it is the nutritional intake that is critical.[84]

Reduced tri-iodothyronine (T_3) levels are linked to a reduction in energy expenditure during starvation and are adaptive in nature, so that substitution of thyroid hormone is not appropriate in anorexia nervosa.[78]

Weight loss and malnutrition

Body weight

The severity of weight loss may be recorded as follows.

1. As a percentage of an 'average' body weight to be found in tables for normal populations according to age and height (e.g. the *Metropolitan Life Insurance Tables*).

2. As a percentage drop from the patient's own weight before the onset of her illness (her 'healthy' weight).

3. Using the Quetelet body mass index

$$BMI = \frac{weight \ (kg)}{(height \ (m))^2}.$$

A BMI between 20 and 25 is regarded as healthy. A BMI of 15 or less indicates a need for hospitalization. A BMI between 10 and 12 represents the lower limit of human survival.

Physical examination

Wasting is variable but may be extremely severe, resulting in a skull-like appearance of the head, stick-like limbs, and flat breasts, buttocks, and abdomen. The hands and feet feel cold and readily turn blue in winter. The skin is dry with an excess of downy hair (lanugo) covering the cheeks, the nape of the neck, the forearms, and the legs. Heartbeat is slow (50–60 beats/min) and the blood pressure is low (e.g. 90/60 mmHg) with orthostatic lability. During the routine physical examination muscle power should be tested to detect proximal myopathy, as explained below.

Differential diagnosis of classical anorexia nervosa

The diagnosis of anorexia nervosa is usually straightforward, especially as the modern diagnostic criteria are objective. Wasting diseases such as inflammatory bowel disease (Crohn's disease or ulcerative colitis), thyrotoxicosis, and diabetes mellitus may sometimes be mistaken for anorexia nervosa, but they can be identified through specific investigations. Occasionally there is an interaction between such a medical illness and anorexia nervosa, when a patient wishes to perpetuate the weight loss caused by the former. Rarely, anorexia nervosa may be mimicked by a cerebral tumour altering the function of the hypothalamus.

In middle-aged or older patients there may be diagnostic difficulty with a major depressive or schizophrenic illness. The weight loss in a severe depressive illness results from loss of appetite and the patient's ideas that she does not deserve food. A schizophrenic patient may avoid food because of paranoid delusions of being poisoned.

Complications of malnutrition

The complications which are part of the illness, such as amenorrhoea due to hypothalamic–pituitary–gonadal axis failure, have already been discussed. The range of medical complications has been extensively reviewed,[84,85] with recommendations for the investigations needed on presentation of the patient.

Fluid and electrolyte disturbances and cardiovascular complications

Patients who induce vomiting, abuse laxatives, or take diuretics are likely to experience dehydration and various electrolyte disturbances.

Self-induced vomiting

Loss of gastric acid leads to a metabolic alkalosis and hypokalaemia. A low serum level of potassium may lead to cardiac conduction defects and arrhythmias, skeletal muscle weakness, and renal tubular dysfunction.

Laxative abuse

The abuse of laxatives is likely to cause dehydration, metabolic acidosis, hyponatraemia, and hypokalaemia.

The use of diuretics

The use of diuretics such as the thiazide group gives rise to low serum sodium levels which in turn cause fatigue and general weakness. A level below 120 mmol/l may lead to coma. The patient often justifies the use of a diuretic as a treatment for swollen ankles or even 'bloating' of the stomach, which she misinterprets as being due to fluid retention.

Impaired renal function

This may be caused by different mechanisms: pre-renal failure due to dehydration or hypokalaemic nephropathy.

Peripheral oedema

Fluid retention leading to oedema occurs frequently in patients with anorexia nervosa. It is important to distinguish between 'benign' oedema, which often occurs during the course of effective refeeding, and oedema from other causes which may have serious consequences.

'Benign' oedema

'Benign' oedema may occur during inpatient treatment. If the patient accepts a high caloric intake, fluid retention is the rule as shown by a steep upward rise in the weight curve. Peripheral oedema is aggravated by venous stasis in patients who walk about the ward or remain standing for long periods.

Famine oedema

If oedema is detected when the patient first presents clinically, or if it develops without a preceding improvement in food intake, the underlying mechanisms should be carefully investigated in order to avoid the risks of congestive cardiac failure and pulmonary oedema. By the time peripheral oedema is detectable, the amount of fluid retained in the body contributes several kilograms to the patient's weight, thereby concealing the true loss of weight. There is a common misconception that peripheral oedema is usually due to a lowering of plasma albumen, but this is uncommon in anorexia nervosa. Therefore the clinician must look for other reasons.

1. A fall in interstitial fluid pressure has been proposed whereby water seeps from the blood into the interstitial spaces[86] whereas the total exchangeable sodium is likely to remain within the normal range.

2. 'Rebound' oedema following hyponatraemia due to abuse of laxatives or diuretics.

3. Wet beri-beri: vitamin deficiency in anorexia nervosa is uncommon because many patients continue to eat vegetables and fruit. Nevertheless a lack of vitamin B_1 (thiamine) may occur in patients who eat a stereotyped diet, and Wernicke's encephalopathy may follow.[87] Vitamin B_1 deficiency may also manifest itself in congestive cardiac failure with severe oedema from a nutritional cardiomyopathy, precipitated by refeeding without thiamine.

4. Congestive heart failure and pulmonary oedema may occur as a result of general undernutrition leading to a decreased cardiac mass, cardiac output, and volume.

Metabolic disturbances

Hypoglycaemia

Severe hypoglycaemia with plasma glucose levels as low as 1.0 mmol/l is rare in anorexia nervosa but is recognized as a cause of death. Hypoglycaemia may go unrecognized, as a lack of sympathetic nervous response may mask the classical symptoms and signs.

Hypercarotenaemia

This is a benign condition causing an orange-yellow coloration of the skin of the palms, soles, forearms, and the region of the nose. It is partly due to the consumption of large amounts of foods rich in carotenoids, especially carrots, tomatoes, and the green outer leaves of vegetables.

Myopathy

Weakness of specific muscle groups is common and is due to severe protein-energy malnutrition. There is a 'proximal' myopathy, affecting the musculature of the pelvic girdle and the shoulder girdle. The patient first notices an increasing difficulty in climbing stairs. Weakness may also affect the muscles of the head and neck. When the patient is asked to rise from a sitting position, she will tend to push herself up using her hands and arms. She also has difficulty in rising unaided from a squatting position.[88]

There are no characteristic abnormalities in blood chemistry, although creatine kinase and liver enzymes may be elevated and the activity of enzyme carnosinase may be reduced. Myopathic changes are consistently present in muscle biopsy specimens. Histology reveals the 'chequerboard' distribution of muscle fibres but with a selective type 2 fibre atrophy. Electron microscopy reveals the presence of strikingly abundant glycogen granules between the myofibrils and under the sarcolemma.[88]

The detection of myopathy is a clear indication for the patient's admission to hospital and a refeeding programme. After a weight gain of a few kilograms her muscle strength will begin to return and a complete recovery is the rule.

Osteoporosis

A high proportion of patients with anorexia nervosa risk developing osteoporosis and consequent pathological fractures. Significant reduction in bone mineral density of the femoral neck was found in all 20 patients with anorexia nervosa of 6 years or more duration.[89] The favourite method of measuring bone density in the lumbar spine and hip is by dual-energy X-ray absorptiometry. A measurement for all patients with anorexia nervosa of 2 years duration or more is recommended.[90] It is difficult to disentangle the harmful effect of the nutritional deficiency itself from the associated oestrogen deficiency. It is likely that the pathogenesis of osteoporosis in anorexia nervosa differs from that in postmenopausal women. In anorexia nervosa the nutritional deficiency (often including a lack of calcium and vitamin D) leads to a low rate of the recycling of bone through bone formation and resorption, but the balance is disturbed by a relative increase in bone resorption.

On the whole the evidence favours the likelihood of improvement of bone density with nutritional recovery and resumption of menstruation.[89] There is much uncertainty about the best treatment. Although patients are often automatically prescribed oestrogen replacement, the only controlled trial undertaken so far indicated that oestrogen was only effective in severely underweight anorexic patients.[91] Indeed, it has been argued that oestrogen replacement could be harmful in some patients (children with premenarchal onset) and unnecessary in others with an illness of less than 3 years duration.[90] Instead the emphasis should be on encouraging weight gain, with the possible addition of calcium and vitamin D. There is a wider acceptance that patients with a poor prognosis (e.g. who have been ill over 10 years) might benefit from oestrogen replacement.

Disturbed temperature regulation

Disturbances in the control of temperature are evident from clinical observations; the patients frequently complain of feeling cold, and in the winter they have cold and blue extremities and suffer from chilblains. In the severely malnourished patient hypothermia may be a cause of death. Severe malnutrition is accompanied by a low central body temperature, presumably because of a low metabolic rate. Ingestion of a high-calorie meal can cause a significant increase in the central body temperature[92] which causes some patients to complain of heat in the periphery and sweating after food.

Haematological changes

Anorexic patients may develop a significantly lowered haemoglobin level and a reduced haematocrit and white cell count, with a relative decrease in neutrophil leucocytes and an increase in lymphocytes.[93] The anaemia is usually moderate and is normocytic normochromic in type. The mechanism is that of starvation-induced bone marrow hypoplasia. Only occasionally is there an iron deficiency. The anaemia gradually becomes corrected with weight gain. A low platelet count in the blood has also been observed and there may be an associated thrombocytopenic purpura.

Complications arising during rapid refeeding

Acute dilatation of the stomach.

This complication has also been described in anorexia nervosa during the course of refeeding.[94] The patient develops copious vomiting, upper abdominal pain, distension of the upper abdomen, and rapid dehydration. Treatment is by continuous gastric aspiration, and this complication is one of the rare indications for intravenous infusions of glucose and saline. Gastric dilation is best prevented by avoiding a food intake above 2000 cal daily during the first week of refeeding.

Hypophosphataemia

When the illness has been protracted and has led to severe emaciation, the body stores of phosphate become depleted. The fall in serum phosphate is aggravated during refeeding, especially parenteral feeding.[95] Levels of phosphate may fall as low as 0.2 mmol/l. Clinical features are cardiac irregularities with a prolonged QT interval, impairment of consciousness, and delirium. Treatment is with oral phosphates rather than by intravenous administration.

Anorexic mothers as parents

A patient who is improving may conceive despite having a suboptimal weight and still not menstruating.[81] A mother may also develop the illness after having borne children. In a series of eight mothers, nine out of 13 of their children suffered from food deprivation, identified by reductions in weight for age and in height for age as shown on Tanner–Whitehouse charts.[96] The anorexic mothers had no intention of abusing the children and indeed were affectionate towards them. They adopted different ways to ration their children's food intake according to their age. They might prolong breast feeding, dilute the bottle feeds, reduce the amount of food available in the home, confine eating to meal times, forbid the consumption of sweets, and prevent others giving them food. The privation of the children resulted from the anorexic mothers' abnormal concern with body size being extended to their children. An important part of the management was the recognition of the children at risk through tactful enquiries. A whole-family approach should be adopted, focusing on the children's needs for food. The children should be followed up to ensure that they gain weight and catch-up growth is established.[96]

Similar findings have been described by other authors.[83] An elegant observational method has been applied to mothers found to have an eating disorder during the postnatal year.[97] They were video recorded while feeding their 1-year-old infants. In comparison with controls, infants of these mothers were found to be lighter, with the weight being inversely related to both the amount of conflict during meal times and the mother's concern about her own shape. The mother's concern about her body shape led her to want a thinner child.

Anorexia nervosa of early onset

It would be too arbitrary to define an early onset by age limits such as an onset from 8 to 16 years. A more meaningful frame of reference is the onset in relation to the stage of puberty which has been reached by the child.[98] Because puberty is a complex developmental process spanning 2 to 3 years, it is best to name as 'premenarchal' the illness which commences some time after the first signs of puberty and before its completion, as shown by the first menstrual period. In true prepubertal anorexia nervosa the illness begins even earlier, before the very first signs of puberty. Postpubertal anorexia nervosa is when the illness commences after menstruation has been established.

There is much similarity between the clinical features of an illness of early onset and one which is postpubertal. However, there are two important differences. The first is the potential for the illness to interfere with the child's pubertal development. The second is the impact of an early onset with particularly heart-rending consequences for the child's family. It follows that the management of the family is of supreme importance, and the clinician should be prepared for parental reactions which may sometimes detract from a rational plan of treatment.

The clinical presentation is variable. Often there are precipitating events such as a family bereavement or a physical illness leading to weight loss. The onset is likely to be insidious[22], with the parents noticing nothing amiss except for non-specific features, which are nevertheless important. Symptoms of depression and irritability are common.[16,99] Some children cannot describe feelings of depression, but tearfulness may be obvious. They withdraw from friends and may refuse to go to school. Others express ideas of being undeserving of love or food. Increasingly these youngsters have been found to injure themselves, especially by scratching with their nails or cutting the skin of the wrists and forearms with sharp objects, and occasionally by knocking and bruising the head. In a severe depression the child may say she hears voices calling her 'bad', but further questioning indicates that these are not true hallucinations but vivid expressions of her own thoughts. Another common presentation is with complaints of bodily symptoms, especially headaches, abdominal discomfort, and a wide range of gastrointestinal symptoms, which inevitably elicit physical investigations.

At some stage, however, the parents observe that their child is avoiding food and is reluctant to eat at normal meal times. She resorts to deviousness and secrecy. The omission of school meals often goes undetected. Eventually it is noticed that she has become thinner and may have lost a great deal of weight. Resistance is met when attempts are made to reverse the loss of weight. Even a young child may become preoccupied with the caloric values of foods. Methods of inducing weight loss additional to food avoidance may become evident. The child is likely to exercise excessively—jogging, walking, or cycling long distances. An attempt to reduce the excess activity may lead to solitary exercising in the bedroom, including press-ups or running on the spot. Other patients may induce vomiting or take laxatives even after small meals, but overeating typical of bulimia nervosa is rare in young children.[100]

Weight loss

Because of the early onset while the child should still be growing in stature, there is a failure to gain the weight which normally accompanies the growth spurt. Later there occurs an actual loss of weight and, because the child has not yet reached her optimum weight, a very low weight indeed may result—25 kg or even less. Symptoms of malnutrition ensue including tiredness, constipation, and sensitivity to cold with cold extremities.

The psychological disorder

Even younger children are likely to disclose that they are fearful of becoming fat, a disturbance similar to the overvalued idea held by older patients. A minority of patients will disclose their reluctance to develop personal, sexual, or social maturity, in a manner which fits into Crisp's model. A few may express reluctance to have menstrual periods. A girl may say she is indifferent whether she menstruates or not, but would like to develop breasts so as not to lag behind other girls in her class. The reluctance to 'grow up' may be expressed in social terms, with the patient saying that she could not imagine herself ever leaving home or her mother. On the other hand most girls are keen to reach a normal stature.

Severe depression was found in 69 per cent of youngsters in the Göteborg study.[16] In the same series one-third of the patients had an obsessive–compulsive personality disorder, and 8 per cent developed hand-washing and other compulsions.

Physical examination

Physical examination will reveal a varying degree of wasting, affecting the limbs, the abdomen, the buttocks, and the facial appearance. The extremities are blue and cold, and ischaemic changes may lead to gangrene affecting the toes. Other physical changes are similar to those in the adult, except for the addition of a delay in puberty.

Delay or arrest of puberty

The illness may adversely affect pubertal development depending on its time of onset. If the onset is truly prepubertal the child will not yet have shown the first signs of puberty, such as the appearance of pubic hair and breast buds. When the illness begins during the course of puberty these early signs may have appeared, but the breasts will show early growth only (Tanner stages 1 or 2), and the child will not yet have menstruated. The effects on pubertal development can be divided into those affecting growth and stature, breast development, and menstrual function.[98]

1. **Growth in stature** may have become arrested. In a series of 20 patients with a premenarchal onset, only two of them had reached the 50th centile in height. With successful treatment and weight gain, catch-up growth of 2 to 5 cm may be achieved, but only in patients aged 17 or less.[98]

2. **Breast development**: in the same series only six patients had normal breasts and as many as 10 had infantile breasts. After prolonged weight gain, eight of the 14 patients showed a considerable response in breast growth.[98]

3. **Menstrual function**: a prepubertal or premenarchal onset of the illness will cause a delay in the onset of menstruation, defined as primary amenorrhoea. In the series already referred to only four of the 20 patients had menstruated by the age of 16 years. A further three began their periods between 16 and 18 years of age, and four at ages ranging from 18 to 25. The remaining patients had prolonged amenorrhoea.

The above series consisted of selected patients in whom pubertal delay was severe, whereas marked pubertal delay has seldom been reported in other series in which only delayed menstruation has been remarked upon.

A young boy who develops anorexia nervosa is also likely to become preoccupied with fatness and accordingly avoids food in order to lose weight. The endocrine disorder in the male similarly consists of a disturbance of the hypothalamic–pituitary–gonadal axis. With a prepubertal onset, the penis and scrotum remain infantile, there is only a scanty growth of pubic and facial hair, and the voice may not break.

Special investigations

Pelvic ultrasound monitoring of the ovaries and uterus is a useful method of ascertaining regression and recovery in children with anorexia nervosa.[101] On first testing, and in the presence of low weight and amenorrhoea, ovarian volume and uterine volume were found to be reduced in comparison with normal pubertal girls. In the latter the normal range of ovarian volume is 3.95 ± 1.7 cm[3] and uterine volume is 14.8 ± 7.6 cm.[3] On retesting the patients 18 months after the first scan those who were menstruating showed significantly larger ovarian and uterine volumes than those with amenorrhoea. The authors concluded that for ovarian and uterine maturity to occur it is necessary to achieve a mean weight of 48 kg and a mean weight-to-height ratio of 96.5 per cent, higher targets than are usually set. They also found that pelvic ultrasound scanning helped to motivate the children to accept a higher body weight.

Differential diagnosis of early-onset anorexia nervosa

Frequent bodily complaints, loss of weight, and abnormalities of growth lead these children to be referred to paediatricians for special investigations. It has been proposed that young anorexic boys should be investigated by means of neuroimaging, so as not to miss occult intracranial tumours masquerading as early anorexia nervosa.[61] The diagnosis of anorexia nervosa should be distinguished from atypical eating disorders in childhood.[99]

1. **Pervasive refusal syndrome** is characterized by a child, usually aged between 11 and 15, refusing to eat, drink, walk, talk, or take care of herself. Anxiety, phobic responses, and depression are also present.

2. **Selective eating** is the term applied to a child who restricts food intake to two or three different foods, such as biscuits, crisps, or potatoes, but usually remains in good health.

3. **Food avoidance emotional disorder**: this condition is one in which food avoidance is attributable to an emotional disturbance in the absence of a dread of fatness, a necessary criterion for the diagnosis of anorexia nervosa.

4. **Food fads and food refusal**: the refusal to eat is usually intermittent and physical health is not compromised.

Classification

ICD-10[102] (including patients with premenarchal onset[98])

1. Body weight is maintained at least 15 per cent below that expected for health. Prepubertal children may fail to gain the weight expected during the growth spurt. Weight loss is caused by avoidance of 'fattening' foods, possibly with the addition of self-induced vomiting, purgative abuse, excessive exercise, or the use of appetite suppressants.

2. The patient holds the overvalued idea of a dread of fatness and keeps her weight below a self-imposed threshold.

3. There is an endocrine failure manifest in women as amenorrhoea and in men as a loss of sexual interest and potency.

4. If the onset is premenarchal, the sequence of pubertal events is delayed: growth is arrested; in girls the breasts do not develop and

there is a primary amenorrhoea; in boys the genitals remain juvenile.

DSM-IV[103]

1. Refusal to maintain body weight above the minimally normal weight for age and height (e.g. weight less than 85 per cent of that expected).

2. Intense fear of gaining weight or becoming fat, even though underweight.

3. Disturbance in the way in which one's body weight or shape is experienced.

4. In postmenarchal females, there is amenorrhoea of at least three menstrual cycles.

DSM-IV subdivides anorexia nervosa as follows.

1. Restricting type, without regular binge-eating or 'purging' behaviour (in the United States this term includes self-induced vomiting and the misuse of diuretics as well as laxatives).

2. Binge-eating/purging type.

Anorexia nervosa in males

The relative rarity of anorexia nervosa in the male might lead one to surmise that the disorder is likely to differ between the sexes in its aetiology, clinical manifestations, and prognosis. The first study that examined this premise in a sizeable series of male patients found remarkable similarities between the sexes as regards the age of onset and the specific features of the psychopathology.[104] For example, the male patients tended to select a diet which was low in fattening foods and resorted to subterfuges to dispose of food, such as self-induced vomiting and purging, and strenuous exercising. They expressed a fear of fatness and considered themselves overweight, even when they were thin. Other investigators were also struck by these surprising similarities.[105]

Of course there are fundamental biological differences which inevitably alter the manifestations of the endocrine disorder in the male and, to a lesser extent, the nutritional disorder. Testicular function, as gauged by the urinary output of testosterone, is disturbed in male patients when they are emaciated. Refeeding leads to at least a partial correction of this abnormality.[104] The body composition of the mature male differs from that in the female; he has a lower reserve of adipose tissue so that protein depletion occurs more rapidly when he loses weight.

The relative resistance of the male against developing anorexia nervosa remains a mystery. It is even unclear whether the sex difference is likely to be due to biomedical factors or psychosocial differences. It has been suggested that young females often become preoccupied with 'fatness' because of its reproductive, biological, and social significance, whereas young males are more concerned with their musculature and its significance for strength, dominance, and masculinity.[105] These differences are linked with the frequency of dieting among adolescent girls and its rarity in boys.[106]

In a series of male patients with 'primary' anorexia nervosa most of the patients reported problems with sexuality.[107] Sexual anxieties had been present with respect to heterosexual as well as homosexual behaviour. One quarter had had homosexual contacts or admitted homosexual tendencies. Almost all were relieved by the loss of libido following weight loss. The authors concluded that males with atypical gender role behaviour had an increased risk for developing anorexia nervosa in adolescence.

There are only a few follow-up studies of anorexia nervosa in males. In the best study available, 27 patients were followed up for a minimum of 2 years and a mean of 8 years.[106] Expressed in the terms of the Morgan–Russell categories of general outcome, a good outcome was found in 44 per cent, an intermediate outcome in 26 per cent, a poor outcome in 30 per cent, and no deaths. Only a few predictors of outcome were identified: disturbed relationships with a parent in childhood led to a poor outcome, and the occurrence of previous sexual activity was associated with a good outcome. The outcome in males was remarkably similar to that in females.[106]

Course and prognosis

The natural outcome is defined as the long-term results of the illness or disease process. The clinical prognosis is the difficult task of forecasting the future course and final outcome of the illness in an individual patient.

Outcomes from follow-up studies in anorexia nervosa

There have been comprehensive appraisals of follow-up studies in anorexia nervosa[108] which have put forward criteria for the near-perfect follow-up study, which in practice are seldom fully met. Among the easier criteria are precision in the diagnostic features, the use of standardized interviews, 100 per cent success in tracing the patients, and a sufficiently long follow-up to determine eventual outcome. An arbitrary interval of at least 4 years was previously set[24] and most recent studies have adhered to this recommendation. Several groups of investigators have adopted the same measures of outcome based on the Morgan–Russell scales.[109] Their use gives rise to three possible categories of general outcome based on body weight and menstrual function: 'good', 'medium', and 'poor'.

In a review comparing three British studies and one Swedish study,[110] each with a mean follow-up of 5 to 6 years, it was found that the patients treated in Bristol had a better outcome than those treated at the Maudsley Hospital in London. The explanation is one of selection bias already mentioned: the Maudsley patients had all required inpatient treatment, whereas in the Bristol series the majority were outpatients. The third British study, from St George's Hospital, London, showed a quality of outcome intermediate between the other two.

The Swedish study was extended by two later follow-ups at 15 and 33 years, and showed a trend in two directions. On the one hand, the percentage of good outcomes gradually increased, while the percentage of poor outcomes diminished. On the other hand, the death rates increased with time; after 33 years the total mortality from anorexia nervosa or suicide was 18 per cent. Slow recovery was the rule: only 29 per cent of patients recovered in less than 3 years of illness, another 35 per cent within 3 to 6 years, and the remainder took much longer with recovery after 12 years being rare.[110] The Maudsley series of patients was also extended to a mean follow-up of 20 years. There was a reduction in the percentage of patients with a poor outcome, but an increase in the mortality rate close to that of the Swedish study.[111]

Prognostic predictors of outcome

In the long-term Maudsley study a poorer outcome was predicted by an older age of onset, a longer duration of illness, the presence of neurotic traits in childhood, personality problems, and the occurrence of relationship difficulties within the family.[111]

Comparison of mortality rates

In a review of 42 studies the aggregate annual mortality rate from anorexia nervosa was found to reach 0.56 per cent on average.[112] Complications of anorexia nervosa accounted for 54 per cent of deaths, suicide for 27 per cent, and other causes for 19 per cent. When the death rate is expressed as a percentage per annum a fair measure of consistency has been found in different parts of the world, especially when allowance is made for selection biases: in Denmark 0.5 per cent per annum (younger patients),[113] in Sweden 0.75 per cent per annum,[110] in the United States 0.66 per cent per annum,[114] and in the United Kingdom 0.75 per cent per annum.[111]

Follow-up studies in early-onset anorexia nervosa

In a series of 34 children with a mean age of onset of 11.7 years treated at Great Ormond Street Hospital, London, a good outcome was obtained in 60 per cent, but there was a mortality rate of 7 per cent over a mean follow-up of 7.2 years.[115] In a series of 60 patients in Berlin with a mean age of onset of 14.7, followed up for at least 4 years, recovery occurred in 68 per cent of patients but there was a 6.6 per cent mortality over a mean of 4.8 years.[116] In both studies a somewhat higher mortality rate was found than in the Danish study already mentioned.

Conclusions

Theander[117] has provided good advice and useful definitions:

> Clinical experience has repeatedly shown that patients with anorexia nervosa can recover after a period of illness amounting to more than ten years.

> A distinction should be made between a 'chronic' illness and a long-standing illness. The word 'chronic' should be restricted to a continuous illness of more than 15 years' duration because up to then the patient is still capable of a full recovery. The term 'protracted' is preferable for an illness of prolonged duration but not as long as 15 years.

Treatment

Review of evidence

There have been regrettably few controlled trials evaluating the effectiveness of treatment in anorexia nervosa. This contrasts with a much larger number of controlled studies in bulimia nervosa. The reasons are not surprising. Most controlled trials in anorexia nervosa encounter serious practical and ethical difficulties arising from the severity and prolonged nature of the illness, and a variable compliance on the part of patients.

Inpatient treatment

Treatment as an inpatient in a specialized eating disorder unit is most likely to restore the patient's weight to a near-normal level within 3 months or less. There have been no controlled studies comparing different treatment programmes. A possible exception is a study comparing a strict operant conditioning programme while refeeding the patients with a 'lenient' programme which was introduced later.[118] No significant difference was found in the rate of weight gain between the two treatments. The value of a specialized eating disorder unit in inducing weight gain has been demonstrated from a series of 17 patients admitted to the Maudsley Unit in 1990. They had previously been admitted elsewhere and information on their previous weights was obtained. In the case of the Maudsley admissions the mean weight rose from 65.8 per cent average body weight (ABW) to 90.4 per cent ABW; in comparison the admissions elsewhere only led to a mean weight rise from 64.4 to 75 per cent ABW.

Day hospital treatment

Once again there is a paucity of controlled trials of day programmes. An exception is the comparison of inpatient and day treatment carried out in Edinburgh.[119] A traditional inpatient programme, aimed strictly at weight gain, was compared with a more permissive day programme stressing open communication and patient autonomy. The day programme consisted of intensive psychological treatments and was available on 4 days each week. Thirty-two patients who would have merited admission to hospital were randomly allocated to the day programme or the inpatient programme. Although statistically significant differences were not found between the two methods of treatment, the author reported interesting trends as gauged by the categories of outcome using the Morgan–Russell scales. The only advantage conferred by inpatient treatment was a slightly greater weight gain. In contrast, the day programme was more popular with the patients who preferred to have a greater say in the rate of weight gain. There was also an impression of a greater return of personal autonomy in the day-patients. A criticism of this study is that the two programmes were imperfectly matched in terms of the therapeutic input and enthusiasm of the two teams.

Comparison of outpatient treatments and hospital admission

An ambitious study, conducted at St George's Hospital, London, aimed at evaluating the advantages of different treatment settings[120]. There were three treatment groups and one control group:

(1) inpatient treatment on average lasting 4 months, followed by 12 sessions of outpatient psychotherapy;

(2) outpatient treatment combining individual and family therapy over the course of 12 sessions spanning several months;

(3) outpatient group therapy consisting of 10 group meetings for the patients and 10 group meetings for the parents separately at monthly intervals;

(4) a control group who were given only a 'one-off' but detailed evaluation.

The two outpatient treatment groups received in addition four sessions of dietary counselling.

Ninety patients were randomly allocated to one or other of the four treatment options above. The authors have stressed the serious methodological difficulties. Patients might drop out of the treatment when it did not conform with what they wanted; for example, out of

30 patients offered inpatient treatment, only 18 accepted it. Among the 20 patients allocated to a one-off evaluation, the majority sought treatment elsewhere.

The patients' progress was re-evaluated at the end of 1 year. The clearest finding was that patients allocated to any one of the three active treatment options fared better than those allocated to the one-off evaluation session. There were fewer clear-cut differences between the patients in the three different treatment groups. The inpatients tended to achieve a more rapid and higher weight gain towards the end of their admission, but at the 1-year follow-up the weights were similar in all three treatment groups. The patients' improvement in their socio-economic status was greatest in the individual–family therapy group.

Family therapy

Family therapy is the main treatment which has been evaluated in anorexia nervosa. A controlled trial of family therapy was undertaken at the Maudsley Hospital on a series of 57 patients.[121] The principles of the family therapy have been incorporated in the Maudsley model.[49] One assumption is that the family is ineffective in helping the patient eliminate her symptoms, or might contribute to their maintenance. It was also considered essential to correct the patient's starvation by assisting the parents to take control jointly of their child's eating until her weight had returned to normal. The effects of the family therapy were compared with a control individual therapy. In order to reduce any ethical objections to the random allocation to two different treatments, the risks were minimized by first ensuring that the patients' weight loss had been corrected by admission to the Eating Disorders Unit. The trial was of outpatient family therapy administered for 1 year. The patients were assessed after treatment for 1 year and 5 years later by a researcher who was not involved in the treatment.[121,122]

In order to increase the homogeneity of the groups undergoing treatment, the patients were subdivided into three groups according to recognized prognostic criteria.

- Group 1: age of onset less than 19 years, duration of illness less than 3 years.

- Group 2: age of onset less than 19 years, duration more than 3 years.

- Group 3: age of onset 19 years or older.

After entry into the appropriate subgroup the patients were randomly allocated to one or other therapy.

The control treatment was a supportive and problem-centred individual therapy with elements of cognitive, interpretative, and strategic therapies. Body weight was recorded daily during inpatient treatment and at each subsequent outpatient attendance and during follow-up. The Morgan–Russell scales were utilized to obtain categories of general outcome and measures of adjustment along five dimensions: nutritional status, menstrual function, mental state, psychosexual adjustment, and socio-economic status. An 'average outcome score' was calculated as the mean of the scores on the five scales.

1. Group 1 (early age of onset, short history): a tendency for the patients to lose weight on discharge from hospital was reversed more readily in those who had been allocated to family therapy, and the superiority of family therapy was demonstrated by a higher weight at the end of treatment ($p < 0.02$) (Fig. 2). The

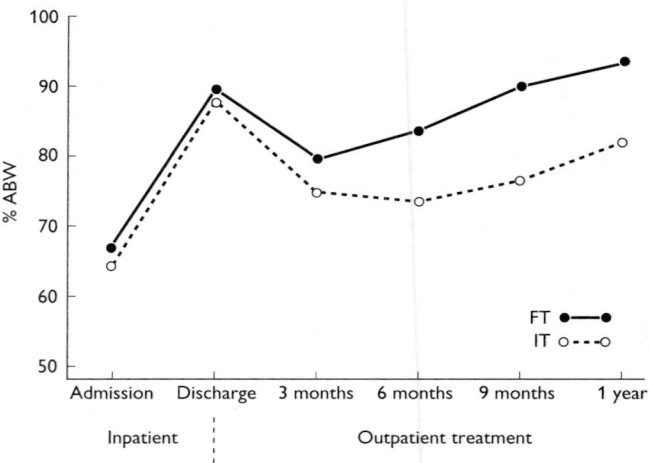

Fig. 2 Group of patients whose illness had an early onset and was of short duration. The mean weight charts are shown during inpatient treatment and thereafter when an outpatient psychotherapy is provided. FT, family therapy; IT, individual therapy; ABW, average body weight.

superiority of family therapy was also demonstrated on the Morgan–Russell scales in terms of more good outcome categories and a higher average outcome score.

2. Group 2 (early age of onset with long duration of illness): the effect of the two therapies did not differ significantly among these patients.

3. Group 3 (late age of onset): in this group of patients the effect of the two therapies was reversed (Fig. 3). Individual therapy led to a significantly greater weight gain when comparing levels at the 6-month follow-up.

From this study it can be concluded that family therapy was more effective than individual therapy in patients whose illness had begun before the age of 19 years and had lasted less than 3 years. A more tentative finding was the greater value of individual supportive therapy in older patients.

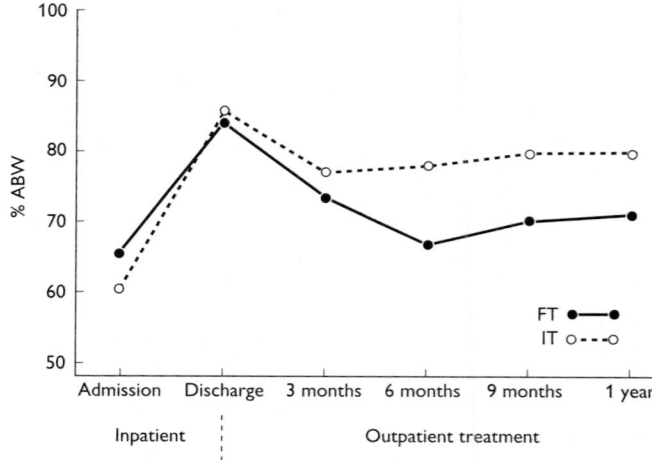

Fig. 3 Patients with a relatively late onset of anorexia nervosa. The mean weight charts are shown during inpatient treatment and thereafter when an outpatient psychotherapy is provided. FT, family therapy; IT, individual therapy; ABW, average body weight.

Enduring benefits from family therapy

The patients who took part in the original controlled trial of family therapy were followed up 5 years after the end of treatment, in order to determine the levels of improvement from the illness and any evidence of long-term benefit from family therapy.[122] Follow-up information was obtained on all 57 patients, but three had died.

The patients' clinical status was ascertained, as before, by their weight and their status on the Morgan–Russell scales. A good or intermediate outcome was found in 34 out of 54 patients at the 5-year follow-up compared with 22 out of 54 at the end of treatment. This overall improvement was mainly attributable to the natural outcome of anorexia nervosa. Within two of the patient groups, however, significant benefits attributable to the previous psychological treatments were still evident.

- Early-onset/short-history group: within this group the patients who had received family therapy achieved a mean weight of 103 per cent ABW, whereas those who had had individual therapy reached a mean weight of 94 per cent ABW. However, this difference was no longer statistically significant. On the Morgan–Russell scales a significant improvement after family therapy was still discernible in terms of the higher proportion of patients who had achieved a 'good' outcome and a higher average outcome score.

- Late-onset group: the late outcome of this group was better than expected, with almost three-quarters having a 'good' or 'intermediate' outcome. When comparing the effects of family and individual therapy, the results were similar to those found at the end of treatment. On the Morgan–Russell dimensional scales the patients who had been in individual therapy obtained a higher average outcome score.

In conclusion, the patients in the early-onset/short-history group showed the best outcome at the end of 5 years, as was predictable from these prognostic indicators. The more important finding was that the benefits of family therapy endured until the 5-year follow-up. Most of the patients with a late onset of illness progressed reasonably well and it was confirmed that the individual supportive therapy had conferred benefits still detectable at 5 years.

Components of family therapy found to the beneficial in adolescent patients

The finding that family therapy is effective in younger patients with anorexia nervosa has led to a search for the effective components of this therapy. Most family therapists consider that it is important to understand the way the family functions; however, some prefer a symptom-oriented approach with an emphasis on helping the parents to manage their child's problem.[49]

The relative importance of the two components of family therapy was investigated by comparing conjoint family therapy with family counselling.[123] In conjoint family therapy the whole family was seen together in the treatment sessions. In family counselling the parents were seen together and given advice on how best to manage their daughter's eating problem; the same therapist also saw the patient for counselling and support. In conjoint family therapy it is possible to observe and interpret family transactions. In family counselling, however, the therapist can only discuss ways in which the family might modify its behaviour but cannot intervene directly in the 'whole' family system. The two treatments share the therapeutic advice to sustain a united parental approach aimed at establishing control of their child's eating pattern. The design was that of an outpatient controlled clinical trial with random allocation between conjoint family therapy and family counselling.

It emerged that the benefits of conjoint family therapy and family counselling were similar, with considerable gains in weight. The family counselling actually produced a somewhat better weight gain, but the differences were not statistically significant. With both treatments there were considerable improvements in the Morgan–Russell average outcome scores when assessed at the end of 32 weeks' treatment. When separated according to the form of treatment the differences were not statistically significant. This finding suggests that the simpler family treatment—family counselling—is as effective as family therapy, at least as far as weight gain is concerned.

Advice on management

It is not possible for the clinician to confine his treatment of anorexia nervosa to those methods which have been proved to be effective.

Main obstacle to treatment: the patient's avoidance of treatment

The avoidance of treatment by the patient is part and parcel of anorexia nervosa. There have been attempts to predict the likely level of the patient's compliance with treatment. For example, a 'transtheoretical model of change' is aimed at improving the patient's motivation by overcoming ambivalence while at the same time avoiding confrontation.[124] Different stages in the patient's approach to treatment have been recognized: precontemplation, contemplation, preparation, action, maintenance, and relapse. Motivational enhancement therapy is at an early stage of development but a practical guide is available.[125]

At our present level of knowledge it is simplest to ascertain the patient's attitude to treatment through the mental state examination. A revealing question is to ask her at the initial interview what weight she would be willing to reach. At this stage it is best to refrain from challenging the patient's weight threshold, even though it will be well below a reasonable therapeutic goal. Having ascertained the limited degree of compliance on the patient's part, the clinician needs to develop a strategy to improve it gradually as treatment proceeds. It is poor clinical practice to place all the onus on the patient herself for accepting or rejecting a package of treatment at the first interview, or even at a later stage. 'Engaging' the patient in treatment is an essential part of most psychotherapeutic methods including cognitive-behavioural therapy.[126] Another tactic for improving the patient's co-operation is to enlist the help of close members of the family. In the case of young patients it is essential to form a therapeutic alliance with the parents. Young patients are likely in any case to require a form of family treatment.

The stepped-care approach

The principle of stepped-care is that with an early presentation of anorexia nervosa the clinician should first apply relatively simple remedies. Only if they fail should more vigorous and time-consuming treatments be provided. In practice, however, the patient who has avoided treatment as long as possible may first be seen when weight loss is already substantial and abnormal attitudes entrenched. If this happens it is not possible to follow a graduated sequence and a short cut may be needed to a more vigorous method including admission to hospital. Admission is also indicated in the presence of 'famine' oedema or proximal myopathy.

In the event of a truly early presentation it will be appropriate for the patient's treatment to be overseen by her general practitioner. A minimal approach should still include dietary education as to the value of nutritious (high-caloric) foods and forging an alliance with the patient's family. The patient should be asked to attend once a week to be weighed with the clear message that she must arrest the weight loss and gradually return to a healthy weight determined by the clinician and not by her.

Outpatient psychotherapies

In the event of a patient's weight loss not exceeding 20 per cent of her healthy weight, it may be possible to obtain a therapeutic response by outpatient treatment including attendance at non-specialist clinics in general psychiatry or child/adolescent psychiatry. The feasibility of this approach will depend on the availability of appropriate psychotherapeutic resources. The clinician should not imagine any conflict between the psychotherapeutic approach and weighing the patient. It is never justified to accept apparent compliance with psychotherapy if the patient's weight continues to decline.

Models of psychotherapy

Hilde Bruch: 'a sparrow in a golden cage'

Bruch developed her aetiological model of anorexia nervosa as the child becoming involved with her family in such a way that she fails to achieve a sense of independence. Thus a paralysing sense of ineffectiveness pervades all her thinking and activities. Bruch used this model to provide an entry into the psychotherapy. She engaged her patient in a dialogue which became central for the resolution of her conflicts. Patients are often receptive and reassured when the therapist does not criticize them for behaviours associated with their illness. They may even obtain a relief from the implication that in some way the families are to blame for the anorexia nervosa. Using this model the therapist will engage his patient in the therapeutic metaphor in which she is seen as 'a sparrow in a golden cage'. She is then encouraged to think of ways of fulfilling her own needs and desires, rather than relying on others, and seek an autonomy that frees her from the tyranny of anorexia nervosa.[25]

Crisp's model of anorexia nervosa as a flight from growth

Crisp has explained in detail how the programme of treatment is based on his model of anorexia nervosa as a refuge from puberty which the patient has found overwhelming. The youngster reverses her pubertal development by limiting her intake of food.[127,128] His treatment initially involves an intensive inpatient programme lasting 10 to 12 weeks followed by outpatient treatment for up to 6 years. The advantage of this extensive programme is that it enables the patient to accept gradually an increase in weight while facing up to the feelings of panic and helplessness that originally led her to arrest her puberty through self-starvation. This interpretation is presented to the patient and to her family so that they come to see the psychotherapy as a way of solving the problems.

The model is a useful one even within a more limited outpatient psychotherapeutic setting. Some patients will readily identify their distress when overwhelmed by powerful sexual feelings or when confronted with personal and social responsibilities perceived as the result of growing up. The aims of the psychotherapy are to support the patient while she is beginning to abandon the psychobiological regression of anorexia nervosa. In addition she is encouraged to broaden her perception of herself in ways that are no longer wholly dependent on her physical appearance but include an improved sense of competence and self-esteem. She is helped to tackle personal and social problems from which she had previously escaped so that she can address her own and her parents' concerns about sexuality.

Cognitive-behavioural therapy

Although a strictly cognitive-behavioural model for the aetiology of anorexia nervosa has not yet been recognized, a theory for faulty cognitions maintaining the illness has been put forward by Fairburn et al.[129] The argument for examining the role of faulty cognitions in anorexia nervosa is inescapable. The original description of perceptual and conceptual disturbances in anorexia nervosa was put forward by Bruch in 1962.[6] It was appreciated that faulty attitudes to body size contributed in part to the patient's determination to reduce her food intake and lose weight.[56] These observations led to the first development of a cognitive-behavioural therapy for anorexia nervosa.[130] Despite the appeal of a therapy based on a cognitive-behavioural approach, there have been virtually no controlled clinical trials of this therapy. The current evidence of its benefit relies therefore on clinical impressions and case reports.[126]

Cognitive-behavioural therapy has much in common with other methods of treatment including the refeeding programme which will be described under inpatient treatment. It relies on building a positive therapeutic alliance between therapist and patient.

The patient's weight and food intake is monitored at each session and she is told her weight at each session. She is encouraged to think of food as medication and to follow a meal plan. She is encouraged to keep a daily written record of all food and liquid consumed. The patient is educated in the disturbances of bodily and psychological function consequent on the state of starvation. The content of the therapy may be divided into two 'tracks'. The first track includes an examination of the behaviours adopted by the patient in order to reduce her weight or maintain it at a low level. The second track is more concerned with psychological themes such as self-esteem, perfectionism, interpersonal functioning, and family conflicts. By asking the patient to give her reasons for specific behaviours, the therapist discovers faulty beliefs and assumptions on her part. For example, the 'anorexic wish' is the patient's wish to recover from her disorder without gaining weight. She is gently persuaded that this is an impossible aim because her real psychological difficulties will remain inaccessible so long as her experiences are clouded by starvation and dieting. The patient also expresses a fear of 'losing control'. By 'losing control' she means that she will run the risk of overeating and become fat. It is explained to the patient that her rigid 'control' over eating deprives her completely of choice, and that far from being in control the reality is the converse. It is also useful for the therapist to analyse the pros and cons of maintaining the disorder of anorexia nervosa. She often feels more uncomfortable at confronting the hidden rewards of remaining thin, for example succeeding in losing weight when everyone else fails.

Having ascertained the particular meanings of attitudes and behaviours for the patient, she is helped to find more adaptive ways of achieving healthier goals, including more relaxed normal eating and weight gain.

Family treatments

Family therapy and family counselling have already been discussed, but additional practical advice will now be given.

Family therapy

The frequency of the sessions is determined by clinical need; it averaged 10.5 over the course of 1 year in the Maudsley trial. There are three stages to the therapy.

1. The first phase begins with a family meal. The parents are urged to identify their future joint attitude to the feeding pattern that should be adopted by their daughter. With a younger patient the therapist assumes that the parents would initially need to take control of their child's eating. With an older patient a preliminary discussion should lead to a decision either to control her eating or to adopt the attitude that her eating was none of their business.

2. During the second phase the parents are urged to be present together at each meal so that they can reinforce each other's efforts in the practical task of ensuring an improved food intake and a steady weight gain.

3. When the patient's weight is under control, responsibility for continued weight gain is handed back to her. Discussions can then commence on more normal family concerns. With an adolescent patient the main focus is on achieving increased autonomy. With an older patient the central theme is how to establish healthy relationships with her parents without the eating disorder as a medium for communication.

Family counselling

As in family therapy the parents are given direct advice on how to manage their daughter's eating problem. The patient herself is provided with individual educative therapy. The therapist provides counselling about abnormal attitudes to weight and emphasizes the weight issue until steady progress has been made.[123] This method is often preferred by the patient and her parents, largely because it is almost devoid of overt confrontation. It is also easier to gain access to the patient's fears and conflicts.

Day treatment

The Edinburgh controlled trial of a day-patient programme has already been discussed.[119] At the Toronto Hospital a day-hospital programme for eating disorders utilizing group treatment has been established since 1985.[131] The programme originally operated on 5 days each week, but since 1994 it has been reduced to 4 days per week. The goals are as follows:

(1) a normalization of disturbed eating behaviour and weight gain;

(2) the identification of psychological and familial processes that serve to perpetuate the eating disorder.

Two meals (lunch and dinner) and a snack are provided during the treatment hours. The staff take turns in supervising the patients during meal times. The psychological treatment consists of intensive group therapy divided between disturbed behaviours around eating and weight, and more general conflicts.

The clinical advantages of day treatment are a reduction in the dependence of patients who still have to maintain themselves in a functioning state outside the hospital. The group treatments carry the advantage of providing an atmosphere of mutual support while permitting interventions through group pressures. There are few contraindications to this treatment, but patients with medical or suicidal risks are admitted instead to inpatient care. For some patients day treatment does not provide as strong a sense of containment as might be found on an inpatient unit. When patients succeed in reducing their disturbed eating behaviours they may 'act out' by self-harm. The clinical staff may find their skills severely taxed by the continuous staff–patient interaction.

Inpatient treatment

At one time inpatient programmes were run on behavioural principles, but in recent years 'lenient' programmes have found favour.[118] The great advantage of treating a patient in a specialist eating disorders unit programme is the certainty that considerable benefit will accrue, including a substantial gain in weight, if the patient can be persuaded to remain in hospital.[132]

Nursing care

Inpatient treatment will include a wide range of psychotherapeutic interventions (individual, group, and family) as well as occupational therapy and an educational programme. But the sheet anchor of successful treatment is a well-trained nursing staff working as a team. The role of the medical staff is subsidiary and consists of maintaining a high level of expectation that the patient's weight will be restored to a normal (or healthy) level. It is necessary to give the nursing staff moral support so that they can develop their confidence and skills.

There are two main components to the nurses' treatment: their psychotherapeutic input and their supervisory role. The latter is less important and should never be draconian. The nursing team establish a relationship of trust with the patient. They get to know each patient as an individual with her own personal needs and concerns. The nurses should also be acutely aware of the anorexic patient's tendency to avoid food and to exercise excessively. It is preferable for the treatment programme to stress the supportive aspects of the nurse's relationship with her patient rather than the undoubted need for careful supervision. The nurse will come to rely on the daily weight record to monitor the success of her treatment as the weight chart should show a smoothly rising curve. All meals are taken in the ward; thus the anorexic patients constitute a group in which peer interactions take place. The meal is taken in the presence of one or more nurses also seated at the table. From the beginning of the treatment the patient learns that she is expected to consume all the food placed before her.

Dietary care

It is not only the patient who tends to underestimate the food requirements to restore her weight to normal. Metabolic studies have demonstrated that for each kilogram of weight gain a surplus calorie balance of 7500 cal is needed.[133] It is prudent to begin with a modest calorie intake of 1200 to 1500 cal daily during the first 7 days in order to avoid the rare but dangerous complication of acute gastric dilatation. Thereafter the caloric intake is gradually increased and may rise to 4000 cal daily. The best diet is that consisting of a wide range of foods avoiding any preferences for 'safe' foods and including carbohydrate and fat-containing foods. Concentrated foods (e.g. Build-up, Complan, Carnation Breakfast Food) added to milk may be used to achieve a high caloric intake. The aim is to achieve a positive energy balance of 1500 to 2250 cal daily, leading to a daily weight gain of 200 to 300 g.

Assessment of progress

Weighing should be a standardized daily procedure before breakfast after the patient has emptied her bladder and while she wears light night clothes. A paradoxical psychological improvement, with a diminution in concern with body size and shape, occurs with weight gain. The improvement is partly through the correction of malnutrition and partly the result of the 'exposure treatment' whereby the patient gradually accepts a higher body weight.

Drug treatment

Exceptionally the patient's tension and depression do not improve and there is a continued resistance to food. It may then be helpful to prescribe moderate doses of chlorpromazine (not more than 300 mg daily), carefully avoiding a fall in blood pressure which is a risk in the emaciated patient. In the case of persistent depression, treatment with an antidepressant may be indicated. However, antidepressants are often ineffective in the presence of malnutrition, and by themselves do not assist the patient to gain weight.

General measures

Inevitably the patient will find it irksome to forego home visits for the whole period of weight gain. Therefore interesting and therapeutic activities should be provided through group meetings, occupational therapy, and social interactions. Visiting is generally encouraged unless the patient's restlessness is such that visiting parents are subjected to emotional appeals to be taken home. They may then be asked to postpone their visits or reduce their duration.

The aim is to restore body weight to a healthy level within 8 to 10 weeks; a further period (usually 2 weeks) in hospital is needed to allow the patient to test her ability to maintain her weight by eating in the general dining room or at home on leave days. It is important to effect a smooth transition to further treatment as a day patient or out-patient.

Compulsory treatment in anorexia nervosa

The management of patients reluctant to accept essential therapeutic goals requires that they should be gradually engaged in a genuine alliance.[134] However, there remains a minority of patients with whom this strategy fails and whose health becomes endangered. For them, compulsory treatment should be considered. A compulsory admission to hospital is indicated not only when patients threaten suicide or suffer from a life-threatening malnutrition, but also when they fail to respond to simpler measures such as outpatient treatment or day care, or in the event of avoiding treatment altogether. Ill health persisting over the course of several months or the development of serious physical complications (e.g. water and electrolyte imbalance, hypo-

glycaemia, and myopathy) should also elicit compulsory admission if the patient cannot be persuaded to accept inpatient treatment.

In the United Kingdom the Mental Health Act Commission[135] has recently (1997) clarified many of the doubts in the minds of clinicians and social workers called upon to consider a compulsory admission under the Mental Health Act 1983. It recognized that anorexia nervosa is a mental disorder within the meaning of the Act and that in some patients their ability to consent may be compromised by fears of obesity or denial of the consequences of their actions. The Mental Health Act Commission concluded that when the patient's health is seriously threatened by food refusal she may be detained in hospital so as to treat the self-imposed starvation. The Commission went as far as to state that nasogastric feeding can be a medical process forming an integral part of the treatment for anorexia nervosa, notwithstanding that nasogastric feeding is seldom required even in patients who are compulsorily admitted.

In a study of the use of compulsory treatment in patients admitted to the Eating Disorders Unit of the Bethlem Royal and Maudsley Hospital, as many as 81 patients (16 per cent) were detained. Section 3 of the Mental Health Act, valid for up to 6 months, was the most frequently applied section.[136] The compulsorily admitted patients were compared with a population of voluntary patients. The need for a compulsory admission was found to have two dimensions—the presence of a severe illness and a rejection of treatment, the latter in part due to abnormal personality traits. The compulsory patients gained at least as much weight as the voluntary patients but required a longer admission for them to return to a near-normal weight. It was thought likely that the compulsory patients presented a selected group by virtue of a more entrenched reluctance to accept treatment. Accordingly it was predicted that in the long term they would fare less well than voluntary patients. It was possible to determine the mortality rate of these patients through the National Register which provided the data at a mean of 5.7 years after the index admission. Ten out of 79 detained patients had died in comparison with two out of 78 voluntary patients, a statistically significant difference. The deaths among the compulsory patients were all due to anorexia nervosa or one of its nutritional complications. Thus the mortality rate among compulsory patients was extremely high at 2.17 per cent per annum. It was concluded that this high mortality was due to the selection factors.

Therefore the evidence points to the usefulness of a compulsory admission in appropriate circumstances in so far as the patients responded well in the short term. Nevertheless, a patient who has required a compulsory admission carries a higher risk, so that it is essential to safeguard her through a long period of observation.

References

1. Gull, W.W. (1874). Anorexia nervosa (apepsia hysterica, anorexia hysterica). *Transactions of the Clinical Society of London*, **7**, 22–8.
2. Lasègue, C. (1873). De l'anorexie hystérique. *Archives Générales de Médicine*, **21**, 385–403.
3. Brumberg, J.J. (1988). *Fasting girls: the emergence of anorexia nervosa as a modern disease.* Harvard University Press, Cambridge, MA.
4. Bell, R.M. (1985). *Holy anorexia.* University of Chicago Press.
5. Rampling, D. (1985). Ascetic ideals and anorexia nervosa. *Journal of Psychiatric Research*, **19**, 89–94.
6. Bruch, H. (1962). Perceptual and conceptual disturbances in anorexia nervosa. *Psychosomatic Medicine*, **24**, 187–94.
7. Russell, G.F.M. (1970). Anorexia nervosa: its identity as an illness and its

treatment. In *Modern trends in psychological medicine* (ed. J. Harding Price), pp. 131–64. Butterworths, Norwich.

8. Garner, D.M. and Garfinkel, P.E. (1979). The Eating Attitudes Test: an index of the symptoms of anorexia nervosa. *Psychological Medicine*, **9**, 273–9.

9. Williams, P., Hand, D., and Tarnopolsky, A. (1982). The problem of screening for uncommon disorders—a comment on the Eating Attitudes Test. *Psychological Medicine*, **12**, 431–4.

10. Johnson-Sabine, E., Wood, K., Patton, G., Mann, A., and Wakeling, A. (1988). Abnormal eating attitudes in London schoolgirls—a prospective epidemiological study: factors associated with abnormal response on screening questionnaires. *Psychological Medicine*, **18**, 615–22.

11. Hoek, H.W. (1991). The incidence and prevalence of anorexia nervosa and bulimia nervosa in primary care. *Psychological Medicine*, **21**, 455–60.

12. Garner, D.M. and Garfinkel, P.E. (1980). Socio-cultural factors in the development of anorexia nervosa. *Psychological Medicine*, **10**, 647–56.

13. Szmukler, G.I., Eisler, I., Gillies, C., and Heyward, M.E. (1985). The implications of anorexia nervosa in a ballet school. *Journal of Psychiatric Research*, **19**, 177–82.

14. Crisp, A.H., Palmer, R.R.L., and Kalucy, R.S. (1976). How common is anorexia nervosa? A prevalence study. *British Journal of Psychiatry*, **128**, 549–54.

15. Mann, A.H., Wakeling, A., Wood, K., Monck, E., Dobbs, R., and Szmukler, G.I. (1983). Screening for abnormal attitudes and psychiatric morbidity in an unselected population of 15-year-old schoolgirls. *Psychological Medicine*, **13**, 573–80.

16. Råstam, M., Gillberg, C., and Garton, M. (1989). Anorexia nervosa in a Swedish urban region. A population based study. *British Journal of Psychiatry*, **155**, 642–6.

17. Theander, S. (1970). Anorexia nervosa: a psychiatric investigation of 94 female patients. *Acta Psychiatrica Scandinavica*, Supplement 214.

18. Jones, D.L., Fox, M.M., Babigian, H.M., and Hutton, H.E. (1980). Epidemiology of anorexia nervosa in Monroe County, New York: 1960–1976. *Psychological Medicine*, **42**, 551–8.

19. Szmukler, G.I., McCance, C., McCrone, L., and Hunter, D. (1986). Anorexia nervosa: a psychiatric case register study from Aberdeen. *Psychological Medicine*, **16**, 49–58.

20. Willi, J., Giacometti, G., and Limacher, B. (1990). Update on the epidemiology of anorexia nervosa in a defined region of Switzerland. *American Journal of Psychiatry*, **147**, 1514–17.

21. Lucas, A.R., Beard, C.M., O'Fallen, W.M., and Kurland, L.T. (1991). 50-year trends in the incidence of anorexia nervosa in Rochester, Minn: a population-based survey. *American Journal of Psychiatry*, **148**, 917–22.

22. Fosson, A., Knibbs, J., Bryant-Waugh, R., and Lask, B. (1987). Early onset anorexia nervosa. *Archives of Disease in Childhood*, **62**, 114–18.

23. Fenwick, S. (1880). *On atrophy of the stomach and on the nervous affections of the digestive organs*. p. 107. Churchill, London.

24. Morgan, H.G. and Russell, G.F.M. (1975). Value of family background and clinical features as predictors of long-term outcome in anorexia nervosa: four-year follow-up study of 41 patients. *Psychological Medicine*, **5**, 355–71.

25. Bruch, H. (1978). *The golden cage: the enigma of anorexia nervosa*. Open Books, London.

26. Williams, P. and King, M. (1987). The 'epidemic' of anorexia nervosa: another medical myth? *Lancet*, **i**, 205–7.

27. Russell, G.F.M. (1993). Social psychiatry of eating disorders. In *Principles of social psychiatry* (ed. D. Bhugra and J. Leff), pp. 273–97. Blackwell Science, Oxford.

28. Fombonne, E. (1995). Anorexia nervosa, no evidence of an increase. *British Journal of Psychiatry* **166**, 462–71.

29. Russell, G.F.M. (1979). Bulimia nervosa: an ominous variant of anorexia nervosa. *Psychological Medicine*, **9**, 429–48.

30. Russell, G.F.M. (1995). Anorexia nervosa through time. In *Handbook of eating disorders: theory, treatment and research* (ed. G. Szmukler, C. Dare, and J. Treasure), pp. 5–17. Wiley, Chichester.

31. Campbell, P.G. (1995) What would a causal explanation of the eating disorders look like? In *Handbook of eating disorders: theory, treatment and research* (ed. G. Szmukler, C. Dare, and J. Treasure), pp. 49–64. Wiley, Chichester.

32. Garfinkel, P.E. and Garner, D.M. (1982). *Anorexia nervosa: a multi-dimensional perspective*. Brunner–Mazel, New York.

33. Birnbaum, K. (1923). *Der Aufbau der Psychose*, pp. 6–7. Springer, Berlin.

34. Patton, G.C., Johnson-Sabine, E., Wood, K., Mann, A., and Wakeling, A. (1990). Abnormal eating attitudes in London schoolgirls—a prospective epidemiological study: outcome at twelve-month follow-up. *Psychological Medicine*, **20**, 383–94.

35. Crisp, A.H. (1970). Premorbid factors in adult disorders of weight, with particular reference to primary anorexia nervosa (weight phobia). A literature review. *Journal of Psychosomatic Research*, **14**, 1–22.

36. Wig, N.N. (1983). DSM-III: a perspective from the Third World. In *International perspectives on DSM-III: diagnostic and statistical manual of mental disorders* (ed. R.L. Spitzer, J.B.W. Williams, and A.E. Skodol), pp. 79–89. American Psychiatric Press, Washington, DC.

37. Prince, R. (1985). The concept of culture-bound syndromes: anorexia nervosa and brain-fag. *Transcultural Psychiatric Research Review*, **22**, 117–21.

38. DiNicola, V.F. (1990). Anorexia multiforme: self-starvation in historical and cultural context. *Transcultural Psychiatric Research Review*, **27**, 165–96, 245–86.

39. Bryant-Waugh, R. and Lask, B. (1991). Anorexia nervosa in a group of Asian children living in Britain. *British Journal of Psychiatry*, **158**, 229–33.

40. Mynors-Wallis, L., Treasure, J., and Chee, D. (1992). Life events and anorexia nervosa: differences between early and late onset cases. *International Journal of Eating Disorders*, **4**, 369–75.

41. Beumont, P.J.V., Abraham, S.F., and Simson, K.G. (1981). The psychosexual histories of adolescent girls and young women with anorexia nervosa. *Psychological Medicine*, **11**, 131–40.

42. Tiller, J. and Treasure, J. (1998). Eating disorders precipitated by pregnancy. *European Eating Disorders Review*, **6**, 178–87.

43. Sloan, G. and Leichner, P. (1986). Is there a relationship between sexual abuse or incest and eating disorders? *Canadian Journal of Psychiatry*, **31**, 656–60.

44. Palmer, R.L., Oppenheimer, R., Dignon, A., Chaloner, D.A., and Howells, K. (1990). Childhood sexual experiences with adults reported by women with eating disorders: an extended series. *British Journal of Psychiatry*, **156**, 699–703.

45. McClelland, L., Mynors-Wallis, L., Fahy, T., and Treasure, J. (1991). Sexual abuse, disordered personality and eating disorders. *British Journal of Psychiatry*, **158** (Supplement 10), 63–8.

46. Wonderlich, S.A., Brewerton, T.D., Jocic, Z., Dansky, B.S., and Abbott, D.W. (1997). Relationship of childhood sexual abuse and eating disorders. *Journal of the American Academy of Child and Adolescent Psychiatry*, **36**, 1107–15.

47. Minuchin, S., Baker, L., Rosman, B.L., Liebman, R., Milman, L., and Todd, T.C. (1975). A conceptual model of psychosomatic illness in children: family organization and family therapy. *Archives of General Psychiatry*, **32**, 1031–8.

48. Selvini Palazzoli, M. (1974). *Self-starvation. From the intrapsychic to the transpersonal approach to anorexia nervosa* (trans. A. Pomerans), pp. 202–16. Human Context Books, London.

49. Dare, C. and Eisler, I. (1997). Family therapy for anorexia nervosa. In *Handbook of treatment for eating disorders* (2nd edn) (ed. D.M. Garner and P.E. Garfinkel), pp. 307–24. Guilford Press, New York.

50. Heron, J.M. and Leheup, R.F. (1984). Happy families? *British Journal of Psychiatry*, **145**, 136–8.

51. Janet, P. (1903). L'obsession de la honte du corps. In *Les obsessions et la psychasthénie*, Vol. 1, Section 5. Germer Gaillière, Paris.

52. Wonderlich, S.A., Swift, W.H., Slotnick, H.B., and Goodman, S. (1990). DSM-III-R personality disorders in eating disorder subtypes. *International Journal of Eating Disorders*, **9**, 607–16.

53. Casper, R.C. (1990). Personality features of women with good outcome from restricting anorexia nervosa. *Psychosomatic Medicine*, **52**, 156–70.

54. O'Dwyer, A.-M. (1999). Studies of the relationship between obsessive–compulsive disorder and anorexia nervosa. MD Thesis, Trinity College, Dublin.

55. Simmonds, K. (1916). Über kachexie hypophysaren ursprungs. *Deutsche Medizinische. Wochenschrift*, **42**, 190–1.

56. Russell, G.F.M. (1977). The present status of anorexia nervosa. *Psychological Medicine*, **7**, 363–7.

57. Anand, B.K. and Brobeck, J.R. (1951). Localization of a 'feeding center' in the hypothalamus of the rat. *Proceedings of the Society for Experimental Biology and Medicine*, **77**, 323–4.

58. Hetherington, A.W. and Ranson, S.W. (1940). Adiposity in the rat. *Anatomical Record*, **78**, 149–72.

59. Schweiger, U., Tuschl, R.J., Laessle, R.G., Broocks, A., and Pirke, K.M. (1989). Consequences of dieting and exercise on menstrual function in normal weight young women. In *The menstrual cycle and its disorders* (ed. K.M. Pirke *et al.*), pp. 142–9. Springer Verlag, Berlin.

60. Diamond, E.F. and Averick, N. (1966). Marasmus and the diencephalic syndrome. *Archives of Neurology*, **14**, 270–2.

61. DeVile, C.H., Sufraz, R., Lask, B., and Stanhope, R. (1995) Occult intracranial tumours masquerading as early onset anorexia nervosa. *British Medical Journal*, **311**, 1359–60.

62. Ploog, D.W. and Pirke, K.M. (1987) Psychobiology of anorexia nervosa. *Psychological Medicine*, **17**, 843–59.

63. Gordon, I., Lask, B., Bryant-Waugh, R., Christie, D., and Timimi, S. (1997). Childhood-onset anorexia nervosa: towards identifying a biological substrate. *International Journal of Eating Disorders*, **22**, 159–65.

64. Holland, A.J., Hall, A., Murray, R., Russell, G.F.M., and Crisp, A.H. (1984). Anorexia nervosa: a study of 34 twin pairs and one set of triplets. *British Journal of Psychiatry*, **145**, 414–19.

65. Holland, A.J., Sicotte, N., and Treasure, J. (1988). Anorexia nervosa: evidence for a genetic basis. *Journal of Psychosomatic Research*, **32**, 561–71.

66. Strober, M., Lampert, C., Morrell, W., Burroughs, J., and Jacobs, C. (1990). A controlled family study of anorexia nervosa: evidence of familial aggregation and lack of shared transmission with affective disorders. *International Journal of Eating Disorders*, **9**, 239–53.

67. Blundell, J.E. and Bill, A.J. (1991). Serotonin, eating disorders and the satiety cascade. In *Serotonin-related psychiatric syndromes: clinical and therapeutic links* (ed. G.B. Cassano and H.S. Asikal), pp. 125–9. Royal Society of Medicine Services, London.

68. Kaye, W.H., Gwirtsman, J.E., George, D.T., Jimerson, D.C., and Ebert, M.H. (1988). CSF-5HIAA concentrations in anorexia nervosa: reduced values in underweight subjects normalize after weight gain. *Biological Psychiatry*, **23**, 102–5.

69. Kaye, W.H., Gwirtsman, H.E., George, D.T., and Ebert, M.H. (1991). Altered serotonin activity in anorexia nervosa after long-term weight restoration: does elevated CSF-5HIAA correlate with rigid and obsessive behavior? *Archives of General Psychiatry*, **48**, 556–62.

70. O'Dwyer, A.-M., Lucey, J.V., and Russell, G.F.M. (1996). Serotonin activity in anorexia nervosa after long-term weight restoration: response to D-fenfluramine challenge. *Psychological Medicine*, **26**, 353–9.

71. Ward, A., Brown, N., Lightman, S., Campbell, I.C., and Treasure, J. (1998). Neuroendocrine, appetitive and behavioural responses to D-fenfluramine in women recovered from anorexia nervosa. *British Journal of Psychiatry*, **172**, 351–8.

72. Samuel-Lajeunesse, B. (1994). Troubles du comportement alimentaire: aspects sémiologiques. In *Les conduites alimentaires* (ed. B. Samuel-Lajeunesse and C. Foulon), pp. 83–109. Masson, Paris.

73. Slade, P.D. and Russell, G.F.M. (1973). Awareness of body dimensions in anorexia nervosa: cross-sectional and longitudinal studies. *Psychological Medicine*, **3**, 188–99.

74. Hsu, L.K.G. and Sobkiewicz, T.A. (1989). Body image disturbance: time to abandon the concept for eating disorders? *International Journal of Eating Disorders*, **10**, 15–30.

75. Hsu, L.K.G. and Lee, S. (1993). Is weight phobia always necessary for a diagnosis of anorexia nervosa? *American Journal of Psychiatry*, **150**, 1466–71.

76. Szmukler, G.I., Andrewes, D., Kingston, K., Chen, L., Stargatt, R., and Stanley, R. (1992). Neuropsychological impairment in anorexia nervosa before and after refeeding. *Journal of Clinical and Experimental Neuropsychology*, **14**, 347–52.

77. Crisp, A.H., Chen, C., Mackinnon, P.C.B., and Corker, C. (1973). Observations of gonadotrophic and ovarian hormone activity during recovery from anorexia nervosa. *Postgraduate Medical Journal*, **49**, 584–90.

78. Fichter, M.M. and Pirke, K.M. (1995). Starvation models and eating disorders. In *Handbook of eating disorders: theory, treatment and research* (ed. G. Szmukler, C. Dare, and J. Treasure), pp. 83–107. Wiley, Chichester.

79. Treasure, J.L., Gordon, P.A.L., King, E.A., Wheeler, M., and Russell, G.F.M. (1985). Cystic ovaries: a phase of anorexia nervosa. *Lancet*, **ii**, 1379–82.

80. Russell, G.F.M. and Treasure, J. (1989). The modern history of anorexia nervosa: an interpretation of why the illness has changed. *Annals of the New York Academy of Sciences*, **575**, 13–30.

81. Namir, S., Melman, K.N., and Yager, J. (1986). Pregnancy in restrictor-type anorexia nervosa: a study of six women. *International Journal of Eating Disorders*, **5**, 837–45.

82. Treasure, J.L. and Russell, G.F.M. (1988). Intrauterine growth and neonatal weight gain in babies of women with anorexia nervosa. *British Medical Journal*, **296**, 1038.

83. Van Wezel-Meijler, G. and Wit, J.M. (1989). The offspring of mothers with anorexia nervosa: a high-risk group for undernutrition and stunting? *European Journal of Pediatrics*, **49**, 130–5.

84. Sharp, C.W. and Freeman, C.P.L. (1993). The medical complications of anorexia nervosa. *British Journal of Psychiatry*, **162**, 452–62.

85. Treasure, J. and Szmukler, G. (1995). Medical complications of chronic anorexia nervosa. In *Handbook of eating disorders: theory, treatment and research* (ed. G. Szmukler, C. Dare, and J. Treasure), pp. 197–220. Wiley, Chichester.

86. Passmore, R. and Eastwood, M.A. (1986). *Human nutrition and dietetics*. Churchill Livingstone, Edinburgh.

87. Handler, C.E. and Pirkin, G.D. (1982). Anorexia nervosa and Wernicke's encephalopathy: an undiagnosed association. *Lancet*, **ii**, 771–2.

88. McLoughlin, D.M., Spargo, E., Wassif, W.S., *et al.* (1998). Structural and functional changes in skeletal muscle in anorexia nervosa. *Acta Neuropathologica*, **95**, 632–40.

89. Treasure, J.L., Fogelman, I., Russell, G.F.M., and Murby, B. (1987). Reversible bone loss in anorexia nervosa. *British Medical Journal*, **295**, 474–5.

90. Serpell, L. and Treasure, J. (1997). Osteoporosis—a serious health risk in chronic anorexia nervosa. *European Eating Disorders Review*, **5**, 149–57.

91. Klibanski, A., Biller, B.M.K., Schoenfeld, D.A., Herzog, D.B., and Saxe, V.C. (1995). The effects of oestrogen administration on trabecular bone loss in young women with anorexia nervosa. *Journal of Clinical Endocrinology and Metabolism*, **80**, 898–904.

92. Wakeling, A. and Russell, G.F.M. (1970). Disturbances in the regulation of body temperature in anorexia nervosa. *Psychological Medicine*, **1**, 30–9.

93. Rieger, W., Brady, J.P., and Weisberg, E. (1978). Hematologic changes in anorexia nervosa. *American Journal of Psychiatry*, **135**, 984–5.

94. Russell, G.F.M. (1966). Acute dilation of the stomach in a patient with anorexia nervosa. *British Journal of Psychiatry*, **112**, 203–7.

95. Beumont, P.J.V. and Large, M. (1991). Hypophosphataemia, delirium and cardiac arrhythmia in anorexia nervosa. *Medical Journal of Australia*, **155**, 519–22.

96. Russell, G.F.M., Treasure, J., and Eisler, I. (1998). Mothers with anorexia nervosa who underfeed their children: their recognition and management. *Psychological Medicine*, **28**, 93–108.

97. Stein, A., Woolley, H.P., Cooper, S.D., and Fairburn, C.G. (1994). An observational study of mothers with eating disorders and their infants. *Journal of Child Psychology and Psychiatry*, **35**, 733–48.

98. Russell, G.F.M. (1985). Premenarchal anorexia nervosa and its sequelae. *Journal of Psychiatric Research*, **19**, 363–9.

99. Lask, B. and Bryant-Waugh, R. (1992). Early onset anorexia nervosa and related eating disorders. *Journal of Child Psychology and Psychiatry*, **33**, 281–300.

100. Lask, B. and Bryant-Waugh, R. (1986). Childhood onset anorexia nervosa. In *Recent advances in paediatrics* (ed. R. Meadow), Vol. 8, pp. 21–31. Churchill Livingstone, Edinburgh.

101. Lai, K., de Bruyn, R., Lask, B., Bryant-Waugh, R., and Hankins, M. (1994). Use of pelvic ultrasound in childhood onset anorexia nervosa. *Archives of Disease in Childhood*, **71**, 228–31.

102. World Health Organization (1992). *International statistical classification of diseases and related health problems, 10th revision*. WHO, Geneva.

103. American Psychiatric Association (1994). *Diagnostic and statistical manual of mental disorders* (4th edn). American Psychiatric Association, Washington, DC.

104. Beumont, P.J.V., Beardwood, C.J., and Russell, G.F.M. (1972). The occurrence of the syndrome of anorexia nervosa in male subjects. *Psychological Medicine*, **2**, 216–31.

105. Crisp, A.H. and Burns, T. (1990). Primary anorexia nervosa in the male and female: a comparison of clinical features and prognosis. In *Males with eating disorders* (ed. A.E. Andersen), pp. 77–99. Brunner–Mazel, New York.

106. Burns, T. and Crisp, A.H. (1990). Outcome of anorexia nervosa in males. In *Males with eating disorders* (ed. A.E. Andersen), pp. 163–86. Brunner–Mazel, New York.

107. Fichter, M.M. and Daser, C. (1987). Symptomatology, psychosexual development and gender identity in 42 anorexic males. *Psychological Medicine*, **17**, 409–18.

108. Steinhausen, H.-C., Rauss-Mason, C., and Seidel, R. (1991). Follow-up studies of anorexia nervosa. A review of four decades of outcome research. *Psychological Medicine*, **21**, 447–54.

109. Morgan, H.G. and Hayward, A.E. (1988). Clinical assessment of anorexia nervosa. *British Journal of Psychiatry*, **152**, 367–71.

110. Theander, S. (1985). Outcome and prognosis in anorexia nervosa and bulimia: some results of previous investigations, compared with a Swedish long-term study. *Journal of Psychosomatic Research*, **19**, 493–508.

111. Ratnasuriya, R.H., Eisler, I., Szmukler, G.I., and Russell, G.F.M. (1991). Anorexia nervosa: outcome and prognostic factors after 20 years. *British Journal of Psychiatry*, **158**, 495–502.

112. Sullivan, P.F. (1995). Mortality in anorexia nervosa. *American Journal of Psychiatry*, **152**, 1073–4.

113. Tolstrup, K., Brinch, M., Isager, T., Nielsen, S., Nystrup, J., and Severin, B. (1985). Long-term outcome of 151 cases of anorexia nervosa. The Copenhagen anorexia nervosa follow-up study. *Acta Psychiatrica Scandinavica*, **71**, 380–7.

114. Eckert, E.D., Halmi, K.A., Marchi, P., Grove, W., and Crosby, R. (1995). Ten-year follow-up of anorexia nervosa: clinical course and outcome. *Psychological Medicine*, **25**, 143–56.

115. Bryant-Waugh, R., Knibbs, J., Fosson, A., Kaminski, Z., and Lask, B. (1988). Long-term follow-up of patients with early onset anorexia nervosa. *Archives of Disease in Childhood*, **63**, 5–9.

116. Steinhausen, H.-C. and Seidel, R. (1993). Outcome in adolescent eating disorders. *International Journal of Eating Disorders*, **14**, 487–96.

117. Theander, S. (1992). Chronicity in anorexia nervosa: results from the Swedish long-term study. In *The course of eating disorders* (ed. W.

Herzog, H.-C. Deter, and W. Vandereycken), pp. 198–213. Springer-Verlag, Berlin.

118. Touyz, S.Q., Beumont, P.J.V., Glaun, D., Phillips, T., and Cowie, I. (1984). A comparison of lenient and strict operant conditioning programmes in refeeding patients with anorexia nervosa. *British Journal of Psychiatry*, **144**, 517–20.

119. Freeman, C. (1992). Day patient treatment for anorexia nervosa. *British Review of Bulimia and Anorexia Nervosa*, **6**, 3–9.

120. Crisp, A.H., Norton, K., Gowers, S., *et al.* (1991). A controlled study of the effect of therapies aimed at adolescent and family psychopathology in anorexia nervosa. *British Journal of Psychiatry*, **159**, 325–33.

121. Russell, G.F.M., Szmukler, G.I., Dare, C., and Eisler, I. (1987). An evaluation of family therapy in anorexia nervosa and bulimia nervosa. *Archives of General Psychiatry*, **44**, 1047–56.

122. Eisler, I., Dare, C., Russell, G.F.M., Szmukler, G., le Grange, D., and Dodge, E. (1997). Family and individual therapy in anorexia nervosa—a 5-year follow-up. *Archives of General Psychiatry*, **54**, 1025–30.

123. Le Grange, D., Eisler, I., Dare, C., and Russell, G.F.M. (1992). Evaluation of family treatments in adolescent anorexia nervosa: a pilot study. *International Journal of Eating Disorders*, **12**, 347–57.

124. Prochaska, J.O. and Di Clemente, C.C. (1992). The transtheoretical approach. In *Handbook of psychotherapy integration* (ed. J.C. Norcross and M.R. Goldfried), pp. 300–34. Basic Books, New York.

125. Treasure, J. and Ward, A. (1997). A practical guide to the use of motivational interviewing in anorexia nervosa. *European Eating Disorders Review*, **5**, 102–14.

126. Garner, D.M., Vitousek, K.M., and Pike, K.M. (1997). Cognitive–behavioural therapy for anorexia nervosa. In *Handbook of treatment for eating disorders* (2nd edn) (ed. D.M. Garner and P.E. Garfinkel), pp. 94–144. Guilford Press, New York.

127. Crisp, A.H. (1980). *Anorexia nervosa: let me be*. Academic Press, London.

128. Crisp, A.H. (1997). Anorexia nervosa as flight from growth: assessment and treatment based on model. In *Handbook of treatment for eating disorders* (2nd edn) (ed. D.M. Garner and P.E. Garfinkel), pp. 248–77. Guilford Press, New York.

129. Fairburn, C.G., Shafran, R., and Cooper, Z. (1999). A cognitive-behavioural theory of anorexia nervosa. *Behaviour Research and Therapy*, **37**, 1–13.

130. Garner, D.M. and Bemis, K.M. (1982). A cognitive-behavioural approach to anorexia nervosa. *Cognitive Therapy and Research*, **6**, 123–50.

131. Kaplan, A.S. and Olmsted, M.P. (1997). Partial hospitalisation. In *Handbook of treatment for eating disorders* (2nd edn) (ed. D.M. Garner and P.E. Garfinkel), pp. 354–60. Guilford Press, New York.

132. Andersen, A.E., Bowers, W., and Evans, K. (1997). In-patient treatment of anorexia nervosa. In *Handbook of treatment for eating disorders* (2nd edn) (ed. D.M. Garner and P.E. Garfinkel), pp. 327–53. Guilford Press, New York.

133. Russell, G.F.M. and Mezey, A.G. (1962). An analysis of weight gain in patients with anorexia nervosa treated with high calorie diets. *Clinical Science*, **23**, 449–61.

134. Goldner, E.M., Birmingham, C.L., and Smye, V. (1997). Addressing treatment refusal in anorexia nervosa: clinical, ethical, and legal considerations. In *Handbook of treatment for eating disorders* (2nd edn) (ed. D.M. Garner and P.E. Garfinkel), pp. 450–61. Guilford Press, New York.

135. Mental Health Act Commission (1997). *Guidance on the treatment of anorexia nervosa under the Mental Health Act 1983*, pp. 1–6. Mental Health Act Commission, Nottingham.

136. Ramsay, R., Ward, A., Treasure, J., and Russell, G.F.M. (1999). Compulsory treatment in anorexia nervosa: short-term benefits and long-term mortality. *British Journal of Psychiatry*, **175**, 147–53.

4.10.2 Bulimia nervosa

Christopher G. Fairburn

Introduction

Origins of the concept

The history of the diagnosis bulimia nervosa begins as recently as 1979. It was in this year that Russell published his now seminal paper 'Bulimia nervosa: an ominous variant of anorexia nervosa'[1] in which he described 30 patients (28 women and two men), seen between 1972 and 1978, who had three major features in common. First, they had recurrent episodes of uncontrolled overeating; second, they regularly used self-induced vomiting or laxatives as means of weight control; and third, they had a morbid fear of becoming fat. Russell described many other features shared by these patients, including a history of anorexia nervosa (present in 80 per cent), the presence of severe depressive symptoms, and the fact that in most cases their body weight was in the healthy range. He noted that the disorder tended to run a chronic course and that it was 'extremely difficult to treat'. Finally, he suggested that this clinical picture should be viewed as a syndrome, distinct from anorexia nervosa, and he proposed the term 'bulimia nervosa'.

It is difficult to exaggerate the importance of Russell's paper. Its greatest contribution was perhaps its prescience in that it separated a subgroup of patients from among the range of eating disorders seen in clinical practice that was just starting to become more common, it identified its central features, and it gave it an appropriate name. In the late 1970s there was beginning to be interest in subdividing patients with anorexia nervosa into those who simply restrict their eating and those who also intermittently overeat, vomit, or take laxatives (see Chapter 4.10.1). There had also been scattered reports of an anorexia-nervosa-like state in which overeating was the dominant feature, and terms such as 'bulimarexia' and the 'dietary chaos syndrome' had been suggested. None of these reports, however, provided the detailed clinical description or the clarity of conceptualization that were the hallmark of Russell's paper.

Events since 1980

Events gathered pace in the 1980s. In 1980 a syndrome termed 'bulimia' was included in DSM-III.[2] This was intended to denote the type of patient that Russell had described, although its diagnostic criteria proved to be overly inclusive. In 1987, the criteria were refined and brought more in line with Russell's original concept. The syndrome was also renamed bulimia nervosa.[3] Also in the early 1980s evidence mounted that bulimia nervosa might be common and this led to a spate of studies of its prevalence. At the same time reports were published describing the successful treatment of these patients, the two most promising approaches being a specific form of cognitive-behavioural therapy and the use of antidepressant drugs. By the mid-1980s, both treatments had been tested in the first of what has become a large series of controlled trials.

Now, two decades later, the diagnosis bulimia nervosa is included in both DSM-IV[4] and ICD-10,[5] its prevalence is established, aspects of its aetiology are beginning to be understood, and much has been learned about its treatment.

Diagnosis and classification

Bulimia nervosa is one of the two main eating disorders recognized in DSM-IV and ICD-10. The other is anorexia nervosa (see Chapter 4.10.1). Three features must be present to make a diagnosis of bulimia nervosa.

1. Recurrent episodes of 'binge eating' (defined below).

2. The regular use of extreme methods of weight control (e.g. highly restrictive dieting, self-induced vomiting, the misuse of laxatives and diuretics, or overexercising).

3. A characteristic set of attitudes to shape and weight, at the heart of which is the judging of self-worth in terms of shape and weight. These attitudes are expressed as an intense dissatisfaction with shape and weight, a fear of weight gain and fatness, and, in many cases, a pursuit of weight loss and thinness.

In addition to the three required diagnostic features, there is an exclusionary criterion. This is that the person must not meet diagnostic criteria for anorexia nervosa. In practice, this means that the patient must not fulfil the low-weight criterion for anorexia nervosa (a body mass index below 17.5). The principal diagnostic criteria for anorexia nervosa and bulimia nervosa are summarized in Table 1.

Both DSM-IV and ICD-10 acknowledge the existence of eating disorders other than anorexia nervosa and bulimia nervosa. These may be described as 'atypical eating disorders'.[6] They have been poorly characterized and little has been written about them. Many appear to be incomplete expressions of anorexia nervosa or bulimia nervosa (either in severity or form), but others are qualitatively different. In DSM-IV, all eating disorders other than anorexia nervosa and bulimia nervosa are placed in the single category 'eating disorder not otherwise specified'. In ICD-10, various additional eating disorder categories are recognized (e.g. atypical anorexia nervosa, atypical bulimia nervosa, overeating associated with other psychological disturbances), although these concepts have never been adequately defined or differentiated. Figure 1 illustrates the relationship between anorexia nervosa, bulimia nervosa, and the atypical eating disorders.

In DSM-IV, a provisional new eating disorder diagnosis was intro-

Table 1 Principal diagnostic criteria for anorexia nervosa and bulimia nervosa

---

Anorexia nervosa
Characteristic extreme concerns about shape and weight (extreme fear of fatness and weight gain, determined pursuit of thinness and weight loss)
Active maintenance of an unduly low weight (BMI < 17.5)
Amenorrhoea

Bulimia nervosa
Characteristic extreme concerns about shape and weight (extreme fear of fatness and weight gain, determined pursuit of thinness and weight loss)
Recurrent binge eating
Extreme weight control behaviour (e.g. strict dieting, self-induced vomiting, misuse of laxatives or diuretics)
Does not fulfil diagnostic criteria for anorexia nervosa

BMI, body mass index.

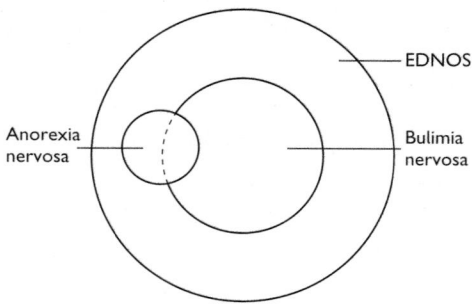

Fig. 1 A Venn diagram illustrating the relationship between the diagnoses anorexia nervosa, bulimia nervosa, and eating disorder not otherwise specified (EDNOS). (Reproduced with permission from C.G. Fairburn and G.T. Wilson (1993). Binge eating: definition and classification. In *Binge eating: nature, assessment and treatment* (ed. C.G. Fairburn and G.T. Wilson), pp. 3–14. Guilford Press, New York.)

duced which is termed binge eating disorder. It is placed in an appendix designed for possible future diagnostic concepts. Patients with binge eating disorder have recurrent episodes of binge eating, like those seen in bulimia nervosa, but they do not fulfil the diagnostic criteria for either anorexia nervosa or bulimia nervosa. This is a controversial category about which much remains to be learned.[7,8]

Clinical features

The great majority of patients with bulimia nervosa are female and most are in their twenties (although the age range is between 10 and 60 years). In considering the psychopathology of the disorder, a distinction may be drawn between its 'specific' and 'general' features. The former comprises features that are largely peculiar to eating disorders (e.g. self-induced vomiting), whereas the latter consists of features seen in other psychiatric conditions (e.g. depressive symptoms). The clinical features of bulimia nervosa are similar in men and women[9] and in those with and without a history of anorexia nervosa.

Specific psychopathology

Dieting and binge eating

The eating habits of patients with bulimia nervosa are characterized by strict dieting punctuated by repeated episodes of binge eating (Fig. 2). The dieting is extreme, in that little tends to be eaten, and it is governed by multiple self-imposed dietary rules. These rules tend to be applied to all aspects of eating, including when to eat, what to eat, and how much to eat. As a result, the food eaten (when not binge eating) is restricted in quantity and range.

Recurrent episodes of 'binge eating' interrupt this dieting. (The term binge eating denotes discrete episodes of eating that have two characteristics—first an unusually large amount of food is eaten, given the circumstances, and second there is a sense of loss of control at the time.[10]) The frequency and regularity of the binges varies. Some patients have episodes almost every day, whereas in others the episodes are intermittent. In DSM-IV, it is specified that the binges should occur on average at least twice a week, but this is an arbitrary figure that has little discriminatory value. Among those patients in whom the

binge eating is frequent, the binges have few, if any, obvious triggers, although there may be circumstances under which binge eating is more likely (e.g. when alone at home). Among patients in whom the binge eating is less frequent, the binges often have clear precipitants. These tend to be of three overlapping types: first there is breaking a personal dietary rule (e.g. exceeding a daily calorie limit or eating a banned food), second there are situations which intensify concerns about shape and weight (e.g. receiving an adverse comment about appearance), and third there is the occurrence of negative moods (often as a result of interpersonal events). All three encourage the temporary abandonment of dietary control.

The amount of food eaten during binges varies, both from patient to patient and from episode to episode. Typical episodes involve the consumption of 4200 to 12 600 kJ (1000–3000 kcal).[11] The food eaten generally comprises items that are otherwise being avoided. Thus binges tend to be composed of energy-dense high-fat items such as chocolate, ice-cream, and pastries. Binges come to an end as a result of the combined influence of exhaustion, extreme fullness, a diminution of the drive to eat, and the running out of food supplies. In about three-quarters of patients they are immediately followed by measures designed to counteract the effects of the overeating, the most common being self-induced vomiting and the taking of laxatives or diuretics.

The binges are a source of considerable distress. They magnify patients' fears of weight gain and fatness, and they are a source of shame and self-disgust. For this reason most binges occur in private and are kept secret from others. It is the binge eating that eventually drives these people to seek help.

Purging and other forms of weight control

In DSM-IV bulimia nervosa is subdivided into two types, a purging and non-purging type. In the purging type there is self-induced vomiting or the misuse of laxatives or diuretics, or both, whereas in the non-purging type purging is either not present or it is infrequent. The majority of patients seen in clinical practice have the purging form of the disorder and it has been the focus of most research.

Self-induced vomiting is the most common form of purging. In most patients it only takes place after binge eating. It is generally achieved by stimulating the gag reflex, using the fingers or some other long object, although in more established cases it can be accomplished with no mechanical aid. The vomiting is repeated until patients think that they have retrieved all the food that they can. Patients become extremely distressed if they are unable to vomit after binge eating: indeed, if they foresee that they may not have the opportunity to vomit, they tend not to binge. A minority of patients also induce vomiting at other times, for example following smaller episodes of overeating (subjective episodes) or ordinary meals or snacks.

The misuse of laxatives or diuretics is somewhat less common than self-induced vomiting. It takes two forms: one is to compensate for specific episodes of binge eating, like self-induced vomiting, and the other is as a general method of weight control (like dieting), in which case it is not tied to particular episodes of overeating. The number of laxatives or diuretics taken varies considerably, sometimes far exceeding the recommended dose.

None of these methods of purging is an effective method of weight control. Self-induced vomiting results in the retrieval of only about half to two-thirds of what has been eaten,[12] the taking of laxatives has a minimal effect on food absorption,[13] and diuretic taking has none. As a result, a significant proportion of each binge is absorbed. The

Day/date ...... Tuesday   25th April ......

Time	Food and drink consumed	Place	*	V/L	Context
7.20	Glass orange juice / Bran Flakes (small bowl) / Black coffee	kitchen			Determined to do well today — good start
10.30	Diet Coke	office			
12.50	Salad sandwich / Diet Coke	canteen			Doing well
3.20	Small piece of fruit cake	office — at desk	*		Offered slice of birthday cake. Nibbled it and then hid it in my pocket. Couldn't cope with idea of eating it.
3.30	Glass water	"			
3.40	Glass water	"			
6.45	Black coffee	kitchen			Hungry. Bored — nothing I want to do.
8.45	Fish & chips / 1 packet crisps	fish & chip shop	* / *		Thought I could handle a small portion. Was v. wrong. Ate the lot. Went
9.10	Sausage & chips / 1 packet crisps / Salad cream +++ / Mars bar / Diet Coke	kitchen / " / " / " / "	* / * / * / *	V	across the road to another shop and bought more. Took it home. Stuffed myself. Disgusting food. Disgusted with self. Cried.
11.30	Glass water	kitchen			Thirsty. Another bad day.

Fig. 2 A monitoring record illustrating the eating habits of a patient with bulimia nervosa.

patient's weight is largely a product of her undereating and overeating, with the two tending to cancel each other out.

Other forms of weight control behaviour are practised by some patients, including overexercising, the spitting out of food, and the taking of repeated enemas or saunas. Overexercising is the most common of these, but it is not nearly as prominent or as obviously pathological as in anorexia nervosa. A minority of patients ruminate, that is repeatedly regurgitate and re-chew food that has been eaten. They may then either re-swallow the food or spit it out. This behaviour is not well understood.

Attitudes to shape and weight

A characteristic set of attitudes to shape and weight is the other distinctive element of the specific psychopathology of bulimia nervosa. Equivalent attitudes are found in anorexia nervosa, and their presence is required to make either diagnosis. These attitudes are often described as the 'core psychopathology' of eating disorders. They are characterized by an overconcern with shape and weight in which there

is a fear of weight gain and fatness that is generally accompanied by a pursuit of weight loss and thinness. Underlying this psychopathology is the tendency to judge self-worth largely, or even exclusively, in terms of shape and weight. Whereas it is usual to evaluate self-worth on the basis of perceived performance in a variety of domains (such as interpersonal relationships, work, sport, artistic ability, etc.), people with anorexia nervosa or bulimia nervosa evaluate themselves primarily in terms of their shape and weight. These attitudes and values constitute a good example of an overvalued idea.

Most features of bulimia nervosa can be understood as being secondary to these attitudes to shape and weight. The dieting, purging, and overexercising are obvious secondary features. In addition, there are direct behavioural expressions of these concerns. For example, many patients repeatedly weigh themselves and scrutinize their appearance in mirrors. Others avoid any knowledge of their weight while being acutely sensitive about their appearance. Some avoid others seeing their body and some even avoid seeing it themselves. This can have a major impact on social and sexual relationships. In the most extreme cases, there is a loathing of body shape (body image disparagement). Unlike in anorexia nervosa, misperception of body shape is rarely seen.

The concerns about shape and weight, and therefore eating, affect others in the patient's immediate environment. Meals are often times of tension and social events which involve eating may be avoided. The feeding of children may be affected,[14–16] and this can result in growth impairment[17] (see Chapter 9.3.4).

General psychopathology

General psychiatric symptoms are prominent in bulimia nervosa, more so than in anorexia nervosa.[18,19] The nature of the comorbid symptoms also differs. Depressive features are particularly striking: indeed, the level of depressive symptoms in bulimia nervosa is equivalent to that seen in major depressive disorder. Depressed mood, feelings of hopelessness and worthlessness, poor concentration, guilt, and suicidal ideation are seen. Anxiety symptoms are also encountered, many of which are directly related to the eating disorder; for example, there is often pronounced anxiety about eating in public. Obsessive–compulsive features are sometimes present, although they are less common than in anorexia nervosa. Similarly, social functioning is less impaired.

A subgroup of patients with bulimia nervosa have 'impulse-control' problems, such as the overconsumption of alcohol or drugs, or repeated self-harm. Some of these patients also meet diagnostic criteria for borderline personality disorder. The prevalence of such features varies according to treatment setting: they are unusual in community samples,[20] whereas they are more frequent among patients seen in specialist treatment centres.[21]

Much more common than frank personality disorders are two traits which are also seen in anorexia nervosa.[22] The first is low self-esteem. This generally antedates the eating disorder, although it is often exaggerated by it. Many patients with bulimia nervosa describe long-standing doubts about their worth and ability, irrespective of their accomplishments. The second is perfectionism, that is, imposing on oneself inordinately high personal standards in a range of domains (e.g. work, sport, personal conduct). Since many of these standards are unachievable, it is common for these patients to give long histories of having viewed themselves as perpetually failing.

Physical features

There are few physical abnormalities in bulimia nervosa.[23,24] Body weight is unremarkable in the majority of patients and thus features of starvation are rarely seen. Nevertheless, menstrual abnormalities or amenorrhoea are present in about a quarter of patients. These are likely to be secondary to the disturbed eating since they generally respond to the successful correction of the eating disorder. On laboratory testing endocrine abnormalities are sometimes encountered and these tend to be mild versions of those found in anorexia nervosa.

Frequent purging, and especially the combination of vomiting and laxative misuse, results in fluid and electrolyte abnormalities in some patients. These abnormalities are varied in nature but most often consist of some combination of hypokalaemia, hyponatraemia, and hypochloraemia. The patients appear to accommodate to these abnormalities since medically serious complications (e.g. cardiac arrhythmias) are much less common than might otherwise be expected given the laboratory findings. Some patients experience intermittent oedema, particularly if there is a sudden decrease in the extent of their purging.

Localized physical abnormalities include erosion of the dental enamel (especially from the lingual surfaces of the front teeth) among those who have vomited for many years, traumatic calluses on the knuckles of the hand of those who use their fingers to induce the gag reflex (Russell's sign), and enlargement of the salivary glands, especially the parotids, probably as a result of chronic inflammation. A small proportion of patients have raised serum amylase levels usually due to an increase in the salivary isoenzyme.

Relationship to other disorders

Anorexia nervosa

Bulimia nervosa has many features in common with anorexia nervosa particularly the characteristic attitudes to shape and weight, and the forms of behaviour that arise as a result. In most cases, bulimia nervosa is preceded either by frank anorexia nervosa (in about a quarter of cases) or an anorexia-nervosa-like state. Movement from bulimia nervosa to anorexia nervosa is unusual although it occurs, and some patients remain on the cusp between the two disorders.

There is some evidence of co-aggregation between bulimia nervosa and anorexia nervosa with increased rates of both disorders among the relatives of probands with either condition.[25] There is substantial overlap in the risk factors for anorexia nervosa and bulimia nervosa.[26,27]

Obesity

Few patients with bulimia nervosa are overweight or frankly obese. However, there is evidence of raised rates of parental and premorbid obesity.[27] Obesity is an unusual sequel of the disorder although this may be because those at most risk of obesity are less likely to recover[28] and so continue to suppress their weight.

Depression

Depressive symptoms are common in bulimia nervosa and they may antedate the eating disorder.[19,27] Most family studies have found a raised rate of affective disorder among the relatives of these patients but the balance of evidence suggests that the increase in risk is largely confined to the relatives of those probands who are themselves depressed.[25]

Anxiety disorders

Little is known about the relationship between bulimia nervosa and the various anxiety disorders. These disorders are common among patients with bulimia nervosa, and they may antedate the disorder.[19,29] There has been just one family genetic study of the relationship between an anxiety disorder and bulimia nervosa. It found that there was an increased risk of obsessive–compulsive disorder among the relatives of these patients, but this was confined to those probands who themselves had a history of the disorder.[30]

Alcohol abuse

There is a raised rate of alcohol and drug abuse among patients with bulimia nervosa. It rarely antedates the eating disorder but this is to be expected given the age of onset of substance abuse disorders. There is also a raised rate of substance abuse disorders among the relatives of these patients. Once again it seems that this is largely confined to those probands who themselves have a history of substance abuse.[30]

Personality disorders

It is hazardous making personality disorder diagnoses among those with eating disorders. This is because eating disorders have their onset in adolescence and they directly affect many of the characteristics upon which personality is judged. Thus there is a risk of overestimating the presence of personality disturbance. Nevertheless, some patients with bulimia nervosa do seem to have a coexisting personality disorder, the most common form being borderline personality disorder.[18] Little is known about the rate of personality disturbance among the relatives of these patients.

Diabetes mellitus

It was thought that eating disorders were over-represented among those with type I diabetes mellitus. This is probably not the case. Controlled studies in which eating disorder features have been assessed by interview rather than self-report questionnaire (the preferred method and one which minimizes the risk of false-positive ratings) have found no evidence of increased risk.[31,32]

Epidemiology

The fact that it took Russell[1] more than 6 years (1972–1978) to collect 30 cases of bulimia nervosa suggested that the disorder was not common. Therefore it is remarkable that within a few years of the publication of Russell's paper it was evident that bulimia nervosa was an important source of psychiatric morbidity among women.

In the early 1980s large numbers of previously undetected cases were identified using the media.[33,34] These were remarkably similar to Russell's cases, except that almost all were female and a small proportion had a history of anorexia nervosa. Most had kept their eating disorder secret for many years, and because of shame and hopelessness few had sought help. Many thought that they were the only person with this type of eating disorder. Simultaneously, however, and doubtless partly as a result of the media attention, there was also a sharp increase in the number of people requesting treatment for bulimia nervosa (Fig. 3) such that it was soon the most common type of eating disorder seen in clinical practice. This remains true today.[35,36]

The marked increase in the number of patients with bulimia nervosa stimulated interest in the prevalence of the disorder. By 1989 over 50 prevalence studies had been conducted, many of which had yielded unrealistically high prevalence figures as a result of using weak assessment and sampling procedures. Gradually methods improved with the result that estimates of the prevalence of bulimia nervosa decreased to more modest and consistent levels with the point prevalence among young adult women (aged 16 to 35 years) being in the region of 1 per cent.[37,38] A similar figure has been obtained for lifetime prevalence.[39] The prevalence of bulimia nervosa among men is not known. Among patient samples, male cases are most unusual. Little is known about the presence of bulimia nervosa in non-Western cultures although it is thought to be uncommon.

There have been few estimates of the incidence of bulimia nervosa,

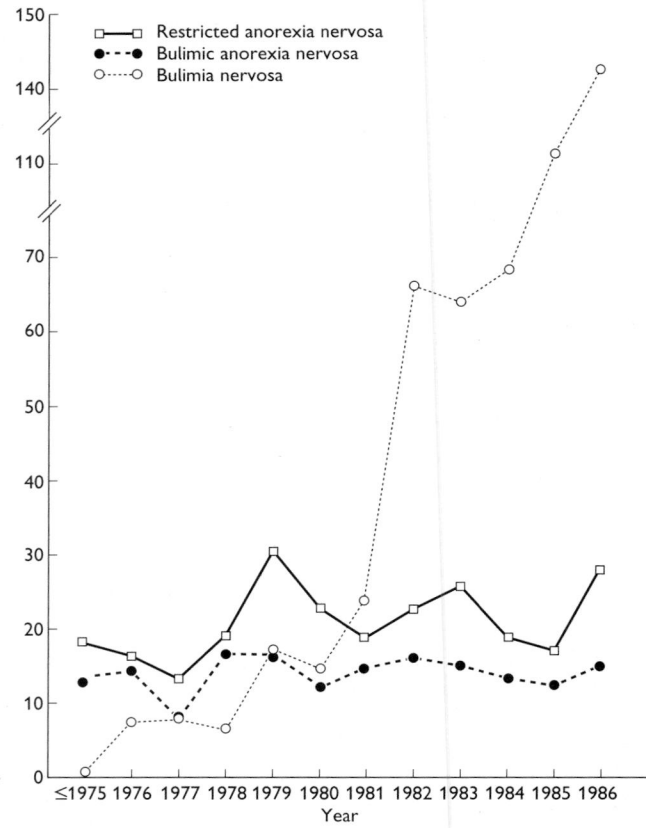

Fig. 3 Rates of referral to a major eating disorder centre in Toronto (1975–1986). (Reproduced with permission from D.M. Garner and C.G. Fairburn (1988). Relationship between anorexia nervosa and bulimia nervosa: diagnostic implications. In *Diagnostic issues in anorexia nervosa and bulimia nervosa* (ed. D.M. Garner and P.E. Garfinkel). Brunner–Mazel, New York.)

and since these have been based upon clinic rather than community samples, they are likely to underestimate the true figures. Even today, many people with bulimia nervosa do not seek help. The lack of reliable community-based incidence figures also makes it impossible to know whether the disorder has become more common since the 1970s or whether the upsurge in cases in the early 1980s was as a result of undetected cases being more likely to seek treatment. Data from the assessment of women in different birth cohorts[40] suggest that the disorder has become much more common (Fig. 4), although other explanations for the apparent increase cannot be ruled out. It is of note that systematic searches of the psychiatric literature prior to the mid-1970s have uncovered very few cases of the disorder.[41]

Aetiology

Development of the disorder

As noted in Chapter 4.10.1, anorexia nervosa generally starts in mid-adolescence with a period of voluntary dietary restriction which proceeds to get out of control. As a result body weight falls and a state of starvation develops. Shape and weight concerns may predate the onset of the dieting or develop as weight is lost.

Bulimia nervosa starts in a similar way although the age of onset is

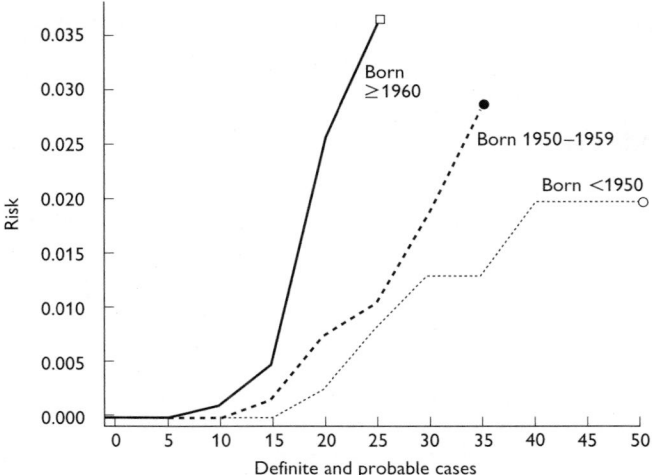

Fig. 4 Lifetime cumulative risk of bulimia nervosa among different birth cohorts of female twins. (Reproduced with permission from K.S. Kendler *et al.* (1991). The genetic epidemiology of bulimia nervosa. *American Journal of Psychiatry*, **148**, 1627–37.)

typically some years later, and shape and weight concerns usually antedate the dieting. The dietary restriction resembles that seen in anorexia nervosa and it leads to weight loss sufficient to result in anorexia nervosa in about a quarter of cases. (As a result of referral bias, this proportion is higher in cases seen in specialist centres.) In the remaining cases there is also weight loss but it is less extreme. After a variable length of time (generally within 3 years) dietary control breaks down with the patient's dieting becoming punctuated by episodes of overeating. At first, the episodes of overeating may be modest in size and intermittent, but gradually they become larger and more frequent. As a result, the lost weight is regained and body weight returns to near its original level. By this point the disorder tends to be self-perpetuating. At some stage in this sequence of events, self-induced vomiting and laxative misuse may be adopted to compensate for the overeating. In practice, however, both forms of behaviour have the opposite effect since belief in their effectiveness encourages a relaxation of control over eating. In those who vomit this phenomenon is exaggerated by the discovery that the process is easier after eating large amounts of food.

Predisposing factors and processes

There are many risk factors for the development of bulimia nervosa[27,42] and these overlap with those for anorexia nervosa.[26] The risk factors may be usefully divided into a number of categories.

1. Demographic factors: these are being female, adolescent, and living in a Western society.

2. Exposure to an immediate social environment that encourages dieting: this includes being brought up in a family in which there is intense interest in shape, weight, and eating as a result of one or more members either having some degree of eating disorder or having a medical condition that affects eating or weight (such as diabetes mellitus). Extreme occupational or recreational pressures to diet also appear to be associated with increased risk (e.g. ballet dancing[43]), although there may also be an element of self-

selection. Another important influence is parental and childhood obesity, the rates of which are substantially increased in bulimia nervosa. Both are likely to sensitize individuals to their appearance and weight, and thereby make them prone to diet. There is also some evidence that puberty occurs comparatively early which may also magnify concerns about shape.

3. Exposure to factors that increase the risk of psychiatric disturbance in general and depression in particular: these include a family history of psychiatric disorder, especially depression, and a range of adverse childhood experiences including parenting deficits and sexual and physical abuse.[27,44,45] It was thought that sexual abuse was especially common among those who develop bulimia nervosa, but the balance of evidence suggests that the rate is no higher than that among those who develop other psychiatric disorders.[27,46] There is some evidence that those who report such a history have more general psychiatric symptoms than those who do not.[46]

4. Perfectionism and low self-esteem: both traits are common antecedents of anorexia nervosa and bulimia nervosa. Typically these factors interact, resulting in feelings of incompetence and ineffectiveness.

5. Family history of substance abuse: there is a raised rate of substance abuse in the families of patients with bulimia nervosa.[30] It is not clear how this increases the risk of bulimia nervosa. Clinical observations suggest that some of those who develop bulimia nervosa learn to modulate their mood by consuming large quantities of food, alcohol, or psychoactive drugs.

An important question is how those with anorexia nervosa are able to maintain strict control over their eating whereas this is not true of those with bulimia nervosa. The explanation is unclear but several processes may be of relevance. First, perfectionism is even more pronounced in anorexia nervosa[42] and it may enhance self-control. Second, the vulnerability to obesity found in bulimia nervosa may somehow undermine dietary restraint. Third, the mood lability of bulimia nervosa may also disrupt restraint.

The contribution of genetic factors

The magnitude of inherited influences is unclear. Several studies have found an increased rate of anorexia nervosa and bulimia nervosa among the relatives of probands with bulimia nervosa,[25] whereas other studies have found either no increase or only an increase in atypical eating disorders.[30] The findings of the first twin series of note suggested that the inherited contribution was minimal.[47] More recent studies from the Virginia Twin Registry have yielded inconsistent findings with estimates of heritability varying from negligible[48] to 55 per cent[40] to 83 per cent.[49] A number of factors are likely to have contributed to the variability in the findings, including the small sample sizes (which render twin models unstable) and the difficulty making lifetime diagnoses of bulimia nervosa. It is also of note that, in contrast with other psychiatric disorders, the findings suggest that there may be violations of the equal environments assumption that underpins twin studies.[48,49]

The nature of any inherited vulnerability is a matter of speculation. The liability appears not to be shared with that for other psychiatric disorders,[25] although there is evidence suggestive of shared familial transmission between anorexia nervosa and obsessive–compulsive personality disorder,[30] a construct which overlaps with that of perfectionism. It is possible that there is an inherited abnormality in the regulation of weight and eating habits in view of the raised rates of parental and childhood obesity. This may include susceptibility to adverse consequences of dieting. Dieting is known to affect 5-hydroxytryptamine neurotransmission particularly among women,[50] and there is evidence of abnormalities in brain 5-hydroxytryptamine function in women who have recovered from bulimia nervosa. For example, one study found that acutely lowering brain 5-hydroxytryptamine function resulted in the temporary reappearance of bulimic symptoms[51] and another found abnormal levels of cerebrospinal fluid 5-hydroxyindoleacetic acid.[52] The molecular genetic studies of eating disorders are focusing on the genes involved in 5-hydroxytryptamine neurotransmission but no consistent findings have emerged.[25]

Maintaining factors and processes

Once established, bulimia nervosa tends to run a chronic course with the proviso that it tends to improve over the long term (see below). There are a number of processes which account for its self-perpetuating character which are discussed in Chapter 4.10.1. They include the ongoing influence of the extreme concerns about shape and weight; the form of these patient's dieting, which encourages binge eating; the mood-modulating effect of binge eating; and the fact that the loss of control over eating perpetuates fears of weight gain.

Assessment

The identification of patients with bulimia nervosa is not difficult so long as the diagnosis is considered. This is important because the shame that characterizes the disorder leads many people to delay seeking help—the average delay between onset and presentation is about 5 years—and when they do present for treatment, some do so indirectly. Thus they may complain of depression, substance abuse, menstrual disturbance, or gastrointestinal symptoms, rather than the eating disorder itself. The best policy is for psychiatrists always to keep in mind the possibility of bulimia nervosa when assessing female patients aged between 16 and 35 years. Negative responses to the following two questions should suffice to exclude the disorder.

1. Do you have any problems with your eating?
2. Do you have any problems controlling your eating, i.e. problems with binge eating?

Patients who present directly complain of having lost control over eating and their assessment is generally straightforward.

The best established measure of eating disorder features is the Eating Disorder Examination.[53] This interview is widely regarded as the 'gold standard' measure of eating disorders,[54] and it may be used either for routine clinical assessment or for research purposes. It defines all key terms and generates operational eating disorder diagnoses. Various self-report questionnaires are available but they provide a more basic level of assessment and they cannot be used to make a clinical diagnosis. The leading self-report measures are the Eating Disorder Inventory[55] and the self-report version of the Eating Disorder Examination.[56]

No assessment is complete without weighing the patient. This needs to be done with considerable sensitivity because of these patients' concerns about their weight. A physical examination is not essential unless the patient is underweight (or there are other medical indications), nor are laboratory tests required except in those cases in which there is reason to suspect that there might be fluid or electrolyte disturbance.

Treatment

Given that bulimia nervosa has only recently been described, there has been a remarkable amount of research on its treatment. Over 50 randomized controlled trials have been completed.[57] Although almost all these studies have been 'efficacy' rather than 'effectiveness' studies, there are reasons to think that their findings are of direct relevance to routine patient care not least because the patients studied have been similar to those seen in clinical practice.[58] Nevertheless, there is a definite need for effectiveness research particularly now that main treatment options are clear.

Studies of pharmacological treatment

A variety of drugs have been tested as possible treatments for bulimia nervosa including antidepressants, appetite suppressants, anticonvulsants, and lithium. Only antidepressants have shown promise.

Antidepressant medication

All the major classes of antidepressant drug have been evaluated, including tricyclic antidepressants, monoamine oxidase inhibitors, selective serotonin uptake inhibitors, and atypical antidepressants. The findings have been relatively consistent and may be summarized as follows (adapted from Wilson and Fairburn[57]).

1. Antidepressant drugs are more effective than placebo at reducing the frequency of binge eating and purging. On average, among treatment completers there is about a 60 per cent reduction in the frequency of binge eating and a cessation rate of about 20 per cent. The therapeutic effect is more rapid than that seen in depression. There is generally little change in the placebo group. The drop-out rate varies but averages about 30 per cent.

2. The longer-term effects of antidepressant drugs remain largely untested. Almost all of the studies to date have been of their short-term use (16 weeks or less). The findings of the few longer-term studies suggest that outcome is poor whether or not patients remain on medication.

3. Few studies have evaluated the effects of antidepressant drugs on features other than binge eating and purging. Mood improves as the frequency of binge eating declines but this effect is common to all treatments for bulimia nervosa. Antidepressant drugs do not appear to modify the patient's extreme dieting which may account for the apparently poor maintenance of change.

4. The different antidepressant drugs seem to be equally effective, although there have been no direct comparisons of different drugs.

5. With one exception, there have been no systematic dose–response studies. The exception showed that fluoxetine at a dose of 60 mg/day, but not 20 mg/day, was more effective than placebo.

6. Patients who fail to respond to one antidepressant drug may respond to another. There have been no drug augmentation studies.

7. No consistent predictors of response have been identified. Pretreatment levels of depression appear not to be related to outcome.

8. The mechanism(s) whereby antidepressant drugs exert their 'antibulimic' effects is not known. The apparent comparability of different classes of drug implicates a common mechanism but this is unlikely to be their antidepressant action since the response is too rapid and the level of depression does not predict outcome.

Studies of psychological treatment

Cognitive-behavioural therapy

The most intensively studied psychological treatment is a specific form of cognitive-behavioural therapy. This was the first promising treatment described[59] and it remains the leading treatment for the disorder. The treatment and its rationale are described in Chapter 6.3.2.2.

Cognitive-behavioural therapy is conducted on an outpatient basis and involves 15 to 20 sessions over about 5 months. It is suitable for all patients bar the small minority (less than 5 per cent) who require hospital admission.

The findings of the studies of cognitive-behavioural therapy (over 20 controlled trials) are summarized below (adapted from Wilson and Fairburn[57]).

1. The drop-out rate with cognitive-behavioural therapy (about 15 per cent) is about half that seen with antidepressant drugs. The treatment is also more acceptable to these patients than treatment with medication.

2. Cognitive-behavioural therapy has a substantial effect on the frequency of binge eating and purging. On average, among treatment completers there is about an 80 per cent reduction in the frequency of binge eating, and a cessation rate of about 60 per cent.

3. The effects of cognitive-behavioural therapy appear to be well maintained. Most of the recent studies have included a 6 to 12 month follow-up period. The relapse rates are low.

4. Cognitive-behavioural therapy affects most aspects of the psychopathology of bulimia nervosa including the binge eating, purging, dietary restraint, and the overevaluation of shape and weight. In common with other treatments, the level of depression decreases as the frequency of binge eating declines. Social functioning and self-esteem also improve.

5. Cognitive-behavioural therapy is more effective than delayed treatment (that is, a waiting list control group), other psychological treatments (other than possibly interpersonal psychotherapy; see below), and antidepressant drugs at reducing the frequency of binge eating and purging. Among the other psychological treatments studied have been supportive psychotherapy, focal psychotherapy, supportive–expressive psychotherapy, interpersonal psychotherapy, hypnobehavioural treatment, stress management, nutritional counselling, behavioural versions of

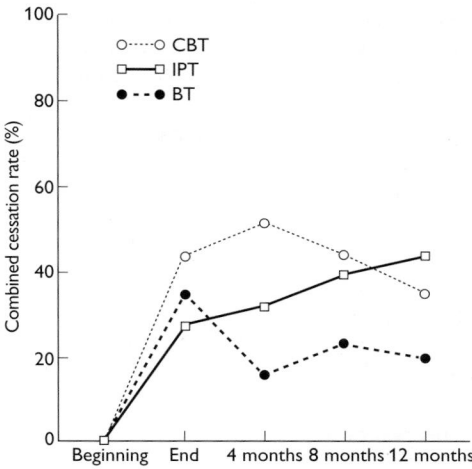

Fig. 5 Rates of abstinence from both binge eating and purging among patients with bulimia nervosa allocated to cognitive-behavioural therapy (CBT), behaviour therapy (BT), and interpersonal psychotherapy (IPT). (Reproduced with permission from C.G. Fairburn *et al.* (1993). Psychotherapy and bulimia nervosa: the longer-term effects of interpersonal psychotherapy, behaviour therapy and cognitive behaviour therapy. *Archives of General Psychiatry*, **50**, 419–28.)

cognitive-behavioural therapy, and exposure with response prevention.

6. No consistent predictors of response to cognitive-behavioural therapy have been identified. Severity of symptoms at presentation, a history of anorexia nervosa, low self-esteem, and the presence of borderline personality disorder have been associated with worse outcome in some studies but not others. Initial response (over the first 4 weeks of treatment) is emerging as a useful predictor of subsequent outcome.

7. The mechanism(s) of action of cognitive-behavioural therapy have yet to be established. It seems that the cognitive procedures are required for progress to be maintained since behavioural versions of the treatment are associated with a greater risk of relapse (as illustrated in Fig. 5).

8. There is evidence that the combination of cognitive-behavioural therapy and antidepressant drugs may be more effective than cognitive-behavioural therapy alone in reducing anxiety and depressive symptoms.

9. Simpler forms of cognitive-behavioural therapy show promise. These include brief versions of the treatment designed for use in primary care and cognitive-behavioural self-help in which patients follow a cognitive-behavioural self-help programme either on their own (pure self-help) or with the guidance of a therapist (guided self-help).[60,61]

Interpersonal psychotherapy

Interpersonal psychotherapy is the leading alternative to cognitive-behavioural therapy. This treatment was originally devised by Klerman *et al.*[62] as a treatment for depression (see Chapter 6.3.3). It is a focal psychotherapy, the main emphasis of which is to help patients identify and modify current interpersonal problems. The treatment is both non-directive and non-interpretative and, as adapted for bulimia nervosa,[63] it pays little attention to the patient's eating disorder. It is therefore very different to cognitive-behavioural therapy. In a comparison of cognitive-behavioural therapy, interpersonal psychotherapy and a behavioural version of cognitive-behavioural therapy, interpersonal psychotherapy was found to be the least effective of the three treatments at the end of treatment but the proportion of responders continued to increase such that it was as effective as cognitive-behavioural therapy by 8 and 12 month follow-up[64] (see Fig. 5), and indeed, 5 years later.[63] The marked difference between the two treatments in their procedures and temporal influence suggested that, although they were equivalent in their eventual effects, each treatment operated through specific mechanisms. A recent large-scale replication of the cognitive-behavioural therapy versus interpersonal psychotherapy comparison has confirmed these findings.

Exposure with response prevention

This is an adaptation of the behavioural treatment for obsessive–compulsive disorder (see Chapter 4.8) in which patients with bulimia nervosa are presented with cues that generally precede binge eating or vomiting and are then prevented from engaging in their usual response. It was advocated in the 1980s both as a treatment in its own right and as an element of cognitive-behavioural therapy. It is difficult to administer for a number of reasons: patients find it aversive; it is procedurally complex; and the sessions are time-consuming. The studies of its use suggest that it conveys no benefit over standard cognitive-behavioural therapy.[57,65]

Management of bulimia nervosa

Given the large number of patients with bulimia nervosa and the scarcity of therapists with training in the treatment of eating disorders, a 'stepped care' approach to management has been advocated. With such an approach a simple treatment is used first and only if this proves insufficient is a more complex and specialized intervention provided. Four steps may be distinguished.

Step 1

Having established the diagnosis, the first decision is whether the patient may be treated on an outpatient basis. The great majority (over 95 per cent of referrals to non-specialist centres) may be managed this way. Exceptions are patients whose level of depression is so severe that they cannot make use of psychological treatment, significant risk of suicide, and physical complications necessitating inpatient or day patient care. Severe substance abuse requires treatment in its own right, although this can sometimes be integrated with the treatment of the eating disorder. For example, it is possible to adapt cognitive-behavioural therapy for bulimia nervosa so that it addresses at the same time the patient's substance abuse.

Step 2

If the patient is suitable for outpatient treatment, guided cognitive-behavioural self-help is the next step. In this context, this involves following a cognitive-behavioural self-help programme under the guidance of a 'facilitator' (a non-specialist therapist). Three cognitive-behavioural self-help books are available,[66–68] two of which are direct translations of cognitive-behavioural therapy for bulimia nervosa. There is evidence to support the use of all three books and it is a matter

of preference which is used. All three provide information about bulimia nervosa together with a self-help programme. The role of the facilitator is not to provide treatment as such, as in a conventional 'therapist-led' treatment, but rather to support and encourage the patient to follow the programme. Thus, this is a 'programme-led' form of treatment, and it is this characteristic that makes it suitable for dissemination. The treatment generally takes about 4 months and involves 8 to 10 meetings with the facilitator, each lasting up to 30 min. It is best if the first few appointments are weekly.

Step 2 may take place in a variety of settings including primary care. A third to a half of patients show substantial change, and their progress appears to be well maintained. No consistent predictors of outcome have been identified. Patients who obtain little benefit (and usually this is obvious within 4 to 6 weeks) need to move on to step 3, although it would not be inappropriate to recommend as an interim step a brief trial of an antidepressant drug with those patients who are willing to consider drug treatment (see step 3).

Research on the treatment of binge eating disorder suggests that there may be a subgroup of patients who will respond to 'pure self-help', that is following a cognitive-behavioural self-help programme with no outside support.[69] In clinical situations in which there will be a delay before therapist/facilitator-led treatment can be provided, pure self-help may have a role. At the very least it provides patients with sound information about the disorder. No adverse effects of pure or guided self-help have been identified, and failure to respond does not seem to affect response to subsequent treatment.

Step 3

Patients who do not benefit from cognitive-behavioural self-help should receive full cognitive-behavioural therapy (see Chapter 6.3.2.2). In most cases this should be provided on its own, but it may be worthwhile adding an antidepressant drug under any one of the following three circumstances: if significant depressive symptoms are interfering with compliance, if depressive symptoms are persisting despite an improvement in eating habits, and if progress is limited. The drug of choice is fluoxetine (60 mg). This can be started without intermediate lower doses and it should be taken in the morning.

Step 4

The fourth step is essentially pragmatic since there are few research findings of relevance. To guide the choice of treatment, reasons for non-response need to be carefully considered. Explanations include failure of cognitive-behavioural therapy, poorly administered cognitive-behavioural therapy, poor patient compliance (which itself needs to be explained), and the influence of outside events.

There are a number of different treatment options under these circumstances, the choice of which depends upon the outcome of the reassessment and the resources available. They include the following.

- Stop treatment and arrange to re-evaluate the patient after an interval of some months. This can be justified on at least two grounds. First, bulimia nervosa has a general tendency to improve over time (see below). Spontaneous improvement may therefore occur. Second, patients and therapists can show 'burn-out' after sustained periods of therapeutic work. A break can often be helpful. Deciding to stop treatment should be a joint decision and it is not appropriate with patients who are distressed or with those whose physical or psychological well being is a cause for concern.

- Change antidepressant drug. As noted above, there is evidence that some patients respond to a change in antidepressant drug. If there is going to be a response to a second-line drug, it is likely to be rapid (within a few weeks). No guidelines are available to govern the choice of drug.

- Embark upon a new psychological treatment. While one obvious choice is interpersonal psychotherapy, there are no grounds for supposing that patients who fail to respond to cognitive-behavioural therapy will respond to interpersonal psychotherapy. Indeed, there is emerging evidence that this is not the case. An alternative strategy is to change the form of cognitive-behavioural therapy. The re-evaluation of the patient may have resulted in the identification of problems that might be amenable to cognitive-behavioural procedures outside the realm of mainstream cognitive-behavioural therapy for bulimia nervosa. For example, those with extreme concerns about shape might benefit from more emphasis on body image[70] and those with markedly low self-esteem might respond to an approach which focuses on negative self-evaluation.[71]

- Arrange for day patient or inpatient treatment. In a small minority of cases outpatient treatment proves not to be sufficient, either because the disorder is resistant to treatment or because the patient's life circumstances are interfering with progress. In such cases day patient or inpatient treatment can be useful. Generally this involves a combination of approaches including elements of cognitive-behavioural therapy. Both day patient treatment and inpatient treatment should be followed by treatment on an outpatient basis designed to ensure that progress is maintained.

Course and outcome

Much remains to be learned about the course and outcome of bulimia nervosa. It is clear from epidemiological studies that many people do not present for treatment. The course of their disorder is completely unknown. Those who do present tend to do so after a considerable period of time indicating that among this subgroup the disorder has a tendency to run a protracted course. Conversely, the findings of the treatment studies indicate that the outcome is considerably better than Russell originally suggested, although it must be stressed that even with cognitive-behavioural therapy, the most effective treatment, only about half the patients make a full recovery.

There have been few studies of long-term course or outcome. The studies with longer periods of follow-up have identified proportionately fewer cases at reassessment.[72] At 10-year follow-up, about 10 per cent meet diagnostic criteria for bulimia nervosa and a further 15 per cent have an atypical eating disorder.[73,74] There is no evidence that bulimia nervosa evolves into any other psychiatric disorder, and anorexia nervosa is a very unusual outcome. Body weight barely changes over time and, in contrast with anorexia nervosa, the mortality rate appears not to be raised. The disorder tends to improve during pregnancy but subsequent relapse is common.[75,76] No robust predictors of course or outcome have been identified.

Thus, if one takes a long-term perspective, there seems to be a trend towards recovery. Whether this is an inherent property of bulimia nervosa, whether it is age-related, or whether it reflects the influence of treatment is not known.

References

1. Russell, G.F.M. (1979). Bulimia nervosa: an ominous variant of anorexia nervosa. *Psychological Medicine*, **9**, 429–48.

2. American Psychiatric Association (1980). *DSM-III: diagnostic and statistical manual of mental disorders*. American Psychiatric Association, Washington, DC.

3. American Psychiatric Association (1987). *DSM-IIIR*. American Psychiatric Association, Washington, DC.

4. American Psychiatric Association (1994). *Diagnostic and statistical manual of mental disorders* (4th edn). American Psychiatric Association, Washington, DC.

5. World Health Organization (1992). *International statistical classification of diseases and related health problems, 10th revision*. WHO, Geneva

6. Fairburn, C.G. and Walsh, B.T. (1995). Atypical eating disorders. In *Eating disorders and obesity: a comprehensive handbook* (ed. K.D. Brownell and C.G. Fairburn), pp. 135–40. Guilford Press, New York.

7. Fairburn, C.G., Welch, S.L., and Hay, P.J. (1993). The classification of recurrent overeating: the 'binge eating disorder' proposal. *International Journal of Eating Disorders*, **13**, 155–9.

8. Castonguay, L.G., Eldredge, K.L., and Agras, W.S. (1995). Binge eating disorder: current state and future directions. *Clinical Psychology Review*, **15**, 865–90.

9. Carlat, D.J., Camargo, C.A., Herzog, P.H., and Herzog, D.B. (1997). Eating disorders in males: a report on 135 patients. *American Journal of Psychiatry*, **154**, 1127–32.

10. Fairburn, C.G. and Wilson, G.T. (1993). Binge eating: definition and classification. In *Binge eating: nature, assessment and treatment* (ed. C.G. Fairburn and G.T. Wilson), pp. 3–14. Guilford Press, New York.

11. Walsh, B.T. (1993). Binge eating in bulimia nervosa. In *Binge eating: nature, assessment and treatment* (ed. C.G. Fairburn and G.T. Wilson), pp. 37–49. Guilford Press, New York.

12. Kaye, W.H., Weltzin, T.E., Hsu, L.K.G., McConaha, C.W., and Bolton, B. (1993). Amount of calories retained after binge eating and vomiting. *American Journal of Psychiatry*, **150**, 969–71.

13. Bo-Linn, G.W., Santa Ana, C.A., Morawski, S.G., and Fordtran, J.S. (1983). Purging and calorie absorption in bulimic patients and normal women. *Annals of Internal Medicine*, **99**, 14–17.

14. Lacey, J.H. and Smith, G. (1987). Bulimia nervosa: the impact of pregnancy on mother and baby. *British Journal of Psychiatry*, **150**, 777–81.

15. Stein, A., Woolley, H., Cooper, S., and Fairburn, C.G. (1994). An observational study of mothers with eating disorders and their infants. *Journal of Child Psychology and Psychiatry*, **35**, 733–48.

16. Stein, A. and Fairburn, C.G. (1989). Children of mothers with bulimia nervosa. *British Medical Journal*, **299**, 777–8.

17. Stein, A., Murray, L., Cooper, P.J., and Fairburn, C.G. (1996). Infant growth in the context of maternal eating disorders and maternal depression: a comparative study. *Psychological Medicine*, **26**, 569–74.

18. Braun, D.L., Sunday, S.R., and Halmi, K.A. (1994). Psychiatric comorbidity in patients with eating disorders. *Psychological Medicine*, **24**, 859–67.

19. Brewerton, T.D., Lydiard, R.B., Herzog, D.B., Brotman, A.W., O'Neil, P.M., and Ballenger, J.C. (1995). Comorbidity of Axis I psychiatic disorders in bulimia nervosa. *Journal of Clinical Psychiatry*, **56**, 77–80.

20. Welch, S.L. and Fairburn, C.G. (1996). Impulsivity or comorbidity in bulimia nervosa. A controlled study of deliberate self-harm and alcohol and drug misuse in a community sample. *British Journal of Psychiatry*, **169**, 451–8.

21. Lacey, J.H. (1993). Self-damaging and addictive behaviour in bulimia nervosa. A catchment area study. *British Journal of Psychiatry*, **163**, 190–4.

22. Vitousek, K. and Manke, F. (1994). Personality variables and disorders in anorexia nervosa and bulimia nervosa. *Journal of Abnormal Psychology*, **103**, 137–47.

23. Mitchell, J.E. (1995). Medical complications of bulimia nervosa. In *Eating disorders and obesity: a comprehensive handbook* (ed. K.D. Brownell and C.G. Fairburn), pp. 271–5. Guilford Press, New York.

24. Mitchell, J.E., Pomeroy, C., and Adson, D.E. (1997). Managing medical complications. In *Handbook of treatment for eating disorders* (ed. D.M. Garner and P.E. Garfinkel), pp. 383–93. Guilford Press, New York.

25. Strober, M., Lilenfeld, L.R., Kaye, W., and Bulik, C. (2000). Genetic factors in anorexia nervosa and bulimia nervosa. In *Feeding problems and eating disorders* (ed. P.J. Cooper and A. Stein). Harwood, Switzerland, in press.

26. Fairburn, C.G., Cooper, Z., Doll, H.A., and Welch, S.L. (1999). Risk factors for anorexia nervosa: three integrated case–control comparisons. *Archives of General Psychiatry*, **56**, 468–76.

27. Fairburn, C.G., Welch, S.L., Doll, H.A., Davies, B.A., and O'Connor, M.E. (1997). Risk factors for bulimia nervosa: a community-based case–control study. *Archives of General Psychiatry*, **54**, 509–17.

28. Fairburn, C.G., Norman, P.A., Welch, S.L., O'Connor, M.E., Doll, H.A., and Peveler, R.C. (1995). A prospective study of outcome in bulimia nervosa and the long-term effects of three psychological treatments. *Archives of General Psychiatry*, **52**, 304–12.

29. Bulik, C.M., Sullivan, P.F., Fear, J.L., and Joyce, P.R. (1997). Eating disorders and antecedent anxiety disorders: a controlled study. *Acta Psychiatrica Scandinavica*, **96**, 101–7.

30. Lilenfeld, L.R., Kaye, W.H., Greeno, C.G., *et al.* (1998). A controlled family study of anorexia nervosa and bulimia nervosa. *Archives of General Psychiatry*, **55**, 603–10.

31. Fairburn, C.G., Peveler, R.C., Davies, B., Mann, J.I., and Mayou, R.A. (1991). Eating disorders in young adults with insulin dependent diabetes: a controlled study. *British Medical Journal*, **303**, 17–20.

32. Peveler, R.C., Fairburn, C.G., Boller, I., and Dunger, D. (1992). Eating disorders in adolescents with IDDM. A controlled study. *Diabetes Care*, **15**, 1356–60.

33. Fairburn, C.G. and Cooper, P.J. (1982). Self-induced vomiting and bulimia nervosa: an undetected problem. *British Medical Journal*, **284**, 1153–5.

34. Fairburn, C.G. and Cooper, P.J. (1984). Binge-eating, self-induced vomiting and laxative abuse: a community study. *Psychological Medicine*, **14**, 401–10.

35. Turnbull, S., Ward, A., Treasure, J., Jick, H., and Derby, L. (1996). The demand for eating disorder care. *British Journal of Psychiatry*, **169**, 705–12.

36. Millar, H.R. (1998). New eating disorder service. *Psychiatric Bulletin*, **22**, 751–4.

37. Fairburn, C.G. and Beglin, S.J. (1990). Studies of the epidemiology of bulimia nervosa. *American Journal of Psychiatry*, **147**, 401–8.

38. van Hoeken, D., Lucas, A.R., and Hoek, H.W. (1998). Epidemiology. In *Neurobiology in the treatment of eating disorders* (ed. H.W. Hoek, J.L. Treasure, and M.A. Katzman), pp. 97–126. Wiley, Chichester.

39. Garfinkel, P.E., Lin, E., Goering, P., *et al.* (1995). Bulimia nervosa in a Canadian community sample: prevalence and comparison of subgroups. *American Journal of Psychiatry*, **152**, 1052–8.

40. Kendler, K.S., MacLean, C., Neale, M., Kessler, R., Heath, A., and Eaves, L. (1991). The genetic epidemiology of bulimia nervosa. *American Journal of Psychiatry*, **148**, 1627–37.

41. Russell, G.F.M. (1997). The history of bulimia nervosa. In *Handbook of treatment for eating disorders* (ed. D.M. Garner and P.E. Garfinkel), pp. 11–24. Guilford Press, New York.

42. Palmer, R.L. (1998). Aetiology of bulimia nervosa. In *Neurobiology in the treatment of eating disorders* (ed. H.W. Hoek, J.L. Treasure, and M.A. Katzman), pp. 143–59. Wiley, Chichester.

43. Garner, D.M., Garfinkel, P.E., Rockert, W., and Olmsted, M.P. (1987). A prospective study of eating disturbances in the ballet. *Psychotherapy and Psychosomatics*, **48**, 170–5.

44. Schmidt, U., Tiller, J., and Treasure, J. (1993). Setting the scene for eating disorders: childhood care, classification and course of illness. *Psychological Medicine*, **23**, 663–72.

45. Welch, S.L., Doll, H.A., and Fairburn, C.G. (1997). Life events and the onset of bulimia nervosa: a controlled study. *Psychological Medicine*, **27**, 515–22.

46. Fallon, P. and Wonderlich, S.A. (1997). Sexual abuse and other forms of trauma. In *Handbook of treatment for eating disorders* (ed. D.M. Garner and P.E. Garfinkel), pp. 394–414. Guilford Press, New York.

47. Treasure, J. and Holland, A. (1991). Genetic vulnerability to eating disorders: evidence from twin and family studies. In *Child and youth psychiatry: European perspectives* (ed. H. Remschmidt and M.H. Schmidt), pp. 59–67. Hogrefe and Huber, New York.

48. Hettema, J.M., Neale, M.C., and Kendler, K.S. (1995). Physical similarity and the equal-environment assumption in twin studies of psychiatric disorders. *Behavior Genetics*, **25**, 327–35.

49. Bulik, C.M., Sullivan, P.F., and Kendler, K.S. (1998). Heritability of binge-eating and broadly defined bulimia nervosa. *Biological Psychiatry*, **44**, 1210–18.

50. Cowen, P.J., Anderson, I.M., and Fairburn, C.G. (1992). Neurochemical effects of dieting: relevance to changes in eating and affective disorders. In *The biology of feast and famine* (ed. G.H. Anderson and S.H. Kennedy), pp. 269–84. Academic Press, San Diego, CA.

51. Smith, K.A., Fairburn, C.G., and Cowen, P.J. (1999). Symptomatic relapse in bulimia nervosa following acute tryptophan depletion. *Archives of General Psychiatry*, **56**, 171–6.

52. Kaye, W.H., Greeno, C.G., Moss, H., *et al.* (1998). Alterations in serotonin activity and psychiatric symptoms after recovery from bulimia nervosa. *Archives of General Psychiatry*, **55**, 927–35.

53. Fairburn, C.G. and Cooper, Z. (1993). The Eating Disorder Examination (12th edition). In *Binge eating: nature, assessment and treatment* (ed. C.G. Fairburn and G.T. Wilson), pp. 317–60. Guilford Press, New York.

54. Garner, D.M. (1995). Assessment of eating disorder psychopathology. In *Eating disorders and obesity* (ed. K.D. Brownell and C.G. Fairburn), pp. 117–21. Guilford Press, New York.

55. Garner, D.M. (1991). *Eating disorder inventory*, Vol. 2. Psychological Assessment Resources, Odessa, FL.

56. Fairburn, C.G. and Beglin, S.J. (1994). Assessment of eating disorders: interview or self-report questionnaire? *International Journal of Eating Disorders*, **16**, 363–70.

57. Wilson, G.T. and Fairburn, C.G. (1998). Treatments for eating disorders. In *A guide to treatments that work* (ed. P.E. Nathan and J.M. Gorman), pp. 501–30. Oxford University Press, New York.

58. Wilson, G.T. (1998). The clinical utility of randomised controlled trials. *International Journal of Eating Disorders*, **24**, 13–29.

59. Fairburn, C.G. (1981). A cognitive behavioural approach to the management of bulimia. *Psychological Medicine*, **11**, 707–11.

60. Fairburn, C.G. and Carter, J.C. (1997). Self-help and guided self-help for binge-eating problems. In *Handbook of treatment for eating disorders* (ed. D.M. Garner and P.E. Garfinkel), pp. 494–9. Guilford Press, New York.

61. Pasquale, L., Sciuto, G., Cocchi, S., Ronchi, P., and Bellodi, L. (1994). A family study of obsessive compulsive, eating and mood disorders. *European Psychiatry*, **9**, 33–8.

62. Klerman, G.L., Weissman, M.M., Rounsaville, B.J., and Chevron, E.S. (1984). *Interpersonal psychotherapy of depression*. Basic Books, New York.

63. Fairburn, C.G. (1997). Interpersonal psychotherapy for bulimia nervosa. In *Handbook of treatment for eating disorders* (ed. D.M. Garner and P.E. Garfinkel), pp. 278–94. Guilford Press, New York.

64. Fairburn, C.G., Jones, R., Peveler, R.C., Hope, R.A., and O'Connor, M. (1993). Psychotherapy and bulimia nervosa: the longer-term effects of interpersonal psychotherapy, behaviour therapy and cognitive behaviour therapy. *Archives of General Psychiatry*, **50**, 419–28.

65. Bulik, C.M., Sullivan, P.F., Carter, F.A., McIntosh, V.V., and Joyce, P.R. (1998). The role of exposure with response prevention in the cognitive-

behavioural therapy for bulimia nervosa. *Psychological Medicine*, **28**, 611–23.

66. Cooper, P.J. (1995). *Bulimia nervosa and binge eating: a guide to recovery*. Robinson, London.

67. Fairburn, C.G. (1995). *Overcoming binge eating*. Guilford Press, New York.

68. Schmidt, U. and Treasure, J. (1993). *Getting better bit(e) by bit(e)*. Erlbaum, Hove.

69. Carter, J.C. and Fairburn, C.G. (1998). Cognitive-behavioral self-help for binge eating disorder: a controlled effectiveness study. *Journal of Clinical and Consulting Psychology*, **66**, 616–23.

70. Rosen, J.C. (1997). Cognitive-behavioural body image therapy. In *Handbook of treatment for eating disorders* (ed. D.M. Garner and P.E. Garfinkel), pp. 188–201. Guilford Press, New York.

71. Fennell, M.J.V. (1997). Low self-esteem: a cognitive perspective. *Behavioural and Cognitive Psychotherapy*, **25**, 1–25.

72. Keel, P.K. and Mitchell, J.E. (1997). Outcome in bulimia nervosa. *American Journal of Psychiatry*, **153**, 313–21.

73. Collings, S. and King, M. (1994). Ten-year follow-up of 50 patients with bulimia nervosa. *British Journal of Psychiatry*, **164**, 80–7.

74. Keel, P.K., Mitchell, J.E., Miller, K.B., Davis, T.L., and Crow, S.J. (1999). Long-term outcome of bulimia nervosa. *Archives of General Psychiatry*, **56**, 63–9.

75. Fairburn, C.G., Stein, A., and Jones, R. (1992). Eating habits and eating disorders during pregnancy. *Psychosomatic Medicine*, **54**, 665–72.

76. Morgan, J.F., Lacey, H.J., and Sedgwick, P.M. (1999). Impact of pregnancy on bulimia nervosa. *British Journal of Psychiatry*, **174**, 135–40.

4.10.3 Obesity

Albert Stunkard and Thomas A. Wadden

Introduction

The task of the psychiatrist in the management of obesity has changed radically over the years. At one time psychiatrists were accorded a major responsibility for what limited treatment of obesity there was. As it became apparent, however, that obesity was far more than the eating disorder that it had appeared, a responsibility for the treatment of obesity shifted to general practitioners and commercial weight-loss organizations. There appeared to be little role for the psychiatrist. As this chapter makes clear, psychiatrists can play a part in the treatment of obesity. But, in order to do so, they must understand this complex disorder. What follows is an attempt to provide such an understanding.

Obesity is a condition characterized by excessive accumulation of fat in the body. In clinical practice, overweight (weight corrected for height) is used as a surrogate for body fat. This practice is reasonable because body weight and fat are highly correlated, especially at greater degrees of obesity.[1]

Unlike many 'real' diseases, and like hypertension, obesity represents one arm of a distribution curve of body weight, with no physiologically defined cut-off point. In the future, the diagnosis of obesity and body fat distribution may be based on newer methods of measurement. Until that time, for most practical purposes, the eyeball test is sufficient: if a person looks fat, the person is fat.

The origins of obesity go far back into prehistory when the ability to store fat contributed to the survival and evolution of hominids.[2] Since food storages were ubiquitous for humans under usual conditions, selection favoured those who could effectively store calories in times of surplus. This capacity was so highly regarded, particularly for women, that the first representation of the human figure, the so-called Venus of Willendorf which was produced 25 000 years ago, depicted an immensely obese woman.

This ability to store large amounts of fat, so valuable in surviving famine in prehistory, has become maladaptive in the Western world today, where most people have more than enough to eat. Under these circumstances, our biological heritage in today's culture of abundance has given rise to widespread obesity with its devastating sequelae.

Clinical features

It is becoming evident that obesity is one of today's major health hazards.[3] It has been estimated that 300 000 deaths a year in the United States can be attributed to obesity, a figure second only to smoking as a potentially preventable cause of death.[4]

The physical signs of obesity are primarily the direct physical consequence of the increase in body weight and the encompassing mass of fatty tissue. The most serious manifestation of this fatty tissue is caused by pressure on the thorax combined with pressure on the diaphragm from below by large intra-abdominal accumulations of fat. The resultant reduction in respiratory capacity may produce dyspnoea on even minimal exertion. In severely obese people, this condition may progress to the so-called Pickwickian syndrome, characterized by hypoventilation with consequent hypercapnia and hypoxia, and finally somnolence.

Visceral obesity has been associated with three disorders (insulin resistance, dyslipidaemias, and hypertension) in what has been termed the 'metabolic syndrome' and which is a strong risk factor for coronary heart disease.[5] Obesity may lead to a variety of orthopaedic disturbances, including low back pain and aggravation of osteoarthritis. Even mild degrees of obesity may be associated with amenorrhoea and other menstrual disturbances. Other conditions strongly associated with obesity are gallbladder disease, endocrine disturbances, and several cancers.

Previously, reports of emotional disturbance among the obese have flooded the literature. Carefully conducted studies, however, have shown little difference in psychopathology between obese and non-obese people in the general population, and the view that obese people have a specific personality disorder is no longer held. Many obese people report that they overeat when they are emotionally upset, but many non-obese people report similar experiences.

Although the differences in psychopathology are relatively small for the obese population as a whole, for certain subgroups the differences may be quite significant.[6] Prominent among them are teenage and young women of upper and middle socio-economic status. Obesity is uncommon among these women, and the sanctions against it are far stronger than they are against other people. These women are the ones against whom prejudice and discrimination are regularly directed, often with devastating effect.

One of the two forms of psychopathology specific to obesity is disparagement of the body image. Obese people with this disturbance characteristically feel that their bodies are grotesque and loathsome and that others view them with hostility and contempt. This feeling is closely associated with self-consciousness and impaired social functioning. The disorder occurs in only a minority of obese people, those who have been obese since childhood, who also have low self-esteem and manifest other indications of psychopathology. In the group with body image disparagement, neurosis is closely related to obesity, and this group contains a majority of obese people with specific eating disorders.

The second form of psychopathology specific to obesity is eating disorders. The more established one is binge eating disorder, characterized by the consumption of large amounts of food in a short period of time, a subjective sense of loss of control during the binge, and distress after it.[7,8] Unlike patients with bulimia nervosa, these patients do not engage in compensatory behaviours such as vomiting or laxative abuse to prevent the weight gain after a binge, and the binge accordingly may contribute to excessive caloric intake. Binge eating disorder increases in prevalence with increasing body weight and afflicts about 10 to 20 per cent of people entering treatment programmes for obesity. As many as 50 per cent of obese binge eaters suffer from depression, compared with 5 per cent of obese people who do not binge.

The night-eating syndrome, characterized by morning anorexia, evening hyperphagia, and insomnia, appears to be a manifestation of an altered circadian rhythm, precipitated by stressful life experiences.[9] People with the night-eating syndrome show frequent night-time awakenings during which they consume high carbohydrate snacks, evidently in an effort to increase the production of serotonin with its sleep-inducing capabilities. Neuroendocrine disturbances occur in the night-eating syndrome: hypomelatoninaemia may impair sleep, and a failure of the night-time rise in plasma leptin may contribute to hunger and night eating.

Classification

Obesity is classified on the basis of (a) the extent of overweight and (b) the fat distribution. The standard classification of obesity, that of the World Health Organization (**WHO**), is based on a measure of body weight adjusted for height, the body mass index:[1]

$$\text{body mass index} = \frac{\text{weight (kg)}}{(\text{height (m)})^2}.$$

The WHO classifications for body mass index are as follows: underweight, less than 18.50; normal weight, 18.50 to 24.99; grade I overweight, 25.00 to 29.99; grade II overweight, 30.00 to 39.99; grade III overweight, over 40.00.

Body fat distribution plays as important a part in the complications of obesity as does the total amount of body fat.[1,5] Visceral fat, that contained within the abdominal wall, is the source of most of the comorbidity associated with obesity. By contrast, fat located around the hips and thighs conveys minimal health risks. In clinical practice, these two distributions are considered 'upper-body' and 'lower-body' fat. This distinction is based on the waist-to-hip ratio, calculated from the waist circumference (halfway between the lower rib margin and the iliac crest) and the hip circumference (at the level of the great trochanter). Upper-body obesity is defined as a waist-to-hip ratio of more than 1.0 for men and 0.8 for women. Risk, however, is directly proportional to the size of the waist-to-hip ratio, independent of gender;

the greater mortality and morbidity of men is a function of their greater waist-to-hip ratio.

Epidemiology

The prevalence of obesity in Western Europe, using the WHO criteria noted above (a body mass index of over 30), is 14 per cent for men and 16 per cent for women. It is higher in both Eastern Europe (17 per cent for men and 30 per cent for women)[10] and the United States (19.5 per cent for men and 25.0 per cent for women).[11] Although there are fewer data from the developing world, rates of obesity appear to be lower.

The world is in the midst of an epidemic of obesity, with the prevalence rising rapidly, both in countries in which the prevalence had been relatively low and in those in which it had been high. There has been a dramatic increase in the prevalence of obesity during the past decade, which has nearly doubled in some countries, including the United Kingdom. Age and gender are positively, and socio-economic status negatively, associated with obesity.[12]

Aetiology

In one sense, the aetiology of obesity is well understood: consuming more calories than are expended as energy. In another sense, the answer is most elusive. The causes of obesity may be found in the regulation of body weight, which is primarily the regulation of body fat, and we still have only an imperfect understanding of how this regulation is achieved.

Body weight is regulated with great precision. During a lifetime, the average person consumes at least 60 million kcal. A gain or loss of 9 kg, representing 72 000 kcal, would represent an error of no more than 0.001 per cent. A physiological basis for the negative feedback that controls this regulation has recently been discovered: the protein leptin.[13] Leptin is formed in adipose tissue cells in direct proportion to the lipid content of the cell and is transported to the brain where it serves as a signal of the extent of adipose tissue stores. In the brain it acts to suppress the action of neuropeptides that mediate food intake, such as neuropeptide Y, and stimulates energy expenditure through increasing physical activity and the action of the sympathetic nervous system.

If body weight is regulated with such precision, why does obesity develop? One suggestion is that obesity results from an elevation of the set-point about which body weight is regulated, and that the aetiology of obesity is to be found in the sources of this elevated set-point. Three such sources are genetic, environmental, and regulatory.

Genetic determinants

The existence of numerous forms of genetic obesity in experimental animals and the ease with which adiposity can be produced by the selective breeding of farm animals has long suggested that genetic factors play an important role in obesity in animals. Striking advances during the past decade have made it clear that genetic factors play an important role in human obesity.[14]

The first studies, using the classic twin method, estimated very high levels of heritability, with the percentage of the variance in body weight accounted for by genetic influences reaching 70 per cent. Even studies of identical twins separated at birth, a method that avoids some of the bias in classic twin studies, estimated a comparably high heritability.[15] These studies are still widely cited but there is a growing belief that they overestimate the influence of heredity. Thus the results of adoption studies and complex segregation analysis agree that the heritability of body weight is about 33 per cent, and this value is now viewed as more reasonable than that of the twin studies.[16] Genetic influences appear to play at least as important a role in the distribution of body fat as in the determination of total body fat or weight.[14] There is currently an intensive search for the genes that determine obesity.[17]

Environmental determinants

The fact that genetic influences may account for no more than one-third of the variation in body weight means that the environment must exert an enormous influence. Striking evidence of this influence is the dramatic increase in the prevalence of obesity throughout the world during the past decade.

An important environmental determinant of obesity is socio-economic status which is inversely related to the prevalence of obesity among women; longitudinal studies in both the United Kingdom and the United States indicate that this relationship is causal.[12] Growing up in a lower-class environment is clearly a risk factor for the development of obesity.

Food intake is a major environmental influence on obesity. After years of uncertainty about the contribution of food intake to the development of obesity, the introduction of the doubly labelled water method to measure energy expenditure, and therefore energy intake, has made it clear that obesity is associated with increased food intake.[18]

Another environmental factor promoting obesity is a sedentary lifestyle. During the past century, as the prevalence of obesity has doubled, food intake has actually decreased. The decrease in physical activity accounts for this paradoxical increase in obesity. For genetically predisposed people, decreased physical activity means increased body weight. Surprisingly, the early home environment, which has been blamed for producing obesity, appears to play no role in obesity in adult life.

Genes and environment

Genetic and environmental determinants of obesity are not in conflict. It is not a question of genes versus environment but rather genes and environment. Neither acts alone. Clinical outcomes are determined instead by the combination of genetic vulnerability and adverse environment. Only those genetically predisposed people who are exposed to adverse environmental conditions are clinically affected, as with obesity.

Regulatory determinants

Four determinants of obesity may be classified by their effect on the regulation of body weight: adipose tissue, brain damage, medication, and psychological factors.

Adipose tissue

Adipose tissue is the organ primarily affected in obesity. Adults of average weight have approximately 25 billion fat cells whereas severely obese people may have as many as 150 billion fat cells, as well as an increase in the size of the cells. Genetic influences play a role in excessive proliferation of fat cells, which occurs particularly in people who have been obese since childhood. When weight is lost, it is solely by a decrease in fat cell size; fat cell number appears to be irreversible. As a result, when fat cell size is reduced to normal levels by dieting, people with excessive numbers of fat cells remain significantly obese.

Brain damage

A small number of people become obese as a result of brain damage from infections and tumours, particularly craniopharyngiomas. Although the tumour itself does not affect food intake, its surgical removal frequently results in damage to the hypothalamus, overeating, and obesity. Most of the patients are children who are presented with a lifelong challenge. Fortunately they may respond to appetite suppressant medications.

Medication

A growing contribution to the prevalence of obesity is the increasing use of medications. Some, such as steroid hormones, contribute not only to obesity but also to altered body fat distribution. More important is the growing use of psychotropic medication that has significantly increased the prevalence of iatrogenic obesity. Lists of psychotropic agents involved in the increase in body weight are shown in Tables 1 and 2.[19]

As many as half of all patients on tricyclic antidepressants discontinue desperately needed treatment because of weight gain, which may reach 2 kg/month. A major reason for the popularity of selective serotonin-reuptake inhibitors is that they are less likely to produce weight gain than are the tricyclic antidepressants. Weight gain with lithium is particularly troublesome because it is usually prescribed for bipolar patients on a chronic basis; weight gains may reach 10 kg over a 2- to 6-year period. Neuroleptic medication also leads to weight gain and, since it must often be used chronically, presents serious problems. Among the traditional neuroleptics, low-potency agents such as chlorpromazine produce larger weight gain than the high-potency ones such as haloperidol. Hopes for the new 'atypical' antipsychotic medications have been dimmed by weight gain, which is often very severe with olanzapine and risperidone.

Psychological factors

Psychological problems are mentioned because for many years they were ascribed a causal role in obesity. As noted above, the current view is that these problems are not causes, but instead consequences of the societal pressures to which obese people are subjected.

Course and prognosis

Obesity is one of the most refractory disorders in medicine. Left untreated, most obese adults continue to gain weight, at a rate of approximately 1 kg/year. Similarly, children and adolescents should not be expected to grow out of their obesity. If, for example, an obese

Table 1 Antidepressant drugs and body weight

Tendency to increase appetite and body weight			May decrease appetite and facilitate weight loss
Greatest	**Intermediate**	**Least**	
Amitryptiline	Imipramine	Amoxapine	Fluoxetine
	Trimipramine	Desipramine	Bupropion
	Nortriptyline	Trazodone	
	Doxepin	Tranylcypromine (MAOI)	
	Phenelzine (MAOI)		

MAOI, monoamine oxidase inhibitor.
Reproduced with permission from J.G. Bernstein (1992). Management of psychotropic drug-induced obesity. In *Obesity* (ed. P. Bjorntropp and B.N. Brodoff), pp. 445–52. Lippincott, Philadelphia, PA.

child does not slim down by the end of adolescence, the odds of him or her doing so as an adult are 28 to 1 against. Obesity must be treated seriously.

Treatment of obesity

The goals of obesity treatment have changed dramatically in the past decade.[20] The traditional goal of reduction to 'ideal' weight has been supplanted by one of reduction of as little as 5 to 15 per cent.[21] This recommendation is based on two facts. First, most obese people are able to lose only 7 to 15 per cent of initial weight, even with state-of-the-art treatment. Second, such weight losses often produce significant improvements in hypertension, hypercholesterolaemia, type II diabetes, depression, and body image dissatisfaction.[23] Obese people must be helped to appreciate the medical benefits of modest weight losses and to eschew the frequently unattainable weight losses demanded by cosmetic concerns. Realistic treatment expectations are critical to long-term weight management.

Selecting treatment

The selection of an appropriate weight reduction therapy begins with the evaluation of the patient's obesity-related health risk. Heavier patients typically have more health complications and a greater mortality, particularly if they have a large waist-to-hip ratio and hypertension, hypercholesterolaemia, or type II diabetes. Table 3 summarizes the characteristics of people with a greater or lesser need for weight loss.[22] Women generally have less need than men because women typically carry excess weight in their lower body. Similarly, the risks of obesity are reduced in older as compared with younger indi-

viduals. Thus, after conducting a risk appraisal, the practitioner may find him- or herself trying to ease weight preoccupation in a 60-year-old female who carries 10 extra kilograms in her hips and thighs, while exhorting a 25-year-old male with a rotund belly and family history of diabetes to take his weight more seriously.

Treatment options

The treatment algorithm in Fig. 1 shows that there are numerous options for obesity. Therapy is selected on the basis of the patient's body mass index, risk profile, and prior history of weight-reducing efforts. Generally, the more obese the patient and the greater the health complications, the more aggressive the intervention selected. Thus an individual with a body mass index over 40 kg/m$^{(2)}$, and a history of yo-yo dieting, will probably require long-term treatment by appetite suppressant medication and, if this is ineffective, gastric surgery.

The psychiatrist's role

After identifying an appropriate therapy, practitioners must determine their role in treating the patient's obesity. Psychiatrists and other mental health professionals can assume primary responsibility for this treatment which is best carried out with the aid of a structured treatment manual, such as Brownell's *The LEARN Program for Weight Control.*[24]

Most psychiatrists will prefer not to direct the patient's weight-loss effort because it reduces the time available for other problems and may confuse the therapeutic agenda. Their time is better spent trying to resolve problems that arise in treatment, particularly problems in adherence to the therapeutic regimen. Such problems may range from the relatively straightforward ones of management of depression to those deriving from personality disorders. A growing task facing the

Table 2 Antipsychotic drugs and body weight

Tendency to increase appetite and body weight			May decrease appetite and facilitate weight loss
Greatest	**Intermediate**	**Least**	
Chlorpromazine	Trifluoperazine	Haloperidol	Molindone
Thioridazine	Perphenazine	Loxapine	
Mesoridazine	Thiothixene		

Reproduced with permission from J.G. Bernstein (1992). Management of psychotropic drug-induced obesity. In *Obesity* (ed. P. Bjorntropp and B.N. Brodoff), pp. 445–52. Lippincott, Philadelphia, PA.

psychiatrist is helping to manage the patient in whom the use of psychotropic medications has given rise to excessive weight gain. Unfortunately there are no magic bullets. The psychiatrist is confined to reducing the amount of medication to the lowest effective dose and to encourage the patient to adopt standard weight control strategies, with the help of a nutritionist or a structured programme. Prior to instituting treatment with a weight-promoting agent, consultation with a psychiatrist knowledgeable about these problems is desirable.

The psychiatrist should be aware of the standard treatments for obesity: (a) behaviour modification, (b) pharmacotherapy, and (c) surgery. Moreover, psychiatrists who deal with obese patients should know the self-help and commercial programmes in their area and develop professional relationships with them. Weight Watchers is the most popular programme. It appears to produce only modest weight losses because of relatively short-term attendance. However, its programme of sound nutrition and behaviour change, combined with low treatment fees, makes this approach attractive to people with a moderate degree of health risk. Unfortunately, few outcome data on commercial weight-loss programmes are available.

Behaviour modification

Behavioural weight control is designed to produce slow but steady weight loss by helping patients make gradual changes in their eating and exercise habits.[24,25] It has three distinguishing features. First, it is goal oriented. The objectives of treatment are clearly specified in weekly homework assignments which patients complete and discuss at the next meeting. Second, treatment is designed to change behaviour *per se* and to establish new skills. Thus, it differs from traditional psychodynamic psychotherapy which, with obese patients, might be more likely to explore the adverse emotional consequences of obesity or emotional conflicts which precipitate eating. Third, treatment is process oriented. It trains patients in analysing their eating and exercise

Table 3 Some modifiers of BMI-associated morbidity and/or mortality risk

Abaters	Augmenters
Lower-body (femoral-gluteal) fat distribution pattern	Upper-body (abdominal) fat distribution pattern
Ostensibly good health	Impaired health
Absence of obesity-related risk factors	Presence of one or more obesity-related risk factors
Middle-aged or elderly	Young adult (20–45 years of age)
Female	Male
Absence of a family history of obesity-relevant illness	Presence of a family history of obesity-relevant illness
Obesity of brief duration	Obesity of prolonged duration
Membership of a race not known to be vulnerable to obesity-associated problems	Membership in a race known to be vulnerable to obesity-associated health problems (e.g. NIDDM vulnerability in obese Pima Indians)
Above normal stature	Below normal stature

NIDDM, non-insulin-dependent diabetes mellitus.
Reproduced with permission from T.B. Van Itallie and E.A. Lew (1992). Assessment of morbidity and mortality risk in the overweight patient. In *Treatment of the seriously obese patient* (ed. T.A. Wadden and T.B. Van Itallie), pp. 3–32. Guilford Press, New York.

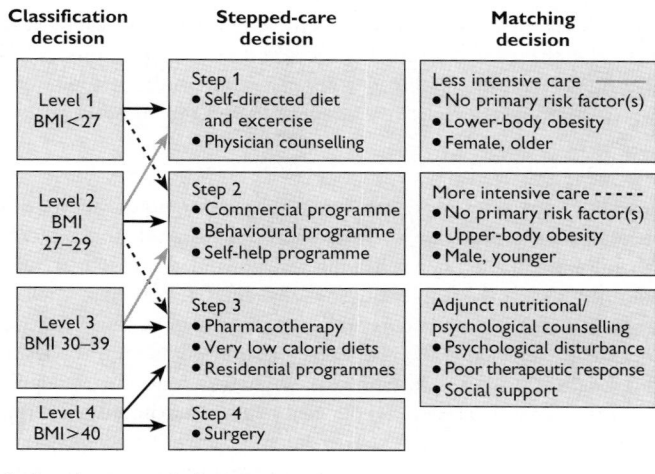

Fig. 1 A conceptual scheme showing a three-stage process for selecting a treatment for obesity. The first stage (the classification decision) divides people into four levels based on body mass index. This level dictates which of four steps is appropriate in the second stage (the stepped-care decision) to determine the least intensive, costly, and risky approach among the treatment alternatives. The solid arrow between the two boxes identifies the treatment most likely to be appropriate. The third stage (the matching decision) is used to make a final treatment selection, based on the patient's need for weight reduction, because of comorbid conditions or other risk factors. The arrow (between boxes) with open circles indicates a reduced need for weight reduction because of the absence of risk factors. The arrow with closed circles shows the more intensive treatment option, appropriate for people with a significant comorbid condition. For example, the appropriate treatment for patients with a body mass index of 27 to 29 kg/m² who do not have health complications would be a commercial programme or self-help approach. In contrast, pharmacotherapy may be considered for people with a body mass index of 29 kg/m² and type II diabetes. Patients with significant psychiatric problems, or who want more support in changing diet and exercise habits, can be referred for adjunctive care. (Courtesy of Dr T.A. Wadden and Dr K. Brownell.)

habits, in determining the behaviours that need to be modified and strategies for changing them. The two most important behaviours to be modified are diet and physical activity.

Diet

Patients keep extensive records of their food intake throughout treatment. In the initial weeks, they record daily the types and amounts of foods eaten and their caloric value. They are instructed to eat a diet that they like but to reduce consumption of high-fat and high-sugar foods.[24] Most patients can decrease their intake by 500 to 700 kcal/day simply by reducing their portion sizes, which have become excessively large in industrialized nations. This reduction is usually sufficient to induce a weight loss of 0.5 kg/week for the first 12 to 16 weeks. In the United States, the Food Guide Pyramid, the ADA Exchange Lists (developed jointly by the American Diabetes Association and the American Dietetic Association), and similar materials provide guidance for people who report that they do not know what to eat or do not have a structured meal plan.

More rapid weight loss is produced by very low calorie diets.[2,26,27] Very low calorie diets, which traditionally provided only 400 to

800 kcal/day, are today more frequently used as part of a meal replacement plan that provides 1000 to 1200 kcal/day. Three or four servings of a liquid diet are combined with an evening meal of food. This approach produces weight losses as great as 15 kg in 16 weeks.[28]

Physical activity

In addition to decreasing energy intake, behaviour modification helps obese people to increase their physical activity and, thus, energy expenditure. The first step is helping patients understand that exercise does not have to be unpleasant and that lifestyle activities, such as leisurely walking, using stairs rather than escalators, and reducing dependence on energy-saving devices, are sufficient to improve health and weight.[29] As a result, new exercise guidelines no longer require patients to exercise at 60 to 80 per cent of their maximum heart rate for 20 to 40 min at a time.[30] Lower-intensity activity is acceptable, as are multiple brief bouts of physical activity performed throughout the day.[31] The goal is to accumulate approximately 30 min/day of moderate-intensity physical activity on most days of the week.

Patients are instructed to identify their position on an activity continuum, ranging from completely sedentary to extremely active, and to then progress to the next step. For many obese people, this may mean starting with no more than a 5-min walk at a slow pace and then increasing the duration and intensity of their activity. It is helpful for them to identify the activity they will engage in and when, where, and how they will perform it. Thus, they should leave the office with a concrete plan, such as, 'I'm going to walk 4 days this week, on Monday, Wednesday, Friday, and Sunday. During the weekdays, I'll walk for 30 min during my lunch hour in the park. On Sunday, I'll walk in my neighbourhood for 45 min after breakfast'. Patients should keep a log of their physical activity which they review at their next treatment visit.[24]

Treatment mechanics and outcome

Behaviour modification is typically delivered in small groups (of 10 to 12 people) in which participants discuss homework assignments and related issues. Groups usually meet weekly (for 60 to 90 min) for 16 to 26 weeks. Weight losses average 7 to 10 per cent of initial weight.[20] Longer therapy is associated with greater losses but the average rarely exceeds 15 per cent of initial weight, even in treatment of 40 to 52 weeks.[32] Patients regain approximately one-third of their weight loss in the year following therapy, with increasing regain over time.[20] Five years after treatment, a majority of patients have returned to their baseline weight.

Perri et al.[33] have shown that weight regain can be minimized by increasing patient–provider contact following the period of acute weight reduction. Patients who had alternate-week contact with their provider, by telephone or mail, maintained their full end-of-treatment weight loss for 12 months. Electronic mail and the Internet are likely to provide even more efficient methods of supporting patient weight maintenance efforts.

Pharmacological treatment of obesity

The pharmacological treatment of obesity has been a source of both great hope and controversy. In 1992, interest in pharmacotherapy increased with the report from Weintraub et al.[34] that low doses of fenfluramine (30 mg/day) combined with phentermine (15 mg/day), produced substantial weight losses that were maintained for as long as 3 years. This interest was dashed by the report in 1997 that fenfluramine and dexfenfluramine, when taken in combination with phentermine, were associated with cardiac valvular damage. They were promptly withdrawn from the market.[35]

Intensive pharmaceutical research now under way will probably produce safe and effective medication for weight control within the next few years. Already two new medications, sibutramine[36] and orlistat,[37] have been approved for long-term use in several countries.

Patient selection

Weight-loss medications are usually reserved for patients with a body mass index over 30 kg/m² who have failed to reduce with conservative approaches. They may also be appropriate for patients with a body mass index over 27 kg/m² who have a comorbid condition which will be improved with weight loss. Weight-loss medications are inappropriate for lactating or pregnant women, as well as for people with eating disorders (i.e. anorexia nervosa and bulimia nervosa).[38]

Approved weight-loss medications

Table 4 shows prescription weight-loss medications approved for use in the United States and/or the European Union. With the exception of sibutramine, these agents have been approved for only short-term use (up to 3 months), and there are no long-term data on their safety and efficacy.[39]

Sibutramine

Sibutramine (Meridia) and its metabolites inhibit the reuptake of norepinephrine and serotonin (and dopamine to a very limited degree).[36] Sibutramine induces weight loss by decreasing food intake (apparently by enhancing satiety). In a 12-month double-blind study, it produced losses of 7 to 8 per cent of initial weight, compared with a loss of only 1 to 2 per cent for placebo-treated patients. Maximum weight loss was achieved in the first 6 months and was maintained from months 6 to 12.

Sibutramine's most common side-effects are mild, infrequent, and usually transitory: headache, dry mouth, constipation, and insomnia. Of potentially greater concern are increases of 4 to 5 beats/min in heart rate and 1 to 2 mmHg in blood pressure. Sibutramine is contraindicated in people with uncontrolled hypertension, a history of coronary artery disease, congestive heart failure, arrhythmias, or stroke, and in people taking monoamine oxidase inhibitors. It is not recommended in combination with selective serotonin reuptake inhibitors for depression or migraine headaches.

Orlistat

Orlistat is a gastric and pancreatic lipase inhibitor which blocks the absorption of approximately one-third of the fat calories contained in a meal[37] which are lost in the stool. Diets containing 30 per cent or more calories from fat produce oily stools, flatulence with discharge, and faecal urgency. Orlistat has no discernible central nervous system effects.

In randomized trials, orlistat produced average weight losses of 10.2 per cent of initial weight in 6 to 12 months compared to 6.1 per cent for placebo. There was good maintenance of weight loss at 24 months in patients who continued medication. In addition to inducing weight loss, orlistat independently reduces serum lipids, presumably by blocking fat absorption.

Table 4 Weight loss medications currently approved by the United States Food and Drug Administration

Medication	Drug Enforcement Agency schedule	Trade name	Dosage (mg)	Daily dose range (mg)
Noradrenergic agents				
Benzphetamine	III	Didrex	25, 50	25–150
Phendimetrazine	III	Anorex and others	35	70–210
Diethylproprion	IV	Tenuate, Tepanol	25, 75 (slow release)	75
Mazindol	IV	Mazanor, Sanorex	1, 2	1–3
Phentermine				
resin	IV	Ionamin	15, 30	15–30
hydrochloride	IV	Adipex-P and others	37.5	18.75–35
hydrochloride	IV	Fastin and others	30	30
Phenylpropanolamine	Over the counter	Dexatrim and others	25, 75	25–75
Noradrenergic/serotonergic agents				
Sibutramine	IV	Meridia	5, 10, 15	5–15

All medications except sibutramine are approved for short-term use only (i.e. 3 months or less). Sibutramine has been approved for long-term use. Adapted from Bray.[39]

Orlistat's principal side-effect consists of the adverse gastrointestinal events described above, which have the favourable effect of inducing a reduction of fat intake. Orlistat has no effect on serum levels of vitamins E and K and only moderately reduces serum levels of vitamins A, β-carotene, and vitamin D. Nevertheless, patients who take orlistat are advised to take a multivitamin supplement that includes fat-soluble vitamins.

Pharmacotherapy and weight-loss maintenance

The greatest strength of pharmacotherapy, particularly as compared with behaviour modification, resides in maintaining rather than inducing weight loss.[39] Studies of a year or longer showed that patients maintained a loss of 5 to 10 per cent of initial weight, as long as they remained on medication,[20] superior to the results with behaviour modification alone. Since these medications can be readily prescribed by primary care doctors, pharmacotherapy will make weight reduction available to large numbers of patients.

Weight regain occurs when appetite suppressant medications are terminated,[40,41] leading to the proposal that these medications be used indefinitely. This recommendation recognizes that obesity is a chronic disorder, which requires long-term care, in the same manner that hypertension and diabetes often necessitate long-term pharmacotherapy. Moreover, long-term weight reduction achieved with pharmacotherapy could eliminate the need for medications used chronically to control the weight-related complications of hypertension, diabetes, and hyperlipidaemia.

Surgery

Surgery is an option for people with a body mass index over 40 kg/m² who have failed to reduce using more conservative approaches, as well as those with a body mass index as little as 35 kg/m², if significant comorbid conditions are present.[23,42,43]

There are two major surgical procedures for the treatment of obesity. In the vertical banded gastroplasty, a vertical staple line is placed just below the gastro-oesophageal junction to create a small pouch (15 to 30 ml) with a narrow opening (10 mm in diameter) to the remaining stomach.[44] The pouch drastically reduces the amount of food which can be eaten at a given meal.

In the gastric bypass, the staple line is vertical, placed just below the gastro-oesophageal junction to create a horizontal pouch which is attached to a loop of the small bowel, permitting nutrients to bypass the remainder of the stomach and the duodenum. Patients lose 25 per cent of their initial weight in the first 1 to 2 years, with the gastric bypass producing somewhat larger losses.[44] An important new development is the use of laparoscopic surgery for obesity, for which data are still limited. This method of limiting the extent of the surgical wound is highly desirable.

Weight loss is associated with significant improvements in health-related complications, particularly glycaemic control, hypertension, sleep apnoea, and mobility. Improvements in psychological status have also been reported.[45] Both vertical banded gastroplasty and the gastric bypass are associated with good maintenance of weight loss as long as 5 years after surgery.

Obesity surgery should be confined to centres which specialize in the procedures and have extensive experience with them. The operative mortality in such centres does not exceed 0.5 per cent.

Preserving patient self-esteem

One of the most important services that psychiatrists can provide obese individuals is an opportunity to discuss their feelings of sadness and frustration concerning their weight. It is imperative that the physician, through words and deeds, helps patients to maintain self-esteem as they struggle with the challenge of weight control.

References

1. Bray, G.A., Bouchard, C., and James, W.P.T. (1998). Definitions and proposed current classification of obesity. In *Handbook of obesity* (ed. G.A. Bray, C. Bouchard, and W.P.T. James), pp. 31–41. Dekker, New York.
2. Brown, P.J. (1991). Culture and the evolution of obesity. *Human Nature*, **2**, 31–57.
3. Pi Sunyer, F.X. (1993). Medical hazards of obesity. *Annals of Internal Medicine*, **119**, 655–60.

4. McGinnis, J.M. and Foege, W.H. (1993). Actual causes of death in the United States. *Journal of the American Medical Association*, **270**, 2207–12.

5. Bjorntorp, P. (1993). Visceral obesity: a 'civilization syndrome'. *Obesity Research*, **1**, 206–22.

6. Stunkard, A.J. and Wadden, T.A. (1992). Psychological aspects of severe obesity. *American Journal of Clinical Nutrition*, **55**, 524S–32S.

7. Spitzer, R.L., Devlin, M., Walsh, T.B., *et al.* (1992). Binge eating disorder: a multisite field trial of the diagnostic criteria. *International Journal of Eating Disorders*, **11**, 191–203.

8. Spitzer, R.L., Yanovski, S.Z., Wadden, T.A., *et al.* (1993). Binge eating disorder: its further validation in a multisite trial. *International Journal of Eating Disorders*, **13**, 137–53.

9. Birketvedt, G.S., Florholmen, J., Sundsfjord, J., *et al.* (1999). The night eating syndrome: behavioral and neuroendocrine characteristics. *Journal of the American Medical Association*, **282**, 657–63.

10. Seidell, J.C. and Rissanan, A.M. (1998). Time trends in the worldwide epidemic of obesity. In *Handbook of obesity* (ed. G.A. Bray, C. Bouchard, and W.P.T. James), pp. 79–91. Dekker, New York.

11. Brown, P.J. (1991). Culture and the evolution of obesity. *Human Nature*, **2**, 31–57.

12. Sobal, J. and Stunkard, A.J. (1989). Socioeconomic status and obesity. *Psychological Bulletin*, **105**, 260–75.

13. Wickelgren, I. (1998). Obesity: how big a problem? *Science*, **280**, 1364–7.

14. Bouchard, C. (ed.) (1994). *The genetics of obesity*. CRC Press, Boca Raton, FL.

15. Stunkard, A.J., Harris, J.R., Pedersen, N.L., and McClearn, G.E. (1990). The body mass index of twins who have been reared apart. *New England Journal of Medicine*, **322**, 1483–7.

16. Vogler, G.P., Sorensen, T.I.A., Stunkard, A.J., *et al.* (1995). Influence of genes and shared family environment on adult body mass index assessed in an adoption study by a comprehensive path analysis. *International Journal of Obesity*, **19**, 40–5.

17. Perusse, L., Chagnon, Y.C., Weisnagel, J., and Bouchard, C. (1999). The human obesity gene map: the 1998 update. *Obesity Research*, **7**, 111–29.

18. Schoeller, D.A. and Field, C.R. (1991). Human energy metabolism: what have we learned from the doubly labelled water method? *Annual Review of Nutrition*, **11**, 355–73.

19. Bernstein, J.G. (1992). Management of psychotropic drug-induced obesity. In *Obesity* (ed. P. Bjorntorp and B.N. Brodoff), pp. 445–52. Lippincott, Philadelphia, PA.

20. Wadden, T.A. (1998). New goals of obesity treatment: a healthier weight and other ideals. *Primary Psychiatry*, **5**, 45–54.

21. World Health Organization (1998). *Obesity: preventing and managing the global epidemic*. WHO, Geneva.

22. Van Itallie, T.B. and Lew, E.A. (1992). Assessment of morbidity and mortality risk in the overweight patient. In *Treatment of the seriously obese patient* (ed. T.A. Wadden and T.B. Van Itallie), pp. 3–32. Guilford Press, New York.

23. NHLBI Obesity Education Initiative Expert Panel (1998). Clinical guidelines on the identification, evaluation, and treatment of overweight and obesity in adults—the evidence report. *Obesity Research*, **6**, 51S–209S.

24. Brownell, K.D. (1991). *The LEARN program for weight control*. American Health Publishing Company, Dallas, TX.

25. Wing, R.R. (1998). Behavioral approaches to the treatment of obesity. In *Handbook of obesity* (ed. G.A. Bray, C. Bouchard, and W.P.T. James), pp. 855–73. Dekker, New York.

26. National Task Force on the Prevention and Treatment of Obesity (1993). Very low calorie diets. *Journal of the American Medical Association*, **270**, 967–74.

27. Wadden, T.A. and Bartlett, S.J. (1992). Very low calorie diets: an overview and appraisal. In *Treatment of the seriously obese patient* (ed. T.A. Wadden and T.B. Van Itallie), pp. 44–79. Guilford Press, New York.

28. Wadden, T.A., Vogt, R.A., Andersen, R., *et al.* (1997). Exercise in the treatment of obesity: effects of four interventions on body composition, resting energy expenditure, appetite and mood. *Journal of Consulting and Clinical Psychology*, **65**, 269–77.

29. Andersen, R.E., Wadden, T.A., Bartlett, S.J., Zemal, B., Verde, T.J., and Franckowiak, S.C. (1992). Effects of lifestyle activity vs. structured aerobic exercise in obese women: a randomizing trial. *Journal of the American Medical Association*, **281**, 335–40.

30. Pate, R.R., Pratt, M., Blair, S.N., *et al.* (1995). A Recommendation from the Centers for Disease Control and Prevention and the American College of Sports Medicine. *Journal of the American Medical Association*, **273**, 402–7.

31. Jakicic, J.M., Wing, R.R., Butler, B.A., and Robertson, R.J. (1995). Prescribing exercise in multiple short bouts versus one continuous bout: effects on adherence, cardiorespiratory fitness, and weight loss in overweight women. *International Journal of Obesity*, **19**, 893–901.

32. Wadden, T.A., Foster, G.D., and Letizia, K.A. (1994). One-year behavioral treatment of obesity: comparison of moderate and severe restriction and the effects of weight maintenance therapy. *Journal of Consulting and Clinical Psychology*, **62**, 165–71.

33. Perri, M., McAllister, D., Grange, J., *et al.* (1988). Effects of four maintenance programs on the long-term management of obesity. *Journal of Consulting and Clinical Psychology*, **56**, 529–34.

34. Weintraub, M., Sundaresan, P., Madan, M., *et al.* (1992). Long-term weight control study I (weeks 0 to 34). *Clinical Pharmacology and Therapeutics*, **51**, 586–94.

35. Bowen, R., Glicklich, A., Kahn, M., *et al.* (1997). Cardiac valvulopathy associated with exposure to fenfluramine or dexfenfluramine: US Department of Health and Human Services Interim Public Health Recommendations November 1997. *Morbidity and Mortality Weekly Report*, **46**, 1061–6.

36. Lean, M.E.J. (1997). Sibutramine—a review of clinical efficacy. *International Journal of Obesity*, **21**, 30S–6S.

37. Sjostrom, L., Rissanen, A., Andersen, T.E., *et al.* (1998). Randomized placebo-controlled trial of orlistat for weight loss and prevention of weight regain in obese patients. *Lancet*, **352**, 167–72.

38. National Task Force on the Prevention and Treatment of Obesity (1996). Long-term pharmacotherapy in the management of obesity. *Journal of the American Medical Association*, **276**, 1907–15.

39. Bray, G.A. (1998). Pharmacologic treatment of obesity. In *Handbook of obesity* (ed. G.A. Bray, C. Bouchard, and W.P.T. James), pp. 953–75. Dekker, New York.

40. Stunkard, A.J. (1982). Minireview: anorectic agents lower a body weight set point. *Life Sciences*, **30**, 2043–55.

41. Craighead, L., Stunkard, A.J., and O'Brien, R. (1981). Behavior therapy and pharmacotherapy for obesity. *Archives of General Psychiatry*, **38**, 763–8.

42. Kral, J. (1995). Surgical interventions of obesity. In *Eating disorders and obesity: a comprehensive handbook* (ed. K.D. Brownell and C. Fairburn), pp. 510–15. Guilford Press, New York.

43. Grace, D.M. (1992). Gastric restriction procedures for treating severe obesity. *American Journal of Clinical Nutrition*, **55**, 556S–9S.

44. Sugarman, H.J., Starkey, J.V., and Birkenhauer, R. (1987). A randomized prospective trial of gastric bypass versus vertical banded gastroplasty for morbid obesity and their effects on sweets versus non-sweets eaters. *Annals of Surgery*, **205**, 613–24.

45. Stunkard, A.J., Stinnet, J.L., and Smoller, J. (1986). Psychological and social aspects of the surgical treatment of obesity. *American Journal of Psychiatry*, **143**, 417–29.

4.11 Sexuality, gender identity, and their disorders

4.11.1 Normal sexual function

R. J. Levin

Introduction

Normal sexual function means different things to different people. It is studied by a variety of disciplines: biology, physiology, psychology, medicine (in the domains of endocrinology, gynaecology, psychiatry, urology, and venereology), sociology, ethology, culture, philosophy, psychoanalysis, and history. There is often little liaison or cross-fertilization between these disciplines and each has its own literature and terminology. Some are regarded as 'hard science', suggesting hypotheses that can be supported or rejected by experiment, observation, or quantitative factual evidence. Others are looked on as 'soft science', where individual and anecdotal evidence are the norm and are encouraged.

As space is limited, this chapter will characterize 'normal sexual activity' in the Western world mainly from biological, physiological, and psychological aspects but will ocasionally utilize other disciplines when they yield insights not available from the 'harder sciences.'

Biological determinants of normal sexual function

Humans are the highest evolved primates. A number of our anatomical/biological features have been described[1,2] as strongly enhancing our sexual behaviour when compared with other primates, although recent studies have shown that the bonobos (pygmy chimpanzees) also use sex for reasons unconnected with reproduction.[3]

In brief, these features are as follows.

1. The relative hairlessness of our bodies allows well-defined visual displays (see point 6 below) and enhanced tactile skin sensitivity.

2. The clitoris, which is an organ whose sole function is for inducing female sexual arousal/pleasure.

3. Orgasms, in both male and female, provide intense euphoric rewards for undertaking sexual arousal to completion. The female is able to have multiple serial orgasms.

4. The largest penis among primates, whether flaccid or erect—the latter acting as a good sexual stimulator of the female genitalia.

5. Concealed (cryptic) ovulation which induces males to undertake coitus more frequently to create pregnancy and prevent cuckolding.

6. Well-defined visual sexual displays in the female that are not linked to season or fertility (i.e. breasts, pubic hair, buttocks, and lips). The everted mucous membranes of the lips serve both as a surface display, and for haptic stimulation during kissing and sucking.

7. Ability of the female to undertake sexual arousal and coitus independent of season, hormonal status, or ovulation. Human females (unlike other primates) can and often do willingly partake of sexual activity and coitus when they are menstruating, pregnant, or menopausal.

8. Development of large mammary glands during puberty which act as visual sexual signals in most cultures.

These biological determinants are augmented by sociocultural factors.

1. Language, art, and music for erotic stimulation.

2. Facial adornment with make-up to heighten appearance.

3. Clothing, especially of the female, such as brassières to redefine the shape of breasts, corsets to redefine the shape of the body, and high-heeled shoes to elongate the legs and thrust out the buttocks. A study of young females has shown how they manipulate body signals at discotheques in Austria. Around ovulation they dress to expose significantly more flesh area than at other times of their menstrual cycle.[4] Young adult males use tight trousers to create a genital 'bulge' and to emphasize firm rounded buttocks, the latter being a highly sexually attractive feature to young women.

4. Perfumes and scents to enhance body aroma.

The last three features (2, 3, and 4) use artificial means to enhance normal sexual signals.[1] These biological and sociocultural factors give human sexual activity an increased appetitiveness and make it more rewarding.

Sexuality as a social construct and the concept of sexual scripting

Laqueur[5] suggests that while the sexual biology remained unchanged, its expression has been influenced over the centuries by culture, social class, ethnic group, and religion. This concept, that human sexuality is a social construct, has been strongly argued by Foucault[6] and promoted by other social constructionist authors.[7] Gagnon and Simon[8] introduced the concept of 'sexual scripting'. Scripts organize and determine the circumstances under which sexual activity occurs, they are involved in 'learning the meaning of internal states, organizing the sequences of specific sexual acts, decoding novel situations, setting limits on sexual responses and linking meanings from non-sexual aspects of life to specifically sexual experience'. Money[9] employed a similar construction in his development of 'love maps' for the individual. While patterns of behaviour are influenced by society and social forces, there is a dearth of evidence to show that sexual identity, orientation, or sexual mechanisms are also influenced.

Modelling normal sexual function—the sex survey

One obvious way of describing normal sexual function is to ask people what they do. Two classic sex surveys were conducted by Kinsey and his coworkers who reported the results of interviews with 12 000 males in 1948[10] and 8000 females in 1953.[11] Their technique of sampling was to interview everyone in specific cooperating groups (clubs, hospital staff, universities, police force, school teachers, etc.). This gave samples of convenience but not a valid sampling of the population. Despite their age and faulty sampling, however, there are still many interesting data in these surveys. In the sexual climate of the 1950s many of the findings were regarded as highly controversial. Clement[12] has reviewed the subseqent studies of human heterosexual behaviour up to 1990.

Surveys give a selective picture of sexual function. Results depend on the formulation of the questions, they rely on self-reports, and they represent only those prepared to describe their sexual behaviour. It is known, for example, that females tend to under-report their premarital sexual experiences[12] while males tend to over-report their lifetime partners.[13] Berk et al.[14] studied the recall by 217 university students of their sexual activity over a 2-week period assessed by questionnaires answered 2 weeks after the recording period, and by daily diaries kept over the same 2 weeks. Subjects reported more sexual activity in the questionnaires than in their diaries. Women reported giving and having more oral sex than the men. Clearly, data from questionnaire surveys should be treated cautiously.

A survey tells only what is frequent and not necessarily what is normal, but the most frequent practices often become identified with normal sexual behaviour. Surveys also vary in the range of behaviours that are asked about, for example coitus without condoms is important in the age of AIDS. Surveys have one great disadvantage, the facts that they produce are often 'perishable'; many aspects of the sex surveys of the pre-pill era, or more recently the pre-AIDS era, are now of use only in a historical or comparative basis.

Two recent well-organized surveys based on samples of the whole population have been undertaken, one in the United States and the other in the United Kingdom. In both surveys, questions about masturbation were disliked by the respondents. In the American survey these questions were asked in a separate self-adminstered questionnaire, while in the British survey they were abandoned.

The American survey[15] was conducted face to face with 3159 selected individuals who spoke English in representative households by 220 trained interviewers (mainly women). Nearly 80 per cent of the individuals chosen agreed to be interviewed. Men thought about sex often, more than 50 per cent having erotic thoughts several times a day, while females thought about sex from a few times a week to a few times a month. The frequency of partnered sex had little to do with race, religion, or education. Only three factors mattered: age, whether married or cohabiting, and how long the couple had been together. Fourteen per cent of males reported having no sex in the previous year, 16 per cent had sex a few times in the year, 40 per cent a few times a month, 26 per cent two to three times a week, and 8 per cent four times a week. The percentages were similar for women. The youngest and the oldest people had the least sex with a partner; those in their twenties had the most. Of the women aged 18 to 59 years, approximately one in three said they were uninterested in sex, and one woman in five said sex gave her no pleasure. Unlike frequency, reported sexual practices do depend on race and social class. Most practices other than vaginal coitus were not very attractive to the vast majority. In women aged 18 to 44 years of age, 80 per cent rated vaginal coitus as 'very appealing' and an additional 18 per cent rated it as 'somewhat appealing'. Among men 85 per cent regarded vaginal coitus as 'very appealing'. The most appealing activity second after coitus was watching the partner undress, and this was appealing to more men (50 per cent) than women (30 per cent). This reflects the greater voyeuristic nature of men and their willingness to pay to look at women undressing or undressed.

In regard to oral sex, both men and women liked receiving more than giving. This practice varied markedly with race and education, with higher reported rates among better educated white people than among less educated and black people. Some 68 per cent of all women had given oral sex to their partner and 19 per cent experienced active oral sex the last time they had intercourse. Seventy-three per cent of all women had received oral sex from the partner, and 20 per cent had received it the last time they had had intercourse. Corresponding experiences were reported by men.

This survey, unlike most earlier ones, asked about anal sex. Of females aged 18 to 44, 87 per cent thought it not at all appealing, and only 1 to 4 per cent thought it very or somewhat appealing. In males of the same age 73 per cent thought it not at all appealing and rather more than women thought it very or somewhat appealing. Similar reports were obtained from women and men aged 44 to 59.

Regarding masturbation, older people (over 54 years old) had lower rates than at any other age, indicating that they do not use masturbation to compensate for an overall decrease in sexual activity with their partners.

In the United Kingdom survey[16] 18 876 people were interviewed by 488 interviewers (of whom 421 were women). The sampling used one person per adddress and the acceptance rate was 71.5 per cent. Questions were asked about the frequency of vaginal coitus, oral sex, and anal sex, but not masturbation. The median number of occasions of sex with a man or woman was five times a month for females aged 20 to 29 and males aged 25 to 34, but declined to a median of two per month for males aged 55 to 59. More than 50 per cent of the females in the 55 to 59 age group reported no sex in the last month, but in this age group females are more likely than men to have no regular partner because they are widowed, separated, or divorced.

Vaginal coitus was reported by nearly all females and males by the age of 25. Fifty-six per cent of males and 57 per cent of females reported vaginal coitus in the previous week, and non-penetrative sex was practised by 75 per cent men and 82 per cent of women. Twenty-five per cent of males had genital stimulation in the previous 7 days. Cunnilingus and fellatio were common but less practised than vaginal coitus. Of men and women aged 18 to 44, 60 per cent had oral sex in the previous year but in the 45- to 59-year-old group this fell to 30 per cent for women and 42 per cent for men. This and other sex surveys suggest that the practice of oral sex has increased since the 1950s and 1960s. Anal coitus was infrequent; approximately 14 per cent of the males and 13 per cent of the females had ever undertaken it, and only 7 per cent of males or females had practised it in the previous year.

Modelling the human sexual response cycle

A direct way of investigating normal sexual function is to observe and measure the body changes that take place when men and women become sexually aroused. From these data, models have been constructed of the normal sequence of changes during sexual arousal and coitus. The first models described a simple sequence of increasing arousal and excitement culminating in rapid discharge by orgasm, displayed graphically as an ascent, peak, and then descent.[17] As the investigations became more sophisticated, understanding of the body responses grew and the models became more detailed and complex.[5,10,11,18,19]

The EPOR model—a human sexual response cycle model

The most successful model was that formulated by Masters and Johnson.[20] In the laboratory, they observed the changes that took place in the male and female body and especially the genitals during sexual arousal to orgasm either by masturbation or by natural or artificial coitus with a plastic penis that allowed internal filming of the female genitalia. After studying approximately 7500 female and 2500 male arousals to orgasm in some 382 female and 312 male volunteers over 11 years they proposed a four-phase linear, sequential, and incremental model of the human sexual response cycle (Fig. 1). The phases were described as the excitation (**E**) phase (stimuli from somatogenic or psychogenic sources raise sexual tensions), the plateau (**P**) phase (sexual tensions intensified), the orgasmic (**O**) phase (involuntary pleasurable climax), and finally the resolution (**R**) phase (dissipation of sexual tensions). The great success of this EPOR model was its wide compass; it could characterize the sexual responses of women and men, both heterosexual and homosexual, ranging from simple petting to vaginal or anal coitus with orgasm. However, it had several weaknesses.

Modifying the EPOR model into the DEOR model

The first weakness of the EPOR model is that it was derived from the study of a highly selected group of American men and women volunteers who could arouse themselves to orgasm in a laboratory, on demand, and allow themselves to be watched/filmed or measured for scientific and altruistic (or perhaps exhibitionistic) purposes. The second weakness was the lack of interobserver agreement about the changes observed and of confirmation of their sequential reliability. Robinson[21] examined the E phase and P phase, and concluded convincingly that the P phase was simply the final stage of the E phase. Helen Kaplan,[22] a New York sex therapist, proposed that before the E

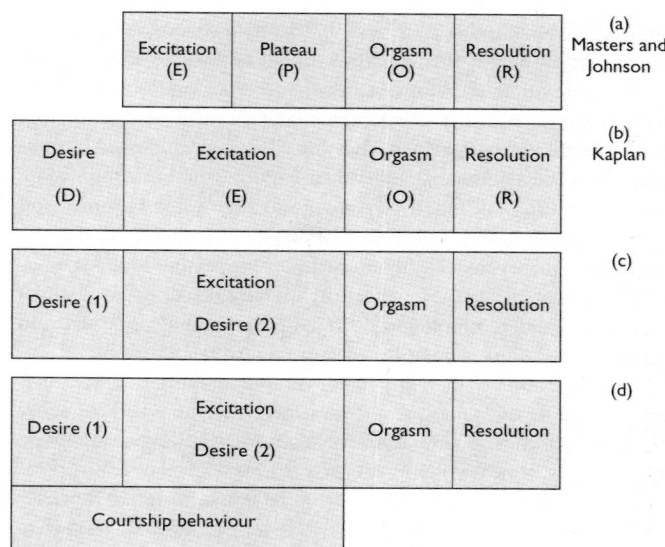

Fig. 1 The development of the linear-sequence human sexual response model from (a) the original EPOR model of Masters and Johnson[20] through (b) the DEOR model of Kaplan[22] to (c) the proposed modification with desire phase 1 (before initiation of the excitation phase and desire phase 2 during excitation phase) and finally (d) with added courtship behaviour.

phase there should be a 'desire phase' (D phase). This proposal came from her work with women who professed to have no desire to be sexually aroused, even by their usual partners. She suggested that the desire must occur before sexual arousal can begin. Kaplan's subjects were attending a clinic and no studies were ever conducted with a control normal population (either women or men) to investigate whether this 'self-evident' fact was true. Despite this, the EPOR model gradually became replaced by the desire, excitation, orgasmic, and resolution phase (**DEOR**) model. While this is the currently accepted model, the centrality of the desire phase in women remains uncertain (Fig. 1). In a survey of non-clinic sexually experienced women in Denmark, about a third reported that they never experienced spontaneous sexual desire[23] and in an American survey women reported periods of several months when they lacked interest in sex.[15] The other problem with the desire phase is its location in the sequential DEOR model. Sexual desire that appears to be spontaneous (but presumably must still be activated by a learned trigger) should obviously be placed at the beginning of the model (Fig. 1(b)), but what of sexual desire created when the person is sexually aroused by another? Where do we place this sexual desire, at the early stages of the excitation phase (Fig. 1(c)? Courtship behaviour, which begins the initiation of sexual activity, is also difficult to position in regard to the DEOR (Fig. 1(d)).

Courtship (mating) behaviour—activity initiating normal sexual behaviour

With the exception of rape, humans initiate sexual activity with courtship behaviour. Sometimes courtship activity precedes the desire phase, sometimes it occurs during the desire phase, and sometimes in the excitation phase (Fig. 1(d)).

Evolutionary psychology attempts to explain the strategies of mating.[24] Its message is not always palatable to modern sensitivities about sexual equality. It is argued that women invest more in their offspring than men,[25] that this investment is a scarce resource that men compete for, and that men can enhance their reproductive strategy by mating frequently. Most men are first visually atttracted to a possible female sexual partner. They look for youthfulness and physical attractiveness in the form of regular features, smooth complexion, optimum stature, and good physique, and they value virginity and chastity. Partner variety is highly desired. Women, however, need to obtain high-quality mates with abundant resources and look for emotional and financial status and security. Clearly the strategies conflict giving rise to different preferences in mate choice and casual sex, and different levels of investment or commitment to relationships.[26]

Once the chosen female (or male) accepts the initiation of courtship behaviour, the subsequent stages form a stereotyped sequence which is found in many different cultures.The stages are look, approach, talk, touch, synchronize, kiss (caress), sex play, coitus.[27] It is a sequence that the poet Ovid knew in the first century BC. Morris[1] characterized human courtship behaviour into 12 basic stages: eye to body, eye to eye, voice to voice, hand to hand, arm to shoulder, arm to waist, mouth to mouth, hand to head, hand to body, mouth to breast, hand to genitals, genitals to genitals. Similar hierarchies have been constructed extending the behaviour further to oral–genital contacts.

Although kissing has been described as 'an inhibited rehearsal for intercourse and other sexual practices'[28] and is usually undertaken in the courtship behaviour well before genital activity occurs, it is sometimes thought of as more intimate than coitus. Prostitutes, for example, traditionally do not kiss their clients on the mouth, reserving the activity for their private sexual behaviour. Nicolson[29] has speculated that kissing may be a mechanism by which semiochemicals (similar to pheromones) are exchanged between humans to induce bonding.

Common extragenital changes during sexual arousal

In both males and females effective sexually arousing stimuli cause a number of physiological changes.[20,30] There is increased respiration, heart rate, and blood pressure, nipple erection, often sweating, and a maculopapular skin rash ('sex flush'). Muscle tension increases and the pupils dilate. All these changes become more intense as arousal increases. Following orgasm the changes dissipate rapidly (R phase); without orgasm they dissipate more slowly.

The endocrinology of normal sexual function

Males

Androgens

The major steroids influencing normal sexual function in males are the androgens secreted by the testes mainly as testosterone with much smaller quantities of androstenedione. The adrenal cortex also manufactures and secretes androgens but this amounts only to 2 per cent of the total. Of the testosterone, 95 per cent is bound to plasma protein; only the unbound fraction is an active virilizing hormone.

The development of the masculine musculature, bone growth, genitals, and pubic and axillary hair is androgen dependent. The mechanism of the hormonal masculinization of the brain in rodents involves the aromatization of testosterone, but in humans the role of aromatization is uncertain.[31]

Androgens and male sexual behaviour

The possible involvement of androgens in adult human male sexual behaviour has been examined many times (see Levin[32] for references). Removal of testosterone by castration usually leads to a decrease in sexual activity and drive in the majority of subjects within 12 months. There is, however, large individual variations, and some castrates retain sexual activity and interest for years.[33] Factors such as adrenal androgens, the availability of sexual partners, and attitude to the operation influence the response. In castrates and in hypogonadal males, replacement of testosterone restores sexual interest and activity.

Everitt and Bancroft[34] proposed two systems in the brain that control erections. The first is an androgen-dependent system subserving sexual desire and arousability and assessed by measuring spontaneous erections during sleep (nocturnal penile tumescence). Nocturnal penile tumescence is impaired in androgen insufficiency and can be restored by androgen replacement. The second system, which is androgen independent, is involved in the erectile response to visual erotic stimuli. It is claimed to be unaffected in hypogonadal men.[34] More recently, however, Bancroft[35] reported that the original proposal was an oversimplification resulting from the use of a single measure of penile response. When other measures are taken, the erectile responses to visual erotic stimuli are affected by androgens in terms of the duration, degree of rigidity, and speed of the detumescence, all measures which had not been used in the earlier studies. Despite these laboratory findings, androgen replacement in androgen-deficient men affects nocturnal penile tumescence more than the erections due to visual erotic stimuli.

Gonadotrophin secretion and control

The control of gonadotrophin secretion in the adult male is by hormonal negative-feedback circuits: luteinizing hormone by testosterone and follicle-stimulating hormone by inhibin (secreted from the Sertoli cells). In the adult male oestrogens are produced by the testis. They exert powerful negative feedback on gonadotrophin secretion (100 times more potent than testosterone) but their amounts are very small and they are not thought to play any significant physiological role. Prolactin is secreted in the male, but it has no proven reproductive function. However, pathologically high levels of prolactin (hyperprolactinaemia) are accompanied by disturbances of sexual function, especially erectile dysfunction. The cause is unknown.

Females

Oestrogen, progesterone, and androgen

In the female, oestrogen, progesterone, and androgens are involved in differentiating and maintaining genital and breast tissues and in influencing normal sexual function. Fetal genital development, unlike that of the male, does not appear to need hormonal stimulation as the development of female genital structures are the fetal prototype or default programme.[36] During puberty, ovarian oestrogen and progesterone together with androgens from the adrenal cortex induce growth and functional changes in the internal and external genitalia, breast, and nipples. Oestrogens induce growth in the fallopian tubes, uterus, vagina, and breasts and lay down subcutaneous fat largely in the breast, hip, and thigh regions to create the rounded contours of the female body that are highly attractive to the male. The fat laid down is enough to supply the energy for a pregnancy and the subseqent lactation. Androgens in the female are responsible for the development of the clitoris, nipples, pubic, and axillary hair, and probably the labia and periurethral glans.

Role of hormones in female sexuality

While over 60 studies have been undertaken to examine whether the changing hormonal levels of the menstrual cycle influence the sexual arousal of the female,[37] neither oestrogen or progesterone have been found convincingly to play a direct role in influencing the sexual activity of the human female apart from their indirect functions in the maintenance of the structures and functions of the female genitals, especially the vagina.

Androgens, secreted by the female's adrenal cortex, have a concentration 10 times less than those in the male. The variation of the androgen levels in the plasma during the menstrual cycle is small and it is the free androgen level that must be taken into account. Androgens maintain the adult female pubic and axillary hair, clitoris, and probably labia and periurethral glans. The role of androgens in female sexuality is controversial and not clear cut.[38] Some propose that, as in the male, it is the major hormonal influence on the female libido. Removal of the adrenals has been shown to reduce desire and ability to reach orgasm. Excess androgens stimulates libido but in pharmacological not physiological doses. Such doses affect the structure and sensitivity of the clitoris (an androgen-sensitive tissue), so the effects on sexuality might not be brain mediated.

Sexual behaviour during the menstrual cycle

Despite numerous studies it is still uncertain whether female sexual behaviour is influenced by the hormonal changes in the menstrual cycle. Meuwissen and Over[37] surveyed 64 published studies. A significant number showed a premenstrual peak in sexual desire and activity, others a postmenstrual peak, either at menstruation or ovulation. (The latter studies often used poor methodology to determine the time of ovulation.)

Male genital functions during normal sexual arousal

While the DEOR model characterizes the general sexual arousal of humans, a more specific detailed physiological model in males is that of excitation, erection, emission, and ejaculation with orgasm. Each of these is served by separate mechanisms. Although ejaculation and orgasm usually occur together, they also have separate mechanisms.

Excitation

Sexual excitation can occur by psychogenic or somatogenic stimuli. In various circumstances arousal can become linked to or greatly enhanced by association with non-sexual objects such as feminine garments of underwear.

Erection: the conversion of the flaccid urinary penis to the rigid sexual penis

The three lengthwise erectile chambers of the penis are arranged with a side-by-side dorsal pair of corpora cavernosa above the single ventral corpus spongiosum. The corpora cavernosa are covered by the tunica albuginea, a 2-mm thick fibrous membrane which is resistant to stretch. The corpus spongiosum surrounds the length of the penile urethra and is enlarged at its base to form the urethral bulb and distally to create the glans penis. While it becomes engorged with blood during arousal it is not involved in the rigidity of the erection but merely protects the urethra from closure. The unaroused penis is flaccid because the pudendal arterial blood flow into the erectile tissues is limited by the high sympathetic constrictive tone in the smooth muscle of the vessels of corpus cavernosum. On sexual arousal, the sympathetic tone is reduced, the neural innervation of the arteries and cavernosal chambers is activated to release vasoactive intestinal peptide (**VIP**), a peptidergic vasodilator neurotransmitter that directly relaxes smooth muscle and nitric oxide, the nitrergic neurotransmitter. Nitric oxide activates the enzyme cyclic guanylase in the smooth-muscle cells of the cavernous tissue and blood-vessel endothelium to produce cyclic guanosine monophosphate (**cGMP**), the second messenger that relaxes the muscle.

The vasodilatation of the arterial supply by VIP together with the relaxation of the vessels of the cavernosal tissue allows them to fill under arterial pressure stretching the chambers until they become stiff against their covering of unyielding tunica albuginea, and the veins (emissary) that pass obliquely through the tunica become occluded greatly reducing penile vascular drainage The flaccid urinary penis has been converted into the erect rigid sexual penis some 7 to 8 cm longer. The rigidity is essential for successful vaginal penetration and to stimulate its walls (especially the anterior) during penile thrusting. The striated muscles of the pelvic region, namely the ischiocavernosus and bulbocavernosus, are not normally involved in creating penile erection,[39] although they can be voluntarily contracted in bursts to aid its rigidity. The engorged corpus spongiosum is less rigid than the cavernosal chambers making the glans of the penis softer and less damaging to the female labia and vagina. Concomitant with the enhanced penile blood flow is a huge increase in the sensitivity of the glans, especially its coronal ridge, to touch and friction.

Internal genitals

The genital fluids of the testes, epididymis, and accessory genital glands of the male are involved in emission. These glands are the bulbo-urethral (Cowper's gland), the prostate (approximately 30 per cent of the total volume of the ejaculate), and the paired seminal vesicles (approximately 60 per cent of the volume of the ejaculate). The fluids from all these together with that of the glands of Littré that line the penile urethra, constitute the ejaculate or semen which has a characteristic odour and forms a coagulum in contact with air.

Emission

This phase begins with the movement of the various genital fluids into the ducts initiated by the neurally induced contraction of smooth muscles in the capsules of the testes, epididymis, and seminal vesicles. The secretions spurt into the prostatic urethra, and the sphincter of the bladder neck closes to prevent reflux into the bladder. When this happens the male experiences the sensation of 'ejaculatory inevitability' and knows that he will ejaculate within a second or two and that conscious suppression of the ejaculatory reflex is now impossible. The contractions of the smooth muscle of the glandular capsules together with the peristalsis of the vas deferens and urethra pushes the semen along into the penile urethra.

Ejaculation

Within a second or two later the ischiocavernosus and the bulbocavernosus muscles of the perineal region contract clonically initially at about one per 0.8 s squeezing the urethra and forcing out the ejaculate. As ejaculation proceeds, the interval between each striated muscle contraction gets longer and their force weaker until they gradually die out.[39] Their number can vary between 5 and 60. Most of the ejaculate is expressed in the first half dozen contractions. If the striated muscles are paralysed the semen is squeezed out only by the smooth muscle peristaltic contractions which produce a dribbling ejaculate with no projectile force and little pleasurable quality.

Male orgasm

Supreme ecstatic pleasure is experienced just before the striated contractions occur and is then associated, throbbingly, with each subsequent contraction slowly decreasing in intensity and dying away as do the contractions. This is the human orgasm. Orgasm is felt as an intense pleasurable throbbing in the penis and pelvic area and can last from 5 to 60 s. Kinsey et al.[11] marshalled the evidence showing that orgasm and ejaculation were separate mechanisms. Briefly, orgasm occurs without ejaculation in preadolescent males, in some adult males orgasm does not occur until a few seconds after ejaculation, a few adult males are anatomically incapable of ejaculation but have orgasms, and males who have been prostatectomized cannot have ejaculations but some can have orgasms.

The intensity of orgasm varies with the duration of the sexual arousal (the longer it is maintained the greater the subsequent orgasm), the erotic excitement and novelty of the arousing stimuli, and previous ejaculation, especially the interval from the last one (initial ejaculations have usually better orgasms than subsequent ones). Males have a refractory period after ejaculation and usually cannot have an erection or another ejaculation until some time has passed. This varies with age and can be anything from minutes, when young, to hours or days when older.[20] It is not known where this inhibitory mechanism resides but animal work suggests that it may be in the brain rather than the spinal cord. Some men claim to be able to learn to inhibit ejaculation and yet have repeated serial orgasms.[40]

Although it has been stated that the larger the ejaculate volume is, the greater is the pleasure,[20] the studies were flawed because they used men who increased semen volume by abstaining from ejaculation for days. This confounds the effects of semen volume with that of ejaculatory abstinence which itself enhances subsequent sexual pleasure. Semen volume does not appear to be either the trigger for ejaculation or the arbiter of pleasure. Drugs can induce a dry ejaculation but the pleasure of the orgasm is unimpaired,[39] and in young boys the pleasure of the early dry orgasm is not noticeably changed when semen is added to the ejaculation around puberty.[41]

Female genital functions during normal sexual arousal

External

Labia

The external female genitalia consist of the outer (majora) and inner (minora) labia containing erectile tissue that surround the vaginal introitus. Normally the outer labia meet and cover the introitus, but in some women the inner labia protrude even when they are sexually unaroused. Sexual arousal creates vasocongestion especially in the labia minora which protrude through the majora adding approximately 1 to 2 cm to the length of the vagina. The labia minora become erotically sensitive to touch and friction when engorged.

Clitoris

Although the clitoris is the homologue of the penis, its precise anatomical structure is still uncertain. The most recent description by O'Connell et al.[42] is of a triplanar complex of erectile tissue with a midline shaft lying in the medial sagittal plane about 2 to 4 cm long and 1 to 2 cm wide, which bifurcates internally into paired curved crura 5 to 9 cm long, and externally is capped with a glans about 20 to 30 mm long with a similar diameter. Two vaginal bulbs of erectile tissue are closely applied on either side of the urethra. The shaft's erectile tissue consists of two corpora cavernosa surrounded by a fibrous sheath (tunica albuginea) and the whole is covered by a clitoral hood formed in part by the fusing of the two labia minora. The uncertainty concerns the location and extent of the female corpus spongiosum. Some describe it as wrapped around the urethra, others state that the vaginal (vestibular) bulbs on either side of the vaginal wall are spongiosus tissue and unite ventrally to the urethral meatus to form a thin strand of erectile tissue ending in the glans. Recent studies by van Turnhout et al.[43] have clarified the situation. They confirmed by dissections in fresh cadavers that the bilateral vestibular bulbs terminate into the glans clitoridis.

With sexual arousal, the blood flow to the clitoris is increased probably by a mechanism involving its vipergic (VIP) and nitrinergic (nitric oxide) innervation leading to its tumescence (swelling) but, contrary to many inaccurate descriptions, without true erection (i.e. without rigidity). The enhancement of its blood flow is paralleled by an increased sensitivity to touch and friction especially of the glans.

Periurethral glans

There is a triangular area of mucous membrane that surrounds the urethral meatus, extending from just below the glans of the clitoris to the entrance of the vagina. This area has been called the 'periurethral glans'[30] and is thought to be capable of erotic stimulation, especially during penile thrusting, as it is known that the tissue is pushed and pulled into the vagina by the movement.[30] The periurethral glans is actually part of the corpus spongiosum if we accept the findings of van Turnhout et al.[43] which suggest that it is the homologue of the the male glans. The extent, mobility, density of innervation, and sensitivity of this erotic site may explain why some women find it easy to reach orgasm during penile thrusting alone.

Internal

Vagina

In sexual quiescence this is a potential space with an H-shaped cross-section and an elongated S-shaped longitudinal section culminating in a cul-de-sac, the anterior wall of which is penetrated by the cervix. The anterior and posterior walls touch but their film of basal vaginal fluid prevents adhesion. This basal fluid is a mixture of fluids from the vagina itself (basal transudate) with uterine and cervical secretions. The squamous epithelial lining of the vagina actively transports sodium ions from the vaginal fluid back into the blood. As fluid follows this ion movement osmotically the vagina is continually producing and reabsorbing its own fluid.[30]

On sexual arousal, the blood supply to the vaginal walls is increased by the liberation of VIP from the vipergic neural innervation while the venous vessels are probably constricted by the release of the vasoconstrictor neuropeptide Y.[30,44] Within seconds this creates blood-vessel engorgement and a plasma transudate leaks out of the capillaries and percolates between the cells of the epithelium saturating its small reabsorptive capacity. The newly formed vaginal fluid creates a lubricating film on the vaginal surface which is essential for painless penile penetration. Poor or inadequate lubrication can lead to dyspareunia and subsequent sexual dysfunction. On cessation of sexual arousal or after orgasm the blood flow returns to the basal level and the fluid is reabsorbed back into the blood following the continuous absorption of sodium ions by the epithelial cells.

Coitus and the vagina

The cul-de-sac of the vagina is expanded during sexual arousal and the cervix is lifted clear of its posterior wall (vaginal tenting).[20] In the ventral–ventral ('missionary') coital position, penile penetration and thrusting stretches and stimulates the structures of the anterior vaginal wall which include the urethra, the 'G spot' (see below), and Halban's fascia. All these are thought to be capable of creating erotic excitement when so stimulated, giving rise to a significant part of the sexual pleasure experienced by most women during coitus.

The erotic structures of the anterior vaginal wall: urethra, 'G spot', and Halban's fascia

The urethra, approximately 4 cm long, is invested with erectile tissue which becomes engorged on sexual arousal.[30,42] Ultrasound imaging during coitus has shown that the thrusting penis stretches the urethra.[45] There is an area a few centimetres from the introitus, at or around the junction of the urethra with the bladder, that becomes swollen and on maintained pressure stimulation can induce orgasm. This urethral area was first identified by Grafenberg[46] but the observation was overlooked until its rediscovery by Ladas et al.[47] who named it the 'G spot' in recognition of the original discoverer. Anatomically, it probably represents the 'paraurethral' or 'periurethral' glands often refered to as the 'female prostate'. In some women these produce at orgasm a small amount of fluid secretion loosely referred to as the 'female ejaculate' (see Levin[30] for references). These glands are in the space between the bladder trigone and the neck of the urethra[48] which is filled with fibroelastic mesenchymal lamina rich in vascular lacunae and contains nerve fibres and pseudocorpuscular terminals.[49] This area is known as Halban's fascia[49] and when stimulated by pressure (penile or digital) creates intense sexual pleasurable feelings.[48,49]

Female orgasm

As in the male, the female orgasm creates supreme ecstatic pleasure usually accompanied by throbbing striated muscle contractions, especially of the ischiocavernous and bulbospongiosus muscles, but other pelvic striated muscles can also be involved.[20] The induction of orgasm in women by coital stimulation alone is not as frequent as that in the male, about half not achieving orgasm unless clitoral stimulation is also used. The reason for this difference is ascribed either to the greater inhibitory education about sexual pleasure experienced by women or the lack of correct genital stimulation. A major difference between males and females is that females can be multiorgasmic because they do not have a refractory period after orgasm.[20,30] There is mounting evidence that, unlike the unitary concept of the DEOR model, the erotic stimulation of different genital sites (especially the anterior vaginal wall compared with the clitoris) induces different types of orgasmic response both subjectively and physiologically.[44,47,48,50]

Summary

Normal human sexual function can be characterized simply by its biological mechanisms which are of obvious importance, not least to reproduction. The mechanisms have changed little over the centuries, but their expression as behaviour, when moulded by historical time, social class, ethnic grouping, religion, and society, creates the changing complex concept of human sexuality. Indeed, it has been said that human sexuality is more about fertilizing relationships than eggs! While we have increased hugely our knowledge about many of the mechanisms involved in human sexuality, the impact of successful oral therapy for erectile dysfunction being an obvious example, those in the brain are still largely unexplored. What creates human sexual desire and sexual excitement and what causes them to fade away are fascinating questions that may be available to study with the new refined technologies of brain imaging and neuropsychopharmacology. The future holds fascinating prospects.

References

1. Morris, D. (1967). *The naked ape.* Jonathan Cape, London.
2. Diamond, J. (1997). *Why is sex fun? The evolution of human sexuality.* Weidenfield and Nicolson, London.
3. Heltne, P.G. and Marquardt, L.A. (ed.) (1989.) *Understanding chimpanzees.* Harvard University Press, Cambridge, MA.
4. Grammer, K., Dittami, J., and Fischman, B. (1998). Changes in female sexual advertisement according to menstrual cycle. http://evolution.humb.univie.ac.at/electronic/estro.jpg
5. Laqueur, T. (1990). *Making sex: body and gender from the Greeks to Freud.* Harvard University Press, Cambridge, MA.
6. Foucault, M. (1980). *The history of sexuality.* Vintage, New York.
7. Tiefer, L. (1992). Historical, scientific, clinical and feminist criticism of the 'the human sexual response cycle' model. *Annual Review of Sex Research*, **2**, 1–23.
8. Gagnon, J.H. and Simon, W. (1973). *Sexual conduct: the social sources of human sexuality.* Aldine, Chicago, IL.
9. Money, J. (1986). *Lovemaps: clinical concepts of sexual/erotic health and pathology, paraphilia, and gender transposition in childhood, adolescence, and maturity.* Irvington, New York.
10. Kinsey, A.C., Pomeroy, W.B., and Martin, C.E. (1948). *Sexual behaviour in the human male.* W.B. Saunders, Philadelphia, PA.

11. Kinsey, A.C., Pomeroy, W.B., Martin, C.E., and Gebhard, P.H. (1953). *Sexual behaviour in the human female.* W.B. Saunders, Philadelphia, PA.

12. Clement, U. (1990). Surveys of heterosexual behaviour. *Annual Review of Sex Research*, **1**, 45–74.

13. Einon, D. (1994). Are men more promiscuous than women? *Ethology and Sociobiology*, **15**, 131–43.

14. Berk, R., Abramson, P.R., and Okami, P. (1995). Sexual activities as told in surveys. In *Sexual nature, sexual culture* (ed. P.R. Abramson and S.D. Pinkerton), pp. 371–86. University of Chicago Press.

15. Michael, R.T., Gagnon, J.H., Laumann, E.O., and Kolata, G. (1994). *Sex in America—a definitive survey.* Little, Brown, London.

16. Wellings, K., Field, J., Johnson, A.M., and Wadsworth, J. (1994). *Sexual behaviour in Britain.* Penguin, Harmondsworth.

17. Van de Velde, Th.H. (1923). *Ideal marriage, its physiology and technique.* Heinemann, London.

18. Bullough, V.L. (1994). *Science in the bedroom—a history of sex research.* Basic Books, New York.

19. Porter, R. and Hall, L. (1995). *The facts of life: the creation of sexual knowledge in Britain, 1650–1950.* Yale University Press, New Haven, CT.

20. Masters, W.H. and Johnson, V.E. (1966). *Human sexual response.* Little, Brown, Boston, MA.

21. Robinson, P. (1976). *The modernization of sex.* Cornell University Press, Ithaca, NY.

22. Kaplan, H. (1979). *Disorders of sexual desire.* Simon and Schuster, New York.

23. Garde, K. and Lunde, I. (1980). Female sexual behaviour. A study in a random sample of 40-year-old women. *Maturitas*, **2**, 225–40.

24. Buss, D.M. (1994). *The evolution of desire: strategies of human mating.* Basic Books, New York.

25. Trivers, R.L. (1972). Parental investment and sexual selection. In *Sexual selection and the descent of man 1871–1971* (ed. B. Campbell), pp. 136–79. Aldine, Chicago, IL.

26. Grammar, K. (1989). Human courtship behaviour: biological basis and cognitive processing. In *The sociobiology of sexual and reproductive strategies* (ed. A.E. Rasa, C. Vogel, and E. Voland), pp. 147–69. Chapman & Hall, London.

27. Perper, T. (1985). *Sex signals. The biology of love.* ISI Press, New York.

28. Phillips, A. (1993). *On kissing, tickling and being bored.* Harvard University Press, Cambridge, MA.

29. Nicholson, B. (1984). Does kissing aid human bonding by semiochemical addiction? *British Journal of Dermatology*, **111**, 623–7.

30. Levin, R.J. (1992). The mechanisms of human female sexual arousal. *Annual Review of Sex Research*, **3**, 1–48.

31. Feder, H. (1984). Hormones and sexual behaviour. *Annual Reviews of Psychology*, **35**, 165–200.

32. Levin, R.J. (1994). Human male sexuality: appetite and arousal, desire and drive. In *Appetite: neural and behavioural bases* (ed. C.R. Legg and D. Booth), pp. 127–63. Oxford University Press.

33. Bremer, J. (1959). *Asexualisation: a follow up of 244 cases.* Macmillan, New York.

34. Everitt, B.J. and Bancroft, J. (1992). Of rats and men: the comparative approach to male sexuality. *Annual Review of Sex Research*, **2**, 77–118.

35. Bancroft, J. (1995). Are the effects of androgens on male sexuality noradrenergically mediated? Some consideration of the human. *Neuroscience and Neurobehavioural Reviews*, **19**, 325–30.

36. Wilson, J. (1978). Sexual differentiation. *Annual Review of Physiology*, **40**, 279–306.

37. Meuwissen, I. and Over, R. (1992). Sexual arousal across phases of the human menstrual cycle. *Archives of Sexual Behaviour*, **21**, 165–73.

38. Hutchinson, K.A. (1995). Androgens and sexuality. *American Journal of Medicine*, **98** (Supplement 1A), 111–15S.

39. Gerstenberg, T.C., Levin, R.J., and Wagner, G. (1990). Erection and ejaculation in man. Assessment of the electromyographic activity of the bulbocavernosus and ischiocavernosus muscle. *British Journal of Urology*, **65**, 395–402.

40. Robbins, M.A. and Jensen, G.D. (1978). Multiple orgasm in males. *Journal of Sex Research*, **14**, 21–6.

41. Langfeldt, T. (1990). Early childhood and juvenile sexuality, development and problems. In *Handbook of sexology*, Vol. 7 (ed. M.E. Perry), pp. 179–200. Elsevier, Amsterdam.

42. O'Connell, H.E., Hutson, J.M., Anderson, C.R., and Plenter, R.J. (1998). Anatomical relation between urethra and clitoris. *Journal of Urology*, **159**, 1892–7.

43. van Turnhout, A.A. W. M., Hage, J.J., and van Diest, P.J. (1995). The female corpus spongiosum revisited. *Acta Obstetrica Scandinavica*, **74**, 762–71.

44. Levin, R.J. (1998). Sex and the human female reproductive tract—what really happens during and after coitus. *International Journal of Impotence Research*, **10** (Supplement 1), S14–21.

45. Riley, A.J., Lees, W.R., and Riley, E.J. (1992). An ultrasound study of human coitus. In *Sex matters* (ed. W. Bezemer, P. Cohen-Kettenis, and K. Slob), pp. 29–32. Excerpta Medica, Amsterdam.

46. Grafenberg, E. (1960). The role of urethra in female orgasm. *International Journal of Sexology*, **3**, 145–8.

47. Ladas, A.K., Whipple, B., and Perry, J.D. (1982). *The G spot and other recent discoveries about human sexuality.* Holt, Rinehart, Winston, New York.

48. Tordjman, G. (1984). Similarities of the sexual responses of men and women. In *Emerging dimensions of sexology* (ed. T.T. Segraves and E.W. Haeberle), pp. 317–30. Praeger, New York.

49. Minh, H.-N., Smadja, A., and De Sigalony, J.P. (1979). Le fascia de Halban: son role dans la physiologie sexuelle. *Gynaecologie*, **30**, 267–73.

50. Hoch, Z. (1986). Vaginal erotic sensitivity by sexological examination. *Acta Obstetrica et Gynaecologica Scandinavica*, **65**, 767–73.

4.11.2 The sexual dysfunctions

Stanley E. Althof and Patricia Schreiner-Engel

Introduction

Men and women have always been curious about sexual life: its inherent mysteries, drives, intentions, oddities, and the all too common sexual problems. Treatment rituals, folk remedies, advice, and sex manuals have been discovered among the writings of the ancient Greek physicians, Islamic and Talmudic scholars, and Chinese and Hindu practitioners. The venerable Indian text *The Kama Sutra*[1] offered sage advice and illustrated the varied coital positions. Even today the public's insatiable curiosity about sexual life, especially 'how to' enhance, improve, restore, or cure problems, is the focus of every monthly women's magazine, television and radio programmes, books, videos, and Internet sites where one finds tests measuring sexual satisfaction, advice, techniques for problem-solving, sexual aides to add 'sizzle', and folk remedies to increase desire, arousal, or (prolong) orgasm.

This chapter is a psychiatric overview of the common male and female sexual dysfunctions, their prevalence and aetiology. Additionally, this chapter provides a schema for understanding sexual problems, methods for accurately assessing them, and discussions of current treatment modalities.

The first attempt at describing and classifying sexual disorders began with Richard von Krafft-Ebing[2] and his *Psychopathia Sexualis*, which influenced medical and legal practice for more than three-quarters of a century. Attempts to develop databases to quantify normal and abnormal sexual acts soon followed, and ultimately led to the seminal contributions of Havelock Ellis[3] and Albert Kinsey.[4,5]

Historically, treatments of sexual dysfunctions were based on prevailing salient ideologies: psychoanalytical, behavioural, Masters and Johnson, neo-Masters and Johnson, and the current psychobiological. Prior to 1950 psychoanalytical concepts guided clinicians in their understanding and treatment of sexual problems. Sexual symptomatology was linked to constellations of unresolved, unconscious conflict(s) occurring during specific developmental periods.[6] Psychoanalytical notions were heterosexist and male-centred, as is clearly evident in the construction of the controversial concept of penis envy and the psychological interpretation given to the classification of women's orgasm as either clitoral or vaginal.

In the late 1950s the behavioural perspective gained ascendancy; sexual problems were understood to be learned (conditioned) anxiety responses.[7,8] Interventions, loosely modelled on classical conditioning paradigms, sought to extinguish the anxiety or performance demands that interfered with normal sexual function.

In 1966 Masters and Johnson reported the first results of laboratory observations of male and female sexual arousal and orgasm.[9] Initially they described the physiology of these phases of functioning, and later highlighted the deleterious influence of performance anxiety (the fear of future sexual failure based upon previous failures, which can contribute to all sexual dysfunctions including those with primary organic aetiologies), the impact of relationship factors, and the significance of biological factors on the development of sexual dysfunctions.[10] Their work foreshadowed the later integration of medical and psychological interventions.

The neo-Masters and Johnson era was heralded by the publication of Helen Singer Kaplan's book, *The New Sex Therapy*.[11] She integrated psychoanalytical theory with Masters and Johnson's cognitive-behavioural understanding of sexual dysfunction. Distinguishing between recent and remote aetiological causations, she recommended behavioural approaches for the former and reserved traditional psychodynamic methods for the latter.

The mid-1980s ushered in the current psychobiological era. This period is distinguished by the medicalization of treatment approaches, primarily for male sexual dysfunction.[12] Scientific investigations of cellular chemistry have elucidated the pathophysiology of male sexual arousal problems and have led to the introduction of new oral treatments, such as sildenafil.

Model for understanding sexual response

For heuristic purposes, the sexual response cycle can be divided into four phases of functioning: desire, arousal, orgasm, and satisfaction. Dysfunctions of sexual response found in both DSM-IV[13] and ICD-10[14] mirror this theoretical model, but also include another dimension, that of sexual pain disorders. These ideas are an elaboration of Masters and Johnson's psychophysiological research as well as the independent theoretical contributions of Kaplan[15] and Lief.[16] Two assumptions underlie this model: (1) each phase of sexual function has relatively discrete underlying psychophysiological mechanisms; and (2) disturbances in one phase do not necessarily denote dysfunctions in another. This conceptualization, however, does not preclude a dysfunction in one area precipitating secondary impairments in another

phase. For example, the loss of erectile capacity may eventually dampen a man's interest in engaging in any sexual activity. The strength of this four-phase model is that it directs clinicians to focus on the aetiology and behavioural manifestations of the primary dysfunction and its specific treatments.

Since multiple biological and psychological influences may effect any phase of the sexual response cycle, careful assessment is required before any treatment approach is initiated. The complex interaction between the social, interpersonal, intrapsychic, hormonal, neurological, and vascular aspects is often not fully appreciated by clinicians and results in treatment efforts that fail. For instance, a graduated behavioural intervention employing dilators to treat a woman with vaginismus may not succeed because the clinician is not sufficiently aware of the marital discord in her relationship. This patient may be able to eventually insert the dilators but not be able to engage in coitus with her husband. Or, for example, the clinician may correctly diagnose a clinical depression in a man complaining of low sexual desire, but fail to discover that the patient also has abnormally low levels of testosterone.

Epidemiology

The best and most current study regarding the prevalence of sexual dysfunction was performed by Laumann *et al.*[17] who studied a random probability sample of 3442 American individuals aged between 18 and 59 years. Summarizing the findings among the female participants, 33 per cent reported a lack of interest in sex, 17 per cent had difficulty with arousal, 24 per cent were unable to reach orgasm, 21 per cent said that sex was not pleasurable, and 14 per cent complained of pain with coitus. Among the male participants 16 per cent reported a lack of sexual interest, 10 per cent identified erectile difficulties, 29 per cent complained of ejaculating too quickly, and 17 per cent acknowledged anxiety about performance. One major criticism of this study is that it did not survey individuals above the age of 59. Also, it is unclear whether the complaints of respondents would meet the diagnostic criteria for each sexual dysfunction. There have also been numerous surveys of sexual problems in non-random samples collected from magazine surveys,[18] community samples,[19] and clinical populations. The prevalence rates of sexual complaints in these groups were found to be higher than those reported by Laumann *et al.* Because these surveys did not employ similar diagnostic criteria or methodology, comparisons between studies are difficult.

General criteria for sexual dysfunction within ICD-10 and DSM-IV

Although ICD-10 and DSM-IV share the basic nomenclature and model for sexual dysfunction, ICD-10 differs from DSM-IV in the specificity of diagnoses. This can be seen in Tables 1 to 9. For example, ICD-10 requires that the subject be unable to participate in a sexual relationship as he or she would wish, that the dysfunction occurs frequently although it may be absent on some occasions, and that the dysfunction has been present for at least 6 months. Both ICD-10 and DSM-IV require that the dysfunction not be entirely attributable to any other mental or physical disorder.

Unlike ICD-10, DSM-IV requires that the dysfunction cause marked distress or interpersonal difficulty. Additionally, for each DSM-IV sexual disorder, the clinician is required to make three judgements: whether the dysfunction is lifelong or acquired, whether it is of a generalized or specific type, and whether it is due to psychological or combined biological and psychological factors.

Disorders of sexual desire

Sexual desire is an extraordinarily complicated aspect of human life and thus requires a multifaceted approach to its understanding.[20] Levine[21,22] has proposed a tripartite model wherein sexual desire is conceptualized as the product of the mind's capacity to integrate three separate elements: drive, wish, and motive. Drive is the neurophysiological generator inducing the internal phenomenon labelled as 'horniness or randiness'. Wish is the cognitive component through which intellectual motives are translated into behaviours, for example 'it's our anniversary, so we should make love'. Motive refers to a combination of affective, transferential, and attachment response that impel one to engage in or avoid sexual experiences.

In men, the biological component underlying sexual desire is circulating levels of testosterone and, more specifically, bioactive or free testosterone. Schiavi et al.[23] found that men with hypoactive sexual desire had significantly lower levels of testosterone than matched controls. In women, however, hormone-behavioural relationships are more difficult to identify because baseline levels of androgens are substantially lower and less variable than men's and thus more difficult to measure. Measurement is further complicated in women because endocrine profiles are considerably altered during periods of menstruation, pregnancy, lactation, and the menopause. Schreiner-Engel and Schiavi[24] failed to find significant differences in mean levels of free testosterone in young women with hypoactive sexual desire compared to matched controls.

Aetiology

Clinicians theorize that strong negative emotions (anger, dysthymia, guilt, shame) result in diminished sexual desire; however, empirical studies supporting these ideas are generally lacking. One exception is Schreiner-Engel and Schiavi's report[24] that men and women with generalized hypoactive sexual desire had higher lifetime prevalences of depressive disorder which had preceded the development of the sexual disorder. Many clinicians also believe that situational sexual desire disorders may have their origin in the deterioration of a couple's nonsexual relationship. Stuart et al.[25] found that hypoactive sexual desire was associated with lower levels of marital satisfaction and lower feelings of romantic love toward the partner. Finally, a history of childhood sexual abuse or gender identity conflict has been associated with generalized hypoactive sexual desire in some women.[26,27]

Diagnosis

The diagnosis of sexual desire disorders is complicated because no objective criteria of normal sexual desire have ever been established.[26,28] Both DSM-IV and ICD-10 require the clinician to render a subjective judgement about whether a deficiency, lack of interest, or absence of sexual desire exists (Table 1). Hypoactive sexual desire is not diagnosed simply because one partner complains that the other is

Table 1 DSM-IV and ICD-10 diagnostic criteria for desire disorder

DSM-IV: Hypoactive sexual desire (302.71)

A. Persistently or recurrently deficient (or absent) sexual fantasies and desire for sexual activity. The judgement of deficiency or absence is made by the clinician, taking into account factors that affect sexual functioning, such as age and the context of the person's life.

B. The disturbance causes marked distress or interpersonal difficulty.

C. The sexual dysfunction is not better accounted for by another Axis I disorder (except another sexual dysfunction) and is not due exclusively to the direct physiological effects of a substance (e.g. a drug of abuse, a medication) or a general medical condition.

ICD-10: Lack or loss of sexual desire (F52.0)

A. The general criteria for sexual dysfunction (F52) must be met.

B. There is a lack or loss of sexual desire, manifest by diminution of seeking out sexual cues, of thinking about sex with associated feelings of desire or appetite, or of sexual fantasies.

C. There is a lack of interest in initiating sexual activity either with a partner or as solitary masturbation, resulting in a frequency of activity clearly lower than expected, taking into account age and context, or in a frequency very clearly reduced from previous much higher levels.

lacking desire, and it is not diagnosed when it fails to cause marked distress. There are cases where two individuals each with low desire have a mutually satisfying sexual relationship.

Assessment

In evaluating male patients with hypoactive sexual desire, the clinician should routinely obtain a total and free testosterone level and consider procuring a prolactin level. In both male and female patients, a thorough medical and pharmacological history should be elicited. This strategy will identify temporal relationships between the dysfunction and the onset of endocrinological disease, medication use, medical treatment, or substance abuse.

Sexual desire is assessed by enquiring into the patient's quality and quantity of sexual imagery in daytime fantasies and night dreams, desire to engage in sexual behaviour both alone and with a partner, and frequency of sexual activity, alone or with a partner. For DSM-IV and ICD-10, the individual's life context must be considered, namely age, health, and partner status.

Psychological and relational factors that require assessment include:

(1) quality of the relationship;

(2) feelings about the partner, e.g. positive regard, anger, or loss of respect;

(3) impact of extramarital liaisons;

(4) sexual orientation incompatibility between the self and partner;

(5) history of childhood or adult sexual trauma;

(6) negative parental transferences and current or prior history of affective disorder;

(7) life circumstances that result in negative emotions, e.g. business failures, death of relatives.

Treatment

Psychotherapeutic interventions for hypoactive sexual desire are generally combinations of behavioural, cognitive, psychodynamic, and marital techniques. No specific treatment regimens have been agreed upon anecdotally by clinicians, nor have any been validated by scientific study. Outcome studies of eclectic treatments demonstrate that 50 to 70 per cent of men and women with disorders of sexual desire appear to achieve modest gains immediately following therapy. However, a marked deterioration in desire is noted at 3-year follow-up.[29–31] Half of the individuals who report success after treatment do not maintain heightened desire 3 years later. Paradoxically, however, couples in these studies report improved and sustained levels of sexual satisfaction despite the regression in levels of sexual desire.

There are reports that testosterone may be helpful to certain groups of women in restoring sexual desire, such as surgically menopausal women.[32] Davidson et al.[33] proposed that androgens may act to facilitate and maintain sensitivity to or pleasurable awareness of both sexual thoughts and activity. In a review of empirically validated treatments for sexual dysfunction Heiman and Meston[34] state: 'Although testosterone has been shown to increase sexual desire in men and women, its effect may be limited to these individuals with abnormally low levels of bioavailable testosterone. No controlled studies in which the effect of testosterone on humans who had adequate testosterone levels but low desire was directly tested.' Segraves and Althof[35] echo this statement by saying, 'There is no pharmacotherapy for primary psychological hypoactive sexual desire with established efficacy'.

Disorders of sexual aversion

These disorders are considered extreme forms of desire disorders differentiated by the emotion of intense aversion to or disgust with sexual activity, rather than the more typical lack of interest in sexual behaviour. The ICD-10 and DSM-IV criteria can be found in Table 2. There is generally a phobic element seen that leads clinicians to consider a traumatogenic aetiology more often than the other factors proposed for generalized hypoactive sexual desire. These may include early sexual abuse, painful experiences with coitus, or the perception of being assaulted by the partner.

Treatment

Pharmacological and psychological interventions tend to mirror the interventions for hypoactive sexual desire.

Disorders of sexual arousal in men

Erectile dysfunction

The past two decades have witnessed major scientific advances in elucidating the pathophysiology of male sexual arousal disorder, commonly referred to as erectile dysfunction or impotence. Oral agents,

Table 2 DSM-IV and ICD-10 diagnostic criteria for sexual aversion disorder

---

DSM-IV: Sexual aversion disorder (302.79)

A. Persistent or recurrent extreme aversion to, and avoidance of, all (or almost all) genital sexual contact with a sexual partner.

B. The disturbance causes marked distress or interpersonal difficulty.

C. The sexual dysfunction is not better accounted for by another Axis I disorder (except another sexual dysfynction)

ICD-10: Sexual aversion (F52.1)

A. The general criteria for sexual dysfunction (F52) must be met.

B. The prospect of sexual interaction with a partner produces sufficient aversion, fear, or anxiety that sexual activity is avoided, or, if it occurs, is associated with strong negative feelings and an inability to experience any pleasure.

C. The aversion is not the result of performance anxiety (reaction to previous failure of sexual response).

---

like sildenafil, are one consequence of these scientific efforts; gene therapy may be a future intervention. Table 3 illustrates DSM-IV and ICD-10 diagnostic criteria for this disorder.

The terms impotence and erectile dysfunction had been used interchangeably to denote the inability of a man to achieve or maintain erection sufficient to permit satisfactory sexual intercourse. Social scientists object to the impotence label because of its pejorative implications and lack of precision.[36] The NIH Consensus Development Conference[37] advocated the label 'erectile dysfunction' be used in its place, and defined it as the 'inability of the male to achieve an erect

Table 3 DSM-IV and ICD-10 diagnostic criteria for erectile dysfunction

---

DSM-IV: Male erectile disorder (302.72)

A. Persistent or recurrent inability to attain, or to maintain until completion of the sexual acitivity, an adequate erection.

B. The disturbance causes marked distress or interpersonal difficulty.

C. The erectile dysfunction is not better accounted for by another Axis I disorder (other than a sexual dysfunction) and is not due exclusively to the direct physiological effects of a substance (e.g. a drug of abuse, a medication) or a general medical condition.

ICD-10: Failure of genital response (F52.2)

A. The general criteria for sexual dysfunction (F52) must be met.

B. Erection sufficient for intercouse fails to occur when intercourse is attempted. The dysfunction takes one of the following forms:

(1) full erection occurs during the early stages of lovemaking but disappears or declines when intercourse is attempted (before ejaculation if it occurs);

(2) erection does occur, but only at times when intercourse is not being considered;

(3) partial erection, insufficient for intercourse, occurs, but not full erection;

(4) no penile tumescence occurs at all.

penis as part of the overall multifaceted process of male sexual function'. This definition de-emphasizes intercourse as the *sine qua non* of sexual life and gives equal importance to other aspects of male sexual behaviour.[38]

Theory

Lifelong or primary erectile dysfunction is understood as a man's developmental failure to become comfortable with adult forms of sexuality, for example unresolved sexual identity or Oedipal conflicts. Acquired or secondary erectile dysfunction is thought to result from interpersonal struggles, for instance marital discord, or intrapsychic phenomena. Until recently, clinicians of virtually all theoretical persuasions considered some form of anxiety, usually performance anxiety, to be responsible for the development and maintenance of lifelong and acquired erectile dysfunction.

Barlow[39] challenged this established concept by experimentally manipulating anxiety and cognitive interference in functional and dysfunctional men. In functional men anxiety facilitated arousal; yet, it had just the opposite effect in dysfunctional men. Cognitive interference, however, facilitated arousal in dysfunctional men and inhibited it in functional men. From these results, Barlow developed a preliminary working model of psychogenic dysfunction which stated:

> …that cognitive interference processes interacting with anxiety are responsible for sexual dysfunction, specifically inhibited sexual excitement in men and women and possibly other related forms of sexual dysfunction. The nature of these cognitive processes in dysfunctional subjects seems to revolve largely around focusing on or attending to task irrelevant contexts. This focus then becomes driven by the physiological aspects of arousal that clinicians more commonly refer to as anxiety which in turn results in further deterioration in sexual performance. On the other hand, sexually functional subjects focus on and process erotic cues without difficulty. Anxiety may enhance this processing (up to a point) and therefore may facilitate sexual arousal.[39]

Alternatively, Bancroft[40] postulates the existence in the central nervous system of both excitatory and inhibitory systems operating in parallel, which provide dual control over sexual response and consequently sexual behaviour. The inhibitory system of this model is further divided into two independent dimensions: threat of performance failure, and the threat of performance consequences. Bancroft suggests that the inhibitory system is adaptive in protecting the individual from danger or other negative consequences associated with sexual response.

Assessment

Erectile dysfunction can be understood as an interactive phenomenon where psychological and physiological factors are conceptualized as dynamically additive. This interactive model captures the ever-changing influences of biology and emotional life. Regardless of the precipitating causes, changes in both domains occur over time. This model encompasses both the psychological impact that the dysfunction has upon the man's and couple's sexual equilibrium as well as the fluctuating influences of medication, lifestyle, and disease.

A Process of Care (**POC**) guide for appropriately assessing and treating erectile dysfunction has been developed by a multidisciplinary panel of experts in family medicine, internal medicine, endocrinology, psychiatry, psychology, and urology.[41] The authors outline six phases.

1. Establishing the diagnosis.

2. Discussing the initial findings, discussing referral, beginning the education process.

3. Modifying reversible causes of erectile dysfunction.

4. Implementing first-line treatment: psychotherapy, oral erectogenic agents, vacuum constriction devices.

5. Implementing second-line treatment: self-injection therapy, transurethral therapy.

6. Implementing third-line treatment: implantation of a penile prosthesis.

Each phase is discussed below.

Phase 1 concentrates on establishing the diagnosis of primary erectile dysfunction. This is accomplished through a conjoint effort of a mental health clinician and a urologist. However, the urological history and examination are beyond the scope of this chapter. By enquiry, the mental health clinician identifies the onset and course of the dysfunction. The patient is asked to rate the current quality of his erections on a scale of zero to 10 (with 10 being the best quality erection) under a variety of circumstances: upon awakening and with fantasy, masturbation, foreplay, intercourse, and different partners. Unusual and/or disturbing life circumstances coincident with the development of the dysfunction are elicited. Other relevant parameters of sexual life are queried including sexual drive, frequency of lovemaking, orgasmic difficulties, and sexual satisfaction. On occasion it is important to enquire about gender identity and paraphilia, as conflicts in these realms may produce erectile dysfunction. The magnitude of performance anxiety is assessed, as are the circumstances that disrupt cognitive focus. The quality of the couple's non-sexual relationship is examined, as are conflicts emanating from other sources, for example work, finances, partner's health, and difficulties with parents or children. It is important to evaluate the patient's motivation for resuming coitus and his past use of other treatment options, such as sex therapy or self-injection treatment. Obstacles to effectively utilizing psychotherapeutic or medical treatment alternatives are evaluated at this point.

Because erectile dysfunction impacts on the man, his partner, and their non-sexual relationship, any evaluation that does not include talking with the partner separately from the patient risks missing vital information. Not infrequently the partner offers the clinician factual information that the patient omitted, for example 'Did he tell you about…his drinking problem, not getting a promotion, his affair, our daughter's drug problem, his mother's death, my mastectomy?' The possibility of the partner having a sexual dysfunction is assessed, as are attitudes that are antithetical to resuming sexual life. This interview may also provide the partner with reassurance by dispelling groundless self-recriminations and faulty self-attributions.

In phase 2 of the POC model the clinician reviews the initial findings, discussing referral if indicated, and beginning the educational process. An in-depth discussion of all relevant treatment options with the benefits and limitations of each is provided. Improving the patient's/couple's understanding of their problem, reviewing their expectations for treatment, and correcting unrealistic hopes engenders a sense that the patient and doctor are working together, thereby enhancing patient compliance.

At this point additional diagnostic testing is often indicated to further clarify and exclude aetiology, to gratify the man's wish to know what is causing the dysfunction, or for medicolegal reasons. These tests may include testosterone level, nocturnal penile tumescence testing, dynamic-infusion cavernosometry/cavernosography, or duplex ultrasonography.

Treatment

Phase 3 of the POC model focuses on modifying reversible causes of the erectile dysfunction, such as offending prescription and/or nonprescription (including recreational) drugs, habitual behaviours such as cigarette smoking, alcohol abuse, partner conflict, lifestyle patterns such as workaholism that may diminish intimacy, specific endocrinological conditions, and pelvic trauma or anatomical defect. Sometimes simple changes in medication or lifestyle are sufficient to reverse the dysfunction.

The POC model then delineates successive psychotherapeutic and medical interventions based on efficacy, degree of reversibility, and invasiveness. There are three first-line treatments recommended in phase 4, including individual and/or couple psychotherapy, oral erectogenic agents, and vacuum constriction devices.

Psychotherapy/sexual counselling

Psychotherapy aims to restore a man's potency to the optimal level possible within the limits of his physical well being and life circumstances. The goal is to surmount the psychological and relational barriers that preclude mutual sexual satisfaction. Psychodynamically oriented therapists view the dysfunction as a metaphor in which the man/couple are trying simultaneously to conceal and express conflictual aspects of themselves or their relationship. In symbolic terms the dysfunction contains a compromised solution to one of life's dilemmas.[42] Alternatively, behaviour therapists understand the dysfunction as a maladaptive response to interpersonal or environmental situations, or past experiences.

To date, no treatment interventions based on the recent theoretical formulations of Barlow[39] (about the role of anxiety and cognitive processing in arousal disorders) and of Bancroft[40] (about the coexistence of mental excitation and inhibition of sexual arousal) have been reported. But as these notions are further elaborated, they may be translated into innovative treatment concepts.

Sex therapy today involves integrating medical and psychotherapeutic interventions. The conventional role of the mental health clinician in the treatment of erectile dysfunction had been to treat those with psychogenic erectile problems. Now with the advent of efficacious, reversible, and safe medical therapies the role of the clinician has expanded to include helping men/couples, regardless of the aetiology of the dysfunction, make use of these new interventions. Thus, the clinician provides assistance in overcoming the resistances to utilizing medical treatments that may help patients and partners develop a satisfying sexual relationship.[43] Sometimes attitudinal or psychological resistances need to be worked through prior to beginning a medical intervention. If not overcome, these forces can render the best-intentioned treatment efforts ineffectual. The therapist can also help the couple to cultivate a romantic ambience and engage in conversations that will physically and psychologically prepare them to become lovers again. Frequently the therapist can also assist the couple in accepting the changes that may have occurred in their lives, for example menopause, disability, illness, or other life stresses.

Many men with erectile dysfunction can achieve a significant recovery in sex therapy; those with acquired disorders typically fare better than those with lifelong problems. In an excellent review of the treatment studies for erectile dysfunction, Mohr and Beutler[44] wrote that the 'component parts of these treatments typically include behavioural, cognitive, systemic and interpersonal communications interventions. Averaging across studies, it appears that approximately two-thirds of the men suffering from erectile failure will be satisfied with their improvement at follow-up ranging from six weeks to six years.'

All studies with long-term follow-up note a tendency for men to suffer temporary relapses. Hawton et al.[29] reported that 75 per cent of couples experienced 'recurrence of, or continuing difficulty with the presenting sexual problem'; but that this caused little or no concern for 34 per cent of these couples. Patients indicated that they now discussed the difficulty with the partner, practised the techniques learned during therapy, accepted that difficulties were likely to recur, and read books about sexuality. These techniques proved to be effective coping strategies. Hawton et al.[45] suggest that a positive treatment outcome is associated with better pretreatment communication, general sexual adjustment (especially when the female partner is interested in and enjoys sex and has no psychiatric history), and with the couple's willingness to complete treatment homework.

Interventions for relapse prevention are seldom reported but should be considered. Routinely requesting patients/couples to return for 'booster sessions' may help to maintain the initial positive gains. Also helping couples understand that a temporary relapse is likely and providing them with coping strategies may enable them to regain their sexual confidence.

Oral treatments

The introduction of sildenafil citrate (Viagra™) in the United States could best be characterized as 'a happening'. In the first 90 days after its approval it became the most prescribed medication with 3 million prescriptions written; 5 months later approximately 90 per cent of those prescriptions had been refilled. Sildenafil acts by inhibiting the enzyme that breaks down cyclic guanosine monophosphate (cGMP). It enhances the man's ability to achieve a natural erection, providing that he is being adequately stimulated mentally and physically. Unlike other medical treatments such as self-injection, transurethral or vacuum therapy, sildenafil does not induce an erection irrespective of the man's degree of arousal. Taken on an empty stomach, sildenafil works in approximately 1 h. The only contraindication to sildenafil is the concomitant use of nitrate medications or a diagnosis of retinosa pigmentosa. Depending on the aetiology of the dysfunction, the efficacy of sildenafil ranges between 40 per cent and 70 per cent.[46] In clinical trials the most common side-effects included headache (16 per cent), facial flushing (10 per cent), dyspepsia (7 per cent), nasal congestion (4 per cent), and abnormal vision (red/blue colour vision changes or blurry vision) (3 per cent).

There are several other oral agents under investigation. Apomorphine (TAP) works centrally on the medial preoptic area to produce erection. Early data suggest a significant improvement in erectile activity over placebo. The main side-effect appears to be nausea, which is counteracted by an oral antiemetic. Other oral agents are vasomax

(Zonagen™) and another unnamed type 5-phosphodiesterase inhibitor developed by the ICOS corporation. Insufficient data are available at present to evaluate the efficacy of these drugs.

Yohimbine, a natural herb made from African tree bark, has been used for years by men with various forms of erectile dysfunction. Anecdotal reports are positive but there are few objective, placebo-controlled studies that validate the use of yohimbine. It has often been given to patients who insisted on an oral agent or used as a placebo.

Vacuum systems

Vacuum pump systems are manufactured by numerous companies (UroHealth, Mission, Post-t-Vac) and consist of several components: a clear plastic cylinder, a hand pump, a lubricant, and tension rings. Battery operated systems are available for men who are unable to manually pump the device. To create an erection the man places the clear plastic tube over his lubricated penis. Pumping creates an erection by producing a negative pressure 'vacuum' to draw blood into the corpora. The tension band is positioned on the base of the penis to maintain the erection. Approximately 90 per cent of men are able to achieve erections sufficient for intercourse with the vacuum pump; drop-out rates are approximately 20 per cent.[47]

The common side-effects associated with vacuum tumescence therapy are haematoma, ecchymosis, petechiae, pain, numbness of the penis, pulling of scrotal tissue into the cylinder, and blocked and painful ejaculation.[47] Blood dyscrasias, penile bends, or anticoagulant therapy are relative contraindications.

Self-injection therapy and transurethral therapy

Phase 5 of the POC guidelines recommends the second-line treatments of self-injection therapy and transurethral therapy. Of the three medications commonly used for self-injection therapy (papaverine hydrochloride, phentolamine, and prostaglandin E_1), only prostaglandin E_1 has received the United States Food and Drugs Administration approval for this indication. The two commercial preparations of prostaglandin E_1 used most frequently by the majority of clinicians are Edex™ (Schwarz Pharma) and Caverjet™ (Pharmacia-Upjohn).

Transurethral therapy allows prostaglandin E_1 to be applied directly to the urethral mucosa through an innovative, drug-delivery system developed by the Vivus Corporation. Known as MUSE™ (medicated urethral system for erection), a pellet of prostaglandin E_1 is placed on to the urethral mucosa and transferred to the corpora cavernosum through vascular channels resulting in an erection. The major advantage of this treatment method is that it obviates the need to inject the penis.

Only one intervention, the implantation of a penile prosthesis, comprises phase 6 of the POC model and is viewed as a third-line treatment for erectile dysfunction. Details about this intervention are also beyond the scope of this chapter.

Disorders of sexual arousal in women

Typically, female arousal disorders are diagnosed in women with complaints of diminished lubrication or painful intercourse. There is considerable ambiguity regarding this diagnosis because, with the exception of postmenopausal women in whom diminished lubrication is a normal physiological change, symptoms of female arousal disorder are frequently subsumed under desire and/or orgasmic disorders

Table 4 DSM-IV and ICD-10 diagnostic criteria for female sexual arousal disorder

DSM-IV: Female sexual arousal disorder (302.79)

A. Persistent or recurrent inability to attain, or to maintain until completion of the sexual activity, an adequate lubrication–swelling response of sexual excitement.

B. The disturbance causes marked distress or interpersonal difficulty.

C. The sexual dysfunction is not better accounted for by another Axis I disorder (other than a sexual dysfunction) and is not due exclusively to the direct physiological effects of a substance (e.g. a drug of abuse, a medication) or a general medical condition.

ICD-10: Lack of sexual enjoyment (F52.11)

A. The general criteria for sexual dysfunction (F52) must be met.

B. Genital repsonse (orgasm and/or ejaculation) occurs during sexual stimulation, but is not accompanied by pleasurable sensations or feelings of pleasant excitement.

C. There is no manifest and persistent fear or anxiety during sexual activity.

ICD-10: Failure of genital response (F52.2)

A. The general criteria for sexual dysfunction (F52) must be met.

B. There is failure of genital response, experienced as failure of vaginal lubrication, together with inadequate tumescence of the labia. The dysfunction takes one of the following forms:

  (1)   general: lubrication fails in all relevant circumstances;
  (2)   lubrication may occur initially but fails to persist for long enough to allow comfortable penile entry;
  (3)   situational lubrication occurs only in some situations (e.g. with one partner but not another, or during masturbation, or when vaginal intercourse is not being contemplated).

(Table 4). Additionally, the definition of female sexual arousal disorder reflects the overemphasis of physical function (lubrication and pelvic vasocongestion) over psychological excitement and/or pleasure. The correlation between physical and mental arousal is at best inconsistent and often puzzling. For instance, Palace[48] evaluated the effects of heightened autonomic arousal, noting that it significantly increased both physiological and subjective sexual arousal. These findings indicate that heightening autonomic arousal in an actual sexual setting might be useful for increasing sexual excitement. The use of this strategy, however, has not been reported.

Assessment

Assessment of female arousal disorders begins with separating out problems of desire and orgasm that disguise themselves as arousal difficulties. Relationship satisfaction is assessed, and queries about current life stressors are posed. The clinician enquires about what forms of sexual activity the woman finds arousing, both in fantasy and behaviour, by herself and with a partner. As with men who have erectile dysfunction, the patient is asked to judge her subjective arousal employing a rating scale of zero to 10 (with 10 being the most aroused) to a wide range of conventional stimuli such as undressing, being touched, touching the partner, kissing, breast stimulation, manual genital stimulation, oral genital stimulation, intercourse in various positions, etc. The course of the disorder's development and the phenomenology of the problem in the women are assessed. It is essential to establish that the woman is receiving adequate cognitive and physical sexual stimulation. Too often hurried attempts at intercourse without adequate preparation and foreplay result in symptoms of an arousal disorder. The clinician should explore whether cultural, social, or religious ideas may be interfering with the development of arousal. The symptom may be a reflection of relationship dissatisfaction, sexual orientation incongruity, preoccupation with other life tasks (childbearing), fatigue, or depression. It is always worthwhile asking about the patient and partner's attribution concerning the onset and maintenance of the problem, and what forms of self-help they have attempted. Finally, enquiries regarding treatment expectations are posed, unrealistic expectations are challenged, and sensible goals negotiated.

An integrated medical–psychological approach is essential in assessing sexual arousal disorders in women. This is best accomplished through the conjoint efforts of a gynaecologist and mental health clinician. Gynaecological aspects of assessment can be found in other texts and are beyond the scope of this chapter.

Treatment

Few empirically validated or anecdotal reports of psychological treatment interventions can be found for arousal disorders in women.[34] Spence[26] has proposed that clinicians employ techniques to facilitate increased arousal, such as fantasy training, use of erotic materials, attention-focusing skills, Kegel exercises (voluntary relaxation and contraction of the pubococcygeus muscle), and enhancing the partner's sexual skills. Concomitantly, she suggests techniques to reduce factors that may inhibit sexual arousal, such as cognitive restructuring, relaxation training, systematic desensitization of anxiety-provoking situations, and addressing the relationship issues that generate negative affects. No treatment data is available on her strategy. The lack of reported treatment studies for this female disorder may reflect the paucity of patients presenting with an arousal disorder clearly attributable to a psychological cause; most arousal complaints appear to be the result of inadequate lubrication.

Thus most female arousal disorders are initially treated with topical lubricants. Chronic medical conditions and medications that may be responsible for decreasing arousal must be carefully evaluated.

The advances in elucidating the pathophysiology of erectile response in men has recently led to renewed efforts to investigate the physiology of female arousal. Several clinical studies are under way to determine whether oral agents may have a role in the treatment of this disorder.

Orgasmic disorders in women

Orgasm is the reflexive culmination of arousal manifested by rhythmic vaginal wall contractions and the release of muscular tension accompanied by varying degrees of pleasure. Achieving orgasm reliably, usually highly valued by women, is associated with enhanced self-esteem,

Table 5 DSM-IV and ICD-10 diagnostic criteria for anorgasmia

DSM-IV: Female orgasmic dysfunction (302.73)

A. Persistent or recurrent delay in, or absence of, orgasm following a normal sexual excitement phase. Women exhibit wide variability in the type or intensity of stimulation that triggers orgasm. The diagnosis of female orgasmic disorder should be based on the clinician's judgement that the woman's orgasmic capacity is less than would be reasonable for her age, sexual experience, and the adequacy of sexual stimulation she receives.

B. The disturbance causes marked distress or interpersonal difficulty.

C. The orgasmic dysfunction is not better accounted for by another Axis I disorder (other than a sexual dysfunction) and is not due exclusively to the direct physiological effects of a substance (e.g. a drug of abuse, a medication) or a general medical condition.

ICD-10: Orgasmic dysfunction (F52.3)

A. The general criteria for sexual dysfunction (F52) must be met.

B. There is orgasmic dysfunction (either absence or marked delay of orgasm) which takes one of the following forms:

(1) orgasm has never been experienced in any situation;

(2) orgasmic dysfunction has developed after a period of relatively normal response:

(a) general: orgasmic dysfunction occurs in all situations and with any partner;

(b) situational: for women, orgasm does occur in certain situations (e.g. when masturbating or with certain partners).

confidence in one's femininity, and the desire to increase sexual activity.[49] The persistent and recurring difficulty achieving orgasm is labelled anorgasmia. Table 5 lists the diagnostic criteria for anorgasmia set forth in DSM-IV and ICD-10.

Diagnostic concerns

DSM-IV cautions that 'the diagnosis of female orgasmic disorder be based on the clinician's judgement that the woman's orgasmic capacity is less than would be reasonable for her age, sexual experience, and the adequacy of sexual stimulation she receives'. These variables lead to diagnostic confusion and little agreement as to what constitutes an orgasmic disorder. Anorgasmia is clearly the diagnosis for a woman who has never achieved orgasm under any circumstances; 10 to 15 per cent of women fall into this category. However, as orgasm achieved solely with intercourse is elusive and masturbation is not widely accepted in women, diagnosing orgasmic conditions becomes more problematic. Kaplan estimated that only one-third of women are able to regularly achieve orgasm through intercourse alone; therefore, two-thirds of adult women cannot be labelled anorgasmic. For some women, manual and/or oral stimulation is often the only means of reaching orgasm, while for others self-stimulation with a vibrator is their sole method of climaxing. Whether or not reliance on only one means of achieving orgasm constitutes a dysfunction is not clear. Adding to the confusion is the media's constant reinforcement of unrealistically high expectations for achieving orgasms from sexual encounters. Both men and women are led to believe that women can easily and regularly achieve multiple orgasms from penile thrusting alone, and all sexual activity should lead to orgasm for the woman as well as the man. The clinician's dilemma is to distinguish between normal variation and dysfunction.

Theory

The most popular theory, although soundly debunked for years, has been Freud's notion that sexual maturity in a woman requires that she give up clitoral sensitivity for vaginal responsiveness. Thus, women who could not achieve orgasm with penile thrusting alone were considered neurotic. Masters and Johnson's psychophysiological research clearly demonstrated that no distinction can be made between vaginal and clitoral orgasms, and that the sensitivity of clitoral/vaginal neuropathways naturally varied among women.

Fisher[50] characterized anorgasmic women as having an increased need to control situations involving high arousal where they might lose control. He believed these women were defending against disappointments with their fathers, which was transferred to their current love object. Although clinicians may question the psychodynamic basis for Fisher's conclusions, none the less many concur that the 'fear of losing control' constitutes a major issue underlying anorgasmia. Other psychological explanations include fear of impregnation, guilt regarding sexual impulses, fear of rejection by one's partner, and fear of vaginal damage by penile thrusting.

The strength and tone of a woman's pubococcygeus muscle has been proposed as a contributing factor in the development of anorgasmia. However, psychophysiological research has demonstrated that the correlation between pubococcygeus muscle tone and orgasmic capacity is low. For some women it is possible that focusing on increasing the tone and strength of the pubococcygeus muscle may idiosyncratically improve their orgasmic ability by eliminating outside distractions.[51]

Assessment

The clinician first establishes whether the patient has ever experienced an orgasm and, if so, how reliably and under what circumstances it occurred, for example by masturbation with her hand or other means, with a partner's hand or mouth, with intercourse, etc. Some women will be unsure what an orgasm feels like. They may be actually having orgasms, albeit mild ones, but not labelling their sensations as such; they were expecting earth-shattering spasms. For women who do have orgasms on occasion, the clinician enquires about whether a particular fantasy is necessary in order to achieve an orgasm, such as being forced to have sex. Questions concerning the woman's ability to relax, sustain, and heighten her arousal and the degree to which she can concentrate on her bodily sensations are asked. If any of these difficulties are present, the clinician explores them further. If orgasmic ability has been lost, the life events/circumstances temporally related to orgasmic cessation are reviewed, for example divorce, job relocation. Societal/religious attitudes that may interfere with excitement are noted, for instance sexual pleasure is not the prerogative of good girls. Finally, questions concerning the partner are posed, including the quality of their non-sexual relationship and his degree of sexual skill, technique, and willingness to please her. Medically, neurological dysfunctions such as spinal cord injury and the use of medications known to impair

orgasmic function, such as serotonin-selective reuptake inhibitors, antihypertensives, central nervous system stimulants, tricyclic antidepressants, and monoamine oxidase inhibitors,[52] should be excluded.

Treatment

Several studies[27,53–55] have documented the success of masturbatory training programmes in facilitating orgasm in women who have never achieved orgasm. Directed masturbation consists of a series of home exercises, which begin with self-exploration and move towards increased genital stimulation.[56] Initial success rates range from 70 to 90 per cent, depending on whether women were treated individually, in couples, groups, or exposed to videotapes or books describing masturbatory training. Kuriansky and Sharpe[57] reported that 15 per cent of their subjects were not able to sustain orgasmic attainment at a 2-year follow-up.

Sensate focus is used as a means of densensitizing performance anxiety or sensitizing the woman to pleasurable bodily areas and erotic sensations. Partners take turns caressing one another in a progressive way from non-sexual touching to sexual stroking of the other's body. The success rate of this treatment alone is less than that of directed masturbation, however; in combination the two treatments appear to have a synergistic effect.[34]

Success in achieving orgasm(s) is highest with a self-induced orgasm, decreases with partner-induced orgasm using manual or oral stimulation, and is lowest with intercourse without simultaneous manual stimulation. Immediately post-therapy, Kuriansky et al.[53] reported that 89 per cent of women achieved orgasm by themselves, 21 per cent within the 'context of a partner encounter', and 16 per cent with intercourse alone. Heiman and Meston[34] reported a two- to threefold increase in coital orgasm at a 3-month follow-up.

The long-term results of treatment for female orgasmic dysfunction have to be evaluated in the context of two facts: first, over time women demonstrate an increased capacity to achieve orgasm with partner stimulation as well as with coital activity; women who drop out of treatment programmes also report improved orgasmic functioning 2 years after seeking therapy. Second, prognosis appears more positive for women with lifelong orgasmic dysfunction than for women who acquire the dysfunction after a period of normal functioning. The poorer outcome for an acquired orgasmic dysfunction is thought to be due to psychological or relationship causes not addressed in masturbatory training programmes. Thus, assessment of these factors is important prior to embarking on a masturbatory training programme. In fact, Heiman and Meston[34] suggest that 'some combination of sex education, sexual skills training, communication on general and sexual issues, body image, and...directed masturbation' appear to be most efficacious in resolving orgasm disorders.

Orgasmic disorders in men

There are two orgasmic disorders in men: rapid ejaculation and delayed ejaculation. Rapid or premature ejaculation is characterized as ejaculation occurring without voluntary control and with minimal sexual stimulation. Delayed ejaculated is defined as the persistent and recurrent difficulty of the man achieving orgasm. The diagnostic criteria for these dysfunctions are presented in Tables 6 and 7.

Rapid ejaculation

It is evident from the examination of the criteria of ICD-10 and DSM-IV that rapid ejaculation can be diagnosed by two different dimensions: ejaculatory latency or voluntary control. According to ICD-10, ejaculation must occur 'within 15 seconds of the beginning of intercourse,' while DSM-IV is equivocal on duration, stating that 'ejaculation occurs with minimal sexual stimulation before, on, or shortly after penetration'. ICD-10 makes no mention of voluntary control, while DSM-IV notes that ejaculation occurs 'before the person wishes'. Both nosologies, however, require the man to be distressed for at least 6 months, and both require the clinician to make a judgement regarding the independence of this condition from other mental, behavioural, or physiological disorders.

Treatment research has been hampered by the lack of a scientifically sound and universally acceptable definition as to which criterion, ejaculatory latency or voluntary control, should be used to diagnose rapid ejaculation. Thus, one finds 'noncomparability across studies, uninterpretability of studies which do not provide their operational definition, inability to generalize from research results,…and lack of data on rapid ejaculation among homosexual couples.[58] The most frequently cited variable is ejaculatory latency, defined as the time

Table 6 DSM-IV and ICD-10 diagnostic criteria for male orgasmic disorder

DSM-IV: Male orgasmic disorder (302.74)

A. Persistent or recurrent delay in, or absence of, orgasm following a normal sexual excitement phase during sexual activity that the clinician, taking into account the person's age, judges to be adequate in focus, intensity, and duration.

B. The disturbance causes marked distress or interpersonal difficulty.

C. The orgasmic dysfunction is not better accounted for by another Axis I disorder (except another sexual dysfunction) and is not due exclusively to the direct physiological effects of a substance (e.g. a drug of abuse, a medication) or a general medical condition.

ICD-10: Orgasmic dysfunction (F52.3)

A. The general criteria for sexual dysfunction (F52) must be met.

B. There is orgasmic dysfunction (either absence or marked delay of orgasm) which takes one of the following forms:

(1) orgasm has never been experienced in any situation;
(2) orgasmic dysfunction has developed after a period of relatively normal response:
   (a) general: orgasmic dysfunction occurs in all situations and with any partner;
   (b) situational: for men, one of the following can be applied:
     (i) orgasm occurs only during sleep, never during the waking state;
     (ii) orgasm never occurs in the presence of the partner;
     (iii) orgasm occurs in the presence of the partner but not during intercourse.

Table 7 DSM-IV and ICD-10 diagnostic criteria for rapid ejaculation

DSM-IV: Premature ejaculation (302.75)

A. Persistent or recurrent ejaculation with minimal sexual stimulation before, on, or shortly after penetration and before the person wishes it. The clinician must take into account factors that affect duration of the excitement phase, such as age, novelty of the sexual partner or situation, and recent frequency of sexual activity.

B. The disturbance causes marked distress or interpersonal difficulty.

C. The premature ejaculation is not due exclusively to the direct effects of a substance (e.g. withdrawal from opiods).

ICD-10: Premature ejaculation (F52.4)

A. The general criteria for sexual dysfunction (F52) must be met.

B. There is an inability to delay ejaculation sufficiently to enjoy lovemaking, manifest as either of the following:

(1) occurrence of ejaculation before or very soon after the beginning of intercourse (if a time limit is required, before or within 15 seconds of the beginning of intercourse);
(2) ejaculation occurs in the absence of sufficient erection to make intercourse possible.

C. The problem is not the result of prolonged abstinence from sexual activity.

from intromission to orgasm, but these studies use very different operational definitions of time, ranging from less than 1 min to 5 min; similar problems exist when the number of coital thrusts are counted. Those who oppose defining rapid ejaculation in quantitative terms argue that the salient parameter should be voluntary control.[59,60] They contend that men who make no attempt to control ejaculation may be considered selfish but are not necessarily dysfunctional. The problem in using this definition lies in deciding what is meant by voluntary control.

Theory

The prevailing opinions regarding the aetiology of rapid ejaculation have typically assumed that the dysfunction was either psychological or learned, depending upon the theorists' assumptions about how the mind operates. Some believe that a lowered ejaculatory threshold stems from anxiety, general hostility toward women, interpersonal conflicts with a particular partner, or conditioning patterned on furtive masturbation practices, early hurried sexual experiences with prostitutes, or hasty lovemaking in the backseat of a car. Once established, performance anxiety was thought to maintain the rapid ejaculatory pattern.

Anxiety is not a singular concept, however. Anxiety may refer to a phobic response such as being fearful of the dark wet unseen vagina. It may also refer to affect, such as the end result of conflict resolution where two contradictory urges are at play, for example the man is angry at his partner but feels guilty about directly expressing his hostility. Anxiety may refer as well to a preoccupation with sexual failure and poor performance. As the man contemplates another sexual experience, his anxiety leads to an avoidance of any future sexual opportunity. McCarthy[60] suggests that this performance anxiety has two discrete dimensions: a cognitive component where the man watches himself, thus removing himself from awareness of his arousal level, as well as an emotional component consisting of fear of failure.

Strassberg et al.[61,62] and Gospodinoff[63] independently speculate that a subgroup of men who rapidly ejaculate may have an underlying neurophysiological vulnerability that explains some of the failures of psychological treatment. They argue that increased penile sensitivity[64] and a constitutionally more rapid bulbocavernousnes reflex create the biological vulnerability. Rowland et al.,[65] however, were unable to find evidence of increased penile sensitivity in rapid ejaculators.

Separating rapid ejaculation into lifelong and acquired groups may prove helpful in clarifying the aetiology of the dysfunction. A subgroup of lifelong rapid ejaculators may have a biological vulnerability, while those with acquired symptoms may not. The development of rapid ejaculation requires an examination of recent psychosocial stressors, medication, or surgery. It is often a consequence of erectile failure. Men develop performance anxiety regarding their erectile reliability and rush intercourse thinking that they have limited time to 'complete the act'. With these thoughts, this additional dysfunction appears and men become even more anxious about sexual interactions.

Assessment

Rapid ejaculation is best assessed along both dimensions of ejaculatory latency following vaginal penetration and degree of voluntary control. Questions are asked about how long it takes the man to reach orgasm under each of the following circumstances: with masturbation, partner hand and/or mouth stimulation, and intercourse. Some men have inordinately high expectations, for instance 'I should be able to last 45 minutes', and falsely label themselves as rapid ejaculators. Education often reverses this misattribution. The man's level of sexual experience is reviewed, as is the duration of his current relationship. Young inexperienced men routinely ejaculate quickly, while men anxious to please new partners often encounter transient problems. Factors that improve and worsen performance are noted, such as coital positions. Next, the man's degree of voluntary control is examined, and which factors improve or worsen it are noted, such as distraction. The clinician reviews whether the dysfunction occurs under all circumstances or only with specific partners. If this is an acquired disorder it is important to ascertain the life events temporally related to the onset of the problem, for example mother-in-law coming to live with the family. It is also necessary to gauge whether rapid ejaculation is the primary problem or is secondary to erectile dysfunction, in other words whether it occurred after the man began having difficulty achieving an erection. The quality of the non-sexual relationship is also studied, with particular attention to the partner's response to the dysfunction and her level of expectation. Finally, it is worthwhile enquiring about the partner's sexual functioning because sometimes rapid ejaculation disguises a partner's dysfunction, that is to say it is an adaptive response to the partner's sexual aversion.

Organic factors are seldom implicated; however, trauma to the sympathetic nervous system during surgery for aortic aneurysm, pelvic fracture, prostatitis, and urethritis can induce rapid ejaculation. Additionally, drug withdrawal from narcotics or trifluoperazine have been associated with this symptom.[66]

Treatment

Since the early 1970s, an array of individual, conjoint, and group therapy approaches employing behavioural strategies, such as the stop–start, squeeze technique, progressive sensate focus exercises, masturbatory exercises, and 'quiet vagina' with the female astride, have evolved as the treatments of choice for rapid ejaculation.[10,15,59,60,67–70]

Behavioural treatment often begins with the man alone, having him repeatedly stimulate himself to midrange levels of excitement before pausing. After several repetitions he is permitted to ejaculate. The aim of this exercise is to help him learn intermediate levels of excitement and begin to slow down his arousal.

The stop–start procedure involves the man repeatedly being brought to high levels of excitement, initially through stimulation by his partner's hand or mouth and later by vaginal thrusting, but stopping prior to ejaculation.[69] This pause allows the man's arousal to decrease and thereby delays orgasm. This behavioural sequence is repeated several times, after which the man is permitted to ejaculate. Subsequently, Masters and Johnson[10] modified the procedure by introducing a squeeze technique. At the point when stimulation is stopped, the man's glans penis is squeezed firmly but quickly by the partner, which is thought to lower arousal more effectively. Often a partial loss of erection occurs.

Sensate focus exercises are designed to allow the man to develop an awareness of his arousal level by lessening the demand characteristics of the sexual experience. In a slow graduated fashion the man and his partner take turns giving and receiving pleasure. Initially, the touching is restricted to non-genital/non-breast stimulation; upon achieving ejaculatory control these areas are also pleasured.

'Quiet vagina' is an extension of the stop–start manoeuvre to include intercourse. After successful hand stimulation the woman sits astride or lies on top of the man and, without any thrusting or rhythmic movement, envelopes his penis in her vagina. The aim of this exercise is to desensitize the man to the wet warm sensations of the vagina. After the man masters the 'quiet vagina' for a prolonged period of time, movement by the woman is slowly introduced. The man directs her to stop when his excitement has increased. The couple sit/lie quietly until his arousal decreases, whereupon they resume the exercise. This is repeated several times before the man is eventually allowed to ejaculate.

It is crucial for the therapist to monitor the partners' needs and responses during therapy. The female partner may feel used and unimportant. This must be acknowledged, while helping her to focus on the ultimate goal of pleasurable sex for both partners. Also, the therapist must monitor both patient and partner for the emergence of any resistances that will sabotage treatment.

McCarthy[60] delineates three foci of a cognitive-behavioural psychotherapeutic approach:

(1) challenging self-defeating ideas about sexuality or women, while replacing them with facilitating thoughts about ejaculatory control, sexuality, and intimacy;

(2) learning the behavioural skill of identifying the point of ejaculatory inevitability through the use of the stop–start technique and alternating intercourse positions or thrusting movements;

(3) establishing a co-operative, intimate, and satisfying relationship.

Levine[59] advocates an integrated approach where the man or couple seek to understand the hidden meaning(s) of the rapid ejaculation, appreciate the interference of performance anxiety, and, when ready, embark on a series of behavioural tasks. He cautions clinicians to be aware of the man or couple's need for a symptom and how rare it is to find 'simple cases' of rapid ejaculation.

It has been found that the impressive treatment success rates of 60 to 95 per cent reported by Masters and Johnson can not be replicated and are not sustainable.[10,29,31] Success rates dwindle to 25 per cent 3 years after behavioural treatment.[30,31] These data suggest that behavioural clinicians may have failed to recognize psychodynamic causes of the disorder, or to develop long-term strategies that allow patients to maintain their initial therapeutic gains. The efficacy of using periodic booster or maintenance sessions after the termination of the original treatment has not been investigated.

Psychopharmacological treatments

Clinicians have long been aware that several classes of drugs impede or eliminate orgasm. These include monoamine oxidase inhibitors, tricyclic and serotonergic antidepressants (phenelzine, pargyline, mebanazine, imipramine, amitripyline, fluoxetine, clomipramine, desipramine), antipsychotics (amoxapine, thioridazine, chlorpromazine, chlorprothizine, mesoridazine, perphenazine, trifluoperazine, and haloperidol), and α-adrenoceptor blocking agents such as phenoxybenzamine and guanethidine.[71]

Several investigators have conducted double-blind randomized placebo-controlled studies using strict dosages in a carefully selected population to determine whether clomipramine and the serotonin-selective reuptake inhibitors (fluoxetine, fluvoxamine, paroxetine, and sertraline) are biologically and psychologically efficacious in delaying ejaculation.[66,72,73] All these studies have confirmed the efficacy of these drugs in significantly delaying ejaculation. However, the medication improvements were lost when the men discontinued treatment and, in general, their ejaculatory latencies returned to baseline. One exception has been reported by McMahon[72] who used a novel method of dosing and withdrawing sertraline. After 7 months two-thirds of the sample population maintained their treatment gains. Side-effects were generally mild, dose-related, and tended to diminish with time; dry mouth, headache, drowsiness, and gastrointestinal upset were most frequently observed.

Although criteria for deciding which patients to provide with psychological, pharmacotherapy, or combined treatment do not yet exist, several points are relevant to this clinical decision.[74] The ideal candidate for initial drug therapy would be a man with several years of sexual experience and a lifelong pattern of rapid ejaculation who is free of substance abuse, depression, and psychosis and who is capable of developing stable, satisfying, non-sexual relationships. Drug therapy can also be considered for those patients who have not profited from a competently conducted psychological treatment. In contrast, men/couples with a relatively recent onset of acquired rapid ejaculation and some degree of psychological mindedness might do better with a psychological intervention in the long run. Also, pharmacotherapy should not be a first-line consideration for the young or inexperienced man who, in his first few sexual encounters, experiences rapid ejaculation. Reassurance and education are likely to be more worthwhile. In time, and with more experience, these men can be expected to develop increased confidence and learn to control ejaculation. Caution is warranted in offering drug therapy alone to men where the symptom clearly reflects intrapsychic or interpersonal conflict. Rapid symptom removal may disrupt the individual's or couple's emotional equilibrium.

Delayed ejaculation

This dysfunction, once referred to as retarded ejaculation, incompetent ejaculation, partner anorgasmia, or absent ejaculation, is much rarer among men than women. Delayed ejaculation can present as the inability to attain orgasm under any circumstance, the inability to achieve orgasm in a partner's presence or with her stimulation, or the inability to attain orgasm with intercourse. Unlike anorgasmia, these distinctions are quite evident.

Diseases associated with delayed ejaculation include spinal cord injury and a variety of neurological conditions. Additionally, many classes of drugs are associated with ejaculatory delay, including antihypertensive agents, serotonin-selective reuptake inhibitors, tricyclic antidepressants, phenothiazines, and the benzodiazepines.[75,76]

Theory

Two antithetical points of view exist for understanding this dysfunction: the inhibition and desire deficit models. Under the inhibition model behaviourists assume that the man is not receiving sufficient stimulation to reach his orgasmic threshold. Dynamic clinicians who ascribe to the inhibition model assume that the symptom is a conscious or unconscious expression of the man's aggression, in other words he is withholding or depriving his partner of something she desires.

Apfelbaum,[77] explaining the desire-deficit model, suggests that delayed ejaculation is a desire dysfunction disguised as a performance disorder. Enigmatically, such men achieve firm erections although subjectively, Apfelbaum contends, these men neither desire sexual intercourse nor are aroused.

Assessment

Assessment begins by reviewing the conditions under which the man is able to ejaculate, for example during sleep, spontaneously, with masturbation, with partner's hand or mouth stimulation, or infrequently with intercourse. The course of the problem is documented, and variables that improve or worsen performance are noted, such as the need for unconventional fantasies. Questions concerning the man's ability to relax, sustain, and heighten arousal and the degree to which he can concentrate on sensations are posed. Troubling factors are noted, and attempts to identify what precipitates and reinforces the problem are made, such as a lifelong need to suppress spontaneous emotional expression. If orgasmic attainment had been possible previously, the life events/circumstances temporally related to orgasmic cessation are reviewed, for example following a heart attack the man is too frightened to permit full arousal. Societal/religious attitudes that may interfere with excitement are noted, such as the 'spilling of seed' as a sin. Finally, questions concerning the quality of the non-sexual relationship are posed and problems explored.

Treatment

Treatment efforts are guided by the assumptions underlying the contrary theoretical models of causation. Proponents of the inhibition model aim to increase excitement through prolonged, intense, rough stimulation or by interpreting the man's aggressive impulses. Masters and Johnson[10] reported a low failure rate of 17.6 per cent using a

Table 8 DSM-IV and ICD-10 diagnostic criteria for dyspareunia

---

DSM-IV: Dyspareunia (302.76)

A.   Recurrent or persistent genital pain associated with sexual intercourse in either a male or a female.

B.   The disturbance causes marked distress or interpersonal difficulty.

C.   The disturbance is not caused exclusively by vaginismus or lack of lubrication, is not better accounted for by another Axis I disorder (except another sexual dysfunction), and is not due exclusively to the direct physiological effects of a substance (e.g. a drug of abuse, a medication) or a general medical condition.

ICD-10: Non-organic dyspareunia (F52.6)

A.   The general criteria for sexual dysfunction (F52) must be met.

In addition, for women:

B.   Pain is experienced at the entry of the vagina, either throughout sexual intercourse or only when deep thrusting of the penis occurs.

C.   The disorder is not attributable to vaginismus or failure of lubrication; dyspareunia of organic orgin should be classified according to the underlying disorder.

In addition, for men:

B.   Pain or discomfort is experienced during sexual response. (The timing of the pain and the exact localization should be carefully recorded.)

C.   The discomfort is not the result of local physical factors. If physical factors are found, the dysfunction should be classified elsewhere.

---

treatment combination of sensate focus, vigorous non-coital penile stimulation, and modifications of intercourse technique. Schnellen[78] reported that 81 per cent of men who were anorgasmic prior to treatment were successful in reaching orgasm through vibrator stimulation.

Apfelbaum[77] criticizes the inhibition model, stating that increased intense stimulation is a demanding and coercive strategy that heightens performance anxiety. His treatment efforts are aimed at having the men acknowledge their lack of both desire to have intercourse and arousal during intercourse. His model mirrors the conventional therapy for female anorgasmia, focusing on decreasing demand and helping the patient focus on heightening erotic sensations. No outcome statistics on Apfelbaum's model have been presented.

Sexual pain disorders

Sexual pain disorders are divided into two dysfunctions: non-organic dyspareunia and vaginismus. Dyspareunia, genital pain in either a male or female, is characterized by recurrent and persistent genital pain before, during, and after sexual activity. Exclusively a female dysfunction, vaginismus is an involuntary spasm of the musculature of the outer third of the vagina which makes penetration difficult or impossible. Non-organic dyspareunia and vaginismus may only be diagnosed in the absence of detectable physical pathology. However, when the aetiology is entirely physical there is likely to be a conditioned psychological response that may require subsequent psychological intervention after medical treatment.[79] Tables 8 and 9 list the DSM-IV and ICD-10 diagnostic criteria for sexual pain disorders.

Dyspareunia is currently the only female sexual dysfunction in which organic factors are hypothesized to play a major role. Abarbanel[80] has devised a useful tripartite classification of medical aetiologies associated with dyspareunia: anatomical, pathological, and iatrogenic. Anatomical factors comprise congenital or developmental impairments such as a rigid hymen or vaginal atrophy. Pathological factors include acute and chronic infections of the genital tract, such as endometriosis. Iatrogenic factors are conditions induced by a physician usually as a consequence of a surgical procedure such as episiotomy.

Pain during and after sexual activity is always the presenting problem in dyspareunia, although penetration is not always necessary to induce pain. It ranges from mild to unbearable and is experienced in a number of anatomical areas ranging from very specific localizations in the vulvar vestibule to a general burning or ache traversing the entire pelvic region.[81] These authors criticize the traditional dualistic conceptualization of dyspareunia as either organic or psychogenic, and suggest that it be conceptualized in a more sophisticated dynamic, interactive, and biopsychosocial schema.

Dyspareunia in men is a rare condition generally associated with organic factors such as Peyronie's disease, prostatitis, or sexually transmitted diseases. Pain is reported to occur in the penis with erection and during and after ejaculation.

Vaginismus is not necessarily limited to sexual situations. Typically, women with this disorder have been unable to insert tampons or permit insertion of a speculum during gynaecological examination. Interestingly, many women with vaginismus are quite capable of becoming sexually aroused, lubricating, and experiencing orgasm. Leiblum *et al.*[82] write, 'What is so striking in so many of these cases is the number of years the couple tolerates the difficulty before seeking treatment,…because of ambivalence about resolving the problem…often,

Table 9 DSM-IV and ICD-10 diagnostic criteria for vaginismus

DSM-IV: Vaginismus (306.51)

A.   Recurrent or persistent involuntary spasm of the musculature of the outer third of the vagina that interferes with sexual intercourse.

B.   The disturbance causes marked distress or interpersonal difficulty.

C.   The disturbance is not better accounted for by another Axis I disorder (e.g. somatization disorder) and is not due exclusively to the direct physiological effects of a general medical condition.

ICD-10: Non-organic vaginismus (F52.5)

A.   The general criteria for sexual dysfunction (F52) must be met.

B.   There is spasm of the perivaginal muscles, sufficient to prevent penile entry or make it uncomfortable. The dysfunction takes one of the following forms:

(1)   normal response has never been experienced;

(2)   vaginismus has developed after a period of relatively normal response:

    (a)   when vaginal entry is not attempted, a normal sexual response may occur;

    (b)   any attempt at sexual contact leads to generalized fear and efforts to avoid vaginal entry (e.g. spasm of the adductor muscles of the thighs).

it is the desire to have children that ultimately propels the couple to seek assistance'.

Vaginismus is hypothesized to be the body's expression of the psychological fear of penetration, but is also characterized as a psychosomatic disorder, a phobia, a conditioned response, and a conversion reaction.[82] A spectrum of aetiological factors, such as specific traumas, interpersonal and intrapsychic conflict, penetration anxiety, and multiple organic pathologies, may cause this dysfunction. Vaginismus may be triggered by real or imagined attempts at penetration. After several unsuccessful and painful attempts at intercourse a pernicious pattern develops. Anticipatory fear of pain now coupled with feelings of inadequacy, leads to further experiences of vaginismus.

Theory

Meana *et al.*[81] and Meana and Binik[83] suggest that dyspareunia be reconceptualized from a sexual dysfunction involving pain to a pain syndrome resulting in sexual dysfunction. Such a reconceptualization would focus on the target symptom (pain) and on the potential underlying mechanisms, rather than on possible psychological theories that have no empirical support.

Vaginismus is most likely multicausal and overdetermined in aetiology.[82] The precipitating events range from specific childhood or adult trauma to unconscious conflict, although attempts to link vaginismus to childhood or adult sexual abuse have not been empirically validated. Analytically oriented therapists have speculated that vaginismus reflects the woman's rejection of the female role, as a resistance against a male sexual prerogative, a defence against her father's real or fantasized incestual threat, and attempts to ward off her own castration images.[84] Spence[26] suggests that fears of pregnancy, strict religious adherence, disgust regarding genitalia, partner dissatisfaction, and irrational beliefs about anatomy underlie the development of vaginismus. Finally, learning theorists understand the dysfunction as a conditioned fear reaction reinforced by the belief that penetration can only be accomplished with great difficulty and will result in pain and discomfort.

Assessment

A medical evaluation by a specialist in gynaecological pain is always necessary. This evaluation must include a careful examination for subtle anatomical, pathological, or iatrogenic factors. Then the mental health clinician should review the locus of the pain, its onset, the average duration of a pain episode, and the degree of interference of the symptom with sexual life.[83] With vaginismus it is important to assess the conditions under which any penetration of the vagina can occur: tampon insertion, speculum examination, physician's finger, woman's finger(s) during masturbation, and partner's finger(s). The couple's sexual style is investigated in terms both of the amount of time devoted to psychological and physical preparation for lovemaking and of the degree of physical aggressiveness used during intercourse. Childhood and adult histories of sexual coercion/abuse are relevant, as are negative cultural/religious attitudes toward sexuality. The consequences of the pain disorder require assessment in terms of the development of secondary avoidance symptoms. Finally, the overall quality of the couple's non-sexual relationship is explored with specific questions about the partner's response to the symptom.

Treatment

Medical interventions for dyspareunia target the disease entity believed to be causing the pain, and include such dissimilar interventions as intravaginal application of oestrogen cream or anaesthetic ointment, surgical repair of the vulvar region, and the extraction of abnormal growths in the adjacent viscera.[85] When dyspareunia has been a long-standing problem medical correction is seldom sufficient treatment, regardless of physical pathology; the psychological fear of the pain recurring persists.[86,87] Fordney[86] reported that 16 out of 18 women who underwent medical procedures for dyspareunia did not improve until completing a course of sex therapy. Similarly, Schover *et al.*[87] noted that the factors that predicted the best post-surgical outcome for a group of women with vulvar vestibulitus were their willingness to engage in psychological treatment, higher socio-economic status, and specific localized areas of vulvar pain.

Vaginismus is typically treated through a combination of the following:

(1) banning intercourse;

(2) *in vivo* graduated self-insertion of dilators of increasing size;

(3) systematic desensitization;

(4) Kegel exercises (see above);

(5) interpretation of resistance and psychodynamic fears.

Masters and Johnson[10] reported a 100 per cent success rate in their treatment of 29 women. Similarly, Scholl reported that 83 per cent of his sample successfully completed therapy and were having intercourse at the 1-year follow-up.[88] Spence[26] suggests that more treatment sessions are required when women have experienced the dysfunction over extended periods of time, have undergone surgery, have thoughts that they are anatomically abnormal, or have negative attitudes toward their genitals. Fewer treatment sessions were related to a strong desire for pregnancy, the presence of an assertive husband, and the woman's knowledge about sexuality.

Conclusions

Mental health clinicians generally avoid asking patients about their sexual life because they themselves are anxious, believe sexual problems occur infrequently, fear being inappropriate, or judge themselves poorly prepared to manage potential problems. It is hoped that this chapter will provide clinicians with the knowledge and motivation to help couples with these all too prevalent problems. Sexual disorders are readily treatable, and their resolution can be gratifying both to the interested clinician and the troubled individual and/or couple.

References

1. Vatsayana (1964). *The Kama Sutra.* Grove Press, New York.
2. von Krafft-Ebing, R. (1894). *Psychopathia sexualis* (7th edn) (trans. C.G. Chaddock). F.A. Davis, Philadelphia, PA.
3. Ellis, H. (1936). *Studies in the psychology of sex.* Modern Library, New York.
4. Kinsey, A., Pomeroy, W., and Martin, C. (1948). *Sexual behavior in the human male.* W.B. Saunders, Philadelphia, PA.

5. Kinsey, A., Pomeroy, W., Martin, C., and Gebhard, P. (1953). *Sexual behavior in the human female.* W.B. Saunders, Philadelphia, PA.

6. Meyer, J. (1976). Psychodynamic treatment of the individual with a sexual disorder. In *Clinical management of sexual disorders* (ed. J. Meyer), pp. 265–75. Williams and Wilkins, Baltimore, MD.

7. Lazarus, A. (1963). The treatment of chronic frigidity by systematic desensitization. *Journal of Nervous and Mental Diseases,* **136**, 272–8.

8. Wolpe, J. (1958). *Psychotherapy by reciprocal inhibition.* Stanford University Press, Stanford, CA.

9. Masters, W. and Johnson, V. (1966). *Human sexual response.* Churchill Livingstone, London.

10. Masters, W. and Johnson, V. (1970). *Human sexual inadequacy.* Little, Brown, Boston, MA.

11. Kaplan, H.S. (1974). *The new sex therapy: active treatment of sexual dysfunctions.* Brunner–Mazel, New York.

12. Tiefer, L. (1995). *Sex is not a natural act and other essays.* Westview Press, Boulder, CO.

13. American Psychiatric Association (1994). *Diagnostic and statistical manual of mental disorders* (4th edn). American Psychiatric Association, Washington, DC.

14. World Health Organization (1993). *The ICD-10 classification of mental and behavioural disorders: diagnostic criteria for research.* World Health Organization, Geneva.

15. Kaplan, H.S. (1977). Hypoactive sexual desire. *Journal of Sex and Marital Therapy,* **3**, 3–9.

16. Lief, H. (1977). Inhibited sexual desire. *Medical Aspects of Human Sexuality,* **7**, 94–5.

17. Laumann, E.O., Gagnon, J.H., Michael, R.T., and Michaels, S. (1994). *The social organization of sexuality.* University of Chicago Press, Chicago, IL.

18. Hite, S. (1976). *The Hite report: a nationwide survey of female sexuality.* Dell, New York.

19. Frank, E., Anderson, C., and Rubinstein, D. (1978). Frequency of sexual dysfunction in 'normal' couples. *New England Journal of Medicine,* **299**, 111–15.

20. Lief, H. (1988). Foreword. In *Sexual desire disorders* (ed. S. Leiblum and R. Rosen), pp. vii–xiii. Guilford Press, New York.

21. Levine, S.B. (1984). An essay on the nature of sexual desire. *Journal of Sex and Marital Therapy,* **10**, 83–96.

22. Levine, S.B. (1988). Intrapsychic and individual aspects of sexual desire. In *Sexual desire disorders* (ed. S. Leiblum and R. Rosen), pp. 21–44. Guilford Press, New York.

23. Schiavi, R.C., Schreiner-Engel, P., White, D., and Mandeli, J. (1988). Pituitary–gonadal function during sleep in men with hypoactive sexual desire and normal controls. *Psychosomatic Medicine,* **50**, 304–18.

24. Schreiner-Engel, P. and Schiavi, R.C. (1986). Lifetime psychopathology in individuals with low sexual desire. *Journal of Nervous and Mental Disorders,* **174**, 646–51.

25. Stuart, F.M., Hammond, D.C., and Pett, M.A. (1987). Inhibited sexual desire in women. *Archives of Sexual Behavior,* **16**, 91–106.

26. Spence, S. (1991). *Psychosexual therapy. A cognitive–behavioral approach.* Chapman & Hall, London.

27. Bancroft, J. (1989). *Human sexuality and its problems.* Churchill Livingstone, Edinburgh.

28. Leiblum, S. and Rosen, R. (1988). *Sexual desire disorders.* Guilford Press, New York.

29. Hawton, K., Catalan, J., Martin, P., and Fagg, J. (1986). Long-term outcome of sex therapy. *Behavior Research and Therapy,* **24**, 665–75.

30. DeAmicus, L., Goldberg, D.C., LoPiccolo, J., Friedman, J., and Davies, L. (1985). Clinical follow-up of couples treated for sexual dysfunction. *Archives of Sexual Behavior,* **14**, 467–89.

31. Hawton, K. (1995). Treatment of sexual dysfunctions by sex therapy and other approaches. *British Journal of Psychiatry,* **167**, 307–14.

32. Sherwin, B. and Gelfand, M. (1987). The role of androgen in the maintenance of sexual functioning in oophorectomized women. *Psychosomatic Medicine,* **49**, 397–409.

33. Davidson, J.M., Kwan, M., and Greenleaf, W. (1982). Hormonal replacement and sexuality in men. *Clinics in Endocrinology and Metabolism,* **2**, 599–624.

34. Heiman, J. and Meston, C. (1997). Empirically validated treatment for sexual dysfunction. *Annual Review of Sex Research,* **8**, 148–94.

35. Segraves, R. and Althof, S. (1997). Psychotherapy and pharmacotherapy of sexual dysfunctions. In *A guide to treatments that work* (ed. P. Nathan and J. Gorman), pp. 447–71. Oxford University Press, New York.

36. Rosen, R. and Leiblum, S. (1992). *Erectile disorders: assessment and treatment.* Guilford Press, New York.

37. National Institutes of Health (1992). *Consensus development conference statement on impotence.* NIH, Bethesda, MD.

38. Althof, S. and Seftel, A. The evaluation and treatment of erectile dysfunction. *Annual Review of Psychiatry,* in press.

39. Barlow, D. (1986). Causes of sexual dysfunction: the role of anxiety and cognitive interference. *Journal of Consulting and Clinical Psychology,* **54**, 140–8.

40. Bancroft, J. Central inhibition of sexual response in the male: a theoretical model. Submitted to *Neuroscience and Biobehavioral Review.*

41. Rosen, R., Goldstein, I., Heimanm, J., *et al.* (1998). *A process of care model: evaluation and treatment of erectile dysfunction.* Robert Wood Johnson Medical School Center for Continuing Education, Piscataway, NJ.

42. Althof, S. (1989). Psychogenic impotence: treatment of men and couples. In *Principles and practice of sex therapy: update for the 1990s* (ed. S. Leiblum and R. Rosen), pp. 237–65. Guilford Press, New York.

43. Althof, S. (1999). New roles for mental health clinicians in the treatment of erectile dysfunction. *Journal of Sex Education and Therapy,* **23**, 229–31.

44. Mohr, D. and Beutler, L. (1990). Erectile dysfunction: a review of diagnostic and treatment procedures. *Clinical Psychology Review,* **10**, 123–50.

45. Hawton, K., Catalan, J., and Faff, J. (1992). Sex therapy for erectile dysfunction: characteristics of couples, treatment outcome, and prognostic factors. *Archives of Sexual Behavior,* **21**, 161–75,

46. Goldstein, I., Lue, T., Padma-Nathan, H., *et al.* (1998). Oral sildenafil in the treatment of erectile dysfunction. *New England Journal of Medicine,* **338**, 1397–404.

47. Althof, S. and Turner, L. (1992). Self injection therapy and external vacuum devices in the treatment of erectile dysfunction. In *Erectile disorders: assessment and treatment* (ed. R. Rosen and S. Leiblum), pp. 283–312. Guilford Press, New York.

48. Palace, E.M. (1995). Modification of dysfunctional patterns of sexual response through autonomic arousal and false physiological feedback. *Journal of Consulting and Clinical Psychology,* **63**, 604–15.

49. Levine, S. and Rosenblatt, E. (1997). Sexual disorders. In *Psychiatry* (ed. A. Tasman, J. Kay, and J. Lieberman), pp. 1173–201. W.B. Saunders, New York.

50. Fisher, S. (1973). *The female orgasm.* Basic Books, New York.

51. Heiman, J. and Grafton-Becker, V. (1989). Orgasmic disorders in women. In *Principles and practice of sex therapy: update for the 1990s* (ed. S. Leiblum and R. Rosen), pp. 51–88. Guilford Press, New York.

52. Sadock, V. (1989). Normal human sexuality and sexual dysfunctions. In *Comprehensive textbook of psychiatry,* Vol. 5 (ed. H. Kaplan and B. Sadock), pp. 1045–61. Williams and Wilkins, Baltimore, MD.

53. Kuriansky, J.B., Sharpe, L., and O'Connor, D. (1982). The treatment of anorgasmia: long-term effectiveness of a short-term behavioral group therapy. *Journal of Sex and Marital Therapy,* **8**, 29–43.

54. McMullen, S. and Rosen, R.C. (1979). Self-administered masturbation training in the treatment of primary orgasmic dysfunction. *Journal of Consulting and Clinical Psychology,* **47**, 912–18.

55. Riley, A.J. and Riley, E.J. (1978). A controlled study to evaluate directed masturbation in the management of primary orgasmic failure in women. *British Journal of Psychiatry,* **133**, 404–9.

56. Barbach, L. (1980). *Women discover orgasm.* Free Press, New York.

57. Kuriansky, J. and Sharpe, L. (1981). Clinical and research implications of the evaluation of women's group therapy for anorgasmia: a review. *Journal of Sex and Marital Therapy*, **7**, 268–77.

58. Grenier, G. and Byers, S. (1995). Rapid ejaculation: a review of conceptual, etiological, and treatment issues. *Archives of Sexual Behavior*, **24**, 447–72.

59. Levine, S. (1992). *Sexual life, a clinician's guide.* Plenum, New York.

60. McCarthy, B. (1989). Cognitive–behavioral strategies and techniques in the treatment of early ejaculation. In *Principles and practice of sex therapy: update for the 1990s* (ed. S. Leiblum and R. Rosen), pp 141–67, Guilford Press, New York.

61. Strassberg, D., Kelly, M., Carroll, C., and Kircher J. (1987). The psychophysiological nature of premature ejaculation. *Archives of Sexual Behavior*, **16**, 327–36.

62. Strassberg, D., Mahoney, J.M., Schaugaard, M., and Hale, V.E. (1990). The role of anxiety in premature ejaculation: a psychophysiological model. *Archives of Sexual Behavior*, **19**, 251–8.

63. Gospodinoff, M. (1989). Premature ejaculation: clinical subgroups and etiology. *Journal of Sex and Marital Therapy*, **15**, 130–4.

64. Fanciullacci, F., Colpi, G., Beretta, G., and Zanollo, A. (1988). Cortical evoked potentials in subjects with true premature ejaculation. *Andrologia*, **20**, 326–30.

65. Rowland, D., Haensel, S., Blom, J. and Slob, A. (1993). Penile sensitivity in men with premature ejaculation and erectile dysfunction. *Journal of Sex and Marital Therapy*, **19**, 189–97.

66. Althof, S. (1995), A new method of treating rapid ejaculation: drug therapy. *Psychiatric Clinics of North America*, **18**, 85–94.

67. Kaplan, H.S. (1989). *PE: how to overcome premature ejaculation.* Bruner/Maxel, New York.

68. Halvorsen, J. and Metz, M. (1992). Sexual dysfunction, part II: classification, etiology and pathogenesis. *Journal of the American Board of Family Practice*, **5**, 177–92.

69. Semans, J. (1956). Premature ejaculation: a new approach. *Southern Medical Journal*, **49**, 353–7.

70. St Lawrence, J. and Madakasira, S. (1992). Evaluation and treatment of premature ejaculation: a critical review. *International Journal of Psychiatry*, **22**, 77–97.

71. Segraves, R. (1998). Antidepressant induced sexual dysfunction. *Journal of Clinical Psychiatry*, **43**, 48–54.

72. McMahon, C. (1998). Treatment of premature ejaculation with sertraline hydrochloride: a single-blind placebo controlled crossover study. *Journal of Urology*, **159**, 1935–8.

73. Waldinger, M., Hengeveld, M., Zwinderman, A., and Oliver, B. (1998). Effect of SSRI antidepressants of ejaculation: a double-blind, randomized, placebo-controlled study with fluoxetine, fluoxamine, paroxetine and sertraline. *Journal of Clinical Psychopharmacology*, **18**, 274–81.

74. Althof, S. (1995). Pharmacological treatment for rapid ejaculation: preliminary strategies, concerns and questions. *Sex and Marital Therapy*, **10**, 247–51.

75. Segraves, R.T. (1995). Psychopharmacological influences on human sexual behavior. *American Psychiatric Press Review of Psychiatry*, **14**, 697–718.

76. Segraves, R.T. (1995). Antidepressant-induced orgasm disorder. *Journal of Sex and Marital Therapy*, **21**, 192–201.

77. Apfelbaum, B. (1989). Retarded ejaculation: a much misunderstood syndrome. In *Principles and practice of sex therapy: update for the 1990s* (ed. S. Leiblum and R. Rosen), pp. 168–206, Guilford Press, New York.

78. Schnellen, T. (1968). Induction of ejaculation by electrovibration. *Fertility and Sterility*, **19**, 566–9.

79. Sarrel, P. and Sarrel, L. (1989). Dyspareunia and vaginismus. In *Treatment of psychiatric disorders*, Vol. 3 (ed. American Psychiatric Association Task Force on Treatments of Psychiatric Disorders), pp. 2291–8. American Psychiatric Press, Washington, DC.

80. Abarbanel, A. (1978). Diagnosis and treatment of coital discomfort. In *Handbook of sex therapy* (ed. J. LoPiccolo and L. LoPiccolo). Plenum, New York.

81. Meana, M., Binik, Y., Khalife, S., Bergeron, S., Pagidas, K., and Berkley, K. (1996). Dyspareunia: more than bad sex. *Pain*, **71**, 211–12.

82. Leiblum, S., Pervin, L., and Campell, E. (1989). The treatment of vaginismus success and failure. In *Principles and practice of sex therapy: update for the 1990s* (ed. S. Leiblum and R. Rosen), pp. 113–40. Guilford Press, New York.

83. Meana, M. and Binik, Y. (1997). Dyspareunia: sexual dysfunction or pain syndrome? *Journal of Nervous and Mental Disease*, **185**, 561–9.

84. Drenth, J. (1988). Vaginismus and the desire for a child. *Journal of Psychosomatic Obstetrics and Gynecology*, **9**, 125–38.

85. Meana, M. and Binik, Y. (1994). Painful coitus: a review of female dyspareunia. *Journal of Nervous and Mental Disease*, **182**, 264–72.

86. Fordney, D. (1978). Dyspareunia and vaginismus. *Clinics in Obstetrics and Gynecology*, **21**, 205–21.

87. Schover, L., Youngs, D., and Cannata, R. (1992). Psychosexual aspects of the evaluation and management of vulvar vestibulitis. *American Journal of Obstetrics and Gynecology*, **167**, 630–6.

88. Scholl, G. (1988). Prognostic variables in treating vaginismus. *Obstetrics and Gynecology*, **72**, 231–5.

4.11.3 The paraphilias

Gene G. Abel and Candice A. Osborn

Sexuality serves a variety of purposes. Among these are perpetuation of the species, expression of feeling and bonding between pairs, and gratification. Sexuality may be expressed in a normal or abnormal fashion, with the definition of normal contingent upon societal rules and definitions. Paraphilias are deviantly expressed sexual interests and behaviours that do not represent culturally defined normal sexual interests.

People generally govern themselves in accordance with social prescriptions which serve to determine sexual activity within their culture. Paraphilic behaviours stem from exaggerations of normal sexual behaviour and represent unusual response to, reaction to, and/or interpretation of normal socially endorsed sexual behaviour.

Generally, personal values, religious beliefs, and the legal system prohibit individuals from acting out paraphilic urges. Attempting to identify, classify, diagnose, and treat individuals with paraphilias can be problematic because admitting to paraphilic interests is often in direct conflict with the values and rules of most societal groups.

Clinical features

Efforts to understand the occurrence of paraphilic behaviour through traditional population sampling are often inconsistent with what is seen in clinical practice. One problem with using traditional methodological approaches to understand paraphilic behaviour is that it is impossible to obtain a random sample reflecting the occurrence of paraphilias in the general population. This is because many paraphilias involve chargeable felonies and thus would be under-reported in such

Table 1 Sexual behaviour of 5873 paraphilic males

Behaviour category	Percentage of individuals evaluated
Exhibitionism	13
Public masturbation	10
Fetishism	12
Frotteurism	10
Voyeurism	19
Zoophilia	8
Obscene telephone calls	6
Necrophilia	0
Masochism	2
Coprophilia/urophilia	2
Child molestation	35
Rape	3
Sadism	2
Transvestic fetishism	6

a sample. Therefore the nearest we can come to understanding the occurrence of the paraphilias is through closely scrutinizing clinical samples of individuals seeking assessment and/or treatment.

In clinical environments, understanding paraphilias requires examining a representational subsection of individuals. A sample of 5873 adult males undergoing clinical evaluation for suspected inappropriate sexual interests throughout North America was collected from over 190 assessment centres and over 800 clinicians. Data from this sample appear in Table 1. Of this sample, 3270 (55.7 per cent) admitted to at least one paraphilic behaviour. Child molestation was the most common (61.5 per cent), with exhibitionism, public masturbation, fetishism, frotteurism, and voyeurism present in 17 to 33 per cent of the sample. Transvestic fetishism, obscene telephone calling, and zoophilia occurred in 10 to 14 per cent, while other paraphilias and rape of adults were less frequently reported.

Onset of paraphilic behaviour is early, ranging from ages 13 to 26 years, with most initiating paraphilic activity prior to age 20. This suggests that early intervention with juvenile sex offenders is warranted. Behaviours that can be carried out with a low likelihood of apprehension (fetishism, zoophilia, and voyeurism) occur at the earliest ages. Because child molesters are not only individuals who molested other children or siblings when they were younger, but also those who molested their own or others' children when they were older, the average age of onset for child molestation is later than that for other paraphilias.

The frequency with which paraphiliacs commit their crimes must be cautiously interpreted because, irrespective of the specific category of paraphilia, there are some paraphiliacs within each category who commit an enormous number of inappropriate sexual acts. Therefore clinicians can better appreciate the relative frequency of acts by examining median numbers of paraphilic sex acts, rather than the average number of paraphilic acts committed. Since individuals from the sam-

ple mentioned above who reported committing over 1000 paraphilic acts were unlikely to be precise in their estimates, categorization of paraphilic acts was given an upper limit of 999 in data analysis. Reported total mean acts committed were high (Table 2): more than 50 for exhibitionism, public masturbation, voyeurism, obscene telephone calls, masochism, coprophilia, and sadism, approximately 45 for child molestation, and 20 for those who had raped adults. Reported total median acts committed were significantly lower.

The number of victims for those with a paraphilia paralleled total acts completed, so that those with the highest total number of acts concomitantly had the highest number of victims. Child molesters, on average, had eight victims and reported molesting each victim approximately five times.

There is a common misconception that paraphiliacs commit only one type of sex crime and do not extend inappropriate sexual behaviour into other paraphilic categories. Various studies have demonstrated crossing of diagnoses, i.e. the paraphiliac has previously or concomitantly participated in a variety of paraphilic acts.[1,2] This sample of male paraphiliacs reported numerous paraphilic interests. Forty-six per cent reported involvement in one paraphilia, 22 per cent in two, 13.8 per cent in three, 7.9 per cent in four, 4.4 per cent in five, 3 per cent in six, 1.4 per cent in seven, 0.6 per cent in eight, 0.7 per cent in nine, 0.2 per cent in 10, 0 per cent in 11, and 0.1 per cent in 12 . Table 3 reflects the propensity that any one category of paraphilia will be comorbid with another. The number of individuals with at least one paraphilia was quite large; consequently a chi-square test was used to determine which other paraphilias were comorbid. In Table 3, paraphilic categories that were positively correlated at a statistically significant level ($p \leq 0.001$) are denoted by a plus sign, and paraphilic categories that were negatively correlated at a statistically significant level ($p \leq 0.001$) are denoted by a minus sign. For example, analyses of exhibitionism determined that this paraphilia is significantly associated with public masturbation, frotteurism, voyeurism, zoophilia, obscene telephone calls, coprophilia/urophilia, child molestation, and transvestitic fetishism. Categories that were most commonly significantly correlated with other paraphilias were transvestic fetishism (comorbid with 12 other paraphilias), followed by public masturbation, fetishism, and obscene telephone calls (11), sadism (10), frotteurism, voyeurism, zoophilia, and child molestation (nine), exhibitionism and coprophilia (eight), masochism (seven), and rape (six). Necrophilia occurred in only nine of the 3270 adult males with a specific paraphilic interest.

Classification

For diagnostic classification purposes, all the paraphilias consist of sexually arousing fantasies, sexual urges, and/or overt sexual behaviours directed towards non-human objects, towards the suffering, humiliation, and/or degradation of oneself or one's partner, and towards children and/or other partners who cannot and/or are not willing to give consent to sexual activity.[3] In order to receive a paraphilic diagnosis in DSM-IV a patient must have experienced one of the preceding behaviours for a period of 6 months or longer, and the behaviour must cause clinically significant distress or impairment in social, occupational, and/or other significant areas of the individual's

Table 2 Sexual behaviour characteristics of 3270 paraphilic males

Behavioural category	Age of onset (years)	Total acts		Number of victims	
		Mean	Median	Mean	Median
Exhibitionism	20	90	12	64	10
Public masturbation	18	89	20	60	15
Fetishism	13	211	60	NA	NA
Frotteurism	17	47	10	40	10
Voyeurism	16	54	10	28	4
Zoophilia	14	17	3	NA	NA
Obscene telephone calls	20	71	11	47	5
Necrophilia	22	30	4	NA	NA
Masochism	17	131	20	NA	NA
Coprophilia/urophilia	18	53	10	NA	NA
Child molestation	26	45	7	8	2
Rape	20	36	3	23	1
Sadism	21	72	10	NA	NA
Transvestic fetishism	17	8	2	NA	NA

NA, data not available.

functioning. As in the rest of ICD-10, impairment is not a criterion for the diagnosis of paraphilia.

Current classification is based on previous identification of the paraphilic behaviour within clinical environments. The paraphilias described in this chapter are Paedophilia, Exhibitionism, Fetishism, Frotteurism, Masochism, Sexual Sadism, Transvestic Fetishism, Voyeurism, and other problematic sexual behaviours that are classified as Paraphilia Not Otherwise Specified (Paraphilia NOS). The most commonly seen paraphilias have their own diagnostic codes, while those less commonly seen are classified under Paraphilia NOS.

Table 3 Crossing of sexual behaviour by 3270 paraphilic males

	Exhibitionism	Public masturbation	Fetishism	Frotteurism	Voyeurism	Zoophilia	Obscene telephone calls	Necrophilia	Masochism	Coprophilia/ urophilia	Child molestation	Rape	Sadism	Transvestic fetishism
Exhibitionism		+		+	+	+	+			+	—			+
Public masturbation	+		+	+	+	+	+		+	+	—		+	+
Fetishism		+		+	+	+	+		+	+	—	+	+	+
Frotteurism	+	+	+		+	+	+					+	+	+
Voyeurism	+	+	+	+		+	+				—		+	+
Zoophilia	+	+	+	+	+				+	+	+			+
Obscene telephone calls	+	+	+	+	+				+	+	—	+	+	+
Necrophilia														
Masochism		+	+		+		+			+			+	+
Coprophilia/ urophilia	+	+	+		+	+	+		+				+	+
Child molestation	—	—	—		—	+	—					—	—	—
Rape		+	+				+				—		+	+
Sadism		+	+	+	+		+		+	+	—	+		+
Transvestic fetishism	+	+	+	+	+	+	+		+	+	—	+	+	

+ Statistically significant ($p \leq 0.001$) likelihood of crossover.
— Statistically significant ($p \leq 0.001$) unlikelihood of crossover.

Table 4 Crossing of age and gender groupings by 2010 male child molesters

	Adolescent females	Adolescent female family	Child females	Child female family	Adolescent males	Adolescent male family	Child male	Child male family
Adolescent females		+	—	—			—	—
Adolescent female family	+		—	+	—			
Child females	—	—		—	—	—		
Child female family	—	+	—		—		—	
Adolescent males		—	—	—		+	+	+
Adolescent male family			—		+		+	+
Child male	—	—		—	+	+		+
Child male family	—				+	+	+	

+ Statistically significant ($p \leq 0.05$) likelihood of crossover.

— Statistically significant ($p \leq 0.05$) unlikelihood of crossover.

Paedophilia

Child molestation is the most common paraphilia brought to the attention of mental health providers. For this reason, it behoves the clinician to become especially knowledgeable about child molestation. Paedophilia involves sexual contact with a child at least 5 years younger than the perpetrator, with the perpetrator being at least 16 years of age or older. Paedophilia involves boys, girls, or both sexes of children; activities are limited to incest, non-incest, or both; sexual interest in children is either exclusive (only being sexually attracted to children and not being attracted to adults) or non-exclusive (attracted to both children and adults). The DSM-IV code for paedophilia is 302.2 and the ICD-10 code is F65.4.[3,4]

Paedophilia must be distinguished from child molestation. From an early age paedophiles have a sexual interest in children which is compulsive and recurrent in nature. Not all paedophiles are child molesters, although the majority are. Some paedophiles have fantasies and urges, but never become involved with a child. The term child molestation applies to individuals who are sexually involved with children. Not all child molesters are paedophiles. Some child molesters molest children, not because of paedophilia, but because of the absence of an appropriate sexual partner, the use of mind altering drugs, brain damage with concomitant poor impulse control, or mental retardation. In other cases, individuals sexually molest children in an attempt to cope with uncomfortable problematic feelings, or to seek revenge against a loved one of the child.

Child molestation committed by teenage or younger children is especially perplexing. Sexual exploration is common in childhood and adolescence. To explore another person's body, children frequently select younger children, since they do not resist such exploration and are less likely to report fondling or bodily examinations. The majority of child molestations by juveniles are not true paedophilic acts but, in the heat of the courtroom, such acts are frequently described by prosecuting attorneys as paedophilia, predatory acts, or rape.[5]

Paedophilia often begins in the early to middle teens and generally persists throughout adulthood. Paedophiles, like other paraphiliacs, do not plan to develop a paraphilic interest, but appear to do so by default. At younger ages they fail to appreciate the relevance of their sexual interest in young children. However, by the time they reach their early twenties, they begin to perceive that their sexual interest in children has persisted, despite their maturation, and are shocked by the realization that they are sexually aroused by children. Most paedophiles have adult sexual interest as well as sexual interest in children; in our sample of 5873 adult males undergoing clinical evaluation, only 6.6 per cent had an exclusive sexual interest in children. When that interest involves adolescent boys or girls it is called ephebophilia. When the child is 13 or younger, it is called paedophilia.

As a youth, a paedophile can easily associate with children without drawing attention to him- or herself. As the paedophile matures, however, it becomes problematic to be around children. Some paedophiles love children and attempt to help them in a variety of circumstances, without ever intending to sexually molest or harm them. Many put themselves in close proximity to children by participating in youth work. Other paedophiles establish relationships with children in their communities or neighbourhoods, and can thereby avoid detection while developing a relationship with a child.

Children are naive, making it easy to socialize with them and to determine which reinforcers motivate them to respond to adult requests. Consequently, the paedophile usually develops a non-sexual relationship with the child in order eventually to justify being alone with the child. Being alone and isolated with the child eventually allows the paedophile to initiate sexual touching without detection. Most paedophiles molest children well known to them; only about 10 per cent molest children who are strangers (Table 4).

Paedophiles, like other paraphiliacs, develop cognitive distortions and justifications for their behaviour. These cognitive distortions may include the following: 'Children should be allowed to make decisions regarding with whom they are sexual'; 'If the child does not report you, the child is enjoying the experience and wants it to continue'; 'Fondling and caressing the genitals of a child can be a form of sexual education to the child'; 'The only way a child can be hurt is if physical force is used with the child'. Child molesters are especially adept at convincing themselves that their behaviour is appropriate and does not injure their victim.

The most problematic issue for the paedophile is evading arrest. The greatest threat of others becoming aware of his molesting is the child revealing the molestation to others. Child molesters may attempt to convince the child that it was he or she who initiated the sexual act, not the molester. As the victim becomes older, the molester may say,

'Well I didn't really want to do this, but you seemed so interested in learning about sex', or 'Yes, I thought it was peculiar that you wanted to get involved in sexual touching, but I really liked you, so I went along with it'. The child molester has to convince the child that revealing the molestation would be harmful not only to the molester, but to the child and the child's family. This is especially problematic when the child attempts to break off the relationship involving molestation.

Child molesters report molesting a variety of children of various ages, genders, and relationships to them (Table 4). The clinician evaluating a known child molester can determine whether to suspect that the child molester is molesting other children within or outside the family by examining this table. Cases where a child molester is statistically likely to cross from one type of child victim to another, are indicated by a plus sign; when it is statistically unlikely that a child molester will molest a child in another category, this is represented by minus sign. For example, those who molest adolescent females are statistically more likely to be concurrently molesting an adolescent female in the family, but are statistically less likely to have molested a young female child under 14, a female child under 14 in the family, a male child under 14, and a male child under 14 in the family. Therefore this table will serve as a guide to the various types of child molestation that a child molester is likely or unlikely to have committed.

Of those children molested, 18 per cent are reportedly biological children, 26 per cent are stepchildren or children of a live-in partner, 2 per cent are foster children, 3 per cent are adopted children, 5 per cent are grandchildren, 11 per cent are younger brothers or sisters, 16 per cent are nieces or nephews, 36 per cent are children of neighbours or acquaintances, 4 per cent are children left in the care of the molester, and 11 per cent are strangers. In other words, child molesters infrequently molest children unknown to them but, rather, molest children in their family or children they meet through neighbours or acquaintances.

Sex between a child and an adult is always unethical, since a child cannot give informed consent to such activities. In order to give consent, one has to be on an equal power base with the sexual partner, which is impossible where children are concerned because adults seeking sexual contact with children are larger and more powerful, as well as being seen by the child as someone whom they must obey. Additionally, perpetrators often have a parental or other position of authority with respect to the child, so that the child cannot give consent. To give informed consent, a child must be knowledgeable about and understand to what he or she is giving consent, but since children are naive about sexual activities, they cannot appreciate the activities molesters want them to participate in or the possible consequences they may suffer as a result of participation. Children are not aware that, if found out, they may be questioned by police, interviewed repeatedly by victim support services, ostracized by other children for having been molested, and required to provide testimony in open court against the person who molested them.[6]

Therapists find it difficult to treat child molesters for a number of reasons. Since paedophiles have a sexual interest in children and such sexual interests are so disparate from the sexual interest of the therapist, many therapists doubt the veracity of a child's accusations and succumb to the rationalizations and justifications for false accusations used by the paedophile and/or the paedophile's lawyer. Therapists and the general public sometimes prefer to not think about the possibilities of paedophiles being around children, including the thought that paedophiles may pose a potential risk to their own children.

In contrast, some therapists view the paedophile as a devil, whose behaviour is sinful. These therapists fail to realize that true paedophiles do not plan to become paedophiles, but instead find themselves with sexual interests disparate from the society in which they live. Therefore many therapists find themselves repulsed by the paedophile and thus unable to be objective in their evaluation and treatment.

Exhibitionism

Exhibitionists are characterized by recurrent compulsive urges to expose their genitals to another person, usually an adult (DSM-IV code 302.4; ICD-10 code F65.2).[3,4] Exhibitionists have strong sexual urges to expose themselves that become so intense that they find themselves sexually aroused and making concerted efforts to expose themselves to particular individuals. Although a few exhibitionists expose themselves to males, this is infrequent; exhibitionism is generally perpetrated by males against females.

As part of the sequence of behaviours leading to exposure, exhibitionists begin by seeking settings where women are present, preferably settings that will not lead to their being identified and/or arrested. Once the female and setting are identified, the exhibitionist begins fantasizing, not about exposing himself, but about having some type of sexual interaction with the victim. His intent is not to frighten the victim, although many victims *are* frightened as they are unclear as to the motives of the exhibitionist. Many exhibitionists report altered states of consciousness, feeling as if they are transcendentally carrying out exposing themselves to the victim. As a victim approaches, the exhibitionist may attract the attention of the victim by stepping out from behind the cover of bushes and exposing his penis. Other variations include taking away books or newspapers from in front of his penis or, in some cases, suddenly appearing totally nude in front of the victim. Once the woman sees the exhibitionist's penis, the exhibitionist begins an extensive set of cognitive distortions that redefine the experience for him. For example, if the female appears to be frightened, the exhibitionist may interpret the startled look on her face as evidence that she is overwhelmed by her own sexual feelings which have surfaced as the result of seeing him and his penis. If the victim retreats and then looks back to assure herself that she is not being followed, the exhibitionist fantasizes that her sexual interest in him is so strong that she wants a second look. If the victim laughs at the inappropriateness of the man's actions, the exhibitionist will fantasize that, far from laughing at him, she is enjoying the sensual pleasure of seeing his penis. Almost irrespective of the victim's response, the perpetrator interprets her behaviour to mean an acceptance of him and a clear sexual interest in him. Some exhibitionists masturbate during the course of exposing themselves, while others wait until after exposing, masturbating later to fantasies of sexual intercourse with the victim as a partner.

One variation of typical exhibitionist behaviour is committed by individuals who completely disrobe and show themselves to females without attempts to masturbate during or after the experience. Aggressive angry feelings towards others appear to lead to this behaviour. According to the self-report of these exhibitionists, from their vantage point this is not a sexual experience even though they behaviourally appear nude before the individual.

Frequently, exhibitionists expose themselves many times daily to a series of women until their fear of apprehension, or guilt about the inappropriateness of their behaviour, leads them to stop. Then they may cease exposing themselves for weeks and/or months, later initiating a new series of exposures.

Exhibitionism is comorbid with a number of other paraphilias (Table 3), especially public masturbation. However, because DSM-IV criteria do not recognize the occurrence of public masturbation as distinguished from exhibitionism, clinicians must diagnose public masturbation as a paraphilia not otherwise specified.[3]

Fetishism

The hallmark of fetishism is long-standing compulsive sexual interest in non-living objects that are used to generate sexual excitement. Fetishism is an exaggeration of normal sexual interest (DSM-IV code 302.81; ICD-10 code F65.0).[3,4] Males without fetishistic interests report sexual interest and attraction to objects worn by their sexual partners such as brassières, panties, garter belts, hose, shoes, and boots. Typically, they purchase these objects for their sexual partners because it adds to their sexual arousal. However, fetishism is an extreme exaggeration of an attachment to objects. Fetishists can become sexually aroused to unusual acts, such as blowing up balloons or imagining triangles turning in space, and may go to extremes to obtain fetishistic objects (e.g. breaking into homes to steal, touch, and masturbate with women's underwear). In some cases, fetishists will become excited by specific parts of their partner's anatomy (e.g. feet or breasts); this variant of fetishism is called partialism. In other cases the fetishist is excited by the sight of a person with an amputation (apotemnophilia). It has been reported that, rarely, the person may even request an amputation.[7]

Fetishism begins at an early age and does not require the active participation of a partner. Consequently, fetish objects can be paired and associated with masturbation and orgasm hundreds of times before others become aware of their influence over an individual's sexual interest. As the fetish object becomes more ingrained in an individual's sexual arousal pattern, the fetishist finds it difficult to relate sexually without the inclusion of the object. Sexual partners are initially naive to the extent of the fetishist's attachment to these objects. As relationships progress, however, fetishists' interests in fetish objects become more dominant, with conflict usually erupting over the extent to which use of the fetish object intrudes into the relationship.

Frotteurism

Frotteurism involves uninvited touching or rubbing against another person for sexual gratification (DSM-IV code 302.89; ICD-10 indicates that frotteurism should be coded under Other Disorders of Sexual Preference F65.8).[3,4] Frotteurs carry out paraphilic behaviour in crowded environments such as bus terminals, subways, sporting events, crowded bars, etc. Fantasy is an extensive part of frotteurism, since frotteurs are able to convince themselves that touching behaviour will not offend victims and, furthermore, victims will find touching pleasurable. Initially, the nature of crowded environments is used as an excuse for being in close proximity to potential victims. For example, subway passengers typically stand close to the tracks when waiting for a train. Frotteurs stand 2 to 3 metres back from the crowd, searching to identify potential victims. Once a female is identified, the frotteur moves behind her and extends his arms toward her waist to prevent others from getting in front of him. As the subway train door opens, he pushes himself near the victim and waits for the carriage to fill up and,

thus, justifies touching her during the train trip. If the train begins to move and the frotteur is not close enough to the desired victim, he will push his way through the crowd to position himself next to her. He then fantasizes that he is in a sexual relationship with the victim. Younger and more naive women are usually selected, whereas older women who stereotypically may seem more assertive are avoided.

The frotteur rubs up against the buttocks, thighs, breasts, or vaginal area with his hand, his leg, his pelvic area, or with a newspaper or some other object. Despite being in a crowded public setting, while rubbing a complete stranger, he finds it easy to fantasize a close sexual relationship with the victim and can get an erection in seconds. Sometimes he will push his erect penis, underneath his clothes, up against the woman's thighs or buttocks.

Some frotteurs wear plastic wrap around their penises during episodes of frottage so that their trousers will not be stained by ejaculate and they can proceed to work. Such evidence of forward-planning by the frotteur is used by the police to bring about conviction of such individuals, once they are apprehended.

Frotteurs frequently have a host of rationalizations or justifications for their behaviours. These include: 'Other men do it, so why can't I?'; 'She really enjoyed it, so it is in no way a sexual crime'; 'I don't actually attack the woman, so there is no injury or emotional harm to her'; 'Women who are in crowds expect this kind of behaviour'; 'I have been doing this for years and have never been reported, so women must enjoy it or do not care about my doing it'.

Eventual consequences, or lack of them, can reinforce continuation of the behaviour. When police arrest a frotteur, female victims often refuse to file charges because the process is time consuming. Furthermore, the legal consequences of frotteurism are usually minimal. Frequently, a small fine is imposed, and the individual is free to continue the behaviour. Frotteurs operate in crowded situations to help conceal their behaviour, while exhibitionists avoid crowds, since crowds increase the likelihood of arrest.

Masochism

Masochists have persistent interest in sexual activities that demean, humiliate, or cause suffering to themselves, and they actively participate in sexual activities to reach this goal (DSM-IV code 302.83; in ICD-10 sadomasochism is coded as F65.5).[3,4] Masochists generally have a few partners with whom they become repetitively involved. Since masochism requires dominance and control by another individual, it is a paraphilia that cannot be forced upon others. Masochists frequently demonstrate some transient interest in masochism to an uncommitted sexual partner hoping that, if they become involved on a sustained basis, that partner will acquire a sexual interest in tying them up, spanking them, or whipping them. In reality, this is an exceedingly difficult interest for a new partner to acquire and, as a result, masochists sometimes join sadomasochistic clubs where it is easier to find a partner to hurt them.

A dangerous variant of masochism is autoerotic asphyxiation (hypoxyphilia), in which individuals are sexually aroused by suffocating themselves, hanging themselves, or in some way cutting off their source of oxygen while masturbating.[8,9] These individuals frequently rig equipment to temporarily hang themselves and set up what they view as a failsafe system to disrupt the hanging experience should they lose consciousness. Unfortunately, these systems sometimes fail and the individual dies. Some individuals engage in transvestic fetishism during the asphyxiation episode.

Sexual sadism

Sexual sadism involves achieving sexual arousal by repeatedly inflicting psychological or physical suffering on a consenting or non-consenting partner (DSM-IV code 302.84; in ICD-10 sadism is coded with masochism as F65.5).[3,4] Sadists are not simply interested in subduing their partners for sex, but instead prefer inflicting pain far in excess of what would be necessary to accomplish compliance with sexual activity. Sexual sadists, like sexual masochists, attempt to develop an ongoing relationship with a sexual partner who enjoys the experience or is reluctant to report the experience to others. In these relationships, the sadist generally accelerates his or her sadistic behaviour when their prior sadistic behaviour with their partner is tolerated. As these relationships persist, more extensive sadistic assault is required to produce the fright and fear that sadists want to see in their partners.

Sadists will attempt to drown their partners, hang or suffocate them, and/or brutally whip, spank, or beat them in order to become aroused. The partner often initially sees this sadistic behaviour as simply sexual play but, as time progresses and the sadistic assaults become increasingly severe, the partner–victim realizes the seriousness of the sadist's sexual interest. Attempts to block or convince the sadist to stop the behaviour are usually ineffective, the relationship deteriorates, and the sadist goes on to locate and develop a new sexual partner.

Transvestic fetishism

The transvestic fetishist shares many commonalities with fetishism, effeminate egodystonic homosexuality, and transsexualism (the last two are non-paraphilias). The transvestic fetishist is usually a heterosexual male who is sexually aroused by cross-dressing and fantasizing himself as an alluring female (DSM-IV code 302.3; in ICD-10 the term is fetishistic transvestism, and the code is F65.1).[3,4] Fetishisim and transvestic fetishism are similar in that individuals in both categories have a sexual preference for adult females, but differ in that the fetishist is usually attracted to inanimate objects and generally does not cross-dress wearing the fetish item but holds or fondles it during masturbation. Effeminate egodystonic homosexuals and male-to-female transsexuals have a sexual preference for adult males. The manner in which individuals walk, sit, and stand reflects their gender motor behaviour. Fetishists have masculine gender motor behaviour, as do transvestic fetishists when not cross-dressing. Effeminate egodystonic homosexuals frequently show feminine gender motor behaviour, while transsexuals frequently display exaggerated feminine gender motor behaviour, almost a caricature of a stereotypical female. Male fetishists, transvestic fetishists, and effeminate egodystonic homosexuals all view themselves as having a male sexual identity, whereas transsexuals view themselves as having a female sexual identity, i.e. as a female trapped in a male's body.

The transvestic fetishist frequently partially cross-dresses but, when viewed by the average adult male, is seen as a male wearing women's garments. As transvestic fetishism continues, the male becomes more adept at cross-dressing and begins to venture outside the privacy of his home into public settings. The long-time transvestic fetishist, the effeminate egodystonic homosexual, and the male-to-female transsexual may look very similar owing to their somewhat exaggerated stereotypical female make-up and clothes. However, the sexual behaviour of transsexuals is markedly different from that of the other three categories in that the transsexual generally has a low sex drive and is more intrigued by assuming the role of a female, or indeed becoming a female, while the others enjoy assuming a feminine role concurrent with maintaining a masculine sexual identity.

Transvestic fetishists initially conceal their sexual behaviours and, early in dating experiences, will frequently hide their proclivities to cross-dress. As their behaviour becomes more long-standing, however, they begin to share their erotic feelings while cross-dressed and will attempt to include this behaviour in their sexual interaction with their female partners. The dilemma develops when the female partner is offended by the transvestic fetishist's cross-dressing behaviour and a major conflict may develop, with the female partner demanding cessation of the cross-dressing behaviour. Although temporary acceptance of a partner's transvestic fetishism can occur for a few years, eventually the adult female partner appreciates the strength of her male partner's sexual attraction to cross-dressing, as opposed to being intimate with her, and divorce is a common outcome.

Voyeurism

Voyeurism is amongst the most common of the paraphilias. Voyeurs seek situations where they can watch others disrobe, have sexual intercourse, or carry out some type of intimate sexual interaction (DSM-IV code 302.82; ICD-10 code F65.3).[3,4] Voyeurism begins at an early age, does not involve actually touching another person, and is usually carried out in a concealed fashion, and so it is difficult to apprehend the perpetrators. A voyeur may be arrested infrequently or not at all. When arrest does occur, since the voyeur is clothed and has made no attempt to touch anyone, he can frequently justify his presence without generating suspicions of misbehaviour; if conviction does occur, the charge is considered a misdemeanour, generating a low fine and little actual consequence to the perpetrator. The inquisitive nature of boys (females are rarely voyeurs), combined with the mysterious secretive nature of sex, can lead individuals to attempt to gain sexual knowledge by surreptitious voyeuristic activity. Because of the ease with which these behaviours are carried out, coupled with the likelihood of escape from negative consequences, voyeurism can become an ingrained, frequent, and highly reinforced learned behaviour before significant consequences occur to the perpetrator.

Voyeurism, like most of the paraphilias, is an extension and exaggeration of normal sexual behaviour. Normally, we enjoy watching our sexual partners undress and are excited by watching them become aroused as they participate in sexual activity with us. The voyeur becomes aroused by this behaviour so frequently as a youth that it becomes entrenched, with sexual arousal and satisfaction being difficult to achieve in the absence of this particular stimulus. Furthermore, risk of apprehension and potential newness of each observed victim contribute to the magnification of the voyeur's excitement. Voyeurs choose environments where there is a high likelihood of satisfying their sexual interests, such as peering into apartment buildings or crowded residential neighbourhoods. Once a voyeur has found an environment where his efforts are particularly successful, he is very likely to return to that situation repeatedly. He approaches windows of homes, conceals himself in department store dressing rooms, and in some cases installs equipment in his own home so that he can 'peep' on those who visit him. As time passes without arrest, the voyeur becomes bolder in his behaviour, in some cases entering the homes of his victims and watching them while they sleep.

Paraphilia not otherwise specified

DSM-IV (code 302.9) and ICD-10 (code F65.9) both list specific conditions considered to be paraphilias because they are frequent clinical conditions that the general psychiatrist is likely to encounter in clinical treatment.[3,4] However, there are other clinical conditions that are considered paraphilic in nature, but are not elaborated in detail in diagnostic categories because they are less commonly seen. Problematic sexual behaviours classified in DSM-IV under Paraphilia NOS and in ICD-10 as Other Disorders of Sexual Preference F65.9 do not meet criteria for any of the specifically classified paraphilias.

Obscene telephone calls (telephone scatologia)

Obscene telephone callers are generally heterosexual males who, during their teenage years, call females known or unknown to them to carry out sexually provocative conversations. These individuals may make hundreds of calls before being apprehended, generally by the Caller ID technology that automatically lists the telephone number of the caller.

Necrophilia

Necrophilia is an exceedingly infrequent paraphilic behaviour. Of 5873 men evaluated for possible paraphilia, only nine reported being sexually attracted to sexual activities with the body of a dead female. Table 3 indicates that necrophilia is infrequently comorbid with other paraphilias. This suggests that necrophilia may not be a true paraphilia, but instead a reflection of another major psychiatric disorder.

Partialism

Partialism involves an exaggerated sexual interest in a specific part of the body. Heterosexual males have an exaggerated sexual arousal to breasts and buttocks, the body parts that most easily discriminate males from females. Homosexuals, likewise, are attracted to the genitals, buttocks, and chest areas of other males, areas of the body that discriminate males from females. Partialism may also involve an exaggerated sexual interest in a portion of the body less likely to be a culturally supported sexualized part of the body, such as leg muscles, feet, or hands.

Public masturbation

Public masturbation involves individuals who expose their penises in public places with the intent of reaching sexual climax. Public masturbation appears to lie between exhibitionism and voyeurism, in that it has diagnostic characteristics of both these activities.[10]

Individuals involved in public masturbation recurrently go to public settings such as cinemas, bars, and/or the carparks of shopping centres. In these public settings, they conceal the fact that their penis is outside their clothing and masturbate while watching females. Public masturbators appear to need the stimulation of viewing women unknown to them to achieve sexual arousal. Arousal is also increased by knowledge of the risk of apprehension when masturbating in a public setting. Unlike the exhibitionist, the public masturbator is unwilling to display his penis to a victim. Typically, public masturbators are criminally charged with public indecency or treated as if they are exhibitionists, because the criminal justice system does not distinguish between the behaviour of public masturbators and exhibitionists.

Public masturbators usually rationalize their behaviours through beliefs that they are not harming their victims because they are not actually exposing themselves to them. However, during the act of public masturbation many victims easily perceive that the public masturbator is masturbating and report his activities to the authorities. Public masturbation is comorbid with a number of paraphilias.

Coprophilia/urophilia

Individuals with coprophilia (sexual interest in faeces) and/or urophilia (sexual interest in urine) generally incorporate faeces and/or urine into their sexual activities. Coprophiliacs and/or urophiliacs are either heterosexual or homosexual males whose early developmental histories involve their developing a sexual attraction and interest that they attempt to incorporate into their sexual interactions. Frequently, however, sexual partners are repulsed by this, and the behaviour is incorporated exclusively into masturbatory activities.

Zoophilia

Zoophilia is an activity that involves becoming sexually aroused by repetitively carrying out sexual activities with animals. Zoophiles usually have other sexual outlets, but participate in zoophilia because of the ease of accessing animals for sexual purposes and the low risk of apprehension for such activity. Therapists frequently view zoophilia as a trivial problem that serves as a butt for jokes. In actuality, zoophilia is a more serious paraphilia than suspected because of the consequences of the learned behaviour.

Zoophiles begin by experimenting with sexual activity with animals. As they become successful at masturbating animals, penetrating them for intercourse, or, in some cases, getting male animals to penetrate them, zoophiles learn to ignore a number of stimuli that would normally be inconsistent with sexual arousal, such as faeces, fur, and the animal's ferocity. Therefore it is not surprising that zoophiles have a high frequency of comorbid paraphilic behaviours. When the zoophile's family becomes aware of his behaviour, they are often shocked by its bizarre nature.

Diagnosis and differential diagnosis

The most cost-effective method of diagnosing paraphilias is to conduct a comprehensive psychiatric history, to use psychophysiological assessment methods to determine sexual interest, and to differentiate organic or psychiatric disorders that can impact on an individual's sexual interest and activity. Interviewing the potential paraphiliac, especially a paraphiliac who has been involved in felonies, requires a non-judgemental clinician. The first step in the interview process is to obtain a client's consent to assessment, with special reference to laws that may legally require the therapist to break confidentiality should a paraphiliac reveal a specific victim that he has sexually abused or a victim he plans to molest. This issue is relevant when a child molester reveals specific names of children that he or she has molested. To proceed with the interview without first explaining this mandatory reporting requirement would be unethical.

The major objective of the initial interview is for the therapist to identify core issues which will motivate a patient to change his or her paraphilic activity. The major obstacle to an effective interview is that the paraphiliac is frequently ashamed regarding his sexual assaults or behaviours, and for years has practised concealing from others the very nature of his sexual interest. Unfortunately, many therapists have been taught that if patients fail to reveal the nature of their problems, then it is their fault that they do not receive treatment. Such training can lead to the paraphiliac not revealing a serious sexual problem and the therapist not attempting to uncover the problem; as a consequence, the patient is not helped and the therapist does not attempt to assist the patient in revealing his or her paraphilic interest. Thus, more individuals are victimized.

A number of methods can be used by the therapist to increase the likelihood of the paraphiliac revealing his or her true sexual interest. Therapists should explain that the more knowledgeable they are about the activities or allegations that led to the referral, the more they will be able to help the patient. The therapist should review all available records before seeing the patient so as to understand the problems that led to his referral. The therapist needs to attempt to block the patient from taking a strong position of innocence, from which he may have to retreat later in the assessment. Should the patient adamantly deny culpability, the therapist should ask questions about whether the victim might have misunderstood the patient's actions. When the patient initially denies inappropriate behaviour, the interviewer should focus on other aspects of the psychological history rather than going into details regarding the allegations. Sometimes the patient's denial is reduced after the interviewer pauses and explains the many components of treatment available and the effectiveness of treatment. The average paraphiliac is frequently unaware of treatment that can help control deviant behaviour; thus, providing details about treatment components helps the paraphiliac to appreciate that there are effective treatment options and that he should, therefore, actively participate in his treatment. A key component of the initial assessment is delineating the client's sexual fantasies during masturbation or sexual activity. Often patients will reveal these fantasies, thereby presenting an opportunity for therapists to appreciate what they find most erotic. Interviewers must avoid reacting emotionally to clients' sexual behaviours. No matter what that behaviour might involve, communication of disapproval of such activity by the therapist obstructs the gathering of critical information needed to help the patient.

A common error is for therapists to ask about only a limited number of paraphilias, usually the paraphilia for which the patient was referred for evaluation. Crossing of diagnoses, or having a variety of paraphilias, is fairly common and therefore the therapist should ask about all paraphilias. When paraphilias are revealed by the client, the therapist should find out the age of onset of such behaviour, the age at which the behaviour stopped, the age and gender of victims, the specific nature of the relationship between the client and his or her victims, the degree of force used during the commission of paraphilic acts, the extent to which the paraphilias occupy the client's fantasy life, and the client's current control over urges to carry out paraphilic behaviour.

It is also helpful for the therapist to use leading questions. Rather than asking if the individual has exposed himself, the therapist might ask 'How often have you exposed yourself?' By querying the client this way, the interviewer gives the message that it is acceptable that such exhibitionism has transpired and gives the patient responsibility for correcting the interviewer if he or she has never been involved in such activity. Near the close of the interview, it is helpful to ask a catch-all question such as: 'What other sexual behaviour have you been interested or involved in that might be problematic if known to others?'

The patient, if accused of paraphilic interest but denying it, usually pressures the therapist to agree with his position of innocence. The therapist should clarify that the purpose of the evaluation is to determine the likelihood of such behaviour, based upon information that is gathered during the psychological interview, psychophysiological assessment, paper-and-pencil testing, and review of records. Only after such information has been collected can the therapist offer an opinion to the patient. At the end of the first interview it is helpful to explain to the patient the importance of being as honest as possible during all phases of the assessment. Clinical interviewing of alleged paraphiliacs is difficult to balance. The goals of the therapist should be to do no harm, to help the patient understand his or her possible sexual interest, and to explore what can be done to help him or her lead a life of closer intimacy with adult partners without injury.

Psychophysiological assessment

Paraphiliacs differ from other psychiatric patients because they have deviant sexual interest. Currently, there are three psychophysiological assessment methods that can be used to evaluate possible paraphilic interest.

Penile plethysmography

Penile plethysmography involves direct measurement of changes occurring in penile circumference or volume when patients are presented with slides, audiotaped vignettes, or videotaped vignettes depicting paraphilic and non-paraphilic sexual behaviour. Penile plethysmography has the advantage of high face validity because one can conclude that if the patient gets erections to unique or unusual sexual interests during such assessment, he probably has considerable interest in this category.[11]

When penile plethysmography reveals aberrant interest in the laboratory, patients can be confronted with their deviant responses, regardless of whether they admit to or deny deviant activities and/or interests outside the laboratory. Paraphiliacs frequently admit paraphilic interests that were either previously concealed or denied during such confrontations.

Patients use a variety of tactics to conceal their sexual interest. There are a number of drawbacks to using penile plethysmograpy for the clinical assessment of deviant sexual response. One central issue is whether or not arousal responses seen in the laboratory are equal to similar arousal in the real world. Individuals undergoing psychophysiological assessment often deny any and all deviant sexual interest, and so penile plethysmography frequently involves measuring possible sexual interest that the patient has absolutely denied. This can be problematic when attempting to delineate deviant sexual interests through penile plethysmography. Recently, penile plethysmography has come under greater scrutiny because slides depicting nude children are frequently used to assess paedophilic interest. The use of nude slides is considered unethical and illegal in some countries such as the United States. Another problematic issue is the necessity of obtaining two separate rooms to complete penile plethysmographic assessments, one for the patient and the other for a highly skilled clinician to administer the plethysmographic evaluation. Finally, there have also been frequent concerns expressed by patients undergoing penile plethysmography regarding possible risk of disease transmission from wearing the genital transducer that is utilized to measure arousal.

Polygraphy

A second means of assessing deviant behaviour involves the clinical usage of polygraphs.[12] Clinical usage has increasingly included 'full disclosure polygraphs', in which patients are asked a series of pointed questions to specify all of their paraphilic interests and activities. In addition, polygraphy is often used during the maintenance phase of treatment, when it is necessary to ask patients whether they have continued involvement in various paraphilic behaviours.

The advantages of polygraphs are that they can be used to assess a wide variety of paraphilic behaviours and, most importantly, to assess recidivism of paraphilic behaviours post-treatment. Also, polygraphy can be used with males or females. Drawbacks include the extensive training needed to become a certified polygrapher and problems with validity and reliability. In many countries polygraphs are not allowed to be used in the courtroom as evidence of criminal activity.

Visual reaction time

The newest method of clinical assessment involves testing visual reaction time to quantify the amount of time that an individual attends to various categories of slides as a measure of sexual interest in those categories.[13] Various methods of measuring visual reaction time have been developed since the early 1940s. The major advantage of this system is that it can be used with males and females, adults and juveniles, without the necessity of showing nude slides. Slides of clothed males and females of various ages are presented to the patient. Patients are confronted when their visual reaction time suggests high sexual interest in a category for which they have previously denied sexual interest.

Organic disease and the differential diagnosis of paraphilias

Mental retardation

Mental retardation causes serious limitations to patients not only because of their cognitive deficits, but also because of the unusual environment in which they live and develop. Families and institutions become frustrated with the mentally retarded individual's limitations and the subsequent economic, social, and emotional burden placed on others. The mentally retarded individual's sex education is dramatically different from that of non-retarded people. Families fear the consequences of involvement of their mentally retarded daughters or sons in any sexual activity and, as a consequence, the message to the mentally retarded is simply never to be sexual.

The mentally retarded person's intellectual limitations make it difficult to access those individuals identified as most attractive. However, because these individuals do nevertheless possess a biologically based sex drive, they find themselves having sexual desire but not having sexual outlets for their expression. Furthermore, intellectual limitations often lead the mentally retarded to spend more time with other retarded people or with children, where they feel more of an intellectual compatibility and hence find it easier to relate to these people. This may lead to sexual interaction with a child but does not necessarily lead to paedophilia, although it might if this interaction is repeated over time. In other cases, mentally retarded individuals may develop an interest in sexual behaviours which do not involve social interaction with a partner, such as fetishism, exhibitionism, or zoophilia.

Studies indicate that paraphilic recidivism for the mentally retarded is almost twice that of the non-retarded individual.[14] This may result from poor quality of treatment for the mentally retarded paraphiliac, limitations in learning resulting from the mental retardation, or the fact that mentally retarded individuals are easier to apprehend since their concealment skills are less effective than the non-retarded.

Obsessive–compulsive disorders

Expanded public attention to the issues of child molestation appears to have led to an increased incidence of individuals with obsessive–compulsive disorders seeking evaluation driven by their fear that they may molest a child. These individuals deny sexual interest in children, and fail to show evidence of sexual interest in children in psychophysiological assessments. Therefore these patients should be treated for their obsessive–compulsive symptoms.

Organic mental syndromes

Organic brain disease resulting from strokes or brain injuries can profoundly effect the sexual behaviour of the patient. Since one of the primary functions of the cortex is to inhibit impulsivity, cortical injuries frequently lead to impulsive behaviour.

Examination of paraphilacs for organic disease varies from treatment centre to treatment centre. When organic disease is suspected, outlying centres refer cases to larger medical facilities for more extensive evaluation. Consequently there have been no random studies of the prevalence of organic disease in paraphiliacs. However, specific medical centres report a relatively high occurrence of organic disease in paraphiliacs. Abnormal hormonal levels are found in 74 per cent of paraphiliacs, soft neurological signs in 27 per cent, chromosomal abnormalities in 24 per cent, seizure disorders in 9 per cent, dyslexia in 9 per cent, abnormal electroencephalograms in 4 per cent, major psychiatric disorders in 4 per cent, and mental retardation in 4 per cent.[15]

Factors suggesting the need for more extensive organic evaluations include the following.

- The paraphilic individual reports altered states of consciousness or seizure-like symptoms prior to committing paraphilic acts.

- The paraphilic individual uses excess aggression during the commission of crime.

- The paraphilic act is atypical of this category of paraphilia.

- The paraphilic individual has abnormal body habits.

- The paraphilic individual's history suggests attention-deficit disorder, dyslexia, or mental retardation.

- The paraphilic individual displays sadistic or aggressive behaviour concomitant with problems of sexual identity or transvestic fetishism.

Aetiology and epidemiology

Aetiology

Theoretical perspectives regarding the aetiology of paraphilias have evolved and shifted as Western society's understanding of mental disorders has increased. In the nineteenth century, paraphilic behaviour was considered sinful, as an expression of evil by the ungodly. As psychiatrists began to elucidate the organic factors causing mental illnesses, the idea of paraphilic behaviour strictly as the expression of sin gave way to the belief that organic disease was responsible for inappropriate sexual behaviour, such as that evolving from central nervous system complications of syphilis. By the early twentieth century, Freudian theory had identified paraphilic interests as inappropriately expressed unconscious conflicts. Dynamic theories have recently been combined with the cognitive-behavioural learning model, creating a more strongly unified theory to explain factors involved in paraphilic behaviour.

Combined dynamic and cognitive-behavioural model

According to psychoanalytic theory, initial paraphilic acts are direct consequences of misplaced sexual and aggressive drives. These drives would normally be channelled into appropriate gender-specific behaviour. However, in the paraphiliac, these sexual and aggressive drives are distorted by anxiety generated by fear of castration and separation from the mother. Inappropriate resolution of the Oedipal complex within the phallic stage of psychosexual development results in identification with the opposite gender parent. Identification with the opposite gender parent causes the child to make inappropriate object choices for libidinal cathexis. As a result, the child goes on to express a paraphilic interest that reflects his initial inappropriate identification with the opposite gender parent.

The cognitive-behavioural learning model views the earliest choice or use of inappropriate objects or behaviour for sexual gratification as a somewhat random event, idiosyncratic to the individual, based upon the child's unique early experiences. Both theoretical orientations see the expression of such early interest in paraphilic objects or behaviour as resulting from the extent to which a child anticipates the consequence of acting on paraphilic interests. If the child is well socialized and has learned appropriate means of expressing sexual behaviour, or if anxiety or the fear of negative consequences resulting from expression of a paraphilic interest is dominant, the initial paraphilic interest is not expressed by the youth. In contrast, when the expression of the earliest interest is unassociated with anxiety or anticipated negative consequences, the child expresses his first paraphilic behaviour. Often, the earliest experiences are found intriguing because of their novelty and uniqueness alone.

Both the psychoanalytic and cognitive-behavioural models agree that, as time passes, the child's use of these paraphilic behaviours, fantasies, or images becomes paired and associated with the pleasurable experience of masturbation and orgasm. The association of paraphilic stimuli with sexual pleasure profoundly accelerates the child's use of paraphilic images, along with ensuring their repeated pairing and reinforcement by the power of genital pleasure and orgasm.

Within the majority of cultures, sexual behaviour is considered to be a private activity that individuals should not discuss and that they should feel guilty for expressing. Aberrant sexual interests, which qualify as any sexual interests other than those that are traditionally accepted within the society, are especially proscribed. Because traditional societal rules and mores play such a large role in identifying what constitutes appropriate versus inappropriate sexual interest, the child learns that his interest in paraphilic stimuli and/or behaviour must be secretive, internalized, and concealed from others. The child with paraphilic interest surreptitiously begins to repetitively pair and associate paraphilic images with orgasm. When a child's paraphilic acts are discovered by others, and he or she is confronted by parents or authorities, the child is initially successful at denying or concealing his or her ongoing interest. The child becomes more clandestine in the use of paraphilic stimuli, with further pairings of each paraphilic stimulus with orgasm, along with added reinforcement from the excitement and anxiety of committing a forbidden act.

By the time the young adult's paraphilic interests are apparent to others, there have been hundreds to thousands of associations between paraphilic stimuli and sexual pleasure. The young adult feels trapped by his or her paraphilic interest. Confrontation by others regarding the inappropriateness of the paraphilic behaviour is appreciated but, at the same time, the use of paraphilic stimuli may have become so ingrained that attempts by the individual to achieve sexual pleasure or orgasm without them are unsuccessful. The individual feels trapped by his own chronic use of paraphilic stimuli and unable to escape into satisfactory sexual experiences without the use of the paraphilic images, fantasies, or behaviour.[16]

The abused-abuser hypothesis

An intriguing hypothesis for the aetiology of child molestation is that being molested by an adult when a child or adolescent may subsequently lead the victim to become a victimizer; this is called the abused-abuser hypothesis for child sexual abuse. A number of theories have been proposed regarding how such victimization could cause the victimization of others.[17,18] If abused as a youth, the child may recall these experiences with great clarity and associate them with masturbation and orgasm, thereby developing an interest in child–adult sex. An emotionally deprived child abused by an adult who views the child in a positive light and showers him with gifts could himself see the experience as personally reinforcing and therefore continue similar behaviour into adulthood by molesting children himself. A further explanation is identification with the aggressor, in which a fearful victim learns to cope with victimization by becoming a child molester and thus no longer fears being abused.

The abused-abuser hypothesis probably emanated from early studies in which child molesters, when questioned about their prior sexual experiences with adults, reported a high incidence of having been abused as children. However, subsequent studies of the early sexual experiences of incarcerated child molesters, compared with the early sexual experiences of incarcerated non-child-molesting sex offenders and incarcerated non-sex offenders, revealed that the prevalence of abuse in childhood within all three groups was not significantly different. This suggests that other factors must be responsible for determining the eventual consequences to and for the victims of child molestation.

The abused-abuser hypothesis appears to be more relevant when examining juvenile sex offenders. When juveniles molest younger children, those younger child victims are prone to carry out similar sexual behaviour with peers or even younger children. With juvenile victims, the abused-abuser hypothesis appears to have greater relevance to the aetiology of child molestation.

Ethnological model

Ethnology has provided another explanation for an individual's sexual interest in children.[19] The purpose of intercourse, from an ethnological point of view, is 'to get one's genes in the gene pool'. Therefore the average male tends to be attracted to individuals more feminine and somewhat younger than him to maximize the likelihood of sexual behaviour perpetuating his genes. Although sexual experiences with individuals older or more masculine than him may be sexually pleasurable, from an ethnological perspective such activity will not lead to procreation and the maintenance of the species. Therefore the average adult male will be more sexually attracted to females somewhat younger than him.

However, the ethnological process is imperfect, with some individuals being attracted to adolescent females (ephebophilia) or younger children (paedophilia). According to ethnological theory, the majority of males will be attracted to adult females somewhat younger than they are, but there will always be some individuals who are attracted to adolescent or much younger females and males.

Epidemiology

The paraphilias are predominantly disorders of males, but do occasionally occur in females. The estimate is that the male-to-female ratio is approximately 30 to 1. The higher prevalence of paraphilias in males probably results from the higher testosterone levels in males compared with females, leading to greater sexual drive at an earlier age.

Estimating the incidence and prevalence of paraphilic behaviour is problematic for various reasons. First, it is difficult to obtain a representative sample of paraphiliacs upon which to base such estimates. Second, it is difficult to determine if information such as frequency of paraphilic behaviour would be more accurate if gathered from samples obtained from clinical populations or from the general population. Both groups present challenges in attempts to elucidate epidemiological characteristics of the paraphilias. For example, in clinical populations it is common to see paraphiliacs who engage in a variety of paraphilic behaviours, even if they restrict those behaviours to one type of paraphilic diagnostic classification. To compound this problem, most paraphiliacs seen within the clinical environment do not fully divulge the extent of their paraphilic activities because they are afraid of criminal recourse. In the general population the accurate reporting of paraphilic interests and behaviours is influenced by the fact that paraphilias are socially undesirable and therefore are underreported. Furthermore, most paraphiliacs fear arrest and prosecution by the criminal justice system; therefore, whether they are being assessed in a clinical environment or are being questioned as part of a survey sample, paraphiliacs are extremely adept at hiding the nature of their paraphilic interests.[10]

Despite the problems indicated above, several studies have described and clarified some of the epidemiological characteristics of the paraphilias. A study of 561 subjects voluntarily seeking assessment and/or treatment of their sexual interests within a psychiatric setting found that the average number of paraphilic crimes and victims was substantial.[20] Participants had been involved in 291 737 paraphilic incidents with 195 408 victims. Additionally, each of the 560 partici-

pants were diagnosed following assessment and evaluation. Categories of paraphilic diagnoses are as follows: 19 per cent were diagnosed as paedophiles interested in extrafamilial girls; 13 per cent were diagnosed as paedophiles interested in extrafamilial boys; 13 per cent were diagnosed as incestuous paedophiles with an interest in girls; 4 per cent were diagnosed as incestuous paedophiles with an interest in boys; 11 per cent were diagnosed as rapists of adult females; 12 per cent were diagnosed as exhibitionists; 5 per cent were diagnosed as voyeurs; 5 per cent were diagnosed as frotteurs; 3 per cent were diagnosed as transsexuals; 3 per cent were diagnosed as transvestites; 2 per cent were diagnosed as sadists; 2 per cent were diagnosed as egodystonic homosexuals; the few remaining participants had carried out minor paraphilic behaviours.

Utilizing data gathered from samples selected from general populations, three studies have provided information on the incidence and frequency of paraphilic behaviour. One study was conducted to assess the frequency of men's erotic fantasies during masturbation and intercourse.[21] Of the 94 males in this study who reported sexual fantasies, 62 per cent fantasized about sexual encounters with young girls, 33 per cent fantasized about raping adult females, 12 per cent fantasized about sadomasochistic encounters, 5 per cent fantasized about zoophilic encounters, and 3 per cent fantasized about sexual encounters with young boys. The other two studies were conducted with college students and were undertaken to investigate paraphilic sexual interests. One of these studies involved 193 male participants who were questioned regarding sexual interest in children.[22] Of these 193 participants, 21 per cent reported sexual attraction to children, 9 per cent fantasized about sexual encounters with a child, 5 per cent reported masturbation fantasies of sex with children, and 7 per cent responded that there was a likelihood of their becoming sexually involved with children if they could find a way to avoid criminal consequences for such activity. The second study involved 60 participants who were questioned about paraphilic interests, especially child molestation.[23] Of the 60 participants, a total of 65 per cent of this sample indicated involvement in a paraphilia; 3 per cent reported sexual encounters with girls under 12, 42 per cent reported voyeurism, 8 per cent indicated participation in telephone scatalogia, 35 per cent in frotteurism, 2 per cent in exhibitionism, and 5 per cent in coercive sexual encounters. These studies are limited because the samples are homogeneous and the participants were not questioned about every form of paraphilic interest. However, the three studies strongly indicate that males often fantasize about paraphilic behaviour and that these same males report engaging in paraphilic activities.

Treatment

Cognitive-behavioural treatment

For the last 10 to 15 years, treatment for paraphiliacs has focused on two primary areas: cognitive-behavioural treatment and pharmacological treatment. Cognitive-behavioural treatment has generally focused on the following:

- techniques to reduce or block inappropriate sexual arousal and/or to increase or maintain non-deviant appropriate sexual arousal[6,24–35]

- improving pro-social behaviour, including assertiveness training, anger-management training, social skills training, intimacy skills training, etc.[36–39]

- cognitive therapy to address distorted thinking patterns that the paraphiliac has used to justify his inappropriate sexual behaviour, as well as the establishment of empathy for the individuals he has victimized[36,40–43]

- relapse prevention, a long-term maintenance therapy which helps offenders to identify and manage more effectively situations that place them at risk of reoffending, to establish or improve social support systems, to develop a methodology for evaluating the effectiveness of their treatment, and to maintain a balanced lifestyle.[44–53]

Pharmacological treatment

Pharmacological treatment for the paraphilias has been increasingly important in the last 20 years. Three categories of medication have proved effective for treating paraphiliacs: antiandrogens, hormonal agents, and selective serotonin reuptake inhibitors (**SSRI**s).

Antiandrogens

Ciproterone acetate has proved quite effective because of its antiandrogenic, antigonadotrophic, and progestational effects.[54] This agent blocks intracellular testosterone uptake as well as the intracellular metabolism of antiandrogens. As a consequence, it drastically reduces circulating testosterone and therefore reduces the paraphiliac's sexual drive. The oral dosage is usually 50 to 200 mg/ day but it is also available in an intramuscular form, requiring a dosage of 200 to 400 mg once every 1 or 2 weeks. Side-effects include liver damage, gynaecomastia (usually temporary and reversible), and reduction of sexual drive, fantasies, erections, frequency of masturbation, and sexual intercourse. This drug was first used in 1971, and a number of studies have shown it to be highly effective at reducing recidivism.[55] Ciproterone acetate is available throughout Europe and Canada, but is not available in the United States.

Hormonal agents

Medroxyprogesterone acetate is the primary hormonal agent that has been used in the United States, since initially reported by Heller *et al.*[56] Its effect results from the acceleration of testosterone-A-reductase in the liver which accelerates testosterone metabolism and thereby reduces testosterone levels. Medroxyprogesterone acetate also reduces plasma testosterone through the pituitary axis. It is not an antiandrogen. Significant side-effects have included liver damage, fatigue, weight gain, hot and cold flushes, headaches, gallbladder disease, diabetes, and thrombophlebitis. Historically, the dose was 300 to 400 mg of the injectable form of medroxyprogesterone acetate, but in recent years lower doses have been found to be equally effective without causing so many side-effects that the medication is discontinued by the paraphiliac. An alternative to injectable medroxyprogesterone acetate can be administered orally. Generally doses of less than 200 mg daily by mouth are effective at helping the paraphiliac gain control over his behaviour.

More recently studies have been reported using **luteinizing hormone-releasing hormone (LHRH) agonists**, which initially accelerate the production of testosterone through the hypothalamic–pituitary axis but then exhaust the axis and result in a dramatic reduction in testosterone to castrated levels. Since these drugs initially cause an acceleration of testosterone production, the non-steroidal antiandrogen flutamide is usually concomitantly administered at a dose of 250 mg three times daily for the first month of LHRH agonist use. After that, flutamide can be discontinued. The LHRH agonists have the advantage of not being true steroids, but polypeptides, and therefore do not cause many of the steroidal effects while still resulting in a dramatic reduction of testosterone and increased control over paraphilic urges.

Since it was reported that **SSRIs** were effective in managing the treatment of exhibitionism, a number of authors have report their effectiveness in the treatment not only of other paraphiliacs, but also of those with hypersexuality.[57,58] The exact mechanism of action of the SSRIs is not completely understood, but it is suspected that their effectiveness results from a reduction of sexual drive and of the obsessive ruminations that accompany paraphiliacs' behaviour. The most extensively investigated SSRI has been sertraline, with the mean dose being 130 mg daily. Fluvoxamine, fluoxetine, and paroxetine have all been found to be effective in treating both the paraphilias and males with non-paraphilic hypersexuality.

The main limitation of ciproterone acetate, medroxyprogesterone acetate, the LHRH agonists, and SSRIs is that they are only effective during clinical administration; to date, there is insufficient evidence to suggest persistent effectiveness following discontinuation of the medication. The SSRIs show great promise because of their greater ease of administration, lower cost, and lower side-effect profiles. These medications are traditionally prescribed as an adjunct to cognitive-behavioural treatment.

Evaluating the effectiveness of treatment

A review of evidence

A number of factors make assessing the effectiveness of treatment outcome with paraphiliacs problematic.

1. Many paraphilias, such as paedophila and rape, are felonies. The accurate determination of recidivism requires that the paraphiliac reports his own commission of another felony, and thereby risks prolonged incarceration.

2. Quantification of treatment effectiveness requires a control group that either receives no treatment or receives a treatment that is not specific to sex offenders. Such a control group would be unethical because, without treatment, individuals in the control group would be allowed, albeit indirectly, potentially to commit additional felonies, which would pose a threat to the general population. Attempts to select a naturally occurring control group are also problematic, since assignment to a treatment or control group cannot be randomized, and therefore treatment outcome may be considerably influenced by the control group selection process.

3. Paraphilic treatment programmes are frequently implemented within the prison environment. As a consequence, established

criteria for behavioural improvement are based upon some measure of treatment responsiveness from within the prison environment rather than treated and non-treated groups being released from prison and the recommission rate determined.

4. A subgroup of paraphiliacs fit classification and diagnostic criteria consistent with concomitant psychopathy.[59] Recent studies have shown that individuals with paraphilic sexual interests and psychopathy do not respond well to treatment, and in fact are made worse. When treatment involves paraphiliacs with concomitant psychopathy, treatment outcome can become problematic since paraphiliacs without psychopathy may improve, while paraphiliacs with psychopathy become worse, and the net effect shows minimal response to treatment across the total group. Hence, this problem contaminates treatment outcome results with paraphiliacs.

5. Until recently, treatment outcome variance has resulted from criteria of recidivism varying from study to study (e.g. self-reported recidivism versus charges for sex crimes versus incarcerations for sex crimes). However, outcome variants can also result from variation in the length of follow-up efforts. Recidivism studies based upon a 4-year follow-up period yield markedly better outcomes than studies with 10 or 25 years of follow-up. Outcome studies cannot provide reliable information to clinicians or researchers if they are not designed to control for the factor of the paraphiliac's opportunity to recommit a paraphilic act. Survival curves have been utilized recently as one method of controlling for this problem, but older outcome studies have been impervious to this issue.[60]

6. Great variation exists regarding the specific populations of paraphiliacs being studied. Some outcome studies involve responsiveness to treatment within prison settings, where individuals' sex crimes have been severe enough to warrant incarceration, while other studies are conducted on outpatient populations, where the extent of perpetrators' paraphilic acts did not warrant incarceration. Comparison of treatment outcome data from different studies, because of disparity between groups of sex-offending populations, makes effective outcome investigations very difficult to carry out, with results from one study to the next often not yielding sufficient data for prediction purposes.

These limitations make it difficult to determine the overall effectiveness of treatment, especially for treatment implemented within prison settings. Treated inmates are usually released from prison into a probation and/or parole setting, where accurate reporting of additional offences would lead not only to a new charge, but also to incarceration for the remainder of their probation and/or parole time, or to extended incarceration time. Marshall et al.[61] describe outcome related to a cognitive-behavioural approach to the treatment of predominantly paedophiles. Their findings are important because not only did they review police records regarding recidivism, but owing to the rural nature of the setting where many of the paedophiles in their investigation were treated, it was possible to corroborate reports from local legal authorities and various social services who were contacted to evaluate new alleged cases of child molestation. Results of this work indicate that after cognitive-behavioural treatment recidivism was reduced by 20 per cent below baseline rates of untreated offenders. They also reported that when a re-offender was apprehended, on average he had molested two further victims. Therefore these findings also

suggest that, since recidivism was reduced by 20 per cent, treatment of 100 paedophiles resulted in stopping 20 child molesters, who had a high likelihood of re-offending without treatment, from molesting the 40 children they might have assaulted if they had not been treated.

Advice about management

Clinicians providing treatment for paraphilias should not approach case management as if once treatment is delivered, follow-up is no longer important. Sex offending should be viewed as a chronic condition that requires surveillance of the offender and periodic maintenance therapy post-treatment in order to ensure the protection of the public.

Probation and parole officers are an exceedingly important part of treatment maintenance. Officers of the court have the authority and responsibility to ensure that sex offenders maintain their treatment contacts and fulfil probation and/or parole requirements. Mental health providers have historically avoided working with the court system in order to maintain complete independence within the patient–therapist relationship, hence protecting that relationship from outside sources of influence. However, complete independence from the legal system is inappropriate given the realities that sex offenders frequently are treated when on probation or parole. The consequences of treatment failure are vastly different for sex offenders than for individuals with neurotic or personality dysfunctions and, in many cases, are much more serious even than in individuals with psychotic conditions. Under the latter conditions, the usual victim is the patient himself, not a member of the general public. When working with paraphiliacs, the mental health provider must assume a new and challenging role of working with the legal system to ensure compliance with treatment and the safety of the public. Regular meetings with probation officers that provide updates of therapeutic progress help the sex offender understand the importance of completing psychological treatment and complying with probation and/or parole requirements.

Surveillance of sex offenders is especially critical because the therapist spends only a brief amount of time with the offender. Some sex offenders are exceedingly adept at convincing their therapist that they are following through on treatment and avoiding environments that in the past have acted as antecedents to sex offending. It is strongly recommended that a surveillance team be developed by the sex offender and the therapist to include five people, at least one of whom comes from the patient's family, one from the patient's work site, and one from the patient's social environment. With the assistance of the therapist, the offender teaches the surveillance team those behavioural precursors that previously may have led to an increased risk of re-offence. The surveillance team, with the assistance of the therapist, develops a surveillance check list that identifies these antecedent behaviours. The offender then teaches the surveillance team how to check specifically on each of these potential antecedents to sex-offending behaviour. Following adequate training, the surveillance team members provide the therapist, on a bimonthly basis, with their observations of the offender based upon this checklist, so that the therapist can be alerted to behaviours that suggest an offender's increased risk of recidivism.[62]

In general, the average sex offender can be successfully treated on an outpatient basis with intensive treatment occurring once or twice per week for approximately 90 sessions. Upon completion of the intensive portion of treatment, the offender can go into a maintenance phase of treatment when he is seen as frequently as once a week, or as infrequently as once every 3 months, depending upon the severity of the individual case. A number of factors increase the need for more frequent therapeutic visits and, in some cases, day-patient, residential treatment, or institutionalized treatment. A number of factors also necessitate the institution of medication, one-to-one supervision by the patient's family, or the use of electronic monitoring or house arrest.

Factors that increase the need for more frequent visits, or more invasive treatment procedures, include a high baseline frequency of the deviant behaviour. Additionally, some behaviours, although infrequent, are potentially so dangerous to the victim that treatment must be intensive and extensive. The sadistic offender, the brutal rapist, the aggressive paedophile, and the brain-damaged sex offender are a few examples of these more dangerous perpetrators. Finally, when there is no independent surveillance of the offender, when there is a lack of involvement from the offender's family or friends, when denial by patients precludes their viewing themselves as having a dangerous sexual behaviour, and/or when the victims are less able to defend themselves (e.g. institutionalized, retarded, or psychiatrically ill potential victims), more rapid intrusive therapy is indicated.

With the combination of currently available medications, the incorporation of surveillance groups, and limited access of potential victims, most sex offenders can be treated on an outpatient basis. However, given the realities of the criminal justice system and the illegality of sex-offending behaviour, many sex offenders are incarcerated before or during the initial phase of their treatment. Economic concerns, which are abundant with sex offenders for whom incarceration has historically been considered a preferable option, should be closely scrutinized because of the limited resources currently available for imprisoned sex offenders and the immense cost of imprisonment. The assessment and management of sex offenders is considered further in Chapter 11.4.2.

Possibilities for prevention

There are two aspects of preventing sexual violence that show considerable promise.

First, paraphilias begin at an early age and fantasies involving paraphilic behaviour are often used by adolescents for years prior to the commission of a paraphilic act. Categories of sexual fantasies that lead to paraphilias are well known. Therefore, paraphilias could be prevented through an educational approach that would teach adolescents the eventual consequences of the chronic use of paraphilic fantasy, which can steer the adolescent into chronic paraphilic behaviour. During the last 20 years there has been a major shift in the scope of educational programmes regarding drug and alcohol abuse to include educating young people about the dangers of drug and alcohol abuse, as well as increasing surveillance regarding drug trafficking within schools. A similar approach is applicable regarding the use of paraphilic fantasies and paraphilic behaviour.

A second major opportunity for prevention involves the identification of potential youth workers who have strong predilections toward involving themselves sexually with children. Individuals seeking employment that would bring them into contact with young children should be screened for paedophilic interests. In the past, criminal background checks, arrest records, searches of databases containing the names of those accused of child molesting, and psychological testing have been used to identify potential child molesters. The recent development of visual reaction time as a means of identifying paedophiles provides an efficient means of screening for paedophilia.[63] Seminaries, boys and girls clubs, youth sports activities, and institutions providing assistance to youth are all sources through which paedophiles may work to obtain access to children. Screening for paedophilia would prevent paedophiles from putting themselves in close proximity of children and therefore prevent child molestation. Since only the minority of applicants to such programmes are actually paedophiles, methodologies that ensure high specificity (i.e. having an exceedingly low false-positive rate) are essential for such screening purposes.

Further reading

Ames, M.A. and Houston, D.A. (1990). Legal, social and biological definitions of pedophilia. *Archives of Sexual Behavior*, **19**, 333–42.

Bradford, J.M.W. and Greenberg, D.M. (1996). Pharmacological treatment of deviant sexual behavior. *Annual Review of Sex Research*, **7**, 283–307.

Feierman, J. (ed.) (1990). *Pedophilia: biosocial dimensions*. Springer-Verlag, New York.

Langevin, R., Bain, J., Wortzman, G., Hucker, S., Dickey, R., and Wright, P. (1988). Sexual sadism: brain, blood, and behavior. *Annals of the New York Academy of Sciences*, **528**, 163–71.

Laws, D.R. (ed.) (1989). *Relapse prevention with sex offenders*. Guilford Press, New York.

Marshall, W.L., Laws, D.R., and Barbaree, H.E. (1990). *Handbook of sexual assault: issues, theories and treatment of the offender*. Plenum Press, New York.

Rosen, I. (1996). *Sexual Deviation* (3rd edn). Oxford University Press.

Ryan, G.D. and Lane, S.L. (1991). *Juvenile sexual offending: causes, consequences, and correction*. Lexington Books, Lexington, MA.

Salter, A.C. (1988). *Treating child sex offenders and victims: a practical guide*. Sage, Newbury Park, CA.

References

1. Abel, G.G., Becker, J.V., Cunningham-Rathner, J., Mittelman, M.S., and Rouleau, J.L. (1989). Multiple paraphilic diagnoses among sex offenders. *Bulletin of the American Academy of Psychiatry and the Law*, **16**, 153–68.

2. Bradford, J.M., Boulet, J., and Pawlak, A. (1992). The paraphilias: a multiplicity of deviant behaviors. *Canadian Journal of Psychiatry*, **37**, 104–8.

3. American Psychiatric Association (1994). *Diagnostic and statistical manual of mental disorders* (4th edn). American Psychiatric Association, Washington, DC.

4. World Health Organization (1992). *International statistical classification of diseases and related health problems, 10th revision*. WHO, Geneva

5. Okami, P. (1996). Evolution, psychopathology, and sexual offending: Aping our ancestors. *Sexual Abuse: Journal of Research and Treatment*, **8**, 337–8.

6. Abel, G.G., Becker, J.V., and Cunningham-Rathner, J. (1984). Complications, consent and cognitions in sex between children and adults. *International Journal of Law and Psychiatry*, **7**, 89–103.

7. Money, J., Jobaris, R., and Furth, G. (1977). Apotemnophilia: two cases of self-demand amputation as a paraphilia. *Journal of Sex Research*, **13**, 115–25.

8. Blanchard, R. and Hucker, S.J. (1991). Age, transvestism, bondage, and concurrent paraphilic activities in 117 fatal cases of autoerotic asphyxia. *British Journal of Psychiatry*, **159**, 371–7.

9. Byard, R.W., Hucker, S.J., and Hazelwood, R.R. (1990). A comparison of typical death scene features in cases of fatal male and autoerotic asphyxia with a review of the literature. *Forensic Science International*, **48**, 113–21.

10. Abel, G.G. and Osborn, C.A. (1992). The paraphilias: the extent and nature of sexually deviant and criminal behavior. *Psychiatric Clinics of North America*, **15**, 675–87.

11. Zuckerman, M. (1972). Physiological measures of sexual arousal in the human. In *Handbook of psychophysiology* (ed. N.S. Greenfield and R.A. Sternbach), pp. 709–40. Holt, Rinehart, Winston, New York.

12. Abrams, S. (1989). *The almost complete polygraph handbook*. Lexington Books, Lexington, MA.

13. Abel, G.G., Lawry, S.S., Karlstrom, E.M., Osborn, C.A., and Gillespie, C.F. (1994). Screening tests for pedophilia. *Criminal Justice and Behavior*, **21**, 115–31.

14. Schoen, J. and Hoover, J.H. (1990). Mentally retarded sex offenders. *Journal of Offender Rehabilitation*, **16**, 81–91.

15. Langevin, R. and Watson, R.J. (1996). Major factors in the assessment of paraphiliacs and sex offenders. *Journal of Offender Rehabilitation*, **23**, 39–70.

16. Abel, G.G. and Blanchard, E.B. (1974). The role of fantasy in the treatment of sexual deviation. *Archives of General Psychiatry*, **30**, 467–75.

17. Garland, R.J. and Dougher, M.J. (1990). The abused/abuser hypothesis of child sexual abuse: a critical review of theory and research. In *Pedophilia: biosocial dimensions* (ed. J.R. Feierman). Springer-Verlag, New York.

18. Freund, K. and Kuban, M. (1994). The basis of the abused abuser theory of pedophilia: a further elaboration of an earlier study. *Archives of Sexual Behavior*, **23**, 553–63.

19. Feierman, J.R. (1990). A biosocial overview of adult human sexual behavior with children and adolescents. In *Pedophilia: biosocial dimensions* (ed. J.R. Feierman), pp. 8–68. Springer-Verlag, New York.

20. Abel, G.G., Becker, J.V., Mittelman, M.S., Cunningham-Rathner, J., Rouleau, J.L., and Murphy, W.D. (1987). Self-reported sex crimes of nonincarcerated paraphiliacs. *Journal of Interpersonal Violence*, **2**, 3–25.

21. Crepault, C. and Coulture, M. (1989). Men's erotic fantasies. *Archives of Sexual Behavior*, **9**, 65–81.

22. Briere, J. and Runtz, M. (1989). University males' sexual interest in children: predicting potential indices of 'pedophilia' in a non-forensic sample. *Child Abuse and Neglect*, **13**, 65–75.

23. Templeman, T.L. and Stinnett, R.D. (1991). Patterns of sexual arousal and history in a 'normal' sample of young men. *Archives of Sexual Behavior*, **20**, 137–50.

24. Abel, G.G. and Osborn, C.A. (1996). Pedophilia. In *Synopsis of treatments of psychiatric disorders* (2nd edn) (ed. G.O. Gabbard and S.D. Atkinson), pp. 821–8. American Psychiatric Press, Wahsington, DC.

25. Maletzky, B.M. (1980). Self-referred versus court-referred sexually deviant patients: success with assisted covert sensitization. *Behavior Therapy*, **11**, 306–14.

26. McConaghy, N. (1990). Assessment in treatment of sex offenders: the Prince of Wales programme. *Australian and New Zealand Journal of Psychiatry*, **24**, 175–81.

27. Serber, M. (1970). Shame aversion therapy. *Journal of Behavior Therapy and Experimental Psychiatry*, **1**, 213–15.

28. Smith, T.A. and Wolfe, R.W. (1988). Treatment model for sexual aggression. *Journal of Social Work and Human Sexuality*, **7**, 149–64.

29. Marshall, W.L. and Lippins, K. (1977). The clinical value of boredom: a procedure for reducing inappropriate sexual interests. *Journal of Nervous and Mental Disease*, **165**, 283–7.

30. Barlow, D.H., Agras, W.S., Abel, G.G., Blanchard, E.B., and Young, L.D. (1975). Case histories and shorter communications: biofeedback and reinforcement to increase heterosexual arousal in homosexuals. *Behaviour Research and Therapy*, **13**, 45–50.

31. Kremsdorf, R.B., Holman, M.L., and Laws, D. (1980). Orgasmic reconditioning without deviant imagery: a case report with a paedophile. *Behaviour Research and Therapy*, **18**, 203–7.

32. Maletzky, B.M. (1985). Orgasmic reconditioning. In *Dictionary of behaviour therapy techniques* (ed. A.S. Bellack and M. Hersen), pp. 157–8. Pergamon Press, New York.

33. Konrad, S.D. and Wincze, J.P. (1976). Orgasmic reconditioning: a controlled study on the effects upon the sexual arousal and behaviour of adult male homosexuals. *Behavior Therapy*, **7**, 155–6.

34. Marques, J. (1970). Orgasmic reconditioning: changing sexual object choice through controlling masturbation fantasies. *Journal of Behavioral Therapy and Experimental Psychiatry*, **1**, 263–71.

35. Leonard, S.R. and Hayes, S.C. (1983). Sexual fantasy alternation. *Journal of Behavioral Therapy and Experimental Psychiatry*, **3**, 241–9.

36. Abel, G.G., Becker, J.V., Cunningham-Rathner, J., Rouleau, J.L., Kaplan, M., and Reich, J. (1984). *The treatment of child molesters*. Behavioral Medicine Institute of Atlanta, GA.

37. Marshall, W.L. (1971). A combined treatment method for certain sexual deviations. *Behaviour Research and Therapy*, **9**, 293–4.

38. Whitman, W.P. and Quinsey, V.L. (1981). Heterosocial skill training for institutionalized rapists and child molesters. *Canadian Journal of Behavioral Science*, **13**, 105–14.

39. Quinsey, V.L., Chaplin, T.C., Maguire, A.M., and Uphold, D. (1989). The behavioral treatment of rapists and child molesters. In *Behavioral approaches to crime and delinquency: application, research and theory* (ed. E.K. Morris and C.J. Braukmann), pp. 363–82. Plenum Press, New York.

40. Abel, G.G., Mittelman, M.S., and Becker, J.V. (1985). Sex offenders: results of assessment and recommendations for treatment. In *Clinical criminology: the assessment and treatment of criminal behaviour* (ed. M.H. Ben-Aron, S.J. Hucker, and C.D. Webster), pp. 191–205. M&M Graphics, Toronto.

41. Lange, A. (1986). *Rational-emotive therapy: a treatment manual*. Florida Mental Health Institute, Tampa, FL.

42. Murphy, W.D. (1990). Assessment and modification of cognitive distortions in sex offenders. In *Handbook of sexual assault: issues, theories and treatment of the offender* (ed. W.L. Marshall, D.R. Laws, and H.E. Barbaree), pp. 331–42. Plenum Press, New York.

43. Knopp, F.H. (1984). *Retraining adult sex offenders: methods and models*. Safer Society Press, Syracuse, NY.

44. George, W.H. and Marlatt, G. (1989). Introduction. In *Relapse prevention with sex offenders* (ed. D.R. Laws), pp. 2–3. Guilford Press, New York.

45. Nelson, C., Miner, M., Marques, J., Russell, K., and Achterkirchen, J. (1989). Relapse prevention: a cognitive–behavioral model for treatment of the rapist and child molester. *Journal of Social Work and Human Sexuality*, **7**, 125–43.

46. Pithers, W.D. (1990). Relapse prevention with sexual aggressors. In *Handbook of sexual assault: issues, theories and treatment of the offender* (ed. W.L. Marshall, D.R. Laws, and H.E. Barbaree), pp. 343–61. Plenum Press, New York.

47. Pithers, W.D., Kashima, K.M., Cumming, G.F., and Beal, L.S. (1988). Relapse prevention a method of enhancing maintenance of change in sex offenders. In *Treating child sex offenders and victims* (ed. A.C. Salter), pp. 131–70. Sage, Newbury Park, CA.

48. Pithers, W.D., Kashima, K.M., Cumming, G.F., Beal, L.S., and Buell, M.M. (1988). Relapse prevention of sexual aggressors. In *Human sexual aggression: current perspectives* (ed. R. Prentky and V. Quinsey), pp. 244–59. New York Academy of Sciences (special volume of *Annals of the New York Academy of Sciences*).

49. Barnard, G.W., Fuller, A.K., Robbins, L., and Shaw, T. (1989). *The child molester: an integrated approach to evaluation and treatment*. Brunner–Mazel, New York.

50. Hall, R.L. (1989). Self-efficacy ratings. In *Relapse prevention with sex offenders* (ed. D.R. Laws), pp. 137–45. Guilford Press, New York.

51. Jenkins-Hall, K.D. and Marlatt, G.A. (1989). Apparently irrelevant decisions in the relapse process. In *Relapse prevention with sex offenders* (ed. D.R. Laws), pp. 47–55. Guilford Press, New York.

52. Marques, J.D. and Nelson, C. (1989). Elements of high risk situations

for sex offenders. In *Relapse prevention with sex offenders* (ed. D.R. Laws), pp. 35–44. Guilford Press, New York.

53. Russell, K., Sturgeon, V.H., Miner, M.H., and Nelson, C. (1989) Determinants of the abstinence violation effect in sexual fantasies. In *Relapse prevention with sex offenders* (ed. D.R. Laws), pp. 63–75. Guilford Press, New York.

54. Bradford, J.M.W. (1983). Research in sex offenders. *Psychiatric Clinics of North America*, **6**, 715–33.

55. Laschet, U. and Laschet, L. (1971). Psychopharmacotherapy of sex offenders with cyproterone acetate. *Pharmakopsychiatrie Neuropsychopharmakologie*, **4**, 99–104.

56. Heller, C.G., Laidlaw, M.W., Harvey, H.T., and Nelson, D.L. (1958). The effects of progestational compounds of the reproductive processes of the human male. *Annals of the New York Academy of Sciences*, **71**, 649–55.

57. Bianchi, M.D. (1990). Fluoxetine treatment of exhibitionism. *American Journal of Psychiatry*, **147**, 1089–90.

58. Kafka, M.P. and Prentky, R. (1992). A comparative study of non paraphilic sexual addictions and paraphilias in men. *Journal of Clinical Psychiatry*, **53**, 345–50.

59. Rice, M. (1997). Violent offender research and indications for the criminal justice system. *American Psychologist*, **52**, 414–23.

60. Prentky, R.A., Lee, A.F.S., Knight, R.A., and Cerce, D. (1997). Recidivism rates among child molesters and rapists: a methodological analysis. *Law and Human Behavior*, **21**, 635–59.

61. Marshall, W.L., Laws, D.R., and Barbaree, H.E. (1990). Outcome of comprehensive cognitive–behavioral treatment programs. In *Handbook of sexual assault: issues, theories and treatment of the offender* (ed. W.L. Marshall, D.R. Laws, and H.E. Barbaree), pp. 363–82. Plenum Press, New York.

62. Abel, G.G. and Rouleau, J.L. (1990). Male sex offenders. In *Handbook of outpatient treatment of adults* (ed. M.E. Thase, B.A. Edelstein, and M. Hersen), pp. 271–90. Plenum Press, New York.

63. Abel, G.G., Huffman, J., Warberg, B., and Holland, C.L. (1998). Visual reaction time and plethysmography as measures of sexual interest in child molesters. *Sexual Abuse: Journal of Research and Treatment*, **10**, 81–95.

4.11.4 Gender identity disorder in adults

Richard Green

History

The behavioural phenomenon of transsexualism of gender identity disorder is ancient. It has been recorded for centuries and in a broad range for cultures.[1] The behavioural picture is comparable to that seen clinically in the second half of the twentieth century.

In the first half of the twentieth century medical reports of sex reassignment surgery were described in Europe, primarily in Switzerland.[2] Additionally, in the 1930s a wide-selling biography *Man into Woman* was published describing a Dutch painter who underwent a series of surgical sex reassignment procedures.[3] Contemporary interest in transsexualism surged in 1952 when George Jorgensen, an American soldier serving in Denmark, remained there after his tour of duty and underwent hormonal and surgical treatment to become Christine Jorgensen.[4] The resultant international publicity yielded hundreds of people worldwide applying to the Danish doctors for similar treatment.[5] It also brought forth thousands of people in many countries requesting that doctors there perform sex change surgery.

By the mid-1960s there were surgeons scattered worldwide who were performing sex reassignment. Then in the United States at the Johns Hopkins Hospital and the University of Minnesota Hospitals and in the United Kingdom at the Charing Cross Hospital comprehensive sex reassignment programmes commenced. Extensive publicity was given to the Johns Hopkins programme as initially reported in the *New York Times* in 1966. It described the rationale for the programme and in the words of its Director, 'if the mind cannot be changed to fit the body, then perhaps we should consider changing the body to fit the mind'.[6]

In 1966 the first professional text on transsexualism was written by Harry Benjamin, widely acknowledged as the 'father of transsexualism'.[7] In 1969 the first interdisciplinary text was edited by Green and Money.[6] During the past 30 years the recognition of transsexualism or gender identity disorder as a treatable condition requiring psychiatric, endocrine, and surgical intervention has been accepted.

Epidemiology

The prevalence of gender identity disorder in adults is estimated from a comprehensive appraisal in The Netherlands at 1 in 10 000 males and 1 in 30 000 females.[8] At nearly all clinical centres the ratio of male-to-female patients ranges from 3:1 to 4:1, in favour of males. In some East European centres the ratio is reversed, an unexplained difference.[9]

Diagnosis

Diagnostic criteria of gender identity disorder as enumerated in DSM-IV[10] include a stated desire to be the other sex, a desire to live and be treated as the other sex, or the conviction that he or she has the typical feelings and reactions of the other sex. In adults the disturbance is manifested by symptoms such as the preoccupation of getting rid of primary and secondary sexual characteristics and the request for hormone surgery or procedures to alter physically the sexual characteristics to simulate the other sex. ICD-10 also notes that the transsexual identity should be present persistently for at least 2 years and not be a symptom of another mental disorder such as schizophrenia.[11] Both sets of diagnostic criteria note that the condition is not associated with chromosomal abnormality or a physically intersexed condition.

Origins

The search for the origins of transsexualism continues with a gradually increasing bias towards those that are physiological. Some 20 years ago there was a false prophet in the guise of the HY antigen, the antigenic influence on the Y chromosome believed to be influential in the development of the testes. A series of male transsexuals studied in Germany were found to be lacking this antigen and the tentative conclusion reached was that its absence resulted in a failure to masculinize the brain in the direction of a male identity.[12] However, the author's collaborative effort to replicate that study was not successful as all the male transsexuals we studied in the United States appeared to have normal HY antigen.[13]

A more recent finding from The Netherlands implicates the brain region known as the bed nucleus of the stria terminalis. In a series of six male transsexuals studied at postmortem over a 10-year period the size of the nucleus was comparable to that of typical females and not males.[14] The nucleus size is believed to be affected prenatally by sex hormone levels. A criticism of this study is that the long-term oestrogen treatment for these males may have altered the size of the nucleus. In response the researchers argue that males treated with antimale hormone drugs or oestrogen for prostate cancer do not have an alteration in the nucleus size from typical males. Another criticism is that the long time of collection, a 10-year period, before the brains were studied may have resulted in an artefactual shrinkage of the nucleus.

Research with male transsexuals has revealed what might be indirect markers reflecting biological distinctions for male transsexuals. In agreement with other researchers' findings that male homosexuals have a greater likelihood of having older brothers,[15] our homosexually orientated male transsexuals also have more older brothers. A theory behind this finding is that there is a progressive immunization with each pregnancy against the male fetus by the pregnant mother perhaps reflecting antigenicity of the HY antigen.[15]

A higher ratio of aunts to uncles on the mother's side has also been found in our male transsexuals, a finding previously reported for a sample of male homosexuals.[16] A theory here is that a semilethal factor has been operant in one generation (uncles) that in the subsequent generation influences brain development resulting in an atypical behavioural pattern (homosexual or transsexual development).[17] Another theory invokes genomic imprinting.[16] We also find that both male and female transsexuals are more often non-right-handed. This in the male may reflect central nervous system dysfunction or hormonal differences prenatally and in the female similar central nervous system dysfunction or masculinization.[18] Typically males are more often non-right handed compared with females.

For female transsexuals, a series of reports indicates a higher rate of polycystic ovarian disease.[19] Women with polycystic ovarian disease secrete higher levels of androgen than typical females. However, nearly all patients with polycystic ovarian disease are not transsexual and the majority of female transsexuals do not have polycystic ovarian disease.

Treatment

Prior to recognition of transsexualism as a disorder deserving medical and psychiatric attention many patients self-mutilated or committed suicide out of despair.[7] Transsexual patients are helped by sympathetic assessment and intervention. However, transsexuals can be difficult patients to manage or treat. It is a rare disorder in which patients make their own diagnosis, 'I am transsexual', and prescribe their own treatment, 'I want sex-change hormones and surgery'. Patients can be demanding and impatient for the therapist's acquiescence to their tailor-made programme. They may be resentful for having to see a psychiatrist, holding the opinion that the desire for hormonal treatment and surgery should be sufficient, and psychiatric agreement should be unnecessary.

Some patients are manipulative and will threaten self-mutilation or suicide if their demands and time schedules for demands are not met. Patients need to know that psychological stability is a key ingredient to successful negotiation of the cross-gender living trial period 'Real Life

Test' (see below) and recommendation for surgery, and that suicidal behaviour is a contraindication to going forward.

During the past 30 years medical doctors and psychologists specializing in the treatment of transsexualism have worked to develop effective intervention strategies. Early on there was some optimism that extensive, prolonged psychotherapy could modify the patient's gender identity to conform to the patient's birth sex. However, in the vast majority of cases, this was not possible.[20]

During the past 20 years one project undertaken by the Harry Benjamin International Gender Dysphoria Association, the professional body dedicated to the study and treatment of transsexualism, has been setting an extensive series of requirements for evaluation and treatment of gender identity disordered people. This set of guidelines is known as the *Standards of Care*.[21] Their principal purpose is to assure that people presenting with dissatisfaction continuing to live in the sex role to which they were born undergo comprehensive psychiatric evaluation and enter into an appropriate treatment programme. The programme includes, in addition to ongoing psychiatric or psychological monitoring, possibly endocrine therapy and, depending on the outcome of the graduated trial period of cross-gender living, possibly sex reassignment surgical procedures. The philosophy of treatment is to do reversible procedures before those that are irreversible. Thus clothing change, name change, and cross-gender role socialization, would precede, in selected cases, endocrine treatment with its gradual somatic changes followed, in carefully selected cases, by surgical treatment.

The crux of the screening and evaluation of those people given the opportunity to demonstrate that they will benefit from cross-gender living, perhaps culminating in surgical treatment, is known as the 'Real Life Test'. This requires that patients who state their need to assume the other gender role live full-time for at least a year and preferably 2 years in that role. The test includes high doses of cross-sex hormones and full-time employment or full-time student status in the new role for at least a year. If patients can demonstrate to themselves and mental health experts that they have successfully negotiated the 'Real Life Test' and are adjusting better socially in this new gender role, they can be referred for surgery.

Hormonal effects

Response to hormonal treatment is variable between patients. This is particularly notable and potentially problematic for males. As with people born female, breast development spans a continuum. Patients may erroneously believe that more hormone will result in greater breast development. They neglect the fact that people born female have quite adequate female hormone production but the limiting factor is tissue response. In addition to breast development, male patients report increased hip and buttock fat, skin softening, and loss of sex drive and erection capacity.

Androgen treatment to the female results in voice deepening, facial hair growth, general body hair growth, menses cessation, clitoral hypertrophy, and increased sex drive.

Cross-sex hormonal effects are more pronounced in females. The deepening voice and beard growth and perhaps scalp hair loss can metamorphose the female's appearance dramatically. For the male, vocal retraining is required and perhaps surgical alteration of the larynx to effect a woman's voice. Extensive facial hair electrolysis is usually mandatory.

Surgery

Genital surgical treatment for the male patient includes penectomy, orchidectomy, and creation of a neovagina. The neovagina may be created from penile skin, perhaps augmented by other skin, or from a portion of large intestine.[22] The cosmetic result is usually very good.

The extent of sexual responsivity with the neovagina is anecdotal. Many patients report the subjective experience of orgasm but describe it in a different form from that experienced prior to surgery as a male. No physiological measures of the sexual response cycle have been reported with postoperative transsexual patients.[23]

Female transsexuals undergo bilateral mastectomy, and usually hysterectomy and ovariectomy. Genital surgery is an option taken by perhaps only half because of the limitations of phalloplasty. Two major approaches are utilized. One is creation of a micropenis from the androgen enlarged clitoris with relocation of the urethra to enable micturition while standing. Prosthetic testes can be incorporated into the labia sutured together. The microphallus will not permit vaginal penetration for intercourse but is erotically sensitive. Alternatively, phalloplasty involves major surgical interventions with scarring at donor sites such as the arm. The neophallus is not as close cosmetically to a natural penis as many patients want. It can be made more rigid with an implant and a conduit for urine may be surgically created.[24] A procedure transplanting and anastomosing a nerve from the arm to that enervating the clitoris offers promise of erotic sensation along the length of the neophallus.

Sex reassignment outcome

Follow-up reports on operated transsexuals are generally quite favourable. An early review of several follow-up studies,[25] reported on 283 male-to-female transsexuals. Results were judged satisfactory for 71 per cent, uncertain for 17 per cent, and unsatisfactory for 8 per cent. For 83 female-to-male transsexuals results were judged satisfactory for 81 per cent, uncertain for 13 per cent, and unsatisfactory for 6 per cent. A more recent report of a series from a Canadian centre considered reassignment successful in 46 of 50 male-to-female transsexuals and successful in all 61 female-to-male transsexuals.[26] In The Netherlands, of 55 male-to-female transsexuals, none regretted surgery and none had significant doubts regarding their reassignment status as women. Of 25 female-to-male transsexuals, at least 90 per cent were judged successful.[27] In another comprehensive review of the English language literature over a 10-year period for operated transsexuals, at least 90 per cent of male-to-female transsexuals were judged to be satisfactory or successful and over 95 per cent of female-to-male transsexuals were similarly judged successful.[28] The criteria for success in some studies include objective measures of psychological and vocational status, in others the criterion is limited to an absence of regret over the reassignment process.

One study is notable because it effected some randomization of treatment conditions.[29] It reported on 40 male-to-female transsexuals approved for surgery at the Charing Cross Hospital, London. As patients qualified for surgery they were randomly assigned to two groups. Half of the patients were operated on in 3 months and the other half were kept on a waiting list for about 2 years. All patients completed a standardized assessment at acceptance for surgery and at the end of 2 years of follow-up. The group that received the earlier surgery showed significant improvement in a range of psychometric measures and maintained employment. The unoperated group showed no improvement in psychological testing and deteriorated in employment.

Family management

Transsexual patients are often married and have children. When possible, the family should become part of the treatment process. Typically relations are strained with the marital partner of the transsexual and divorce is usual. Particularly when children are involved an effort should be made to deal with the feelings of betrayal or abandonment from the transsexual's spouse that contaminate the continuing relationship between transsexual parent and children. Often there is concern by the parents that the patient's transsexualism will impact adversely on the children. There is concern specifically in areas of gender identity of the children and peer group reactions to the knowledge that one of their age mate's parents is transsexual. However, in the author's research of children of transsexuals, totalling 34, who were living with or in regular contact with the transsexual parent, there were no instances of gender identity disorder in the children and no instances of peer group alienation that were especially problematic.[30] Children typically have many questions about the transsexual transformation of that parent that can be answered by the clinician, perhaps with the transsexual present.

The third sex

A recent development in the pattern of patients presenting clinically are those with a transgendered identity, popularly known as 'the third sex'. These males or females do not request 'sex change'. Rather, they want, if male, to be demasculinized and, if female, to be defeminized. Thus males want castration and penectomy but no oestrogen treatment and no neovagina, and females want mastectomy, perhaps hysterectomy, but no androgen treatment and no neophallus.

These patients pose a dilemma for clinicians. The crux of patient management for gender identity disorder is the 'Real Life Test' (see above), including cross-sex hormonal treatment, the prelude to possible surgical alteration. Reversible procedures precede those that are irreversible in this management strategy. But with these third-sex patients, no 'Real Life Test' is possible. They do not have a trial period. Guidelines for testing the rationality and stability of their requests need to evolve from the body of clinicians currently attempting management of this unique population.

Transsexual patient subgroups

Professionals not experienced in the treatment of large numbers of transsexual patients are often unaware that a substantial minority, perhaps a third of male-to-female transsexuals, are not sexually orientated to male partners. Many but not all of these patients have been previously married and are fathers, and many will be bisexual or remain sexually attracted to females only after reassignment surgery. Both younger and older male-to-female transsexuals may live as lesbian women after surgery. By contrast, a much smaller number of female-to-male transsexuals are sexually attracted to male partners or live as gay men after reassignment surgery. About 95 per cent are sexually attracted to female partners only.

In addition to the subtypes of transsexuals based on their sexual orientation, a substantial number of male transsexual patients evolve through a diagnostic phase more closely fitting fetishistic transvestism. These patients have been more masculine in general lifestyle and appearance than other male transsexuals, cross-dressing has been sexually arousing, and they have usually been heterosexually oriented. However, with the passage of time gender dysphoria increases and fetishistic components of cross-dressing diminish or disappear. Many have been sexually aroused by fantasies of themselves as women.[31] There is some evidence that males evolving through a fetishistic cross-dressing phase, presenting as somewhat older at gender identity clinics, have a poorer prognosis after surgery. This is marginally evident in some follow-up studies. Primarily, it is the progression through the 'Real Life Test' that becomes the critical management guideline for patients, irrespective of their background.

Gender identity as a disorder

A growing movement among transsexual people argues for removal of gender identity disorder from the psychiatric and medical lists of disorders or diseases. These advocates argue that their sexual identity is normal male or female and that surgical correction of their anatomical anomaly is all that is required to allow them to live as normal men or women. Their condition is depicted as distinctive from the recognized traditional forms of mental disorder such as schizophrenia or major depression. Furthermore, carrying a psychiatric diagnosis is stigmatizing.

One argument for inclusion of transsexualism in the diagnostic manual of disorders is that it follows the criteria of other entries, that is subjective distress and social disadvantage. Another considers third-party payment for treatment. It is unlikely that insurance carriers, private or governmental, would be prepared to fund intervention for a non-medical condition that could be dismissed as merely 'cosmetic'.

Legal issues

Part of the 'Real Life Test' of cross-gender living includes employment in the desired gender role. However, transsexuals may be the object of employment discrimination based on their transsexualism. In the United States transsexuals are not given legal protection against discrimination under Title VII, the federal antisex discrimination law.[32] Other potential sources of protection such as the Americans with Disabilities Act specifically exclude them. In the United Kingdom, in 1997, a ruling on an English case before the European Court of Justice held that antisex discrimination law, to which all European Union members were subject, did include transsexuals. Thus discrimination in employment was illegal sex discrimination.[33]

Changing sex on one's birth certificate can be an important step in the life of the postoperative transsexual. In its absence, the person's legal sex may remain in the preoperative status, and pose obstacles to a full life after treatment. Marriage is a key issue here. In the United

Kingdom, postoperative transsexuals cannot have a new birth certificate issued and change their legal sex. Thus a postoperative male-to-female transsexual cannot marry a male and a female-to-male transsexual cannot marry a female. Efforts to have the United Kingdom law declared in violation of the Human Rights Charter before the European Court have failed.[34] In the United States more than half the states permit birth certificate change, as do most Western European countries.[32]

References

1. Green, R. (1966). Transsexualism: mythological, historical and cross-cultural aspects. Appendix to *The transsexual phenomenon* (H. Benjamin). Julian Press, New York.
2. Abraham, F. (1931). Genital alteration in two male transvestites. *Zeitschrift Sexualwissenschaft*, **18**, 223–6.
3. Hoyer, N. (1933). *Man into woman: an authentic record of a change of sex*. E.P. Dutton, New York.
4. Hamburger, C., Sturup, G., and Dahl-Iversen, E. (1953). Transvestism: hormonal, psychiatric and surgical treatment. *Journal of the American Medical Association*, **12**, 391–6.
5. Hamburger, C. (1953). The desire for change of sex as shown by personal letters from 465 men and women. *Acta Endocrinologica*, **14**, 361–75.
6. Green, R. and Money, J. (ed.) (1969). *Transsexualism and sex reassignment*. Johns Hopkins Press, Baltimore, MD.
7. Benjamin, H. (1966). *The transsexual phenomenon*. Julian Press, New York.
8. Kesteren, P., Gooren, L., and Megens, J. (1996). An epidemiological and demographic study of transsexuals in The Netherlands. *Archives of Sexual Behavior*, **25**, 589–600.
9. Godlewski, J. (1988). Transsexualism and anatomic sex ratio reversal in Poland. *Archives of Sexual Behavior*, **17**, 547–8.
10. American Psychiatric Association (1994). *Diagnostic and statistical classification of diseases and related health problems* (4th edn). American Psychiatric Association, Washington, DC.
11. World Health Organization (1992). *International statistical classification of diseases and related health problems, 10th revision*. WHO, Geneva.
12. Eicher, W., Spoljar, M., Cleve, H., Murken, J., Richter, K., and Stengel-Rutkowski, S. (1979). H-Y antigen in trans-sexuality. *Lancet*, **ii**, 1137–8.
13. Wachtel, S., Green, R., Simon, N., *et al.* (1986). On the expression of H-Y antigen in transsexuals. *Archives of Sexual Behavior*, **15**, 49–66.
14. Zhou, J., Hoffman, M., Gooren, L., and Swaab, D. (1995). A sex difference in the human brain and its relation to transsexuality. *Nature*, **378**, 68–70.
15. Blanchard, R. (1997). Birth order and sibling sex ratio in homosexual versus heterosexual males and females. *Annual Review of Sex Research*, **8**, 27–67.
16. Green, R. and Keverne, E.B. The disparate maternal aunt–uncle ratio in male transsexuals: an explanation invoking genomic imprinting. *Journal of Theoretical Biology*, in press.
17. Turner, W. (1995). Homosexuality, type 1: an Xq 28 phenomenon. *Archives of Sexual Behavior*, **24**, 109–34.
18. Springer, S. and Deutsch, G. (1993). *Left brain, right brain* (4th edn). W.H. Freeman, New York.
19. Futterweit, W., Weiss, R., and Fagerstrom, R. (1986). Endocrine evaluation of 40 female-to-male transsexuals: increased frequency of polycystic ovarian disease in female transsexualism. *Archives of Sexual Behavior*, **15**, 69–78.
20. Pomeroy, W. (1975). The diagnosis and treatment of transvestites and transsexuals. *Journal of Sexual and Marital Therapy*, **1**, 215–24.
21. Harry Benjamin International Gender Dysphoria Association (1981). *The standards of care for gender identity disorder*. Symposion, Düsseldorf.
22. Schrang, E. (1998). Male-to-female feminizing genital surgery. In

Current concepts in transgender identity (ed. D. Denny), pp. 315–33. Garland, New York.

23. Green, R. (1998). Sexual functioning in post-operative transsexuals. *International Journal of Impotence Research*, **10** (Supplement 1), 22–4.

24. Laub, D., Eicher, W., and Laub, D. (1989). Penis construction in female-to-male transsexuals. In *Plastic surgery in the sexually handicapped* (ed. W. Eicher, F. Kubli, and F. Herms), pp. 113–28. Springer-Verlag, New York.

25. Pauly, I. (1981). Outcome of sex reassignment surgery for transsexuals. *Australian and New Zealand Journal of Psychiatry*, **15**, 45–51.

26. Blanchard, R., Steiner, B., Clemensen, L., and Dicky, R. (1989). Prediction of regrets in postoperative transsexuals. *Canadian Journal of Psychiatry*, **34**, 43–5.

27. Kuiper, B. and Cohen-Kettenis, P. (1988). Sex reassignment surgery. A study of 141 Dutch transsexuals. *Archives of Sexual Behavior*, **17**, 439–57.

28. Green, R. and Fleming, D. (1991). Transsexual surgery follow up: status in the 1990s. In *Annual review of sex research* (ed. J. Bancroft, C. Davis, and D. Weinstein). Society for the Scientific Study of Sex, Mount Vernon, IA.

29. Mate-Cole, C., Freschi, M., and Robin, A. (1990). A controlled study of psychological and social change after surgical gender reassignment in selected male transsexuals. *British Journal of Psychiatry*, **157**, 261–4.

30. Green, R. (1998). Transsexuals' children. *International Journal of Transgenderism*, **2**, 1–7.

31. Blanchard, R. (1989). The classification and labelling of non-homosexual gender dysphorics. *Archives of Sexual Behavior*, **18**, 315–34.

32. Green, R. (1992). *Sexual science and the law*. Harvard University Press, Cambridge, MA.

33. *P* v. *S and Cornwall* (1996). ECRI-2143 C-13/94.

34. Cossey (1989). ECHR (16/1989/176/232), Vol. 184, Series A.

4.12 Personality disorders

4.12.1 Introduction to personality disorders

Juan López-Ibor

Psychiatry and abnormal behaviours

Psychiatry is the study of mental disorders. In this chapter we consider how and up to what point personality disorders should be considered as psychiatric disorders.

Descriptions of individuals with behavioural characteristics of a negative moral or social value exist in every culture. At times, most societies have established institutions in which all types of marginalized people have been confined, as recorded by Foucault in his *Histoire de la Folie à l'Âge Classique*.[1]

In 1575, the first description of individual character from a clinical perspective was contributed by the physician Juan Huarte de San Juan in his *Examination of Wits*.[2]

A distinction between immoral behaviour and mental illness was established in France at the end of the eighteenth century, coinciding with the birth of modern psychiatry,. For this reason the Marquis de Sade was expelled from the Chârenton Hospital even though he had been admitted by an order (*lêttre de cachet*) from King Louis XVI because, in words of the director, 'he is not ill, his only madness is vice'.[1] The same reasoning was applied in the case of a man who, in an attack of rage, threw a woman into a well; Pinel[3] considered that he was not mentally ill since his ability to judge was clear and intact and he presented no delusional ideas, although his behaviour was characteristic of a mental patient. Consequently, this murderer was diagnosed as *manie sans délire* and his madness was classified as **reasoning madness** (*folie raisonnante*). This same idea was expressed 150 years latter by Cleckley[4] who proposed that the social maladaptation of psychopaths is of such high degree that they should considered as psychotic—personality disorder is a mask of sanity.

Prichard, in his *Treatise on Insanity and Other Disorders Affecting the Mind*,[5] defined the concept of **moral insanity** from which, together with the moral degeneration described by Morel,[6] the modern concepts of **psychopathy** and **personality disorders** are derived.

Difficulties in the study of personality disorders

Two factors have prevented the development of scientific knowledge in this field: first the negative evaluation of the concept of moral insanity, and second the dualism inherent in psychopathology.

The stigma of personality disorder

The diagnosis of personality disorder generally implies the idea of untreatability and frequently leads to a lack of proper medical care. This attitude is the expression of a negative, moralizing, and, according to Tyrer *et al.*,[7] delusional attitude of the doctor towards the patient.

The preparation of the Green Book on *The Health of the Nation* in the United Kingdom raised a problem of great interest with respect to personality disorders.[8] On the one hand, they have a prevalence between 7 and 13 per cent in the general population and of 20 to 30 per cent in general medical practice. On the other hand, they rarely appear in isolation and when associated with other disorders their prognosis worsens and they have an impact on length of stay and treatment cost. They are frequently associated with alterations of eating behaviour, alcohol and substance abuse, tobacco abuse, accidents, HIV infections, other mental disorders, antisocial behaviour, and sexual promiscuity. In addition, their demands on health services are atypical in the sense that such patients usually appear with great urgency, in moments of crisis, and with poor tolerance of any kind of authority, including that of the doctor himself.

Cusack and Malaney[9] posed the question as to whether patients with antisocial personality disorders are 'bad' or 'mad'. They attempted to establish differential criteria in order to show that if patients with an antisocial personality disorder are not 'mad', then they must be considered as 'bad' and therefore must be delivered to the judicial system, after diagnosis and treatment for any secondary symptomatology.

Dualism in psychopathology

Dualism has been present in psychiatry since its origins as specialty. According to Griesinger:[10]

> It is time that [mental medicine] should be cultivated as a branch of brain pathology and of [the study of] the nervous system in general, and to apply serious diagnostic methods used in all branches of medicine. ... Besides this purely medical element, mental medicine has another essential one and which gives a special and proper character to this part of the healing art; it is the

psychological study of the aberrations of the intelligence observed in mental illnesses.

The radical separation between mental–brain illnesses and 'aberrations of intelligence' is fundamental to modern psychopathology. Schneider[11] distinguished between psychoses as pathological conditions of the brain (disease or defective structure) and variations of the psychic life. Abnormal personalities, personality disorders, and neurotic disorders belong to the second category.

Schneider[12] defines some **abnormal personalities**, in the statistical sense, which include those individuals whose form of feeling, experience, and behaving differs to a certain degree from what is considered to be normal for most individuals in a social group. Some of these are **psychopathic personalities** who, as a result of their abnormality, suffer or make others suffer. It should be stressed that, according to Schneider's definition of personality and the dualism of his psychopathological system, the only possible criterion for defining a clinical condition in the absence of brain pathology is suffering—pathos. Schneider had to add suffering inflicted on others (social suffering) in order to be able to include certain kinds of abnormal personalities characterized by the absence of personal suffering (heartless psychopaths, sociopaths).

The criteria of induced suffering which characterizes some psychopathic personalities, defined following Schneider, is not generally acceptable in medicine and it is surprising that this has been little criticized. As pointed out by López-Ibor,[13] the clue lies in Schneider's definition of personality which excludes any biological substratum. Nowadays it is impossible to maintain such a reductionist perspective, and it is through the study of changes in this biological substratum that the morbid character of personality disorders can be understood.

Models of personality

The study of the personality has been based on two types of model—categorical and dimensional.

Categorical models

Categorical models consider discontinuous personality categories. This type of model is used in DSM-IV[14] and ICD-10[15] because of the need for a specific diagnostic, i.e. a categorical approach.

In modern nosology the categorization of illness is based on the presenting symptoms and not on their aetiopathology, and says nothing about the nature of the disorders themselves. In the case of personality disorders, the categorization does not affirm or deny that they are disorders or illnesses, nor does it indicate where the symptoms differ from non-morbid behaviour patterns.

There is a high comorbidity among personality disorders and between personality disorders and other mental disorders. The main problem is to determine the exact nature of this comorbidity. In comorbid cases, the personality disorder could be a predisposing factor, a consequence, or an attenuated form of the mental disorder, or it could be independent of the mental disorder. The fact that the association between a mental disorder and a personality disorder is not always fortuitous has been shown by the observation that effective treatment of the former can lead to the disappearance of the latter, as has been demonstrated in the treatment of obsessive–compulsive patients with pharmacotherapy and behavioural therapy.[16]

The better a personality disorder is understood and the more biological correlations are found in it, the more likely it is to be transferred from Axis II to Axis I of DSM-IV, i.e. to be classified as a 'real' disorder. Epileptic personality, depressive personality, cyclothymic personality, and even schizothymic personality are now classified as Axis I disorders in ICD-10.

Dimensional models

Jung[17] made the first important contribution to the dimensional concept of the personality, based on the concept of trait or disposition. A trait implies a disposition, a permanent inclination towards behaving in a determinant way. Traits are dimensions along which persons can be classified. The various dimensional models are based on the supposition that we all share the same personality structure, differing only in the various combinations of traits. These models have benefited from innovative statistical techniques which enable the different qualities of an individual character to be grouped around factors of correlation or dimensions.

The main problem is to define the number of dimensions that define personality and to establish whether or not these traits are universal. Eysenck[18] identified three basic types of personality—extraversion–introversion, neuroticism, and psychoticism—each including many levels of traits. The problem is solved by establishing correlations between the dimensions and biological, cultural, and genetic factors. For Eysenck and Eysenck,[19] the concept of arousal level is essential. Individuals have an optimal activation level of specific systems of the central nervous system—the better they feel, the better they will perform. This approach has been developed by many authors including Zuckermann,[20] who described sensation-seeking behaviour, Oreland et al.,[21] and Siever and Davis,[22] who proposed new traits and dimensions.

Cloninger[23] initially proposed three dimensions: novelty-seeking, harm avoidance, and reward dependence. More recently, Cloninger[24] has attempted to overcome the dichotomy between dimensional and categorical models by using four temperamental dimensions (novelty-seeking, harm avoidance, reward dependence, and persistence), which are life-long and stable, and three character dimensions (self-direction, co-operation, and self-transcendency) which are variable and susceptible to environmental influences and development.

The five-factor model, based on factorial studies and individual differences,[25] has been widely accepted. It comprises the personality dimensions openness, conscientiousness, extraversion, agreeableness, and neuroticism, known by the acronym OCEAN. About 40 per cent of individual personality differences can be explained in terms of heredity.[26] In the five-factor model the same proportion does not apply to each factor; openness to experience appears to have the greatest hereditary input, whereas conscientiousness appears to have the least.

Personality disorders versus personality variants

It is necessary to establish a clear distinction between personality disorders and personality variants, and to view the former as true morbid entities. ICD-10 allows us to differentiate, at least theoretically, personality disorders that appear in the chapter on mental disorders from personalities relevant for medicine in Chapter Z. Personality disorders should be characterized by the presence of symptoms, and relevant personalities by their traits. Symptoms are used as diagnostic criteria in a categorical classification, while psychological traits can be classified according to dimensions.

Personality variants relevant to medicine, although not morbid, play an important role in the aetiopathogenesis of illnesses or are important for prognosis and rehabilitation. The study of the variants of personality also reminds the practitioner of the necessity to identify the uniqueness of the patient's personality.[27]

Biological substrates of personality and personality disorders

Many investigators have concluded that there appears to be a high genetic component in the aetiology of schizoid, depressive, psychopathic, and introversive traits.

Personality disorders and major psychiatric disorders

Personality disorders have been considered as belonging to the spectrum of major psychiatric disorders. However, it must be remembered that external events, such as brain damage (organic personality disorders), or the psychological impact of a catastrophic event may also lead to personality changes. Severe psychiatric disorders may have a repercussion on the personality of the patient, and other illnesses may also have this effect. For example, chronic pain (of organic nature) can be accompanied by a profound personality change (algogenic psychosyndrome). Hypochondria or dissociative symptoms and traits may become relevant only after the patient has suffered an illness, or a problem related to diagnosis or treatment, or a problem involving the patient–physician relationship.

According to the hypothesis of a spectrum of disorders, personality disorders can often be treated by the same method as those applied to the major psychiatric disorders to which they are related. Patients with anxious or avoidant personality disorder may respond to anxiolytic medication, patients with borderline personality disorder may respond to lithium and antidepressives, patients with schizotypal personality disorder may respond to antipsychotic agents, and patients with disorders characterized by poor impulse control may respond to antidepressives with a selective serotonergic action.

Impulsivity and personality disorders

According to Santayana,[28] humans can be described as beings 'constitutionally inclined to resist impulses and to take long-term perspectives'. On the basis of this principle, two types of psychiatric disorders can be considered: those characterized by excessive impulsivity, and those characterized by excessive control of impulses. Behaviours leading to sociopathy and to the commission of certain types of offence belong to the first category. The term 'impulsive madness' was used in German literature. Jaspers[29] published an article on impulsive madness, referring it to homesickness and uprooting.

The balance between social and individual norms is related to the origin of mental disorders. Durkheim[30] introduced the concept of **anomia** when describing a particular form of suicide in individuals who perceive that their own norms and values are no longer relevant and that their relation to the community is weak or non-existent. However, the opposite may also occur. Kraus[31] coined the term hypernomia for premorbid personality traits of depressive patients, which consist in an exaggerated form of adaptation to social norms. This personality type is the converse of the impulsive madness that can be characterized as **hyponomic**.

We have proposed the term **dysnomic** for obsessive patients who show a distorted adaptation to social norms.[32,33] For example, patients with obsessions and compulsions related to cleanliness usually appear to be extremely dirty because of their fear of contamination and their unrealistic compulsions, which are based more on 'magic' control than on efficient behaviour oriented towards concrete goals.

The common link in the psychopathology of obsessive–compulsive disorders and the group of impulsive disorders experienced by the **impulsivists**[34] is poor control of the impulses, in the sense that novel interior or exterior experiences are not converted into adequate behavioural patterns. Rather, obsessives abandon actions uncompleted and impulsivists behave in a disorganized manner (acting out). In both cases, 'the insignificant substitutes the significant'.[35] From a neurobiological point of view, there are serotonergic deficits in both cases, although of different types. The function of serotonin is to modulate the impulse to act.

Psychoneuroendocrinological research in personality disorders

Coccaro et al.[36] found a blunted prolactin response to stimulation with fenfluramine in patients with personality disorders with physical aggression and motor impulsivity. Moreno et al.[37] obtained similar results in patients with a borderline personality disorder and impulsive suicidal behaviour, and a blunted response to prolactin after stimulation with clomipramine in pathological gamblers.

Insel et al.[38] observed that behavioural changes (increase in anxiety and obsessive–compulsive symptoms) and physiological changes (variations in body temperature) occurred after the administration of methylchlorphenylpiperazine to patients with obsessive–compulsive disorders. This suggested a hypersensibility to serotonin receptors, compensating a presynaptic function deficit.

Studies by the author's group have provided some clarification of this problem.[39–44] First, unlike patients with impulsive disorders, patients with obsessive–compulsive disorders do not have a blunted prolactin response to the clomipramine challenge test when compared with the control group. However, if the sample of patients is divided according to the depressive symptoms present, those with a pure obsessive–compulsive disorder without depression have a high response to CMI. The presence of a secondary depression produces a blunting of the prolactin response as observed in depressive disorders in general.

Recent research has revealed the impact of social conditions on the neuroendocrine regulation of the individual, particularly with respect to the adaptation to stressful situations. In our sample of patients with a borderline personality disorder and impulsive suicidal behaviour we have found high basal concentrations of cortisol (suggesting a high level of stress) and a very blunted response to the stimulus (suggesting a reduced capacity to respond to external stimulus) compared with the control group. We have found the same pattern in heroin-dependent individuals receiving naltrexone maintenance treatment.

A clue to the interpretation of these results lies in the work of Sapolsky,[45] who has studied the adaptation to stress of baboons in the Serengeti savannah in Africa. Males of a lower rank have consistently high concentrations of the stress hormone hydrocortisone in their blood, whereas the concentration is lower in the dominant males. However, in the dominant males hydrocortisone concentrations increase rapidly at times of stress and decrease once the situation is resolved, whereas the lower-order males, who live in a permanent state of stress, are unable to initiate more adaptive resources (increase hydrocortisone secretion) when new stressful events appear. These patterns are the consequence and not the cause of the rank (if the opposite were true, the baboons who were physiologically better able to respond to stressful situations would achieve a higher rank). During periods of revolution, members of the colony hold successively different ranks and, although there is always one dominant animal, the stability of the society is lost and with it the stress-adapted physiology of the dominant males who show prolonged increased hydrocortisone concentrations like the rest of the group. When calm is established again, the normal pattern related to the hierarchical rank of the baboons is restored regardless of what their cortisol secretion pattern was prior to the revolution.

Impulsivity has been correlated with a low platelet monoamine oxidase (**MAO**) activity. Carrasco et al.[46] have studied two groups of professions characterized, at least in principle, by their impulsivity, extraversion, and sensation- and novelty-seeking traits—bullfighters and bomb-disposal officers. They were compared with pathological gamblers and with non-impulsive controls. Their psychological traits were assessed using a series of questionnaires and their platelet MAO activity was measured. The bomb-disposal officers did not differ from the control group, which shows that the process used to select them is very effective. However, bullfighters obtained the highest scores in the traits of impulsivity, extraversion, and sensation-seeking and had reduced platelet MAO activity. Pathological gamblers obtained the highest impulsivity score and the lowest platelet MAO activity of all groups. In addition, the range of MAO concentration in the gamblers was very narrow and all of them showed low MAO activity, whereas in the bullfighters this range was as large as in the controls and many of them had normal values.

This finding suggest that normal impulsive and sensation-seeking behaviours, present for example in the bullfighters, correlate with a diminished platelet MAO activity, which represents a dimensional marker of a temperamental trait. However, in the morbid forms of the behaviour, as in the case of pathological gamblers, the relation with platelet MAO represents a non-dimensional alteration resulting from a pathological change of serotonergic activity, among other factors.

Cosmetic psychopharmacology?

Kamer[47] has described how a selective serotonin uptake inhibitor used for the treatment of depression and for other psychiatric alterations can remove personality traits in some people. He has considered traits previously considered as an expression of human misery or, in some cases, as the consequence of negative childhood experiences. Kamer even questions whether there could be a 'pandemic' of cosmetic psychopharmacologies which would lead to the disappearance of phenomena such as anguish which are essential for personal realization in the arts, religion, and creativity. In the light of present knowledge, it can be deduced that the characteristics of personality disorders do not have to be present in the traits of a normal personality. The disappearance of clinical symptoms as a result of pharmacological treatment directed at potentiating the serotonergic metabolism of, for example, a violent or obsessive patient is not the same as modifying personality traits which contribute to determining that an ambitious, artistically oriented, and aggressive young male becomes a bullfighter.

Cosmetic psychopharmacology does not exist. What does exist is the treatment of personality disorders, which are real illnesses characterized by symptoms and by a biological substrate. These disorders are amenable to treatment, although further research on many aspects is still required. In the past, these disorders would have been considered as a form of moral degeneration.

References

1. Foucault, M. (1961). *Folie et déraison. Histoire de la folie à l'âge classique.* Plon, Paris.
2. Huarte de San Juan, J. (1575). *Examen de ingenios para las ciencias.* Reprinted by Esteban de Torre, Madrid, 1977.
3. Pinel, P.H. (1809). *Traité médico-philosophique sur l'alienation mentale.* Brosson, Paris.
4. Cleckley, H. (1941). *The mask of sanity.* Henry Kimpton, London.
5. Prichard, J.C. (1835). *A treatise on insanity and other disorders affecting the mind.* Sherwood, Gilbert and Piper, London.
6. Morel, B. (1859). *Traité des dégénérescences physiques, intellectuelles et morales de l'espèce humaine.* Paris.
7. Tyrer, P., Casey, P., and Ferguson, B. (1991). Personality disorder in perspective. *British Journal of Psychiatry*, **159**, 463–71.
8. Norton, K. (1992). Health of the nation: personality disorders. *British Medical Journal*, **304**, 255–6.
9. Cusack, J.R. and Malaney, K.R. (1992). Patients with antisocial personality disorder. Are they bad or mad? *Postgraduate Medicine*, **91**, 341–4, 349–52, 355.
10. Griesinger, W. (1872). *Gesammelte Abhandlungen.* Vol. I, *Psychiatrische und nervenpathologische Abhandlungen.* Reprinted by Bonset, Amsterdam, 1968.
11. Schneider, K. (1971). *Klinische Psychopathologie* (9th edn). Thieme Verlag, Stuttgart.
12. Schneider, K. (1950). *Die psychopathischen Persönlichkeiten* (9th revised edn). Deuticke, Vienna.
13. López-Ibor, J.J. (1966). *Las neurosis como enfermedades del ánimo.* Gredos, Madrid.
14. American Psychiatric Association (1994). *Diagnostic and statistical manual of mental disorders* (4th edn). American Psychiatric Association, Washington, DC.
15. World Health Organization (1992). *The ICD-10 classification of mental and behavioural disorders—clinical descriptions and diagnostic guidelines.* World Health Organization, Geneva..
16. Ricciardi, J.N., Baer, L., Jenike, M.A., Fischer, S.C., Sholtz, D., and Buttolph, M.L. (1992). Changes in DSM-III-R axis II diagnoses following treatment of obsessive–compulsive disorder. *American Journal of Psychiatry*, **149**, 829–31.
17. Jung, C.J. (1966). *Two essays of analytical psychology.* Princeton University Press.
18. Eysenck, H.J. (1970). *The structure of human personality.* Methuen, London.
19. Eysenck, H.J. and Eysenck, M.W. (1985). *Personality and individual differences: a natural science approach.* Plenum Press, New York.
20. Zuckermann, M. (1979). *Sensation seeking: beyond the optimal level of arousal.* Erlbaum, Hillsdale, NJ.
21. Oreland, L., Wiberg, A., Åsberg, M., *et al.* (1981). Platelet MAO activity

and monoamine metabolism in CSF in depressed and suicidal patients and in healthy controls. *Psychiatric Research*, **4**, 21–9.

22. Siever, L.J. and Davis, K.L. (1991). A psychobiological perspective on the personality disorders. *American Journal of Psychiatry*, **148**, 1647–58.

23. Cloninger, C.R. (1987). A systematic method for clinical description and classification of personality variants. *Archives of General Psychiatry*, **44**, 573–88.

24. Cloninger, C.R. (1996). A psychobiological model of temperament and character. Fundamental findings for use in clinical practice. In *New research in psychiatry* (ed. H. Häfner and E.M. Wolpert), pp. 95–112. Hogrefe and Huber, Göttingen.

25. McCrae, R.R. and John, O.P. (1992). An introduction to the five-factor model and its applications. *Journal of Personality*, **60**, 175–213.

26. Loehlin, J.C. (1992). *Genes and environment in personality development*. Sage, Newbury Park, CA.

27. Janca, A., Kastrup, M., Katschnig, H., López-Ibor, J.J., Jr, Mezzich, J., and Sartorius, N. (1996). The ICD-10 multiaxial system for use in adult psychiatry: structure and applications. *Journal of Nervous and Mental Disease*, **184**, 191–2.

28. Santayana, G. (1905–6). The life of reason. In *Selected critical writings of George Santayana*, Vol. 2 (ed. N. Henfrey), pp. 189–234. Cambridge University Press.

29. Jaspers, K. (1909). *Heimweh und Verbrechen*, Vogel, Leipzig.

30. Durkheim, E. (1951). *Suicide*. Free Press, Glencoe, IL.

31. Kraus, A. (1977). *Sozial Verhalten und Psychosen manisch-depressiver*. Enke, Stuttgart.

32. López-Ibor, J.J., Jr (1991). Obsessive–compulsive disorder and other disorders. *European Neuropsychopharmacology*, **1**, 275–9.

33. López-Ibor, J.J., Jr (1993). *La personalidad en medicina y sus trastornos*. Instituto de España, Real Academia Nacional de Medicina, Madrid.

34. Lacey, J.H. and Evans, C.D.H. (1986). The impulsivist: a multi-impulsive personality disorder. *British Journal of Addiction*, **81**, 641–9.

35. Janet, P. (1903). *Les obsessions et la psychasthenie*. Alcan, Paris.

36. Coccaro, E.F., Siever, L.J., Klar, H.M., *et al.* (1990). Serotonergic studies in patients with affective and personality disorders: correlates with suicidal and impulsive agressive behavior. *Archives of General Psychiatry*, **46**, 587–99.

37. Moreno, I., Saíz-Ruiz, J., and López-Ibor, J.J., Jr (1991). Serotonin and gambling dependence. *Human Psychopharmacology, Clinical and Experimental*, **6**, 9–12.

38. Insel, T., Mueller, E.A., and Altermann, I. (1985). Obsessive–compulsive disorder and serotonin. Is there a connection? *Biological Psychiatry*, **20**, 1174–88.

39. López-Ibor, J.J., Saíz Ruiz, J., and Moral Iglesias, L. (1989). Neuroendocrine challenges in the diagnosis of depressive disorders. *British Journal of Psychiatry*, **154**, 73–6.

40. López-Ibor, J.J., Jr, Viñas Pifarré, R., and Saíz Ruiz, J. (1990). Bases biológicas del trastorno obsesivo compulsivo. *Actas Lusoespañolas de Neurologia, Psiquiatria y Ciencias Afines*, **18**, 306–16.

41. López-Ibor, J.J., Jr, Lana, F., and Saíz, J. (1991). Serotonin, impulsiveness and aggression in humans. In *Serotonin related psychiatric syndromes: clinical and therapeutic links* (ed. G.B. Cassano and H.S. Akiskal), pp. 35–9. Royal Society of Medicine, London.

42. López-Ibor, J.J., Jr (1992). Serotonin and psychiatric disorders. *International Journal of Clinical Psychopharmacology*, **7**, 5–11.

43. López-Ibor, J.J., Jr, Saíz Ruiz, J., and Moreno Oliver, I. (1992). Ludomanía: estudio clínico y terapéutico-evolutivo de un grupo de jugadores patológicos. *Actas Lusoespañolas de Neurologia, Psiquiatria y Ciencias Afines*, **20**, 189–97.

44. Saíz, J., López-Ibor, J.J., Jr., Viñas, R., and Hernández, M. (1992). The clomipramine challenge test in obsessive compulsive disorder. *International Journal of Clinical Psychopharmacology*, **7**, 41–2.

45. Sapolsky, R.M. (1990). Adrenocortical function, social rank, and personality among wild baboons. *Biological Psychiatry*, **15**, 862–78.

46. Carrasco, J.L., Saíz-Ruiz, J., Moreno, I., and López-Ibor, J.J., Jr (1992).

Baja actividad de la monoamino oxidasa plaquetaria en el juego patológico. *Anales de Psiquiatría*, **8**, 72.

47. Kamer, P.D. (1993). *Listening to Prozac*. Viking, New York.

4.12.2 General clinical description of personality disorders

Armand W. Loranger

During the past two decades there has been an unprecedented interest in the personality disorders. This is due in no small measure to the introduction in 1980 of the American Psychiatric Association's multi-axial classification system.[1] This influential nosology assigned a separate axis to the personality disorders. An indication of the dramatic impact of that innovation is a statistic on diagnostic practice at a leading university hospital in the United States.[2] There was a more than twofold increase in the diagnosis of personality disorders (19.1 per cent to 49.2 per cent) when 5143 consecutive admissions during the last 5 years of DSM-II (1975–1979) were compared with 5771 patients admitted during the initial 5 years of DSM-III (1981–1985). The increase was not due to artefacts like a change in the theoretical orientation of the staff, differences in the pathways of referral, demographics of the patient population, or reimbursement formulas. This was demonstrated when the transition from one classification system to the other occurred at midyear in 1980. When the first and last 6 months of that year were compared, the statistics were very similar (16.6 to 52.4 per cent).

Of no small significance is the fact that 97 per cent of the patients with a personality disorder also had other psychiatric conditions, typically anxiety, mood, alcohol, drug, and eating disorders. Presumably in the pre-DSM-III era, clinicians believed that such Axis I diagnoses usually provided an adequate description of a patient's current illness, and a sufficient explanation for the subjective distress or social and occupational impairment that often accompanied it. This raises the interesting question of whether personality disorders were previously underdiagnosed, or are now overdiagnosed. Although a definitive answer is not immediately forthcoming, the question does bring to the fore some fundamental issues about the nature of personality disorders.

According to DSM-III and its revisions, personality disorders are characterized by maladaptive traits that cause subjective distress or significant impairment in social or occupational functioning. The behaviour is deeply ingrained and inflexible, displayed in a wide range of personal and social situations, enduring rather than episodic, and has its onset by adolescence or early adulthood. Although these requirements also describe certain features of some mental state or Axis I disorders, they are not absolutely essential for their diagnosis.

Not all the mentally ill have personality disorders, but like everyone else they do have personalities. Since many of the criteria used to diagnose personality disorders are exaggerations of traits observed in the general population, there may be a temptation to lower the threshold for a particular criterion and label a trait pathological, when it is within the broad, somewhat arbitrary, limits of normality. This may be more likely to occur when the classification system requires that a decision regarding the presence or absence of a personality disorder be made for all patients.

It is sometimes difficult, even for the experienced clinician, to disentangle personality disorders from other psychiatric conditions. The availability of a separate axis for personality disorders may bias the decision-making process in that direction. This may be compounded by the error introduced by trait-state artefacts,[3] a phenomenon known to astute clinicians long before it was discovered by psychometricians. It is not always easy to penetrate the symptoms of other disorders, and to reconstruct a patient's premorbid personality. A common example is the depressed patient who appears introverted, but whose family and acquaintances are quick to point out that he is actually quite extraverted when his usual self. Clinicians may succumb to such artefacts when they view a patient in the midst of an episode of illness.

This is not to suggest that most personality disorders are merely Axis I disorders masquerading as Axis II. For example, I do not share the view of some that borderlines are merely misclassified bipolar II disorders. However, the more prominent that anxiety or an abnormal mood are in the clinical picture, the greater the potential for error. All other things being equal, there is less likelihood of misdiagnosing an antisocial or schizoid disorder than a borderline or avoidant one. In dealing with egosyntonic conditions, it is usually not necessary to rule out anxiety and mood disorders as the reason for the clinical presentation. However, with egodystonic disorders, there are circumstances when the ultimate diagnostic decision may have to await the successful treatment of the Axis I disorder, in order to determine whether there is any residue of what previously appeared to be the manifestations of a personality disorder.

Little is known about the other reasons for the frequent co-occurrence of personality disorders and mental state disorders.[4] In the absence of epidemiological data, it is possible that the current statistics on the subject, which are derived from treated cases, may overstate the relationship. Those with two disorders may be more likely to seek treatment than those with only one. For patients with similar disorders, for example social phobia and avoidant personality, the explanation may reside in overlapping symptomatology, shared aetiologies, or an imperfect nosology.

One disorder may also create a greater vulnerability to another, as does, for example, AIDS with pneumonia. The situation is further complicated by conditions like substance abuse and eating disorders, where the chronology of their appearance, and therefore the direction of the putative causal connection with personality, is not always readily identifiable. Some Axis I and Axis II distinctions are also somewhat arbitrary, particularly when the disorders have a wide range of severity or are viewed as part of a spectrum. ICD-10 lists schizotypal under schizophrenia and related conditions, while DSM-IV considers it a personality disorder.

The term 'comorbidity' is frequently used to describe the association of personality disorders with other psychiatric conditions. If the term is meant to imply the presence of a distinctly different clinical entity, this is probably ill-advised. At the present time, in the absence of more definitive data on the subject, the expression 'co-occurrence' is probably preferable. The added presence of a personality disorder is often but not invariably associated with a poorer response to the treatment of mental state disorders like anxiety and depression.[5] But there are also reports suggesting that the presence of some specific personality disorders, for example the dependent type, may augur a more favourable response to treatment, perhaps due to greater compliance.[5]

It is debatable whether reserving a separate axis for personality disorders has actually led to their overdiagnosis. Still it is worth considering the pros and cons of having a different kind of Axis II. Personality disorders might be returned to the primary axis where they were in DSM-II, and still are in ICD-10. Axis II could then be used to provide a concise description of the most salient premorbid personality traits of all patients, with the possible exception of those with a personality disorder. Implicitly this would revive a distinction made in early twentieth-century German psychiatry. Traits were considered pathogenic when they were aetiologically linked to the principal manifestations of the clinical syndrome, as with personality disorders. They were pathoplastic when they merely coloured or modified the expression, course, or outcome of a clinical syndrome. Consider, for example, two patients with unipolar depression, one introverted, modest, and conscientiousness, the other extraverted, exhibitionistic, and dependent. The comprehension and management of their depressions would likely present quite different challenges to the clinician.

Such an alternative classification would not be without problems of its own. Like the current system it might be susceptible to trait-state artefacts. A more formidable hurdle, perhaps, would be determining the array of normal traits that should be used to characterize a patient's personality, as well as the method of assessing them. One would soon encounter the considerable divide that separates clinicians from psychologists devoted to the study of normal personality, most notably the conspicuous lack of integration and cross-fertilization of ideas.

Psychiatrists generally favour categorical classification systems, while students of normal personality usually prefer dimensional taxonomies. Categorical classification has a long clinical tradition, and it has proved to be a very effective shorthand form of communication. Ideally, a category should not only specify the defining features of a disorder, but it should also have points of rarity with normality and other disorders. Personality disorders like many other mental as well as physical disorders do not always conform to this ideal, but that does not negate the usefulness of categorical classification. Advocates of dimensional taxonomies also argue that because many abnormal personality traits exist on a continuum with normality, dichotomizing them diminishes the reliability of diagnosis. There is no inherent reason, however, that clinicians have to choose between dimensional and categorical classifications. Dimensions can be used to supplement categorical information, witness their long-standing use in the diagnosis of mental retardation and hypertension.

The methods of assessment employed by clinicians and personality psychologists often differ. The delineation of the personality disorders emerged primarily from clinical observation. Therefore, the interview approximates the clinical diagnostic process more than the self-administered questionnaires favoured by many psychologists. However, there are data from the pre-DSM-III era[6] and the field trials of DSM-III and ICD-10[7] indicating that clinicians tend to agree less about the diagnosis of personality disorders than they do about many other mental disorders. This has been the inspiration for the development of several semistructured clinical interviews to improve diagnostic reliability. These instruments were primarily intended to encourage investigators to employ more uniform methods of case identification in their research, in order to facilitate the comparison and generalization of results. The interviews, however, also have heuristic value, and some clinicians have found them useful in their practice.

Perhaps the most widely used and extensively tested semistructured interview of this kind is the International Personality Disorder Examination (**IPDE**)[8,9] It was developed for international and cross-cultural use, as part of the World Health Organization (**WHO**) instrumentation package, and is available in separate modules[10] based on either ICD-10[11] or DSM-IV.[12] The 67 items for ICD-10 and 99 items for DSM-IV are arranged topically under six headings: Work, Self, Interpersonal relationships, Affects, Reality testing, and Impulse control. In addition to diagnoses, the interview provides dimensional scores for each disorder based on its diagnostic criteria, regardless of whether the subject has the disorder. There is a detailed item-by-item scoring manual that defines the scope and meaning of each criterion, and that provides anchor points for scoring. The interview takes into account the age at onset and the duration of the behaviour, and it requires substantiation of responses with anecdotes and examples. The scoring also has provision for information from informants. At the conclusion of the interview, the final algorithmic integration of the scores is done clerically or with a personal computer. The IPDE is designed for use by experienced clinicians, namely those capable of making independent psychiatric diagnoses. It is available in more than 20 languages, and training in its use is available at WHO centres around the world. Table 1 displays a sample item from the interview.

The IPDE was subjected to a worldwide field trial that involved 716 patients examined by 58 psychiatrists and clinical psychologists at 14 clinical facilities in Austria, England, Germany, India, Japan, Kenya, Luxembourg, The Netherlands, Norway, Switzerland, and the United States. The inter-rater agreement and temporal stability of the interview were comparable to that reported with similar instruments for the psychoses, anxiety, mood, and substance use disorders. This was true despite the fact that the IPDE was subjected to an unusually exacting test with culturally and linguistically diverse patients in North America, Europe, Africa, and Asia. Although the WHO study was not epidemiological in nature, it did provide evidence that the personality disorders in DSM and ICD, despite their obvious origins in European and American psychiatry, were present, identifiable, and clinically meaningful, in a variety of nations and cultures. Not surprisingly, the study also found that dimensional measures were more reliable than categorical ones, additional evidence in support of the argument for retaining both methods of assessment.

The literature suggests that self-administered personality questionnaires are especially prone to false–positive diagnoses and should not be used to make psychiatric diagnoses.[13] This does not undermine their potential value as screening instruments.[14] Nor does it diminish their usefulness as economical, objective measures of the traits that underlie a particular diagnostic category. Indeed, if future nosologies should include an axis for listing normal premorbid personality traits, it is inevitable that the optimal method of assessment would be some form of personality questionnaire. A number of such inventories already exist, but because of the terminology and constructs they employ, many of them do not appeal to clinicians, or they are wedded to a particular theory of personality not favoured by some.

The author recently developed such a personality questionnaire

Table 1 Sample item from the International Personality Disorder Examination (IPDE)

Is excessively devoted to work and productivity to the exclusion of leisure activities and friendships (not accounted for by obvious economic necessity)
DSM–IV obsessive–compulsive disorder: Criterion 3

Do you spend so much time working that you don't have any time left for anything else?
If yes: Tell me about it.

Do you spend so much time working that you (also) neglect other people?
If yes: Tell me about it.

The examiner should be alert to the use of rationalizations to defend the behaviour. The fact that work itself is pleasurable to the subject should not influence the scoring. There is no requirement that the subject actually enjoy the work, although that is often the case. Personal ambition, high economic aspirations, or inefficient use of time are unacceptable excuses. Exoneration due to economic necessity should be extended only when supported by convincing examples. Allowance should be made for short-term unusual circumstances, e.g. physicians in training who have little or no control over their work schedule. Avoidance of interpersonal relationships or leisure activities for reasons other than devotion to work is not within the scope of the criterion.

2   Excessive devotion to work and productivity that usually prevents any significant pursuit of both leisure activities and interpersonal relationships.

1   Excessive devotion to work and productivity that occasionally prevents any significant pursuit of both leisure activities and interpersonal relationships. Excessive devotion to work and productivity that usually prevents any significant pursuit of either leisure activities or interpersonal relationships but not both.

0   Denied or rarely or never leads to exclusion of leisure activities or interpersonal relationships.

with the clinician in mind, but one which also maintains a link with the extensive literature on normal personality traits. It consists of 375 items, each with seven response options, and it assesses 25 normal traits as well as the dimensions underlying each of the 10 DSM-IV personality disorders. It also measures seven broad personality constructs derived from a factor analysis of the combined normal and personality disorder scales. To make the inventory acceptable to a greater number of psychiatrists and psychologists, the normal traits were selected without reference to any particular theory of personality. A collaborative group of clinicians considered the traits meaningful and potentially useful. The scales measuring the traits were refined and developed through extensive field-testing with 2000 subjects in the general population, and several hundred non-psychotic psychiatric patients. To acquaint the reader with the kind of normal traits with potential relevance to clinical practice, Table 2 describes the lower-order or more specific traits, and Table 3 presents the higher-order or more general constructs, that were derived from a factor analysis of the combined normal and DSM-IV personality disorder scales.

The history of medicine is replete with diseases that have shed light on normal physiology, and discoveries regarding normal physiology that have informed and advanced the understanding of pathology. It would be surprising if a similar potential for mutual enrichment were not latent in the increased integration of research on normal and abnormal personality. This should enhance our understanding of the

Table 2 Proposed list of clinically relevant normal personality traits

Aestheticism	Enjoys art, music, natural beauty, style, fashion
Ambition	Strives for success, status, fame, influence, power
Anxiety	Apprehensive, worrisome, nervous, tense, jittery
Assertiveness	Expresses contrary opinions, protective of self-interest, dominates others
Conventionality	Traditional, conservative, conforming
Depression	Unhappy, dissatisfied, sad, anhedonic, pessimistic, guilty, low self-esteem
Dutifulness	Conscientious, dependable, persistent, loyal, hard-working
Energy	Active, busy, engaged
Excitement	Easily bored, craves stimulation, thrill-seeking
Exhibitionism	Attention-seeking, self-dramatizing, thrives on being noticed
Flexibility	Adaptable, adjusts to novelty and change, responsive to influence
Hostility	Criticizes, demeans, offends others, assaultive
Impulsiveness	Acts on the spur of the moment without foresight or planning
Intellect	Has intellectual interests and curiosity, and values mental activity
Irritability	Impatient, easily annoyed, quick tempered, low frustration tolerance
Modesty	Humble, unassuming, unpretentious, self-effacing
Moodiness	Emotionally labile, prone to short-lived fluctuations in mood
Orderliness	Neat, methodical, meticulous, thorough, careful
Self-indulgence	Poor control of eating, drinking, spending, sexual urges
Self-reliance	Handles decisions and tasks without help, emotional needs not excessive
Sincerity	Earnest, genuine, candid, truthful, guileless
Sociability	Seeks out people, enjoys talking to them, engages in group activities
Tolerance	Comfortable with diversity, does not attempt to impose own views on others
Trustfulness	Not wary or suspicious, has faith and confidence in others
Warmth	Displays affection, sympathetic, empathic, helps others, has close relationships

Table 3 Broad personality constructs derived from factor analysis of 25 normal traits and 10 DSM–IV personality disorder dimensions

Neuroticism	**Extraversion**	**Narcissism**
Anxiety	Sociability	Ambition
Depression	Warmth	Assertiveness
Moodiness	Avoidant PD (−)	Exhibitionism
Self-reliance (−)	Schizoid PD (−)	Modesty (−)
Avoidant PD	Schizotypal PD (−)	Sincerity (−)
Borderline PD	**Disagreeableness**	Histrionic PD
Dependent PD	Flexibility (−)	Narcissistic PD
Sensation-seeking	Hostility	**Conscientiousness**
Excitement	Irritability	Ambition
Impulsiveness	**Openness**	Dutifulness
Self-indulgence	Aestheticism	Energy
Antisocial PD	Conventionalism (−)	Orderliness
Borderline PD	Intellect	
Histrionic PD	Tolerance	

(−), trait reversed; PD, personality disorder.

origins and organization of personality, its disorders, and their biological substrate.

References

1. American Psychiatric Association, Committee on Nomenclature and Statistics (1980). *Diagnostic and statistical manual of mental disorders* (3rd edn). American Psychiatric Association, Washington, DC.
2. Loranger, A.W. (1990). The impact of DSM-III on diagnostic practice in a university hospital: a comparison of DSM-II and DSM-III in 10 914 patients. *Archives of General Psychiatry*, **47**, 672–5.
3. Loranger, A.W., Lenzenweger, M.F., Gartner, A.F., *et al.* (1991). Trait-state artifacts and the diagnosis of personality disorders. *Archives of General Psychiatry*, **48**, 72–8.
4. Lyons, M.J., Tyrer, P., and Gunderson, J. (1997). Heuristic models of comorbidity of Axis I and Axis II disorders. *Journal of Personality Disorders*, **11**, 260–9.
5. Tyrer, P., Gunderson, J., Lyons, M., and Toben, M. (1997). Extent of comorbidity between mental state and personality disorders. *Journal of Personality Disorders*, **11**, 242–59.
6. Spitzer, R.L. and Fleiss, J.L. (1974) A re-analysis of reliability of psychiatric diagnosis. *British Journal of Psychiatry*, **125**, 341–7.
7. Sartorius, N., Kaelber, C.T., Cooper, J.E., *et al.* (1993). Progress toward achieving a common language in psychiatry: results from the field trial of the clinical guidelines accompanying the WHO classification of mental and behavioral disorders in ICD-10. *Archives of General Psychiatry*, **50**, 115–24.
8. Loranger, A.W., Sartorius, N., Andreoli, A., *et al.* (1994). The World Health Organization/Alcohol, Drug Abuse and Mental Health Administration international pilot study of personality disorders. *Archives of General Psychiatry*, **51**, 215–24.
9. Loranger, A.W., Sartorius, N., and Janca, A. (ed.) (1997). *Assessment and diagnosis of personality disorders*. Cambridge University Press.
10. Loranger, A.W. (1999). *International Personality Disorder Examination (IPDE), DSM-IV and ICD-10 interviews*. PAR Psychological Assessment Resources, Odessa, FL.
11. World Health Organization (1993). *The ICD-10 classification of mental and behavioural disorders: diagnostic criteria for research*. World Health Organization, Geneva.
12. American Psychiatric Association (1994). *Diagnostic and statistical manual of mental disorders* (4th edn). American Psychiatric Association, Washington, DC.
13. Loranger, A.W. (1992). Are current self-report and interview measures adequate for epidemiological studies of personality disorders? *Journal of Personality Disorders*, **6**, 313–25.
14. Lenzenweger, M.F., Loranger, A.W., Kornfine, L., and Neff, C. (1997). Detecting personality disorders in a nonclinical population: application of a two-stage procedure for case identification. *Archives of General Psychiatry*, **54**, 345–51.

4.12.3 Specific types of personality disorder

Jose Luis Carrasco and Dusica Lecic-Tosevski*

Cluster A personality disorders

Paranoid personality disorder (JLC)

This disorder is characterized by pervasive suspiciousness, mistrust, and hypersensitivity to criticism and hostility. Paranoid individuals live an isolated emotional life because they fear the malevolent intent of others. As a rule, paranoid people are ready to counter-attack, provoking repeated confrontations. In this way, they induce hostility and resentment in others.

The term paranoia may lead to some confusion if it is not properly delimited. Paranoid had been used as an adjective to label various delusional representations or syndromes. Kraepelin[1] differentiated paranoia as a distinct condition characterized by chronic and highly systematized delusional ideas (see Chapter 4.4). Schneider[2] described people with this paranoid personality as fanatic psychopaths, stressing their intensity and rigidity in confrontation with others. He denied any relationship with paranoia. Freud[3] and other psychoanalysts construed the paranoid character as a pattern of mistrust and feeling of being attacked, based on distortions and externalization of the person's inner world.

Paranoid personality disorder was included in DSM-III with criteria of suspiciousness, mistrust, hypersensitivity, and restricted affectivity. This last criterion does not appear in DSM-IV and ICD-10, since restricted affectivity is neither necessary nor specific for paranoid personalities. Instead, emphasis is placed on mistrust and sensitivity to setbacks. The DSM-IV criteria for paranoid personality disorder are shown in Table 1.

Epidemiology

The prevalence of paranoid personality disorder is estimated at about 0.5 to 1 per cent in the general population and at 10 to 20 per cent among psychiatric patients. The disorder is more commonly diagnosed in males.

Aetiology

This personality disorder has a familial relationship with delusional disorders and with schizophrenia,[4] and has been included in the so-called schizophrenic spectrum.[5] Deficits in cortical dopamine activity may be associated with a poor conceptual organization that could in turn be responsible for suspiciousness and distorted interpretations.[6]

Mistrust and lack of confidence may reflect deficits arising in early developmental stages and resulting in a lack of basic self-confidence.[7] Lack of protective care and affective support in childhood could perhaps facilitate the development of paranoid features.

* The contributions of each author are indicated by **JLC** and **DLT** respectively.

Table 1 DSM-IV diagnostic criteria for paranoid personality disorder

A. A pervasive distrust and suspiciousness of others such that their motives are interpreted as malevolent, beginning by early adulthood and present in a variety of contexts, as indicated by four (or more) of the following

   (1) Suspects, without sufficient basis, that others are exploiting, harming, or deceiving him or her

   (2) Is preoccupied with unjustified doubts about the loyalty or trustworthiness of friends or associates

   (3) Is reluctant to confide in others because of unwarranted fear that the information will be used maliciously against him or her

   (4) Reads hidden demeaning or threatening meanings into benign remarks or events

   (5) Persistently bears grudges, i.e. is unforgiving of insults, injuries, or slights

   (6) Perceives attacks on his or her character or reputation that are not apparent to others and is quick to react angrily or to counterattack

   (7) Has recurrent suspicions, without justification, regarding fidelity of spouse or sexual partner

B. Does not occur exclusively during the course of Schizophrenia, a Mood Disorder With Psychotic Features, or another Psychotic Disorder and is not due to the direct physiological effects of a general medical condition.

Note If criteria are met prior to the onset of Schizophrenia, add 'Premorbid', e.g. 'Paranoid Personality Disorder (Premorbid)'.

Clinical picture

Paranoid individuals do not often ask for help from psychiatrists. They have no wish to be cured; instead, they believe that they have to be protected from other people's hatred and attacks. Subjects with this personality disorder suspect that others are acting to harm, exploit, or deceive them. These suspicions are based not on objective evidence, but on internal conviction and an attempt to find a rational explanation for the supposed wrongs.

Paranoids are reluctant to confide in others; they tend to feel that others are plotting against them, and that the enemy may be found in unexpected places. They do not readily tell others about their suspicions. The disorder may be manifested by irritability, unusual defensive or self-protective behaviours (e.g. locking doors and closing windows and curtains to avoid being spied on, and hiding papers or documents), or emotional detachment.

Paranoid people lack confidence in others. They doubt the loyalty or trustworthiness of friends and partners, and check their behaviour repeatedly for evidence of malevolent intentions. They assume that others are not trustworthy, to the extent that they cannot believe it when friends demonstrate their loyalty. They withhold personal or significant information from friends, fearing that it will be used maliciously against them. They do not form close friendships and are often isolated. When in trouble, paranoids do not expect help from friends or others close to them; instead, they expect to be attacked or ignored.

Many of the suspicious and distrustful attitudes of paranoids are perpetuated by their intense interpersonal sensitivity. They react intensely to any comment or event that may relate to them. Hidden meanings that are demeaning and threatening may be read into benign events or the remarks of others. Unintended errors by colleagues or public servants are taken as deliberate attempts to harm or deceive them. Humorous remarks or jokes may be interpreted as attacks on their character. Paranoids are easily hurt, and their pride is easily damaged by minor critical comments or questioning. They are excessively preoccupied with attacks on their reputation or character, and minor slights may arouse major hostility and a counter-attack. They bear grudges and harbour hostile feelings for a long time, and are unwilling to forgive the insults, injuries, or slights that they think they have received.[8]

Pathological jealousy is a common presentation of paranoid individuals. They have unreasonable doubts about the loyalty and faithfulness of their partners, based on little or no evidence. They may try to gather trivial and circumstantial facts to justify their beliefs. To avoid betrayal they attempt to gain complete control of intimate relationships, continuously questioning and challenging partners about their whereabouts and intentions.

The interpersonal world of paranoids is a consequence of their suspiciousness and distrust. They have difficulty in relating to others, especially with close relationships. Hostility is always present and can be manifested as excessive argumentativeness, recurrent complaint and confrontation, or hostile aloofness.[8]. Although they may appear rational, unemotional, and cold, the affect of paranoids is labile and oversensitive and they may be hostile, stubborn, and sarcastic. This mixture of secretive, cold, hostile, and sarcastic behaviours often elicits a hostile response in others which confirms the paranoid person's beliefs.

Paranoids blame others for their shortcomings. They are querulous and quick to counter-attack, so that they may become involved in frequent litigation. Since they do not confide in others, paranoids need self-confidence and a sense of autonomy and independence. They need to control people who might be harmful. While they do not accept criticism, they are highly critical.

One group of paranoids are close to Schneider's 'fanatics'.[2] They have hidden grandiose fantasies of power and negative views of other people, especially those belonging to another group who come to be considered as natural enemies. They simplify issues and avoid any ambiguous perspective. Some form cults or other tightly knit groups with people who share their paranoid belief systems.

Course

Paranoid features may be present in childhood and early adolescence in the form of hypersensitivity, social anxiety, poor peer relationships, and eccentricity. These features sometimes elicit teasing from other children, which in turn may aggravate the paranoid attitudes.

In situations of stress, individuals with paranoid personality disorder may respond with brief psychotic episodes. During these episodes, they may have frank delusional ideas or distorted perceptions. Some paranoid personality disorders are the premorbid state for a delusional disorder or even schizophrenia.

Individuals with this personality disorder may be at increased risk for agoraphobia, obsessive–compulsive disorder, and substance abuse or dependence. This personality disorder is often codiagnosed with schizoid, schizotypal, narcissistic, and avoidant personality disorders.

Differential diagnosis

Paranoid personality disorder should be distinguished from suspicious attitudes towards examination among immigrants, ethnic groups, or political groups. Members of these groups may display defensive and mistrustful behaviours owing to lack of familiarity with the language or the rules of a society, or in response to perceived neglect or rejec-

tion. Their behaviour may elicit further rejection from the majority, thus reinforcing the defensive behaviours.

Paranoid personality disorder is distinguished from delusional disorder, paranoid schizophrenia, and depression with psychotic symptoms, all of which are characterized by periods of persistent psychotic symptoms. Paranoid personality disorder present before the occurrence of these syndromes should be diagnosed as 'premorbid'.

People with schizotypal personality disorder are suspicious, have paranoid ideas, and keep their distance from others. However, they also experience perceptual distortions and magical thinking, and are usually odd and eccentric. Schizoid personality disorder is characterized by aloofness, coldness, and eccentricity, but these individuals usually lack prominent suspiciousness or paranoid ideation. Individuals with **avoidant personality disorder** are hypersensitive and do not confide in others. However, their lack of confidence is based on fear of being embarrassed or found inadequate rather than fear of other people's malicious intentions. Some antisocial behaviour by paranoid individuals originates in a wish for revenge or counter-attack, rather a desire for personal gain as in antisocial personality disorder. Paranoid features are often present in narcissistic individuals who fear that their imperfections could be revealed. The differential diagnosis should be based on the predominance of persistent need of praise versus persistent suspiciousness and distrust.

Treatment

Antidepressant and anxiolytic treatment may be useful for anxiety and depression resulting from a paranoid response to stressful situations. Low-dose antypsychotics may be indicated during brief psychotic episodes or when ideas of reference are present.

Psychological treatment is difficult owing to the lack of insight. The approach is to attempt to gain the patient's confidence, avoiding early confrontation of distorted ideas, followed by a slow gentle attempt at cognitive restructuring.

Schizoid personality disorder (JLC)

Schizoid personality disorder is characterized by a persistent pattern of social withdrawal. Schizoid individuals show discomfort in social interactions and are introverted. They are seen by others as eccentric, isolated, or lonely. DSM-IV diagnostic criteria are shown in Table 2.

This type of personality became recognized in the first two decades of the twentieth century. August Block's description of the shut-in personality and Eugen Bleuler's description of autism distinguished between shy and lonely persons and those who engage in relationships only in fantasy. Psychoanalysts included this term in their writings and developed an approach based on deficient object relations and individuation.[9]

Some schizoid personalities have probably been sweet children who were very easy to care for, although giving less joy to their parents and eliciting less stimulation and fewer expressions of emotion than more expressive children.[7]

Epidemiology

The epidemiology of schizoid personality disorder is not clearly established. Recent studies give a median prevalence of 0.5 to 1 per cent (see Chapter 4.12.5).

Table 2 DSMV-IV diagnostic criteria for schizoid personality disorder

A. A pervasive pattern of detachment from social relationships and a restricted range of expression of emotions in interpersonal settings, beginning by early adulthood and present in a variety of contexts, as indicated by four (or more) of the following

    (1) Neither desires nor enjoys close relationships, including being part of a family

    (2) Almost always chooses solitary activities

    (3) Has little, if any, interest in having sexual experiences with another person

    (4) Takes pleasure in few, if any, activities

    (5) Lacks close friends or confidants other than first-degree relatives

    (6) Appears indifferent to the praise or criticism of others

    (7) Shows emotional coldness, detachment, or flattened affectivity

B. Does not occur exclusively during the course of Schizophrenia, a Mood Disorder With Psychotic Features, another Psychotic Disorder, or a Pervasive Developmental Disorder and is not due to the direct physiological effects of a general medical condition.

Note If criteria are met prior to the onset of Schizophrenia, add 'Premorbid,' e.g. 'Schizoid Personality Disorder (Premorbid)'.

Aetiology

A familial association may exist between schizotypal personality disorder and schizophrenia.

Clinical picture

People with schizoid personality disorder appear cold, reserved, distant, and unsociable. They lack involvement in everyday events and in the concerns of others. They rarely tolerate eye contact, usually give short answers, and appear uneasy when asked about emotions or feelings. However, they may invest much energy in abstract ideas such as those of mathematics or philosophy.

There is a characteristic lack of emotional expression and low energy. Speech is typically slow and monotonous, and seems to lack associated emotion. Affect is excessively serious or constrained, although some inner fear may be detected by an experienced clinician. If they try to be humorous, they usually give a child-like impression. Psychomotor activity tends to be lethargic, lacking gesture and rhythmic movement. They may seem absorbed in insignificant matters, keeping quiet and not annoying anybody, as if in their own world. They do not express joy, anger, sadness, or other emotions. Interpersonal communication tends to be formal and impersonal, although not irrational. Threats, real or imagined, are dealt with by fantasized omnipotence or resignation. Aggressive acts are infrequent.

People with schizoid personality disorder characteristically seem to lack interest in the lives and concerns of others. When in a group, they stay unnoticed and detached, seeming indifferent to critiscism or praise or to the reactions of others. Schizoids are attracted to solitary hobbies, and may be successful in lonely jobs that others find difficult to tolerate. Many prefer working at night. Usually, they do not seem to suffer because of this detachment and they have no desire for closeness or intimacy. They seldom have close friends or relationships, except with immediate relatives. Their sexual lives may be poor or exist only in fantasy, and some postpone mature sexuality indefinitely. They do not usually marry, although some, especially schizoid women, may passively agree to marriage. However, schizoid individuals may make emotional attachments with animals or inanimate objects.

Schizoid personalities lack insight, and generally have a poorly developed sense of identity and a poor capacity for evaluating interpersonal events. They may appear to be self-absorbed and engage in excessive daydreaming. However, some schizoid individuals have original and creative ideas.

Differential diagnosis

Schizoids have better occupational functioning than patients with **schizophrenia** or **schizotypal personality disorder**, and, although isolated, can have successful careers. Schizophrenic patients exhibit delusional thinking or hallucinations and psychotic episodes. Schizotypal individuals show greater eccentricity and oddness than schizoids, and also have perceptual and thought disturbances including magical thinking.

People with **paranoid personality disorder** may also show social detachment and lack close relationships. However, they show more social engagement than schizoids and may have a history of aggressive behavior.

Emotional constrant is also present in **obsessive–compulsive personality disorder**, but obsessional patients are more involved in everyday life and concerns, and may be worried by criticism. People with **avoidant personality disorder** are also detached and aloof. However, although they actively avoid interpersonal contact because of fear of rejection or being found inadequate, they have an intense desire for close relationships.

Course

Schizoid personality disorder is usually apparent in early childhood. As with all personality disorders, it is usually long-lasting; however, it is not necessarily lifelong although there is seldom any rapid or profound change. If their deficits are moderate and social circumstances are favourable, some schizoids achieve social and vocational adaptation.

Although this personality disorder is sometimes a precursor of schizophrenia, the number of schizoid patients who go on to develop schizophrenia is unknown.

Treatment

Because they lack insight and have little motivation for change, schizoids seldom seek treatment. Motivation for change may depend on life circumstances and external pressures.

Low-dose antipsychotic medication is useful in some situations. Antidepressants and psychostimulants have also been used with some positive effects.

The psychotherapy of patients with schizoid personality disorder must be based on gaining a therapeutic alliance. Unlike paranoid patients, they may become involved in therapy and reveal fantasies, imaginary friends, and fears of unbearable dependency. Ambivalence may appear because of fear of dependence on the therapist, who must keep the necessary distance to allow a tolerable relationship for the patient.

Social skills training is sometimes useful in improving their awareness of social cues.

Schizotypal personality disorder (JLC)

Schizotypia is a controversial term in psychiatry. The term was used by Kretschmer[10] to denominate the phenotypic characters that antedated the development of schizophrenia. Nevertheless, the term schizotypal personality disorder was not included in psychiatric classifications until the publication of DSM-IIIR in 1987.[11] Before that date, schizotypal individuals were allocated either with schizoids or with schizophrenics, and were usually labelled as latent schizophrenics or pseudoneurotic schizophrenics. However, the validity of this nosological entity is still controversial and, despite its acceptance in DSM-IV, ICD-10 does not recognize it as a separate personality disorder. Instead, ICD-10 includes the schizotypal syndrome among the psychotic disorders and not as a personality disorder, based on the biological affinities of schizotypal individuals with other schizophrenic patients. DSM-IV diagnostic criteria are shown in Table 3.

Epidemiology

Schizotypal personality disorder is present in 0.5 to 3 per cent of the general population, with no demonstrated differences between sexes. It is more commonly diagnosed in relatives of schizophrenic patients, and the incidence is much in monozygotic than in dizygotic twins (33 per cent versus 4 per cent).[4]

Clinical picture

The essential feature of schizotypal individuals is a pattern of peculiarity and oddness in interpersonal relationships with resulting social detachment and lack of close relationships. Because of their distorted reality processing schizotypal individuals feel intensely uncomfortable in the presence of others. Conversely, others feel uneasy in the presence of schizotypals because of their unusual ways of thinking and expressing emotions.

Like schizoids, schizotypals have a decreased desire for intimate contacts, although they may sometimes express unhappiness about their lack of relationships. As a consequence they do not have close friends or confidants other than relatives. They experience intense anxiety in social situations with unfamiliar people. They can interact if necessary, but they prefer to keep aloof because they feel different and are not interested in the concerns of others. Their anxiety in these situations is not based on feelings of inadequacy or fear of humiliation. Rather, it is due to suspicion of the motivation of others, and therefore it is not alleviated as time passes and the situation becomes more familiar. Thus schizotypals feel progressively worse and more reluctant to confide in other people.

Individuals with schizotypal personality disorder often have ideas of reference, i.e. interpretations of casual events as having specific and unusual meanings related to themselves. However, these ideas do not achieve the pathological conviction of delusions. Similarly, these individuals may be preoccupied with superstitions or paranormal phenomena. They may feel that they may read other people's thoughts or influence their behaviour by the power of thought. Their magical thinking is often manifested by ritualized behaviours aimed at avoiding harmful events.

Perceptual disturbances are frequent in schizotypal personality disorder. An experience of a sixth sense is typical, with the 'ability' to notice someone's presence. Distorted perceptions are present in the

Table 3 DSMV-IV diagnostic criteria for schizotypal personality disorder

A. A pervasive pattern of social and interpersonal deficits marked by acute discomfort with, and reduced capacity for, close relationships as well as by cognitive or perceptual distortions and eccentricities of behaviour beginning by early adulthood and present in a variety of contexts, as indicated by five (or more) of the following

   (1) Ideas of reference (excluding delusions of reference)
   (2) Odd beliefs or magical thinking that influences behaviour and is inconsistent with subcultural norms (e.g. superstitiousness, belief in clairvoyance, telepathy, or 'sixth sense'; in children and adolescents, bizarre fantasies or preoccupations)
   (3) Unusual perceptual experiences, including bodily illusions
   (4) Odd thinking and speech (e.g. vague, circumstantial, metaphorical, overelaborate, or stereotyped)
   (5) Suspiciousness or paranoid ideation
   (6) Inappropriate or constricted affect
   (7) Behaviour or appearance that is odd, eccentric, or peculiar
   (8) Lack of close friends or confidants other than first-degree relatives
   (9) Excessive social anxiety that does not diminish with familiarity and tends to be associated with paranoid fears rather than negative judgements about self

B. Does not occur exclusively during the course of Schizophrenia, a Mood Disorder With Psychotic Features, another Psychotic Disorder, or a Pervasive Developmental Disorder.

Note If criteria are met prior to the onset of Schizophrenia, add 'Premorbid', e.g. 'Schizotypal Personality Disorder (Premorbid)'.

form of sounds perceived as calling voices or shadows transformed into figures and faces.

Thought processing and speech are characteristically affected. Speech may be constructed in an unusual and idiosyncratic way—generally loose, digressive, or vague, but without actual derailment or incoherence. Responses may be either excessively concrete or far too abstract, and words may be used in unusual ways.

The interpersonal relationships of schizotypal individuals are primarily affected by paranoid and suspicious ideation. They may believe that colleagues at work want to damage their reputation. In addition to the social anxiety of these individuals, this leads to a stiff and constricted contact and affect. They are considered odd and eccentric by others: they have peculiar mannerisms, dress in an unusual and unkempt manner, adopt extravagant postures and clothing combinations, do not obey normal social conventions, and generally avoid eye contact.

Course

Schizotypal features may be present in childhood and adolescence in the form of solitariness, academic underachievement, hypersensitivity, and bizarre fantasies. Schizotypals do not seek treatment because of their personality disorder, but rather because of the presentation of associated depression, dysphoria, and anxiety. In response to stressful situations, these patients may experience transient psychotic episodes lasting from minutes to hours. In some cases, clinical symptoms and duration reach the degree of brief psychotic disorder, schizophreniform disorder, or schizophrenia, with the schizotypal personality disorder as the premorbid state. The prevalence of major depressive episodes is notoriously high, as is co-diagnosis with paranoid, schizoid, avoidant, and borderline personality disorders.

Differential diagnosis

Delusional disorder, **schizophrenia**, and **mood disorder with psychotic symptoms** have to be excluded based on the greater intensity and persistence of psychotic symptoms.

In childhood, it can be difficult to distinguish schizotypal personality disorder from other forms of disorders characterized by odd behaviour, isolation, eccentricity, and peculiarities of language. These include **autistic disorder**, **Asperger's disorder**, and some **language disorders**. The differentiation with communication disorders is based on the prominence of language symptoms in these children and the compensatory efforts to communicate by gesture and other means. Autism and Asperger's disorder present an even more intense social isolation and indifference, and stereotyped behaviours and interests.

Paranoid and **schizoid personality disorders** lack the perceptual and speech impairment of schizotypal personality disorder, as well as the marked eccentricity and oddness. **Avoidant personality disorder**, while including social anxiety and isolation, differs from schizotypal personality disorder in that avoidants have an intense desire for closeness which is constrained by fear of rejection. Schizotypals do not have a desire for relationships. **Borderline personality disorder** has a high rate of co-occurrence with schizotypal personality disorder and frequently the two disorders cannot be differentiated. Brief psychotic episodes in people with borderline personality disorder are more dissociative-like and generally follow affective shifts in response to stress or frustration. Social isolation in borderline personality patients is generally due to repeated interpersonal failures rather than a persistent lack of desire for relationships and intimacy.

Finally, schizotypal personality disorder must be diagnosed in the cultural context of the patient. It should be noted that some perceptual peculiarities and magical beliefs may be due to culturally determined characteristics. For example, mind reading, voodoo, shamanism, evil eye, and so on should not be considered as personality disorders in some cultural areas.

Treatment

Low-dose antipsychotic medication may be useful for ideas of reference, perceptual disturbances, and other psychotic-like symptoms. Antidepressants are effective when depressive states are associated.

The psychological management of schizotypals should include a prolonged period of gaining the confidence of the patient. However, a particularly careful approach must be adopted owing to the peculiar thought processing of these patients.

Cluster B personality disorders

Antisocial personality disorder (DLT)

Definition

Antisocial personality disorder is characterized by continuous disregard for the safety of oneself and others and violation of the rights of others, without feeling remorse. Individuals with this disorder are unreliable, manipulative, incapable of lasting relationships, and unable to conform to social norms. The disorder starts early (before the age of 15), is pervasive, and manifests in variety of contexts. Although social deviance is one of the core features of antisocial personality disorder, it is not synonymous with criminality.

Antisocial personality disorder uncomplicated by other disorders is

Table 4 DSMV-IV diagnostic criteria for antisocial personality disorder

A. There is a pervasive pattern of disregard for and violation of the rights of others occurring since age 15 years, as indicated by three (or more) of the following

  (1) Failure to conform to social norms with respect to lawful behaviours as indicated by repeatedly performing acts that are ground for arrest

  (2) Deceitfulness, as indicated by repeated lying, use of aliases, or conning others for personal profit or pleasure

  (3) Impulsivity or failure to plan ahead

  (4) Irritability and aggressiveness, as indicated by repeated physical fights or assaults

  (5) Reckless disregard for safety of self or others

  (6) Consistent irresponsibility, as indicated by repeated failure to sustain consistent work behaviour or honour financial obligations

  (7) Lack of remorse, as indicated by being indifferent to or rationalizing having hurt, mistreated, or stolen from another

B. The individual is at least age 18 years

C. There is evidence of conduct disorder with onset before 15 years

D. The occurrence of antisocial behaviour is not exclusively during the course of Schizophrenia or a Manic Episode.

not often met in clinical settings, except forensic psychiatry. However, owing to its impact on family and social environment, it has major public health significance and has been extensively studied in academic psychiatry, psychoanalysis, law, sociology, theology, and literature.

Historical perspective

Early contributions

Antisocial behaviour resulting from mental disturbance was recognized early, by Pinel, Pritchard, Lombroso, Koch, Kraepelin, and others. It was labelled *manie sans délire*, moral insanity, moral mania, born criminality, and constitutional psychopathic inferiority. The terms used in the past, and still appearing today (sociopathy, psychopathy, deviant, amoral, dissocial and asocial personalities), indicated either disorder of personality or disorder based on behaviour that was unacceptable to the societal norms.

Cleckley's seminal work *The Mask of Sanity*[12] is considered to be the basic text on antisocial personality disorder. Cleckley differentiated psychopathic personality from criminality and social deviance and strongly influenced the DSM-I concept of 'sociopathic personality disturbance' as well as the description of antisocial personality disorder in DSM-II.

Contemporary concepts

Robins' follow-up study *Deviant Children Grown Up*[13] described antisocial personality as beginning before the age of 8 and continuing into adult life, and introduced the child-to-adult continuum of antisocial psychopathology. The classic studies by Glueck[14] and Robins[13] were crucial determinants of the DSM-III approach, which focused on criminal behaviour. Personality traits or traditional symptoms of psychopathy were neglected, and the disorder was conceptualized as synonymous with criminality, which was a major source of criticism of DSM-IIIR. The criteria for DSM-IV (Table 4) were modified and included personality traits as well as the original Cleckley

Table 5 ICD-10 diagnostic criteria for dissocial personality disorder

Personality disorder, usually coming to attention because of a gross disparity between behaviour and the prevailing social norms, and characterized by

- (a) callous unconcern for the feelings of others
- (b) gross and persistent attitude of irresponsibility and disregard for social norms, rules and obligations
- (c) incapacity to maintain enduring relationships, though having no difficulty in establishing them
- (d) very low tolerance to frustration and a low threshold for discharge of aggression, including violence
- (e) incapacity to experience guilt and to profit from experience, particularly punishment
- (f) marked proneness to blame others, or to offer plausible rationalizations, for the behaviour that has brought the patient into conflict with society

There may also be persistent irritability as an associated feature. Conduct disorder during childhood and adolescence, though not invariably present, may further support the diagnosis.

Includes: amoral, antisocial, psychopathic, and sociopathic personality (disorder)

Excludes: conduct disorders, emotionally unstable personality disorder

description. ICD-10 (Table 5) reflects personality traits more than overt criminal behaviour.

According to Cloninger's biosocial theory of personality,[15] antisocial personality disorder is defined as the personality variant characterized by high novelty seeking, low harm avoidance, and low reward dependence, which determines its impulsive-aggressive and socially insensitive temperament. The character trait of uncooperativeness[16] is pronounced, involving lack of empathy, social tolerance, compassion, and moral principles. The uncooperativeness is associated with hostility and depression, frequently leading to serious aggression and/or suicide attempts.

Epidemiology

A prevalence rate of about 3 per cent is consistently found in the general population, and it is more frequent in males than females, with sex ratios ranging from 2:1 to 7:1. It is more common among younger adults, people living in urban areas and lower socio-economic groups.[17] In special settings (substance abuse programmes, probation centres, prisons) prevalence may rise to 75 per cent.

Aetiology

The aetiology of antisocial personality disorder is complex and multifactorial, involving biological, early developmental, and social determinants.

Biological issues

Genetic factors Twin, adoption, and family studies have demonstrated that genetic factors contribute to the development of antisocial personality.[18–20] Having one or both parents with this disorder would be a strong predictor of future antisocial psychopathology. Among the offspring, antisocial personality disorder was diagnosed more often in males than in females. Women manifested an increased rate of hysteria, which suggested that the two conditions might be alternative expressions of the same genetic endowment, belonging to 'spectrum conditions'.[19] Longitudinal studies of hyperactive children have reported high rates of later (adult) antisocial behaviour, and have suggested a 'developmental' relationship between antisocial behaviour and childhood hyperactivity.

Chromosomal abnormalities are found to be an occasional cause of abnormally aggressive behaviour. Three per cent of patients in a maximum security hospital had the XYY karyotype.[21] The finding is not considered particularly significant, as the incidence of this karyotype is much higher in the general population than was originally thought. Swedish studies[22] reported that clients undergoing forensic psychiatric examination after severe criminality display a higher frequency of two long alleles in exon III of the *D4DR* gene compared with controls. These studies await further confirmation.

Biochemical studies Numerous studies of humans and non-human primates have demonstrated associations between hostile–aggressive behaviour and low levels of the serotonin metabolite 5-hydroxyindole-acetic acid in the cerebrospinal fluid.[23,24]

Low platelet monoamine oxidase activity has been used as a biological indicator for vulnerability to the disinhibitory psychopathology present in different forms of psychosocial disorders and manifested as psychopathy, violent suicide attempts, hyperactivity, and alcoholism. The Swedish studies demonstrated a rather strong correlation between the activity of this enzyme and central serotonergic activity.[25] The finding of low levels of adrenaline (epinephrine) in the urine of subjects with persistent criminality,[26] suggests that physiological factors are of importance in the development of criminal behaviour.

Linnoila and Virkkunen[27] have postulated a comprehensive 'low-serotonin syndrome' model. A deficit in serotonin activity at the level of the raphe nuclei would lead to a functional lesion of the suprachiasmatic nucleus and a reduction in serotonergic output to the forebrain, which reduces glucose regulation, promotes dysphoria and alcohol consumption, and initiates aggressive outbursts. They believe that recognition of the syndrome and treatment of such individuals with serotonergic medications may help to reduce alcohol consumption, stabilize blood glucose levels, and prevent aggression.

Cerebral pathology Although no clear organic basis for antisocial personality disorder is known, hyperactivity and attention-deficit disorder may be caused by minimal brain dysfunction indicated by soft neurological signs. Subtle EEG abnormalities[28] and single-photon emission CT[29] findings of a marked frontal hypoperfusion were found in habitual aggressives. It was postulated that the aetiology of pathological persistent aggression might be a disturbance of cerebral physiology caused by an innate or acquired impairment in frontal-lobe function.

Developmental issues

Parental deprivation and deviance during the critical period (rapprochement subphase of separation–individuation) seem to be a critical factor. Robins[13] showed that having a sociopathic or alcoholic father was a powerful predictor of antisocial personality disorder in adult life. However, Glueck and Glueck[30] stressed the importance of inconsistent maternal care. Future antisocial individuals were neglected and 'psychologically undernourished' children. Violent acts witnessed during childhood and/or severe physical abuse caused splitting of their inner world and development of borderline personality organization. Splitting remains the main defence, identity diffusion prevails, and object constancy is never achieved. Severe superego pathology is also present.

Social issues

Social disintegration can cause episodic antisocial behaviour, reflecting a normal adaptation to an abnormal social environment.[31] Severe and chronic criminality can also be facilitated by social influences. However, the multifactorial origin of the antisocial personality disorder and its early onset and manifestations indicate that it cannot be attributed to cultural conflicts and social determinants.

Clinical features and diagnosis

Patients with antisocial personality disorder often wear 'a mask of sanity' and may appear quite normal, charming, and understanding. However, their history reveals disturbed functioning in the domains of behaviour and self-concept, love and sexuality, interpersonal relations, and cognitive style.[32]

Behavioural expression and self-concept

Reckless behaviour unaffected by punishment is typical of antisocial individuals, who are also exploitative, manipulative, demanding, and lacking in a sense of responsibility. An easy-going hedonistic attitude may be interrupted by rage, cruelty, and violence. Lying, truancy, running away from home, thefts, fights, substance abuse, and illegal activities may be typical experiences, beginning in early childhood. Tattoos and scars from self-mutilation are common, as well as a propensity towards substance abuse, delinquency, and criminality.

Affectivity

A disinhibitory syndrome is an essential feature, characterized by an impaired control of impulses and a reduced ability to anticipate the negative consequences of behaviour. Antisocial individuals are egocentric and unable to feel genuine guilt and remorse, and, like neglected children, they exhibit intense and persistent anger that is expressed as a reproach towards various subjects, including the self. They are intolerant of any increase in anxiety without developing additional symptoms or pathological behaviours, and have an incapacity for reflective mourning or sadness. Frequent suicide threats and attempts are also common, as is somatic preoccupation.

Love and sexuality

Unable to love or to comprehend incest taboos, antisocial individuals have a tendency towards Don Juanism, perversion, and polymorphous perverse sexuality. Abuse of partners and children is frequent, as are severe marital difficulties.

Cognitive style

Cognitive peculiarities, such as glibness, plagiarism, and a tendency to confuse intention with action, are present. Superficiality of knowledge, failure to learn from experience, and a paranoid view of the world are typical.

Interpersonal relations

Manipulativeness and parasitic attitudes are common in the unstable interpersonal relationships of antisocial individuals. They are characterized by transient, superficial, and indifferent relations with others, a lack of capacity to invest emotionally in people, and the absence of internalized moral values. They display deficient parenting and social dysfunction, and resistance to authorities is pronounced.

Diagnosis may be difficult, since patients often look composed and deny problems. A complete history, also taken from informants, is necessary. Thorough neurological examination, EEG, and radiological examination may be necessary in order to exclude damage to the central nervous system caused by reckless behaviour. The Psychopathy Check List[22] may be useful for diagnosis.

Comorbidity and differential diagnosis

Antisocial personality disorder is frequently comorbid with **depression**, which usually has atypical features. **Bipolar disorder** (manic phase) and **mental retardation** (learning difficulties) should be excluded. Substance abuse may be comorbid from childhood, and antisocial behaviour may be secondary to premorbid alcoholism type 2. **Atypical schizophrenic disorder** (pseudopsychopathic schizophrenia), **temporal-lobe epilepsy**, or a **limbic-lobe syndrome** should also be excluded.

Kernberg[31] presented a hierarchical differential diagnosis of antisocial behaviour, with the following categories lying on a continuum:

(1) antisocial personality disorder

(2) the syndrome of malignant narcissism

(3) narcissistic personality disorder with antisocial behaviour

(4) other severe personality disorders with antisocial features

(5) neurotic personality disorders with antisocial features

(6) antisocial behaviour as part of a symptomatic neurosis

(7) dissocial reaction.

A careful assessment of the personality structure in each case of antisocial behaviour is necessary in order to determine the level of personality functioning and to choose an appropriate treatment strategy.[33]

Course and prognosis

Antisocial behaviour is most pronounced in early adult years, and gradually decreases with age. A favourable occupation with overcompensation possibilities or a good marriage/partnership may have beneficial effects. Maturation of the personality might also take place. Depression and hypochondriasis develop when acting-out and alloplastic defences are abandoned. Substance abuse and promiscuity are risky behaviours for developing HIV infection.

Treatment

Pharmacotherapy

The primary aim is control of impulsivity and aggression. Medication is also used to deal with incapacitating symptoms, such as anxiety, rage, depression, and somatic complaints.[34] Selective serotonin reuptake inhibitors and lithium may be beneficial in regulating serotonergic function. Antiepileptic drugs, such as carbamazepine and clonazepam could be used for aggressive outbursts, especially if abnormal waves are noted on the EEG. Psychostimulants such as methylphenidate (Ritalin[®]) may be useful if there is evidence of attention-deficit hyperactivity disorder. Benzodiazepines are contraindicated since they might cause behavioural disinhibition. Noncompliance and drug abuse are common problems; therefore drugs should be used judiciously.

Psychotherapy

Outpatient psychotherapy has been very discouraging, and most patients are unresponsive to psychodynamic approaches. Antisocial individuals may wish to escape from honest human relationships because of their fear of intimacy, and this causes difficulties in establishing a therapeutic alliance. They should be encouraged to find alternative defence mechanisms to acting-out, and protected from their self-defeating behaviour. Realistic conditions should be created, limits should be set, and all tertiary gains of treatment (escape from the law, and ongoing parasitic dependence on parents or other social support systems) should be eliminated.

Various treatment modes have been applied, with effectiveness depending on the severity of the disorder. Group treatment may be more beneficial than individual therapy.

Small groups should be homogeneous, preferably with two therapists who share responsibility and lead groups in a non-authoritarian way. **Self-help groups** may be useful and prognostically better, since antisocial individuals accept confrontation with their peers more easily than with therapists–authorities.

A **therapeutic community,** based on the principles outlined by Maxwell Jones[35] with a general social adjustment as a main task, might give positive results. Special programmes should be developed, providing firm structure, supervision, and direct confrontation of interpersonal behaviours and defences. Therapists should have an enthusiastic and non-controlling but firm attitude, and empathic and consistent behaviour. They should try to understand the split-off inner pain of antisocial patients and not punish them. Counter-transference problems are unavoidable, and true ambivalence in the reaction to antisocial patients is considered to be a healthy response.[31]

Borderline personality disorder (DLT)

Definition

Many definitions and meanings have been proposed for borderline personality disorder. This most controversial of all personality disorders is best understood as a heterogeneous syndrome manifested by egosyntonic affective instability and impulsivity (behavioural dyscontrol) and propensity to cognitive–perceptual distortions in the context of a chronically unstable interpersonal relationships.

Historical perspective

Early contributions

Early psychoanalysis did not explicitly deal with borderline personality disorder, although a careful retrospective study of the literature shows that some of Freud's classical patients (e.g. the wolf-man) would have been diagnosed today as typical borderline cases. Stern[36] was the first to use the term 'borderline' in 1938, placing borderline patients on the border between neuroses and psychoses. The concepts of 'ambulatory schizophrenia', 'as-if' personality, 'pseudoneurotic schizophrenia', 'borderline states', and 'psychotic character' paved the way to the contemporary concept of borderline psychopathology. In 1947, Schmideberg[37] first described borderline as a disorder of character which was 'stable in its instability'.

Phenomenological research was started by Grinker et al.,[38] who proposed a borderline syndrome, and by Gunderson and Kolb,[39] who described the distinguishing features of the disorder. Spitzer et al.[40] introduced diagnostic criteria, labelling the condition 'unstable personality'. Their description led to the differentiation of two disorders—schizotypal and borderline—and their official acceptance in DSM-III.

Table 6 DSM-IV diagnostic criteria for borderline personality disorder

A pervasive pattern of instability of interpersonal relationships, self-image, and affects and marked impulsivity beginning by early adulthood and present in a variety of contexts, as indicated by five (or more) of the following

(1) Frantic efforts to avoid real or imagined abandonment. **Note:** Do not include suicidal or self-mutilating behaviour covered in Criterion 5

(2) A pattern of unstable and intense interpersonal relationships characterized by alternating between extremes of idealization and devaluation

(3) Identity disturbance: markedly and persistently unstable self-image or sense of self

(4) Impulsivity in at least two areas that are potentially self-damaging (e.g spending, sex, substance abuse, reckless driving, binge eating). **Note:** Do not include suicidal or self-mutilating behaviour covered in Criterion 5

(5) Recurrent suicidal behaviour, gestures, or threats, or self-mutilating behaviour

(6) Affective instability due to a marked reactivity of mood (e.g. intense episodic dysphoria, irritability, or anxiety usually lasting a few hours and only rarely more than a few days)

(7) Chronic feelings of emptiness

(8) Inappropriate intense anger or difficulty controlling anger (e.g. frequent displays of temper, constant anger, recurrent physical fights)

(9) Transient stress-related paranoid ideation or severe dissociative symptoms

Contemporary concepts

Modern concepts can be summarized in four groups: borderline personality organization, borderline personality disorder, the DSM-III (IV) concept, and borderline as a severe personality dysfunction.

1. Otto Kernberg[41] is one of the most prominent authors in the field and his theory is the most coherent. He proposed the term 'borderline personality organization', a broad concept encompassing all severe personality disorders. Borderline personality organization is a stable permanent state based on three criteria: diffuse identity, primitive defences centred around splitting and intact reality testing. Dahl's[42] concept of a core borderline syndrome is in agreement with Kernberg's theory.

2. Gunderson[43] focused attention on 'borderline personality disorder' as a distinct entity which could be distinguished from both other mental disorders and other personality disorders. Gunderson's descriptive phenomenological designation had a considerable influence on contemporary classifications (DSM-III and DSM-IV).

3. The DSM-III (DSM-IV) definition of borderline personality disorder identifies a narrower group of patients than those covered by Kernberg's construct of a borderline personality organization, and is in line with Gunderson's theoretical position. However, borderline personality disorder has been found to be associated with so many other Axis I and II diagnoses that its validity as an independent diagnostic category is still weak relative to other personality disorders, psychoses in remission, and some affective disorders. It is hoped that the slightly refined DSM-IV criteria (Table 6) will reduce the problems encountered with those in DSM-III.

4. Berelowitz and Tarnopolsky[44] suggested that borderline personality disorder should be regarded as a 'severe personality dysfunc-

tion rather than as a discrete diagnostic entity'. The heterogeneity of borderline features and the wide differences in severity found in patients diagnosed with borderline personality disorder make the categorical diagnosis of limited value. The disorder is best understood as a current position or level of functioning, rather than a fixed type of personality disorder.[45,46]

Akiskal[47] defines the borderline as an attenuated or subclinical variant of affective disorders, belonging to a 'spectrum of disorders' with the same aetiology as proper affective disorders. This interesting hypothesis is still debatable, but it is certain that depression exaggerates and distorts personality characteristics.

Borderline personality disorder has been introduced into ICD-10 as a subcategory of the 'emotionally unstable personality disorder', a phenomenological term that resembles Spitzer's description accepted in DSM-III. However, the descriptions of the two subcategories (impulsive and borderline types) capture two crucial dimensions of borderline personality disorder—impulsivity and affective instability—so that division into subtypes may not be warranted. It is the only personality disorder in the ICD-10 without operational criteria (only research criteria exist), reflecting the state of the art in European psychiatry which, until recently, has not had many dealings with this disorder.

Epidemiology

Borderline personality disorder is common in both inpatient and outpatient settings, and probably in the general population. It is estimated that 11 per cent of all psychiatric outpatients and 19 per cent of all inpatients have this diagnosis.[48] In the community, where less systematic research has been conducted, estimates vary widely from 1.1 to 4.6 per cent, depending on the instrument used.[49] It is significantly more common among women, and among people who are either widowed or unmarried. The highest rates were found in the age range from 19 to 34 years.

Aetiology

The origin of borderline personality disorder is multifactorial. It should be considered a final common pathway for a variety of non-specific predisposing neurobiological, early developmental, and social factors.[50]

Biological issues

Research into the biological mechanism underlying borderline personality disorder is, although promising, still in its infancy. Most theories suggest that an interaction between an innate biological vulnerability to stress (anxiety, affect regulation) and an invalidating parental environment would cause future borderline psychopathology.[36,41]

Family studies of borderline personality disorder support the constitutional psychobiological role. There is increasing evidence that parents of borderline patients have a high incidence of affective disorder and borderline-type behaviours, alcoholism, antisocial personality disorder, and other cluster B personality disorders.[50]

A number of investigators have performed studies on well-diagnosed patients with borderline personality disorder, focusing on biological variables (abnormal dexamethasone suppression test results, shortened rapid eye movement latency, blunted thyrotrophin response, and an abnormal sensitivity to amphetamine). However,

even when positive, these biological markers are non-specific for borderline personality disorder, do not necessarily demonstrate a biological factor, and may not reflect pathogenesis.

Markers for impulsivity are more specific. Coccaro et al.[51] found reduced serotonergic functioning (as measured by the 5-hydroxy-indolacetic acid level in cerebrospinal fluid, or by blunted prolactin response to fenfluramine challenge) in patients who demonstrated impulsive aggression, which is a 'core' feature of borderline personality disorder. Similar findings were obtained for borderline patients with a history of suicide attempts. These data suggest a psychobiological basis for impulsive-aggressive behaviour caused by a deficiency of central serotonergic function.

Andrulonis et al.[52] reported that 38 per cent of borderline patients had a significant organic contribution, such as previous head injury, epilepsy, encephalitis, or a history of childhood emotional deficit disorder. They subdivided borderline patients into organic and functional subtypes, and noted that borderline personality disorder would manifest 'soft' neurological signs.

Developmental issues

Case histories of patients in psychodynamically oriented treatment revealed the presence of developmental conflicts in borderline personality disorder. Masterson[53] emphasized the abandonment fears which originate in traumatic childhood separation experiences. Gunderson[54] identified intolerance of aloneness as a serious psychological deficit which seems to develop from developmental attachment failures.

Kernberg[41] and the object relation theorists believe that a lack of optimal emotional availability on the part of the mother during the rapprochement subphase of separation–individuation may be critical in the development of a future borderline personality. Splitting remains in the internal world of pre-borderline children, identity diffusion prevails, and object constancy is never reached. Superego pathology is evident, with sadistic superego forerunners being predominant.

The role of childhood trauma in the development of borderline personality disorder has been identified as crucial in numerous studies. Zanarini et al.[55] found that childhood experiences of both abuse and neglect were basically ubiquitous among borderline patients, with sexual abuse noted as an important aetiological factor in about 60 per cent of severely disturbed borderline patients.

Paris[56] has elegantly summarized all the aetiological factors mentioned above in his biopsychosocial model of borderline personality disorder. He suggested that there are a number of interacting biological, psychological and social risk factors for the development of borderline personality disorder, such as innate temperament, difficult childhood experiences, and relatively subtle forms of neurological and biochemical dysfunction (which may be either sequelae of these childhood experiences or innate vulnerabilities). Psychological and social stressors would precipitate a transition from innate vulnerability to overt psychopathology.

Clinical features and diagnosis

In a review of 14 research studies, Widiger and Frances[48] found that impulsivity and affective instability, self-damage, identity disturbance, and unstable/intense interpersonal relationships were the most characteristic manifestations of borderline personality disorder. These characteristics are manifested in behaviour and self-concept, affectivity, love and sexuality, cognitive style and interpersonal relationships.[57]

Behaviour and self-concept

Identity diffusion lies at the heart of many phenomena seen in borderline personality disorder. It is clinically manifested by contradictory character traits, temporal discontinuity of the self, lack of authenticity, feeling of emptiness, gender dysphoria, and inordinate ethnic and moral relativism.[57] Self-damaging acts are frequent, manifesting as recurrent suicidal behaviour or self-mutilation, as well as alcohol and substance abuse.

Affectivity

Borderline patients are chronically dysphoric. Their unstable mood is a mixture of depressed affect, anger, loneliness, and emptiness. Impulsive-aggressive behaviour is a core feature of borderline personality disorder.

Love and sexuality

Infatuations are followed by devaluation of love objects. There is a tendency towards promiscuity and perversions.

Cognitive style

Borderline patients are easily suggestible and frequently change their decisions. Things and people are seen in black-and-white terms. They are prone to transient micropsychotic episodes and emotional amnesia, especially in unstructured and stressful situations.

Interpersonal relationships

Interpersonal relationships are unstable, intense, demanding, clinging, and characterized by alternation between extremes of idealization and devaluation, deriving from splitting, which is a clinical marker of borderline personality disorder. Diagnostics can be improved by Kernberg's structural interview[58] and the Diagnostic Interview for Borderline Patients.[59]

Comorbidity and differential diagnosis

Borderline personality disorder is frequently comorbid with **affective disorders** (major depression, dysthymia, and 'double depression'), **anxiety disorders**, **somatization disorder**, **post-traumatic stress disorder**, and **alcohol abuse**. Comorbidity with affective disorders is particularly important. There is an ongoing debate about which condition begins first and may be primary.

Borderline personality disorder has been shown to be associated with most personality disorders, especially with those from the dramatic cluster. A high prevalence of comorbid personality disorders may be a result of insufficient criteria, or of the underlying borderline personality organization of all severe personality disorders. The following traits (a core syndrome of borderline personality disorder) help to discriminate it from other personality disorders: chronic feelings of emptiness, self-mutilation, short-lived psychotic episodes, impulsive acts, manipulative suicide attempts, and extremely demanding involvement in close relationships.

Multiple personality disorder and psychotic-like experiences of **schizotypal personality disorder** should be differentiated from borderline personality disorder.

Course and outcome

Borderline patients often experience profound dysfunction in many important aspects of life including education, jobs, partner relationships, and marriage. Alcohol and psychosexual problems are also frequent.

Repeated suicide attempts and premature death from suicide are frequent complications of borderline personality disorder; therefore suicidal gestures and intentions should be always taken seriously. It has been reported that 8 to 10 per cent per cent of all persons with borderline personality disorder die by suicide.[60]

The long-term outcome of borderline patients has not been studied, but the diagnosis is rarely made in patients aged over 40. It is speculated that neural structures and defence mechanisms mature with age and that these changes, together with social learning, reduce symptomatology.

Treatment

The treatment should be multidimensional, continuous, multimodal, and eclectic. Most frequently, both pharmacotherapy and psychotherapy should be applied.

Pharmacotherapy

Target symptoms of borderline personality disorder, such as affective changes (depression, anxiety, rage, dysphoria), various cognitive disturbances (brief psychotic episodes or interpretative distortions), and impulsive behavioural dyscontrol, should be treated. Stein[61] has summarized possible drug treatments, providing helpful guidelines for clinical practice.

Behavioural dyscontrol is undoubtedly the most serious management problem with borderline personality disorder patients. Neuroleptics and carbamazepine may help some patients, even in the absence of EEG or organic changes. Lithium may be indicated for patients with serious episodes of aggressive behaviour extending over years, especially if there is a family history of classic affective disorder or alcoholism.

Newer psychopharmacological agents, the selective serotonin reuptake inhibitors such as fluoxetine, have shown positive effects in treating a broad spectrum of acute symptoms, including depression, hostility, irritability, anxiety, obsessive–compulsive symptoms, suicidal attempts, and impulsivity.

There are still no clinical predictors in the patient's history as to which drug might be helpful. A pragmatic approach is best, with patients being treated by two or three drugs in a sequential trial in the hope that one will be found that is both beneficial and well tolerated, as Stein[61] has wisely pointed out. Some drugs could cause deterioration and side-effects. Increased behavioural dyscontrol or paradoxical rage reactions have been reported with benzodiazepines and tricyclic antidepressants, which contraindicate their use. Suicidal abuse of drugs and non-compliance may be serious problems.

Psychotherapy

Psychotherapy of borderline patients is often approached with pessimism. Various psychotherapeutical modalities are used, including psychodynamic psychotherapy, supportive psychotherapy, and dialectical–cognitive psychotherapy.

Classical psychoanalysis has been considered to be contraindicated. **Long-term individual psychotherapy** can be helpful to patients with borderline personality disorder. Kernberg[62] recommended a more structured form, expressive psychotherapy (a modified psychoanalytical procedure), involving an active technique focusing on confrontation of maladaptive defences and interpretation of transference, focusing on the 'here and now', without attempting the achievement of a full genetic reconstruction.

Short-term psychotherapy is useful for managing crises or introducing long-term forms of therapy. **Supportive psychotherapy** is suggested for more fragile borderline patients, who are prone to serious regression in treatment. In practice, supportive therapy, with a psychoeducational component, has been the most frequently used form of treatment for borderline personality disorder. It is also possible to combine elements of intensive dynamic therapy with supportive therapy, depending on the ego strength of the patients.[56]

Some authors consider **long-term intermittent treatment** to be the standard method for borderline personality disorder.[63] Another variant of intermittent therapy is crisis intervention. An increasing number of experts see **combined individual and group treatment**, preferably by the same therapist, as a promising development in the treatment of borderline patients. **Dialectical behavioural therapy**[64] can be useful for parasuicidal borderline patients. Intermittent hospitalization, usually for short periods, together with adjunctive treatment may help in crises.

Psychiatrists who intend to treat borderline patients need special training and sensitivity. Countertransference problems are frequent, and regular supervision is necessary.

Histrionic personality disorder (DLT)

Definition

Histrionic personality disorder is a polymorphic concept supported by descriptive literature and clinical tradition, but not so much by valid empirical research. It is characterized by excessive emotionality and attention seeking, and by dramatic, colourful, and extroverted behaviour. Egocentric, dependent, and demanding interpersonal relationships are typical of this disorder, which begins in early adulthood and is present in a variety of contexts.

Historical perspective

Early contributions

Histrionic personality disorder is a descendant of 'hysteria' described by Hippocrates 2400 years ago. It was included in scientific medicine by Kraepelin,[65] who described multiple symptoms, including capricious and inconsistent behaviour, histrionic exaggeration, and a life of illness, which captured the core pattern of the illness.

At the end of the nineteenth century, Charcot and Janet linked hysteria with conversion symptoms. Through the work of Bernheim and Freud, the personality characteristics of patients displaying hysterical phenomena provided an important impetus to the development of psychoanalysis. Freud[66] recognized the relationship between hysterical neurosis and what he called the 'erotic personality, whose major goal in life is the desire to love or above all to be loved'. The first psychoanalytic description of hysterical personality was given by Wittels[67] and refined by Reich,[68] who focused on the oral and genital determinants of the disorder.

Table 7 DSM-IV diagnostic criteria for histrionic personality disorder

A pervasive pattern of excessive emotionality and attention seeking, beginning by early adulthood and present in a variety of contexts, as indicated by five (or more) of the following

(1) Is uncomfortable in situations in which he or she is not the centre of attention
(2) Interaction with others is often characterized by inappropriate sexually seductive or provocative behaviour
(3) Displays rapidly shifting and shallow expression of emotions
(4) Consistently uses physical appearance to draw attention to self
(5) Has a style of speech that is excessively impressionistic and lacking in detail
(6) Shows self-dramatization, theatricality, and exaggerated expression of emotion
(7) Is suggestible, i.e. easily influenced by others or circumstances
(8) Considers relationships to be more intimate than they actually are

Contemporary concepts

Chodoff and Lyons[69] clarified the terminological confusion surrounding hysterical personality, differentiating it from conversion reaction. In DSM-II, the concept was influenced by the psychoanalytic heritage. In DSM-III, the term histrionic personality disorder, coined by Brody and Sata,[70] was used, reflecting the diagnostic importance of external features such as dramatization, emotional instability, and attention-seeking. The change in terminology was in tune with the descriptive tradition of contemporary psychiatry and reliance on observable behavioural phenomena.

DSM-III captured the lower level of hysterics (infantile personality) which showed substantial overlap with borderline personality disorder (ranging from 44 to 95 per cent in various studies).[71] The question of whether the criteria are insufficiently discriminatory or the two disorders represent slightly different manifestations of the same underlying psychopathology remains unresolved.

DSM-IIIR and DSM-IV reduced this problem to some extent by refining the criteria set (Table 7). The concept adopted in ICD-10 (Table 8) is generally congruent with DSM-IV.

Psychoanalytic theorists often distinguish hysterical ('healthier') and histrionic ('sicker') personalities, where the latter has borderline organization and is an exaggeration of the former. Differences between the two concepts are shown in Table 9.

Table 8 ICD-10 diagnostic criteria for histrionic personality disorder

Personality disorder characterized by at least three of the following:

(a) self-dramatization, theatricality, exaggerated expression of emotions
(b) suggestibility, easily influenced by others or by circumstances
(c) shallow and labile affectivity
(d) continually seeking for excitement, appreciation by others, and activities in which the patient is the centre of attention
(e) Inappropriate seductiveness in appearance or behaviour
(f) Overconcern with physical attractiveness

Associated features may include egocentricity, self-indulgence, continuous longing for appreciation, feelings that are easily hurt, and persistent manipulative behaviour to achieve own needs

Includes: hysterical and psycho-infantile personality (disorder)

Table 9 Types of histrionism

Hysterical personality	Histrionic personality[a]
Neurotic personality organization	Borderline personality organization
Integrated identity	Diffuse identity
Predominance of repression	Predominance of splitting
Intact reality testing	Intact reality testing (proneness to distortion)
Integrated superego	Marked superego defects
Strongly bonded families	Disturbed, often broken families
Steady educational and vocational careers	Erratic careers
Capable of maintaining long-term friendships	Chaotic interpersonal relationships
Suggestible in triangular relationships	Diffuse suggestibility
Inauthenticity	Multiple identifications
Changing moods	Frequent dysphoria
Sexual inhibition	Promiscuity, perverse tendencies
Competitiveness with the same sex	Less differentiated behaviour toward sexes
Genital traits	Oral/pregenital traits

[a] Includes hysteroid, hysteriform, oral hysteric, and sick hysteric personality disorders. After Akhtar.[32]

Some authors believe that a common underlying psychopathological process may express itself as histrionic personality disorder and/or somatization disorder in women and as antisocial personality disorder in men,[72] which is in accordance with the 'spectrum' concept.[73] The possibility of organizing histrionic and borderline personality disorders (and possibly antisocial and narcissistic personality disorders) on a continuum of related diagnoses is an intriguing idea deserving empirical research. It could be concluded that histrionic personality disorder comprises a heterogeneous group of patients who can function on any level of the continuum from neurotic to borderline. The best way to diagnose personality disorder would be a label of the specific disorder and the level of its functioning (adding a dimension of severity), which would then determine the choice of therapeutic strategy.[74]

Epidemiology

The prevalence is found to be 2 to 3 per cent of the general population and 10 to 15 per cent in clinical settings.[75] No significant difference has been found in terms of race and education, but it is higher among separated and divorced persons. Clinicians diagnose histrionic personality more often in women than in men, for various reasons:

- different psychosexual development in boys and girls, as claimed by Freud
- the sex bias inherent in the given criteria
- male diagnosticians may elicit responses which might not have been obtained by a woman examiner[69]
- the traits characteristic of this personality are regarded by society as being feminine and thus more acceptable in women than in men.[76]

Further cross-cultural studies are needed to evaluate the importance of cultural influences on sex role stereotypes and emotional expressiveness.

Aetiology

There has been very little empirical investigation of the aetiology of histrionic personality disorder, which is probably multidimensional (biological, developmental, and social).

Biological issues

The increasing evidence that typical hysterical traits, such as emotional expressiveness, extraversion, and reward dependence, are constitutional suggests that there might be an inherited predisposition for the development of this disorder. In his twin study, Torgersen[77] found that the hysterical dimension is genetically influenced among women but not among men. Similar findings have been reported in a family study of somatization disorder, which is historically related to histrionic personality.[78] Some studies suggest that histrionic personality runs in families, but more research is needed in order to establish whether it has a biological or developmental cause.

Cadoret[73] postulated an interesting hypothesis, based on an adoption study, in which hysteria is assumed to be part of the antisocial spectrum, i.e. a different phenotypic manifestation of the antisocial personality genotype.

Developmental issues

Early psychoanalysts thought that histrionic personality disorder was determined by a fixation on the genital phase of infantile development, associated with an incestuous attachment. Later, this idea was challenged,[76] and pregenital oral fixations were considered to be more important. The conflict between oral and genital determinants would be solved if the continuum of hysterical psychopathology mentioned above was shown to exist.

Histrionic individuals, especially those at the sicker end of the continuum, have often had deprived and traumatic childhoods, similar to those of antisocial personalities. Zetzel[79] pointed out that the developmental history of hysterical individuals reveals significant separations in the first four years of life, serious parental psychopathology, much physical illness during childhood, and absence of meaningful sustained relations with either sex.

Clinical features and diagnosis

Lazare et al.[80] were the first to use factor analysis to examine the clustering of traits in hysterical personality. A hysterical factor emerged that included emotionality, oral aggression, exhibitionism, egocentricity, and sexual provocativeness. Diagnosis should not be difficult if behavioural expression, affectivity, love and sexuality, cognitive style, and interpersonal relations[32] are carefully assessed.

Behavioural expression

Histrionic individuals have been described as a caricature of femininity, as pointed out by Easser and Lesser.[81] They are coquettish, inappropriately seductive, and aggressively demanding. These self-centred persons crave novelty and excitement, and are inconsiderate, manipulative, and prone to temper tantrums. Their appearance is exhibitionistic and their behaviour has sexual implications.

Affectivity

Histrionic persons are hyperemotional and impulsive, but their emotional enthusiasm is transient and their mood is labile. They describe their emotions in an inappropriate and exaggerated way. Emotional display is used to obtain attention and desired goals, and to avoid responsibilities and unpleasant affects. However, their emotions are neither constant nor consistent, which often exasperate friends and clinicians. Histrionic individuals are suggestible, demanding, accusative, and guilt inducing. Instead of feeling anxiety or depression in stressful situations, they show inappropriate naiveté or *la belle indifference*.

Love and sexuality

Histrionic personalities are inclined to sexualize all non-sexual relations, often indiscriminately, not only with a chosen partner but also with a wide variety of persons in various social, occupational, and professional relationships. Pseudosexuality is often accompanied by frigidity. A romantic outlook or a superficially adoring attitude often disguises needs for dependency and emotional attachment to a significant protective figure. Sicker individuals may be promiscuous, and may engage in multiple perverse activities.

Cognitive style

Cognitive style is global, impressionistic, and diffuse, and lacks sharpness of detail. Non-verbal communication is better than verbal, speech is inhibited, and education is often superficial. Speech may show malapropisms or slips of the tongue. Histrionic individuals are suggestible and promptly forget affect-laden material. Rather than mature thought and consideration of all facets of a problem, they rapidly 'comprehend' a situation, relying upon intuition.

Interpersonal relationships

The basic belief of histrionic personalities is that others should be impressed, and their basic strategy is dramatization. They blossom when they are the centre of attention and are highly disappointed when they are not, and draw attention to themselves by acting and speaking in a charming flirtatious way. Histrionic individuals quickly respond to others in an intimate way, often treating superficial acquaintances as if they were friends. They have a high level of energy, but their persistent demands and insatiability can be exasperating.

Comorbidity and differential diagnosis

There is current evidence that **somatization disorder** (Briquet's syndrome) and **conversion disorder** can occur in conjunction with histrionic personality disorder, as well as **dissociative disorder** and **brief reactive psychosis**.[32] Differential diagnosis should not be difficult, because histrionic personality disorder is a lifelong disturbance with a chronic course, unlike Axis I disorders which are episodic. **Hypomanic and manic states** may be accompanied by seductive behaviour and exaggerated expression of emotions, but can be distinguished from histrionic personality by their episodic nature and the presence of other characteristic symptoms.

A great deal of overlap has been found between histrionic personality disorder and other **Axis II disorders**, defined by DSM-IIIR criteria; of these, the borderline, narcissistic, antisocial, and dependent personality disorders are the most frequent.

Borderline patients have more chaotic interpersonal relationships, make frequent suicide attempts, and are prone to regressive episodes of a psychotic nature. Histrionic individuals share sexual promiscuity, corruptibility, shallow emotions, and a self-centred attitude with antisocial personalities.[82] However, they do not show sustained, calculated, and ruthless disregard of social norms. Narcissists may also seek attention, but they want to be admired for their superiority while histrionic persons are clinging and dependent. Unlike narcissists, histrionic individuals have empathy for other persons. However, the features of the two disorders can be combined.

Course and prognosis

Depressive symptoms, suicide attempts, and frequent use of medical services are common. Histrionic personality may gradually improve with age, as if a maturation of histrionic infantilism occurs over the years.

Treatment

Pharmacotherapy

Patients with histrionic personality disorder often seek treatment when depressed, or have unexplained somatic complaints and interpersonal difficulties. Target medication may be useful, but it should be brief, and patients should be checked for non-compliance and abuse.

Psychotherapy

Psychotherapy, which may help to stabilize erratic mood, and prevent depressive and other decompensations, is the treatment of choice.

Supportive therapy is indicated for acutely distressed histrionic patients, as well as for those at the sicker end of the continuum. In order to decrease the risk of self-harm or other impulsive acting-out behaviour, a combination of support, judicious medication, and brief hospitalization may be needed.[45]

Psychoanalysis can be used for patients in the healthier part of the histrionic continuum. Histrionic personalities, functioning on the clear borderline level, should be treated by **expressive psychotherapy**.[82]

Identification and clarification of the patient's covert inner feelings is an important part of the therapeutic process. Histrionic patients often develop erotic-idealizing transference. They may be sexually provocative in their relationships with the therapist, who should not reward the exaggerated feelings and should be careful in managing the transference. Patients are often demanding, want to take a special place in the therapist's life, and act out during therapy sessions, threatening to abandon treatment or undertake dangerous actions. Clear limits should be set and demanding dependent behaviour should not be rewarded. The treatment should be carefully planned and goals discussed with the patient, who should express a desire and motivation to change his or her behaviour, and not just to change the external world.

Therapists must be aware of their own narcissistic needs for admiration, which are easily evoked by histrionic patients, and should be supervised in order not to become trapped in a vicious circle of dependence, demanding behaviour, and latent aggressive control.

Narcissistic personality disorder (DLT)

Narcissistic personality disorder is characterized by an exaggerated sense of self-importance with a lack of sustained positive regard for others. Grandiosity (in fantasy or behaviour) and constant craving for admiration and external gratification are additional features of this disorder. They are present in a variety of contexts and begin by early adulthood.

Historical perspective

The term narcissism originates from the Greek myth of Narcissus who was infatuated with his own reflection in the mirror-lake. Its contemporary usage has many meanings and implications, from its colloquial

Table 10 Types of narcissism

Normal	Pathological	Malignant
Infantile	Grandiose self-image	Grandiose self-image
Regression or fixation to infantile narcissistic goals in personality disorders (personality traits)	Low self-esteem	Aggression
	Primitive defences	Paranoid traits
	Superego defects	Explosive traits
	Borderline organization	Antisocial behaviour
		Borderline organization
Adult		
Healthy self-esteem regulated by normal self-structure		
Integrated object representations		
Capacity for deep object relations		
Integrated superego		

After Kernberg.[31,41]

usage denoting self-centred persons, often with pejorative connotations, to a pathological clinical syndrome. Despite the popularity of the construct, there is still considerable disagreement on the aetiology and phenomenology of narcissistic personality disorder. There is little empirical evidence regarding its description, clinical utility, and validity.

Early contributions

Freud[83] described primary (normal) and secondary (pathological) narcissism, the nature of narcissistic object choices, and the narcissistic foundation of the ego ideal as a psychic structure in his seminal paper on narcissism. In 1931, Freud[66] described the narcissistic character type, which is considered to be a pioneering portrayal of narcissistic personality disorder. Jones[84] gave a detailed description of narcissistic individuals, who exhibit a 'God complex' and have some cognitive peculiarities. Reich[68] described the phallic–narcissistic character, with grandiosity used as a defence against underlying inferiority. Fenichel[85] saw the narcissist as 'the Don Juan of achievement', pointing out that some narcissistic individuals may adapt a criminal lifestyle owing to superego defects. Nemiah[86] described 'narcissistic character disorder', which was later elaborated by two leading workers in the field, Heinz Kohut and Otto Kernberg.

Contemporary concepts

Kohut, in *The Analysis of the Self*,[87] described narcissistic personality disorder as presenting a failure to internalize healthy self-esteem; it is a derivative of normal infantile grandiosity, causing a poor self-image against which narcissism develops as a defensive reaction. Kernberg[41] divided narcissism into normal infantile, normal adult, and pathological. This idea is in tune with the continuum of psychopathology (Table 10), in which fixation or regression to infantile narcissistic goals is an important feature of all personality disorders that include narcissistic traits or narcissism as a defensive reaction. Narcissism, in its normal sublimated form, is necessary for the self-esteem essential for a healthy life and a capacity for deep object relations.

A narcissistic personality has a pathological grandiose self which hides a diffuse and aimless inner identity. Kernberg argues that self-hatred, rather than self-love, lies at the root of pathological narcissism,

and distinguishes between narcissism in the broad sense and the specific pathological structures of the narcissistic personality. According to Kernberg, narcissistic patients function on a borderline level. Malignant narcissism,[31] which develops when primitive aggression infiltrates the pathological grandiose self, lies at the extreme end of a continuum. It is a combination of narcissistic personality disorder, antisocial behaviour, egosyntonic aggression or sadism directed against others, and a strong paranoid orientation.

Narcissistic personality disorder was officially accepted in DSM-III. Somewhat refined criteria were adopted in DSM-IV (Table 11), because some studies showed a substantial lack of diagnostic reliability when the DSM-III criteria were used. Narcissistic personality disorder is not included in ICD-10, being mentioned only in the category 'Other specific personality disorders'.

Epidemiology

The prevalence of narcissistic personality disorder in the community has been found to be 0.4 per cent.[49] Its prevalence in clinical populations is estimated to range from 1 to 3 per cent, and is greater among males. It is not yet clear whether this is due to diagnostic bias, more frequent seeking of treatment by males, or the difference in psychosexual development between males and females.

Aetiology

There has been very little empirical investigation of the aetiology of narcissistic personality disorder. It is probably multidimensional, as in other personality disorders, with biological, developmental, and social factors. In the absence of other information, psychoanalytical theory remains the most important of the aetiological explanations.

Biological issues

Although Freud[66] prophesied that biological factors may be important in the aetiology of narcissism, they have yet to be studied. Accord-

Table 11 DSM-IV diagnostic criteria for narcissistic personality disorder

A pervasive pattern of grandiosity (in fantasy or behaviour), need for admiration, and lack of empathy, beginning by early adulthood and present in a variety of contexts, as indicated by five (or more) of the following

(1) Has a grandiose sense of self-importance (e.g. exaggerates achievements and talents, expects to be recognized as superior without commensurate achievements)

(2) Is preoccupied with fantasies of unlimited success, power, brilliance, beauty, or ideal love

(3) Believes that he or she is 'special' and unique and can only be understood by, or should associate with, other special or high-status people (or institutions)

(4) Requires excessive admiration

(5) Has a sense of entitlement, i.e. unreasonable expectations of especially favourable treatment or automatic compliance with his or her expectations

(6) Is interpersonally exploitative, i.e. takes advantage of others to achieve his or her own ends

(7) Lacks empathy, i.e. is unwilling to recognize or identify with the feelings and needs of others

(8) Is often envious of others or believes that others are envious of him or her

(9) Shows arrogant haughty behaviours or attitudes

ing to Cloninger's[15] biosocial model of personality, the narcissistic personality results from high novelty seeking and high reward dependence, which might reflect neurotransmitter involvement.

Developmental issues

Severe frustration with early objects is considered important in the defensive genesis of narcissistic personality disorder. Reich[88] described narcissistic ego-inflation as a defence against narcissistic injuries during both the pre-Oedipal and Oedipal periods of development. Behind the compensatory grandiose self, a hungry and inferior real self resides, as the core problem of narcissistic personality disorder. Nemiah[86] saw the origin of this disorder in high parental expectations and harsh criticism of the child, which become internalized in their developing character. Many narcissistic individuals are gifted and often are the first, if not the only, child in their families. Nemiah proposed that the parents used the child for their own needs, which led the child to seek compensatory admiration and greatness. Since there is often frustration during the vulnerable rapprochement subphase of separation–individuation, splitting of good and bad self and object representatives remains in the inner world, with the typical conflicts of borderline personality organization covered by the protective shield of grandiose self.

Social issues

Some authors have suggested that narcissistic personality disorder is not a psychopathological entity but merely a sociocultural phenomenon related to the contemporary Western 'culture of narcissism'.[89] This approach is probably misleading. Such an explanation may provide a cultural rationalization for some pathological narcissists, but society cannot produce either normal or pathological narcissism as these disorders are complex and are likely to be established during early childhood.[62]

Clinical characteristics and diagnosis

Narcissistic patients seldom approach a psychiatrist, and then usually when depressed or involved in interpersonal problems. The surface functioning of the narcissistic individual may show very little disturbance. However, the inner world of narcissistic patients is extremely pathological, despite their superficially well-adapted behaviour, and this pathology is shown in their self-concept, affectivity, love and sexuality, interpersonal relations and cognitive style.[90]

Behavioural expression and self-concept

A seductive and charming appearance, which is engaging and attractive, masks intense preoccupation with self-regard and an unusual absence of concern for others. Narcissistic individuals may be energetic, capable of consistent work, and socially successful, but this is done in order to obtain admiration. These 'Don Juans of achievement' run from one achievement to another, but their successes provide no inner satisfaction and always end with frustration and a feeling of emptiness. Narcissistic grandiosity is often masked by opposing tendencies (false modesty, social aloofness, and a pretended contempt for status). Pathological lying is frequent.

Affectivity

Narcissistic individuals feel bored when the external glitter wears off and there are no new sources to feed their self-esteem, which is extremely fragile. Lacking emotional depth, they do not have genuine feelings of sadness or longing. Anger and resentment laden with vengeful wishes are frequent as a reaction to injured self-esteem. Chronic intense envy is present, as are defences against such envy, particularly devaluation, omnipotent control, and narcissistic withdrawal. They have frequent mood swings, and hypomanic exaltation is often part of the clinical picture.

Love and sexuality

Narcissistic persons are unable to fall in love, and only have fantasies of ideal love. Sexuality is trivialized, and intercourse is a purely physical pleasure. Promiscuity, perverse fantasies, devaluation of objects, and boredom in relationships are frequent.

Cognitive style

Language is typically used to regulate self-esteem rather than to communicate or understand. Narcissists may be articulate and excellent lecturers, but their knowledge is often shallow and exhibitionistic (so-called 'headline intelligence').

Interpersonal relationships

Interpersonal relationships are frequently parasitic, manipulative, and exploitative. They idealize people whom they expect to feed their narcissism, but deprecate and treat with contempt others (often former idols) from whom they do not expect to receive anything. They lack empathy and concern for others, who are welcome only as an applauding crowd and as mirrors of success.

Typical defence mechanisms (omnipotence, omniscience, intellectualization, rationalization, idealization, and devaluation) are derived from splitting. The Narcissistic Personality Inventory[91] and the semi-structured Diagnostic Interview for Narcissism[92] assess characteristics imputed to pathological narcissism.

Comorbidity and differential diagnosis

Narcissistic personality disorder is often comorbid with major depression, dysthymic disorder, substance abuse, and anorexia nervosa. Patients meeting criteria for narcissistic disorder have a high overlap with **histrionic, borderline, and antisocial personality disorders**, and also with **schizotypal, paranoid, and passive-aggressive personality disorders**.

Narcissistic personality disorder may display some features of bipolar disorder (manic and hypomanic episodes). However, the mood swings are of limited duration and change rapidly, while insight is maintained and the general integrity of the personality is preserved.

Narcissistic personality disorder is strikingly similar to borderline personality disorder. Phenomenologically, grandiosity is the best discriminator between the two disorders.[93] In narcissistic personality disorder, there is also better impulse control, greater social adjustment and anxiety tolerance, less frequent suicide attempts, and less danger of regressive fragmentation and psychotic episodes.

Narcissistic individuals, especially those manifesting malignant narcissism, may demonstrate antisocial behaviour. However, antisocial individuals are more impulsive and less capable of concentrating on work and career, and they are devoid of guilt feelings. Similarities with histrionic and obsessive–compulsive personalities are superficial, since people with these disorders have a capacity for empathy and a concern and love for others.

Course and prognosis

Patients often become depressed or defensively hypomanic during middle age, when their internal life gradually deteriorates owing to a vicious circle of frustrations and disappointments and diminishing narcissistic supplies. They may cynically withdraw into 'splendid isolation', away from the 'empty' external world. Hypochondriasis and anxiety disorders are frequent complications.

Treatment

Pharmacotherapy

At times antiaxiety agents and antidepressants, especially selective serotonin reuptake inhibitors, may be helpful for alleviating target symptoms (mood swings, anxiety, narcissistic rage and depression).

Psychotherapy

Individual psychotherapy is the treatment of choice for narcissistic patients. Various approaches can be used.

In Kohut's self-psychology approach[87] transference is used as both a diagnostic and a therapeutic tool. Idealizing transference is supported and left uninterpreted until optimal disillusionment gradually develops through the therapist's unintended but inevitable empathic failures. At this point the patient may integrate his or her own and the therapist's realistic limitations.

Modell's approach[94] focuses on a therapeutic relationship within an ego-psychology object relations model. At first, the narcissistic idealization and the patient's incapacity to absorb interpretations are respected in a 'holding' function. Later, the grandiose self is gradually interpreted, and the treatment largely corresponds to that of Kernberg.

Kernberg[41,62] suggests that the approach should vary according to the degree of disturbance. Psychoanalysis is suggested for some well-functioning narcissistic patients, and expressive psychotherapy is indicated for narcissistic pathology with overt borderline features. A systematic analysis is made of both the grandiose self, which presents itself pervasively in the transference, and the patient's use of primitive defences, especially devaluation and idealization. Supportive therapy is indicated for malignant narcissism. Sometimes it may be needed as a preparatory period for expressive psychotherapy. Group therapy may be combined with individual therapy, during which peer confrontation of grandiosity and a shared 'special relationship' with the therapist might be useful. Hospital admission is required only in severe depressive decompensations.

The treatment of narcissistic individuals inevitably arouses serious countertransference problems, because of the emotional detachment, demanding behaviour, and devaluative actions of narcissistic patients. The therapist should have worked through his or her own narcissism and retain an empathic and non-judgemental attitude.

Cluster C personality disorders

Avoidant personality disorder (JLC)

Avoidant personality disorder was first introduced into psychiatric classification in DSM-III.[11] Before this, such patients were included among the schizoid or dependent patients. The emphasis on avoidant behaviour as a consequence of an intense sensitivity to rejection led to the differentiation of this new personality type. Before this, such people had been described as 'hyperaesthetic shut-in individuals',[10] phobic personalities,[95] or active-detached personalities.[96]

The characteristic behaviour of the avoidant personality is active

Table 12 DSM-IV diagnostic criteria for avoidant personality disorder

A pervasive pattern of social inhibition, feelings of inadequacy, and hypersensitivity to negative evaluation, beginning by early adulthood and present in a variety of contexts, as indicated by four (or more) of the following

(1) Avoids occupational activities that involve significant interpersonal contact, because of fears of criticism, disapproval, or rejection
(2) Is unwilling to get involved with people unless certain of being liked
(3) Shows restraint within intimate relationships because of the fear of being shamed or ridiculed
(4) Is preoccupied with being criticized or rejected in social situations
(5) Is inhibited in new interpersonal situations because of feelings of inadequacy
(6) Views self as socially inept, personally unappealing, or inferior to others
(7) Is unusually reluctant to take personal risks or to engage in any new activities because they may prove embarrassing

isolation from the social environment. Unlike schizoids, who are characterized by passive social isolation, avoidant subjects turn inward to protect themselves because they are extremely sensitive to rejection.[97] They desire interpersonal relationships but they avoid any chance of disapproval. Thus, only relationships that are likely to lead to complete non-critical acceptance are established. The extreme sensitivity to criticism is based on intense feelings of inferiority, poor self-concept and low self-esteem. This disorder is termed anxious personality disorder in ICD-10, since anxiety is considered to be the basic affective feature. The DSM-IV criteria for avoidant personality disorder are shown in Table 12.

Epidemiology

The prevalence of avoidant personality disorder is estimated to be less than 1 per cent in the general population, but almost 10 per cent in clinical populations. No differences between sexes are found.

Aetiology

Some familial transmission is possible, perhaps involving learning and identification, but genetic transmission may also be involved.[98] The biological mechanisms involved in anxiety disorders and social phobia may have a role in the development of this personality disorder. It has been suggested that hypersensitivity of brain areas involved in the separation-anxiety response and overactivity of serotonin limbic neuronal circuits may underlie the avoidant temperament trait.[98]

Psychosocial factors mediate the extent to which biological vulnerability is expressed. Children who are belittled, criticized, and rejected by parents have decreased self-esteem, resulting in social avoidance. These problems are reinforced and perpetuated at school and may generate the expectation of rejection from everyone.[97]

Clinical picture

Avoidant people are characterized by extreme shyness. They appear distant from others and do not express wishes, demands, or opinions. However, this behaviour contrasts with an extreme internal need for warmth and closeness. This contradiction is explained by an exaggerated sensitivity to rejection by others. People with this personality disorder are easily hurt and humiliated by comments from others, which they misinterpret as degrading and disapproving. They tend to be shy, quiet, and inhibited. They say nothing rather than risk being wrong, and they react strongly to any possible indications of mockery or criticism. They usually appear anxious, self-doubting, and insecure when speaking, often use self-defeating expressions, and try to please others. Their tense and fearful demeanour may elicit ridicule from others which confirms their insecurity. They are concerned with reacting to scrutiny by blushing or crying, which is a cause of further interpersonal avoidance. These patients often choose occupations where no social interaction is needed, and strongly avoid talking in public. The avoidant person lacks intimate relationships with friends or sexual partners unless they anticipate non-critical acceptance.

Patients with avoidant personality disorder perceive themselves as inept and inadequate, and assume that they are unattractive. They tend to see others as negative and potentially harmful. They are inattentive and repeatedly distracted by intrusive thoughts, but they attend intensely to signals of rejection. These people tend to make negative evaluations of situations and exaggerate risk. They have a low tolerance for dysphoric affects which they avoid by escaping. Escape from reality through fantasy is their usual way of satisfying their needs and relieving frustration.

At interview they may be quite open if they feel accepted. This happens when good rapport is made, which is often easier in clinical than in social situations. However, social limitation outside the office may be intense. Avoidant patients usually feel ashamed about many aspects of their lives and are excessively self-critical, although most of the concerns expressed seem to be trivial.

Course

Avoidant personality disorder may follow childhood fear of strangers and shyness and isolation during school years. However, most shyness in childhood gradually dissipates in adolescence. When it evolves into avoidant personality disorder, the shyness may worsen in adolescence when social and interpersonal relationships become more complex and demanding. The disorder tends to remit or to become less evident in older people.

Avoidant personality disorder is often associated with depressive episodes, dysthymia, and anxiety disorders, particularly social phobia.

Differential diagnosis

It is often difficult to differentiate avoidant personality disorder and social phobia of the generalized type. Impairment and distress due to the phobic situations is more intense in social phobia, which may have started in middle adulthood rather than adolescence. It is not clear whether the disorders are alternative manifestations of the same condition, or are separate disorders.

Hypersensitivity to rejection and criticism, low self-esteem, and feelings of inadequacy are also features of dependent personality disorder. While the avoidant patient avoids contact, the dependent patient focuses on being cared for. However, the disorders often co-occur and must be diagnosed together.

Schizoid and schizotypal personality disorder are also characterized by social isolation. However, avoidants want to have relationships and suffer for their isolation, while schizoids and schizotypals accept isolation.

People with paranoid personality disorders lack confidence in others. However, avoidants do not confide in others because they fear being found inadequate, whereas paranoids fear malicious intent.

Treatment

Anxiety and hypersensitivity to rejection may improve with anxiolytic medication, β-blockers, monoamine oxidase inhibitors, and antidepressant medication. Medication should be combined with psychological treatment based on reinforcing assertiveness and self-esteem, and restructuring cognitive distortions concerning the self and others. Conscious and unconscious dependency needs should be addressed.

Dependent personality disorder (JLC)

Individuals with this disorder show a persistent and global pattern of behaviours directed at avoidance of the loss of intimate others. To attain this goal, they relinquish their own needs, opinions, expression of feelings, and even their self-identity. In exchange, they get others to take over responsibility for major areas of their lives and to protect them. Their self-concept is characterized by weakness and helplessness, while others are perceived as powerful and protective.

These people were formerly included in different classificatory categories. They belong to the abulic type of Kraepelin and of Schneider[2] and were considered as immature personalities.

Aetiology

According to Freud,[99] the dependent personality was the manifestation of fixation in the oral phase of psychosexual development. Abraham believed that the disorder originated in an excess of oral gratification and protection.[95,100] More recent studies have ruled out these hypotheses and suggested that the excessive concern with oral satisfaction, passivity, self-doubt, and dependence are related to deprivation rather than overgratification in the oral phase.

Diagnosis

Dependent personality was recognized first in DSM-III.[11] The description has changed little in DSM-IV (Table 13) and ICD-10.[101] The crucial feature in both systems is the urgent need of patients to be cared for by others, with dependence, attachment, and fear of abandonment. Lack of self-confidence was required in DSM-III, but was eliminated from recent classifications because it is not specific to this disorder.

Clinical picture

Dependent patients are passive. They rarely express needs or feelings, especially those that are sexual or aggressive. They tend to avoid responsibilities or decisions in major areas of their lives, such as work and financial or interpersonal relationships. Instead they get others, particularly family or partner, to decide for them or to provide continuous guidance. They depend on others (often one other person, usually the partner or a parent) to decide where they should go, what they should do, and even which clothes they should wear. They manifest self-doubt, pessimism, and a need for affection. They lack aggressiveness and appear helpless. The dependent patient avoids jobs that demand taking responsibility and managing others, and becomes anxious when forced into such situations. These patients seek intensely for companionship and do not tolerate being alone. They may function at an adequate level if in a close and protective relationship, but when left alone they are unable to survive. They believe that they are incapable

Table 13 DSM-IV diagnostic criteria for dependent personality disorder

A pervasive and excessive need to be taken care of that leads to submissive and clinging behaviour and fears of separation, beginning by early adulthood and present in a variety of contexts, as indicated by five (or more) of the following

(1) Has difficulty making everyday decisions without an excessive amount of advice and reassurance from others

(2) Needs others to assume responsibility for most major areas of his or her life

(3) Has difficulty expressing disagreement with others because of fear of loss of support or approval. **Note** Do not include realistic fears of retribution

(4) Has difficulty initiating projects or doing things on his or her own (because of a lack of self-confidence in judgement or abilities rather than a lack of motivation or energy)

(5) Goes to excessive lengths to obtain nurturance and support from others, to the point of volunteering to do things that are unpleasant

(6) Feels uncomfortable or helpless when alone because of exaggerated fears of being unable to care for himself or herself

(7) Urgently seeks another relationship as a source of care and support when a close relationship ends

(8) Is unrealistically preoccupied with fears of being left to take care of himself or herself

of functioning independently and require constant assistance. They do not initiate projects, but wait for others who, they believe, will do them better. However, dependent individuals can perform such tasks for other people whom they want to please and to whom they want to attach themselves.

They accept unpleasant tasks, are self-sacrificing, and tolerate verbal, physical, or sexual abuse. Abusive relationships may be accepted as long as the attachment is preserved and is not excessively distorted.

An excessive and unrealistic fear of abandonment is constant in dependent individuals. When an intimate relationship is terminated by separation or death, dependent individuals urgently seek another person who will provide the care and support they seek. Thus they become rapidly and indiscriminately attached to other persons when left alone.

These people are pessimistic, self-doubting, and have low self-esteem. They belittle their capacities and successes and present themselves as inept. They take criticism as a proof of their ineptness and confirmation of their lack of self-confidence.

Epidemiology

Recent studies have found a median prevalence of 0.7 per cent (see Chapter 4.12.5). Although dependent personality disorder is diagnosed more frequently in women, structured interviews have not shown significant differences between the sexes. Cultural factors may affect the reported prevalence, as passivity, politeness, and submission are normal in some societies.

Course

Dependent personality features present in adolescence may evolve positively in adulthood or lead to a personality disorder. Dependent individuals are at increased risk of depressive, anxiety, and adjustment disorders, particularly in relation to loss of close relationships. Dependent personality disorder may follow separation anxiety in

childhood, or chronic physical illnesses in childhood requiring long periods of care and attention.

Differential diagnosis

Dependent personality disorder has some similarities with histrionic personality disorder. Histrionic patients, like dependent patients, adjust their conduct to please other people. Their lives are centred in these others. However, people with histrionic personality disorder obtain attention and care by seductive or manipulative behaviours, whereas people with dependent personality disorder wait passively for others to care for them.[7]

Like people with avoidant personality disorder, dependent individuals may feel devastated by minor criticism or lack of attention from others. However, they lack the sense of embarrassment and social shyness of the avoidant, and fear loneliness or abandonment.

People with dependent and borderline personality disorders share an excessive fear of abandonment. However, borderline individuals react to separation with feelings of emptiness and rage, and are demanding, in contrast with the submissive and appeasing attitude of dependent individuals, which is directed towards finding another person to provide support.

Dependent personality disorder must be differentiated from normal dependent behaviours in specific life situations; for example, elderly people with chronic or debilitating disease may become dependent.

Treatment

Pharmacological treatment is indicated only when depressive or anxiety symptoms are present, especially when associated with separation or loss.

In psychotherapy, the therapist must avoid the development of excessively dependent attachments. Self-confidence and self-esteem should be enhanced and the patient helped to enjoy the feeling of personal autonomy and independence. Cognitive restructuring and social skills training are often useful in bringing these changes about.

Obsessive–compulsive (anankastic) personality disorder (JLC)

While DSM-IV labels this personality disorder as obsessive–compulsive personality disorder (Table 14), ICD-10 prefers the term anankastic, previously used in European psychiatry to refer to fearful, insecure, and compulsive individuals. The cardinal feature of this disorder is an exaggerated and pervasive attempt to control. Anankastic patients need to control those who are close to them, to control every uncertainty, and to control their own thoughts and emotions. The anankastic lacks an internal sense of security and tries to make the external world totally predictable. The anankastic is afraid of his own internal aggressive drives and avoids free emotional expression. Others perceive this kind of personality as characterized by inflexibility and stubborn inefficiency.

Epidemiology

The prevalence of obsessive–compulsive personality disorders is about 1 per cent in community samples and up to 10 per cent in psychiatric patients, especially those with depressive and anxiety disorders. It is most frequent among males. Some obsessive–compulsive traits are sanctioned in some cultures, and a personality disorder should not be

Table 14 DSM-IV diagnostic criteria for obsessive–compulsive personality disorder

A pervasive pattern of preoccupation with orderliness, perfectionism, and mental and interpersonal control, at the expense of flexibility, openness, and effciency, beginning by early adulthood and present in a variety of contexts, as indicated by four (or more) of the following

(1) Is preoccupied with details, rules, lists, order, organization, or schedules to the extent that the major point of the activity is lost
(2) Shows perfectionism that interferes with task completion (e.g. is unable to complete a project because his or her own overly strict standards are not met)
(3) Is excessively devoted to work and productivity to the exclusion of leisure activities and friendships (not accounted for by obvious economic necessity)
(4) Is overconscientious, scrupulous, and inflexible about matters of morality, ethics, or values (not accounted for by cultural or religious identification)
(5) Is unable to discard worn-out or worthless objects even when they have no sentimental value
(6) Is reluctant to delegate tasks or to work with others unless they submit to exactly his or her way of doing things
(7) Adopts a miserly spending style toward both self and others; money is viewed as something to be hoarded for future catastrophes
(8) Shows rigidity and stubbornness

diagnosed unless the traits are markedly beyond the average for the culture.

Aetiology

Biological factors and learning seem to be involved in the aetiology of obsessive–compulsive personality disorder. The personality may be partly inherited.[102] Early psychodynamic theories linked obsessive personality to the anal phase of psychosexual development between the ages of 2 and 4, when libidinal drives come into conflict with parental attempts to socialize the child, especially in sphincter control and toilet training. Later psychoanalytic theory[103] emphasized earlier manifestations of the child's autonomy versus parental wishes. The expression of drives and emotions, including anger, is shaped by parental responses and may evoke shame and criticism. According to this theory, as children, obsessional patients were often praised for what they did as opposed to who they were. Feelings were relegated to the realm of weakness and shame. The child could avoid criticism by focusing on tasks and displacing anger. By adopting moralistic attitudes towards anger, the child gained affection and attention from the parents.

This dynamic sequence is reinforced in societies which are strongly influenced by the Protestant work ethic, in families where individual emotions are subordinated to the group, and in societies in which open expression of emotions is discouraged.

Clinical picture

The behaviour of an obsessive–compulsive personality has been consistently described as one of orderliness. The patient is preoccupied with details, and pays attention to rules, procedures, schedules, and punctuality. Patients with obsessional personalities often produce their own detailed lists of symptoms and are annoyed if any item is neglected or misinterpreted. They repeat actions and check for mistakes, despite the inconvenience and annoyance that result from this behav-

iour. As a consequence, their conduct is frequently inefficient. For example, the combination of unproductive perfectionism and rigidity may lead to difficulty in finishing a written report on time because of excessive correction and rewriting. Since this striving for perfection and order is time consuming, other areas of their lives often appear disorganized. One room or one desk drawer may fall into disarray, or parts of their social or family lives may be disorganized.

People with obsessive–compusive personality focus on work and productivity. It is difficult for them to take vacations or even to have free time. They do not enjoy leisure activity, which they may consider a waste of time. Often, they need to take work home to alleviate their anxiety. Hobbies and leisure pursuits become formally organized activities. They insist on perfect performance of sports or games and transform them into a serious task requiring careful organization and hard work. Leisure activities may be an unpleasant experience for the others involved, owing to the insistence on rules and standards.

Stubbornness is another characteristic of these people. They need things to be done in their way, and realistic arguments do not usually make them change their insistence. They need others to submit to their way of doing things, and often believe that no one can do the tasks as perfectly as they can. They give detailed instructions, insisting that their way is the only way of doing things, and are irritated if others suggest alternatives. Therefore, they generally insist in doing everything themselves and are unable to delegate, which increases their inefficiency at work. Paradoxically, their stubbornness is associated with doubt. Indecisiveness is a constant characteristic unless they have structured guidelines. They fear making mistakes or misjudgements, and delay repeatedly until they have enough data to take what they consider the only right decision. When rules do not dictate the correct answer to a problem or when procedures for tasks are not laid down, decision-making or task initiation may become a lengthy and painful process.

People with this personality disorder are characterized by excessive conscientiousness and scruples. They are inflexible about matters of morality, ethics, or values. Moral principles and standards of performance have to be followed rigidly, and respect for authority and rules is absolute. Failure to do these things leads to irritation, anger, and self-criticism.

These people are stingy and mean, and often live with standards far below their actual socio-economic status. They dislike spending, believing that money should be saved in case of future difficulties. They have great difficulty in discarding worn-out or worthless objects, believing that they might be useful some day. They may hoard objects such as newspapers or broken appliances, even when they have no sentimental value.

These people are humourless and lack spontaneity of emotional expression. Usually they do not express anger directly. However, they are often angry in situations in which they are unable to control the behaviour of themselves or others. Anger is generally manifested by indirect aggressive acts (such as leaving a small tip or not providing minor help when expected). Their management of anger is closely related to their attitude of dominance–submission toward authority figures. They may be excessively submissive to a person in authority whom they respect, but obstructive with an authority figure whom they do not respect.

The affect of the obsessive person is controlled and stilted. It is not flat or blunted, but constricted. They do not laugh or cry, and feel uncomfortable with people who express their feelings. Their mood is usually serious but may appear anxious or depressed. In a clinical interview they may sit in a stiff unnatural posture, and seldom make spontaneous comments about their emotions. They usually relate their history in a pedantic and circumstantial manner. If interrupted by a question from the doctor, they have to finish their monologue before answering. When asked about feelings, they answer with lists of facts and circumstances. They can label emotions and feelings, but are unable to display them.

In summary, obsessive personalities love order, neatness, and sameness, and hates novelty, spontaneity, and change. They need control, security, and certainty, and avoid creativity, art, and excitement. They mitigate anxiety by following strict rules and repress emotional expression by avoiding spontaneity. They fear their inner fragile and aggressive emotional world.

Course

Like other personality disorders, obsessive–compulsive personality disorder is present in early adulthood and tends to be persistent and constant. However, some adolescents with marked obsessive traits become warm, loving, and tender adults . On the other hand, intense obsessional traits in adolescence are occasionally a premorbid stage of schizophrenia ('pseudoneurotic schizophrenia'). The developmental relationship between obsessive–compulsive personality disorder and obsessive–compulsive disorder is controversial. In the past it was suggested that most obsessive–compulsive personality disorder evolved to a full obsessive–compulsive disorder, indicating that the two syndromes were expressions of the same basic disorder. More recent investigations[104] indicate that most obsessive–compulsive disorder patients do not have a comorbid obsessive–compulsive personality disorder. A variety of psychiatric disorders may present in a patient with obsessive personality, but depressive and anxiety disorders are the most common, followed by phobic, somatoform, and obsessive–compulsive symptoms. Hypochondriacal syndromes are commonly found in obsessive individuals when they lose control of situations.

Persons with this personality disorder may do well in jobs that demand working with detail, order, and structured procedures, and may adjust to interpersonal relationships with submissive spouses. However, they are particularly vulnerable to unexpected changes in their occupational and social environment. Late-onset depression is a common occurrence in obsessive–compulsive personalities.

Differential diagnosis

The main difficulty in diagnosing obsessive–compulsive personality disorder is to differentiate it from obsessive–compulsive disorder. The latter diagnosis is made when occupational and personal functioning is severely impaired as a consequence of doubt, indecisiveness, hoarding, or any other obsessive behaviour. In many, but not all, cases of obsessive personality, the traits and behaviours are egosyntonic and no resistance is present, in contrast with obsessive–compulsive disorder.

The perfectionism of obsessive personalities may be present in narcissistic personality disorder. However, narcissistic individuals tend to believe that they have achieved perfection, while obsessive individuals tend to be highly critical of their own achievements.

Social detachment and the lack of empathy and warmth may suggest schizoid personality disorder. However, obsessive individuals constrain their emotional expression to keep control of a situation, while schizoids lack the fundamental capacity for affective display or intimacy.

Not all individuals with obsessive traits have obsessive–compulsive personality disorder. Obsessive traits can be adaptive in some situations; it is only when they are maladaptive, inflexible, and persistently cause functional impairment that a personality disorder be diagnosed.

Treatment

Pharmacological treatment may be tried in patients with anxiety and distress due to intense doubts, indecisiveness, and scruples. Benzodiazepines may alleviate tension in these cases. Antidepressants with a serotonergic profile sometimes improve mood and global functioning.

Psychological treatment, focusing on perfectionism, rigidity, scrupulousness, and intolerance of failure, is the main therapeutic approach. Repressed aggression, guilt, and dependency needs should be addressed using a psychodynamic approach.

Other personality disorders (not included in DSM-IV)

Passive-aggressive (negativistic) personality disorder (DLT)

Definition

Passive-aggressive disorder was not included in DSM-IV because of the many unsolved problems related to its concept in previous classifications. Instead, it is placed in Appendix B of DSM-IV where it is alternatively called negativistic personality disorder. Research criteria are proposed which are expected to be empirically evaluated and to determine the validity and reliability of this diagnosis (Table 15).

Resistance to demands for adequate social and occupational performance and negativistic attitude are considered to be central features of passive-aggressive personality disorder. A pervasive pattern of argumentativeness, oppositional behaviour, and defeatist attitudes are typical, and are thought to be a covert manifestation of underlying aggression which is expressed passively and indirectly. Passive-aggressive personalities have interpersonal and cognitive dysfunction

Table 15 DSM-IV research criteria for passive–aggressive personality disorder

A. A pervasive pattern of negativistic attitude and passive resistance to demands for adequate performance, beginning by early adulthood and present in variety of contexts, as indicated by four (or more) of the following

  (1) Passively resists fulfilling routine social and occupational tasks
  (2) Complains of being misunderstood and unappreciated by others
  (3) Is sullen and argumentative
  (4) Unreasonably criticizes and scorns authority
  (5) Expresses envy and resentment toward those apparently more fortunate
  (6) Voices exaggerated and persistent complaints of personal misfortune
  (7) Alternates between hostile defiance and contrition

B. Does not occur exclusively during major depressive episodes and is not better accounted for by dysthymic disorder and severe impairment in terms of self-image, global mental health, and ability to function at work and in intimate relationships.[105]

Historical perspective

Early contributions

Passive-aggressive personality disorder was officially included in DSM-I as the passive-aggressive personality 'trait disturbance' depicted as an immature reaction to military stress by helpless, passive, and obstructive resistant behaviour of Second World War soldiers facing extreme demands. However, many clinical theorists at the beginning of the twentieth century[106] described certain dispositions and characteristics that parallel the contemporary description of passive-aggressive disorder.

Contemporary concepts

Passive-aggressive personality survived though DSM-II and DSM-III, despite resistance towards its inclusion in these classifications. The original descriptions were relatively narrow yet descriptively clear and clinically relevant. According to Kernberg[62] this diagnosis has been a useful grab-bag for personality disorders that do not fit easily into any other major category.

There has been much debate as to whether passive aggression constitutes a personality disorder, a defence mechanism, or a specific maladaptive personality trait (coping style).[107] Surprisingly, empirical literature on the subject is scarce, although passive-aggressive behaviour has been widely recognized by clinicians. An overlap with other personalities has been shown, and it has never been included as a separate category in the *International Classification of Diseases*. The passive-aggressive dimension, as assessed by self-reports, is always high in depressed patients and is state-dependent.[108] Perhaps it would be best to conceptualize passive aggression as a continuum: a passive-aggressive defence mechanism may be normal in some situations, it could be a trait of many personality disorders, and when pronounced and long-lasting it should be designated as passive-aggressive personality disorder.

Epidemiology

The population prevalence ranges from 0.9 to 3 per cent, but in those cases in which a secondary co-occurring diagnosis was assigned, the secondary frequency of passive-aggressive personality disorder was about 10 per cent.[106] Some studies found a higher prevalence in women and others in men.

Aetiology

The cause of the disorder is multidimensional, comprising biological, psychoanalytical, behavioural, interpersonal, and social learning perspectives.

Biological issues

Early authors, such as Kraepelin, Bleuler and Schneider, considered passive-aggressive personality to be constitutionally determined. Millon[109] has noted that oppositional disorder of childhood and adolescence may be related to passive-aggressive personality disorder in adulthood, suggesting that there may be specific genetic and/or metabolic factors contributing to a lifelong pattern of erratic moods and angry irritability. However, this interesting hypothesis of a psychopathology continuum is still speculative and should be supported by empirical research.

Developmental issues

Ambivalence is considered to be a core conflict of passive-aggressive personalities, which originates from fixation to the biting or sucking stages of the oral phase of psychosexual development. Some authors consider masochism to be another precursor of the passive-aggressive personality. Suffering arises when the individual obstructs the movement and attainment of goals in others and then experiences overwhelming unconsious guilt.[62] Masochistic tendencies observed in the passive-aggressive personality may cause self-defeating life attitudes and frequent depressive episodes.

Behavioural issues

According to the behavioural model, passive-aggressive behaviour is the expression of anger in maladaptive verbal and non-verbal ways that do not lead to rewarding problem-solving.[107] Failure to learn appropriate assertive behaviour would be the main aetiological factor.[109] Cognitive theorists[110] believe that the passive-aggressive personality results from faulty cognition and unconscious assumptions that things in life always go wrong.

Social issues

Millon's biosocial theory describes the passive-aggressive personality as active–ambivalent, resulting from environmental experiences to which the person has been exposed.[111] The primary social factor influencing the development of passive-aggressive patterns would be contradictory parental attitudes in childhood which, being conflicting and incompatible, prevent the child from expressing his feelings directly and thus urge him to develop passive resistance.

Clinical characteristics and diagnosis

Clinical manifestations of passive-aggressive personality disorder can be divided into four domains: behaviour, affectivity, cognitive style, and interpersonal relationships. A longitudinal history of these typical features is usually sufficient for diagnosis.

Behaviour

Passive-aggressive personalities seek novel and stimulating situations in impulsive ways, while remaining unpredictable.[15] Procrastination and inefficiency are behaviours used to avoid responsibility, which they show by stubborn resistance to the fulfilment of expectations and claiming forgetfulness.

Affectivity

Passive-aggressive individuals easily become irritable, gloomy, and despondent; they are resentful, sullen and discontent with life. The affective pattern is characterized by turning anger against the self, which may take form of self-destructive behaviour. Hostility, although covert, is never entirely concealed and may be detected by the therapist. Accumulated anger may be expressed by verbal acting-out, after which passive-aggressive individuals feel guilty and gloomy. Since they have difficulties in expressing emotions directly, they are prone to diffuse somatic complaints, hypochondriasis, and psychosomatic disorders.

Interpersonal relationships

Interpersonal relationships are contrary and stormy. Interpersonal ambivalence is a core feature of passive-aggressive personality disorder. Negativism is particularly expressed towards authorities, with whom they are never satisfied and whom they criticize constantly. They find fault with those on whom they depend, and yet do not extricate themselves from dependent relationships and passive roles. The argumentative self-detrimental behaviour of passive-aggressive personalities is often experienced by others as punitive and manipulative. Negative verbal comments, which are often caustic, and irritable and moody patterns of communication are typical.

Cognitive style

Passive-aggressive individuals are cynical, sceptical, hypercritical, and mistrustful. Disillusioned with life, discouraged, discontented with themselves and with others, they are also pessimistic about the future. They persistently complain and blame others for their own bad luck, feeling themselves to be misunderstood martyrs and victims of destiny.

Typical defence mechanisms of passive-aggressive personalities are centred around repression and manifested as turning their anger against themselves, sadomasochistic behaviour, denial, rationalization, and acting-out.

Comorbidity and differential diagnosis

Passive-aggressive personality disorder is frequently comorbid with major depression, dysthymic disorder, anxiety, panic disorder, and hypochondriasis. Patients with depressive disorders are more aware of their feelings of inferiority and more likely to feel guilty, and their depressed mood is continuous rather than erratically hostile and moody, as in passive-aggressive personality.

Comorbidity with many personality disorders (histrionic, borderline, obsessive–compulsive, dependent, narcissistic) is also frequently observed. People with these personality disorders may use passive aggression as a defence mechanism. Suicide attempts are not as frequent as in histrionic and borderline personality disorders, and features of passive-aggressive personality are less dramatic, affective, openly aggressive, and severe.

Course and prognosis

There are insufficient data on the course and prognosis of passive-aggressive personality disorder. When passive-aggressive people are able to control their anger, they may experience anxiety, panic states, depressive episodes, chronic depression, and psychosomatic disorders. They are prone to alcohol abuse, and their careers are erratic and stunted despite their abilities (frequent changes of jobs are common). Suicide attempts may complicate this disorder.

Treatment

Pharmacotherapy

Target symptoms, such as depression, anxiety, and somatic complaints, should be treated. Benzodiazepines may be warranted and helpful in the initial period of psychotherapy. The side-effects of medication are often the reason for complaints about their psychiatrist's inefficiency. Non-compliance is frequent, reflecting resistance to the therapist. Abuse of medicaments should be controlled and considered seriously.

Psychotherapy

Psychotherapy is the treatment of choice. Various modes are used, including supportive, psychodynamic, behavioural assertiveness training, and the paradoxical approach in group or individual settings. The goal of treatment should be to help the patient escape from the vicious

circle of self-defeating behaviour and develop a mature way of expressing anger and other feelings. The sessions can become a battleground and struggle for control, in which the patient opposes, criticizes, and resents the therapist on whom he or she wants to be dependent. It is very important for a therapist not to engage in a sadomasochistic power game with passive-aggressive patients; therefore humiliating and critical comments should be avoided.

Paradoxical approaches may be useful for overcoming resistance and achieving more compliance by the patients. Symptom prescription is a particularly useful strategy. Behavioural therapy techniques, such as assertiveness training or behavioural contracting, may be beneficial.

Self-defeating (masochistic) personality disorder (JLC)

Individuals with masochistic personality disorder persistently seek humiliation and failure, and submit to the will of others.

The term masochism was introduced to psychiatry by Krafft-Ebing in 1882. Its derived from a character in a novel by the German author Leopold von Sacher-Masoch, a man who endured torture, scorn, and humiliation from a woman. Later, Freud conceptualized masochism as the result of aggressive instinct directed towards the self instead of an external object. Reich[68] described the masochistic character as a person who suffered deep frustrations in early developmental stages and needed to express this frustration through suffering inflicted by the love 'objects'. Thus defiance is always present in the masochistic search for love. According to Horney,[112] helplessness and victimization may be a masochistic way of expressing hostility by making others feel shameful. Masochistic suffering may also be used to avoid reproach and responsibility and as a way of restoring a sign of personal value.

Clinical picture

People with self-defeating personality disorder avoid pleasurable experiences and undermine their achievements. They neglect their appearance and live below their means. They accept and endure humiliation, expecting that others will sympathize with them. In this way, they fulfil their expectation that submission will bring love and care. They prefer to relate to people who abuse them and consider those who consistently treat them well to be boring.

These people fail to accomplish tasks of which they are capable and adopt an inferior role. When making appropriate demands, they feel that they are taking advantage of others and adopt an apologetic manner. For them, success is inversely related to inner security. Successful relationships do not make them feel confident, but increase their fears. They tend to believe that all experiences involve future frustration and pain. They may respond to positive personal events with depression and behaviour that negates their accomplishments. They look for people who will respond to their behavior with disdain, rejection, or cruelty.

People with self-defeating personality disorder do not defend themselves against expressions of disgust and resentment directed towards them and rarely accuse or reproach others. They do not feel confident and are not assertive. They fear that optimism may lead to greater problems.

They are not worried by these attitudes. Rather, masochists believe that by exaggerating their weaknesses and inefficiency they will protect themselves from aggression by others. They feel protected when someone needs something from them, and many non-assertive masochists engage in self-sacrifice for their own protective feelings rather than for the welfare of others. What seems to be a comprehensive and self-sacrificing attitude reflects a lack of confidence and empathy.

The mood of these individuals is usually dysphoric, fluctuating between anxiety and sadness.

Differential diagnosis

Since masochistic personality disorder is not included in DSM-IV, little research has been done on comorbidity or on the validity or specificity of this diagnosis.

Self-defeating attitudes, low self-esteem, and depression may be found in individuals with dependent, borderline and depressive personality disorders. Some of the characteristics are also found in avoidant personality disorder.

Masochists are prone to mood disorder and dysthymia. Anxiety disorders are frequent. Their fears of abandonment are a persistent source of anxiety. Hypochondriasis and somatization are also common, sometimes as a way of obtaining attention.

Treatment

Antidepressants and anxiolytics may be useful to alleviate a dysphoric state. Psychological treatment should take into account that masochistic patients sometimes induce an aggressive countertransference as a response to their own wish to be hurt. The therapist should gradually clarify the behaviours which provoke hostile responses and seek to reward adaptive interpersonal behaviours. Training in assertiveness and social skills is sometimes helpful.

Sadistic personality disorder (DLT)

Sadistic personality disorder is a controversial category which is not included in either DSM-IV or ICD-10. Some authors, especially those working with perpetrators of abuse, support its inclusion in the diagnostic nomenclature, believing that it is a valid clinical entity which deserves special treatment.

Sadistic personality disorder has substantial precedent within the psychodynamic literature. Sadism as a term describing desire to inflict pain upon the sexual object was originally used by Krafft-Ebing,[113] after the writings of the Marquis de Sade. Later, many psychoanalysts dealt with various forms of sadistic behaviour that are different and distinct from sexual sadism,[68,95,114] stressing its instinctual basis as well as its interrelationship with masochism. Various stages (Oedipal, pre-Oedipal) were mentioned as being important in the development of sadistic defences or personality styles. The object-relations theorists later shifted the concept of sadism to environmental and interpersonal factors. Sadomasochism was conceptualized as a type of object relationship that defends against frank object loss.

Like the early psychoanalysts, Kernberg[41] connects two dispositions (sadistic and masochistic) into a sadomasochistic character, which includes 'help-rejecting complainers' and often has underlying borderline personality organization. In tune with this, other authors consider sadistic personality disorder to be complementary to self-defeating personality disorder, because the person who is prone to abusing others is likely to be masochistic (or self-defeating) and the person who is repeatedly abused is likely to be sadistic.[115]

Aetiology

Gay, one of the chief investigators of this disorder, found that subjects with sadistic personality disorder often had a history of significant childhood loss and physical, emotional, or sexual abuse during childhood.[116] She noted that, despite their significant psychopathology, sadistic individuals are surprisingly highly functioning, with steady employment and intense long-lasting relationships. They consider abuse of the partner and children as egosyntonic and consistent with culturally accepted patriarchal values.

Clinical picture

Sadistic individuals demonstrate a long-standing maladaptive pattern of cruel, demeaning, and aggressive behaviour towards others in order to cause suffering and pain and to establish dominance and control. They are extremely antagonistic to the point of being ruthless and brutal. Sadistic persons are fascinated by violence, weapons, injuries, and torture, and are most frequently encountered in forensic settings among child and partner abusers.

Differential diagnosis

The major distinction for the diagnosis of sadistic personality disorder is from antisocial personality disorder. Widiger et al.[117] note that the sadistic person may simply represent an aggressive (antagonistic) subtype of psychopathy. Intimidation and sadistic control of others, as well as a fascination with weapons, martial arts, and torture, may be manifested by both antisocial and sadistic individuals. Moreover, both disorders may display 'malignant narcissism',[31] with an admixture of narcissistic, antisocial, sadistic, and paranoid features. Such a characterological constellation is frequent among murderers and therefore is considered to be of great forensic significance.[118] Widiger et al.[117] state that making a distinction between antisocial personality disorder and the sadistic personality disorder may be as meaningless as trying to determine whether a person is psychopathic or antisocial.

Epidemiology

Existing data[119] suggest that sadistic personality disorder is relatively uncommon, although it may have a higher prevalence in specific forensic populations. Several studies found a high overlap with narcissistic, paranoid, and antisocial personality disorders, which raised the possibility that sadistic personality disorder may not be a distinct entity. Indeed, all these personality dimensions may occur together, comprising the syndrome of 'malignant narcissism' mentioned above.

Course

No data are available on the course of this disorder.

Treatment

Sadistic individuals seldom seek treatment, and are usually encountered in forensic settings. No treatment has been successful for this disorder. Since the aetiology is probably multifactorial, there should be multiple approaches to treatment. The primary aim of treatment is control of cruelty and malignant aggression. As with antisocial personalities, selective serotonin reuptake inhibitors and lithium may be beneficial in regulating the serotonergic function that probably underlies the aggressive action, and carbamazepine and clonazepam may act to regulate ictal aggressive outbursts.

Psychotherapy is usually difficult because these individuals lack any desire to change and because there may be serious countertransference problems for the therapists. Small groups may be helpful because there is a dissolution of transference and peer confrontation is accepted more easily. The therapist should beware of becoming involved in a sadomasochistic game of control with the patient. Supervision of the therapist is necessary.

Status

Sadistic personality disorder has not been accepted as an official diagnosis. It was placed in an appendix to DSM-IIIR for research purposes, but there have been relatively few studies with systematic data collection. It was not included in DSM-IV, since the proposed criteria lacked empirical support and critical review. Critics of sadistic personality disorder as a distinct entity were concerned because of its potential use in mitigating responsibility for violent crime. Its proponents, strongly supporting its inclusion in diagnostic nomenclature, believe that better understanding of the phenomenology and aetiology of sadistic behaviour, or uncontrolled aggression and violence, might be useful in the development of effective interventions, thus decreasing the widespread societal problem of domestic violence, abuse, and murder, or severe distress and suffering in others.[115] However, it is clear that more systematic research is needed to determine whether sadistic behaviour is a separate personality disorder.

Depressive personality disorder (JLC)

This personality disorder is not included in ICD-10 or DSM-IV, although it is considered as a subject for further study in the latter. However, the concept of depressive personality was well recognized in previous decades (e.g. by Kraepelin and Schneider). Depressive personality was seen as a pattern of brooding, pessimism, and low self-confidence,[2] and as a tendency to physical lassitude and suffering. Phenomenological accounts[120] emphasize dependency, orderliness, and adherence to social conventions. The psychoanalytic concept of masochism[82] overlaps to some extent with the classical depressive personality. More recently, Akiskal[121] has discussed the depressive personality as part of a spectrum of affective disorders, reviving Kretschmer's ideas[10] on the role of temperament as the base from where psychiatric disorders develop.

Aetiology

Psychological and biological factors have been suggested as causes of depressive personality disorder. Early losses, inadequate attention from parents, and a punitive superego have been postulated by psychoanalytic authors. Others have suggested that a depressive temperament is genetically related to affective disorder.

Clinical picture

People with depressive personality disorder are submissive, quiet, introverted, and unassertive. Their cognitive style is marked by pessimism, dejection, and self-reproach. They appear gloomy, joyless, cheerless, and unhappy. They are serious and lack a sense of humour. They do not believe that they deserve to be happy. They have a negative view of the past and present and do not expect things to improve. They anticipate failure and dwell on their negative perspective of life. They have a low tolerance to shortcomings and failures, which are seen as confirming their own pessimistic assumptions. They are prone to guilt and judge themselves severely. Their self-esteem is low and they feel inadequate. They focus on the failings of others and are critical of themselves.

Epidemiology

No data are available on the frequency of this disorder in the population.

Differential diagnosis

Some clinicians doubt whether a distinction can be made between between depressive personality disorder and dysthymic disorder. The diagnosis of depressive personality disorder emphasizes cognitive and behavioural aspects rather than the depressed mood. Also, dysthymia, although chronic, has a fluctuating course.

Dysthymic patents generally experience their symptoms as egodystonic, while people with depressive personality disorder think that they have a realistic view of their situation. People with depressive personality disorder may meet the criteria for dependent personality disorder and self-defeating personality disorder, and it is difficult to distinguish between these disorders.

Course

Patients with depressive personality disorder have depressive episodes and dysthymia more frequently than other individuals, and may have difficulties in adapting to stressful or uncertain situations.

Treatment

Antidepressants may be useful when the person is at higher risk for developing a depressive episode. Psychological treatment may be helpful, since these people have a good capacity for introspection and reality testing. Cognitive approaches can help patients to understand their negative views and derogatory attitudes. These patients usually establish a good therapeutic relationship with the clinician.

Personality changes

Enduring personality changes after traumatic experiences (JLC)

ICD-10 has two categories for personality changes: those occurring after catastrophic situations, and those starting after psychiatric illness. Either diagnosis should be made only when there is evidence of a definite personality change, including cognition, behaviour, and interpersonal relationships. The changes must not be a manifestation of a current mental disorder or the residue of a previous mental disorder. It must not be an exacerbation of a pre-existing personality disorder.

The **aetiology** of the personality change presumably relates to the extreme existential experience of the catastrophic situation or the psychiatric illness.

Examples of catastrophic experiences include life in concentration camps, experiences of disaster, and prolonged exposure to other life-threatening situations. Personality changes following short-term exposure to life-threatening situations, such as a car accident, should not be included in this group, since such changes probably depend on a previous psychological vulnerability. In ICD-10, the symptoms of personality change after catastrophic experiences include hostility and mistrust of the environment, social withdrawal, feelings of emptiness or hopelessness, estrangement, and alertness or feeling on the edge.

When the personality change follows a mental disorder, the cause is related to the stressful experience and the perceived damage to the patient's self-image arising from the disease. Other people's attitudes towards the illness, the subjective emotional experience, and previous psychological adjustment are also important. Features of the personality change after mental disorders include feelings of being stigmatized and consequent withdrawal, passivity, and loss of interests, dependence, excessive demandingness and complaining, and dysphoric–labile mood.

Personality change due to a general medical condition (JLC)

This category, which is included in both ICD-10 and DSM-IV, describes syndromes affecting global features of behaviour, cognition, and emotions, and secondary to the physiological effects of general medical diseases.

The essential feature is a change in personality after a general medical disease. In childhood before a stable pattern of personality has been established, a marked deviation from normal development suggests the diagnosis.

A central feature is loss of control over the expression of emotions and impulses. Affect is commonly labile and shallow, although persistent mild euphoria or apathy may be present, especially when the frontal lobes are affected. The elevated mood of these patients is hollow and silly, unlike that of hypomania. Patients may appear childish, expansive, and disinhibited, but they may admit to not feeling happy. Other are indifferent and apathetic.

Exaggerated expressions of rage and aggression are usually present, often out of proportion to any stressor. Loss of impulse control is also shown in social and sexual disinhibition, inappropriate jokes, and overeating.

Aetiology

In most cases this disorder is associated with structural damage to the brain. Head trauma, cerebral neoplasms, vascular accidents, multiple sclerosis, Huntington's disease, and complex partial epilepsy may all cause personality change, especially when affecting frontal and temporal lobes. Systemic diseases involving the central nervous system, including endocrine disorders, AIDS, lupus erythematosus and chronic metal poisoning, may have the same effect.

Patients with this disorder generally have a clear sensorium but may be inattentive and have some mild cognitive dysfunction. They do not show intellectual deterioration.

Differential diagnosis

In dementia, personality change is accompanied by intellectual deterioration. However, personality change may predate the dementia. Distinction from schizophrenia and other personality disorders is based on the clinical history and the presence of a general medical disease capable of causing personality change.

Treatment

If possible, treatment is directed to the causative condition. Pharmacological treatment of specific symptoms may be useful when depression or inappropriate anger is present.

References

1. Kraepelin, E. (1921). *Manic-depressive insanity and paranoia.* Livingstone, Edinburgh.
2. Schneider, K. (1950). *Psychopathic personalities* (9th edn). Cassell, London.
3. Freud, S. (1911). Psychoanalytic notes upon an autobiographical account of a case of paranoia. In *Collected papers*, Vol. 3. Hogarth Press, London, 1925.
4. Perry, J.C. and Vaillant, G.E. (1989). Personality disorders. In *Textbook of psychiatry* (ed. H.I. Kaplan and B.J. Sadock), pp. 1352–87. Williams and Wilkins, Baltimore, MD.
5. Kendler, K.S., Masterson, C.C., Ungaro, R., and Davis, K.L. (1984). A family history study of schizophrenia related personality disorders. *American Journal of Psychiatry*, **141**, 424–7.
6. Seiver, L.J. and Davis, K.L. (1991). A psychobiological perspective on the personality disorders. *American Journal of Psychiatry*, **148**, 1647–58.
7. Millon, T. (1997). *Disorders of personality: DSM-IV and beyond* (2nd edn). Wiley, New York.
8. American Psychiatric Association (1994). *Diagnostic and statistical manual of mental disorders* (4th edn). American Psychiatric Association, Washington, DC.
9. Sullivan, H.S. (1953). *The interpersonal theory of psychiatry.* Norton, New York.
10. Kretschmer, E. (1936). *Physique and character.* Kegan Paul, Trench, Trubner, London.
11. American Psychiatric Association (1987). *Diagnostic and statistical manual of mental disorders* (3rd edn revised). American Psychiatric Association, Washington, DC.
12. Cleckley, H. (1941). *The mask of sanity.* Mosby, St Louis, MO.
13. Robins, L.N. (1966). *Deviant children grown up: a sociological and psychiatric study of sociopathic personality.* Williams and Wilkins, Baltimore, MD.
14. Glueck, S. (1959). *Predicting delinquency and crime.* Harvard University Press, Cambridge, MA.
15. Cloninger, C.R. (1987). A systematic method for clinical description and classification of personality variants. *Archives of General Psychiatry*, **44**, 573–88.
16. Cloninger, C.R. (1995). The psychobiological regulation of social cooperation. *Nature Medicine*, **1**, 14–15.
17. de Girolamo, G. and Reich, J.H. (1993). *Personality disorders.* WHO, Geneva.
18. Crowe, R.R. (1974). An adoption study of antisocial personality. *Archives of General Psychiatry*, **31**, 785–91.
19. Cadoret, R.J. (1978). Psychopathology in adopted-away offspring of biologic parents with antisocial behaviour. *Archives of General Psychiatry*, **35**, 176–84.
20. Dinwiddie, S.H. (1994). Psychiatric genetics and forensic psychiatry: a review. *Bulletin of the American Academic Psychiatry and Law*, **22**, 327–42.
21. Jacobs, P.A., Brunton, M., and Melville, M.M. (1965). Aggressive behaviour and subnormality. *Nature*, **208**, 1351–2.
22. Garpenstrand, H., Jonas, E., Hallman, J., and Oreland, L. Frequent occurrence of individuals carrying two long alleles of the dopamine D4 receptor gene in a group of forensic psychiatric clients. Submitted for publication.
23. Coccaro, E.F., Siever, L.J., Klar, H.M., *et al.* (1989). Serotonergic studies in patients with affective and personality disorders. *Archives of General Psychiatry*, **46**, 587–99.

24. Dee Higley, J., Mehlman, P.T., Taub, D.M., *et al.* (1992). Cerebrospinal fluid monoamine and adrenal correlates of aggression in free-ranging rhesus monkeys. *Archives of General Psychiatry*, **49**, 436–41.

25. Oreland, L. and Hallman, J.(1995). The correlation between platelet MAO activity and personality: short review of findings and a discussion on possible mechanisms. In *Progress on brain research*, 106, *Current neurochemical and pharmacological aspects of biogenic amines* (ed. P.M. Yu, K.F. Tipton, and A.A. Boulton), pp. 77–84. Elsevier, Amsterdam.

26. Magnusson, D. and Ohman, A. (1987). *Psychopathology: an interactional perspective*. Academic Press, Orlando, FL.

27. Linnoila, V.M.I. and Virkkunen, M. (1992). Aggression, suicidality and serotonin. *Journal of Clinical Psychiatry*, **53** (Supplement), 46–51.

28. Williams, D. (1969). Neural factors related to habitual aggression. *Brain*, **92**, 503–20.

29. Kuruoglu, A.C., Arikan, Z., Vural, G., Karatas, M., Arac, M., and Isik, E. (1996). Single photon emission computerised tomography in chronic alcoholism. *British Journal of Psychiatry*, **169**, 348–54.

30. Glueck, B. and Glueck, E. (1956). *Physique and delinquency*. Harper, New York.

31. Kernberg, O. (1989). The narcissistic personality disorder and the differential diagnosis of antisocial behaviour. *Psychiatric Clinics of North America*, **12**, 553–70.

32. Akhtar, S. (1992). *Broken structure*. Aronson, Northvale, NJ.

33. Hare, R.D. (1983). A research scale for the assessment of psychopathy in criminal populations. *Personality and Individual Differences*, **1**, 111–17.

34. Stein, G. (1992). Drug treatment of personality disorders. *British Journal of Psychiatry*, **161**, 167–84.

35. Jones, M. (1952). *Social psychiatry: a study of therapeutic communities*. Tavistock Publications, London.

36. Stern, A. (1938). Psychoanalytical investigation and therapy in borderline group of neuroses. *Psychoanalytic Quarterly*, **7**, 467–89.

37. Schmideberg, M. (1947). The treatment of psychopathic and borderline patients. *American Journal of Psychotherapy*, **1**, 45–71.

38. Grinker, R., Werble, B., and Drye, R.C. (1968). *The borderline syndrome*. Aronson, New York.

39. Gunderson, J.G. and Kolb, J.E. (1978). Discriminating features of borderline patients. *American Journal of Psychiatry* **135**, 792–6.

40. Spitzer, R., Endicott, J., and Gibbon, M. (1979). Crossing the border into borderline schizophrenia: the development of criteria. *Archives of General Psychiatry* **36**, 17–24.

41. Kernberg, O.F. (1975). *Borderline conditions and pathological narcissism*. Aronson, New York.

42. Dahl, A.A. (1990). Empirical evidence for a core borderline syndrome. *Journal of Personality Disorders*, **4**, 192–202.

43. Gunderson, J.G. (1984). *Borderline personality disorder*. American Psychiatric Press, Washington, DC.

44. Berelowitz, M. and Tarnopolsky, A. (1993). The validity of borderline personality disorder: an updated review of recent research. In *Personality disorder reviewed* (ed. P. Tyrer and G. Stein), pp. 90–112. Gaskell, London.

45. Quality Assurance Project (1991). Treatment outlines for borderlines, narcissistic and histrionic personality disorders. *Australian and New Zealand Journal of Psychiatry*, **25**, 392–403.

46. Divac-Jovanovic, M., Svrakic, D., and Lecic-Tosevski, D. (1993). Personality disorders: model for conceptual approach and classification. Part I: general model. *American Journal of Psychotherapy*, **47**, 558–71.

47. Akiskal, H.S. (1981). Subaffective disorders: dysthymic, cyclothymic and bipolar II disorders in the 'borderline realm'. *Psychiatric Clinics of North America*, **4**, 25–46.

48. Widiger, T.A. and Frances, A. (1989). Epidemiology, diagnosis, and comorbidity of borderline personality disorder. In *American Psychiatric Press review of psychiatry*, Vol. 8 (ed. A. Tasman, R.E. Hales, and A.J. Frances), pp. 8–24. American Psychiatric Press, Washington, DC.

49. Zimmerman, M. and Coryell, W.H. (1990). Diagnosing personality disorders in the community. *Archives of General Psychiatry*, **47**, 527–31.

50. Stone, M.H. (1980). *The borderline syndromes. Constitution, personality and adaptation*. McGraw-Hill, New York.

51. Coccaro, E.F., Siever, L.J., Klar, H.M., Maurer, G., Cochrane, K., and Cooper, T.B. (1989). Sertonergic studies in patients with affective and personality disorders: correlates with suicidal and impulsive aggressive behaviour. *Archives of General Psychiatry*, **46**, 587–99.

52. Andrulonis, P.A., Gluesch, B.C., Stroebel, C.F., *et al.* (1982). Borderline personality disorder subcategories. *Journal of Nervous and Mental Disease*, **170**, 670–9.

53. Masterson, J.F. (1976). *Psychotherapy of the borderline adult: a developmental approach*. Brunner–Mazel, New York.

54. Gunderson, J.G. (1996). The borderline patient's intolerance of aloneness: insecure attachment and therapist availability. *American Journal of Psychiatry*, **153**, 752–8.

55. Zanarini, M.C., Williams, A.A., Lewis, R.E., *et al.* (1997). Reported pathological childhood experiences associated with the development of borderline personality disorder. *American Journal of Psychiatry*, **154**, 1101–6.

56. Paris, J. (1994). *Borderline personality disorder—a multidimensional approach*. American Psychiatric Press, Washington, DC.

57. Akhtar, S. (1984). The syndrome of identity diffusion. *American Journal of Psychiatry* **141**, 1381–5.

58. Kernberg, O.F. (1981). Structural interviewing. *Psychiatric Clinics of North America*, **4**, 169–95.

59. Gunderson, J.G., Kolb, J.E., and Austin, V. (1981). The Diagnostic Interview for Borderline Patients. *American Journal of Psychiatry*, **138**, 896–903.

60. Gunderson, J.G. and Phillips, K.A. (1995). Personality disorders. In *Comprehensive textbook of psychiatry* (5th edn) (ed. H.I. Kaplan and B.J. Sadock), pp. 1438–41. Williams and Wilkins, Baltimore, MD.

61. Stein, G. (1992). Drug treatment of personality disorders. *British Journal of Psychiatry*, **161**, 167–84.

62. Kernberg, O.F. (1984). *Severe personality disorder—psychotherapeutic strategies*. Yale University Press, New Haven, CT.

63. McGlashan, T.H. (1986). The Chestnut Lodge follow-up study. III: Long-term outcome of borderline patients. *Archives of General Psychiatry*, **43**, 20–30.

64. Linehan, M.M., (1987). Dialectical behavior therapy: a cognitive behavioral approach to parasuicide. *Journal of Personality Disorders*, **1**, 328–33.

65. Kraepelin, E. (1913). Hysterical insanity. In *Lectures on clinical psychiatry* (trans. T. Johnstone), pp. 249–58. William Wood, New York.

66. Freud, S. (1931). Libidinal types. In *Standard edition of the complete psychological works of Sigmund Freud*, Vol. 21 (ed. J. Strachey), p. 266. Hogarth Press, London, 1961.

67. Wittels, F. (1930). The hysterical character. *Medical Review of Reviews*, **36**, 186–90.

68. Reich, W. (1933). *Character analysis* (3rd edn) (trans. V.R. Carfagno). Farrar, Straus and Giroux, New York.

69. Chodoff, P. and Lyons, H. (1958). Hysteria: the hysterical personality and hysterical conversion. *American Journal of Psychiatry*, **114**, 734–40.

70. Brody, E.B. and Sata, L.S. (1967). Personality disorders: traits and pattern disturbances. In *Comprehensive textbook of psychiatry* (ed. A.M. Friedman and H.I. Kaplan), pp. 932–50. Williams and Wilkins, Baltimore, MD.

71. Pfohl, B. (1991). Histrionic personality disorder: a review of available data and recommendations for DSM-IV. *Journal of Personality Disorders*, **5**, 150–66.

72. Lilienfeld, S., Van Valkenburg, C., Larntz, K., and Akiskal, H. (1986). The relationship of histrionic personality disorder to antisocial personality and somatisation disorders. *American Journal of Psychiatry*, **143**, 718–22.

73. Cadoret, R.J. (1978). Psychopathology in adopted-away offspring of biologic parents with antisocial behaviour. *Archives of General Psychiatry*, **35**, 176–84.

74. Divac-Jovanovic, M., Svrakic, D., and Lecic-Tosevski, D. (1993).

Personality disorders: model for conceptual approach and classification. Part I: General model. *American Journal of Psychotherapy*, **47**, 558–71.

75. Zimmerman, M. and Coryell, W.H. (1990). Diagnosis personality disorders in the community. *Archives of General Psychiatry*, **47**, 527–31.

76. Marmor, J. (1953). Orality in the hysterical personality. *Journal of the American Psychoanalytic Association*, **1**, 656–71.

77. Torgersen, S. (1980). The oral, obsessive and hysterical personality syndromes. A study of hereditary and environmental factors by means of the twin method. *Archives of General Psychiatry*, **37**, 1272–7.

78. Cloninger, C., Martin, R., Guze, S., and Clayton, P. (1986). A prospective follow-up and family study of somatisation in men and women. *American Journal of Psychiatry*, **143**, 873–8.

79. Zetzel, E. (1968). The so-called good hysteric. *International Journal of Psychoanalysis*, **49**, 256–60.

80. Lazare, A., Klerman, G., and Armor, D. (1966). Oral, obsessive, and hysterical personality patterns. *Archives of General Psychiatry*, **14**, 624–30.

81. Easser, B.R. and Lesser, S.R. (1965). Hysterical personality: a re-evaluation. *Psychoanalytic Quarterly*, **34**, 390–405.

82. Kernberg, O. (1988). Hysterical and histrionic personality disorders. In *The personality disorders and neuroses* (ed. A. Cooper, A. Frances, and M. Sacks), pp. 231–41. J.B. Lippincott, Philadelphia, PA.

83. Freud, S. (1914). On narcissism: an introduction. In *Standard edition of the complete psychological works of Sigmund Freud*, Vol. 14 (ed. J. Strachey), pp. 67–103. Hogarth Press, London, 1957.

84. Jones, E. (1913). The God complex. In *Essays in applied psycho-analysis*, Vol. 2, pp. 244–65. Reprinted by International Universities Press, New York.

85. Fenichel, O. (1945). *The psychoanalytic theory of neurosis*. Norton, New York.

86. Nemiah, J.C. (1961). *Foundations of psychopathology*. Oxford University Press, New York.

87. Kohut, H. (1971). *The analysis of the self*. International Universities Press, New York.

88. Reich, A. (1960). Pathological forms of self-esteem regulation. *Psychoanalytic Study of the Child*, **15**, 215–32.

89. Lasch, C. (1978). *The culture of narcissism: American life in an age of diminishing expectations*. Norton, New York.

90. Akhtar, S. (1989). Narcissistic personality disorder. Descriptive features and differential diagnosis. *Psychiatric Clinics of North America*, **12**, 505–29.

91. Raskin, R. and Hall, C.S. (1981). The Narcissistic Personality Inventory (NPI) in a psychiatric sample. *Journal of Clinical Psychology*, **40**, 140–2.

92. Gunderson, J., Ronningstam, E., and Bodkin, A. (1990). The Diagnostic Interview for Narcissistic Patients. *Archives of General Psychiatry*, **47**, 676–80.

93. Ronningstam, E. and Gunderson, J. (1991). Differentiating borderline personality disorder from narcissistic personality disorder. *Journal of Personality Disorders*, **5**, 225–32.

94. Modell, A. (1976). 'The holding environment' and the therapeutic action of psychoanalysis. *Journal of the American Psychoanalytic Association*, **24**, 285–307.

95. Fenichel, O. (1945). *The psychoanalytic theory of the neuroses*. Norton, New York.

96. Millon, T. (1973). *Theories of psychopathology and personality* (2nd edn). W.B. Saunders, Philadelphia, PA.

97. Millon, T. (1981). *Disorders of personality: DSM-III Axis II*. Wiley, New York.

98. Cloninger, C.R. (1986). A unified biosocial theory and its role in the development of anxiety states. *Psychiatric Development*, **3**, 167–226.

99. Freud, S. (1915). Some character types met with in psychoanalytic work. In *Collected papers* (ed. J. Strachey), Vol. 4, pp. 42–9. Hogarth Press, London, 1925.

100. Abraham, K. (1970). Notes on the psycho-analytical investigation and treatment of manic depressive insanity and allied conditions. In *Selected papers of Karl Abraham*, pp. 418–502. Hogarth Press, London.

101. World Health Organization (1992). *The ICD-10 classification of mental and behavioural disorders—clinical descriptions and diagnostic guidelines*. World Health Organization, Geneva.

102. Clifford, C.A., Murray, R.M., and Fulker, D.W. (1984). Genetic and environmental influences on obsessional traits and symptoms. *Psychological Medicine*, **14**, 791–800.

103. Erikson, E. (1959). Growth and crises of the healthy personality. In *Psychological issues* (ed. G.S. Klein). International Universities Press, New York.

104. Baer, L. and Jenike, M.A. (1992). Personality disorders in obsessive compulsive disorder. *Psychiatric Clinics of North America*, **15**, 803–12.

105. Drake, R.E. and Vaillant, G.E. (1985). A validity study of axis II of DSM-III. *American Journal of Psychiatry*, **142**, 553–8.

106. Millon, T. (1993). Negativistic (passive-aggressive) personality disorder. *Journal of Personality Disorders*, **7**, 78–85.

107. Perry, J.C. and Flannery, R.B. (1982). Passive-aggressive personality disorder: treatment implications of a clinical typology. *Journal of Nervous and Mental Diseases*, **170**, 164–73.

108. Lecic-Tosevski, D. and Divac-Jovanovic, M. (1996). Effects of dysthymia on personality assessment. *European Personality*, **11**, 244–8.

109. Millon, T. (1981). *Disorders of personality. DSM-III: Axis II*. Wiley, New York.

110. Murray, E.J. (1988). Personality disorders: a cognitive view. *Journal of Personality Disorders*, **2**, 37–43.

111. McCann, J.T. (1988). Passive-aggressive personality disorder: a review. *Journal of Personality Disorders*, **2**, 170–9.

112. Horney, K. (1945). *Our inner conflicts*. Norton, New York.

113. Krafft-Ebing, R. (1989). *Psychopathia sexualis* (10th edn). Enke, Stuttgart.

114. Menninger, K.A. (1938). *Man against himself*. Harcourt, Brace, New York.

115. Simons, R.C. (1987). Self-defeating and sadistic personality disorders: needed additions to the diagnostic nomenclature. *Journal of Personality Disorders*, **1**, 161–7.

116. Gay, M. and Fiester, S. (1991). Sadistic personality disorder. In *Psychiatry* (ed. R. Michaels). J.B. Lippincott, Philadelphia, PA.

117. Widiger, T.A., Frances, A.J., Spitzer, R.L., and Williams, J.B.W. (1988). The DSM-III-R personality disorders: an overview. *American Journal of Psychiatry*, **145**, 786–95.

118. Stone, M.H. (1989). Murder. *Psychiatric Clinics of North America*, **12**, 643–52.

119. Fiester, S.J. and Gay, M. (1995). Sadistic personality disorder. In *The DSM-IV personality disorders* (ed. W.J. Livesley), pp. 329–40. Guilford Press, New York.

120. Tellenbach, H. (1980). *Melancholia*. Duquesne University Press, Pittsburgh, PA.

121. Akiskal, H.S. (1989). Validating affective personality types. In *The validity of psychiatric diagnosis* (ed. L. Robins), pp. 217–27. Raven Press, New York.

4.12.4 Diagnosis and classification of personality disorders

James Reich and Giovanni de Giralamo

Definitions of personality disorders

There has been considerable interest in the study of personality and personality disorder (PD) since early times and in many different cultures. However, as noted by Tyrer *et al.*,[1] 'The categorization of personality disorder did not receive any firm support until the time of

Schneider'. Schneider[2] regarded abnormal personalities as 'constitutional variants that are highly influenced by personal experiences' and identified 10 specific types or classes of 'psychopathic personality'. The classification system proposed by Schneider has deeply influenced subsequent classification systems:[1] of the ten types of PD identified by Schneider, eight are closely related to similar types of PD as classified in DSM-III.[3] Many of these categories are also represented in DSM-IV[4] and ICD-10.[5]

Personality is defined in the second edition of the WHO *Lexicon of Psychiatric and Mental Health Terms*[6] as 'The ingrained patterns of thought, feeling, and behaviour characterising an individual's unique lifestyle and mode of adaptation, and resulting from constitutional factors, development, and social experience'. Personality disorders, according to the ICD-10 diagnostic guidelines:[5]

…comprise deeply ingrained and enduring behaviour patterns, manifesting themselves as inflexible responses to a broad range of personal and social situations. They represent either extreme or significant deviations from the way the average individual in a given culture perceives, thinks, feels, and particularly, relates to others. Such behaviour patterns tend to be stable and to encompass multiple domains of behaviour and psychological functioning. They are frequently, but not always, associated with various degrees of subjective distress and problems in social functioning and performance.

For example, a dependent PD in a favourable environment might not cause dysfunction, but nevertheless might be considered a disorder since it is clinically identical to the same disorder that usually causes dysfunction.

DSM-IV[4] defines a PD as 'an enduring pattern of inner experience and behaviour that deviates markedly from the expectations of the individual's culture'. The pattern is manifested in two or more of the following areas: cognition, affectivity, interpersonal functioning, and impulse control. The pattern is inflexible and pervasive across a broad range of situations, has an early onset, is stable and leads to significant distress or impairment.

Personality traits, according to DSM-IV,[4] 'are enduring patterns of perceiving, relating to and thinking about the environment and oneself that are exhibited in a wide range of social and personal contexts. Only when personality traits are inflexible and maladaptive and cause significant functional impairment or subjective distress do they constitute PDs.'

ICD and DSM classifications of personality disorders

Table 1 lists the specific PDs as classified in ICD-9,[7] ICD-10, DSM-IIIR,[8] and DSM-IV.

In the ICD-10 classification, which does not have a multiaxial system for the separate recording of the personality status, PD can be diagnosed together with any other mental disorder, if present. Although a multiaxial system for ICD-10 is being developed, this will not include a separate axis for PDs, as in DSM-IV.

Despite the importance given to behavioural manifestations for the classification and assessment of PDs, personality traits and attitudes are also considered when a diagnosis is made. The ICD-10 diagnostic

guidelines subdivide PDs 'according to clusters of traits that correspond to the most frequent or conspicuous behavioural manifestations'. As stressed by Widiger and Frances,[9] the reliance on behavioural indicators can improve inter-rater reliability, which reduces the amount of inferential judgement required for the diagnosis, but it does not ensure that the same diagnosis will be made at different times. Moreover, the diagnosis of a PD cannot be based on a single behaviour, as any given behaviour may have multiple causes (e.g. situational and role factors).

There have been four studies that have explored the diagnostic categories for PDs contained in ICD-10 and compared them with the DSM classification. The first[10] was carried out among 177 American clinicians who found some degree of overlap between the different categories. When the authors compared the diagnostic categories in ICD-10 with those in DSM-IIIR, they found that only anankastic (ICD) and obsessive–compulsive (DSM) PDs showed a high level of correspondence. The second study[11] looked at 52 outpatients and compared DSM-IIIR to ICD-10. It found fair concordance for the diagnosis of 'any PD', but poor agreement for individual PDs; the ICD-10 tended to overdiagnose PDs relative to DSM-IIIR. The third report[12] compared ICD-10 and DSM-IV in 58 patients with panic disorder. There was good agreement for the presence of 'any PD', and a reasonable agreement between individual diagnoses (κ ranged from 0.51 to 0.83.), with a tendency for ICD-10 to overdiagnose PDs relative to DSM-IV. In the fourth study,[13] ICD-10 criteria were found to have satisfactory inter-rater reliability in a sample of homeless adults.

In the American taxonomic system, a multiaxial classification was first introduced in DSM-III. With the development of DSM-IIIR, more than 100 changes in the classification of PDs were introduced compared with DSM-III.[14,15] While the multiaxial and categorical style of classification was maintained, the diagnostic criteria were revised to form a list of symptoms for each PD, of which only a certain number were required for a diagnosis to be reached. In DSM-IIIR, each category of PD comprised seven to ten criteria, with the presence of four to six criteria required for diagnosis. DSM-IIIR contained 11 PDs (see Table 1), plus two new disorders (self-defeating PD and sadistic PD) that were not included in DSM-III but were considered as diagnostic categories needing further study. As in DSM-III, the 11 PDs were divided into three clusters:

- cluster A (the 'odd' or 'eccentric' cluster), which included paranoid, schizoid, and schizotypal PD;

- cluster B (the 'dramatic' or 'erratic' cluster), which included histrionic, narcissistic, antisocial, and borderline PDs;

- cluster C (the 'anxious' cluster), which included avoidant, dependent, obsessive–compulsive, and passive–aggressive PDs.

One study in the United States examined changes in personality diagnoses using DSM-III versus DSM-IIIR.[16] For some categories there was a considerable difference in the frequency of diagnosis: for example, there was an 800 per cent increase in the rate of schizoid PD and a 350 per cent increase in the rate of narcissistic PD diagnosed by the clinicians when DSM-IIIR criteria were applied.

DSM-IV was designed to be a conservative evolution from DSM-IIIR; however, some differences in diagnoses between DSM-IIIR and DSM-IV can be expected.[17] In general, the different DSMs should not be considered interchangeable unless there is specific data supporting agreement of a diagnosis across systems. As shown in Table 1, DSM-IV includes 11 PDs as in the DSM-IIIR classification; slight changes were

Table 1 Comparison of different classification systems of personality disorders: ICD-9, ICD-10, DSM-IIIR, and DSM-IV

ICD-9	ICD-10	DSM-IIIR	DSM-IV
Paranoid personality disorder	Paranoid personality disorder	Paranoid personality disorder	Paranoid personality disorder
Schizoid personality disorder	Schizoid personality disorder	Schizoid personality disorder	Schizoid personality disorder
Personality disorder with predominantly sociopathic or asocial manifestations	Dissocial personality disorder	Antisocial personality disorder	Antisocial personality disorder
	Emotionally unstable personality disorder		
(a) Explosive personality disorder	(a) Impulsive type	(a) —	(a) —
(b) —	(b) Borderline type	(b) Borderline personality disorder	(b) Borderline personality disorder
Histrionic personality disorder	Histrionic personality disorder	Histrionic personality disorder	Histrionic personality disorder
Anankastic personality disorder	Anankastic personality disorder	Obsessive–compulsive personality disorder	Obsessive–compulsive personality disorder
—	Anxious (avoidant) personality disorder	Avoidant personality disorder	Avoidant personality disorder
—	Dependent personality disorder	Dependent personality disorder	Dependent personality disorder
Affective personality disorder Asthenic personality disorder	Other specific personality disorders	Passive-aggressive personality disorder Schizotypal personality disorder Narcissistic personality disorder Self-defeating personality disorder Sadistic personality disorder	— Schizotypal personality disorder Narcissistic personality disorder — — Personality disorder not otherwise specified

introduced in the diagnostic criteria, and a new category 'PD not otherwise specified' added. Passive-aggressive, self-defeating, and sadistic PDs (provisionally included in DSM-IIIR) were dropped. The overall effect of these changes will be to increase the concordance between the DSM-IV and the ICD-10 classification systems compared with that between DSM-IIIR and ICD-10. DSM-IV also includes the three clusters present in DSM-IIIR.

Similarities and differences between ICD-10 and DSM-IV

Table 1 shows that for seven categories of PD (paranoid, schizoid, dissocial/antisocial, histrionic, anankastic/obsessive–compulsive, anxious/avoidant, and dependent), there is a specific correspondence between ICD-10 and DSM-IV. For three categories, there are differences in nomenclature between the two systems; in particular ICD-10 uses the term 'anankastic' instead of 'obsessive–compulsive', to avoid the erroneous implication of an inevitable link between this type of personality and obsessive–compulsive disorder. ICD-10 also uses the term ' dissocial' instead of 'antisocial', to prevent any possible connotation of stigmatization, and the term 'anxious' instead of 'avoidant'. Moreover, while DSM-IV classifies borderline PD as a specific category, ICD-10 includes it as a subcategory of emotionally unstable PD. Narcissistic and passive-aggressive PDs (present in DSM-IV) are included in ICD-10 under the category of 'other specific PDs'. Finally, while DSM-IV includes schizotypal PD as a PD, ICD-10 classifies it in the overall group of 'Schizophrenia, schizotypal and delusional disorders', to highlight the contiguity between this disorder and the schizophrenia group disorders, as shown by genetic and clinical studies. DSM-IV has the category 'Personality disorders not otherwise specified', while ICD-10 has the category 'Other specific personality disorders'.

Categorical versus dimensional styles of classification

In general, researchers involved in the assessment of personality traits tend to use dimensional measures based on normal populations. In contrast, those concerned with personality types and, even more, clinicians concerned with PDs, tend to employ categorical concepts and assessment measures based on these concepts.[15]

Each of the two approaches has specific advantages and disadvantages. The drawbacks of the categorical approach are represented by the difficulty of classifying patients who are at the boundary of different categories or who do not meet the diagnostic criteria for any specific PD, but who still have significant pathology. Other points that should be addressed include the wide variation of symptomatology found within each given category, the need for heterogeneous categories, such as 'mixed' and 'atypical', the need to simplify necessarily complex conditions, the need to define valid cut-off points, and the use of a nominal rather than an ordinal scale.

On the other hand, a dimensional approach may not be appropriate when dealing with severe clinical problems and may not permit findings from different cultures to be compared easily. Those in favour of a dimensional approach argue that PDs differ from normal variations in personality only in terms of degree, and to some extent this is supported by empirical data.[18,19]

Moreover, it is still unclear whether normal and abnormal personality traits are the same or whether they are qualitatively different. Two main findings seem to support the latter hypothesis: first, normal personality traits are at least moderately heritable, while abnormal personality traits appear less heritable; second, the prevalence rates of PDs found in surveys are much greater than would be expected from the prevalence rates of normal personality traits in the general population. Some researchers[20] have even suggested that an extreme form of a normal personality trait is not necessarily pathological. Although some authors argue that there is no difference between normal and abnormal personality traits,[18] this is still an area of open inquiry. It is possible that different models may be appropriate in different situations.

Controversial diagnostic categories

Some diagnostic categories of PD have raised important conceptual problems and have stimulated an active discussion among various researchers. They include borderline PD, histrionic PD, and dissocial (antisocial) PD.

Borderline PD has, for many years, been a debated diagnostic concept. It did not appear in ICD-9 and the term was rarely used in Europe; on the other hand, it became quite popular in the United States. A review of over 70 papers published on this topic, mainly between 1980 and 1986, concluded that the weight of evidence supported the validity of this category.[21] However, more recent studies have found that borderline PD constitutes a very heterogeneous category with unclear boundaries, overlapping with many different disorders but without a specific association with any of them.[22,23]

Histrionic PD has also been criticized for compromising validity by including female social norms to diagnose women as having the disorder. The fact that histrionic PD is frequently diagnosed in women is used to support this conclusion. However, there is no evidence of this

disorder being overdiagnosed by experienced clinicians. Moreover, it is not necessarily a sign of bias for a disorder to occur more frequently in one sex; major depression is also more common in women, while dissocial PD is more common in men. A recent study has demonstrated that there is no evidence that diagnostic thresholds used in women are any different than those used in men.[24]

The concept of dissocial (antisocial) PD has been used for over 180 years,[25] and yet it has remained a difficult concept. This is because of the difficulty in drawing a dividing line between normal and abnormal behaviour that is independent of local cultural values and societal norms. Blackburn[26] has been the most critical exponent among those who have stressed the 'normative' aspect of this diagnosis. He has suggested that the concept of dissocial PD 'remains a "mythical entity"'…Such a concept is little more than a moral judgement masquerading as a clinical diagnosis. Given the lack of demonstrable scientific or clinical utility of the concept, it should be discarded.' Similar views were expressed by Lewis[25] and Shepherd and Sartorius,[27] who stated that 'antisocial personality disorder…is peculiarly susceptible to misunderstanding and misuse'. Although the diagnosis of dissocial PD has the greatest empirical support and highest inter-rater reliability, it has been criticized for compromising validity for reliability by emphasizing easily identifiable criminal and delinquent behaviour. In particular, DSM-III criteria for antisocial PD have been criticized because they do not give prominence to the traditional personality traits of psychopathy (e.g. incapacity to experience guilt, to learn from experience, or to maintain enduring relationships) and emphasize different aspects of criminality and irresponsibility. In addition, the diagnostic criteria are cumbersome. Similar problems have also been reported with DSM-IIIR criteria for antisocial PD.[28] DSM-IV criteria have moved more towards Hare's concept of psychopathy, apparently without any loss of reliability.[29]

Assessment methods for personality disorders

Table 2 shows the main methods currently available for assessing all PDs. Additional instruments for assessing specified PDs have also been developed—some of the methods listed are new, while others have been revised two or three times.[30,31] The following points related to these methods need to be mentioned.

1. The interview measures have generally shown a satisfactory inter-rater reliability, while test–retest reliability has not been well established. However, three methods do show some evidence of good test–retest reliability—the Personality Assessment Schedule (**PAS**),[32] the International Personality Disorder Examination (**IPDE**),[33] and the SCID-II.[34] In the assessment of this particular group of disorders, the stability over time is especially important,[35–37] as personality characteristics tend to be long-lasting.

2. Many of the methods have been standardized on psychiatric inpatient or outpatient populations; their applicability in epidemiological community studies is largely unknown.[38,39]

3. The various measures tend not to agree with each other on specific diagnoses.[29–31] A measurement on one standardized instrument is not necessarily the same as the measurement on another.

4. Some authors, mostly developers of interview instruments, have

Table 2 Assessment methods for all personality disorders

Name of the instrument	Author(s)[a]	Method of assessment	Number of items	Time required (min)
Diagnostic Interview for Personality Disorders (DIPD)	Zanarini	Semistructured interview with patient using DSM-IIIR criteria	101	60–120
International Personality Disorder Examination (IPDE)	Loranger et al.	Semistructured interview with patient using ICD-10 and DSM-IIIR criteria	157	150
Millon Clinical Multiaxial Inventory (MCMI)	Millon	Self-report by patient using DSM-IIIR criteria	175	20–30
Personality Assessment Schedule (PAS)	Tyrer et al.	Semistructured interview with informant(s) using DSM-IIIR criteria	24	60
Personality Diagnostic Questionnaire–Revised (PDQ-R)	Hyler and Reider	Self-report by patient or informant(s) using DSM-IIIR criteria	152	30
Personality Interview Questions II (PIQ-II)	Widiger	Semistructured interview with patient using DSM-III criteria	375	60–120
Schedule for Normal and Abnormal Personality Disorders (SNAP)	Clark	Self-report by patient using DSM-III and dimensional criteria	106	10
Standardized Assessment Personality (SAP)	Pilgrim and Mann	Semistructured interview with informant(s) using ICD-10 and DSM-IIIR criteria	NA	10–15
Structured Clinical Interview for DSM-IIIR Personality Disorders (SCID-II)	Spitzer and Williams	Semistructured interview with patient using DSM-IIIR criteria	120	60–90
Structured Interview for DSM-III Personality Disorders (SIPD)	Pfohl et al.	Semistructured interview with patient or informant(s) using DSM–III criteria	136	90
Tridimensional Personality Questionnaire (TPQ)	Cloninger	Self-report by patient	100	20–30
Wisconsin Personality Inventory (WISPI)	Klein	Self-report by patient using DSM-III criteria	360	20

NA, not applicable.

[a] For specific references to each instrument please see de Girolamo and Reich[30] and Reich.[31]

stated that self-report measures are not as valid for the measurement and study of personality as interview measures. These arguments tend to be based on the finding that self-report instruments do not agree well with interview instruments, and that a PD diagnosis cannot be made without a clinical interview. The first argument does not hold water, since none of the interview instruments agree well with each other either. Whether self-report instruments can reliably diagnose a PD (as opposed to personality traits) is an open question. However, dimensional interview instruments have high test–retest reliability (some for as long as 30 years) and have been, and will continue to be, a valuable component of personality research, especially where the focus is on dimensions.[40] Self-report instruments measuring DSM disorders tend to disagree with each other in a similar way to the interview instruments. In conclusion, the instrument chosen for any given clinical or research endeavour should reflect the ability of the individual instrument to meet the specific needs of the project.

5. Standardized testing of personality and clinician impression do not tend be in good agreement. This is due both to the tendency of instruments to report more disorders and for clinicians to use idiosyncratic criteria in their diagnoses.[41,42] Standardized measures are a must, however, if the data is to be used for research or public policy purposes.

6. Most personality measurement instruments are affected by the comorbid presence of a non-personality emotional disorder (Axis I disorder in the DSM system). Some structured interviews try to correct for this by asking patients about times when they were not suffering from an Axis I disorder; however, when the Axis I disorder is chronic, this may be difficult to achieve.[33,34] This problem also affects the ability of questionnaires to differentiate between current Axis I disorders and PDs, as this self-judgement of patients who are suffering from a psychiatric condition is frequently impaired.[33] The PDE, PAS, and SCID-II may be less affected by this problem.

7. There is disagreement among experts about the use of informants. Many authors have argued that, besides the patient, a key informant should also be interviewed, given the likelihood that many patients will not reply reliably to questions about their personality and the possibility that informant ratings will differ substantially from patient ones.[33,43] However, even if an informant is interviewed, it is often unclear which source to use to score the test if the interviewee and informant disagree. This tends to reduce their value.

8. Discriminant validity refers to the ability of a diagnostic system and measurement system to diagnose non-overlapping disorders. Discriminant validity is not high with the ICD-10 and DSM-IV PDs.[44] This means that it is the rule, rather the exception, that multiple personality diagnoses will be made: some studies have provided evidence of this assumption. For instance, in four studies that examined personality comorbidity in a total of 568 patients, the average percentage of multiple diagnoses was 85 per cent.[45] To what extent this reflects the real coexistence of different disorders—with distinct patterns of symptoms, correlates, and course—or if it is simply the effect of an insufficient discriminant validity of current diagnostic systems has still to be clarified.

References

1. Tyrer, P., Casey, P., and Ferguson, B. (1991). Personality disorder in perspective. *British Journal of Psychiatry*, **159**, 463–71.

2. Schneider, K. (1923). *Die Psychopathischen personlichkeiten*. Springer, Berlin.

3. American Psychiatric Association (1980). *Diagnostic and statistical manual of mental disorders* (3rd edn). American Psychiatric Press, Washington, DC.

4. American Psychiatric Association (1994). *Diagnostic and statistical manual of mental disorders* (4th edn). American Psychiatric Association, Washington, DC.

5. World Health Organization (1992). *International statistical classification of diseases and related health problems, 10th revision*. WHO, Geneva.

6. World Health Organization (1994). *Lexicon of psychiatric and mental health terms* (2nd edn). WHO, Geneva.

7. World Health Organization (1977). *International classification of diseases, injuries and causes of death, ninth revision*. WHO, Geneva.

8. American Psychiatric Association (1987). *Diagnostic and statistical manual of mental disorders* (3rd edn, revised). American Psychiatric Press, Washington, DC.

9. Widiger, T.A. and Frances, A. (1985). Axis II personality disorders: diagnostic and treatment issues. *Hospital and Community Psychiatry*, **36**, 619–27.

10. Blashfield, R.K. (1991). An American view of the ICD-10 personality disorders. *Acta Psychiatrica Scandinavica*, **82**, 250–6.

11. Sara, G., Raven, P., and Mann, A. (1996). A comparison of DSM-III-R and ICD-10 personality disorder criteria in an outpatient population. *Psychological Medicine*, **26**, 151–60.

12. Starcevic, V., Bogojevic, G., and Kelin, K. (1997). Diagnostic agreement between the DSM-IV and ICD-10-DCR personality disorders. *Psychopathology*, **30**, 328–34.

13. Merson, S., Tyrer, P., Duke, P., and Henderson, F. (1994). Interrater reliability of ICD-10 guidelines for the diagnosis of personality disorders. *Journal of Personality Disorders*, **8**, 89–95.

14. Gorton, G. and Akhtar, S. (1990). The literature on personality disorders, 1985–88: trends, issues and controversies. *Hospital and Community Psychiatry*, **41**, 39–51.

15. Widiger, T.A., Frances, A., Spitzer, R.L., and Williams, J.B.W. (1988). DSM-III-R Personality disorders: an overview. *American Journal of Psychiatry*, **145**, 786–95.

16. Morey, L.C. (1988). Personality disorders in DSM-III and DSM-III-R: convergence, coverage and internal consistency. *American Journal of Psychiatry*, **145**, 573–7.

17. Coolidge, F.L. and Segal, D.L. (1998). Evolution of personality disorder diagnosis in the *Diagnostic and Statistical Manual of Mental Disorders*. *Clinical Psychology Review*, **19**, 583–99.

18. Livesley, W.J., Schroeder, M.L., Jackson, D.N., and Jang, K.L. (1994). Categorical distinctions in the study of personality disorders: implications for classification. *Journal of Abnormal Psychology*, **103**, 6–17.

19. Schroeder, M.L. and Livesley, W.J. (1991). An evaluation of DSM-III-R personality disorders. *Acta Psychiatrica Scandinavica*, **84**, 512–59.

20. Birtchnell, J. (1988). Defining dependence. *British Journal of Medical Psychology*, **61**, 111–23.

21. Tarnopolsky, A. and Berelowitz, M. (1987). Borderline personality: a review of recent research. *British Journal of Psychiatry*, **151**, 724–34.

22. Fyer, M.R., Frances, A.J., Sullivan, T., Hurt, S.W., and Clarkin, J. (1988). Comorbidity of borderline personality disorder. *Archives of General Psychiatry*, **45**, 348–52.

23. Nurnberg, G.H., Raskin, M., Levine, P.E., Pollack, S., Siegel, O., and Prince, R. (1991). The comorbidity of borderline personality disorder and other DSM-III-R axis II personality disorders. *American Journal of Psychiatry*, **148**, 1371–7.

24. Funtowicz, M.N. and Widiger, T.A. (1995). Sex bias in the diagnosis of personality disorders: a different approach. *Journal of Psychopathology and Behavioral Assessment*, **17**, 145–65.

25. Lewis, A. (1974). Psychopathic personality: a most elusive category. *Psychological Medicine*, **4**, 133–40.

26. Blackburn, R. (1988). On moral judgments and personality disorders. The myth of psychopathic personality. *British Journal of Psychiatry*, **153**, 505–12.

27. Shepherd, M. and Sartorius, N. (1974). Personality disorder and the International Classification of Diseases. *Psychological Medicine*, **4**, 141–6.

28. Hare, R.D., Hart, S.D., and Harpur, T.J. (1991). Psychopathy and the DSM-IV criteria for antisocial personality disorder. *Journal of Abnormal Psychology*, **100**, 391–8.

29. Widiger, T.A., Cadoret, R., Hare, R., *et al.* (1996). DSM-IV Antisocial personality disorder field trial. *Journal of Abnormal Psychology*, **105**, 3–16.

30. de Girolamo, G. and Reich, J.H. (1993) *Personality disorders*. WHO, Geneva.

31. Reich, J.H. (1989). Update on instruments to measure DSM-III and DSM-III-R personality disorders. *Journal of Nervous and Mental Disease*, **177**, 366–70.

32. Tyrer, P., Casey, P., and Gall, J. (1983). Relationship between neurosis and personality disorder. *British Journal of Psychiatry*, **142**, 404–8.

33. Loranger, A.W., Sartorius, N., Andreoli, A., *et al.* (1994). The International Personality Disorder Examination: the World Health Organization/Alcohol, Drug Abuse, and Mental Health Administration international pilot study of personality disorders. *Archives of General Psychiatry*, **51**, 215–24.

34. Ouimette, P.C. and Klein, D.N. (1995). Test–retest stability, mood–state dependence and informant–subject concordance in the SCID-Axis II questionnaire in a non clinical sample. *Journal of Personality Disorders*, **9**, 105–11.

35. Tyrer, P. (1987). Problems in the classification of personality disorder. *Psychological Medicine*, **17**, 15–20.

36. Tyrer, P. (1987). Measurement of abnormal personality: a review. *Journal of the Royal Society of Medicine*, **80**, 637–9.

37. Tyrer, P. (1990). Diagnosing personality disorders. *Current Opinion in Psychiatry*, **3**, 182–7.

38. Zimmerman, M. (1994). Diagnosing personality disorders. A review of issues and research methods. *Archives of General Psychiatry*, **51**, 225–45.

39. Jackson, H.J., Gazis, J., Rudd, R.P., and Edwards, J. (1991). Concordance between two personality disorder instruments with psychiatric inpatients. *Comprehensive Psychiatry*, **32**, 252–60.

40. Clark, L.A., Livesley, W.J., and Morey, L. (1997). Special feature: personality disorder assessment: the challenge of construct validity. *Journal of Personality Disorders*, **11**, 205–31.

41. Blashfield, R.K. and Herkov, M.J. (1996). Investigating clinician adherence to diagnosis by criteria: a replication of Morey and Ochoa (1989). *Journal of Personality Disorder*, **10**, 219–28.

42. Perry, J.C. (1992). Problems and considerations in the valid assessment of personality disorders. *American Journal of Psychiatry*, **149**, 1645–53.

43. Dodwell, D. (1988). Comparison of self-ratings within informant-ratings of pre-morbid personality on two personality rating scales. *Psychological Medicine*, **18**, 495–502.

44. Bornstein, R.F. (1998). Reconceptualizing personality disorder diagnosis in the DSM-IV: the discriminant validity challenge. *Clinical Psychology: Science and Practice*, **5**, 333–43.

45. Widiger, T.A. and Rogers, J.H. (1989). Prevalence and comorbidity of personality disorders. *Psychiatric Annals*, **19**, 132–6.

4.12.5 Epidemiology of personality disorders

Giovanni de Girolamo and Patrizia Dotto

Introduction

Only recently has the epidemiology of personality disorder (**PD**) begun to be scientifically investigated. This development has taken place because a number of standardized instruments to assess personality and PD in an empirical fashion have been developed, in parallel with the refinement of a valid and reliable diagnostic system based on a categorical approach.

The need for the epidemiological investigation of PD seems justified for several reasons.

1. As seen in recent epidemiological surveys, PDs are frequent and have been found in different countries and sociocultural settings.

2. PDs can seriously impair the life of the affected individual and can be highly disruptive to societies, communities, and families.

3. Personality status is often a major predictive variable in determining the outcome of psychiatric disorders and the response to treatment.

In this chapter we review the epidemiological literature on PDs up to the end of 1998, focusing on studies carried out since the development of the DSM-III. First, community prevalence studies of PD are reviewed. We then look at the prevalence of individual PDs in the community. Finally, we consider the prevalence of PDs in clinical populations, and in special settings (e.g. primary care, prisons, etc.).

Community epidemiological studies of unspecified personality disorders

Until the development of the DSM-III diagnostic criteria for PD and the subsequent availability of standardized assessment instruments, epidemiological studies aimed at assessing the prevalence rate of PDs were hampered by severe methodological limitations, including differences in sampling methods and in diagnostic criteria, the known unreliability of PD diagnoses based on clinical judgement, and the lack of standardized assessment methods. Since 1980, eight studies have ascertained the prevalence rate of PDs in different community samples using assessment instruments specific for PD; they are shown in Table 1.

In these studies, the sample sizes ranged between 200 and 1646 subjects, with an average sample of 564; all surveyed individuals (all randomly selected) were evaluated by means of a specific PD assessment instrument, mainly a structured interview. While most studies were carried out in one stage, Lenzenweger *et al.*[3] first screened a large sample of university students with a self-administered Axis II inventory, and then interviewed a subgroup of 258 subjects using the International Personality Disorder Examination. The median prevalence rate of any PDs in these eight studies is 10.5 per cent.

In the surveys considered here the rate of PDs decreases in older age groups; although the sex ratio is different for specific types of PD (e.g. more antisocial PDs among males, more dependent and anxious PDs among females), the overall rates of PD are about equal for both sexes. Finally, prevalence rates are generally higher in urban populations and lower socio-economic groups.

Community epidemiological studies of specified personality disorders

Table 2 lists the median prevalence rates for specified PDs based on studies that surveyed different types of randomly selected community

Table 1 Prevalence rates of personality disorders in epidemiological surveys

Reference	Country	Sample size	Sample features	Diagnostic criteria	Assessment method	PD prevalence rate (%)
Casey and Tyrer[1]	UK	200	Urban and rural residents	ICD-9	PAS	13.0
Klein et al.[2]	USA	229	Urban and rural residents	DSM-IIIR	PDE	14.8
Lenzenweger et al.[3]	USA	1646	18- to 19-year-old university students	DSM-IIIR	IPDE	6.7
Moldin et al.[4]	USA	302	Urban residents	DSM-IIIR	PDE	7.3
Maier et al.[5]	Germany	447	Unscreened sample of 109 families	DSM-IIIR	SCID	10.0
Reich et al.[6]	USA	235	Urban residents	DSM-III	PDQ	11.1
Samuels et al.[7]	USA	762	Urban residents	DSM-III	SPE	5.9
Zimmerman and Coryell[8]	USA	697	Non-patient relatives of psychiatric patients and healthy controls	DSM-III	(a) PDQ (b) SIPD	(a) 10.3 (b) 13.5

PAS, Personality Assessment Schedule; PDE, Personality Disorder Examination; IPDE, International Personality Disorder Examination; SCID, Structured Clinical Interview for DSM-IIIR Personality Disorders; PDQ, Personality Diagnostic Questionnaire; SIPD, Structured Interview for DSM-IIIR Personality Disorders.

samples. We will comment on some of the findings. The second column shows the number of studies on which the median prevalence rate is based.

Table 2 Median prevalence rates of specified personality disorders in epidemiological surveys

PD category	Number of studies (N)	Median prevalence rate (%)
Paranoid personality disorder	8	0.6
Schizoid personality disorder	9	0.4
Schizotypal personality disorder	8	0.6
Antisocial (dissocial) personality disorder	18	1.9
Borderline personality disorder	9	1.6
Histrionic personality disorder	8	2
Narcissistic personality disorder	7	0.2
Obsessive–compulsive (anankastic) personality disorder	8	1.7
Avoidant (anxious) personality disorder	7	0.7
Dependent personality disorder	8	0.7
Passive–aggressive personality disorder	7	1.7

Paranoid personality disorder

The median prevalence rate of paranoid PD is 0.6 per cent. In the study by Baron[9] paranoid PD was remarkably more common among relatives of schizophrenic probands (7.3 per cent) than among relatives of control probands (2.7 per cent).

Schizoid personality disorder

There have been nine studies evaluating the prevalence of schizoid PD in the community, with a median prevalence rate of 0.4 per cent. Baron[9] reported a rate of 1.6 per cent of schizoid PD among relatives of schizophrenic probands, but no cases among relatives of control probands.

Schizotypal personality disorder

The median prevalence rate of schizotypal PD is 0.6 per cent. However, in the study by Baron[9] schizotypal PD was remarkably more common among relatives of schizophrenic probands (14.6 per cent) than among relatives of control probands (2.1 per cent). This result provides additional support for the specific relationship between schizophrenia and schizotypal PD.

Antisocial (dissocial) personality disorder

Antisocial is the most studied PD. Its prevalence has been assessed in 18 epidemiological surveys, with a median sample size of 3359 subjects; six studies used the Diagnostic Interview Schedule as the assessment instrument. Antisocial PD seems to have a prevalence of around 1.9 per cent in the general population and to be more frequent among males than females, with sex ratios ranging from 2:1 to 7:1. It is also more common among younger adults, those living in urban areas, and the lower socio-economic classes. People with a diagnosis of antisocial PD are also high users of medical services.

Borderline personality disorder

Borderline PD has been investigated in nine studies. Swartz et al.[10] carried out a study among 1541 community subjects (between 19 and 55 years of age) at the North Carolina site of the Epidemiologic Catchment Area (ECA) Program, using a diagnostic algorithm derived from the Diagnostic Interview Schedule (**DIS**). They found a rate of 1.8 per cent for borderline PD; the disorder was significantly more common among females, the widowed, and the unmarried. There was a trend towards an increase in the diagnosis in younger, non-white, urban, and poorer respondents. The highest rates were found in the 19 to 34 age range, with the rates declining with age. All borderline respondents had also a DIS DSM-III Axis I lifetime diagnosis.

Although some believe there is a preponderance of females with borderline PD, they do not always take into account a preponderance of females in the populations studied. There were two studies that did not find a higher female prevalence.

Histrionic personality disorder

Histrionic PD has the highest median prevalence rate (2 per cent). A study by Nestadt et al.,[11] carried out at the Baltimore (Maryland) site of the Epidemiologic Catchment Area Program, ascertained the prevalence of histrionic PD in the community. The authors found a prevalence of 2.1 per cent in the general population, with virtually identical rates in men and women. No significant differences were found in terms of race and education, but the prevalence was significantly higher among separated and divorced persons. It should be noted that the study derived the diagnosis from instruments not originally intended to diagnose personality disorders; it might be possible that, in some cases, this study has identified personality traits rather than 'true' PDs.

Narcissistic personality disorder

No cases of narcissistic PD were found in four studies. However, Reich et al.[6] and Lenzenweger et al.[3] found rates of 0.4 per cent and 1.2 per cent respectively, whereas Klein, in a sample of 229 subjects, found a very high rate (3.9 per cent).

Obsessive–compulsive (anankastic) personality disorder

The median prevalence rate of obsessive–compulsive PD, obtained from eight studies, was found to be 1.7 per cent. The rate of compulsive PD was especially high in a study in which the Personality Diagnostic Questionnaire was used (6.4 per cent).[3] However, lower rates were reported with structured interviews. A community study, carried out at the Epidemiologic Catchment Area Program Baltimore site, found a prevalence of 1.7 per cent.[12] Males had a rate about five times higher than females. The disorder was also more frequent among white, highly educated, married, and employed subjects, and it

Table 3 Median prevalence rates of PDs among psychiatric patients in prospective studies including more than 100 subjects

Diagnostic category	Number of studies (N)	Median sample (N)	Median prevalence rate (%)
Alcohol and substance abuse [13–20]	8	327	56
Affective disorders [21–27]	7	176	57
Anxiety disorders [28–32]	5	200	41
Any Axis I disorders [33–44]	12	133	50

was associated with anxiety disorders. However, the study derived the diagnosis from an interview originally not intended to diagnose PDs. This could mean that adaptive obsessive–compulsive traits, rather than a 'true' PD, were identified.

Avoidant (anxious) personality disorder

A total of seven studies have investigated the prevalence of avoidant PD in community samples, with a median prevalence rate of 0.7 per cent.

Dependent personality disorder

In eight studies in which the frequency of dependent PD was assessed, the median prevalence rate was 0.7 per cent.

Passive-aggressive personality disorder

The median prevalence rate of passive-aggressive PD, obtained from seven studies, was found to be quite high (1.7 per cent); interestingly, this type of PD has not been included either in DSM-IV or in ICD-10.

Epidemiological studies of personality disorders carried out in psychiatric settings

Table 3 lists the median prevalence rates for any PDs found in 32 studies carried out in inpatient and outpatient psychiatric samples and published between 1981 and 1998. Only those prospective studies that surveyed homogeneous clinical samples (either inpatients or outpatients) of more than 100 subjects have been considered for this analysis. The second column shows the number of studies on which the median prevalence rate is based.

In these studies subjects have been directly evaluated for the purpose of obtaining PD rates, by means of a standardized assessment instrument specific for PDs. Several other studies, which have evaluated only the prevalence of specified PDs in clinical samples, are not shown here.

In general, the prevalence of PDs among psychiatric outpatients and inpatients is quite high, with a majority of studies ($n = 17$) showing a PD prevalence rate higher than 50 per cent of the sample. However, it is difficult to draw more definite conclusions from these studies, because of substantial differences in sampling, diagnostic criteria, assessment methods, availability of mental health services, prevalence of Axis disorders, and sociocultural factors.

There are, however, some consistencies across studies that deserve consideration. The most prevalent PD seems to be borderline, both in inpatient and in outpatient settings. The next most common PDs are schizotypal and histrionic. These three disorders are also characterized by the lowest social functioning. They are especially common in inpatient settings, as their symptomatology often results in the patient being admitted to hospital due to their suicidal behaviour, substance abuse, and cognitive–perceptual abnormalities. In outpatient settings, dependent and passive-aggressive PD are also common.

Especially in inpatient settings, many people who meet the criteria for one PD also meet the criteria for other PDs.[45,46] The highest comorbidity rate appears to occur with borderline PD, with the frequent coexistence of borderline and histrionic PDs, followed by antisocial, schizotypal, and dependent PDs.

With regard to comorbidity between PDs and Axis I disorders, the most common and best-studied patterns are between substance abuse and PDs, affective disorders and PDs, and anxiety disorders and PDs (particularly borderline, antisocial, avoidant, and dependent PDs). Other clinically significant associations have been found between bulimia nervosa and borderline PD, as well as between anorexia and avoidant PD.[47] High rates of PD (especially borderline and antisocial PDs) have also been detected in patients with selected medical conditions, such as HIV-positive patients.[48]

Some studies have assessed the treated prevalence of PD using administrative data (e.g. discharge figures, psychiatric case register data, etc.). In the United States, using data from the 1993 National Hospital Discharge Survey, Olfson and Mechanic[49] found that almost 12 per cent of patients discharged from public general hospitals had a diagnosis of PD, compared with 11 per cent of patients from non-profit hospitals and 5 per cent of patients from proprietary general hospitals. In England and Wales, 7.6 per cent of all admissions and 8.5 per cent of first admissions over a 1-year period were diagnosed as having PDs.[50]

Some investigations, which compared the hospital admission rates for PD over time, allow us to assess the impact of diagnostic changes. In Denmark, sex- and age-standardized rates of first-admitted borderline patients significantly increased during the 16-year interval between 1970 and 1985, and this might be explained in terms of a change in diagnostic habits.[51] In the United States, comparing the diagnoses given to inpatients in a large university-affiliated mental hospital in the last 5 years of the DSM-II era ($n = 5143$) with those given in the first 5 years of the DSM-III era ($n = 5771$), a marked increase (from 19 per cent to 49 per cent) was found in the diagnosis of PD, together with a decrease in the diagnosis of schizophrenia and a corresponding increase in the diagnosis of affective disorders.[52]

The epidemiological findings in treated samples are especially important if we bear in mind that the presence of a PD among those suffering from other mental disorders can be a major predictor of the natural history and treatment outcome. Therefore an important clinical implication of these findings is that patients in treatment because of severe Axis I disorders must be carefully assessed with an assessment instrument specific for PDs, because of the high likelihood of diagnosing a PD and the subsequent need to adjust their treatment accordingly.

Epidemiological studies of personality disorders carried out in other settings

A few epidemiological studies on PDs have been carried out among patients attending primary healthcare settings; in these studies between 5 and 8 per cent of patients have been identified as having a primary diagnosis of PD.[45] When the assessment is made independently of the primary diagnosis, however, the average prevalence rate can rise several-fold because of state effects. There are also indications that people showing certain PDs are high users of medical services.

In other institutional settings, such as prisons, several studies have found very high rates of PDs. In the United Kingdom, two large-scale studies have recently been completed; in the first, carried out among 750 prisoners representing a 9 per cent cross-sectional sample of the entire male unconvicted population, a PD was diagnosed in 11 per cent of the sample.[53] In the second study, a representative sample of the entire prison population of England and Wales was evaluated; a subsample was assessed with the SCID-II administered by a clinician.[54] The prevalence rates for any PD were 78 per cent for male remand prisoners, 64 per cent for male sentenced prisoners, and 50 per cent for female prisoners. High rates of borderline and antisocial PDs have also been found in a sample ($n = 805$) of women felons entering prison in a North American State.[55]

Conclusions

Up to 20 years ago, the epidemiology of PDs had not received the same amount of attention as that of many other psychiatric disorders. Since then the situation has changed, and we now have data on the prevalence of PD in the community and in psychiatric facilities. Community data come primarily from eight studies, with a total sample of 4518 subjects from three countries (Germany, the United Kingdom, and the United States). There are excellent national and cross-national epidemiological data on antisocial personality disorder based on the same diagnostic methods. There are almost no data on other PDs from countries other than the United States, the United Kingdom, and Germany.

One important methodological problem is that some PDs have a very low prevalence rate. Consequently, epidemiological surveys carried out among the general population may require very large samples in order to identify a sufficient number of cases to study demographic correlates and the association of PD with other psychiatric disorders. Future studies should try to address this problem and provide us with more definite epidemiological data. These data will also be invaluable in showing the validity of current classifications and in better delineating the boundaries between different PDs.

References

1. Casey, P.R. and Tyrer, P.J. (1986). Personality, functioning and symptomatology. *Journal of Psychiatric Research*, **20**, 363–74.

2. Klein, D.L., Riso, L.P., Donaldson, S.K., *et al.* (1995). Family study of early-onset dysthymia. *Archives of General Psychiatry*, **52**, 487–96.

3. Lenzenweger, M.F., Loranger, A.W., Korfine, L., and Neff, C. (1997). Detecting personality disorders in a nonclinical population. Application of a 2-stage procedure for case identification. *Archives of General Psychiatry*, **54**, 345–51.

4. Moldin, S.O., Rice, J.P., Erlenmeyer Kimling, L., and Squires Wheeler, E. (1994). Latent structure of DSM-III-R Axis II psychopathology in a normal sample. *Journal of Abnormal Psychology*, **103**, 259–66.

5. Maier, W. (1992). Prevalences of personality disorders (DSM-III-R) in the community. *Journal of Personality Disorders*, **6**, 187–96.

6. Reich, J.H., Yates, W., and Nduaguba, M. (1989). Prevalence of DSM-III personality disorders in the community. *Social Psychiatry*, **24**, 12–16.

7. Samuels, J.F., Nestadt, G., Romanoski, A.J., Folstein, M.F., and McHugh, P.R. (1994). DSM-III personality disorders in the community. *American Journal of Psychiatry*, **151**, 1055–62.

8. Zimmerman, M. and Coryell, W.H. (1990). Diagnosing personality disorder in the community. *Archives of General Psychiatry*, **47**, 527–31.

9. Baron, M. (1985). A family study of schizophrenic and normal control probands: implications for the spectrum concept of schizophrenia. *American Journal of Psychiatry*, **142**, 447–55.

10. Swartz, M., Blazer, D., George, L., and Winfield, I. (1990). Estimating the prevalence of borderline personality disorder in the community. *Journal of Personality Disorders*, **4**, 257–72.

11. Nestadt, G., Romanoski, A.J., Chahal, R., *et al.* (1990). An epidemiological study of histrionic personality disorder. *Psychological Medicine*, **20**, 413–22.

12. Nestadt, G., Romanoski, A.J., Brown, C.H., *et al.* (1991), DSM-III compulsive personality disorder: an epidemiological survey. *Psychological Medicine*, **21**, 461–71.

13. Barber, J.P., Frank, A., Weiss, R.D., *et al.* (1996). Prevalence and correlates of personality disorder diagnoses among cocaine dependent outpatients. *Journal of Personality Disorders*, **10**, 297–311.

14. Brooner, R.K., King, V.L., Kidorf, M., Schmidt, C.W., Jr, and Bigelow, G.E. (1997). Psychiatric and substance use comorbidity among treatment-seeking opioid abusers. *Archives of General Psychiatry*, **54**, 71–80.

15. Driessen, M., Veltrup, C., Wetterling, T., John, U., and Dilling, H. (1998). Axis I and axis II comorbidity in alcohol dependence and the two types of alcoholism. *Alcoholism Clinical and Experimental Research*, **22**, 77–86.

16. Marlowe, D.B., Husband, S.D., Bonieskie, L.M., Kirby, K.C., and Platt, J.J. (1997). Structured interview versus self-report test vantages for the assessment of personality pathology in cocaine dependence. *Journal of Personality Disorders*, **11**, 177–90.

17. Morgenstern, J., Langenbucher, J., Labouvie, E., and Miller, K.J. (1997). The comorbidity of alcoholism and personality disorders in a clinical population: prevalence rates and relation to alcohol typology variables. *Journal of Abnormal Psychology*, **106**, 74–84.

18. Nace, E.P., Davis, C.W., and Gaspari, J. (1991). Axis II comorbidity in substance abusers. *American Journal of Psychiatry*, **148**, 118–20.

19. Rousanville, B.J., Kranzler, H.R., Ball, S., Tennen, H., Poling, J., and Triffleman, E. (1998). Personality disorders in substance abusers: relation to substance use. *Journal of Nervous and Mental Disease*, **186**, 87–95.

20. Verheul, R., Hartgers, C., Van Den Brink, W., and Koeter, M.W.J. (1998). The effect of sampling, diagnostic criteria and assessment procedures on the observed prevalence of DSM-III-R personality disorders among treated alcoholics. *Journal of Studies on Alcohol*, **59**, 227–36.

21. Charney, D.S., Nelson, J.C., and Quinlan, D.M. (1981). Personality traits and disorder in depression. *American Journal of Psychiatry*, **138**, 1601–4.

22. Flick, S.N., Roy Byrne, P.P., Cowley, D.S., Shores, M.M., and Dunner, D.L. (1993). DSM-III-R personality disorders in a mood anxiety disorders clinic: prevalence, comorbidity, and clinical correlates. *Journal of Affective Disorders*, **27**, 71–9.

23. Garyfallos, G., Adamopoulou, A., Voikli, M., Saitis, M., Kirtsos, P., and Moutzoukis, C. (1994). DSM-III-R personality disorders among patients with depressive and/or anxiety disorders. *Journal of Personality Disorders*, **8**, 320–32.

24. Patience, D.A., McGuire, R.J., Scott, A.I.F., and Freeman, C.P.L. (1995). The Edinburgh primary care depression study: personality disorder and outcome. *British Journal of Psychiatry*, **167**, 324–30.

25. Pilkonis, P.A. and Frank, E. (1988). Personality pathology in recurrent depression: nature, prevalence, and relationship to treatment response. *American Journal of Psychiatry*, **145**, 435–41.

26. Shea, M.T., Pilkonis, P.A., Beckham, E., *et al.* (1990). Personality disorders and treatment outcome in the NIMH Treatment of Depression Collaborative Research Program. *American Journal of Psychiatry*, **147**, 711–17.

27. Spalletta, G., Troisi, A., Saracco, M., Ciani, N., and Pasini, A. (1996). Symptom profile, Axis II comorbidity and suicidal behaviour in young males with DSM-III-R depressive illnesses. *Journal of Affective Disorders*, **39**, 141–8.

28. Jansen, M.A., Arntz, A., Merckelbach, H., and Mersch, P.P.A. (1994). Personality disorders and features in social phobia and panic disorder. *Journal of Abnormal Psychology*, **103**, 391–5.

29. Reich, J.H., Perry, J.C., Shera, D., *et al.* (1994). Comparison of personality disorders in different anxiety disorder diagnoses: panic, agoraphobia, generalized anxiety, and social phobia. *Annals of Clinical Psychiatry*, **6**, 125–34.

30. Sanderson, W.C., Wetzler, S., Beck, A.T., and Betz, F. (1994). Prevalence of personality disorders among patients with anxiety disorders. *Psychiatry Research*, **51**, 167–74.

31. Skodol, A.E., Oldham, J.M., Hyler, S.E., *et al.* (1995). Patterns of anxiety and personality disorders comorbidity. *Journal of Psychiatric Research*, **29**, 361–74.

32. Tyrer, P., Casey, P., and Gall, J. (1983). Relationship between neurosis and personality disorder. *British Journal of Psychiatry*, **142**, 404–8.

33. Alnaes, R. and Torgersen, S. (1988). DSM-III symptom disorders (axis I) and personality disorders (Axis II) in an outpatient population. *Acta Psychiatrica Scandinavica*, **78**, 348–55.

34. Berger, J. (1985). Private practice: the first five years. *Canadian Journal of Psychiatry*, **30**, 566–71.

35. Cutting, J. (1986). Personality and psychosis: use of the standardized assessment of personality. *Acta Psychiatrica Scandinavica*, **73**, 87–92.

36. Grilo, C.M., Levy, K.N., Becker, D.F., Edell, W.S., and McGlashan, T.H. (1996). Comorbidity of DSM-III-R Axis I and II disorders among female inpatients with eating disorders. *Psychiatric Services*, **47**, 426–9.

37. Grilo, C.M., McGlashan, T.H., Quinlan, D.M., Walker, M.L., Greenfeld, D., and Edell, W.S. (1998). Frequency of personality disorders in two age cohorts of psychiatric inpatients. *American Journal of Psychiatry*, **155**, 140–2.

38. Jackson, H.J. (1991). Diagnosing personality disorders in psychiatric inpatients. *Acta Psychiatrica Scandinavica*, **83**, 206–13.

39. Mors, O. and Sorensen, L.V. (1994). Incidence and comorbidity of personality disorders among first ever admitted psychiatric patients. *European Psychiatry*, **9**, 175–84.

40. Oldham, J.M., Skodol, A.E., Kellman, H.D., *et al.* (1995). Comorbidity of Axis I and Axis II disorders. *American Journal of Psychiatry*, **152**, 571–8.

41. Pfhol, B. (1986). DSM-III personality disorders: diagnostic overlap and interconsistency of individual DSM-III criteria. *Comprehensive Psychiatry*, **27**, 21–34.

42. Pilgrim, J. and Mann, A. (1990). Use of the ICD-10 version of the Standardized Assessment of Personality to determine the prevalence of personality disorder in psychiatric in-patients. *Psychological Medicine*, **20**, 985–92.

43. Reich, J.H. (1987). Sex distribution of DSM-III personality disorders in psychiatric outpatients. *American Journal of Psychiatry*, **144**, 485–8.

44. Tyrer, P., Merson, S., Onyett, S., and Johnson, T. (1994). The effect of personality disorder on clinical outcome, social networks and

adjustment: a controlled clinical trial of psychiatric emergencies. *Psychological Medicine*, **24**, 731–40.

45. de Girolamo, G. and Reich, J.H. (1993). *Personality disorders*. WHO, Geneva.

46. Dolan, B., Evans, C., and Norton, K. (1995). Multiple Axis-II diagnoses of personality disorder. *British Journal of Psychiatry*, **66**, 107–12.

47. Skodol, A.E., Oldham, J.M., Hyler, S.E., Kellman, H.D., Doidge, N., and Davies, M. (1993). Comorbidity of DSM-III-R eating disorders and personality disorders. *International Journal of Eating Disorders*, **14**, 403–16.

48. Golding, M. and Perkins, D.O. (1996). Personality disorder in HIV infection. *International Review of Psychiatry*, **8**, 253–8.

49. Olfson, M. and Mechanic, D. (1996). Mental disorders in public, private nonprofit, and proprietary general hospitals. *American Journal of Psychiatry*, **153**, 1613–19.

50. Department of Health and Social Security (1985). *Mental illness hospitals and units in England. Results from the Mental Health Inquiry. Statistical bulletin*. HMSO, London.

51. Mors, O. (1988). Increasing incidence of borderline states in Denmark from 1970–1985. *Acta Psychiatrica Scandinavica*, **77**, 575–83.

52. Loranger, A.W. (1990). The impact of DSM-III on diagnostic practice in a university hospital. *Archives of General Psychiatry*, **47**, 672–5.

53. Brooke, D., Taylor, C., Gunn, J., and Maden, A. (1996). Point prevalence of mental disorder in unconvicted male prisoners in England and Wales. *British Medical Journal*, **313**, 1524–7.

54. Singleton, N., Meltzer, H., Gatward, R., Coid, J., and Deasy, D. (1998). *Psychiatric morbidity among prisoners in England and Wales*. Office of National Statistics, London.

55. Jordan, B.K., Schlenger, W.E., Fairbank, J.A., and Caddell, J.M. (1996). Prevalence of psychiatric disorders among incarcerated women. II. Convicted felons entering prison. *Archives of General Psychiatry*, **53**, 513–19.

4.12.6 Aetiopathogenesis of personality disorders (from genes to biodevelopmental processes)

Adolf Tobeña

The scaffolding of personality: a trait structure for normal and abnormal temperaments?

A productive science of personality has evolved in recent decades around two main postulates.

1. A small number of dimensions (factors) provide a basic framework for describing the rich variety of human personality. These factors are high-level traits, derived from models based on investigations characterized by careful consistent measures of individual variations in behaviour, feeling, and thinking.[1–4]

2. These general factors of temperament reflect the operation of particular brain systems that are probably multifaceted and multipurpose.[5–7]

This global outline of the structure of personality depends on the assumption that genetic and developmental dispositions combine with critical nurturing and social conditioning to form the tapestry of human uniqueness within temperamental clusters. (Throughout this chapter, the terms 'temperament' and 'personality' are used interchangeably because of the continuing debate on how to distinguish between them.) In other words, personality types are expressed through relatively clear-cut and stable traits that are accessible to objective measurement at behavioural, emotional, and cognitive levels. These depend, in turn, upon the specific and early organization of particular neurocognitive and neuroendocrine systems.

The first of the postulates mentioned above has received a good deal of support from most of the psychometric research assessing durable trends for individual personality profiles within and across particular cultures.[3,4] Currently, there is an increasing consensus that five 'superfactors' (broad traits) may capture the essential features of all traits used to describe normal personality. These superfactors are neuroticism, extraversion, agreeableness/friendliness, conscientiousness, and intellectual openness.

Despite some dissent regarding the exact nature and definition of these superfactors,[8,9] a five-dimensional structure is advocated by many researchers.[3,4,10] Based on the pioneering programme of research developed by Hans Eysenck at the Institute of Psychiatry, London, neuroticism and extraversion always appear in the dimensional 'menu' which some consider to be the basis of the modern science of personality. However, the remaining three superfactors—conscientiousness (reliability), friendliness (against aggressiveness/hostility), and intellectual curiosity (openness/creativity)—are obvious departures from the three-dimensional structure proposed by Eysenck that included only one more, very controversial, superfactor (psychoticism) to encompass the whole of 'personality space'. It seems improbable that these controversies can be resolved by using psychometric techniques alone.

Determination of the biological substrates for these personality dimensions was neglected by those researchers who preferred a purely psychometric/behavioural approach, although some early theories tried to root behavioural trait variations within biological concepts.[1] These attempts can be traced back as far as Pavlov, but for a long time they were either speculative or very rudimentary. Changes began when several models were produced which focused on certain brain systems and subsystems as possible sites for the factors and traits underlying normal and abnormal temperaments.[5,6,11,12] Currently, this particular area is growing steadily, and is the most exciting and fruitful field of personality research.

Progress made in various fields of basic neuroscience has made it possible to relate a variety of biological markers to the results of paper-and-pencil tests or cognitive-behavioural tests in normal temperaments. Biological screening has increasingly been applied to patients with personality disorders, using the clinical clusters defined in DSM-IV or ICD-10.[6,11] As well as these attempts to build consistent psychobiological profiles of normal and abnormal temperaments, an increasing convergence of other evidence has suggested that categorical and dimensional models for diagnosing personality disorders should be integrated.[13–15]

To give a broad overview of an area that may have enormous implications for understanding the aetiopathogenesis of personality disorders, we shall first discuss recent studies that have tried to find genetic evidence for personality traits that are both behaviourally consistent and biologically well established. Previous work using classical (familial or twin) methods found substantial heritability estimates for several personality traits.[16,17] The new data may support the view that some traits contribute to the basic structuring of personality via particular neuroendocrine systems. We shall also explore the possible origins of other basic traits within biodevelopmental processes mediating enduring neural and cognitive organization.

Because of the limitations of space, our approach is deliberately selective, citing supportive evidence rather than performing a systematic assessment of the field. For reasons of convenience and possible clinical relevance, we have selected some of the traits that demonstrate solid biological foundations, although they are not necessarily prominent in the progressively powerful and elegant dimensional solutions for normal and abnormal temperaments. In other words, the following discussion is centred on several primary factors instead of the constellation of superfactors.

A genetic marker for novelty/sensation-seeking behaviour?

In January 1996 two independent teams reported that a particular chromosomal 'locus' was associated with a well-established trait of human temperament—the hunger for novelty and excitement that lies behind impulsivity or sensation-seeking behaviour.[18–20] A polymorphism in the sequence of the gene expressing the D4 dopamine receptor (D4DR), located on the short arm of chromosome 11, explained 10 per cent of the genetic variance due to this trait. Individuals with the longer repeat allele at exon III of the *D4DR* gene scored higher in novelty-seeking behaviour (explorers, risk-seekers), whereas those with the shorter allele had lower scores (prudent, cautious). The first of these studies[19] investigated a heterogeneous sample of young Israelis, and showed the association to be independent of ethnicity (Ashkenazim versus Sephardim), sex, or age. The second study, carried out in the United States,[20] used a random sample of people who had initially been recruited in a search for chromosomal regions possibly associated with sexual orientation; this sample mainly comprised white men, although some ethnic minorities were also included. The personality questionnaires used in the two studies were also different: the Israelis were evaluated using Cloninger's Tridimensional Personality Questionnaire (**TPQ**),[21] which gives direct scores of novelty-seeking behaviour, whereas the American study used the Revised NEO Personality Inventory[22] which measures the five superfactors mentioned above, from which scores for novelty-seeking were derived. The results of the two studies were highly concordant. The American sample had the additional advantage of including intra- and extrafamilial comparisons as the sample contained many pairs of siblings.

Despite the small explanatory power of this reported association, the link between temperamental variability for one trait and a chromosomal polymorphism was the first evidence for a direct relationship between a putative 'genetic marker' and a core dimension of normal personality. In this case, the potential genetic marker appeared promising because of the amount of basic clinical research linking dopaminergic function with the regulation of stimulus-seeking, sensitivity to incentives, and impulse control behaviour. In theory, if similar degrees of explained variance were assignable to other sound gene markers, a substantial part of the heritability of the trait could be explained.

Subsequent studies in Finland,[23] Sweden,[24,25] and New Zealand[26] failed to replicate these early findings. However, the heterogeneity of the samples could explain the disparate results. Although further research is required, it may be useful to remember that previous work, mostly with twins, consistently established that novelty-seeking behaviour was moderately heritable (40 to 50 per cent). In any case, it is important to reiterate that such an association, if confirmed, only accounts for part of the genetic variance in a normal dimension of temperament.

Genetic markers for fearfulness/anxiety?

Shortly afterwards, the same American team[27] reported new data that suggested an association between the neuroticism trait and a chromosomal region linked to the serotonin neurotransmitter system, which is involved in modulating anxiety-related traits. The 5-hydroxytryptamine transporter protein (5-HTT) that promotes the reuptake of serotonin in cell membranes is encoded by a gene located in the q12 segment of chromosome 17. The particular region governing the transcriptional control of the protein shows a polymorphism that influences its expression and functioning. Individuals carrying the short variant of the polymorphism show a reduced efficiency of serotonin reuptake compared with those possessing the longer variant. The study measured several of these parameters in the lymphoblasts of two independent samples totalling more than 500 volunteers who had been recruited for different studies; it also included the subsample that had been used in the previous study of the relationship between the *D4DR* gene and the novelty-seeking behavioural trait.

Using two different personality questionnaires (NEO and Cattell's 16PF Personality Inventory) and estimated scores on various dimensions of Cloninger's TPQ, the evidence showed that subjects who carried the short variant in the 5-HTT gene polymorphism had higher neuroticism (NEO), anxiety (16PF), and harm-avoidance (TPQ) scores. The results were equally consistent across and within pedigrees. Comparison of the relatedness effects was made possible because the sample contained a substantial number of siblings.

Across the three personality measures, the 5-HTT polymorphism contributed a modest 3 to 4 per cent of the total variance and 7 to 9 per cent of the genetic variance in anxiety-related traits. However, such a modest association may have widespread implications if confirmed by further research. It was suggested that, if other genes contributed similar dosage effects to anxiety traits, approximately 10 to 15 genes might be involved in the heritability of neuroticism.

Furthermore, the implication of the serotonin transporter protein in the potential genetic predisposition towards anxiety/emotionality traits agrees with other data. Serotonergic neurotransmission is involved in several brain functions with little or no relationship with anxiety regulation, but there is a large body of evidence linking serotonergic brain function with the modulation of some adaptive responses to serious conflict and emotionally demanding situations.[5,7,11] Moreover, many drugs currently used to treat anxiety, depressive, and personality disorders depend on some kind of restoration of serotonergic function. Therefore, although the exact role of the brain serotonergic subsystems in the modulation of emotionality is far from established, it is rather improbable that the neurohormonal changes that participate in individual adaptations to serious emotional conflicts would not include serotonin. Such defensive adaptations require the participation of other central neuromodulators with equally, or even more, prominent roles than serotonin, the corticotrophin-releasing factor–ACTH regulatory cascade, γ-aminobutyric acid, neuropeptide Y, and substance P.[5,7,11,12] Further studies are required to determine whether this particular polymorphism in the 5-HTT gene contributes to the general tendency for individuals who score higher on neuroticism, in different personality tests, to be at higher risk for personality disorders (within anxiety/affective clusters).

In the case of the genetics of neuroticism there are other lines of evidence, mainly from animal research, that can be used to support the claim of a possible genetic basis for emotionality. This evidence is derived from studies of the psychogenetics of emotional susceptibility in animals, which is currently culminating in a search for chromosome loci. In many biological and behavioural tests, comparisons of several reactive and non-reactive strains of mice and rats have produced consistent results, and have narrowed the search for a possible genetic locus using different methods of chromosomal mapping. Thus, in recent work with progeny obtained by crossing two strains of mice selected for activity and defecation in an open-field test, three loci which explained most of the genetic variance in emotionality were found on chromosomes 1, 12, and 15 of the murine genome.[28]

These data have been confirmed both directly[29] and indirectly using another strategy that measured fear responses towards particular stimuli.[30–32] The same segment of chromosome 1 was again identified as a relevant 'locus' for emotional susceptibility in mice. Finally, several research programmes are under way to determine whether there is concordance in the chromosomal marking of emotionality in various strains of rats that differ in emotional susceptibility: the Maudsley reactive (**MR**) versus the Maudsley non-reactive (**MNR**) strains, and the Roman high-avoider (**RHA**) versus the Roman low-avoider (**RLA**) lines. These strains represent a particularly interesting assay because of the very large body of evidence showing their usefulness as animal models of 'temperamental' styles.[33–35]

Biodevelopmental basis for affiliative traits?

Affiliation (social attachment, friendliness, gregariousness, empathy, etc.) is another core trait that can be measured consistently in personality questionnaires. Poor or distorted affiliative behaviour is the most predictive marker for a reliable diagnosis of personality disorder.[11,13,36] Deficits or alterations in affiliative tendencies may show a variety of clinical manifestations: extreme aloofness and detachment, manipulative, non-empathic or exploitative attitudes, and even definite asocial or antisocial tendencies.

These behavioural styles appear, in different degrees and combinations, in several clinical categories of abnormal temperament. They could reflect alterations in the functioning of neuroendocrine systems specialized in mediating affective attachments, possibly including subsystems for social reward and social distress.[37] In this respect, an impressive amount of evidence has been gathered from the behavioural neurosciences (mostly in animals but recently in humans as

well) showing that prosocial behaviours, such as sexuality, maternal nurturing, friendliness/gregariousness, separation distress, social bonding, and group play, share some neurochemical controls. Central oxytocin and opioid systems are among the more relevant of these modulatory controls, because several types of attachments (mother–infant bonds, young peer bonds, pair-mating bonds, in-group tendencies, etc.) are dramatically altered when the functions of oxytocinergic or opioid systems in the brain are modified.[37,38] Other centrally acting neuropeptides, such as prolactin and vasopressin, may also contribute to particular types of species-specific social bonding. In addition, both the central regulatory monoaminergic systems and the corticotrophin–adrenal cascades that mediate stress adaptations help to organize responses to everyday social challenges.[37]

The application of these ideas to personality measurement is still in its infancy and requires the development of reliable biological markers. However, theory and research in the psychobiology of social attachments[12,39–42] has linked the impact of early rearing practices (secure/nurturing mothering versus peer rearing or isolation) with the future organization and functioning of several neuroendocrinological systems. This research has mainly explored the function of the central modulatory monoamines noradrenaline (norepinephrine), dopamine, and serotonin, and the hypophyseal–adrenal axis responses to social challenges. The evidence has shown that socially deprived monkeys differ physiologically, behaviourally, and cognitively from mother-reared infants in almost every aspect of what it means to be a social monkey; if the privation extends over the first 6 to 9 months of postnatal life, most effects persist into the adulthood. According to Kraemer:[41] 'The way in which socially deprived individuals orient to and respond physiologically to social stressors is altered and the kind of behavioural differences that seem to be the most important are those usually assigned to the domain of "temperament"'.

With the addition of the central neuropeptide systems that specifically modulate affiliative tendencies, the study of some crucial experiences during early infancy (and probably adolescence) may provide clues to the clarification of the role that developmental processes play in shaping attachment styles. Neural organization depends, to a great extent, on critical environmental inputs to produce enduring behavioural and cognitive adaptation in all domains. Therefore ontogenic factors must be particularly important in modelling social behaviour and in sustaining profiles of affiliative versus non-affiliative temperaments, in the same way as has already been demonstrated for other temperamental traits. For instance, in reactive/fearful monkeys, maternal and even grandparental rearing practices can significantly modify future neuroendocrine and behavioural adaptations.[42] More recently, parallel data have been obtained in rats.[43]

These findings do not exclude the participation of genetic dispositions in attachment styles. Some authors have suggested that the operation of 'communicative' or 'affiliative' genes could prime individual tendencies through different sorts of emotional affects.[44] However, it is important to remember that we are dealing with genetically based dispositions that can be environmentally malleable, although the complex interactions have still to be elucidated. There is a paucity of data on the putative genetic basis of attachment styles. When a molecular approach has been used in some rodent species to establish a genetic link (within the domain of the oxytocin receptor gene) with conspicuous social behaviour, such as monogamous pair-bonding, the results have been mainly inconclusive.[45] However, recent data for the vasopressin V1a receptor have yielded promising results.[46]

Biodevelopmental processes for aggressiveness?

Aggressiveness is another core personality trait that has a well-founded biodevelopmental basis. Current dimensional descriptions of the structure of personality do not always include aggressiveness as a high-level factor, but it is embedded in other traits such as impulsiveness, poor control, or even psychotic behaviour. However, aggressiveness is a major behavioural trait that has to be taken into account in the routine management of mental disorders, and it is also a prevalent characteristic in personality disorders (generally as an excess, but sometimes because of its absence). In the past, it was extremely difficult to prove that individual variations in aggressive behaviour might be correlated with neurohormonal characteristics. However, this was because of inadequate methods of quantifying biological and behavioural variations.[47]

In humans, the link between aggressive styles and familial/subcultural problems is very strong, and suggests that lower socio-economic status, increased rates of abuse, coercive family interactions, and neglect or other adversities contribute to violent behaviour from infancy to adolescence and into adulthood.[48] But this cannot obscure the effects of enduring biological dispositions that could, in part, result from the influence of socio-environmental insults to the developing brain. However, intensive research in behavioural neuroendocrinology and molecular neuroscience using animal models has shown that aggressive temperaments are associated with both genetic disposition and critical developmental processes, which affect the function of neuroregulatory controls that either promote or inhibit aggression.[49,50]

Therefore it is not surprising that an association between a specific gene and an aggressive disorder in humans has been reported.[51] The males of a Dutch family that carried a mutation of the gene for monoaminoxidase A (**MAO-A**) had a record of many severe aggressive incidents. An investigation in mice has shown that ablating the gene for MAO-A resulted in the 'knockout' mutants being much more aggressive.[52] MAO plays an important part in the breakdown of serotonin and other central monoamines, and previous research in humans had found consistent relationships between impulsive or 'poorly controlled' behavioural styles and low-MAO activity,[18] a feature also seen in sensation-seekers.[18,53]

Other genetically altered animals have been produced that are highly aggressive and typically show deficits in serotonin function. For example, mice deficient in α-calcium–calmodulin-dependent kinase II (α-**CaMKII**) show decreased fear responses and increased defensive aggression associated with low serotonin levels.[54] Moreover, knockout mice that do not express the serotonin 5-HT1B receptors are much quicker to attack intruders,[55] an action that can be blocked with targeted serotonergic drugs.

All this adds to the evidence obtained from mentally ill patients presenting aggressive outbursts and from chronic offenders in prisons, which shows an inverse relationship between serotonergic function and violent attacks directed towards others or themselves.[47,56] Taken together, the data appear to suggest that preserved brain serotonin function helps to attenuate aggressive impulses, probably by blocking other neuroregulatory systems that promote aggression such as androgens, insulin, vasopressin, and perhaps substance-P.[57,58]

Vasopressin is involved in the establishment of pair-bonds and ter-

Table 1 Summary of behavioural phenotypes in α-CaMKII mutant mice

Behavioural phenotype	Heterozygote	Homozygote
Fear-related responses	Decrease	Decrease
Offensive aggression	Normal	Decrease
Defensive aggression	Increase	Decrease
Pain sensitivity	Normal	Increase
Startle response	Normal	Increase
Vigilance	Normal	Increase
Mating	Decrease	Decrease
Maze learning	Normal	Decrease

Reproduced with permission from C. Chen et al. (1994). Abnormal fear response and aggressive behaviour in mice deficient for alpha–calcium–calmodulin–leinase II. Science, **266**, 291–4.

ritorial tendencies in mammals, and promotes aggressive behaviour when social/dominance challenges are perceived. There is evidence from adolescent and juvenile hamsters showing that proserotonergic interventions attenuate vasopressin-induced attacks.[48,57] More recently, a study of patients with personality disorders[59] has shown that cerebrospinal fluid levels of vasopressin were positively correlated with a life history of aggression, and with attacks against persons in particular. This was a more powerful relationship than the negative one usually obtained from measurements of serotonergic function and aggression.

A working scheme and other relevant traits

All the evidence seems consistent with previous research in animals, which has shown that Brattelboro rats (a genetically defective line lacking the vasopressin receptor gene) are less fearful, more aggressive, and less prone to forming strong infant–mother bonds,[37] and that in the two Roman rat lines selectively bred for differential fearfulness RHAs are more aggressive and more avid incentive-seekers then their RLA counterparts.[35] Thus temperamental styles in animals show differential clustering of behavioural traits, which correspond to specific (and complex) neurohormonal profiles. Sometimes a specific genetic modification is sufficient to promote a fully differentiated temperament, as in the case of the mice lacking α-CaMKII mentioned above[54] (Table 1).

It is possible that this may also hold for particular temperamental clusters in humans. However, we have already established that, when trying to explain the genetic contribution to basic ('universal') personality traits, a multigenic/interactional approach was necessary to explain just part of the measured variance in each trait. Nevertheless, this contribution can be very important, as most of the systematic research involving twins has yielded estimates of just over 40 per cent for the genetic input to typical personality traits, with modest estimations of around 7 per cent assignable to the so-called shared (familial/cultural) environment.[10,60]

Despite this, non-shared environmental influences (from the womb onwards) and genetic–environmental interactions make a well-known contribution to each individual temperament.[61,62] These complex influences may act first by modelling the development of basic neuroendocrine regulatory systems that cope with both natural and social challenges, and second by shaping the neurocognitive architecture that results in an autonomous and particular lifestyle. An interactional approach along these lines is now laying the foundation for a better description of the different factors that contribute to building the typical profiles of normal or abnormal personalities.

Such a general scheme must include other factors, in addition to the basic ones considered so far. For instance, the recent detection of a substantial genetic contribution to the baseline level of happiness,[63] which all individuals show throughout life independently of the events or episodes that they encounter, must be important for personality diagnoses, because such a 'calibration point' has a direct relationship with the affective tone of optimism or pessimism.[11,64]

Moreover, other traits and measures in the domain of cognitive performance (e.g. attention spans and oscillations, perceptual/appraisal reliability, typical thinking styles, and memory biases) or of character (e.g. religiosity/transcendence, conservatism, self-directness/self-esteem, and the drive to achieve/enthusiasm) should be incorporated into the whole description of personality structure. This is essential if the aim is to produce a general framework powerful enough to contain the complex categories that clinicians have tried to construct on the basis of systematic observation for more than a century. Cloninger[13,65,66] has advanced a proposal along these lines, which may function as an initial useful step to guide future work.

Conclusion: a complex approach to the aetiopathogenesis of personality disorders

Although the evidence discussed so far is only preliminary, it could have a major impact on the reconceptualizing of the approach that has been applied in psychiatry to the detection and categorization of the elusive profiles of normal and abnormal personalities.[7] It is clear that anchoring some temperamental traits to a strong genetic or biodevelopmental base will not provide a complete, or even improved, solution to the problems encountered in the aetiology and diagnosis of personality disorders. Many additional steps will have to be worked out and the task ahead is hard. But in view of the increasing links that are being established between core personality traits and some genetic/developmental mechanisms, the task of building a framework which would allow improved identification and differentiation of abnormal personalities no longer seems hopeless. In fact, such research is opening up many new avenues for understanding the effects of different factors (innate dispositions, neurodevelopmental organization, neurocognitive architecture, critical social transitions, and repeated stress episodes) on an individual's vulnerability to developing a personality disorder.

Hence, the use of behaviourally well-defined and biologically well-established personality dimensions must be the starting point for achieving the fine-tuned diagnoses increasingly required in modern medicine. Complexity in measurement will increase, but there is no other way of obtaining data that are sufficiently valid to allow understanding of the classical personality disorders. It is hoped that advances in the psychometric detection of the more salient 'clinical' profiles within each of the personality subspaces (at the level of either

traits or dimensions), together with a refinement of the neurocognitive and neurohormonal data, will produce much better solutions.

Some of the old-established and very consistent categories of personality disorders will be confirmed, but it is possible that unexpected 'types' of abnormal personalities, with clinical relevance, will emerge. In this new framework it may be easier to detect at an early stage those 'exceptional' and 'charismatic', although pathological, personalities who often impose great social costs and dramatic consequences not only for themselves but also for the group or the society in which they live.[67]

References

1. Eysenck, H.J. (1967). *The biological basis of personality.* Charles Thomas, London.
2. Eysenck, H.J. (1995). *Genius: the natural history of creativity.* Cambridge University Press, New York.
3. Goldberg, L.R. (1993). The structure of phenotypic personality traits. *American Psychologist*, **48**, 26–34.
4. McRae, R.R. and Costa, P.T. (1997). Personality trait structure as a human universal. *American Psychologist*, **52**, 509–16.
5. Gray, J.A. (1997). *The psychology of fear and stress.* Cambridge University Press, New York.
6. Cloninger, C.R. (1987). A systematic method for clinical description and classification of personality variants. *Archives of General Psychiatry*, **44**, 573–88.
7. Kandel, E.R. (1998). A new intellectual framework for psychiatry. *American Journal of Psychiatry*, **155**, 457–69.
8. Block, J. (1995). A contrarian view of the five-factor approach to personality description. *Psychological Bulletin*, **117**, 187–215.
9. McKenzie, J. (1998). Fundamental flaws in the five-factor model: a reanalysis of the seminal correlation matrix from which the 'openness to experience' factor was extracted. *Personality and Individual Differences*, **24**, 475–80.
10. Bouchard, T.J. (1994). Genes, environment and personality. *Science*, **262**, 1700–1.
11. Siever, L.J. and Davis, K.L. (1991). A psychobiological perspective on the personality disorders. *American Journal of Psychiatry*, **148**, 1647–58.
12. Kagan, J. (1994). *Galen's prophecy: temperament in human nature.* Harper and Collins, London.
13. Cloninger, C.R., Svrakic, D.M., and Przybeck, T.R (1993). A psychobiological model of temperament and character. *Archives of General Psychiatry*, **50**, 975–90.
14. Blackburn, R. and Coid, J.W. (1998). Psychopathy and the dimensions of personality disorders in violent offenders. *Personality and Individual Differences*, **25**, 129–45.
15. Widiger, T.A. and Frances, A.J. (1994). Towards a dimensional model for personality disorders. In *Personality disorders and the five-factor model of personality* (ed. P.T. Costa and T.A. Widiger). American Psychological Association Press, Washington, DC.
16. Tellegen, A., Lykken, D.T., Bouchard, T.J., Wicox, K.J., Segal, N.I., and Rich, S. (1988). Personality similarity in twins reared apart and together. *Journal of Personality and Social Psychology*, **54**, 1031–9.
17. Plomin, R., Owen, M.J., and McGuffin, P. (1994). The genetic basis of complex human behaviors. *Science*, **264**, 1733–9.
18. Zuckerman, M. (1994). Behavioral expressions and biosocial bases of sensation seeking. Cambridge University Press.
19. Ebstein, E.P., Novick, O., Umansky, R. *et al.* (1996). Dopamine D4 receptor (D4DR) exon III polymorphism associated with the human personality trait of novelty seeking. *Nature Genetics*, **12**, 78–80.
20. Benjamin, J., Li, L., Greenberg, B.D., Murphy, D.L., and Hamer, D.H. (1996). Population and familial association between the D4 dopamine receptor gene and measures of novelty seeking. *Nature Genetics*, **12**, 81–4.

21. Cloninger, C.R., Przybeck, T.R., and Svrakic, D.M. (1991). The Tridimensional Personality Questionnaire: US normative data. *Psychological Reports*, **69**, 1047–57.

22. Costa, P.T. and McCrae, R.R. (1992). *Revised NEO Personality Inventory and NEO Five Inventory*. Psychological Assessment Resources, Odessa, FL.

23. Malhotra, A.K., Virkkunen, M., Rooney, W., Egger, M., Linnoila, M., and Goldman, D. (1996). The association between the dopamine D4 receptor (DRD4) 16 aminoacid repeat polymorphism and novelty seeking. *Molecular Psychiatry*, **1**, 388–91.

24. Jönson, E.G., Nöthen, M.M., Gustavsson, J.P., *et al.* (1997). Lack of evidence for allelic association between personality traits and the dopamine D4 receptor gene polymorphism. *American Journal of Psychiatry*, **154**, 697–9.

25. Jönson, E.B., Nöthen, N.M., Gustavsson, J.P., *et al.*(1998). Lack of association between dopamine D4 receptor gene and personality traits. *Psychological Medicine*, **28**, 985–9.

26. Sullivan, P.F., Fifield, W.J., Kennedy, M.A., Mulder, R.T., Sellman, J.D., and Joyce, P. (1998). No association between novelty seeking and the type 4 dopamine receptor gene (DRD4) in two New Zealand samples. *American Journal of Psychiatry*, **155**, 98–101.

27. Lesch, K.P., Bengel, D., Heils, A., *et al.* (1996). Association of anxiety related traits with a polymorphism in the serotonin transporter gene regulatory region. *Science*, **274**, 1527–31.

28. Flint, J., Carley, R., DeFries, J.C., *et al.* (1995). A simple genetic basis for a complex psychological trait in laboratory mice. *Science*, **268**, 1432–5.

29. Gershenfield, H.K., Neumann, P.E., Mathis, C., Crawley, J.N., Xiaouhua, L., and Paul, S.M. (1997). Mapping quantitative trait loci for open field behavior in mice. *Behavior Genetics*, **27**, 201–10.

30. Flint, J. (1997). Freeze. *Nature Genetics*, **17**, 250–1.

31. Caldarone, B., Saavedra, B., Tartaglia, K., Wehner, J.M., Dudek, B.C., and Flaherty, L. (1997). Quantitative trait loci analysis affecting contextual conditioning in mice. *Nature Genetics*, **17**, 335–7.

32. Wehner, J.M., Radcliffe, R.A., Rosmann, S.T., *et al.* (1997). Quantitative trait locus analysis of contextual fear conditioning in mice. *Nature Genetics*, **17**, 331–4.

33. Whatley, S.A., Perret, C.W., Zamani, R., and Gray, J.A. (1992). Analysis of relative mRNA levels and protein patterns in brains of rat stems bred for differing levels of emotionality. *Behavior Genetics*, **22**, 403–13.

34. Fernández Teruel, A., Escorihuela, R.M., Castellano, B., González, B., and Tobeña, A. (1997). Neonatal handling and environmental enrichment effects on emotionality, novelty/reward seeking and age-related cognitive and hippocampal impairments: focus on the Roman rats. *Behavior Genetics*, **27**, 513–26.

35. Driscoll, P., Escorihuela, R.M., Fernández-Teruel, A. *et al.* (1998). Genetic selection and differential stress responses: the Roman lines/strains of rats. *Annals of the New York Academy of Sciences*, **851**, 521–30.

36. Livesley, W.J. (1987). A systematic approach to the delineation of personality disorders. *American Journal of Psychiatry*, **144**, 772–7.

37. Panksepp, J., Nelson, E., and Bekkedal, M. (1997). Brain systems for the mediation of social-separation distress and social reward: evolutionary antecedents and neuropeptide intermediaries. *Annals of the New York Academy of Sciences*, **807**, 78–100.

38. Pedersen, C.A., Caldwell, J.D., Jirikowski, G.F., and Insel, T.R (ed.) (1992). Oxytocin in maternal, sexual and social behaviors. *Annals of the New York Academy of Sciences*, **652**.

39. Bowlby, J. (1988). *A secure base*. Basic Books, New York.

40. Kagan, J. and Snidman, N. (1991). Temperamental factors in human development. *American Psychologist*, **46**, 856–62.

41. Kraemer, G.W. (1997). Psychobiology of early social attachment in rhesus monkeys. In *The integrative neurobiology of affiliation* (ed. C.S. Carter, I.I. Lederhendler, and B. Kirpatrick). *Annals of the New York Academy of Sciences*, **807**, 401–18.

42. Suomi, S.J. (1991). Uptight and laid-back monkeys: individual differences in the response to social challenges. In *Plasticity and development* (ed. S.E. Brauth, W.S. Hall, and R.J. Dooling), pp. 27–56. MIT Press, Cambridge, MA.

43. Liu, D., Diorio, J., Tannenbaum, B., *et al.* (1997). Maternal care, hippocampal glucocorticoid receptors and hypothalamic–pituitary–adrenal responses to stress. *Science*, **277**, 1659–62.

44. Buck, R. and Ginsburgh, B. (1997). Communicative genes and the evolution of empathy: selfish and social emotions as voices of selfish and social genes. *Annals of the New York Academy of Sciences*, **807**, 481–3.

45. Insel, T.R., Young, L., and Wang, Z. (1997). Molecular aspects of monogamy. *Annals of the New York Academy of Sciences*, **807**, 302–16

46. Young, L.J., Wilson, R., Maguire, K.G., MacGregor, G.R., and Jusel, T.R. (1999). Increased affiliative response to vasopressin in mice expressing the V1a receptor from a monogamous vole. *Nature*, **400**, 766–8.

47. Volavka, I. (1995). *Neurobiology of violence*. American Psychiatric Association Press, Washington, DC.

48. Ferris, C.F. and Grisso, T. (ed.) (1996). Understanding aggressive behavior in children. *Annals of the New York Academy of Sciences*, **794**.

49. Gartner, J. and Whitaker-Azmitia, P.M. (1996). Developmental factors influencing aggression: animal models and clinical correlates. *Annals of the New York Academy of Sciences*, **794**, 113–20.

50. De Kloet, E.R., Korte, S.M., Rots, N.Y., and Kruk, M.R. (1996). Stress hormones, genotype and brain organization: implications for aggression. *Annals of the New York Academy of Sciences*, **794**, 179–91.

51. Brunner, H.G., Nelen, M., Breakefiled, X.O., Ropers, H.H., and Van Oost, B.A. (1994). Abnormal behavior associated with a point mutation in the structural gene for monoamine oxidase A. *Science*, **262**, 578–80.

52. Cases, O., Seif, I., Gromsby, J., *et al.* (1995). Aggressive behavior and altered amounts of brain serotonin and noradrenaline in mice lacking MAO-A. *Science*, **268**, 1763–6.

53. Arqué, J.M., Unzeta, M., and Torrubia, R. (1988). Neurotransmitter systems and personality measurements: a study in psychosomatic patients and healthy subjects. *Neuropsychobiology*, **19**, 149–57.

54. Chen, C., Rainnie, D.G., Greene, R.W., and Tonegawa, S. (1994). Abnormal fear response and aggressive behavior in mice deficient for alpha-calcium–calmodulin-kinase II. *Science*, **266**, 291–4.

55. Saudou, F., Amarada, G., Dierich, A., *et al.* (1994). Enhanced aggressive behavior in mice lacking 5-HT1b receptor. *Science*, **265**, 1875–8.

56. Coccaro, E.F., Kavoussi, R.J., Trestman, R.L., Gabriel, S.M., Cooper, T.G., and Siever, L.J. (1997). Serotonin function in human subjects: intercorrelation among central 5-HT indices and aggressiveness. *Psychiatry Research*, **73**, 1–14.

57. Ferris, C.F., Meloni, R.H., Koopel, G., Perry, K.W., Fuller, R.W., and Delville, Y. (1997). Vasopressin/serotonin interactions in the anterior hypothalamus control aggressive behavior in golden hamsters. *Journal of Neuroscience*, **17**, 4331–40.

58. De Felipe, C., Herrero, J.F., O'Brien, J.A., *et al.* (1998). Altered nociception, analgesia and aggression in mice lacking the receptor for substance P. *Nature*, **392**, 394–7.

59. Coccaro, E.F., Kavoussi, R.J., Hauger, R.L., Cooper, T.B., and Ferris, C.F. (1998). Cerebrospinal fluid vasopressin levels: correlates with aggression and serotonin function in personality-disordered patients. *Archives of General Psychiatry*, **55**, 708–14.

60. Loehlin, J.C. (1992). *Genes and environment in personality development*. Sage, Newbury Park, CA.

61. Sokol, D.K., Moore, C.A., Rose, R.J., Williams, C.J., Reed, T., and Christian, C. (1995). Intrapair differences in personality and cognitive ability among young monozygotic twins distinguished by chorion type. *Behavior Genetics*, **25**, 457–66.

62. McGue, M. and Bouchard, T.J. (1998). Genetic and environmental influences on human behavioral differences. *Annual Review of Neuroscience*, **21**, 1–24.

63. Lykken, D.T. and Tellegen, A. (1996). Happiness is a stochastic phenomenon. *Psychological Science*, **7**, 186–9.

64. Torrubia, R., Avila, C., Moltó, J., and Grande, I. (1995). Testing for stress and happiness: the role of the behavioral inhibition system. In *Stress and emotion: anxiety, anger and curiosity*, Vol. 15 (ed. A.C.D.

Spielberger, I.G. Sarason, J. Brebner, E. Greenglass, P. Langani, and A.M. O'Roark), pp. 189–211. Taylor and Francis, Washington, DC.

65. Cloninger, C.R., Adolfsson, R., and Svrakic, N.M. (1996). Mapping genes for human personality. *Nature Genetics*, **12**, 3–4.

66. Svrakic, D.M., Whitehead, C., Przybeck, T.R., and Cloninger, R. (1993). Differential diagnoses of personality disorders by the seven factor model of personality disorders. *Archives of General Psychiatry*, **50**, 991–9.

67. Henry, D., Geary, D., and Tyrer, P. (1993). Adolf Hitler: a re-assessment of his personality status. *Irish Journal of Psychological Medicine*, **10**, 148–51.

4.12.7 Management of personality disorder

Peter Tyrer and Kate Davidson

Introduction

This is a difficult subject, in both clinical and research terms, and at the outset it is important to identify the main difficulties in determining best practice for this group of conditions. The following account supplements the sections on treatment that form part of the descriptions of specific types of personality disorders in Chapter 4.12.3 and expresses rather different views.

Categorization and description of personality disorder

The classification of personality disorder has been developed in relative isolation from investigations of management. The consequence is a sad example of clinical inutility; the standard descriptions of ICD-10 and DSM-IV appear to have face validity but are shown to be extremely limited when discussing specific treatments. Thus a specific question 'What are the different management strategies for dependent and histrionic personality disorder?' is met with a deafening silence from all those who wish to quote from evidence-based practice rather than making *ex cathedra* statements. A large part of the problem of deciding on the treatment of individual personality disorders follows from the degree of overlap between the various personality disorders and other mental state disorders. This is discussed below in the section on comorbidity, but covers a much greater area than the presence of several disabilities at a single point in time.

Methodological difficulties in evaluating the efficacy of treatment

The requirements for establishing whether a treatment is effective for personality disorders are than exacting than for mental state disorders. These can usefully be described under four headings:

- duration of treatment
- comorbidity
- adherence to treatment
- outcome measures.

Duration of treatment

For most mental state disorders it is relatively easy to choose the period over which efficacy has to be demonstrated. For conditions that develop suddenly (e.g. panic), treatment trials could be for a very short time indeed. For others, particularly when maintenance treatment is being evaluated, at least 6 months may be necessary to establish continued efficacy. In the case of personality disorders, which by definition have a prolonged course, at least 2 years is desirable before one can judge the efficacy of a treatment. To our knowledge no studies have used this length of follow-up in their judgement of efficacy. Such a requirement is not a purist position; if a treatment for personality disorder appears to be effective over a shorter period, this may be due to change in a concurrent (comorbid) condition. In addition, for a treatment is to be judged efficacious in personality disorder its effects should be lasting.

Comorbidity

Comorbidity has been defined as 'the presence of any distinct clinical entity that has existed or that may occur during the clinical course of a patient who has the index disease under study'.[1] The key word here is 'distinct'. True comorbidity implies the presence of two completely separate disorders in the same person which are not causally related to each other in any way. Co-occurrence ranges from true comorbidity to the presence of the same disorder in two or more different forms.[2]

Comorbidity is the norm for most personality disorders both with other personality disorders or with mental state disorders. Borderline personality disorder is a major offender in this regard. Only about one in 20 of such disorders constitutes the pure condition,[3] and multiple comorbidity with four or more disorders is more common.

In deciding on the efficacy of any treatment for personality disorder it is impossible to be certain whether observed improvement is in the personality disorder or in a comorbid condition. As personality disorders are generally more persistent than mental state disorders, it is reasonable to suppose that improvement is more likely to be due to a change in comorbid condition than a change in the personality disorder. This problem is made worse because personality assessment is often confounded, or 'contaminated', by the effect of a concurrent mental state disorder. Thus personality status apparently changes during the presence of a mental state disorder such as depression, only to return to the baseline normal subsequently.[4,5] Apparent improvement in a personality disorder following a treatment may be entirely due to improvement in a concurrent mental state disorder.

In view of these problems, a treatment for a personality disorder should ideally be tested in patents who have that personality disorder only. As these patients are uncommon and atypical, it is difficult to interpret the data from clinical trials.

Adherence to treatment

People with personality disorders do not usually form good relationships with therapists. Although this is in keeping with their problems with relationships elsewhere, it can be a major problem in any form of therapy. The problem is particularly marked with psychotherapy, in which long-held views are challenged by the therapist. The consequence is that many patients drop out of care, and sometimes no amount of therapeutic skill can maintain them in care.[6] In long-term follow-up studies continued contact with the patient is almost a therapeutic achievement in itself.[7]

Any study of personality disorder is likely to have a large proportion of drop-outs and this complicates the interpretation of the effects of treatment. The exception is when patients are treated in restricted settings such as prisons and other closed facilities,[8] but as these circumstances are abnormal it is difficult to generalize from them.

Therefore treatments that aid adherence to an appropriate intervention are likely to be of value in personality disorder. The evidence suggests that cognitive and behavioural approaches, particularly those that work in a collaborative way, are helpful in this regard as both primary and adjunctive therapies.[9–12]

Outcome measures

The choice of outcome measures is a problem in the assessment of all psychiatric disorders, but difficulty is particularly great in studies of personality disorders. These disorders affect both the individual and society, and a range of outcomes can be measured to cover these possibilities. Forensic psychiatrists and the general public usually consider that the outcome of mentally disordered offenders is best measured by the frequency of reoffending. This is an easily measured and reliable statistic, but it does not necessarily record symptomatic or personality change, and may be distorted by a range of other factors (e.g. patients who spend a long time in hospital or prison are not likely to reoffend). Changes in symptoms also have limited use since they may be a consequence of changes in mental state disorders quite independent of personality. Repeated measures of personality status also have disadvantages since, as noted earlier, they may be affected by changes with concurrent mental state disorder. Personality also changes with ageing without treatment.[13]

Because of these difficulties, global outcome measures are often used to determine the degree of improvement in personality disorders in long-term follow-up studies, although a battery of measurements is normally used in short-term treatment studies. Unfortunately, there is no standardized set of measures of global outcome. It is reasonable to take into account symptomatic change, social functioning, quality of life, incidents of societal conflict (e.g. police contacts), and reports from informants. Even these may not correctly reflect change in personality status. Thus a person whose personality disorder does not change in any basic way may find an environmental niche in which the personality disturbance does not manifest itself as conflict. Such a person would show improvement on all the items listed above, but the improvement would be a consequence of environmental change, not of personality alteration.

Minimum requirements for establishment of efficacy

The evidence base for effectiveness of treatment in personality disorders is also exacting.[14] The requirements are as follows.

1. The treatment should be effective when used in the pure form of the personality disorder (in an explanatory trial) and subsequently in other forms of the disorder in which comorbidity is more common (pragmatic trial).

2. Efficacy cannot be established satisfactorily unless the treatment is tested in a randomized controlled trial.

3. A suitable control treatment or management needs to be tested against the experimental treatment.

4. Efficacy should only be determined after a period of at least 6 months because of the long duration of personality disorder.

Because of the difficulties of meeting these requirements there has been a tendency for investigators to abandon them.

Dynamic psychotherapy

Since the time of Freud and Jung, the treatment of personality disorders has been regarded as a fundamental component of therapy. However, from classical descriptions it is clear that psychoanalysts were mainly treating neurotic disorder with associated personality pathology (from the cluster C group) when ostensibly treating personality disorder. No evidence of efficacy of treatment of personality disorder *per se* has been claimed for this approach until recently, and even now the view of Andrews[15] that dynamic psychotherapy 'has not been demonstrated to be superior to placebo in the treatment of the neuroses and personality disorders' is probably the consensus.

However, there has been considerable interest in the dynamic psychotherapy of borderline personality disorder in the last 20 years. As discussed in Chapter 4.12.3, borderline personality disorder is not typical of other personality disorders and patients often seek treatment for it repeatedly. Because it is associated with intense anger and emotion, the normal processes of psychoanalysis, involving interpretation, transference, and countertransference, are not considered suitable for this group and more subtle approaches are needed.[6,16]

Kernberg and his colleagues at the Menninger Clinic[17,18] developed an approach which was neither supportive nor openly confrontational, but which aimed to tackle patients' core psychopathology which is inchoate and confused and is quickly converted to aggression. This approach—expressive psychotherapy—has been extended further by Masterson[19] as confrontative psychotherapy which anticipates the difficulties often found when therapy ceases. Kohut[20] adopts an approach that identifies the inner functioning of borderline and narcissistic personalities and how they have developed in response to trauma in childhood and adolescence. None of these approaches has been formally evaluated with a control group.

The only formal evaluation of two forms of dynamic psychotherapy, short-term dynamic psychotherapy and brief adaptational psychotherapy, was carried out by Winston *et al.*[21] but specifically excluded patients with borderline and narcissistic pathology. The results essentially showed no differences between treatments, but they were both better than a waiting-list control group which suggests that these approaches have some value. Group psychotherapies using similar approaches are being evaluated at the Cassel Hospital in the United Kingdom at present.

Cognitive therapies

Cognitive–analytical therapy

Cognitive–analytical therapy combines cognitive and analytical approaches and has been applied to the treatment of personality disorders, particularly the borderline group.[22] The clinical manifestations of this condition are postulated to be a set of partially dissociated 'self-states' which account for the clinical features of this disorder. Such patients typically describe rapid switching from one state of mind to another, experiencing intense uncontrollable emotions or alternatively feeling muddled or emotionally cut off. Such 'dissociative states' (different from the conditions of similar name formerly linked to hysteria) are said to be activated by severe external threats and to be maintained by repetitions of threat and reinforcement by memories or situations which are similar to the original source of threat.

Cognitive–analytical therapy is concerned with the identification of these different self-states and helping patients to identify 'reciprocal role procedures', or patterns of relationships which are learned in early childhood and are relatively resistant to change.[22] The patient is taught to observe and try to change damaging patterns of thinking and behaviour which relate to these self-states and to become more self-aware. The therapist's role is to gather information about the patient's experience of relationships and the different states he or she experiences, including interpretation where necessary.

Cognitive therapy

Cognitive therapy has expanded dramatically from its original use in the treatment of depression to a wide range of other conditions, including personality disorder. Its application to personality disorder is not surprising. Although there are important differences between cognitive therapy in Axis I and Axis II disorders, there are probably more common features. In both groups of conditions cognitive therapy is a goal-directed problem-solving therapy that focuses on teaching specific cognitive and behavioural skills to improve present function and may also be helpful in preventing relapse. The therapeutic focus is to define the patient's presenting problems, to set goals, and to modify dysfunctional thinking and associated behaviours which prevent adaptive functioning. The clinician teaches the patient to identify and modify dysfunctional thoughts and beliefs through the use of specific cognitive techniques such as Socratic questioning.

Several differences in cognitive and related therapies for mental state disorders and for personality disorders have been emphasized.[9,23–25] One of these differences is on the emphasis and attention paid to the therapeutic relationship. In cognitive therapy for personality disorder, more emphasis is placed on establishing and maintaining a therapeutic alliance, as interpersonal difficulties which occur in the patient's life outside therapy are also likely to arise within therapy. This is based on the hypothesis that the patient's maladaptive beliefs are consistent across a wide range of settings and therefore are also likely to be manifest in therapeutic relationships.

One of the goals of cognitive therapy with personality-disordered patients is to take advantage of these interpersonal difficulties in treatment by identifying and modifying the beliefs underlying them and, by extension, other relationships. Patients are encouraged to test out their beliefs and assumptions about others by using the therapeutic relationship as a 'relationship laboratory', and are helped to learn new and more adaptive strategies for relating to others. In comparison with the treatment of Axis I disorders, cognitive therapy with personality-disordered individuals usually takes more sessions and spans a longer time because the problems are pervasive and long-standing.

Although people with personality disorders can recognize difficulties, they experience the problems as egosyntonic[26] (i.e. accepted as normal because they are an intrinsic part of usual functioning). As a result, alternative and potentially more adaptive beliefs about the self, others, and the world need to be identified and evaluated to see if they are indeed more adaptive and embraced as a consequence. These alternative more adaptive beliefs require to be systematically reviewed and reinforced, and new behaviours and ways of relating to others need to be practised repeatedly if changes are to be consolidated.[10] To achieve these changes, the therapist usually has to adopt a more directive approach than in cognitive therapy for depression and other Axis I disorders, and throughout will be more concerned with identifying and overcoming cognitive, emotional, and behavioural avoidance which maintains core beliefs. Many of the maladaptive patterns of behaviour and beliefs are likely to have their origin in childhood experience, and therefore cognitive therapy for personality disorders is more concerned with historical data than is cognitive therapy for Axis I disorders. Young[27] has emphasized the importance of establishing the core beliefs or schemas that can be traced through recalling memories that contribute to these beliefs, and thereby to the expression of personality.

A major problem with all forms of psychotherapy for personality disorders is the high level of drop-out from treatment. In cognitive therapy care has to be taken not to alienate the patient by aggressive introduction of new belief structures. By gentle introduction of ways of encouraging patients to challenge their maladaptive core beliefs, it is possible to deflect criticism that the therapist wishes to introduce a 'model system' of beliefs that may not be congruent with the patient's own perceptions. Patients are requested to keep log books to record new ways of behaving as they attempt to change their 'schema-driven' behaviours, and to keep records of evidence which support more adaptive beliefs about themselves and others. Although most of the techniques designed to change beliefs are focused on present-day function, historical and developmental perspectives may be incorporated as explained above. Restructuring of the meaning of earlier memories by methods such as psychodrama[28] have been found to be useful in that the emotional impact of the schema can be evoked. This may facilitate changes in, or reassessment of, the core belief. Although there are some differences in the cognitive therapeutic approach for personality disorders and for mental state disorders, there are also many common features. In particular, the collaborative empirical approach involving the patient's views at all stages is an important common element.

The models of treatment for personality disorder proposed by Beck and Freeman[23] and by Linehan[11] have in common an attempt to integrate biological and psychosocial factors. All models of treatment recognize the importance of building a secure therapeutic relationship, but transference and countertransference issues in therapy are not given specific focus in cognitive treatment strategies, except in Ryle's cognitive analytical therapy.[29] Cognitive therapists have yet to develop a cognitive model of these reactions which may interfere with the aim of developing a collaborative working relationship.

Cognitive therapy for personality disorder is still at an experimental phase of development. Although the patient's overt problems are the initial focus of treatment, the therapist utilizes hypotheses about the underlying mechanisms that create these problems in order to aid understanding.[30] This formulation allows therapy to proceed with a coherent strategy rather than following a piecemeal approach to symptoms and problems. The development of cognitive models of personality disorder helps to guide the therapist in understanding this group of often diverse patients and provides a framework in which to formulate problems and intervene.

Dialectic behaviour therapy

Most of the reported work with cognitive therapy in personality disorder has been open and uncontrolled,[10,24] and there have been no controlled studies apart from those of Marsha Linehan, notably a study carried out in the late 1980s in which a special form of cognitive behaviour therapy— dialectical behaviour therapy—was compared with the usual treatment in a group of repeatedly parasuicidal female patients with borderline personality disorder.[31] However, the main treatment outcome chosen was not resolution of the personality disorder but reduction in the frequency of self-harm episodes. The hypothesis that dialectical behaviour therapy was effective in reducing self-harm was supported.

This treatment has been used systematically only in the treatment of borderline personality disorder. According to Linehan,[11] borderline personality disorder is primarily a dysfunction of emotional regulation which is assumed to have resulted from biological irregularities combined with certain dysfunctional environments. Others in contact with the patient are postulated as reinforcing this dysfunction by discounting or, in Linehan's preferred term, 'invalidating' their emotional experiences. Borderline patients are emotionally vulnerable and have difficulty in regulating patterns of responses associated with emotional states. The maladaptive behaviours which form part of the borderline syndrome can be viewed as either the product of emotional dysregulation or as attempts by the individual at regulating intense emotional states by maladaptive problem-solving strategies. Dialectical behaviour therapy, as its name suggests, contains within it the notion of opposites; common themes that emerge in therapy with borderline patients, such as acceptance of things as they are (so that there is no need for suicidal action), and change (from former maladaptive types of response) may appear incompatible but are synthesized in the therapy.

The essentials of dialectical behaviour therapy[11] are manualized weekly individual psychotherapy, group psychoeducational behavioural skills training, and telephone consultation when considered necessary. Therefore the content comprises a variety of problem-solving techniques including teaching the patient skills to help regulate emotions and tolerate distress, methods for validating the patient's perceptions, and behavioural and psychological versions of meditation skills. Therapists are also trained in case management. Linehan[11] also describes 'core mindfulness skills' which are aimed at teaching the patient to observe, describe, and take part in events and responses to events without separating him- or herself or dissociating from what is happening. The treatment encourages patients to take a non-judgemental approach to events and interactions and to do what is effective in situations rather than what they may feel is the 'right' thing to do.

The results of this intensive programme are impressive in the short term, with a dramatic reduction in self-harming behaviour in the first few months of treatment, but are less satisfactory in the longer term.[32] This inability to maintain initial improvement suggests that the treatment is more focused on reducing a single behavioural outcome (parasuicide) rather than altering personality status *per se*. There are considerable difficulties in extrapolating from this work with a highly selected group to personality disorders in general. Borderline personality disorder is very different from other disorders in the group, with egodystonic rather than egosyntonic features (i.e. the patient is distressed by symptoms and behaviour and wants to have them removed), and has a different natural history with a high rate of spontaneous resolution. Many of the features of borderline personality disorder are seen in other personality disorders and its status as a separate homogeneous disorder has long been disputed.[33]

Some of the features of dialectical behaviour therapy (e.g. group behavioural skills training) are used in other psychological treatments (milieu therapy, therapeutic communities) but it is difficult to see how the treatment could be extended to involve those with personality disorders who are generally non-compliant with any form of treatment. The treatment has been extended to those with substance misuse[12] but not to other personality disorders beyond borderline and, to a lesser extent, the antisocial group.

However, the general principles of dialectical behaviour therapy can be used in a much less labour-intensive way. In a recent randomized controlled trial a manualized brief cognitive treatment for patients with personality disturbance within the flamboyant cluster (dissocial, histrionic, borderline, impulsive) was tested in those with a history of repeated self-harm.[34] Patients were randomly assigned to treatment as usual or manualized cognitive therapy. In contrast with Linehan's treatment,[31] the patients treated received only brief therapy from a six-chapter treatment manual and between two and six sessions of treatment. The manual contained information and examples of problem solving and cognitive strategies aimed at reducing problems, emotional disturbance, and the risk of further self-harm. The results of this study demonstrated the feasibility of a brief manualized cognitive treatment in parasuicidal patients in that there was a trend in favour of the cognitive treatment reducing the rate of self-harm and a significant reduction in levels of depressive symptoms over the 6-month follow-up. However, because of the small numbers in the study ($n = 34$), few definitive conclusions could be drawn.

Therapeutic community treatments

The term 'institutionalization' is relatively recent [35] but the damaging effects of mental hospitals on patients has been recognized for much longer, at least since the early years of this century.[36] In the period after the Second World War, hospitals were organized in a less hierarchical and dehumanized way to avoid or reverse these adverse effects.

There has been some confusion regarding the term 'therapeutic community'. In the formal usage the term describes an intensive form of treatment in which every aspect of the environment is part of a setting in which behaviour can be challenged and modified, essentially through the group pressure. This is very different from approaches which attempt to prevent the dehumanizing effects of mental hospitals by creating a general therapeutic and democratic atmosphere[37] (see Chapter 6.3.9)

Milieu therapy

The term milieu therapy has been used to describe an environment which is in some way therapeutic. The therapeutic component may be supportive, or it may be challenging. It is often difficult to define exactly what is the 'milieu' component of the therapy. People kept in a hospital cannot offend outside, but this is not a success for the hospital environment. Prisons do the same, without any pretence at therapy. It is suggested that this term is now outmoded and, whenever it is being considered, should be replaced by an attempt to describe a specific intervention.

Community supervision

Many people with personality disorder are reluctant to change and will only take part in a treatment programme under duress. This is a particular concern with personality disorders that lead to antisocial behaviour. Because of this there have been moves to introduce community supervision of those with antisocial personality disorder or judged to have a serious risk of reoffending. Although the procedure has not been evaluated formally, it has been suggested that people with these disorders who are discharged under some form of community supervision are less likely to reoffend than those who do not receive such supervision.[38] These results are difficult to interpret as the patients were not randomized to type of care.

There is also a dispute as to who should carry out community supervision and the form that it should take. Most studies have been carried out on patients who are subject to particular sections of mental health legislation[39] and therefore supervised by health workers. It has also been suggested that probation officers could carry out this role under the criminal justice rather than the mental health system. This type of intervention has a simple measure of outcome—reconviction—but this is not necessarily correlated with improvement in the personality disorder. Measures of behavioural change, improvement in relationships, or formal personality assessment should also be included. Currently there is much dispute as to whether some form of community supervision of severe personality disorder should be introduced by legislation, and it is regrettable that there is no hard evidence of efficacy on which to base action, although community supervision has face validity.

Drug treatment

Drugs are often used for treating personality disorders although it is important to note that none are licensed for the treatment of these conditions. As with other forms of treatment, borderline personality disorder constitutes the largestest group in which drug treatment is being used and is therefore worth examining separately. Again, it is important to note that borderline personality disorder is one of the most heterogeneous of all groups within the personality classification and includes extensive comorbidity with other personality disorders as well as with mental state disorders, particularly mood and stress-related disorders.

Borderline personality disorder

Antipsychotic drugs

The antipsychotic drugs have been tested in the treatment of borderline personality disorder using more rigorous methodology than any other treatments. Despite this, the results are equivocal. Two studies published in 1986[8,40] showed in randomized placebo-controlled trials that low doses of haloperidol and thiothixene were effective in reducing typical borderline behaviour and associated symptoms. These symptoms included depression, and as amitriptyline was one of the

comparison drugs in one of these studies[8] it is of particular interest that haloperidol was superior to this drug in reducing depressive symptoms. However, since these apparently clear-cut findings were published, further studies have failed to show the same level of efficacy.[41] When treatment is extended, the gains of antipsychotic drugs over placebo disappear after about 16 weeks. One of the major problems of antipsychotic drugs, even in the low dosage used to treat borderline personality disorder, is their propensity to create adverse effects which leads to low compliance with therapy. Although in a secure penitentiary[8] it may be possible to ensure that all patients take their drugs at the appropriate times, in most other settings it is necessary to allow patients to maintain their own motivation to take treatment. The possibility of giving antipsychotic drugs in low-dose depot injections has been considered, although not in borderline personality disorders (see below), but is unlikely to command wide appeal.

Antidepressants

Tricyclic antidepressants, mainly in the form of amitriptyline, have been compared with other treatments, including placebo, in the treatment of borderline personality disorder[8,42] but the results are difficult to interpret. Some patients show extremely good response to this treatment, whereas others show no benefit whatsoever.[42]

There are some suggestions that selective serotonin reuptake inhibitors (SSRIs) might also be effective, with one randomized controlled trial using fluoxetine showing superiority over placebo and another suggesting that SSRIs reduce impulsiveness.[43,44] This is of particular interest because of the apparent differences between SSRIs and tricyclic antidepressants, although neither of these studies involved a tricyclic antidepressant comparison. In one of the early controlled studies,[45] the monoamine oxidase inhibitor tranylcypromine was compared with alprazolam, carbamazepine, and trifluoperazine. The results were equivocal, which is not surprising as the sample only included 45 patients, and some gains from all treatments were judged to be present. However, since no placebo control was included this could only be speculative.

The results of these studies are very difficult to interpret because of the unsatisfactory status of borderline personality disorder. The evidence of efficacy in the short term, disappearing in the longer term, suggests that improvement is more likely to be a consequence of successful treatment of a mental state disorder rather than the personality component.

Other personality disorders

Flamboyant group

Low dosage of antipsychotic drugs has been recommended for the treatment of antisocial (now called dissocial) personality disorder for many years,[46] and these recommendations have included treatment by depot injection. Most of these reports are anecdotal and no control comparisons have been made. Mood stabilizers have also been considered for the treatment of personality disorder. Carbamazepine was one of the comparison drugs used in the study by Cowdry and Gardner[45] and lithium has been shown to reduce anger and impulsiveness in those with antisocial personality disorder[47] but this study has never been replicated. Similar benefits for lithium were shown in the treatment of alcohol dependence, probably because this condition is often associated with personality disorder (although personality was not mentioned in the study).[48] Similar anti-aggressive action of lithium has been demonstrated in learning disability.[49]

Odd and eccentric group (cluster A)

There is limited evidence that antipsychotic drugs may also be effective in the odd or eccentric cluster of personality disorders (schizoid, schizotypal, and paranoid). This is generally unsatisfactory evidence, and the only controlled trial[40] included both borderline and schizotypal personality disorder in its selection criteria. No studies of drug treatment in paranoid personality disorder have been published, and indeed this condition seems to have escaped formal assessment of all therapeutic interventions. A mistrust of treatment given by others is probably an intrinsic part of the condition.

Anxious fearful cluster (cluster C)

There is a strong association between neurotic disorder and what is commonly known as the cluster C group of personality disorders, comprising dependent, obsessive–compulsive, and anxious (avoidant) personality disorders. There is considerable overlap between the criteria for many neurotic disorders and these disorders within the cluster C group, and this is particularly prominent with social phobia and avoidant personality disorder.[50,51] The evidence that antidepressants are effective in avoidant personality disorder[52] should be taken with a degree of scepticism; it is more likely that the antidepressants have been effective in treating social phobia.

A retrospective study[53] compared the outcome of the treatment of depression with monoamine oxidase inhibitors and tricyclic antidepressants in those who also had concurrent personality disorder and found that tricyclic antidepressants were in general superior. In the Nottingham Study of Neurotic Disorder,[54] in which drug treatment, mainly in the form of tricyclic antidepressants, was compared with cognitive-behavioural therapy and self-help in patients with neurotic disorder over 2 years, it was found that those who had a concurrent personality disorder had better symptomatic outcome if they were treated in the drug group whereas those with no personality disorder fared better with self-help.

In a study of antidepressant drug treatment with fluvoxamine in obsessive–compulsive disorder, it was found that those with concurrent obsessive–compulsive personality disorder had a better outcome.[55] It was difficult to know if this was a consequence of better response or better adherence to treatment in those with personality disorders.

Conclusion

Although there have been several controlled trials involving psychotropic drugs and placebo in the treatment of personality disorder, none of them satisfy the full requirements for establishment of efficacy set out at the beginning of this chapter. This does not mean that drugs are ineffective in personality disorder, but there is no satisfactory evidence that would allow specific recommendations to be made. Since most patients receiving drug treatment have a mental state disorder independent of their personality status, further studies, such as those of Ansseau et al.,[55] in which patients with mental state disorders being treated with drugs also have their personality status assessed would be helpful in elucidating the role of personality in treatment response.

Summary of treatments claimed to be effective in personality disorder

Psychological treatments

Dynamic psychotherapy

Although dynamic psychotherapy and psychoanalysis have used personality disorder (mainly the less serious variety) as their stock-in-trade for treatment over many years, there is little evidence to suggest clear gains for this approach in its treatment. Nevertheless, the absence of evidence is largely related to the absence of adequate research, and there are several approaches that may be of value for borderline personality disorder in particular, but the consensus is that the brief forms of psychotherapy are likely to be the most valuable in these conditions and that conventional psychotherapeutic approaches are not efficacious.[56]

Cognitive therapy

It is too early to assess the claims for cognitive therapy. The technique may have particular value in increasing adherence to treatment through the collaborative approach that is used.

Democratic therapeutic community

This approach was developed to treat antisocial personality disorders. There are severe methodological problems in evaluating this method and no definite conclusions can be drawn regarding its efficacy.

Drug treatment

Neuroleptic drugs

Neuroleptic (antipsychotic) drugs have almost an established place in the treatment of some forms of personality disorder, particularly the antisocial, borderline, narcissistic, and histrionic types. There is some evidence of efficacy in schizotypal personality disorder. Although the effectiveness of these compounds is certainly not striking, it has been better documented than most other treatments.

Antidepressant drugs

All three groups of antidepressants—monoamine oxidase inhibitors, tricyclic and associated antidepressants, and SSRIs—have been claimed to be of some value in the treatment of personality disorder. The evidence for this is less clear than for the neuroleptic (antipsychotic) drugs, but this is partly because of the difficulty of separating personality from depression, which is so often associated with personality disturbance. The evidence taken as a whole suggests that these drugs may be of some value, particularly in the treatment of the anxious/fearful cluster of personality disorders and the borderline group.

Mood stabilizers

Lithium and carbamazepine have been investigated in the management of personality disorder. Although studies to date have not been methodologically sound and the work needs to be replicated, such evidence that exists suggests better efficacy than most other forms of management.

Other drugs

Although a number of other drug groups, including benzodiazepines, anticonvulsants, anticholinergics, and antilibidinal drugs, have all been claimed to have some effect on personality disorders, the evidence is not strong enough to justify further discussion. Also, there is some evidence that benzodiazepines in the presence of personality disorder hinder the effects of other forms of treatment and may lead to addiction.[57]

Linking treatment to diagnosis in personality disorder

As indicated above, the current classification of personality disorder is controversial and generally unhelpful to the clinician. In particular, the extent of apparent comorbidity between groups of disorders is an illusion of multiple diagnosis, varying from complete independence in some disorders to such close interdependence in others that they could be given the same name.[58]

This explains why in this chapter discussion of treatment has generally followed the simple classification based on the three clusters of personality disorder that have persistently been identified in factor analytical studies and cluster analysis.[59–62]

- The flamboyant or dramatic group, comprising antisocial (dissocial), borderline, impulsive, histrionic, and narcissistic personality disorders (cluster B in DSM).
- The odd or eccentric group, comprising paranoid, schizoid, and schizotypal personality disorders (cluster A).
- The anxious or fearful group, comprising the dependent, anxious (avoidant), and obsessive–compulsive (anankastic) personality disorders (cluster C). Sometimes the obsessive–compulsive group is assigned to a separate cluster, as it can be effectively separated from cluster C.

Although it has been argued that, as personality disorder is primarily manifested by difficulties in interpersonal relationships, it should be classified in these terms rather than as separate categories,[63] there are sufficient differences between the main clusters to justify separate examination. In particular, in the United Kingdom there is a medicolegal requirement to identify those with 'psychopathic disorder' who, under successive Mental Health Acts since 1979, may be compulsorily admitted for treatment if they have 'a persistent disorder or disability of mind (whether or not including subnormality of intelligence) which results in abnormally aggressive or seriously irresponsible conduct on the part of the patient, and requires or is susceptible to medical treatment'.[39] There is an urgent need to modernize this definition.

Management

Some general principles of management apply to all personality disorders although the consequences of ignoring them will be greater for the flamboyant cluster of personality disorders than for others.

Consistency

One of the reasons why those with personality disorders create so many problems in therapy is that they are able to detect and exploit inconsistency in their treatment. Often this is merely a way of deflecting attention away from fundamental problems associated with the personality disorder, but they are nonetheless effective in creating a screen that prevents other issues from being addressed. Clearly the fewer the people involved in care, the less are the chances of creating inconsistency, and keeping the number of main workers down to two or three is a sound goal.

Constancy

It is helpful to avoid changes in staff as far as possible. This is of particular relevance in the treatment of borderline personality disorder in which changes in therapists often re-enact the problems of loss and despair that the patient experiences so commonly in relationships.

Adequate inpatient support

Staff involved in hospital care often believe that people with personality disorders should be kept out of hospital. This belief is based on the observation that such people exploit the opportunities offered by admission and create circumstances whereby it is difficult to discharge them. Much of this opinion is ill founded. Patients with comorbid mental state and personality disorders actually have better outcomes if they have a hospital-oriented programme of care than treatment in the community, whereas the opposite is true in the absence of personality disorder.[64] People with personality disorders have fewer attachment and support figures in the community than others,[64] and few community teams can provide the level of support needed when function begins to disintegrate. Few services desire to treat this group of difficult patients and refuse them because they are 'not suitable', but this opinion should carry little weight.

Joint working

Although it is advisable to keep the number of therapists to a minimum in the care of those with personality disorder, there are disadvantages in having a lone therapist. This has led to problems in implementing the Care Programming Approach,[65] especially when the worker is less experienced. Planned sharing of cases between two or three therapists, each with a clearly demarcated role, helps to maintain a treatment programme.[11]

Perhaps the most important error in management is failure to recognize personality disorder when other psychiatric disorders are more prominent and may seem to be the only presenting problem. This is becoming recognized in the development of treatment protocols. This problem is encountered widely in the mental health services among people presenting to emergency psychiatric clinics,[66] in services for the homeless mentally ill,[67] and among heavy users of psychiatric services[68] and those with multiple admissions.[69] In all these settings, personality disorder is often not recognized early enough. This is to some extent understandable as the assessment of personality disorder is difficult in, for example, a busy emergency clinic. Nevertheless, failure to achieve a predicted response is often due to an earlier failure to detect the presence of personality disorder.

Further developments

It is unlikely that many studies will ever be carried that satisfy the four requirements of minimum evidence of efficacy described at the beginning of this chapter. This is because such explanatory trials would be so far removed from usual psychiatric practice that their results will be difficult to translate into such practice. There is also continuing uncertainty about the best ways of classifying personality disorder and widespread dissatisfaction with the current categorical system.[70] The arguments in favour of a dimensional system of classification extending from normal personality through to higher levels of personality disorder[71] are becoming more powerful. The problem of comorbidity between personality disorders is accentuated by evidence that the more severe personality disorders are associated with greater comorbidity.[72] It may be better to regard comorbidity as a measure of severity, thereby combining the advantages of categorical and dimensional systems.[73] It seems increasingly likely that it is severity of personality disturbance rather than a specific categorical label that will be more important in selecting patients for treatment studies.

The problem of adherence to treatment will be more difficult to overcome. Because personality disorders are usually ingrained egosyntonic, it is highly unlikely that patients will continue treatment effectively either with regular medication or with frequent sessions of psychological treatment. However, it may be less difficult to improve compliance with psychological treatment than with drug treatment. Combined drug and psychological treatments may be of value as there is no reason to believe that these would be antagonistic in the treatment of personality disorder. The collaborative approach of cognitive therapy seems well suited to the treatment of personality disorder and could improve adherence to all modes of treatment.

It would be very useful if there was a better theoretical basis for the treatment of personality disorder. Apart from schema theory, there is little rationale for any current treatment of personality disorder. Despite these somewhat gloomy and sceptical views it is important to note that for the first time in the history of personality disorder people the condition is no longer regarded as untreatable. We expect that effective treatments will be found in the course of the next 30 years and, if this happens, it will help greatly in removing the pejorative views that are currently attached to these conditions.

References

1. Feinstein, A. (1970). The pre-therapeutic classification of comorbidity in chronic disease. *Journal of Chronic Diseases*, **23**, 455–62.
2. Tyrer, P. (1996). Comorbidity or consanguinity. *British Journal of Psychiatry*, **168**, 669–71.
3. Fyer, M.R., Frances, A.J., Sullivan, T., *et al.* (1988). Co-morbidity of borderline personality disorder. *Archives of General Psychiatry*, **45**, 348–52.
4. Coppen, A.L. and Metcalfe, H. (1965). The effect of a depressive illness on MMPI scores. *British Journal of Psychiatry*, **111**, 236–9.
5. Stuart, S., Simons, A.D., Thase, M.E., and Pilkonis, P. (1992). Are personality assessments valid in acute major depression? *Journal of Affective Disorders*, **24**, 281–9.
6. Adler, G. (1979). The myth of the alliance with borderline patients. *American Journal of Psychiatry*, **136**, 642–5.
7. Stone, M.H., Hurt, S.W., and Stone, D.K. (1987). The PI 500: long-term follow-up of borderline patients meeting DSM-III criteria—1. Global outcome. *Journal of Personality Disorders*, **1**, 291–8.
8. Soloff, P.H., George, A., Nathan, R.S., *et al.* (1986). Progress in pharmacotherapy of personality disorders: a double blind study of amitriptyline, haloperidol and placebo. *Archives of General Psychiatry*, **43**, 691–7.
9. Davidson, K. (1993). A new cognitive therapy for borderline and anti-social personality disorders. *Proceedings of the 3rd International Conference of Disorders of Personality*, Vol. 1, p. 15.
10. Davidson, K. and Tyrer, P. (1996). Cognitive therapy for anti-social and borderline personality disorder: single case study series. *British Journal of Clinical Psychology*, **35**, 413–29.
11. Linehan, M.M. (1992). *Cognitive therapy for borderline personality disorder*. Guilford Press, New York.
12. Linehan, M.M. (1995). Combining pharmacotherapy with psychotherapy for substance abusers with borderline personality disorder: strategies for enhancing compliance. *NIDA Research Monograph*, **150**, 129–42.
13. Tyrer, P. and Seivewright, H. (1999). Studies of outcome. In *Personality disorders: diagnosis, management and course* (2nd edn) (ed. P. Tyrer). Butterworth Heinemann, Oxford.
14. Tyrer, P. (1998). Drug treatment of personality disorder. *Psychiatric Bulletin*, **22**, 242–4.
15. Andrews, G. (1991). The essential psychotherapies. *British Journal of Psychiatry*, **162**, 447–51.
16. Higgitt, A. and Fonagy, P. (1992). Psychotherapy in borderline and narcissistic personality disorder. *British Journal of Psychiatry*, **161**, 23–43.
17. Kernberg, O.F., Burstein, E., Coyne, L., *et al.* (1972). Psychotherapy and psychoanalysis: final report of the Menninger Foundation's psychotherapy research project. *Bulletin of the Menninger Clinic*, **36**, 1–275.
18. Kernberg, O.F. (1984). *Severe personality disorders: psychotherapeutic strategies.* Yale University Press, New Haven, CT.
19. Masterson, J.F. (1976). *Treatment of the borderline adult.* Brunner–Mazel, New York.
20. Kohut, H. (1977). *The restoration of self.* International Universities Press, New York.
21. Winston, A., Pollack, J., McCullough, L., *et al.* (1994). Brief psychotherapy of personality disorders. *American Journal of Psychiatry*, **151**, 190–4.
22. Ryle, A. (1997). The structure and development of borderline personality disorder: a proposed model. *British Journal of Psychiatry*, **170**, 82–7.
23. Beck, A.T. and Freeman, A. (1990). *Cognitive therapy of personality disorders.* Guilford Press, New York.
24. Benjamin, L.S. (1993). *Interpersonal diagnosis and treatment of personality disorders.* Guilford Press, New York.
25. Beck, J.S. (1996). Cognitive therapy for personality disorders. In *Frontiers of cognitive therapy* (ed. P.M. Salkovskis). Guilford Press, New York.
26. Alexander, F. (1930). The neurotic character. *International Journal of Psychoanalysis*, **11**, 291–311.
27. Young, J.E. (1994). *Cognitive therapy for personality disorders: a schema-focused approach* (revised edn). Practitioner's Resource Series, Professional Resource Press, Sarasota, FL.
28. Edwards, D.J.A. (1990). Cognitive therapy and the restructuring of early memories through guided imagery. *Journal of Cognitive Psychotherapy*, **4**, 33–50.
29. Ryle, A. (1997). *Cognitive analytical therapy and borderline personality disorder: the model and the method.* Wiley, Chichester.
30. Persons, J.B. and Bertagnolli, A. (1994). Cognitive–behavioural treatment of multiple-problem patients: application to personality disorder. *Clinical Psychology and Psychotherapy*, **1**, 279–85.
31. Linehan, M.M., Armstrong, H.E., Suarez, A., Allmon, D., and Heard, H.L. (1991). Cognitive–behavioral treatment of chronically parasuicidal borderline patients. *Archives of General Psychiatry*, **48**, 1060–4.
32. Linehan, M.M., Heard, H.L., and Armstrong, H.E. (1993). Naturalistic follow-up of a behavioural treatment for chronically parasuicidal borderline patients. *Archives of General Psychiatry*, **50**, 971–4.
33. Akiskal, H.S., Hirschfeld, R.M.A., and Yerevanian, B.I. (1983). The relationship of personality to affective disorders: a critical review. *Archives of General Psychiatry*, **40**, 801–10.

34. Evans, K., Tyrer, P., Catalan, J., *et al.* (1999). Manual-assisted cognitive–behaviour therapy (MACT): a randomised controlled trial of a brief intervention with bibliotherapy in the treatment of recurrent deliberate self-harm. *Psychological Medicine*, **29**, 19–25.

35. Barton, R. (1959). *Institutional neurosis*. John Wright, Bristol.

36. Manning, N. (1989). *The Therapeutic Community Movement: charisma and routinization*. International Library of Group Psychotherapy and Group Process, Routledge and Kegan Paul, London.

37. Clark, D.H. (1965). The therapeutic community concept: practice and future. *British Journal of Psychiatry*, **106**, 947–54.

38. Walker, N. and McCabe, S. (1973). *Crime and insanity in England*, Vol. 2. Edinburgh University Press.

39. *Mental Health Act (England and Wales)* (1983). Department of Health, London.

40. Goldberg, S.C., Shulz, S.C., Shulz, P.M., Resnick, R.J., Haymer, R.M., and Friedel, R.O. (1986). Borderline and schizotypal personality disorders treated with low dose thiothixene versus placebo. *Archives of General Psychiatry*, **43**, 680–6.

41. Cornelius, J.R., Soloff, P.H., Perel, J.M., *et al.* (1993). Continuation pharmacotherapy of borderline personality disorder with haloperidol and phenelzine. *American Journal of Psychiatry*, **150**, 1843–8.

42. Soloff, P.H. (1994). Is there any drug treatment of choice for the borderline patient? *Acta Psychiatrica Scandinavica*, **89** (Supplement 379), 50–5.

43. Salzman, C., Wolfson, A.N., Schatzberg, A., *et al.* (1995). Effect of fluoxetine on anger in symptomatic volunteers with borderline personality disorder. *Journal of Clinical Psychopharmacology*, **15**, 23–9.

44. Yerkes, R.J., van der Mast, R.C., Kerkhof, A.J., *et al.* (1998). Platelet serotonin, monoamine oxidase activity, and [3H]paroxetine binding related to impulsive suicide attempts and borderline personality disorder. *Biological Psychiatry*, **43**, 740–6.

45. Cowdry, R.W. and Gardner, D.L. (1988). Pharmacotherapy of borderline personality disorder: alprazolam, carbamazepine, trifluoperazine and tranylcypromine. *Archives of General Psychiatry*, **45**, 111–19.

46. Bennie, E.H. and Kinnell, H.G. (1975). Dangerous offenders. *Lancet*, **ii**, 1303.

47. Sheard, M.H., Marini, J.L., Bridges, C.I., and Wagner, E. (1976). The effect of lithium on impulsive aggressive behavior in man. *American Journal of Psychiatry*, **133**, 1409–13.

48. Merry, J., Reynolds, C.M., Bailey, J., and Coppen, A. (1976). Prophylactic treatment of alcoholism by lithium carbonate. *Lancet*, **ii**, 481–2.

49. Tyrer, S.P., Walsh, A., Edwards, D.E., Berney, T.P., and Stephens, D.A. (1984). Factors associated with a good response to lithium in aggressive mentally handicapped subjects. *Progress in Neuropsychopharmacology and Biological Psychiatry*, **8**, 751–5.

50. Herbert, J.D., Hope, D.A., and Bellack, A.S. (1992). Validity of the distinction between generalized social phobia and avoidant personality disorder. *Journal of Abnormal Psychology*, **101**, 332–9.

51. Tyrer, P. (1996). Diagnostic anomalies in social phobia. *International Clinical Psychopharmacology*, **11** (Supplement 3), 29–33.

52. Deltito, J.A. and Stam, M. (1989). Psychopharmacological treatment of avoidant personality disorder. *Comprehensive Psychiatry*, **30**, 498–504.

53. Shawcross, C.R. and Tyrer, P. (1985). Influence of personality on response to monoamine oxidase inhibitors and tricyclic antidepressants. *Journal of Psychiatric Research*, **19**, 557–62.

54. Tyrer, P., Seivewright, N., Ferguson, B., *et al.* (1993). The Nottingham Study of Neurotic Disorder: effect of personality status on response to drug treatment, cognitive therapy and self-help over two years. *British Journal of Psychiatry*, **162**, 190–226.

55. Ansseau, M., Troisfontaines, B., Papart, P., and von Frenckell, R. (1991). Compulsive personality as predictor of response to serotonergic antidepressants. *British Medical Journal*, **303**, 760–1.

56. Dowson, J.H. and Grounds, A.T. (1995). *Personality disorders: recognition and clinical management*. Cambridge University Press.

57. Tyrer, P. (1989). Risks of dependence on benzodiazepine drugs: the importance of patient selection. *British Medical Journal*, **298**, 102–4.

58. Lyons, M.J., Tyrer, P., Gunderson, J., *et al.* (1997). Heuristic models of comorbidity of axis I and axis II disorders. *Journal of Personality Disorders*, **11**, 260–9.

59. Walton, H.J. and Presly, A.S. (1973). Use of a category system in the diagnosis of abnormal personality. *British Journal of Psychiatry*, **122**, 259–68.

60. Tyrer, P. and Alexander, J. (1979). Classification of personality disorder. *British Journal of Psychiatry*, **135**, 163–7.

61. Cloninger, C.R. (1987). A systematic method for clinical description and classification of personality variants. *Archives of General Psychiatry*, **44**, 573–88.

62. Mulder, R.T. and Joyce, P.R. (1995). Temperament and the structure of personality disorder symptoms. *Psychological Medicine*, **27**, 99–106.

63. Rutter, M. (1987). Temperament, personality and personality disorder. *British Journal of Psychiatry*, **150**, 443–58.

64. Tyrer, P., Merson, S., Onyett, S., and Johnson, T. (1994). The effect of personality disorder on clinical outcome, social networks and adjustment: a controlled clinical trial of psychiatric emergencies. *Psychological Medicine*, **24**, 731–40.

65. North, C., Ritchie, J., and Ward, K. (1993). *Factors influencing the implementation of the care programming approach*. HMSO, London.

66. Breslow, R.E., Klinger, B.I., and Erickson, B.J. (1996). Acute intoxication and substance abuse among patients presenting to a psychiatric emergency service. *General Hospital Psychiatry*, **18**, 183–91.

67. North, C.S., Thompson, S.J., Pollio, D.E., Ricci, D.A., and Smith, E.M. (1997). A diagnostic comparison of homeless and nonhomeless patients in an urban mental health clinic. *Social Psychiatry and Psychiatric Epidemiology*, **32**, 236–40.

68. Kent, S., Fogarty, M., and Yellowlees, P. (1995). Heavy utilization of inpatient and outpatient services in a public mental health service. *Psychiatric Services*, **46**, 1254–7.

69. Geller, J.L., Fisher, W.H., McDermeit, M., and Brown, J.M. (1998). The effects of public managed care on patterns of intensive use of inpatient psychiatric services. *Psychiatric Services*, **49**, 327–32.

70. Clark, L.A., Livesley, W.J., Schroeder, M.L., and Irish, S.L. (1996). Convergence of two systems for assessing personality disorders. *Psychological Assessment*, **8**, 294–303.

71. Livesley, W.J., Jang, K.L., and Vernon, P.A. (1998). Phenotypic and genetic structure of traits delineating personality disorder. *Archives of General Psychiatry*, **55**, 941–8.

72. Dolan, B.M., Norton, K., and Warren, F.M. (1996). Cost-offset following specialist treatment of severe personality disorder. *Psychiatric Bulletin*, **20**, 413–17.

73. Tyrer, P. and Johnson, T. (1996). Establishing the severity of personality disorder. *American Journal of Psychiatry*, **153**, 1593–7.

4.13 Habit and impulse control disorders

4.13.1 Impulse control disorders

Susan L. McElroy, Lesley M. Arnold, and DeAnna A. Beckman

This chapter first reviews impulse control disorders as mental disorders, and then considers the available research on the clinical features, epidemiology, psychiatric comorbidity, biology, and treatment response of various recognized and putative impulse control disorders (except for trichotillomania and pathological gambling, which are reviewed in Chapters 4.13.2 and 4.13.3 respectively). It is concluded that impulse control disorders are legitimate mental disorders.

Definitions of impulse control disorders

Historically, impulse control disorders have been defined as harmful behaviours performed in response to irresistible impulses.[1] In DSM-IV, an impulse control disorder is defined as the failure to resist an impulse, drive, or temptation to commit an act that is harmful to the individual or to others.[2,3] DSM-IV also stipulates that for most impulse control disorders, the individual feels an increasing sense of tension or arousal before committing the act and then experiences pleasure, gratification, or relief at the time of committing the act. In the text describing these disorders, DSM-IV states that after the act, there may or may not be genuine regret, self-reproach, or guilt. In ICD-10,[4] these conditions are classified as habit and impulse disorders and defined as repeated acts that have no clear rational motivation that generally harm the patient's own interests and those of other people. ICD-10 further states that the behaviours are associated with impulses to action that cannot be controlled.

In DSM-IV, impulse control disorders are listed in a residual category, 'Impulse control disorders not elsewhere classified', which includes intermittent explosive disorder, kleptomania, pathological gambling, pyromania, trichotillomania, and impulse control disorders not otherwise specified. Examples of impulse control disorders not otherwise specified are compulsive buying or shopping (also called buying mania or oniomania), repetitive self-mutilation, psychogenic excoriation (also called compulsive skin picking), and onychophagia (severe nail-biting).[1] In ICD-10, habit and impulse disorders are also listed as a residual category. Similar to DSM-IV, it includes pathological gambling, pathological fire-setting (pyromania), pathological stealing (kleptomania), trichotillomania, other habit and impulse disorders (which includes intermittent explosive (behaviour) disorder), and habit and impulse disorder, unspecified.

Intermittent explosive disorder

Definition and clinical features

Intermittent explosive disorder is defined in DSM-IV as several discrete episodes of failure to resist aggressive impulses that result in serious assaultive acts or destruction of property (criterion A). Also, the degree of aggression expressed during an episode is grossly out of proportion to any precipitating psychosocial stressors (criterion B) and the explosive episodes are not better accounted for by another mental disorder or due to the direct physiological effects of a substance or a general medical condition (criterion C). ICD-10 lists intermittent explosive disorder under 'Other habit and impulse disorders', but does not provide specific guidelines for its diagnosis.

Some authorities continue to doubt the validity of intermittent explosive disorder as an independent diagnostic entity, seeing loss of control of aggressive impulses (also called explosive rage, rage outbursts, or episodic dyscontrol) instead as a non-specific symptom that occurs in a wide range of psychiatric and medical disorders.[2] By contrast, other authorities argue that intermittent explosive disorder is in fact a distinct mental disorder that is an important cause of violent behaviour, that the DSM criteria for intermittent explosive disorder are too narrow, and that clinically significant milder forms of intermittent explosive disorder exist that should be nosologically recognized.[5]

Although there are few systematic studies of the phenomenology of intermittent explosive disorder, there are numerous clinical reports of people with rage outbursts which are described as explosive, uncontrollable, unpremeditated, and brief, provoked by minor stimuli, and associated with various psychological and physical symptoms, especially changes in mood, awareness, and sympathetic arousal.[5] For example, of 27 subjects with DSM-IV intermittent explosive disorder,[6] all reported aggressive impulses or violent urges prior to their aggressive acts which were variously described as the 'need to attack', the 'need to defend oneself', the 'need to strike out', an 'adrenalin rush', 'seeing red', or the 'urge to kill someone'. Most subjects described tension with the impulses and relief that was sometimes pleasurable with the acts. Most subjects also reported that affective symptoms accompanied their aggressive episodes. The most common affective symptoms associated with the impulses and acts were manic-like, and included irritability/rage, increased energy, and racing thoughts. After performance of the acts, the most frequent affective symptoms were depressed mood and fatigue. Approximately one-half of subjects stated that their episodes were associated with some degree of loss of or change in awareness, and one-third reported that their episodes were often preceded or accompanied by physical symptoms (e.g. tingling, tremor, palpitations, chest tightness, or head pressure).

Epidemiology and course

Although intermittent explosive disorder is presumed to be rare, its prevalence is unknown. However, in a recent study of the prevalence of various impulse control disorders in a psychiatric outpatient population, intermittent explosive disorder was the second most common current (3.8 per cent) and lifetime (6.2 per cent) impulse control disorder diagnosis (after compulsive buying).[7]

Intermittent explosive disorder is probably more common in men than women. Many cases of intermittent explosive disorder begin in adolescence and follow a chronic or episodic course.[6]

Associated psychopathology and comorbidity

Intermittent explosive disorder often co-occurs with other psychiatric disorders. For example, of 46 impulsive violent offenders (n = 24) and fire-setters (n = 22) in one study,[8] 33 (72 per cent) of whom met the DSM-III criteria for intermittent explosive disorder, 44 (96 per cent) had a lifetime diagnosis of alcohol abuse, 41 (89 per cent) had border-line personality disorder, 24 (52 per cent) had a mood disorder, and nine (20 per cent) had antisocial personality disorder. Of 27 subjects with DSM-IV intermittent explosive disorder evaluated with the Structured Clinical Interview for DSM-IV,[6] 25 (93 per cent) met life-time criteria for a mood disorder (with 15 (55 per cent) meeting criteria for a bipolar disorder), 13 (48 per cent) for a substance use disorder, 13 (48 per cent) for an anxiety disorder (with six (22 per cent) meeting criteria for obsessive–compulsive disorder), six (22 per cent) for an eating disorder, and 12 (44 per cent) for an impulse control disorder other than intermittent explosive disorder.[6]

Family studies

Family studies suggest that relatives of probands with intermittent explosive disorder have high rates of substance abuse, violent behaviour, and possibly mood disorders. Of 54 impulsive violent offenders and fire-setters (29 (54 per cent) of whom had DSM-III intermittent explosive disorder and 52 (96 per cent) of whom had alcohol abuse), 41 (81 per cent) had first- or second-degree relatives with alcoholism and 35 (65 per cent) had alcoholic fathers.[9] In a family history study of patients with temper outbursts meeting the first two DSM-III criteria for intermittent explosive disorder, adopted patients were significantly less likely than non-adopted patients to have a family history of temper outbursts.[10] Of 25 subjects with DSM-IV intermittent explosive disorder evaluated via the family history method, 20 (80 per cent) had at least one first-degree relative with a substance use disorder, 14 (56 per cent) a mood disorder, and 14 (56 per cent) an impulse control disorder.[6] Eight (32 per cent) of subjects had a first-degree relative with probable intermittent explosive disorder.

Biology

A consistent finding in biological psychiatric research has been abnormalities in serotonergic function in people with impulsive aggression, including those with intermittent explosive disorder. For example, mean platelet [^{3}H] 5-hydroxytryptamine (serotinin) uptake was significantly lower in 15 male outpatients with episodic aggression than in 15 non-aggressive comparison subjects.[11] Similarly, in a study of 58 violent offenders and impulsive fire-setters, 33 (57 per cent) of whom had DSM-III intermittent explosive disorder, lower cerebrospinal fluid concentrations of 5-hydroxyindoleacetic acid were found in the impulsive offenders and fire-setters than in the non-impulsive offenders and normal control subjects.[8]

Treatment response

Clinical experience suggests that intermittent explosive disorder may be less responsive to insight-oriented and more responsive to cognitive-behavioural therapies, particularly those stressing anger management.[1] Medications reported effective in intermittent explosive disorder or apparent intermittent explosive disorder, some in controlled trials, include antiepileptics (e.g. phenytoin, carbamazepine), thymoleptics (e.g. tricyclics, serotonin reuptake inhibitors, lithium, valproate), β-blockers, psychostimulants, and even antiandrogens.[1,6,12] Also, serotonin reuptake inhibitors, mood stabilizers, and antiepileptics may be effective for impulsive-aggressive behaviour in personality-disordered patients.[13]

Kleptomania

Definition and clinical features

Kleptomania is defined in DSM-IV as follows:

- recurrent failure to resist impulses to steal objects that are not needed for personal use or for their monetary value (criterion A);
- increasing sense of tension immediately before committing the theft (criterion B);
- pleasure, gratification, or relief at the time of committing the theft (criterion C);
- the stealing is not committed to express anger or vengeance and is not in response to a delusion or a hallucination (criterion D);
- the stealing is not better accounted for by conduct disorder, a manic episode, or antisocial personality disorder (criterion E).

In ICD-10, kleptomania (or pathological stealing) is defined as the repeated failure to resist impulses to steal objects that are not acquired for personal use or monetary gain.

Two modern studies[14-16] have systematically examined the phenomenology of sizeable groups of people with DSM-defined kleptomania. In the first,[14] 20 patients with DSM-IIIR kleptomania were referred for clinical evaluation. All 20 patients described irresistible impulses or urges to steal, and tension relief either during or shortly after the act of theft (as required by the DSM-IIIR criteria). Although most patients described the impulses as senseless, intrusive, and uncomfortable, and many tried to resist them, half reported pleasurable feelings during the act of theft, variously described as 'a rush' or 'a high'. All patients reported instances of impulsive stealing, but some also described premeditated stealing, the aim of which was often to relieve the impulses to steal. Several patients developed rules for their stealing behaviour—for instance, stealing only from work or from certain types of shops (e.g. drug stores but not department stores), or stealing certain items but not others (e.g. jewellery but not clothing). All patients stated that they considered their stealing to be wrong, and most, but not all, reported guilt or remorse after stealing.

In the second study,[15,16] 37 people fulfilling DSM-IV criteria for kleptomania recruited through newspaper advertisement were interviewed and compared with 50 shoplifters interviewed directly after apprehension. When asked to rate their last theft on a number of variables, persons with kleptomania reported more inner tension before the theft and greater relief and impulsivity during the theft than the shoplifters. However, the shoplifters also rated high on these variables. Also, both groups reported similar degrees of planning, thrill, vengeance, need, pleasure, and psychiatric imbalance on a visual analogue scale. The authors concluded that there were no 'absolute borders' between 'pure' DSM-IV kleptomania and other forms of shoplifting.

Epidemiology and course

Although kleptomania is presumed to be rare, its prevalence is unknown. Available studies suggest that only a small portion of shoplifters (from none to 8 per cent) represent true cases of kleptomania.[17] However, it has been argued that these rates may be spuriously low because psychiatric evaluations may not have always been sufficiently thorough, operational diagnostic criteria were rarely used, and kleptomania may have been under-represented in the samples due to selection bias (i.e. people with repeated apprehensions were more likely to be legally rather than psychiatrically referred). Also, kleptomania is a secret disorder (i.e. afflicted people hide their symptoms).

Kleptomania is probably more common in women than in men.[17] Many cases begin in adolescence or early adulthood, and often follow an episodic or a chronic course.

Associated psychopathology and comorbidity

Kleptomania often co-occurs with other psychiatric disorders. Of 20 patients with DSM-IIIR kleptomania evaluated with the Structured Clinical Interview for DSM-IIIR,[14] all 20 patients met criteria for a lifetime mood disorder (with 12 (60 per cent) having a bipolar disorder), 16 (80 per cent) for at least one anxiety disorder (with nine (45 per cent) having obsessive–compulsive disorder, eight (40 per cent) having panic disorder, and eight (40) per cent having social phobia), 12 (60 per cent) for an eating disorder, 10 (50 per cent) for a substance use disorder, and eight (40 per cent) for at least one other impulse control disorder. Of 37 people recruited by newspaper advertisement with DSM-IV-defined kleptomania, 30 (81 per cent) reported current psychiatric problems.[15] Specifically, 54 per cent had 'hereditary psychiatric illness', 43 per cent had 'more general problems related to food intake and body weight', and 22 per cent had alcohol misuse or abuse. Conversely, high rates of impulsive or compulsive stealing, including kleptomania, ranging from 12 to 79 per cent, have been found in women with eating disorders.[17]

The relationship between kleptomania and personality disorders has not been systematically studied. Of 20 patients with kleptomania, none met the DSM-IIIR criteria for antisocial personality disorder (other types were not assessed).[14] By contrast, in a study of 72 female 'psychopaths' who also met DSM-IIIR criteria for borderline personality disorder, 96 per cent of the subjects described compulsions to carry out at least one form of deviant behaviour, including stealing.[18] These behaviours were often described as 'impossible to resist' and

followed by 'relief'. These subjects, however, were probably not representative of individuals with personality disorders in general.

Family studies

Of 103 first-degree relatives of 20 patients with DSM-IIIR-defined kleptomania evaluated blindly by the family history method,[14] 22 (21 per cent) had a major mood disorder, 21 (20 per cent) had a substance use disorder, and 13 (13 per cent) had an anxiety disorder, including seven (7 per cent) with obsessive–compulsive disorder. Also, two (2 per cent) had apparent kleptomania.

Biological studies

There are no biological studies of kleptomania.

Treatment response

Various types of cognitive-behavioural therapy may be effective in kleptomania.[17] There are also successful reports of the use of psychoanalytic psychotherapy, but there are negative reports as well.

Medical treatments with antidepressant or mood-stabilizing properties may be effective in kleptomania. These treatments include tricyclics, serotonin reuptake inhibitors, trazodone, lithium, valproate, and electroconvulsive therapy.[14,16] There is also one case report of a patient with kleptomania responding to high doses of the opioid antagonist naltrexone (100 to 150 mg/day).[19]

Pyromania

Definition and clinical features

Pyromania is defined in DSM-IV as follows: deliberate and purposeful fire-setting on more than one occasion (criterion A) that is associated with tension or affective arousal before the act (criterion B), fascination with, interest in, curiosity about, or attraction to fire and its situational contexts (criterion C), and pleasure, gratification, or relief when setting fires, or when witnessing or participating in their aftermath (criterion D). Also, the fire-setting is not done for monetary gain, as an expression of sociopolitical ideology, to conceal criminal activity, to express anger or vengeance, to improve one's living circumstances, in response to a delusion or hallucination, or as a result of impaired judgement (criterion E), and is not better accounted for by conduct disorder, a manic episode, or antisocial personality disorder (criterion F). In ICD-10, pyromania (or pathological fire-setting) is defined as multiple acts of, or attempts at, setting fire to property or other objects, without apparent motive, and by a persistent preoccupation with subjects related to fire and burning. The essential features are as follows:

- repeated fire-setting without any obvious motive such as monetary gain, revenge, or political extremism

- an intense interest in watching fires burn

- reported feelings of increasing tension before the act, and intense excitement immediately after it has been carried out.

Although the authors were unable to locate any systematic reports of a group of people with rigorously diagnosed pyromania, there are numerous case reports of people with repetitive fire-setting behaviour who would probably meet the DSM-IV or ICD-10 criteria for pyromania. For example, in what is still probably the largest study of pathological fire-setting, in 1951, Lewis and Yarnell[20] evaluated 1145 of 2000 American case records of males 16 years of age and older from the National Board of Fire Underwriters (selection criteria were otherwise not clearly specified). They concluded that 688 of these males were best classified as 'pyromaniacs' as 'they set fires for no practical reason and received no material profit from the act, their only motive being to obtain some sort of sensual satisfaction'. Although Lewis and Yarnell did not provide quantitative data summarizing these 688 cases, they stated that 50 of these subjects 'approached true pyromania', in that they were able to give a 'classical description of the irresistible impulse'. Specifically, before they set fires, these subjects described 'mounting tension; … restlessness; the urge for motion; … conversion symptoms such as headaches, palpitations, ringing in the ears, and the gradual merging of their identity into a state of unreality'.

Epidemiology and course

The prevalence of pyromania is unknown. Although there are numerous studies of fire-setting behaviour, few of these studies systematically assessed pyromania in their subjects. Those that have used variable definitions of pyromania and reported widely discrepant rates, ranging from none to 60 per cent.[2,20] For example, in their 1951 study of 1145 adult males with pathological fire-setting, Lewis and Yarnell[20] reported that 688 (60 per cent) could be classified as having broadly defined pyromania, but only 50 (4 per cent) as having the 'true' disorder.

Pyromania is probably more common in men than women and usually begins in adolescence or early adulthood.[20] How often childhood fire-setting represents pyromania is unknown. Clinical descriptions indicate that the course of pyromania may be episodic or chronic, but its course into old age is unknown.

Associated psychopathology and comorbidity

There are no studies of the psychiatric comorbidity of a group of people with well-defined pyromania. However, there are case reports of people with apparent pyromania who have comorbid mood, obsessive–compulsive, eating, paraphilic, and possibly psychotic disorders.[20,21] Also, of 22 impulsive fire-setters, 21 (95 per cent) met the DSM-IIIR criteria for dysthymia or major depression, 20 (91 per cent) for alcohol abuse, 15 (68 per cent) for intermittent explosive disorder, 17 (77 per cent) for borderline personality disorder, and three (14 per cent) for antisocial personality disorder.[8] Also, 16 (73 per cent) had a history of at least one suicide attempt.

Family studies

There are no family history studies of pyromania, but studies of impulsive fire-setters suggest elevated familial rates of substance use disorders.[9]

Biological studies

There are no biological studies of pyromania, but studies of impulsive fire-setters suggest they have abnormalities in central serotonergic neurotransmission.[8]

Treatment response

There are no systematic treatment studies of pyromania. There is one case report of two men in both of whom pyromania appeared to be part of a paraphilia and responded to antiandrogen medication.[21] Clinical reports on the treatment of pathological fire-setting in general stress use of various psychological interventions (e.g. cognitive-behavioural, psychoeducational, supportive, and insight-oriented) to address the fire-setting, and appropriate treatment of any comorbid psychiatric disorders.

Compulsive buying

History and clinical description

People who are compulsive buyers usually report irresistible or uncontrollable impulses to buy or shop, which they describe as senseless, intrusive, and persistent, mounting tension or anxiety with the impulses, and relief of tension and/or pleasurable feelings (e.g. 'a high', 'a buzz', or 'a rush') with the act of buying or shopping.[22–25] Although compulsive buying is not classified in DSM-IV or ICD-10 as a mental disorder, modern studies suggest that it causes significant morbidity, including personal distress, functional impairment, and financial problems (e.g. indebtedness, bankruptcy).

Epidemiology and course

Compulsive buying has an estimated prevalence of 2 to 8 per cent.[25] Indeed, in a recent study of the prevalence of various impulse control disorders in a psychiatric outpatient population, compulsive buying was the most common current (5.6 per cent) and lifetime (9.0 per cent) impulse control disorder diagnosis.[7]

Compulsive buying is probably more common in women than men.[22–25] It may begin in adolescence or adulthood and usually has either an episodic or a chronic course.

Associated psychopathology and comorbidity

Compulsive buying often co-occurs with Axis I and II disorders. Combining four comorbidity studies of 123 compulsive buyers, 66 (54 per cent) had a lifetime mood disorder, 61 (50 per cent) an anxiety disorder, and 40 (33 per cent) a substance use disorder.[22–25] Of 46 compulsive buyers assessed using both a structured interview and a self-report instrument in one study, 27 (59 per cent) met criteria for at least one personality disorder through a consensus of both instruments, most commonly obsessive–compulsive (22 per cent), borderline (15 per cent), and avoidant (15 per cent) types.[23]

Family studies

In a comparison study of the family history of psychiatric disorders (evaluated via the family history method) of first-degree relatives of 33 compulsive buyers who volunteered for a medication trial versus that of 22 comparison subjects, significantly more relatives of compulsive buyers had depression, alcoholism, or drug abuse.[25] Relatives of compulsive buyers were also more likely to have any, or more than one, psychiatric disorder. Although not assessed in the comparison relatives, compulsive buying was identified in 13 (9.5 per cent) of the first-degree relatives of the compulsive buyers.

In another study, of 18 compulsive buyers evaluated with the family history method, 17 (94 per cent) had at least one first-degree relative with a mood disorder, 11 (61 per cent) a substance use disorder, three (17 per cent) an anxiety disorder, and three (17 per cent) (two of whom were sisters) compulsive buying.[24]

Biological studies

There are no studies of the biology of compulsive buying.

Treatment response

Isolated reports of psychoanalytic and insight-oriented psychotherapy in compulsive buying have mostly been unsuccessful.[24] There is one report, however, of two patients with compulsive buying who each responded to behaviour therapy (cue exposure plus response prevention) after failing clomipramine treatment.[26]

Antidepressant and mood-stabilizing medications may be effective in compulsive buying, including serotonin reuptake inhibitors, tricyclics, bupropion, lithium, and valproate.[24] For example, in a 9-week, open-label trial of fluvoxamine (up to 300 mg/day), nine of 10 compulsive shoppers were described as improved, in that they were less preoccupied with shopping, spent less time shopping, and spent less money.[27] There is also one report of two patients with compulsive buying who responded to high doses of the opioid antagonist naltrexone (100 mg/day).[19]

Repetitive self-mutilation

Clinical description

Repetitive self-mutilation, also called deliberate self-harm or self-injurious behaviour, is the repeated, direct destruction of body tissue without suicidal intent.[28–30] Examples include skin cutting, skin burning, self-hitting, severe skin scratching, and even bone breaking. A wide range of body parts are mutilated, such as arms, legs, abdomen, head, chest, and genitals.

Although recommendations that repetitive self-mutilation be included as a formal impulse control disorder not elsewhere classified in DSM-IV were rejected because of concerns that it was usually a symptom of borderline personality disorder, numerous clinical studies suggest that this syndrome does in fact meet the DSM-IV and ICD-10 concepts of impulse control disorders, and as such, may exist in the absence of borderline personality disorder.[28–30] Specifically, repetitive self-mutilation is characterized by intrusive, recurrent, and irresistible impulses to harm oneself without suicidal intent that are associated with increasing tension, anxiety, anger, or other dysphoric states, along with relief of the uncomfortable affect with or shortly after the act of self-harm. In addition, the act of self-harm is often not associated with pain and performed privately.

Epidemiology and course

The prevalence of narrowly defined repetitive self-mutilation is unknown. Available studies, however, suggest that repetitive self-mutilation is more common in women than men, usually begins early in life (e.g. late childhood, adolescence, and early adulthood), and may persist for 10 to 15 years.

Associated psychopathology and comorbidity

Repetitive self-mutilation often co-occurs with other Axis I and II psychiatric disorders, especially mood, substance use, eating, psychotic, and borderline personality disorders. For example, in a 1983 review of 56 cases from the literature of patients with the 'deliberate self-harm syndrome', 45 per cent of patients were depressed, 41 per cent were psychotic, and 36 per cent were substance abusers.[28] In another evaluation of 54 psychiatric inpatients with 'self-injurious behaviour', eating disorders were the most common associated ICD-10 Axis I diagnosis, present in 54 per cent of patients, followed by substance use (33 per cent), affective disorders (20 per cent), and schizophrenic disorders (18 per cent).[29] Borderline and histrionic were the most frequent personality disorders, present in 52 and 23 per cent of the group, respectively. However, 22 per cent of patients did not fulfil criteria for any personality disorder.

Family history

No family history studies of repetitive self-mutilation have been conducted.

Biological studies

Preliminary biological studies in repetitive self-mutilation suggest derangement in central serotonergic and possibly endogenous opioid systems. In a study of 21 patients with major depression, the five patients who exhibited self-aggressive behaviours had significantly lower cerebrospinal fluid 5-hydroxyindoleacetic acid concentrations than the other 16 patients.[31] Similarly, in a controlled study of 42 personality- disordered subjects, 26 of whom had repetitive self-mutilation, lower serotonergic activity (as measured by platelet imipramine binding sites) was correlated with greater severity of self-mutilation.[32] In a study of the endogenous opioid system, patients with habitual self-mutilation had higher mean plasma metenkephalin concentrations than control subjects.[33]

Treatment response

There are no controlled treatment studies of narrowly defined repetitive self-mutilation. Psychological modalities that may be beneficial include cognitive-behavioural, psychoeducational, supportive, and insight-oriented therapies.[30] Regarding medical treatments, agents with antidepressant, mood-stabilizing, or antipsychotic properties may be helpful.[30,34]

Psychogenic excoriation

Clinical description

Psychogenic excoriation (also called neurotic excoriation, pathological or compulsive skin picking, and dermatotillomania) is excessive scratching, picking, gouging, or squeezing of the skin sometimes in response to an itch or other skin sensation or to remove a lesion on the skin (for example *acné excorié*).[35–37] Most patients use fingernails to excoriate the skin, but the teeth and instruments (for example tweezers, nail files, pins, or knives) are also used. Psychogenic excoriation causes substantial distress in patients, with most experiencing functional impairment and many reporting medical complications, some severe enough to warrant surgery.

Although not recognized as a distinct DSM-IV or ICD-10 disorder, psychogenic excoriation resembles an impulse control disorder in that patients often find themselves acting automatically and sometimes experience an increase in tension prior to scratching with transient relief or pleasure immediately afterwards. It also has compulsive features, in that it is repetitive, ritualistic, anxiety reducing, often resisted, and egodystonic. Moreover, some patients describe obsessions about an irregularity on the skin or preoccupations with having smooth skin.

In a recent study of the phenomenology of a group of 34 adults with psychogenic excoriation,[36] 27 (79 per cent) met DSM-IV criteria for impulse control disorder not otherwise specified. Many of these patients also had either body dysmorphic disorder ($n = 11$) or obsessive–compulsive disorder ($n = 4$). Only symptoms in a minority of patients ($n = 2$) met criteria for obsessive–compulsive disorder alone. Moreover, 29 (85 per cent) subjects reported skin sensations related to the excoriation, most commonly, idiopathic pruritus. Fourteen (41 per cent) subjects reported primary pruritus (i.e. pruritus that occurred prior to any excoriation) and met criteria for undifferentiated somatoform disorder.

Epidemiology and course

Psychogenic excoriation occurs in about 2 per cent of dermatology clinic patients, predominately in women.[35–37] The disorder may begin in adolescence or adulthood, and the mean duration of symptoms has ranged from 5 to 18 years, with a better prognosis for patients who have had the symptoms for less than 1 year.

Associated psychopathology and comorbidity

Psychogenic excoriation often co-occurs with mood and anxiety disorders. Of 34 adults with psychogenic excoriation evaluated with the Structured Clinical Interview for DSM-IV, lifetime mood disorders were diagnosed in 27 (79 per cent) of subjects, with the most common types being major depressive disorder (in 13 (38 per cent)) and bipolar disorder type II (in nine (26 per cent)).[36] Lifetime anxiety disorders were diagnosed in 19 (59 per cent) subjects, with the most common types being panic, generalized anxiety, and specific phobia (all appearing in seven (21 per cent)). The comorbidity of psychogenic excoriation and personality disorders has not been systematically studied.

Family studies

Of 56 first-degree relatives of 34 patients with psychogenic excoriation evaluated via the family history method, 17 (30 per cent) had a mood disorder, 28 (50 per cent) a substance use disorder, three (5 per cent) an anxiety disorder, one (2 per cent) hypochondriasis, one (2 per cent) an eating disorder, one (2 per cent) pathological gambling, and four (7 per cent) attention-deficit hyperactivity disorder.[36]

Treatment response

Various behavioural treatments (e.g. habit reversal) may be effective in psychogenic excoriation.[38] One controlled trial found that fluoxetine (mean dose of 55 mg/day) may be beneficial.[35] Other serotonin reuptake inhibitors and the tricyclic doxepin (which has been hypothesized to have antipruritic properties due to its antihistaminic effects) may also be effective.[37]

Onychophagia

Clinical description

Onychophagia is repetitive and excessive nail-biting.[37,39] The cuticles and skin around the nails are also frequently bitten, picked, or clipped. Onychotillomania, the excessive picking, clipping, or tearing of the nail, may be a variant.

Although not classified as a psychiatric disorder in DSM-IV or ICD-10, onychophagia resembles an impulse control disorder in that the behaviour is often automatic, irresistible, and associated with an increase of tension before and transient relief or pleasure during or immediately after its enactment.[37,39] It also has compulsive features in that it is repetitive, resisted, and associated with relief of anxiety.

Epidemiology and course

Nail-biting may affect 28 to 33 per cent of children between the ages of 7 and 10 years, 45 per cent of adolescents, 20 to 25 per cent of late adolescents and young adults, and 5 to 10 per cent of adults over the age of 30 years.[39] Boys and girls are affected equally until after the age of 10 years, when nail-biting becomes more common in boys.

Associated psychopathology and comorbidity

Onychophagia may be associated with mood, anxiety, and substance use disorders. Of 25 adult subjects who underwent a medication trial for onychophagia, 17 (68 per cent) had a lifetime Axis I psychiatric disorder—despite the exclusion of subjects with obsessive–compulsive disorder, a primary major affective disorder, current substance abuse, or psychosis.[39] Specifically, 11 (44 per cent) subjects met DSM lifetime criteria for major depression, five (20 per cent) for dysthymic disorder, six (24 per cent) for substance abuse, six (24 per cent) for generalized anxiety disorder, and three (12 per cent) for phobic disorder. Four subjects (16 per cent) had at least one personality disorder, including dependent, avoidant, passive-aggressive, histrionic, and obsessive–compulsive types.

Family studies

In one study, monozygotic twins had a 66 per cent concordance of nail-biting compared with 34 per cent in dizygotic twins.[40] In another, of 112 family members of 25 subjects entering a medication trial for onychophagia, seven (6 per cent) had severe nail-damaging behaviour, four (4 per cent) were severe nail-biters, and three (3 per cent) picked or chewed their hands or feet.[39] Two (2 per cent) members had probable obsessive–compulsive disorder, two (2 per cent) had eating disorders, one (1 per cent) had compulsive gambling, two (2 per cent) had probable mood disorder, and two (2 per cent) received psychiatric hospital admissions for unknown reasons.

Treatment response

Various cognitive-behavioural therapies (especially habit reversal, but also self-monitoring, use of bitter tasting substances, competing responses, and negative practice training) are probably effective in onychophagia.[38] Only one study has evaluated the pharmacological treatment of onychophagia. This double-blind cross-over study demonstrated that clomipramine (mean dose 120 mg/day) was significantly better than desipramine (mean dose 135 mg/day) in eliminating nail-biting, reducing nail-biting severity and impairment, and in improving overall clinical progress.[39]

Conclusion

Although some authors continue to doubt the diagnostic legitimacy of the impulse control disorders, the modern literature contains increasing numbers of reports of different types of irresistible impulses responding to treatment with medications with thymoleptic, antiepileptic, and, more recently, opioid antagonistic properties as well as to therapies with cognitive-behavioural orientations. The consistency of the 'structure' of the irresistible impulse (a core disturbance of impulsivity and compulsivity) together with reports of it responding to psychopharmacological agents and cognitive-behavioural therapies, regardless of its 'content' (the specific behaviour performed), strongly suggest that it is as a valid psychopathological symptom and that impulse control disorders are legitimate mental disorders that are in fact related.

References

1. McElroy, S.L., Keck, P.E. Jr, Hudson, J.I., and Pope, H.G., Jr (1995). Disorders of impulse control. In *Impulsivity and aggression* (ed. H. Hollander and D.J. Stein), pp. 109–36. Wiley, Chichester.

2. Bradford, J., Geller, J., Lesieur, H.R., Rosenthal, R., and Wise, M. (1996). Impulse control disorders. In *DSM-IV sourcebook* (ed. T.A. Widger, A.J. Frances, H.A. Pincus, *et al.*), Vol. 2, pp. 1007–31. American Psychiatric Press, Washington, DC.

3. American Psychiatric Association (1994). *Diagnostic and statistical manual of mental disorders* (4th edn). American Psychiatric Association, Washington, DC.

4. World Health Organization (1992). *International statistical classification of diseases and related health problems, 10th revision*. WHO, Geneva

5. Coccaro, E.F., Kavoussi, R.J., Berman, M.E., and Lish, J.D. (1998). Intermittent explosive disorder—revised: development, reliability, and validity of research criteria. *Comprehensive Psychiatry*, **39**, 1–10.

6. McElroy, S.L., Soutullo, C.A., Beckman, D.A., Taylor, P.J. Jr, and Keck, P.E. Jr (1998). DSM-IV intermittent explosive disorder: a report of 27 cases. *Journal of Clinical Psychiatry*, **59**, 203–10.

7. Zimmerman, M., Mattia, J.I., Younken, S., and Torres, M. (1998). *The prevalence of the DSM-IV impulse control disorders in psychiatric outpatients*, NR 265, p. 139. American Psychiatric Association Annual Meeting, 30 May–4 June, Toronto.

8. Virkkunen, M., DeJong, J., Bartko, J., and Linnoila, M. (1989). Psychobiological concomitants of history of suicide attempts among violent offenders and impulsive fire setters. *Archives of General Psychiatry*, **46**, 604–6.

9. Linnoila, M., DeJong, J., and Virkkunen, M. (1989). Family history of alcoholism in violent offenders and impulsive firesetters. *Archives of General Psychiatry*, **46**, 613–16.

10. Mattes, J.A. and Fink, M. (1990). A controlled family study of adopted patients with temper outbursts. *Journal of Nervous and Mental Disorders*, **178**, 138–9.

11. Brown, C.S., Kent, T.A., Bryant, S.G., *et al.* (1989). Blood platelet uptake of serotonin in episodic aggression. *Psychiatry Research*, **27**, 5–12.

12. Barratt, E.S., Stanford, M.S., Felthous, A.R., and Kent, T.A. (1997). The effects of phenytoin on impulsive and premeditated aggression: a controlled study. *Journal of Clinical Psychopharmacology*, **17**, 341–9.

13. Coccaro, E.F. and Kavoussi, R.J. (1997). Fluoxetine and impulsive aggressive behavior in personality-disordered subjects. *Archives of General Psychiatry*, **54**, 1081–8.

14. McElroy, S.L., Pope, H.G., Jr, Hudson, J.I., Keck, P.E., Jr, and White, K.L.

15. Sarasalo, E., Bergman, B., and Toth, J. (1996). Personality traits and psychiatric and somatic morbidity among kleptomaniacs. *Acta Psychiatrica Scandinavica*, **94**, 358–64.

16. Sarasalo, E., Bergman, B., and Toth, J. (1997). Theft behavior and its consequences among kleptomaniacs and shoplifters—a comparative study. *Forensic Science International*, **86**, 193–205.

17. McElroy, S.L., Keck P.E., Jr, Pope, H.G.J., and Hudson, J.I. (1991). Kleptomania: clinical characteristics and associated psychopathology. *Psychological Medicine*, **21**, 93–108.

18. Coid, J.W. (1991). An affective syndrome in psychopaths with borderline personality disorder? *British Journal of Psychiatry*, **162**, 641–50.

19. Kim, S.W. (1998). Opioid antagonists in the treatment of impulse-control disorders. *Journal of Clinical Psychiatry*, **59**, 159–64.

20. Lewis, N.D.C. and Yarnell, H. (1951). Pathological firesetting (pyromania). *Nervous and mental disease monograph 82*. Coolidge Foundation, New York.

21. Bourget, D. and Bradford, J. (1987). Fire fetishism, diagnostic and clinical implications: a review of two cases. *Canadian Journal of Psychiatry*, **32**, 459–62.

22. Christenson, G.A., Faber, R.J., and de Zwaan, M. (1994). Compulsive buying: descriptive characteristics and psychiatric comorbidity. *Journal of Clinical Psychiatry*, **55**, 5–11.

23. Schlosser, S., Black, D.W., Repertinger, S., and Freet, D. (1994). Compulsive buying. Demography, phenomenology, and comorbidity in 46 subjects. *General Hospital Psychiatry*, **16**, 205–12.

24. McElroy, S.L., Keck, P.E., Jr, Pope, H.F., Jr, Smith, J.M.R., and Strakowski, S.M. (1994). Compulsive buying: a report of 20 cases. *Journal of Clinical Psychiatry*, **55**, 242–8.

25. Black, D.W., Repertinger, S., Gaffney, G.R., and Gabel, J. (1998). Family history and psychiatric comorbidity in persons with compulsive buying: preliminary findings. *American Journal of Psychiatry*, **155**, 960–3.

26. Bernik, M.A., Akerman, D., Amaral, J.A.M.S., and Braun, R.C.D.N. (1996). Cue exposure in compulsive buying. *American Journal of Psychiatry*, **57**, 90.

27. Black, D.W., Monahan, P., and Gabel, J. (1997). Fluvoxamine in the treatment of compulsive buying. *Journal of Clinical Psychiatry*, **58**, 159–63.

28. Pattison, E.M. and Kahan, J. (1983). The deliberate self-harm syndrome. *American Journal of Psychiatry*, **140**, 867–72.

29. Herpertz S. (1995). Self-injurious behavior. Psychopathological and nosological characteristics in subtypes of self-injurers. *Acta Psychiatrica Scandinavica*, **91**, 57–68.

30. Favazza, A.R. (1998). The coming of age of self mutilation. *Journal of Nervous and Mental Disease*, **186**, 259–68.

31. Lopez-Ibor, J.J. Jr, Saiz-Ruiz, J., and Perez de los Cobos, J.C. (1985). Biological correlates of suicide and aggressivity in major depressions (with melancholia): 5-hydroxyindolacetic acid and cortisol in cerebrospinal fluid, dexamethasone suppression test and therapeutic response to 5-hydroxytryptophan. *Neuropsychobiology*, **14**, 67–74.

32. Simeon, D., Stanley, B., Frances, A., Mann, J.J., Winchel, R., and Stanley, M. (1992). Self-mutilation in personality disorder: psychological and biological correlates. *American Journal of Psychiatry*, **149**, 221–6.

33. Coid, J., Allolio, B., and Rees, L.H. (1983). Raised plasma metenkephalin in patients who habitually mutilate themselves. *Lancet*, **ii**, 545–6.

34. Khouzam, H.R. and Donnelly, N.J. (1997). Remission of self-mutilation in a patient with borderline personality disorder during risperidone therapy. *Journal of Nervous and Mental Disease*, **185**, 348–9.

35. Simeon, D., Stein, D.J., Gross, S., Islam, N., Schmeidler, J., and Hollander, E. (1997). A double-blind trial of fluoxetine in pathologic skin picking. *Journal of Clinical Psychiatry*, **58**, 341–7.

36. Arnold, L.M., McElroy, S.L., Mutasim, D.F., Dwight M.M., Lamerson, C.L., and Morris E.M. (1998). Characteristics of 34 adults with psychogenic excoriation. *Journal of Clinical Psychiatry*, **59**, 509–14.

37. Arnold, L.M. Dermatology. In *Psychiatric care of the medical patient* (2nd edn) (ed. A. Stoudemire, B.S. Fogel, and D. Greenberg). Oxford University Press, New York, in press.

38. Peterson, A.L., Campise, R.L., and Azrin, N.H. (1994). Behavioral and pharmacological treatments for tic and habit disorders: a review. *Developmental and Behavioral Pediatrics*, **15**, 430–41.

39. Leonard, H.L., Lenane, M.C., Swedo, S.E., Rettew, D.C., and Rapoport, J.L. (1991). A double-blind comparison of clomipramine and desipramine treatment of severe onychophagia (nail biting). *Archives of General Psychiatry*, **48**, 821–7.

40. Bakwin, H. (1971). Nail-biting in twins. *Developmental Medicine and Child Neurology*, **13**, 304–7.

4.13.2 Trichotillomania

Gary Christenson

Trichotillomania denotes the pulling out of one's own hair. Tricho-cryptomania refers to breaking off the hair and can be conceptualized as a similar condition.

Definition

Both DSM-IV[1] and ICD-10[2] define trichotillomania similarly. Recurrent pulling out of one's hair must result in noticeable hair loss. An increasing sense of tension is experienced before hair pulling (or when attempting to resist the behaviour according to DSM-IV) and pleasure, gratification, or relief results from pulling out hair. Hair pulling should not be better accounted for by another mental disorder or be due to a dermatological or other medical condition. DSM-IV requires that the disturbance causes clinically significant distress or impairment in functioning.

Not all patients, particularly children, report mounting tension, tension reduction, or gratification when pulling out hair.[3] Additionally, a patient may have a completely denuded scalp yet deny much stress or impaired functioning. Therefore the term trichotillomania is typically used to refer to the minimum criteria of visible hair loss secondary to hair pulling, which is not attributable to psychotic thinking or a medical condition.

Clinical features

Hair pulling sites

Scalp hair is pulled out in approximately 80 per cent of cases, resulting in diverse patterns of bald patches and/or hair thinning.[3] One pattern of hair loss, tonsure (Fig. 1), is characterized by a circular denuded patch over the top of the scalp.

Most patients pull from multiple hair sites. The most common sites, in descending order of frequency, are the scalp, eyelashes, eyebrows, pubis, face, and the extremities.[4] Rarely, hair is additionally pulled from spouses, children, or pets. Children may pull hair from dolls.[3]

Associated features

Hair pulling is typically accomplished by grasping individual hairs between the thumb and index finger,[3] although some patients utilize tweezers or other devices to pull out hair. Hair which is coarse, kinky, or in other ways texturally distinct may be preferentially targeted. For some patients the examination of the hair in general, or root in particular, is an important aspect of their behaviour. Half of hair pullers rub the pulled hair over their lips or bite off the hair end or root; approximately 10 per cent admit to hair ingestion (trichophagy).[4]

Trichotillomania is typically painless.[4] Increased pain tolerance (and/or thresholds) has been proposed as a permissive factor to the development of trichotillomania, but this has not been verified. A minority of patients describe pain as pleasurable.[3]

A distinction between 'automatic' versus 'focused' hair pulling has been proposed.[4] Automatic hair pulling occurs with little or no awareness, and as a parallel behaviour to other mental or behavioural activity. Automatic hair pulling typically occurs during 'sedentary contemplative' activities such as reading, watching TV, working at a desk, driving, speaking on the phone, or lying in bed at night. In contrast, during 'focused' hair pulling attention is centred on the hair pulling itself. Focused hair pulling may involve certain rules (for example symmetrical pulling) or goals (for example obtain a hair with intact root) and shares greater similarities to compulsions. Of all patients with tri-

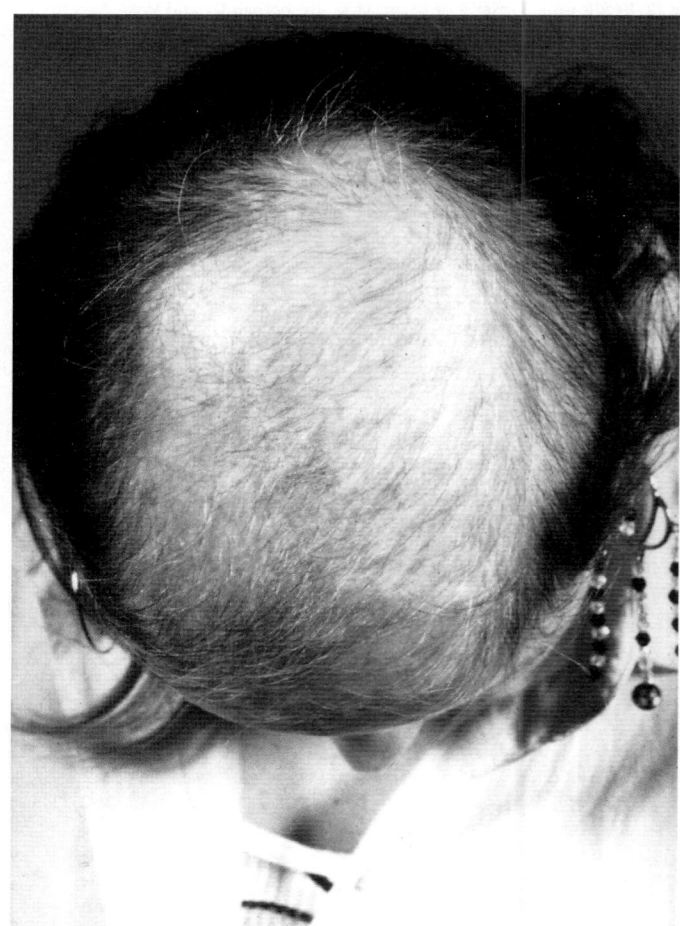

Fig. 1 Tonsure pattern of hair loss in trichotillomania.

chotillomania 75 per cent report their primary style of hair pulling as being automatic, with the remainder reporting the focused style as primary.[3] However, many, if not most, patients report engaging in both styles to some degree.[3]

Sex ratio

In clinical samples, approximately 90 per cent of adult hair pullers are female, although this observation may be biased by referral patterns.[3] One large epidemiological survey of freshman college students noted a female to male ratio of 2.3 to 1.[5] The sex ratio in young children may be even greater.[3]

Avoidant behaviours

Hair pullers may avoid situations which could reveal hair loss.[3] Swimming, wind, well-lit conditions, or environments in which others might look down upon the scalp (e.g. sports ground seating, restaurants) are often avoided. Hair stylists may be avoided as well as doctors. Some hair pullers isolate themselves from intimate relationships or, if entered into a relationship, never reveal the real reason for their hair loss. Hair pullers often spend excessive amounts of time styling their hair. Wigs, scarves, and hats are used to conceal hair loss. Wide-rimmed glasses, false eyelashes, or extensive make-up are applied in cases of lash or brow pulling.

Comorbidity

Psychiatric comorbidity is frequent in trichotillomania.[3,4] Half of patients have past or present episode of major depression. Generalized anxiety disorder is found in over one-quarter of patients. The prevalence of obsessive–compulsive disorder in trichotillomania has been reported to range between 13 per cent to 27 per cent, a rate far greater than that expected in the general population.[3] Other anxiety disorders, eating disorders, and chemical dependency are common. There is no specific personality disorder associated with trichotillomania. Whether or not another psychiatric disorder is present, low self-esteem, a diminished sense of attractiveness, shame, and embarrassment are common.[3,6]

Trichotillomania by definition results in dermatological consequences (namely thinned or denuded hair). A distinct histopathological profile is evident on biopsy.[7] Recurrent pulling or scratching can lead to erythema, scabbing, or infection.[3] Hair regrowth may be grey, white, thick, and/or curly. Dermal scarring occurs infrequently.[6] Repetitive pulling has occasionally resulted in musculoskeletal and neurological problems such as carpal tunnel syndrome.[6] Trichobezoars (hair balls) can develop secondary to hair ingestion. Although rare in adults,[4] a high index of suspicion should be maintained for the presence of trichobezoars in young hair pullers.[3] Untreated trichobezoars are associated with high rates of morbidity and mortality.[3]

Classification

Trichotillomania is currently classified as an impulse-control disorder in both DSM-IV[1] and ICD-10.[2] Such disorders are characterized by the presence of mounting tension before the behaviour and pleasure or relief during or after the behaviour. They are egosyntonic (that is to say

they are consistent with the will of the patient at the time). Although most individuals with trichotillomania describe such traits, the breadth of phenomenological experience with trichotillomania has led to proposals that trichotillomania is better described as a tic or a habit,[6] an obsessive–compulsive spectrum disorder,[8] or an affective spectrum disorder.[9] Additionally, it has even been proposed that trichotillomania is not a disorder *per se*, but one of many behavioural symptoms of anxiety, depression, or a more general state of tension.[4,6]

Differential diagnosis

The diagnosis of trichotillomania in adults is usually straightforward since patients usually admit to pulling out hair.[3] However, young children may not admit to hair pulling and may never have been observed pulling out hair.[3,10] Dermatological conditions such as alopecia areata may then be mistakenly diagnosed.[9] Scalp biopsy will differentiate between trichotillomania and other dermatological conditions.[7]

The diagnosis of trichotillomania should not be made if hair pulling occurs in response to a delusion or hallucination.[1,2] Hair pulling typically is not associated with obsessions or specific rules as in obsessive–compulsive disorder.[4] DSM-IV[1] excludes hair pulling from the diagnosis of stereotypic movement disorder; whereas in ICD-10[2] the diagnosis of stereotypic movement disorder with hair pulling can be made, but it should generally be reserved for hair pulling accompanying other stereotypies in the context of mental retardation or developmental delay.

Epidemiology

There are no systematic studies of the prevalence of trichotillomania in the general population. Most attempts at estimating prevalence have used college populations.[3] In the largest study, the lifetime prevalence was estimated to be 0.6 per cent for strict DSM-IIIR criteria and 2.5 per cent (3.4 per cent female; 1.5 per cent male) when more broadly defined.[5]

Aetiology

Dynamic explanations

The current literature tends to ignore dynamic theory in favour of behavioural and biological models. However, dynamic formulations for trichotillomania have included disturbances in the mother–infant bond, early mother deprivation, hair acting as a transitional object, renouncement of adulthood, denial of femininity, attempts at masculinization, attempts to resolve the Oedipal conflict, symbolic castration, autoaggression, masochism, autoerotism, and hair pulling equating to a masturbatory equivalent.[11] Loss or perceived loss is frequently reported as being associated with the onset of trichotillomania.[3] Such losses have been due to injury, isolation, decreased attention, or loss of contact with friends, parents, or other family members. Mothers of patients with trichotillomania have been characterized as ambivalent, competitive, and mutually dependent on their daughters, and fathers characterized as passive and emotionally distant.[12]

Serotonin dysregulation

A connection between trichotillomania and serotonin dysregulation is hypothesized due to the similarities between trichotillomania and obsessive–compulsive disorder.[13] Reports of the efficacy of the serotonin-reuptake inhibitors in the treatment of trichotillomania supports this hypothesis, as does a correlation between the trichotillomania response to serotonergic drugs and baseline serotonin metabolite levels.[14] Challenge of trichotillomania subjects to the serotonergic partial agonist *m*-chlorophenylpiperazine results in a mild euphoria, a response typical of conditions characterized by impulse control, but not the typical endocrine, behavioural, and emotional responses observed in obsessive–compulsive disorder.[14] The dopaminergic and opioid systems, have also been hypothesized to be important in trichotillomania.[14]

Brain localization

The repetitive nature of trichotillomania as well as its similarity to tics and grooming behaviours implies a potential involvement of orbitofrontal–basal ganglia brain circuitry.[14] Volumetric magnetic resonance imaging studies demonstrate a reduced left putamen volume but no caudate abnormalities.[14] Baseline glucose hypermetabolism of the right superior parietal lobe, bilateral cerebellum, and whole brain, as well as a negative correlation between anterior cingulate and orbitofrontal metabolism and serotonin-reuptake inhibitor (clomipramine) treatment response, has been observed using positron emission tomography.[15] Studies of neurospsychological testing have been inconsistent, but they suggest a possible visuospatial dysfunction mediated by corticostriatal pathways.[14] The onset of trichotillomania in very young children has been observed to be associated with streptococcal infection, and has been hypothesized to occur when antistreptococcal antibodies crossreact with the basal ganglia.[9]

Ethological parallels

Abnormal grooming behaviours in other species include canine acral lick in dogs, feline psychogenic alopecia in cats, and feather picking in birds. Grooming in animals is often considered to be a fixed-action pattern, a complex innate behavioural sequence mediated by deep brain structures such as the basal ganglia. Inappropriate fixed-action patterns, referred to as displacement behaviours, are observed in situations characterized by heightened physiological stress or arousal. The conceptualization of trichotillomania as a displacement behaviour is supported by phenomenological similarities to animal displacement behaviours as well as similar treatment responses of both trichotillomania and animal grooming disorders to serotonin-reuptake inhibitors and opiate antagonists.[16]

Course and prognosis

Trichotillomania usually develops in childhood or adolescence with a mean age of onset around 13 years.[3,4] Claims that trichotillomania is usually self-limited in childhood are only partially substantiated.[3] Prognosis may be better if the duration of trichotillomania at inter-

vention is 6 months or less. Otherwise, the disorder typically takes on a chronic waxing and waning course. Prognosis following treatment has been poorly studied. However, patients with comorbid borderline personality disorder or anxiety disorders appear to be more resistant to treatment.[9]

Treatment

Medication

Controlled studies[16,17]

Only three published and two abstracted medication treatment studies of trichotillomania incorporate controlled or comparison methodologies. All are limited by small sample sizes and a brief duration of treatment.

Evidence for the effectiveness of the serotonin-reuptake inhibitor clomipramine derives from two studies utilizing crossover paradigms: one demonstrating clomipramine's superiority over desipramine and another which concluded that clomipramine was equally efficacious when compared to the serotonin-selective reuptake inhibitor fluoxetine. However, fluoxetine proved ineffective in two other placebo-controlled studies.

Naltrexone, an opiate antagonist, is the only other agent to have been studied in a controlled fashion. Compared with placebo, naltrexone was statistically superior on a number of outcome measures. Potential explanations for its usefulness include drug-induced decreased pain thresholds, reduced reward via internal opioid pathways, as well as effects on opioid-regulated fixed-action patterns.

Uncontrolled observations[16,17]

The negative controlled studies of fluoxetine conflict with multiple open studies and case reports of the effectiveness of this agent. The other serotonin-selective reuptake inhibitors paroxetine, fluvoxamine, sertraline, and citalopram as well as venlafaxine (which has strong but not exclusive serotonergic properties), have limited support as useful treatments for trichotillomania. The mixed indirect and direct serotonin agonist fenfluramine was noted to be initially useful in combination with a serotonin-reuptake inhibitor and then as a single agent.

Lithium was found to be useful for a small series of trichotillomania patients, some of whom were characterized by emotional instability. Case studies have reported the usefulness of antidepressants including the tricyclics amitriptyline, desipramine, and imipramine, the tetracyclic mianserin, the monamine oxidase inhibitor isocarboxazid, and the serotonin receptor antagonists trazodone and nefazodone. The anxiolytics buspirone and clonazepam have also been helpful, as has the progestin levonorgestrel.

Neuroleptics have occasionally been useful in cases associated with psychosis and autism. Augmentation of serotonin-reuptake inhibitors with haloperidol, pimozide, and risperidone as well as the atypical antipsychotic olanzapine have also been efficacious. The presence of comorbid tics may be a predictor of the treatment response to neuroleptic augmentation.

Patients with trichotillomania sometimes report pruritis or other skin sensations at the site of pulling. The addition of topical steroid (fluocinolone) to serotonin-reuptake inhibitors has been useful in these circumstances. Topical capsaicin assisted in the behavioural treatment of a patient with trichotillomania, in which the drug assisted the patient's awareness of the pulling via a heightened pain sensation.

Medication continuation[16,17]

Few reports comment on the utility of long-term treatment with medications. A moderate success with selective serotonergic agents has been reported to surpass 4 years of treatment, although medication changes and additional treatment approaches were often required. Other reports suggest that any positive effects of serotonergic drugs are likely to be short-lived. The long-term efficacy of other agents has not been addressed.

Behavioural therapy

Many behavioural techniques are effective for treating trichotillomania.[18,19] However, most of the behavioural literature is limited to case reports and case series lacking randomized controlled methodologies. Behavioural approaches have included self-monitoring, therapist praise, token economy, differential reinforcement of other behaviours, relaxation training, rational emotive therapy, self-instruction, and covert desensitization. Punishment/aversive techniques include self-administered rubber band snaps, faradic shock, aromatic ammonia inhalation, hand slaps, and response cost. The mildly aversive techniques of overcorrection and facial screening have been used with the developmentally disabled. Painting aversive-tasting substances on to the thumb has been successful in treating both thumb sucking and hair pulling when these behaviours covaried in young children. Aversive techniques have generally been used only when other approaches have failed, or where the patient has a limited capability in co-operating with the treatment plan (very young children and the developmentally disabled). Very short haircuts have also been effective in ameliorating trichotillomania, but this is generally discouraged due to the potential negative effects on the patients self-esteem.

Habit reversal

Habit reversal is the only behavioural technique to have been evaluated using a controlled, randomized group design.[19,20] Habit reversal is a multicomponent treatment package comprising the principal components of behaviour monitoring, relaxation, and competing-response training. A competing response is a behaviour that is incompatible with hair pulling. The patient performs the competing response (e.g. clenching a fist for 3 min), when faced with urges to pull hair or when catching themselves pulling out hair. Habit reversal was shown to be substantially superior to a comparison technique (negative practice) in a study of 34 patients.[20] More than a 90 per cent reduction in hair pulling was noted at 4 months. However, several aspects of this study's methodology have been criticized. Variations on habit reversal in both individual and group formats remain the most popular treatment for adults with trichotillomania.

Other treatment approaches

A broad variety of hypnotic techniques has been reported as being effective in the treatment of trichotillomania in single case and case series reports.[21] Traditional psychodynamic techniques have been less frequently described as beneficial.[6]

Treatment management

The relative paucity of treatment studies of trichotillomania preclude any convenient treatment algorithm.[16] However, several aspects of an individual case can be useful in considering an appropriate treatment.

Psychiatric comorbidity

Consideration of comorbid conditions in treatment selection is important, since treatment of the comorbid condition itself is often indicated and trichotillomania may be a manifestation of the comorbid condition rather than a separate issue in some cases. Treatment with a serotonin-reuptake inhibitor is recommended in cases of comorbid depression, obsessive–compulsive disorder, panic disorder, social phobia, and/or bulimia nervosa. The use of anxiolytics is reasonable in cases of generalized anxiety. Lithium should be considered in cases of mood instability. The presence of tics is a reasonable indication to consider a dopamine antagonist, probably as an augmentor to a selective serotonergic agent. The risks of extrapyramidal symptoms and tardive dyskinesia need to be considered in such circumstances.

Individual phenomenology

The presence of a predominately automatic or habitual style of hair pulling may be less responsive to medication. In these cases, behavioural techniques, particularly habit reversal, are preferable initial interventions. Hypnosis likely plays a role here as well. Focused and/or ritualized hair pulling indicates a trial of a serotonin-reuptake inhibitor. Hair pulling associated with pain might be addressed with a trial of naltrexone or topical capsaicin. Topical steroids may be a useful adjunct when pruritus is present. If an infectious cause of pruritus is suspected topical antibiotics may also assist in treatment.

Motivation

Habit reversal and self-hypnosis are two interventions that require a high degree of motivation and compliance. Although these issues are also pertinent to pharmacotherapy, medication often presents an easier mode of intervention in cases of low motivation.

Age

Although children with trichotillomania have responded to pharmacotherapy, medication response in this age group appears to be less robust.[6,10] Behavioural approaches should be considered first. Older children and adolescents may be appropriate candidates for habit-reversal therapy. However, younger children cannot be expected to possess the understanding necessary for habit reversal. In such cases alternate behavioural treatments should be tailored to the individual. Younger patients are much more likely to be affected by family dynamics centred around the patient's hair pulling.[6] Parents should be active but not overly involved in treatment.

Capability of co-operation

In addition to young children, patients with developmental delays and mental retardation may be unable to actively participate in their treatment. Medications may be a useful first approach, but several behavioural approaches (for example facial masking, token economies) can also be tailored for these populations.[18] Ethical issues must be considered when any aversive technique is considered.

Multiple interventions

No studies have yet addressed whether combined treatment approaches are superior to single-treatment paradigms.

Treatment resistance

Treatment resistance is best addressed by re-evaluating motivation and compliance and combining treatment approaches. In the case of serotonin-selective reuptake inhibitors, augmentation with dopamine antagonists (for instance naltrexone) and topical steroids have all been reported as having improved the treatment response.[16,17]

Prevention of recurrence

Although no formal studies have investigated the utility of prevention strategies, limited follow-up data suggests that continued treatment, including modulation of the original intervention, are typically required.[16,17]

References

1. American Psychiatric Association (1994). *Diagnostic and statistical manual of mental disorders* (4th edn). American Psychiatric Association, Washington, DC.
2. World Health Organization (1992). *International statistics and classification of diseases and related health problems* (10th revision). World Health Organization, Geneva.
3. Christenson, G.A. and Mansueto, C.S. (1999). Trichotillomania: descriptive characteristics and phenomenology. In *Trichotillomania* (ed. D. Stein, G. Christenson, and E. Hollander), pp. 1–41. American Psychiatric Press, Washington, DC.
4. Christenson, G.A., Mackenzie, T.B., and Mitchell, J.E. (1991). Characteristics of 60 adult chronic hair pullers. *American Journal of Psychiatry*, **148**, 365–70.
5. Christenson, G.A., Pyle, R.L., and Mitchell, J.E. (1991). Estimated lifetime prevalence of trichotillomania in college students. *Journal of Clinical Psychiatry*, **52**, 415–17.
6. O'Sullivan, R.L., Keuthan, N.J., Christenson, G.A., Mansueto, C.S., Stein, D.J., and Swedo, S.E. (1997). Trichotillomania: behavioral symptom or clinical syndrome. *American Journal of Psychiatry*, **154**, 1442–9.
7. Muller, S.A. (1990). Trichotillomania: a histopathologic study in sixty-six patients. *Journal of the American Academy of Dermatology*, **23**, 56–62.
8. McElroy, S.L., Hudson, J.I., Pope, H.G., Keck, P.E., and Aizley, H.G. (1992). The DSM-IIIR impulse control disorders not elsewhere classified: clinical characteristics and relationships to other psychiatric disorders. *American Journal of Psychiatry*, **149**, 318–27.
9. Swedo, S.E. and Leonard, H.L. (1992). Trichotillomania. An obsessive compulsive spectrum disorder? *Psychiatric Clinics of North America*, **15**, 777–90.
10. Reeve, R. (1999). Hair pulling in children and adolescents. In *Trichotillomania* (ed. D. Stein, G. Christenson, and E. Hollander), pp. 201–24. American Psychiatric Press, Washington, DC.
11. Koblenzer, C.S. (1999). Psychoanalytic perspectives in trichotillomania. In *Trichotillomania* (ed. D. Stein, G. Christenson, and E. Hollander), pp. 125–45. American Psychiatric Press, Washington, DC.
12. Greenberg, H.R. and Sarner, C.A. (1965). Trichotillomania: symptom and syndrome. *Archives of General Psychiatry*, **12**, 482–9.
13. Swedo, S.E., Leonard, H.L., Rapoport, J.L., Lenane, M.C., Goldberger, E.L., and Cheslow, D.L. (1989). A double-blind comparison of clomipramine and desipramine in the treatment of trichotillomania (hair pulling). *New England Journal of Medicine*, **321**, 497–501.
14. Stein, D.J., O'Sullivan, R.L., van Heerden, B., Seedat, S., and Niehaus, D. (1998). The neurobiology of trichotillomania. *CNS Spectrum*, **3**, 47–51.
15. Swedo, S.E., Rapoport, J.L., Leonard, H.L., Schapiro, M.B., Rapoport, S.I., and Grady, C.L. (1991). Regional cerebral glucose metabolism in women with trichotillomania. *Archives of General Psychiatry*, **48**, 828–33.
16. Christenson, G.A. and O'Sullivan, R.L. (1996). Trichotillomania: rational treatment options. *CNS Drugs*, **6**, 23–34.
17. O'Sullivan, R.L., Christenson, G.A., and Stein, D.J. (1999). Pharmacotherapy of trichotillomania. In *Trichotillomania*. (ed. D. Stein, G. Christenson, and E. Hollander), pp. 93–123. American Psychiatric Press, Washington, DC.
18. Friman, P.C., Finney, J.W., and Christophersen, E.R. (1984). Behavioral treatment of trichotillomania: an evaluative review. *Behavior Therapy*, **15**, 249–65.
19. Keuthan, N.J., Aronowitz, B., Badenoch, J., and Wihelm, S. (1999). Behavioral treatment for trichotillomania. In *Trichotillomania*. (ed. D. Stein, G. Christenson, and E. Hollander), pp. 147–66. American Psychiatric Press, Washington, DC.
20. Azrin, N.H., Nunn, R.G., and Frantz, S.E. (1980). Treatment of hairpulling (trichotillomania): a comprehensive study of habit reversal and negative practice training. *Journal of Behavior Therapy and Experimental Psychiatry*, **11**, 13–20.
21. Robiner, W.N., Edwards, P.E., and Christenson G.A. (1999). Hypnosis in the treatment of trichotillomania. In *Trichotillomania* (ed. D. Stein, G. Christenson, and E. Hollander), pp. 167–99. American Psychiatric Press, Washington, DC.

4.13.3 Special psychiatric problems relating to gambling

Emanuel Moran

Introduction

Gerolamo Cardano (1501–1576), in his treatise *Liber de Ludo Alae* (*The Book on Games of Chance*),[1] used his own experience of gambling to formulate the laws of probability. He was a physician and scholar in Milan, who gambled heavily himself. In the chapter on 'The utility of play, and losses', he drew attention to:

> …the danger that it may become a settled habit…For then a man is carried away into playing for high stakes…so that he no longer has control of his own mind. As a result he throws out large sums of money and may be said to abandon them rather than play for them.

Cardano stated that gambling 'ought to be discussed by a medical doctor like one of the incurable diseases' and referred to it as a 'natural evil'. However, at a behavioural level, gambling is an activity with the following elements.

1. A contract between two or more people, which is based on a forecast of the outcome of an uncertain event involving random processes.

2. Property, referred to as the stake, is transferred between those taking part, so that some gain at the expense of others.

3. The property transfer depends on the outcome or result of the uncertain event, which has been forecast.

4. Participation is voluntary and not necessarily related to gaining property, but may be used to obtain an experience.

Cardano emphasized that, 'the most fundamental principle of all in gambling is simply equal conditions'. However, gambling is usually organized on a commercial basis with a promoter, who may be at a distance, as in fruit/slot machine gambling. Promoters make their profit by setting the odds in their favour, with an inbuilt disadvantage to the others taking part.

Clinical features

Gambling misuse can usually be recognized by the presence of any of the following features.

1. Concern about gambling, which is considered to be excessive either in terms of the money spent or the time devoted.

2. Intermittent or continuous preoccupation with gambling and the development of tolerance and craving for it.

3. Loss of control over gambling and 'chasing of losses', despite the realization that damage is resulting.

4. Disorder affecting the person who is gambling and the family:

   (a) financial disturbances, such as debt and shortage;

   (b) social disturbances, such as loss of employment and friends, running away from home, eviction, marital problems, divorce, behaviour disorders in the children of the family, criminality and imprisonment;

   (c) psychological disturbances, such as depression and attempted suicide.

Classification

In the past, this syndrome has been referred to as compulsive gambling. However, it is not a true obsessive–compulsive state but a heterogeneous group of conditions, characterized by excessive gambling resulting in disturbance for those involved. The term 'pathological gambling' is more appropriate, since it is not based on any assumptions concerning the underlying processes.[2]

ICD-10[3] describes pathological gambling as a form of behaviour under 'habit and impulse disorders'. On the other hand, DSM-IV[4] implies a homogeneous disease entity and provides criteria for its recognition under 'impulse-control disorders not elsewhere classified'. The ICD-10 approach is preferable.

A total of five varieties of pathological gambling can be recognized.[2,5]

1. Symptomatic gambling occurs in mental illness, usually depression, which is the primary disorder.

2. Neurotic gambling occurs as a response to an emotional problem, particularly in a disturbed relationship in marriage or during adolescence.

3. Impulsive gambling is characterized by loss of control for varying periods and is particularly liable to be associated with tolerance, craving, and dependence on the activity.

4. Psychopathic gambling is part of the generalized disturbance of behaviour that characterizes antisocial personality disorder.

5. Subcultural gambling arises out of the person's background, which is one of socially accepted heavy gambling.

Diagnosis

In general, pathological gambling is most easily recognized in men. This seems to be due to the fact that, for various social reasons, horse-race and greyhound-race betting and gaming are more frequently patronized by men. These types of gambling have a high turnover of money and therefore the consequences of excess become evident more quickly.

Women are more likely to gamble on lotteries, bingo, and football pools. These may not involve such large sums of money. When excess occurs, the presentation is much more subtle with disturbances in the social sphere rather than through the accumulation of large debts. However, the situation has changed considerably in recent years with the vast increase of interest in lotteries in various parts of the world.

While pathological gambling is seen at all ages, an increasing number of children and young people are presenting with difficulties as a result of excessive gambling. This is in spite of the fact that most jurisdictions treat gambling as an adult activity and those under the age of 18 years tend to be prohibited from taking part. In the 1980s, excessive gambling among children and young people was largely seen in the setting of fruit/slot machine gambling. This has often been available to children on the dubious pretext that it is an 'amusement with prizes' rather than gambling, which it clearly is. Since the appearance of various national and state lotteries, and their ready availability in public places, heavy gambling on these by children and young people has occurred. Many, who have gambled heavily in childhood and adolescence, have subsequently gone on to pathological gambling in adulthood.

Aetiology and epidemiology

The nature of gambling

Gambling with its winnings and losses provides an opportunity for operant conditioning.[6] The most effective learning schedule is one of intermittent variable ratio reinforcement. This unpredictable contingency of reinforcement is exploited by gambling promoters. Since it produces a stable and persistent response, the long-term net gain or loss to those who gamble is almost irrelevant. Within this setting, a large win when gambling is first started ('beginner's luck') may produce the predisposition to pathological gambling.

The speed of turnover of the event, which is the basis of the gamble, varies from being very rapid in gaming such as roulette at one extreme, to being rather more slow in other types of gambling such as lotteries. The former are therefore more likely to be taken to excess, but the situation is also affected by the size of the possible prize. The advent of national and state lotteries with very large jackpot prizes makes these types of gambling appear attractive. Even though the chances of winning these are extremely small, they encourage excess.[7]

While limited skill may be applied in certain types of gambling, this is usually over-rated. Indeed, much of the supposed skill implies an unrealistic ability to control the uncertain event that is the subject of the gamble.[8] If a win occurs, such notions appear to be confirmed and encourage further gambling.

Traditionally, the most that can be lost in gambling is the money staked. However, new types have recently appeared. Thus, in spread-betting, winnings and losses are multiples of the money staked. In gambling on the Internet, often operated by unscrupulous promoters, the money is staked via credit cards. These have introduced new possibilities for excess, especially in the setting of 'chasing losses'.

Social pressures

The experience of risk provides amusement, thrill, and excitement and may therefore be pleasurable. These experiences make gambling so attractive. This has led to it being organized commercially, so that it is not usually available on the basis of what Cardano[1] referred to as 'equal conditions', but with an inbuilt disadvantage to those who gamble. In reality, the stake money is used to purchase an experience, with winnings as an occasional bonus. A few, who gamble professionally, are able also to win money regularly because they have sources of information that reduce the uncertainty, as in betting on horses and dogs, and their gambling is planned and deliberate.[9]

Yet, those who gamble are encouraged by the promoters to think that it is a form of investment and will lead to the accumulation of wealth. In addition, they are often given dubious information, which it is claimed will enable them to improve their chances of winning. All this inevitably incites people to gamble more and eventually leads to pathological gambling.[10,11]

In the United Kingdom, public policy has operated on the principle of providing gambling facilities on the basis of unstimulated demand, since this limits the level of pathological gambling.[12] Recently, this principle has been eroded because governments have increasingly relied on national and state lottery takings for revenue purposes. One of the most insidious aspects of this has been the promotion of the idea that lotteries, in particular, and gambling, in general, are ways for those taking part to make money.[7]

Also, the advent of large lotteries has made this heavily promoted form of gambling available in public places, whereas, previously, commercial gambling involving large sums of money has generally been confined to licensed premises. This has resulted in children becoming involved.[13]

Predisposing factors

In the presence of social pressures, predisposed individuals are propelled towards pathological gambling. Some of the factors involved in this predisposition are discussed below.

Morbid risk-taking

Since gambling is a type of risk-taking, it lends itself to be used by those who, for reasons related to their personality, have a high need for risk. They spend large sums of money on the intangible commodity of risk, which may easily pass unnoticed because it is fleeting.

This morbid propensity to take risks shows itself in other ways. Thus, the incidence of attempted suicide appears to be about eight times the expected rate among those who gamble pathologically.[5]

Other personality factors

Freud[14] asserted that gambling resembles masturbation, is a substitute for it, and is resorted to in the context of unresolved Oedipal difficulties. Also, pathological gambling may be a manifestation of self-punishment, with an unconscious desire to lose arising from a psychological mechanism that has been referred to as 'psychic masochism'.[15]

Those who gamble pathologically appear to have other predisposing personality traits. They view their behaviour as being largely determined by factors outside their personal control. They also tend towards greater impulsivity.[5,16]

Learning processes

Apart from the winnings and losses, the gambling situation itself may affect learning. As far as the random processes inherent in gambling are concerned, all participants, even a total failure, stand on an equal footing. This may be the only circumstance in which some people have this experience. Gambling may therefore provide a means of dealing with morbid anxiety in the presence of feelings of inferiority, leading to a conditioned avoidance reaction. In this situation, there is more likely to be psychological dependence on gambling and loss of control.[17,18]

Mental disorder

Pathological gambling may occur in any mental disorder. However, it is most commonly associated with depression. More usually, a neurotic type of depression occurs after a bout of heavy gambling with large losses. In symptomatic pathological gambling, the depression is primary and a response to the tension and feelings of guilt that occur in depression. This latter situation is similar to alcohol misuse and shoplifting, as part of the depressive syndrome. Pathological gambling may also be a manifestation of antisocial personality disorder.

Misuse of alcohol and pathological gambling can occur together; either may be the primary disorder and either may lead to the other.

Constitutional and physical factors

Twin studies have demonstrated that the likelihood of pathological gambling occurring in a person is influenced, to an important degree, by inherited factors and/or experiences shared during childhood.[19]

There also appears to be a significant association between pathological gambling and genetic abnormalities involving the dopamine reward pathways.[20] Disturbances of serotonergic, noradrenergic, and dopaminergic neurotransmitter systems have all been implicated in the aetiology of pathological gambling. This is particularly so in relation to the arousal, behavioural initiation, behavioural disinhibition, and reward/reinforcement mechanisms that are evident in this condition.[21]

Course and prognosis

The natural history of pathological gambling is one characterized by exacerbations and remissions, often related to life events. Important elements in this are relationships within the family, especially with the spouse/partner. An example of this is the not infrequent sequence of an exacerbation of heavy gambling in the husband, coterminous with the wife's first pregnancy.

The outlook in pathological gambling is usually determined by the integrity of the underlying personality. In those in whom the condition appears as a symptom of a neurotic disorder or depression, the prognosis depends on that of the underlying disorder.

Management and treatment

Pathological gambling involves a whole way of life, which has many ramifications. If its management is to be successful, there need to be major changes in the lifestyle of the person concerned. It is best dealt with by a team approach involving at least a psychiatrist, psychologist, and social worker.

Assessment of the problem

It is important to obtain a detailed appraisal of the extent and amount of gambling occurring, as well as a detailed history of the development of the gambling from its early beginnings. Since the history is often chequered, a more accurate account can usually be obtained if the person being assessed provides the information by means of a detailed written narrative. This can subsequently be amplified and used as the basis of discussion.

In addition, an attempt should be made to obtain some indication of the person's motivation. Many who seek help for pathological gambling appear not to recognize the need even to restrict their gambling. Indeed, many of these people readily admit that they enjoy it and only want assistance for the problems that have resulted. It is important to emphasize that, at least initially, there must be an immediate period of total abstinence.

Management of the finances

Excessive gambling is usually associated with a disturbed appreciation of the value of money. Because of this and the continued temptation to gamble, it is wise for the family finances to be controlled, at least for some time, by the spouse/partner or some trusted person. Regular income from wages or salaries should be paid into a bank account over which the spouse/partner or trusted person has sole control. As the period of abstinence from gambling continues, the person who has been gambling pathologically needs to become gradually involved in working jointly with whoever controls the finances.

In addition, there is a need to obtain a detailed statement of all the outstanding debts, as well as an inventory of the income and outgoings of the person seeking help and his or her family. In terms of this information, the person who has been gambling pathologically needs to be encouraged to draft a realistic plan of repayment. Since debts are often considerable, the repayments may have to continue over many years. This can obviously only be achieved by encouraging the person concerned to discuss the whole matter with the creditors involved. However, it is important that the repayments should be consistent with the person's regular income and circumstances. There is a considerable danger that in the first flush of enthusiasm, unrealistic repayments will be contemplated, which may result in temptations to gamble in order to maintain them.

Counselling

On the basis of information obtained during the course of the assessment, there must be some discussion of the nature of the activity of gambling. Attention needs to be drawn to some of the snares involved, such as exaggerated ideas of the importance of skill (information from tipsters and various dubious numbers systems), as well as the subtle ways in which loss of control can occur. This will involve discussion about the processes of habit formation and may best be dealt with by a clinical psychologist.

The person whose gambling has become pathological and the spouse/partner should be encouraged to review their social relationships. In doing so, the involvement of a social worker can be helpful. This is especially so if there have been serious marital problems that predated the pathological gambling. In particular, the couple need to consider how they spend their spare time, what friends they cultivate, and what interests they pursue. It is often within specific settings that incitement to gambling has occurred in the past, and the couple need to make very careful arrangements to avoid such situations or, at least, to be prepared for them. They may be helped in achieving their objective if they draw up a joint contract, which spells out in detail those types of behaviour to be avoided as well as those to be encouraged. This needs to be reviewed regularly.

Gamblers Anonymous

This form of self-help for pathological gambling is organized in regular local groups. As well as meetings for those who have a problem with gambling, there are also separate ones for their spouses/partners. Quite apart from the valuable work done in the group setting, Gamblers Anonymous provides a useful means of establishing alternative social contacts to those that were associated with gambling. Indeed, in some people, Gamblers Anonymous may be the vehicle through which all the necessary help can be provided. Even if this is not the case, Gamblers Anonymous still provides a valuable form of support for the individual and the family.

Psychological treatments

A variety of psychological treatments have been advocated but, in general, their long-term efficacy has not been established. A good outcome has been reported after a cognitive-behavioural approach.[22] Also, controlled gambling, rather than permanent abstinence, has led to a reported successful outcome after behavioural treatment.[23]

Psychiatric treatments

Specialist treatment from a psychiatrist and/or a psychotherapist for a neurotic disorder or severe depression may be required, if these clearly underlie the pathological gambling.

Prevention

In view of the nature of gambling and the importance of the social causation of pathological gambling, it is vital that it should be seen to be an activity that requires moderation. Public policies concerning the availability of gambling facilities and incitements to participate should reflect this.

Unfortunately, the recent increasing reliance of governments and states on lotteries for revenue purposes and the rapid development of Internet gambling make it difficult to be optimistic that this will be done.

References

1. Ore, O. (1953). *Cardano the gambling scholar.* Princeton University Press, Princeton, NJ.

2. Moran, E. (1970). Varieties of pathological gambling. *British Journal of Psychiatry*, **116**, 593–7.

3. World Health Organization (1992). *International statistical classification of diseases and related health problems, 10th revision*. WHO, Geneva.

4. American Psychiatric Association (1994). *Diagnostic and statistical manual of mental disorders* (4th edn). American Psychiatric Association, Washington, DC.

5. Moran, E. (1970). Clinical and social aspects of risk-taking. *Proceedings of the Royal Society of Medicine*, **63**, 1273–7.

6. Skinner, B.F. (1966). *Science and human behaviour*. Macmillan, New York.

7. Clotfelter, C.T. and Cook, P.J. (1991). *Selling hope: state lotteries in America*. Harvard University Press, Cambridge, MA.

8. Moran, E. (1975). Pathological gambling. In *Contemporary psychiatry: selected reviews from the British Journal of Hospital Medicine* (ed. T. Silverstone and B. Barraclough), *British Journal of Psychiatry Special Publication No.9*, pp. 416–28. Royal College of Psychiatrists, London.

9. Lowe, J. and Clark, T. (1999). *The Which? guide to gambling*. Consumers' Association, London.

10. Moran, E. (1979). An assessment of the report of the Royal Commission on gambling 1976–78. *British Journal of Addiction*, **74**, 3–9.

11. Volberg, R.A. (1994). The prevalence and demographics of pathological gamblers: implications for public health. *American Journal of Public Health*, **84**, 237–41.

12. Moran, E. (1993). The growing presence of pathological gambling in society: what we know now. In *Gambling behaviour and problem gambling* (ed. W.R. Eadington and J.A. Cornelius), pp. 135–41. University of Nevada, Reno, NV.

13. Office of the National Lottery (1998). *Gambling and problem gambling among young people in England and Wales*. Office of the National Lottery, London.

14. Freud, S. (1961). Dostoevsky and parricide. In *Standard edition of the complete psychological works of Sigmund Freud*, Vol. 21 (ed. J. Strachey), p. 177. Hogarth Press, London.

15. Bergler, E. (1970) *The psychology of gambling*. International Universities Press, New York.

16. Steel, Z. and Blaszczynski, A. (1998). Impulsivity, personality disorders and pathological gambling severity. *Addiction*, **93**, 895–905.

17. Moran, E. (1970). Gambling as a form of dependence. *British Journal of Addiction*, **64**, 419–27.

18. Wray, I. and Dickerson, M.G. (1981). Cessation of high frequency gambling and withdrawal symptoms. *British Journal of Addiction*, **76**, 528–31.

19. Eisen, S.A., Lin, N., Lyons, M.J., *et al.* (1998). Familial influences on gambling behaviour: an analysis of 3359 twin pairs. *Addiction*, **93**, 1375–84.

20. Cummings, D.E. (1998). The molecular genetics of pathological gambling. *CNS Spectrums: International Journal of Neuropsychiatric Medicine*, **3**, 20–37.

21. DeCaria, C.M., Begaz, T., and Hollander, E. (1998). Serotonergic and noradrenergic function in pathological gambling. *CNS Spectrum: International Journal of Neuropsychiatric Medicine*, **3**, 38–47.

22. Sylvain, C., Ladouceur, R., and Boisvert, J.M. (1997). Cognitive and behavioural treatment of pathological gambling: a controlled study. *Journal of Consulting and Clinical Psychology*, **65**, 727–32.

23. Blaszczynski, A., McConaghy, N., and Frankova, A. (1991). Control versus abstinence in the treatment of pathological gambling: a two to nine year follow-up. *British Journal of Addiction*, **86**, 299–306.

4.14 Sleep–wake disorders

4.14.1 Introduction to sleep–wake disorders

Gregory Stores

Introduction

A sound working knowledge of the diagnosis, significance, and treatment of sleep disorders is essential in all branches of clinical psychiatry. Unfortunately, however, psychiatrists and psychologists share with other specialties and disciplines an apparently universal neglect of sleep and its disorders in their training. Surveys in the United States and Europe point to the consistently meagre coverage of these topics in their courses at both undergraduate and postgraduate levels.[1] Others have argued for better teaching, research, and clinical provision.[2]

The following account is an introductory overview of normal sleep, the effects of sleep disturbance, sleep disorders and the risk of failure to recognize them in psychiatric practice, assessment of sleep disturbance, and the various forms of treatment that are available. The aim is to provide a background for the other chapters in this section.

Benca (Chapter 4.14.5) describes how sleep disturbance is commonly a feature of a wide range of psychiatric conditions in adults. The same point is made by Stores (Chapter 9.2.9) regarding psychiatric disorders in children and adolescents. A number of practical implications for clinical practice follow from these associations and the various other ways in which sleep disorders and psychiatric conditions are linked.

- Psychiatrists need to be familiar with the field of sleep disorders medicine whatever the age group of their patients.

- Detailed enquiries about sleep should be a basic part of the assessment of any patient.

- The possibility of psychiatric disorder should routinely be considered in any patient with a sleep complaint.

- Physiological sleep studies are unnecessary as a guide to diagnosis, choice of treatment or prognosis for most psychiatric disorders, although such investigations may be very important in the diagnosis of sleep disorders (see later).

- Whether accompanied by a psychiatric illness or not, sleep disturbance should be treated early and vigorously to prevent the development or the exacerbation of a psychological disturbance, or to limit its duration.

Basic aspects of normal sleep

Well before clinicians took an interest in such problems, accurate literary descriptions of sleep disorders were provided by Shakespeare[3] and Dickens.[4] In fact, the scientific study of sleep and its disorders is largely confined to the last several decades. Over that time, much has been established about the physiology of sleep (including phylogenetic differences and developmental changes from infancy to old age), the wide variety of ways in which sleep can become disordered causing adverse psychological and physical effects, and the methods by which sleep disorders can be treated by pharmacological and other means. These essentially interdisciplinary advances have displaced earlier speculative accounts including those in psychiatry concerning the significance of dreams, for example. They are well described in recent textbooks of sleep disorder medicine.[5,6] Only general points are mentioned here, with special reference to psychiatry where possible.

The nature of sleep

Behaviourally, sleep is a reversible state of reduced awareness of and responsiveness to the environment. Usually (but not necessarily) sleep occurs when lying down, quietly, with little movement.

Physiologically, sleep has characteristic features which distinguish it from other states of relative inactivity. Within sleep two physiologically distinct states have been defined, i.e. non-rapid eye movement (**NREM**) sleep and rapid eye movement (**REM**) sleep. Both NREM and REM sleep are active processes. Wakefulness is maintained by cortical noradrenaline (norepinephrine), dopamine, and acetylcholine from terminals of brainstem neurones. For sleep to occur, activity in the ascending reticular activating system must diminish. In addition, however, NREM sleep depends on activity especially in the basal forebrain systems, while the pons is primarily responsible for the control of REM sleep. Serotonin and γ-aminobutyric acid neurones, as well as various peptides, are involved in NREM sleep; acetylcholine is essentially involved in the generation of REM sleep.

The functions of sleep

Debate continues about the various theories about sleep, each of which has emphasized physical and psychological restoration and recovery, energy conservation, memory consolidation, discharge of emotions, brain growth, and other various biological functions including maintenance of immune systems. No one theory accounts for all the complexities of sleep and it seems likely that sleep serves multiple purposes.[7]

From the practical point of view, the most obvious observation is that both physical and psychological impairment follows persistent sleep disturbance. Animals totally deprived of sleep for very long periods die with loss of temperature regulation and multiple system failure. As described later, the adverse effects of chronic partial sleep deprivation (considered to be common in modern society) on mood, behaviour, and cognitive function can be substantial with various consequences for personal, social, occupational, and family functioning.

The physiological changes that have been studied in humans following sleep disturbance have been relatively crude (aspects of electroencephalographic, autonomic, biochemical, and endocrine function mainly in relation to experimental sleep loss). Either no change has been observed or the changes have reversed fairly promptly when sleep patterns have returned to normal. The apparently more subtle neurophysiological changes underlying the various neuropsychological deficits and psychiatric disturbance are difficult to define at present.

Sleep stages

Conventionally, standardized criteria[8] are used to identify different sleep stages according to their characteristic physiological features especially in the electroencephalographam (**EEG**), electro-oculogram, and electromyogram.

NREM sleep is divided into four stages of increasing depth. **Stage I** occurs at sleep onset or following arousal from another stage of sleep. The EEG is low voltage with mixed frequencies and reduced alpha activity compared with the awake state. Vertex sharp waves are seen in the EEG and slow rolling eye movements occur. This stage represents 4 to 5 per cent of the main sleep period. **Stage II** contains more slow activity, and sleep spindles and K complexes are seen. It accounts for 45 to 55 per cent of overnight sleep. **Stage III** (4–6 per cent of total sleep time) contains yet more slow EEG activity. **Stage IV** is characterized by the slowest activity and constitutes 12 to 15 per cent of sleep. The combination of Stages III and IV is called slow-wave sleep (**SWS**) or delta sleep. This is considered to be the deepest form of sleep from which awakening is particularly difficult. The arousal disorders (confusional arousals, sleep walking, and sleep terrors) arise from SWS.

REM sleep is physiologically very different. Brain metabolism is highest in this stage of sleep with a low voltage, mixed frequency, non-alpha EEG. Spontaneous rapid eye movements are seen and electromyogram activity is virtually absent in skeletal musculature. Heart rate, blood pressure, and respiration are all variable, body temperature regulation ceases temporarily, and penile and clitoral tumescence occurs. REM sleep usually takes up 20 to 25 per cent of total sleep time. Most dreams, including nightmares, occur in REM sleep.

Sleep architecture

NREM and REM sleep alternate cyclically throughout the night starting with NREM sleep lasting about 80 min followed by about 10 min of REM sleep. This 90-min **sleep cycle** is repeated three to six times each night. Each REM period typically ends with a brief arousal or transition into light NREM sleep.

In successive cycles the amount of NREM sleep decreases and the amount of REM sleep increases. SWS is usually confined to the first two sleep cycles. The diagrammatic representation of overnight sleep structure is known as a hypnogram, a simplified form of which is shown in Fig. 1.

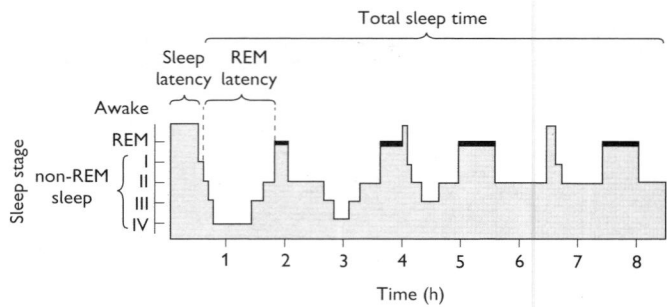

Fig. 1 Diagram of an overnight hypnogram in a young adult

This conventional sleep staging is concerned with the macrostructure of sleep but there is increasing interest in the microstructural fragmentation of sleep by frequent, brief arousals (seen mainly in the EEG) lasting a matter of seconds without obvious clinical accompaniments. This subtle type of sleep disruption, overlooked by conventional sleep staging, is increasingly associated with impairment of daytime performance, mood, and behaviour, more so than any one stage of sleep.[9]

Circadian sleep–wake rhythms

The timing of sleep (but not its amount) is regulated by a circadian 'clock' in the suprachiasmatic nucleus of the hypothalamus. Without an environmental cue to time of day (or *zeitgeber*), the duration of the endogenous 'free running' sleep–wake cycle in humans has generally been considered to be about 25 h, although doubt has been cast on this recently with the suggestion that the intrinsic circadian pacemaker is close to 24 h in human adults consistent with other species.[10] From an early age the individual's sleep–wake rhythm has to synchronize with the 24-h day–night rhythm. The main *zeitgeber* by which this is achieved ('entrainment') is sunlight, but social cues, such as meal times and social activities, are also important, as well as ambient temperature or noise level, and internal body signals such as hunger, temperature, and hormonal changes.

The suprachiasmatic nucleus also controls other biological rhythms including body temperature and cortisol production with which the sleep–wake rhythm is normally synchronized. In contrast, growth hormone in adults is locked to the sleep–wake cycle and is released with the onset of SWS, whatever its timing.

Melatonin is related to the light–dark cycle rather than the sleep–wake cycle. It is secreted by the pineal gland during darkness and suppressed by exposure to bright light. It influences circadian rhythms via the suprachiasmatic nucleus pacemaker which, in turn, regulates melatonin secretion by relaying light information to the pineal gland. Its widespread popularity as a sleep-promoting agent is not justified by what little is known about its action and clinical effectiveness.[11]

Changes with age

Changes in basic aspects of sleep are prominent from birth to old age, although individual differences are seen at all ages. As in other biological variables, any one sleep measure at a given age will show a relatively normal (bell-shaped) distribution. Changes of clinical significance include the following.

- **Total sleep time** decreases with age. Average daily values are as follows: newborns, 16 to 18 h; young children, 10 h; adolescents, 8 h; adults, 7.5 h and possibly less than this in elderly people. This total amount of sleep includes daytime napping in children up to the age of 3 years and often again in old age.

- **NREM sleep** shows an overall decrease across the lifespan. SWS is particularly prominent in young children who sleep very soundly. Its decline begins in early adolescence and continues throughout adulthood.

- The **proportion of REM sleep** declines from 50 per cent or more of total sleep time in the newborn (more than this in premature babies) to 20 to 25 per cent by 2 years. This figure remains fairly constant throughout the rest of life. The high level of REM sleep in very early life suggests a role in cerebral maturation but at present its true significance remains unclear.

- **NREM–REM sleep cycles** occur at intervals of 50 to 60 min in infants who often enter REM at the start of their sleep period. This interval between sleep cycles remains until adolescence when the periodicity changes to 90 to 100 min, which persists into adult life. The amounts of NREM and REM in each sleep cycle is about equal in early infancy. Afterwards NREM sleep (especially SWS) predominates in the earlier cycles and REM sleep in the later cycles.

- **Continuity of sleep** is greatest in early childhood (as mentioned previously) and least at the extremes of age. Infants are easily wakened and so are the elderly who also wake spontaneously more often. Fragmentation of sleep by brief arousals without actual waking is described as particularly common in the elderly (see Chapter 4.14.5) as confirmed in a recent cross-sectional study which also showed a gradual increase in brief arousals in healthy subjects from teenage to old age.[12]

- **Circadian sleep–wake rhythms** change considerably in early development. Full-term neonates show 3- to 4-h sleep–wake cycles. Sleep periods have largely shifted to the night and wakefulness to daytime by 12 months, except for napping which gradually diminishes and has usually stopped by about 3 years of age. However, a physiological tendency towards an afternoon nap remains throughout the rest of life. Although repeated brief waking at night is more common in infancy and early childhood than later, it remains a normal occurrence throughout life increasing in frequency again in old age. The clinical problem arises when there is difficulty returning to sleep after such awakenings.

Psychological effects of sleep disturbance

Bonnet[9] has comprehensively reviewed the clinical and experimental evidence that sustained sleep disturbance can have serious adverse psychological effects. The term sleep disturbance covers the following.

- Loss of sleep (i.e. shortened duration).

- Impaired quality of sleep (disruption of sleep architecture at either the macro- or microstructural level of sleep, or both).

- Inappropriate timing of the sleep period in relation to sleep–wake rhythms (as in the various circadian sleep rhythm disorders such as jet lag, shift work, or the more persistent forms seen in clinical practice).

Experimental studies of **total sleep loss** demonstrate a progressive deterioration in cognitive function, mood, and behaviour related to length of sleep loss. However, inter- and also intraindividual differences in susceptibility are seen reflecting such factors as motivation, personality, and usual sleep requirements. Task characteristics, timing of the task in relation to the circadian sleep–wake rhythm, and physical environmental factors, such as noise and other distracting stimuli, are also important.

Variations for similar reasons are reported in **partial sleep deprivation** experiments which (like those concerning fragmentation of sleep) are much closer to real-life sleep disturbance caused by social activities, job demands and other aspects of modern lifestyle. These studies raise the issues of how much sleep is needed for optimal daytime functioning and whether these requirements are not being met. It has been argued that there is a 'national sleep debt' in the United States (and other Western countries) and that by sleeping longer than they do habitually, many people would increase their performance and improve their well being during the day.[13] This view has been contested.[14]

Whatever the size of the sleep deprivation problem in the community, experimental evidence does suggest that a consistent reduction of the total sleep time by more than about 1 to 2 h compared with the individual's unrestricted sleep period is likely to affect daytime performance and behaviour. This is in keeping with the suggestion that the first few overnight NREM–REM sleep cycles (core sleep) are the most important part of sleep for brain restitution rather than either NREM or REM sleep individually.[15] As already mentioned, however, continuity of sleep is important, as well as timing of the sleep phase.

The usual subjective effects of sleep disturbance are mood changes, especially irritability, and complaints of fatigue and poor concentration. More dramatic effects are described with prolonged and severe sleep disturbance such as disorientation, illusions, hallucinations, persecutory ideas, and inappropriate behaviour with impaired awareness (automatic behaviour) caused by frequent microsleeps. Psychometric studies have shown that sleep disturbance can produce a range of cognitive impairments, again depending on its duration and individual susceptibility. Sustained attention (vigilance) is particularly vulnerable and possibly divergent intelligence or creativity.[16] A recent meta-analysis of research findings in adults indicated that the mean level of functioning of sleep-deprived subjects was equivalent to only the ninth percentile of non-sleep deprived subjects. In addition, however, mood was more affected by sleep deprivation than cognitive performance and much more than psychomotor function, which, however, was still significantly worse than in the non-sleep-deprived groups.[17]

The experimental findings are in keeping with the results from studies of various occupational groups, including junior hospital doctors[18] and drivers of various types of vehicle,[19] in which reduced performance or accidents are associated with sleep disturbance. The common and increasing practice of shiftwork is contrary to the fundamental biorhythm of sleeping at night and being awake during the day, and is often accompanied by a reduction in total sleep time and poor-quality sleep. It is not surprising that working shifts commonly results in loss of well being, physical complaints, and impaired productivity and safety. Similarly, the distribution over the 24-h period of road accidents (especially those not involving other vehicles) and other mishaps at work, corresponds to that of the levels of sleep tendency assessed objectively. Even industrial and engineering disasters have been attributed to sleep loss and impaired performance on the part of key personnel.[20]

Additional evidence that sleep disturbance affects daytime function comes from neuropsychological studies of certain sleep disorders. The impaired performance on prolonged and complex tasks of subjects with narcolepsy has been shown to be secondary to the effects of their daytime sleepiness rather than to an intrinsic neurological deficit. In adult patients with obstructive sleep apnoea, attention and memory impairments (like the depression and irritability commonly reported by these patients) are also largely attributable to daytime sleepiness and the limitations that this imposes. However, there is some evidence that their deficits in more complicated 'executive functions' (formulating goals, planning and carrying out plans effectively) are not necessarily reversed when their sleepiness is relieved by treatment. This might be the result of irreversible anoxic brain damage in the later stages of the condition.[21] Clearly, early detection and treatment of this condition is essential to prevent this happening.

Both clinical and polysomnographic recovery from short periods of sleep disturbance occurs after much less sleep than that originally lost, for example, after one night's sleep following sleep loss over several days and nights. Reversal of the effects of prolonged sleep disturbance in real life is likely to be complicated, for example, by the emotional consequences of the disturbance.

Almost all the above observations about the psychological effects of sleep disturbance have been made on adult subjects or patients. The area is largely unexplored in other age groups but there is no reason why the general principles should not apply in children[22] and the elderly. In one recent study of children with nocturnal asthma, it was possible to demonstrate that an improvement in the physiological quality of sleep (achieved by better asthma control) was associated with improvements in some aspects of daytime psychological function.[23]

Another group on whom further research is particularly required are people with mental retardation. Neglect of this group, despite the strong evidence of their very high rates of sleep disturbance,[24] is reflected in their omission from the section concerned with mental and neurological disorders in the *International Classification of Sleep Disorders* (described below). The available literature provides good reason to believe that the sleep disorders, especially in the more severely retarded groups, not only affect the majority but also are unusually severe and long lasting because of lack of appropriate advice and treatment. The sleep disturbance is a problem in its own right, and is often associated with various cognitive and behavioural abnormalities which might, at least partly, be the consequence of the sleep disturbance.

Improvement in the duration or the quality of sleep may be one of the few ways of improving the psychological well being of people with mental retardation (and that of their carers) whose basic condition itself cannot be improved. Contrary to the common supposition by both professionals and relatives, success can usually be achieved (even in severe and long-standing problems[25]) given an accurate diagnosis of the type of sleep disorder, which may be predominantly behavioural or physical in type depending on the cause of the mental retardation.

Sleep disturbance in the aetiology of psychiatric illness

General aspects

These reports that aspects of psychological function can be adversely influenced by sleep disturbance support the idea that psychiatry patients with disturbed sleep may well have additional problems arising from their sleep disorder which, therefore, requires early detection and treatment in its own right. Various 'psychotic' and other abnormal psychological phenomena were mentioned earlier resulting from prolonged and severe sleep disturbance, but these are soon reversed when normal sleep is restored. It remains an open question how often sleep disturbance is a primary cause of psychiatric illness. Evidence is patchy, tentative, and in need of clarification.

- Over a wide age range, patients with a prior history of insomnia have been found consistently to be at significantly increased risk for severe depression.[26–28] This could be interpreted in different ways including that sleep disturbance and the depression have a common underlying pathology or that the sleep problems are an early sign of depression.

- A less fundamental role (but again implying preventative possibilities) is the suggestion that sleep deprivation late in pregnancy and in labour and childbirth at night might trigger postnatal depression.[29]

- Abnormal circadian sleep–wake rhythms have been implicated in various depressive disorders including seasonal affective disorder. Light therapy has been used to correct the abnormality and relieve the depression.[30]

- Disordered REM sleep mechanisms have (questionably) been considered as fundamental in the development of post-traumatic stress disorder symptoms.[31]

- Some forms of attention-deficit–hyperactivity disorder in children are attributed to persistent sleep disturbance.

- In a proportion of patients with schizophrenia, narcolepsy has been reported as the cause of their psychotic symptoms.[32]

In addition to the clinical sleep disorders which it is thought are important in the pathogenesis of psychiatric illness, much attention has been paid to polysomnographic abnormalities which seem to indicate underlying neurophysiological mechanisms (see Chapter 4.14.5). An understanding of these mechanisms might help explain related observations such as the seemingly paradoxically therapeutic effect of sleep deprivation in some forms of depression.

REM sleep changes (especially reduced REM latency) in particular, but also reduction in SWS, have been closely linked with certain types of severe depression.[33] However, the meaning of reduced REM latency remains obscure,[34] not helped by the fact that it is not specific to depressive illness. It has also been described in schizophrenia, borderline personality disorder, eating disorder, post-traumatic stress disorder and panic disorder, as well as during recovery from sleep loss, in narcolepsy and the Kleine–Levin syndrome.

A potentially more promising approach than considering types of psychiatric illness separately is to examine abnormalities of sleep physiology associated with particular phenomena occurring in a range of psychiatric disorders. Sleep-onset REM abnormalities have been considered in this way in relation to several neuropsychiatric disorders in which psychotic phenomena occur. The suggestion is that some forms of psychosis are a manifestation of brainstem pathology as indicated by the REM sleep abnormalities.[35]

Disorders of sleep

Sleep complaints

The starting point for the clinician is the patient's sleep complaint. They are of three basic types:

- not enough sleep or unrefreshing sleep (insomnia)

- sleeping too much (excessive daytime sleepiness)

- disturbed episodes during or otherwise related to sleep (parasomnias)

The detailed accounts later in this section are organized in relation to these main types of sleep complaint: insomnias (Chapter 4.14.2), excessive daytime sleepiness (Chapter 4.14.3), and parasomnias (Chapter 4.14.4). In recognition of the frequency with which sleep disturbance complicates physical and mental illness, additional accounts are then provided of sleep disturbance associated with psychiatric conditions (Chapter 4.14.5) and with medical disorders (Chapter 4.14.6). Sleep problems in childhood and adolescence are discussed in Chapter 9.2.9, with a separate account regarding preschool children in Chapter 9.2.8. The relationship between mental retardation and sleep disturbance are considered above, and common sleep problems in the elderly (which are common and troublesome[36]) are discussed in Chapter 8.6.

Whatever the clinical setting in which sleep complaints are investigated, the aim is to identify the specific sleep disorder from the many other conditions that can give rise to such complaints. Some sleep disorders may cause more than one type of complaint and a patient may have more than one sleep disorder. The question arises which scheme to use for the classification of sleep disorders.

DSM and ICD classification systems

Both these systems provide schemes for classifying a range of sleep disorder but they do so in different ways. DSM-IV allocates sleep disorders to three broad categories: primary sleep disorders, sleep disorders related to mental disorders, and other sleep disorders. In ICD-10, classification of sleep disorders is different and appears in three locations: under mental disorders, under diseases of the nervous system and sense organs, and under symptoms, signs, and ill-defined conditions. Apart from this dispersal of sleep disorders across the whole classification scheme, the major distinction between 'the specific disorders of non-organic origin' and 'the sleep disturbances' presupposes more about the specific pathophysiologies underlying the various sleep disorders than is justified at present.

International Classification of Sleep Disorders–Revised

Elaborate classification schemes developed by enthusiastic experts can be daunting to the non-specialist. However, despite its apparent complexity, there is much in favour of using the *International Classification*

Table 1 *International Classification of Sleep Disorders — Revised* (1997): classification outline

Dyssomnias
- A. Intrinsic sleep disorders
- B. Extrinsic sleep disorders
- C. Circadian rhythm sleep disorders

Parasomnias
- A. Arousal disorders
- B. Sleep–wake transition disorders
- C. Parasomnias usually associated with REM sleep
- D. Other parasomnias

Sleep disorders associated with mental, neurological, or other medical disorders
- A. Associated with mental disorders
- B. Associated with neurological disorders
- C. Associated with other medical disorders

Proposed sleep disorders

of Sleep Disorder system (developed from wide international consultation) especially to standardize diagnosis in clinical work and research.

The revised *International Classification of Sleep Disorders* (**ICSD-R**)[37] is the latest in a number of attempts to organize rationally the various ways in which sleep can be disturbed. The 80 or more different sleep disorders, occurring in adults and children, are grouped as shown in Table 1.

- Dyssomnias are primary sleep disorders which cause either difficulty getting off to sleep or remaining asleep (insomnia) or excessive sleepiness during the day. They are divided into intrinsic sleep disorders (originating from within the body), extrinsic sleep disorders (caused by external factors) and circadian rhythm sleep disorders (related to the timing of sleep within the 24-h period).

- Parasomnias (disorders which intrude into the sleep process) are subdivided according to the phase of sleep with which they are associated: arousal disorders (arising from NREM sleep); sleep–wake transition disorders, and parasomnias usually associated with REM sleep. Other parasomnias are those which do not fall into these three categories.

- The sleep disorders associated with mental, neurological or other medical disorders are not primarily sleep disorders but psychiatric or medical disorders in which sleep disturbance is a major feature.

- Conditions that need further assessment before each can be convincingly seen as a disorder in their own right are called proposed sleep disorders.

ICSD-R contains useful summaries of each of these sleep disorders including main features, associated features, and possible complications, course, predisposing factors, prevalence, age at onset, sex ratio, familial patterns, polysomnographic and other laboratory features and differential diagnosis. Diagnostic, severity, and duration criteria are also provided. Each sleep disorder is given a unique code number. By means of a three-axis system, a patient's condition and treatment needs can be characterized in terms of the ICSD diagnosis of his or her sleep disorder, investigations performed, and particular abnormalities demonstrated, plus any accompanying medical and psychiatric disorders. A glossary of basic terms and concepts is also provided.

The advantages of this system over the DSM and ICD systems are that it provides a more comprehensive, logically structured, and regularly revised account of sleep disorders which is based on the latest information provided by clinicians and researchers in the field of sleep disorders medicine. As described above, it also provides valuable structured summaries of individual sleep disorders as well as criteria for comprehensive diagnosis in the individual case. It is generally much more informative about sleep and its disorders than other systems.

Sleep disorders mistaken for psychiatric conditions

Sleep disorders manifest themselves in many ways. Failure to realize this can result in the misdiagnosis of primary sleep disorders as primarily psychiatric conditions.

Prominent examples of this mistake are seen in the **circadian rhythm sleep disorders**. These disorders are also important causes of insomnia (see Chapter 4.14.2) and/or excessive daytime sleepiness (see Chapter 4.14.3). Therefore they can also be important in the aetiology of psychological dysfunction caused by sleep disturbance. Collectively, circadian rhythm sleep disorders are common. They are caused either by malfunction of the endogenous systems (the 'biological clock' described earlier) involved in the regulation of sleep–wake rhythm, or by environmental effects on these systems (as in jet lag or shift work). Because of their basically biological nature, this group of sleep disorders requires treatment to produce physiological readjustment to the basic sleep–wake mechanism (e.g. chronotherapy schedules, bright-light therapy, or melatonin).[38]

Probably the most common circadian rhythm sleep disorder is the **delayed sleep phase syndrome** which is thought to affect a particularly high proportion of adolescents (see Chapter 9.2.9). Its main features are long delays in getting off to sleep and great difficulty in waking up in the morning. Both problems are often misconstrued as difficult 'adolescent' behaviour, but in fact they reflect disturbed sleep physiology and require measures to correct this physiological disturbance rather than recriminations or other psychological pressures. Persistence of the delayed sleep phase syndrome readily gives rise to psychological complications including depression, which has been described in a high proportion of people with the condition.[39] In some cases the origin of the abnormal sleep pattern can be traced to psychological difficulties. The situation can become complicated if alcohol or other substances are used either to get to sleep at night or to keep awake during the day.

The **advanced sleep phase syndrome** consists of a troublesome inability to stay awake in the evening and early morning waking. It is generally thought to be uncommon, but may be encountered in the elderly whose sleep may be further disturbed by other aspects of the normal ageing process and the effects of physical or psychiatric illness (Chapter 4.14.5). In the absence of such complications, the early morning waking of advanced sleep phase syndrome is not accompanied by evidence of major depression.

In the **non-24-hours sleep–wake syndrome** the time at which the individual goes to sleep and wakes up is consistently delayed by 1 to 2 h each night in succession. This condition (mainly described in blind patients) is rare in the general population. The same may be true of the **irregular sleep–wake pattern**, but increasingly less so in view of its occurrence in patients with degenerative brain disease including dementia (see Chapter 4.14.5). The absence of a regular daily routine in such patients, and others with this form of sleep disorder, is thought to contribute to characteristic lack of consistency in the times of going to sleep and waking up from day to day, with sleep broken up into three or more short periods in each 24 h. This degree of sleep disorganization is highly likely to produce psychological effects, which might be mistaken for a primary psychiatric illness, or to increase the degree of cognitive or behavioural disturbance of patients with a degenerative disorder.

The remaining circadian rhythm sleep disorders, caused by environmental factors, also have psychological effects which need to be distinguished from primary psychiatric disorders. The effects of **jet lag** are usually transient, but travellers who frequently cross several time zones on each flight can develop chronic sleep disturbances with potentially serious effects on mood and performance, sometimes exacerbated by their use of alcohol or sedatives. The effects of **night shift work** pose a greater problem. Increasing numbers of people are working shifts which involve being active at the times when their biological clock is indicating that they should be asleep. Many fail to adapt, resulting in chronic sleep disturbance, high accident rates, physical and psychiatric illness, and impaired social relationships, again often complicated by self-treatment by means of alcohol or other substances.

All causes of excessive daytime sleepiness provide good examples of the potential misinterpretation of sleep disorders as primarily psychiatric conditions. Long delays (often years) commonly occur in the diagnosis of **narcolepsy**, partly because physicians may be unfamiliar with the condition. In the meantime, the patient's sleepy behaviour is often misconstrued as laziness, disinterest, or even psychiatric disorder including depression. The accompanying feature of cataplexy is open to similar misinterpretation. These diagnostic problems have been described in both adults and children with narcolepsy. It has also been claimed that, because a sleep history has not been taken routinely, patients with a psychotic variant of narcolepsy may be misdiagnosed as schizophrenic.[32] Misdiagnosis of an essentially psychological disorder also occurs in the **Kleine–Levin syndrome**, especially in its classical form where excessive sleepiness occurs episodically in association with a number of behavioural disturbances which can be quite bizarre. Severe degrees of **obstructive sleep apnoea** cause serious problems in daytime performance and behaviour, the physical origins of which may well not be recognized. **Automatic behaviour** and **sleep drunkenness**, both of which may occur in very sleepy people, are also easily misinterpreted as primarily psychological conditions.

The **parasomnias** can be another source of diagnostic difficulty. **Headbanging**, **arousal disorders**, and other dramatic parasomnias (see Chapter 4.14.4) in children may well be interpreted by concerned parents as suggestive of psychological disturbance. Health-care professionals often share this concern which, however, is rarely justified. **Sleep-related violence**, occurring mainly in adults, may well be taken to mean that the patient is psychiatrically disturbed, but the more usual explanation is a sleep disorder (especially **sleepwalking** or **REM sleep behaviour disorder**) in which the patient acts violently without malicious intent.[40] **Sleep paralysis** may also be misconstrued as a psychotic disorder when accompanied by hallucinatory experiences.[41] **Parasomnias that are secondary to physical conditions** can also be mistaken for psychological disturbance. Nocturnal epilepsy is a prime example, especially mesial frontal seizures because of the bizarre movements and dramatic vocalizations.[42]

In addition to sleep disorders being mistaken for psychiatric disorder, the opposite problem arises occasionally, i.e. some patients simulate excessive daytime sleepiness in order to avoid a psychologically troubling situation. Similarly, even in childhood, apparent parasomnias during sleep have sometimes been shown by polysomnography to occur when the patient is actually awake.[43]

Detection and assessment of sleep disturbance

As suggested earlier, evidence of a sleep disturbance should be actively sought in members of the general population and the various groups, including psychiatric patients, who are at special risk of sleep disorders. Otherwise, many instances of even severe sleep disturbance will continue to go unrecognized and untreated. For a more detailed account of basic assessment see Naylor and Aldrich.[44]

Sleep history

Routinely, all patients should be asked the following screening questions.

- Do you sleep long enough or well enough?
- Are you very sleepy during the day?
- Is your sleep disturbed at night?

Ideally, a bed partner or other relative would also be asked the same questions because the existence or severity of some forms of sleep disturbance are not known to the patient. In the case of children, parents are the main source of information but teachers' observations about daytime sleepiness or disturbance are also important.

If the answer to any of these enquiries is positive, a detailed sleep history is required. As traditional clinical history-taking schedules pay little attention to sleep, additional sleep-related enquiries will need to be made covering the following points about the sleep problem.

- Precise nature of the sleep complaint, its onset, development, and current patterns.
- Medical or psychological factors at the onset of the sleep problem or which might have maintained it.
- Patterns of occurrence of the symptoms—factors making them better or worse, weekdays compared with weekends, or work compared with holiday periods.
- Effects on mood, work, social life, other family members.
- Past and present treatments for sleep problems and their effects.
- Past and present medication or other treatments for other illness or disorder.

In addition, detailed information is required concerning the following.

- The patient's typical 24-h sleep—wake schedule: this can usefully start with the evening meal, followed by preparation for and timing of bedtime, time and process of getting to sleep, events during the night, time and ease of waking up and getting up, level of alertness, and mental state and behaviour during the day.
- An attempt should be made to establish the duration, continuity,

and timing of the patient's overnight sleep as these are the most important aspects of sleep for daytime functioning. It is also important to identify events of particular diagnostic significance (e.g. loud snoring).

- Sleep hygiene (see Chapter 4.14.2).

Compilation of a sleep history can be aided by the use of a preliminary sleep questionnaire. Some are general in their scope[45] while others are directed to particular aspects such as sleepiness,[46] including the effect of excessive sleepiness on daytime function in a number of important real-life situations.[47]

Sleep diary

Systematic recording each day over 2 weeks or more, using a standardized format, avoids the bias or distortion of retrospective generalizations.

- From recording times of going to bed, getting to sleep, awake periods during the night, final awakening, and getting up, estimates can be made of total sleep time, sleep efficiency (proportion of time in bed the patient is actually asleep), and number of awakenings.
- The occurrence and nature of night-time episodes of disturbed behaviour can be determined.
- Daytime events including sleepiness can be assessed.
- Previously unrecognized patterns of occurrence of these sleep phenomena may become apparent including temporal patterns, shift of the sleep phase, or relationships to stressful events or other factors.

Histories

Medical and psychiatric history should include past and current treatment details (in view of the wide range of illnesses or disorders and their treatment with which sleep disturbance is associated). Social history should include occupational, marital, and recreational factors (drinking, smoking, drug use) which may affect sleep. Family history is often positive, for example in arousal disorders and narcolepsy.

Review of systems

Breathing difficulties and nocturia, for example, are associated with sleep disturbance. Severe obstructive sleep apnoea can cause cardiopulmonary complications.

Physical and mental state examination

Particular attention should be paid to the following.

- Evidence of any systemic illness including cardiorespiratory disease or neurological disorder, such as Parkinson's disease or stroke, which may disturb sleep (see Chapter 4.14.6).
- Obesity, oral and pharyngeal abnormalities, retrognathia, or midface deformity (predisposing to upper airway obstruction).
- Depression or other psychiatric disorder.
- Intellectual impairment, especially features of dementia or mental retardation (including specific retardation syndromes) in view of their strong association with sleep disturbance.

Video and actigraphy

Video recordings can be very instructive in the parasomnias, sometimes revealing a very different clinical picture than that provided in the clinic. Home video systems can be used where admission to hospital is not feasible. Similarly, monitoring of body movements by means of wrist-watch-like devices (actigraphy) can be used at home, if necessary, to quantify basic circadian sleep–wake patterns for example.[48]

Polysomnography

Physiological sleep studies are necessary for diagnosis in only the minority of sleep disorders. Traditionally this has entailed admission to a sleep laboratory. However, especially where such facilities are difficult to obtain or where the laboratory situation is unacceptable to patients (including some children or patients who are psychiatrically disturbed), home polysomnography[49] using portable systems is very useful, although the procedure has yet to be fully standardized and for some disorders is best seen as only a screening procedure. Recording in the home environment has the further advantage that, if the patient is allowed to adapt to the recording procedure before bedtime, the results from a single night's recording will be representative of the patient's habitual sleep. In contrast, because 'first night effects' are prominent in laboratory recordings, more than one night of polysomnography is required to allow adaptation to take place.

Basic polysomnography entails the recording of an EEG, an electro-oculogram, and an electromyogram. This allows sleep to be staged and a hypnogram to be compiled. Usually the recording is made overnight but it may be extended during the day if appropriate. Basic measures obtained from this information are as follows.

- Sleep continuity: total time in bed (TIB); total sleep time (TST); total time awake; number of awakenings; sleep efficiency (TIB/TST × 100).

- NREM measures: actual and percentage time in Stages I–IV; total SWS.

- REM measures: REM latency; actual and percentage time in REM sleep; total REM sleep.

Polysomnography can be extended to additional physiological measures, especially the following.

- Respiratory variables (and video/audio recordings) for sleep-related breathing problems.

- Additional EEG channels (combined with video) if nocturnal epilepsy is suspected.

- Anterior tibialis electromyogram for the detection of periodic limb movements in sleep (**PLMS**).

The main indications for polysomnography[50] are as follows.

- The investigation of excessive daytime sleepiness including the diagnosis of sleep apnoea, narcolepsy, or PLMS.

- The diagnosis of parasomnias where their nature is unclear from the clinical details, where polysomnography findings contribute essentially to the diagnosis (e.g. REM sleep behaviour disorder (Chapter 4.14.4)), where the possibility of epilepsy exists, or where there may be more than one parasomnia present.

- An objective check on the accuracy of the sleep complaint, or response to treatment.

Table 2 Examples of treatment approaches for sleep disorders

General principles
Explain the problem, reassure where appropriate, and provide support
Encourage good sleep hygiene
Where possible treat any underlying condition causing the sleep disturbance
Medical
Psychiatric
Safety or protective measures (especially for dangerous parasomnias)
Specific measures
Behavioural treatment (mainly for insomnia or childhood sleeplessness)
Positive associations
Modification of inappropriate behaviour
Sleep consolidation
Chronobiological (for circadian sleep–wake rhythm disorders)
Sleep phase rescheduling
Light therapy
Medication
Hypnotics (selectively and short term)
Stimulants (excessive sleepiness)
Melatonin (some circadian rhythm disorders)
Physical measures
Continuous positive airway pressure (OSA)
Surgery
Adenotonsillectomy (OSA)
Uvulopalatopharyngoplasty (some adults with OSA)

OSA, obstructive sleep apnoea.

Other investigations

Further laboratory investigations may be appropriate depending on the nature of the sleep problem and the purpose of the assessment.

- The multiple sleep latency test, involving the recording of basic polysomnography variables, quantifies the degree of daytime sleepiness by measuring the time a patient takes to fall asleep during five opportunities to do so during the day. In adults a mean sleep latency of 5 min or less indicates pathological sleepiness (usually of organic origin); 5 to 10 min is a grey area which usually includes excessive sleepiness associated with primary psychiatric disorder; while longer than 10 min is normal. These values do not apply to children, whose sleep tendency varies with age (Chapter 9.2.9).

- HLA typing for the investigation of narcolepsy, and nocturnal penile tumescence monitoring in the differential diagnosis of organic versus psychogenic impotence, are examples of other specific tests that may be appropriate depending on the clinical problem.

- Formal psychometric assessment or, in children, developmental assessment may be appropriate.

Treatment approaches for sleep disorders

In clinical practice the pharmacological approach to treatment is generally overemphasized, especially the use of hypnotic–sedative drugs. Table 2 provides some indication of the wide range of available types of treatment, as well as general principles of management, for adults and children. They are arranged roughly in order of the frequency of their use in the comprehensive management of sleep disorders in general. An appropriate choice from this range requires an accurate diagnosis of the underlying sleep disorder. Further details are provided in later contributions to this section. Claims for the effectiveness of these various measures are based on widespread clinical experience and reports. Few randomized controlled clinical trials have been published as yet.

References

1. Stores, G. and Crawford, C. (1998). Medical student education in sleep and its disorders. *Journal of the Royal College of Physicians of London*, **32**, 149–53.
2. Dement, W.C. and Mitler, M.M. (1993). It's time to wake up to the importance of sleep disorders. *Journal of the American Medical Association*, **269**, 1548–50.
3. Furman, Y., Wolf, S.M., and Rosenfeld, D.S. (1997). Shakespeare and sleep disorders. *Neurology*, **49**, 1171–2.
4. Cosnett, J.E. (1992). Charles Dickens: observer of sleep and its disorders. *Sleep*, **15**, 264–7.
5. Kryger, M.H., Roth, T., and Dement, W.C. (ed.) (1994). *Principles and practice of sleep medicine* (2nd edn). W.B. Saunders, Philadelphia, PA.
6. Ferber, R. and Kryger, M. (ed.) (1995.) *Principles and practice of sleep medicine in the child*. W.B. Saunders, Philadelphia, PA.
7. Rechtschaffen, A. (1998). Current perspectives on the function of sleep. *Perspectives in Biology and Medicine*, **41**, 359–89.
8. Rechtschaffen, A. and Kales, A. (ed.) (1968). *A manual of standardised terminology, techniques and scoring system for sleep stages of human subjects*. UCLA Brain Information Service/Brain Research Institute, Los Angeles, CA.
9. Bonnet, M.H. Sleep deprivation. In *Principles and practice of sleep medicine* (2nd edn) (ed. M.H. Kryger, T. Roth, and W.C. Dement), pp. 50–67. W.B. Saunders, Philadelphia, PA.
10. Czeisler, C.A., Duffy, J.F., Shanahan, T.L., *et al.* (1999). Stability, precision and near 24 hour period of the human pacemaker. *Science*, **284**, 2177–81.
11. Kryger, M.H. (1997). Controversies in sleep medicine: melatonin (editorial). *Sleep*, **20**, 898.
12. Boselli, M., Parrino, L., Smerieri, A., and Terzano, M.G. (1998). Effect of age on EEG arousals in normal sleep. *Sleep*, **21**, 351–7.
13. Bonnet, M.H. and Arand, D.L. (1995). We are chronically sleep deprived. *Sleep*, **18**, 908–11.
14. Harrison, Y. and Horne, J.A. (1995). Should we be taking more sleep? *Sleep*, **18**, 901–7.
15. Horne, J.A. (1988). *Why we sleep*. Oxford University Press.
16. Horne, J.A. (1988). Sleep loss and 'divergent' thinking ability. *Sleep*, **11**, 528–36.
17. Pilcher, J.J. and Huffcutt, A.I. (1996). Effects of sleep deprivation on performance: a meta-analysis. *Sleep*, **19**, 318–26.
18. Leonard, C., Fanning, N., Attwood, J., and Buckley, M. (1998). The effect of fatigue, sleep deprivation and onerous working hours on the physical and mental well being of pre-registration house officers. *Irish Journal of Medical Science*, **167**, 22–5.
19. Dinges, D.F. (1995). An overview of sleepiness and accidents. *Journal of Sleep Research*, **4** (Supplement 2), 4–14.
20. Mitler, M.M., Carskadon, M.A., Czeisler, C.A., Dement, W.C., Dinges, D.F., and Graeber, R.C. (1988). Catastrophes, sleep and public policy: consensus report. *Sleep*, **11**, 100–9.
21. Bédard, M.A., Montplaisir, J., Malo, J., Richer, F., and Rouleau, I. (1993). Persistent neuropsychological deficits and vigilance impairment in sleep apnea syndrome after treatment with continuous positive airway pressure (CPAP). *Journal of Clinical and Experimental Neuropsychology*, **15**, 330–41.
22. Stores, G. (1999). Children's sleep disorders: modern approaches, developmental effects, and children at special risk. *Developmental Medicine and Child Neurology*, **41**, 568–73.
23. Stores, G., Ellis, A.J., Wiggs, L., Crawford, C., and Thomson, A. (1998). Sleep and psychological disturbance in nocturnal asthma. *Archives of Disease in Childhood*, **78**, 413–19.
24. Stores, G. (1992). Annotation: sleep studies in children with a mental handicap. *Journal of Child Psychology and Psychiatry*, **33**, 1303–17.
25. Wiggs, L. and Stores, G. (1998). Behavioural treatment for sleep problems in children with severe learning disabilities and challenging daytime behaviour: effects on sleep patterns of mother and child. *Journal of Sleep Research*, **7**, 119–26.
26. Ford, D.E. and Kamerow, D.B. (1989). Epidemiologic study of sleep disturbances and psychiatric disorders: and opportunity for prevention. *Journal of the American Medical Association*, **262**, 1479–84.
27. Breslau, N., Roth, T., Rosenthal, L., and Andreski, P. (1996). Sleep disturbance and psychiatric disorders: a longitudinal epidemiological study of young adults. *Biological Psychiatry*, **39**, 411–18.
28. Livingston, G., Blizard, B., and Mann, A. (1993). Does sleep disturbance predict depression in elderly people? A study in inner London. *British Journal of General Practice*, **43**, 445–8.
29. Wilkie, G.T. and Shapiro, C.M. (1992). Sleep deprivation and the postnatal blues. *Journal of Psychosomatic Research*, **36**, 309–16.
30. Chesson, A.L., Littner, M., Davila, D., *et al.* (1999). Practice parameters for the use of light therapy in the treatment of sleep disorders. *Sleep*, **22**, 641–8.
31. Reynolds, C.F. (1989). Sleep disturbance in posttraumatic stress disorder: pathogenetic or epiphenomenal? *American Journal of Psychiatry*, **146**, 695–6.
32. Douglass, A.B., Shipley, J.E., Haines, R.F., Scholten, R.C., Dudley, E., and Tapp, A. (1993). Schizophrenia, narcolepsy, and HLA-DR15, DQ6. *Biological Psychiatry*, **34**, 773–80.
33. Kupfer, D.J. (1995). Sleep research in depressive illness: clinical implications—a tasting menu. *Biological Psychiatry*, **38**, 391–403.
34. Le Bon, O., Staner, L., Murphy, J.R., Hoffman, G., Pull, C.H., and Pelc, I. (1997). Critical analysis of the theories advanced to explain short REM sleep latencies and other sleep anomalies in several psychiatric conditions. *Journal of Psychiatric Research*, **31**, 433–50.
35. Howland, R.H. (1997). Sleep-onset rapid eye movement periods in neuropsychiatric disorders: implications for the pathophysiology of psychosis. *Journal of Nervous and Mental Disease*, **185**, 730–8.
36. Ancoli-Israel, S., Poceta, J.S., Stepnowsky, C., Martin, J., and Gehrman, P. (1997). Identification and treatment of sleep problems in the elderly. *Sleep Medicine Reviews*, **1**, 3–17.
37. American Sleep Disorders Association (1997). *International Classification of Sleep Disorders, Revised: diagnostic and coding manual*. American Sleep Disorders Association, Rochester, MN.
38. Wagner, D.R. (1990). Circadian rhythm sleep disorders. In *Handbook of sleep disorders* (ed. M.J. Thorpy), pp. 493–527. Marcel Dekker, New York.
39. Regestein, Q.R. and Monk, T.H. (1995). Delayed sleep phase syndrome: a review of the clinical aspects. *American Journal of Psychiatry*, **152**, 602–8.
40. Broughton, R.J. and Shimizu, T. (1997). Dangerous behaviors by night. In *Forensic aspects of sleep* (ed. C.M. Shapiro and A. McCall Smith), pp. 63–83. Wiley, Chichester.
41. Stores, G. (1998). Sleep paralysis and hallucinosis. *Behavioural Neurology*, **11**, 109–12.
42. Stores, G., Zaiwalla, Z., and Bergel, N. (1991). Frontal lobe complex partial seizures in children: a form of epilepsy at particular risk of misdiagnosis. *Developmental Medicine and Child Neurology*, **33**, 998–1009.
43. Molaie, M. and Deutsch, G.K. (1997). Psychogenic events presenting as parasomnia. *Sleep*, **20**, 402–5.

44. Naylor, M.W. and Aldrich, M.S. (1994). Approach to the patient with disordered sleep. In *Principles and practice of sleep medicine* (2nd edn) (ed. M.H. Kryger, T. Roth, W.C. Dement), pp. 413–17. W.B. Saunders, Philadelphia, PA.

45. Douglass, A.B., Bornstein, R., Nino-Murcia, G., *et al.* (1994). The Sleep Disorders Questionnaire I: creation and multivariate structure of SDQ. *Sleep*, **17**, 160–7.

46. Johns, M. (1998). Rethinking the assessment of sleepiness. *Sleep Medicine Reviews*, **2**, 3–15.

47. Weaver, T.E., Laizner, A.M., Evans, L.K., *et al.* (1997). An instrument to measure functional status outcomes for disorders of excessive sleepiness. *Sleep*, **20**, 835–43.

48. Sadeh, A., Hauri, P.J., Kripke, D.F., and Lavie, P. (1995). The role of actigraphy in the evaluation of sleep disorders. *Sleep*, **18**, 288–302.

49. Broughton, R.J. (1994). Ambulant home monitoring of sleep and its disorders. In *Principles and practice of sleep medicine* (2nd edn) (ed. M.H. Kryger, T. Roth, and W.C. Dement), pp. 978–83. W.B. Saunders, Philadelphia, PA.

50. Indications for Polysomnography Task Force, American Sleep Disorders Association Standards of Practice Committee (1997). Practice parameters for the indications for polysomnography and related procedures. *Sleep*, **20**, 406–22.

4.14.2 Insomnias

Colin A. Espie

Introduction

Most people's experiences of poor sleep are memorable, because sleeplessness and its daytime consequences are unpleasant. There are those, however, for whom insomnia is the norm. Persistent and severe sleep disturbance affects at least one in ten adults and one in five older adults, thus representing a considerable public health concern. Sleep disruption is central to a number of medical and psychiatric disorders, and insomnia is usually treated by general practitioners. Therefore differential diagnosis is important, and respiratory physicians, neurologists, psychiatrists, and clinical psychologists need to be involved. The purpose of this chapter is to summarize current understanding of the insomnias, their appraisal, and treatment. Particular emphasis will be placed upon evidence-based practical management.

Clinical features

Insomnia often remains unreported, and finally presents when a poor sleep pattern is well established.[1] Alcohol has long been a first-line self-administered sleep aid, and recent years have seen an increasing use of 'over-the-counter' preparations and 'self-help' strategies. The clinical presentation is commonly of a frustrated patient, trapped in a vicious circle of anxiety and poor sleep, who reports having 'tried everything'.[2]

There may be concern about the pattern of sleep. This is the most quantifiable aspect of self-report relating to, for example, length of time taken to fall asleep, frequency and duration of wakenings, or total amount of sleep. A poorly established sleep pattern can lead to unpredictability of what sleep will be like on any given night. Patients often report poor quality of sleep, and subjective perceived quality can be a critically important outcome variable. Typical reports relate to light sleep and sleep felt to be unrestorative. Although it may be unclear how such complaints relate to EEG sleep architecture, the clinician should not overlook qualitative report as it may reflect underlying pathophysiology. Concerns are often expressed also about the daytime effects of poor sleep. These can be cognitive effects, such as fatigue, sleepiness, and impairments in performance, or emotional effects, such as irritability and anxiety.[2,3]

Classification

The *International Classification of Sleep Disorders* (**ICSD-R**)[4] was revised in 1997 and provides the most comprehensive account of sleep disorders, both for descriptive purposes and for differential diagnosis (see Chapter 4.14.1). ICSD-R describes insomnias as disorders of initiating and maintaining sleep. Patients may have either sleep-onset problems or wakenings from sleep, or both of these. Table 1 summarizes the principal classifications that relate to insomnia. As can be seen, sleeplessness requires careful assessment of concomitant symptomatology in order to reach a valid diagnosis.

Diagnosis and differential diagnosis

Severity of insomnia is judged along dimensions of frequency, intensity, and duration, as well as impact on daytime functioning and quality of life. Generally, the criteria for severe and chronic insomnia are a minimum duration of 6 months with problems presenting at least four nights per week. Restlessness, irritability, anxiety, daytime fatigue, and tiredness commonly accompany such presentations. Mild and moderate insomnia may be diagnosed where problems are less intrusive.

Most patients presenting with insomnia have psychophysiological difficulty initiating and/or maintaining sleep. Usually marked functional effects and somatized tension associated with sleep are evident. The patient reports extreme tiredness while being unable to sleep satisfactorally. This contrasts with the circadian disorders where, in delayed sleep-phase syndrome, the patient may not feel sleepy until late in the normal sleep period, and in advanced sleep-phase syndrome, may waken early and be unable to return to sleep. Taking a history, incorporating screening questions on restlessness, limb movements, and breathing can help to diagnose obstructive sleep apnoea syndrome, periodic limb movement disorder, and restless legs syndrome, although full polysomnographic evaluation is usually also required.[5] However, polysomnography is not essential for the diagnosis of insomnia, for which sleep diary monitoring (see Chapter 4.14.1) is usually the most useful form of assessment.[2] Wrist actigraphy is an inexpensive objective evaluation, which estimates sleep/wakefulness based upon body movement.[6] Continuous recordings can be made over five to ten consecutive 24-h periods. It is useful in identifying sleep state misperception and charted data can be

Table 1 The classification and differential diagnosis of the insomnias within ICSD-R

Classification	Sleep disorder	Essential features: Complaint of insomnia plus. . .
Dyssomnia (intrinsic)	Psychophysiological insomnia	Learned sleep-preventing associations, conditioned arousal
	Sleep state misperception	Sleep duration and quality appear normal
	Idiopathic insomnia	Insomnia typically begins in childhood or from birth
	Obstructive sleep apnoea syndrome	Excessive sleepiness, obstructed breathing in sleep, associated symptoms include snoring and a dry mouth
	Periodic limb movement disorder	Excessive sleepiness, repetitive limb muscle movements in sleep
	Restless legs syndrome	Unpleasant 'creeping' sensation in legs relieved by movement
Dyssomnia (extrinsic)	Inadequate sleep hygiene	Daily living activities inconsistent with maintaining good-quality sleep and alertness
	Adjustment sleep disorder	Identifiable stressor, disorder expected to remit
	Hypnotic-dependent sleep disorder	History of hypnotic use, withdrawal syndrome including exacerbation of insomnia
	Stimulant-dependent sleep disorder	Use or withdrawal of stimulant
	Alcohol-dependent sleep disorder	Attempts to withdraw from alcohol ingestion at bedtime
Circadian rhythm disorder	Delayed sleep-phase syndrome	Phase delay of major sleep episode, initial insomnia, excessive sleepiness in morning
	Advanced sleep-phase syndrome	Phase advance of major sleep episode, inability to stay awake, early wakening

inspected for circadian anomalies, as in delayed sleep-phase syndrome and advanced sleep-phase syndrome.

Extrinsic causes of insomnia are reported in Table 1 and should not be overlooked. In particular, hypnotic dependent sleep disorder is associated with benzodiazepine drugs where withdrawal leads to exacerbation of the primary problem.[7] This can be mistaken for a severe underlying insomnia and hence reinforce hypnotic dependency.

A wide range of psychiatric conditions, particularly affective disorders, have associated sleep symptomatology (see Chapter 4.14.5). For example, a primary diagnosis of psychophysiological insomnia cannot be made where diagnostic criteria for DSM-IV Axis I or Axis II disorders are fulfilled. Similar caveats apply to insomnia associated with medical disorders (see Chapter 4.14.6).

Epidemiology

Insomnia affects one-third of adults occasionally, and 9 to 12 per cent on a chronic basis.[8] It is more common in women, in shift workers, and in patients with medical and psychiatric disorders. Prevalence amongst older adults has been estimated at up to 25 per cent[9] and sleepiness and hypnotic drugs are risk factors for injury and fracture.[10] Although in the United Kingdom there was a decline in prescription of benzodiazepines between 1983 and 1996, the rate of decline for anxiolytic prescription (54 per cent) has been greater than

that for hypnotic prescription, which reduced from 11.7 million to 8.4 million (a 28 per cent reduction) in that time period.[11] Insomnia continues to be associated with significant health-economic costs.[12]

Aetiology

Many patients report having been marginal light sleepers before developing insomnia.[4] There is evidence that insomniacs internalize anxiety and are prone to repetitious worry,[13–15] and some suggestion that sleep disturbance often arises during life change or stress.[16] Indeed, adjustment sleep disorder may represent a normal transient disruption of sleep. Secondary factors, such as anxiety over sleep and faulty conditioning, may then exacerbate and maintain the insomnia.

Course and prognosis

There has been little research on the natural course of insomnia. However, untreated psychophysiological insomnia can last for decades, and may gradually worsen over time.[4] One long-term study of untreated insomnia indicated that insomnia tends to persist[17] and there is a developmental trend for sleep pattern to deteriorate, with increasing age.[18,19] Delayed sleep-phase syndrome and insufficient sleep hygiene can be associated with lifestyle problems and may ameliorate as these are resolved. Although insomnia tends to persist if untreated, prognosis with effective treatment can be very good.

Treatment

A review of the evidence

Drug therapy

Traditionally, insomnia was treated pharmacologically. Barbiturates were superseded by benzodiazepine compounds during the 1960s and 1970s. These drugs were safer in overdose, were thought to have fewer side-effects, and to be less addictive. Controlled studies have demonstrated that a considerable number of benzodiazepines, of short to intermediate half-life, are effective hypnotic agents.

However, from the mid-1970s potential problems became apparent, both during administration and withdrawal. Longer-acting hypnotics were prone to carry-over effects of morning lethargy and sleepiness (e.g. flurazepam), and shorter acting drugs to 'rebound insomnia' and elevated daytime anxiety; all part of a withdrawal syndrome.[7,20] Furthermore, tolerance develops with frequent administration leading either to increased dosing or switching to alternative medication. Although benzodiazepines used for short periods or intermittently can maintain effectiveness, these are not the treatment of choice in chronic insomnia, and are contraindicated in older adults and where insomnia may involve sleep-related breathing disorder (such as obstructive sleep apnoea syndrome).[21,22] A number of benzodiazepine compounds have been removed from the market in the United Kingdom, United States, and elsewhere.

Nevertheless prescribing of hypnotics remains high.[11] A recent study of older people found that trends in the duration of hypnotic use show a remarkably stable pattern, with drug use commenced after 1989 being as likely to become chronic as that which commenced before.[23] Such findings reflect the overwhelming demand for treatment and the limited progress made thus far in introducing non-pharmacological alternatives on a wide scale (see also Chapter 6.5).

Psychological therapy

Psychological treatment has been investigated in over 50 controlled studies in the past 20 years, involving over 2000 patients. These studies have mainly evaluated the efficacy of cognitive-behavioural therapy. Two meta-analyses have reported effect sizes (measured in standardized z scores) of 0.87 for reductions in sleep latency, and significant effects have been found for number and duration of wakenings (0.53–0.65) and sleep quality (0.94).[24,25] A recent review concludes that 70 to 80 per cent of patients benefit from cognitive-behavioural therapy.[1] Furthermore, cognitive-behavioural therapy appears equally efficacious in older adults. A controlled outcome study of 139 chronic insomniacs treated with cognitive-behavioural therapy in general practice, reported mean reductions of 62 min per night in sleeplessness (sleep latency and night wakenings combined) maintained 12 month post-treatment.[26] Total time slept had also increased by 34 min per night on average. The demonstration of durable effects is of critical importance; a feature notably lacking in the pharmacological literature on insomnia.

Within the cognitive-behavioural therapy model, a number of strategies have strong empirical support. Behavioural procedures such as stimulus control and sleep restriction, and cognitive strategies such as paradoxical intention and thought restructuring have been extensively investigated [2,27,28] and are outlined briefly below.

Melatonin, light therapy, and exercise

The pineal hormone melatonin has been the subject of highly publicized claims. However, scientific research has been limited. A recent controlled study in older sleep maintenance insomniacs yielded some support for sleep-promoting effects, but concluded that melatonin replacement was not as efficacious as hypnotics or bright light treatment.[29] The use of melatonin continues to be controversial, and at best it may be useful for reducing sleep latency.[30]

Bright light is a potent marker for human circadian rhythms, and has been known for some time to enable the resetting of such rhythms in advanced sleep-phase syndrome and delayed sleep-phase syndrome.[31] The results of studies investigating the efficacy of bright light against psychological treatments for psychophysiological insomnia are awaited. A limiting factor to the value of light therapy is that continued treatment may be required to maintain therapeutic effects.

Athletic people sleep well, although this may be more to do with behavioural patterning than aerobic fitness. Nevertheless, there is evidence that exercise can have positive effects upon sleep quality, particularly if taken late afternoon or early evening, and in otherwise relatively fit individuals.[32]

Advice about management

General perspective

Non-pharmacological treatment using cognitive-behavioural therapy procedures should be preferred over pharmacological treatment, in cases of severe persistent insomnia. Hypnotic agents should be recommended only for short-term or occasional use. The practitioner should be aware of morning-after effects, and potential problems of withdrawal and dependency. There is also increasing evidence that psychological intervention may facilitate reduction or discontinuation of medication in hypnotic-dependent insomniacs when a supervised taper is integrated into treatment[33,34] There is very limited support for the use of melatonin or exercise as treatments of choice, although light therapy seems effective for circadian disorders.

Using cognitive–behavioural therapies

Brief descriptions of effective management strategies are presented in Tables 2 and 3. The following text provides explanation of underlying psychological models and further information on implementation.

Sleep education and sleep hygiene

The simple provision of information ameliorates the sense of being out of control. Inaccurate attributions are challenged and misunderstandings corrected by understanding what sleep is, how common insomnia can be, how sleep changes with age, good sleep hygiene practices, and some facts about sleep loss. Similarly, sleep hygiene provides patients with a starting point for self-management. These techniques are best construed as introductory and will not of themselves treat insomnia effectively.

Table 2 Summary description of sleep hygiene and education components for the treatment of chronic insomnia

Components of sleep education

The need for sleep and its functions
Sleep patterns across the lifespan
Sleep as a process with stages/phases
Factors adversely affecting sleep
The effects of sleep loss
The concept of insomnia
Measuring sleep and sleep problems

Components of sleep hygiene treatment

Bedroom comfortable for sleep
Regular exercise, timing, and fitness
Stable and appropriate diet
Undesirable effects of caffeine and other stimulants
Moderation of alcohol consumption
Other common 'self-help' strategies

Stimulus control treatment

Stimulus control increases the bedroom's cueing potential for sleep. For good sleepers, the pre-bedtime period and the stimulus environment trigger positive associations of sleepiness and sleep. For the poor sleeper, however, the bedroom triggers associations with restlessness and lengthy night-time wakening via a stimulus–response relationship, thereby continuing to promote wakefulness and arousal. The model is similar to phobic conditions where a conditioned stimulus precipitates an anxiety response.

Treatment involves removing from the bedroom all stimuli which

Table 3 Summary description of cognitive–behavioural components for the treatment of chronic insomnia

Components of stimulus control and sleep restriction treatment

Define individual sleep requirements
Establish parameters for bedtime period (threshold time and rising time)
Eliminate daytime napping
Differentiate rest from sleep
Schedule sleep periods with respect to needs
Establish 7 day per week compliance
Remove incompatible activity from bedroom environment
Rise from bed if wakeful (>20 min)
Avoid recovery sleep as 'compensation'
Establish stability from night to night
Adjust the sleep period as sleep efficiency improves

Components of cognitive intervention

Identify thought patterns and content that intrude
Address (mis)attributions connecting sleep and waking life
Establish rehearsal/planning time in early evening
Relaxation and imagery training
Distraction and thought blocking
Develop accurate beliefs/attributions about sleep and sleep loss
Challenge negative and invalid thoughts
Eliminate 'effort' to control sleep
Motivate to maintain behaviour and cognitive change
Utilize relapse-prevention techniques

are potentially sleep-incompatible. Reading and watching television, for example, are confined to living-rooms. Sleeping is excluded from living areas and from daytime, and wakefulness is excluded from the bedroom. The individual is instructed to get up if not asleep within 20 min or if wakeful during the night. Conceptually, stimulus control is a reconditioning treatment which forces discrimination between daytime and sleeping environments.

Sleep restriction therapy

Sleep restriction restricts sleep to the length of time which the person is likely to sleep. This may be equivalent to promoting 'core sleep' at the expense of 'optional sleep'.[35] Sleep restriction primarily aims to improve sleep efficiency. Since sleep efficiency is the ratio of time asleep to time in bed, it can be improved either by increasing the numerator (time spent asleep) or by reducing the denominator (time spent in bed). Insomniacs generally seek the former, but this may not be necessary, either biologically or psychologically. Sleep restriction first involves recording in a sleep diary and calculating average nightly sleep duration. The aim, then, is to obtain this average each night. This is achieved by setting rising time as an 'anchor' each day and delaying going to bed until a 'threshold time' which permits this designated amount of sleep. Thus the sleep period is compressed and sleep efficiency is likely to increase.

Cognitive control

This technique aims to deal with thought material in advance of bedtime and to reduce intrusive bedtime thinking. The insomniac is asked to set aside 15 to 20 min in the early evening to rehearse the day and to plan ahead for tomorrow; thus putting the day to rest. It is a technique for dealing with unfinished business and may be most effective for rehearsal, planning, and self-evaluative thoughts which are important to the individual and which, if not dealt with, may intrude during the sleep-onset period.

Thought suppression

Thought-stopping and articulatory suppression attempt to interrupt the flow of thoughts. No attempt is made to deal with thought material *per se* but rather to attenuate thinking. With articulatory suppression the patient is instructed to repeat, subvocally, the word 'the' every 3 seconds. This procedure is derived from the experimental psychology literature. Articulatory suppression is thought to occupy the short-term memory store used in the processing of information. The type of material most likely to respond is repetitive but non-affect-laden thoughts, not powerful enough to demand attention. Additionally, this technique may be useful during the night to enable rapid return to sleep.

Imagery and relaxation

There is a wide range of relaxation methods including progressive relaxation, imagery training, biofeedback, meditation, hypnosis, and autogenic training, but little evidence to indicate superiority of any one approach. Furthermore, there is little evidence to support the presumption that insomniacs are hyperaroused in physiological terms or that relaxation has its effect through autonomic change. At the cognitive level, these techniques may act through distraction and the promotion of mastery. During relaxation the mind focuses upon alternative themes such as visualized images or physiological responses. In meditation the focus is upon a 'mantra' and in self-hypnosis upon positive self-statements. Relaxation may be effective for thought processes that are anxiety-based, confused, and which flit from topic to topic.

Cognitive restructuring

Cognitive restructuring challenges faulty beliefs which maintain wakefulness and the helplessness which many insomniacs report. It appears to work through appraisal by testing the validity of assumptions against evidence and real-life experience. As an evaluative technique, it may be effective with beliefs that are irrational but compelling. If such thoughts, for example 'I am going to be incapable at work tomorrow', are not challenged, they will create high levels of preoccupation and anxiety and sleep is unlikely to occur. With cognitive restructuring, the insomniac learns alternative responses to replace inaccurate thinking.

Paradoxical intention

Finally, the technique of paradoxical intention is useful in situations where performance anxiety has developed, i.e. where the effort to produce a response inhibits that response itself. The paradoxical instruction is to allow sleep to occur naturally through passively attempting to remain quietly wakeful rather than attempting to fall asleep. Paradox may be regarded as a decatastrophizing technique since it appears to act upon the ultimate anxious thought (of remaining awake indefinitely) initially by focusing on and enhancing this thought (a habituation model) and then subjecting it to appraisal through rationalization and experience. By intending to remain awake, and failing to do so, the strength of the sleep drive is re-established, and performance effort is reduced.

Possibilities for prevention

There is insufficient knowledge of the natural course of transient sleep disorders. Mention has been made of adjustment sleep disorder and of the association of life events and stressors with the onset of insomnia. Systematic research is required to establish the 'setting conditions' for the secondary maintenance of insomnia beyond an initial normative reaction to events. Perhaps there is an interaction with a predisposing tendency to light sleep, or with introspection and worry.

The establishment and maintenance of a regular routine, both prebedtime and in terms of sleep schedule, seem to be important preventive factors. Such chronobehavioural functioning can be at risk of disruption by, for example, jet lag, shift work, weekend patterns differing from weekday, adolescent lifestyle, and retirement. Adherence to, and/or reinstatement of, an adaptive pattern seems crucial.

It is important not to underestimate the importance of attitudes and beliefs in the presentation of insomnia. Exaggerated or emotionally and mentally arousing thoughts should be dealt with promptly. Sleep loss can be distressing, but patients should be reminded that nature seeks to restore equilibrium. What they need do is provide the conditions under which sleep can occur rather than attempt directly to control the sleep process. Expectations are important also, since it is the breach of these which generally give rise to anxiety. More often than not sleep-related expectations are unrealistic and require reappraisal.

Finally, prevention should be extended to the known extrinsic causes of certain sleep disorders. Where alcohol, stimulants, or proprietary drugs interfere with sleep and the recovery of the normal sleep process, attention should be paid to these factors. Better still, patients should be encouraged to seek advice early rather than go down the path of self-administered treatment. Avoiding the use of hypnotic agents, both in general practice and during acute admissions to hospital, would substantially reduce the number of iatrogenic cases of chronic insomnia.

References

1. Morin, C.N., Hauri, P.J., Espie, C.A., Spielman, A., Buysse, D., and Bootzin, R.R. Nonpharmacologic treatment of insomnia: report of a task force of the American Sleep Disorders Association Standards of Practice Committee. *Sleep*, in press.
2. Espie, C.A. (1991). *The psychological treatment of insomnia*. Wiley, Chichester.
3. Monk, T.H. (1991). *Sleep, sleepiness and performance*. Wiley, New York.
4. American Sleep Disorders Association (1997). *International classification of sleep disorders, revised: diagnostic and coding manual*. American Sleep Disorders Association, Rochester, MN.
5. Reite, M., Buysse, D., Reynolds, C., and Mendelson, W. (1995). The use of polysomnography in the evaluation of insomnia. *Sleep*, **18**, 58–70.
6. Sadeh, A., Hauri, P.J. Kripke, D.F., and Lavie, P. (1995). The role of actigraphy in the evaluation of sleep disorders. *Sleep*, **18**, 288–302.
7. Gillin, J.C., Spinwebber, C.L., and Johnson, L.C. (1989). Rebound insomnia: a critical review. *Journal of Clinical Psychopharmacology*, **9**, 161–72.
8. Ford, D.E. and Kamerow, D.B. (1989). Epidemiologic study of sleep disturbances and psychiatric disorders. *Journal of the American Medical Association*, **262**, 1479–84.
9. Foley, D.J., Monjan, A.A., Brown, S.L., Simonsick, E.M., Wallace, R.B., and Blazer, D.G. (1995). Sleep complaints among elderly persons: an epidemiologic study of three communities. *Sleep*, **18**, 425–33.
10. Wysowski, D.K., Baum, C., Ferguson, W.J., Lundin, F., Ng, M.J., and Hammerstrom, T. (1996). Sedative-hypnotic drugs and the risk of hip fracture. *Journal of Clinical Epidemiology*, **49**, 111–13.
11. Department of Health (1997). *Benzodiazepines: number of prescriptions (thousands) and net ingredient costs (£ thousands) 1983–1996*. Report, Statistics Division 1E. Department of Health, London.
12. Chilcott, L.A. and Shapiro, C.M. (1996). The socioeconomic impact of insomnia: an overview. *Pharmacoeconomics*, **10**, 1–14.
13. Edinger, J.D., Stout, A.L., and Hoelscher, T.J. (1988). Cluster analysis of insomniacs' MMPI profiles: relation of subtypes to sleep history and treatment outcome. *Psychosomatic Medicine*, **50**, 77–87.
14. Kales, A. and Vgontzas, A.N. (1992). Predisposition to and development and persistence of chronic insomnia: importance of psychobehavioral factors. *Archives of Internal Medicine*, **152**, 1570–2.
15. Buysse, D.J., Reynolds, C.F., Kupfer, D.J., *et al.* (1994). Clinical diagnoses in 216 insomnia patients using the International Classification of Sleep Disorders (ICSD), DSM-IV and ICD-10 categories: a report from the APA/NIMH DSM-IV field trial. *Sleep*, **17**, 630–7.
16. Shealy, E.S., Kales, A., Monroe, L.J., Bixler, E.O., Chamberlin, K., and Soldatos, C.R. (1981). Onset of insomnia: role of life-stress events. *Psychosomatic Medicine*, **43**, 439–51.
17. Mendelson, W.B. (1995). Long-term follow-up of chronic insomnia. *Sleep*, **18**, 698–701.
18. Morgan, K. and Clarke, D. (1997). Risk factors for late-life insomnia in a representative general practice sample. *British Journal of General Practice*, **47**, 166–9.
19. Bliwise, D.L. (1997). Sleep and ageing. In *Understanding sleep: the evaluation and treatment of sleep disorders* (ed. M.R. Pressman and W.C. Orr), pp. 441–64. American Psychological Association, Washington, DC.
20. Kales, A., Soldatos, C.R., Bixler, E.O., and Kales, J.D. (1983). Rebound insomnia and rebound anxiety: a review. *Pharmacology*, **26**, 121–37.

21. National Institutes of Health (1984). Drugs and insomnia: the use of medication to promote sleep. *Journal of the American Medical Association*, **18**, 2410–14.

22. National Institutes of Health (1991). Consensus development conference statement: the treatment of sleep disorders of older people. *Sleep*, **14**, 169–77.

23. Morgan, K. and Clarke, D. (1997). Longitudinal trends in late-life insomnia: implications for prescribing. *Age and Ageing*, **26**, 179–84.

24. Morin, C.M., Culbert, J.P., and Schwartz, M.S. (1994). Non-pharmacological interventions for insomnia: a meta-analysis of treatment efficacy. *American Journal of Psychiatry*, **151**, 1172–80.

25. Murtagh, D.R. and Greenwood, K.M. (1995). Identifying effective psychological treatments for insomnia: a meta-analysis. *Journal of Consulting and Clinical Psychology*, **63**, 9–89.

26. Espie, C.A., Brindle, S.J., Tessier, S., Harvey, L., and McColl, J.H. A controlled trial of non-pharmacological treatment of chronic insomnia. *Behaviour Research and Therapy*, in press.

27. Morin, C.M. (1993). *Insomnia: psychological assessment and management*. Guilford Press, New York.

28. Espie, C.A. (1993). The practical management of insomnia: behavioural and cognitive techniques. *British Medical Journal*, **306**, 509–11.

29. Hughes, R.J., Sack, R.L., and Lewy, A.J. (1998). The role of melatonin and circadian phase in age-related sleep-maintenance insomnia: assessment in a clinical trial of melatonin replacement. *Sleep*, **21**, 52–68.

30. Mendelson, W.B. (1997). A critical evaluation of the hypnotic efficacy of melatonin. *Sleep*, **20**, 916–19.

31. Czeisler, C.A., Johnson, M.P., Duffy, J.F., Brown, E.N., Ronda, J.M., and Kronauer, R.E. (1990). Exposure to bright light and darkness to treat physiologic maladaptation to night work. *New England Journal of Medicine*, **322**, 1253–8.

32. Singh, N.A., Clements, K.M., and Fiatarone, M.A. (1997). A randomized controlled trial of the effect of exercise on sleep. *Sleep*, **20**, 95–101.

33. Espie, C.A., Lindsay, W.R., and Brooks, D.N. (1988). Substituting behavioural treatment for drugs in the treatment of insomnia: an exploratory study. *Journal of Behaviour Therapy and Experimental Psychiatry*, **19**, 51–6.

34. Morin, C.M., Colecchi, C.A., Ling, W.D., and Sood, R.K. (1995). Cognitive behaviour therapy to facilitate benzodiazepine discontinuation among hypnotic-dependent patients with insomnia. *Behaviour Therapy*, **26**, 733–45.

35. Horne, J.A. (1988). *Why we sleep*. Oxford University Press.

4.14.3 Excessive sleepiness

Michel Billiard

Excessive sleepiness is not a homogeneous concept. It can manifest itself as recurrent and refreshing daytime sleep episodes; recurrent but not refreshing daytime sleep episodes; abnormal lenghthening of night sleep with a major difficulty waking up in the morning and more or less constant excessive sleepiness; or periods of a week or so of almost permanent sleep, recurring over several months.

According to the *International Classification of Sleep Disorders* (**ICSD-R**),[1] disorders of excessive sleepiness are classified as dyssomnias, intrinsic or extrinsic, and as disorders associated with medical or psychiatric disorders. However, in this chapter a more clinical classification will be used, with reference firstly to the types of excessive sleepiness that are provoked by insufficient sleep or by medications, and secondly to the disorders of excessive sleepiness that may be primary or secondary to a pathological process (Table 1). In this chapter disorders of the circadian rhythm of sleep, such as shift work disorder, jet lag, and delayed or advanced sleep phase syndrome, which are responsible for both insomnia and excessive sleepiness, will not be addressed except as causes of excessive sleepiness.

Epidemiology

Contrary to common thinking, excessive sleepiness is neither exceptional nor rare. Epidemiological surveys conducted in the 1980s all agree with a prevalence of excessive sleepiness of between 3 and 5 per cent.[2–7] Yet most physicians are not aware of excessive sleepiness as a pathological process. Thus, there is a definite need to identify those subjects suffering from excessive sleepiness, to evaluate them adequately, and to treat them.

Table 1 Disorders of wakefulness

| Provoked | Pathological | | Circadian |
	Primary	Secondary	
Insufficient sleep syndrome	Obstructive sleep apnoea–hypopnoea syndrome	Hypersomnia associated with Neurological disorders	Shift work sleep disorder
Hypersomnia secondary to drug intake	Upper airway resistance syndrome	Infectious disorders Metabolic disorders Endocrine disorders Mood disorders	Time zone change syndrome Delayed and advanced sleep phase syndromes
	Narcolepsy		
	Idiopathic hypersomnia Polysymptomatic Monosymptomatic	Post-traumatic hypersomnia	Non-24-h sleep–wake syndrome
	Recurrent hypersomnia		
	Periodic limb movement disorder		

Morbidity

Excessive sleepiness is much more severe than one would expect. Excessive sleepiness, whether caused by voluntary or involuntary sleep deprivation or by psychiatric or organic disorders, includes diminished mental and physical health, increased morbidity, and lowered productivity, and increases the incidence of road, rail, maritime, aircraft, nuclear industry, hospital, and military accidents.[8]

Clinical work-up and laboratory tests

Some subjects may seek a diagnosis because of discomfort or embarrassment caused by excessive sleepiness. Other subjects are brought to the outpatient clinic by their spouse or partner because they fall asleep while driving or at the end of a meal or in a friend's company. Many of these subjects have difficulty in accepting the fact that they are abnormally sleepy. Finally, some subjects are referred after an accident or are recognized as abnormally sleepy while hospitalized for a medical or psychiatric disorder.

Whatever the circumstance of the first visit, the subject should be interviewed on the history of the symptom, the type and severity of the excessive sleepiness, the associated symptoms, diurnal and nocturnal, the familial and professional consequences, the past and current treatments, and the personal and familial medical past-history. In addition the subject should complete a self-administered behavioural scale, the Epworth Sleepiness Scale,[9] involving self-assessment of the likelihood of falling asleep under a variety of conditions with various activity levels. The subject will then undergo a physical and psychological examination.

Laboratory tests will be performed according to the clinical impression. These include nap studies and/or prolonged polysomnographic recordings. Two basic nap approaches are available to assess the level of daytime sleepiness: multiple daytime naps with instructions to try to fall asleep as rapidly as possible (e.g. multiple sleep latency test),[10] and multiple daytime recordings with instruction to attempt to stay awake (maintenance of wakefulness test).[11] Prolonged polysomnographic recordings, obtained by either traditional laboratory polysomnographic monitoring or ambulatory recordings at home or in the laboratory, provide a good picture of the actual time asleep within the 24-h period.

Aetiology and treatment

Provoked disorders of wakefulness

Insufficient sleep syndrome

According to ICSD-R[1] the insufficient sleep syndrome is defined as a disorder that occurs in an individual who persistently fails to obtain sufficient nocturnal sleep required to support normally alert wakefulness.

Although no epidemiological studies are available, this syndrome is likely to be widespread, especially in lorry drivers, physicians, working mothers, students, and executives. The main symptoms are excessive sleepiness in the afternoon and early evening, late awakening or the necessity for an afternoon nap on rest days, a consistent decrease of diurnal performances, in particular relating to tasks requiring sustained attention, and irritability, depression, nervousness, gastro-intestinal problems, muscle aches, and visual disturbances. Diagnosis of this syndrome is relatively easy provided that a thorough interview is conducted. The most rational treatment is an increase of the time spent asleep, either by spending more time in bed at night, or by taking one or two naps per day.

Hypersomnia secondary to drug intake

A wide spectrum of medications may be responsible for excessive sleepiness: some, such as slow and intermediate half-life hypnotics and anxiolytics, affect patients quite consistently, and others affect certain subjects only. Positive diagnosis requires a thorough listing of all medications taken by the patient.

Anxiolytics and hypnotics

These include benzodiazepines, non-benzodiazepine hypnotics such as zopiclone and zolpidem, and non-benzodiazepine anxiolytics such as meprobamate and buspirone. Benzodiazepines have sedative effects in humans, but this effect varies with dose, administration (single or repeated dose), age of subject, and state of the subject (normal, anxious, or depressed). Two recent non-benzodiazepine hypnotics (zopiclone and zolpidem) induce either no sleepiness at all or limited sleepiness in the morning immediately after awakening. Buspirone seems to induce less sleepiness than the benzodiazepines.

Neuroleptics

Neuroleptics have a sedative effect. However, the degree of sedation varies widely from subject to subject. Empirically, three-quarters of patients treated with neuroleptic phenothiazines experience sleepiness in a dose-dependent manner. Sleepiness tends to vanish with time.

Antidepressants

Tricyclic antidepressants have sedative effects. These effects are associated with the blockade of histamine H_1 and postsynaptic α-adrenergic receptors. They are responsible for an alteration of information processing, psychomotor performance, and car-handling ability.

Excessive sleepiness is observed in some patients treated with trazodone, mianserine, fluoxetine, fluvoxamine, and paroxetine. Excessive sleepiness is among the undesirable effects of lithium.

Antiepileptic drugs

Phenobarbitone, carbamazepine, phenytoin, valproic acid, progabide, and ethosuccinimide induce sleepiness, especially at the beginning of the course.

Antihistaminic drugs

H_1 antihistamines have sedative effects. The intensity of this effect depends on the molecule, the dose administered, and the subject. Several medications such as neuroleptics with a phenothiazine structure, tricyclic antidepressants, mianserine, flunarizine, and hydroxyzine, have antihistaminic properties.

Miscellaneous

In addition to the above-mentioned medications some cardiovascular medications such as clonidine, α-methyl dopa, and prazosine, and some anticholinergic molecules such as scopolamine and progestative medications may induce excessive sleepiness.

Pathological disorders of wakefulness

Primary disorders of wakefulness

Sleep-induced respiratory disturbances

These are the most frequent causes of pathological sleepiness. They include the obstructive sleep apnoea syndrome, the sleep hypopnea syndrome, and the upper airway resistance syndrome.

Obstructive sleep apnoea syndrome This syndrome was first described by Guilleminault *et al.*[12] It is most frequent in 50-year-old males. According to Young *et al.*[13] the prevalence of sleep-disordered breathing accompanied by excessive daytime sleepiness in North America is 4 per cent in men and 2 per cent in women.

Clinical features include night-time and daytime symptoms. Night-time symptoms are represented by loud snoring, apnoeic episodes ending with sonorous breathing resumption, nocturia, severe fatigue upon awakening, and sometimes headache. Daytime symptoms are dominated by excessive sleepiness which varies in intensity among patients. Other symptoms include irritability, negligence, loss of concentration, loss of libido, impotence, and sometimes depression.

Patients are often obese or mildly obese. High blood pressure is a frequent feature. The ear, nose, and throat examination usually reveals a narrow upper airway due to close-set posterior tonsillar pillars, an abnormally long and hypotonic soft palate, a hypertrophic uvula, or macroglossia.

Obstructive sleep apnoea syndrome is associated with occasional arrhythmias and conduction disturbances, systemic hypertension, pulmonary hypertension, functional cognitive impairment, and cardiac or cerebral ischaemic manifestations.

Polysomnography aids **diagnosis** by allowing the identification of apnoeas and of their types (obstructive, central, or mixed), as well as the consequences of apnoeas on heart rate, oxygen saturation, and degree of somnolence.

There are several possible approaches to **treatment**. Continuous positive airway pressure at night is the most widely used treatment. A modification of continuous positive airway pressure where bilevel positive pressure is applied with higher pressure during inspiration may be more useful for patients requiring high continuous positive airway pressure levels, since it reduces the average pressure and the work of breathing during the night. Good compliance requires proper preparation for the patient and an adaptation period.

Surgical procedures include uvulopalatopharyngoplasty and bimalleolar advancement. The former leads to an improvement of symptoms but is not very efficient on the apnoeas; the latter is more efficient but is also more aggressive.

Oral appliances are suitable in mild obstructive sleep apnoea syndromes.

Weight loss may improve obstructive sleep apnoea syndrome. Avoidance of alcohol and sedatives should be recommended

Obstructive sleep hypopnoea syndrome Manifestations and consequences are less severe than in the obstructive sleep apnoea syndrome.

Upper airway resistance syndrome First described by Guilleminault *et al.*,[14] the upper airway resistance syndrome differs from the obstructive sleep apnoea syndrome and the sleep hypopnoea syndrome by the absence of a consistent number of apnoeas and the absence of oxygen desaturation.

Symptoms are very much the same as in the obstructive sleep apnoea syndrome with loud snoring, fatigue on awakening, and excessive daytime sleepiness. However, snoring may be absent and special physical features such as high arched palate, malocclusion of the jaw type II, mandibular instability, or micrognathia may direct the diagnosis.

Positive **diagnosis** requires oesophageal pressure monitoring and quantification of airflow using a face-mask with a pneumotachometer to document the so-called crescendo (a sequence of breaths with progressively increasing inspiratory efforts indicated by progressively negative peak and inspiratory pressure) and a simultaneous decrease in tidal volume compared with preceding breaths without increase efforts.

Treatment is not yet well codified. Continuous positive airway pressure is useful but often not well tolerated. Uvulopalatopharyngoplasty is rarely efficient. Oral appliances should to be tested. Bimandibular advancement is an appropriate procedure when facial abnormalities are present.

Narcolepsy

First described in 1877[15] and given its name by Gelineau in 1880,[16] narcolepsy is not a rare condition. According to most recent evaluations its prevalence is 0.21 to 0.26 per 1000,[17,18] i.e. slightly less than the prevalence of multiple sclerosis.

The two cardinal symptoms of narcolepsy are excessive daytime sleepiness culminating in recurrent daily irresistible and refreshing episodes of sleep, and cataplexy, a sudden loss of muscle tone triggered by an emotional factor, most often a positive one, such as laughter, compliments, or dry humour, and less often a negative one, such as stress or anger. Cataplexy occurs with a frequency anywhere between once a year or less to several times a day. The loss of tone may be total, causing the subject to fall, but much more frequently it is partial when the subject is unable to articulate words, has a strange feeling in the face, or experiences unlocking of the knees. It may last from a split second to several minutes. Other symptoms are not necessary for the diagnosis. Hypnagogic (at sleep onset) or hypnopompic (at sleep offset) hallucinations are somesthetic, auditory, or sometimes visual. The impression of a human presence in the room is frequent. Hypnagogic hallucinations are sometimes so frightening that the subject keeps a weapon on the bedside table or a dog in the room for reassurance. Sleep paralysis is an inability to move the arms, legs, and head or to breathe normally. It is often associated with an hypnagogic hallucination. It is terrifying, and may last for 10 min or more. Finally, narcoleptic subjects experience disturbed nocturnal sleep with recurrent awakening, sleeptalking, and frequently rapid eye movement (**REM**) sleep behaviour disorder.

Diagnosis of narcolepsy is based on clinical features. However, there are cases where there is uncertainty due to rare or atypical cataplexies. In these cases laboratory tests (polysomnography and HLA typing) are particularly helpful. Polysomnography includes monitoring of night sleep followed by the multiple sleep latency test procedure. Night sleep is characterized by increased Stage I sleep, increased number of awakenings, and often a sleep-onset REM period. The multiple sleep latency test typically shows a mean sleep latency less than 7 min over the five sessions of the test and two sleep-onset REM periods at least. However, subjects with typical narcolepsy may show only one or even no sleep-onset REM period in some cases. HLA typing shows an association with HLA DR15-DQ6 (DRB1*1501–DQB1*0602) in 96 to 98 per cent of Caucasian patients and in 60 per cent of African-American patients.

The **natural history** of narcolepsy is chronic. Excessive daytime sleepiness is lifelong, although subjects cope with it more easily after retirement. Cataplexy may vanish with age in some subjects. Hypnagogic hallucinations and sleep paralysis are most often temporary. Poor sleep does not show a tendency to improve.

The mainstay of **treatment** is pharmacological, although taking naps may alleviate excessive daytime sleepiness, and refraining from emotion may prevent cataplexy. Excessive daytime sleepiness is treated by stimulants (methylphenidate, methamphetamine, mazindol, pemoline) or by modafinil, a new drug with awakening properties. Cataplexy and other REM-related symptoms, hypnagogic hallucinations, and sleep paralysis respond to tricyclic or selective serotonin reuptake inhibitor antidepressants. Poor sleep may be improved by the use of hypnotics.

Idiopathic hypersomnia

In comparison with narcolepsy, which is characterized by well-defined clinical, polysomnographic and immunogenetic features, idiopathic hypersomnia is not as well delineated. Its first description dates back to 1976,[19] almost a century after that of narcolepsy. No prevalence study has ever been conducted. However, from the different series published so far the ratio of idiopathic hypersomnia to narcolepsy could be as low as 10 per cent or even less.[20] There are two forms of idiopathic hypersomnia:[19] one is referred to as polysymptomatic and is characterized by nocturnal sleep of prolonged duration (as much as 10 h or more), signs of sleep drunkenness on awakening, and constant or recurrent excessive daytime sleepiness leading to unrefreshing prolonged naps, and the other is referred to as monosymptomatic, with excessive daytime sleepiness but no abnormally long sleep periods or sleep drunkenness.

The **diagnosis** of idiopathic hypersomnia is mainly based on clinical features and the absence of associated symptoms such as cataplexy, snoring at night, or depression. Polysomnography is necessary to exclude other sleep disorders, especially the upper airway resistance syndrome. Nocturnal sleep recording shows a sleep of normal quality with few awakenings and a normal proportion of the different sleep stages. Sleep apnoeas and periodic movements in sleep are absent. The multiple sleep latency test is not very demonstrative in showing a mean sleep latency of 8 to 10 min. On the other hand, continuous polysomnography with the subject free to switch on and off the light at his or her own convenience shows most prolonged night sleep followed by one or two naps of long duration. Sleep-onset REM periods are not a feature of the condition.

The **natural history** of idiopathic hypersomnia is chronic. It is a lifelong disorder with no tendency to remit spontaneously. Complications are mostly social and professional as is the case in narcolepsy.

Treatment of idiopathic hypersomnia relies on the same drugs as those used in narcolepsy. In contrast with narcolepsy, naps are not refreshing and should be avoided.

Recurrent hypersomnia

In 1936 Levin[21] described a syndrome of periodic somnolence and morbid hunger occurring exclusively in males, starting in the second decade, and characterized by attacks of somnolence lasting several days or weeks, associated with abnormal behaviour, including overeating and sexual disinhibition, and various mental features such as irritability, mild confusion, incoherent speech, and at times hallucinations. In 1942 Critchley and Hoffmann[22] reported two more cases and coined the eponymous term **Kleine–Levin syndrome**.

Kleine–Levin syndrome is a rare condition; in our case statistics there were 19 subjects with this condition compared with 336 narcoleptics. Adolescent males are most commonly affected, but female cases are not unknown.

Excessive sleep develops either abruptly or gradually. The subject retires to his or her bedroom and almost refuses to leave it. Sleep is either calm or agitated. Abnormal behaviours, overeating, and sexual disinhibition are generally viewed as compulsive. Patients eat all food within sight, even if it is of poor quality. Manifestations of hypersexuality, indiscriminate sexual advances regardless of age and sex, and/or overt masturbation are reported in one-third of males and less often in females. Mental disturbances are of varying types. Irritability is the most frequent symptom, then a feeling of unreality, and less often confusion and/or visual or auditory hallucinations. The duration of episodes varies from 1 day to 3 to 4 weeks and the interval between episodes varies from less than a month to several months. Between episodes physical examination is normal. There is no consistent personality disorder.

Positive **diagnosis** of the Kleine–Levin syndrome is based on clinical features and not on laboratory investigations.

According to Critchley,[23] the **natural history** of the Kleine–Levin syndrome follows a decreasing course and attacks eventually cease. However, cases have been reported in which the symptoms have persisted for over 20 years.

Treatment includes symptomatic and preventive measures. The former are oriented towards cessation of the hypersomniac episodes, and rely on stimulant or awakening drugs, the effectiveness of which does not generally exceed a few hours or so. The latter have to be considered when hypersomniac episodes are frequent enough to disturb personal and family life. Positive results have been recorded with carbamazepine, valpromide, and lithium carbonate.

Periodic limb movement disorder

In some patients with excessive sleepiness the most conspicuous abnormality is the occurrence of periodic limb movements in sleep (**PLMS**) consisting of repetitive stereotypic dorsiflexion of the big toe accompanied by flexion of the ankle, and sometimes the knee and the thigh. The movements recur at intervals of 10 to 90 s and last for 0.5 to 5 s. The periodic limb movement index is the number of movements per hour of total sleep time as determined by polysomnography. An index of 5 or more is regarded as abnormal.

However, recent articles cast some doubt on the responsibility of PLMS in causing excessive sleepiness,[24,25] and there is no evidence that anti-PLMS medications are useful in alleviating excessive sleepiness in these subjects.[26]

Secondary disorders of wakefuless

Hypersomnia associated with neurological conditions

Brain tumours Brain tumours of specific location may result in excessive sleepiness in the absence of raised intracranial pressure. Excessive sleepiness is typically permanent. This is the case with some tumours affecting the posterolateral hypothalamus (gliomas, hamartomas, suprasellar craniopharyngiomas more than metastases or malignant lymphomas), the pineal gland (pinealomas, teratomas, astrocytomas), and the upper brainstem.

Of special interest are the cases of brain tumours involving hypothalamic or mesencephalic regions and presenting as narcolepsy with irresistible sleep episodes, cataplexy, and sometimes hypnagogic hallucinations and/or sleep paralysis.

Post-stroke hypersomnia The clinical spectrum of hypersomnia is heterogeneous. It includes sleep-like behaviour, yawning, stretching, 'presleep' behaviours, inversion of the sleep–wake cycle, loss of heteroactivation (awakening difficulties), loss of autoactivation (apathy), etc.

Clinical symptoms depend upon location of the pathological process: hemispheric, thalamic, mesencephalic, or pontine. Most frequently they are paramedian thalamopeduncular infarcts or bilateral paramedian thalamic infarcts. Paramedian thalamic infarcts are characterized by hypersomnia, deep coma, or akinetic mutism associated with ocular motility abnormalities. Bilateral paramedian thalamic infarcts are characterized by disturbances of consciousness and behaviour, leading eventually to thalamic dementia. Hypersomnia may be transiently present. Large hemispheric strokes may also induce excessive sleepiness.

Neurodegenerative diseases A number of neurodegenerative disorders may be associated with several sleep complaints, particularly insomnia and excessive sleepiness. Such disorders include Parkinson's disease, Alzheimer's disease, multiple system atrophy, and progressive supranuclear palsy. Several mechanisms may be involved, including alteration of systems responsible for the sleep–wake regulation by neurochemical changes found in these disorders, sleep-related respiratory disturbances, which are greater in patients with autonomic disturbance, dysfunction within the circadian system, sleep changes associated with medications, or mood disorders.

Neuromuscular diseases Sleep-related disturbances of breathing are most frequently responsible for excessive sleepiness. This is the case in poliomyelitis, motor neurone disease, myasthenia gravis, metabolic myopathies, muscular dystrophies, and polyneuropathies. Among the postulated causative mechanisms are weakness of the diaphragm and the intercostal muscles, weakness of the pharyngeal muscles, increasing the tendency of the upper airway to collapse during sleep, scoliosis, and facial and cranial dysmorphisms. In myotonic dystrophy central nervous system lesions, as well as obstructive and central sleep apnoeas, may play a role.

Hypersomnia associated with infectious disorders

Excessive sleepiness occurring during the acute phase of a bacterial or viral infection, without any other symptom of central nervous system involvement, is commonplace in medicine. Its mechanism may involve certain cytokines.

There are other conditions, also presenting with excessive sleepiness, which may be life threatening. The most frequent of these is African trypanosomiasis (sleeping sickness) caused by the haemoflagellate *Trypanosoma brucei*. The incubation period of the parasite lasts about 2 weeks. Systemic manifestations become apparent during the haematogenous dissemination of the trypanosome. They include an irregular fever and generalized lymphadenopathy, particularly of the posterior cerebral chain. The parasite enters the central nervous system after a delay of up to several years. Cerebral trypanosomiasis can be explosive, with seizures, coma, and eventually death, or more frequently it may

be progressive with abnormal sleepiness, headaches, and tremor of the hands. Positive diagnosis is based on a history of a stay in an endemic zone, the presence of inflammatory signs, and finding the trypanosomes in the blood, aspirate of lymph nodes, or cerebrospinal fluid. Curative treatment consists of melarsoprol or pentamidine. Prophylaxis is the preferred treatment of the disease.

European tick-borne encephalitis occurs mainly in Eastern Europe. It is characterized by two stages, one viraemic and the second one referred to as nervous. Hypersomnia is common during the second stage.

Encephalitis lethargica first appeared in France and Vienna in 1917. It then spread rapidly through Western Europe and affected thousands of people. Two main varieties were encountered: the common somnolent form and the hyperkinetic form. Sporadic cases of encephalitis lethargica are sometimes encountered today.[27]

Hypersomnia associated with metabolic or endocrine disorders

Excessive somnolence is the first manifestation of portal systemic encephalopathy. It can either vanish under the effect of treatment or give way to obtundation or coma.

Hypersomnia may develop as a consequence of sleep apnoea, often associated with hypothyroidism or acromegaly.

Hypersomnia associated with mood disorders

Insomnia is a frequent feature of mood disorder and excessive sleepiness is rarely encountered. However, hypersomnia in depressed patients is often referred to in literature,[28–32] although the reported rates vary from study to study and it cannot be ascertained from index or behavioural observations whether these subjects experience true daytime sleepiness and/or excessive sleep, or simply spend more time in bed than normal subjects. Thus objective measures of excessive daytime sleepiness or prolonged sleep monitoring are required. However, in comparison with subjective studies the number of objective studies is rather limited.[33–35] From these studies it appears that some subjects complaining of excessive sleepiness associated with a mood disorder display evidence of objective excessive sleepiness or increased total sleep time at night or during the day. However, a large number of them spend a considerable time in bed during day and night, with polysomnography not documenting actual sleep, a behaviour referred to as 'clinophilia' from the Greek κλινη (bed) and φιλεω (love).

Post-traumatic hypersomnia

Any abnormal daytime sleepiness developing within a year after a head trauma may be considered as post-traumatic sleepiness. Lesions involving the brainstem (tegmentothalamic region, pontine tegmentum) or posterior hypothalamus are responsible for hypersomnia. Typical obstructive sleep apnoea syndrome may develop shortly after brain trauma.[36] Post-head-injury syndrome or post-concussion syndrome is also a possibility, although insomnia is more frequent than hypersomnia in this syndrome.

Disorders of the circadian rhythm of sleep (see also Chapters 4.14.1, 4.14.2, and 9.2.9)

The major feature of these disorders is a misalignment between the patient's sleep pattern and that which is desirable or regarded as the societal norm. As a consequence sleep episodes and the corresponding wake periods occur at inappropriate times. Therefore the patient complains of insomnia and/or sleepiness.

Shift work sleep disorder and **jet lag syndrome** consist of symptoms of insomnia and/or excessive sleepiness that occur as transient phenomena related to work schedules or rapid travel across a number of time zones.

Delayed and advanced sleep phase syndromes are disorders in which the major sleep episode is either delayed or advanced relative to the desired clock time, and the non-24-h sleep–wake syndrome consists of a chronic steady pattern comprising delays of 1 to 2 h in sleep onset and wake times. These syndromes are associated with an abnormal departure of the individual circadian rhythm of sleep from synchronizer control.

Treatment of these disorders utilizes various approaches including sleep hygiene, scheduling of naps, chronotherapy, light exposure, and melatonin therapy.

Conclusion

Excessive sleepiness has many manifestations and aetiologies, and its consequences are far from negligible. Treatments are effective, provided that the aetiology is well recognized.

References

1. American Sleep Disorders Association (1997). *International classification of sleep disorders, revised: diagnostic and coding manual*. American Sleep Disorders Association, Rochester, MN.
2. Bixler, E.D., Kales, A., Soldatos, C.R., Kales, J.D., and Healy, S. (1979). Prevalence of sleep disorders in the Los Angeles metropolitan area. *American Journal of Psychiatry*, **136**, 1257–62.
3. Lavie, P. (1981). Sleep habits and sleep disturbances in industrial workers in Israel. *Sleep*, **4**, 147–58.
4. Franceschi, M., Zamproni, P., Crippa, D., and Smirne, S. (1982). Excessive daytime sleepiness: a 1-year study in an unselected inpatient population. *Sleep*, **5**, 239–47.
5. Partinen, M. and Rimpelä, M. (1982). Sleeping habits and sleep disorders in a population of 2016 Finnish adults. *The yearbook of health education research 1982*, pp. 253–60. The National Board of Health, Helsinki, Finland.
6. Lugaresi, E., Cirignotta, F., Zucconi, M., Mondini, S., Lenzi, P.L., and Coccagna, G. (1983). Good and poor sleepers: an epidemiological survey of the San Marino population. In *Sleep–wake disorders: natural history, epidemiology and long-term evolution* (ed. C. Guilleminault and E. Lugaresi), pp. 1–12. Raven Press, New York.
7. Billiard, M., Alperovitch, A., Perot, C., and Jammes, A. (1987). Excessive daytime somnolence in young men: prevalence and contributing factors. *Sleep*, **10**, 297–305.
8. National Commission on Sleep Disorders Research (1992). *Wake up America: a national sleep alert. Executive summary and executive report*. Report of the National Commission on Sleep Disorders Research. DHSS Publication. US Government Printing Office, Washington, DC.
9. Johns, M.W. (1991). A new method for measuring daytime sleepiness: The Epworth Sleepiness Scale. *Sleep*, **14**, 540–5.
10. Carskadon, M. and Dement, W.C. (1977). Sleep tendency: an objective measure of sleep loss. *Sleep Research*, **6**, 200.
11. Mitler, M.M., Gujavarty, S., and Browman, C.P. (1982). Maintenance of wakefulness test: a polysomnographic technique for evaluating treatment efficacy in patients with excessive somnolence. *Electroencephalography and Clinical Neurophysiology*, **53**, 658–61.
12. Guilleminault, C., Tilkian, A., and Dement, W.C. (1976). The sleep apnea syndromes. *Annual Review of Medicine*, **27**, 465–84.
13. Young, T., Palta, M., Dempsey, J., Skatrud, J., Weber, S., and Badr, S. (1993). The occurrence of sleep-disordered breathing among middle-aged adults. *New England Journal of Medicine*, **328**, 1230–5.
14. Guilleminault, C., Stoohs, R., Clerk, A., Simmons, J., and Labanowski, M. (1992). From obstructive sleep apnea syndrome to upper airway resistance syndrome—consistency of daytime sleepiness. *Sleep*, **15**, S13–S16.
15. Westphal, C. (1877). Eigentümliche mit Einschlafen verbundene Anfälle. *Archiv für Psychiatrie Nervenkrankheiten*, **7**, 631–5.
16. Gelineau, J. (1880). De la narcolepsie. *Gazette des Hôpitaux*, **55**, 626–8, 635–7.
17. Hublin, C., Kaprio, J., Partinen, M., *et al.* (1994). The prevalence of narcolepsy: an epidemiological study of the Finnish twin cohort. *Annals of Neurology*, **35**, 709–16.
18. Ondzé, B., Lubin, S., Lavandier, B., Kohler, F., Mayeux, D., and Billiard, M. (1998). Frequency of narcolepsy in the population of a French 'département'. *Journal of Sleep Research*, **7** (Supplement 2), 193.
19. Roth, B. (1976). Narcolepsy and hypersomnia. *Schweizer Archiv für Neurologie und Psychiatrie*, **119**, 31–41.
20. Billiard, M. and Besset, A. (1998) L'hypersomnie idiopathique. In *Le sommeil normal et pathologique* (2nd edn) (ed. M. Billiard), pp. 292–8. Masson, Paris.
21. Levin, M. (1936). Periodic somnolence and morbid hunger: a new syndrome. *Brain*, **59**, 494–504.
22. Critchley, M. and Hoffman, H.L. (1942). The syndrome of periodic somnolence and morbid hunger (Kleine–Levin syndrome). *British Medical Journal*, **i**, 137–9.
23. Critchley, M. (1962). Periodic hypersomnia and megaphagia in adolescent males. *Brain*, **85**, 627–56.
24. Mendelson, W.B. (1996). Are periodic leg movements associated with clinical sleep disturbance? *Sleep*, **19**, 219–23.
25. Nicolas, A., Lespérance, P., and Montplaisir, J. (1998). Is excessive daytime sleepiness with periodic leg movements during sleep a specific diagnostic category? *European Neurology*, **40**, 22–6.
26. Montplaisir, J., Boucher, S., Gosselin, A., Poirier, G., and Lavigne, G. (1996). Persistence of repetitive EEG arousals (K-alpha complexes) in RLS patients treated with L-dopa. *Sleep*, **19**, 196–9.
27. Howard, R.S. and Lees, A.J. (1987). Encephalitis lethargica. A report of four recent cases. *Brain*, **110**, 19–33.
28. Detre, T., Himmelhoch, J., Swartzburg, M., Anderson, C.M., Byck, R., and Kupfer, D.J. (1972). Hypersomnia and manic–depressive disease. *American Journal of Psychiatry*, **128**, 1303–5.
29. Michaelis, R. and Hofmann, E. (1973). Zur Phänomenologie und Atiopathogenese der Hypersomnie bei endogenphasischen Depressionen. In *The nature of sleep* (ed. U.J. Jovanovic), pp. 190–3. Gustav Fischer, Stuttgart.
30. Claghorn, J.L., Mathew, R.J., Weinman, M.L., and Hruska, N. (1981). Daytime sleepiness in depression. *Journal of Clinical Psychiatry*, **42**, 342–3.
31. Garvey, M.J., Mungas, D., and Tollefson, G.D. (1984). Hypersomnia in major depressive disorders. *Journal of Affective Disorders*, **6**, 283–6.
32. Southmayd, S.E., Cairns, J., Delva, N.J., Letemendia, F.J.J., and Brunet, D.G. (1986). Awake, perchance asleep? *British Journal of Psychiatry*, **148**, 748–9.
33. Shimizu, A., Hiyama, H., Yagasaki, A., Takahashi, H., Fujiki, A., and Yoshida, I. (1979). Sleep of depressed patients with hypersomnia: a 24 h study. *Waking and Sleeping*, **3**, 335–9.
34. Nofzinger, E.A., Thase, M.E., Reynolds, C.F., *et al.* (1991). Hypersomnia in bipolar depression: a comparison with narcolepsy using the multiple sleep latency test. *American Journal of Psychiatry*, **148**, 1177–81.
35. Billiard, M., Dolenc, L., Aldaz, C., Ondze, B., and Besset, A. (1994). Hypersomnia associated with mood disorders: a new perspective. *Journal of Psychosomatic Research*, **38** (Supplement 1), 41–7.
36. Guilleminault, C., Faull, K.F., Miles, L., and Van den Hoed, J. (1983). Posttraumatic excessive daytime sleepiness: a review of 20 patients. *Neurology*, **33**, 1584–9.

4.14.4 Parasomnias

Carlos H. Schenck and Mark W. Mahowald

In all of us, even in good men, there is a lawless, wild-beast nature which peers out in sleep.

Plato, *The Republic*

Relevance of parasomnias to psychiatrists

Parasomnias are defined as undesirable physical phenomena accompanying sleep that involve skeletal muscle activity and/ or autonomic nervous system changes.[1] Parasomnias can be objectively diagnosed by means of polysomnography (i.e. the physiological monitoring of sleep), and can be successfully treated in the majority of cases.[2–4] Understanding of the parasomnias, based on polysomnographic documentation, has expanded greatly over recent years, as new disorders have been identified, and as known disorders have been recognized to occur more frequently, across a broader age group, and with more serious consequences than previously understood.[2–6] There are at least eight reasons why parasomnias should be of interest to psychiatrists.

1. Parasomnias can be misdiagnosed and inappropriately treated as a psychiatric disorder.

2. Parasomnias can be a direct manifestation of a psychiatric disorder, e.g. dissociative disorder.

3. The emergence and/or recurrence of a parasomnia can be triggered by stress.

4. Psychotropic medications can induce the initial emergence of a parasomnia, or aggravate a pre-existing parasomnia.

5. Parasomnias can cause psychological distress or can induce or reactivate a psychiatric disorder in the patient or bed partner on account of repeated loss of self-control during sleep and sleep-related injuries.

6. Familiarity with the parasomnias will allow psychiatrists to be more fully aware of the various medical and neurological disorders that can be associated with disturbed (sleep-related) behaviour and disturbed dreaming.

7. Parasomnias present a special opportunity for interlinking animal basic science research (including parasomnia animal models) with human (sleep) behavioural disorders.

8. Parasomnias carry forensic implications. Psychiatrists are often asked to render an expert opinion in medicolegal cases pertaining to sleep-related violence.

Classification of parasomnias

Parasomnias can be classified according to whether the signs or symptoms are primary phenomena of sleep itself, or whether they are secondary phenomena derived from various underlying disorders, with sleep facilitating the nocturnal manifestation of these disorders.[7]

Table 1 contains such a classification, and provides a context (along with other sources[1,8,9]) for the parasomnias to be covered in this chapter. Parasomnias demonstrate how sleep and wakefulness are not mutually exclusive states. Features of rapid eye movement (**REM**) sleep, non-REM sleep, and wakefulness can occur simultaneously, and with rapid oscillations.[10] Status dissociatus represents the most extreme form of state dissociation.[11]

Clinical evaluation of parasomnias

The evaluation of complex and violent nocturnal behaviours at our centre (Minnesota Regional Sleep Disorders Center) includes the following.[2,12]

1. Clinical sleep–wake interview, with review of medical records, and review of a patient questionnaire that covers sleep–wake, medical, psychiatric, and alcohol/chemical use and abuse history, review of systems, family history, and past or current physical, sexual, and emotional abuse.

2. Psychiatric and neurological interviews and examinations, including psychometric testing.

3. Extensive overnight polysomnographic monitoring at a hospital sleep laboratory, with continuous audiovisual recording. Figures 1 and 2 show the polysomnography montage: electro-oculogram, EEG, chin and four-limb electromyograms, ECG, and nasal–oral

Table 1 Classification of parasomnias: primary and secondary sleep phenomena

Primary sleep phenomena

Non-REM sleep
   Disorders of arousal: sleepwalking/sleep terrors/confusional arousals

REM sleep
   REM sleep behaviour disorder (RBD)
   Dream anxiety attacks (nightmares)

Miscellaneous (including mixed non-REM/REM sleep)
   Parasomnia overlap disorder (sleepwalking/sleep terrors/RBD)
   Nocturnal sleep-related eating disorders
   Restless legs syndrome/periodic limb movements in sleep
   Obstructive sleep apnoea-related parasomnias
   Rhythmic movement disorders
   Status dissociatus
   Bruxism

Secondary sleep phenomena

Central nervous system
   Seizures (conventional, unconventional)
   Headaches
Psychiatric
   Nocturnal dissociative disorders
   Nocturnal panic attacks
   Nocturnal bulimia nervosa
   Post-traumatic stress disorder
Cardiopulmonary (arrhythmias, asthma, etc.)
Gastrointestinal (gastro-oesophageal reflux etc.)

Malingering

Modified from Mahowald and Ettinger.[7]

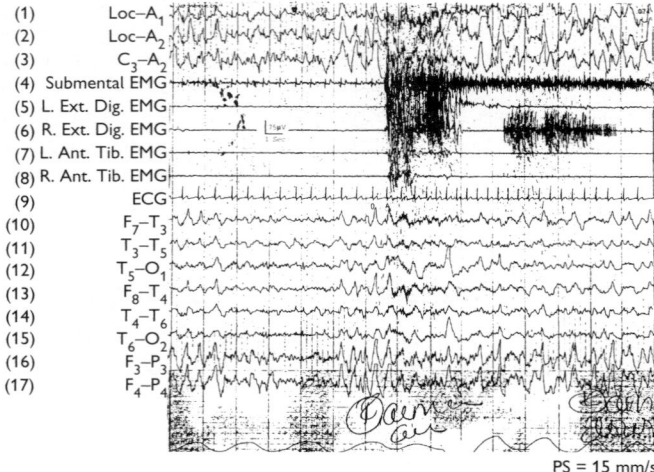

(1) Loc–A₁
(2) Loc–A₂
(3) C₃–A₂
(4) Submental EMG
(5) L. Ext. Dig. EMG
(6) R. Ext. Dig. EMG
(7) L. Ant. Tib. EMG
(8) R. Ant. Tib. EMG
(9) ECG
(10) F₇–T₃
(11) T₃–T₅
(12) T₅–O₁
(13) F₈–T₄
(14) T₄–T₆
(15) T₆–O₂
(16) F₃–P₃
(17) F₄–P₄

PS = 15 mm/s

Fig. 1 Polysomnogram of a disordered arousal, with the persistence of sleep, in a 23-year-old man with a history of sleepwalking and sleep terrors. After a behavioural arousal from slow-wave sleep (with arm lifted up and then down), the EEG shows irregular delta and theta activity and superimposed faster frequencies. Immediately preceding the arousal, there is a cluster of three high-amplitude delta waves (channel 3). Electro-oculogram, channels 1, 2; EEG, channels 3, 10–17; EMG, electromyogram. (Reproduced with permission from C.H. Schenck et al. (1998). Analysis of polysomnographic events surrounding 252 slow-wave sleep arousals in thirty-eight adults with injurious sleepwalking and sleep terrors. *Journal of Clinical Neurophysiology*, **15**, 159–66.)

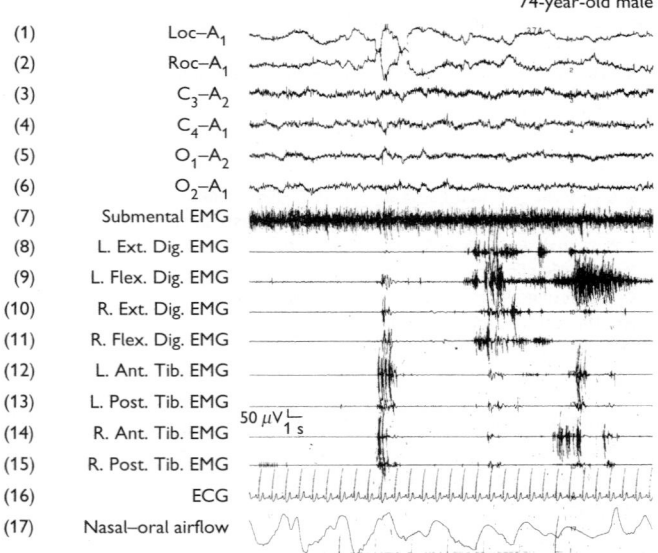

74-year-old male

(1) Loc–A₁
(2) Roc–A₁
(3) C₃–A₂
(4) C₄–A₁
(5) O₁–A₂
(6) O₂–A₁
(7) Submental EMG
(8) L. Ext. Dig. EMG
(9) L. Flex. Dig. EMG
(10) R. Ext. Dig. EMG
(11) R. Flex. Dig. EMG
(12) L. Ant. Tib. EMG
(13) L. Post. Tib. EMG
(14) R. Ant. Tib. EMG
(15) R. Post. Tib. EMG
(16) ECG
(17) Nasal–oral airflow

50 μV | 1 s

Fig. 2 Polysomnogram of disordered rapid eye movement (REM) sleep in a man with REM sleep behaviour disorder who eventually developed Parkinson's disease. There is complete loss of 'REM-atonia', as the submental electromyogram (EMG) shows continuous muscle tone (channel 7). The appearance of a rapid eye movement (channels 1, 2) signals the onset of excessive muscle twitching in the upper/lower extremity EMGs (channels 8–15). The EEG (channels 3–6) shows the typical low-voltage fast-frequency desynchronized activity of REM sleep. ECG rate (channel 16) remains constant despite generalized muscle twitching, which is a common finding in REM sleep behaviour disorder. Electro-oculogram: channels 1, 2.

airflow (with full respiratory monitoring whenever indicated). Polysomnographic paper speeds of 15 to 30 mm/s are employed in order to detect epileptiform activity. Urine toxicology screening is performed whenever indicated.

4. Daytime multiple sleep latency testing, if there is a complaint or suspicion of excessive daytime sleepiness or fatigue (methods discussed in Chapter 4.14.3).

Causes of sleep-related injury

A report on a series of 100 consecutive adults presenting to a multidisciplinary sleep disorders centre on account of sleep-related injury identified five causes[2]:

(1) sleepwalking/sleep terrors (N = 54; 33 males, 21 females; mean age of onset, 5 years (range, 3–58));

(2) REM sleep behaviour disorder (N = 36; 35 males, one female; mean age of onset, 57 years (range, 13–73));

(3) dissociative disorders (N = 7; one male, six females; mean age of onset, 21 years (range, 12–27));

(4) nocturnal seizures (N = 2);

(5) obstructive sleep apnoea/periodic limb movements (N = 1).

For the entire group of 100 adults, the mean age of parasomnia onset was 31 years (range, 3–77), the mean age at referral was 44 years (range, 18–79), 71 per cent were male and 29 per cent were female, the positive diagnostic yield from polysomnographic studies was 91 per cent, and the sleep-related injuries included ecchymoses, lacerations, and fractures in 95 per cent, 30 per cent, and 9 per cent of patients respectively.

Non-REM sleep parasomnias: sleepwalking and sleep terrors

The polysomnographic correlates of sleepwalking and sleep terrors were first identified in the 1960s and 1970s by Gastaut and Broughton,[13,14] Kales *et al.*,[15] and Fisher *et al.*[16] from France, Canada, and the United States. Sleepwalking and sleep terrors typically arise from delta non-REM (slow-wave) sleep, and usually affect children, but adults can also be afflicted and suffer from sleep-related injuries and adverse social consequences.[2,17–22]

Clinical findings

Sleepwalking is characterized by complex, automatic behaviours, such as aimlessly wandering about, nonsensically carrying objects from one place to another, rearranging furniture, inappropriately eating, urinating in cupboards, going outdoors, and on rare occasion driving a car.[23,24] The eyes are usually wide open and have a glassy stare, and there may be some mumbling. However, communication with a sleepwalker is usually poor or impossible. Frenzied or aggressive behaviour, the wielding of weapons (knives, guns), or the calm suspension of judgement (e.g. leaving via a bedroom window, wandering far outdoors) can result in inadvertent injury or death to self or others. Homicidal sleepwalking can occur.[23]

Sleepwalking episodes usually emerge 15–120 min after sleep onset, but can occur throughout the entire sleep period in adults. The duration of each episode can vary widely. The following is a wife's description.[2]

> He seems to have the strength of 10 men and shoots straight up from bed onto his feet in one motion. He's landed clear across the room on many occasions and has pulled down curtains (bending the rods), upset lamps, and so forth. He's grabbed me and pulled on me, hurting my arms, because he's usually dreaming that he's getting me out of danger...He's landed on the floor so hard that he's injured his own body...There are low windows right beside our bed and I'm afraid he'll go through them some night.

Sleep terrors are characterized by sudden loud terrified screaming and prominent autonomic nervous system activation (tachycardia, tachypnoea, diaphoresis, mydriasis) that usually appears early in the sleep period, although episodes in adults can occur at any time of the night. The individual may sit up rapidly while screaming, and engage in frenzied activity and become injured.

Childhood sleepwalking and sleep terrors are characterized by complete amnesia for the events. In adult sleepwalking and sleep terrors, there can be subsequent recall of the behavioural episode, and also recall of dream-like mentation that usually involves being threatened by imminent danger.[2,25] The distinction between sleep terrors and agitated sleepwalking in adults is often blurred, with both states being admixed in response to a perceived threat.[22]

The prevalence of sleepwalking has been estimated to be as high as 17 per cent in childhood (peaking at age 4–8 years), and recent data indicate a higher prevalence in adults (4–10 per cent) than previously recognized.[26–28] The prevalence of sleep terrors is approximately 3 per cent in children and 1 per cent in adults.[1] A familial–genetic basis for sleepwalking and sleep terrors is well established.[28,29] Non-injurious sleepwalking has no gender preference,[1] but injurious sleepwalking is more predominant in males.[2] Sleep terrors may be more common in males.[1] 'Confusional arousals' comprise another category of 'disorder of arousal', and represent partial manifestations of sleepwalking and sleep terrors.[1]

Polysomnographic findings

Sleepwalking/sleep terror episodes arise abruptly during arousals from delta non-REM sleep.[13–16] In a systematic study of 38 adults with injurious sleepwalking/sleep terrors,[22] three postarousal EEG patterns were detected: diffuse, rhythmic delta activity; diffuse delta and theta activity, with some alpha and beta activity; and prominent alpha and beta activity. Thus, the postarousal EEG can show the persistence of sleep, the admixture of sleep and wakefulness, or complete wakefulness. Figure 1 shows the polysomnogram of a disordered arousal from slow-wave sleep.

Although the sleep architecture (i.e. distribution of sleep stages) is usually normal in sleepwalking/sleep terrors, the 'microstructure' of non-REM sleep in adult sleepwalking/sleep terrors can be perturbed, with increased microarousals and increased rate of the 'cyclic alternating EEG pattern'.[2,19,21]

Association with medical and psychiatric risk factors

Sleepwalking and sleep terrors may be triggered by obstructive sleep apnoea, periodic limb movements, nocturnal seizures, medical and neurological disorders, febrile illness, alcohol use or abuse, sleep deprivation, pregnancy, menstruation and psychotropic medications—especially lithium carbonate and anticholinergic agents.[4,30,31]

A strong association between sleepwalking/sleep terrors and psychopathology in adults was suggested by an early literature, but polysomnographic monitoring was not conducted and there were considerable methodological problems. The recent literature reporting polysomnogram-confirmed cases has indicated that most adult cases are either not associated or else not closely associated with a psychiatric disorder, although stress can play a promoting role.[2,4,17,18,20] Genetic–constitutional factors appear to be predominant in adult and childhood sleepwalking/sleep terrors.[32]

Treatment

Treatment (especially in childhood) is usually not necessary, other than identifying and minimizing any identified risk factors. In cases involving sleep-related injury, pharmacological treatment is necessary and can be life-saving. A benzodiazepine such as clonazepam (0.25–1.5 mg) taken 1 h before sleep onset is usually effective. Alprazolam, diazepam, imipramine, and paroxetine can also be used. Teaching a patient self-hypnosis can be effective in milder cases of adult or childhood sleepwalking/sleep terrors.[33] Treatment of any concurrent psychiatric disorder does not usually control sleepwalking/sleep terrors.[2,20]

REM sleep behaviour disorder

Although various aspects of REM sleep behaviour disorder have been identified by European, Japanese, and American investigators since 1966,[34] REM sleep behaviour disorder was not formally recognized and named until 1985,[35] and it was incorporated within the international classification of sleep disorders in 1990.[1] A typical clinical presentation of REM sleep behaviour disorder is contained in the description of the index case.[35]

> A 67-year-old dextral man was referred because of violent behaviour during sleep...4 years before referral..he experienced the first 'physically moving dream' several hours after sleep onset; he found himself out of bed attempting to carry out a dream. This episode signaled the onset of an increasingly frequent and progressively severe sleep disorder; he would punch and kick his wife, fall out of bed, stagger about the room, crash into objects, and injure himself...his wife began to sleep in another room 2 years before referral. They remain happily married, believing that these nocturnal behaviours are out of his control and discordant with his waking personality.

Mammalian REM sleep, REM atonia, and paradox lost

REM sleep in mammals involves a highly energized state of brain activity, with both tonic (i.e. continuous) and phasic (i.e. intermittent) activations occurring across a spectrum of physiological parameters.[34] REM sleep has two major synonyms: 'active sleep,' because of the high level of brain activity during REM sleep, and 'paradoxical sleep,' because of the nearly complete suppression of muscle tone despite the high level of brain activity. This generalized skeletal muscle atonia ('REM atonia') is one of the three defining features of mammalian REM sleep, besides rapid eye movements and a desynchronized EEG.

Table 2 Findings in 96 patients with chronic REM sleep behaviour disorder (RBD)

Categories	Percentage (N)	Comments
Gender		
Male	87.5 (84)	Mean age of RBD onset (N = 90):
Female	12.5 (12)	52 years (range 9–81)
		Mean age at polysomnography:
		58 years (range 10–83)
Chief complaint		
Sleep injury	79.2 (76)	Ecchymoses (76); lacerations
		(32); fractures (7)
Sleep disruption	20.8 (20)	
Altered dream	87.5 (84)	More vivid, intense, action filled,
process and		violent (reported as severe
content		nightmares)
Dream-enacting	87.5 (84)	Talking, laughing, yelling,
behaviours		swearing, gesturing, reaching,
		grabbing, arm flailing,
		punching, kicking, sitting,
		jumping out of bed, crawling,
		running
Clonazepam treatment		
Efficacy (N = 67)		
Complete	79.1 (44/67)	Rapid control of problematic
Partial	11.9 (8/67)	sleep behaviours *and*
Total	91.0 (61/67)	altered dreams, sustained for
		up to 9 years

Modified from Schenck et al.[36]

The loss of the customary paradox of REM sleep in REM sleep behaviour disorder bears serious clinical consequences: 'paradox lost' means loss of safe sleep.

Animal model of REM sleep behaviour disorder

In 1965, Jouvet and Delorme reported from France that experimental pontine lesions in cats caused permanent loss of REM atonia, and the cats displayed attack and exploratory behaviours during REM sleep that resembled dream enactment (oneirism). This experiment established the animal model of REM sleep behaviour disorder.[36]

Clinical and polysomnographic findings

Between 1982 and 1991, 96 patients at our centre were diagnosed with chronic REM sleep behaviour disorder. (There is an acute form of REM sleep behaviour disorder that can emerge during withdrawal from ethanol or sedative–hypnotic abuse and with anticholinergic and other drug intoxication states.[34]) Data on this series[36] are contained in Table 2, and are concordant with the published world literature.[12] The older male predominance in REM sleep behaviour disorder is striking, although females and virtually all age groups are represented. Approximately half of REM sleep behaviour disorder cases are closely associated with neurological disorders, predominantly neurodegenerative disorders (especially parkinsonism) and narcolepsy. In fact, REM sleep behaviour disorder may be the first sign of a neurological disorder whose other (classic) manifestations may not emerge until several years after the onset of REM sleep behaviour disorder. Thus, routine neurological evaluations are indicated in the long-term management of REM sleep behaviour disorder. The prevalence of REM sleep behaviour disorder is unknown. The course is usually progressive; spontaneous remissions are very rare. Patients with REM sleep behaviour disorder usually have calm and pleasant personalities, and do not display irritability or anger while awake. Figure 2 depicts a typical polysomnogram of REM sleep behaviour disorder.

Association of REM sleep behaviour disorder with psychiatric disorders and stress

Psychiatric disorders are rarely associated with REM sleep behaviour disorder.[12,36] Fluoxetine treatment of obsessive–compulsive disorder,[37] or cessation of use or abuse of REM-suppressing agents (viz. ethanol, amphetamine, cocaine, imipramine[38]) can trigger REM sleep behaviour disorder. Tricyclic antidepressants, monoamine oxidase inhibitors, selective serotonin reuptake inhibitors, and venlafaxine can induce or aggravate REM sleep behaviour disorder. In four cases, major stress involving divorce, automobile accident, sea disaster, or public humiliation triggered REM sleep behaviour disorder.[2,12]

Diagnosis of REM sleep behaviour disorder

The diagnostic criteria of REM sleep behaviour disorder are as follows.[1,34]

1. Polysomnographic abnormality during REM sleep: elevated submental electromyographic tone and/or excessive phasic submental and/or limb electromyographic twitching.

2. Documentation of abnormal REM sleep behaviours during polysomnographic studies, or a history of injurious or disruptive sleep behaviours.

3. Absence of EEG epileptiform activity during REM sleep.

Treatment of REM sleep behaviour disorder

Clonazepam is remarkably effective in controlling both the behavioural and the dream-disordered components of REM sleep behaviour disorder, at a usual bedtime dose of 0.5 to 1.0 mg. The long-term efficacy and safety of chronic, nightly clonazepam treatment of REM sleep behaviour disorder has been established.[3] Other treatments include carbamazepine, melatonin, L-dopa, imipramine, etc. Maximizing the safety of the sleeping environment should always be encouraged.

Parasomnia overlap disorder: sleepwalking/sleep terrors/REM sleep behaviour disorder

A group of 33 patients has been reported with polysomnogram-documented sleepwalking, sleep terrors, and REM sleep behaviour disorder.[5] The mean age was 34 years, the mean age of parasomnia onset was 15 years (range:1–66 years), and 70 per cent were male. An idiopathic subgroup (N = 22) had a significantly earlier mean age of parasomnia onset (9 years) than a symptomatic subgroup (27 years) (N = 11) whose parasomnia began with either a neurological disorder (N = 6), nocturnal paroxysmal atrial fibrillation (N = 1), post-traumatic stress disorder/major depression (N = 1), chronic ethanol/amphetamine abuse and withdrawal ($N = 1$), or mixed disorders (schizophrenia, brain trauma, substance abuse ($N = 2$)). The rate of psychiatric disorders was not elevated; group scores on various psychometric tests were not elevated. Forty-five per cent ($N = 15$) had previously received psychological or psychiatric therapy for their parasomnia, without benefit. Treatment, usually with clonazepam, was effective for most patients. The natural history is not yet known.

An experimental animal model is applicable to combined sleepwalking/sleep terrors/REM sleep behaviour disorder (as cited[36]): cats who receive kainic acid injections into the midbrain display 'hallucinatory-type' behaviours in wakefulness, with complete unresponsiveness to environmental stimuli, which are identical to the oneiric behaviours displayed in the cat model of REM sleep behaviour disorder.

Nocturnal sleep-related eating disorders

The 'night-eating syndrome' was first reported in 1955. Over the next 35 years, this condition received scant attention in the literature, until a series of 19 cases with polysomnographic data was published.[31] Reports from various countries have now been published.[4,31,39–42]

Clinical findings

Pathological sleep-related eating has characteristic features, as identified in a series of 38 consecutive adults presenting to a multidisciplinary sleep disorders centre.[4] In this series, the mean age of onset of sleep-related eating was 27 years (range 5–44), the mean age at referral was 39 years (range 18–65), 66 per cent ($N = 25$) were female, 71 per cent ($N = 27$) had nightly eating episodes, 71 per cent ($N = 27$) had careless sloppy nocturnal eating, 68 per cent ($N = 26$) had high-caloric nocturnal binging, and 53 per cent ($N = 20$), 32 per cent ($N = 12$), and 16 per cent ($N = 6$) reported being partially conscious, totally unconscious, or fully conscious respectively during nocturnal eating. Patient concerns related to nocturnal eating included weight gain in 71 per cent ($N = 27$), abdominal distention in 58 per cent ($N = 22$), loss of control in 55 per cent ($N = 21$), and injuries (burns, lacerations) in 34 per cent ($N = 13$).

Thick substances, such as milkshakes, peanut butter, and brownies, are preferentially consumed. Excessive weight gain is common. Nocturnal eating is not associated with hunger or thirst, the consumption of alcohol, or with purging.

Sleep-related eating is most commonly associated with sleepwalking, but also with restless legs syndrome, obstructive sleep apnoea, narcolepsy, cessation of alcohol, opiate, or cocaine abuse, triazolam/midazolam use or abuse, cessation of cigarette smoking, stress (particularly involving separation anxiety), bulimia nervosa, dissociative states, psychotropic medications (especially lithium and anticholinergics), and various medical/neurological disorders (e.g. autoimmune hepatitis, encephalitis, migraines).

Prescribing a monoamine oxidase inhibitor to a patient with sleep-related eating can be hazardous, since indiscriminate food consumption at night could jeopardize the mandatory dietary restrictions of monoamine oxidase inhibitor treatment.

Treatment

Treatment is directed at controlling the underlying sleep disorder.[4] For cases associated with sleepwalking and restless legs syndrome/periodic limb movements of sleep, either monotherapy or combined therapy utilizing dopaminergic agents (including bupropion), benzodiazepines, and opiates can be effective, whereas psychological treatments are usually ineffective.

Sleep-related eating disorders share much in common with the 'nocturnal eating syndrome' in adults;[1,41,42] the latter, in fact, may represent the subgroup of patients with sleep-related eating disorders who ate during full consciousness. However, the 'night eating syndrome' typically involves compulsive eating before the onset of sleep, namely a presleep eating disorder.

Nocturnal dissociative disorders

A nocturnal dissociative disorder with polysomnographic monitoring was first reported in 1976 by Rice and Fisher[43] in a man with daytime and night-time fugues that began after his father's death. Another polysomnogram-documented case was described by Fleming in 1987 in a woman with a history of being physically and sexually assaulted.[44] A series of eight cases was reported in 1989.[44]

Clinical manifestations

The onset may be sudden or gradual, and the course is chronic. There usually is a history of repeated physical and sexual abuse in childhood and/or adulthood. In a series of eight cases, seven were female who also had daytime states of dissociation with self-mutilating behaviours, such as genital cutting, self-burning, and punching through windows.[44] One male patient had exclusively nocturnal episodes in which he acted like a jungle cat.

A typical spell during polysomnographic monitoring involves complex and lengthy behaviours that emerge during well-established EEG wakefulness, after a prior episode of sleep.[44] The nocturnal episodes appear to be re-enactments of previous assaults.

Treatment

Treatment involves long-term therapy of the dissociative disorder and of any associated psychiatric disorders, usually initiated in a specialized inpatient setting. Bedtime administration of benzodiazepines may aggravate a nocturnal dissociative disorder.

Restless legs syndrome

Restless legs syndrome, first described in 1945 by Ekbom from Sweden, is a chronic disorder that often results in severe insomnia, and can be incapacitating.[1,29,45] It is characterized by unpleasant and at times painful sensations in the lower extremities that emerge during periods of inactivity, particularly during the transition from wakefulness to sleep. These abnormal sensations are relieved by movement or stimulation of the legs, such as walking, stomping the feet, rubbing or squeezing the legs, taking hot showers, or applying hot packs or ointments to the legs.

Both the restless legs syndrome and the therapeutic interventions just described are incompatible with successful entry into sleep. The more severely affected individuals cannot easily sit still while watching television or a film, or during protracted car or plane journeys. Restless legs syndrome is quite common, affecting up to 10 per cent of the general population, and tends to become more prevalent with increasing age. It affects males and females equally. Childhood cases may masquerade as attention-deficit disorder with hyperactivity or as 'growing pains'.

Most cases of restless legs syndrome are either idiopathic or have a familial basis. Caffeine, fatigue, or stress may worsen the symptoms. There is no evidence that restless legs syndrome is related to psychiatric disorders. However, neuroleptic-induced akathisia can mimic restless legs syndrome.

Nearly all patients with restless legs syndrome have periodic limb movements of non-REM sleep (formerly called nocturnal myoclonus).[1] Periodic limb movements are characterized by movements of the legs every 15 to 40 s, namely slow dorsiflexion, that may or may not be associated with arousals. Excessive arousals during sleep can result in daytime fatigue or sleepiness.

Restless legs syndrome can usually be diagnosed by history alone, and polysomnographic monitoring is not usually indicated. The syndrome is one of the major organic causes of insomnia, and commonly responds to treatment that includes use of antiparkinsonian medications, benzodiazepines (especially clonazepam), and opiates. Combinations of these drugs are often necessary. Since restless legs syndrome is a chronic disorder that often worsens with advancing age, long-term treatment is usually warranted.

Differential diagnosis of dream-enacting behaviours and other parasomnias

A history of dream-enacting behaviours does not automatically implicate REM sleep behaviour disorder. Other diagnoses include sleepwalking/sleep terrors, nocturnal dissociative disorders, with the 'dreams' being wakeful memories of past abuse, nocturnal complex seizures, with the 'dreams' being the seizure equivalents,[46] obstructive sleep apnoea, with apnoea-induced arousals from REM sleep being associated with violent behaviours and vivid REM-related dreams,[30] intoxication states, and malingering.

Other parasomnias of interest to psychiatrists include sexual parasomnias,[47] nocturnal panic attacks, which arise from Stages II and III non-REM sleep,[48] nocturnal paroxysmal dystonia,[1] nocturnal frontal-lobe epilepsy,[46] episodic nocturnal wanderings,[46] rhythmic movement disorders of non-REM and REM sleep,[1] and obstructive sleep apnoea with complex interactions with various parasomnias.[30]

Forensic guidelines for psychiatrists

The legal implications of automatic behaviour have long been discussed and debated. With regard to sleep-related automatic behaviours, the objective identification of a sleep disorder does not establish causality for any given deed. Guidelines have been developed to assist in determining the role of a sleep disorder in an act of violence.[49]

The American Academy of Neurology and other professional organizations have developed guidelines for expert witnesses, with the most stringent being as follows.

1.   The expert should be willing to submit his or her testimony for peer review.

2.   The expert must be impartial and be willing to prepare his or her testimony for use by either or both the plaintiff or defendant. Ideally, the expert should assume the role of 'friend of the court'.

References

1. American Sleep Disorders Association (1990). *International classification of sleep disorders: diagnostic and coding manual.* American Sleep Disorders Association, Rochester, MN.
2. Schenck, C.H., Milner, D.M., Hurwitz, T.D., Bundlie, S.R., and Mahowald, M.W. (1989). A polysomnographic and clinical report on sleep-related injury in 100 adult patients. *American Journal of Psychiatry*, **146**, 1166–73.
3. Schenck, C.H. and Mahowald, M.W. (1996). Long-term, nightly benzodiazepine treatment of injurious parasomnias and other disorders of disrupted nocturnal sleep in 170 adults. *American Journal of Medicine*, **100**, 548–54.
4. Schenck, C.H., Hurwitz, T.D., O'Connor, K.A., and Mahowald, M.W. (1993). Additional categories of sleep-related eating disorders and the current status of treatment. *Sleep*, **16**, 457–66.
5. Schenck, C.H., Boyd, J.L., and Mahowald, M.W. (1997). A parasomnia overlap disorder involving sleepwalking, sleep terrors, and REM sleep behavior disorder in 33 polysomnographically confirmed cases. *Sleep*, **20**, 972–81.
6. Ohayon, M.M., Caulet, M., and Priest, R.G. (1997). Violent behavior during sleep. *Journal of Clinical Psychiatry*, **58**, 369–76.
7. Mahowald, M.W. and Ettinger, M.G. (1990). Things that go bump in the night: the parasomnias revisited. *Journal of Clinical Neurophysiology*, **7**, 119–43.
8. Kryger, M.H., Roth, T., and Dement, W.C. (ed.) (1994). *Principles and practice of sleep medicine* (2nd edn). W.B. Saunders, Philadelphia, PA.
9. Broughton, R.J. (1999). Behavioral parasomnias. In *Sleep disorders medicine: basic science, technical considerations, and clinical aspects* (2nd edn) (ed. S. Chokroverty), pp. 635–60. Butterworth Heinemann, Boston, MA.
10. Mahowald, M.W. and Schenck, C.H. (1992). Dissociated states of wakefulness and sleep. *Neurology*, **42** (Supplement 6), 44–52.
11. Mahowald, M.W. and Schenck, C.H. (1991). Status dissociatus—a perspective on states of being. *Sleep*, **14**, 69–79.
12. Schenck, C.H. and Mahowald, M.W. (1996). REM sleep parasomnias. *Neurologic Clinics*, **14**, 697–720.
13. Gastaut, H. and Broughton, R. (1965). A clinical and polygraphic study of episodic phenomena during sleep. *Recent Advances in Biological Psychiatry*, **7**, 197–222.
14. Broughton, R. (1968). Disorders of sleep: disorders of arousal? *Science*, **59**, 1070–8.
15. Kales, A., Jacobson, A., Paulson, J., Kales, J.K., and Walter, R. (1966). Somnambulism: psychophysiological correlates. I. All-night EEG studies. *Archives of General Psychiatry*, **14**, 586–94.
16. Fisher, C., Kahn, E., Edwards, A., and Davis, D. (1973). A psychophysiological study of nightmares and night terrors. I. Physiological aspects of the stage 4 night terror. *Journal of Nervous and Mental Disease*, **157**, 75–98.
17. Kavey, N.B., Whyte, J., Resor, S.R. and Gidro-Frank, S. (1990). Somnambulism in adults. *Neurology*, **49**, 749–52.
18. Crisp, A.H., Matthews, B.M., Oakey, M., and Crutchfield, M. (1990). Sleepwalking, night terrors, and consciousness. *British Medical Journal*, **300**, 360–2.
19. Blatt, I., Peled, R., Gadoth, N., and Lavie, P. (1991). The value of sleep

recording in evaluating somnambulism in young adults. *Electroencephalography and Clinical Neurophysiology*, **78**, 407–12.

20. Llorente, M.D., Currier, M.B., Norman, S.E., and Mellman, T.A. (1992). Night terrors in adults: phenomenology and relationship to psychopathology. *Journal of Clinical Psychiatry*, **53**, 392–4.

21. Zucconi, M., Oldani, A., Ferini-Strambi, L., and Smirne, S. (1995). Arousal fluctuations in non-rapid eye movement parasomnias: the role of cyclic alternating pattern as a measure of sleep instability. *Journal of Clinical Neurophysiology*, **12**, 147–54.

22. Schenck, C.H., Pareja, J.A., Patterson, A.L., and Mahowald, M.W. (1998). Analysis of polysomnographic events surrounding 252 slow-wave sleep arousals in thirty-eight adults with injurious sleepwalking and sleep terrors. *Journal of Clinical Neurophysiology*, **15**, 159–66.

23. Broughton, R., Billings, R., Cartwright, R., *et al.* (1994). Homicidal somnambulism: a case report. *Sleep*, **17**, 253–64.

24. Schenck, C.H. and Mahowald, M.W. (1995). A polysomnographically-documented case of adult somnambulism with long-distance automobile driving and frequent nocturnal violence: parasomnia with continuing danger as a non-insane automatism? *Sleep*, **18**, 765–72.

25. Kavey, N.B. and Whyte, J. (1993). Somnambulism associated with hallucinations. *Psychosomatics*, **34**, 86–90.

26. Bixler, E.O., Kales, A., Soldatos, C.R., Kales, J.D., and Healey, S. (1979). Prevalence of sleep disorders in the Los Angeles metropolitan area. *American Journal of Psychiatry*, **136**, 1257–62.

27. Klackenberg, G. (1982). Somnambulism in childhood—prevalence, course and behavior correlates. A prospective longitudinal study (6–16 years). *Acta Paediatrica*, **71**, 495–9.

28. Hublin, C., Kaprio, J., Partinen, M., Heikkila, K., and Koskenvuo, M. (1997). Prevalence and genetics of sleepwalking: a population-based twin study. *Neurology*, **48**, 177–81.

29. Kales, A., Soldatos, C.R., Bixler, E.O., *et al.* (1980). Hereditary factors in sleepwalking and night terrors. *British Journal of Psychiatry*, **137**, 111–18.

30. Mahowald, M.W. and Schenck, C.H. (1998). Parasomnias including the restless legs syndrome. *Clinics in Chest Medicine*, **19**, 183–202.

31. Schenck, C.H., Hurwitz, T.D., Bundlie, S.R., and Mahowald, M.W. (1991). Sleep-related eating disorders: polysomnographic correlates of a heterogeneous syndrome distinct from daytime eating disorders. *Sleep*, **14**, 419–31.

32. Crisp, A.H. (1996). The sleepwalking/night terrors syndrome in adults. *Postgraduate Medical Journal*, **72**, 599–604.

33. Hurwitz, T.D., Mahowald, M.M., Schenck, C.H., Schluter, J.L., and Bundlie, S.R. (1991). A retrospective outcome study and review of hypnosis as treatment of adults with sleepwalking and sleep terror. *Journal of Nervous and Mental Disease*, **179**, 228–33.

34. Mahowald, M.W. and Schenck, C.H. (1994). REM sleep behavior disorder. In *Principles and practice of sleep medicine* (2nd edn) (ed. M.H. Kryger, T. Roth, and W.C. Dement), pp. 574–88. W.B. Saunders, Philadelphia, PA.

35. Schenck, C.H., Bundlie, S.R., Ettinger, M.G., and Mahowald, M.W. (1986). Chronic behavioral disorders of human REM sleep: a new category of parasomnia. *Sleep*, **9**, 293–308.

36. Schenck, C.H., Hurwitz, T.D., and Mahowald, M.W. (1993). REM sleep behaviour disorder: an update on a series of 96 patients and a review of the world literature. *Journal of Sleep Research*, **2**, 224–31.

37. Schenck, C.H., Mahowald, M.W., Kim, S.W., O'Connor, K.A., and Hurwitz, T.D. (1992). Prominent eye movements during NREM sleep and REM sleep behavior disorder associated with fluoxetine treatment of depression and obsessive–compulsive disorder. *Sleep*, **15**, 226–35.

38. Schenck, C.H., Hurwitz, T.D., and Mahowald, M.W. (1988). REM sleep behavior disorder. *American Journal of Psychiatry*, **145**, 652.

39. Schenck, C.H. and Mahowald, M.W. (1994). Review of nocturnal sleep-related eating disorders. *International Journal of Eating Disorders*, **15**, 343–56.

40. Spaggiari, M.C., Granella, F., Parrino, L., Marchesi, C., Melli, I., and

41. Terzano, M.G. (1994). Nocturnal eating syndrome in adults. *Sleep*, **17**, 339–44.

41. Manni, R., Ratti, M.T., and Tartara, A. (1997). Nocturnal eating: prevalence and features in 120 insomniac referrals. *Sleep*, **20**, 734–8.

42. Winkelman, J.W. (1998). Clinical and polysomnographic features of sleep-related eating disorder. *Journal of Clinical Psychiatry*, **59**, 14–19.

43. Rice, E. and Fisher, C. (1976). Fugue states in sleep and wakefulness: a psychophysiological study. *Journal of Nervous and Mental Disease*, **163**, 79–87.

44. Schenck, C.H., Milner, D.M., Hurwitz, T.D., Bundlie, S.R., and Mahowald, M.W. (1989). Dissociative disorders presenting as somnambulism: polysomnographic, video and clinical documentation (8 cases). *Dissociation*, **2**, 194–204.

45. Montplaisir, J., Godbout, R., Pelletier, G., and Warnes, H. (1994). Restless legs syndrome and periodic limb movements during sleep. In *Principles and practice of sleep medicine* (2nd edn) (ed. M.H. Kryger, T. Roth, and W.C. Dement), pp. 589–97. W.B. Saunders, Philadelphia, PA.

46. Mahowald, M.W. and Schenck, C.H. (1997). Sleep disorders. In *Epilepsy: a comprehensive textbook* (ed. J. Engel Jr and T.A. Pedley), pp. 2705–15. Lippincott–Raven, Philadelphia, PA.

47. Fenwick, P. (1996). Sleep and sexual offending. *Medicine, Science and the Law*, **36**, 122–34.

48. Shapiro, C.M. and Sloan, E.P. (1998). Nocturnal panic—an underrecognized entity. *Journal of Psychosomatic Research*, **44**, 21–3.

49. Mahowald, M.W. and Schenck, C.H. (1999). Sleep-related violence and forensic medicine issues. In *Sleep disorders medicine: basic science, technical considerations, and clinical aspects* (2nd edn) (ed. S. Chokroverty), pp. 729–39. Butterworth Heinemann, Boston, MA.

4.14.5 Psychiatric sleep–wake disorders

Ruth M. Benca

Introduction

Sleep complaints are commonly reported by psychiatric patients, and polysomnographic studies show objective evidence of disturbed sleep associated with all major psychiatric disorders.[1,2] In fact, sleep disturbance is a primary or associated feature included in the diagnostic criteria for most psychiatric illnesses. It is likely that psychiatric disorders disrupt sleep through the increased anxiety and arousal which accompanies most acute episodes of illness. Increasing evidence, however, suggests that neural systems affected by psychiatric disorders are also involved in sleep regulation, which may explain associations between specific sleep abnormalities and particular disorders.

Psychiatric medications may also contribute to sleep problems; many drugs cause sedation or worsen insomnia. Antidepressants can precipitate parasomnias, such as rapid eye movement (**REM**) sleep behaviour disorder, or periodic movements in sleep. Psychiatric patients also suffer from primary sleep disorders, and accurate diagnosis is often difficult because of the overlap between symptoms of psychiatric and sleep disorders.

As discussed in Chapter 4.14.1, sleep deprivation can also affect psychological function, and it is possible that disturbed sleep may exacerbate and/or precipitate episodes of psychiatric illness. For example, manic episodes are not uncommonly triggered by sleep deprivation.

Psychiatric patients with significant sleep complaints should be evaluated similarly to other patients with sleep problems. In particular, they should be assessed for primary sleep disorders or other medical causes of sleep problems, since it cannot be assumed that all sleep disturbance in a psychiatric patient is caused by the psychiatric illness. Assessment is considered in Chapter 4.14.1.

For sleep problems determined as being related to the underlying psychiatric disorder, several general treatment approaches should be considered. First, many psychiatric patients may have poor sleep habits related to their illness, or lack social structure or support. They may also abuse substances which further interfere with sleep. Principles of good sleep hygiene should be discussed with every patient. Anxious patients or those with insomnia may also benefit from additional behavioural treatments such as relaxation training, or stimulus control (see Chapter 4.14.2). Since sleep problems may worsen with exacerbations of the psychiatric illness, initial approaches should be aimed at treating the underlying disorder. Lastly, symptomatic treatment of sleep disturbance with hypnotics or other medications should be considered.

Sleep abnormalities associated with clinical syndromes of adult psychiatry and specific approaches to treatment are summarized below.

Mood disorders

Depressed patients most commonly report insomnia, with difficulty falling asleep, prolonged and/or frequent waking during the night, and early morning awakening. They frequently complain of daytime fatigue and they may also experience vivid or disturbing dreams. A minority of depressives report hypersomnia, particularly those with bipolar disorders or seasonal affective disorder (winter depression);[3] symptoms may include prolonged periods of nocturnal sleep, difficulty awakening in the morning, and daytime napping.

Manic patients may show profound insomnia during episodes of illness, and tend to report feeling a decreased need for sleep. Manic episodes are often preceded by insomnia and can be triggered by sleep loss.[4]

Most psychiatric sleep studies have been performed on patients with major depression and have demonstrated a number of sleep abnormalities,[1] which are traditionally grouped into three general categories.[5]

1. **Sleep disruption**: depressed patients tend to show prolonged latency to sleep onset, increased amounts of wakefulness during sleep and/or early morning awakening; these result in reduced sleep efficiency and reduced total sleep time.

2. **Loss of slow-wave sleep** (**SWS**): when compared with age-matched normal controls, depressives have fewer total minutes of SWS and decreased SWS percentage of total sleep. Analysis of sleep EEG has shown decreased delta wave activity, with relative loss of delta activity in the first versus second non-REM (NREM) sleep period of the night.

3. **Changes in REM sleep**: depressives typically show alterations in the timing and amount of REM sleep. The most widely reported finding has been the reduced latency to REM sleep onset. Other findings include an increased proportion of REM sleep occurring in the first third of the night, and an increased REM sleep percentage of total sleep. There is often an increase in the total number and/or density of rapid eye movements across the night.

The sleep abnormalities listed above are not necessarily seen in all depressed patients, but represent the most consistently reported differences between groups of depressed patients and normal controls reported in the literature.[1] Although sleep is generally most disturbed during acute episodes of depression, sleep abnormalities often continue during periods of clinical remission. Reduced REM sleep latency and loss of SWS may be 'trait' markers since they persist in remitted patients, whereas other parameters, such as increased REM density and reduced sleep efficiency, may be 'state' markers since they are more abnormal during acute depression.[6]

Patients with mood disorders other than major depression have been less well studied. Manic patients show similar sleep abnormalities to depressives.[7,8] Dysthymic patients or those with subclinical depression tend to be indistinguishable from normal controls, however.

Although objective sleep changes, particularly REM sleep abnormalities, are most consistently found in depressed patients, no sleep parameters have been found to be sensitive or specific enough to be useful by themselves for clinical diagnosis. As described below, most psychiatric patients show disturbed sleep continuity. Reduced REM sleep latency, which is probably the most specific sleep marker for depression, is found in a variety of other conditions, including other psychiatric disorders, narcolepsy, following withdrawal from REM sleep-suppressing agents (e.g. antidepressants, benzodiazepines, or alcohol), and during recovery from chronic sleep deprivation. Nevertheless, the association of certain sleep abnormalities with depression suggests that they may be useful for identifying neurobiological systems involved in sleep and depression.

At present, the pathophysiological mechanisms for sleep changes in depression are not specifically known. A relative imbalance in cholinergic versus monoaminergic activity may occur in depression,[9] and increased cholinergic activity could account for the abnormalities in REM sleep and loss of SWS. In fact, depressives show a more rapid induction of REM sleep following administration of cholinergic drugs.[10,11] Changes in sleep patterns could also be due to circadian rhythm abnormalities, specifically, a phase advance in the circadian rhythm of REM sleep relative to the sleep–waking cycle.[12] Recent neuroimaging studies have suggested abnormalities in prefrontal and limbic regions in depressives,[13] and these areas also appear to be activated in REM sleep.[14]

One of the more intriguing links between sleep and mood has been the observation that sleep deprivation has antidepressant effects in patients with mood disorders.[15,16] Various therapies, including total sleep deprivation, partial sleep deprivation, and REM sleep deprivation have all been reported to reduce depressive symptoms in a majority of patients, although relapse tends to occur following recovery sleep.

Treatment

For patients whose sleep disturbance is thought to be related to a mood disorder, primary treatment should be directed at the mood disorder itself. The choice of antidepressant treatment is often influenced by the sleep complaint; patients with severe insomnia are usually prescribed sedating antidepressants (e.g. tricyclics, trazodone, nefazodone, or mirtazepine), whereas patients with hypersomnia may be given more activating medications (e.g. selective serotonin reuptake inhibitors (**SSRIs**) or buproprion). When activating medications are used in patients with insomnia, sedating antidepressants and/or hypnotics may be added to improve sleep. There is little evidence, however, to suggest that antidepressant response is dependent on eliminating insomnia. For example, a recent study found that fluoxetine and nefazodone were equally effective antidepressants, even though patients treated with fluoxetine continued to show evidence of insomnia whereas nefazodone improved sleep quality.[17]

In contrast, since sleep loss can trigger or exacerbate mania, insomnia should be monitored carefully in bipolar patients and treated aggressively during episodes of hypomania or mania. Hypersomnolent patients, usually those with bipolar depression and/or seasonal affective disorder, may require additional treatment with light therapy (see Chapter 6.2.9.2) and, possibly, stimulant medication.

In addition to their activating or sedating effects, sleep-related side-effects of antidepressants include exacerbation or precipitation of primary sleep disorders, such as restless legs syndrome, periodic leg movements, and REM sleep behaviour disorder.[18–20] These effects have been reported primarily in conjunction with use of REM sleep-suppressing agents (e.g. tricyclics and SSRIs).

Anxiety disorders

Insomnia is strongly associated with the symptom of anxiety; most acute episodes of insomnia are triggered by stressful events or situations. Patients with anxiety disorders typically complain of difficulty sleeping. Sleep studies have been performed for various categories of anxiety disorders, including generalized anxiety disorder, panic disorder, post-traumatic stress disorder, and obsessive–compulsive disorder. Most groups of patients show evidence of sleep disruption, as evidenced by prolonged latency to sleep onset, increased time awake during the sleep period, early morning awakening, decreased sleep efficiency and reduced total sleep. Changes in REM sleep or SWS are not typically observed. Additional sleep abnormalities have been reported in conjunction with specific anxiety disorders.

Panic disorder

Most patients with panic disorder experience at least one sleep-related panic attack, and one-third or more of patients have recurrent nocturnal panic attacks.[21] Data from the few sleep panic attacks that have been recorded suggests that they occur more commonly during NREM sleep, at the transition to SWS.[22,23] Symptoms of sleep panic attacks are essentially the same as those which occur during daytime attacks. Typically, patients report waking in a state of intense fear or anxiety, commonly with palpitations, shortness of breath, choking sensation, chest discomfort, and chills or hot flushes. They do not usually report dreaming just before the attacks. Unlike night terrors, which are characterized by incomplete arousal from sleep, patients having a sleep panic attack are awake and alert immediately after the attack begins. Patients with frequent sleep panic attacks may become fearful of going to sleep, which can contribute further to their insomnia.

Post-traumatic stress disorder

Recurrent, distressing dreams of the traumatic event is one of the diagnostic features of post-traumatic stress disorder, which has led to investigation of possible REM sleep abnormalities.[24] Sleep studies performed in post-traumatic stress disorder patients have yielded quite variable findings regarding REM sleep. There are reports of depression-like REM sleep changes, most notably increases in phasic REM sleep.[25,26] However, several recent studies have failed to document changes in sleep architecture in comparison to control subjects.[27,28]

Treatment

Anxiolytic drugs tend to have sedative–hypnotic effects, albeit at somewhat higher doses. Patients whose anxiety disorders are treated with benzodiazepines are frequently given a larger dose at bedtime for sleep induction and maintenance. For those treated with activating antidepressants (SSRIs), additional treatments for insomnia may be required, including behavioural therapy, hypnotics, or sedating antidepressants.

Schizophrenia

Some of the earliest psychiatric sleep studies were performed in schizophrenic patients because of the similarities between psychosis and dreaming. Although no evidence for REM sleep 'intrusions' into wakefulness has been documented, it is of interest that frontal brain regions (e.g. dorsolateral prefrontal cortex) which seem to be affected in schizophrenia are also relatively inactivated during REM sleep.[14] Schizophrenics often suffer from disturbed sleep, particularly during acute exacerbations of illness. Behavioural and illness factors such as social withdrawal, paranoid delusions and general behavioural disorganization can lead to increased nocturnal wakefulness and daytime napping. Underlying central nervous system abnormalities in dopaminergic and serotonergic systems may also contribute to sleep abnormalities.

Objective studies of sleep in groups of schizophrenic patients have generally shown significant sleep disruption;[1,29] frankly psychotic patients may have profound insomnia. A number of studies have suggested that schizophrenics, even in the absence of depression, may show reduced REM sleep latency.[30–32] In general, REM sleep abnormalities, if present, are not as robust as those reported in depression. Some studies have also reported decrements in SWS amounts in schizophrenia, particularly in relationship to negative symptoms and abnormalities in prefrontal cortex.[33,34] A study of drug-naive schizophrenics, however, failed to find changes in SWS or REM sleep,[35] suggesting the possibility that chronic neuroleptic treatment might contribute to sleep abnormalities seen in other studies.

There are a number of case reports which suggest that some individuals with narcolepsy and hypnagogic hallucinations may be misdiagnosed with schizophrenia. On the other hand, sleep disorders such as narcolepsy or obstructive sleep apnoea can certainly occur in patients along with schizophrenia. It should, therefore, not be assumed that hypersomnolence in a patient with a psychotic disorder is simply due to nocturnal sleep disruption without further investigation.

Treatment

Most antipsychotic drugs have sleep-promoting effects, particularly the low-potency neuroleptics (e.g. chlorpromazine) and clozapine. In fact, hypersomnolence can be a significant side-effect of these medications. Attention to sleep hygiene and behavioural factors is particularly important in schizophrenia, since behavioural disorganization can be profound in these patients.

Eating disorders

Patients with eating disorders may have a variety of sleep complaints, and some studies have documented objective sleep abnormalities.[36] Those with anorexia nervosa may report excess energy and symptoms of insomnia, particularly during periods of weight loss, whereas those with bulimia nervosa may experience hypersomnia, typically following eating binges. Comorbid depression is not uncommon in patients with eating disorders, and polysomnographic investigations of sleep patterns were motivated at least in part to determine if common biological markers could be identified in patients with depression and eating disorders. One of the major problems with this work has been the age of the subjects studied; patients with eating disorders are typically young. A number of investigations have failed to document significant sleep changes in subjects with eating disorders,[37-39] but this is also true for most sleep parameters in young depressives.[1] In studies that have documented sleep abnormalities, patterns of sleep disturbance have generally been similar to those seen in depression: sleep continuity disruption, loss of SWS, and reduced REM sleep latency.[40,41]

Sleep-related eating disorders have been increasingly recognized, both in patients with known eating disorders as well as in individuals with no apparent histories of daytime eating abnormalities, although the latter is probably less common. Bulimics frequently binge late in the evening or during the night, and up to a third have episodes of binge-eating which occur during sleep.[42] In sleep-related eating, the individual may partially arouse sometime after sleep onset and consume a large amount of high-calorie food; sometimes the foods consumed during these episodes is not typical of what is eaten during the daytime, and patients may be unusually sloppy or careless while eating. There may be little or no recollection of the eating episode the following day. Many of these patients have prior histories of sleepwalking, and polysomnographic studies have documented SWS parasomnias in half or more of patients studied.[43,44] Sleep-related eating has also been reported in association with other sleep disorders (e.g. periodic limb movements, narcolepsy, and obstructive sleep apnoea), substance abuse (e.g. benzodiazepine and alcohol abuse) and other psychiatric disorders (mood and anxiety disorders).[43,45] (See also Chapter 4.10.3.)

Treatment

Eating disorders are often treated with SSRIs, which may further contribute to insomnia as described above in the section on mood disorders. For patients with sleep-related eating, clonazepam may help to prevent the nocturnal arousals. Treatment of other primary sleep disorders, such as periodic movements, which may be contributing to arousals may reduce nocturnal eating episodes. Behavioural treatments have not been reported to be successful, but measures to limit access to food at night may need to be considered in some situations.

Normal and pathological ageing

As discussed in Chapter 4.14.1, ageing is typically accompanied by a number of alterations in sleep patterns. Sleep generally becomes more shallow and disrupted, with prolonged latency to sleep onset, more frequent arousals during sleep, reduced sleep efficiency, loss of SWS, and decreased amounts of total sleep; these changes are frequently accompanied by an increase in daytime napping. In addition, a number of primary sleep disorders, such as sleep apnoea and periodic movements in sleep, occur with increased frequency in older adults.

Sleep is further disrupted in patients with dementia,[46] and the degree of sleep disturbance is probably related to the severity of the dementia. Demented patients may experience episodes of confusion and agitation during the sleep period, often referred to as 'sundowning'.[47] Objective sleep studies have shown that in comparison with 'healthy' aged subjects, those with dementia show further prolongation of sleep latency, reduced sleep efficiency, and loss of total sleep time.[1] Several studies have suggested that individuals with Alzheimer's disease, the most common cause of dementia, also show decrements in SWS and REM sleep,[48-50] the latter finding perhaps related to deterioration of central cholinergic systems. Sleep–waking or rest–activity patterns across the 24-h day are also more disrupted in comparison to age-matched control subjects.

Treatment

Environmental/behavioural reinforcement of the 24-h rest–activity cycle may help normalize patterns for some individuals; measures include increasing daytime light exposure and activity, and avoidance of daytime napping. For patients with nocturnal agitation, low doses of antipsychotic medications such as haloperidol or risperidone may be required.

Substance abuse

Most psychoactive substances affect sleep, either as a result of acute ingestion/intoxication or withdrawal.[51,52] In general, drugs of abuse tend to cause either sedation or stimulation; withdrawal effects are usually opposite of acute effects. Patients with histories of substance abuse frequently complain of sleep abnormalities, even after prolonged periods of abstinence; this may be related to chronic and irreversible effects of drugs on sleep, and/or the possibility that sleep disturbance may indicate a vulnerability for substance abuse. The effects of some of the more commonly abused substances are reviewed below, although it is important to keep in mind that many patients abuse multiple substances, often with differing effects on sleep.

Alcohol

Alcohol is frequently used for its sedative–hypnotic effects. Acutely, it decreases latency to sleep, increases SWS, and can mildly suppress REM sleep during the first part of the night. During the second half of the night, however, it can cause sleep disruption and increase REM sleep. Chronic alcoholics tend to show loss of SWS and sleep disruption; they frequently complain of significant insomnia. During alcohol withdrawal, sleep is characterized by even greater prolongation of sleep latency, reduction of total sleep, and loss of SWS. Increased REM sleep pressure, indicated by increased REM density and/or increased REM sleep amount may also be seen, particularly in more severe cases of withdrawal.

Nicotine

Although few studies have been performed on effects of nicotine on sleep, available data suggest that nicotine use may promote insomnia. Cigarette smokers often report sleep-onset insomnia, and use of nicotine patches or gum has been associated with increased sleep disruption.

Opiates

Although opiates lead to analgesia and subjective feelings of drowsiness, their objective acute effects on sleep in both naive users and addicts include generalized sleep disruption, with decreases in sleep efficiency, total sleep, SWS, and REM sleep. Exceptions are patients in acute pain or with restless legs syndrome, whose sleep is generally improved with opiates. Opiate withdrawal is also accompanied by insomnia, although little data is available on the objective effects on sleep.

Sedative—hypnotic drugs

Benzodiazepines and barbiturates have similar effects on sleep, including decreased latency to sleep, increased total sleep, reduced stage 1, REM, and SWS volumes, and increased stage 2 proportion of sleep. Withdrawal effects on sleep are similar to those seen following alcohol withdrawal, and drugs with shorter half-lives cause more severe rebound insomnia.

Stimulants

Stimulants include various classes of compounds, ranging from the xanthines (caffeine and theophylline) to amphetamines, methylphenidate, pemoline, and cocaine; some of these agents are highly addictive. They all cause increased wakefulness, sleep loss, and decreased SWS. The more potent agents, such as amphetamines and cocaine, can also suppress REM sleep. Stimulant abusers can sometimes induce prolonged bouts of wakefulness, followed by bouts of sleep. Alcohol and/ or sedatives are frequently used to counteract stimulant effects and promote sleep. Stimulant withdrawal is characterized by increases in total sleep and REM sleep (REM sleep rebound).

Treatment

In general, patients with histories of substance abuse should not be given sedative—hypnotic drugs. Treatment must be based on substance withdrawal and maintenance of abstinence. Patients should be educated in principles of sleep hygiene and comorbid psychiatric disorders treated. Sedating antidepressants may be helpful for those who continue to suffer from significant sleep disruption.

References

1. Benca, R.M., Obermeyer, W.H., Thisted, R.A., and Gillin, J.C. (1992). Sleep and psychiatric disorders: a meta-analysis. *Archives of General Psychiatry*, **49**, 651–68.
2. Benca, R.M. (1996). Sleep in psychiatric disorders. In *Sleep disorders* (ed. M.S. Aldrich), pp. 739–64. W.B. Saunders, Philadelphia, PA.
3. Rosenthal, N.E., Sack, D.A., Gillin, J.C., *et al.* (1984). Seasonal affective disorder. A description of the syndrome and preliminary findings with light therapy. *Archives of General Psychiatry*, **41**, 72–80.
4. Wehr, T.A., Sack, D.A., and Rosenthal, N.E. (1987). Sleep reduction as a final common pathway in the genesis of mania. *American Journal of Psychiatry*, **144**, 201–4.
5. Reynolds, C.F., III, and Kupfer, D.J. (1987). Sleep research in affective illness: state of the art circa 1987. *Sleep*, **10**, 199–215.
6. Thase, M.E., Fasiczka, A.L., Berman, S.R., Simons, A.D., and Reynolds, CFr. (1998). Electroencephalographic sleep profiles before and after cognitive behavior therapy of depression. *Archives of General Psychiatry*, **55**, 138–44.
7. Linkowski, P., Kerkhofs, M., Rielaert, C., and Mendlewicz, J. (1986). Sleep during mania in manic-depressive males. *European Archives of Psychiatry and Neurological Sciences*, **235**, 339–41.
8. Hudson, J.I., Lipinski, J.F., Keck, P.E., *et al.* (1992). Polysomnographic characteristics of young manic patients: comparison with unipolar depressed patients and normal control subjects. *Archives of General Psychiatry*, **49**, 378–83.
9. Janowsky, D.S., Davis, J.M., El-Yousef, M.K., and Sekerke, H.J. (1972). A cholinergic–adrenergic hypothesis of mania and depression. *Lancet*, **ii**, 632–5.
10. Sitaram, N., Nurnberger, J.I., Jr., Gershon, E.S., and Gillin, J.C. (1980). Faster cholinergic REM sleep induction in euthymic patients with primary affective illness. *Science*, **208**, 200–2.
11. Gillin, J.C., Sutton, L., Ruiz, C., *et al.* (1991). The cholinergic rapid eye movement induction test with arecoline in depression. *Archives of General Psychiatry*, **48**, 264–70.
12. Wehr, T.A. and Wirz-Justice, A. (1981). Internal coincidence model for sleep deprivation and depression. In *Sleep 1980* (ed. W.P. Koella), pp. 26–33. Karger, Basel.
13. Soares, J.C. and Mann, J.J. (1997). The functional neuroanatomy of mood disorders. *Journal of Psychiatric Research*, **31**, 393–432.
14. Maquet, P., Peters, J., Aerts, J., *et al.* (1996). Functional neuroanatomy of human rapid-eye-movement sleep and dreaming. *Nature*, **383**, 163–6.
15. Wu, J.C. and Bunney, W.E. (1990). The biological basis of an antidepressant response to sleep deprivation and relapse: review and hypothesis. *American Journal of Psychiatry*, **147**, 14–21.
16. Leibenluft, E. and Wehr, T.A. (1992). Is sleep deprivation useful in the treatment of depression? *American Journal of Psychiatry*, **149**, 159–68.
17. Rush, A.J., Armitage, R., Gillin, J.C., *et al.* (1998). Comparative effects of nefazodone and fluoxetine on sleep in outpatients with major depressive disorder. *Biological Psychiatry*, **44** (1), 3–14.
18. Bakshi, R. (1996). Fluoxetine and restless legs syndrome. *Journal of Neurological Science*, **142**, 151–2.
19. Dorsey, C.M., Lukas, S.E., and Cunningham, S.L. (1996). Fluoxetine-induced sleep disturbance in depressed patients. *Neuropsychopharmacology*, **14**, 437–42.
20. Schenck, C.H., Mahowald, M.W., Kim, S.W., O'Connor, K.A., and Hurwitz, T.D. (1992). Prominent eye movements during NREM sleep and REM sleep behavior disorder associated with fluoxetine treatment of depression and obsessive–compulsive disorder. *Sleep*, **15**, 226–35.
21. Mellman, T.A. and Uhde, T.W. (1989). Sleep panic attacks: new clinical findings and theoretical implications. *American Journal of Psychiatry*, **146**, 1204–7.
22. Hauri, P.J., Friedman, M., and Ravaris, C.L. (1989). Sleep in patients with spontaneous panic attacks. *Sleep*, **12**, 323–37.
23. Mellman, T.A. and Uhde, T.W. (1989). Electroencephalographic sleep in panic disorder. *Archives of General Psychiatry*, **46**, 178–84.

24. Ross, R.J., Ball, W.A., Sullivan, K.A., and Caroff, S.N. (1989). Sleep disturbance as the hallmark of posttraumatic stress disorder. *American Journal of Psychiatry*, **146**, 697–707.

25. Ross, R.J., Ball, W.A., Dinges, D.F., *et al.* (1994). Rapid eye movement sleep disturbance in posttraumatic stress disorder. *Biological Psychiatry*, **35**, 195–202.

26. Mellman, T.A., Nolan, B., Hebding, J., Kulick-Bell, R., and Dominguez, R. (1997). A polysomnographic comparison of veterans with combat-related PTSD, depressed men, and non-ill controls. *Sleep*, **20**, 46–51.

27. Hurwitz, T.D., Mahowald, M.W., Kuskowski, M., and Engdahl, B.E. (1998). Polysomnographic sleep is not clinically impaired in Vietnam combat veterans with chronic posttraumatic stress disorder. *Biological Psychiatry*, **44**, 1066–73.

28. Lavie, P., Katz, N., Pillar, G., and Zinger, Y. (1998). Elevated awaking thresholds during sleep: characteristics of chronic war-related posttraumatic stress disorder patients. *Biological Psychiatry*, **44**, 1060–5.

29. Keshavan, M.S., Reynolds, C.F., III, and Kupfer, D.J. (1990). Electroencephalographic sleep in schizophrenia: a critical review. *Comprehensive Psychiatry*, **31**, 34–47.

30. Benson, K.L. and Zarcone, V.P., Jr. (1993). Rapid eye movement sleep eye movements in schizophrenia and depression. *Archives of General Psychiatry*, **50**, 474–82.

31. Hudson, J.I., Lipinski, J.F., Keck, P.E., Jr, *et al.* (1993). Polysomnographic characteristics of schizophrenia in comparison with mania and depression. *Biological Psychiatry*, **34**, 191–3.

32. Zarcone, V.P., Benson, K.L., and Berger, P.A. (1987). Abnormal rapid eye movement latencies in schizophrenia. *Archives of General Psychiatry*, **44**, 45–8.

33. Ganguli, R., Reynolds, C.F., III, and Kupfer, D.J. (1987). Electroencephalographic sleep in young never-medicated schizophrenics. *Archives of General Psychiatry*, **44**, 36–44.

34. van Kammen, D.P., van Kammen, W.B., Peters, J., Goetz, K., and Neylan, T. (1988). Decreased slow-wave sleep and enlarged lateral ventricles in schizophrenia. *Neuropsychopharmacology*, **1**, 265–71.

35. Lauer, C.J., Schreiber, W., Pollmacher, T., Holsboer, F., and Krieg, J.C. (1997). Sleep in schizophrenia: a polysomnographic study on drug-naive patients. *Neuropsychopharmacology*, **16**, 51–60.

36. Benca, R.M. and Casper, R.C. (1994). Sleep in eating disorders. *In Principles and practice of medicine* (2nd edn) (ed. M.H. Kryger, T. Roth, and W.C. Dement), pp. 927–33. W.B. Saunders, Philadelphia, PA.

37. Hudson, J.I., Pope, H.G., Jr, Jonas, J.M., *et al.* (1987). Sleep EEG in bulimia. *Biological Psychiatry*, **22**, 820–8.

38. Lauer, C.J., Krieg, J.-C., Riemann, D., Zulley, J., and Berger, M. (1990). A polysomnographic study in young psychiatric inpatients: major depression, anorexia nervosa, bulimia nervosa. *Journal of Affective Disorders*, **18**, 235–45.

39. Levy, A.B., Dixon, K.N., and Schmidt, H. (1987). REM and delta sleep in anorexia nervosa and bulimia. *Psychiatry Research*, **20**, 189–97.

40. Delvenne, V., Kerkhofs, M., Appelboom Fondu, J., Lucas, F., and Mendlewicz, J. (1992). Sleep polygraphic variables in anorexia nervosa and depression: a comparative study in adolescents. *Journal of Affective Disorders*, **25**, 167–72.

41. Levy, A.B., Dixon, K.N., and Schmidt, H. (1988). Sleep architecture in anorexia nervosa and bulimia. *Biological Psychiatry*, **23**, 99–101.

42. Gupta, M.A. (1991). Sleep-related eating in bulimia nervosa—an underreported parasomnia disorder. *Sleep Research*, **20**, 182.

43. Schenck, C.H., Hurwitz, T.D., Bundlie, S.R., and Mahowald, M.W. (1991). Sleep-related eating disorders: polysomnographic correlates of a heterogeneous syndrome distinct from daytime eating disorders. *Sleep*, **14**, 419–31.

44. Winkelman, J.W. (1998). Clinical and polysomnographic features of sleep-related eating disorder. *Journal of Clinical Psychiatry*, **59**, 14–19.

45. Spaggiari, M.C., Granella, F., Parrino, L., Marchesi, C., Melli, I., and Terzano, M.G. (1994). Nocturnal eating syndrome in adults. *Sleep*, **17**, 339–44.

46. Bliwise, D.L. (1993). Sleep in normal aging and dementia. *Sleep*, **16**, 40–81.

47. Vitiello, M.V., Bliwise, D.L., and Prinz, P.N. (1992). Sleep in Alzheimer's disease and the sundown syndrome. *Neurology*, **42** (Supplement 6), 83–94.

48. Prinz, P.N., Peskind, E.R., Vitaliano, P.P., *et al.* (1982). Changes in the sleep and waking EEGs of nondemented and demented elderly subjects. *Journal of the American Geriatrics Society*, **30**, 86–92.

49. Bliwise, D.L., Tinklenberg, J., Yesavage, J.A., *et al.* (1989). REM latency in Alzheimer's disease. *Biological Psychiatry*, **25**, 320–8.

50. Vitiello, M.V., Prinz, P.N., Williams, D.E., Frommlet, M.S., and Ries, R.K. (1990). Sleep disturbances in patients with mild-stage Alzheimer's disease. *Journal of Gerontology*, **45**, M131–8.

51. Gillin, J.C. (1994). Sleep and psychoactive drugs of abuse and dependence. In *Principles and practice of sleep medicine* (2nd edn) (ed. M.H. Kryger, T. Roth, and W.C. Dement), pp. 934–42. W.B. Saunders, Philadelphia, PA.

52. Obermeyer, W.H. and Benca, R.M. (1996). Effects of drugs on sleep. *Neurologic Clinics of North America*, **14**, 827–40.

4.14.6 Medical sleep–wake disorders

Sudhansu Chokroverty

Introduction

As medical factors can cause or contribute to psychiatric illness, medical assessment of patients is important in psychiatry. This needs to include the possibility of medically induced sleep disturbance in view of the aetiological role that such disturbance can have in psychiatric illness (Chapter 4.14.1). The need to consider this possibility is particularly important for psychiatrists involved in liaison work with medical specialties, whatever the age of the patients but especially the elderly. Neurological disorders may cause disruption of sleep/wakefulness by directly affecting the neurones that promote sleep/wakefulness; general medical disorders may affect them indirectly through metabolic, toxic, or anoxic disturbances, or medications used in their treatment. The main sleep complaints in neurological and other medical diseases are insomnia and hypersomnia, but parasomnias, sleep-related breathing problems, and circadian rhythm sleep disorders are also seen. Further details are available in the literature.[1–4]

Neurological disorders and sleep–wake disturbances

Neurodegenerative disorders

Alzheimer's disease

Sleep disturbances in Alzheimer's disease may be related to the severity of dementia and possibly to the associated periodic limb movements in sleep (**PLMS**) or sleep-related respiratory dysrhythmias. The presenting complaints include insomnia, inversion of sleep rhythm, and in some cases, excessive daytime sleepiness. 'Sundowning' is a major problem, characterized by episodes of confusion accompanied by partial or complete inversion of sleep rhythm with increased wakefulness at night and excessive daytime sleepiness. Mechanisms of sleep disturbances in Alzheimer's disease include degeneration of the neurones of the suprachiasmatic nuclei. Other factors include associated depression, PLMS, general medical disorders, medication effects, and environmental factors.

Parkinson's disease

Sleep difficulties are noted in 70 to 90 per cent of patients with Parkinson's disease,[2,3] and include difficulty in initiating and maintaining sleep causing sleep fragmentation, with frequent arousals and excessive daytime sleepiness. Sleep problems in Parkinson's disease arise from a combination of factors: an inability to turn over at night or on awakening in the middle of the night, leg cramps and jerks, dystonic spasm of the limbs or face, back pain, excessive nocturia, difficulty in getting out of bed unaided, and re-emergence of tremor and rigidity in sleep. Sleep disruption is more common in advanced than in early Parkinson's disease.

Antiparkinsonian medications may induce either peak-dose dyskinesias (mainly choreiform) or end-of-dose dyskinesia (mostly dystonic), causing disruption and fragmentation of sleep. Other abnormal movements which may occur after prolonged L-dopa therapy are myoclonus, akathisia, and PLMS which may cause sleep-initiating problems. Vivid or frightening dreams (nightmares) and sometimes psychosis can occur after long-standing dopaminergic treatment, causing sleep maintenance problems and excessive daytime sleepiness.

Sleep disruption in Parkinson's disease can also be caused by depression, dementia, sleep apnoea, restless legs syndrome, REM behaviour disorder (see Chapter 4.14.4), other parasomnias (sleep walking, sleep talking), and circadian rhythm disturbances. Sleep-related respiratory dysrhythmias (e.g. obstructive, central, or mixed apnoeas or hypopnoeas) may be more common in Parkinson's disease patients than in age-matched elderly controls.[2,3]

Other degenerative disorders

Sleep disturbance is present in almost all cases of **progressive supranuclear palsy**,[2,3] with reduced total sleep time, prolonged sleep latency, marked diminution of sleep spindles, reduced REM sleep time with abnormal rapid eye movements, disordered sleep architecture, and frequent awakenings. Some patients may develop REM behaviour disorder.

Insomnia with difficulty in initiation and maintenance of sleep, and sleep fragmentation are common complaints in **Huntington's disease**, especially in moderate to severe cases.

Progressive deterioration of sleep has been documented in many patients with **torsion dystonia**. Sleep disorders also occur in **spinocerebellar ataxias**, **multiple system atrophy (Shy–Drager syndrome)**, and **degenerative diseases of the motor neurones**.

Tourette's syndrome has many sleep-related features similar to those noted in degenerative disorders. The tics frequently persist in sleep, mostly in NREM stages 1 and 2. Sleep disturbances, including parasomnias and respiratory disturbances, occur in about 44 to 80 per cent of patients. Some patients may have a history of somnambulism, night terrors, nocturnal enuresis, and confusional arousal.

Stroke and sleep–wake disturbance

Sleep disturbances have been described in patients with cerebral hemispheric, paramedian thalamic, and brainstem infarctions. Associated depression and immobility with repeated awakenings may be responsible for insomnia in some patients, and there is an increased frequency of sleep apnoea in both infratentorial and supratentorial strokes. It is important to make a diagnosis of sleep apnoea in stroke patients because of the possible adverse effects on the long-term outcome, and because effective treatment is available for sleep apnoea. Brainstem infarction may cause the Ondine's curse syndrome in which patients become apnoeic during sleep but their voluntary breathing control during wakefulness remains intact.

Sleep and epilepsy

Sleep affects epilepsy and epilepsy affects sleep.[5] Certain types of clinical seizure (as well as interictal discharges) occur mainly, and sometimes exclusively, during sleep. Examples include mesial frontal seizures, benign centrotemporal (Rolandic) epilepsy of childhood, and tonic seizures in the Lennox–Gastaut syndrome in people with mental retardation (learning disability). Electrical status epilepticus during slow-wave sleep is associated with psychological deterioration. The short-lasting form of nocturnal paroxysmal dystonia is now increasingly recognized as a form of frontal-lobe epilepsy. The distinction between nocturnal seizures and other parasomnias (Chapter 4.14.4) is important because of their different significance and management requirements.

In turn, high rates of sleep disturbance have been reported in both adults and children with epilepsy. Depending on the type of epilepsy, this may be the result of disruption of sleep by seizures or interictal discharges, antiepileptic medication, or the various neurological disorders that can be associated with having seizures.

Neuromuscular disorders

Sleep disturbances have been described in many patients with neuromuscular disorders including **myotonic dystrophy**, **motor neurone disease**, **neuromuscular junctional disorders**, and **polyneuropathies**. Sleep disturbance has generally been secondary to involvement of the respiratory muscles, the phrenic and intercostal nerves, or the neuromuscular junctions of the respiratory and oropharyngeal muscles. The most common complaint is excessive daytime sleepiness resulting from repeated arousals and sleep fragmentation associated with apnoeas, hypopneas, and hypoventilation. Similar sleep disturbance is also seen in the acute convalescent stages of **poliomyelitis**.

Sleep and headache syndromes

Cluster headache and chronic paroxysmal hemicrania are most often related to sleep, and migraine may occur both during sleep and wakefulness. Cluster headache is predominantly noted in men and is a severe unilateral headache which occurs more frequently during sleep at night than during the daytime. The headache is characterized by severe excruciating pain around one eye and on the same side of the temple, accompanied by increased lacrimation, conjunctival injection, nasal stuffiness, rhinorrhea, and increased sweating from the forehead on the same side of the face. Polysomnographic recording documents occurrence of cluster headache out of REM sleep. Attacks usually last a few hours. Sleep apnoea, particularly REM-related sleep apnoea, may trigger cluster headache and there may be an increased prevalence of sleep apnoea in this condition. These patients also suffer from sleep maintenance insomnia because of awakening with cluster headache.

Other neurological conditions

Sleep disturbances have been noted in many patients with **multiple sclerosis** and these have been related to a combination of factors such as sleep-related breathing disturbances, immobility, leg-muscle spasms, pain, nocturia, and medication. Sleep complaints include insomnia and excessive daytime sleepiness.

Sleep disturbances in the form of insomnia, hypersomnia, or circadian rhythm dysfunction may occur after **traumatic brain injuries**, but adequate studies including sleep studies in such patients have not been documented.

Fatal familial insomnia is a recently described rare autosomal dominant prion disease.[6] This is a rapidly progressive disease with a clinical course running from 7 to 48 months with an average of 12 months. The clinical manifestations include impaired control of sleep–wake cycle including circadian rhythm, autonomic, and neuroendocrine dysfunction in addition to somatic neurological, cognitive, and behavioural manifestations. From the very beginning of the illness, profound sleep disturbances, particularly severe insomnia, are noted.

Idiopathic recurrent stupor is characterized by recurrent episodes of stupor without any metabolic, toxic, or structural brain dysfunction.[7] The episodes of stupor vary from 1 to 6 per week and the duration ranges between 2 and 120 h. The characteristic feature is that the patients are all briefly arousable from the stupor. Endozepine-4 in plasma and cerebrospinal fluid is markedly elevated in all patients. Following intravenous administration of flumazenil (0.5–1.0 mg), a benzodiazepine-receptor antagonist, the clinical manifestations and the EEG abnormalities all rapidly reverse to the normal state.

The **Kleine–Levin syndrome** is discussed in Chapter 9.2.9.

Sleep–wake dysfunction in other medical disorders

Cardiovascular diseases

Patients with **acute myocardial infarction** may suffer from sleep disturbances. Anginal pain may disturb the patient, causing frequent awakenings and impaired sleep efficiency. Sleep disturbance associated with periodic breathing and hypoxaemia has been described in patients with **congestive cardiac failure**. Cheyne–Stokes respiration commonly associated with congestive cardiac failure may cause hypoxaemia, hypercapnia, sleep disruption due to repeated arousals, excessive daytime sleepiness, and impaired cognitive function. It is important to diagnose sleep apnoea syndrome in congestive cardiac failure as treatment with nocturnal oxygen administration or continuous positive airway pressure titration may improve the patient. **Systemic hypertension** is associated with a high prevalence (22–48 per cent) of sleep apnoea and related symptoms. Treatment of obstructive sleep apnoea can reduce daytime as well as night-time blood pressure.

Respiratory diseases

Sleep disturbances in patients with **bronchial asthma** include early morning awakening, difficulty in maintaining sleep, and excessive daytime sleepiness, often with a combination of insomnia and hypersomnia.[4] In **chronic obstructive pulmonary disease** sleep efficiency is reduced, sleep onset is delayed, and awakenings increase with frequent stage shifts and arousals. Cardiac arrhythmias may occur, particularly during sleep. In some patients, chronic obstructive pulmonary disease may coexist with obstructive sleep apnoea syndrome, when it is known as overlap syndrome. Sleep disturbances may also be related to medication (e.g. methylxanthines), increased nocturnal cough, and accumulation of bronchial secretions leading to hypoxaemia and hypercapnia.

Gastrointestinal diseases

Patients with **peptic ulcer** may have repeated arousals and awakenings as a result of episodes of nocturnal epigastric pain. Gastro-oesophageal reflux disease (**reflux oesophagitis**) may cause difficulty in initiating sleep, frequent awakenings, and fragmentation of sleep related to the symptoms of retrosternal burning pain due to repeated spontaneous reflux episodes.

Endocrine diseases

Upper airway obstructive and central sleep apnoeas related to impaired central respiratory drive have been described in **myxoedema**. Both central and obstructive sleep apnoeas causing excessive daytime sleepiness and sleep fragmentation have been noted in **diabetes mellitus**, especially when associated with autonomic neuropathy. Central sleep apnoea has been noted in **acromegaly**; it responds to treatment with octreotide, a long-acting somatostatin analogue.

Chronic renal failure

Sleep complaints are common in chronic renal failure with or without dialysis. They include insomnia, excessive daytime sleepiness, and disturbed nocturnal sleep with reversal of day and night sleep rhythm. Restless legs syndrome and PLMS are common in uraemic patients. Many patients with chronic renal failure have sleep apnoea syndrome, mainly obstructive in nature, the cause of which is uncertain.

Other medical conditions

Sleep disturbance is very common in the **fibromyalgia syndrome**. The most prominent complaints in these patients consist of non-restorative sleep which is associated with non-specific polysomnographic abnormalities of sleep fragmentation, increased awakenings, decreased sleep efficiency, and also alpha-NREM sleep which, however, is not specific to this condition. PLMS has been documented in many patients. Treatment of this condition, which is unsatisfactory, combines tricyclic antidepressants with short-term intermittent treatment with zolpidem, an exercise programme, education, and reassurance.

Sleep disturbances are not uncommon in haematological disorders. **Paroxysmal nocturnal haemoglobinuria** may disturb sleep as a result of increased levels of plasma haemoglobin in the middle of the night and the early hours of the morning. Obstructive sleep apnoea and reduced oxygen saturation during sleep, causing sleep disturbance, have been described in patients with **sickle cell disease**.

Almost half of patients with **AIDS** develop neurological manifestations which include HIV encephalopathy causing dementia, seizures, focal or diffuse central nervous system dysfunction, and sleep disturbances as well as myelopathy, peripheral neuropathy, and polyradiculopathy. Sleep disturbances have been reported in many AIDS patients as part of the manifestation of AIDS encephalopathy. Sleep apnoea with sleep fragmentation and excessive daytime sleepiness in addition to sleep initiation and maintenance difficulties has been reported but no large study has been carried out. Sleep dysfunction has also been reported in seropositive patients without the full AIDS syndrome.

Dermatological disorders may cause sleep disruption because of pruritus and painful skin diseases.[8] Patients may have sleep-initiating and sleep-maintenance insomnia.

The neurological manifestations of African sleeping sickness (**trypanosomiasis**) are characterized by delusions, hallucinations, personality changes, and reversal of sleep–wake rhythm. The patient remains somnolent in the daytime and progresses gradually into the stage of stupor or coma. Disruption of the circadian sleep–wake rhythm is the most prominent finding in polysomnography. Circadian disruption of plasma cortisol, prolactin, and sleep–wake rhythms are noted in the most advanced stages, and these findings suggest selective changes in the suprachiasmatic nucleus. The diagnosis of trypanosomiasis is based on history and confirmation of the organism in the blood, bone marrow, cerebrospinal fluid, lymph-node aspirates, or a scraping from the chancre.

Sleep–wake disorders in intensive care unit patients

Insomnia, hypersomnia, and sleep-related respiratory dysrhythmia are common in the acute medical, surgical, and neurological disorders for which the patients are admitted to the intensive care unit. These disturbances may be intense in severely ill patients requiring life-saving cardiorespiratory support. The noise, bright light, and constant activity in the unit interfere with sleep, and the drugs used in intensive care may add to this. A reversible confusional state may develop 3 to 7 days after admission secondary to sleep deprivation. In the surgical intensive care unit additional factors interfering with sleep include anaesthesia, pain, and metabolic disturbances or infection. REM behaviour disorder may occur in patients admitted to the intensive care unit. Intensive care unit patients often have excessive daytime sleepiness as a result of night sleep disturbance.

Medication-related sleep–wake disturbances

Many medications cause sleep–wake disturbances[9,10] (Table 1).

Drugs for general medical disorders

Antihistamines (H$_1$ blockers), used to treat allergies, cause drowsiness. However, antihistamines are not recommended as hypnotics because of inadequate knowledge about their efficacy and safety as

Table 1 Medications causing sleep–wake disorders

Drugs used to treat general medical disorders
Antihistamines, analgesics, antiemetics, angiotensin-converting enzyme inhibitors, β-blockers, bronchodilators, theophylline, appetite suppressants, sleeping pills

Drugs for treating neurological disorders
Anticonvulsants, antiparkinsonian medications

Drugs used to treat psychiatric disorders
Antidepressants, neuroleptics

Miscellaneous agents (drugs of abuse and alcohol)
Amphetamines, cocaine, LSD, mescaline, marijuana, ethanol

Over-the-counter medications
Nasal decongestants, anorectics, caffeine, sleeping pills

hypnotics as well as their daytime sedation and anticholinergic effects.

Analgesics affect sleep–wake function. Narcotics (e.g. morphine, codeine, and other opioids), which are used to relieve severe pain and to induce sleep, can cause central nervous system sedation. Aspirin also may have a mild hypnotic effect.

Antiemetics (e.g. metaclopramide, domperidone, the phenothiazines, and the anticholinergic scopolamine) may produce drowsiness as a common side-effect. Domperidone has the least side-effect.

Angiotensin-converting enzyme inhibitors, used as hypotensive agents, may affect sleep adversely causing impairment of performance and mood. β-**Blockers** such as propranolol, metaprolol, and pindolol, which are used to treat hypertension, cardiac arrhythmias, and angina, may cause difficulty in initiating sleep and increase awakenings and frequent nightmares. **Bronchodilators**, used to treat chronic obstructive pulmonary disease and bronchial asthma, may cause insomnia. Theophylline may cause sleep fragmentation and increased wakefulness during sleep. **Anorectics** (**appetite suppressants**) increase catecholaminergic activity and hence act as central nervous system stimulants causing insomnia.

Sleeping pills, such as barbiturates, benzodiazepines, tranquillizers, and zolpidem may have opposite effects after prolonged use, and an abrupt withdrawal may disrupt sleep due to severe withdrawal effects. Transient disruption of sleep after cessation of a hypnotic is common. There is individual variation and susceptibility to the withdrawal effects. All the hypnotics, particularly long-acting ones, may affect daytime function. The short-acting drugs may cause rebound insomnia, daytime anxiety, and amnesia. Although benzodiazepines affect cognition and memory, they are relatively safe, they have low risk of abuse, and their side-effects are predictable. All hypnotics have respiratory depressing effects, particularly in patients with chronic obstructive pulmonary disease, bronchial asthma, and sleep apnoea. Sleeping medications should be used cautiously in older people as these may easily induce side-effects because of alteration of metabolism and drug absorption in the elderly.

Drugs used to treat psychiatric disorders

Antidepressants such as tricyclics, monoamine oxidase inhibitors, and others (trazodone, fluoxetine, bupropion, ritenserin, and lithium) may cause sleep disruption, alter sleep architecture, and suppress REM sleep. Sedative antidepressants (e.g. amitryptiline (Elavil[®]), doxepin, and trazodone) may be used to treat insomnia, especially if associated with depression. Most tricyclic antidepressants may cause daytime sedation. Monoamine oxidase inhibitors have alerting properties and so they should be used preferably in the morning or early afternoon. Trazodone, a sedative antidepressant, increases SWS but is a weak REM suppressant. Fluoxetine has an alerting effect and can suppress REM sleep at high doses. Lithium increases SWS and has a mild REM suppressant effect. Sudden withdrawal of these REM-suppressant medications may cause REM rebound.

Neuroleptics such as haloperidol, phenothiazines, and thioridazine are used to treat schizophrenia and other psychotic conditions. Some of these drugs, particularly phenothiazines, may cause drowsiness and impairment of performance. All neuroleptics may produce serious side-effects in combination with hypnotics, alcohol, or antihistaminic agents.

Drugs used for neurological disorders

Some anticonvulsants, especially benzodiazepines and barbiturates, cause sedation. Well-controlled studies documenting effects of anticonvulsants on sleep architecture are lacking. Effective seizure control results in reduction of sleep disturbance due to the reduction of seizures and not to any specific effect of anticonvulsants on sleep architecture. Antiparkinsonian medications, such as L-dopa may cause nocturnal hallucinations and agitated confusion disturbing sleep at night. Dopaminergic agonists such as pergolide may cause nightmares.

Miscellaneous agents

Stimulant drugs of abuse (e.g. amphetamines and cocaine) produce insomnia. Amphetamines increase wakefulness, suppress REM sleep, and delay sleep onset. Cocaine reduces REM sleep and increases sleep latency and REM latency. On cessation, this may cause REM rebound. Hallucinogens, such as lysergic acid diethylamide and mescaline, may produce a state resembling dreaming. Marijuana, through its active ingredient tetrahydrocannabinol, may cause sedation at lower doses and hallucination at higher doses. Tetrahydrocannabinol increases slow-wave sleep and reduces REM sleep. Drugs of abuse mostly alter the amount and timing of REM sleep and produce REM rebound on discontinuation.

Alcohol has profound effects on sleep/wakefulness. Acute administration of alcohol, a central nervous system sedative, will cause shortening of sleep onset and increase slow-wave sleep, reducing REM sleep. However, after the initial sedative effects and as the blood alcohol level falls, the patient has repeated awakenings causing sleep fragmentation and REM rebound. REM rebound is also noted on discontinuation after several nights of alcohol consumption. The sedative action of alcohol may be due to facilitation of γ-aminobutyric acid function and inhibition of glutamate. Alcohol, barbiturates, and tricyclic antidepressants may also produce REM behaviour disorder and other complex phenomena.

Over-the-counter medications

Nasal decongestants and anorectics, which are stimulants (e.g. pseudoephedrine, phenylpropranolamine), will cause insomnia. Caffeine, which is present in coffee, tea, colas, and chocolate, also is a stimulant and may cause insomnia. Over-the-counter sleeping pills are widely used for the induction of sleep. The active ingredients in these agents are antihistamines (diphenhydramine and doxylamine) and are the most commonly used antihistamines in over-the-counter preparations. They are H_1 blockers and have undesirable anticholinergic effects (e.g. dryness of mouth, palpitation, dilatation of pupils, tachycardia, difficulty in urination) and cause daytime sedation.

Principles of management of medical sleep–wake disorders

The first step is an accurate diagnosis and treatment of the primary medical disorder. Without this, treatment of secondary sleep disturbances is unlikely to be successful. Treatment of the primary condition may improve sleep disturbance. If not, it is often difficult to manage sleep disturbance. Sleep hygiene measures should be instituted followed by more specific treatment for the sleep complaints such as insomnia, hypersomnia, circadian rhythm sleep disorders, and parasomnia.

Management of insomnia in medical sleep–wake disorders includes judicious use of hypnotics for transient or short-term insomnia. Hypnotics should be avoided in patients with sleep apnoea syndrome and used cautiously in patients with renal, hepatic, or pulmonary diseases.

Treatment of sleep-related breathing disorders includes general measures of avoidance of sedatives, hypnotics, and alcohol which can aggravate sleep-related breathing disorders, and use of nasal continuous positive airway pressure or bilevel positive airway pressure in selected patients with medical sleep–wake disorders. In patients with neuromuscular disorders associated with obstructive sleep apnoea or sleep hypoventilation, intermittent positive-pressure ventilation using a nasal mask during sleep is the best treatment.

In most cases REM behaviour disorder responds dramatically to small doses of clonazepam by mouth at night. Restless legs syndrome–PLMS associated with medical or neurological disorders should be treated in the same way as idiopathic restless legs syndrome–PLMS. Four groups of drugs have been found to be useful in such conditions: dopaminergic agents, benzodiazepines, gabapentine, and opioids.[11]

For treatment of patients with dementias and confusion associated with sleep disturbances, certain general principles as outlined in Table 2 should be instituted.

Treatment of Parkinson's disease has not been found to improve sleep consistently. In those with reactivation of parkinsonian symptoms during sleep at night, adjustment in the timing and choice of medication may be helpful. Dopamine agonists (e.g. bromocriptine, pergolide) or longer-acting preparations of L-dopa taken near bedtime may benefit sleep in some patients. Antihistamines such as diphenhydramine may promote sleep in addition to the modest antiparkinsonian effect. A small dose of L-dopa/carbidopa, with a second dose later at night if the patient awakens, may sometimes help those with insomnia. Nocturnal dyskinesias related to L-dopa causing insomnia may respond to a reduction in the dose of dopamine agonists or by addition of a small dose of benzodiazepine. Clonazepam at bedtime may benefit those patients with nocturnal hallucinations and nightmares. In patients with psychosis and severe nocturnal hallucinations, clozapine or newer drugs such as olanzapine may be used with con-

Table 2 Treatment of sleep disturbances in patients with dementias and confusion

---

Institute regular sleep schedule as much as possible

Eliminate alcohol and caffeine in the evening

Try an intermediate-acting benzodiazepine or zolpidem for not more than three times per week to treat insomnia

Reduce or eliminate medications that may contribute to sleep disturbances or sleep-related respiratory dysrhythmias

Treat associated depression with a sedative antidepressant

Treat associated conditions that may interfere with sleep (e.g. pain due to arthritis and other causes)

Discourage patients from taking daytime naps

Encourage regular exercise (e.g. walking)

For extreme agitation use small doses of haloperidol (0.5–1 mg twice or thrice daily) or thioridazine (25 mg thrice daily)

In selected patients, use bright-light therapy in the evening

---

siderable benefit. During clozapine treatment the usual precautions of monitoring blood count and testing liver function should be taken.

References

1. Chokroverty, S. (1999). Approach to the patient with sleep complaints. In *Sleep disorders medicine: basic science, technical considerations and clinical aspects* (2nd edn) (ed. S. Chokroverty), pp. 275–85. Butterworth Heinemann, Boston, MA.

2. Chokroverty, S. (1999). Sleep, breathing and neurological disorders. In *Sleep disorders medicine: basic science, technical considerations and clinical aspects* (2nd edn) (ed. S. Chokroverty), pp. 509–71. Butterworth Heinemann, Boston, MA.

3. Chokroverty, S. (1996). Sleep and degenerative neurologic disorders. *Neurology Clinics*, **14**, 807–26.

4. Chokroverty, S. (1999). Sleep disturbances in other medical disorders. In *Sleep disorders medicine: basic science, technical considerations and clinical aspects* (2nd edn) (ed. S. Chokroverty), pp. 587–617. Butterworth Heinemann, Boston, MA.

5. Chokroverty, S. and Quinto, C. (1999). Sleep and epilepsy. In *Sleep disorders medicine: basic science, technical considerations and clinical aspects* (2nd edn) (ed. S. Chokroverty), pp. 697–727. Butterworth Heinemann, Boston, MA.

6. Montagna, P., Cortelli, P., Tinuper, S., *et al.* (1994). Fatal familial insomnia. A disease that emphasizes the role of the thalamus in the regulation of sleep and vegetative functions. In *Fatal-familial insomnia: inherited prion diseases, sleep and the thalamus* (ed. C. Guilleminault, E. Lugaresi, P. Montagna, and P. Gambetti). Raven, New York.

7. Tinuper, P., Montagna, P., Plazzi, G., *et al.* (1994). Idiopathic recurring stupor. *Neurology*, **44**, 621–5.

8. Aoki, T., Kushimoto, H., Hishikawa, Y., *et al.* (1991). Nocturnal scratching and its relationship to the disturbed sleep of itchy subjects. *Clinical Experimental Dermatology*, **16**, 268–72.

9. Obermeyer, W.H. and Benca, R.M. (1996). Effects of drugs on sleep. *Neurologic Clinics*, **14**, 827–40.

10. Nicholson, A.N., Bradley, C.M., and Pascoe, P.A. (1994). Medications: effect on sleep and wakefulness. In *Principles and practice of sleep medicine* (2nd edn) (ed. M.H. Kryger, T. Roth, and W.C. Dement), pp. 364–72. W.B. Saunders, Philadelphia, PA.

11. Hening, W.A., Allen, R., Walters, A.S., and Chokroverty, S. (1999). Motor functions and dysfunctions in sleep. In *Sleep disorders medicine: basic science, technical considerations and clinical aspects* (2nd edn) (ed. S. Chokroverty), pp. 441–507. Butterworth Heinemann, Boston, MA.

4.15 Suicide

4.15.1 Epidemiology and causes of suicide

Jouko K. Lonnqvist

Definition of suicide and the reliability of suicide statistics

Suicidal behaviour or suicidality can be conceptualized as a continuum ranging from suicidal ideation to suicide attempts and completed suicide. A developmental process which leads to suicidal ideation, self-destructive behaviour, in some cases even to suicide, and its consequences to the survivors is often referred to as a suicidal process. There is no single unanimously accepted definition of suicide, although in most proposed definitions it is considered as a fatal act of self-injury (self-harm) undertaken with more or less conscious self-destructive intent, however vague and ambiguous. Since the deceased cannot testify as to his or her intent, the conclusions about this must be drawn by inference. The evidence required for this inference depends on many factors, for example the mode of death, the use of autopsy, age, gender, social and occupational status, and the social stigma of suicide in the person's culture. The assessment of suicide intent is always based on a balance of probabilities.

Besides the conceptual problems, there are differences in operational definitions of suicidal behaviour which may lead to lack of uniformity of case definition and difficulties in comparing suicide statistics. The reliability of suicide statistics is influenced by whether suicide is ascertained by legal officials as in the United Kingdom and Ireland, or by medical examiners as elsewhere in Europe. In general, suicides tend to be undercounted, whereas non-suicidal deaths are very rarely misidentified as suicides. Most misclassified suicides fall into the category of undetermined deaths and are more like suicides than accidents. Underestimation is reasoned to be less than 10 per cent in the more developed countries, which allows rate comparisons between countries and over time. Despite problems in the recording of suicide, reports on suicide rates among different cultures or people suggest a true variation in suicide mortality.[1,2]

The suicide process and the act of suicide

Suicide is a mode of death usually consequent to a complex and multi-faceted behaviour pattern. It is typically seen as the fatal outcome of a long-term process shaped by a number of interacting cultural, social, situational, psychological, and biological factors. Suicide is a rare, shocking, and very individual final act, which often leaves the survivors helpless. The suicide process model is used to organize and clarify the complexity of factors associated with suicide (Fig. 1).

Suicide is usually preceded by years of suicidal behaviour or feelings, and plans and warnings. In about half of all suicides a previous attempt is found in the person's history, which offers, in theory, an opportunity for suicide intervention wherever suicide attempts occur. Male suicide attempts are more violent and the first attempt more likely to end in death. Particularly among males, suicide prevention ought to begin earlier in the course of the suicide process. Successful

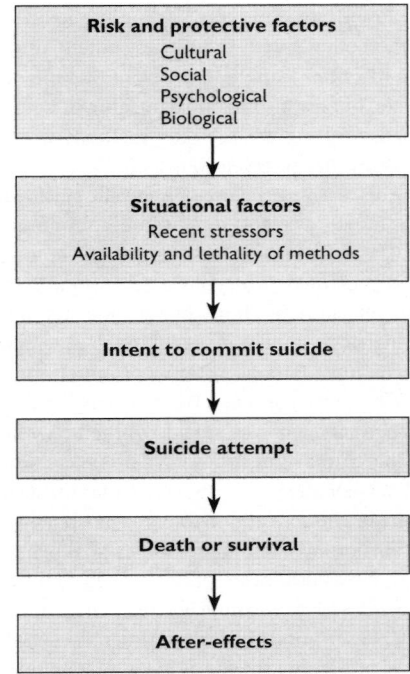

Fig. 1 Risk and protective factors.

suicide prevention calls for sensitive understanding of suicidal intent and active early intervention.[3]

Various risk or protective factors underlie suicidal behaviour, and the changing balance of these helps to explain the fluctuation of suicide risk over the course of time. An appearance of suicidality means either an intensified effect of risk factors or a weakened effect of protective factors. For example, a separation from someone close may precipitate a suicidal imbalance in a vulnerable person due to the adverse life event as a stressor and the broken social network as a loss of social support.

The treating personnel and relatives of the suicide victim tend to overemphasize the meaning of the most recent events in the course of the suicide process. A precipitating factor may well be decisive in explaining the precise timing of suicide in the long course of a person's suicide process. Often, however, it also allows a simple and rational explanation in the face of the complexity of suicide. The guilt feelings of survivors are often dealt with by rationalization or projective accusations.

The choice of a specific method takes place at the very end of the suicide process and represents the last possibility to intervene. Availability is a major factor affecting this choice. Hanging is universally available and it is the most common suicide method globally. In many countries the ready access to firearms makes them potentially dangerous, especially among male adolescents and young adults. Restricting access to handguns might be expected to reduce the suicide rate of young people. Previously domestic gas was frequently used as a suicide method, and detoxfication resulted in a significant decrease in suicide rates. Restrictive availability measures may also be important in the clinical treatment of individual suicidal patients. Restriction in availability of dangerous means is a strategy based on the fact that suicidal crises are often brief, suicidal acts are often impulsive, and the long-term suicide rate of serious suicide attempts is remarkably low.[4–8]

The lethality of the suicide act is related to the severity of the intent to die and the degree of mutilation caused by the act, and how quickly a method can cause death. Firearms, carbon monoxide, and hanging are active suicide methods with the highest potential to cause death. Jumping from a height or leaping in the front of a moving vehicle are more passive ways, but are also highly damaging in nature. Poisoning, drowning, or wrist cutting are typically methods which leave more time for help seeking and intervention.

Imitation means learning the use of a specific suicide method from a model which is overtly available in a culture, community, institution, or mass media. The risk of imitation emerges if an emotionally loaded suicide model is presented in detail on television.[9] Imitation may have a significant effect on the choice of a suicide method, especially at schools, in psychiatric hospital wards, and in the general population of young people. The most famous example of imitation is the effect of Goethe's novel *The Sorrows of Young Werther*, which was widely read in Europe about 200 years ago. The suicide of the hero was imitated to such an extent that authorities in several European countries banned the novel. The 'Werther effect' also appeared after the death of Marilyn Monroe; the suicide rate rose about 10 per cent over the next 10 days. Despite suggestions of media influence on suicidal behaviour, contradictory findings have also been presented. Recommendations for reporting of suicide have encouraged avoidance of repetitive and excessive reports, descriptions of technical details, simplified explanations for suicide, presenting suicide as means of coping with personal problems, or glorifying suicide victims.[10] Experiences from subway suicides in Vienna show that well-considered media guidelines changed the style of suicide reporting in Austrian newspapers, which probably led to a marked decrease in the imitation effect and consequently also in subway suicides.[11]

Most suicides are solitary and private, but a few result from a pact between people to die together. Suicide pacts are exceptional, accounting for less than 1 per cent of all suicides, and their incidence seems to be declining.

Suicide always has a major impact on the survivors. Suicide is a threatening event not only among close family members, but also in the surrounding population, including treating personnel and the people at the victim's workplace. The major challenges after a suicide, in addition to a normal mourning process, are dealing with shame and guilt feelings, and the crisis of survivors. Sharing of the traumatic experience and social support should be arranged immediately and continued, if necessary, at least for the first 6 months after the suicide and with the help of mental health professionals.

Epidemiology and public health aspects of suicide

Every year more than one million people commit suicide, accounting for 1 to 2 per cent of total global mortality. Suicide is a leading cause of premature death, especially among young adults. It is the fifth highest cause of years of life lost in the developed world. In many Westernized countries suicide is a more frequent cause of death than traffic accidents. According to World Health Organization (**WHO**) statistics, the annual world-wide incidence of completed suicide was 16 per 100 000 persons in 1995. This means that globally 1 per 6000 persons commits suicide every year.

The long-term trend in suicide mortality has been increasing. The rank order of suicide mortality in the European region in 1990 to 1991 shows 19 countries with suicide rates above the mean for the region: Lithuania, the Russian Federation, Latvia, Estonia, Hungary, Slovenia, Finland, Belarus, Kazakstan, Ukraine, Croatia, Austria, Switzerland, Denmark, Czech Republic, France, Belgium, Republic of Moldova, Slovakia, and Bulgaria. Most of the countries with high suicide mortality are located in Eastern Europe. The lowest suicide rates (below 10 per 100 000) in the WHO's European region are found in the following 15 countries: Azerbaijan, Armenia, Albania, Greece, Georgia, Tajikistan, Uzbekistan, Turkmenistan, Malta, the United Kingdom, Spain, Portugal, Ireland, Italy, and The Netherlands. Outside this region suicide mortality has been exceptionally high (above 40 per 100 000) in Sri Lanka during the civil war, and is also high (above 16 per 100 000) in Japan. Suicide rate is moderate (10–16 per 100 000) in China, Cuba, Canada, Singapore, Australia, New Zealand, Mauritius, the United States, and Uruguay. Everywhere, the male suicide rate is two to four times higher than the female rate; China is the only exception with a very high female suicide rate.[12]

The suicide rate of elderly people has been higher than in the younger age groups almost universally. In addition, in many Western countries the suicide rate for people aged 65 years and over has been declining for decades. This change is associated with the growth of the general well being and the better social and health services.

Traditionally the incidence of suicide has been low in the younger age group (15–24), but during the past 20 to 30 years the suicide rate has been rising in many Western countries, especially among young males. The suicide rate of the young male adults is nowadays almost at the same level as the rate of middle-aged men. Alcohol misuse has been suggested as one possible causal factor for the increase of suicide rate. Other risk factors of adolescent suicides are school problems, a family history of suicidal behaviour, poor communication, and stressful life events. The most recent adolescent suicide statistics have been encouraging in many countries. In the United States the rate reached a peak in 1987, remained fairly constant for several years, and began to decline in 1996.

A long list of major public health concerns in the field of suicidology has emerged in the Western world in the 1990s:

- suicidal ideation and suicide attempts are surprisingly common in the general population

- the high, and in many countries rapidly rising, rate of suicides among adolescents and young adults

- unemployment as a major risk factor for suicide in Europe

- easy access to lethal suicide methods such as psychotropic or analgesic drugs, guns, and motor vehicles

- high alcohol consumption and increasing substance misuse

- undertreatment of major psychiatric disorders such as depression and schizophrenia

- suicide models projected by the mass media.

These findings indicate that rapid growth and continuous changes in society are simultaneously causing instability and disturbing the development of integration. Some regions and groups of people are inevitably affected negatively by this development, and large numbers of people are thus moving towards a greater risk of suicide.

Scores of special and comprehensive suicide prevention programmes have been launched both locally and nationally during the last 10 years. Everywhere, suicide research has come to be seen as an elementary component of suicide prevention. Only critical research can identify new and specific high-risk groups, and properly evaluate specific interventions and suicide prevention activities in general.[13] Suicide prevention is considered in Chapter 4.15.4.

Determinants of suicide

Usually, suicide has no single cause. It is the endpoint of an individual process, in which several interacting determinants or risk factors can be identified (Tables 1 and 2). Risk factors are by their nature cultural, social, situational, psychological, biological, and even genetic.

Cultural factors in suicide

Culture defines basic attitudes towards life and death, and also towards suicide in society. A hundred years ago suicide was illegal in many European countries. Similarly, most churches overtly opposed suicide and allowed suicide victims to be buried only outside the cemetery. Religion was also a major integrating force between individuals and the community. In a modern secularized society, religion is still a meaningful and protective factor for many individuals in a suicidal crisis. Church plays an important role in suicide prevention in many countries, by arranging crisis services for suicidal people and support for survivors. Western culture has had a tendency to emphasize the individuals's free will and the shouldering of responsibility for one's life, while egoistic and anomic trends in society have intensified and altruism has almost disappeared. Such changes may have increased the

Table 1 Risk factors for suicide: sociodemographic variables

Gender	Male
Age	Elderly
Social status	Low
Educational status	Low
Marital status	Unmarried, separated, divorced, widowed
Residential status	Living alone
Employment status	Unemployed, retired, insecure employment
Economic status	Weak (males)
Profession	Farmer, female doctor, student, sailor
Special subpopulations	Students, prisoners, immigrants, refugees, religious sects
Special institutions	Hospitals, prisons, army
Region	Uneven distribution locally by urban–rural, residential, or subcultural area
Season and time	Spring and autumn, weekend, evening, anniversary
Life events	Adverse life events such as losses and separations, criminal charges
Social support	Low
Social integration	Lacking

incidence of suicide in society. The cultural background of suicide is a deep structure inhereted over the generations. Cultural factors also prevent rapid changes in suicidal behaviour, which is evident among immigrants, whose mode and rate of suicide usually lie somewhere between the original and the host cultures.[14]

Sociological theories on suicide

Classic sociology views suicide as a social, not an individual, phenomenon. The suicide victim's moral predisposition to commit suicide, not

Table 2 Clinical determinants of suicide

Family history	Suicidal behaviour, mental disorders
Mental disorders	Any disorder, depression, substance use disorders, personality disorders, schizophrenia
Contact with psychiatric services	Any contacts, recent contacts, post-discharge period, psychotropic drugs
Psychiatric symptoms	Hopeless, helpless, depressive, psychotic, delirious, anxious, aggressive, introversive
Suicidal behaviour	Previous suicide attempts, suicidal ideations, death wishes, indirect gestures
Physical health	Severe physical illness such as cancer, AIDS, stroke, and epilepsy; permanent sickness
Availability of suicide methods	Easy access to lethal methods

his or her individual experiences, is felt to be the crucial factor. Moral predisposition means the degree to which the victim is involved in more or less integrated groups and in the values of those groups. Suicides are seen as a disturbance or symptom of a relationship between society and individuals. In 1897 Durkheim published his famous work on suicide and described four basic types. Anomic suicide reflects a situation where an individual is no longer guided by the society due to its weakness, like the suicide of an unemployed and rejected alcoholic without any support from society. Altruistic suicide is illustrated by a society which can exert a strong influence on an individual's decision to sacrifice his or her life, as did the captain of the *Titanic*, for example. Egoistic suicide is an individualistic decision of a person no longer dependent on others' control or opinion such as a person who has arranged an assisted suicide. Fatalistic suicide is seen as a result of strict rules in a society which have proved decisive for the destiny of an individual, for example the suicide of a person held as a slave.[15] There are also newer social theories of suicide which stress more the joint effects of social factors. The concept of social isolation has been clinically useful in understanding the socio-ecological and social–psychiatric background of suicide.[16,17] Some sociologists have underlined the individual meanings associated with suicide.

Life events and social support

The life situation preceding suicide is typically characterized by an excess of adverse life events and recent stressors. Usually, the sum effect of events is overwhelming and more important than a single life event. Job problems, family discord, somatic illness, financial trouble, unemployment, separation, and death and illness in the family are the most common life events preceding suicide. Somatic illness and retirement are age-specifically connected with the suicides of elderly men, while separation, financial troubles, job problems, and unemployment are more common among younger men. Severely disabling somatic illness is a very important risk factor for suicide in elderly male patients, especially when associated with signs of distress and depression. In general, suicide among men is more often related to recent stressors than it is among women. The excess of specific stressors among men implies a subjective lack of success or failures in achievements expected in the social roles of adult life.

In most cases life events are not accidental, but are usually also dependent on the individual's own behaviour. Personality features, even mental disorders, often explain the difficulties the victim has had. Among male alcoholics life stress is connected with family discord and separations in all age groups. Other sources of stress in alcoholic male suicides are unemployment and financial troubles, whereas in depressive non-alcoholic male victims life stress is associated more with somatic illness. Among alcoholic males, adverse life events and living alone clearly have an enhancing effect on suicidality, which should be taken into account when treating alcohol misuse. In the extreme case of a rejected suicidal alcoholic husband of a divorcing wife, all available social support should be mobilized for both sides. Among females life events as psychosocial stress are less strongly connected with suicide. Depression and adverse interpersonal life events are more frequent contributors to female than male suicides.[18,19]

Psychology of suicide

Early psychological theories of suicide focused on the concept of the self. A classical example is Freud's theory assuming that self-destructive behaviour in depression represents aggression directed against a part of the self that has incorporated a loss or rejection of a love object. In his later theory of suicide Freud presented the construction of the dual instincts, where Eros is a life-sustaining and life-enhancing drive in constant interaction with Thanatos, the aggressive death instinct.

Later psychodynamic thinking on suicide focused more on the self in relation to others. Suicide was seen as an aggressive attack against the 'bad mother', a failure of the separation–individuation transition, a failure to achieve adaptation in situations of confusion and loss of control, an expression of narcissistic rage and an inability to tolerate feelings of shame, an effort to re-establish control over a chaotic inner world, or as a need to regain feelings of self-esteem by merging with a lost loved object through death. Failures in the developmental and adaptational processes are reflected in negative self-images and distorted cognitive schemas, leading to such feelings as depression, hopelessness, rage, shame, guilt, and anxiety. It is widely held that psychological pain is found as a common element at the core of all suicidal behaviours; suicide occurs when the individual can no longer endure the pain. Most recent psychological theories of suicide accept a multiaxial causation of suicide resulting from an interaction of predisposing and precipitating factors.[20] A person moves towards a suicidal crisis depending on the stressors and precence or absence of protective factors in his or her life.

Neurobiological determinants of suicide

Suicide often aggregates in families. Relatives of patients who commit suicide are themselves more likely to commit suicide than relatives of patients who do not commit suicide. Liability to suicidal behaviour may be a familially transmitted trait which is independent on the specific mental disorders.

Results of adoption studies suggest that genetic factors rather than familial environmental factors are the determinants of familial concordance for suicidal behaviour. Among biological relatives of adopted suicide victims there is a higher incidence of suicide than among the relatives of non-suicide controls or among the adoptive relatives of the suicide victims. Also identical twins have a higher concordance for suicide, attempted suicide, and suicide ideation compared with nonidentical twins.[21]

Patients who have seriously attempted suicide by violent means have low levels of the serotonin metabolite 5-hydroxyindole acetic acid in their cerebrospinal fluid.[22] These and other biochemical changes are discussed in Chapter 4.15.3.

Basic characteristics of the suicide victim

Persons at greatest risk of suicide are usually middle-aged or older, non-married men with poor social and economic position, and a family history of mental disorders and suicidal behaviour. Usually they are living alone, and often unemployed or with insecure employment. They also typically have marked recent life stress and a weak social network. Most suffer from depression and many have a comorbid substance abuse or personality disorder. Almost all elderly victims have comorbid physical illness or are permanently disabled. Most have previously contacted health care, and communicated their suicidal tendencies at least indirectly, although usually without receiving adequate

Table 3 Rank order of suicide in mental disorders

Suicide attempt

Anorexia nervosa

Major depression

Mood disorders not otherwise specified

Reactive psychoses

Bipolar disorder

Dysthymia

Schizophrenia

Anxiety disorders

Personality disorders

Substance use disorders

Table 4 Major findings on mental disorders in five psychological autopsy studies[24–28] on completed suicides using DSM-III or DSM-IIIR criteria

Disorder	Percentage
Depressive disorders	36–90
Alcohol dependence or abuse	43–54
Drug dependence or abuse	4–45
Schizophrenic disorders	3–10
Organic mental disorders	2–7
Personality disorders	5–44

psychiatric treatment. Half of them have previously attempted suicide.

Mental disorders and suicide

Virtually all mental disorders carry an increased risk of suicide, except for mental retardation and dementia. The suicide risk in functional mental disorders is double that in substance use disorders, which in turn carry double the risk of suicide compared to organic disorders. The greatest risk of suicide among all clinical states is in attempted suicide, which carries about 40 times the expected value (Table 3). In anorexia nervosa and major depression the risk is about 20-fold, and in other mood disorders and psychoses about 10 to 15 times higher than expected. In anxiety, personality, and substance use disorders the suicide risk is at lower levels, but about five to 10 times higher than the expected value. In subtance disorders the risk is dependent on the type of disorder, being clearly lowest in alcohol, cannabis, and nicotine abusers.[23]

Psychological autopsy studies have been used to construct an overall view of suicide by collecting all available relevant information on the victim's life preceding his or her death. In five psychological autopsy studies[24–28] mental disorders of suicide victims have been assessed using DSM-III or DSM-IIIR diagnoses and large unselected samples. Although the range of figures for individual suicides is wide, the victim received at least one diagnosis on Axis I in 86 to 98 per cent of these suicides and at least one diagnosis on Axis II in 5 to 44 per cent. In all five studies depressive disorders and substance use disorders were frequent and comorbidity was common (Table 4).

In two recent European psychological autopsy studies[25,28] from Finland and Northern Ireland the distribution of the principal diagnoses was similar (Table 5). The most common psychiatric diagnoses in suicide were major depression (30–31 per cent) and alcohol dependence (17–24 per cent). All other single diagnoses formed less than 10 per cent of all suicides. As a principal diagnosis, major mood disorders together comprised 42 to 36 per cent and substance use disorders 19 to 30 per cent of all suicides. Comorbidity was a major finding in both samples. The most commonly observed comorbidity

pattern in suicide has been substance use disorder with major depression.

The mortality risk for suicide in major depression is 20 times that expected, and 15- to 20-fold in all affective disorders. Every sixth death among depressive people treated as psychiatric patients is by suicide.[29] The risk of suicide varies across the subclasses of depression, and is related to the selection of suicidal patients for the various types of treatment. The risk is highest for depressive inpatients, even during the postdischarge period, and much lower among psychiatric outpatients, although clearly lowest for those treated for depression in primary care.[30]

Table 5 Principal DSM-IIIR Axis I and II diagnoses of male and female suicide victims in Finland and Northern Ireland

Diagnosis	Finland (%) (n = 229)	Northern Ireland (%) (n = 118)
Major depression	30	31
Depressive disorder not otherwise specified	9	—
Dysthymia	—	1
Bipolar disorder	3	4
Alcohol dependence	17	24
Alcohol misuse	2	4
Other substance use disorders	—	2
Schizophrenia	7	6
Schizoaffective disorder	3	1
Other psychoses	3	4
Anxiety disorders	1	5
Adjustment disorder	3	3
Organic mental disorders	2	1
Other Axis I disorders	2	2
Personality disorder	9	3
No diagnosis	2	10
Insufficient information for assessment	7	—

Depression of suicide victims seems to differ qualitatively from that of living controls; it seems to be more severe and accompanied more often by insomnia, anhedonia, self-neglect, and impaired memory. Moreover, suicide risk in follow-up is higher in depression associated with such symptoms as insomnia, anhedonia, diminished concentration, and anxiety. Of the various subjective qualities of depression, hopelessness or negative anticipation is most widely accepted as the best predictor of suicide. Inadequate and inefficient antidepressant treatment of depressed suicide victims has been a persistent finding in several studies. Less than half of suicide victims with major depression have been in contact with psychiatric care at the time of suicide. However, there is some evidence that good monitoring and maintenance treatment in high-risk groups of patients may be able to decrease their suicide rates.[31]

At the individual level, misuse of alcohol or drugs complicates the suicidal process. Alcohol and drugs, often combined, are a major risk or a precipitating factor for suicide. They may intensify the suicidal intent, offer a constantly available suicide method, worsen the somatic status of the victim and increase the risk of complications after the attempt. Alcohol impairs judgement and lowers the threshold to suicide. Alcohol is detected in about every third case at the moment of suicide.[32] The lifetime risk of suicide has been estimated at 7 per cent for alcohol dependence, with only slight variation over the life.[33] The suicide rate in alcoholism is about six times higher than that in the general population.[23] In drug dependence or abuse it is 15 to 20 times higher than expected.[23,34] In some countries, the level of alcohol consumption seems to be associated directly with the suicide rate, especially among young males and adolescents.[35]

The suicide risk in schizophrenia appears to be almost 10 times higher than in the general population.[23] The lifetime risk of suicide in schizophrenia is estimated to be at least 4 per cent, and in selected follow-up studies has been as high as 10 to 13 per cent.[33] The great majority of schizophrenic patients commit suicide in the active phase of the disorder after having suffered depressive symptoms. Suicide in schizophrenia is thus less of a surprise; it is typically preceded by a previous attempt, and suicidal intent has been communicated at least as often as in non-schizophrenic suicides.[36] Undertreatment, comorbidity, treatment non-compliance, and a high frequency of non-responders are also common problems among schizophrenic suicide victims. Adequacy of comprehensive care is crucial for suicide prevention in schizophrenia, especially among actively psychotic patients with recent suicidal behaviour and depressive symptoms.[37]

Most of the suicide victims with personality disorder, especially with borderline personality disorder, have also comorbid depressive disorder or substance abuse. This kind of comorbidity is very frequent among the young suicide victims.[25,26]

Mental disorders, particularly depressive disorders, substance abuse, and antisocial behaviour have an important role in the adolescent suicides. The diagnostic distribution of mental disorders among them is surprisingly similar to that of the young and even middle-aged adults.[38]

References

1. Lönnqvist, J. (1977). Suicide in Helsinki: an epidemiological and socialpsychiatric study of suicides in Helsinki in 1960–61 and 1970–71. *Monographs of Psychiatria Fennica*, No. 8.
2. Sainsbury, P. and Jenkins, J.S. (1982). The accuracy of officially reported suicide statistics for purposes of epidemiological research. *Journal of Epidemiology and Community Health*, **36**, 43–8.
3. Isometsä, E.T. and Lönnqvist, J.K. (1998). Suicide attempts preceding completed suicide. *British Journal of Psychiatry*, **173**, 531–6.
4. Ohberg, A., Lonnqvist, J., Sarna, S., Vuori, E., and Penttila, A. (1995). Trends and availability of suicide methods in Finland: proposals for restrictive measures. *British Journal of Psychiatry*, **166**, 35–43.
5. Kreitman, N. (1976). The coal gas history: UK suicide rates 1960–1971. *British Journal of Preventive and Social Medicine*, **30**, 83–90.
6. Ohberg, A., Lonnqvist, J., Sarna, S., and Vuori, E. (1996). Violent methods associated with high suicide mortality among the young. *Journal of American Academy of Child and Adolescent Psychiatry*, **35**, 144–53.
7. Lewis, G., Hawton, K., and Jones, P. (1997). Strategies for preventing suicide. *British Journal of Psychiatry*, **171**, 351–4.
8. Hawton, K., Fagg, J., Simkin, S., Harris, L., and Malmberg, A. (1998). Methods used for suicide by farmers in England and Wales. *British Journal of Psychiatry*, **173**, 320–4.
9. Schmidtke, A. and Schaller, S. (1998). What do we know about media effects on imitation of suicidal behaviour: state of the art. In *Suicide prevention: a holistic approach* (ed. D. DeLeo, A. Schmidtke, and R.F.W. Diekstra), pp. 121–37. Kluwer, Dordrecht.
10. The Center for Disease Control and Prevention (1994). Program for the prevention of suicide among adolescents and young adults. *Morbidity and Mortality Weekly Report*, **43**, 3–7.
11. Sonneck, G., Etzersdorfer, E., and Nagel-Kuess, S. (1994). Imitative suicide on the Viennese subway. *Social Science and Medicine*, **38**, 453–7.
12. World Health Organization (1997). *Atlas of mortality in Europe*. WHO Regional Publications, European Series, No. 75. World Health Organization, Geneva.
13. Prevention of Suicide (1996). *Guideline for the formulation and implementation of national strategies*. United Nations, New York.
14. Neeleman, J., Halpern, D., Leon, D., and Lewis, G. (1997). Tolerance of suicide, religion and suicide rates: an ecological and individual study in 19 Western countries. *Psychological Medicine*, **27**, 1165–71.
15. Durkheim, E. (1897). *Le suicide, etude de sociologie*. Alcan, Paris. (English translation: *Suicide*. Routledge and Kegan Paul, London, 1952.)
16. Maris, R.W. (1981). *Pathways to suicide*. Johns Hopkins University Press, Baltimore, MD.
17. Maris, R.W. (1997). Social and familial risk factors in suicidal behavior. *Psychiatric Clinics of North America*, **20**, 519–50.
18. Heikkinen, M.E., Isometsä, E.T., Marttunen, M.J., Aro, H.M., and Lonnqvist, J.K. (1995). Social factors in suicide. *British Journal of Psychiatry*, **167**, 747–53.
19. Lewis, G. and Slogget, A. (1998). Suicide, deprivation, and unemployment: record linkage study. *British Medical Journal*, **317**, 1283–6.
20. Farberow, N.L. (1997). The psychology of suicide: past and present. In *Suicide: biopsychosocial approaches* (ed. A.J. Botsis, C.R. Soldatos, and C.N. Stefanis), pp. 147–63. Elsevier, Amsterdam.
21. Roy, A., Nielsen, D., Rylander, G., Sarchiapone, M., and Segal, N. (1999). Genetics of suicide in depression. *Journal of Clinical Psychiatry*, **60** (Supplement 2), 12–17.
22. Mann, J.J., Oquendo, M., Underwood, M.D., and Arango, V. (1999). The neurobiology of suicide risk: a review for the clinician. *Journal of Clinical Psychiatry*, **60** (Supplement 2), 7–11.
23. Harris, E.C. and Barraclough, B. (1997). Suicide as an outcome for mental disorders. A meta-analysis. *British Journal of Psychiatry*, **170**, 205–28.
24. Rich, C.L., Young, D., and Fowler, R.C. (1986). San Diego suicide study: I. Young vs old subjects. *Archives of General Psychiatry*, **43**, 577–82.
25. Henriksson, M.H., Aro, H.A., Marttunen, M.J., *et al.* (1993). Mental disorders and comorbidity in suicide. *American Journal of Psychiatry*, **150**, 935–40.
26. Cheng, A.T.A. (1995). Mental illness and suicide. A case–control study in East Taiwan. *Archives of General Psychiatry*, **52**, 594–603.

27. Conwell, Y., Duberstein, P.R., Cox, C., Herrmann, J.H., Forbes, N.T., and Caine, E.D. (1996). Relationship of age and axis I diagnoses in victims of completed suicide: a psychological autopsy study. *American Journal of Psychiatry*, **153**, 1001–8.

28. Foster, T., Gillespie, K., and McClelland, R. (1997). Mental disorders and suicide in Northern Ireland. *British Journal of Psychiatry*, **170**, 447–52.

29. Wulsin, L.R., Vaillant, G.E., and Wells, V.E. (1999). A systematic review of the mortality of depression. *Psychosomatic Medicine*, **61**, 6–17.

30. Simon, G.E. and VonKorff, M. (1998). Suicide mortality among patients treated for depression in an insured population. *American Journal of Epidemiology*, **147**, 155–60.

31. Isometsä, E.T., Henriksson, M.M., Aro, H.M., Heikkinen, M.E., Kuoppasalmi, K.I., and Lonnqvist, J.K. (1994). Suicide in major depression. *American Journal of Psychiatry*, **151**, 530–6.

32. Ohberg, A., Vuori, E., Ojanperä, I., and Lonnqvist, J. (1996). Alcohol and drugs in suicides. *British Journal of Psychiatry*, **169**, 75–80.

33. Inskip, H.M., Harris, E.C., and Barraclough, B. (1998). Lifetime risk of suicide for affective disorder, alcoholism and schizophrenia. *British Journal of Psychiatry*, **172**, 35–7.

34. Fombonne, E. (1998). Suicidal behaviours in vulnerable adolescents: time trends and their correlates. *British Journal of Psychiatry*, **173**, 154–9.

35. Mäkelä, P. (1996). Alcohol consumption and suicide mortality by age among Finnish men, 1950–1991. *Addiction*, **91**, 101–12.

36. Heila, H., Isometsä, E., Henriksson, M.H., Heikkinen, M., Marttunen, M., and Lonnqvist, J. (1997). Suicide and schizophrenia: a nationwide psychological autopsy study on age- and sex-specific clinical characteristics of 92 suicide victims with schizophrenia. *American Journal of Psychiatry*, **154**, 1235–42.

37. Heilä, H., Isometsä, E., Henriksson, M.H., Heikkinen, M., Marttunen, M., and Lonnqvist, J. (1999). Suicide victims with schizophrenia in different treatment phases and adequacy of antipsychotic medication. *Journal of Clinical Psychiatry*, **60**, 200–8.

38. Marttunen, M.J., Aro, H.M., Henriksson, M.M., and Lonnqvist, J.K. (1991). Mental disorders in adolescent suicide: DSM-III-R axes I and II diagnoses in suicides among 13- to 19-year-olds in Finland. *Archives of General Psychiatry*, **48**, 834–9.

4.15.2 Attempted suicide and deliberate self-harm: epidemiology and risk factors

A. J. F. M. Kerkhof and E. Arensman

Introduction

Attempted suicide and deliberate self-harm are terms used to describe behaviours through which people inflict acute harm upon themselves, poison themselves, or try do so, with non-fatal outcome. These behaviours are somehow linked to, but do not result in, death. Common to these behaviours is that they occur in conditions of emotional turmoil. In former days attempted suicides were often regarded as failed suicides. However, this view did not appear to be correct, and the great majority of patients in fact do not try to kill themselves. Therefore the term deliberate self-harm was introduced to describe the behaviour without implying any specific motive.[1] But this too has some disadvantages because there is a temporal association between non-fatal and fatal suicidal behaviour; many people who kill themselves have

attempted suicide before or have displayed deliberate self-harm. Thus Kreitman *et al.*[2] introduced the concept of parasuicide to describe behaviour that, mostly without the intention to kill oneself, communicates a degree of suicidal intent. However, both terms, deliberate self-harm and parasuicide, are still somewhat confusing, because in practice they include people who really have the intent of killing oneself but survive the attempt. The difficulty of finding a good terminology for these behaviours is reflected in differences in research populations in empirical studies: some studies are limited to self-poisoning only (overdose), a few studies are restricted to self-injury (wrist cutting) only, some to self-poisoning and self-injury combined, and some studies include behaviours in which due to last-moment intervention from others, there was no actual self-harm inflicted at all.

In this chapter we will use the terms attempted suicide and deliberate self-harm interchangeably to refer to non-fatal suicidal behaviours in which there may have been an intention to die, however ambiguous this intention may have been, and irrespective of other intentions that may have been operating at the same time. It should be stressed that in attempted suicide/deliberate self-harm many motives may play a role simultaneously, even contradictory motives such as the hope of being rescued and the wish to continue living. Intentions may vary from attention seeking or communication of despair, appeal for help, to a means for stress reduction. Common to these behaviours is that they are motivated by change: people want to bring about changes in their present situation through the actual or intended harm or unconsciousness inflicted upon the body. Attempted suicide/deliberate self-harm may be defined as follows.[3]

> An act with non-fatal outcome, in which an individual deliberately initiates a non-habitual behaviour that, without intervention from others, will cause self-harm, or deliberately ingests a substance in excess of the prescribed or generally recognised therapeutic dosage, and which is aimed at realising changes which the subject desired via the actual or expected physical consequences.

This definition covers deliberate non-fatal suicidal behaviours. Not included are accidental cases of self-poisoning, accidental overdoses of opiates, or self-harmful acts by persons who do not anticipate the consequences of their actions. It does not include automutilation, which is a habitual, often obsessive act of inflicting (minor) self-harm, mostly without a conscious intent of changing the present situation, as with certain persons with learning disability.

Clinical features

Non-fatal suicidal behaviours can have very different motivations, varying from an intention to die to a cry for help. These behaviours may be well prepared or carried out impulsively, and may have different physical consequences. The degree of lethality and the degree of medical seriousness of the consequences thus depend upon intention, preparation, knowledge, and expectations of the method chosen, and sometimes upon coincidental factors, such as intervention from others.

It is often difficult to assess the true intent of non-fatal suicidal behaviour. Because of fear for consequences, such as admission to a psychiatric hospital, or because of psychological defence mechanisms, people sometimes deny or conceal their intention to die. They also may exaggerate their intention to die in order to receive help. Sometimes people engage in potentially highly lethal self-destructive behaviour without any wish to die, for example when they do not have adequate knowledge of the medication used. People who present at a general hospital with minor self-injury or minor self-poisoning may have had strong intentions to die, but had insufficient knowledge of the lethality of the method. Therefore one cannot always reliably infer what the precise meaning of the behaviour was, either from its overt characteristics, or from the person's self-report.

Epidemiology

In the 1960s and 1970s, there was a sharp increase in the numbers of people treated in hospitals in Europe, the United States, and Australia because of intentional overdoses or self-injury. In the 1980s several studies showed a stabilization.[4,5] In the early 1990s these numbers increased further in some regions.[6] The absolute number of persons treated for attempted suicide in general hospitals, however, does not adequately reflect the size of the problem. These numbers should be calculated against the size and the characteristics of the population in the areas that are being served by the hospitals. Furthermore, in some countries suicide-attempt patients are treated by general practitioners when there is no need for hospital admission. In many instances simple emergency attendance for overdosing is not even registered. There are no national registrations that reliably monitor trends in attempted suicide treated in general hospitals. Studies on attempted suicide concern the United States, Canada, Western Europe, and Australia. Few studies originate from other parts of the world.

Changes over time

In Edinburgh and Oxford, in the United Kingdom, there has been continuous monitoring of attempted suicides over a long period of time, where characteristics of persons attempting suicide have been related to the corresponding population.[5–7] In these two cities trends in attempted suicide rates have been documented reliably. After a period of stabilization in the 1980s a marked increase was observed. Between 1985 and 1995 the rates of deliberate self-harm in Oxford increased by 62 per cent in males and 42 per cent in females. The increase in deliberate self-harm has been most marked among young males. This appeared to be related to considerable excess of substance abuse in males.

In Canada the parasuicide rate was estimated to be around 304 per 100 000.[8] In the United States National Institute of Mental Health's Epidemiological Catchment Area study (1980–1985) it was found that 2.9 per cent of the respondents had made a suicide attempt at some point of time.[9]

So far only one international multicentre study into attempted suicide has been conducted taking into consideration the methodological pitfalls outlined above. The World Health Organization (**WHO**) initiated a collaborative multicentre study in 16 regions areas in Europe, using the same methodology, definition and case-finding criteria.[10] The findings were related to the size and characteristics of the corresponding general population in order to investigate rates, trends, risk factors, and social indicators. Most of the epidemiological data pre-

sented here have been drawn from that study for the years 1989 to 1992.[11]

Differences between countries

Obviously there are enormous differences in suicide attempt rates between different areas in Europe: For females the rates vary between 542 and 72 per 100 000 (age 15+) in Cergy-Pontoise, France, and Guipuzcoa, San Sebastian, Spain, respectively—a sevenfold difference. Oxford ranks second with 368, followed by Bordeaux with 248, Helsinki with 247, and Stockholm with 232. Low rates are found in the Italian and Spanish centres, in Würzburg, Germany, and in Innsbruck, Austria. The average female suicide attempt rate for all centres combined is 193 per 100 000 females aged 15 years and older. Even within a country there appear to be differences between catchment areas. In Sweden, the urban catchment area of Stockholm had a rate of 232, whereas the much less urbanized catchment area of Umea had a rate of 145. During the study period (1989–1992) the female attempted suicide rate decreased by 14 per cent on average in all centres.

For males the rates vary between 327 in Helsinki and 46 in Guipuzcoa, Spain, again a sevenfold difference. Oxford again ranks second with 264, followed by Cergy-Pontoise, France, with 252. Low rates are found in the two Italian centres (Padova and Emilia-Romagna) and in Würzburg, Germany. The male average suicide attempt rate for all centres combined was 140 per 100 000 males of 15 years and older. Within Sweden the difference in rates between Stockholm (154) and Umea (92) is remarkable. During the study period (data for 1989–1992), the male attempted suicide rate decreased by 17 per cent on average in all centres.

Differences between catchment areas in suicide attempt rates in the WHO/EURO project have been studied in relation to socio-economic characteristics of these areas.[12] No correlations were found with most of the social and economical factors supposedly related to suicide attempt rates, such as population density, urban–rural distribution, proportion working in agriculture forestry or fishery, sex ratio, percentage aged 40 and over, number of people per household, percentage people living alone, percentage single parent families, per capita income, unemployment rate, life expectancy, mortality rate, infant mortality, crimes per year per 1000, and per capita alcohol consumption. Only two characteristics of the catchment areas seemed to be related to suicide attempt rates: the percentage of divorced people in the area and the percentage receiving social security. Family stability, and the percentage of the population relying on welfare, both seem to be related to the frequency of attempted suicide, but the interpretation of these findings is difficult, since one would expect the other related social indicators of societal cohesion to covary as well.

It is important, however, to realize that the characteristics mentioned above relate to regions or countries, and do not relate to individuals. On the individual level characteristics such as unemployment do play an important role, but that does not mean that on a sociological level unemployment rates explain high attempted suicide rates in a region.[13,14] This relationship holds only for some regions and not for others, as is documented repeatedly.[15]

Cultural variation in attempted suicide has been documented from India,[16] Sri Lanka,[17] and Pakistan,[18] and from ethnic groups within Western societies, such as the Inuit in Canada.[19] Neeleman et al.[20] studied ethnic differences in parasuicide in Camberwell, London, and found considerable differences between the deliberate self-harm rates for white people and for British-born Indian females and African-Caribbeans[20]. Indian females had a particularly high rate, 7.8 times that of white females. Marriage problems seem to be related to attempted suicide in Asian countries such as India, Pakistan, Sri Lanka, and China. Young married women may have serious difficulties after moving in with their husbands' extended families. Dowry problems and problems with in-laws are thought to be precipitants of attempted suicide among young married women. In Asian countries the methods used in attempted suicide reflect differences in accessibility. Self-poisoning with organophosphate pesticides and other household poisons is prevalent. As in the Western world attempted suicide/deliberate self-harm behaviours appear to reflect feelings of hopelessness and helplessness in adverse living conditions with no prospect of improvement. Women tend to be more powerless to bring about changes in their living conditions. In Sri Lanka the continuous warfare, poverty, and the lack of opportunities at home and abroad frustrates the young who are relatively well educated.[17]

Sex and age

In all but one centre (Helsinki) of the WHO Multicentre Study into Parasuicide the female attempted suicide rates were higher than the male suicide attempt rates. On average the rates of females were 1.5 times higher than those for men.

The highest average rates were found for young females of aged 15 to 24 years (283 per 100 000), followed by 25 to 34 years (262), and 35 to 44 years (235). High rates for females age between 15 and 24 years were found in Cergy-Pontoise, France (766), and Oxford (629).

For males, highest average rates were found in the 25 to 34 age group (199), followed by the 35 to 44 group (169), and young males aged 15 to 24 years (168). The rate in males aged 25 to 44 years was particularly high in Helsinki (459). High rates among young males (15–24 years) were found in Helsinki (372), Cergy-Pontoise, France (337), and Oxford (314).

Sociodemographic characteristics

Single and divorced people were over-represented among suicide attempters in the WHO/EURO study.[11] In Leiden, a region in the western part of The Netherlands, the rates of attempted suicide were highest among divorced women (248 per 100 000) and divorced men (191) and lowest for the widowed (39 for women, 16 for men).[21] Compared with the general population those with low levels of education, the unemployed, and the disabled are significantly overrepresented among suicide attempters. About 22 per cent of the male and 15 per cent of the female suicide attempters in the Dutch region areas were unemployed versus 3 per cent and 2 per cent for the male and for the female corresponding general population (15–64 years). About 57 per cent had a low level of formal education, the majority had no vocational training. When expressed in rates per 100 000 for the Dutch part of the study it appeared that the unemployed (322 for males, 455 for females) and the disabled (113 for males, 205 for females) had much higher rates than the employed (27 for males, 31 for females). Those who completed primary education only had rates of 160 per 100 000 compared to 27 per 100 000 for those with higher vocational training or university education.[21] These findings support data from the United Kingdom, where socio-economic deprivation (low social class and unemployment) repeatedly appear as characteristics of the parasuicide populations.[22]

These findings indicate that suicide attempters disproportionately have had low education, and have high levels of unemployment, poverty, and divorce. The findings may be partly related to underlying common causes, such as the presence of psychiatric disorders, but they also suggest the influence of sociological factors impacting on a relatively economically deprived group in society with a greater share of adversity.[15] Socio-economic deprivation is a well-established determinant of psychiatric morbidity and attempted suicide.[23,24] In contrast with completed suicide, where the presence of psychiatric disorders is well documented (up to 95 per cent of suicides may have suffered from a psychiatric disorder), psychiatric disorders are much less frequent among those who attempt suicide or deliberately harm themselves. Among those who engage in suicidal behaviour for the first time in their lives, the prevalence of psychiatric disorders may be rather low; among repeaters, psychiatric morbidity is considerable.[25]

Methods

Methods used in suicide attempts are mostly 'non-violent'. In the WHO Multicentre Study 64 per cent of males and 80 per cent of females used self-poisoning. Cutting, mostly wrist cutting, was employed in 17 per cent of male cases and 9 per cent of female cases. There are some differences between European countries in the use of particular methods. In Szeged (Hungary) for example, 19 per cent of males and 15 per cent of females used poisoning with pesticides, herbicides, or other toxic agricultural chemicals. In Sor-Trondelag, Norway, higher percentages attempted suicide by deliberate alcohol overdose (6 per cent of males, and 5 per cent of females). In general, somewhat older men used the method of jumping or jumping in front of a moving object. In the Oxford studies between 1985 and 1995, 88 per cent of all episodes involved self-poisoning, 8 per cent involved self-injury, and 4 per cent involved both. There was an increase in the use of paracetamol from 31 per cent of poisoning cases in 1985 to 50 per cent in 1995.[6] There was also an increase in antidepressant overdoses, and a decrease in overdoses of minor tranquillizers and sedatives. The differences in methods between countries may be related to differences in the accessibility of certain methods. Until recently, paracetamol was available in large quantities in the United Kingdom, unlike other European countries.[26] The ingestion of alcohol during or before the act sometimes can be considered to be a part of the actual method of attempted suicide (when used to bring about unconsciousness, or to increase the risk of a fatal outcome), as part of the preparation (to lower the treshold for engaging in an attempt because of disinhibition), or as a long-term risk factor. Hawton et al. [27,28] found that 22 to 26 per cent of attempted suicide patients had consumed alcohol at the time of the attempt (males more frequent than females), and that 44 to 50 per cent had consumed alcohol during the 6 h before the episodes, this again being more common in males than in females. About 28 per cent of attempted suicide patients in Oxford could be labelled substance misusers (alcohol and drugs).

General population self-report surveys

A number of surveys have been conducted to estimate the prevalence of attempted suicide. Most of these surveys concerned adolescents and were administered anonymously. Most questionnaire studies revealed that between 1 and 4 per cent of respondents had attempted suicide at some point in time,[29,30] but some studies even reported 20 per cent.[31] However, the validity of some of these findings is questionable; the prevalence of lifetime attempted suicide among non-respondents is not known, the influence of social desirability is not known, and the wording of the questions is rather important.

Lifetime prevalence

Based upon the rates from the WHO/EURO study the lifetime prevalence of medically treated suicide attempts should be around 3 per cent for females and 2 per cent for males, with some variations between countries and regions. Suicide attempts that did not lead to medical treatment at a hospital or general practitioner's surgery are very difficult to study, because of the limited validity of self-report data.

Classification

As previously mentioned, there is a considerable variety of behaviours within the broad category of non-fatal suicidal behaviour. A review of classification studies[25] revealed three types of suicide attempt(er)s: a 'mild' type, a 'severe' type, and a 'mixed' type in between.

The mild type of non-fatal suicidal behaviour encompasses mostly relatively non-violent methods followed by non-serious physical injury. Young age, living together, few precautions to prevent discovery, low level of suicidal preoccupation, low suicidal intent, interpersonal motivation are all characteristics associated with mild forms of attempted suicide/deliberate self-harm. The severe category consists mostly of relatively hard methods followed by serious physical consequences. Older age (over 40), many precautions to prevent discovery, high level of suicidal preoccupation, high suicidal intent, self-directed motivation, often relocated, previous attempted suicides, depression, drug dependence, a high degree of overall dysfunctioning, poor physical health, and previous psychiatric treatment are all characteristics associated with the concept of 'severe' attempted suicide/deliberate self-harm. The risk of repetition is greater in the severe type. In between, in the mixed type of attempted suicide/deliberate self-harm, the attempts and the attempters show mixed characteristics, which makes this type harder to distinguish in medical practice.

In order to refine further the classification of attempted suicide/deliberate self-harm, Arensman[32] included psychological and personal history variables and these characteristics were studied in relation to recurrent non-fatal suicidal behaviour in a follow-up period of 1 year. She validated the mild type, approximately 40 per cent of the total sample, as being predominantly younger than 30 years of age, single, living alone or with parents, and having minor injuries because of the index attempt. The mean number of previous attempts was 3.7 attempts. The repetition rate in the follow-up period for this group was 27 per cent. In the older age group, two groups were distinguished: a moderate group, and a group with an extremely high risk for non-fatal repetition was identified. The high-risk group, consisting of approximately 28 per cent of the total sample, suffered more physical injury as a consequence of their attempted suicide/deliberate self-harm. The high-risk group consisted predominantly of females in the age group 30 to 49 years who were divorced or separated, living alone, and who were economically inactive. Most had made previous attempts (mean number of five previous attempts). They had histories of traumatic life events and experiences that mostly started early in life. A high percentage reported physical, sexual, and mental maltreatment by parents in childhood and early adolescence, followed by physical and mental maltreatment by partners later in life. The females in this group more often were divorced and the total number of times they were divorced or had cohabited with a partner was significantly higher. The high-risk group had highest scores on depression, hopelessness, and expression of state-anger. Two thirds of this high-risk group could be diagnosed as having borderline personality disorder, which accounts for the patterns of unstable personal relationships and affective instability. In the follow-up at least 75 per cent engaged in repeated non-fatal suicidal behaviours.

The moderate group was characterized by low levels of physical injury following their non-fatal suicidal behaviour, they were predominantly aged at least 30 years and married, and scored intermediate on measures of depression, hopelessness, and anger. The mean number of previous attempts was 2.3, and 33 per cent made one or more repeated attempt in the follow-up. Surprisingly, this classification into three types of non-fatal suicidal behaviours did not correspond to the levels of reported suicide intent nor to the levels of the different motivations reported (to die, to appeal, to lose consciousness, revenge), underlining the difficulty of classifying attempted suicide according to intentions.

Aetiology

The last psychological step towards attempted suicide is always set in conditions of emotional turmoil, an emotional crisis. Essential in crisis is the absence of any positive outlook towards the future. People completing suicide do not expect any improvement of their situation in the near or distant future. People attempting suicide without fatal outcome indicate that their future is hopeless, but they still seem to have a faint hope, however ambiguous this may be, that the future might improve. In this way attempted suicide may be conceived as a self-invented form of crisis intervention. Studies into the cognitive functioning of suicide attempters indeed show a global and stable form of negative anticipations and absence of positive anticipations towards the future, probably as a consequence of disturbances in their autobiographical memory, i.e. an overgeneral memory.[33] Whenever these anticipations remain overgenerally negative after an attempt, it is likely that hopelessness will increase and that this behaviour will occur again.[34]

Precipitants

Difficulties or conflicts that may bring the person to believe that his or her future is without hope can trigger the psychological crisis resulting in attempted suicide/deliberate self-harm. Attempted suicide often is precipitated by disharmony with key figures, work-related problems, financial difficulties, or physical illnesses. Long-standing relationship problems or feelings of loneliness are especially common. People displaying attempted suicide/deliberate self-harm have weak social support systems,[33] and they report relational difficulties as major problems in life. They show deficits in interpersonal problem solving, and they are well aware of that. Their future holds no promise. Their emotional status can best be described as a state of learned helplessness, a situation of a blocked escape, in which no solution exists for a perceived insurmountable adversity. This leads to the question as to why these persons have developed such helpless attitudes.

Long-term vulnerability factors

The conflicts suicidal patients experience in the days before attempted suicide/deliberate self-harm are not different from the same conflicts they have experienced over and over again. Not only recent life events, but also the life events that occurred in their past are important.[32] Many suicide attempters, males as well as females, have had traumatic childhood experiences, including physical and emotional neglect, broken homes, other unstable parental conditions, violence, sexual and physical abuse, incest, parents who had psychiatric treatment, who were alcoholics and/or addicted to opiates. Women who have been abused have a much greater probability of becoming a repeater later. In addition they often develop poor relationships, lack self-esteem, and experience overwhelming feelings of helplessness and hopelessness. Any trigger, for example an argument with a friend, may be sufficient to provoke suicidal ideation and behaviour.

Attempted suicide/deliberate self-harm patients not only suffer from helplessness with regard to interpersonal conflicts, they also tend to be powerless in other domains of life. The attempted suicide/deliberate self-harm population disproportionately consists of unemployed persons, from low social classes, with low educational levels, economically deprived, divorced, disabled, addicted, incarcerated, and/or lonely. Many have received in- or outpatient psychiatric treatment. These findings are somewhat complicated by the fact that many of these vulnerability factors are strongly interrelated. Unemployment, addiction, and unstable partnership relations all may be caused by psychiatric diseases. For example, unemployment and attempted suicide may both be a consequence of addiction. However, it is not fair to assume that most of the economic deprivation of suicidal patients is explained by their psychiatric condition. The considerable differences between nations in the prevalence of attempted suicide support the importance of socio-economic conditions.

Course and prognosis

Repetition is one of the core characteristics of suicidal behaviour. Among those who commit suicide up to 40 per cent attempted before.[35] Among suicide attempters 'repeaters' are probably commoner than 'first-evers'. Between 30 and 60 per cent of suicide attempters made previous attempts, and between 15 and 25 per cent did so within the last year.[3,5,36,37]

Risk of suicide after attempted suicide/deliberate self-harm

Prospectively, suicide attempters have a high risk of committing suicide. Between 10 and 15 per cent eventually die because of suicide.[35] Mortality by suicide is higher among suicide attempters who have made previous attempts.[38,39] The risk of suicide after attempted suicide/deliberate self-harm for males is nearly twice the female risk, the risk being particularly high in the first year.[40,41] Alcohol and drug abuse and related social deterioration are risk factors for subsequent suicide,[42] as are psychiatric diagnosis (affective disorders, schizophrenia, personality disorders), and a highly lethal non-impulsive index suicide attempt.

Repetition of non-fatal suicidal behaviour

Risk of repeated suicidal behaviour is highest during the first year after a suicide attempt, and especially within the first 3 to 6 months.[37,39,43] In the WHO/EURO Multicentre Study on Parasuicide it was found that at least 54 per cent of attempters had attempted before, 30 per cent at least twice. Prospectively, 30 per cent of suicide attempters made at least one repeated attempt in a 1-year follow-up.[44,45]

It is hoped for that knowledge of antecedents or risk factors may foster early identification of persons at risk, and improvement of treatment. Many studies have tried to identify risk factors or antecedents and some of these by now are well known. Sociodemographic risk factors associated with repetition are belonging to the age group of 25 to 49 years, being divorced, unemployed, and coming from low social class. Psychosocial characteristics of repeaters are substance abuse, depression, hopelessness, powerlessness, personality disorders, unstable living conditions/living alone, criminal records, previous psychiatric treatment, and a history of stressful traumatic life events, including broken homes and family violence, especially physical and mental maltreatment by partners. Prospectively, a history of previous attempts is one of the most powerful predictors of future non-fatal suicide attempts.[25,46,47]

Conclusions

Attempted suicide/deliberate self-harm are major problems in many contemporary societies. They seem to reflect the degree of powerlessness and hopelessness of young people with low education, low income, unemployment, and difficulties in coping with life stress. As such, non-fatal suicidal behaviour should be a major concern for politicians. There are substantial differences between communities in the prevalence of attempted suicide. This suggests that some communities better meet the needs of their underprivileged youngsters than others do, but we barely understand the differences between communities and nations. Preventive action therefore is difficult to design. There is a need for a better nationwide continuous registration of attempted suicide and related socio-economic conditions. There is also a need for better mental health care management of suicide attempters, and for experimental studies on the prevention of repetition. Although we know that persons with suicide attempts are at high risk for future fatal and non-fatal suicidal behaviour, we still need to develop better means to help them.

References

1. Morgan, H.G., Barton, J., Pottle, S., Pocock, H., and Burns-Cox, C.J. (1976). Deliberate self-harm: a follow-up study of 279 patients. *British Journal of Psychiatry*, **128**, 361–8.
2. Kreitman, N., Philip, A.E., Greer, S., and Bagley, C.R. (1969). Parasuicide. *British Journal of Psychiatry*, **115**, 746–7.
3. Platt, S., Bille-Brahe, U., Kerkhof, A., *et al*. (1992). Parasuicide in Europe: the WHO/EURO Multicentre Study on Parasuicide. I. Introduction and preliminary analysis for 1989. *Acta Psychiatrica Scandinavica*, **85**, 97–104.
4. Hawton, K. and Fagg, J. (1992). Trends in deliberate self-poisoning and self-injury in Oxford, 1976–1990. *British Medical Journal*, **304**, 1409–11.

5. Platt, S., Hawton, K., Kreitman, N., Fagg, J., and Foster, J. (1988). Recent clinical and epidemiological trends in parasuicide in Edinburgh and Oxford: a tale of two cities. *Psychological Medicine*, **18**, 405–18.

6. Hawton, K., Fagg, J., Simkin, S., Bale, E., and Bond, A. (1997). Trends in deliberate self-harm in Oxford, 1985–1995. *British Journal of Psychiatry*, **171**, 556–60.

7. Kreitman, N. (1977). *Parasuicide*. Wiley, London.

8. Sakinofsky, I. (1996). The epidemiology of suicide in Canada. In *Suicide in Canada* (ed. A.A. Leenaars, S. Wenckstern, I. Sakinovsky, D. Dyck, M. Kral, and R. Bland). University of Toronto Press.

9. Moscicki, E.K., O'Carroll, P., Rae, D.S., Locke, B.Z., Roy, A., and Regier, D.A. (1988). Suicide attempts in the Epidemiologic Catchment Area Study. *Yale Journal of Biology and Medicine*, **61**, 259–68.

10. Kerkhof, A.J.J.M., Schmidtke, A., Bille Brahe, U., De Leo, D., and Lönnqvist, J. (1994). *Attempted suicide in Europe*. DSWO-Press/World Health Organization, Leiden and Copenhagen

11. Schmidtke, A., Bille Brahe, U., De Leo, D., *et al.* (1996). Attempted suicide in Europe: rates, trends and sociodemographic characteristics of suicide attempters during the period 1989–1992. Results of the WHO/EURO Multicentre Study on Parasuicide. *Acta Psychiatrica Scandinavica*, **93**, 327–38.

12. Bille-Brahe, U., Andersen, K., Wasserman, D., *et al.* (1996). The WHO-EURO Multicentre Study: risk of parasuicide and the comparability of the areas under study. *Crisis*, **17**, 32–42.

13. Platt, S. (1984). Unemployment and suicidal behaviour: a review of the literature. *Social Science and Medicine*, **19**, 93–115.

14. Platt, S. and Dyer, J. (1987). Psychological correlates of unemployment among male parasuicides in Edinburgh. *British Journal of Psychiatry*, **151**, 27–32.

15. Adam, K.S. (1990). Environmetal, psychosocial, and psychoanalytic aspects of suicidal behavior. In *Suicide over the life cycle* (ed. S.J. Blumenthal and D.J. Kupfer), pp. 39–96. American Psychiatric Press, Washington, DC.

16. Latha, K.S., Bhat, S.M., and D'Souza, P. (1996). Suicide attempters in a general hospital unit in India: their socio-demographic and clinical profile—emphasis on cross-cultural aspects. *Acta Psychiatrica Scandinavica*, **94**, 26–30.

17. Eddleston, M., Rezvi Sheriff, M.H., and Hawton, K. (1998). Deliberate self harm in Sri Lanka: an overlooked tragedy in the developing world. *British Medical Journal*, **317**, 133–5.

18. Khan, M.M., Islam, S., and Kundi, A.K. (1996). Parasuicide in Pakistan: experience at a university hospital. *Acta Psychiatrica Scandinavica*, **94**, 264–7.

19. Kirmayer, L.J., Malus, M., and Boothroyd, L.J. (1996). Suicide attempts among Inuit youth: a community survey of prevalence and risk factors. *Acta Psychiatrica Scandinavica*, **94**, 8–17.

20. Neeleman, J., Jones, P., van Os, J., and Murray, R.M. (1996). Parasuicide in Camberwell—ethnic differences. *Social Psychiatry and Epidemiology*, **31**, 284–7.

21. Arensman, E., Kerkhof, A.J.F.M., Hengeveld, M., and Mulder, J. (1995). Medically treated suicide attempts: a four year monitoring study of the epidemiology in The Netherlands. *Journal of Epidemiology and Commmunity Health*, **49**, 285–9.

22. Hawton, K. and Catalan, J. (1982). *Attempted suicide. A practical guide to its nature and management*. Oxford University Press.

23. Gunnell, D.J., Peters, T.J., Kammerling, R.M., and Brooks, J. (1995). Relation between parasuicide, suicide, psychiatric admissions, and socioeconomic deprivation. *British Medical Journal*, **311**, 226–30.

24. Congdon, P. (1996). Suicide and parasuicide in London; a small-area study. *Urban Studies*, **1**, 137–58.

25. Arensman, E. and Kerkhof, A.J.F.M. (1996). Classification of attempted suicide: a review of empirical studies, 1963–1993. *Suicide and Life-Threatening Behaviour*, **26**, 46–67.

26. Gunnell, D., Hawton, K., Murray, V., *et al.* (1997). Use of paracetamol for suicide and non-fatal poisoning in the UK and France: are

restrictions on availability justified? *Journal of Epidemiology and Community Health*, **51**, 175–9.

27. Hawton, K., Fagg, J., Simkin, S., Harris, L., Bale, E., and Bond, A. (1997, 1998). *Deliberate self-harm in Oxford, 1996, 1997. Reports from the Oxford Monitoring System for Attempted Suicide*. Warneford Hospital, Oxford.

28. Hawton, K., Simkin, S., and Fagg, J. (1997). Deliberate self-harm in alcohol and drug misusers: patient characteristics and patterns of clinical care. *Drug and Alcohol Review*, **16**, 123–9.

29. Paykel, E.S., Myers, J.K., Lindentall, J.J., and Tanner, J. (1974). Suicidal feelings in the general population: a prevalence study. *British Journal of Psychiatry*, **124**, 460–9.

30. Kienhorst, C.W.M., de Wilde, E.J., Diekstra, R.F.W., and Wolters, W.H.G. (1991). Construction of an index for predicting suicide attempts in depressed adolescents. *British Journal of Psychiatry*, **159**, 676–82.

31. Rubinstein, J.L., Heeren, T., Housman, D., Rubin, C., and Stechler, G. (1989). Suicidal behavior in 'normal' adolescents: risk and protective factors. *American Journal of Orthopsychiatry*, **59**, 59–71.

32. Arensman, E. (1997). Attempted suicide: epidemiology and classification. Unpublished Ph.D. Dissertation, University of Leiden, The Netherlands.

33. Williams, J.M.G. (1997). *The cry of pain*. Penguin, Harmondsworth.

34. MacLeod, A.K., Rose, G.S., and Williams, J.M.G. (1993). Components of hopelessness about the future in parasuicide. *Cognitive Therapy and Research*, **17**, 441–55.

35. Maris, R.W. (1992). The relationship of nonfatal suicide attempts to completed suicide. In *Assessment and prediction of suicide* (ed. R.W. Maris, A.L. Berman, J.T. Maltsberger, and R.I. Yufit), pp. 362–80. Guilford Press, New York.

36. Kreitman, N. and Casey, P. (1988). Repetition of parasuicide: an epidemiological and clinical study. *British Journal of Psychiatry*, **153**, 792–800.

37. Hawton, K. and Fagg, J. (1995). Repetition of attempted suicide: the performance of the Edinburgh predictive scales in patients in Oxford. *Archives of Suicide Research*, **1**, 261–72.

38. Hawton, K. and Catalan, J. (1981). Psychiatric management of attempted suicide patients. *British Journal of Hospital Medicine*, **26**, 365–8.

39. Hawton, K. and Fagg, J. (1988). Suicide and other causes of death, following attempted suicide. *British Journal of Psychiatry*, **152**, 359–66.

40. Nordstrom, P., Samuelsson, M., and Asberg, M. (1995). Survival analysis of suicide risk after attempted suicide. *Acta Psychiatrica Scandinavica*, **91**, 336–40.

41. Suokas, J. and Lonnqvist, J. (1991). Outcome of attempted suicide and psychiatric consultation: risk factors and suicide mortality during a five year follow-up. *Acta Psychiatrica Scandinavica*, **84**, 545–9.

42. Cullberg, J., Wasserman, D., and Stefansson, C.G. (1988). Who commits suicide after a suicide attempt? An 8 to 10 year follow-up in a suburban catchment area. *Acta Psychiatrica Scandinavica*, **77**, 598–603.

43. Goldacre, M. and Hawton, K. (1985). Repetition of self-poisoning and subsequent death in adolescents who take overdoses. *British Journal of Psychiatry*, **146**, 395–8.

44. Kerkhof, A.J.F.M., Arensman, E., Bille-Brahe, U., *et al.* (1998). Repetition of attempted suicide: results from the WHO/EU Multicentre Study on Parasuicide. Paper presented at the VIIth European Symposium on Suicide and Suicidal Behaviour, Ghent, Belgium.

45. Arensman, E., Kerkhof, A., Dirkzwager, A., *et al.* (1999). Prevalence and risk factors for repeated suicidal behaviour: results from the WHO/EURO Multicentre Study on Parasuicide, 1989–1992. Submitted for publication.

46. van Egmond, M. and Diekstra, R.F.W. (1989). The predictability of suicidal behaviour: the results of a meta-analysis of published studies. In *Suicide and its prevention* (ed. R.F.W. Diekstra, R. Maris, S. Platt, A. Schmidtke, and G. Sonneck), pp. 37–61. Brill, Leiden.

47. Kreitman, N. and Foster, J. (1991). Construction and selection of

predictive scales, with special reference to parasuicide. *British Journal of Psychiatry*, **159**, 185–92.

4.15.3 Biological aspects of suicidal behaviour

Lawrence Amsel and J. John Mann

From metaphors to models: historical developments in the study of biological correlates of suicidal behaviour

Of all the pathological states that psychiatrists deal with, suicide seems to be most of the mind and least of the brain. As such, suicidal behaviours might seem to be beyond the competence of the current state of neurobiological modelling. Yet, suicide was treated as a biomedical concept 150 years ago by Jean Esquirol (1772–1840), a partisan in the French Revolution. By borrowing concepts from Linnaeus' plant taxonomy, he devised a categorization of mental illness, the *Treatise on Insanity* (1838). Esquirol devoted a chapter to suicide, thus becoming the forerunner of the biological approach to the study of suicide.

Over the last 30 years the modelling of suicidal behaviour has undergone a transformation through the influence of psychometrics, phenomenological psychiatry, neurobiology, epidemiology, genetics, and cognitive psychology. In addition, the emergence of the biopsychosocial approach to health problems in general, has introduced a more comprehensive, multifaceted approach to the study and modelling of suicidal behaviour. The biological study of suicide has also moved from focusing on suicidal ideation as primarily related to depression to focusing on suicidal acts as primarily related to the biology of aggression and impulsivity.

Modelling suicidal behaviours

Requirements for constructing a biological model

The requirements for a model in the biological study of suicide are that it is clinically explanatory, biologically correlated, and testable in both clinical and biological studies.[1] Ideally, it would also be predictive of those at high risk for suicide. Obviously, to be meaningful such a model must account for, or at least be consistent with, the wealth of epidemiological and clinical information available about suicide. Moreover, its component clinical phenomena should have corresponding biological mechanisms that can be studied in a standard biomedical paradigm.

The stress diathesis model

A parsimonious model meeting the above criteria has been proposed by our group.[1] (Fig. 1) It is based on the following key observations.

1. Over 90 per cent of suicides occur in the context of a psychiatric disorder.

2. The overwhelming majority of persons with psychiatric disorders do not make suicide attempts.

3. The objective severity of symptoms is not predictive of suicidal behaviours.

4. In a factor analysis, a combination of aggression and impulsivity was the most important predictive factor for suicidality.

5. Familial grouping of suicidal behaviour seems to indicate an inherited suicidal trait independent of the inheritance of particular diagnosis.

In addition there are the following intriguing biological findings: (1) suicide attempters and completers seem to have a dysfunction of the serotonergic system, similar to that found in aggressive or violent subjects; (2) abnormalities of the prefrontal cortex appear to be involved in suicide, and have long been known to be involved in aggression, disinhibition, and violence.

Based on these observations, the model postulates two independent components in suicidal behaviour that work in concert. The first consists of lifelong stable traits that comprise a diathesis, which predisposes to aggressive/impulsive behaviour in response to stressful circumstances or powerful emotions. This tendency might be conceived as a lowered threshold for motor activation, a diminution in natural inhibitory circuits, or as a volatile cognitive decision style.

This diathesis may be necessary but insufficient for suicide. Most people with this trait will never make a suicide attempt. Rather, it is a behavioural tendency to cope with powerful feelings by taking action—action that is often definitive, aggressive, and impulsive.

One biological correlate of this diathesis appears to be an overall diminution in serotonergic activity. Numerous elements can contribute to this diathesis, including genetics, early life experiences, chronic illness, chronic alcoholism, substance abuse, and even possibly cholesterol levels. Some factors operate via the serotonergic system.

The second component of the model is an acute stressor that supplies an intense desire to end one's life. Whether this is brought about by life circumstances, a psychiatric illness, or both, it results in the drive or desire to end the noxious experience. Psychological autopsy studies demonstrate that a psychiatric illness is almost always part of this stressor. Patients have portrayed the mental anguish of depression as worse than any experience of physical pain, and it is often accompanied by a sense of hopelessness.

Yet, the majority of psychiatric patients and of persons experiencing a major loss do not make suicide attempts. It seems that there are powerful protective inhibitory circuits that prevent most persons

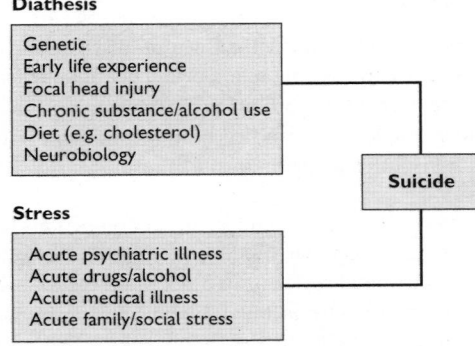

Fig. 1 A stress diathesis model of suicide.

undergoing severe psychological stress from acting on these intense feelings, just as there are inhibitory circuits that preventing overt, outwardly directed aggression under most circumstances. An eloquent description of this restraint system is contained in Hamlet's soliloquy. Upon finding his father murdered and his own succession challenged, Hamlet has the stressor but not the diathesis. After convincing himself that suicide might be a reasonable option he notes his hesitation:

> Thus conscience does make cowards of us all;
> And thus the native hue of resolution
> Is sicklied o'er with the pale cast of thought,
> And enterprises of great pith and moment
> With this regard their currents turn awry,
> And lose the name of action. (*Hamlet*, Act III, Scene 1)

Suicide and suicide attempts occur in those relatively uncommon circumstances when both components coexist—someone with the aggressive/impulsive diathesis is undergoing a severe psychological stressor.

Postmortem brain studies of suicide victims

The serotonergic system in postmortem brain

There is considerable converging evidence that serotonin-system dysfunction is correlated with suicidal behaviours. Serotonin neurones have their cell bodies in the dorsal raphe nucleus, while their axons innervate most of the brain including the ventral prefrontal cortex. Postmortem study of the concentration of serotonin and its major metabolite, 5-hydroxyindoleacetic acid (**5-HIAA**), in brain tissue has limitations such as the postmortem loss of these substances. Because most of this decline takes place in the first 2 h postmortem, results from different studies are comparable. Of seven studies that examined the postmortem brainstem, five found modest but significant reductions of serotonin or 5-HIAA in suicide victims compared to controls, while two studies found no changes.[2] Studies of other brain regions including the prefrontal cortex have generated results that are more equivocal. The reductions in serotonin or 5-HIAA are independent of psychiatric diagnosis, and, despite early reports to the contrary, are independent of suicide method. Thus these reductions appear to be related specifically to the suicidal status of the subjects studied.[3]

Receptor and transporter binding studies in the prefrontal cortex

Receptors tend to be more stable than neurotransmitters in the postmortem brain, and have become an important neurobiological tool for studying the function of the various neurotransmitter systems. Postmortem studies employ radiolabelled ligands specific for a particular receptor or transporter in order to measure its density (B_{max}) and affinity (K_D).

Of 18 studies reported, 12 found significant reductions in the presynaptic serotonin-transporter binding sites (**SERT**) in suicide victims, either in the frontal cortex or in other brain regions. One study found a significant increase in SERT binding in the frontal cortex, while five found no change in the brain regions that were examined.[2]

We have pointed out that these seemingly contradictory findings are not unexpected given the many confounding factors that can add artefacts or mask a difference in receptor density.[3,4] First, the radioligands used in these studies such as [3H]imipramine, [3H]paroxetine, and [3H]cyanoimiprimine have different affinities (K_D) for different receptors/transporters. Binding to non-transporter sites may explain discrepant results in the literature. Second, there are two high-affinity binding sites for [3H]paroxetine.[5] One of these sites, for which binding is dependent on Na^+ and Cl^-, is believed to represent the serotonin transporter. Binding to the other site is independent of Na^+ and Cl^-, and it probably does not function as a reuptake transporter. We showed that the number of actual SERT sites is not altered in Brodmann area 9 in suicide subjects. Rather, it is the non-transporter SERT-like binding sites that are fewer. While the specific function of these sites is not known, their density may be a valid index of the integrity of presynaptic serotonin nerve terminals. Ventral prefrontal cortex, however, does exhibit fewer SERT sites in suicide victims.

Third, there is evidence of an increased binding to SERT sites with an increase in the postmortem time interval in the suicide group but not the control group.[4] Given all of these potential confounds, the positive findings of reduced SERT and SERT-like protein complexes are more compelling.

Some, but not all, studies have found an increase in the concentration of the postsynaptic serotonin receptor 5-HT$_{2A}$ in the brains of suicide victims compared to controls. If this finding is ultimately verified, it would be consistent with an upregulation of postsynaptic receptors due to a decrease in serotonin activity. However, thus far, six studies have found significant increases in 5-HT$_{2A}$ in suicidal subjects, while seven other studies have failed to find a difference.[4,6]

As with SERT there are a number of issues in these studies that may account for the inconsistent findings. The first is the type of ligand used. Both Laruelle and Hrdina (reviewed by Arango *et al.*[7]) used the more selective ligand [3H]ketanserin, and found significant differences. Second, depression even without suicidality may cause an increase in 5-HT$_{2A}$ receptor density, while treatment with antidepressants may cause downregulation.[2] Thus, unless studies control for mood state and treatment status, the 5-HT$_{2A}$ receptor results can be misleading.

There have also been contradictory findings among six studies of the postsynaptic 5-HT$_{1A}$ receptor: two found an increased density in the suicide group, two failed to find an increase, one found the increase only for the subgroup of non-violent suicides, and one found a trend that was not significant.[2] Lopez *et al.*[8] found reduced 5-HT$_{2A}$ binding and reduced mRNA for the receptor in the hippocampus of suicides. Also, in a hippocampal rat model, the 5-HT$_{1A}$ receptor interacts with the hypothalamic–pituitary–adrenal axis, and is sensitive to chronic stress, which causes its downregulation via corticosteroids.[9]

Distal to the receptor, Pacheco *et al.*[10] reported that in the prefrontal cortex of suicide victims there were alterations in the functioning of second-messenger signal transduction. The phosphoinositide signalling mechanism and G-protein levels are significantly reduced.

Taken together, these findings point to a specific anomaly in the serotonergic system. This deficit is reflected in the decreased presynaptic binding and possibly in a compensatory postsynaptic increase in receptor density.

Quantitative morphometric studies of brainstem nuclei

The dorsal raphe nucleus and median raphe nuclei supply most of the serotonin innervation to the cortex. Using an antibody to tryptophan hydroxylase, which selectively stains serotonin neurones, and a computer-aided imaging system, cells in the brainstems of suicide victims and controls have been counted and morphologically analysed.[11] Suicides have a mean cell density in the dorsal raphe nucleus of 120 neurones/mm, while controls have 80 neurones/mm^2. The critical factor, however, is the total cell number, which does not appear to be reduced. If this is correct, this net reduction in serotonin activity appears to be associated with dysfunctional cells and not with actual cell loss. Stockmeier et al.[12] measured the binding of [^{3}H]8-hydroxy-2-(di-n-propyl)aminotetralin (**8-OH-DPAT**), an agonist which, in the dorsal raphe nucleus, binds specifically to a 5-HT$_{1A}$ autoreceptor. They found significantly elevated binding within the dorsal and ventrolateral subnuclei of the dorsal raphe nucleus in suicide victims with major depression, which may reflect upregulation in response to diminished serotonergic activity.

Noradrenergic system

The findings in the noradrenergic system have not been as robust as the serotonergic findings, and it has been more difficult to correlate the neurochemistry with specific behaviours. There are fewer noradrenergic neurones arrayed at a lower density in the locus coeruleus of suicide victims, but no morphological anomalies.[13]

Interestingly, despite the reduction in cell number there is reported to be an increase in tyrosine hydroxylase, the rate-limiting enzyme of noradrenaline (norepinephrine) metabolism. This could indicate a highly active system depleting noradrenaline and compensating with accelerated biosynthesis of the neurotransmitter. This interpretation is supported by the findings of elevated noradrenaline and fewer α_1-adrenergic receptors in the cortex of suicide victims. Most studies also report an upregulation in α_2-adrenergic autoreceptors, also believed to occur in response to depletion.[2]

Finally, most studies find the β-adrenergic receptors elevated in the prefrontal cortex of suicide victims. However, we have found that β$_1$-adrenergic receptor binding is actually decreased, and thus the elevation in β-receptors previously reported is probably due to elevated β$_2$ adrenergic receptors.[3]

While the findings in the noradrenergic system require further study, they point to a chronic stress response, which depletes noradrenaline. In this regard, the connection between chronic stress, depression, suicide, and the hypothalamic–pituitary–adrenal axis warrants more study.[14]

Neurobiological studies of suicide attempters

Levels of homovanillic acid and 5-hydroxyindoleacetic acid in cerebrospinal fluid

Suicide attempts represent a more varied type of behaviour than completed suicides, yet neurobiological studies of suicide attempters have shown a remarkable consistency in pointing to a serotonergic dysfunction. In a meta-analysis, which included 20 research reports, Lester[15] concluded that there is strong evidence of decreased cerebrospinal fluid levels of 5-HIAA in subjects who had previously made a suicide attempt compared to diagnostically matched non-attempters. Moreover, in three out of five studies, low cerebrospinal-fluid 5-HIAA was also able to predict future suicidal behaviour in subjects with depression or schizophrenia. Lester did not, however, find enough evidence to substantiate a relationship between suicide attempt status and the levels of homovanillic acid or 3-methoxy-4-hydroxphenylglycol (**MHPG**), a metabolite of noradrenaline, in cerebrospinal fluid.

Nordström et al.[16] found that the risk of completed suicide within 1 year after a suicide attempt was 2.5 times greater in those depressed patients whose cerebrospinal fluid level of 5-HIAA was in the lower half of the group.

The association between lowered 5-HIAA cerebrospinal fluid levels and suicidality has not been convincingly shown for bipolar disorder, but it does hold for people with unipolar depression, schizophrenia, and those with personality disorders. It therefore appears to represent a biochemical marker for suicidality, and is largely independent of diagnosis.[2]

Not all depressed people who attempt suicide have low 5-HIAA cerebrospinal fluid levels, however, raising the question as to whether there are biologically defined subtypes of suicide attempters. We found that 5-HIAA was lower in depressed subjects who made the most serious suicide attempts, i.e. those attempts that were planned and resulted in the highest lethality.[2]

These findings are consistent with both human and animal studies that show an association between low cerebrospinal fluid levels of 5-HIAA and greater lifetime aggressivity and impulsivity. Thus, low serotonergic activity is associated with both suicidal acts and externally directed aggression.

Fenfluramine and other neuroendocrine challenge studies

Another index of serotonergic function is the fenfluramine challenge test. Fenfluramine is a serotonin-releasing agent, as well as a reuptake inhibitor, that may also directly stimulate postsynaptic 5-HT receptors. Because the release of serotonin causes a measurable increase in serum prolactin levels, the fenfluramine challenge test provides an indirect probe of central serotonergic functioning. Most studies have found that depressed subjects have a blunted prolactin response to fenfluramine challenge compared to controls.[17] Flory et al.[18] have shown that the blunted response is a trait marker that persists after the depression remits.

Four studies have now reported an association between a prolactin response to fenfluramine and a history of suicide attempts.[3] We have reported that the degree of prolactin blunting distinguishes depressed subjects with serious past suicide attempts from depressed subjects with less serious attempts. Interestingly, New et al.[19] found a blunted prolactin response in subjects with a history of either suicide attempts or repeated self-mutilatory behaviours. While any neuroendocrine challenge involves several interacting neurophysiological systems, there is mounting evidence that the prolactin response to fenfluramine is indeed mediated primarily by serotonin.[3,17] Thus the fenfluramine challenge test supplies independent evidence for the role of serotonin in suicidal behaviour.[2]

Coccaro et al.[20] have shown that blunted prolactin response correlated with scores on three scales of aggression and impulsivity, as well as correlating with a direct laboratory measure of aggressive behaviour, the Point-Subtraction Aggression Paradigm (**PSAP**). Moeller et al.[21] also used the PSAP in conjunction with ipsapirone, a specific 5-HT$_{1A}$ agonist, and found that subjects with a high aggression score had a significantly blunted temperature response to ipsapirone compared with those with a lower score.

Finally, Coccaro et al.[22] also found that a blunted prolactin response predicted impulsive personality disorder traits in the first-degree relatives of patients with a primary DSM-III diagnosis of a personality disorder. This was a more sensitive parameter for identifying this familial trait than the presence of impulsive or aggressive behaviours in the proband.

Platelet function in suicide attempters

Platelets contain a 5-HT$_{2A}$ receptor that is genetically, pharmacologically, and mechanistically the same as the 5-HT$_{2A}$ receptor in the central nervous system. Moreover, it is coupled to the same phosphoinositide second-messenger system as the 5-HT$_{2A}$ receptor in the central nervous system.[17] Serotonin induces a change in platelet shape and aggregation. Platelets also have serotonin transporter sites, which are pharmacologically the same as central nervous system reuptake sites, and mediate platelet accumulation of serotonin.

A number of studies using the radioligands [^{3}H]ketanserin or [^{3}H]lysergic acid diethylamide have found platelet 5-HT$_{2A}$ receptor density (B_{max}) to be increased in depressed patients, while a study by Cowen et al.[23] found no changes. We also found no difference between the depressive and control groups, but found a positive correlation between receptor density and lethality of recent suicide attempt.[24] A subsequent study by Pandey[17] found that receptor density was increased in suicidal subjects independent of their psychiatric diagnosis; Pandey further reported that the increased 5-HT$_{2A}$ density was significantly higher in subjects with a recent attempt compared with those with past suicide attempts. This may be consistent with the findings of Biegon et al.,[25] who reported a normalization of platelet 5-HT$_{2A}$ density after successful antidepressant therapy, and it raises the intriguing possibility that platelet 5-HT$_{2A}$ receptor number is a state-dependent marker of suicidality.

In addition to changes in the density of 5-HT$_{2A}$ receptors, we reported that mean physiological responsivity of individual 5-HT$_{2A}$ receptors, as measured by serotonin-amplified platelet aggregation, was decreased in subjects with a history of high-lethality suicide attempts.[24]

Cholesterol studies

A meta-analysis of treatment trials intended to lower cholesterol and encompassing 119 000 person-years found a 70 per cent increase in mortality by accident, violence, or suicide among the treatment groups.[26] Observational studies have shown a relative risk for suicide as high as 4.2-fold in the low cholesterol group. Moreover, in a case–control study, 331 individuals admitted to psychiatric unit for suicidality were found to have significantly lower cholesterol levels than a matched sample.[27]

Although there is no absolute evidence of causality in these associations, in the face of considerable convergent evidence, Kaplan et al.[27] have proposed the cholesterol–serotonin hypothesis. The hypothesis is that low cholesterol results in reduced serotonergic function and thereby predisposes individuals to impulsive behaviours associated with the risk of accident or suicide.

Genetics of suicide

Familial transmission of suicidal behaviour

There is an accumulating consensus that suicidal behaviour has a significant genetic component independent of the inheritance of psychiatric illness. First-degree relatives of people who attempt suicide have a higher rate of suicide attempts, antisocial personality disorder, assaultive behaviour, and substance abuse.[28] Half of the mothers of suicidal adolescents report a personal history of a suicide attempt. On the other hand, mood disorders in first-degree relatives are not associated with suicidality in the proband.

Looking at 100 completed suicides, Farberow and Simon[28] found that 6 per cent had a parent who had also completed suicide. This is 8.8 times the expected rate. In a cohort of 5845 inpatients, Roy et al.[29] found that 243 (4.2 per cent) had a family history of completed suicide. Almost half the subjects (48 per cent) with familial suicide made a suicide attempt, compared to only 21 per cent of the 5602 patients without a family history. Moreover, this relationship was true across a wide variety of diagnoses.

Egeland studied 26 Amish suicides that occurred between 1880 and 1980, and found that suicides were largely confined to four families with heavy loading for both affective disorder and suicidality. However, the family loading for affective disorder alone did not account for the suicides, because there were Amish pedigrees with equal numbers of affective illness but not a single suicide in 100 years.[30]

In an analysis combining 399 twin pairs from several studies, Roy et al.[29] found that the concordance rate for suicide was 13 per cent in monozygotic twins and less than 1 per cent in dizygotic twins. While these studies are compelling, one can never be sure that those behaviours are not simply transmitted by parenting or through modelling, or other environmental or psychological factors. To overcome these objections Wender et al.[31] conducted an adoption study. The biological relatives of the adoptees who had committed suicide had six times the rate of suicide compared to biological relatives of matched non-suicidal adoptees. Taken together these studies supply substantial evidence of a genetically inherited risk factor for suicide that is independent of the inheritance of psychiatric diagnosis.

Candidate gene studies: a polymorphism in the gene for tryptophan hydroxylase

Tryptophan hydroxylase is the rate-limiting enzyme in the synthesis of serotonin. There is a polymorphism in intron 7 of the gene for this enzyme, named L and U, giving rise to three genotypes: L/L, L/U, U/U.[32] In Finnish alcoholics with impulse dyscontrol, Nielsen et al.[32] found that low cerebrospinal fluid levels of 5-HIAA and a history of suicide attempts correlated with the L allele.

However, the association between these genotypes and the potential phenotypes has proven to be more complex and elusive. In another study with Finnish offenders, Nielsen et al.[33] were able to replicate the association between the L allele and suicidality, but not the association with 5-HIAA in cerebrospinal fluid. We found an association between the U allele and suicidality in major depression, and Manuck et al.[34]

found an association of the *U* allele with a blunted prolactin response to fenfluramine and aggressive behaviour in a non-psychiatric sample. Although these two studies appear to contradict Nielsen's earlier findings, the association between a particular genotype and its phenotypic expression may turn out to depend on complex interactions of genes, which may differ by diagnosis, ethnicity, sex, or be a combination of all three. In any case, much research in this area can be expected.

Towards a biological assay to predict suicide risk

Given the remarkable progress that has been made in the biological study of suicide in a relatively short time, it seems reasonable to predict that biological assays will one day help us identify those at high risk for suicide. Suicidal behaviour is an affair of the brain as well as of the mind.

References

1. Mann, J.J., Waternaux, C., Haas, G.L., and Malone, K.M. (1999). Towards a clinical model of suicidal behavior in psychiatric patients. *American Journal of Psychiatry*, **156**, 181–9.
2. Mann, J.J. and Arango, V. (1998). Neurobiology of suicidal behavior. In *The Harvard Medical School guide to suicide assessment and intervention* (ed. D.G. Jacobs), pp. 98–114. Jossey-Bass, San Francisco, CA.
3. Mann, J.J. (1998). The neurobiology of suicide. *Nature Medicine*, **4**, 25–30.
4. Arango, V. and Underwood, M.D. (1997). Serotonin chemistry in the brain of suicide victims. In *Review of suicidology* (ed. R. Maris, M. Silverman, and S. Canetto), p. 237–50. Guilford Press, New York.
5. Mann, J.J., Henteleff, R.A., Lagattuta, T.F., Perper, J.A., Li, S., and Arango, V. (1996). Lower ^{3}H-paroxetine binding in cerebral cortex of suicide victims is partly due to fewer high-affinity, non-transporter sites. *Journal of Neural Transmission*, **103**, 1337–50.
6. Weinberger, D.R., Berman, K.F., and Zec, R.F. (1986). Physiologic dysfunction of dorsolateral prefrontal cortex in schizophrenia. *Archives of General Psychiatry*, **43**, 114–24.
7. Arango, V., Underwood, M.D., and Mann, J.J. (1997). Postmortem findings in suicide victims: implications for *in vivo* imaging studies. *Annals of the New York Academy of Sciences*, **836**, 269–87.
8. Lopez, J.F., Palkovits, M., Arató, M., Mansour, A., Akil, H., and Watson, S.J. (1992). Localization and quantification of pro-opiomelanocortin mRNA and glucocorticoid receptor mRNA in pituitaries of suicide victims. *Neuroendocrinology*, **56**, 491–501.
9. Lopez, J.F., Vazquez, D.M., Akil, H., and Watson, S.J. (1994). Effect of imipramine administration and swim stress on the hypothalamic pituitary adrenal axis. *Endocrine*, **2**, 723–8.
10. Pacheco, M.A., Stockmeier, C.A., Meltzer, H.Y., Overholser, J.C., Dilley, G.E., and Jope, R.S. (1996). Alterations in phosphoinositide signaling and G-protein levels in depressed suicide brain. *Brain Research*, **723**, 37–45.
11. Arango, V., Underwood, M.D., Gubbi, A.V., and Mann, J.J. (1995). Localized alterations in pre- and postsynaptic serotonin binding sites in the ventrolateral prefrontal cortex of suicide victims. *Brain Research*, **688**, 121–33.
12. Stockmeier, C.A., Shapiro, L.A., Dilley, G.E., Kolli, T.M., Friedman, L., and Rajkowska, G. (1998). Increase in serotonin-1A autoreceptors in the midbrain of suicide victims with major depression—postmortem evidence for decrease serotonin activity. *Journal of Neuroscience*, **18**, 7394–401.
13. Arango, V., Underwood, M.D., and Mann, J.J. (1996). Fewer pigmented locus coeruleus neurons in suicide victims: preliminary results. *Biological Psychiatry*, **39**, 112–20.
14. López, J.F., Vázquez, D.M., Chalmers, D.T., and Watson, S.J. (1997). Regulation of 5-HT receptors and the hypothalamic–pituitary–adrenal axis. Implications for the neurobiology of suicide. *Annals of the New York Academy of Sciences*, **836**, 106–34.
15. Lester, D. (1995). The concentration of neurotransmitter metabolites in the cerebrospinal fluid of suicidal individuals: a meta-analysis. *Pharmacopsychiatry*, **28**, 77–9.
16. Nordström, P., Samuelsson, M., Asberg, M., *et al.* (1994). CSF 5-HIAA predicts suicide risk after attempted suicide. *Suicide and Life-Threatening Behaviour*, **24**, 1–9.
17. Pandey, G.N. (1997). Altered serotonin function in suicide. Evidence from platelet and neuroendocrine studies. *Annals of the New York Academy of Sciences*, **836**, 182–3.
18. Flory, J.D., Mann, J.J., Manuck, S.B., and Muldoon, M.F. (1998). Recovery from major depression is not associated with normalization of serotonergic function. *Biological Psychiatry*, **43**, 320–6.
19. New, A.S., Trestman, R.L., Mitropoulou, V., *et al.* (1997). Serotonergic function and self-injurious behavior in personality disorder patients. *Psychiatry Research*, **69**, 17–26.
20. Coccaro, E.F., Kavoussi, R.J., Trestman, R.L., Gabriel, S.M., Cooper, T.B., and Siever, L.J. (1997). Serotonin function in human subjects: intercorrelations among central 5-HT indices and aggressiveness. *Psychiatry Research*, **73**, 1–14.
21. Moeller, F.G., Allen, T., Cherek, D.R., Dougherty, D.M., Lane, S., and Swann, A.C. (1998). Ipsapirone neuroendocrine challenge: relationship to aggression as measured in the human laboratory. *Psychiatry Research*, **81**, 31–8.
22. Coccaro, E.F., Silverman, J.M., Klar, H.M., Horvath, T.B., and Siever, L.J. (1994). Familial correlates of reduced central serotonergic system function in patients with personality disorders. *Archives of General Psychiatry*, **51**, 318–24.
23. Cowen, P.J., Charig, E.M., Fraser, S., and Elliott, J.M. (1987). Platelet 5-HT receptor binding during depressive illness and tricyclic antidepressant treatment. *Journal of Affective Disorders*, **13**, 45–50.
24. McBride, P.A., Brown, R.P., DeMeo, M., Keilp, J., Mieczkowski, T., and Mann, J.J. (1994). The relationship of platelet 5-HT$_2$ receptor indices to major depressive disorder, personality traits, and suicidal behavior. *Biological Psychiatry*, **35**, 295–308.
25. Biegon, A., Hanau, M., Greenberger, V., and Segal, M. (1989). Aging and brain cholinergic muscarinic receptor subtypes: an autoradiographic study in the rat. *Neurobiology of Aging*, **10**, 305–10.
26. Muldoon, M.F., Manuck, S.B., and Matthews, K.A. (1990). Lowering cholesterol concentrations and mortality: a quantitative review of primary prevention trials. *British Medical Journal*, **301**, 309–14.
27. Kaplan, J.R., Muldoon, M.F., Manuck, S.B., and Mann, J.J. (1997). Assessing the observed relationship between low cholesterol and violence-related mortality. Implications for suicide risk. *Annals of the New York Academy of Sciences*, **836**, 57–80.
28. Farberow, N.L. and Simon, M.D. (1969). Suicides in Los Angeles and Vienna. An intercultural study of two cities. *Public Health Reports*, **84**, 389–403.
29. Roy, A., Rylander, G., and Sarchiapone, M. (1997), Genetics of suicide. Family studies and molecular genetics. *Annals of the New York Academy of Sciences*, **836**, 135–57.
30. Egeland, J.A. and Sussex, J.N. (1985). Suicide and family loading for affective disorders. *Journal of the American Medical Association*, **254**, 915–18.
31. Wender, P.H., Kety, S.S., Rosenthal, D., Schulsinger, F., Ortmann, J., and Lunde, I. (1986). Psychiatric disorders in the biological and adoptive families of adopted individuals with affective disorders. *Archives of General Psychiatry*, **43**, 923–9.
32. Nielsen, D.A., Goldman, D., Virkkunen, M., Tokola, R., Rawlings, R., and Linnoila, M. (1994). Suicidality and 5-hydroxyindoleacetic acid

concentration associated with a tryptophan hydroxylase polymorphism. *Archives of General Psychiatry*, **51**, 34–8.

33. Nielsen, D.A., Virkkunen, M., Lappalainen, J., *et al.* (1998). A tryptophan hydroxylase gene marker for suicidality and alcoholism. *Archives of General Psychiatry*, **55**, 593–602.

34. Manuck, S.B., Flory, J.D., Ferrell, R.E., Dent, K., Mann, J.J., and Muldoon, M.F. (1999). Aggression and anger-related traits associated with a polymorphism of the tryptophan hydroxylase gene. *Biological Psychiatry*, **45**, 603–14.

4.15.4 Treatment of suicide attempters and prevention of suicide and attempted suicide

Keith Hawton

Introduction

In considering the treatment and prevention of suicidal behaviour it is important to take account of recent trends in suicide and attempted suicide, particularly in individual countries. These have been reviewed in other chapters in this section. While the term 'attempted suicide' is being used in this chapter it is important to recognize that this includes any acts of non-fatal self-poisoning or self-injury, irrespective of the motive or intention. It is known, for example, that in many cases the primary aim is not death but some other outcome, such as demonstrating distress to other people, seeking a change in other people's behaviour, or temporary escape.[1] Treatment and prevention strategies must be considered with this in mind.

Suicide prevention has been incorporated within the World Health Organization Health for All strategy[2] and has received substantial support from the United Nations.[3] In recent years several countries have developed national suicide prevention programmes.[4] Increased suicide rates in young people have probably been a stimulus behind this trend. However, suicide rates in most countries remain higher in older people than in younger people and prevention programmes must include this increasingly large sector of society.

Treatment of suicide attempters

Suicide attempts occur for a wide range of reasons.[5,6] This means that a broad range of treatments are required since the needs of individual patients will vary widely (Table 1).

Characteristics of suicide attempters which are relevant to treatment needs

Repetition of attempts and risk of suicide

Repetition of attempts is common, with 15 to 25 per cent repeating suicidal acts within a year. Repetition is associated with a greater risk of eventual suicide.[5] The frequency of occurrence of suicide following attempted suicide varies from country to country, depending on the overall characteristics of the patient population. In countries where the patient population tends to be extremely young, as in the United

Kingdom, the suicide rate is likely to be lower than in countries, such as those in Scandinavia, where a larger proportion of the patient population is somewhat older. Clearly, prevention of repetition of suicidal behaviour and especially of suicide is a major aim in treating suicide attempters.

Psychiatric and personality disorders

A range of psychiatric disorders are found in suicide attempters. Depression and alcohol abuse are particularly common. While treatment directed at the underlying causes of such disorders, where possible, will be important in managing attempted-suicide patients, often the disorders themselves will require specific treatment. In addition, substantial proportions of patients, particularly males, have personality disorders. Effective treatment of such individuals may require intensive therapies.

Life events and difficulties

Certain problems are particularly common in suicide attempters, including difficulties in interpersonal relationships, especially with partners and with other family members, employment problems, particularly in males, and financial difficulties. Life events frequently precede suicidal acts.[7,8] Disruption in a relationship with a partner is the most frequent of these. Treatment will often need to include helping people deal with such events and difficulties.

Poor problem-solving skills

Many suicide attempters have difficulties in problem-solving, particularly in dealing with difficulties in interpersonal relationships.[9] These difficulties are more marked in suicide attempters than in patients with psychiatric disorders who have not carried out a suicidal act. Suicide attempters also often tend to adopt a passive approach to problem-solving. Attention to problem-solving skills is therefore often regarded as an important element in treating these patients.

Impulsivity and aggression

There is a strong link between suicidal behaviour and both impulsivity and aggression. There is also accumulating evidence that hypofunction of brain serotonergic systems is linked to aggression (and possibly impulsivity) and also to suicidal behaviour[10] (see Chapter 4.15.3). It is unclear whether this represents a state phenomenon associated with psychiatric disturbance or a trait phenomenon, but current evidence

Table 1 Characteristics of suicide attempters which determine treatment needs

Risk of repetition of attempts
Risk of suicide
Psychiatric disorder (especially depression and substance abuse)
Personality disorders
Life events and difficulties
Poor problem-solving skills
Impulsivity and aggression
Hopelessness
Low self-esteem
Motivational problems and poor compliance with treatment

points towards the latter. Therefore interest has recently focused on altering serotonergic function, especially with antidepressants.

Hopelessness and low self-esteem

Hopelessness, or pessimism about the future, is very important in suicidal behaviour, having been shown to be a key factor linking depression with suicidal acts, being an important predictor of repetition of suicidal behaviour, and a risk factor for eventual suicide.[5] Low self-esteem is another important characteristic. There is likely to be a link between low self-esteem and a tendency to experience hopelessness when faced by adverse circumstances. Treatment of low self-esteem and vulnerability towards experiencing hopelessness may require cognitive-behavioural therapy.

Motivational problems and poor compliance with treatment

Management of suicide attempters is complicated by the fact that some patients are poorly motivated to engage in aftercare. This is also likely to affect compliance with medication and other treatments. The style of organization of general hospital psychiatric services will be an important factor in determining whether continuity of care, which is likely to aid compliance, can be achieved.

General overview of treatments

As will be apparent from the range of factors described above, the treatment of suicide attempters draws on psychosocial and pharmacological approaches. While these are considered separately below, in some patients both will be appropriate. This might be the case, for example, where a patient suffers from depression with biological features in the setting of employment and financial difficulties—then treatment with an antidepressant might be combined with problem-solving therapy.

Psychosocial treatments

A range of psychosocial therapies have been evaluated in suicide attempters in randomized controlled clinical trials. The efficacy of these approaches has been examined in a systematic review of the world-wide literature,[11] and the findings from this review and some further studies are summarized below.

Problem-solving

In the series of trials that have been conducted so far to evaluate the effectiveness of brief problem-solving therapy there has been a trend towards reduction of repetition of self-harm episodes, but the total number of subjects included has been insufficient for the combined trials to have the power to detect clinically significant levels of reduction in repetition at a statistically significant level. Nevertheless, this approach seems to be promising, particularly as it is reasonably easily taught and can be used by clinicians from different professional backgrounds. Evidence of other positive outcomes, such as improvement in problems and changes in problem-solving skills, has been convincingly demonstrated in these studies.

Problem-solving involves helping patients define their problems accurately, deciding on appropriate goals, using a stepwise approach to

dealing with the problems and working on the patient's cognitions or beliefs when these interfere with the process[12] (see Chapter 6.3.1).

Intensive care plus outreach

Several trials have been conducted which share two common factors, namely community outreach either for all patients, or for those that have not attended treatment sessions, together with a relatively intense treatment programme. Overall these studies have failed to show convincing evidence of effectiveness in reducing repetition of attempts compared with less intensive routine care. One study in which non-attenders at outpatient appointments were followed up at home by a nurse who tried to encourage them to attend their appointments did, however, have promising results in that the proportion of patients in the experimental group who attended appointments was significantly greater than in the control group, and there was a near significant reduction in the rate of repetition of suicide attempts during the year after entry to the study.[13] The results of this study suggest that outreach could be a useful component or treatment for this population, perhaps reserved for patients who are poorly compliant with aftercare.

Outreach may be essential in treatment of patients in remote rural areas in developing countries. This approach has been utilized with some success in Sri Lanka.[14]

Provision of emergency cards

In the United Kingdom there has recently been interest in providing suicide attempters with cards which indicate how they might get emergency help at times of crisis. Two initial relatively small studies of this approach, one involving adults and the other young adolescents, have produced encouraging results, but a larger evaluation is required. Provision of emergency cards requires there to be a 24-h service that can deal with emergency calls. In order to prevent misuse of the service it is probably wise for there to be careful selection of patients who are offered this facility.

Intensive psychotherapy

One trial has been conducted in which an intensive form of psychological treatment known as dialectical behaviour therapy was evaluated.[15] Female patients with borderline personality disorders who had a history of repeated self-harm were offered a year of individual and group cognitive–behavioural therapy aimed at addressing the patients' problems of motivation and strengthening their behavioural skills, particularly in relation to interpersonal difficulties. Compared with routine care this approach seemed to result in a reduction in repetition of self-harm as well as a number of other positive outcomes during the year of therapy. The reduction in self-harming behaviour continued 6 months after therapy ended. Further evaluation of this approach in other centres is required. Investigations are also needed to determine if it is effective in male patients and in adolescents, and whether it can be delivered in an abbreviated form. However, it is a promising if labour-intensive approach that may be helpful for what is a particularly difficult group of patients.

Other psychosocial approaches

The importance of continuity of care was emphasized in a study from Germany in which patients who were followed up by the same therapist who assessed them in hospital after their attempts were more likely to attend treatment sessions than patients who were offered treatment with a different therapist than the one they saw in hospital.[16] However, there was a paradoxically higher repetition rate in the former group, but this seems to have been the result of a failure of the randomization procedure to produce balanced groups in terms of risk factors. The same investigators found that monthly therapy for a year did not produce any difference in outcome compared with 3 months of weekly therapy, although the details of the content of therapy were not provided. The most useful and relevant finding is that continuity of care for suicide attempters increases compliance. Therefore, it is helpful if treatment for many patients can be provided by clinicians who are working in general hospital services for suicide attempters.

Pharmacological treatments

There have been surprisingly few treatment studies of the effectiveness of pharmacological agents in suicide attempters. This perhaps reflects the problems of compliance with therapy which were noted earlier.

Antidepressants

Two trials which included the older antidepressants nomifensine and mianserin failed to show any benefit of the antidepressants in terms of repetition of attempts.

A recent trial from The Netherlands in which paroxetine was compared with placebo in patients who were all repeaters of self-harm but who did not suffer from current depressive disorder showed apparent benefits for a subgroup of patients who received paroxetine, namely those who had a history of between one and four episodes of self-harm. Patients with a history of five or more episodes did not seem to benefit.[17] The findings of this study are clearly of interest (although *post hoc* subgroup analyses of this kind must be treated with caution), particularly in the light of the evidence from another recent investigation that the selective serotonin reuptake inhibitor (**SSRI**) fluoxetine seemed to decrease self-reported aggression in a short-term trial.[18] Clearly this is an area where much further work is required, although variable compliance with long-term medication may be a limiting factor.

Neuroleptics

A trial in which the depot neuroleptic flupenthixol was administered monthly in a dose of 20 mg for 6 months to repeaters of self-harm and compared with placebo in similar patients appeared to show that the active drug was effective in reducing the recurrence of self-harm.[19] This study requires replication. However, in patients who repeat self-harm frequently and are willing to receive a depot this approach might be worth trying. It might also be worth using one of the atypical oral neuroleptics in patients who are likely to comply with oral treatment.

Management in clinical practice

Given the paucity of firmly proven effective treatments for attempted suicide patients, how is the clinician dealing with this heterogeneous patient population to proceed? Before a treatment plan can be formulated a careful assessment must be carried out. The key factors that should be covered are listed in Table 2. For the purpose of formulating a management plan it is particularly useful to draw up a problem list which summarizes the patient's current difficulties. This should be done in collaboration with the patient as far as possible.

During the assessment it is crucial to estimate the risk of suicide or of another non-fatal attempt. However, accurate assessment is far from easy. One element of suicide risk is the degree of suicidal intent involved in the current attempt. Useful factors to consider are listed in Table 3. Clinicians should consider the use of the valuable Beck Suicidal Intent Scale,[20] which covers these items. Factors known to be associated with risk of a further attempt are listed in Table 4. It should be noted that while individuals who score positive on several of these factors will have considerably increased risk of repetition, a substantial proportion of those who repeat will not show these characteristics, i.e. the predictive value of scales to predict repetition is modest.

Risk factors for suicide following attempted suicide are shown in Table 5. Because suicide is less common than non-fatal repetition the predictive value of such items is even more limited.

The treatment plan should be drawn up on the basis of the patient's needs and risks. Inpatient psychiatric treatment will usually be indicated for patients with severe psychiatric disorders, especially where immediate risk of suicide appears to be high.

Major psychiatric disorders should be treated in the usual way, but with particular care about use of medication which might be toxic in overdose. Specific treatment should be provided for alcohol and drug

---

Table 2 The assessment of attempted-suicide patients

Factors that should be covered
Life events that preceded the attempt
Motives for the act, including suicidal intent and other reasons
Problems faced by the patient
Psychiatric disorder
Personality traits and disorder
Alcohol and drug misuse
Family and personal history
Current circumstances
    Social (e.g. extent of social relationships)
    Domestic (e.g. living alone or with others)
    Occupation (e.g. whether employed)
Psychiatric history, including previous suicide attempts

Assessments that should be made
Risk of a further attempt
Risk of suicide
Coping resources and supports
What treatment is appropriate to the patient's needs
Motivation of patient (and significant others where
    appropriate) to engage in treatment

Table 3 Factors that suggest high suicidal intent

Act carried out in isolation
Act timed so that intervention unlikely
Precautions taken to avoid discovery
Preparations made in anticipation of death (e.g. making will, organizing insurance)
Preparations made for the act (e.g. purchasing means, saving up tablets)
Communicating intent to others beforehand
Extensive premeditation
Leaving a note
Not alerting potential helpers after the act
Subsequent admission of suicidal intent

Table 4 Factors associated with risk of repetition of attempted suicide

Previous attempt(s)
Personality disorder
Alcohol or drug abuse
Previous psychiatric treatment
Unemployment
Lower social class
Criminal record
History of violence
Age 25–54 years
Single, divorced, or separated

abuse; indeed, a suicide attempt is sometimes the first occasion that abuse may come to the attention of the clinician.

The bulk of this patient population can be managed in the community. Brief problem-solving therapy will be appropriate for those patients who have clear problems such as in interpersonal relationships, employment, or social adjustment. This approach is readily taught to clinicians from different backgrounds and of varying levels of experience and can therefore be made readily available. Outreach programmes (e.g. home visiting) may be helpful to increase the proportion of patients who receive treatment, but are probably not necessary for all patients. This approach will often be an essential part of treatment in rural settings in developing countries. If possible there should be continuity of therapy in terms of the same person who saw the patient in hospital after their attempt providing aftercare as this is likely to result in better compliance with therapy. Provision of an emergency card to allow patients to avail themselves of emergency help may be useful for a subgroup of patients but not all. Longer-term cognitive-behavioural therapy or dynamic psychotherapy may be required for patients whose attempts are related to traumas such as sexual abuse or to personality disorder. People who are repeaters of suicide attempts may also require more intensive treatment, especially those who frequently repeat. If resources permit, the use of a programme based on dialectical behaviour therapy, possibly using a group format for at least part of treatment, might be considered. If frequent repeaters are willing to accept neuroleptic medication, low-dose oral or intramuscular phenothiazines may be worth trying.

Family therapy may be required for young adolescents, and also for

Table 5 Factors associated with risk of suicide after attempted suicide

Older age (females only)
Male gender
Unemployed or retired
Separated, divorced, or widowed
Living alone
Poor physical health
Psychiatric disorder (particularly depression, alcoholism, schizophrenia, and 'sociopathic' personality disorder)
High suicidal intent in current episode
Violent method involved in current attempt (e.g. attempted hanging, shooting, jumping)
Leaving a note
Previous attempt(s)

patients with difficulties in relation to children. The needs of young children of attempters must be considered because there is a substantial association between parental attempted suicide and abuse or neglect of children.

Prevention of suicide and attempted suicide

A wide diversity of individuals are at risk of suicidal behaviour and it occurs in relation to a wide range of problems and situations.[6] For example, suicide may occur in the context of long-term difficulties extending back to childhood, acute severe life events, or, and perhaps most importantly, acute or long-term and relapsing mental illness. Because of this the range of potential prevention strategies is also wide.

While ethical issues in relation to suicide prevention are not dealt with in detail in this chapter, they are none the less highly important. Opinions will vary, for example, about whether suicide should always be prevented. This particularly relates to suicides occurring in the context of terminal and/or painful physical illnesses, and relapsing and debilitating mental illnesses. The ethics of suicide prevention overlap those of assisted suicide and euthanasia. Psychiatrists are increasingly likely to be drawn into debate and controversy about the ethical aspects of these issues, particularly in relation to severe and chronic mental illness, and mental health aspects of assisted suicide and euthanasia in people with severe physical illnesses. The reader is referred to an article by Burgess and Hawton[21] which provides a detailed consideration of this important topic.

Cultural and ethnicity issues are also very important when considering prevention strategies. For example, while suicide rates are generally relatively low in young females in the United Kingdom, this is not the case in young Asian females of the Hindu faith, in which rates are relatively high and greater than in their male peers.[22] The issues surrounding such deaths are often related to cultural clashes regarding values and expectations between young Asian females and their parents.

General principles of prevention

Broadly there are two approaches to suicide prevention.[23] As described by Rose[24] in the context of prevention of health problems in general, one can distinguish between population preventive strategies, which aim to decrease risk in the population as a whole, and high-risk preventive strategies, in which specific groups that are at increased risk are targeted. High-risk strategies often appear more attractive and realistic (e.g. identification of psychiatric patients at high risk). However, risk factors for many disorders are widely spread in the population and so the high-risk strategy tends to exclude a large number of people at moderate risk and is often ineffective in reducing the burden of a disease at the population level. On the other hand, population strategies may appear more difficult to achieve (e.g. generally improving the mental health of the population) but are more likely to be effective in reducing population levels of disease (see also Chapter 7.4). The main population and high-risk strategies in the prevention of suicide and attempted suicide which are considered here are shown in Table 6.

Table 6 Strategies for prevention of suicide and attempted suicide

Population strategies

Reducing availability of means for suicide
Educating of primary care physicians
Influencing media portrayal of suicide
Education of the public about mental illness and its treatment
Educational approaches in schools
Befriending agencies and telephone helplines
Addressing the economic factors associated with suicidal behaviour

High-risk strategies

Patients with psychiatric disorders
The elderly
Suicide attempters
High-risk occupational groups
Prisoners

Population strategies

Reducing availability of means for suicide

This is the most widely discussed population strategy.[25] It is based on evidence that if the availability and/or danger of a popular method for suicide changes then this tends to have an impact on suicide rates. The general principles of prevention through reducing availability of means are, first, that many suicidal acts occur impulsively and therefore if a dangerous means is available this is more likely to result in death and, secondly, that the eventual suicide rate in survivors of serious attempts is remarkably low.[26] Also the common adage that if people are intent on committing suicide they will find a means is not entirely correct (see below).

The most cited evidence for the effectiveness of this approach is the reduction in suicides in the United Kingdom which occurred in the 1960s and early 1970s when toxic coal gas supplies were gradually replaced with non-toxic North Sea gas.[27] Prior to this time coal gas poisoning through people placing their head in a gas oven was the most common method of suicide in the United Kingdom. As North Sea gas was gradually introduced the suicide rate dropped steadily, eventually being reduced by approximately a third. It is estimated that as many as 6000 deaths may have been prevented by this change. The effect also illustrates the point that when one method of suicide is no longer available people do not automatically immediately turn to another method, or if they do it may be to one that is less likely to cause death. Thus, it was some years before the suicide rate rose again, this being related to an increase in deaths from poisoning with carbon monoxide from car exhausts. Another factor that may well have been relevant to the decline in suicides during the 1960s and early 1970s was the reduction in prescribing of barbiturates, these being replaced by far less toxic benzodiazepines.

Reversal of the recent increase seen in many countries in deaths from carbon monoxide poisoning is likely to occur as more car exhausts are produced with catalytic converters. Indeed there is already evidence in the United Kingdom that a reversal in this trend has started to occur, with a consequent decline in suicide rates, particularly in young males.[28]

The widespread availability of guns in certain countries, particularly the United States, has been proposed as an important reason for their relatively high suicide rates. Guns are used in more than half of all suicides in the United States and their use for suicide correlates with the holding of gun licences in households.[29] Some controversy surrounds the question of whether restricting availability of guns leads to a reduction in suicide rates, but the weight of evidence seems to indicate that it does.[30]

Given the very strong link between suicide and depression, and the risk of death from overdose of some of the older antidepressants, there has been much debate about whether more extensive use of less toxic newer antidepressants would prevent suicides. This is not a simple question, since some patients respond better to the older tricyclic antidepressants. Another consideration concerns the cost of the newer antidepressants compared with the older varieties. Also it is very important to remember that most people who are taking antidepressants do not kill themselves with their antidepressants but use other methods. This and the probable selective prescribing of SSRIs to people judged to be at risk probably accounts for the finding that suicide rates were higher in patients taking fluoxetine than patients taking other and in some cases more toxic antidepressants.[31] Nevertheless, common sense dictates that patients known to be at risk, and especially those with a history of suicidal behaviour, should be prescribed the less toxic preparations.

In the United Kingdom and some other countries there has been particular concern about deaths from paracetamol self-poisoning. A clear relationship between both fatal and non-fatal overdoses of paracetamol and availability has been shown for the United Kingdom and France.[32] Countries which have fewer tablets per pack seem to have a lower rate of mortality from paracetamol self-poisoning. This has resulted in legislation in the United Kingdom to reduce in the number of tablets of paracetamol (and aspirin) available per pack. It is too early to say whether or not this has been effective.

Much attention has also been paid to improving safety at popular sites for suicide. This includes erecting suicide barriers on bridges, multistorey car parks, and other sites. If environmental changes are made such that a popular suicide site becomes safer this does not mean that people at risk automatically move to using another site.

Clinicians involved in the development of suicide prevention strategies should look very carefully for local patterns which might provide clues about potentially effective measures for reducing access to methods. This could include, for example, ensuring that psychiatric inpatient units are free of hooks, pipes, and other objects or structures from which patients could hang themselves, secure fencing of railway lines or waterways close to psychiatric hospitals, and making local popular sites for suicide safer (e.g. suicide barriers on bridges). In addition attention should be paid to common dangerous methods of self-poisoning. Specific strategies may be required depending on local patterns. For example, ready availability of organophosphates and other toxic pesticides in some Asian countries, especially Sri Lanka,[33] appears to be a major factor in many suicides.

Education of primary care physicians

Much of the attention regarding improved detection of individuals at risk has concerned the management of depression in general practice. This was stimulated by findings that showed that many people who died by suicide or who attempted suicide had seen their general practitioners shortly before these acts. Thus, Barraclough et al.[34] found that 63 per cent of suicides had seen their general practitioners in the month before death and 36 per cent in the week before death. Changes in the profile of suicides in recent years have resulted in somewhat fewer patients having seen their general practitioners shortly before death (although this could of course reflect improved detection and treatment of other patients at risk). Thus, Vassilas and Morgan[35] found that 48 per cent of individuals aged 35 years and over who died by suicide and 20 per cent of those aged less than 35 years had seen their general practitioners in the month before death.

The main evidence that an educational programme for general practitioners might be effective in influencing suicide rates comes from a study conducted on the Swedish island of Gotland.[36] The 18 general practitioners on the island, which has a population of approximately 54 000, were offered an intensive educational programme consisting of lectures on depression in adults, children, adolescents, and the elderly, examination of local treatment practices, discussion of long-term treatment strategies, consideration of various aspects of suicide and suicide risk, and group discussions of case reports. In the year following this programme the suicide rate dropped significantly, prescribing of antidepressants by general practitioners increased, referrals to psychiatry, especially for depression, decreased, the amount of time lost from work for depression decreased, as did psychiatric admissions. Unfortunately this effect was fairly short-lived in that suicide rates rose again in subsequent years, which the authors attributed to some of the general practitioners having left the island. They also suggested that such programmes need to be repeated.[37] It is also important to note that the suicide rate only declined in females. The evidence in this study was based on relatively small numbers, at least with reference to suicide, although the effects on the management and outcome of depression are perhaps more impressive.

While the Gotland study has generated a lot of debate about suicide prevention in primary care, detection of people most at risk in general practice is extremely difficult because a large number of patients share risk factors, and because suicide is a rare event. The most pragmatic view is that effective detection and treatment of depression (and other psychiatric disorders) in primary care are extremely important aims in their own right and that they might also have benefits in terms of preventing some suicides.

Psychiatrists involved in designing suicide prevention strategies might ensure that there are effective local educational programmes for clinicians in primary care and other settings regarding detection and treatment of people with mental disorders.

Influencing media portrayal of suicidal behaviour

Dramatic reporting and portrayal of suicidal behaviour by the media can facilitate suicidal acts in other people.[38] This has been shown in the United States for both newspaper and television reporting of suicides.[39,40] The most dramatic demonstration of the potential power of the media in this regard is probably the effect found for a six-part fictional television series in Germany in which the railway suicide of a 19-year-old student was shown (in all six episodes).[41] In the weeks following this series there was a dramatic increase in railway suicides, particularly in young males, with no compensatory decrease in suicides by other methods. When the television series was shown again a similar but less marked effect was found, which appeared to be in keeping with the somewhat smaller audience viewing figures compared to the first occasion.

The possible influence of the media on attempted suicide has been less studied. There is, however, evidence that portrayal of suicide in films on television resulted in an increase in attempted suicide referrals to general hospitals in the New York area.[42] Recently, portrayal of a paracetamol overdose in a very popular television drama in the United Kingdom appeared to result in a marked short-term increase in general hospital referrals for self-poisoning, especially overdoses of paracetamol, with clear evidence that the impact on paracetamol overdoses was in viewers of the episode.[43]

Therefore it is not surprising that there is much support for changing the way suicidal behaviour is presented in the media. For example, it has been suggested that reports of actual suicides should be straightforward, non-dramatic, and not include details of the method used (since the main media impact seems to be on actual methods for suicidal behaviour). In particular, dramatizing suicidal behaviour in popular television series should be avoided. Producers of programmes should be encouraged to seek advice from experts when contemplating including a suicidal act in a programme. Advertisements for helplines and other means of obtaining help should be shown following any programmes which include detailed discussion of suicidal behaviour.

In each country, consideration should be paid to the development of consensus statements about media policies, which could be produced by joint working parties including representatives of the press, clinical and voluntary agencies, and experts in the field of suicidal behaviour. More difficult is the potentially valuable task of encouraging a policy whereby the media can be used to portray effective coping strategies for people in distress. Such a strategy will need to encompass local cultural factors. Psychiatrists developing suicide prevention strategies might examine the practices of their local media with regard to reporting of suicides and, if necessary, hold meetings with media producers to explain the dangers of dramatic and extensive reporting, and also to explore how the media might help in prevention.

Education of the public about mental illness and its treatment

In view of the very strong link between suicide and mental illness, effective treatment of psychiatric disorder must be a central theme in suicide prevention. However, detection of people with disorder will depend on the awareness that they and those around them have regarding the signs and symptoms of disorder, and their willingness to seek appropriate help. These important stages in receiving effective help will depend on attitudes towards mental illness and knowledge of its nature and the feasibility of treatment. In the United Kingdom, the Defeat Depression Campaign[44] and the Changing Minds 'Stigma Campaign'[45] represent major efforts to tackle the public's attitude and knowledge about depression and other mental disorders. At this stage, evidence is lacking as to whether or not they have been successful. Psychiatrists and their colleagues in other countries might consider similar campaigns where these are not already in place, although the method of delivery of messages will clearly depend on local factors. Potential strategies include leaflets in hospital and doctors' waiting rooms, workshops for the public, and articles in the local press or other media.

Educational approaches in schools

There have been three broad approaches to trying to prevent suicide through school-based programmes. The first of these includes teaching about the facts of suicide. Worrying evidence from the United States that such a programme appeared to lead to a small increase in pupils' ratings of the acceptability of suicide as an option compared with the ratings of pupils who did not receive the programme[46] suggests that this is not a wise approach.

Because suicidal behaviour in young people and others often appears to be related to poor problem-solving skills, a second school-based strategy has been the development of educational programmes in schools about life skills and problem-solving.[47] Given the early age at which suicidal behaviour begins, such programmes probably have to be targeted at extremely young school children, possibly with booster sessions later on. It is likely that the requirements of females from such programmes may differ those of males.[48]

A third approach is to train teachers, possibly with the assistance of screening questionnaires, in the detection of children and adolescents at risk of psychiatric disorder and possible suicidal behaviour. Pupils that are so detected will then need referral to an appropriate agency for further assessment and possible treatment. Such an approach is currently under investigation.[46] (Suicide in children and adolescents is considered further in Chapter 9.2.10.)

For psychiatrists and others involved in developing local prevention strategies it is important to recognize that this is a highly sensitive area and one where the most effective (and least risky) approach is at present unclear.

Befriending agencies and telephone helplines

A very important component of suicide prevention policy in many countries is the support provided by largely volunteer staffed befriending agencies and especially telephone helplines. The best known of these is the Samaritans, which was founded in London in 1953 by Chad Varah.[49] Befrienders International is the main international organization which facilitates the development of such services. A key principle on which such services are based is that people in distress and at risk of suicide will benefit from being able to discuss their problems with someone entirely confidentially. Recently, more assertive outreach programmes, in which volunteers meet up with distressed individuals such as in prisons and in remote areas, have been added to the traditional telephone service. In the United Kingdom and elsewhere the use of e-mail counselling is gaining momentum.

One example of how such befriending has developed in a fashion to take account of local needs is the outreach programme by the Sumithrayo in Sri Lanka.[14] In some senses this service overlaps that of mental health services in that people admitted to hospital because of suicidal behaviour are followed up back in their own villages, where efforts are made to generate community support through engaging families and friends in providing help.

The effectiveness of these approaches is largely unknown. Clearly, conducting controlled trials to examine their efficacy is very difficult. Naturalistic studies have produced conflicting evidence about the effectiveness of the Samaritans in the United Kingdom.[50,51] An examination of changes in suicide rates in areas with and without crisis intervention services in the United States suggested that suicide rates in young white females may have been reduced in areas where such services were developed.[52] Given the large numbers of contacts made with the Samaritans in the United Kingdom (4.5 million in 1998), it is clear that the service is valued by people in distress whether or not it has a major preventive impact on suicide.

Volunteer-run telephone helpline and similar services benefit greatly from the support and advice of local clinicians, who should regard them as a potentially valuable element in a local suicide prevention strategy.

Addressing the economic factors associated with suicidal behaviour

The association between suicidal behaviour and unemployment and poverty suggests that in order for suicide rates to change markedly these important socio-economic factors must be modified. The big increase in suicide rates during the economic depression of the late 1920s and early 1930s and the statistical association between suicide risk and unemployment would support this. Clearly such factors are increasingly a reflection of the global economic situation, but the strategies of individual governments, particularly in relation to the employment prospects for young people, may be influential. The main role of psychiatrist should probably be in highlighting these factors. Responsibility for suicide prevention tends to be laid at the door of psychiatry as if suicide is nearly always entirely the result of mental illness. The considerable evidence, however, that changes in the economic environment can exert a powerful influence on suicide rates indicates that governments with serious intentions to reduce suicide rates should address these issues.[23]

High-risk strategies

There are a wide range of possible prevention strategies which can be targeted at high-risk groups. Here some of the more important examples of such groups and relevant strategies will be discussed.

Patients with psychiatric disorders

One obvious approach to preventing suicide in people with known psychiatric disorders is to try and use recognized risk factors for suicide in each disorder to identify high-risk patients. The main psychiatric disorders in series of people who have died by suicide when examined using the psychological autopsy approach are depression (approximately two-thirds), severe alcohol abuse (approximately 15 per cent), and schizophrenia (5–10 per cent). The main risk suicide risk factors identified in these three disorders include, for example, previous attempts, family history of suicidal behaviour, and living alone. One difficulty in using a risk-identification approach, however, is that the risk factors identified from studies of groups of individuals who have died from suicide are often misleading when applied to individual patients. Also there is the issue that when applying such factors a relatively large number of individuals will appear to be at risk when they may not in fact be so.[53,54] In clinical practice it is important to be aware of patients who because of their individual characteristics are at long-term high risk and also the acute situations which may temporarily increase the risk in patients, be they ones at long-term risk or not. The most pragmatic approach, therefore, is to ensure that proven effective treatments for patients with these conditions are available and also to be particularly cautious at times of obvious high risk. There are particular periods of risk of suicide for patients with psychiatric disorders. One of these is during the first few weeks after discharge from psychiatric hospital.[55] This emphasizes the necessity for continuity of care at this critical time, and especially the clear identification of a key worker who gets to know the patient before discharge from hospital and provides him or her with early support after discharge. Other risk times may be following the break-up of a relationship or other significant loss, during periods of marked hopelessness, shortly after discharge from hospital, and following recent suicidal behaviour by another patient or someone else close to the individual.

Important strategies in preventing suicide in patients with affective disorders include very active treatment of individual episodes of illness, use of lithium and other mood stabilizers for patients with recurrent bipolar disorders,[56] and use of long-term antidepressants in patients with frequent relapses of depressive disorders. The risk factors in schizophrenia indicate that risk is greatest not so much during acute episodes but between episodes when patients may have insight and feel hopeless about their circumstances and prospects.[57] Continuity of care is likely to be a particularly important factor in preventing suicides in such patients at risk, with care being continued energetically during periods of remission. Community psychiatric nurses have a very important role with such patients. The use of the newer atypical neuroleptics might also be beneficial.[58]

Direct treatment of abuse is likely to be the best preventive strategy for patients with substance abuse disorders, with care taken to manage episodes of depression. The particularly high risk in the weeks following a break-up of a relationship for patients with severe alcohol abuse[59] again points to the need for continuity of support in the community.

Studies of suicides indicate that comorbidity is particularly common, especially the combination of depression with alcohol abuse and/or personality disorder.[60] Clearly the prevention of suicide in such patients is a challenging task, especially as compliance with treatment is often less good than in patients with single disorders. Effective prevention is likely to depend on close integration of care between different statutory care agencies.

Another important element in prevention in this population is education in suicide risk assessment and management procedures for clinical staff at all levels of seniority. These might be incorporated in educational programmes for risk assessment in general.

Elderly people

In planning suicide prevention in the elderly population, account must taken of the relative immobility of many older people. In a region of Italy, introduction of a telephone service to provide support and access to emergency help for elderly persons at risk has been associated with an encouraging decline in elderly suicides in the area.[61] This might serve as a model for other countries.

Suicide attempters

In view of the clear association between non-fatal suicidal behaviour and subsequent suicide, establishment of adequate services for suicide attempters, including the provision of careful assessments of patients in the general hospital and offering treatments for which at least some indicators of benefit are available (see above), is an important element in any national suicide prevention strategy. There is good evidence that non-medical staff can carry out assessments and arrange aftercare as safely and effectively as psychiatrists. Models for ideal services exist, such as that published by the Royal College of Psychiatrists in the United Kingdom.[62] Similar policies might be developed for general hospitals in other countries.

High-risk occupational groups

Certain occupational groups are known to be at relatively high risk of suicide. In the United Kingdom these include farmers, veterinary surgeons, dental practitioners, medical practitioners, pharmacists, and female nurses.[63,64] It is interesting to note that all these groups have relatively easy access to dangerous methods for suicide. Prevention of suicide in such occupational groups is an important consideration, although each group makes a relatively small contribution to the overall national suicide rate and prevention through detection of those most at risk encounters the usual difficulties of prevention of relatively rare behaviour using rather crude risk factors. It is probably more important to have general strategies for improving care in individual groups. In doctors, for example, there are some particular difficulties about confidentiality and therefore providing easy means of doctors getting confidential help is important. In farmers, improving the knowledge and attitudes of farming communities towards psychiatric disorder, and removing access to firearms at times of risk, are likely to be important.[65]

Prisoners

There are relatively high suicide rates in prisoners, especially young males held on remand.[66] While one aspect of prevention is through ensuring that prisons and police cells are safe in terms of absence of structures from which inmates can hang themselves, there are a range of other potentially useful and humane strategies. These include careful assessments of new inmates using risk-assessment procedures, training of staff with regard to both assessment skills and attitudes towards mental health problems and suicide prevention, in-reach programmes by befriending organizations such as the Samaritans, and ready access to psychiatric and psychological services. Clinicians involved in local suicide prevention programmes should include prisons in their considerations. (Suicide in prison is considered further in Chapter 11.8.)

Conclusions

The pathways to suicidal behaviour are often long and complex. Therefore, treatment and prevention of suicidal behaviour require attention to a range of broad and specific strategies. A variety of treatments have been developed, evaluations of which provide some guidelines for clinical practice, but there is a major need for large-scale treatment studies which will provide definitive results.

While there are general strategies for suicide prevention which are probably relevant to most communities (e.g. reducing the availability of means for suicide), specific local cultural factors will necessitate emphasis on particular strategies in certain countries. There is a general trend towards establishment of suicide prevention programmes in many countries. This is to be welcomed, not only because of the potential benefits in terms of suicide prevention, but also because of the likely benefits for the broader population of individuals with mental health problems.

It is too soon to know the extent to which national suicide prevention programmes are effective. The most impressive programme is probably that which has been developed in Finland. It is based on information from a detailed national study of all suicides in one year and includes a wide range of elements.[67] The recent decline in the Finnish suicide rate has been attributed to the programme.[68] National suicide targets were set in the early 1990s in the United Kingdom,[69] since when suicide rates have also declined.[64] Thus, while prevention strategies are difficult to evaluate[70] and have been assessed rather pessimistically by some authors,[71] there is now reason to be more optimistic that programmes for prevention of suicide on a national scale can be effective.

References

1. Bancroft, J., Hawton, K., Simkin, S., Kingston, B., Cumming, C., and Whitwell, D. (1979). The reasons people give for taking overdoses: a further inquiry. *British Journal of Medical Psychology*, **52**, 353–65.

2. World Health Organization (1994). *Ninth general programme of work covering the period 1996–2000*. World Health Organization, Geneva.

3. United Nations (1996). *Prevention of suicide guidelines for the formulation and implementation of national strategies*. United Nations, New York.

4. Taylor, S.J., Kingdon, D., and Jenkins, R. (1997). How are the nations trying to prevent suicide? An analysis of national suicide prevention strategies. *Acta Psychiatrica Scandinavica*, **95**, 457–63.

5. Hawton, K. and Catalan, J. (1987). *Attempted suicide: a practical guide to its nature and management* (2nd edn). Oxford University Press.

6. Hawton, K. and Van Heeringen, C. (ed.) (2000). *The international handbook of suicide and attempted suicide*. Wiley, Chichester.

7. Paykel, E.S., Prusoff, B.A., and Myers, J.K. (1975). Suicide attempts and recent life events: a controlled comparison. *Archives of General Psychiatry*, **32**, 327–33.

8. Bancroft, J., Skrimshire, A., Casson, J., Harvard-Watts, O., and Reynolds, F. (1977). People who deliberately poison or injure themselves: their problems and their contacts with helping agencies. *Psychological Medicine*, **7**, 289–303.

9. Williams, J.M.G. and Pollock, L.R. (2000). The psychology of suicidal behaviour. In *The international handbook of suicide and attempted suicide* (ed. K. Hawton and C. Van Heeringen), pp. 79–93. Wiley, Chichester,

10. Mann, J. and Träskman-Bendz, L. (2000). Biological aspects of suicidal behaviour. In *The international handbook of suicide and attempted suicide* (ed. K. Hawton and C. Van Heeringen), pp. 65–77. Wiley, Chichester.

11. Hawton, K., Arensman, E., Townsend, E., *et al.* (1998). Deliberate self-harm: a systematic review of the efficacy of psychosocial and pharmacological treatments in preventing repetition. *British Medical Journal*, **317**, 441–7.

12. Hawton, K. and Kirk, J. (1989). Problem-solving. In *Cognitive behaviour therapy for psychiatric problems: a practical guide* (ed. K. Hawton, P. Salkovskis, J. Kirk, and D.M. Clark), pp. 406–26. Oxford University Press.

13. Van Heeringen, C., Jannes, S., Buylaert, W., Henderick, H., De Bacquer, D., and Van Remoortel, J. (1995). The management of non-compliance with referral to out-patient after-care among attempted suicide patients: a controlled intervention study. *Psychological Medicine*, **25**, 963–70.

14. Ratnayeke, L. (1998). Suicide in Sri Lanka. In *Suicide prevention: the global context* (ed. R.J. Kosky, H.S. Eshkevari, R.D. Goldney, and R. Hassan), pp. 139–42. Plenum, New York.

15. Linehan, M.M., Armstrong, H.E., Suarez, A., Allmari, D., and Heard, H.L. (1991). Cognitive-behavioral treatment of chronically parasuicidal borderline patients. *Archives of General Psychiatry*, **48**, 1060–4.

16. Torhorst, A., Moller, H.J., Burk, F., Kurz, A., Wachtler, C., and Lauter, H. (1987). The psychiatric management of parasuicidal patients: a controlled clinical study comparing different strategies of outpatient treatment. *Crisis*, **8**, 53–61.

17. Verkes, R.J., Van der Mast, R.C., Hengeveld, M.W., Tuyl, J.P., Zwinderman, A.H., and Van Kempen, G.M.J. (1998). Reduction by paroxetine of suicidal behavior in patients with repeated suicide attempts but not major depression. *American Journal of Psychiatry*, **155**, 543–7.

18. Coccaro, E.F. and Kavoussi, R.J. (1997). Fluoxetine and impulsive aggressive behavior in personality-disordered subjects. *Archives of General Psychiatry*, **54**, 1081–8.

19. Montgomery, S.A., Montgomery, D.B., Jayanthi-Rani, S., Roy, D.H., Shaw, P.J., and McAuley, R. (1979). Maintenance therapy in repeat suicidal behaviour: a placebo controlled trial. *Proceedings of the 10th International Congress for Suicide Prevention and Crisis Intervention*, pp. 227–9.

20. Beck, A.T., Schuyler, D., and Herman, I. (1974). Development of Suicidal Intent Scales. In *The prediction of suicide* (ed. A.T. Beck, H.L.P. Resnik, and D.J. Lettieri), pp. 45–56. Charles Press, Philadelphia, PA.

21. Burgess, S. and Hawton, K. (1998). Suicide, euthanasia and the psychiatrist. *Philosophy, Psychiatry and Psychology*, **5**, 113–26.

22. Soni Raleigh, V. and Balarajan, R. (1992). Suicide and self-burning among Indians and West Indians in England and Wales. *British Journal of Psychiatry*, **161**, 365–8.

23. Lewis, G., Hawton, K., and Jones, P. (1997). Strategies for preventing suicide. *British Journal of Psychiatry*, **171**, 351–4.

24. Rose, G. (1992). *The strategy of preventive medicine*. Oxford University Press.

25. Clarke, R. and Lester, D. (1989). *Suicide: closing the exits*. Springer-Verlag, New York.

26. O'Donnell, I., Arthur, A.J., and Farmer, R.D.J. (1994). A follow-up study of attempted railway suicides. *Social Science and Medicine*, **38**, 437–42.

27. Kreitman, N. (1976). The coal gas story: UK suicide rates 1960–1971. *British Journal of Preventive and Social Medicine*, **30**, 86–93.

28. Kendell, R.E. (1998). Catalytic converters and prevention of suicides. *Lancet*, **352**, 1525.

29. Kellermann, A.L., Rivara, F.P., Somes, G. *et al.* (1992). Suicide in the home in relation to gun ownership. *New England Journal of Medicine*, **327**, 467–72.

30. Youth Suicide by Firearms Task Force (1998). Consensus statement on youth suicide by firearms. *Archives of Suicide Research*, **4**, 89–94.

31. Jick, S.S., Dean, A.D., and Jick, H. (1995). Antidepressants and suicide. *British Medical Journal*, **310**, 215–18.

32. Gunnell, D., Hawton, K., Murray, V., *et al.* (1997). Use of paracetamol for suicide and non-fatal poisoning in the UK and France: are restrictions on availability justified? *Journal of Epidemiology and Community Health*, **51**, 175–9.

33. Eddleston, K., Resvi Sherriff, M.H., and Hawton, K. (1998). Deliberate self-harm in the developing world—an overlooked tragedy. *British Medical Journal*, **317**, 133–5.

34. Barraclough, B.M., Bunch, J., Nelson, B., and Sainsbury, P. (1974). A hundred cases of suicide: clinical aspects. *British Journal of Psychiatry*, **12**, 355–73.

35. Vassilas, C.A. and Morgan, H.G. (1993). General practitioners' contact with victims of suicide. *British Medical Journal*, **307**, 300–1.

36. Rutz, W., von Knorring, L., and Walinder, J. (1989). Frequency of suicide on Gotland after systematic postgraduate education of general practitioners. *Acta Psychiatrica Scandinavica*, **80**, 151–4.

37. Rutz, W., von Knorring, L., and Walinder, J. (1992). Long-term effects of an educational program for general practitioners given by the Swedish Committee for the Prevention and Treatment of Depression. *Acta Psychiatrica Scandinavica*, **85**, 83–8.

38. Schmidtke, A. and Schaller, S. (1998). What do we know about media effects on imitation of suicidal behaviour: state of the art. In *Suicide prevention: a holistic approach* (ed. D. De Leo, A. Schmidtke, and R.F.W. Diekstra), pp. 121–37. Kluwer, Dordrecht.

39. Phillips, D.P. (1974). The influence of suggestion on suicide: substantive and theoretical implications of the Werther effect. *American Sociological Review*, **39**, 340–54.

40. Phillips, D.P. and Carstersen, L.L. (1986). Clustering of teenage suicides after television news stories about suicide. *New England Journal of Medicine*, **315**, 685–9.

41. Schmidtke, A. and Häfner, H. (1988). The Werther effect after television films: new evidence for an old hypothesis. *Psychological Medicine*, **18**, 665–76.

42. Gould, M.S. and Shaffer, D. (1986). The impact of suicide in television movies. Evidence of imitation. *New England Journal of Medicine*, **315**, 690–4.

43. Hawton, K., Simkin, S., Deeks, J.J. *et al.* (1999). Overdoses on television may influence self-poisoning behaviour: a time-series and questionnaire

study of self-poisoning presentations to hospitals before and after an overdose in a television drama. *British Medical Journal*, **318**, 972–7.

44. Paykel, E.S., Tylee, A., Wright, A., Priest, R.G., Rix, S., and Hart, D. (1997). The Defeat Depression Campaign: psychiatry in the public arena. *American Journal of Psychiatry*, **154**, 59–66.

45. Byrne, P. (1999). Stigma of mental illness. Changing minds, changing behaviour. *British Journal of Psychiatry*, **174**, 1–2.

46. Shaffer, D. (1994). Implications for education: prevention of youth suicide. In *The prevention of suicide* (ed. R. Jenkins, S. Griffiths, I. Wylie, K. Hawton, G. Morgan, and A. Tylee), pp. 163–73. HMSO, London.

47. Diekstra, R. and Hawton, K. (ed.) (1987). *Suicide in adolescence*. Nijhoff, The Hague.

48. Overholser, J., Evans, S., and Spirito, A. (1990). Sex differences and their relevance to primary prevention of adolescent suicide. *Death Studies*, **14**, 391–402.

49. Varah, C. (1980). *The Samaritans in the '80s*. Constable, London.

50. Bagley, C.R. (1968). The evaluation of a suicide prevention scheme by an ecological method. *Social Science and Medicine*, **2**, 1–14.

51. Jennings, C., Barraclough, B.M., and Moss, J.R. (1978). Have the Samaritans lowered the suicide rate? A controlled study. *Psychological Medicine*, **8**, 413–22.

52. Lester, D. (1974). Effect of suicide prevention centers on suicide rates in the United States. *Health Service Reports*, **89**, 37–9.

53. Murphy, G.E. (1984). The prediction of suicide: why is it so difficult? *American Journal of Psychotherapy*, **38**, 341–9.

54. Hawton, K. (1987). Assessment of suicide risk. *British Journal of Psychiatry*, **150**, 145–53.

55. Goldacre, M., Seagroatt, V., and Hawton, K. (1993). Suicide after discharge from psychiatric inpatient care. *Lancet*, **342**, 283–6.

56. Tondo, L., Jamison, K.R., and Baldessarini, R.J. (1997). Effect of lithium maintenance on suicidal behavior in major mood disorders. In *The neurobiology of suicide: from the bench to the clinic* (ed. D.M. Stoff and J.J. Mann), pp. 339–51. Annals of the New York Academy of Sciences, New York.

57. De Hert, M. and Peuskens, J. (2000). Psychiatric aspects of suicidal behaviour: schizophrenia. In *The international handbook of suicide and attempted suicide* (ed. K. Hawton and C. Van Heeringen), pp. 121–34. Wiley, Chichester.

58. Meltzer, H.Y. and Okayli, G. (1995). Reduction of suicidality during clozapine treatment of neuroleptic-resistant schizophrenia: impact on risk benefit assessment. *American Journal of Psychiatry*, **152**, 183–90.

59. Murphy, G.E., Armstrong Jr, J.W., Hermele, S.L., Fischer, J.R., and Clendenin, W.W. (1979). Suicide and alcoholism: interpersonal loss confirmed as a predictor. *Archives of General Psychiatry*, **36**, 65–9.

60. Henriksson, M.M., Aro, H.M., Marttunen, M.J., *et al.* (1993). Mental disorders and comorbidity in suicide. *American Journal of Psychiatry*, **150**, 935–40.

61. De Leo, D., Carollo, G., and Dello Buono, M. (1995). Lower suicide rates associated with a TeleHelp/TeleCheck service for the elderly at home. *American Journal of Psychiatry*, **152**, 632–4.

62. Royal College of Psychiatrists (1994). *The general hospital management of adult deliberate self-harm. Council Report CR32*. Royal College of Psychiatrists, London.

63. Charlton, J., Kelly, S., Dunnell, K., Evans, B., and Jenkins, R. (1993). Suicide deaths in England and Wales: trends in factors associated with suicide deaths. *Population Trends*, **71**, 34–42.

64. Kelly, S. and Bunting, J. (1998). Trends in suicide in England and Wales, 1982–96. *Population Trends*, **92**, 29–41.

65. Hawton, K., Simkin, S., Malmberg, A., Fagg, J., and Harriss, L. (1998). *Suicide and stress in farmers*. HMSO, London.

66. Dooley, E. (1994). Prisons. In *The prevention of suicide* (ed. R. Jenkins, S. Griffiths, I. Wylie, K. Hawton, G. Morgan, and A. Tylee), pp. 104–8. HMSO, London.

67. Upanne, M. (1998). Implementation of the Suicide Prevention Strategy in Finland: first follow-up. In *Suicide prevention: a holistic approach* (ed. D. De Leo, A. Schmidtke, and R.F.W. Diekstra), pp. 219–23. Kluwer, Dordrecht.

68. Ohberg, A. and Lönnqvist, J. (1997). Suicide trends in Finland 1980–1995. *Psychiatrica Fennica*, **28**, 11–23.

69. Department of Health (1992). *The health of the nation: a strategy for health in England*. HMSO, London.

70. Goldney, R.D. (1998). Suicide prevention is possible: a review of recent studies. *Archives of Suicide Research*, **4**, 329–39.

71. Gunnell, D. and Frankel, S. (1994). Prevention of suicide: aspirations and evidence. *British Medical Journal*, **308**, 1227–33.

4.16 Culturally related syndromes

Wolfgang G. Jilek

The concept of 'culture-bound syndromes' or 'culture-specific disorders'

In the most comprehensive treatises on comparative psychiatry[1] and transcultural psychiatry,[2] 'culture' is defined as comprising the ideas, values, habits, and other patterns of behaviour which a human group transmits from one generation to another, or as the whole complex of traditional experiences, concepts, system of values, and behavioural rules in a society. The 8th edition of Kraepelin's textbook, published in 1909,[3] is the first well-known manual of psychiatry describing conditions which are today recognized as culturally related syndromes, namely *latah*, *koro*, and *amok*. In the past, some authors designated culturally related syndromes by the term 'exotic', a Eurocentric label not applicable to a disorder such as anorexia nervosa (see Chapter 4.10.1) that is closely related to Western culture and to Westernizing cultural influences. The concept of 'culture-bound reactive syndromes' was introduced into psychiatric literature in the 1950s and 1960s by Yap[4] who also made the first attempt to order some of these conditions, known under a great variety of folk names, in a diagnostic classification scheme. A list of 168 so-called culture-bound syndromes was compiled in a glossary by Hughes;[5] DSM-IV[6] contains a glossary with 25 entries. These listings also include colloquial and local names for some well-known ubiquitous conditions. The *ICD-10 Diagnostic Criteria for Research*[7] briefly describe 12 examples of 'culture-specific disorders' and suggest diagnostic codes, while also stating that these conditions cannot be easily accommodated in established psychiatric classifications. Indeed, attempts at a nosological classification of culturally related syndromes have never been quite satisfactory due to (i) the overlap of diagnostically relevant symptoms and (ii) the fact that the various indigenous terms for similar syndromes are charged with different culture-specific meanings and traditional interpretations that codetermine the illness behaviour of the patient and the reaction of the human environment. In recent years the concept of 'culture-bound syndromes' has been the focus of a debate between universalists, who interpret these conditions as cultural elaborations of universal neuropsychological or psychopathological phenomena,[8] and cultural relativists, who see them as generated by, and expressive of, distinctive features of a particular culture.[9] The present overview is not guided by either of these ideologically influenced paradigms. It describes representative examples of culturally related syndromes, and defines these as clusters of symptoms and behaviours that can be plausibly related to cultural emphases and to specific stress situations which are typical of particular populations.

ICD-10 and DSM-IV codes will be cited for the purpose of clinical and research statistics with reference to conditions for which folk labels are not too ambiguous. A question mark preceding a code indicates 'possible but questionable' use of that code.

Local folk idioms of distress

Susto, espanto, miedo

These colloquially equivalent Spanish terms, implying an experience of fright or scare, are widely used among Hispanic populations of the Western hemisphere for a great variety of symptoms.[10] The conditions so labelled frequently resemble neurotic or somatoform disorders, but may also be caused by organic pathology. These folk diagnostic labels may be given to all kinds of complaints if (i) the complaints are associated with a frightening experience of the patient, (ii) it is generally assumed that this experience caused the soul to separate from the body, either spontaneously or through supernatural forces, and (iii) the diagnosis of *susto*, *espanto*, or *miedo* is confirmed by a trusted folk healer.

Nervios, nerves

The Spanish term *nervios* is often used among Hispano-American and Caribbean populations, as is the English term nerves among rural Anglo-American groups, to denote chronic dysphoric mood states with various somatic manifestations, especially in postmenopausal women under psychosocial stress because of family problems, loneliness, loss, and privation, as are commonly also encountered in other cultures.

Ataque de nervios

This Spanish term is mainly used among Hispanic populations of Central and North America and the Caribbean with reference to women showing a brief episode of behavioural discontrol as an immediate reaction to an emotionally traumatizing experience.[11] The symptoms are those of an acute dissociative state or panic attack.

Hwa-byung

This term, denoting 'fire illness' in traditional Chinese and Korean medicine, is commonly used among Korean populations to describe a chronic depressive condition in older women who experience marked feelings of anger under ongoing psychosocial stress and present with somatic complaints, specifically the sensation of an imaginary epigastric mass.[12] In Korea it is commonly considered an indication for treatment by female shamanic healers.

Culturally stereotyped reactions to extreme environmental conditions ('arctic hysteria')

'Arctic hysteria' is a vague general term used by outside observers for often dramatic behavioural reactions shown by indigenous inhabitants of arctic and subarctic areas in stress situations, in which the person affected experiences a temporary state of dissociated consciousness induced by acute anxiety.[13] Physical deprivation, mineral and vitamin deficiencies, and the psychological stresses of surviving in an extreme climate have been adduced to explain phenomena of 'arctic hysteria'. In traditional aboriginal culture, participation in shamanic group seances facilitated the occurrence of dissociative states in anxiety-arousing situations.

The following conditions are widely known, but nowadays are quite rare.

- *Pibloktoq* (Inuit, 'crazy'): an attack of motor agitation in which the person, usually a younger woman, engages in wild seemingly dangerous action—without, however, leaving the zone of relative safety—followed by collapse, sleep, and amnesia or rather disavowal. (ICD-10, F44.7; DSM-IV, 300.15)

- *Kayak-svimmel* (Danish, 'kayak dizziness'): this has been experienced by seal-hunting Greenlanders in situations of social isolation and sensory deprivation when sitting in a kayak for hours, waiting for seals to surface. Typical prodromal syndromes are dizziness and a sensation of cold ascending from below as if the kayak was filling with icy water. This precipitates an attack of panic anxiety in which the hunter feels immobilized and is subject to frightening illusional perceptions. (ICD-10, F41.0; DSM-IV, 300.01)

- *Windigo, witiko, witigo* (Algonkian name of mythical monster): fanciful reports of so-called *windigo* psychoses with cannibalistic urges among northern Canadian Indian populations have aroused much sensational interest in the past. Today the term *windigo* is used by the northern Ojibwa to signify a depressed mood of deep sorrow and hopelessness.[14] (ICD-10, F32; DSM-IV, ?296.2)

Syndromes related to a cultural emphasis on fertility and procreation

'Genital shrinking' syndrome (*koro, suo-yang*)

The Malayo-Indonesian term *koro* and the Mandarin Chinese term *suo-yang* (Cantonese *suk-yang*) denote 'shrinking of the penis'.

The 'genital shrinking' syndrome is a transient state of acute anxiety associated with vegetative symptoms, in which the affected male subjectively experiences a shrinking of his penis and the affected female a shrinking of her breasts and/or labia; the sufferers anticipate not only impotence or sterility but, in the case of complete genital retraction, certain death. Moreover, the immediate human environment of the sufferers is convinced of the same outcome and this explains the 'life saving' measures commonly taken, such as holding on to the sufferer's genitals manually or with special instruments. The 'genital shrinking' syndrome came to the attention of European psychiatry in the late nineteenth century through reports of colonial physicians working in Southeast Asia and through the growing interest in traditional Chinese medicine. Chinese traditional medicine interprets *suo-yang* as *yin–yang* imbalance due to a deficiency of the 'warm' male principle *yang* and an excess of the 'cold' female principle *yin*, so that vitalizing *yang* remedies are indicated. For the theorists of psychoanalysis *koro* served as the concrete example of Oedipal castration anxiety, while some pioneers of transcultural psychiatry saw in *suo-yang* the paradigm of a true culture-bound syndrome, assuming that the disorder itself was generated by the suggestive effect of traditional Chinese concepts.[15] However, it has since been ascertained that the typical 'genital shrinking' syndrome also occurs not infrequently among Asian and African populations without Chinese cultural influence.[2] Complaints of genital shrinking are also occasionally verbalized by Western patients and such cases are increasingly published since *koro* has become widely known. Nevertheless, these cases are different from the culturally related 'genital shrinking' syndrome as (i) they are associated with other, usually chronic, neurotic, psychotic, or organic conditions and (ii) the patient's ethnocultural group in Western society does not share the belief in the reality of genital disappearance and ensuing death. *Koro/suo-yang* is the only culturally related syndrome that has occurred in major epidemic outbreaks. Epidemics of 'genital shrinking'[16] have been observed repeatedly in recent decades—in Singapore, Thailand, Northeast India, and South China precipitated by collective anxieties over perceived threats to security or even survival of the afflicted population, and in Nigeria precipitated by fears of magic robbing of the genitals. (ICD-10, F48.8; DSM-IV, 300.81, ?300.01)

'Semen loss' syndrome (*shen-k'uei, dhat, jiryan, sukra prameha*)

Known in the traditional medicine of China as *shen-k'uei* ('weakness of kidneys'), in the Ayurvedic medicine of India as *dhat* (from the Sanskrit *dhatu*, essential body substance) or *jiryan*, and in Sri Lanka as *sukra prameha*, 'semen loss' is not an uncommon complaint among young men of these countries where a high premium is placed on reproductive capability and semen is considered a most precious elixir of life. The presented symptoms have a hypochondriac quality; they usually include general weakness, lack of energy and concentration, impaired sexual functions, and vague somatic troubles, all associated with an anxious and dysphoric mood state and typically attributed to the imagined loss of sperm in urine or to natural nocturnal emissions.[17] Many of these patients consult practitioners of traditional medicine as well as medical doctors; as immigrants they are also increasingly seen in European and North American clinics. (ICD-10, F48.8; DSM-IV, 300.81)

Syndromes related to a cultural emphasis on learnt dissociation

Latah-type reactions

In recent years *latah* reactions have been cited by cultural relativists as a paradigm of culturally conditioned behaviour[18] and by biopsychological universalists as cultural elaborations of the neurophysiological startle reflex.[19] *Latah* reactions have impressed famous neuropsychiatrists who interpreted them according to the focus of their research—Gilles de la Tourette[20] as a variant of his neurological syndrome and Kretschmer[21] as a phylogenetic mechanism. The complete *latah* syndrome consists of an exaggerated startle response to stimuli that are individually and culturally specific, often triggered by unexpected visual or acoustic perceptions, improper words, touching, or tickling, which causes sudden involuntary movements and inarticulate, often coprolalic, utterances; the *latah*-afflicted person instantly enters a transient dissociative state in which echopraxia and echolalia are manifested, as are hypersuggestibility and often command obedience.[2] Because of the characteristic echo symptoms, *latah* reactions are known in French psychiatry as *névroses d'imitation*. However, automatic imitation behaviour has also repeatedly been observed in absolutely normal indigenous people during their first contact with Europeans, as reported in 1845 by Darwin[22] from Tierra del Fuego and more recently from remote areas of Melanesia[23] and East Africa.[24] The typical *latah* syndrome occurs mostly in females over two geographical zones of epidemiological distribution.[25]

1. Southeast Asian zone: Malaysia, Indonesia (*latah*, 'nervous, ticklish'), Thailand (*bah-tschi*, 'tickle-crazy'), Burma (Myanmar) (*yaun*, 'ticklish'), and the Philippines (*mali-mali*).

2. North Eurasian zone: Ainu people of Hokkaido and Sakhalin (*imu*, 'startle'), aboriginal peoples of Mongolia and Siberia (Russian, *miryachit*), and in the past among the Sami of northernmost Europe ('Lapp panic').

The varied ethnic groups of these two *latah* zones have no other culture traits in common than (i) learnt dissociation, which is practised from early youth onwards in religious, social, and therapeutic ceremonies, trance rituals and shamanic seances, and (ii) learning by imitation and coping by copying the behaviour of persons who appear to be more powerful. Sporadic occurrence of *latah* symptoms has been reported among some males in Arabic–Islamic populations of North Africa and Yemen, and among South African Bantu people. While European cases are rarely encountered elsewhere, the endemic and familiar incidence of so-called jumping, a reaction similar to *latah*, among males of French-Canadian background in certain rural areas of Maine, New Hampshire, and Quebec, attracted scientific interest from the 1870s to the 1960s.[26] (ICD-10, F44.88; DSM-IV, 300.15)

Amok-type reactions

The term *amok* was originally derived from the Portuguese–Indian name *amuco* referring to heroic warriors ready to die in battle, and was immortalized in Malayan epics, similar to the *berserkr* in ancient Norse sagas. Today, 'running amok'—likewise 'going berserk'—has become a colloquial label for any episode of apparently unprovoked randomly aggressive and homicidal behaviour usually engaged in by attention-craving angry young men, often under substance influence. Such acts have become quite common in modern Western society and have to be seen in the context of the media popularization of macho 'Rambo' and other killer types. Although such behaviour has certain features in common with the *amok* reaction observed in Malayo-Indonesian men, it does not represent the specific dissociative syndrome described under this term by experienced clinicians.[2,27] Typical *amok* reactions are preceded by a prodromal state of dysphoria and tension experienced in conjunction with interpersonal or situational problems, especially feelings of slight or loss of 'face'. An upsetting incident, often seemingly trivial, then triggers an altered state of consciousness with changes in visual perception and threatening illusions causing fear and rage, followed by a sudden kinetic discharge starting the *amok* run during which randomly aggressive, destructive, and homicidal acts are committed. The *amok* run ends with suicide; alternatively, the exhausted perpetrator is overpowered and falls into a stupor or deep sleep, afterwards claiming amnesia for his deeds. Typical *amok* reactions have been presented as specific to the male ethos of Malayo-Indonesian culture,[28] but they also occur among other ethnocultural groups of Southeast Asia. In times of rapid social change and armed conflict, series of *amok* acts have been committed by young recruits in the Philippines and in Laos.[29] Cases of *amok* very similar to the Malayo-Indonesian syndrome have been diagnosed in Papua New Guinea[30] and these must be differentiated from the non-violent pseudo-*amok*, the psychodramatic 'wild man behaviour' of New Guinea highlanders. In historical analysis, *amok* in Southeast Asia appears to have changed from a glorified warrior ethos and means of social protest in the precolonial era, to a dissociative reaction which in more recent times is mainly found in marginal figures or as an episode during the course of a chronic neurotic, psychotic, or cerebro-organic disorder.[31] (ICD-10, F44.88; ?F68.8; DSM-IV, 300.15)

Syndromes related to a cultural emphasis on presenting a physical appearance pleasing to others (*taijin-kyôfu* reactions)

In contrast to the condition commonly diagnosed in Western psychiatry as social phobia (ICD-10, F40.1; DSM-IV, 300.23), with which it has some features in common, the Japanese form of anthropophobia *taijin-kyôfu* ('fear in relation to others') is not a phobic avoidance of social contacts in order to avoid unpleasant feelings for oneself, rather it is the fear that one's external appearance and behaviour may be disturbing or offending to the other, who as a rule is neither a stranger nor a close relation but a respected acquaintance. Symptoms of *taijin-kyôfu* were mentioned in the eleventh-century Genji saga by Lady Murasaki Shikibu, and detailed clinical descriptions of this condition suggest it to be typical of Japanese culture[32,33] and as paradigmatic for a culturally related syndrome;[34] that it is also not uncommon in Korea[35] may only indicate a cultural relationship. The clinical syndrome *taijin-kyôfu* was introduced into psychiatric literature in the 1920s by Morita as a subtype of the *shinkeishitsu* nervous temperament that he considered to be the main indication for his 'Morita psychotherapy'. The group of *taijin-kyôfu* symptoms include fears of inconveniencing, disturbing, offending, or even insulting the other by blushing, by one's body odour, by staring into the other's face (therefore avoiding eye contact), by one's assumedly defective facial or body features, or by other negative attributes of one's person. As in other delusion-near phobias, the differential diagnostic exclusion of paranoid schizophrenia and persecutory delusional disorder is of prognostic and therapeutic importance. Private clinics in Japan have numerous admissions with *taijin-kyôfu* symptoms that were in the past mostly manifested by young males, but more recently also by young females and older persons, which has been attributed to sociocultural changes associated with an increasingly competitive economic climate.

Syndromes related to acculturative stress

Brain fag

The term brain fag, coined by Nigerian students, refers to a condition first reported in 1959 by Prince among this population.[36] Since then the brain fag syndrome has been recognized in many Nigerian students at home and abroad, and also in students of other African countries who are exposed to the acculturative stress of a Western-type education system emphasizing theoretical book knowledge, quite different from the practical know-how and tribal lore acquired through oral traditions by older generations in Africa. Nevertheless, the older generations expect their students to achieve academic and socio-economic success in modern society and these parental expectations are increasing the emotional pressure on the students. The clinical picture of brain fag is characterized by a variety of symptoms:[36] bothering sensations on or in the head and body, especially aches, burning, and crawling; eye trouble and visual disturbances, especially blurred vision and tears when reading; impaired concentration, difficulty in comprehending and retaining learning material in written or oral presentation; feelings of general weakness, dizzy spells, and daytime fatigue. Depressed mood states are reactive to academic failure and not preceding or underlying this syndrome. It is noteworthy that subnormal intelligence, malnutrition, or physical disease do not account for the brain fag symptoms which are also seen at educational institutions in Europe and North America among African students in satisfactory nutritional and health conditions. The brain fag syndrome is categorically different from the general study stress and examination crises experienced by students from Western or Asian cultures, with their centuries of literary tradition and education systems based on reading and writing, and on memorizing texts for formal examinations. The brain fag syndrome is also clinically different in so far as the mere effort of reading may trigger the symptoms, some of which are quite typical and do not usually occur in Western students under stress, such as the burning heat feeling and the sensation of crawling as if caused by insects on, or by worms under, the skin. The latter are, of course, common reality in tropical Africa; they also play a role as supposedly sick-making agents in folk aetiological concepts of nervous and mental disorders. (ICD-10, F43.0, ?F43.2; DSM-IV, ?309.9)

Bouffée délirante-type reactions

Transient psychotic disorders in general are dealt with in Chapter 4.3.9. The following is a short summary of information indicating that acute transient psychotic and psychosis-like reactions occuring in Afri-

can and African-Caribbean populations are disorders directly related to culture and culture change. These reactions appear to be encountered with increasing frequency in Africa, and are embedded in anxieties over sorcery and witchcraft that persist or even increase under rapid sociocultural changes.[37] Anglophone psychiatrists have described transient psychotic and psychosis-like reactions in Africans under various terms, while their francophone colleagues use the neutral diagnostic label *bouffée délirante* which was introduced into French psychiatry in the 1880s by Magnan and later redefined by French-speaking authors in Africa in accordance with their clinical data.[38] The *bouffée délirante* reactions are of sudden onset and brief duration and occur in Africans, as a rule, in connection with experiences that are charged with culturally validated fears of magic persecution. The clinical picture is characterized by unsystematized paranoid delusions, often also visual and auditory hallucinations, acute and extreme anxiety, and agitation with highly emotionalized, often demonstrative and sometimes dangerous acting-out behaviour in apparent confusion, followed by retrograde amnesia, or rather disavowal. The Nigerian psychiatrist Lambo reported such reactions as frequently shown by Africans under intense fear of bewitchment; he introduced the English term frenzied anxiety and equated it with *bouffée délirante*.[39] As repeatedly stated by Lambo and other researchers who have examined African patients after *bouffée délirante* reactions, the underlying causes for these are not of a toxic–organic nature but sociocultural factors. Among these factors, of paramount importance is the acculturative stress affecting many persons in many parts of contemporary Africa who have become marginalized in society through rapid culture change, as recently again confirmed by an extensive study in Swaziland.[40] Under modern situations of urbanization and Westernizing acculturative pressures the traditional communalistic society is disintegrating and the supportive kin network is breaking down. The individual experiences an increasing economic rivalry and social isolation that intensifies the old fears of witchcraft and sorcery, never obliterated by Christianity, while the traditional protective and remedial resources are no longer readily available. (ICD-10, F23; DSM-IV, 298.8)

Diagnostic pitfalls

Ethnocentric fallacy

Culturally related syndromes have to be conceptionally and clinically differentiated from extracurricular but not pathological ritual behaviour, which is institutionalized in a culture or subculture and sanctioned by a religious or therapeutic ceremonial. As a general statement it can be said that the culturally related syndromes described above (i) are not integral parts of religious or therapeutic ceremonials and (ii) are defined as abnormal behaviour by the indigenous experts who explain these conditions in terms of the particular folk aetiology that determines traditional management. Before diagnosing apparently unusual behaviour or ideas in a person of another cultural group the psychiatrist has to inquire with discerning key informants of that cultural group whether such behaviour and ideas are considered culture congenial or pathological in a given situation. By attaching pathology labels to behaviour and ideas, which in the so-diagnosed person's own cultural group are considered normal in a particular context, the psychiatrist may commit an ethnocentric fallacy by ignoring the foreign culture's norms of behaviour and ideation, religious and other ceremonial practices, and its folk system of explanation.

Altered states of consciousness—normal or abnormal?

In many cultures altered states of consciousness are induced for religious and/or therapeutic purposes and are sanctioned practices in institutionalized ritual activities. These temporarily modified waking states are associated with selectively focused attention, heightened suggestibility, various degrees of anaesthesia or analgesia, blurring of cause and effect distinction, altered time sense, body image changes, and illusional perceptions. The often intense emotional experiences are felt to be ineffable but also to have a special significance; they are given a culture-congenial meaning and are interpreted according to the prevailing belief system. Behaviour in altered states of consciousness during rituals is culturally defined as not under voluntary control and is often not clearly remembered. Nevertheless, such behaviour follows culturally accepted patterns and social rules which are monitored by the officiating functionaries. In religious and therapeutic cult groups, altered states of consciousness depend on the member's motivation and are primarily based on collective and individual suggestion. However, entering an altered state of consciousness is frequently facilitated by induction techniques that utilize the somatopsychic effects of fasting hypoglycaemia and dehydration, sleep deprivation, sensory deprivation, forced hypermotility, kinetic, pain and temperature stimulation and, of great importance, rhythmic acoustic stimulation of a type that appears to exert a direct dissociating effect on the central nervous system.[41]

In most traditional non-Western cultures, and in the West in some fundamentalist Christian groups, altered states of consciousness are induced for religious or healing purposes and are interpreted as either (i) special states that permit close interaction and communication with supernatural or divine entities in order to receive their messages, perceive them in an ecstatic vision, or acquire from them power, inspiration, or healing, or (ii) states of ritual possession in which a supernatural or divine entity acts through the possessed person. These two basic variants of culturally defined and accepted altered states of consciousness have been designated trance and possession-trance, respectively, and their global distribution has been delineated.[42] Trance and possession-trance differ in terms of religious-cultural but not in terms of neuropsychological interpretation. The pathology labelling of such ritual behaviour and its motivating beliefs constitutes a positivistic fallacy, in so far as it considers as psychiatrically abnormal whatever does not fit into the logico-experimental explanatory framework of positive science. Religious or shamanic beliefs and ritual behaviour cannot be judged by the criteria of positive science, for ritual acts are, above all, manifestations of sentiments, as Pareto[43] has shown. Culturally non-approved altered states of consciousness, which are entered into in an idiosyncratic manner and in an inappropriate situational context outside sanctioned religious or other culture-congenial practices, are probably manifestations of underlying psycho- or neuropathology. These abnormal altered states of consciousness are often defined by religious functionaries and traditional healers as afflictions and explained as due to sorcery or witchcraft, or to possession by a sick-making or demoniac spirit. The possessing evil spirit has to be removed from the possessed person according to cultural–religious prescriptions, for example through appeasement or through

exorcism, widely practised in many cultures, such as the *Rituale Romanum* in traditional Christianity. While an exorcistic procedure may well be of help, at least temporarily, in hysteriform and other neurotic conditions, it can be harmful in cases of psychotic or cerebro-organic illness.

Therapeutic approaches to culturally related syndromes

Modern medicine treats the disorders discussed above according to the predominant symptoms with anxiolytic, tranquillizing, or antidepressant medication, and also with parenteral neuroleptics in cases of acute severe agitation. Brief psychotropic chemotherapy usually achieves temporary remission, but it should always be combined with supportive and reassuring counselling that includes family members. Western-type psychotherapy can claim little long-term success in dealing with the culturally related syndromes described in this chapter. These syndromes are the domain of traditional therapeutic resources and in most cases folk healers are already involved before a physician or psychiatrist is consulted. In fact, in cases of psychiatric disorder the 'double-tracked' utilization of both traditional and modern medicine is common today among indigenous non-Western populations.

Traditional healing tends to be therapeutically effective in most culturally related functional disorders, and in general in neurotic disorders with anxiety, dysthymia, reactive depressive, psychosomatic, and somatoform symptoms, and also in transient psychotic reactions and in alcohol and drug dependence.[44] There are a great variety of traditional non-Western folk healing procedures, but the following are common and characteristic approaches:

- holistic integration of physical, psychological, spiritual, and social modalities

- ritual–symbolic acts in which images or paraphernalia as culturally validated symbols are skilfully manipulated by the therapist under incantations and invocations

- naming of the affliction and its causation in a divining procedure

- affectivity therapy operating through the arousal of emotional responses rather than through rational 'insight'

- cathartic abreaction facilitated by appropriate sensory stimulation in a psychodramatic scenario

- 'purifying' measures understood to eliminate 'polluting' or otherwise harmful agents or substances

- sacrificial rites to appease supernatural or ancestral powers and solicit their intercession on behalf of the patient, who often also publicly confesses transgressions and vows to rectify wrongs in order to be relieved from guilt or shame

- induction of altered states of consciousness in the shamanic healer to enhance the suggestive effect of his or her performance, and/or in the patients and in participants of group therapeutic ceremonials or healing cults, which serves to facilitate collective suggestion and emotional release.

In most types of traditional folk healing three effective therapeutic principles are present, in contrast with usual Western-type psychotherapy: (i) the culture congeniality of both the therapist and treatment modality, (ii) the primary importance of the therapist's personality characteristics, and (iii) the use of explicit and implicit suggestion.

Although not easy to achieve because of past Western discrimination and pathology labelling of traditional practitioners and in view of the sacred character of some healing rituals, it is possible to establish a close collaborative relationship between physician/psychiatrist and indigenous healers.[45] Such a relationship can be achieved if there is mutual concern regarding patients who utilize both modern and traditional therapeutic resources. Collaboration with knowledgeable traditional practitioners will enlighten the physician/psychiatrist about culture-specific views of normality and illness, thereby helping to prevent diagnostic errors that are due to ethnocentric or positivistic fallacies.

References

1. Murphy, H.B.M. (1982). *Comparative psychiatry.* Springer, Berlin.
2. Pfeiffer, W.M. (1994). *Transkulturelle Psychiatrie* (2nd edn). Thieme, Stuttgart.
3. Kraepelin, E. (1909). *Psychiatrie—Ein Lehrbuch für Studierende und Ärzte* (8th edn), Vol. 1. Barth, Leipzig.
4. Yap, P.M. (1967). Classification of the culture-bound reactive syndromes. *Australian and New Zealand Journal of Psychiatry*, **1**, 172–9.
5. Hughes, C.C. (1985). Glossary of 'culture-bound' or folk psychiatric syndromes. In *The culture-bound syndromes* (ed. R.C. Simons and C.C. Hughes), pp. 469–505. Reidel, Dordrecht.
6. American Psychiatric Association (1994). *Diagnostic and statistical manual of mental disorders* (4th edn). American Psychiatric Association, Washington, DC.
7. World Health Organization (1993). *The ICD-10 classification of mental and behavioural disorders—diagnostic criteria for research.* World Health Organization, Geneva.
8. Simons, R.C. (1985). Sorting the culture-bound syndromes. In *The culture-bound syndromes* (ed. R.C. Simons and C.C. Hughes), pp. 25–38. Reidel, Dordrecht.
9. Kleinman, A.M. (1987). Anthropology and psychiatry: the role of culture in cross-cultural research on illness. *British Journal of Psychiatry*, **151**, 447–54.
10. Rubel, A.J., O'Nell, C.W., and Collado, R. (1985). The folk illness called susto. In *The culture-bound syndromes* (ed. R.C. Simons and C.C. Hughes), pp. 333–50. Reidel, Dordrecht.
11. Oquendo, M. (1994). Differential diagnosis of ataque de nervios. *American Journal of Orthopsychiatry*, **65**, 60–5.
12. Lin, K.-M. (1983). Hwa-byung: a Korean culture-bound syndrome? *American Journal of Psychiatry*, **140**, 105–7.
13. Foulks, E.F. (1972). *The arctic hysterias of the North Alaskan Eskimo.* Anthropological Studies No. 10. American Anthropological Association, Washington, DC.
14. Marano, L. (1982). Windigo-psychosis: the anatomy of an emic-etic confusion. *Current Anthropology*, **23**, 385–412.
15. Yap, P.M. (1965). Koro: a culture-bound depersonalization syndrome. *British Journal of Psychiatry*, **3**, 43–50.
16. Jilek, W.G. (1986). Epidemics of 'genital shrinking' (koro): historical review and report of a recent outbreak in South China. *Curare (Heidelberg)*, **9**, 269–82.
17. Paris, J. (1992). Dhat: the semen loss anxiety syndrome. *Transcultural Psychiatric Research Review*, **29**, 109–18.
18. Kenny, M.G. (1978). Latah: the symbolism of a putative mental disorder. *Culture, Medicine, and Psychiatry*, **2**, 209–31.
19. Simons, R.C. (1996). *Boo! Culture, experience, and the startle reflex.* Oxford University Press, New York.
20. Gilles de la Tourette, G. (1884). Jumping, latah, myriachit. *Archives de Neurologie*, **8**, 68–74.
21. Kretschmer, E. (1958). *Hysterie, Reflex und Instinkt* (6th edn). Thieme, Stuttgart.
22. Darwin, C. (1845). *Naturalist's voyage around the world.* Appleton, New York.
23. Gajdusek, D.C. (1970). Physiological and psychological characteristics of stone age man. *Engineering and Science*, **33**, 26–33, 56–62.
24. Jilek-Aall, L. (1979). *Call mama doctor: African notes of a young woman doctor.* Hancock House, Saanichton, BC, Canada.
25. Winzeler, R.L. (1995). *Latah in Southeast Asia: the history and ethnography of a culture-bound syndrome.* Cambridge University Press.
26. Kunkle, C.E. (1967). The 'jumpers' of Maine: a reappraisal. *Archives of Internal Medicine*, **119**, 355–8.
27. Van Wulfften Palthe, P.M. (1933). Amok. *Nederlandsch Tijdschrift voor Geneeskunde*, **77**, 983–91.
28. Carr, J.E. (1985). Ethno-behaviorism and the culture-bound syndromes: the case of amok. In *The culture-bound syndromes* (ed. R.C. Simons and C.C. Hughes), pp. 199–223. Reidel, Dordrecht.
29. Westermeyer, J. (1972). A comparison of amok and other homicide in Laos. *American Journal of Psychiatry*, **129**, 703–9.
30. Burton-Bradley, B.G. (1975). *Stone age crisis: a psychiatric appraisal.* Vanderbilt University Press, Nashville, TN.
31. Murphy, H.B.M. (1973). History and the evolution of syndromes: the striking case of latah and amok. In *Psychopathology: contributions from the biological, behavioral and social sciences* (ed. M. Hammer, K. Salzinger, and S. Sutton), pp. 33–55. Wiley, New York.
32. Kimura, B. (1993). *Zwischen Mensch und Mensch: Strukturen japanischer Subjektivität.* Wissenschaftliche Buchgesellschaft, Darmstadt.
33. Yamashita, I. (1993). *Taijin kyôfu or delusional social phobia.* Hokkaido University Press, Sapporo.
34. Kirmayer, L.J. (1991). The place of culture in psychiatric nosology: taijin kyôfusho and DSM-III-R. *Journal of Nervous and Mental Disease*, **179**, 19–28.
35. Lee, S.H., Shin, Y.C., and Oh, K.S. (1994). A clinical study of social phobia for 10 years. *Journal of the Korean Neuropsychiatric Association*, **33**, 305–12.
36. Prince, R. (1989). The brain-fag syndrome. In *Textbook of clinical psychology in Africa* (ed. K. Peltzer and P.O. Ebigbo), pp. 276–87. University of Nigeria Press, Enugu.
37. Jilek, W.G. and Jilek-Aall, L. (1970). Transient psychoses in Africans. *Psychiatria Clinica*, **3**, 337–64.
38. Collomb, H. (1965). Bouffées délirantes en psychiatrie africaine. *Psychopathologie Africaine*, **1**, 167–239.
39. Lambo, T.A. (1960). Further neuropsychiatric observations in Nigeria. *British Medical Journal*, **ii**, 1696–704.
40. Guinness, E.A. (1992). Patterns of mental illness in the early stages of urbanization. *British Journal of Psychiatry*, **160** (Supplement 16), 12–72.
41. Jilek, W.G. (1982). *Indian healing: shamanic ceremonialism in the Pacific Northwest today.* Hancock House, Surrey, British Columbia.
42. Bourguignon, E. (1973). Introduction: a framework for the comparative study of altered states of consciousness. In *Religion, altered states of consciousness and social change* (ed. E. Bourguignon), pp. 3–35. Ohio State University Press, Columbus, OH.
43. Pareto, V. (1935). *The mind and society*, Vol. 1, *Non-logical conduct.* Harcourt Brace, New York.
44. Jilek, W.G. (1993). Traditional medicine relevant to psychiatry. In *Treatment of mental disorders* (ed. N. Sartorius, G. De Girolamo, G. Andrews, and G.A. German), pp. 341–90. World Health Organization/American Psychiatric Press, Washington, DC.
45. Jilek, W.G. and Jilek-Aall, L. (1978). The psychiatrist and his shaman colleague: cross-cultural collaboration with traditional Amerindian therapists. *Journal of Operational Psychiatry*, **9**, 32–9.

Index

Page numbers for main references in the text are shown in **bold** type. Page numbers in *italics* refer to tables, figures and boxes. vs. refers to differential diagnosis or comparisons. The alphabetical order of the index is letter-by-letter.

Abbreviations used in subentries:

AIDS	acquired immunodeficiency syndrome	HPA axis	hypothalamic–pituitary–adrenal axis
CJD	Creutzfeldt–Jakob disease	MAOIs	monoamine oxidase inhibitors
CNS	central nervous system	MRI	magnetic resonance imaging
ECT	electroconvulsive therapy	OCD	obsessive–compulsive disorder
EEG	electroencephalography	PET	positron emission tomography
GAD	generalized anxiety disorder	PTSD	post-traumatic stress disorder
5-HIAA	5-hydroxyindoleacetic acid	SPET	single-photon emission tomography
HIV	human immunodeficiency virus	SSRIs	selective serotonin reuptake inhibitors

epidemiology (*contd.*)
  contribution to scientific basis of aetiology **307–19**
  contribution to transcultural psychiatry **12–14**
  experiential variables 314–15, *316*
  how epidemiologists think 315–17, *316*
    coarse observations 317
    inspired hypotheses 315–16
    matrix construction *316*, 317
    theory driven enquiries 317
  levels in research 308, *308*
  measurement of psychiatric symptoms 311–13
    assessment of dementia and depression in elderly 312
    disablement 313
    questionnaires 311, *311*
    standardized psychiatric interviews 311–12
    typical prevalence estimates 312–13, *313*
    validity issues 312
  and molecular genetics 315, 701, 702–4, 707
  needs estimates for populations 1528–9, 1530, 1552
  personality variables 315
  principles of sampling 309–10
  social environment 313–14
  sociodemographic variables 313, *316*
  specifying disorders 310–11
    continuous measures of morbidity 310–11
    diagnostic categories 310
    disablement 311
  and statistics, *see* statistics, and design of experiments
    and surveys
  uses 307–8
    applying population data to individual risk 308
    community diagnosis 307
    completing clinical picture 307
    delineation of syndromes 308
    health services research 308
    prevention 308
    search for causes 308
    secular changes in incidence 307
  see also specific disorders/patient groups
epilepsia partialis Kojewnikow 1982
epilepsy 9, **1153–7**
  aetiology 1154, 1788, 1983–4, *1983*, *1984*
  and antidepressants 730
  and automatism 455, 1092, 1153, 2050
  in childhood and adolescence 1154, 1155, **1787–9**
    acquired aphasia with epilepsy (Landau–Kleffner
      syndrome) **1717**, 1730, 1788, 1813, 1982
    aetiology 1788
    classification 1787
    clinical features and clinical course 1787
    course and prognosis 1788
    diagnosis and differential diagnosis 1787–8
    drug treatment 1905
    epidemiology 1788
    management 1788–9
    in mental retardation 1966, *1981*, 1982
    nocturnal 1803
    post-traumatic 448
    prevention 1789
  classification 1153, *1153*, 1787, *1981*
  cognitive impairment 101–2
  complex partial seizures *1153*, **1153–4**, 1329, 1331
    aetiology 1788
    in childhood 1787, 1788
    complex partial status 1154
    frontal-lobe 1787
    and learning and memory **226**
    and Lewy body dementia 418
    and limbic system 712
    in mental retardation *1981*, 1982, 1985
    and neuronal networks 223, **226**
    and personality 1155
    and psychosis 583, 1155
    and suicide 1156
  diagnosis 1154–5, 1787–8
  drug treatment, *see* antiepileptic drugs
  ECT in intractable epilepsy 1346
  epidemiology 1154, 1788, 1982–3

  frontal-lobe 1787
  and gamma rhythms 225
  generalized seizures *1153*, 1154, *1981*, *1985*
    absence 226, 1154, 1982, 1985
    myoclonic 1154, 1981
    tonic–clonic (grand mal), *see below*
  genetic factors 1788, 1983–4, *1984*
  hysterical seizures 1091–2, 1155
  infantile spasms 1151
  limbic, *see* complex partial seizures (*above*)
  in mental retardation 1155, **1979–88**, *1981*
    in adulthood and old age 1982
    aetiology and pathogenesis 1983–4, *1983*, *1984*
    behavioural disorders caused by antiepileptic drugs
      1986
    behavioural disorders due to epilepsy 1966, *1981*,
      1982
    diagnosis and differential diagnosis 1979–80, *1980*,
      1981
    drug therapy 1984–5, *1985*
    in early childhood 1982
    epidemiology 1982–3
    in infancy 1980–1, *1981*
    in later childhood and adolescence *1981*, 1982
    and mortality 1997
    prognosis 1986
    and pseudoretardation 1984
    surgery 1985–6
    tuberous sclerosis 1151, 1788, 1789, 1966, *1984*
  mesial frontal seizures 1000–1, 1027
  nocturnal 1000–1, 1016, 1027, 1803
  partial seizures 1153–4, *1153*
    complex, *see* complex partial seizures (*above*)
    drug treatment 1331, *1985*
    simple 1153, *1153*, 1329, 1982, 1985
  post-traumatic **447–8**
  prodrome 1153
  pseudoseizures 1091–2, 1155, 1787–8, 1979, 1980, *1980*
  psychiatric consequences **1155–6**
    chronic interictal psychoses 583, 1155
    neuroses 1156
    offending 1156, 2047, 2050
    personality disorder and social development 1155
    postictal psychosis 583, 1155–6
    sexual function 1156
    suicide 1156
  psychomotor 712
  and schizophrenia 583, 592, 1155, 1342
  seizure types **1153–4**
  status epilepticus 1153, 1346, 1787, 1982, 1985, 1997
  surgery 459, 1156, 1985–6
  symptomatic 1154
  syndromes 1153, 1154, 1979, 1980–2, *1981*
  temporal lobe, *see* complex partial seizures (*above*)
  tetanus toxin model 226
  tonic–clonic (grand mal) seizures 1154, *1981*
    in alcohol withdrawal 489
    in ECT 1347
    treatment 1328, 1329, 1332
  transient epileptic amnesia 455
epinephrine (adrenaline) 171, 181, 764, 932
episodic dyscontrol, *see* intermittent explosive disorder
episodic memory 264, 272, 459, 460, 1286
epistasis (gene–gene interaction) 235, 253
epochal menstrual psychosis 1197
epoché 360
Epstein–Barr virus 1112, 1115, 1120, **1172–3**
eptastigmine 1335, *1335*
Epworth Sleepiness Scale 1010
erectile dysfunction 878, *885*, **885–8**
  and ageing 1663
  assessment 886–7
  and dementia 467
  and epilepsy 1156
  Process of Care model 886–7, 888
  theory 886
  treatment 887–8
    in elderly 1664–5

  oral 887–8
  psychotherapy/counselling 887
  self-injection and transurethral therapy 888
  vacuum systems 888
ergot 536
erotomania **665–6**, 2048
errorless learning 274–5
error term 93
error theory of ageing 1612
erythema chronicum migrans 1172
erythropoietic porphyria 1161
espanto 1061
Esquirol, J. E. **18**, 148, 378, 1045
ethics **27–32**
  casuistry and medical know-how 30
  and clinical practice skills 30–1
  codes 27–8, 30
  and counselling 1371–2
  and diagnostic concepts 28–9
  ethical principles 30
  ethical theory 29–31
  and factitious disorder 1128–9
  and health screening programmes 1211
  issues in forensic psychiatry 2016
    assessment of capacity 2103–4
    assessment under status test 2105
    law relating to mental disorder 2099
    psychiatric testimony 2094
    punishment and public protection 2102–3
    risk assessment 2068, 2102
  and medical vs. moral models 28–9
  and neurosurgery 1356–7
  and old age psychiatry 1672–3
  and panic disorder 819–20
  and prevention of mental retardation 1951
  and prevention of suicide 1053
  and surrogate motherhood 1195
  and use of placebos 1273, *1273*
  and value judgements in diagnosis 29
  see also confidentiality
ethnicity
  and adoption 1847
  and alcohol misuse 480
  and child sexual abuse 1827
  and epidemiology in childhood and adolescence 1698
  and hypertension 1157
  and obesity *871*
  and pathways to care 1534, 1535–6, 1604
  and population stratification 241, 703
  and PTSD 766
  and suicide/attempted suicide 1040–1, 1053, 1806, *1807*
  and treatment type and outcome 1537
ethnic minorities
  African–Caribbeans, *see* African–Caribbeans
  alcohol use disorders 510
  clinical assessment issues 76
  and communication in primary care 91–2
  drug misuse 545, 549
  family interventions 1903
  help-seeking 510, 1604
  mental health services **1603–5**
    and anthropological concepts/methods 303–4
    pathways to service utilization 1604
    service models and ways forward 1604–5
    service needs 1531, 1603–4
  mental retardation 1996, 1998–9
  and racism 302, 1605
  staff from 1604–5
  and transcultural psychiatry 12
ethnocentric fallacy 1064–5
ethnography 301, 302, *303*, 304
ethnological model of child molestation 908
ethological approach
  in behavioural assessment 105
  to trichotillomania 988
ethosuximide *1985*, 1986
etic and emic approaches 301, 1587–8
euphoria 58–9, 1150, 1202

incapacity test, need for 2100, 2103, 2105
'incipient lunacy' 323
incontinence 400, 468
incubus syndrome 665
independent assortment 233
Indian hemp 519
individualized treatment plans 1526
individual patient data reviews 1256
individuation process 346–7
inducible gene knockouts 248
infancy
    attachment, *see* attachment
    cognitive development 261–2
    epilepsy and mental retardation 1980–1, *1981*
    language development 262–3, *263*
    and maternal eating disorders 844, 1849
    and phobic avoidance by mother 1205
    and postpartum depression 1204, 1206, 1368, 1709
    sleep 997, 1791–2
    sudden death 1201, 1205
    see also breast feeding; mother–infant relationship;
        neonates
infanticide **1207–8**, **2051**, 2092
infantile amnesia 263
infantile sexuality **325–6**, 332–3
infantile spasms 1151, 1980–1
infant loss **1200–2**
infections **1168–73**
    and aetiology of mental retardation 1949, 1960–1
    and chronic fatigue syndrome 1112, 1115, 1120
    congenital 1949, 1960–1
    and cytokines 230–1
    and delirium 383, 384
    and effects of psychoactive drugs 230
    and exercise 229
    and hypersomnia 1013
    and intravenous drug misuse 475, 522, 525, *525*, 562
    opportunistic in HIV/AIDS 437–8, 1170–1
    paranatal 1949
    and psychosis 582–3
    and seizures 1979
    self-induced 1127
    streptococcal 988, 1150, 1776
    and stress 229, 1070
    see also specific infections
infectious mononucleosis 1172–3
inferior frontal cortex 712, 717
inferotemporal cortex 166, 168
infertility 842, **1195**
infestation, delusions of 58, 61, **661–2**
inflammatory bowel disease **1160**
influenza, maternal 594, 601
informal patients 22, 35, 36, 2021
information-giving model of counselling 1363
information processing approaches 278, **281–6**
    and attention 282–3
    and emotional valence 281–2, 289
    and interpretation 284–6
    and memory 283–4
inhalant abuse, *see* volatile substance abuse
inhaled β-adrenergic agents 1159
inhibin 878
inhibitory interneurones 169, *169*
initial placebo run-in period (IPR) 1271–2, *1272*
injecting drug misuse, *see* intravenous drug misuse
Injury Severity Score 1187
inner speech 280, 577–8
inositol-1,4,5-trisphosphate 189, *190*, 196
in-patient treatment
    in accidental injury 1187–9
    in alcohol dependence 495, 502, 506–7, 509
    in anorexia nervosa 847–8, 851–2
    in attempted suicide in childhood and adolescence 1808
    in childhood emergencies 1922
    in dementia 465
    in depression 729
    in drug misuse 525, 562
    in forensic psychiatry 2112–13, 2125–8

mother and baby 1204, 1207
    in personality disorders 973–4, 976
    and psychiatric nursing 1498–9
    and psychodynamic approach 368–9
    in schizophrenia 627
    in sex offending 2063–4
    see also hospitals
inquiries 2068, 2069, 2100–1, 2126
insane automatism 456, 2022, 2049
insanity defence 28, 1207, 2016, 2022, 2080, 2092
insertional mutations 248, 409, 411–12
insight **67**
    after head injury 449–50
    in body dysmorphic disorder 1121
    and capacity 2104
    in delirium 383
    in delusional disorders 655, 673
    in dementia 398
    in hallucinogen-induced psychosis 538
    and outsight, in group psychotherapy 1453
    in psychoanalysis 1435
    in schizophrenia 574, 578
    triangle of 1423, 1424–5
insomnia 999, **1004–9**
    aetiology 1005, *1005*
    in anxiety disorders 1023
    in childhood and adolescence 1800–1
    childhood-onset/idiopathic 1800
    classification 1004, *1005*
    clinical features 1004
    conditioned 1800
    course and prognosis 1005–6
    in depression 683, 998, 1022–3
    diagnosis and differential diagnosis 1004–5
    in eating disorders 868, 1024
    in elderly 1667–8
    epidemiology 1005
    fatal familial 406, 410, 1028
    in hyperthymia 746
    in mania 1022, 1023
    in neurasthenia 1133
    in opiate withdrawal 524–5
    prevention 1008
    psychophysiological 1005, *1005*
    in puerperium 1202, 1205
    rebound insomnia 1291
    in restless legs syndrome 1019
    in substance misuse 1025, 1030
    treatment 1006–8, 1417
        cognitive–behavioural therapy 1006–8
        drug therapy, *see* hypnotics
        management advice 1006–8
        in medical conditions 1030
        melatonin/light therapy/exercise 1006
        review of evidence 1006
institutionalization, effects of 259
instruments for assessment 71, **78–82**, 115
    of acute stress reactions 753
    of behaviour 106–7
    'bottom-up' and 'top-down' structure 80
    in childhood and adolescence 1697, 1701, 1965–6
    of cognitive and neuropsychological functioning **95–8**,
        97, *98*
    comprehensive 82
    culturally sensitive 1587–8
    of delirium 385, 1634
    of dementia 115, 311, 312, 391, 463, 1334
    of depression 78, 311, 312, 463, 687, 1265
    developments since 1950s 79–80
    of drug misuse 561, *561*, 1265
    of eating disorders 835, 862, 1265
    in epidemiological research **311–13**, 587, 1697
    of hypochondriasis 1099
    inter-rater reliability 78, 79, 105–6
    investigator-based 293–4
    of malingering 1131
    in mental retardation 1938, 1965–6, 1975
    of mental state and behaviour 78–9

of need 82, 106–7, 1527, *1527*
of negative symptoms 81
of outcome 82, 1264–7, 1563
of pain disorders 1110
of personality disorders 81, 924–5, *925*, 956–8, *957*
of PTSD 761
reasons for development 78
of refugees 1599
reliability **159–60**
of risk 2069–70
sensitivity and specificity 162, 311, *311*
of service components 1552–3, *1555*
use by clinicians and lay interviewers 79, 115, 312, 587
validation of screening questionnaires 162
see also specific instruments
insufficient sleep syndrome 1010
insula 165–6, 168, *177*, 179
insulin coma 1343
insulinomas 1180
intellectual impairment category 1941–2
intelligence **64–5**
    and antisocial/violent behaviour 1862, 2030–1, 2071
    assessment 64, *95*, **95–6**, *99*, 442, 1704
    conceptualization 64
    and conduct disorder 1756
    later-onset disorders of 64–5
    and risk of Alzheimer's disease 1621
    and risk of childhood disorder 1698
    and schizophrenia 576, 577, 582, 594, 602, 607
    see also mental retardation
intensive care patients 1029, 1177, 1230
intentional explanations of behaviour 277, 286, 289
intentionality of consciousness 357, 358
intention-to-treat analysis (ITT) 141, 1256
interferon 231
interim hospital orders 2093
interleukin 1 (IL-1) 229, 230–1
INTERMED 1238, *1239*
intermittent explosive disorder **979–80**
    associated psychopathology and comorbidity 980
    biology 980
    definition and clinical features 979–80
    epidemiology and course 980
    family studies 980
    in mental retardation 1993
    treatment response 980
internal objects 348
International Association of Cognitive Psychotherapy 1403
International Classification of Diseases (ICD-10) 110, 116,
    118–24 Appendix
    aims of Chapter V (F) 111
    associated empirical research 114
    characteristics of subchapters of Chapter V (F) 113–14
    childhood and adolescence in 123–4 Appendix, 1687–9,
        1965–6
    comparison with DSM-IV 114–15, 955, *955*, 1075,
        1687–8, *1714*
    comparison with previous versions 112
    culture-bound syndromes in 648, 1061
    development **111–14**
    and epidemiological research 310
    family of documents connected to Chapter V (F) 112–13
        casebooks 112
        Clinical Descriptions and Diagnostic Guidelines 111,
            112, 114, 310, 1687, 1752
        computer diagnosis 113
        Diagnostic Criteria for Research 112, 114, 310, 645–6,
            760–1, 1061, 1687, 1752
        lexica 112
        multiaxial version 82, 112, 114, 1688–9
        Pocket Guide 112
        Primary Health Care (PHC) Version 112, 1583, *1583*
        reference tables 112
        Short Glossary 112
        training material 112
        tutorial 112–13
    mental retardation in 64, 123 Appendix, 1688, *1689*
    and operationalized psychodynamic diagnosis 113